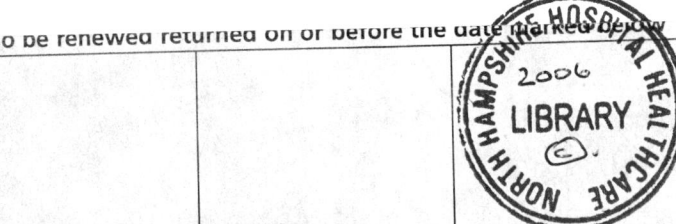

P. J. Frosch

T. Menné

J.-P. Lepoittevin

Editors

Contact Dermatitis

4th Edition

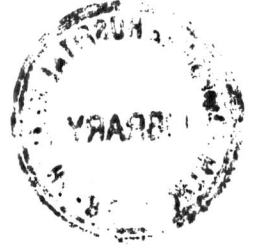

P. J. Frosch
T. Menné
J.-P. Lepoittevin
Editors

Contact Dermatitis

4th Edition

With 345 Figures, 238 in Color
and 180 Tables

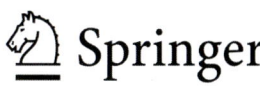
Springer

Frosch, Peter J., Professor
(e-mail: peter.frosch@klinikumdo.de)
Klinikum Dortmund gGmbH, Hautklinik
Lehrstuhl Dermatologie der Universität Witten/Herdecke
Beurhausstr. 40, 44137 Dortmund, Germany

Menné, Torkil, Professor Dr.
(e-mail: TOMEN@gentoftehosp.kbhamt.dk)
Dermatologisk afdeling K, Amtssygehuset Gentofte
2900 Hellerup, Denmark

Lepoittevin, Jean-Pierre, Professor
(e-mail: jplepoit@chimie.u-strasbg.fr)
Laboratoire de Dermato-Chimie
Clinique Dermatologique, CHU
67091 Strasbourg Cedex, France

Originally published under Rycroft, R.J.G.

Library of Congress Control Number: 2005926892

ISBN-10 3-540-24471-9 Springer Berlin Heidelberg New York
ISBN-13 978-3-540-24471-4 Springer Berlin Heidelberg New York

3rd Edition
ISBN 3-540-66842-X
Springer Berlin Heidelberg New York

Springer is a part of Springer Science+Business Media
springer.com
© Springer-Verlag Berlin Heidelberg 2006
Printed in Germany

The use of general descriptive names, registered names, trademarks, etc. in this publication does not imply, even in the absence of a specific statement, that such names are exempt from the relevant protective laws and regulations and therefore free for general use.

Product liability: the publishers cannot guarantee the accuracy of any information about dosage and application contained in this book. In every individual case the user must check such information by consulting the relevant literature.

Editor: Marion Philipp, Heidelberg, Germany
Desk Editor: Ellen Blasig, Heidelberg, Germany
Cover: Frido-Steinen-Broo, EStudio, Calamar, Spain
Typesetting: K. Detzner, 67346 Speyer, Germany

Printed on acid-free paper   24/3151 ML   5 4 3 2 1 0

Dedication

*To Kelly for her
continuous support
of my scientific activities.*

Peter J. Frosch

Preface

It is an unusual event for a textbook covering such a highly specialized field as contact dermatitis to be published in its fourth edition within a time period of 13 years. When the European and Environmental Contact Dermatitis Research Group was founded in 1985, one of the major goals was to edit a textbook of high scientific standard written by renown experts and keep it regularly updated. The greatest danger for a textbook is to become outdated – then it stays on the bookshelf and is rarely consulted. The continuous flow of new medicaments, the fascinating improvements in diagnostic image analysis and ever-changing operative procedures are the reasons for considerable knowledge deficits in old textbooks, often painfully experienced by young colleagues who look for advice in practice.

The sub-specialty of dermatology, contact dermatitis, has shown an impressive development over the last three decades. Scientific research groups have been founded in all major countries, national and international conferences are held at regular intervals, and several journals – peer reviewed and listed in data banks – are exclusively focusing on various aspects of contact dermatitis. The leading journal "*Contact Dermatitis*" has an impact factor of 1.7 and thus belongs in the ten top journals of dermatology.

One parameter of research quality is the number of acquired grants. If one leaves through the journals it is evident that our sub-specialty gets a great share of national and international research funds. A recent example is the multicenter research project on fragrances supported by the European Union with a considerable amount for 6 years.

Modern research in contact dermatitis is more than patch testing! In nearly every issue of "*Contact Dermatitis*" a new allergen is described. Starting with the observation of a keen clinician the culprit is characterized in cooperation with chemists after elaborative bioassay-guided investigations. Contact dermatitis is one of the major problems in occupational skin diseases. There, the differentiation between "irritant" and "allergic" is of high importance and may have profound consequences for the affected individual. In the past, reliable data on epidemiology were very limited. After the foundation of national and international networks and the use of standardized methodology, a highly differentiated picture can now be painted; we know the major professions at risk, as well as the influences of age and various cofactors. This is a solid basis for preventive measures. A new allergen, described in one center, can now be tested on a large scale in a short time period. If the data evaluation shows an unacceptably high rate of sensitization in the exposed population, regulatory measures will be undertaken to protect the consumer. A recent example is the "methyldibromo glutaronitrile story."

These and other issues of importance are covered in depth in the newest edition of this textbook. All chapters have been revised, many of them completely rewritten or considerably expanded. In order to increase the didactic value "core messages" are provided as often as possible. Furthermore, in some clinical chapters instructive case reports are given. As the novice is often lost in the jungle of references many authors have highlighted "Suggested reading" as valuable and pertinent literature.

Many new color figures have been added – most spectacular are those of the "temporary black henna tattoos" – some have to pay a high price with a life-long sensitization to p-phenylenediamine (including multiple cross-reactions) for this fad.

Many of those buying this textbook will also teach. Springer-Verlag and the editors would like to be of assistance in this task and therefore provide a CD-ROM containing all clinical photographs and important diagrams.

The editors are very grateful to all contributors. In times where the impact factor is an important incentive for publishing activities it is often difficult to motivate colleagues to write a book chapter. In our pursuit of continuous improvement we would like to ask all readers to comment and suggest further topics to be covered by the next edition of this textbook.

Last but not least we would like to thank Springer-Verlag, particularly Marina Litterer, for excellent support of this project.

July 2005
The Editors

Foreword to the Third Edition

So here it is, the third edition in nine years. This frequent revision of a textbook is well motivated by the impressive growth of the subspecialty.

The growth has been catalyzed by 1) the formation of national and international groups of clinicians and scientists interested in contact allergy and contact dermatitis; 2) the scientific production each year of 50–100 original articles in the journal Contact Dermatitis alone as well as papers and symposia at the flourishing European conferences; 3) the formation in many clinical departments of special units for environmental and occupational dermatology.

Early textbooks were the result of an amazing one-man/woman effort (Fisher, Cronin) and are still gold-mines of personally collected experiences. The present text emanates from world experts with special knowledge in a particular field. Because of the impressive development in several areas the volume has extended, the number of pages having increased by a third since the first edition.

It goes without saying that the text is primarily clinical. It might be presumed that contact dermatitis could be easily described on half a page. The great variation in clinical pattern, however, is amazing with regard to individual lesions and the grouping of lesions which are regularly influenced by the body region, by the particular irritant or allergen, or by the route and way of exposure, including the various expressions of systemic contact dermatitis. You learn with surprise that discoveries are still being made in this purely clinical field. Read and get wiser!

Historical aspects on contact dermatitis are continuously given in the running text. We need to keep in mind the fundamental knowledge acquired during the last century, not just to remember names of the pioneers but also to acknowledge the scientific buildingstones which form the basis of present progress. During the last two decades major improvements have taken place in the prevention of contact dermatitis e.g. by controlling occupational environments (exposure to water and surfactants); by diminishing the presence of allergens (formaldehyde in clothing, methylisothiazolinones as preservatives, nickel in clothing and jewelry); and by changing the chemistry of allergens (chromates in cement). Read and respect!

Immunological and biotechnical research has recently given important contributions, presented here, so that the pathogenesis of allergic as well as irritant contact dermatitis now is more fully understood. The etiological diagnostics in individual cases has developed, not only by improving the century-old patch test method (new allergens, test reading routines, occlusive and non-occlusive alternatives), but also by introducing new investigative methods, e.g. non-invasive ones for the inflammatory process, and modern analytical techniques for chemicals such as allergens in colophony, fragrances and plastics. The final tables on contact allergens with advice for choice of test vehicle and concentration constitute an enormous source of practical information. Read and do it yourself!

The comprehensive text provides a wealth of information for those particularly interested in and working with patients suffering from contact dermatitis. It should, however, be available to all dermatologists, the disease being a great mimic of other dermatoses. Read and enjoy!

Halvor Möller

Foreword to the Second Edition

The growth of contact dermatitis as a subspecialty of dermatology has been impressive in the past couple of decades. Each new textbook that is published reflects the considerable increase in information coming from many parts of the world. An important advance was made 3 years ago with the appearance of this new comprehensive textbook, brought to fruition from the contributions of nearly all the workers active in this field throughout Europe.

In the Foreword to the first edition, Dr. Etain Cronin described the greatest pitfalls of patch testing as the lack of knowledge in selecting the correct allergen and the difficulty encountered in interpreting the results. It is works such as this that bring together the knowledge of the past, in such a way that the reader/investigator can have readily available the information necessary to study the patients, patch test them, and interpret the results with accuracy and precision. Millions of patients worldwide experience contact dermatitis each year; not nearly enough of them are studied in detail to determine the precise cause of their affliction. In almost no other branch of medicine is it possible to pinpoint a specific, often removable, cause of a recurring, disabling disease. With the assistance of the information that is so prolifically available in this text, physicians will be able to bring help to many of these patients.

The 22 chapters of this volume cover every aspect of contact dermatitis, even including the addresses of physicians worldwide who work in this field. This work brings together dermatologists from many different countries and is an excellent example of what can be accomplished by the cooperation of those from a variety of nationalities and languages; truly a "European union" of contact dermatology!

The editors, including the late Dr. Claude Benezra, worked with devotion and care in the creation of this fine book. Dr. Rycroft, especially, deserves congratulations for bringing everyone together and organizing this textbook, which will surely remain a model of its kind for many years.

Robert M. Adams, M.D.
Department of Dermatology Stanford University
Medical Center
Stanford, CA 94035, USA

Foreword to the First Edition

Ideally every patient with eczema should be patch tested and the importance of this investigation is now universally accepted. The simplicity of the technique belies its many pitfalls, the greatest being to lack the knowledge required to select the correct allergens and to interpret the results. The introduction, nearly 20 years ago, of the journal Contact Dermatitis greatly stimulated the reporting of the clinical side of contact dermatitis but a vast amount of laboratory work has also been published in other journals on the mechanisms and theory of these reactions. The literature on the subject is now quite vast and a comprehensive book on the clinical and research aspects of contact dermatitis has been sorely needed. This textbook was carefully planned to gather together what is known of the subject into a cohesive whole and it has succeeded admirably. It consists of 22 chapters written by 41 contributors, each selected for their special study of particular subjects. Every feature of contact dermatitis has been covered, beginning with its history and even concluding with the names and addresses of those worldwide who have a specific interest in the subject. The text is illustrated and well laid out; it has been broken up into clearly demarcated sections making it easy to read and its information readily accessible. One's own writing concentrates the mind but editing the texts of authors from so many different countries was a task of considerable proportions. The editors are greatly to be congratulated, particularly Dr. Rycroft who has worked tirelessly to mould this multi-authored book into an integrated whole. This Textbook of Contact Dermatitis is an impressive achievement; it will instruct and help all who read it and stimulate many to take a greater interest in this fascinating subject.

Etain Cronin
St John's Institute of Dermatology
St Thomas's Hospital London SE1 7EH, UK

Contents

List of Contributors

Aberer, Werner
(e-mail: Werner.Aberer@klinikum-graz.at)
Umweltdermatologie Univ.-Hautklinik
Auenbruggerplatz 8
8036 Graz
Austria

Agner, Tove
(e-mail: TOAG@gentoftehosp.kbhamt.dk)
Department of Dermatology
Amtssygehuset Gentofte
2900 Hellerup
Denmark

Alanko, Kristiina
(e-mail: Kristiina.Alanko@ttl.fi)
Finnish Institute of Occupational Health
Topeliuksenkatu 41 aA
00250 Helsinki
Finland

Andersen, Klaus E.
(e-mail: kea@dou.dk)
Department of Dermatology
Odense University Hospital
5000 Odense C
Denmark

August, P. J.
Contact Dermatitis Investigation Unit
University of Manchester
Dermatology, Hope Hospital
Stott Lane, Salford, Lancs., M6 8HD
UK

Baadsgaard, Ole
Genmab A/S
Copenhagen
Denmark

Basketter, David
(e-mail: David.Basketter@unilever.com)
Unilever Environmental Safety Laboratory
Colworth House, Sharnbrook, Bredford, MK44 ILQ
UK

Beck, Michael H.
(e-mail: sue.parkinson@srht.nhs.uk)
Contact Dermatitis Investigation Unit
University of Manchester
Dermatology, Hope Hospital
Stott Lane, Salford, Lancs., M6 8HD
UK

Björkner, Bert
Dept. Occupational Dermatology
General Hospital
214 01 Malmö
Sweden

Blomberg von, Mary E.
Department of Pathology
Free University Hospital
De Boelelaan 1117
1081 HV Amsterdam
The Netherlands

Bock, Meike
Universität Osnabrück, Dermatologie
Sedanstrasse 115
49069 Osnabrück
Germany

Boman, Anders
(e-mail: anders.boman@sll.se)
Occupational and Environmental Medicine
Department of Occupational
and Environmental Dermatology
Norrbacka, 171 76 Stockholm
Sweden

Brandão, Francisco M.
(e-mail: mbrandao@hgo.min-saude.pt)
Department of Dermatology
Hospital Garcia de Orta
2800 Almada
Portugal

Bruynzeel, Derk P.
(e-mail: dp.bruynzeel@vumc.nl)
Department of Dermatology
Free University Hospital
De Boelelaan, 1117, 1081 HV Amsterdam
The Netherlands

Bruze, Magnus
(e-mail: magnus.bruze@derm.mas.lu.se)
Department of Occupational
and Environmental Dermatology
University Hospital Malmö
205 02 Malmö
Sweden

Coenraads, Pieter-Jan
(e-mail: p.j.coenraads@med.rug.nl)
Dermatology Department, University Hospital
9700 RB Groningen
The Netherlands

Conde-Salazar, L.
Escuela Nacional de Medicina del Trabajo
Instituto Carlos III
Madrid
Spain

Constandt, Lieve
Stationsstraat 84
8790 Waregem
Belgium

Darsow, Ulf
(e-mail: ulf.darsow@lrz.tum.de)
Klinik und Poliklinik für Dermatologie
und Allergologie am Biederstein, TU München
Biedersteiner Str. 29
80802 Munich
Germany

Diepgen, Thomas L.
(e-mail: Thomas.diepgen@med.uni-heidelberg.de)
Universitätsklinikum Heidelberg
Bergheimer Str. 58
69115 Heidelberg
Germany

Ducombs, Georges
(e-mail: georges.ducombs@wanadoo.fr)
50 Avenue Thiers
33109 Bordeaux
France

Erkek, Emel
A-61 Dermatology, Cleveland Clinic
9500 Euclid Ave., Cleveland, OH 44106
USA

Estlander, Tuula
(e-mail: tuula.estlander@pp.inet.fi)
Suomen Terveystalo and Finnish Institute
of Occupational Health
Mäntypaadentie 13
00830 Helsinki
Finland

Fregert, Sigfrid
Department of Occupational
and Environmental Dermatology
University Hospital
205 02 Malmö
Sweden

Frick, Malin
Department of Occupational Dermatology
General Hospital
214 01 Malmö
Sweden

Frosch, Peter J.
(e-mail: peter.frosch@klinikumdo.de)
Klinikum Dortmund gGmbH, Hautklinik
Lehrstuhl Dermatologie
der Universität Witten/Herdecke
Beurhausstr. 40
44137 Dortmund
Germany

Gefeller, Olaf
Univ. Erlangen Nürnberg
Waldstr. 6
91054 Erlangen
Germany

Geier, Johannes
(e-mail: Jgeier@med.uni-goettingen.de)
IVDK, Universitäts-Hautklinik
Von-Siebold-Str. 3
37075 Göttingen
Germany

Giménez-Arnau, Ana M.
(e-mail: 22505aga@comb.es)
Department of Dermatology, Hospital del Mar
Passeig Maritim 25–29
08003 Barcelona
Spain

Gogniat, Thierry
Rue de la Paix
2300 La Chaux-de-Fonds
Switzerland

Goh, Chee-Leok
(e-mail: nsc@pacific.net.sg)
National Skin Centre
1 Mandalay Road
Singapore 308205

Gonçalo, Margarida
(e-mail: mmgoncalo@netcabo.pt
or mgoncalo@interacesso.pt)
Rua Infanta D. Maria, No 30-30-A-3D
3030-330 Coimbra
Portugal

Goon, Anthony
(e-mail: anthonygoon@nsc.gov.sg)
National Skin Centre
1 Mandalay Road
Singapore 308205

Goossens, An
(e-mail: An.Goossens@uz.kuleuven.ac.be)
Dermatology/Contact allergy, U.Z.K.U. Leuven
Kapucijnenvoer 33
3000 Leuven
Belgium

de Groot, Anton C.
(e-mail: anton.de-groot@planet.nl)
Schipslootweg 5
8351 HV Wapserveen
The Netherlands

Gruvberger, Birgitta
(e-mail: birgitta.gruvberger@derm.mas.lu.se)
Department of Occupational
and Environmental Dermatology
University Hospital Malmö
205 02 Malmö
Sweden

Hannuksela, Matti
(e-mail: Matti.Hannuksela@pp.fimnet.fi)
Paatsamatie 4A3
00320 Helsinki
Finland

Held, Elisabeth
(e-mail: elisabeth-held@dadlnet.dk)
Department of Dermatology
Amtssygehuset Gentofte
2900 Hellerup
Denmark

Hoogstraten van, Ingrid M.W.
Department of Pathology, Free University Hospital
De Boelelaan 1117
1081 HV Amsterdam
The Netherlands

Johansen, Jeanne Duus
(e-mail: jedu@gentoftehosp.kbhamt.dk)
National Allergy Research Centre
Ledreborg Allé 40
2820 Gentofte
Denmark

John, Swen Malte
(e-mail: sjohn@uos.de)
Universität Osnabrück, Dermatologie
Sedanstrasse 115
49069 Osnabrück
Germany

Jolanki, Riitta
(e-mail: riitta.jolanki@ttl.fi)
Section of Dermatology
Finnish Institute of Occupational Health
Topeliuksenkatu 41 aA
00250 Helsinki
Finland

Kimber, Ian
(e-mail: ian.kimber@syngenta.com)
Syngenta Central Toxicology Laboratory
Alderley Park, Macclesfield
Cheshire SK10 4TJ
UK

Krutmann, Jean
(e-mail: krutmann@rz.uni-duesseldorf.de)
Institut für umweltmedizinische Forschung
Auf'm Hennekamp 50
40225 Düsseldorf
Germany

Lachapelle, Jean-Marie
(e-mail: Jean-Marie.Lachapelle@derm.ucl.ac.be)
Clos Chapelle-aux-Champs 30, UCL 3033
1200 Bruxelles
Belgium

Lahti, Arto
(e-mail: arto.lahti@oulu.fi)
Department of Dermatology
PL 5000, 90014 University of Oulu
Finland

Le Coz, Christophe J.
(e-mail: christophe.lecoz@wanadoo.fr)
Unité Dermato-Allergologie
Hôpitaux Universitaires de Strasbourg
1, Place de l'Hôpital
67091 Strasbourg
France

Lepoittevin, Jean-Pierre
(e-mail: jplepoit@chimie.u-strasbg.fr)
Laboratoire de Dermato-Chimie
Clinique Dermatologique, CHU
67091 Strasbourg Cedex
France

Lessmann, Holger
IVDK, Universitäts Hautklinik
Von-Siebold-Str. 3
7075 Göttingen
Germany

Lidén, Carola
(e-mail: carola.liden@smd.sll.se)
Dept. of Occupational and Environmental
Dermatology Stockholm County Council
Norrbacka
17176 Stockholm
Sweden

Lindberg, Magnus
(e-mail: magnus.lindberg@sll.se)
Department of Occupational Dermatology
Norrbacka
17176 Stockholm
Sweden

Lisby, Steen
(e-mail: SLi@genmab.com)
Genmab A/S
Toldbodgade 55B
1253 Copenhagen K
Denmark

Maibach, Howard I.
(e-mail: himjlm@itsa.ucsf.edu)
Department of Dermatology UCSF
School of Medicine
Box 0989, Surge 110
San Francisco, CA 94143–0989
USA

Mang, Renz
(e-mail: mang@uni-duesseldorf.de)
Universitäts-Hautklinik Düsseldorf
Moorenstr. 5
40225 Düsseldorf
Germany

Maqueda, J.
Escuela Nacional de Medicina del Trabajo
Instituto Carlos III
Madrid
Spain

Marot, Lilianne
Université Catholique de Louvain
30, Clos Chapelle-aux-Champs, UCL 3033
1200 Brussels
Belgium

McFadden, John
(e-mail: john.mcfadden@kcl.ac.uk)
St. John's Institute of Dermatology
St. Thomas' Hospital
London SE1 7EH
UK

Mellström, Gunh A.
(e-mail: gunh.mellstrom@alfa.telenordia.se)
Analytical and Pharmaceutical Research
and Development
Astra Pain Control AB
15185 Södertälje
Sweden

Menné, Torkil
(e-mail: TOMEN@gentoftehosp.kbhamt.dk)
Dermatologisk afdeling K, Amtssygehuset Gentofte
2900 Hellerup
Denmark

Morren, M.
Dermatology/Contact allergy, U.Z.K.U. Leuven
Kapucijnenvoer 33
3000 Leuven
Belgium

Muston, Haydn L.
Contact Dermatitis Investigation Unit
University of Manchester
Dermatology, Hope Hospital
Stott Lane
Salford, Lancs., M6 8HD
UK

Nakayama, Hideo
(e-mail: nakayamadermatology@eos.ocn.ne.jp)
Nakayama Dermatology Clinic
Shinyo CK Building 6F, 3–3–5, Kami-Ohsaki
Shinagawa-ku
Tokyo 141–0021
Japan

Nixon, Rosemary L.
Occupational Dermatology Research
and Education Centre
PO Box 132
Carlton South
Victoria 3053
Australia

Olmstead, William
Language and Educational Consultant
Lausanne
Switzerland

Orton, D.
(e-mail: David.ORTON@sbucks.nhs.uk)
Amersham Hospital, Environmental
and Contact Dermatitis Unit
Whielden Street
Amersham, Bucks., HP7 0JD
UK

Palmer, Roy A.
(e-mail: roypalmer@totalise.co.uk)
Department of Photobiology
St. John's Institute of Dermatology
St. Thomas' Hospital
London SE1 7EH
UK

Perrenoud, Daniel
(e-mail: dperreno@chuv.hospvd.ch)
Clinique de Dermato-Venerologie
1011 Chuv-Lausanne
Switzerland

Podmore, Patricia
Altnagelvin Hospital, Anderson House
Skin Department Ward 16
Londonderry BT47 1SB
UK

Pontén, Ann
Dept. Occupat. Dermatol., General Hospital
214 01 Malmö
Sweden

Rast, Hanspeter
Fluhmattstrasse 1, Postfach
6002 Luzern
Switzerland

Redelmeier, Thomas E.
Blumenweg 8
12105 Berlin
Germany

Ring, Johannes
(e-mail: johannes.ring@lrz.tu-muenchen.de)
Klinik und Poliklinik für Dermatologie
und Allergologie am Biederstein, TU München
Biedersteiner Str. 29
80802 Munich
Germany

Rustemeyer, Thomas
(e-mail: T.Rustemeijer@vumc.nl)
Department of Pathology, Free University Hospital
De Boelelaan, 1117
1081 HV Amsterdam
The Netherlands

Rycroft, Richard J.G.
St. John's Institute of Dermatology
St. Thomas's Hospital
London SE1 7EH
UK

Schaefer, Hans
(e-mail: schaefer_berlin@t-online.de)
Blumenweg 8
12105 Berlin
Germany

Scheper, R.J.
(e-mail: rj.scheper@vumc.nl)
Department of Pathology, Free University Hospital
De Boelelaan, 1117
1081 HV Amsterdam
The Netherlands

Schnuch, Axel
(e-mail: aschnuch@med.uni-goettingen.de)
Informationsverbund Dermatologischer Kliniken
Univ. Hautklinik
Von Siebold-Str. 3
37075 Göttingen
Germany

Serup, Jørgen
(e-mail: JS16@bbh.hosp.dk)
Bispebjerg Hospital, Dept. of Dermatology
2100 Copenhagen NV
Denmark

Skudlik, Christoph
(e-mail: cskud@uos.de)
University of Osnabrück, Department
of Dermatology, Environmental Medicine
and Health Theory
Sedanstrasse 115
49069 Osnabrück
Germany

Søsted, Heidi
Dermatologisk afdeling K, Amtssygehuset Gentofte
2900 Hellerup
Denmark

Stege, Helger
Heinrich-Heine University Düsseldorf
Moorenstr. 5
40225 Düsseldorf
Germany

Taylor, James S.
(e-mail: taylorj@ccf.org)
A-61 Dermatology, Cleveland Clinic
9500 Euclid Ave.
Cleveland, OH 44106
USA

Tichelen, van W.I.
Stationsstraat 84
8790 Waregem
Belgium

Tosti, Antonella
Department of Dermatology, University of Bologna
Via G. Massarenti 1
40138 Bologna
Italy

Uter, Wolfgang
(e-mail: wolfgang.uter@rzmail.uni-erlangen.de)
Univ. Erlangen Nürnberg
Waldstr.6
91054 Erlangen
Germany

Veien, Niels K.
(e-mail: veien@dadlnet.dk)
Niels K. Veien, Dermatology Clinic
Vesterbro 99
9000 Aalborg
Denmark

Wahlberg, Jan E.
(e-mail: janewahlberg@spray.se)
Karolinska Hospital
Department of Occupational Dermatology
10401 Stockholm
Sweden

White, Ian R.
(e-mail: ian.white@kcl.ac.uk)
St. John's Institute of Dermatology
St. Thomas' Hospital
London SE1 7EH
UK

Wigger-Alberti, W.
(e-mail: wwigger@proderm.de)
ProDerm
Industriestr. 1
22869 Schenefeld/Hamburg
Germany

Willis, Carolyn M.
(e-mail: carolyn.willis@sbucks.nhs.uk)
Dept. of Dermatology, Wycombe General Hospital
High Wycombe, Bucks. HP11 2TT
UK

Wulfhorst, Britta
(e-mail bwulf@uos.de)
University of Osnabrück, Department
of Dermatology, Environmental Medicine
and Health Theory
Sedanstrasee 115
Osnabrück
Germany

Zimerson, Erik
Dept. of Occupational Dermatology
General Hospital
214 01 Malmö
Sweden

Chapter 1

Historical Aspects

1

JEAN-MARIE LACHAPELLE

Contents

1.1 Introduction

Contact dermatitis, an inflammatory skin reaction to direct contact with noxious agents in the environment, was most probably recognized as an entity even in ancient times, since it must have accompanied mankind throughout history. Early recorded reports include Pliny the Younger, who in the first century A.D. noticed that some individuals experienced severe itching when cutting pine trees (quoted in [1]). A review of the ancient literature could provide dozens of similar, mostly anecdotal, examples and some are cited in modern textbooks, monographs and papers [2–4].

It is interesting to note that the presence of idiosyncrasy was suspected in some cases of contact dermatitis reported in the nineteenth century, many decades before the discovery of allergy by von Pirquet. For instance, in 1829, Dakin [5], describing *Rhus* dermatitis, observed that some people suffered from the disease, whereas others did not. He therefore posed the question: „Can it be possible that some peculiar structure of the cuticule or rete mucosum constitutes the idiosyncrasy?"

The history of contact dermatitis in the twentieth century is indistinguishable from the history of patch testing, which is considered the main tool for unmasking the causative chemical culprits. Nevertheless, starting in the early 1980s, additional tests (within the scope of patch testing) have been introduced, such as the open test, the semi-open test, the ROAT test and its variants, referred to as „use tests". Moreover, prick testing, which has been underestimated for decades in dermato-allergology, has gained in popularity, as an investigatory tool for immediate contact hypersensitivity.

Core Message

■ Historical aspects of contact dermatitis are indistinguishable from those of patch testing and prick testing.

1.2 Historical Aspects of Patch Testing

Historical aspects of patch testing are reviewed by Foussereau [6] and by Lachapelle [7]. A selection of important steps forward has been made for this short survey.

1.2.1 The Pre-Jadassohn Period

During the seventeenth, eighteenth, and nineteenth centuries [6] some researchers occasionally repro-

1

duced contact dermatitis by applying the responsible agent (chemical, plant, etc.) to intact skin. Most of the observations are anecdotal, but some deserve special attention.

In 1847, Städeler [8] described a method devised to reproduce on human skin the lesions provoked by *Anacardium occidentale* (Städeler's blotting paper strip technique), which can be summarized as follows: „Balsam is applied to the lower part of the thorax on an area measuring about 1 cm². Then a piece of blotting paper previously dipped in the balsam is applied to the same site. Fifteen minutes later, the subject experiences a burning sensation, which increases very rapidly and culminates about half an hour after. The skin under the blotting paper turns whitish and is surrounded by a red halo. As the burning sensation decreases, the blotting paper is kept in place for 3 h." This observation is important because it was the first time that any test was actually designed and described in full detail [6].

In 1884, Neisser [9] reviewed a series of eight cases of iodoform dermatitis triggered by a specific influence. Neisser wrote that it was a matter of idiosyncrasy, dermatitis being elicited in these cases by iodoform application. The symptoms were similar to those subsequent to the application of mercurial derivatives, and a spread of the lesions that was much wider than the application site was a common feature to both instances.

In retrospect, this presentation can be considered an important link between casuistical writings of older times and a more scientifically orientated approach of skin reactions provoked by contactants. It was a half-hidden event that heralded a new era, which blossomed at the end of the nineteenth century.

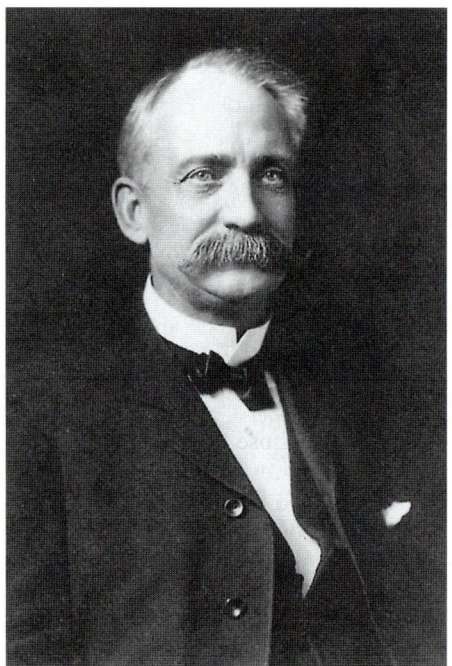

Fig. 1. Josef Jadassohn (1863--1936) (used with the kind permission of the Institut für Geschichte der Medizin der Universität Wien)

> ### Core Message
>
> ■ The first experimental – clinically orientated – attempts to relate contact dermatitis to a causative agent were made during the nineteenth century, both anecdotal and unscheduled.

1.2.2 Josef Jadassohn, the Father of Patch Testing in Dermatology

Josef Jadassohn (Fig. 1) is universally acknowledged as the father of patch testing („*funktionelle Hautprüfung*"), a new diagnostic tool offered to dermatol-

ogists [10]. At the time of his discovery, Jadassohn was a young Professor of Dermatology at Breslau University (Germany); he most probably applied and expanded – in a practical way – observations and interpretations previously made by his teacher Neisser [9]. Summing up the different sources of information available, we can reasonably assume that: (1) the birthday and birthplace of the patch test is Monday, 23 September 1895 at the Fünfter Congress der Deutschen Dermatologischen Gesellschaft held in Graz (Austria), where Jadassohn made his oral presentation „*Zur Kenntnis der medicamentösen Dermatosen*;" (2); the birth certificate is dated 1896, when the proceedings of the meeting were published [11].

As recorded by Sulzberger in 1940 in his classic textbook [12], the key message of Jadassohn's paper was the fact that he recognized the process of delayed hypersensitivity to simple chemicals:

> » In his original publication Jadassohn describes the following two occurrences: A syphilitic patient received an injection of a mercurial preparation and developed a mercurial dermatitis which involved all parts of the skin except a small, sharply demarcated area. It was found that the spared area was the site previously occupied by a mercury plaster which had been

applied in the treatment of a boil.

In a second observation, a patient who had received an injection of a mercurial preparation developed an acute eczematous dermatitis which was confined to the exact sites to which gray ointment (Hg) had been previously applied in the treatment of pediculosis pubis. In this patient, the subsequent application of a patch test (*funktionelle Hautprüfung*) with gray ointment to unaffected skin sites produced an eczematous reaction consisting of a severe erythematous and bullous dermatitis.

When put together, those two observations reflect a double-winged discovery: the local elicitation of a mercury reaction and the local elicitation of refractoriness to reaction.

Concerning the technical aspects of the „*Funktionelle Hautprüfung*," the methodology was quite simple: gray mercury ointment was applied on the skin of the upper extensor part of the left arm and covered by a 5-cm² piece of tape for 24 h. Many comments can be made at this point: (1) from the beginning, the patch test appears as a „closed" or occlusive testing technique, (2) the size of the patch test material is large (2.3–2.3 cm) compared to current materials available, (3) the amount of ointment applied is not mentioned (the technique is therefore considered as qualitative), and (4) the duration of the application is limited in the present case to 24 h.

It should be remembered that soon after developing the patch test, Jadassohn was appointed Professor of Dermatology (1896) at the University of Bern (Switzerland) where he stayed for several years, before coming back (in 1917) to his native Silesia, in Breslau again. One of his major accomplishments there was the observation of a specific anergy in patients suffering from sarcoidosis or Hodgkin's disease, for example.

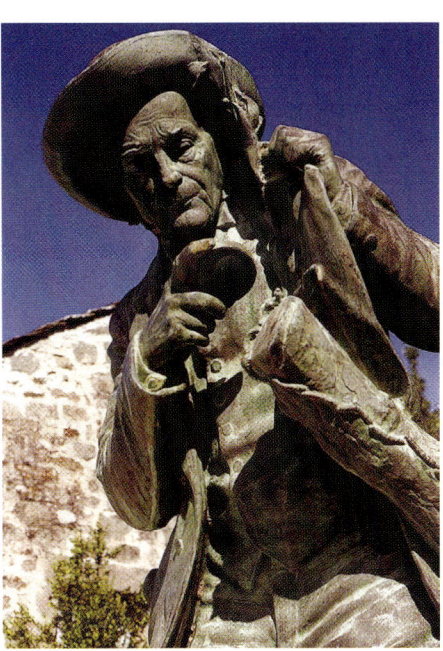

Fig. 2. Jean-Henri Fabre, French entomologist (1823–1915)

1.2.3 Jean-Henri Fabre's Experiments

Another description of a patch test technique was given by the French entomologist Jean-Henri Fabre (1823–1915), who lived in Sérignan-du-Comtat, a village in Provence (Fig. 2). This work was contemporaneous with Jadassohn's experiments, but it is described here because it was not designed primarily for dermatological diagnosis [13]. Fabre reported in 1897 (in the sixth volume of the impressive encyclopedia *Souvenirs entomologiques*, translated into more than 20 languages) that he had studied the effect of processionary caterpillars on his own skin. A square of blotting paper, a novel kind of plaster, was covered by a rubber sheet and held in place with a bandage. The paper used was a piece of blotting paper folded four times, so as to form a square with one-inch sides, which had previously been dipped into an extract of caterpillar hair. The impregnated paper was applied to the volar aspect of the forearm. The next day, 24 h later, the plaster was removed. A red mark, slightly swollen and very clearly outlined, occupied the area that had been covered by the „poisoned" paper.

In these and further experiments he dissected various anatomical parts of the caterpillars in order to isolate noxious ones (barbed hairs) that provoked burning or itching. Rostenberg and Solomon [14] have emphasized the importance to dermatology of Fabre's methodology, so often used in the past

> **Core Message**
>
> ■ A careful analysis of the historical literature clearly indicates that Josef Jadassohn is the initiator of aimed patch testing in dermatology.

1

decades by dermato-allergologists. For instance, many similar attempts were made during the twentieth century to isolate noxious agents (contact allergens and irritants), not only from different parts of plants, woods, and animals, but also from various other naturally occurring substances and industrial products encountered in our modern environment.

In my view, Fabre's experiments are gratifying for an additional reason: they reproduce another common skin reaction of exogenous origin, contact urticaria [15]. It is well known today that a protein, thaumetopoietin (mol. wt. 28 kDa), is responsible for the urticarial reaction. In an attempt to reproduce Fabre's experiments, I applied to my skin caterpillars' barbed hairs, using as patch test material a plastic square chamber designed by Van der Bend, which was kept in place for 2 h. After removal of the patch, two types of reactions were recorded consecutively: (1) at 20 min, an urticarial reaction (considered to be nonimmunological), which faded slowly during the next 2 h, and (2) at day 2, an eczematous reaction, spreading all around the application site and interpreted as an experimentally induced immunological protein contact dermatitis.

Core Message

■ Surprisingly, the first steps of patch testing were introduced – at the same time as Jadassohn's experiments – by an entomologist, J.-H. Fabre, when he was working on processionary caterpillars.

1.2.4 A General Overview of Patch Testing During the Period 1895–1965

It is difficult, in retrospect, to assess the importance of the patch test technique to the diagnosis of contact dermatitis between 1895 and the 1960s. Some points are nevertheless clear: (1) the technique was used extensively in some European clinics, and ignored in others, (2) no consensus existed concerning the material, the concentration of each allergen, the time of reading, the reading score, etc., and (3) differential diagnosis between irritant and allergic contact dermatitis was very often unclear.

It is no exaggeration to say that patch testers were acting like skilled craftsmen [16], though – step by step – they provided new information on contact dermatitis.

When covering this transitional period, we should recall the names of some outstanding dermatologists who directly contributed to our present knowledge and to the dissemination of the patch test technique throughout the world.

1.2.5 Bruno Bloch's Pioneering Work in Basel and in Zurich

Bruno Bloch is considered by the international community as one of the more prominent pioneers in the field of patch testing, continuing and expanding Jadassohn's clinical and experimental work. In many textbooks or papers, patch testing is often quoted as the Jadassohn–Bloch technique.

The major contributions made by Bloch to patch testing are the following:

■ When he was in Basel, he described in 1911 [17] in detail the technique of patch testing. The allergen should be applied to a linen strip which is put on the back, covered with a slightly larger piece of gutta-percha and fixed in place with zinc oxide adhesive plaster; the test should then be left for 24 h. The size of the patch was chosen to be 1 cm². For the first time in the history of patch testing, he graded the stages of the skin reaction from simple erythema to necrosis and ulceration, and stressed that a normal and a sensitized subject differ fundamentally in that only the latter reacts.

■ In collaboration with the chemist Paul Karrer, who first synthesized vitamin C and received the Nobel Prize in 1937, Bloch discovered and successfully synthesized primin, the specific chemical in *Primula obconica* that is responsible for allergic contact dermatitis in persons contacting the common plant [18].

■ He also conceived the concept of cross-sensitization in contact dermatitis by studying the reactivity patterns of iodoform, a commonly used topical medication at that time.

■ He described the first cases of systemic contact dermatitis, illustrated forever by moulages of the Zurich collection (moulageur: Lotte Volger).

■ The idea of developing a standard series of allergens was also developed extensively by Bruno Bloch in Zurich [19]. The substances with which standard tests were made were the following: formaldehyde (1% to 5%), mercury

(1% sublimate or ointment of white precipitate of mercury), turpentine, naphthalene (1%), tincture of arnica, *P. obconica* (piece of the leaf), adhesive plaster, iodoform (powder), and quinine hydrochloride (1%).

As far as we can understand it by consulting various sources of information, Bruno Bloch acted as a group leader for promoting and disseminating the idea of applying a limited standard series in each patient. This was made in close connection with Jadassohn in Breslau (his former teacher when he was in Bern), Blumenthal and Jaffé in Berlin, and – later on – Sulzberger in New York. In Bloch's clinic, Hans Stauffer and Werner Jadassohn worked on determining the adequate concentration and vehicle for each allergen.

Core Message

■ Bruno Bloch's devotion to patch testing methodology at Zurich University led to its expansion and initial standardization (including standard series) throughout the world.

1.2.6 Marion Sulzberger, the Propagator of Patch Testing in North America

Sulzberger was one of the most brilliant assistants of Bruno Bloch in Zurich, and later of Josef Jadassohn in Breslau. In both places, he was considered as the beloved American fellow worker. When Sulzberger came back to New York and became one of the Professors of Dermatology there, he modified considerably the spirit of the discipline, which was at that time very static in the New World. During his entire academic life, he was extremely active and scientifically productive. He introduced the patch test technique, and, since he had a plentiful harvest of trainees during his long career, he disseminated it broadly to the various parts of the United States.

1.2.7 The Influence of Poul Bonnevie in Scandinavian Countries

Poul Bonnevie, a former assistant of Bruno Bloch at Zurich University, was Professor of Occupational

Table 1. The standard series of patch tests proposed by Poul Bonnevie [20]

Allergen	Concentration (%)	Vehicle
Turpentine	50	Olive oil
Colophony	10	Olive oil
Balsam of Peru	25	Lanolin
Salicylic acid	5	Lanolin
Formaldehyde	4	Water
Mercuric chloride	0.1	Water
Potassium dichromate	0.5	Water
Silver nitrate	2	Water
Nickel sulfate	5	Water
Resorcinol	5	Water
Primula obconica	As is	
Sodium perborate	10	Water
Brown soap	As is	
Coal tar	Pure	
Wood tars	Pure	
Quinine chlorhydrate	1	Water
Iodine	0.5	Ethanol
Pyrogallol	5	Petrolatum
p-Phenylenediamine	2	Petrolatum
Aminophenol	2	Petrolatum
Adhesive plaster	As is	

Medicine in Copenhagen. He expanded Bloch's limited standard series of tests and published it in his famous textbook of environmental dermatology [20].

This list (Table 1) can be considered as the prototype of the standard series of patch tests. It was built on the experience gained at the Finsen Institute in Copenhagen regarding the occurrence of positive reactions to various chemicals among patch-tested patients. It is remarkable that the list was used in Copenhagen without any change from 1938 until 1955, which allowed Marcussen to publish, in 1962 [21], a most impressive epidemiological survey concerning time fluctuations in the relative occurrence of contact allergies. Of the 21 allergens listed by Bonnevie, 7 are still present in the standard series of patch tests used currently.

Core Message

■ Poul Bonnevie is the author of the first modern textbook on occupational dermatology. The key role played by a standard series of patch tests for investigating contact dermatitis is obvious in his personal approach.

1

1.2.8 A Controversial Period: The Pros and Cons of a Standard Series

In the 1940s and 1950s, the standard series did not blossom throughout Europe. Some authors refused to adhere to the systematic use of a standard series in all patients and championed the concept of „selected epicutaneous tests." Two former assistants of Bruno Bloch, Hans Stauffer and Werner Jadassohn, were particularly keen on this concept of selection.

Werner Jadassohn (son of Josef), Professor of Dermatology at Geneva University, had a strong influence on many colleagues in this respect. The principle of „choice" or „selection" was based upon a careful recording of anamnestic data, especially in the field of occupational dermatology [22].

A similar view was defended in France by Foussereau [23]; this was a source of intense debates at meetings. This discussion is obsolete nowadays due to a general agreement as regards the practical interest of using standard and additional patch test series in daily practice.

1.2.9 The Founding of Groups

A Scandinavian Committee for Standardization of Routine Patch Testing was formed in 1962. In 1967, this committee was enlarged, resulting in the formation of the International Contact Dermatitis Research Group (ICDRG). The founder members of the ICDRG were H.J. Bandmann, C.D. Calnan, E. Cronin, S. Fregert, N. Hjorth, B. Magnusson, H.I. Maibach, K.E. Malten, C. Meneghini, V. Pirilä, and D.S. Wilkinson. The major task for its members was to standardize at an international level the patch testing procedure, for example the vehicles used for allergens, the concentration of each allergen, and so on.

Niels Hjorth (1919–1990) in Copenhagen was the vigorous chairman of the ICDRG for more than 20 - years. He organized the first international symposium on contact dermatitis at Gentofte, Denmark, in October 1974; this symposium was followed by many others, which led to an increasing interest in contact dermatitis throughout the world, and, consequently, to the establishment of numerous national and/or international contact dermatitis groups. Hjorth's contribution to promoting our knowledge of contact dermatitis was enormous; it is true to say that he ushered in a new era in environmental dermatology. All contributors to this textbook are greatly indebted to him; he showed us the way forward.

1.2.10 The Founding of the European Environmental and Contact Dermatitis Research Group (EECDRG) and the European Society of Contact Dermatitis (ESCD)

During the 1980s, an increasing interest for all facets of contact dermatitis was evident in many European countries. This led some dermatologists and basic scientists to join their efforts to improve knowledge in the field. The European Environmental and Contact Dermatitis Research Group (EECDRG) was born and the first meeting initiated by John Wilkinson, took place at Amersham, England (28 June to 1 July, 1985). Later, two meetings were organized each year. At that time, the members of the group were: K.E. Andersen, C. Benezra, F. Brandao, D. Bruynzeel, D. Burrows, J. Camarasa, G. Ducombs, P. Frosch, A. Goossens, M. Hannuksela, J.M. Lachapelle, A. Lahti, T. Menné, R. Rycroft, R. Scheper, J. Wahlberg, I. White, and J. Wilkinson. The main goal was to perform joint studies to clarify the allergenicity (and/or irritant potential) of different chemicals. Studies were planned following the principles of „new-born" evidence-based dermatology. The adventure was fruitful and many joint papers were published.

From the early days of its founding, the group felt the need to disseminate the acquired expertise to other experienced colleagues. Peter Frosch was the leader of this new policy, by organizing a Symposium in Heidelberg, Germany in May 1988, that – obviously – was a great success. This event was the starting point of the European Society of Contact Dermatitis (ESCD). The new society was involved in the organization of congresses, on a two-year schedule. The first congress took place in Brussels, Belgium in 1992, under the chair of Jean-Marie Lachapelle and has been followed by seven others, so far!

Additional aims of the Society were: the publication of the *Textbook of Contact Dermatitis* (first edition in 1992) and the creation of subgroups of specialists, devoted to the study of specific research projects. The *Journal Contact Dermatitis* is the official publication of the ESCD.

1.2.11 Recent Advances in the Management of Patch Testing

Recent history has forwarded some new insights to reach a better significance of patch test results, either positive or negative. First of all, in case of doubt, additional tests are available, among which the **Repeat-**

ed Open Application Test (ROAT), standardized by Hannuksela and Salo [24] and completed by other variants of use tests, provides a more accurate answer in some difficult cases.

In addition, efforts have been made to determine more precisely the relevance (or non relevance) of positive patch test results [25], which is the ultimate goal in dermato-allergology.

Much attention has been paid to the dose–response relationships in the elicitation of contact dermatitis, a concept that modifies our views in the matter.

1.3 Historical Aspects of Prick Testing

The historical aspects of prick testing are rather difficult to circumscribe.

Blackley [26] was probably the first to suggest that allergens could be introduced into the skin to detect sensitization. Schloss [27] used a scratch technique in studies of food allergy between 1910 and 1920. The „codified" methodology of prick testing was described as early as 1924 by Lewis and Grant, but became widely used only after its modification by Pepys [28], almost exclusively by allergologists and pneumologists.

In dermato-allergology, it was introduced routinely in the late 1980s, in relation to expanding knowledge on contact urticaria, immediate allergy to latex proteins, and also protein contact dermatitis considered a well-defined entity.

Nowadays, it is an undisputed tool of investigation in the field of contact dermatitis.

Core Message

■ Historically, prick testing was developed independently from patch testing; today, it is considered an important tool of investigation in contact urticaria and/or protein contact dermatitis.

References

1. Castagne D (1976) Dermatoses professionnelles provoquées par les bois tropicaux. Thèse de médecine, Bordeaux
2. Avenberg KM (1980) Footnotes on allergy. Pharmacia, Uppsala
3. Mitchell J, Rook AJ (1979) Botanical dermatology. Greengrass, Vancouver
4. Rostenberg A (1955) An anecdotal biographical history of poison ivy. Arch Dermatol 72:438–445
5. Dakin R (1829) Remarks on a cutaneous affection produced by certain poisonous vegetables. Am J Med Sci 4:98–100
6. Foussereau J (1984) History of epicutaneous testing: the blotting–paper and other methods. Contact Dermatitis 11:219–223
7. Lachapelle JM (1996) A century of patch testing. First Jadassohn Lecture (ESCD) Jadassohn's Centenary Congress, London, 9–12 October 1996
8. Städeler J (1847) Über die eigenthümlichen Bestandtheile der Anacardium Früchte. Ann Chemie Pharmacie 63:117–165
9. Neisser A (1884) Über Jodoform-Exantheme. Dtsch Med Wochenschr 10:467–468
10. Adams RM (1993) Profiles of greats in contact dermatitis. I: Josef Jadassohn (1863–1936). Am J Contact Dermat 4:58–59
11. Jadassohn J (1896) Zur Kenntnis der medicamentösen Dermatosen. Verhandlungen der Deutschen Dermatologischen Gesellschaft, V Congress, Vienna (1895). Braumüller, Vienna, pp 103–129
12. Sulzberger MD (1940) Dermatologic allergy. Thomas, Springfield, Ill., p 88
13. Fabre JH (1897) Souvenirs entomologiques, vol 6. Delagrave, Paris, pp 378–401
14. Rostenberg A, Solomon LM (1968) Jean Henri Fabre and the patch-test. Arch Dermatol 98:188–190
15. Lachapelle JM, Frimat P, Tennstedt D, Ducombs G (1992) Précis de Dermatologie Professionnelle et de l'Environnement. Masson, Paris
16. Sézary A (1936) Méthodes d'exploration biologique de la peau. Les tests cutanés en dermatologie. Encyclopédie médico-chirurgicale, Paris, 12010, pp 1–8
17. Bloch B (1911) Experimentelle Studien über das Wesen der Jodoformidiosynkrasie. Z Exp Pathol Ther 9:509–538
18. Bloch B, Karrer P (1927) Chemische und biologische Untersuchungen über die Primelidiosynkrasie. Beibl Vierteljahrsschr Naturforsch Gesell Zürich 72:1–25
19. Bloch B (1929) The role of idiosyncrasy and allergy in dermatology. Arch Dermatol Syphilis 19:175–197
20. Bonnevie P (1939) Aetiologie und Pathogenese der Ekzemkrankheiten. Klinische Studien über die Ursachen der Ekzeme unter besonderer Berücksichtigung des Diagnostischen Wertes der Ekzemproben. Busch, Copenhagen / Barth, Leipzig
21. Marcussen PV (1962) Variations in the incidence of contact hypersensitivities. Trans St Johns Hosp Dermatol Soc 48:40–49
22. Jadassohn W (1951) A propos des tests épicutanés „dirigés" dans l'eczéma professionnel. Praxis 40:1–4
23. Foussereau J, Benezra C (1970) Les eczémas allergiques professionnels. Masson, Paris
24. Hannuksela M, Salo H (1986) The repeated open application test (ROAT). Contact Dermatitis 14:221–227
25. Lachapelle JM, Ale I, Maibach HI (2003) Clinical relevance of patch test reactions. In: Lachapelle JM, Maibach HI (eds) Patch testing/prick testing. A practical guide. Springer, Berlin Heidelberg New York, chap 8, pp 121–130
26. Blackley CH (1873) Experimental research on the causes and nature of catarrhus aestivus. Baillere, Tindall and Cox, London
27. Schloss OM (1920) Allergy in infants and children. Am J Dis Child 19:433–436
28. Pepys J (1975) Skin testing. Br J Hosp Med 14:412

Part I

Basic Features

I

Chapter 2

Mechanisms in Allergic Contact Dermatitis

2

THOMAS RUSTEMEYER, INGRID M.W. VAN HOOGSTRATEN,
B. MARY E. VON BLOMBERG, RIK J. SCHEPER

Contents

2.1 Introduction

During the past few decades, our understanding of why, where, and when allergic contact dermatitis (ACD) might develop has rapidly increased. Critical discoveries include the identification of T-cells as mediators of cell-mediated immunity, their thymic origin and recirculation patterns, and the molecular basis of their specificity to just one or a few allergens out of the thousands of allergens known. Progress has also resulted from the identification of genes that determine T-cell function, and the development of monoclonal antibodies that recognize their products. Moreover, the bio-industrial production of large amounts of these products, e.g., cytokines and chemokines, and the breeding of mice with disruptions in distinct genes (knock-out mice) or provided with additional genes of interest (transgenic mice), have allowed in-depth analysis of skin-inflammatory processes, such as those taking place in ACD.

Although humoral antibody-mediated reactions can be a factor, ACD depends primarily on the activation of allergen-specific T-cells [1], and is regarded as a prototype of delayed hypersensitivity, as classified by Turk [2] and Gell and Coombs (type IV hypersensitivity) [3]. Evolutionarily, cell-mediated immunity has developed in vertebrates to facilitate eradication of microorganisms and toxins. Elicitation of ACD by usually nontoxic doses of small-molecular-weight allergens indicates that the T-cell repertoire is often slightly broader than one might wish. Thus, ACD can be considered to reflect an untoward side-effect of a well-functioning immune system.

Subtle differences can be noted in macroscopic appearance, time course, and histopathology of allergic contact reactions in various vertebrates, including rodents and humans [4]. Nevertheless, essentially all basic features are shared. Since both mouse and guinea pig models, next to clinical studies, have greatly contributed to our present knowledge of ACD, both data sets provide the basis for this chapter.

In ACD, a distinction should be made between induction (sensitization) and effector (elicitation)

2

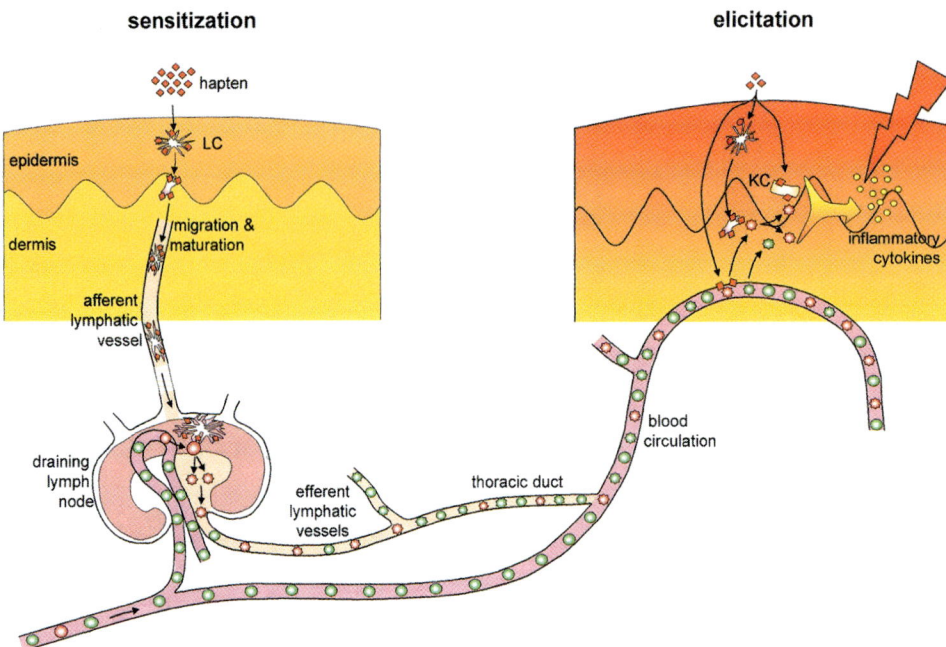

Fig. 1. Immunological events in allergic contact dermatitis (*ACD*). During the induction phase (*left*), skin contact with a hapten triggers migration of epidermal Langerhans cells (*LC*) via the afferent lymphatic vessels to the skin-draining lymph nodes. Haptenized LC home into the T-cell-rich paracortical areas. Here, conditions are optimal for encountering naive T cells that specifically recognize allergen–MHC molecule complexes. Hapten-specific T-cells now expand abundantly and generate effector and memory cells, which are released via the efferent lymphatics into the circulation. With their newly ac- quired homing receptors, these cells can easily extravasate peripheral tissues. Renewed allergen contact sparks off the effector phase (*right*). Due to their lowered activation threshold, hapten-specific effector T-cells are triggered by various haptenized cells, including *LC* and keratinocytes (*KC*), to produce proinflammatory cytokines and chemokines. Thereby, more inflammatory cells are recruited further amplifying local inflammatory mediator release. This leads to a gradually developing eczematous reaction, reaching a maximum within 18–48 h, after which reactivity successively declines

phases [5] (Fig. 1). The induction phase includes the events following a first contact with the allergen and is complete when the individual is sensitized and capable of giving a positive ACD reaction. The effector phase begins upon elicitation (challenge) and results in clinical manifestation of ACD. The entire process of the induction phase requires at least 3 days to several weeks, whereas the effector phase reaction is fully developed within 1–2 days. Main episodes in the induction phase (steps 1–5) and effector phase (step 6) are:

- *Binding of allergen to skin components.* The allergen penetrating the skin readily associates with all kinds of skin components, including major histocompatibility complex (MHC) proteins. These molecules, in humans encoded for by histocompatibility antigen (HLA) genes, are abundantly present on epidermal Langerhans cells (LC).

- *Hapten-induced activation of allergen-presenting cells.* Allergen-carrying LC become activated and travel via the afferent lymphatics to the regional lymph nodes, where they settle as so-called interdigitating cells (IDC) in the paracortical T-cell areas.
- *Recognition of allergen-modified LC by specific T-cells.* In nonsensitized individuals the frequency of T-cells with certain specificities is usually far below 1 per million. Within the paracortical areas, conditions are optimal for allergen-carrying IDC to encounter naive T-cells that specifically recognize the allergen–MHC molecule complexes. The dendritic morphology of these allergen-presenting cells strongly facilitates multiple cell contacts, leading to binding and activation of allergen-specific T-cells.
- *Proliferation of specific T-cells in draining lymph nodes.* Supported by interleukin-1

(IL-1), released by the allergen-presenting cells, activated T-cells start producing several growth factors, including IL-2. A partly autocrine cascade follows since at the same time receptors for IL-2 are up-regulated in these cells, resulting in vigorous blast formation and proliferation within a few days.

- *Systemic propagation of the specific T-cell progeny.* The expanded progeny is subsequently released via the efferent lymphatics into the blood flow and begins to recirculate. Thus, the frequency of specific effector T-cells in the blood may rise to as high as 1 in 1000, whereas most of these cells display receptor molecules facilitating their migration into peripheral tissues. In the absence of further allergen contacts, their frequency gradually decreases in subsequent weeks or months, but does not return to the low levels found in naive individuals.

- *Effector phase.* By renewed allergen contact, the effector phase is initiated, which depends not only on the increased frequency of specific T-cells, and their altered migratory capacities, but also on their low activation threshold. Thus, within the skin, allergen-presenting cells and specific T-cells can meet, and lead to plentiful local cytokine and chemokine release. The release of these mediators, many of which have a pro-inflammatory action, causes the arrival of more T-cells, thus further amplifying local mediator release. This leads to a gradually developing eczematous reaction that reaches its maximum after 18–48 h and then declines.

In the following sections, we will discuss these six main episodes of the ACD reaction in more detail. Furthermore, we will discuss local hyper-reactivity, such as flare-up and retest reactivity, and hyporeactivity, i.e., upon desensitization or tolerance induction.

2.2 Binding of Contact Allergens to Skin Components

2.2.1 Chemical Nature of Contact Allergens

Most contact allergens are small, chemically reactive molecules with a molecular weight less than 500 Da [6]. Since these molecules are too small to be antigenic themselves, contact sensitizers are generally referred to as haptens. Upon penetration through the epidermal horny layer, haptens readily conjugate to epidermal and dermal molecules. Sensitizing organic compounds may covalently bind to protein nucleophilic groups, such as thiol, amino, and hydroxyl groups, as is the case with poison oak/ivy allergens (reviewed in [7, 8]). Metal ions, e.g., nickel cations, instead form stable metal–protein chelate complexes by co-ordination bonds [9].

2.2.2 Hapten Presentation by LC

Sensitization is critically dependent on direct association of haptens with epidermal LC-bound MHC molecules, or peptides present in the groove of these molecules. Both MHC class I and class II molecules may be altered this way, and thus give rise to allergen-specific CD8$^+$ and CD4$^+$ T-cells, respectively. Distinct differences between allergens can, however, arise from differences in chemical reactivity and lipophilicity (Fig. 2), since association with MHC molecules may also result from internalization of the haptens, followed by their intracellular processing as free hapten molecules or hapten–carrier complexes. Lipophilic haptens can directly penetrate LC, conjugate with cytoplasmic proteins and be processed along the "endogenous" processing route, thus favoring association with MHC class I molecules [10]. In contrast, hydrophilic allergens such as nickel ions may, after conjugation with skin proteins, be processed along the "exogenous" route of antigen processing and thus favor the generation of altered MHC class II molecules. Thus, the chemical nature of the haptens can determine the extent to which allergen-specific CD8$^+$ and/or CD4$^+$ T-cells will be activated [11–13].

2.2.3 Prohaptens

Whereas most allergens can form hapten–carrier complexes spontaneously, some act as prohaptens and may need activation, e.g., by light- or enzyme-induced metabolic conversion, or oxidation [14]. A prototype prohapten is *p*-phenylenediamine, which needs to be oxidized to a reactive metabolite, known as Bandrowski's base [15, 16]. Tetrachlorosalicylanilide is a typical photoallergen, which undergoes photochemical dechlorination with UV irradiation, ultimately leading to photoadducts with skin proteins [17]. Reduced enzyme activity in certain individuals, related to genetic enzyme polymorphisms, explains the reduced risk of sensitization to prohaptens that need enzymatic activation [18]. Subsequent chapters of this book will present in extensive detail the numerous groups of molecules that have earned disrepute for causing ACD [19].

2

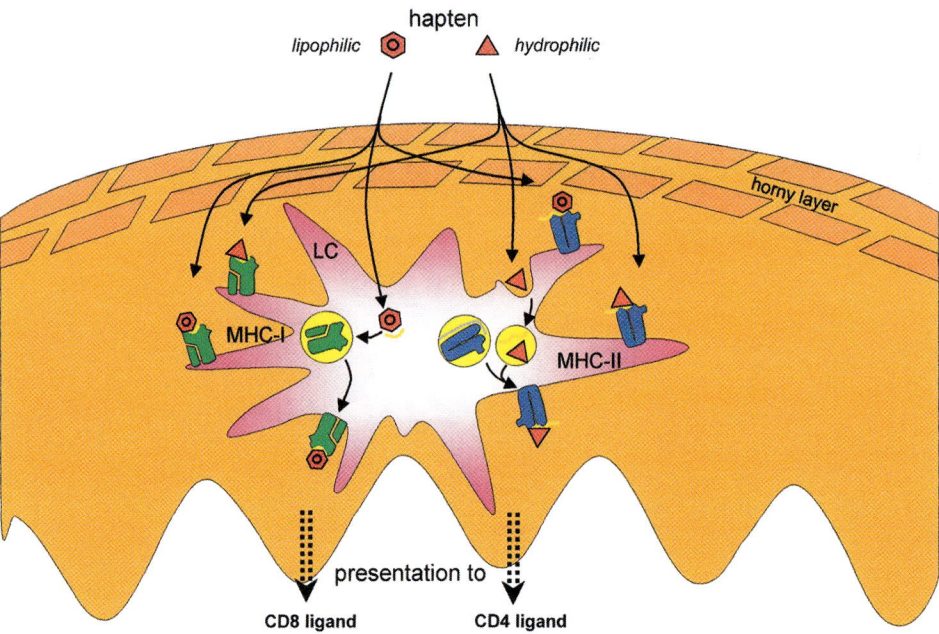

Fig. 2. Hapten presentation by epidermal Langerhans cells (*LC*). Allergen penetrating the epidermis readily associates with all kinds of skin components, including major histocompatibility complex (*MHC*) proteins, abundantly present on epi- dermal *LC*. Both MHC class I and class II molecules may be altered directly or via intracellular hapten processing and, subsequently, be recognized by allergen-specific CD8$^+$ and CD4$^+$ T cells

Core Message

- Allergenicity depends on several factors determined by the very physicochemical nature of the molecules themselves, i.e., their capacity to penetrate the horny layer, lipophilicity, and chemical reactivity. The sensitizing property of the majority of contact allergens can be predicted from these characteristics. Two other factors, however, further contribute to the allergenicity of chemicals, namely their pro-inflammatory activity and capacity to induce maturation of LC.

2.3 Hapten-Induced Activation of Allergen-Presenting Cells

2.3.1 Physiology of Langerhans Cells

LC are "professional" antigen-presenting dendritic cells (DC) in the skin [20]. They form a contiguous network within the epidermis and represent 2% to 5% of the total epidermal cell population [21]. Their principal functions are internalization, processing, transport, and presentation of skin-encountered antigens [22–23]. As such, LC play a pivotal role in the induction of cutaneous immune responses to infectious agents as well as to contact sensitizers [24–26]. LC originate from CD34$^+$ bone marrow progenitors, entering the epidermis via the blood stream [27]. Their continuous presence in the epidermis is also assured by local proliferation [28, 29]. They reside as relatively immature DC, characterized by a high capacity to gather antigens by macropinocytosis, whereas their capacity to stimulate naive T-cells is still underdeveloped at this stage [30]. Their prominent dendritic morphology and the presence of distinctive Birbeck granules were observed long ago [31–33]. In the last decade, their pivotal function in the induction of skin immune responses was explained by high expression of molecules mediating antigen presentation (e.g., MHC class I and II, CD1), as well as of cellular adhesion and costimulatory molecules [e.g., CD54, CD80, CD86, and cutaneous lymphocyte antigen (CLA)] [34–36].

2.3.2 Hapten-Induced LC Activation

Upon topical exposure to contact sensitizers, or other appropriate stimuli (e.g., trauma, irradiation), up to 40% of the local LC become activated [37, 38], leave the epidermis, and migrate, via afferent lymphatic vessels, to the draining lymph nodes [39] (Fig. 3). This process of LC migration results from several factors, including contact allergen-induced production of cytokines favoring LC survival [40–42] and loosening from surrounding keratinocytes [43–45]. Thus, within 15 min after exposure to a contact sensitizer, production of IL-1β mRNA and release of IL-1β protein from LC are induced [46, 47]. In turn, IL-1β stimulates release of tumor necrosis factor-α (TNF-α) and granulocyte-macrophage colony-stimulating factor (GM-CSF) from keratinocytes [47, 48]. Together, these three cytokines facilitate migration of LC

from the epidermis towards the lymph nodes [49]. IL-1β and TNF-α downregulate membrane-bound E-cadherin expression and thus cause disentanglement of LC from surrounding keratinocytes (Fig. 3) [45, 50, 51]. Simultaneously, adhesion molecules are increasingly expressed that promote LC migration by mediating interactions with the extracellular matrix and dermal cells, such as CD54, α$_6$ integrin, and CD44 variants [52–56]. Also, production of the epidermal basement membrane degrading enzyme metalloproteinase-9 is upregulated in activated LC [57].

Next, LC migration is directed by hapten-induced alterations in chemokine receptor levels [58]. Upon maturation, LC downregulate expression of receptors for inflammatory chemokines (e.g., CCR1, 2, 5, and 6), whereas others (including CCR4, 7, and CXCR4) are upregulated (Fig. 3) (reviewed by [59] and [60–62]). Notably, CCR7 may guide maturing LC into the

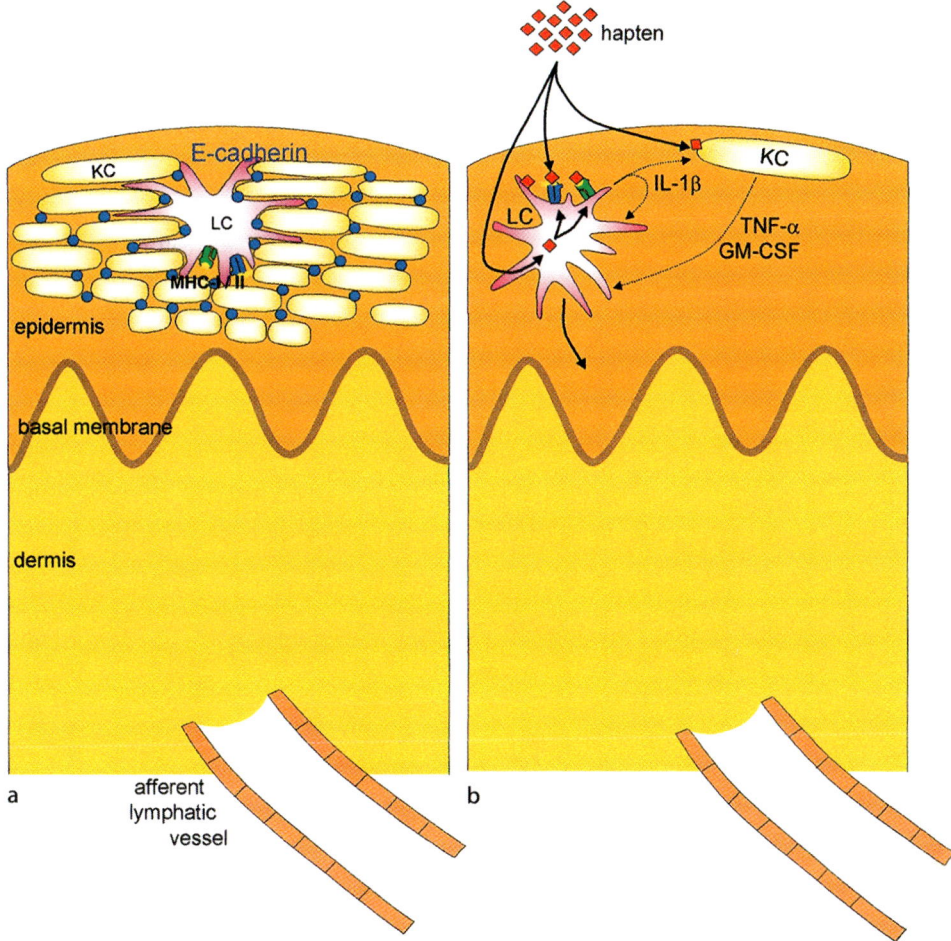

Fig. 3a–d. Hapten-induced migration of Langerhans cells (*LC*). **a** In a resting state, epidermal Langerhans cells (*LC*) reside in suprabasal cell layers, tightly bound to surrounding keratinocytes (*KC*), e.g., by E-cadherin. **b** Early after epidermal hapten exposure, LC produce IL-1β, which induces the release of tumor necrosis factor α (*TNF-α*) and granulocyte-macrophage colony-stimulating factor (*GM-CSF*) from keratinocytes. Together, these three cytokines facilitate migration of LC from the epidermis towards the lymph nodes.

2

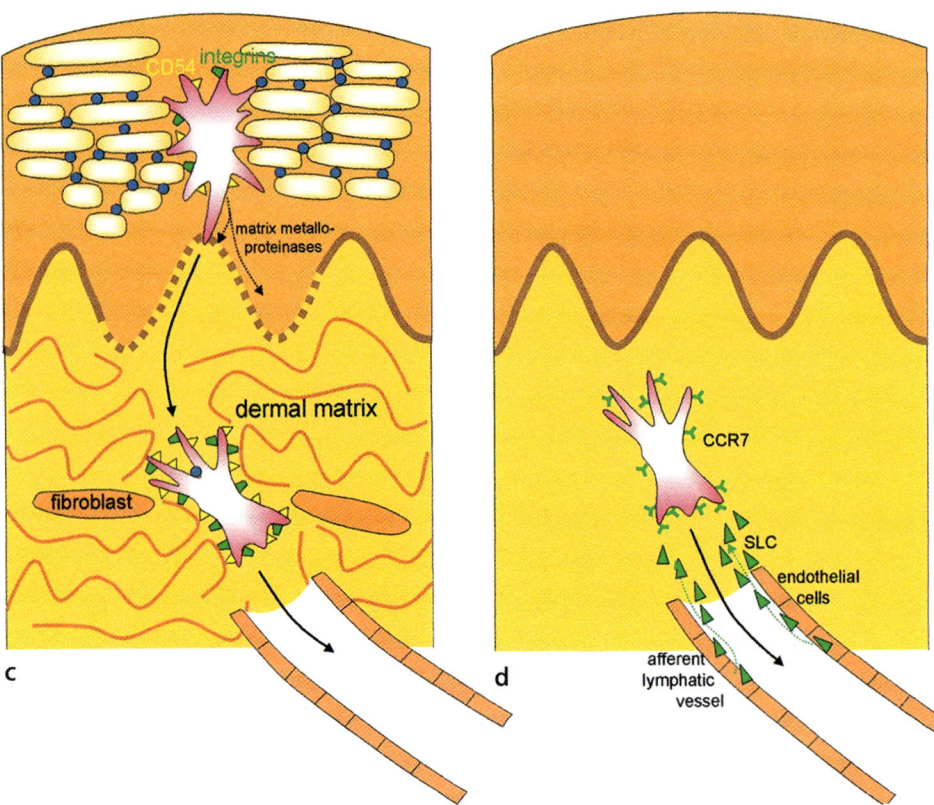

Fig. 3a–d. Hapten-induced migration of Langerhans cells (*LC*). **c** Emigration of LC starts with cytokine-induced disentanglement from surrounding keratinocytes (e.g., by downregulation of E-cadherin) and production of factors facilitating penetration of the basal membrane (e.g., matrix metalloproteinases) and interactions with extracellular matrix and dermal cells (e.g., integrins and integrin ligands). **d** Once in the dermis, LC migration is directed towards the draining afferent lymphatic vessels, guided by local production of chemokines (e.g., secondary lymphoid tissue chemokine, *SLC*) acting on newly expressed chemokine receptors, such as CCR7, on activated LC. Along their journey, haptenized LC further mature as characterized by their increased dendritic morphology and expression of costimulatory and antigen-presentation molecules

draining lymphatics and the lymph node paracortical areas, since one of its ligands (secondary lymphoid tissue chemokine, SLC) is produced by both lymphatic and high endothelial cells [63, 64]. Notably, the same receptor–ligand interactions cause naive T-cells, which also express CCR7, to accumulate within the paracortical areas [65]. Migratory responsiveness of both cell types to CCR7 ligands is promoted by leukotriene C4, released from these cells via the transmembrane transporter molecule Abcc1 (previously called MRP1) [58, 66, 67]. Interestingly, Abcc1 belongs to the same superfamily as the transporter associated with antigen-processing TAP, known to mediate intracellular peptide transport in the "endogenous route" which favors peptide association with MHC class I molecules. Final positioning of the LC within the paracortical T-cell areas may be due to another CCR7 ligand, EBI1-ligand chemokine (ELC), produced by resident mature DC [68]. Along with their migration and settling within the draining lymph nodes, haptenized LC further mature, as char-

acterized by their increased expression of costimulatory and antigen-presentation molecules [69, 70]. In addition, they adopt a strongly veiled, interdigitating appearance, thus maximizing the chances of productive encounters with naive T lymphocytes, recognizing altered self [48, 71, 72].

Core Message

■ Professional antigen-presenting cells of the epidermis, called Langerhans cells, take up penetrated allergens and present them in the context of MHC molecules. Thereby, they are activated and emigrate from the epidermis via afferent lymphatics to the draining lymph nodes, where they can come into contact with naive T lymphocytes.

2.4 Recognition of Allergen-Modified Langerhans Cells by Specific T-Cells

2.4.1 Homing of Naive T-Cells into Lymph Nodes

More than 90% of naive lymphocytes present within the paracortical T-cell areas have entered the lymph nodes by high endothelial venules (HEV) [73]. These cells are characterized not only by CCR7 but also by the presence of a high molecular weight isoform of CD45 (CD45RA) [73, 74]. Entering the lymph nodes via HEV is established by the lymphocyte adhesion molecule L-selectin (CD62L), which allows rolling interaction along the vessel walls by binding to peripheral node addressins (PNAd), such as GlyCAM-1 or CD34 [75–77]. Next, firm adhesion is mediated by the interaction of CD11a/CD18 with endothelial CD54, resulting in subsequent endothelial transmigration. Extravasation and migration of naive T-cells to the paracortical T-cell areas is supported by chemokines such as DC-CK-1, SLC, and ELC produced locally by HEV and by hapten-loaded and resident DC [66, 78–80]. In nonsensitized individuals, frequencies of contact-allergen-specific T-cells are very low, and estimates vary from 1 per 109 to maximally 1 per 106 [73, 81]. Nevertheless, the preferential homing of naive T-cells into the lymph node paracortical areas, and the large surface area of interdigitating cells make allergen-specific T-cell activation likely with only few dendritic cells exposing adequate densities of haptenized-MHC molecules [82, 83].

2.4.2 Activation of Hapten-Specific T-Cells

As outlined in Sect. 2.2, "Binding of Contact Allergens to Skin Components," the chemical nature of the hapten determines its eventual cytoplasmic routing in antigen-presenting cells (APC), and thus whether presentation will be predominantly in context of MHC class I or II molecules (Fig. 2). T cells, expressing CD8 or CD4 molecules, can recognize the hapten-MHC class I or II complex, which in turn stabilizes MHC membrane expression [84, 85]. Chances of productive interactions with T-cells are high since each MHC–allergen complex can trigger a high number of T-cell receptor (TCR) molecules ("serial triggering") [86]. Moreover, after contacting specific CD4[+] T-cells, hapten-presenting DC may reach a stable super-activated state, allowing for efficient activation of subsequently encountered specific CD8[+] T-cells [87]. The actual T-cell activation is executed by TCRξ-chain-mediated signal transduction, followed by an intracellular cascade of biochemical events, including protein phosphorylation, inositol phospholipid hydrolysis, increase in cytosolic Ca^{2+} [88, 89], and activation of transcription factors, ultimately leading to gene activation (Fig. 4) [90].

For activation and proliferation, TCR triggering ("signal 1") is insufficient, but hapten-presenting APC also provide the required costimulation ("signal 2"; Fig. 4) [91, 92]. The costimulatory signals may involve secreted molecules, such as cytokines (IL-1), or sets of cellular adhesion molecules (CAMs) and their counter-structures present on the outer cellular membranes of APC and T-cells (summarized in Fig. 5). Expression levels of most of these CAMs vary with their activational status, and thus can provide positive stimulatory feedback loops. For example, as mentioned above, after specific TCR binding and ligation of CD40L (CD154) on T-cells with CD40 molecules, APC reach a super-activated state, characterized by over-expression of several CAMs, including CD80 and CD86 (Fig. 4) [93, 94]. In turn, these molecules bind to and increase expression of CD28 on T-cells. This interaction stabilizes CD154 expression, causing amplified CD154–CD40 signaling [94, 95].

The activational cascade is, as illustrated above, characterized by mutual activation of both hapten-presenting APC and hapten-reactive T-cells. Whereas this activation protects the APC from apoptotic death and prolongs their life to increase the chance of activating their cognate T-cells, only the latter capitalize on these interactions by giving rise to progeny. As discussed below, to promote T-cell growth, cellular adhesion stimuli need to be complimented by a broth of cytokines, many of which are released by the same APC. Together, elevated expression levels of (co-)stimulatory molecules on APC and local abundance of cytokines overcome the relatively high activation threshold of naive T-cells [96].

The intricate structure of lymph node paracortical areas, the differential expression of chemokines and their receptors, the characteristic membrane ruffling of IDC, and the predominant circulation of naive T lymphocytes through these lymph node areas provide optimal conditions for TCR binding, i.e., the first signal for induction of T-cell activation [97]. Intimate DC–T-cell contacts are further strengthened by secondary signals, provided by sets of cellular adhesion molecules, and growth-promoting cytokines (reviewed in [98, 99]).

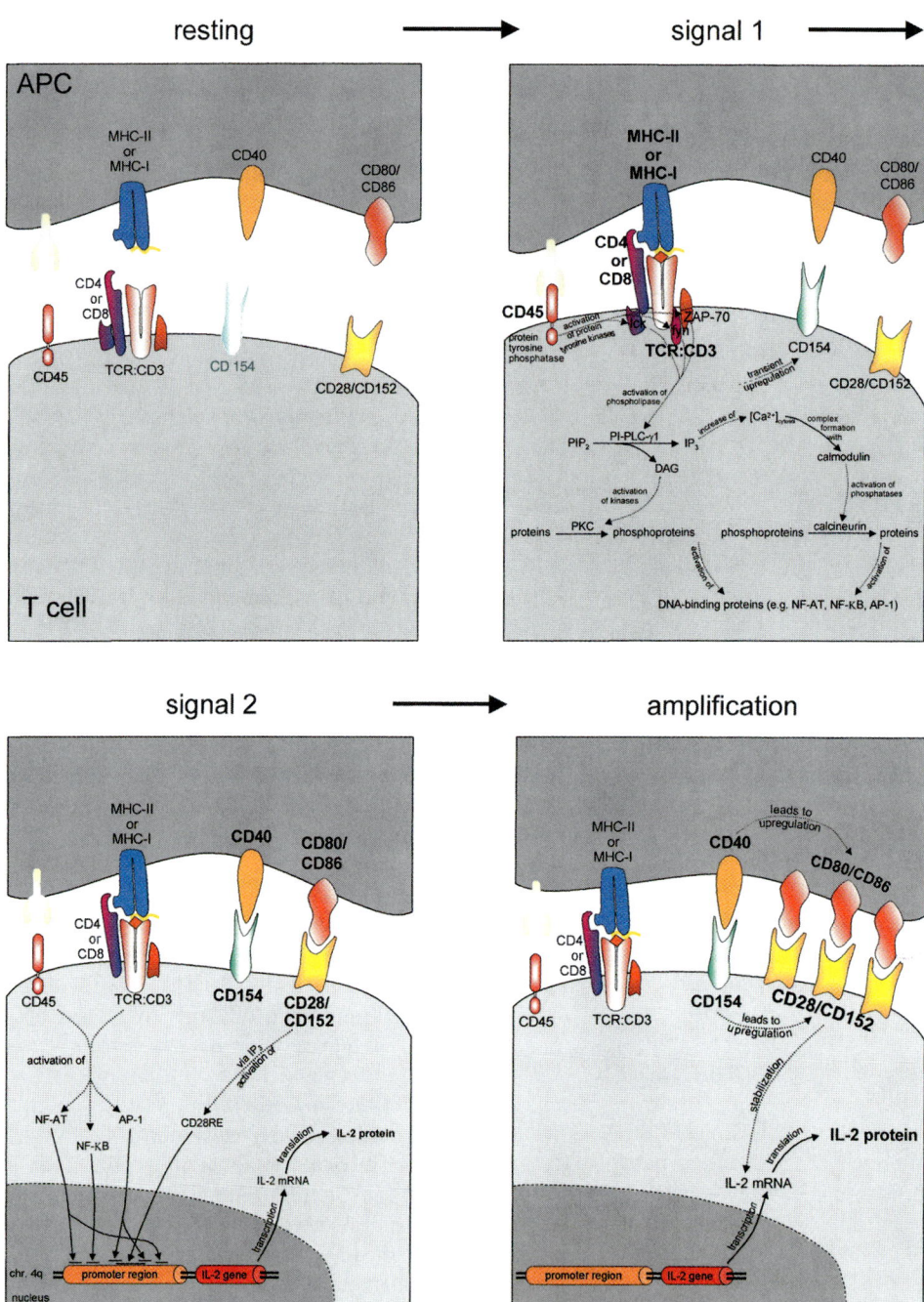

Fig. 4. Activation of hapten-specific T-cells. T-cell receptor (*TCR*) triggering by hapten-major histocompatibility complex (*MHC*) complexes ("*signal 1*") is insufficient for T-cell activation. But "professional" antigen-presenting cells (*APC*), such as Langerhans cells, can provide the required costimulation ("*signal 2*"), involving secreted molecules such as cytokines, or sets of cellular adhesion molecules present on the outer cellular membranes of APC and T-cells. T-cells, stimulated in this way, activate nuclear responder elements (e.g., CD28RE). Together with nuclear transcription factors (*NF*), produced upon TCR triggering, these nuclear responder elements enable transcription of T-cell growth factors, e.g., IL-2. APC–T-cell interaction gives rise to mutual activation ("amplification"): on APC, ligation of CD40 with CD154 molecules on T-cells induces overexpression of several costimulatory molecules, including CD80 and CD86. In turn, these molecules bind to and increase expression of CD28 on T-cells. This interaction stabilizes CD154 expression, causing amplified CD154–CD40 signaling, and preserves strong IL-2 production, finally resulting in abundant T-cell expansion. (*DAG* Diacylglycerol, *IP₃* inositol 1,4,5-trisphosphate, *PI* phosphatidylinositol, *PIP₂* phosphatidylinositol 4,5-bisphosphate, *PKC* protein kinase C, *PLC* phospholipase C)

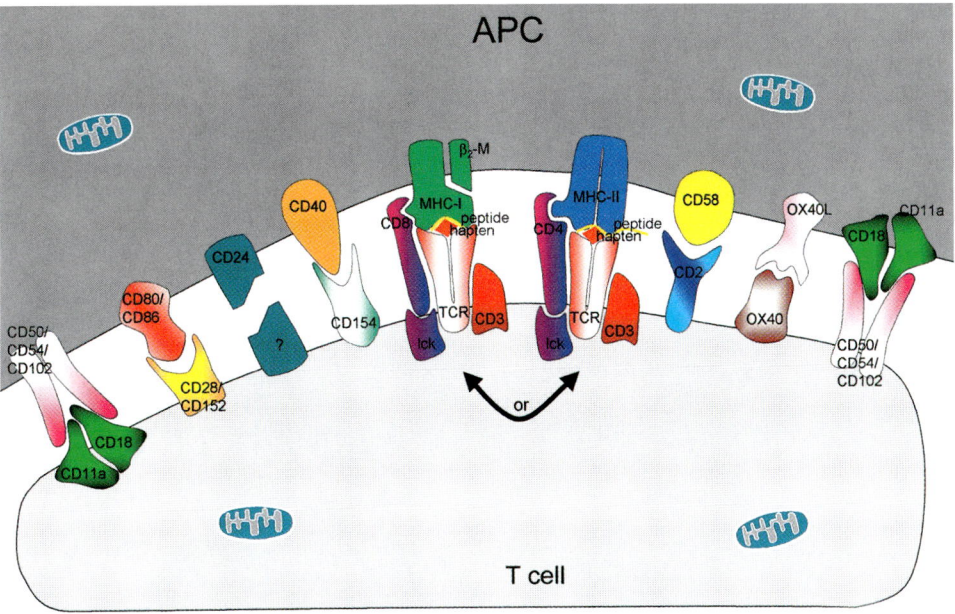

Fig. 5. Antigen-presenting cell and T-cell interaction molecules. On the outer cellular membranes of antigen-presenting cells (*APC*) and T-cells, respectively, sets of interaction molecules are expressed. They include antigen presentation (such as MHC class I and II) and recognition (such as T-cell receptor, TCR/CD8, and CD4 complexes, respectively) and various adhesion molecules

2.5 Proliferation and Differentiation of Specific T-Cells

2.5.1 T-Cell Proliferation

When activated, naive allergen-specific T-cells start producing several cytokines, including IL-2, which is a highly potent T-cell growth factor [100–102]. Within 30 min after stimulation, IL-2 mRNA can already be detected [100, 103]. In particular, ligation of T-cell-bound CD28 receptors augments and prolongs IL-2 production for several days [104]. Simultaneously, the IL-2 receptor α-chain is upregulated, allowing for the assembly of up to approximately 10^4 high-affinity IL-2 receptor molecules per T-cell after 3–6 days [102]. This allows appropriately stimulated T-cells to start proliferating abundantly. This process can be visible as an impressive, sometimes painful lymph node swelling.

2.5.2 T-Cell Differentiation

Whereas their allergen specificity remains strictly conserved along with their proliferation, the T-cell progeny differentiates within a few days into effector cells with distinct cytokine profiles [105, 106]. While naive T-cells release only small amounts of a limited number of cytokines, e.g., IL-2, activated T-cells secrete a broad array of cytokines which, besides IL-2, include IL-4, IL-10, interferon-γ (IFN-γ), and TNF-β ("type-0" cytokine profile) [107–109]. Within a few days, however, T-cell cytokine production can polarize towards one of the three major cytokine profiles, referred to as "type 1" (characterized by a predominant release of IFN-γ and TNF-β), "type 2" (IL-4 and/or IL-10), or "type 3" [transforming growth factor-β (TGF-β); Fig. 6] [110, 111]. Evolutionarily, based on requirements for combating different exogenous microbial infections, these polarized cytokine profiles promote inflammation and cytotoxic effector cell functions (type 1), antibody production (type 2), or anti-inflammatory activities in conjunction with production of IgA (type 3) [112, 113]. The latter excretory antibody excludes microbial entry, e.g., along mucosal surfaces [114]. As outlined above, both CD4+ and CD8+ allergen-specific T-cells may become involved in contact sensitization, and it is now clear that both subsets can display these polarized cytokine profiles and, thereby, play distinct effector and regulatory roles in ACD [115–117].

Polarization of cytokine production depends on several factors, including: (1) the site and cytokine environment of first allergenic contact, (2) the molecular nature and concentrations of the allergen, and (3) the neuroendocrine factors.

Fig. 6. Generation and cross-regulation of different types of T-cells. Depending on the immunological microenvironment, activated naive T cells, which only release low amounts of few cytokines (e.g., IL-2), can differentiate into type-0 cells, secreting a broad array of cytokines, or the more polarized T-cell types 1, 2, or 3, with their characteristic cytokine profiles. By secreting mutually inhibitory cytokines, the latter cell types can interactively regulate their activation and, thereby, control the type of immune response. (*IFN* Interferon, *IL* interleukin, *LT* lymphotoxin, *TGF* transforming growth factor)

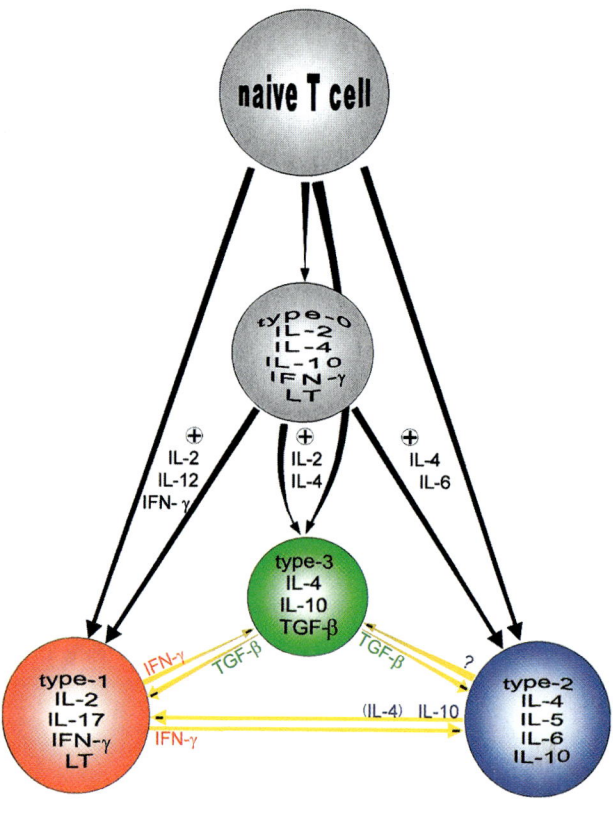

2.5.3 Cytokine Environment

In the skin-draining lymph nodes, allergen-activated LC and macrophages rapidly produce large amounts of IL-12, switching off IL-4 gene expression, thus promoting the differentiation of type-1 T-cells [107, 118, 119]. Notably, this process is reversible, and type-1 T-cells retain high IL-4R expression throughout, leaving these sensitive for IL-4 as a growth factor [120]. On the other hand, functional IL-12R expression remains restricted to type-0 and type-1 cells [121]. Type-2 T-cells, e.g., developing in mucosa-draining lymph nodes, lose the genes encoding the IL-12-R β2 chain and thus, type-2 differentiation is irreversible [121]. Early differentiation of type-1 T-cells is co-promoted by IL-12-induced secondary cytokines, e.g., IFN-γ, released by nonspecific "bystander" lymphocytes, including natural killer (NK) cells, within the lymph nodes [122, 123]. Next, cell-contact-mediated signals provided by APC during priming of naive T-cells constitute a critically important factor in skewing T-cell differentiation [124]: type-1 differentiation of T-cells is strongly stimulated by CD154 triggering through CD40 on APC [125]. In contrast, ligation of CD134L (gp 34; on APC) by CD134 (OX40; on T-cells) promotes the differentiation of type-2 T-cells [126].

Also, CD86 expression on APC contributes to preferential differentiation of naive T-cells towards a type-2 cytokine profile [127–130].

After a few days type-1, but not type-2, T-cells lose functional IFN-γR expression [131, 132] and thus become refractory to the growth inhibitory effects of IFN-γ [133]. Once established, the type-1-differentiated T-cells produce IFN-γ and IL-18, thereby further suppressing development of type-2 T-cells [134]. Thus, considering that contact allergens will mainly enter via the skin, type-1 pro-inflammatory T-cells are thought to represent the primary effector cells in ACD. Nevertheless, in sensitized individuals, type-2 T-cells also play a role, as shown by both IL-4 production and allergen-specific type-2 T-cells in the blood and at ACD reaction sites (see Sect. 2.7, "The Effector Phase of Allergic Contact Dermatitis") [135–137]. Their role may increase along with the longevity of sensitization, since several factors contribute to shifting type-1 to type-2 responses, including reversibility of the former and not of the latter T-cells, as mentioned above [138].

After mucosal contacts with contact allergens, type-2 T-cell responses are most prominent. In the mucosal (cytokine) environment, DC release only small quantities of IL-12, whereas IL-4 and IL-6 production by cells of the mast cell/basophil lineages, macrophages and NK(T) cells is relatively high [139–141], abundantly present within the mucosal layers. Moreover, these tissues, as compared to the skin, contain high frequencies of B-cells, which, when presenting antigen, favor type-2 responses through the abundant release of IL-10 [142, 143]. IL-10 is known to inhibit type-1 differentiation, just as IFN-γ and IL-18 interfere with type-2 T-cell differentiation [106, 144, 145]. Along the mucosal surfaces, T-cells may also develop, exhibiting the third "type-3" T-cell-cytokine profile, characterized by TGF-β production (reviewed by [146]). Since these cells play critical regulatory roles in ACD, they will be described further in Sect. 2.9, "Hyporeactivity: Tolerance and Desensitization."

2.5.4 Nature of the Allergen

A second factor in determining T-cell cytokine-production profiles, although still poorly understood, is the molecular character of the contact allergen itself, and the resulting extent of TCR triggering [106, 147, 148]. For both protein and peptide antigens, high doses of antigen might favor type-2 responses, whereas intermediate/low doses would induce type-1 T-cell responses [106, 149]. To what extent this translates to contact allergens is still unclear. Certainly, endogenous capacities of contact allergens to induce IL-12 by LC, versus IL-4 by mast cells, basophils, or NK(T) cells, will affect the outcome. In this respect, some contact allergens are notorious for inducing type-2 responses, even if their primary contact is by the skin route, e.g., trimellitic acid, which is also known as a respiratory sensitizer [150].

2.5.5 Neuroendocrine Factors

Diverse neuroendocrine factors co-determine T-cell differentiation [151–153]. An important link has been established between nutritional deprivation and decreased T-cell-mediated allergic contact reactions [154]. Apparently, adipocyte-derived leptin, a hormone released by adequately nourished and functioning fat cells, is required for type-1 T-cell differentiation. Administration of leptin to mice restored ACD reactivity during starvation [154]. Also, androgen hormones and adrenal cortex-derived steroid hormones, e.g., dehydroepiandrosterone (DHEA), promote type-1 T-cell and ACD reactivity. DHEA, like testosterone, may favor differentiation of type-1 T-cells by promoting IFN-γ and suppressing IL-4 release [155, 156]. In contrast, the female sex hormone progesterone furthers the development of type-2 CD4+ T-cells and even induces, at least transiently, IL-4 production and CD30 expression in established type-1 T-cells [157, 158]. Type-2 T-cell polarization is also facilitated by adrenocorticotrophic hormone (ACTH) and glucocorticosteroids [159], and by prostaglandin (PG) E$_2$ [160]. PGE$_2$, released from mononuclear phagocytes, augments intracellular cAMP levels, resulting in inhibition of pro-inflammatory cytokine, such as IFN-γ and TNF-α, production [161–164] and thus can influence the development of effector T-cells in ACD.

In healthy individuals, primary skin contacts with most contact allergens lead to differentiation and expansion of allergen-specific effector T-cells displaying the type-1 cytokine profile. The same allergens, if encountered along mucosal surfaces, favor the development of type-2 and/or type-3 effector T-cells. Factors skewing towards the latter profile remain unknown, despite their critical importance for understanding mucosal tolerance induction (see Sect. 2.9, "Hyporeactivity: Tolerance and Desensitization"). For most, if not all, allergens prolonged allergenic contacts, also along the skin route, ultimately lead to a predominance of type-2 allergen-specific T-cells, which may take over the role of type-1 T-cells in causing contact allergic hypersensitivity.

2.6 Systemic Propagation of the Specific T-Cell Progeny

2.6.1 T-Cell Recirculation

From the skin-draining lymphoid tissue, the progeny of primed T-cells are released via the efferent lymphatic vessels and the thoracic duct into the blood where they circulate for several minutes, up to 1 h (Fig. 7) [165, 166]. Like their naive precursors, these effector/memory T-cells can still enter lymphoid tissues upon adhering to HEV within the paracortical areas, because they continue to express L-selectin molecules (see Sect. 2.3, "Recognition of Allergen-Modified Langerhans Cells by Specific T Cells") [167, 168]. However, their lymph node entry via the afferent lymphatics increases as a consequence of their higher capacity to enter peripheral tissues [169, 170]. The latter capacity relates to higher surface densities of adhesion molecules, such as VLA-4, facilitating migration through nonactivated, flat endothelia, e.g., in the skin. Notably, vascular adhesion within peripheral tissues is strongly augmented when expression of vascular adhesion molecules, such as vascular cell adhesion molecule (VCAM), is upregulated, e.g., through cytokines released at inflammatory sites.

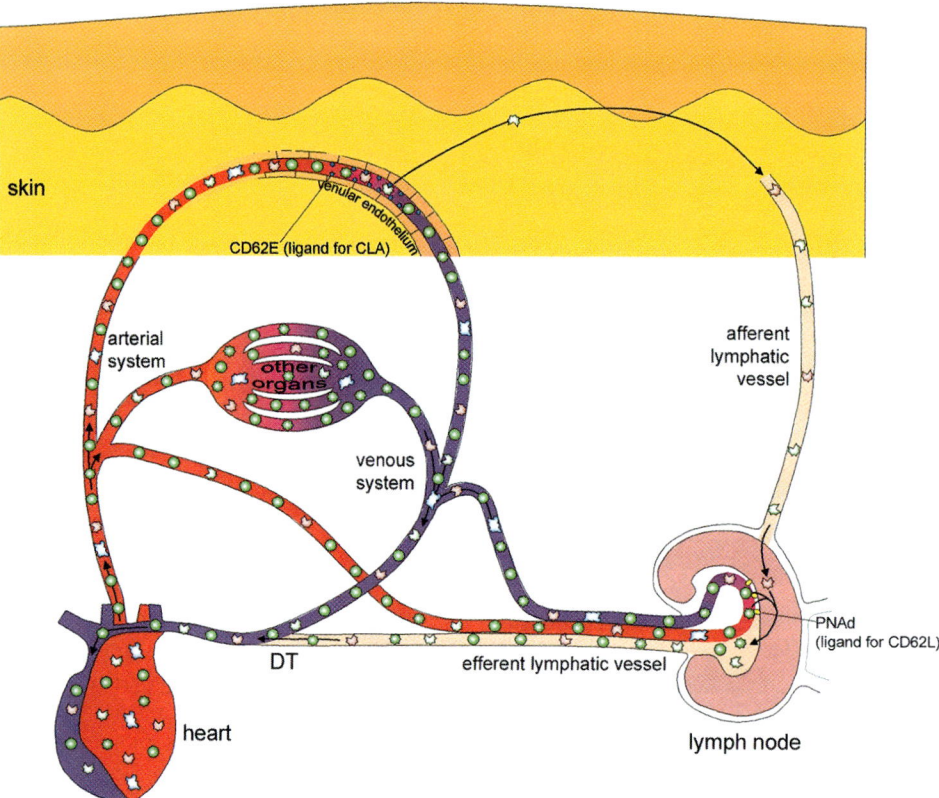

Fig. 7. Systemic propagation of hapten-specific T-cells. From the skin-draining lymphoid tissue, the progeny of primed T-cells is released via the efferent lymphatic vessels and the thoracic duct (*DT*) into the blood and becomes part of the circulation. Like their naive precursors, these effector/memory T-cells can still enter lymphoid tissues by binding to peripheral node addressins (*PNAd*). But increased expression of skin-homing molecules, e.g., cutaneous lymphocyte antigen (*CLA*), facilitates their migration in the skin. Via the afferent lymphatic vessels, cells re-enter draining nodes and the recirculating lymphocyte pool

Similarly, other ligand–counter structure pairs contribute to migration into peripheral tissues. Cutaneous lymphocyte-associated antigen and the P-selectin glycoprotein ligand (PSGL-1; CD162) are overexpressed on effector/memory T-cells, and mediate binding to venules in the upper dermis through the sugar-binding counter structures CD62 E (E-selectin) and CD62P (P-selectin) [171, 172]. Vascular expression of the latter molecules is also greatly increased by local inflammatory reactions [173–175]. Notably, expression of the lymphocyte-bound ligands is highest only for short periods after activation, thus endowing recently activated T-cells with unique capacities to enter skin sites and exert effector functions.

Upon repeated allergenic contacts, therefore, in particular within a few weeks after sensitization, recently activated effector T-cells will give rise to allergic hypersensitivity reactions, as outlined below. However, within lymph nodes draining inflamed skin areas, they can also contribute to further expansion of the allergen-specific T-cell pool.

2.6.2 Different Homing Patterns

Effector/memory T-cells show different recirculation patterns depending on their sites of original priming, e.g., within skin- or mucosa-draining lymphoid tissues [176, 177]. These differences are mediated by distinct vascular adhesion molecules and by the involvement of different chemokine–receptor pairs. First, mucosal lymphoid tissue venules express yet another L-selectin binding molecule, the mucosal addressin MAdCAM-1. The latter molecule mediates preferential binding of lymphoid cells generated within the mucosal lymphoid tissues, showing overexpression of $\alpha_4\beta_7$, a MAdCAM-1 binding integrin [178]. Thus, along the gut, Peyer's patches and lamina propria attract T lymphocyte progeny generated within other mucosal tissues, rather than contact allergen-specific cells derived from skin-draining lymph nodes. As outlined above, the latter are characterized by their high expression of CLA, facilitating preferential homing to the skin through its ligand CD62E [179, 180]. Second, T-cells biased towards production of type-1 cytokines may show a higher propensity to enter skin sites, as compared to mucosal tissues. In mice, the early influx of type-1 T-cells into delayed-type hypersensitivity (DTH) reactions was found to be more efficient than that of type-2 T-cells, although both cell types expressed CLA. Here, CD162, highly expressed by type-1 T-cells, was found to be important for this preferential homing [173, 181, 182]. Moreover, type-1 T-cells express distinct chemokine receptors, notably CCR5 and CXCR3, contributing to skin entry [60, 183, 184]. In contrast, recirculation through mucosal tissues preferentially involves CCR3 and CCR4 [67, 185]. The latter chemokine receptors are not only overexpressed on type-2 cytokine-producing T-cells, but also on basophils and eosinophils. Together, these cells contribute strongly to local immediate allergic hyper-responsiveness. Results obtained thus far favor the view that type-1 T-cells enter skin sites most readily [181, 186]. Their primary function may be in the early control of antigenic pressure, e.g., through amplification of macrophage effector functions. However, subset recirculation patterns are not rigid, and, given the fact that type-1 cells can shift cytokine production towards a type-2 profile, allergic contact skin inflammatory lesions may rapidly be dominated by type-2 allergen-specific T-cells (see Sect. 2.4, "Proliferation and Differentiation of Specific T-Cells").

2.6.3 Allergen-Specific T-Cell Recirculation: Options for In Vitro Testing

The dissemination and recirculation of primed, allergen-specific T-cells throughout the body suggests that blood represents a most useful and accessible source for T-cell-based in vitro assays for ACD. A major advantage of in vitro testing would be the non-interference with the patient's immune system, thus eliminating any potential risk of primary sensitization by in vivo skin testing. Although such tests have found several applications in fundamental research, e.g., on recognition of restriction elements, cross-reactivities and cytokine profile analyses, their use for routine diagnostic purposes is limited. Even in highly sensitized individuals, frequencies of contact allergen-specific memory/effector cells may still be below 1 per 10^3 [117, 187]. Given the relatively small samples of blood obtainable by venepuncture (at only one or a few time points), numbers of specific T-cells in any culture well used for subsequent in vitro testing would typically be below 100 cells/well. For comparison, in vivo skin test reactions recruit at least 1000 times more specific T-cells from circulating lymphocytes passing by for the period of testing, i.e., at least 24 h [165]. The sensitivities required, therefore, for direct in vitro read-out assays, e.g., allergen-induced proliferation or cytokine production, may often exceed the lowest detection limits. However, the observation that in vivo signal amplification may allow for the detection of a single memory/effector T-cell [188–190] suggests that it may be possible to solve sensitivity problems [190].

Appropriate allergen presentation, however, is a major hurdle for in vitro testing, with a broad range of requirements for different allergens with unique solubilities, toxicities, and reactivity profiles. Moreover, in the absence of LC, monocytes are the major source of APC, though their numbers in peripheral blood may vary substantially within and between donors. Of note, optimal APC function is particularly critical for recirculating resting/memory T-cells to respond. In the absence of repeated allergenic contacts, most CD45RO memory cells may finally revert to the naive CD45RA phenotype, with a higher threshold for triggering [191, 192]. Supplementing in vitro test cultures with an appropriate mix of cytokines may, however, compensate for this effect [187, 190].

After antigenic activation the progeny of primed T-cells, i.e., effector/memory cells, are released via the efferent lymphatics into the blood stream. Like their naive precursors, they can again leave the circulation and go into lymphoid organs anywhere in the body, thus rapidly ensuring systemic memory. They differ, however, from naive T-cells in many ways, including increased surface exposure of ligands facilitating entry into the peripheral tissues, such as the skin. On the vascular side, distinct exit patterns from the circulation are determined by tissue-dependent expression of vascular addressins and other adhesion molecules, and locally released chemoattractant molecules, i.e., chemokines. Once inside the tissues, these chemokines and stromal adhesion molecules determine the transit times before recirculating T-cells eventually re-enter the blood stream. Thus, peripheral blood provides a good source for in vitro studies in ACD but, besides budgetary and logistical reasons, theoretical considerations argue against wide-scale applicability of in vitro assays for routine diagnostic purposes.

2

Core Message

■ In the paracortical areas of peripheral lymph nodes mature antigen-presenting cells can activate antigen-specific naive T-cells. This results in the generation of effector and memory T-cell populations, which are mainly released into the blood flow. Upon allergen contact these primed T-cells can elicit an allergic contact dermatitis reaction.

2.7 The Effector Phase of Allergic Contact Dermatitis

2.7.1 Elicitation of ACD

Once sensitized, individuals can develop ACD upon re-exposure to the contact allergen. Positive patch test reactions mimic this process of allergen-specific skin hyper-reactivity. Thus, skin contacts induce an inflammatory reaction that, in general, is maximal within 2–3 days and, without further allergen supply, declines thereafter (Fig. 8). Looked at superficially, the mechanism of this type of skin hyper-reactivity

is straightforward: allergen elicitation or challenge leads to the (epi)dermal accumulation of contact allergen-specific memory/effector T lymphocytes which, upon encountering allergen-presenting cells, are reactivated to release pro-inflammatory cytokines. These, in turn, spark the inflammatory process, resulting in macroscopically detectable erythema and induration. As compared to immediate allergic reactions, developing within a few minutes after mast cell degranulation, ACD reactions show a delayed time course, since both the migration of allergen-specific T-cells from the dermal vessels and local cytokine production need several hours to become fully effective. Still, the picture of the rise and fall of ACD reactions is far from clear. Some persistent issues are discussed below, notably: (1) irritant properties of allergens, (2) role of early-phase reactivity, (3) T-cell patrol and specificity, (4) effector T-cell phenotypes, and (5) downregulatory processes.

2.7.2 Irritant Properties of Allergens

Within a few hours after allergenic skin contact, immunohistopathological changes can be observed, including vasodilatation, upregulation of endothelial adhesion molecules [193, 194], mast-cell degranulation [195, 196], keratinocyte cytokine and chemokine production [197], influx of leucocytes [198, 199], and

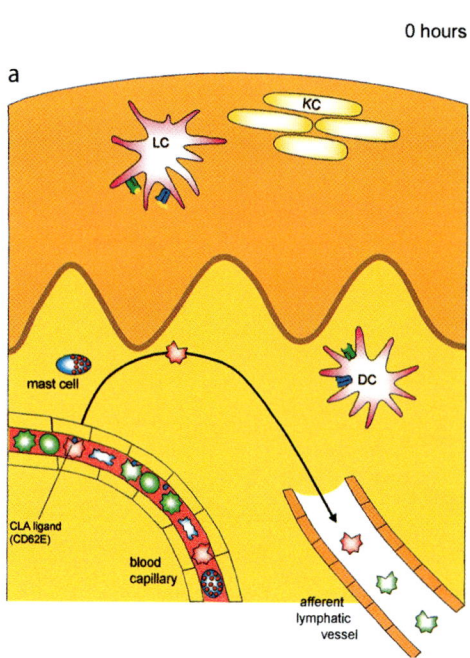
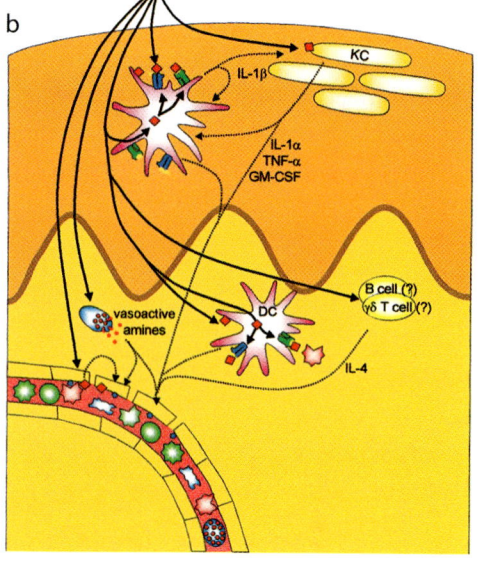

Fig. 8a, b.

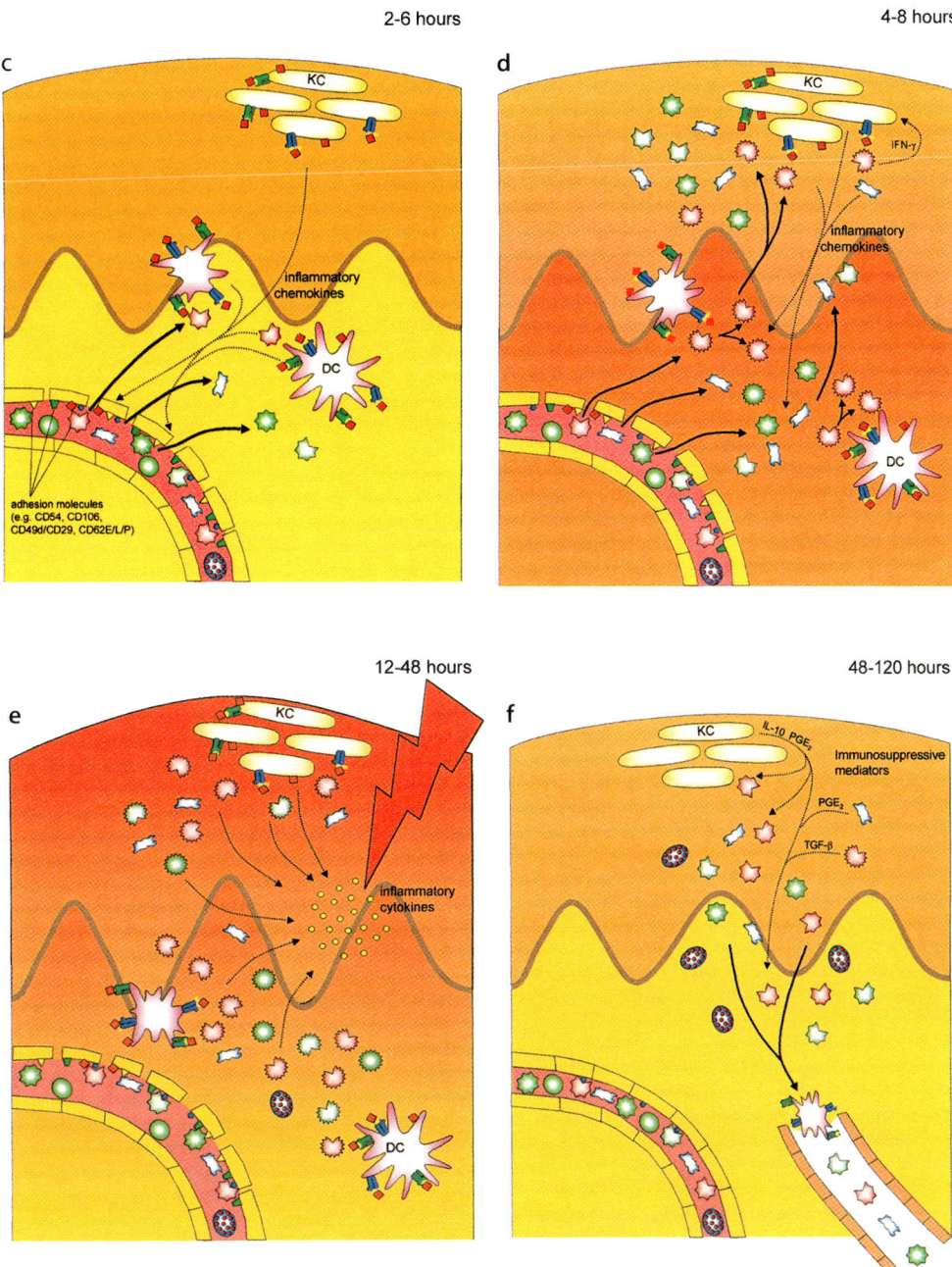

Fig. 8a–f. The effector phase of allergic contact dermatitis. **a** *0 h* In resting skin relatively few randomly patrolling, skin-homing CLA⁺ T-cells are present. **b** *0–4 h* Re-exposure of the contact allergen, binding to (epi)dermal molecules and cells, induces release of proinflammatory cytokines. The effector phase of allergic contact dermatitis. **c** *2–6 h* Influenced by inflammatory mediators, activated epidermal Langerhans cells (*LC*) start migrating towards the basal membrane and endothelial cells express increased numbers of adhesion molecules. Endothelial-cell-bound hapten causes preferential extravasation of hapten-specific T-cells, which are further guided by inflammatory chemokines. **d** *4–8 h* Hapten-activated T-cells re-

lease increasing amounts of inflammatory mediators, amplifying further cellular infiltration. **e** *12–48 h* The inflammatory reaction reaching its maximum, characterized by (epi)dermal infiltrates, edema, and spongiosis. **f** *48–120 h* Gradually, downregulatory mechanisms take over, leading to decreased inflammation and disappearance of the cellular infiltrate. Finally, primordial conditions are reconstituted except for a few residual hapten-specific T-cells causing the local skin memory. (*DC* Dendritic cell, *GM-CSF* granulocyte-macrophage colony-stimulating factor, *IL* interleukin, *IFN* interferon, *KC* keratinocyte, *PG* prostaglandin, *TGF* transforming growth factor, *TNF* tumor necrosis factor)

LC migration towards the dermis [53, 200, 201]. These pro-inflammatory phenomena, which are also observed in nonsensitized individuals [202] and in T-cell-deficient nude mice [203], strongly contribute to allergenicity [5]. Clearly most, if not all, of these effects can also be caused by irritants and, therefore, do not unambiguously discriminate between irritants and contact allergens [204–206]. Probably, true differences between these types of compounds depend on whether or not allergen-specific T-cells become involved. Thus, only after specific T-cell triggering might distinctive features be observed, e.g., local release of certain chemokines, such as CXCL10 (IP-10) and CXCL11 (I-TAC/IP-9) [207]. The latter chemokines are produced by IFN-γ-activated keratinocytes and T lymphocytes [208].

Certainly, pro-inflammatory effects of contact allergens increase, in many ways, the chance of allergen-specific T-cells meeting their targets. The first cells affected by skin contact, i.e., keratinocytes and LC, are thought to represent major sources of pivotal mediators such as IL-1β and TNF-α [46, 209]. First, as described in Sect. 2.3, "Hapten-Induced Activation of Allergen-Presenting Cells", these cytokines cause hapten-bearing LC to mature and migrate towards the dermis [34, 48]. But, these cytokines also cause (over)expression of adhesion molecules on dermal postcapillary endothelial cells, and loosen intercellular junctions. Thereby, extravasation of leucocytes, including allergen-specific T-cells, is strongly promoted [209–212]. Moreover, haptens can stimulate nitric oxide (NO) production of the inducible NO-synthase (iNOS) of LC and keratinocytes [213–215], which contributes to local edema, vasodilatation, and cell extravasation [213, 215].

Histopathological analyses support the view that the major causative events take place in the papillary dermis, close to the site of entry of allergen-specific T-cells, for instance at hair follicles, where haptens easily penetrate and blood capillaries are nearby [216]. Here, perivascular mononuclear cell infiltrates develop, giving the highest chance of encounters between allergen-presenting cells and specific T-cells. Once triggered, extravasated T-cells will readily enter the lower epidermal layers, in which haptenized keratinocytes produce lymphocyte-attracting chemokines, such as CXCL10 (IP-10) [207]. Subsequently, since memory T-cells can also be triggered by "non-professional" APC, including KC, fibroblasts, and infiltrating mononuclear cells, ACD reactivity is amplified in the epidermis [96, 98, 202]. Together, these events result in the characteristic epidermal damage seen in ACD, such as spongiosis and hyperplasia. Notably, in ongoing ACD reactions, the production of chemokines attracting lymphocytes and monocytes/macrophages, in addition to the production of cytokines, adds to the nonspecific recruitment and activation of leucocytes [60, 217, 218]. Thus, like the very early events in the effector phase reaction, the final response to a contact allergen is antigen-nonspecific. It is therefore not surprising that allergic and irritant reactions are histologically alike.

2.7.3 Early Phase Reactivity

The role of an antibody-mediated early phase reaction in the development of ACD is still unclear in humans, although Askenase and his colleagues have generated robust data to support this view in murine models [219–222]. Hapten-specific IgM, produced upon immunization by distant hapten-activated B-1 cells [223, 224], can bind antigen early after challenge [223, 225] and activate complement [226]. The resulting C5a causes the release of serotonin and TNF-α from local mast cells and platelets, leading to vascular dilatation and permeabilization, detectable as an early ear swelling peaking at 2 h [222, 227, 228]. Furthermore, C5a and TNF-α induce the upregulation of adhesion molecules on local endothelial cells [229, 230], thereby contributing to the recruitment of T-cells in hapten challenge sites [222, 230]. In addition, human T-cells were recently found to express the C5a receptor and are chemoattracted to endothelium-bound C5a [231]. However, antibodies against most contact allergens, including nickel, are only occasionally detectable in humans, arguing against humoral mechanisms playing more than a minor role in clinical ACD [232, 233]. Interestingly in mice, immunoglobulin light chains, which have long been considered as the meaningless remnants of a spillover in the regular immunoglobulin production by B cells, were recently discovered to mediate very early hypersensitivity reactions [234]. In addition to an auxiliary role of humoral immunity, similar effects may be mediated by allergen-specific T-cells with an unusual phenotype (CD3⁻CD4⁻CD8⁻Thy1⁺), which recognize the hapten and, within 2 h of hapten application, were found to elicit an early phase response [221]. Also, γδ-T-cells might contribute in a non-antigen-specific, probably non-MHC-restricted manner, to (early) elicitation responses [235–237].

2.7.4 T-Cell Patrol and Specificity of T-Cell Infiltrates

Whereas early nonspecific skin reactivity to contact allergens is pivotal for both sensitization and elicitation, full-scale development of ACD, of course, depends on allergen-specific T-cells within the (epi)dermal infiltrates. In healthy skin there is a constant flow of memory T-cells from the dermis towards the draining lymph nodes: about 200 T-cells $h^{-1} cm^{-2}$ skin [56]. Since just one single antigen-specific T cell can trigger visible skin inflammation [190], randomly skin-patrolling memory/effector T-cells might account for the initiation of the allergen-specific effector phase. However, since frequencies of hapten-specific T-cells in sensitized individuals may still remain below 1 in 1000, this does not seem to be a realistic scenario. Thus, augmented random and/or specific T-cell infiltration accompanies the development of ACD. Apparently, local chemokine release is pivotal in this respect [238]. The question concerning the specificity of ACD T-cell infiltrates has so far received little attention. In a guinea pig model, preferential entry of dinitrochlorobenzene (DNCB)-specific T-cells was observed within 18 h after elicitation of skin tests with DNCB, as compared to nonrelated compounds [239]. Probably, extravasation of hapten-specific T-cells benefits from T-cell receptor-mediated interactions with endothelial MHC molecules, presenting hapten penetrated from the skin. Within minutes after epicutaneous application, hapten can indeed be found in dermal tissues and on endothelial cells [193, 240, 241]. Interestingly, whereas preferential entry may already contribute to extraordinarily high frequencies of allergen-specific T-cells (within 48 h up to 10%) [136, 188], at later stages, when the ACD reaction fades away, the local frequency of allergen-specific T-cells may increase even further, due to allergen-induced proliferation and rescue from apoptosis. Thus, at former skin reaction sites these cells can generate "local skin memory" (see Sect. 2.8, "Flare-up and Retest Reactivity").

2.7.5 Effector T-Cell Phenotypes

The debate on phenotypes of effector T-cells in ACD is ongoing, although recent studies have shed light on longstanding issues [242]. This certainly holds true for expression of membrane molecules determining lymphocyte-migration patterns. Once released from reactive skin-draining lymph nodes to the blood, effector T-cells express increased levels of molecules mediating adhesion to peripheral vascular endothelia, e.g., the cutaneous lymphocyte antigen CLA [243, 244]. Notably, the same molecule is used by precursor LC to find their way to the skin [245]. To what extent other cellular adhesion molecules associated with T-cell differentiation and maturation, in particular the low-molecular-weight CD45 isoforms, contribute to migration into skin-inflammatory foci is still unclear

[246, 247]. Tissue-bound ligand molecules clearly involved in lymphocyte extravasation and extra vascular migration in the skin are fibronectin and collagens [248–251].

Since cutaneous infiltrates show a clear preponderance of CD4$^+$ T-cells, it is not surprising that these cells have most often been held responsible for mediating ACD. Nevertheless, as discussed in Sect. 2.3, "Recognition of Allergen-Modified Langerhans Cells by Specific T Cells," infiltrates contain both allergen-specific CD4$^+$ and CD8$^+$ T-cells [252, 253]. The latter might mediate skin inflammation through killing of hapten-bearing target cells. Indeed, it has become clear that both CD4$^+$ and CD8$^+$ T-cells can act as effector cells in DTH and ACD reactions [254–257]. Thus, neither of these subsets can be regarded simply as regulatory or suppressor cells, although both of these subsets may, depending on the allergen models and read-out assays, play such roles [116, 258].

An essentially similar conclusion holds true for T-cell subsets (whether CD4$^+$ or CD8$^+$), releasing type-1 or type-2 cytokines, or both (type 0) [190]. Whereas type-1 cytokines, in particular IFN-γ, display well-established pro-inflammatory effects [133, 259], IL-4, a hallmark type-2 cytokine, can cause erythema and induration when released in the skin [260, 261]. Indeed, blockage of IL-4 can interfere with ACD [261]. Furthermore, analyses of skin test biopsy samples demonstrate the presence of not only type-1 T-cells, but also allergen-specific type-2 and type-0 T-cells [117, 135, 136]. Entry of type-1 T-cells into skin-inflammatory sites is facilitated by their expression of CCR1, 5, and CXCR3 receptors for IFN-γ-induced chemokines such as MIP-1α, MIP-1β, and IP-10 [60, 262, 263]. Type-2 T-cells overexpress a partially different set of chemokine receptors, including, similar to eosinophils and basophils, CCR3, 4, and 8 [67, 264]. This would explain why local release of mediators commonly associated with immediate allergic reactions, such as eotaxins, preferentially involves type-2 T-cells. Thus, a picture emerges in which ACD reactions can be caused both by allergen-specific type-1 or type-2 T-cells [117, 190, 265]. In retrospect, the downregulatory effects of IL-4 on ACD reactions observed earlier in some mouse models [266] might be ascribed to accelerated allergen clearance rather than to blunt suppression. Still, both with time and repeated allergen pressure, type-2 responsiveness may rapidly take over [267]. Allergen-specific T-cells isolated from skin test sites of sensitized individuals, as compared to blood, showed a strong bias towards type-2 cytokine profiles [135]. Additional local IFN-γ release seems, however, indispensable, since for a broad panel of contact allergens, clinical ACD reactions were characterized by increased expression of mRNA encoding IFN-γ-inducible chemokines [207]. In addition, transgenic mice expressing IFN-γ in the epidermis showed strongly increased ACD reactivity [268].

2.7.6 Downregulatory Processes

Resolution of ACD reactions and risk factors for the development of chronicity are not yet fully understood. Of course, if the allergen source is limited, as with skin testing, local concentrations of allergen usually rapidly decrease, thus taking away the critical trigger of the ACD reaction cascade. Since even ACD reactions due to chronic exposure to allergen seldom result in permanent tissue destruction and scarification, immunoregulatory factors most likely contribute to prevention of excessive cytotoxicity and fatal destruction of the basal membrane. Both IL-1 and heparinase, secreted from activated keratinocytes and T-cells, protect keratinocytes from TNF-α-induced apoptosis [269, 270]. Moreover, activated effector T-cells can undergo activation-induced cell death (AICD) during the resolution phase [271]. Notably, pro-inflammatory type-1 T-cells, expressing high levels of Fas-ligand (CD95L) and low amounts of apoptosis-protecting FAP-1 protein, are more susceptible than type-2 cells to AICD [272]. This may partly explain the shift towards type-2 reactivity that is observed upon prolonged allergen exposure [267]. Moreover, during the late phase of ACD, keratinocytes, infiltrated macrophages, and T-cells start producing IL-10 [273–275], which has many anti-inflammatory activities, including suppression of antigen-presenting cell and macrophage functions [111, 276]. In addition, the release of factors such as PGE_2 and TGF-β, derived from activated keratinocytes and infiltrated leucocytes, e.g., type-3 T-cells, contributes to dampening of the immune response [277, 278]. Release of PGE_2, on the one hand, inhibits production of pro-inflammatory cytokines [164, 279] and, on the other hand, activates basophils [280]. These may constitute up to 5–15% of infiltrating cells in late-phase ACD reactions [281] and are also believed to contribute to downregulation of the inflammatory response [282, 283]. TGF-β silences activated T-cells and inhibits further infiltration by downregulating the expression of adhesion molecules on both endothelial and skin cells [110]. Regulatory cells producing these suppressive mediators might even predominate in skin sites frequently exposed to the same allergen, and which are known to show local (allergen-specific) hypo-responsiveness [284].

ACD reactions can certainly be mediated by classical effector cells, i.e., allergen-specific $CD4^+$ type-1 T-cells which, upon triggering by allergen-presenting cells, produce IFN-γ to activate nonspecific inflammatory cells such as macrophages. However, $CD8^+$ T-cells, and other cytokines including IL-4, can also play major roles in ACD. The conspicuous difference with DTH reactions induced by intradermal administration of protein antigens, i.e., the epidermal infiltrate, can largely be attributed to hapten-induced chemokine release by keratinocytes.

Core Message

■ In sensitized individuals, allergen-specific T-cells migrate to allergen contact sites and release pro-inflammatory mediators, which, subsequently, attract various inflammatory cells. This results in the elicitation of an allergic contact dermatitis reaction within 24–72 h.

2.8 Flare-up and Retest Reactivity

2.8.1 Flare-up Phenomena

Flare-up reactivity of former ACD and patch-test reaction sites is sometimes observed [285–287]. From the basic mechanisms of ACD, it can be inferred that allergen-specific flare-up reactions depend either on local allergen or on T-cell retention at these skin sites. Flare-up reactions due to locally persisting allergen can readily be observed in humans, when, from about 1 week after primary sensitization, sufficient effector T-cells have entered the circulation to react with residual allergen at the sensitization site [288]. This was most likely also the case when a patient was patch tested with different penicillin derivatives, one of which released formaldehyde, (H. Neering, personal communication). Pre-existing allergic reactivity and, thus, positive reactivity to formaldehyde apparently potentiated primary sensitization to penicillin, causing the other, previously negative, penicillin patch test sites to flare up from about 1 week after skin testing. Local allergen retention, however, is usually of short duration only. In experimental guinea pig studies using DNCB, chromium, and penicillin allergens for sensitization, and skin testing at different days before or after sensitization, we never observed allergen retention in the skin to mediate flare-up reactions for periods exceeding 2 weeks (R.J. Scheper et al., unpublished results).

2.8.2 Local Skin Memory

In contrast, allergen-specific T-cells may persist for at least several months in the skin (Fig. 9) [289, 290]. Thus, locally increased allergen-specific hyper-reactivity, detectable through either accelerated "retest" reactivity (after repeated allergenic contacts at the same skin site) or flare-up reactivity (after repeated allergen entry from the circulation, e.g., derived from food), may be observed for long periods of time at former skin reaction sites [291–293]. Typically, the erythematous reactions peak between 2 h and 6 h after contact with the allergen. Histological examination of such previous skin reaction sites shows that the majority of remaining T-cells are CD4$^+$ CCR10$^+$ [290]. The remarkable flare-up reactivity at such sites can be understood by considering that just one specific effector T-cell can be sufficient to generate macroscopic reactivity [188]. Moreover, a very high frequency of the residual T-cells may be specific for the allergen, as discussed in Sect. 2.7, "The Effector Phase of Allergic Contact Dermatitis". Notably, with higher allergen doses, in highly sensitized individuals, unrelated skin test sites may show flare-up reactions [289] and even generalized erythematous macular eruptions can be observed [294]. The latter reactivities are probably a corollary of the fact that recently activated T-cells show strong expression of adhesion and homing molecules, e.g., CLA, and chemokine receptors, such as CCR5, facilitating migration into peripheral tissues and thus allergen-specific T-cell patrol in the skin [244, 263, 295]. Upon allergen entry from the circulation, these allergen-specific T-cells could mediate generalized erythematous reactions [286, 296].

Recently, we have explored the possibilities of exploiting the specific retest/"skin memory" phenomenon in both guinea pig models and humans, for differentiating between concomitant sensitization and cross-reactivity [297–299]. We hypothesized that, with preferential local retention of T-cells reactive to the first allergen used for skin testing, no accelerated retest reactivity would be observed with a second, non-cross-reactive allergen, even when the individual would also be allergic to the latter allergen. But, if retests were made with a second allergen, cross-reactive with the same T-cells, again an accelerated erythematous reaction would be observed. Indeed, this hypothesis was confirmed for several different combinations of contact allergens, in both guinea pigs and humans. Thus, retesting guinea pigs previously sensitized to both methyl methacrylate (MMA) and DNCB, and skin tested with both allergens, showed accelerated retest reactivities with four different methacrylate congeners on the former MMA, but not DNCB, patch test sites [297]. This retest model can also be readily applied in clinical practice to discriminate between cross-reactivity and concomitant

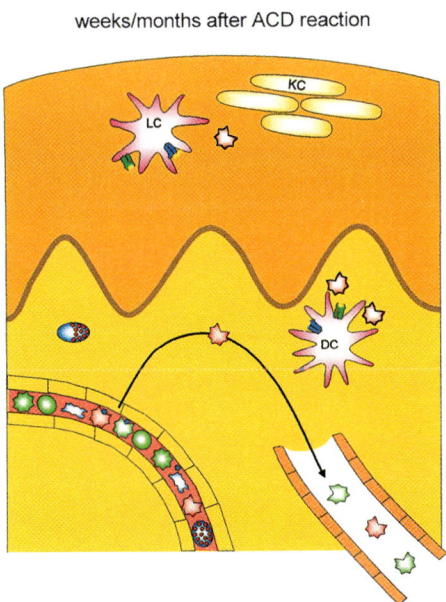
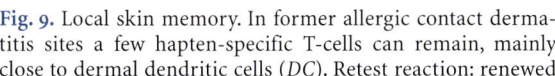
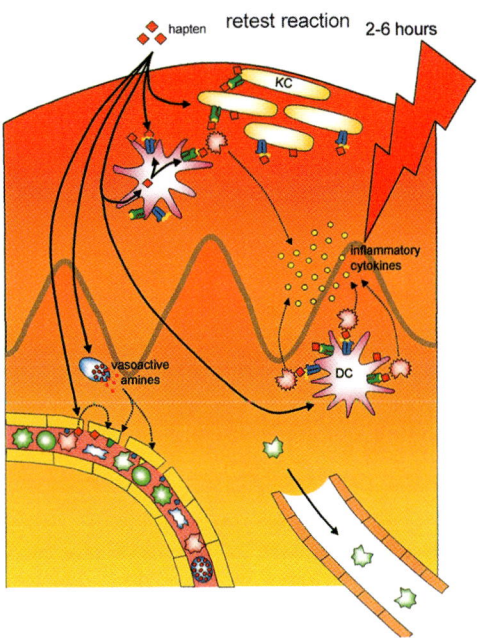

Fig. 9. Local skin memory. In former allergic contact dermatitis sites a few hapten-specific T-cells can remain, mainly close to dermal dendritic cells (*DC*). Retest reaction: renewed hapten contact can induce the rapid onset of an erythematous reaction, sparked off by the residual hapten-specific T-cells. (*KC* Keratinocyte, *LC* Langerhans cell)

2

sensitization. Matura et al. [298] confirmed positive cross-retest reactions for cloprednol and tixocortol pivalate, both belonging to group A corticosteroids, and budesonide, amcinonide, and triamcinolone, all belonging to group B corticosteroids (see also [296]).

> ### Core Message
>
> ■ At skin sites of allergic contact dermatitis reactions, few but allergen-specific T-cells can reside. Upon renewed allergen contact, these cells can cause an accelerated "flare-up" reaction peaking within few hours.

2.9 Hyporeactivity: Tolerance and Desensitization

Of course, uncontrolled development and expression of T-cell-mediated immune function would be detrimental to the host. During evolution, several mechanisms developed to curtail lymph node hyperplasia or to prevent excessive skin damage upon persisting antigen exposure.

2.9.1 Regulation of Immune Responses

First, allergen contacts, e.g., by oral or intravenous administration, may lead to large-scale presentation of allergen by cells other than skin DC (Fig. 10). In the absence of appropriate co-stimulatory signals (as described in Sect. 2.3, "Recognition of Allergen-Modified Langerhans Cells") naive T-cells may be anergized, i.e., turned into an unresponsive state, eventually leading to their death by apoptosis (Fig. 11) [300–303]. With increasing density of MHC–antigen complexes on the surface of APC, multiple levels of T-cell tolerance might be induced, with the characteristic stages called ignorance, anergy, and deletion [304–306]. Unresponsiveness of T-cells induced by allergenic contacts at skin sites where LC/DC functions have been damaged, e.g., by UV irradiation, or are naturally absent, e.g., in the tail skin of mice, may be ascribed to T-cell anergy, frequently associated with TCR/CD4 or CD8 downregulation [307, 308]. Whereas such anergy reflects "passive" unresponsiveness, tolerance by "active" suppression may also be induced under similar circumstances [309]. Actually, even regular epicutaneous allergenic contacts not only induce effector T-cells but also lymphocytes regulating T-cell proliferation (afferently acting regulatory cells) or, with frequent skin contacts, causing decreased skin reactivity (regulatory cells of effector

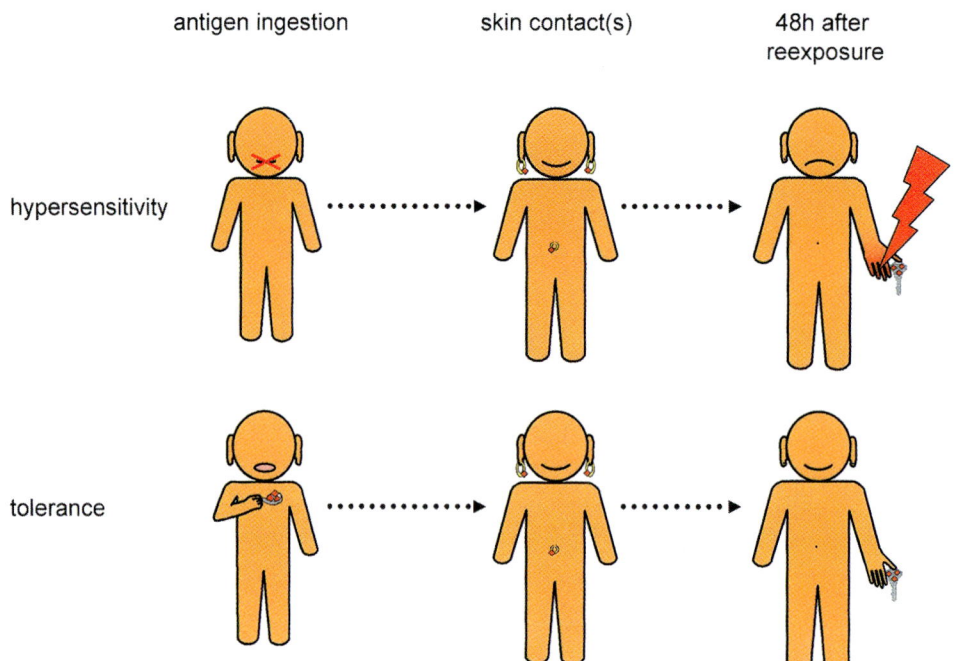

antigen ingestion   skin contact(s)   48h after reexposure

hypersensitivity

tolerance

Fig. 10. Induction of oral tolerance. Hapten ingestion, prior to potential sensitizing skin contact(s), can induce hapten-specific tolerance

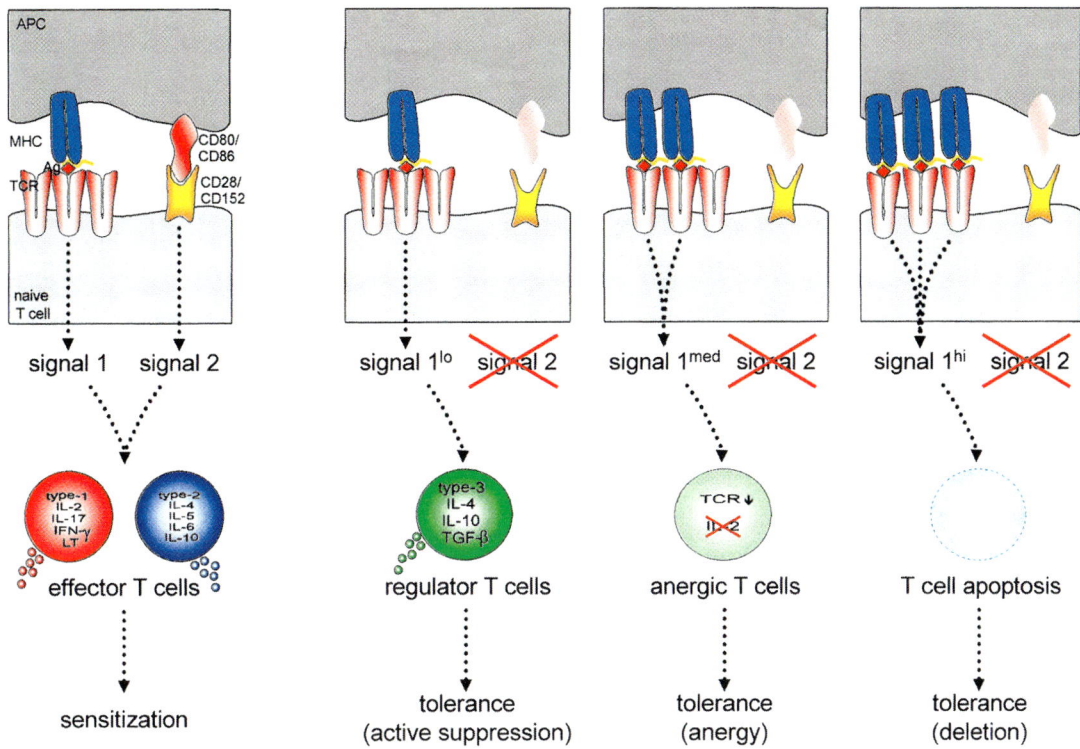

Fig. 11. The character of the APC–T-cell interaction determines the immunological outcome. Sensitization: naive T-cells, activated by antigen-presenting cells (*APC*) providing both hapten-specific ("*signal 1*") and appropriate costimulatory ("*signal 2*") signals, develop into effector T-cells, characterized by type-0, -1, and -2 cytokine secretion profiles. Tolerance: in the absence of appropriate costimulatory signals, immunological tolerance may develop. With increasing density of MHC–hapten complexes on the surface of APC activating "signal 1" T-cell pathways, multiple levels of T-cell tolerance might be induced

phase). Apparently, allergic contact hypersensitivity is the result of a delicate balance between effector and regulatory mechanisms [284, 310].

2.9.2 Cellular Basis of Active Tolerance

Upon preferential stimulation of regulatory cells, e.g., by feeding nonprimed, naive individuals with contact allergens, strong and stable allergen-specific, active tolerance may develop [311–314]. The concept of active regulatory ("suppressor") cells controlling ACD is based on the fact that, in experimental animal models, such allergen-specific tolerance can be transferred by lymphoid cells from tolerant to naive animals [237, 315]. Active suppression, as revealed by these adoptive cell transfers, is a critical event in regulating T-cell responses to contact sensitizers, and to all possible peptide/protein antigens, including bacterial, autoimmune, and graft rejection antigens [316–318].

Like effector T-cells in ACD, regulatory cells are not a single subpopulation of cells. As outlined above,

depending among other things on the nature of the allergen and route of exposure, ACD can be mediated by both CD4$^+$ and CD8$^+$ T-cells, either or both releasing type-1 or type-2 cytokines. Probably, given a predominant effector phenotype for a particular allergen, each of the other phenotypes can act as regulatory cells [319]. Nevertheless, earlier data suggested that type-2 cytokine-producing cells may be the most prominent regulatory cells in ACD, since allergic contact hypersensitivity was found to be enhanced, and tolerance reversed, by appropriately timed treatment with cytostatic drugs, including cyclophosphamide [320–322], preferentially affecting type-2 T-cells [323]. Interferons and IL-12, both impairing type-2 and -3 cells, were also shown to inhibit regulatory cells and to stimulate effector-cell functions in mouse models [324–326]. On the other hand, in particular after mucosal allergen contact stimulation, T-cells predominantly producing TGF-β (type-3 cytokine profile) may act as regulatory cells [327, 328]. These T-cells promote anti-inflammatory immunity, e.g., by switching antibody production to IgA, which mediates secretory immunity and thus contributes to antigen exclusion in the lumen, e.g., of the gastro-intestinal tract [329]. Of note, TGF-β strongly suppresses development of both type-1 and -2 effector T-cells, and can silence T-cells in a semi-naive state [110]. Whether these type-3 T-cells, or their precursors, are more sensitive to cytostatic drugs is not known. Another population of T-cells involved in tolerogenic processes is the group of $CD4^+CD25^+$ T-cells [330].

2.9.3 Regulatory Mechanisms of the Effector Phase

A critical feature of the regulatory principles involving mutual regulation of T-cell subpopulations by type-1 and -2 cytokines, and both of these in turn by TGF-β-producing T-cells, is that their function is observed foremost in primary immune responses (Fig. 6). Regulation may also pertain to the actual ACD reactions, i.e., the effector phase. Several "suppressive" pathways could lead to decreased allergic skin reactivity, including hapten removal by increased blood flow and metabolism by cells of the inflammatory infiltrate. Other regulatory mechanisms can also be involved, such as $CD8^+$ T-cells, acting either as suppressor ($CD28^-CD11b^+$) or cytotoxic ($CD28^+CD11b^-$) T-cells [331, 332], which may downregulate skin reactivity by focusing on allergen-presenting DC as their targets [332].

2.9.4 Redundancy of Tolerance Mechanisms

Besides these types of regulatory T-cells producing different cytokines, or exerting distinct cytotoxicities, other mechanisms may also contribute to immune regulation and tolerance. Apparently, the risk of excessive immune reactivity should be very low. These mechanisms involve allergen-specific T-cells shedding truncated T-cell receptors, acting as antagonists and blocking allergen presentation [333], and high-dose allergen-induced anergic T-cells [307]. Possibly, the latter cells, by actively suppressing DC functions, can function as "active" suppressor cells [307, 334]. Interestingly, DC, becoming suppressive by this mechanism [307] or by suppressive cytokines such as IL-10 and PGE_2 [164, 335, 336], can, in turn, act themselves as suppressor cells by conferring antigen-specific anergy to subsequently encountered T-cells [337–339]. Although, at present, consensus has been reached about a critical role of regulatory/suppressor cells in the development and expression of ACD, the relative contributions of each of the various mechanisms are still far from clear. Potential therapeutic applications of regulatory cells in various disorders, such as allergic contact dermatitis and autoimmune diseases, are currently under investigation.

2.9.5 Induction of Lasting Tolerance Only in Naive Individuals

Both clinical and experimental findings indicate that full and persistent tolerance can only be induced prior to any sensitizing allergen contacts [312, 340, 341]. Upon primary allergenic contacts, naive T-cells differentiate to produce polarized cytokine profiles (Fig. 6). Once polarized, however, T-cell profiles are irreversible, due to loss of cytokine (receptor) genes, or are at least very stable, due to the mutually suppressive activities of T-cell cytokines. An important corollary of the latter concept of active suppression is the bystander effect, in which the response to any antigen can be downregulated by immunosuppressive cytokines acting at a very local tolerogenic microenvironment [342]. The latter was observed for both protein antigens [343, 344] and methacrylate contact allergens [315]. The concept may also explain why even nonsensitizing doses of nickel applied to the skin prevented subsequent tolerance induction by feeding the metal allergen [345]. This may have contributed to incomplete tolerance induction in earlier clinical studies when feeding with poison ivy-/oak-derived allergens [346]. Apparently, the progeny of naive allergen-specific cells, once "on the stage," have been triggered to a "subclinical" degree towards effector cells and become refractory to regulatory cell action. Indeed, to our knowledge, permanent reversal of existing ACD in healthy individuals has, as yet, never been achieved. Nevertheless, as described above, effector cells still seem susceptible, though transiently, to the downregulation of allergen reactivity, as was observed in desensitization procedures [345, 347].

2.9.6 Transient Desensitization in Primed Individuals

For dermatologists, methods by which patients might be desensitized for existing ACD would be a welcome addition to the currently prevailing symptomatic therapies, and investigators have made a wide variety of attempts to achieve this goal. Unfortunately, therapeutic protocols involving ingestion of poison ivy allergen, penicillin, or nickel sulfate were of only transient benefit to the patients [346–350]. Similarly, in animal models, only a limited and transient degree of hyposensitization was obtained by Chase [351] when feeding DNCB-contact-sensitized guinea pigs with the allergen, whereas, to achieve persistent chromium-unresponsiveness in presensitized animals, Polak and Turk [352] needed a rigorous protocol involving up to lethal doses of the allergen. As outlined above, mechanisms underlying specific desensitization in ACD probably depend on direct interference of allergen with effector T-cell function, by blocking or downregulating T-cell receptors, leading to anergy [353]. As the onset of desensitization is immediate, no suppressor mechanisms may initially be involved. Apparently in the absence of LC, MHC class II-positive keratinocytes can serve as APC and are very effective in rendering allergen-specific effector cells anergic [354]. Moreover, at later stages, active suppression may come into play resulting from secondary inactivation of DC function by anergized T-cells [307]. Nevertheless, major problems with in vivo desensitization procedures relate to the refractoriness of effector T-cells to regulatory cell functions, and the rapid replacement of anergized effector cells by naive T-cells from relatively protected peripheral lymphoid tissues, which can be the source of a new generation of effector cells upon sensitizing allergen contacts. The same conclusions can be drawn from attempts to achieve local desensitization. It was found that local desensitization by repeatedly applying allergen at the same skin site did not result from local skin hardening or LC inactivation, as local reactivity to an unrelated allergen at the site was unimpaired [284]. Persistence of cellular infiltrates, in the absence of erythematous reactivity, at a desensitized skin site could reflect local anergy, but also locally active regulatory cells. Upon discontinuation of allergen exposure, however, local unresponsiveness was rapidly (within 1 week) lost. Collectively, these data illustrate the problems encountered in attempting to eradicate established effector-T-cell function, not only in ACD but also in autoimmune diseases [316].

2.10 Summary and Conclusions

Extensive research has led to a better understanding of the mechanisms of ACD. The basic immunology of ACD is now well defined, including T-cell migratory patterns, recognition of distinct allergens, interactions with other inflammatory cells to generate inflammation, and cytokine profiles. But new complexities have emerged. For instance, in contrast to earlier belief, many of the currently known T-cell subpopulations can act either or both as effector and regulatory cells, depending on the nature of the allergen, the route of entry, frequency of exposure, and

many other, still ill-defined factors. In particular, the poor understanding of regulatory mechanisms in ACD still hampers further therapeutic progress. So far, no methods of permanent desensitization have been devised.

Nevertheless, recently defined cellular interaction molecules and mediators provide promising targets for anti-inflammatory drugs, some of which have already entered clinical trials. Clearly, drugs found to be effective in preventing severe T-cell-mediated conditions, e.g., rejection of a vital organ graft, should be very safe before their use in ACD would seem appropriate. To date, prudence favors alternative measures to prevent ACD, be it through legal action to outlaw the use of certain materials or through avoiding personal contact with these materials. In the meantime, for difficult-to-avoid allergens, further studies on the potential value of tolerogenic treatments prior to possible sensitization seem warranted.

Suggested Reading

Janeway CA, Travers P, Walport M, Shlomchik M (2001) Immunobiology, 5th edn. Garland, New York

Roitt I, Delves PJ (2001) Roitt's essential immunology, 10th edn. Blackwell, London

References

1. Bergstresser PR (1989) Sensitization and elicitation of inflammation in contact dermatitis. In: Norris DA (ed) Immune mechanisms in cutaneous disease. Dekker, New York, pp 219–246
2. Turk JL (1975) Delayed hypersensitivity, 2nd edn. North-Holland, Amsterdam
3. Gell PDH, Coombs RRA, Lachman R (1975) Clinical aspects of immunology, 3rd edn. Blackwell, London
4. Mestas J, Hughes CC (2004) Of mice and not men: differences between mouse and human immunology. J Immunol 172:2731–2738
5. Saint-Mezard P, Krasteva M, Chavagnac C, Bosset S, Akiba H, Kehren J, Kanitakis J, Kaiserlian D, Nicolas JF, Berard F (2003) Afferent and efferent phases of allergic contact dermatitis (ACD) can be induced after a single skin contact with haptens: evidence using a mouse model of primary ACD. J Invest Dermatol 120:641–647
6. Bos JD, Meinardi MMHM (2000) The 500 Dalton rule for the skin penetration of chemical compounds and drugs. Exp Dermatol 9:165–169
7. Roberts DW, Lepoittevin J-P (1998) Hapten–protein interactions. In: Lepoittevin J-P, Basketter DA, Goossens A, Karlberg A-T (eds) Allergic contact dermatitis. Springer, Berlin Heidelberg New York, pp 81–1118
8. Eliasson E, Kenna JG (1996) Cytochrome P450 2E1 is a cell surface autoantigen in halothane hepatitis. Mol Pharmacol 50:573–582

9. Budinger L, Hertl M (2000) Immunologic mechanisms in hypersensitivity reactions to metal ions: an overview. Allergy 55:108–115

10. Blauvelt A, Hwang ST, Udey MC (2003) Allergic and immunologic diseases of the skin. J Allergy Clin Immunol 111:S560–S570

11. Kimber I, Dearman RJ (2002) Allergic contact dermatitis: the cellular effectors. Contact Dermatitis 46:1–5

12. Liberato DJ, Byers VS, Ennick RG, Castagnoli N (1981) Region specific attack of nitrogen and sulfur nucleophiles on quinones from poison oak/ivy catechols (urushiols) and analogues as models for urushiol-protein conjugate formation. J Med Chem 24:28–33

13. Kalish RS, Wood JA, LaPorte A (1994) Processing of urushiol (poison ivy) hapten by both endogenous and exogenous pathways for presentation to T cells in vitro. J Clin Invest 93:2039–2047

14. Naisbitt DJ (2004) Drug hypersensitivity reactions in skin: understanding mechanisms and the development of diagnostic and predictive tests. Toxicology 194:179–196

15. Krasteva M, Nicolas JF, Chabeau G, Garrigue JL, Bour H, Thivolet J, Schmitt D (1993) Dissociation of allergenic and immunogenic functions in contact sensitivity to para-phenylenediamine. Int Arch Allergy Immunol 102:200–204

16. Merk HF, Abel J, Baron JM, Krutmann J (2004) Molecular pathways in dermatotoxicology. Toxicol Appl Pharmacol 195:267–277

17. Epling GA, Wells JL, Ung Chan Yoon (1988) Photochemical transformations in salicylanilide photoallergy. Photochem Photobiol 47:167–171

18. Schnuch A, Westphal GA, Muller MM, Schulz TG, Geier J, Brasch J, Merk HF, Kawakubo Y, Richter G, Koch P, Fuchs T, Gutgesell T, Reich K, Gebhardt M, Becker D, Grabbe J, Szliska C, Aberer W, Hallier E (1998) Genotype and phenotype of N-acetyltransferase 2 (NAT2) polymorphism in patients with contact allergy. Contact Dermatitis 38:209–211

19. Patlewicz GY, Basketter DA, Pease CK, Wilson K, Wright ZM, Roberts DW, Bernard G, Arnau EG, Lepoittevin JP (2004) Further evaluation of quantitative structure–activity relationship models for the prediction of the skin sensitization potency of selected fragrance allergens. Contact Dermatitis 50:91–97

20. Wilson NS, Villadangos JA (2004) Lymphoid organ dendritic cells: beyond the Langerhans cells paradigm. Immunol Cell Biol 82:91–98

21. Hoath SB, Leahy DG (2003) The organization of human epidermis: functional epidermal units and phi proportionality. J Invest Dermatol 121:1440–1446

22. Breathnach SM (1988) The Langerhans cell. Centenary review. Br J Dermatol 119:463–469

23. Romani N, Holzmann S, Tripp CH, Koch F, Stoitzner P (2003) Langerhans cells – dendritic cells of the epidermis. APMIS 111:725–740

24. Kimber I, Dearman RJ (2003) What makes a chemical an allergen? Ann Allergy Asthma Immunol 90:28–31

25. Inaba K, Schuler G, Witmer MD, Valinsky J, Atassi B, Steinman RM (1986) Immunologic properties of purified epidermal Langerhans cells. Distinct requirements for stimulation of unprimed and sensitized T lymphocytes. J Exp Med 164:605–613

26. Kimber I, Cumberbatch M (1992) Dendritic cells and cutaneous immune responses to chemical allergens. Toxicol Appl Pharmacol 117:137–146

27. Dieu M-C, Vanbervliet B, Vicari A, Bridon J-M, Oldham E, Ait-Yahia S, Brière F, Zlotnik A, Lebecque S, Caux C (1998) Selective recruitment of immature and mature dendritic cells by distinct chemokines expressed in different anatomic sites. J Exp Med 188:373–386

28. Stingl G, Katz SI, Clement L, Green I, Shevach EM (1978) Immunological functions of Ia-bearing epidermal Langerhans cells. J Immunol 121:2005–2013

29. Czernielewski SM, Demarchez M (1987) Further evidence for the self-reproducing capacity of Langerhans cells in human skin. J Invest Dermatol 88:17–20

30. Streilein JW, Grammer SF (1989) In vitro evidence that Langerhans cells can adopt two functionally distinct forms capable of antigen presentation to T lymphocytes. J Immunol 143:3925–3933

31. Langerhans P (1868) Über die Nerven der menschlichen Haut. Virchows Arch Pathol Anat 44:325–337

32. Birbeck M (1961) An electron microscope study of basal melanocytes and high level clear cells (Langerhans cells) in vitiligo. J Invest Dermatol 37:51–56

33. Braathen LR (1980) Studies on human epidermal Langerhans cells. III. Induction of T lymphocyte response to nickel sulphate in sensitized individuals. Br J Dermatol 103:517–526

34. Kimber I, Dearman RJ, Cumberbatch M, Huby RJ (1998) Langerhans cells and chemical allergy. Curr Opin Immunol 10:614–619

35. Kimber I, Basketter DA, Gerberick GF, Dearman RJ (2002) Allergic contact dermatitis. Int Immunopharmacol 2:201–211

36. Park SH, Chiu YH, Jayawardena J, Roark J, Kavita U, Bendelac A (1998) Innate and adaptive functions of the CD1 pathway of antigen presentation. Semin Immunol 10:391–398

37. Weinlich G, Heine M, Stössel H, Zanella M, Stoitzner P, Ortner U, Smolle J, Koch F, Sepp NT, Schuler G, Romani N (1998) Entry into afferent lymphatics and maturation in situ of migrating murine cutaneous dendritic cells. J Invest Dermatol 110:441–448

38. Richters CD, Hoekstra MJ, van Baare J, Du Pont JS, Hoefsmit EC, Kamperdijk EW (1994) Isolation and characterization of migratory human skin dendritic cells. Clin Exp Immunol 98:330–336

39. Jakob T, Ring J, Udey MC (2001) Multistep navigation of Langerhans/dendritic cells in and out of the skin. J Allergy Clin Immunol 108:688–696

40. Ozawa H, Nakagawa S, Tagami H, Aiba S (1996) Interleukin-1b and granulocyte-macrophage colony stimulating factor mediate Langerhans cell maturation differently. J Invest Dermatol 106:441–445

41. Wong BR, Josien R, Lee SY, Sauter B, Li HL, Steinman RM, Choi YW (1997) TRANCE (Tumor necrosis factor [TNF]-related activation-induced cytokine), a new TNF family member predominantly expressed in T cells, is a dendritic cell-specific survival factor. J Exp Med 186:2075–2080

42. Aiba S, Tagami H (1999) Dendritic cell activation induced by various stimuli, eg exposure to microorganisms, their products, cytokines, and simple chemicals as well as adhesion to extracellular matrix. J Dermatol Sci 20:1–13

43. Inaba K, Schuler G, Steinman RM (1993) GM-CSF – a granulocyte/macrophage/dendritic cell stimulating factor. In: Van Furth R (ed) Hemopoietic growth factors and mononuclear phagocytes. Karger, Basel, pp 187–196

44. Jakob T, Udey MC (1998) Regulation of E-Cadherin mediated adhesion in Langerhans cell-like dendritic cells by

inflammatory mediators that mobilize Langerhans cells in vivo. J Immunol 160:4067–4073

45. Schwarzenberger K, Udey MC (1996) Contact allergens and epidermal proinflammatory cytokines modulate Langerhans cell E-cadherin expression in situ. J Invest Dermatol 106:553–558

46. Enk AH, Katz SI (1992) Early molecular events in the induction phase of contact sensitivity. Proc Natl Acad Sci USA 89:1398–1402

47. Enk AH, Angeloni VL, Udey MC, Katz SI (1993) An essential role for Langerhans cell-derived IL-1b in the initiation of primary immune responses in skin. J Immunol 150:3698–3704

48. Steinman RM, Hoffman L, Pope M (1995) Maturation and migration of cutaneous dendritic cells. J Invest Dermatol 105:2S–7S

49. Wang B, Esche C, Mamelak A, Freed I, Watanabe H, Sauder DN (2003) Cytokine knockouts in contact hypersensitivity research. Cytokine Growth Factor Rev 14:381–389

50. Tang A, Amagai M, Granger LG, Stanley JR, Udey MC (1993) Adhesion of epidermal Langerhans cells to keratinocytes mediated by E-cadherin. Nature 361:82–85

51. Jakob T, Udey MC (1998) Regulation of E-cadherin-mediated adhesion in Langerhans cell like dendritic cells by inflammatory mediators that mobilize Langerhans cells in vivo. J Immunol 160:4067–4073

52. Ma J, Wing J-H, Guo Y-J, Sy M-S, Bigby M (1994) In vivo treatment with anti-ICAM-1 and antiLFA-1 antibodies inhibits contact sensitization-induced migration of epidermal Langerhans cells to regional lymph nodes. Cell Immunol 158:389–399

53. Rambukhana A, Bos JD, Irik D, Menko WJ, Kapsenberg ML, Das PK (1995) In situ behaviour of human Langerhans cells in skin organ culture. Lab Invest 73:521–531

54. Price AA, Cumberbatch M, Kimber I (1997) α6 integrins are required for Langerhans cell migration from the epidermis. J Exp Med 186:1725–1735

55. Weiss JM, Sleeman J, Renkl AC, Dittmar H, Termeer CC, Taxis S, Howells N, Hofmann M, Kohler G, Schöpf E, Ponta H, Herrlich P, Simon JC (1997) An essential role for CD44 variant isoforms in epidermal Langerhans cell and blood dendritic cell function. J Cell Biol 137:1137–1147

56. Brand CU, Hunger RE, Yawalkar N, Gerber HA, Schaffner T, Braathen LR (1999) Characterization of human skin-derived CD1a-positive lymph cells. Arch Dermatol Res 291:65–72

57. Kobayashi Y (1997) Langerhans cells produce type IV collagenase (MMP-9) following epicutaneous stimulation with haptens. Immunol 90:496–501

58. Randolph GJ (2001) Dendritic cell migration to lymph nodes: cytokines, chemokines, and lipid mediators. Semin Immunol 13:267–274

59. Sallusto F, Lanzavecchia A, Mackay CR (1998) Chemokines and chemokine receptors in T-cell priming and Th1/Th2-mediated responses. Immunol Today 19:568–574

60. Zlotnik A, Morales J, Hedrick JA (1999) Recent advances in chemokines and chemokine receptors. Crit Rev Immunol 19:1–47

61. Caux C, Ait-Yahia S, Chemin K, de Bouteiller O, Dieu-Nosjean MC, Homey B, Massacrier C, Vanbervliet B, Zlotnik A, Vicari A (2000) Dendritic cell biology and regulation of dendritic cell trafficking by chemokines. Springer Semin Immunopathol 22:345–369

62. Sallusto F, Palermo B, Lenig D, Miettinen M, Matikainen S, Julkunen I, Forster R, Burgstahler R, Lipp M, Lanzavecchia A (1999) Distinct patterns and kinetics of chemokine production regulate dendritic cell function. Eur J Immunol 29:1617–1625

63. Saeki H, Moore AM, Brown MJ, Hwan ST (1999) Secondary lymphoid-tissue chemokine (SLC) and CC chemokine receptor 7 (CCR7) participate in the emigration pathway of mature dendritic cells from the skin to regional lymph nodes. J Immunol 162:2472–2475

64. Gunn MD, Tangemann K, Tam C, Cyster JG, Rosen SD, Williams LT (1998) A chemokine expressed in lymphoid high endothelial venules promotes the adhesion and chemotaxis of naive T lymphocytes. Proc Natl Acad Sci USA 95:258–263

65. Kim CH, Broxmeyer HE (1999) Chemokines: signal lamps for trafficking of T and B cells for development and effector function. J Leuk Biol 65:6–15

66. Robbiani DF, Finch RA, Jager D, Muller WA, Sartorelli AC, Randolph GJ. (2000) The leukotriene C(4) transporter MRP1 regulates CCL19 (MIP-3beta, ELC)-dependent mobilization of dendritic cells to lymph nodes. Cell 103:757–768

67. Honig SM, Fu S, Mao X, Yopp A, Gunn MD, Randolph GJ, Bromberg JS (2003) FTY720 stimulates multidrug transporter- and cysteinyl leukotriene-dependent T cell chemotaxis to lymph nodes. J Clin Invest 111:627–637

68. Sallusto F, Schaerli P, Loetscher P, Schaniel C, Lenig D, Mackay CR, Qin S, Lanzavecchia A (1998) Rapid and coordinated switch in chemokine receptor expression during dendritic cell maturation. Eur J Immunol 28:2760–2769

69. Cumberbatch M, Dearman RJ, Kimber I (1997) Interleukin 1-beta and the stimulation of Langerhans cell migration – comparisons with tumour necrosis factor alpha. Arch Dermatol Res 289:277–284

70. Heufler C, Koch F, Schuler G (1988) Granulocyte/macrophage colony-stimulating factor and interleukin 1 mediate the maturation of epidermal Langerhans cells into potent immunostimulatory dendritic cells. J Exp Med 167:700–705

71. Furue M, Chang CH, Tamaki K (1996) Interleukin-1 but not tumor necrosis factor a synergistically upregulates the granulocyte-macrophage colony-stimulating factor-induced B7-1 expression of murine Langerhans cells. Br J Dermatol 135:194–198

72. Schuler G, Steinman RM (1985) Murine epidermal Langerhans cells mature into potent immune-stimulatory dendritic cells in vitro. J Exp Med 161:526–546

73. Haig DM, Hopkins J, Miller HRP (1999) Local immune responses in afferent and efferent lymph. Immunology 96:155–163

74. Altin JG, Sloan EK (1997) The role of CD45 and CD45-associated molecules in T cell activation. Immunol Cell Biol 75:430–445

75. Schon MP, Zollner TM, Boehncke WH (2003) The molecular basis of lymphocyte recruitment to the skin: clues for pathogenesis and selective therapies of inflammatory disorders. J Invest Dermatol 121:951–962

76. Von Andrian UH, Mrini C (1998) In situ analysis of lymphocyte migration to lymph nodes. Cell Adh Comm 6:85–96

77. Vestweber D, Blanks JE (1999) Mechanisms that regulate the function of the selectins and their ligands. Physiol Rev 79:181–213

78. Adema GJ, Hartgers F, Verstraten R, de Vries E, Marland G, Menon S, Foster J, Xu Y, Nooyen P, McClanahan T, Bacon

KB, Figdor CG (1997) A dendritic-cell-derived C-C chemokine that preferentially attracts naive T cells. Nature 387: 713–717

79. Ngo VN, Tang LH, Cyster JG (1998) Epstein-Barr virus-induced molecule 1 ligand chemokine is expressed by dendritic cells in lymphoid tissues and strongly attracts naive T cells and activated B cells. J Exp Med 188: 181–191

80. Nagira M, Imai T, Hieshima K, Kusuda J, Ridanpaa M, Takagi S, Nishimura M, Kakizaki M, Nomiyama H, Yoshie O (1997) Molecular cloning of a novel human CC chemokine secondary lymphoid-tissue chemokine that is a potent chemoattractant for lymphocytes and mapped to chromosome 9p13. J Biol Chem 272: 19518–19524

81. Rustemeyer T, von Blomberg BME, de Ligter S, Frosch PJ, Scheper RJ (1999) Human T lymphocyte priming in vitro by dendritic cells. Clin Exp Immunol 117: 209–216

82. Crivellato E, Vacca A, Ribatti D (2004) Setting the stage: an anatomist's view of the immune system. Trends Immunol 25: 210–217

83. Itano AA, Jenkins MK (2003) Antigen presentation to naive CD4 T cells in the lymph node. Nat Immunol 4: 733–739

84. Griem P, Wulferink M, Sachs B, Gonzales JB, Gleichmann E (1998) Allergic and autoimmune reactions to xenobiotics: how do they arise? Immunol Today 19: 133–141

85. Moulon C, Vollmer J, Weltzien H-U (1995) Characterization of processing requirements and metal crossreactivities in T cell clones from patients with allergic contact dermatitis to nickel. Eur J Immunol 25: 3308–3315

86. Li QJ, Dinner AR, Qi S, Irvine DJ, Huppa JB, Davis MM, Chakraborty AK (2004) CD4 enhances T cell sensitivity to antigen by coordinating Lck accumulation at the immunological synapse. Nat Immunol 5: 791–799

87. Schoenberger SP, Toes REM, Vandervoort EIH, Offringa R, Melief CJM (1998) T-cell help for cytotoxic T lymphocytes is mediated by CD40-CD40L interactions. Nature 393: 480–483

88. Gascoigne NR, Zal T (2004) Molecular interactions at the T cell-antigen-presenting cell interface. Curr Opin Immunol 16: 114–119

89. Cantrell D (1996) T cell receptor signal transduction pathways. Annu Rev Immunol 14: 259–274

90. Kuo CT, Leiden JM (1999) Transcriptional regulation of T lymphocyte development and function. Annu Rev Immunol 17: 149–187

91. Davis SJ, van der Merwe PA (2003) TCR triggering: co-receptor-dependent or -independent? Trends Immunol 24: 624–626

92. Trautmann A, Randriamampita C (2003) Initiation of TCR signalling revisited. Trends Immunol 24: 425–428

93. Acuto O, Michel F (2003) CD28-mediated co-stimulation: a quantitative support for TCR signalling. Nat Rev Immunol 3: 939–951

94. Quezada SA, Jarvinen LZ, Lind EF, Noelle RJ (2004) CD40/CD154 interactions at the interface of tolerance and immunity. Annu Rev Immunol 22: 307–328

95. Dong C, Nurieva RI, Prasad DV (2003) Immune regulation by novel costimulatory molecules. Immunol Res 28: 39–48

96. Viola A, Lanzavecchia A (1996) T cell activation determined by T cell receptor number and tunable thresholds. Science 273: 104–106

97. Banchereau J, Steinman RM (1998) Dendritic cells and the control of immunity. Nature 392: 245–252

98. Hommel M (2004) On the dynamics of T-cell activation in lymph nodes. Immunol Cell Biol 82: 62–66

99. Cella M, Sallusto F, Lanzavecchia A (1997) Origin, maturation and antigen presenting function of dendritic cells. Curr Opin Immunol 9: 10–16

100. Gomez J, Gonzalez A, Martinez-A C, Rebollo A (1998) IL-2-induced cellular events. Crit Rev Immunol 18: 185–220

101. Berridge MJ (1997) Lymphocyte activation in health and disease. Crit Rev Immunol 17: 155–178

102. Theze J, Alzari PM, Bertoglio J (1996) Interleukin 2 and its receptors: recent advances and new immunological functions. Immunol Today 17: 481–486

103. Lacour M, Arrighi J-F, Müller KM, Carlberg C, Saurat J-H, Hauser C (1994) cAMP up-regulates IL-4 and IL-5 production from activated CD4$^+$ T cells while decreasing IL-2 release and NF-AT induction. Int Immunol 6: 1333–1343

104. Linsley PS, Ledbetter JA (1993) The role of the CD28 receptor during T cell responses to antigen. Annu Rev Immunol 11: 191–212

105. Mazzoni A, Segal DM (2004) Controlling the Toll road to dendritic cell polarization. J Leukoc Biol 75: 721–30

106. Constant SL, Bottomly K (1997) Induction of Th1 and Th2 CD4$^+$ T cell responses: the alternate approaches. Annu Rev Immunol 15: 297–322

107. Nakamura T, Lee RK, Nam SY, Podack ER, Bottomly K, Flavell RA (1997) Roles of IL-4 and IFN-g in stabilizing the T helper cell type-1 and 2 phenotype. J Immunol 158: 2648–2653

108. O'Garra A (1998) Cytokines induce the development of functionally heterogeneous T helper cell subsets. Immunity 8: 275–283

109. Santana MA, Rosenstein Y (2003) What it takes to become an effector T cell: the process, the cells involved, and the mechanisms. J Cell Physiol 195: 392–401

110. Sallusto F, Geginat J, Lanzavecchia A. (2004) Central memory and effector memory T cell subsets: function, generation, and maintenance. Annu Rev Immunol 22: 745–763

111. Morel PA, Oriss TB (1998) Crossregulation between Th1 and Th2 cells. Crit Rev Immunol 18: 275–303

112. Dabbagh K, Lewis DB (2003) Toll-like receptors and T-helper-1/T-helper-2 responses. Curr Opin Infect Dis 16: 199–204

113. Burkett PR, Koka R, Chien M, Boone DL, Ma A (2004) Generation, maintenance, and function of memory T cells. Adv Immunol 83: 191–231

114. Spahn TW, Kucharzik T (2004) Modulating the intestinal immune system: the role of lymphotoxin and GALT organs. Gut 53: 456–465

115. Bour H, Peyron E, Gaucherand M, Garrigue JL, Desvignes C, Kaiserlian D, Revillard JP, Nicolas JF (1995) Major histocompatibility complex class I-restricted CD8$^+$ T cells and class II-restricted CD4$^+$ T cells, respectively, mediate and regulate contact sensitivity to dinitrofluorobenzene. Eur J Immunol 25: 3006–3010

116. Kimber I, Dearman RJ (2002) Allergic contact dermatitis: the cellular effectors. Contact Dermatitis 46: 1–5

117. Cavani A, Mei D, Guerra E, Corinti S, Giani M, Pirrotta L, Puddu P, Girolomoni G (1998) Patients with allergic contact dermatitis to nickel and nonallergic individuals display different nickel-specific T cell responses. Evidence for the presence of effector CD8$^+$ and regulatory CD4$^+$ T cells. J Invest Dermatol 111: 621–628

118. Kang KF, Kubin M, Cooper KD, Lessin SR, Trinchieri G, Rook AH (1996) IL-12 synthesis by human Langerhans cells. J Immunol 156: 1402–1407

119. Pulendran B (2004) Modulating TH1/TH2 responses with microbes, dendritic cells, and pathogen recognition receptors. Immunol Res 29: 187–196

120. Paul WE, Ohara J (1987) B-cell stimulatory factor-1/interleukin 4. Annu Rev Immunol 5:429–459
121. Rogge L, Barberis-Maino L, Biffi M, Passini N, Presky DH, Gubler U, Sinigaglia F (1997) Selective expression of an interleukin-12 receptor component by human T helper 1 cells. J Exp Med 185:825–831
122. Nakamura T, Kamogawa Y, Bottomly K, Flavell RA (1997) Polarization of IL-4- and IFN-gamma-producing CD4(+) T cells following activation of naive CD4(+) T cells. J Immunol 158:1085–1094
123. Orange JS, Biron CA (1996) An absolute and restricted requirement for IL-12 in natural killer cell IFN-g production and antiviral defense. J Immunol 156:1138–1142
124. Mackey MF, Barth RJ, Noelle RJ (1998) The role of CD40/CD154 interactions in the priming, differentiation, and effector function of helper and cytotoxic T cell. J Leuk Biol 63:418–428
125. Cella M, Scheidegger D, Palmer-Lehmann K, Lane P, Lanzavecchia A, Alber G (1996) Ligation of CD40 on dendritic cells triggers production of high levels of interleukin 12 and enhances T cell stimulatory capacity. J Exp Med 184:747–752
126. Ohshima Y, Tanaka Y, Tozawa H, Takahashi Y, Maliszewski C, Delespesse C (1997) Expression and function of OX40 ligand on human dendritic cells. J Immunol 159:3838–3848
127. Kuchroo V, Prabhu Das M, Brown JA Ranger A, Zamvill MSS, Sobel RA, Weiner HL, Nabavi N, Glimcher LH (1995) B7-1 and B7-2 costimulatory molecules activate differentially the Th1/Th2 developmental pathways. Application to autoimmune disease therapy. Cell 80:707–718
128. Ranger AM, Prabhu Das M, Kuchroo VK, Glimcher LH (1996) B7-2 (CD86) is essential for the development of IL-4 producing cells. Int Immunol 153:1549–1560
129. Schweitzer AN, Borriello F, Wong RCK, Abbas AK, Sharpe AH (1997) Role of costimulators in T cell differentiation – studies using antigen-presenting cells lacking expression of CD80 or CD86. J Immunol 158:2713–2722
130. Rulifson IC, Sperling AI, Fields PE, Fitch FW, Bluestone JA (1997) CD28 costimulation promotes the production of Th2 cytokines. J Immunol 158:658–665
131. Groux H, Sornasse T, Cottrez F, de Vries JE, Coffman RL, Roncarolo MG, Yssel H (1997) Induction of human T helper cell type-1 differentiation results in loss of IFN-g receptor b-chain expression. J Immunol 158:5627–5631
132. Pernis A, Gupta S, Gollob KJ, Garfein E, Coffman RL, Schindler C, Rothman P (1995) Lack of interferon gamma receptor beta chain and the prevention of interferon signaling in Th1 cells. Science 269:245–247
133. Gajewski TF, Fitch FW (1988) Antiproliferative effect of IFN-gamma in immune regulation. I. IFN-gamma inhibits the proliferation of Th2 but not Th1 murine helper T lymphocyte clones. J Immunol 140:4245–4252
134. Yoshimoto T, Takeda K, Tanaka T, Ohkusu K, Kashiwamura S, Okamura H, Akira S, Nakanishi K (1998) IL-12 upregulates IL-18 receptor expression on T cells, TH1 cells, and B cells – synergism with IL-18 for IFN-gamma production. J Immunol 161:3400–3407
135. Werfel T, Hentschel M, Kapp A, Renz H (1997) Dichotomy of blood- and skin-derived IL-4-producing allergen-specific T cells and restricted V beta repertoire in nickel-mediated contact dermatitis. J Immunol 158:2500–2505
136. Probst P, Küntzlin D, Fleischer B (1995) T$_H$2-type infiltrating T cells in nickel-induced contact dermatitis. Cell Immunol 165:134–140
137. Zanni MP, Mauri-Hellweg D, Brander C, Wendland T, Schnyder B, Frei E, von Greyerz S, Bircher A, Pichler WJ (1997) Characterization of lidocaine-specific T cells. J Immunol 158:1139–1148
138. Perez VL, Lederer JA, Lichtman AH, Abbas AK (1995) Stability of Th1 and Th2 populations. Int Immunol 7:869–875
139. Rincon M, Anguita J, Nakamura T, Fikrig E, Flavell RA (1997) Interleukin (IL)-6 directs the differentiation of IL-4 producing CD4+ T cells. J Exp Med 182:1591–1596
140. Yoshimoto T, Bendelac A, Watson C, Hu-Li J, Paul WE (1995) Role of NK1.1+ T cells in a TH2 response and in immunoglobulin E production. Science 270:1845–1847
141. Hiroi T, Iwatani K, Iijima H, Kodama S, Yanagita M, Kiyono H (1998) Nasal immune system – distinctive Th0 and Th1/Th2 type environments in murine nasal-associated lymphoid tissues and nasal passage, respectively. Eur J Immunol 28:3346–3353
142. Banchereau J (1995) Converging and diverging properties of human interleukin-4 and interleukin-10. Behr Inst Mitteil 96:58–77
143. Itoh K, Hirohata S (1995) The role of IL-10 in human B cell activation, proliferation, and differentiation. J Immunol 154:4341–4350
144. Napolitano LM, Buzdon MM, Shi HJ, Bass BL (1997) Intestinal epithelial cell regulation cell regulation of macrophage and lymphocyte interleukin 10 expression. Arch Surg 132:1271–1276
145. Xu H, Banerjee A, Diulio NA, Fairchild RL (1996) T cell populations primed by hapten sensitization in contact sensitivity are distinguished by polarized patterns of cytokine production: interferon gamma-producing (Tc1) effector CD8+ T cells and interleukin (IL)-4/IL-10-producing (Th2) negative regulatory CD4+ T cells. J Exp Med 183:1001–1012
146. Letterio JL, Roberts AB (1998) Regulation of immune responses by TGF-beta. Annu Rev Immunol 16:137–161
147. Hosken NA, Shibuya K, Heath AW, Murphy KM, O'Garra A (1995) The effect of antigen dose on CD4+ T helper cell phenotype development in a T cell receptor phenotype development in a T cell receptor alpha/beta-transgenic model. J Exp Med 182:1579–1584
148. Constant SL, Pfeiffer C, Woodard A, Pasqualini T, Bottomly K (1995) Extent of T cell receptor ligation can determine the functional differentiation of naive CD4+ T cells. J Exp Med 5:1591–1596
149. Bretscher PA, Ogunremi O, Menon JN (1997) Distinct immunological states in murine cutaneous leishmaniasis by immunizing with different amounts of antigen: the generation of beneficial, potentially harmful, harmful and potentially extremely harmful states. Behring Inst Mitt 98:153–159
150. Kanerva L, Hyry H, Jolanki R, Hytonen M, Estlander T (1997) Delayed and immediate allergy caused by methylhexahydrophthalic anhydride. Contact Dermatitis 36:34–38
151. Geenen V, Brilot F (2003) Role of the thymus in the development of tolerance and autoimmunity towards the neuroendocrine system. Ann NY Acad Sci 992:186–195
152. Scholzen T, Armstrong CA, Bunnett NW, Luger TA, Olerud JE, Ansel JC (1998) Neuropeptides in the skin: interactions between the neuroendocrine and the skin immune systems. Exp Dermatol 7:81–96
153. Luger TA, Lotti T (1998) Neuropeptides: role in inflammatory skin diseases. J Eur Acad Derm Venereol 10:207–211
154. Lord GM, Matarese G, Howard LK, Baker RJ, Bloom SR, Lechler RI (1998) Leptin modulates the T-cell immune response and reverses starvation-induced immunosuppression. Nature 394:897–901

155. Morfin R, Lafaye P, Cotillon AC, Nato F, Chmielewski V, Pompon D (2000) 7 alpha-hydroxy-dehydroepiandrosterone and immune response. Ann NY Acad Sci 917: 971–982

156. Cutolo M, Seriolo B, Villaggio B, Pizzorni C, Craviotto C, Sulli A (2002) Androgens and estrogens modulate the immune and inflammatory responses in rheumatoid arthritis. Ann NY Acad Sci 966:131–142

157. Kidd P (2003) Th1/Th2 balance: the hypothesis, its limitations, and implications for health and disease. Altern Med Rev 8:223–246

158. Piccinni MP, Giudizi MG, Biagiotti R, Beloni L, Giannarini L, Sampognaro S, Parronchi P, Manetti R, Annuziato F, Livi C, Romagnani S, Maggi E (1995) Progesterone favors the development of human T helper cells producing Th2-type cytokines and promotes both IL-4 production and membrane CD30 expression in established Th1 cell clones. J Immunol 155:128–133

159. Vieira PL, Kalinski P, Wierenga EA, Kapsenberg ML, Dejong EC (1998) Glucocorticoids inhibit bioactive IL-12P70 production by in vitro-generated human dendritic cells without affecting their T cell stimulatory potential. J Immunol 161:5245–5251

160. Calder PC, Bevan SJ, Newsholme EA (1992) The inhibition of T-lymphocyte proliferation by fatty acids is via an eicosanoid-independent mechanism. Immunology 75: 108–115

161. Uotila P (1996) The role of cyclic AMP and oxygen intermediates in the inhibition of cellular immunity in cancer. Cancer Immunol Immunother 43:1–9

162. Demeure CE, Yang LP, Desjardins C, Raynauld P, Delespesse G (1997) Prostaglandin E-2 primes naive T cells for the production of anti-inflammatory cytokines. Eur J Immunol 27:3526–3531

163. Abe N, Katamura K, Shintaku N, Fukui T, Kiyomasu T, Lio J, Ueno H, Tai G, Mayumi M, Furusho K (1997) Prostaglandin E2 and IL-4 provide naive CD4$^+$ T cells with distinct inhibitory signals for the priming of IFN-gamma production. Cell Immunol 181:86–92

164. Kalinski P, Hilkens CMU, Snijders A, Snijdewint FGM, Kapsenberg ML (1997) IL-12 deficient dendritic cells, generated in the presence of prostaglandin E$_2$, promote type-2 cytokine production in maturing human naive T helper cells. J Immunol 159:28–35

165. von Blomberg BME, Bruynzeel DP, Scheper RJ (1991) Advances in mechanisms of allergic contact dermatitis: in vitro and in vivo research. In: Marzulli FN, Maibach HI (eds) Dermatotoxicology, 4th edn. Hemisphere, New York, pp 255–362

166. Sallusto F, Geginat J, Lanzavecchia A (2004) Central memory and effector memory T cell subsets: function, generation, and maintenance. Annu Rev Immunol 22:745–763

167. Westerman J, Geismar U, Sponholz A, Bode U, Sparshott, Bell EB (1997) CD4$^+$ T cells of both the naive and the memory phenotype enter rat lymph nodes and Peyer's patches via high endothelial venules: within the tissue their migratory behaviour differs. Eur J Immunol 27: 3174–3181

168. Marshall D, Haskard DO (2002) Clinical overview of leukocyte adhesion and migration: where are we now? Semin Immunol 14:133–140

169. Hall JG, Morris B (1965) The origin of cells in the efferent lymph from a single lymph node. J Exp Med 121:901–910

170. Hwang ST (2001) Mechanisms of T-cell homing to skin. Adv Dermatol 17:211–241

171. Pober JS, Kluger MS, Schechner JS (2001) Human endothelial cell presentation of antigen and the homing of memory/effector T cells to skin. Ann NY Acad Sci 941: 12–25

172. Mackay CR (1993) Homing of naive, memory and effector lymphocytes. Curr Opin Immunol 5:423–427

173. Tietz W, Allemand Y, Borges E, Vonlaer D, Hallmann R, Vestweber D, Hamann A (1998) CD4($^+$) T cells migrate into inflamed skin only if they express ligands for E- and P-selectin. J Immunol 16:963–970

174. Rosen Homey B (2004) Chemokines and chemokine receptors as targets in the therapy of psoriasis. Curr Drug Targets Inflamm Allergy 3:169–174

175. Homey B, Bunemann E (2004) Chemokines and inflammatory skin diseases. Ernst Schering Res Found Workshop 4:69–83

176. Tanchot C, Rocha B (1998) The organization of mature T-cell pools. Immunol Today 19:575–579

177. Williams IR (2004) Chemokine receptors and leukocyte trafficking in the mucosal immune system. Immunol Res 29:283–292

178. Telemo E, Korotkova M, Hanson LA (2003) Antigen presentation and processing in the intestinal mucosa and lymphocyte homing. Ann Allergy Asthma Immunol 90: 28–33

179. Picker LJ, Treer JR, Ferguson-Darnell B, Collins PA, Bergstresser PR, Terstappen LWMM (1993) Control of lymphocyte recirculation in man. II. Differential regulation of the cutaneous lymphocyte associated antigen, a tissue-selective homing receptor for skin homing T cells. J Immunol 150:1122–1136

180. Sunderkötter C, Steinbrink K, Henseleit U, Bosse R, Schwarz A, Vestweber D, Sorg C (1996) Activated T cells induce expression of E-selectin in vitro and in an antigen-dependent manner in vivo. Eur J Immunol 26: 1571–1579

181. Austrup F, Vestweber D, Borges E, Lohning M, Brauer R, Herz U, Renz H, Hallmann R, Scheffold A, Radbruch A, Hamann A (1997) P- and E selectin mediate recruitment of T-helper-1 but not T-helper-2 cells into inflamed tissues. Nature 385:81–83

182. Borges E, Tietz W, Steegmaier M, Moll T, Hallmann R, Hamann A, Vestweber D (1997) P-selectin glycoprotein ligand-1 (PSGL-1) on T helper 1 but not on T helper 2 cells binds to P-selectin and supports migration into inflamed skin. J Exp Med 185:573–578

183. Tensen CP, Flier J, Rampersad SS, Sampat-Sardjoerpersad A, Scheper RJ, Boorsma DM, Willemze R (1999) Genomic organization, sequence and transcriptional regulation of the human CXCL 11 gene. Biochim Biophys Acta 1446: 167–172

184. Sallusto F, Kremmer E, Palermo B, Hoy A, Ponath P, Qin SX, Forster R, Lipp M, Lanzavecchia A (1999) Switch in chemokine receptor expression upon TCR stimulation reveals novel homing potential for recently activated T cells. Eur J Immunol 29:2037–2045

185. Baggiolini M (1998) Chemokines and leukocyte traffic. Nature 392:565–568

186. Fuhlbrigge RC, Kieffer JD, Armerding D, Kupper TS (1997) Cutaneous lymphocyte antigen is a specialized form of PSGL-1 expressed on skin-homing T cells. Nature 389: 978–981

187. Rustemeyer T, von Blomberg BME, de Ligter S, Frosch PJ, Scheper RJ (1999) Human T lymphocyte priming in vitro by haptenated autologous dendritic cells. Clin Exp Immunol 117:209–216

188. Milon G, Marchal G, Seman M, Truffa-Bachi P (1981) A delayed-type hypersensitivity reaction initiated by a single T lymphocyte. Agents Actions 11:612–614

189. Marchal G, Seman M, Milon G, Truffa-Bachi P, Zilberfarb V (1982) Local adoptive transfer of skin delayed-type hypersensitivity initiated by a single T lymphocyte. J Immunol 129:954–958

190. Rustemeyer T, von Blomberg BME, van Hoogstraten IMW, Bruynzeel DP, Scheper RJ (2004) Analysis of effector and regulatory immune-reactivity to nickel. Clin Exp Allergy 34(9):1458–1466

191. Bell EB, Sparshott SM, Bunce C (1998) CD4+ T-cell memory, CD45R subsets and the persistence of antigen – a unifying concept. Immunol Today 19:60–64

192. Bell EB, Sparshott SM, Ager A (1995) Migration pathways of CD4 T cell subsets in vivo: the CD45RC- subset enters the thymus via alpha 4 integrin- VCAM-1 interaction. Int Immunol 11:1861–1871

193. Goebeler M, Meinardus-Hager G, Roth J, Goerdt S, Sorg C (1993) Nickel chloride and cobalt chloride, two common contact sensitizers, directly induce expression of intercellular adhesion molecule-1 (ICAM-1), vascular cell adhesion molecule-1 (VCAM-1), and endothelial leukocyte adhesion molecule (ELAM-1) by endothelial cells. J Invest Dermatol 100:759–765

194. Goebeler M, Roth J, Brocker EB, Sorg C, Schulze-Osthoff K (1995) Activation of nuclear factor-kappa B and gene expression in human endothelial cells by the common haptens nickel and cobalt. J Immunol 155:2459–2467

195. Walsh LJ, Lavker RM, Murphy GF (1990) Determinants of immune cell trafficking in the skin. Lab Invest 63:592–600

196. Waldorf HA, Walsh LJ, Schechter NM, Murphy GF (1991) Early molecular events in evolving cutaneous delayed hypersensitivity in humans. Am J Pathol 138:477–486

197. Stoof TJ, Boorsma DM, Nickoloff BJ (1994) Keratinocytes and immunological cytokines. In: Leigh I, Lane B, Watt F (eds) The keratinocyte handbook. Cambridge University Press, Cambridge, pp 365–399

198. Bangert C, Friedl J, Stary G, Stingl G, Kopp T (2003) Immunopathologic features of allergic contact dermatitis in humans: participation of plasmacytoid dendritic cells in the pathogenesis of the disease? J Invest Dermatol 121:1409–1418

199. Houck G, Saeed S, Stevens GL, Morgan MB (2004) Eczema and the spongiotic dermatoses: a histologic and pathogenic update. Semin Cutan Med Surg 23:39–45

200. Silberberg-Sinakin I, Thorbecke GJ, Baer RL, Rosenthal SA, Berezowsky V (1976) Antigen-bearing Langerhans cells in skin, dermal lymphatics, and in lymph nodes. Cell Immunol 25:137–151

201. Hill S, Edwards AJ, Kimber I, Knight SC (1990) Systemic migration of dendritic cells during contact sensitization. Immunology 71:277–281

202. Sterry W, Künne N, Weber-Matthiesen K, Brasch J, Mielke V (1991) Cell trafficking in positive and negative patch test reactions: demonstration of a stereotypic migration pathway. J Invest Dermatol 96:459–462

203. Herzog WR, Meade R, Pettinicchi A, Ptak W, Askenase PW (1989) Nude mice produce a T cell-derived antigen-binding factor that mediates the early component of delayed-type hypersensitivity. J Immunol 142:1803–1812

204. Willis CM, Young E, Brandon DR, Wilkinson JD (1986) Immunopathological and ultrastructural findings in human allergic and irritant contact dermatitis. Br J Dermatol 115:305–316

205. Brasch J, Burgard J, Sterry W (1992) Common pathways in allergic and irritant contact dermatitis. J Invest Dermatol 98:166–170

206. Hoefakker S, Caubo M, van 't Herve EHM, Roggeveen MJ, Boersma WJA, van Joost Th, Notten WRF, Claassen E (1995) In vivo cytokine profiles in allergic and irritant contact dermatitis. Contact Dermatitis 33:258–266

207. Flier J, Boorsma DM, Bruynzeel DP, van Beek PJ, Stoof TJ, Scheper RJ, Willemze R, Tensen CP (1999) The CXCR3 activating chemokines IP-10, MIG and IP-9 are expressed in allergic but not in irritant patch test reactions. J Invest Dermatol 113:574–578

208. Tensen CP, Flier J, van der Raaij-Helmer EM, Sampat-Sardjoepersad S, van den Schors RC, Leurs R, Scheper RJ, Boorsma DM, Willemze R (1999) Human IP-9: a keratinocyte derived high affinity CXC-chemokine ligand for the IP-10/Mig receptor (CXCR3). J Invest Dermatol 112:716–722

209. Kondo S, Sauder DN (1995) Epidermal cytokines in allergic contact dermatitis. J Am Acad Dermatol 33:786–800

210. Wardorf HA, Walsh LJ, Schechter NM (1991) Early cellular events in evolving cutaneous delayed hypersensitivity in humans. Am J Pathol 138:477–486

211. Pober JS, Bevilacqua MP, Mendrick DL, Lapierre LA, Fiers W, Gimbrone MA Jr (1986) Two distinct monokines, interleukin 1 and tumor necrosis factor, each independently induce biosynthesis and transient expression of the same antigen on the surface of cultured human vascular endothelial cells. J Immunol 136:1680–1687

212. Shimizu Y, Newman W, Gopal TV, Horgan KJ, Graber N, Beall LD, van Seventer GA, Shaw S (1991) Four molecular pathways of T cell adhesion to endothelial cells: roles of LFA-1, VCAM-1, and ELAM-1 and changes in pathway hierarchy under different activation conditions. J Cell Biol 113:1203–1212

213. Ross R, Gilitzer C, Kleinz R, Schwing J, Kleinert H, Forstermann U, Reske-Kunz AB (1998) Involvement of NO in contact hypersensitivity. Int Immunol 10:61–69

214. Virag L, Szabo E, Bakondi E, Bai P, Gergely P, Hunyadi J, Szabo C (2002) Nitric oxide-peroxynitrite-poly(ADP-ribose) polymerase pathway in the skin. Exp Dermatol 11:189–202

215. Rowe A, Farrell AM, Bunker CB (1997) Constitutive endothelial and inducible nitric oxide synthase in inflammatory dermatoses. Br J Dermatol 136:18–23

216. Szepietowski JC, McKenzie RC, Keohane SG, Walker C, Aldridge RD, Hunter JA (1997) Leukaemia inhibitory factor: induction in the early phase of allergic contact dermatitis. Contact Dermatitis 36:21–25

217. Yu X, Barnhill RL, Graves DT (1994) Expression of monocyte chemoattractant protein-1 in delayed type hypersensitivity reactions in the skin. Lab Invest 71:226–235

218. Buchanan KL, Murphy JW (1997) Kinetics of cellular infiltration and cytokine production during the efferent phase of a delayed-type hypersensitivity reaction. Immunology 90:189–197

219. Ptak W, Askenase PW, Rosenstein RW, Gershon RK (1982) Transfer of an antigen-specific immediate hypersensitivity-like reaction with an antigen-binding factor produced by T cells. Proc Natl Acad Sci USA 79:1969–1973

220. Van Loveren H, Ratzlaff RE, Kato K, Meade R, Ferguson TA, Iverson GM, Janeway CA, Askenase PW (1986) Immune serum from mice contact-sensitized with picryl chloride contains an antigen-specific T cell factor that transfers immediate cutaneous reactivity. Eur J Immunol 16:1203–1208

221. Ptak W, Herzog WR, Askenase PW (1991) Delayed-type hypersensitivity initiation by early-acting cells that are antigen mismatched or MHC incompatible with late-acting, delayed-type hypersensitivity effector T cells. J Immunol 146:469–475

222. Tsuji RF, Geba GP, Wang Y, Kawamoto K, Matis LA, Aske-nase PW (1997) Required early complement activation in contact sensitivity with generation of local C5-dependent chemotactic activity, and late T cell interferon g: a possible initiating role of B cells. J Exp Med 186:1015–1026

223. Askenase PW, Kawikova I, Paliwal V, Akahira-Azuma M, Gerard C, Hugli T, Tsuji R (1999) A new paradigm of T cell allergy: requirement for the B-1 B cell subset. Int Arch All Appl Immunol 118:145–149

224. Hardy RR, Hayakawa K (1994) CD5$^+$ B cells, a fetal B cell lineage. Adv Immunol 55:297–339

225. Askenase PW, Kawikova I, Paliwal V, Akahira-Azuma M, Gerard C, Hugli T, Tsuji R (1999) A new paradigm of T cell allergy: requirement for the B-1 cell subset. Int Arch Allergy Immunol 118:145–149

226. Feinstein A, Richardson N, Taussig MJ (1986) Immunoglobulin flexibility in complement activation. Immunol Today 7:169–173

227. Van Loweren H, Meade R, Askenase PW (1983) An early component of delayed type hypersensitivity mediated by T cells and mast cells. J Exp Med 157:1604–1617

228. Geba GP, Ptak W, Anderson GA, Ratzlaff RE, Levin J, Askenase PW (1996) Delayed-type hypersensitivity in mast cell deficient mice: dependence on platelets for expression on contact sensitivity. J Immunol 157:557–565

229. Foreman KE, Vaporciyan AA, Bonish BK, Jones ML, Johnson KJ, Glovsky MM, Eddy SM, Ward PA (1994) C5a-induced expression of P-selectin in endothelial cells. J Clin Invest 94:1147–1155

230. Groves RW, Allen MH, Ross EL, Barker JN, MacDonald DM (1995) Tumor necrosis factor alpha is pro-inflammatory in normal human skin and modulates cutaneous adhesion molecule expression. Br J Dermatol 132:345–352

231. Nataf S, Davoust N, Ames RS, Barnum SR (1999) Human T cells express the C5a receptor and are chemoattracted to C5a. J Immunol 162:4018–4023

232. Wilkinson SM, Mattey DL, Beck MH (1994) IgG antibodies and early intradermal reactions to hydrocortisone in patients with cutaneous delayed-type hypersensitivity to hydrocortisone. Br J Dermatol 131:495–498

233. Shirakawa T, Kusaka Y, Morimoto K (1992) Specific IgE antibodies to nickel in workers with known reactivity to cobalt. Clin Exp Allergy 22:213–218

234. Redegeld FA, Nijkamp FP (2003) Immunoglobulin free light chains and mast cells: pivotal role in T-cell-mediated immune reactions? Trends Immunol 24:181–185

235. Salerno A, Dieli F (1998) Role of gamma delta T lymphocytes in immune response in humans and mice. Crit Rev Immunol 18:327–357

236. Szczepanik M, Lewis J, Geba GP, Ptak W, Askenase PW (1998) Positive regulatory gamma-delta T cells in contact sensitivity – augmented responses by in vivo treatment with anti-gamma-delta monoclonal antibody, or anti-V-gamma-5 or V-delta-4. Immunol Invest 27:1–15

237. Dieli F, Ptak W, Sireci G, Romano GC, Potestio M, Salerno A, Asherson GL (1998) Cross-talk between V-beta-8($^+$) and gamma-delta($^+$) T lymphocytes in contact sensitivity. Immunology 93:469–477

238. Tang HL, Cyster JG (1999) Chemokine up-regulation and activated T cell attraction by maturing dendritic cells. Science 284:819–822

239. Scheper RJ, van Dinther-Janssen AC, Polak L (1985) Specific accumulation of hapten-reactive T cells in contact sensitivity reaction sites. J Immunol 134:1333–1336

240. Macatonia SE, Knight SC, Edwards AJ, Griffiths S, Fryer P (1987) Localization of antigen on lymph node dendritic cells after exposure to the contact sensitizer fluorescein isothiocyanate. Functional and morphological studies. J Exp Med 166:1654–1667

241. Lappin MB, Kimber I, Norval M (1996) The role of dendritic cells in cutaneous immunity. Arch Dermatol Res 288:109–121

242. Vana G, Meingassner JG. (2000) Morphologic and immunohistochemical features of experimentally induced allergic contact dermatitis in Gottingen minipigs. Vet Pathol 37:565–80

243. Teraki Y, Picker LJ (1997) Independent regulation of cutaneous lymphocyte-associated antigen expression and cytokine synthesis phenotype during human CD4$^+$ memory T cell differentiation. J Immunol 159:6018–6029

244. Butcher EC, Picker LJ (1996) Lymphocyte homing and homeostasis. Science 272:60–66

245. Strunk D, Egger C, Leitner G, Hanau D, Stingl G (1997) A skin homing molecule defines the Langerhans cell progenitor in human peripheral blood. J Exp Med 185:1131–1136

246. Wroblewski M, Hamann A (1997) CD45-mediated signals can trigger shedding of lymphocyte L-selectin. Int Immunol 9:555–562

247. Burastero SE, Rossi GA, Crimi E (1998) Selective differences in the expression of the homing receptors of helper lymphocyte subsets. Clin Immunol Immunopathol 89:110–116

248. Wahbi A, Marcusson JA, Sundqvist KG (1996) Expression of adhesion molecules and their ligands in contact allergy. Exp Dermatol 5:12–19

249. Dailey MO (1998) Expression of T lymphocyte adhesion molecules: regulation during antigen-induced T cell activation and differentiation. Crit Rev Immunol 18:153–184

250. Oppenheimer-Marks N, Lipsky PE (1997) Migration of naive and memory T cells. Immunol Today 18:456–457

251. Romanic AM, Graesser D, Baron JL, Visintin I, Janeway CA Jr, Madri JA (1997) T cell adhesion to endothelial cells and extracellular matrix is modulated upon transendothelial cell migration. Lab Invest 76:11–23

252. Zanni MP, von Greyerz S, Schnyder B, Brander KA, Frutig K, Hari Y, Valitutti S, Pichler WJ (1998) HLA-restricted, processing- and metabolism-independent pathway of drug recognition by human alpha beta T lymphocytes. J Clin Invest 102:1591–1598

253. Akdis CA, Akdis M, Simon HU, Blaser K (1999) Regulation of allergic inflammation by skin-homing T cells in allergic eczema. Int Arch Allergy Immunol 118:140–4

254. Okazaki F, Kanzaki H, Fujii K, Arata J, Akiba H, Tsujii K, Iwatsuki K (2002) Initial recruitment of interferon-gamma-producing CD8+ effector cells, followed by infiltration of CD4+ cells in 2,4,6-trinitro-1-chlorobenzene (TNCB)-induced murine contact hypersensitivity reactions. J Dermatol 29:699–708

255. Pichler WJ, Schnyder B, Zanni MP, Hari Y, von Greyerz S (1998) Role of T cells in drug allergies. Allergy 53:225–232

256. Kehren J, Desvignes C, Krasteva M, Ducluzeau MT, Assossou O, Horand F, Hahne M, Kagi D, Kaiserlian D, Nicolas JF (1999) Cytotoxicity is mandatory for CD8$^+$ T cell mediated contact hypersensitivity. J Exp Med 189:779–786

257. Mauri-Hellweg D, Bettens F, Mauri D, Brander C, Hunziker T, Pichler WJ (1995) Activation of drug-specific CD4$^+$ and CD8$^+$ T cells in individuals allergic to sulfonamides, phenytoin, and carbamazepine. J Immunol 155:462–472

258. Abe M, Kondo T, Xu H, Fairchild RL (1996) Interferon-gamma inducible protein (IP-10) expression is mediated by CD8$^+$ T cells and is regulated by CD4+ T cells during the elicitation of contact hypersensitivity. J Invest Dermatol 107:360–366

259. Stark GR, Kerr IM, Williams BRG, Silverman RH, Schreiber RD (1998) How cells respond to interferons. Annu Rev Biochem 67:227–264

260. Rowe A, Bunker CB (1998) Interleukin-4 and the interleukin-4 receptor in allergic contact dermatitis. Contact Dermatitis 38:36–39

261. Asherson GL, Dieli F, Sireci G, Salerno A (1996) Role of IL-4 in delayed type hypersensitivity. Clin Exp Immunol 103:1–4

262. Yamada H, Matsukura M, Yudate T, Chihara J, Stingl G, Tezuka T (1997) Enhanced production of RANTES, an eosinophil chemoattractant factor, by cytokine-stimulated epidermal keratinocytes. Int Arch Aller Immunol 114:28–32

263. Moser B, Loetscher M, Piali L, Loetscher P (1998) Lymphocyte responses to chemokines. Int Rev Immunol 16:323–3244

264. Siveke JT, Hamann A (1998) T helper 1 and T helper 2 Cells respond differentially to chemokines. J Immunol 160:550–554

265. Moed H, Boorsma DM, Stoof TJ, von Blomberg BM, Bruynzeel DP, Scheper RJ, Gibbs S, Rustemeyer T (2004) Nickel-responding T cells are CD4+ CLA+ CD45RO+ and express chemokine receptors CXCR3, CCR4 and CCR10. Br J Dermatol 151:32–41

266. Asada H, Linton J, Katz SI (1997) Cytokine gene expression during the elicitation phase of contact sensitivity – regulation by endogenous IL-4. J Invest Dermatol 108:406–411

267. Kitagaki H, Fujisawa S, Watanabe K, Hayakawa K, Shiohara T (1995) Immediate-type hypersensitivity response followed by late reaction is induced by repeated epicutaneous application of contact sensitizing agents in mice. J Invest Dermatol 105:749–755

268. Carroll JM, Crompton T, Seery JP, Watt FM (1997) Transgenic mice expressing IFN-gamma in the epidermis have eczema, hair hypopigmentation, and hair loss. J Invest Dermatol 108:412–422

269. Lider O, Cahalon L, Gilat D, Hershkoviz R, Siegel D, Margalit R, Shoseyov O, Cohen IR (1995) A disaccharide that inhibits tumor necrosis factor alpha is formed from the extracellular matrix by the enzyme heparinase. Proc Natl Acad Sci USA 92:5037–5041

270. Kothny-Wilkes G, Kulms D, Poppelmann B, Luger TA, Kubin M, Schwarz T (1998) Interleukin-1 protects transformed keratinocytes from tumor necrosis factor-related apoptosis-inducing ligand. J Biol Chem 273:29247–2953

271. Orteu CH, Poulter LW, Rustin MHA, Sabin CA, Salmon M, Akbar AN (1998) The role of apoptosis in the resolution of T cell-mediated cutaneous inflammation. J Immunol 161:1619–1629

272. Zhang X, Brunner T, Carter L, Dutton RW, Rogers P, Bradley L, Sato T, Reed JC, Green D, Swain SL (1997) Unequal death in T helper cell (Th)1 and Th2 effectors: Th1, but not Th2, effectors undergo rapid Fas/FasL-mediated apoptosis. J Exp Med 185:1837–1849

273. Enk AH, Katz SI (1992) Identification and induction of keratinocyte-derived IL-10. J Immunol 149:92–95

274. Schwarz A, Grabbe S, Riemann H, Aragane Y, Simon M, Manon S, Andrade S, Luger TA, Zlotnik A, Schwarz T (1994) In vivo effects of interleukin-10 on contact hypersensitivity and delayed-type hypersensitivity reactions. J Invest Dermatol 103:211–216

275. Berg DJ, Leach MW, Kuhn R, Rajewsky K, Muller W, Davidson NJ, Rennick D (1995) Interleukin 10 but not interleukin 4 is a natural suppressant of cutaneous inflammatory responses. J Exp Med 182:99–108

276. Lalani I, Bhol K, Ahmed AR (1997) Interleukin-10 biology, role in inflammation and autoimmunity. Ann Allergy Asthma Immunol 79:469–484

277. Epstein SP, Baer RL, Thorbecke GJ, Belsito DV (1991) Immunosuppressive effects of transforming growth factor beta: inhibition of the induction of Ia antigen on Langerhans cells by cytokines and of the contact hypersensitivity response. J Invest Dermatol 96:832–837

278. Lawrence JN, Dickson FM, Benford DJ (1997) Skin irritant-induced cytotoxicity and prostaglandin E-2 release in human skin keratinocyte cultures. Toxicol Vitro 11:627–631

279. Walker C, Kristensen F, Bettens F, deWeck AL (1983) Lymphokine regulation of activated (G1) lymphocytes. I. Prostaglandin E$_2$-induced inhibition of interleukin 2 production. J Immunol 130:1770–1773

280. Weston MC, Peachell PT (1998) Regulation of human mast cell and basophil function by cAMP. Gen Pharmacol 31:715–719

281. Dvorak HF, Mihm MC Jr, Dvorak AM (1976) Morphology of delayed-type hypersensitivity reactions in man. J Invest Dermatol 64:391–401

282. Marone G, Spadaro G, Patella V, Genovese A (1994) The clinical relevance of basophil releasability. J Aller Clin Immunol 94:1293–1303

283. Lundeberg L, Mutt V, Nordlind K (1999) Inhibitory effect of vasoactive intestinal peptide on the challenge phase of allergic contact dermatitis in humans. Acta Derm Venereol 79:178–182

284. Boerrigter GH, Scheper RJ (1987) Local and systemic desensitization induced by repeated epicutaneous hapten application. J Invest Dermatol 88:3–7

285. Jensen CS, Menne T, Lisby S, Kristiansen J, Veien NK (2003) Experimental systemic contact dermatitis from nickel: a dose-response study. Contact Dermatitis 49:124–132

286. Hindsen M, Bruze M, Christensen OB (2001) Flare-up reactions after oral challenge with nickel in relation to challenge dose and intensity and time of previous patch test reactions. J Am Acad Dermatol 44:616–623

287. Larsson A, Moller H, Björkner B, Bruze M (1997) Morphology of endogenous flare-up reactions in contact allergy to gold. Acta Derm Venereol 77:474–479

288. Skog E (1976) Spontaneous flare-up reactions induced by different amounts of 1,3-dinitro-4-chlorobenzene. Acta Derm Venereol 46:386–395

289. Scheper RJ, von Blomberg BME, Boerrigter GH, Bruynzeel D, van Dinther A, Vos A (1983) Induction of local memory in the skin. Role of local T cell retention. Clin Exp Immunol 51:141–148

290. Moed H, Boorsma DM, Tensen CP, Flier J, Jonker MJ, Stoof TJ, von Blomberg BM, Bruynzeel DP, Scheper RJ, Rustemeyer T, Gibbs S (2004) Increased CCL27-CCR10 expression in allergic contact dermatitis: implications for local skin memory. J Pathol 204:39–46

291. Christensen OB, Beckstead JH, Daniels TE, Maibach HI (1985) Pathogenesis of orally induced flare-up reactions at old patch sites in nickel allergy. Acta Derm Venereol 65:298–304

292. Hindsen M, Christensen OB (1992) Delayed hypersensitivity reactions following allergic and irritant inflammation. Acta Derm Venereol 72:220–221

293. Gawkrodger DJ, McVittie E, Hunter JA (1987) Immunophenotyping of the eczematous flare-up reaction in a nickel-sensitive subject. Dermatology 175:171–177

294. Polak L, Turk JL (1968) Studies on the effect of systemic administration of sensitizers in guinea-pigs with contact

sensitivity to inorganic metal compounds. II. The flare-up of previous test sites of contact sensitivity and the development of a generalized rash. Clin Exp Immunol 3:253–262

295. Qin S, Rottman JB, Myers P, Kassam N, Weinblatt M, Loetscher M, Koch AE, Moser B, Mackay CR (1998) The chemokine receptors CXCR3 and CCR5 mark subsets of T cells associated with certain inflammatory reactions. J Clin Invest 101:746–754

296. Isaksson M, Bruze M (2003) Late patch-test reactions to budesonide need not be a sign of sensitization induced by the test procedure. Am J Contact Dermatol 14:154–156

297. Rustemeyer T, de Groot J, von Blomberg BME, Frosch PJ, Scheper RJ (2002) Assessment of contact allergen cross-reactivity by retesting. Exp Dermatol 11:257–265

298. Matura M (1998) Contact allergy to locally applied corticosteroids. Thesis, Leuven Belgium

299. Inerot A, Moller H (2000) Symptoms and signs reported during patch testing. Am J Contact Dermatol 11:49–52

300. Zinkernagel RM (2004) On "reactivity" versus "tolerance". Immunol Cell Biol 82:343–352

301. Piccirillo CA, Thornton AM (2004) Cornerstone of peripheral tolerance: naturally occurring CD4+CD25+ regulatory T cells. Trends Immunol 25:374–380

302. Rocha B, von Boehmer H (1991) Peripheral selection of the T cell repertoire. Science 251:1225–1228

303. Benson JM, Whitacre CC (1997) The role of clonal deletion and anergy in oral tolerance. Res Immunol 148:533–541

304. Ferber I, Schönrich G, Schenkel J, Mellor AL, Hämmerling GJ, Arnold B (1994) Levels of peripheral T cell tolerance induced by different doses of tolerogen. Science 263:674–676

305. Arnold B, Schönrich G, Hämmerling GJ (1993) Multiple levels of peripheral tolerance. Immunol Today 14:12–14

306. Morgan DJ, Kreuwel HTC, Sherman LA (1999) Antigen concentration and precursor frequency determine the rate of CD8$(^+)$ T cell tolerance to peripherally expressed antigens. J Immunol 163:723–727

307. Shreedhar V, Giese T, Sung VW, Ullrich SE (1998) A cytokine cascade including prostaglandin E2, IL-4, and IL-10 is responsible for UV-induced systemic immune suppression. J Immunol 160:3783–3789

308. Semma M, Sagami S (1981) Induction of suppressor T cells to DNFB contact sensitivity by application of sensitizer through Langerhans cell-deficient skin. Arch Dermatol Res 271:361–364

309. Taams LS, van Eden W, Wauben MHM (1999) Dose-dependent induction of distinct anergic phenotypes: multiple levels of T cell anergy. J Immunol 162:1974–1981

310. Girolomoni G, Gisondi P, Ottaviani C, Cavani A (2004) Immunoregulation of allergic contact dermatitis. J Dermatol 31:264–270

311. Mayer L, Sperber K, Chan L, Child J, Toy L (2001) Oral tolerance to protein antigens. Allergy 56:12–15

312. Van Hoogstraten IMW, Andersen JE, von Blomberg BME, Boden D, Bruynzeel DP, Burrows D, Camarasa JMG, Dooms-Goossens A, Lahti A, Menné T, Rycroft R, Todd D, Vreeburg KJJ, Wilkinson JD, Scheper RJ (1989) Preliminary results of a multicenter study on the incidence of nickel allergy in relationship to previous oral and cutaneous contacts. In: Frosch PJ, Dooms-Goossens A, Lachapelle JM, Rycroft RJG, Scheper RJ (eds) Current topics in contact dermatitis. Springer, Berlin Heidelberg New York, pp 178–184

313. Pozzilli P, Gisella Cavallo M (2000) Oral insulin and the induction of tolerance in man: reality or fantasy? Diabetes Metab Res Rev 16:306–307

314. Weiner HL, Gonnella PA, Slavin A, Maron R (1997) Oral tolerance: cytokine milieu in the gut and modulation of tolerance by cytokines. Res Immunol 148:528–533

315. Rustemeyer T, de Groot J, von Blomberg BME, Frosch PJ, Scheper RJ (2001) Induction of tolerance and cross-tolerance to methacrylate contact sensitizers. Toxicol Appl Pharmacol 176:195–202

316. Miller SD, Sy M-S, Claman HN (1977) The induction of hapten-specific T cell tolerance using hapten-modified lymphoid membranes. II. Relative roles of suppressor T cells and clone inhibition in the tolerant state. Eur J Immunol 7:165–170

317. Polak L (1980) Immunological aspects of contact sensitivity. An experimental study. Monogr Allergy 15:4–60

318. Weiner HL (1997) Oral tolerance: immune mechanisms and treatment of autoimmune diseases. Immunol Today 18:335–343

319. Weigle WO, Romball CG (1997) CD4$^+$ T-cell subsets and cytokines involved in peripheral tolerance. Immunol Today 18:533–538

320. Zembala M, Asherson GL (1973) Depression of T cell phenomenon of contact sensitivity by T cells from unresponsive mice. Nature 244:227–228

321. Boerrigter GH, Scheper RJ (1984) Local administration of the cytostatic drug 4-hydroperoxy-cyclophosphamde (4-HPCY) facilitates cell mediated immune reactions. Clin Exp Immunol 58:161–166

322. Boerrigter GH, de Groot J, Scheper RJ (1986) Intradermal administration of 4-hydoperoxy-cyclophosphamde during contact sensitization potentiates effector T cell responsiveness in draining lymph nodes. Immunopharmacology 1:13–20

323. Mokyr MB, Kalinichenko T, Gorelik L, Bluestone JA (1998) Realization of the therapeutic potential of CTLA-4 blockade in low-dose chemotherapy-treated tumor-bearing mice. Cancer Res 58:5301–5304

324. Knop J, Stremmer R, Neumann C, Dc Maeyer D, Macher E (1982) Interferon inhibits the suppressor T cell response of delayed-type hypersensitivity. Nature 296:775–776

325. Zhang ZY, Michael JG (1990) Orally inducible immune unresponsiveness is abrogated by IFN-gamma treatment. J Immunol 144:4163–4165

326. Claessen AME, von Blomberg BME, de Groot J, Wolvers DAE, Kraal G, Scheper RJ (1996) Reversal of mucosal tolerance by subcutaneous administration of interleukin-12 at the site of attempted sensitization. Immunology 88:363–367

327. Röcken M, Shevach EM (1996) Immune deviation – the third dimension of nondeletional T cell tolerance. Immunol Rev 149:175–194

328. Bridoux F, Badou A, Saoudi A, Bernard L, Druet E, Pasquier R, Druet P, Pelletier L (1997) Transforming growth factor beta (TGF-beta)-dependent inhibition of T helper cell 2 (Th2)-induced autoimmunity by self-major histocompatibility complex (MHC) class II-specific, regulatory CD4+ T cell lines. J Exp Med 185:1769–1775

329. Hafler DA, Kent SC, Pietrusewicz MJ, Khoury SJ, Weiner HL, Fukaura H (1997) Oral administration of myelin induces antigen-specific TGF-beta 1 secreting T cells in patients with multiple sclerosis. Ann NY Acad Sci 835:120–131

330. Cavani A, Nasorri F, Ottaviani C, Sebastiani S, de Pita O, Girolomoni G (2003) Human CD25+ regulatory T cells maintain immune tolerance to nickel in healthy, nonallergic individuals. J Immunol 171:5760

331. Lonati A, Licenziati S, Marcelli M, Canaris D, Pasolini G, Caruso A, de Panfilis G (1998) Quantitative analysis "at

the single cell level" of the novel CD28⁻CD11b⁻ subpopulation of CD8⁺ T lymphocytes. ESDR meeting at Cologne

332. De Panfilis G (1998) CD8⁺ cytolytic T lymphocytes and the skin. Exp Dermatol 7:121–131

333. Kuchroo VK, Byrne MC, Atsumi Y, Greenfeld E, Connol JH, Whitters MJ, O'Hara RM, Collins M, Dorf ME (1991) T cell receptor alpha chain plays a critical role in antigen-specific suppressor cell function. Proc Natl Acad Sci USA 88:8700–8704

334. Kumar V, Sercarz E (1998) Induction or protection from experimental autoimmune encephalomyelitis depends on the cytokine secretion profile of TCR peptide-specific regulatory CD4 T cells. J Immunol 161:6585–6591

335. Kalinski P, Schuitemaker JH, Hilkens CM, Kapsenberg ML (1998) Prostaglandin E₂ induces the final maturation of IL-12 deficient CD1a⁺CD83⁺ dendritic cells. J Immunol 161: 2804–2809

336. Steinbrink K, Wolf M, Jonuleit H, Knop J, Enk AH (1997) Induction of tolerance by IL-10-treated dendritic cells. J Immunol 159:4772–4780

337. Steinbrink K, Jonuleit H, Muller G, Schuler G, Knop J, Enk AH (1999) Interleukin-10-treated human dendritic cells induce a melanoma-antigen-specific anergy in CD8(⁺) T cells resulting in a failure to lyse tumor cells. Blood 93: 1634–1642

338. Taams LS, Boot EPJ, van Eden W, Wauben MHM (2000) 'Anergic' T cells modulate the T-cell activating capacity of antigen-presenting cells J Autoimmun 14:335–341

339. Taams LS, van Rensen AJML, Poelen MC, van Els CACM, Besseling AC, Wagenaar JPA, van Eden W, Wauben MHM (1998) Anergic T cells actively suppress T cell responses via the antigen presenting cell. Eur J Immunol 28:2902–2912

340. Strobel S, Mowat AM (1998) Immune responses to dietary antigens: oral tolerance. Immunol Today 19:173–181

341. Strober W, Kelsall B, Marth T (1998) Oral tolerance. J Clin Immunol 18:1–30

342. von Herrath MG (1997) Bystander suppression induced by oral tolerance. Res Immunol 148:541–554

343. Inobe J, Slavin AJ, Komagata Y, Chen Y, Liu L, Weiner HL (1998) IL-4 is a differentiation factor for transforming growth factor-beta secreting Th3 cells and oral adminis-

tration of IL-4 enhances oral tolerance in experimental allergic encephalomyelitis. Eur J Immunol 28:2780–2790

344. Fowler E, Weiner HL (1997) Oral tolerance: elucidation of mechanisms and application to treatment of autoimmune diseases. Biopolymers 43:323–335

345. Van Hoogstraten IMW, von Blomberg BME, Boden D, Kraal G, Scheper RJ (1994) Non-sensitizing epicutaneous skin tests prevent subsequent induction of immune tolerance. J Invest Dermatol 102:80–83

346. Epstein WL (1987) The poison ivy picker of Pennypack Park: the continuing saga of poison ivy. J Invest Dermatol 88:7–9

347. Morris DL (1998) Intradermal testing and sublingual in desensitization for nickel. Cutis 61:129–132

348. Wendel GD, Stark BJ, Jamison RB, Molina RD, Sullivan TJ (1985) Penicillin allergy and desensitization in serious infections during pregnancy. N Engl J Med 312:1229–1232

349. Panzani RC, Schiavino D, Nucera E, Pellegrino S, Fais G, Schinco G, Patriarca G (1995) Oral hyposensitization to nickel allergy: preliminary clinical results. Int Arch Allergy Immunol 107:251–254

350. Troost RJ, Kozel MM, van Helden-Meeuwsen CG, van Joost T, Mulder PG, Benner R, Prens EP (1995) Hyposensitization in nickel allergic contact dermatitis: clinical and immunologic monitoring. J Am Acad Dermatol 32: 576–583

351. Chase MW (1946) Inhibition of experimental drug allergy by prior feeding of the sensitizing agent. Proc Soc Exp Biol Med 61:257–259

352. Polak L, Turk SL (1968) Studies on the effect of systemic administration of sensitizers in guinea pigs with contact sensitivity to inorganic metal compounds. I. The induction of immunological unresponsiveness in already sensitized animals. Clin Exp Immunol 3:245–251

353. Polak L, Rinck C (1978) Mechanism of desensitization in DNCH-contact sensitive guinea pigs. J Invest Dermatol 70:98–104

354. Gaspari AA, Jenkins MK, Katz SI (1988) Class II MCH-bearing keratinocytes induce antigen-specific unresponsiveness in hapten-specific TH1 clones. J Immunol 141: 2216–2220

Molecular Aspects of Allergic Contact Dermatitis

Jean-Pierre Lepoittevin

Contents

3.1 Introduction

The skin sensitization reaction to a chemical is a multistep process with two principal stages:

- A state of sensitization to a chemical is induced. This may be on first exposure to the chemical or only after many exposures.
- A sensitization response is elicited. This happens when a subject sensitive to a given chemical is exposed to, or challenged with, the same or a related chemical.

Chemical reactions and/or interactions are involved throughout these biological processes which will result in the patient developing delayed hypersensitivity, whether it be during the crossing of the cutaneous barrier (mainly controlled by the physicochemical properties of the allergen), during the formation of the hapten–protein complex (in which chemical bonds are involved) or during the phenomenon of recognition between the antigen and the T-cell receptors (TcR).

For the present purpose, a relatively simple description of the biological mechanism of skin sensitization is sufficient.

At induction, the chemical penetrates or is introduced into the epidermis, beneath the stratum corneum. There it binds to protein, thus modifying the protein's structure. The modified protein is processed and presented, in a form that can be recognized as antigenic, to uncommitted T-cells. Those T-cells whose receptors match the modified protein are stimulated to multiply, producing expanded clones of circulating T-cells capable of recognizing the modified protein. The subject is now sensitized.

At elicitation or challenge, on subsequent exposure to the same chemical, or a cross-reactive chemical, the same, or a similar, protein modification is produced, and the modified protein is recognized by

3

the circulating T-cells which resulted from the induction stage. As a result a chain of biochemical events is initiated, leading to the symptoms of allergic contact dermatitis.

In general the induction of sensitization is partly, but not completely, specific to the compound applied at induction. For example, in a classic study carried out in the 1960s on alkyl catechols with a variety of R chain lengths, Baer et al. [1] found that the magnitude of cross-challenge responses decreased as the difference in R chain length between the two compounds increased. Cross-reactivity is highly relevant to human sensitization; for example, North Americans who have been sensitized by poison ivy, which grows only on the East Coast, react strongly to poison oak which grows only on the West coast [2] and contains similar haptens. Typically humans can become sensitive to industrial chemicals in the workplace, naturally occurring chemicals in the garden and in the countryside, and to chemical components of domestic products.

It follows from the above description of the biological mechanism that, for a chemical to be a sensitizer, it must have the ability to bind to protein so that a nonself antigen can be produced. The evidence indicates that normally this binding occurs by covalent bond formation and one of the earliest structure–activity studies of skin sensitization was reported by Landsteiner and Jacobs in the 1930s [3]. Although the biological mechanism of sensitization was not at that time understood in any detail, they had already come to the view that sensitization to chemicals involved covalent binding to proteins.

Core Message

■ For a chemical to be a sensitizer, it must have the ability first to penetrate the skin and second to bind to epidermal proteins.

3.2 Chemical Basis

Haptens (small molecules with a molecular weight of less than 1,000 Da) interact with proteins by mechanisms leading to the formation of bonds [4]. These bonds, known as chemical bonds, result from electronic interactions between atoms and are characterized by the energy involved that reflects their stability. This energy must be provided to break the bond between the two atoms. In general, a distinction is made between *weak interactions*, involving energy levels from a few joules to around 50 kJ per mole of complex, and *strong interactions*, covalent or co-ordination bonds, with bond energies ranging from 200 to 420 kJ/mol.

3.2.1 Weak Interactions

Weak interactions are normally grouped into three main categories: hydrophobic, dipolar, and some ionic bonds. Although these weak interactions involve modest energy levels and produce complexes of low stability, they are nonetheless of great biological importance, as they control virtually all the phenomena of recognition between receptors and substrates.

Hydrophobic interactions result from the ability of organic molecules to arrange themselves in such a way as to minimize the area of contact with the aqueous medium. This is for example how hydrophobic molecules insert themselves into the phospholipid bilayers of cell membranes and into hydrophobic regions of proteins or membrane receptors. These hydrophobic bonds involve very low energies of about $40-90$ J$\cdot$Å$^{-2}\cdot$mol^{-1} (1 Å$=0.1$ nm), but they play an important role in allergies to very lipophilic haptens, such as the allergens of poison ivy (*Rhus radicans* L.) or poison oak (*Rhus diversiloba* T.). This could also be of importance for the interaction of haptens with lipophilic domains of antigen-presenting cells.

Dipolar interactions are electrostatic interactions between pre-existing or induced dipoles. Electron clouds do not always have a uniform density of charge, and zones of high and low electron density can interact. Dipoles can form when molecules approach one another, the electron clouds deforming at the approach of another cloud, due to repulsion and attraction of charges, and electrons moving to the interior of the cloud, thus creating a dipole. Such interactions (induced dipoles) are known as van der Waals forces, the amount of energy involved being $0.2-2$ kJ/mol. Hydrogen bonds are a special case of dipolar interaction. They occur between a hydrogen atom, linked to an electron-withdrawing atom, and an electron-rich atom. The energy involved can be up to 25 kJ/mol and the bond can form between two different molecules (intermolecular) or within a molecule (intramolecular).

Ionic bonds are electrostatic interactions between pre-existing and generally localized charges on organic molecules or minerals. Such interactions occur, for example, between the charged amino acids in proteins and are therefore important in recognition phenomena.

Core Message

■ Hydrophobic, dipolar, and ionic bonds are weak interactions between atoms. They lead to reversible interactions but may play an important role in biological mechanisms.

3.2.2 Strong Interactions

Strong interactions, mainly *covalent bonds*, are formed by the sharing of a pair of electrons by two atoms and are classically represented in chemical formulae by dashes. When elements are not able to stabilize themselves by a loss or gain of one or two electrons, they do so by sharing electrons with other atoms, the shared electrons stabilizing both partners. Carbon, for example, forms four covalent bonds with four other atoms by sharing its valence electrons. This can be seen in the case of methane, one of the simplest carbon compounds with the composition CH_4, in which the carbon atom forms four covalent bonds with the four hydrogen atoms. Covalent bonds involve energies of the order of 200–420 kJ/mol and are therefore very stable compared with the weak interactions.

Core Message

■ Covalent bonds are strong interactions between atoms. They lead to nonreversible interactions and are therefore considered as the major form of protein modification by haptens.

3.2.2.1 Heterolytic or Nucleophilic–Electrophilic Reactions

The two electrons required for bond formation can be contributed by both partners, in which case it is called a radical reaction, or by one of the atoms that is especially rich in electrons, and shared with another atom poor in electrons. In this latter case, it is referred to as a reaction between a nucleophile (from *nucleus* and *philos*, abbreviated Nu), which is rich in electrons, and an electrophile (from *elektron* and *phi-*

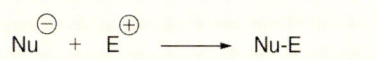

Fig. 1. Principle of nucleophilic–electrophilic reaction. (*E* Electrophile, *Nu* nucleophile)

los, abbreviated E), which is poor in electrons (Fig. 1). These two terms, nucleophile and electrophile, represent the ability of a molecule, or rather an atom of this molecule, to donate or accept electrons to form a covalent bond. Nucleophilic centers are rich in electrons and are therefore negatively charged or partially negatively charged, while electrophilic centers, deficient in electrons, are positively charged or partially positively charged. Nucleophilic atoms can react with electrophilic centers according to several mechanisms (Fig. 2).

Core Message

■ Nucleophiles (electron-rich atoms) can react with electrophiles (electron-poor atoms) to form a stable covalent bond.

3.2.2.2 Homolytic or Radical Reactions

Homolytic or radical reactions arise from the homolytic cleavage of a covalent bond (Fig. 3). The symmetrical sharing of the common electron doublet in the covalence results in each of the two atoms retaining an electron. This leads to the formation of free radicals, which are uncharged atoms, or groups of atoms, containing an uneven number of electrons. Radical reactions are mainly the reactions of molecules with weakly polar or nonpolar bonds (hydrocarbon reactions), and they require a radical inducer, such as ultraviolet radiation (hν) or atmospheric oxygen. The stability of radicals is relative, as they are unstable species and therefore highly reactive. For this reason radical reactions often occur as chain reactions. Again, radicals can react through different mechanisms to form covalent bonds (Fig. 4).

Core Message

■ Radicals can combine to form stable covalent bonds.

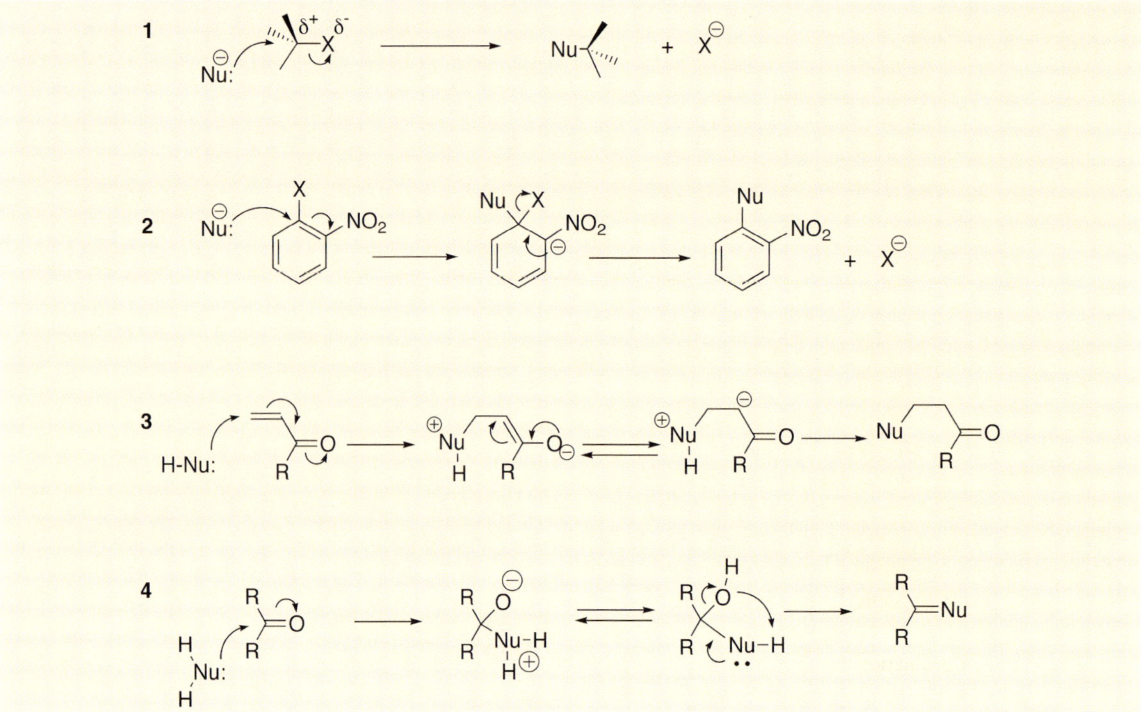

3

Fig. 2. Main nucleophilic reactions involved in allergic contact dermatitis. *1* Nucleophilic substitution on a saturated center. *2* Nucleophilic substitution on an unsaturated center. *3* Michael-type nucleophilic addition. *4* Nucleophilic addition on a carbonyl function

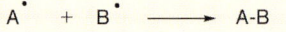

Fig. 3. Principle of radical reaction

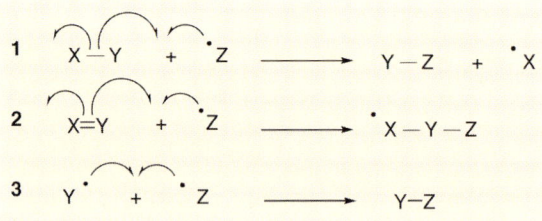

Fig. 4. Main radical reaction mechanisms. *1* Substitution mechanism. *2* Addition mechanism. *3* Termination mechanism

3.2.2.3 Co-ordination Bonds

Another type of relatively strong bond, comparable to covalent bonds, is formed between metals or metal salts and electron-rich atoms (mainly heteroatoms, such as nitrogen, oxygen, sulfur, and phosphorus). These interactions, known as co-ordination bonds, permit these electron-rich groups or "ligands" to transfer part of their electron density to the positively charged metal in order to increase its stability. Co-ordination bonds are characterized by the number of ligands and by the geometry of the complex thus formed, which is both specific for the metal and for its oxidation state. The most common geometries for co-ordination bonds are tetrahedral and square planar for four ligands, trigonal bipyramidal for five, and octahedral for six. It is not unusual for a metal at the same oxidation level or for a metal at two different oxidation levels to have several possible geometries. For example, cobalt II (Co^{2+}) is characterized by a tetrahedral arrangement, nickel II (Ni^{2+}) by a square planar tetra-co-ordinated arrangement (Fig. 5), and chromium III (Cr^{3+}) by a six-ligand octahedral arrangement. It is the number of ligands and the geometry of these co-ordination complexes that determines whether the metals are allergenic and controls cross-reactions.

Core Message

■ Co-ordination bonds are strong interactions between metals and ligands. Co-ordination bonds are characterized by the number of ligands and by the geometry of the complex thus formed, which is specific for both the metal and its oxidation state.

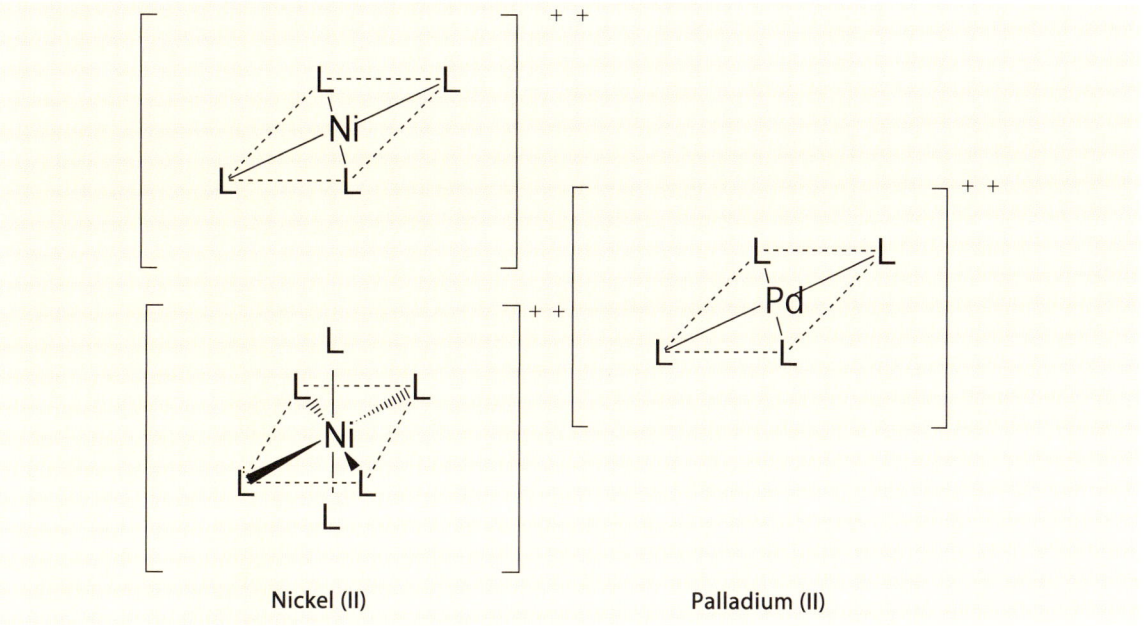

Fig. 5. Example of co-ordination bonds to metal salts

Nickel (II)   Palladium (II)

3.3 Chemical Aspects of Allergic Contact Dermatitis

3.3.1 Reactive Amino Acids

In proteins, the side-chain of several amino acids contain electron-rich or nucleophilic groups capable of reacting with haptens (Fig. 6). Lysine and cysteine are those most often cited, but other amino acids containing nucleophilic hetero-atoms, for example histidine, methionine and tyrosine, have been shown to react with electrophiles. Studies performed in the last few years on the mechanisms involved in the modification of proteins by small xenobiotic molecules have made it possible to demonstrate the involvement of a wide variety of mechanisms, depending on the structure of the hapten.

Core Message

- The lateral chains of several amino acids contain nucleophilic groups.

3.3.2 Reactivity of Haptens

One direct consequence of this diversity is the existence of selectivity in the modification of amino acids (Table 1). Thus, it has been shown that methyl alkanesulfonates, lipophilic methylating agents and strong allergens, modify almost exclusively histidine and methionine residues in proteins [5], while the α-methylene-γ-butyrolactones, the main allergens in plants of the Asteraceae (Compositae) family, mainly modify lysine residues [6]. Similarly, alk-2-ene-γ-sultones have been shown, in several animal models, to be particularly strong skin sensitizers [7, 8], exhibiting sensitization potential down to levels of approximately 1 ppm. Attention was focused on these chemicals in the mid-1970s, when the cause of a 1968 outbreak of contact dermatitis in Scandinavia was traced to 2-chloro-γ-sultones and α,β-unsaturated-γ-sultones, formed as contaminants in a batch of ether sulfate used to formulate dishwashing liquids [9]. Recent studies have shown that these molecules are highly oxophilic and are reactive mainly with tyrosine at physiological pH [10]. However, the sensitizing potential appeared to be associated with the ability to modify some lysine residues [11]. The suspected role of lysine residues was further confirmed with reactivity studies carried out on 5-chloro-2-methylisothiazol-3-one (MCI) and 2-methylisothiazol-3-one (MI), the main components of Kathon CG,

3

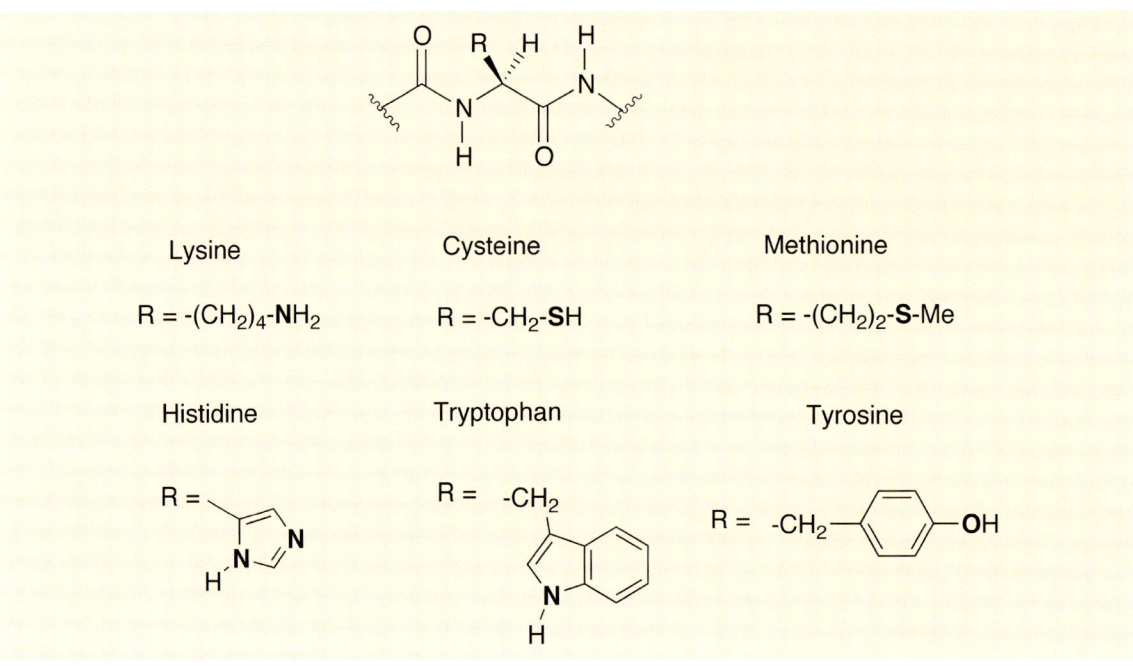

Fig. 6. Main nucleophilic residues on amino acids – reactive atoms are in *bold*

Table 1. Examples of main adducts formed between strong haptens and Human Serum Albumin

Haptens	Main adducts formed

(structures shown below)

R–S(=O)$_2$–O–CH$_3$ HSA-His-CH$_3$

(butyrolactone methylene hapten)   (butyrolactone) Lys-HSA

(cyclic sulfone)   HSA-Tyr $^{\ominus}$O$_3$S   HO $^{\ominus}$O$_3$S   Lys-HSA

Cl–S,N–CH$_3$ (isothiazolone)   HSA-His   S,N–CH$_3$

HSA-Lys–N(H)–C(=O)–CH$_2$–C(=O)–NHCH$_3$

HSA-Lys–N(H)–C(=S)–CH$_2$–C(=O)–NHCH$_3$

a well-known preservative. While both molecules were very reactive toward cysteine residues [12], the strong sensitizer MCI was also shown to react with lysine and histidine residues in proteins [13, 14].

Such studies have also been applied to co-ordination bonds and it has been shown by nuclear magnetic resonance (NMR) that nickel sulfate interacts with histidine residues of peptides bound to the MHC molecule [15].

In recent years, the radical mechanism has gained increasing interest in discussions of the mechanism of hapten-protein binding [16]. This mechanism, which has never been firmly established, has been postulated to explain, for example, the allergenic potential of eugenol versus iso-eugenol [17]. More recently, studies indicating that radical reactions were important for haptens containing allylic hydroperoxide groups (Fig. 7) have been published [18–20].

Core Message

■ Each haptens has its own chemical reactivity pattern towards nucleophilic amino acids. This reactivity pattern depends on the electron density at the reactive site.

3.3.3 Mechanisms of Reactions

The selectivity of haptens for some amino acids is directly related to the electron density at the reaction site (determined by the structure of the molecule) and to the type of chemical reaction that takes place. The chemical reactions can be divided into several groups on the basis of their characteristics and the mechanisms involved in the breaking and forming of bonds. Thus, molecules with very similar structures can give rise to the formation of different intermediates, for example during metabolization, which lead to different reaction mechanisms. The case of eugenol and iso-eugenol is very relevant in this respect.

These two molecules, present in many natural extracts, have very similar structures, but their sensitizing potentials are very different, eugenol being a weak, and iso-eugenol a relatively strong, sensitizer. Studies in the mouse seem to indicate that these two very similar molecules are metabolized in different ways and have different reaction mechanisms [21], which could explain the observed differences in sensitization potential. Eugenol (Fig. 8) could be metabolized to an electrophilic orthoquinone after a demethylation step, whereas iso-eugenol (Fig. 9) could be directly oxidized to a quinonemethide.

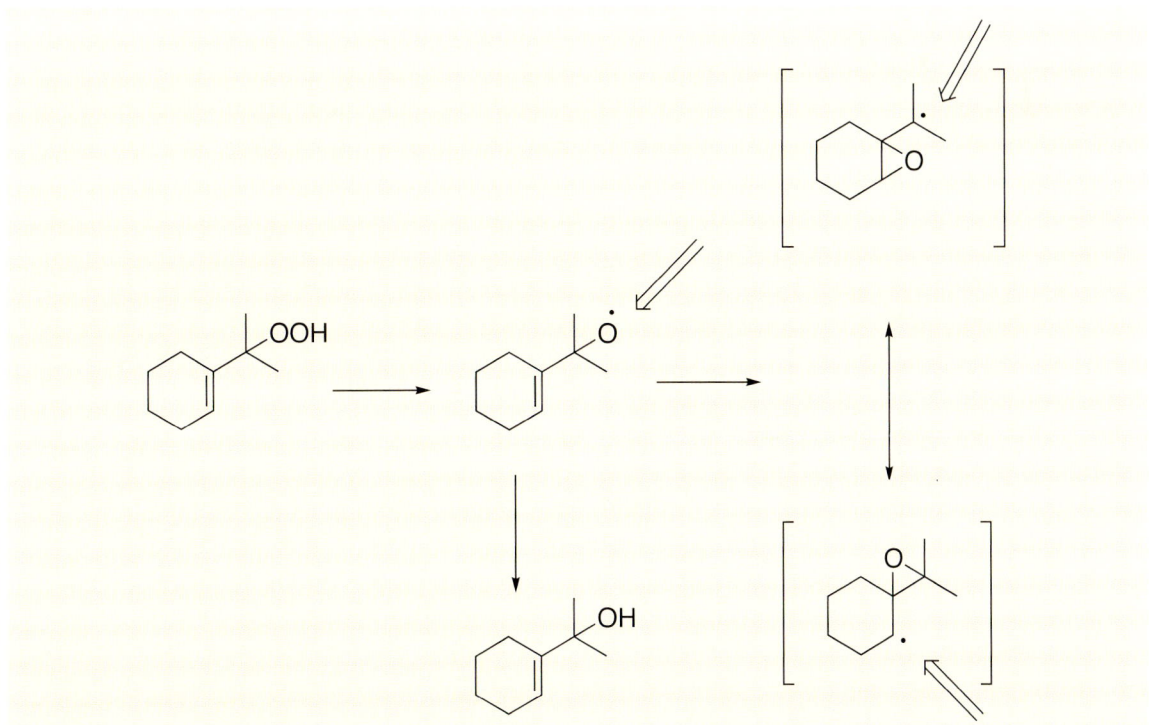

Fig. 7. Example of radical formation from allylic hydroperoxides. *Arrows* indicate major reactive sites

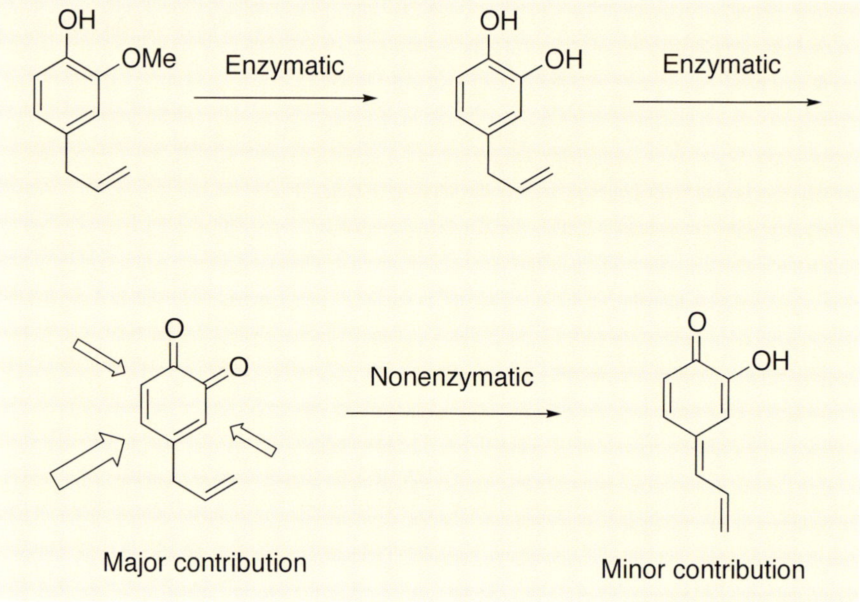

3

Fig. 8.
Proposed mechanism to explain the sensitizing potential of eugenol in mice. *Arrows* indicate major reactive sites

Major contribution   Minor contribution

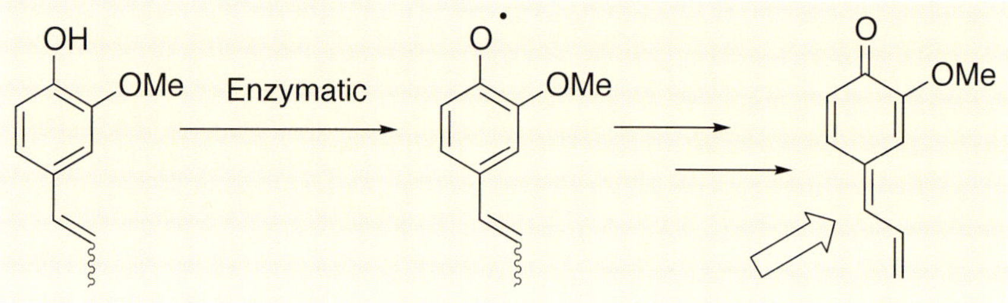

Fig. 9.
Proposed mechanism to explain the sensitizing potential of iso-eugenol in mice. *Arrows* indicate major reactive sites

---

Core Message

■ Even similar haptens can react with proteins through different chemical mechanisms and with different amino acids.

3.4 Modifications of Molecules

3.4.1 Enzymatic Processes – Prohaptens

Far from being an inert tissue, the skin is the site of many metabolic processes, which can result in structural modification of xenobiotics that penetrate it (Fig. 10). These metabolic processes, primarily intended for the elimination of foreign molecules during detoxification, can, in certain cases, convert harmless molecules into derivatives with electrophilic, and therefore allergenic, properties. The metabol-

ic processes are mainly based on oxido-reduction reactions via extremely powerful enzymatic hydroxylation systems, such as the cytochrome P450 enzymes [22] or flavine mono-oxygenase, but monoamine oxidases, which convert amines to aldehydes, and peroxidases seem to play an important role in the metabolism of haptens. When activated by the production of hydrogen peroxide during the oxidative stress following the introduction of a xenobiotic into the skin, peroxidases convert electron-rich aromatic derivatives (aminated or hydroxylated) into quinones, which are powerful electrophiles. In this way, long-chain catechols, responsible for the severe allergies to poison ivy (*Rhus radicans* L.) and poison oak (*Rhus diversiloba* T.), are oxidized in vivo to highly reactive orthoquinones (Fig. 11) [23], though we cannot exclude a radical participation. The same applies to para-phenylenediamine or hydroquinone derivatives, e.g., the allergens from *Phacelia crenulata* Torr. [24], which are converted into electrophilic paraquinones (Fig. 12). Metabolic reactions involving enzymatic hydrolysis can also occur in the skin. It is

Fig. 10.
Principles of primary and secondary metabolization of xenobiotics

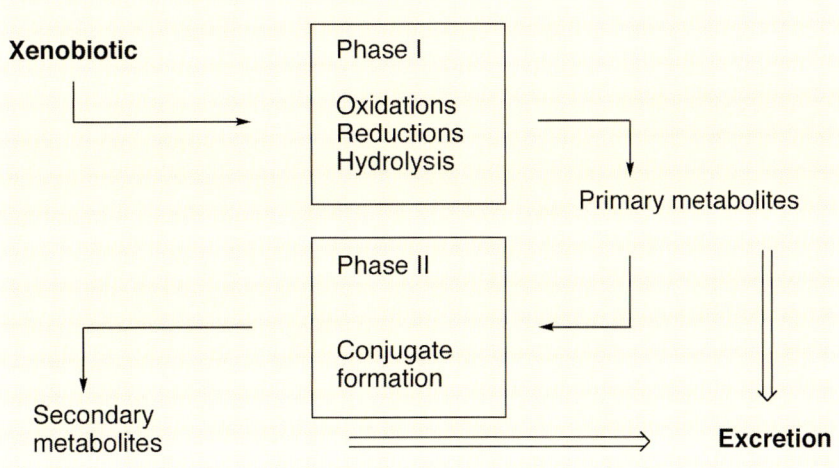

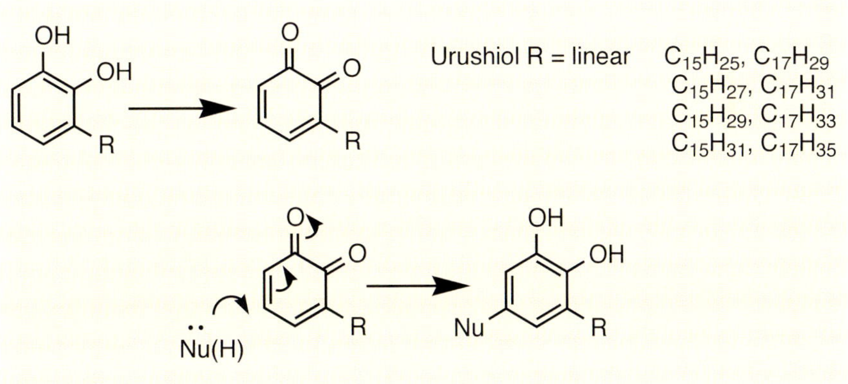

Fig. 11.
Nucleophilic addition to the ortho-quinones derived from urushiol

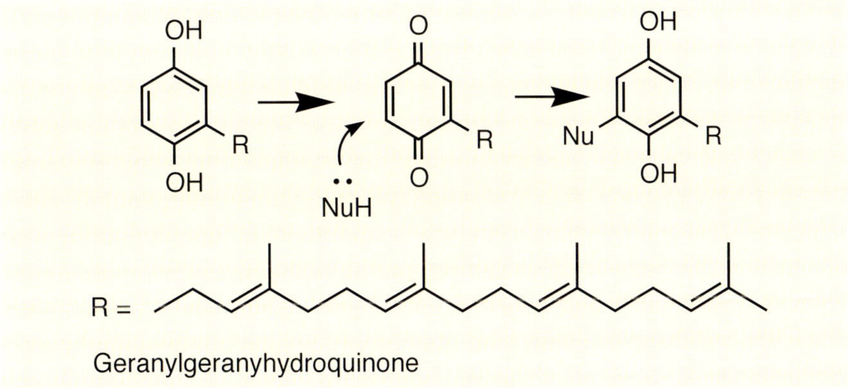

Urushiol R = linear $C_{15}H_{25}$, $C_{17}H_{29}$
$C_{15}H_{27}$, $C_{17}H_{31}$
$C_{15}H_{29}$, $C_{17}H_{33}$
$C_{15}H_{31}$, $C_{17}H_{35}$

Fig. 12.
Nucleophilic addition to the para-quinone derived from geranylgeranyl hydroquinone

R =

Geranylgeranyhydroquinone

thus that tuliposides A and B, found in the bulb of the tulip (*Tulipa gesneriana* L.), are hydrolyzed, releasing the actual allergens, tulipalins A and B [25].

All these molecules, which have themselves no electrophilic properties and cannot therefore be hap- tens but which can be metabolized to haptens, are re- ferred to as *prohaptens* [26, 27], and play an impor- tant role in contact allergy because of their number and their highly reactive nature. The fact that the structure of the metabolized molecule can be far removed from the structure of the initial molecule can make allergologic investigations even more difficult.

Core Message

■ During metabolism and detoxification steps some nonsensitizing molecules can be transformed into reactive haptens. We will refer to theses molecules as prohaptens.

3.4.2 Nonenzymatic Processes – Prehaptens

Nonenzymatic processes, such as reaction with atmospheric oxygen or ultra-violet irradiation, can also induce changes in the chemical structure of molecules. Many terpenes autoxidize at air exposure, producing sensitizing derivatives. In the 1950s it was found that the allergenic activity of turpentine was mainly due to hydroperoxides of the monoterpene Δ^3-carene (Fig. 13) [28]. This is also the case for abietic acid, the main constituent of colophony, which is converted into highly reactive hydroperoxide (Fig. 14) [29] by contact with air. Such an auto-oxidation mechanism has also been demonstrated for another monoterpene, *d*-limonene, found in citrus fruits. *d*-Limonene itself is not allergenic but on air exposure hydroperoxides, epoxides, and ketones are formed, which are strong allergens [30].

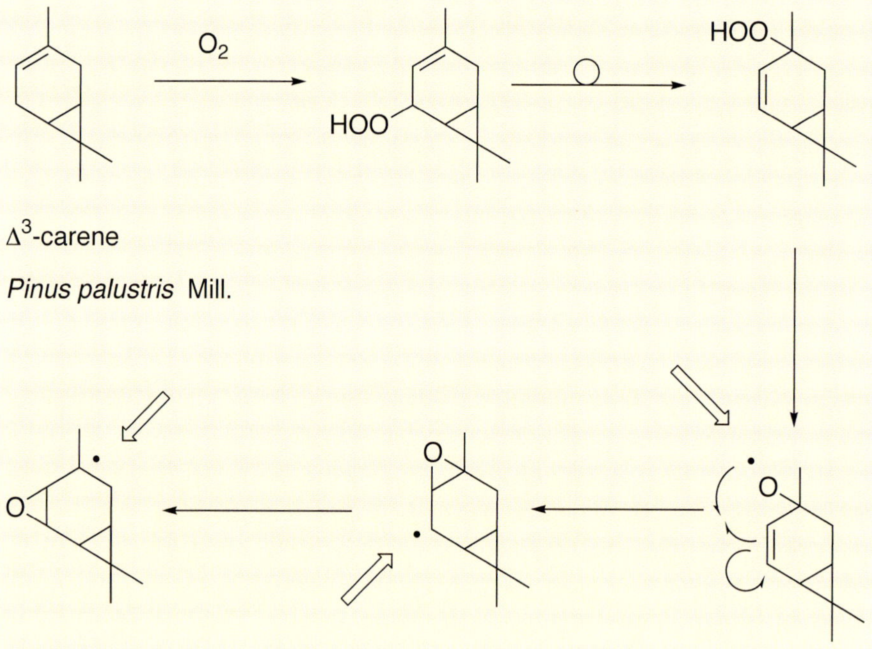

Fig. 13.
Autoxidation of Δ^3-carene to form hydroperoxides and subsequent formation of potentially reactive radicals

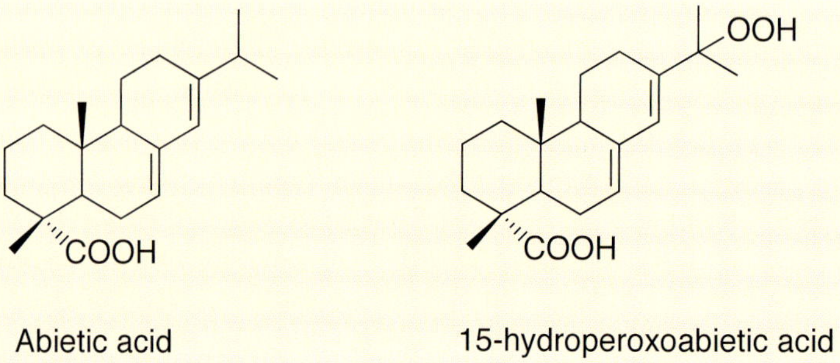

Δ^3-carene

Pinus palustris Mill.

Fig. 14.
Structure of abietic acid and of 15-hydroperoxoabietic acid

Abietic acid

15-hydroperoxoabietic acid

- Haptens, as any molecule, are sensitive to heat, light, and oxygen. Some nonsensitizing molecules can be transformed into sensitizers by chemical modification during storage and handling. By extension, these molecules are often considered as prohaptens but should rather be considered as prehaptens as no enzymatic process is involved.

3.5 Haptens and Cross-allergies

The factors that control molecular recognition during the elicitation stage are primarily the nature of the chemical group and the compatibility of the spatial geometry. Although the identity of the chemical group is very important and serves to define what are commonly called group allergies, it cannot account for all structure–activity relationships. Receptor molecules are highly sensitive to volume and shape, and molecules must have a similar size and spatial geometry to be recognized by the same receptor. Thus, even though the molecules tulipalin A or B and alantolactone (the allergen of *Inula helenium* L.) bear the same chemical group, α-methylene-γ-butyrolactone, they cannot give rise to cross-allergic reac-

tions, as their spatial volumes differ too much. In contrast, isoalantolactone and alantolactone produce a cross-allergic reaction [31], since they share both a *homologous chemical group and spatial volume* (Fig. 15). The term cross-allergy is often misused and should be restricted to the well-defined cases that can be called true cross-allergies [32, 33].

True cross-allergy between a sensitizer A and a triggering agent B can be interpreted in various ways:

- A and B are chemically and structurally similar
- A is metabolized to a compound which is similar to B
- B is metabolized to a compound which is similar to A
- A and B are both metabolized to similar compounds.

The identification of cross-allergic responses can be especially difficult, particularly in humans, in whom the possibility of co- or poly-sensitization should never be ruled out. In addition, the metabolism of molecules can be very complex and two molecules with a priori little in common can be converted to derivatives that have a similar structure. Thus, derivatives of hydroquinones and para-phenylenediamines can be converted into benzoquinone derivatives. It is therefore dangerous to draw conclusions from tests without knowing how the substances used are liable to be metabolized. Many reactions described as dem-

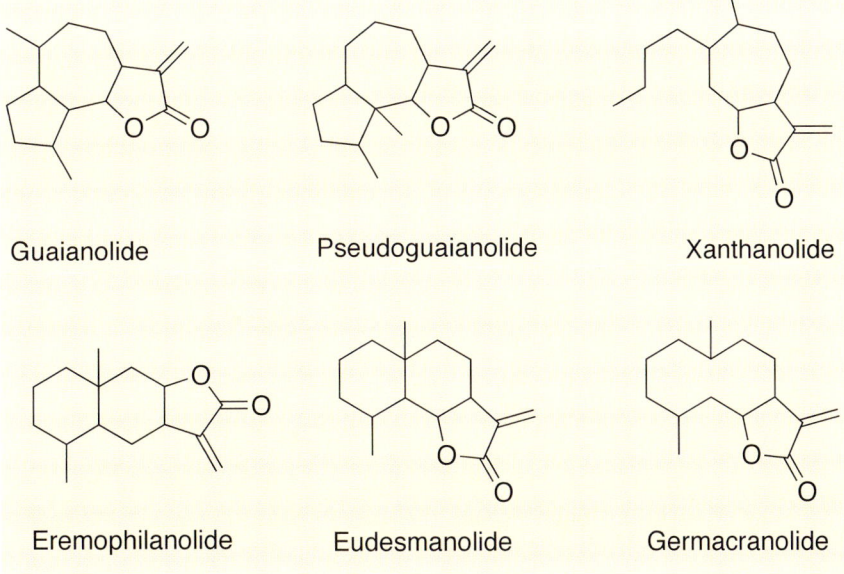

Guaianolide   **Pseudoguaianolide**   **Xanthanolide**

Eremophilanolide   **Eudesmanolide**   **Germacranolide**

Fig. 15.
Main structures of sesquiterpene lactones

onstrating cross-allergy are, without doubt, due to co-sensitization. Experimental studies in animals are often the only means of being really certain of what happens during recognition. The concept of the prohapten is very important in the interpretation of results in allergy studies. As the structure of the metabolized molecule can sometimes be very different from that of the initial molecule, it can be difficult to establish similarities between chemical groups and structures.

3

Core Message

■ Two molecules of different structure but similar in chemical reactivity and molecular shape can activate the same T-cell receptors. This is the base of the so-called cross-reaction phenomenon. A "group sensitization" refers to a series of similar molecules often giving cross-reactions in patients. Cross-reactions are not always easy to distinguish from concomitant sensitization.

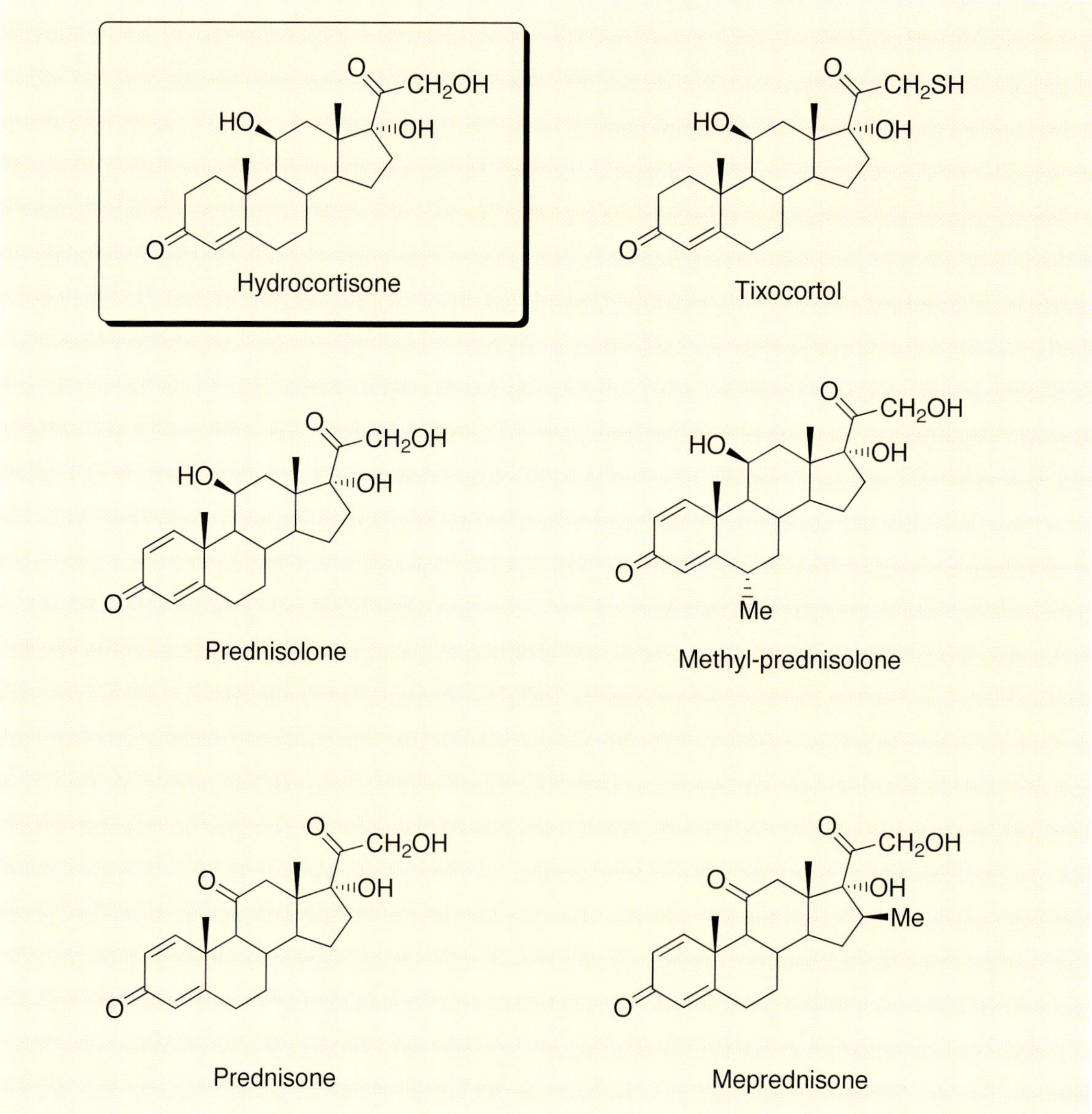

Fig. 16. Chemical structure of main group A corticosteroids

3.6 Some Applications of the Chemical Knowledge

3.6.1 Understanding Cross-reactions Among Corticosteroids

In the last few years, molecular modeling has been shown to be a powerful tool in studies of conformational-dependent drug–receptor interactions and structure–activity relationship analysis [34]. Despite the great potential of this technique, few attempts to analyze cross-reaction patterns in the field of allergic contact dermatitis have yet been reported. One reason may be the heterogeneous population of patients with heterogeneous clinical histories, in which it is somewhat difficult to distinguish between actual cross-reaction and concomitant sensitization. A second reason is that, to be effective, structure–activity relationship studies need data for a wide range of molecules. The clinical investigation of contact dermatitis from corticosteroids, in which a large number of related substances are tested on a large number of patients, represents a good opportunity to carry out such a structure–activity study. From the statistical analysis of the clinical data, it is now possible to advance an experimentally supported hypothesis for cross-reaction patterns. Coopman et al. [35] hypothesized that cross-reactions occur primarily within certain groups of corticosteroids. They distinguished four groups: group A (Fig. 16) consisting of hydrocortisone, tixocortol pivalate, and related compounds; group B consisting of triamcinolone acetonide, amcinonide, and related compounds (Fig. 17); group C consisting of betamethasone, dexamethasone, and related compounds; and group D (Fig. 18) consisting of esters such as hydrocortisone-17-butyrate and clobetasone-17-butyrate. It is now possible to correlate this with conformational characteristics and to establish a molecular basis for cross-reaction patterns in patients sensitized to corticosteroids. This could be invaluable in the prediction of potential cross-reactions to new molecules.

The conformation of corticosteroids from groups A, B, C, and D were analyzed [36]. This study was based on two hypotheses. The first was that all corticosteroids should interact with proteins in a similar way. All corticosteroid molecules were designed to interact with the same type of receptors, and thus should be metabolized in more or less similar ways.

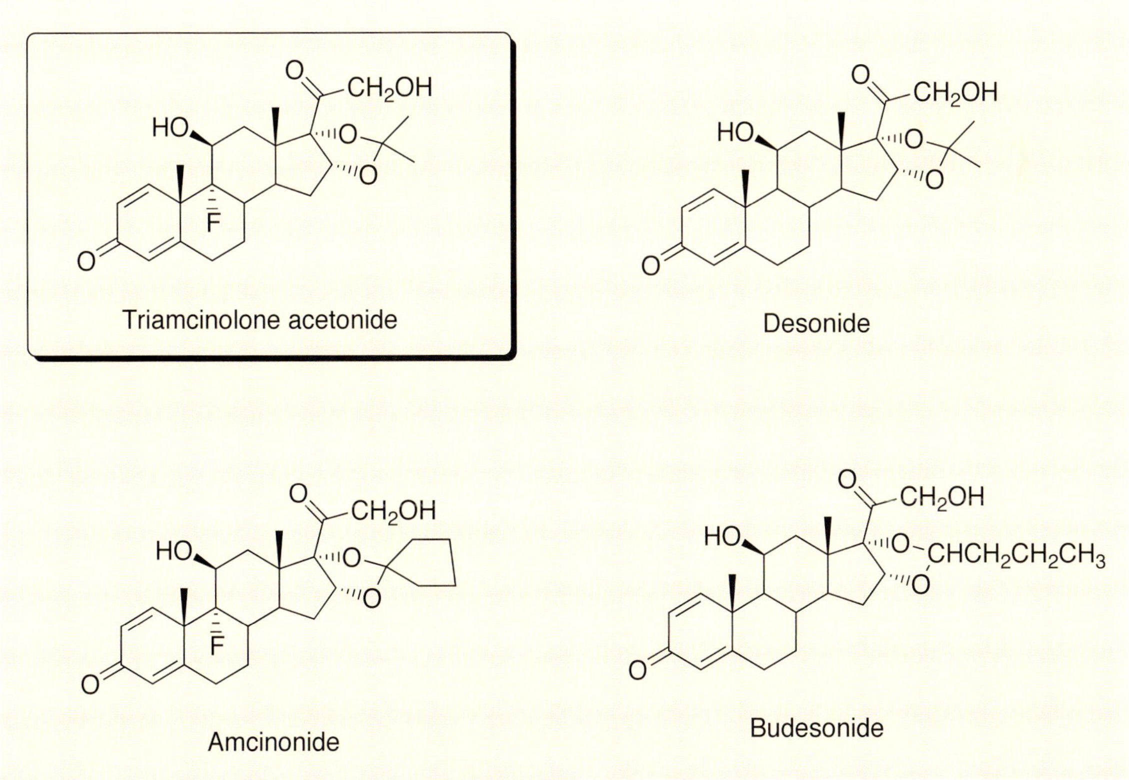

Fig. 17. Chemical structure of main group B corticosteroids

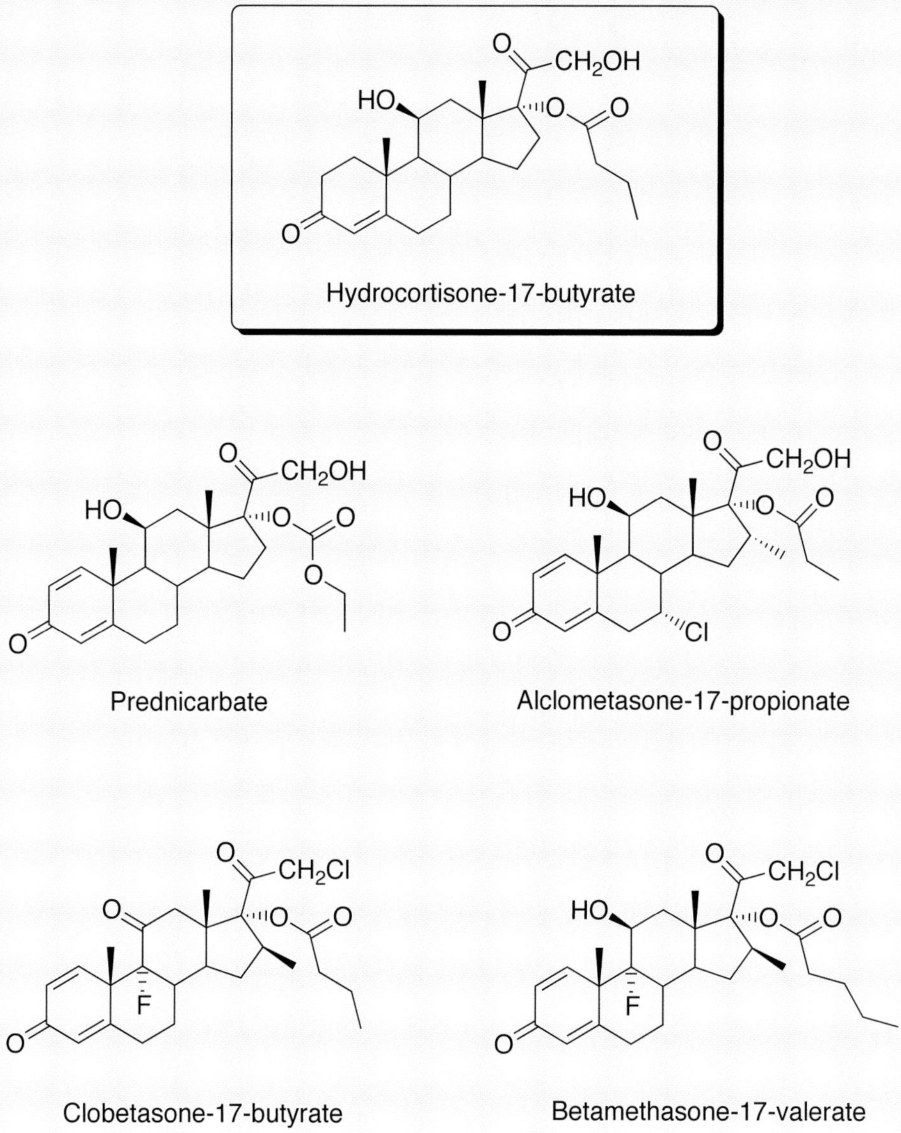

3

Hydrocortisone-17-butyrate

Prednicarbate

Alclometasone-17-propionate

Clobetasone-17-butyrate

Betamethasone-17-valerate

Fig. 18. Chemical structure of main group D corticosteroids

The second hypothesis, based on chemical observations, was that esters at position 21 are readily hydrolyzed to give the free alcohol, while esters at position 17 are more resistant to hydrolysis, due to strong steric hindrance. Thus, for example, tixocortol pivalate was considered as tixocortol with a free thiol group at position 21, and alclometasone-17,21-dipropionate was considered as alclometasone-17-propionate.

All molecules were drawn from energy-minimized building blocks and were then submitted to a multi-conformational analysis in order to achieve the most energetically stable conformation. These con-

formations were then compared for analogies or differences in the van der Waals volumes, which define the electronic shape of the molecule. As expected from the hypothesis, significant group-specific characteristics of volume and shape were found for molecules of group A, B, and D but not for molecules of group C.

Molecular characteristics: the existence of groups A, B, and D, as defined by the analysis of cross-reaction patterns in patients sensitized to corticosteroids, is fully supported by the conformational analysis of these molecules. Molecules of the same group

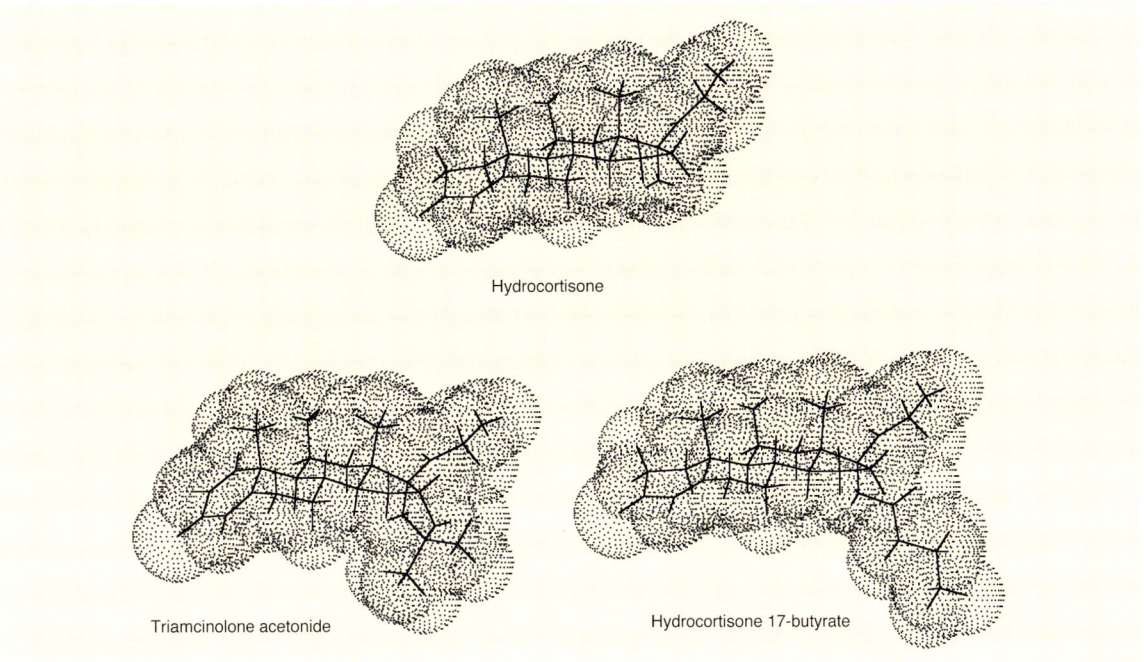

Fig. 19. General electronic shape of hydrocortisone (group A), triamcinolone acetonide (group B), and hydrocortisone 17-butyrate (group D)

have very similar spatial structures, explaining the cross-reactions observed. In addition, molecules from one group are sufficiently different from molecules of another group to explain the lack of cross-reactions observed between groups A, B, and D.

The volume occupied by specific groups on the α face of ring D seems to be critical for the molecular recognition of corticosteroids by receptors of immunocompetent cells, while modifications of other parts of the molecule seem to have little effect on the recognition patterns. Each group represents a well-defined, characteristic shape (Fig. 19) that can be very useful for the prediction of potential cross-reactions of new corticosteroid molecules.

Core Message

■ Four main structural groups have been identified for the cross-reactivity pattern of corticosteroids. These groups correspond to the presence of specific chemical functions on the α face of the D ring and can explain the lack of cross-reactivity between molecules of the different groups.

3.6.2 Use of Structure–Activity Relationships for the Identification of Sensitizers in Complex Mixtures

3.6.2.1 Introduction

Structural alerts consist of total or partial chemical structures known to present allergizing risks. They are defined mainly by analysis of the literature and contact allergy databases and allow detection of a "risk." One expert system based on this approach is currently marketed under the name of DEREK (Deductive Estimation of Risk from Existing Knowledge).

This expert system consists of a "control" program that analyses the structure of the molecules and a database consisting of "rules" in the form of substructures known to be associated with allergizing activity [37]. Examples of "rules" are shown in Table 2 and a comparison of results obtained with the Local Lymph Node Assay and DEREK is listed in Table 3.

Table 2. Examples of rules and chemical structures used by DEREK to predict the sensitizing potential

Chemical function	Substituents	Structure
Aldehydes	R = alkyl, aryl	
Ketones	R, R¹= alkyl, aryl	
Aldehydes, amides, esters and α,β-unsaturated ketones	R = H, C, N, O (not OH) R¹ = not heteroatoms, esters, ketones R² = not aryl except when R = H	
Phenyl esters	R = alkyl, aryl R¹ = any	
Hydroquinones and their O-alkyl precursors	R = H, alkyl R¹ = any	
Catechols and their O-alkyl precursors	R = H, alkyl R¹ = any	
Anhydrides	R = any	
Aromatic primary and secondary amines	R = alkyl, aryl R¹ = any	
Alkyl halides	R = alkyl X = Cl, Br, I	R —X

3.6.2.2 The Case of Oak Moss

One practical application of structure–activity relationship (SAR) and structural alerts has been to speed-up the process of hapten identification in complex mixtures. In the course of investigations on fragrance chemical allergy, a new approach for the identification of fragrance sensitizers present in commercial perfumes and eaux de toilette has developed [38, 39]. The method is based on the combination of bioassay-guided chemical fractionation, chemical analysis and SARs studies (Fig. 20). After a first fractionation and patch-test session, positive fractions are subjected to an extensive chemical analysis in order to identify molecule structures. From the structures, a SARs analysis allows one to select molecules with a sensitizing potential as defined by the presence of structural alerts. These molecules are then directly patch-tested for the identification of the actual sensitizer. This approach avoids iterative fractionation/patch-testing sessions that are time consuming and very often of low benefit. Like commercial eaux de toilette and perfumes, natural extracts contain several hundred different chemicals that are responsible for the complexity of the odor. Among them oak moss absolute, prepared from the lichen *Evernia prunastri* (L.) Arch., is considered a major contact sensitizer and is therefore included in the fragrance mix used for diagnosing perfume allergy. The process of preparing oak moss absolute has changed recently and, even if several potential sensitizers have been identified from former benzene extracts, its present constituents and their allergenic status are not clear. The method developed for the identification of contact allergens present in natural complex mixtures was applied to oak moss absolute. First results showed that atranol and chloroatranol, formed by transesterification and decarboxylation of the lichen depsides atranorin and chloroatranorin during the preparation of oak moss absolute (Fig. 21), were strong elicitants in most patients sensitized to oak moss [40, 41].

Table 3. Demonstration data set. Comparison of the sensitizing potential of a list of chemicals determined using DEREK and the local lymph node assay (*LLNA*)

Chemical[a]	Sensitizer[b]	DEREK[c]	Skin penetration[d]	LLNA[e]
2,4-Dinitrochlorobenzene	+	+	High	+
Formaldehyde	+	+	High	+
Potassium dichromate	+	+	Low	+
Iso-eugenol	+	+	High	+
4-Ethoxymethylene-2-phenyl-2-oxazol-5-one	+	+	High	+
Paraphenylenediamine	+	+	Moderate	+
Ethylenediamine	+	+	High	+
Cinnamic aldehyde	+	+	High	+
Kathon CG	+	+	High	+
Dowicil 200	+	+	Moderate	+
Cobalt chloride	+	+	Low	+
Nickel sulfate	+	+	Low	+
Hexyl cinnamic aldehyde	+	+	High	+
Benzocaine	+	+	Moderate	±
Mercaptobenzothiazole	+	+	High	+
Glutaraldehyde	+	+	High	+
Hydroxyethylacrylate	+	+	Moderate	+
Penicillin G	+	+	Moderate	+
Toluene diamine bismaleimide	+	+	Moderate	+
Eugenol	+	+	High	+
Cocoamidopropylbetaine	+	–	Low	+
Citral	+	+	High	+
Ethyleneglycol dimethacrylate	+	+	High	+
Hydroxycitronellal	+	+	Moderate	+
Diphenylthiourea	+	+	Moderate	+
Methyl salicylate	–	–	High	–
Sodium dodecyl sulfate	–	–	Low	±
Para-aminobenzoic acid	–	+	Low	–
Diethylphthalate	–	–	Low	NT
2-Hydroxypropyl methacrylate	–	+	Moderate	–
Glycerol	–	–	Low	NT
Zinc sulfate	–	–	Low	NT
Isopropanol	–	–	Moderate	NT
Lead acetate	–	–	Low	NT
Olive oil	–	–	Low	–
Tartaric acid	–	–	Moderate	NT
Dimethyl formamide	–	–	High	–

[a] The list of chemicals is from the European Centre for Ecotoxicology and Toxicology of Chemicals (ECETOC)
[b] Classification based on EU criteria
[c] DEREK expert system assessment of the presence of a structural alert for skin sensitization
[d] Expert view on likelihood of skin penetration, including evaluation of log *P* and molecular volume by computation
[e] Result of testing in the LLNA. Data taken from previous publications

Core Message

■ A combination of chemical analysis and SARs allows one to identify candidate molecules for patch-testing. This allows the easiest identification of sensitizers present in complex mixtures such as perfume concentrates or natural extracts.

3.6.3 Development of Quantitative Structure–Activity Relationships

3.6.3.1 Introduction

The main objective of the quantitative structure–activity relationship (QSAR) approach is to define "quantifiers" for a given biological reaction, and then combine these to give a quantitative estimate of the

3

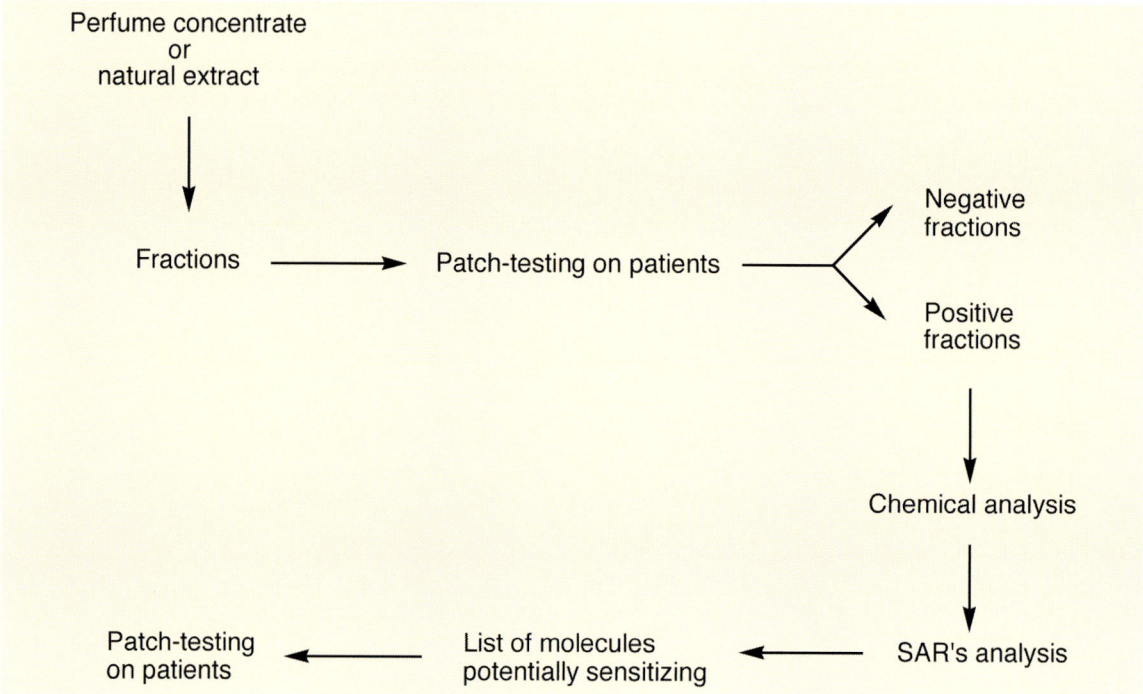

Fig. 20. Principle of SARs based identification of sensitizers in complex mixtures

biological activity. Therefore, it no longer simply answers the question of whether the molecule is potentially sensitizing, but also gives a quite accurate indication of the expected intensity of the biological response. Several approaches have been reported in the literature mainly based on reactivity and lipophilicity parameters. Thus, Roberts and Williams [42] established QSARs using the relative alkylation index mathematical model.

This quantifier gives an estimate of the level of protein modifications by a potentially sensitizing molecule and assumes that the intensity of the biological response is directly related to the level of modification. This is a simple hypothesis taking into account three parameters: the dose of the product applied to the skin, its lipophilicity, and its chemical reactivity. These parameters were chosen because it has been known experimentally for a long time that the sensitizing response increases with an increase in each of these parameters.

It is thus possible to express the relative level of protein modification by the equation:

$$\mathrm{RAI} = a \log k + b \log P + c \log D$$

where a, b, and c represent the relative weight of each parameter. At the present time, these constants are determined experimentally and are only valid for a

series of molecules with the same reaction mechanism and it is for this reason that the RAI is defined as a relative index of alkylation.

This model has been used to evaluate data of various sets of skin sensitizing chemicals [43–46].

A complementary approach is to search for empirical quantitative SARs by application of statistical methods to sets of biological data and structural descriptors.

The development of the local lymph node assay (LLNA) has facilitated the use of QSARs to predict the skin sensitization potential of chemicals because it provides well-defined end-points. The LLNA is described in detail in the literature [47, 48] and a given chemical is tested over a range of concentrations such that a dose–response relationship can be determine from which the sensitizing potential is defined in terms of the concentration required to give a specified stimulation index value. Currently the preference is to estimate the concentration of a chemical required to generate a stimulation index of 3, the $\mathrm{EC_3}$ value [48].

3.6.3.2 Example of Fragrance Aldehydes

As part as a European-Union-funded project on fragrance allergy, QSARs have been developed for sensi-

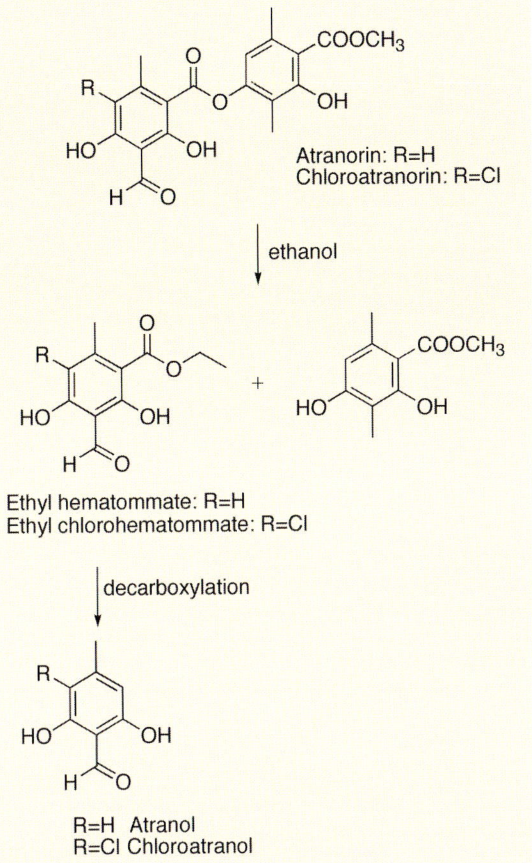

Fig. 21. Formation of atranol and chloroatranol from atranorin and chloroatranorin

tizing aldehydes. Aldehydes are molecules widely used by the fragrance industry because of their floral odor, but it has been known for many years that these molecules may be associated with skin sensitizations. From a chemical point of view, aldehydes can be classified into two main categories with respect to their reaction mechanisms toward amino groups on proteins. So-called saturated aldehydes are suspected to react with lysine residues through formation of Schiff's base, while unsaturated aldehydes, with a carbonyl function conjugated with one or more double bonds, are suspected to react with lysine through a Michael addition. From 71 aldehydes a cluster analysis was used to select subsets of 10 materials from the 2 classes – Schiff base (aliphatic) and Michael addition (α,β-unsaturated) aldehydes. LLNA tests were conducted using a 4:1 acetone:olive oil vehicle to generate dose–response data for the aldehydes in order to determine EC_3 values. The negative logarithm of

this molar EC_3, $\log(1/EC_3)$, was used as a quantitative measure of sensitizing potential and it was investigated how the sensitization potential varied with the chemical reactivity and lipophilicity. Chemical reactivity was modeled using Taft σs^* values. The Taft σs^* constant for a substituent R is a measure of the inductive effect of R. The σs^* values used were taken from the extensive compilation by Perrin et al. [49]. Lipophilicity was modeled by $\log P$ values, computed using $c \log P$.

A QSAR was developed for each of the Michael addition aldehydes and Schiff base aldehydes [50] (Fig. 22).

> ■ Michael addition aldehydes:
> $\log(1/EC_3) = 0.54 + 0.17 \log P + 0.49 R\sigma s^* + 1.31 R\sigma s^*$
> $N=9 R^2=0.741 s=0.184$ F ratio=4.77
> ■ Schiff's base aldehydes:
> $\log(1/EC_3) = 0.25 + 0.28 \log P + 0.86 R\sigma s^*$
> $N=12 R^2=0.825 s=0.172$ F ratio=21.2592

These QSARs illustrate that only molecules reacting through a similar mechanism, i.e., Schiff's base formation or Michael addition, can be correlated. Despite this restriction, a good correlation was found, and these QSARs were further validated with a new set of molecules for which a good quantitative prediction was found.

Core Message

■ Quantitative Structure–Activity Relationships (QSARs) based on reactivity factors and lipophilicity allow one to predict the sensitizing potential of aldehydes.

3.6.4 Identification of Sensitizers by Peptide Binding

3.6.4.1 Introduction

One of the major objectives of this century is the development of "alternative" tests for evaluating the pharmacological and/or toxicological activity of newly developed molecules. Contact allergy is no exception to the rule and many research programs have been started to develop in vitro techniques for the detection of allergizing compounds [51]. To date, despite the considerable effort expended in the last few

3

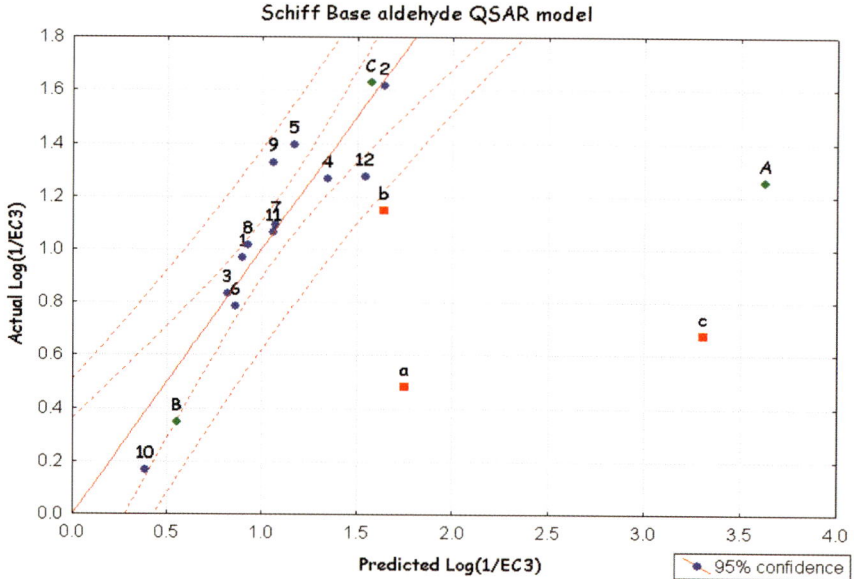

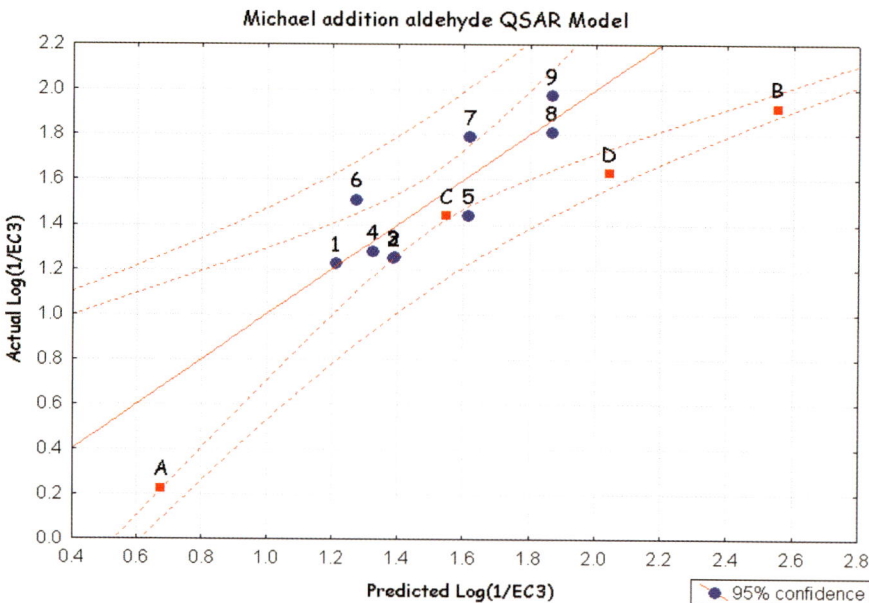

Fig. 22. QSARs for two series of aldehydes (saturated and unsaturated)

years, the complex character of the biological mechanism of allergy has prevented the development of a reliable test. Various promising routes are currently being explored, but are not expected to yield a result for several years.

In parallel with these biological studies, another approach could be based on the quantification of the chemical reactivity of haptens toward nucleophiles such as amino acids, peptides or proteins. This approach is based on the observation already reported by Landsteiner in the 1930s that a correlation exists between the chemical reactivity of a molecule and its sensitizing potential.

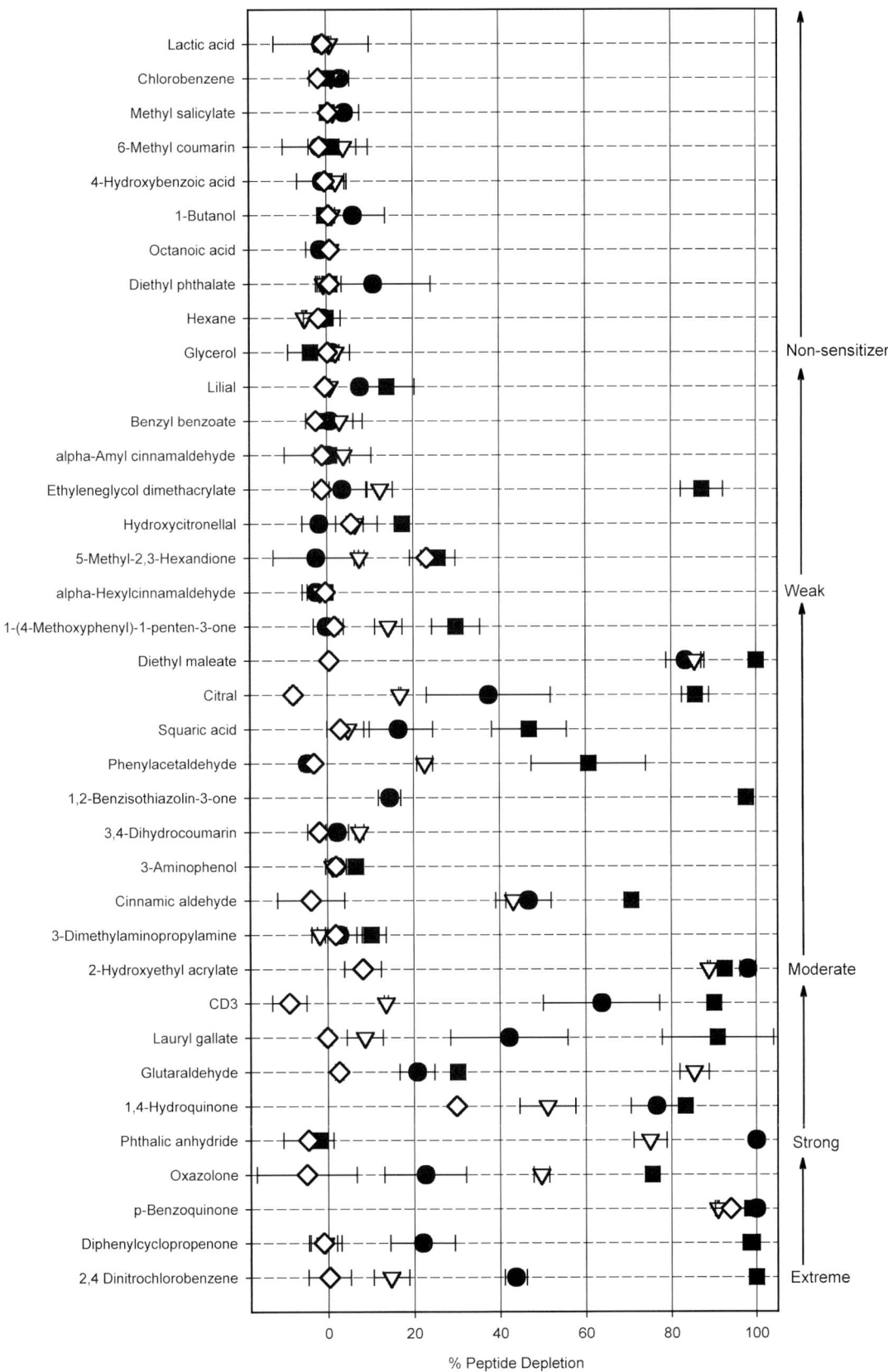

Fig. 23. Histogram of peptide reactivity and LLNA potency (from [52])

3.6.4.2 Peptide Reactivity Model

Since reactivity is a key step in the induction of skin sensitization it was hypothesized that reactivity could be used to screen the sensitization potential of chemicals. Therefore, a chemical-based peptide assay was developed and chemicals representing allergens of different potencies (weak to extreme) along with nonsensitizers were evaluated to determine if reactivity could be used as a potential skin sensitization screening tool [52]. All materials used have been evaluated in the LLNA and each assigned a skin sensitization potency category: extreme, strong, moderate, and weak. These molecules were reacted with glutathione (GSH) and two synthetic peptides containing a cysteine or a lysine, respectively, as reactive function. The depletion of peptides was measured after 24 h and used as a quantifier to assess the reactivity of the molecules. These data demonstrate that a significant correlation exists between a chemical's skin sensitization potency and its ability to react with peptides containing nucleophilic amino acids such as cysteine and lysine (Fig. 23).

Core Message

■ A significant correlation exists between a chemical's skin sensitization potency and its ability to react with peptides containing nucleophilic amino acids such as cysteine and lysine.

3.7 Conclusion

Although many questions are still unanswered or partly answered, the present state of understanding has proven useful in a variety of situations, for example in deciding whether a positive sensitization result is due to the allergenic properties of the compound under consideration or more likely to an allergic impurity.

Current knowledge, in our experience, has led to successful predictions much more often than not. Occasionally, predictions have turned out to be incorrect: most of these cases have led to refinements in our understanding.

Ongoing research into structure–skin sensitization relationships is aimed at clarifying some of the major areas where our understanding is still insufficient to be useful for predictive purposes, in particular pro-electrophile and radical mechanisms.

Suggested Reading

Dupuis G, Benezra C (1982) Allergic contact dermatitis to simple chemicals. Dekker, New York

Lepoittevin JP, Basketter DA, Goossens A, Karlberg AT (eds) (1997) Allergic contact dermatitis: the molecular basis. Springer, Berlin Heidelberg New York

Smith CK, Hotchkiss SAM (2001) Allergic contact dermatitis: Chemical and metabolic mechanisms. Taylor and Francis, London

References

1. Baer H, Watkins RC, Kurtz AP, Byck JS, Dawson CR (1967) Delayed contact sensitivity to catechols. J Immunol 99:307–375
2. Corbett MD, Billets S (1975) Characterization of poison oak urushiol. J Pharm Sci 64:1715
3. Landsteiner K, Jacobs J (1936) Studies on the sensitization of animals with simple chemical compounds. J Exp Med 64:625–639
4. Lepoittevin JP, Berl V (1997) Chemical basis. In: Lepoittevin JP, Basketter DA, Goossens A, Karlberg AT (eds) Allergic contact dermatitis: the molecular basis. Springer, Berlin Heidelberg New York, pp 19–42
5. Lepoittevin J-P, Benezra C (1992) ^{13}C-Enriched methylalkanesulfonates: new lipophilic methylating agents for the identification of nucleophilic amino acids of protein by NMR. Tetrahedron Lett 33:3875–3878
6. Franot C, Benezra C, Lepoittevin J-P (1993) Synthesis and interaction studies of ^{13}C labeled lactone derivatives with a model protein using ^{13}C NMR. Biorg Med Chem 1:389–397
7. Ritz HL, Connor DS, Sauter ED (1975) Contact sensitization of guinea-pigs with unsaturated and halogenated sultones. Contact Dermatitis 1:349–358
8. Goodwin BFJ, Roberts DW, Williams DL, Johnson AW (1983) Relationships between skin sensitization potential of saturated and unsaturated sultones. In: Gibson GG, Hubbard R, Parke DV (eds) Immunotoxicology. Academic, London, pp 443–448
9. Magnusson B, Gilje O (1973) Allergic contact dermatitis from dishwashing liquid containing lauryl ether sulfate. Acta Derm Venereol (Stockh) 53:136–140
10. Meschkat E, Barratt M, Lepoittevin JP (2001) Studies of chemical selectivity of hapten, reactivity and skin sensitization potency. Synthesis and studies on the reactivity towards model nucleophiles of the ^{13}C-labeled skin sensitizers, hex-1-ene- and hexane-1,3 sultones. Chem Res Toxicol 14:110–117
11. Meschkat E, Barratt M, Lepoittevin JP (2001) Studies of chemical selectivity of hapten, reactivity and skin sensitization potency. NMR studies of the covalent binding of the ^{13}C-labeled skin sensitizers, 2-[^{13}C] and 3-[^{13}C]-hex-1-ene- and 3-[^{13}C]-hexane-1,3-sultones to human serum albumin. Chem Res Toxicol 14:118–126
12. Alvarez-Sanchez R, Basketter D, Pease C, Lepoittevin JP (2003) Studies of chemical selectivity of hapten, reactivity and skin sensitization potency. 3. Synthesis and studies on the reactivity towards model nucleophiles of the ^{13}C-labeled skin sensitizers, 5-chloro-2-methylisothiazol-3-one (MCI) and 2-methylisothiazol-3-one (MI). Chem Res Toxicol 16:627–636
13. Alvarez-Sanchez R, Basketter DA, Pease C, Lepoittevin JP (2004) Covalent binding of the 13C-labeled skin sensitizers

5-chloro-2-methylisothiazol-3-one (MCI) and 2-methylis-othiazol-3-one (MI) to a model peptide and glutathione. Bioorg Med Chem Lett 14:365–368

14. Alvarez-Sanchez R, Divkovic M, Basketter D, Pease C, Panico M, Dell A, Morris H, Lepoittevin JP (2004) Effect of glutathione on the covalent binding of the ^{13}C-labeled skin sensitizer 5-chloro-2-methylisothiazol-3-one (MCI) to human serum albumin: identification of adducts by NMR, MALDI-MS and nano-ES MS/MS. Chem Res Toxicol 17(9): 1280–1288

15. Romagnoli P, Labahrdt AM, Sinigaglia F (1991) Selective interaction of nickel with an MHC bound peptide. EMBO J 10:1303–1306

16. Schmidt R, Kahn L, Chung LY (1990) Are free radicals and quinones the haptenic species derived from urushiols and other contact allergenic mono- and dihydric alkyl-benzenes? The significance of NADH, glutathione and redox cyucling in the skin. Arch Dermatol Res 282:56–64

17. Barratt MD, Basketter DA (1992) Possible origin of the skin sensitization potential of eugenol and related compounds. Contact Dermatitis 27:98–104

18. Gäfvert E, Shao LP, Karlberg A-T, Nilsson U, Nilsson JLG (1994) Contact allergy to resin acid hydroperoxides. Hapten binding via free readicals and epoxides. Chem Res Toxicol 7:260–266

19. Mutterer V, Gimenez-Arnau E, Karlberg AT, Lepoittevin JP (2000) Synthesis and allergenic potential of a 15-hydroperoxyabietic acid-like model: trapping of radical intermediates. Chem Res Toxicol 13:1028–1036

20. Giménez-Arnau E, Haberkorn L, Grossi L, Lepoittevin JP (2002) Identification of alkyl radicals derived from an allergenic cyclic tertiary allylic hydroperoxide by combined use of radical trapping and ESR studies. Tetrahedron 58: 5535–5545

21. Bertrand F, Basketter DA, Roberts DW, Lepoittevin J-P (1997) Skin sensitization to eugenol and isoeugenol in mice: possible metabolic pathways involving ortho-quinone and quinone methide intermediates. Chem Res Toxicol 10:335–343

22. Merk HF (1997) Skin metabolism. In: Lepoittevin JP, Basketter DA, Goossens A, Karlberg AT (eds) Allergic contact dermatitis: the molecular basis. Springer, Berlin Heidelberg New York, pp 68–80

23. Dupuis G (1979) Studies of poison ivy. In vitro lymphocytes transformation by urushiol protein conjugates. Br J Dermatol 101:617–624

24. Reynolds G, Rodriguez E (1981) Prenylated hydroquinones: contact allergens from trichomes of *Phacelia minor* and *P. parryi*. Phytochemistry 20:1365–1366

25. Bergmann HH, Beijersbergen JCH, Overeem JC, Sijpesteijn AK (1967) Isolation and identification of α-methylene-γ-butyrolactone: a fungitoxic substance from tulips. Recueil Travaux Chim Pays-Bas 86:709–713

26. Landsteiner K, Jacobs JL (1936) Studies on the sensitization of animals with simple chemicals. J Exp Med 64:625–639

27. Dupuis G, Benezra C (1982) Allergic contact dermatitis to simple chemicals. Dekker, New York

28. Hellerström S, Thyresson N, Blohm SG, Widmark G (1955) On the nature of eczematogenic component of oxidized Δ3-carene. J Invest Dermatol 24:217–224

29. Karlberg AT (1988) Contact allergy to colophony. Chemical identification of allergens. Sensitization experiments and clinical experiments. Acta Fermato Venereol 68 [Suppl 139]:1–43

30. Karlberg AT, Shao L.P, Nilsson U, Gäfvert E, Nilsson JLG (1994) Hydroperoxides in oxidized d-limonene identified as potent contact allergens. Arch Dermatol Res 286:97–103

31. Stampf JL, Benezra C, Klecak G, Geleick H, Schulz KH, Hausen B (1982) The sensitization capacity of helenin and two of its main constituents, the sesquiterpene lactones, alantolactones and isoalantolactone. Contact Dermatitis 8:16–24

32. Baer RL (1954) Cross-sensitization phenomena. In: Mackenna MB (ed) Modern trends in dermatology. Butterworth, London, pp 232–258

33. Benezra C, Maibach H (1984) True cross-sensitization, false cross-sensitization and otherwise. Contact Dermatitis 11:65–69

34. Cohen NC, Blaney JM, Humblet C, Gund P, Barry DC (1990) Molecular modeling software and methods for medicinal chemistry. J Med Chem 33:883–984.

35. Coopman S, Degreef H, Dooms-Goossens A (1989) Identification of cross-reaction patterns in allergic contact dermatitis from topical corticosteroids. Br J Dermatol 121: 27–34

36. Lepoittevin JP, Drieghe J, Dooms-Goossens A (1995) Studies in patients with corticosteroid contact allergy: understanding cross-reactivity among different steroids. Arch Dermatol 131:31–37

37. Barratt MD, Basketter DA, Chamberlain M, Admans GD, Langowski JJ (1994) An expert system rulebase for identifying contact allergens. Toxic In Vitro 8:1053–1060

38. Mutterer V, Giménez Arnau E, Lepoittevin J-P, Johansen JD, Frosch PJ, Menné T, Andersen KE, Bruze M, Rastogi SC, White IR (1999) Identification of coumarin as the sensitizer in a patient sensitive to her own perfume but negative to the fragrance mix. Contact Dermatitis 40:196–199

39. Giménez Arnau E, Andersen KE, Bruze M, Frosch PJ, Johansen JD, Menné T, Rastogi SC, White IR, Lepoittevin J-P (2000) Identification of Lilial® as a fragrance sensitizer in a perfume by bioassay-guided chemical fractionation and structure-activity relationships. Contact Dermatitis 43: 351–358

40. Bernard G, Giménez-Arnau, Rastogi SC, Heydorn S, Duus Johansen J, Menné T, Goossens A, Andersen KE, Lepoittevin JP (2003) Contact allergy to oak moss: search for sensitizing molecules using combined bioassay-guided fractionation, GC-MS and structure-activity relationship analysis, part 1. Arch Dermatol Res 295:229–235

41. Johansen JD, Andersen KE, Svedman C, Bruze M, Bernard G, Giménez-Arnau E, Rastogi SC, Lepoittevin JP, Menné T (2003) Chloroatranol an extremely potent allergen hidden in perfumes – a dose-response elicitation study. Contact Dermatitis 49:180–184

42. Roberts DW, Williams DL (1982) The derivation of quantitative correlations between skin sensitisation and physicochemical parameters for alkylating agents and their application to experimental data for sultones. J Theor Biol 99: 807–825

43. Fraginals R, Roberts DW, Lepoittevin J-P, Benezra C (1991) Refinement of the relative alkylation index (RAI) model for skin sensitization and application to mouse and guinea-pig test data for alkylsulfonates. Arch Dermatol Res 283:387–394

44. Franot C, Roberts DW, Basketter DA, Benezra C, Lepoittevin J-P (1994) Structure-activity relationships for contact allergenic potential of γ,γ-dimethyl-γ-butyrolactone derivatives, part II. Chem Res Toxicol 7:307–312

45. Roberts DW, Basketter DA (1997) Further evaluation of the quantitative structure-activity relationship for skin-sensitizing alkyl transfer agents. Contact Dermatitis 37:107–112

46. Roberts DW, Basketter DA (2000) Quantitative structure-activity relationships: sulfonate esters in the local lymph node assay. Contact Dermatitis 42:154–161

3

47. Basketter DA, Gerberick GF, Kimber I, Loveless SE (1996) The local lymph node assay: a viable alternative to currently accepted skin sensitization tests. Food Chem Toxicol 34:985–997

48. Basketter DA, Lea LJ, Dickens A et al (1999) A comparison of statistical approaches to the derivation of EC3 values from local lymph node assay dose-response. J Appl Toxicol 19:261–266

49. Perrin DD, Dempsey B, Serjeant EP (1981) pKa prediction for organic acids and bases. London, Chapman and Hall, pp 109–126

50. Patlewicz GY, Wright ZM, Basketter DA, Pease CK, Lepoittevin JP, Gimenez-Arnau E (2002) Structure-activity rela-tionships for selected fragrance allergens. Contact Dermatitis 47:219–226

51. Barbier A, Rizova E, Stampf J-L, Lacheretz F, Pistor FHM, Bos JD, Kapsenberg ML, Becker D, Mohamadzadeh M, Knop J, Mabic S, Lepoittevin J-P (1994) Development of a predictive in vitro test for detection of sensitizing compounds (European BRIDGE project). In: Rougier A, Goldberg AM, Maibach HI (eds) In vitro skin toxicology (irritation, phototoxicity, sensitization). Liebert, New York, pp 341–350

52. Gerberick F, Vassallo J, Bailey R, Morrall S, Lepoittevin J-P (2004) Development of peptide reactivity assay for screening allergens. Toxicol Sci 81:332–343

Chapter 4

Mechanisms of Irritant Contact Dermatitis

4

Steen Lisby, Ole Baadsgaard

Contents

4.1 Introduction

Irritant contact dermatitis is an eczematous reaction in the skin of external origin. In contrast to allergic contact dermatitis, no eliciting allergens can be identified. The spectrum of irritant reactions includes subjective irritant response, acute irritant contact dermatitis, chronic irritant contact dermatitis, and chemical burns (Table 1). Irritant contact dermatitis is in its acute form characterized by erythema, infil-

tration, and vesiculation. In its more chronic form, dryness, fissuring, and hyperkeratosis are more pronounced. It is thus clear that the clinical reaction pattern of mild to moderate irritant contact dermatitis is often indistinguishable from the allergic contact dermatitis reaction. Thus, differentiation between these two reaction types is often based solely on patient history and skin allergy tests. Despite the common hallmarks of irritant contact dermatitis, the clinical manifestation of the skin lesions developing following contact with different irritants varies. Factors that may influence the outcome of skin contact with irritants can be divided as follows:

- Exogenous: such as structural and chemical properties of the irritant, exposure to other irritants, and environmental conditions, e.g., temperature and humidity.
- Endogenous: such as body region that is exposed (the scrotum is much more sensitive than, e.g., the upper back), age [1], race [2], and pre-existing skin disease.

Moreover, in addition to the capacity of different irritants to induce clinically different reactions, it has been reported that marked interindividual variation in the threshold for eliciting clinical irritant reaction in skin is present [3].

In the past, the pathogenesis of irritant contact dermatitis was thought to be nonimmunological. However, today it is generally accepted that the immune system plays a key role in eliciting irritant reactions. This has been underscored by human and animal studies demonstrating the importance of sig-

Table 1. Type of irritant reactions

Subjective irritant reaction (stinging)
Acute irritant contact dermatitis
Chronic irritant contact dermatitis
Chemical burn

nal molecules, e.g., cytokines, in eliciting the irritant reaction.

4

> ## Core Message
>
> ■ Irritant contact dermatitis is an eczematous reaction in the skin caused by exposure to external agents/chemicals. Clinically the reaction manifests similar to the allergic contact dermatitis reaction.

4.2 Clinical Spectrum of Irritant Skin Reactions

The spectrum of the clinical appearances of irritant contact dermatitis is extremely broad. It is therefore widely accepted that no single mechanism underlying the development of this disease entity exists. In this chapter, we briefly outline the different clinical reaction types. For more extensive description, the reader is referred to Chap. 15.

> ## Core Message
>
> ■ Irritant contact dermatitis can be divided into different reaction types, including stinging, acute irritant reaction, chronic irritant reaction, and chemical burn.

4.2.1 Subjective Irritant Reaction

The hallmark of this type of irritation is the lack of clinical manifestation. Subjective registration of a burning or stinging feeling following contact with certain chemicals is diagnostic (Table 2). Despite no clinical manifestation, the reaction can be reproduced. Typically, symptoms occur rapidly following exposure (i.e., within seconds to minutes). There seem to be interindividual differences in eliciting this type of reaction, and several studies have classed individuals as sensitive (stingers) and nonsensitive (nonstingers) [4]. One example of immediate stinging is the appliance of a mixture of chloroform and methanol to the skin. In stingers, even when applied to intact skin, a sharp pain develops within seconds to minutes following exposure to the chloroform/ methanol mixture [5].

Table 2. Chemicals involved in subjective skin reactions (adapted from [4])

Immediate stinging potential
    Chloroform
    Methanol
    Hydrochloric acid
    Retinoic acid

Delayed stinging potential
    Weak:
        Aluminum chloride
        Benzene
        Phenol
        Phosphoric acid
        Resorcinol
        Salicylic acid

    Moderate:
        Propylene glycol
        Dimethylsulfoxide
        Benzoyl peroxide

    Severe:
        Crude coal tar
        Lactic acid
        Hydrochloric acid
        Sodium hydroxide
        Amyldimethyl-*p*-aminobenzoic acid

4.2.2 Acute Irritant Contact Dermatitis

This type of reaction is often the result of a single exposure to an irritant. The clinical appearance is very variable and often indistinguishable from the allergic contact dermatitis reactions. The manifestation may vary from a little dryness and redness to severe reactions with edema, inflammation, and vesiculation. Often the clinical reactions are located to areas of exposure and the skin manifestations often disappear within days to weeks.

4.2.3 Chronic (Cumulative) Irritant Contact Dermatitis

This type of reaction develops as a result of cumulative exposures of the skin to irritants. Clinically, this type of reaction is characterized by dryness, redness, infiltration, scaling, fissuring, and vesiculation to only a minor degree. Often this type of irritant contact dermatitis is located on the hands. A hallmark of this type of reaction is its chronicity. Despite removal of irritant exposure, the clinical reaction may continue for several years. Several external factors are known to contribute to elicitation of chronic irritant eczema. These agents include water, detergents, organic solvents, oils, alkalis, acids, oxidizing agents, heat, cold, friction, and multiple microtrauma.

4.2.4 Chemical Burn

Reactions are induced by highly alkaline or acid compounds. These agents can result in severe damage of the skin. The reaction often develops within minutes, and frequently manifests with the appearance of a painful erythema, followed by vesiculation, and the formation of necrotic scars. This type of reaction is often sharply demarcated and may lead to deep tissue destruction even after only a short exposure.

4.3 Skin – the Outpost of the Immune System

To understand the pathogenic mechanisms involved in irritant contact dermatitis, it is important to address the involvement of the different cell types constitutively present within the skin, and the cell types that can be recruited to the site of the irritant reaction as well as the proinflammatory and inflammatory mediators induced by the different cell populations following irritant exposure.

4.3.1 Immunocompetent Cells of the Skin

The outermost part of the skin is the epidermis. Epidermis is mainly composed of keratinocytes, Langerhans cells, and melanocytes. Both keratinocytes and Langerhans cells are involved in immunological processes. In contrast, the immunological importance of the epidermal melanocyte, if any, is not known.

The involvement of the keratinocyte in the skin immune system was first indicated in 1981/1982 by Luger et al. and Sauder et al. who described a keratinocyte-derived cytokine, epidermal-derived thymocyte activating factor (ETAF) [6, 7]. The majority of ETAF activity was later confined to interleukin-1 (IL-1). It has now been demonstrated that the keratinocyte is capable of producing a variety of immunological active cytokines/factors (Table 3), including IL-1, IL-6, IL-8, IL-10, IL-12, granulocyte-macrophage colony-stimulating factor (GM-CSF), tumor necrosis factor-alpha (TNF-α), and transforming growth factor-beta (TGF-β). The involvement of some of these factors in irritant contact dermatitis is reviewed later in this chapter. Beside cytokine expression, keratinocytes can be induced to express or increase expression of major histocompatibility complex (MHC) molecules [8, 9] and cell adhesion molecules such as intercellular adhesion molecule-1 (ICAM-1) [10, 11]. Expression of these molecules, in combination with the release of chemotactic cytokines, and factors involved in the upregulation of E-selectin and vascular

cell adhesion molecule-1 (VCAM-1) on dermal endothelial cells [12], makes the keratinocyte an important player in the induction and maintenance of inflammatory cells within the skin.

The epidermal Langerhans cell is the only cell type in normal epidermis that exhibits all accessory cell functions and thus acts as a complete antigen-presenting cell. The epidermal Langerhans cell was originally described in 1868 by Paul Langerhans [13] and comprises 2–5% of the total epidermal cell population. It is constitutively present in the skin and is localized to the suprabasal part of the epidermis. The Langerhans cell is a dendritic, bone marrow-derived cell characterized by surface expression of type-1a cluster of differentiation (CD1a) antigen, as well as MHC class I, and MHC class II (HLA-DR, -DP, -DQ) molecules. Ultrastructurally, the Langerhans cell contains characteristic intracytoplasmic Birbeck's granules. Beside its capacity to present antigens to T-cells, the Langerhans cell is capable of secreting cytokines such as IL-1β, IL-6, IL-10, IL-12, and TNF-α [14]. The Langerhans cell has been implicated in the immune surveillance of the skin; it is also required for induction of primary immune responses in skin, and as such is suggested to be a key player in allergic contact dermatitis. In addition, recent research has associated this cell type with events occurring during the development of irritant contact dermatitis.

Several dermal antigen-presenting cell subsets have been described including macrophages and dendritic cells. Macrophages are bone marrow-de-

Table 3. Keratinocyte-derived cytokines

Interleukin-1α
Interleukin-1β
Interleukin-3
Interleukin-6
Interleukin-7
Interleukin-8
Interleukin-10
Interleukin-12
Interleukin-15
Interleukin-18
Tumor necrosis factor-α
Transforming growth factor-α
Transforming growth factor-β
Granulocyte colony-stimulating factor
Granulocyte-macrophage colony-stimulating factor
Platelet-derived growth factor
Epidermal cell-derived lymphocyte differentiation inhibiting factor
Keratinocyte lymphocyte inhibitory factor

4

rived cells with a broad range of functions, including antimicrobial activity, anti-tumor activity, regulation of B and T lymphocytes, release of cytokines and processing antigens – thereby functioning as antigen-presenting cells. These cells are characterized by surface expression of Fc-receptors, including CD16 and CDw32, and MHC class II molecules. Furthermore, these cells express LFA-1 (CD11a) and when activated also CD11b.

In ultraviolet-irradiated skin, dermal and epidermal monocyte/macrophage-like cells expressing a HLA-DR$^+$, CD11b$^+$, CD36$^+$ phenotype have been observed [15]. These cells are involved in downregulation of the immune response, revealed by their capacity to preferentially activate CD4$^+$ suppressor-inducer T lymphocytes [16, 17]. In addition, these CD11b$^+$, MHC class II$^+$ cells were found to secrete large amounts of IL-10, in contrast to the residual epidermal Langerhans cells, which secrete mainly IL-12 [18]. Thus, different bone marrow-derived cells of the macrophage or dendritic cell lineage are differently involved in the ongoing immune regulation within the skin during an inflammatory reaction.

In skin diseases, such as mycosis fungoides and contact dermatitis, cells with a similar HLA-DR$^+$, CD36$^+$ phenotype have been detected within the epidermis [19, 20]. Their functional role is underscored by observations that depletion of the epidermal Langerhans cells only partially inhibits an autologous epidermal lymphocyte reaction. Furthermore, when isolated from involved epidermis, HLA-DR$^+$, CD36$^+$ cells exhibit the capacity directly to stimulate autologous T lymphocytes in vitro [21]. In addition, HLA-DR$^+$, CD36$^+$ cells have been observed in the irritant reaction [22]. However, their functional role in the development of an irritant reaction is still unknown.

Core Message

■ Immunocompetence of normal epidermis is restricted to the epidermal Langerhans cell. In irritant contact dermatitis, other dendritic cells are present, and the keratinocytes develop immunoregulatory functions, including but not limited to MHC class II and ICAM-1 expression.

4.3.2 Skin Infiltrating T Lymphocytes

It has been known for several years that many skin diseases are characterized by skin infiltration by T lymphocytes. These T lymphocytes often express a CD3$^+$, CD4$^+$ phenotype, although CD8$^+$ T lymphocytes are also present. While trafficking the skin, these T lymphocytes are capable of releasing a variety of cytokines, including IL-2, IL-4, IL-10, interferon-γ (IFN-γ) and TNF-α. Based on their cytokine secretion, T lymphocytes can be divided into T helper-1-like (Th1-like), Th2-like or Th0-like cells (Table 4). This division was originally suggested in 1986 by Mosmann et al. based on investigation of murine T lymphocyte clones [23]. He distinguished two different subsets of T lymphocyte clones. The first was named Th1 and comprised clones preferentially producing IL-2 and IFN-γ, while the other group of clones was termed Th2 and produced large amounts of IL-4 and IL-5. Following this observation, several studies have included more cytokines in this subdivision and furthermore suggested a similar division of human T lymphocytes. Many of the T lymphocyte-derived cytokines are involved in regulation of inflammatory processes. IL-2 is known as a T lymphocyte growth factor, another cytokine like IFN-γ is involved in the induction or upregulation of cell adhesion molecules [10], and IL-10 downregulates Th1-type cytokine secretion [24] and thus acts as an inhibitory molecule.

In humans, a disease such as atopic eczema is characterized by skin infiltration by T lymphocytes expressing a Th2 like profile in its acute phase whether the skin-infiltrating T lymphocytes in allergic contact dermatitis, psoriasis, and late-phase chronic atopic dermatitis express a Th1 like profile. In irritant contact dermatitis, studies investigating cytokine profiles in the acute reactions have mainly detected increased levels of IL-2 and IFN-γ, thereby indicating a Th1-cytokine profile, as discussed in this chapter.

Recent, it has been demonstrated that T lymphocytes entering the skin often are characterized by increased expression of a surface molecule – cutaneous lymphocyte-associated antigen (CLA) [25]. This molecule participates directly in transendothelial migration of T lymphocytes. The ligand for CLA is E-

Table 4. T helper (Th) lymphocyte cytokine profiles: cytokines predominant in the different groups

Th1	Th2	Th0
IFN-γ	IL-4	INF-γ
IL-2	IL-5	IL-2
TNF-α	IL-6	IL-4
TNF-β	IL-9	TGF-β
	IL-10	
	IL-13	

selectin, which is found to be upregulated in various skin diseases, including contact dermatitis. Other receptor-ligand pairs, such as lymphocyte function-associated antigen (LFA)-1/ICAM-1 and very late antigen-4 (VLA-4)/VCAM-1, are also involved in this process [26]. The importance of CLA has been demonstrated by blocking CLA in vitro, which resulted in inhibition of transendothelial T lymphocyte migration [26]. Furthermore, studies on T lymphocytes from individuals with contact allergic dermatitis have revealed that preferentially CLA$^+$ cells are activated and recruited to the skin [27]. Thus, the importance of CLA as a selective skin homing receptor for T lymphocytes has been established and this molecule seems to play an important role in the recruitment of T lymphocytes to the local inflammatory reaction site in the skin. Despite these observations, the role of CLA expression in irritant contact dermatitis is still not clarified.

Core Message

- Inflammatory skin diseases, including irritant contact dermatitis, are characterized by influx of activated T lymphocytes. In general the skin-infiltrating T lymphocytes express CLA; however, their role in irritant contact dermatitis is unknown. In irritant contact dermatitis, studies investigating cytokine profiles are preferentially performed in the acute reactions and these investigations have detected increased levels of IL-2 and IFN-γ and thereby indicate a Th1-cytokine profile.

4.4 Pathogenesis of Acute Irritant Contact Dermatitis

Research within the field of irritant contact dermatitis has primary been focused on the development of the acute irritant reaction and only to a lesser degree the chronic irritant reaction. For many years researchers have tried to differentiate between the allergic and irritant skin reactions by the means of histopathology or immunohistopathology [28, 29] – as described in Chapter 8. However, only minor differences have been revealed. Until recently, skin irritation was thought to be a nonimmunological reaction in the skin; however, recent work has indeed implicated the immune system in the development and maintenance of irritant-induced skin reactions. In

contrast to allergic skin reactions, no immunological memory seems to be involved in eliciting irritant contact dermatitis and the development of irritant skin reactions does not require prior sensitization.

Although chemical differences exist between different irritants, exposure of the skin to irritants often lead to skin barrier perturbation, skin infiltration by immunocompetent cells, and induction of inflammatory signal molecules.

4.4.1 Skin Barrier Perturbation

One major finding following exposure to skin irritants is perturbation of the skin barrier. The skin barrier is composed of the outermost layer of the epidermis – the stratum corneum. The stratum corneum consists of protein-rich cells, the corneocytes, which are embedded within a continuous lipid-rich matrix. Within the stratum corneum, the barrier function is mainly confined to the inner one-third – included within the compact part of the stratum corneum [30]. The dynamic process of damaging and re-normalization of the skin barrier can be quantified using a noninvasive technique based on the measurement of transepidermal water loss (TEWL). This method has today been accepted as a reliable marker of skin barrier disruption. Much research has been conducted using the anionic surfactant sodium lauryl sulfate (SLS). Application of SLS to human skin results in perturbation of the skin barrier and an increased TEWL measurement as compared to control values [31]. This effect is not only a transient phenomenon. Increased TEWL values have indeed been observed more than 6 days following exposure to SLS [32]. In addition, another study demonstrated that complete recovery of the skin barrier was first obtained more than 3 weeks after irritant challenge [33]. This was demonstrated by re-testing the irritant-treated skin area with the same irritant. Thus, long-lasting perturbation of the skin barrier is observed following SLS challenge of the skin in vivo.

The mechanisms behind the irritant-induced barrier perturbation are not fully understood; however, increased hydration [34] and disorganization of the lipid bilayers of the epidermis [35] have been reported. Although one could argue that disruption of the skin barrier is merely a mechanical change of the skin, several studies have demonstrated the importance of an intact stratum corneum. Disruption of the barrier could actually result in the induction of a danger signal. In support of this, it has been demonstrated that acetone treatment or impeachment of the skin barrier by tape stripping results in increased mitotic activity in the basal keratinocytes [36]. Fur-

4

thermore, studies have indicated that, following disruption of the skin barrier, increased levels of immunological active signal molecules, in particular IL-1α, IL-1β, TNF-α and GM-CSF, are present within the skin [37]. Thus, taken together, perturbation of the skin barrier itself could actually initiate an immunological stress signal leading to the subsequent development of an inflammatory reaction locally in the skin.

Finally, an impaired skin barrier also facilitates skin penetration by the irritant itself, or by other external agents including allergens and bacteria. Thus, perturbation of the skin barrier is thereby implicated in many skin diseases and thought to be a major player in the induction of irritant contact dermatitis.

Core Message

■ One hallmark of irritant exposure is perturbation of the skin barrier. This facilitates penetration by external agents and by itself induces inflammatory signals locally in challenged skin.

4.4.2 Cellular Immunological Changes in Irritant Contact Dermatitis

As described above, the skin, which is the outermost outpost of the immune system, is an organ essential for the initiation and maintenance of contact dermatitis. Although much research has been focused on allergic contact dermatitis, numerous studies have characterized the cellular infiltrate in irritant contact dermatitis, especially the experimentally induced acute irritant reaction. The histological manifestation of the irritant reaction is often impossible to distinguish from the manifestation observed in the contact allergic reaction [28, 29]. In addition, diversity of the histopathological changes is seen following skin exposure to different irritants [38]. However, the cellular infiltrate is characterized mainly by mononuclear cells in particular T lymphocytes belonging to the CD4$^+$ subset [39, 40]. These T lymphocytes detected in irritant contact dermatitis seem to belong to a Th1-like subpopulation, as the major T lymphocyte cytokines detected are IFN-γ and IL-2 [41]. This observation parallels findings in allergic contact dermatitis. Furthermore, a study has shown that in both allergic and irritant skin reactions, an increase in number of CLA$^+$ T lymphocytes is observed in the skin [42]. This study was, however, performed on atopic individuals. Another study also found an increase in CD3$^+$ cells in skin biopsy samples from irritant reactions, however in this study they actually observed a decreased percentage of CLA$^+$ cells as compared to samples from atopic dermatitis skin [43]. Furthermore, the same study found marked expression of integrin α4β7 by T lymphocytes present in the skin [43]. α4β7 is a gut homing marker and skin expression of this molecule suggests that a nonspecific influx of T lymphocytes has occurred and that CLA is not a prerequisite for cutaneous T lymphocyte infiltration [43, 44]. Thus, the precise role of CLA in irritant contact dermatitis is still not clearly understood.

In addition to CLA-positive T cells, new information has implicated cells expressing IL-2 receptor (CD25) in the regulation of inflammation in tissues, including the skin. The CD25-positive T cells seem to be downregulators of inflammation and thus involved in the regulation and termination of inflammatory processes. In allergic contact dermatitis, a decreased number of CD25-positive cells has been observed in involved skin (nickel allergic patch tests) compared to normal skin. However, it is imperative to state that a role for CD25-positive T cells in the development and maintenance of the irritant reaction is currently unknown.

Many studies have implicated the keratinocyte as an important player in the induction of immunological changes observed in irritant contact dermatitis (Fig. 1). The effect of irritants on the epidermal keratinocytes varies depending on the exposure. Strong acids or alkalis often result in necrosis of keratinocytes. In contrast, following damage to the skin barrier by tape-stripping or irritant challenge using SLS, an increased mitotic activity in keratinocytes has been observed [36, 45]. At the histopathological level, irritants exhibit different effects on keratinocyte morphology. Willis et al. [38] evaluated clinical and histological changes in skin following 48 h of exposure to different irritants [38]. Nonanoic acid induced eosinophilic degeneration of keratinocytes with nuclear degeneration and only minimal spongiosis. Croton oil produced considerable spongiosis, and the presence of intracytoplasmic vesicles in the upper dermis was observed. SLS induced minor morphological changes in the keratinocytes and induced parakeratosis, suggesting increased epidermal turnover. Finally, ditranol induced a marked swelling of the keratinocytes in the upper epidermis. Thus, specific changes of keratinocytes can be observed following exposure to structurally different irritants. In addition to inducing morphological changes in the skin, irritants are also capable of upregulating cell surface molecules on epidermal cells. One important observation

Fig. 1.
Keratinocyte responses to
skin irritants

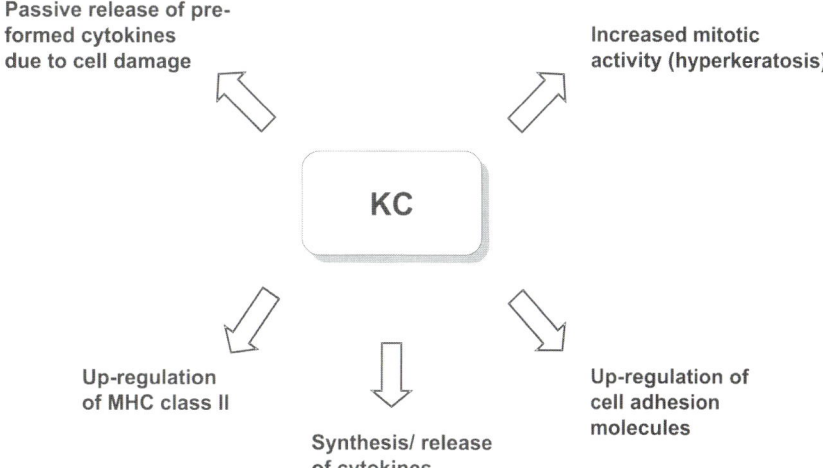

is the capacity to upregulate MHC class II expression on keratinocytes [46]. This upregulation is also observed in the contact allergic reaction. Furthermore, induction of adhesion molecules such as ICAM-1 on keratinocytes has been demonstrated [47] and this molecule, possibly in combination with irritant-induced upregulation of E-selectin on endothelial cells [48], is known to be involved in T lymphocyte accumulation within the skin. Finally, irritant challenge results in the release of several keratinocyte-derived cytokines, as discussed later.

The involvement of the epidermal Langerhans cell in irritant contact dermatitis is still unclear. Some studies have indicated that the number of epidermal Langerhans cells remain unaltered in the skin. In contrast, other studies have demonstrated a decrease in epidermal Langerhans cell numbers following irritant challenge [22, 49–51]. The effect of irritants on Langerhans cell number was long lasting, and full recovery was first obtained 4 weeks following irritant challenge [22]. In support of the latter observation, increased numbers of Langerhans cells have been identified in the afferent lymphatic system following irritant challenge of human skin [52, 53]. However, one must consider that chemically different irritants might have different capacities to modulate Langerhans cell numbers. Accordingly, different effects on Langerhans cell numbers have been observed when comparing SLS and nonanoic acid (NAA) [54].

changes are seen following skin exposure to different irritants. In general, during the acute phase of the irritant reaction, a decrease in epidermal Langerhans cells number is observed, and upregulation of MHC class II and ICAM-1 on keratinocytes is demonstrated.

4.4.3 Epidermal Cytokines Involved in Irritant Contact Dermatitis

As discussed before, both keratinocytes and Langerhans cells exhibit the capacity to secrete a variety of immunologically active cytokines. In irritant contact dermatitis many cytokines have been found to be upregulated as compared to normal, uninvolved skin (Table 5). Although demonstration of increased levels

Table 5. Cytokines upregulated in irritant contact dermatitis

	In vivo	In vitro
Interleukin-1α	[41, 55]	
Interleukin-1β	[56, 57]	
Interleukin-2	[41]	
Interleukin-6	[57, 58]	
Interleukin-8		[59]
Interleukin-10	[56]	
Tumor necrosis factor-α	[60, 61]	[62]
Granulocyte-macrophage colony stimulating factor	[60]	
Interferon-γ	[41, 60]	

Core Message

■ The histological manifestation of the irritant reaction is often impossible to distinguish from the contact allergic reaction. Furthermore, diverse histopathological

4

of cytokines in the irritant reaction is well established both in vivo and in vitro, different results are published in the literature as to which cytokines actually are increased. Many studies have investigated one or two irritants, and generalized from these data. However, today it is known that the application of different irritants to the skin results in the induction of different cytokine profiles. One example is a study by Grängsjö et al. demonstrating that in contrast to SLS, NAA is capable of upregulating IL-6 mRNA in human skin [63]. Similar, several irritants including SLS, but not benzalkonium chloride, have been demonstrated to upregulate TNF-α [58]. The complexity of irritant-induced cytokine profiles in skin is further underscored by the findings that SLS, phenol, and croton oil all upregulate IL-8 whereas only croton oil upregulates GM-CSF [64]. Thus, differences exist in the capability of irritants to induce cytokines. Of the many irritant-inducible cytokines (see Table 5), the pro-inflammatory cytokines IL-1α, IL-1β, and TNF-α are of particular interest.

4.5 Irritant-induced Interleukin-1

Interleukin-1, which was first isolated from monocytes, is now known to be synthesized in several cell types, including keratinocytes. IL-1 exists in two functionally active forms: IL-1α and IL-1β.

In normal skin, IL-1α is constitutively produced by the keratinocytes, and damaging the cell membrane can result in the release of pre-formed IL-1α to the intercellular space. IL-1α is the major form of IL-1 produced by keratinocytes and is secreted as an active molecule. In contrast, IL-1β is secreted as a 31-kDa biologically inactive precursor, which has to be cleaved into an active 17.5-kDa molecule by a protease, not present in resting human keratinocytes. However, in activated keratinocytes, mRNA of IL-1β-converting-enzyme was readily detected following incubation with the hapten urushiol or the irritants phorbol myristate acetate (PMA) or SLS [65]. Thus, even though the keratinocyte is not capable of synthesizing immunological active IL-1β in intact skin, this capacity can be induced by external inflammatory signals. The mechanism for this induction remains unclear. IL-1 is a multifunctional cytokine [66], implicated in T lymphocyte activation and IL-2 production. In addition, IL-1 is involved in upregulation of IL-2 receptors on activated T lymphocytes and is chemotactic for T lymphocytes. IL-1β is also produced by the Langerhans cell and involved in antigen presentation and Langerhans cell migration. Furthermore, IL-1 is capable of inducing other keratinocytes to release or synthesize IL-1 in a paracrine

or even autocrine fashion [67] as well as upregulating other cytokines including epidermal growth factor, IL-6, IL-8, and GM-CSF [68]. Thus, the release of IL-1 can lead to amplification of the ongoing immunological process. In addition to its capacity to regulate other cytokines, IL-1 upregulates cell adhesion molecules on the keratinocyte. In vitro analyses have demonstrated that IL-1 upregulates ICAM-1 expression on keratinocytes, thereby further contributing to the maintenance of the inflammatory cells in the skin.

When analyzing cytokine profiles in the early phases of the allergic as well as irritant reaction in mice, Enk and Katz demonstrated that IL-1β is upregulated as early as 15 min following application of an allergen but not an irritant. Cell depletion studies revealed the Langerhans cell as the cellular source [60]. Furthermore, blocking IL-1β inhibited the elicitation of the allergic reaction, thereby substantiated by the importance of IL-1β. Similar, injection of recombinant IL-1β in vivo led to the development of a clinical reaction, indistinguishable from the contact dermatitis reaction. This observation has supported the hypothesis that expression of IL-1β could differentiate between contact allergic and irritant reactions. However, later studies have indeed found IL-1β in the irritant reaction, though at later time points [56, 57]. Thus, early synthesis of IL-1β seems to be an important initial step in the induction of allergic contact dermatitis, but is not specific for allergic reactions.

> ## Core Message
>
> ■ Both IL-1α and IL-1β have been found to be upregulated in the contact irritant reaction. In murine studies, IL-1β was the first cytokine upregulated and injection of IL-1β in vivo resulted in clinical eczema indistinguishable from the irritant reaction.

4.6 Irritant-induced TNF-α

TNF-α was first described as a molecule exhibiting anti-tumor activity in vivo and in vitro. TNF-α is a highly pleomorphic cytokine [66], produced by a variety of cell types, including T lymphocytes, monocytes, Langerhans cells, fibroblasts, and keratinocytes. TNF-α is synthesized as a 26-kDa pro-peptide. Before secretion the pro-peptide is converted into a 17-kDa protein by metalloproteases [69]. In its active form, TNF-α is composed of three 17-kDa subunits.

TNF-α exerts its function by binding to specific cell surface receptors. Two distinct TNF-α receptors are described. TNF-R1 (414 amino acids) has a molecular weight of approximately 55–60 kDa and TNF-R2 (461 amino acids) is a 75- to 80-kDa receptor. These receptors have similar extracellular structures but distinct cytoplasmic domains. The TNF receptors are expressed on a variety of cells, however mainly the TNF-R1, which is involved in metabolic alterations, cytokine production, and cell death, is expressed on the keratinocytes [70]. TNF-α stimulates the production of collagenase and prostaglandin E_2 by synovial cells and dermal fibroblasts and thus contributes to inflammation and tissue destruction in general. TNF-α increases both MHC class II antigen expression and upregulates the surface expression of ICAM-1 on keratinocytes [71, 72]. Thus, TNF-α is an important cytokine involved in the maintenance of inflammatory processes in the skin. The pro-inflammatory role of TNF-α is stressed by its capacity to induce other inflammatory markers, including IL-1α, IL-6, and the chemoattractant IL-8 [66].

Finally, it has been demonstrated that blocking TNF-α results in inhibition of Langerhans cell migration towards the local lymph nodes following epicutaneously applied allergens or irritants [73, 74]. The importance of TNF-α in irritant contact dermatitis has been further emphasized by studies by Piguet et al. demonstrating that primary irritant reactions to trinitrochlorobenzene (TNCB) could be inhibited in vivo by injection of antibodies to TNF or recombinant soluble TNF receptors [61]. Thus, TNF-α seems to be a key player in the induction of irritant reactions in the skin.

Several irritants exhibit the capacity to upregulate TNF-α in skin. These irritants include dimethylsulfoxide (DMSO), PMA, formaldehyde, phenol, tributylin, and SLS [56, 62, 75]. The list of skin irritants that upregulate TNF-α is still growing, and studies reveal that this upregulation is also found by application of allergens to the skin and when analyzing the irritant capacity of sensitizers, e.g., TNCB, DNTB, and nickel [61, 62]. Although many irritants upregulate TNF-α in skin, no increase in TNF-α expression has been observed following skin application of benzalkonium chloride [58]. Thus, as previously discussed, different irritants interact or regulate the immune system at different levels.

Core Message

■ Several irritants can induce keratinocyte expression of TNF-α both in vitro and in vivo. The importance of irritant-induced TNF-α is stressed by observations by Piguet et al. [61], who could block elicitation of irritant reactions by administration of anti-TNF antibodies.

4.7 Mechanisms of Irritant-induced TNF-α in Keratinocytes

Most previous studies addressing the upregulation of cytokine expression in skin have focused on protein measurements – often by ELISA. In addition, cytokine mRNA expression has been determined by either Northern blotting or reverse transcriptase polymerase chain reaction (RT-PCR). Increased protein and mRNA expression has been interpreted as an increase in synthesis of the investigated cytokine. However, increased mRNA stability or other posttranscriptional modifications have hardly been addressed. The importance of such investigations is stressed by findings that both transcriptional and translational mechanisms were involved the lipopolysaccharide-induced upregulation of TNF-α mRNA in macrophages [76]. Recently it was determined whether transcriptional or posttranscriptional mechanisms are involved in the irritant-induced upregulation of TNF-α in keratinocytes [62]. This study was performed on murine keratinocytes that were transfected with a chloramphenicol acetyl transferase (CAT) reporter construct containing the full-length TNF-α 5´-promoter region. Increased TNF-α promoter activity was indeed observed following in vitro exposure to the irritants PMA and DMSO, strongly suggesting that the PMA- and DMSO-induced upregulation of TNF-α mRNA in keratinocytes is due to increased transcription of the TNF-α gene. These findings were further substantiated by the observation that no significant difference in TNF-α mRNA stability was observed between unstimulated and stimulated keratinocytes [62]. It is generally accepted that the irritant PMA mediates most of its effects via PKCα-dependent signal transduction pathways. Accordingly, it was found that PMA, as well as the common irritants DMSO and SLS, induced an increase in TNF-α mRNA in keratinocytes via a PKC-dependent signaling pathway (Fig. 2).

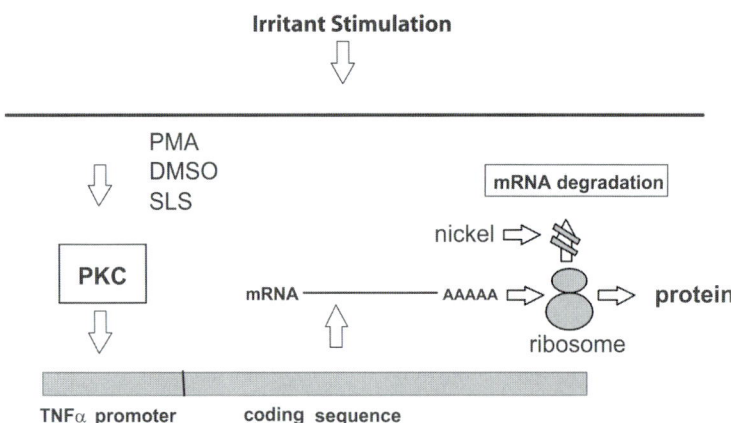

4

Fig. 2. Mechanisms of irritant-induced TNF-α in keratinocytes. Irritants (e.g., PMA, DMSO, SLS) upregulate TNF-α mRNA in keratinocytes via a PKC-dependent signaling pathway resulting in increased mRNA transcription. In contrast, nickel salts mediate their effects by increasing the stability of TNF-α mRNA. Both pathways ultimately lead to increased release of TNF protein. (*DMSO* Dimethylsulfoxide, *PKC* protein kinase C, *PMA* phorbol myristate acetate, *SLS* sodium lauryl sulfate, *TNF* tumor necrosis factor)

It is known that nickel, in addition to being a frequent contact sensitizer, can act as an irritant in nonsensitized animals. Furthermore, nickel exhibits the capacity to upregulate TNF-α mRNA and protein in purified keratinocytes. Inhibitors of PKC and of the cyclic nucleoside-dependent protein kinase were reported not to block this nickel-induced increase in TNF-α mRNA. In addition, this study demonstrated no increase in TNF-α promoter activity following stimulation with nickel. Of particularly interest was the finding that nickel stimulation of keratinocytes in vitro resulted in a pronounced increase in the stability of TNF-α mRNA as compared to unstimulated control cultures [62]. The precise mechanism of the nickel-induced increased stability of TNF-α mRNA remains unclear. One possibility is modification of peptides binding to an AUUUA-sequence in the 3′-region of the mRNA thereby blocking/inhibiting degradation of the mRNA transcript. Another possibility is that nickel stimulation could result in sequestering TNF-α mRNA in the ribosomal compartment, thereby stabilizing the mRNA. Independently of the mechanism, the overall result was an increase in the release of biologically active TNF protein.

Thus, when comparing the irritant effect of nickel in nonsensitized animals with irritants such as DMSO and PMA, different intracellular signaling mechanisms are involved in upregulation of TNF-α peptide expression (Fig. 2).

Core Message

■ Not all skin irritants induce measurable TNF-α. Furthermore, different signaling mechanisms have been described, including direct gene activation (transcription) and stabilization of the TNF-α mRNA (posttranscriptional regulation).

4.7.1 Regulation of the Inflammatory Milieu Locally in Inflamed Skin

As described in this chapter, an upregulation of pro- and inflammatory cytokines is present in the irritant reaction. It is noteworthy that this type of reaction often tends to exhibit a prolonged course, even despite removal of the irritant exposure. Thus, the clinical reaction may continue for several years. Until recently, no explanation for this phenomenon has been forwarded. However, data are now available suggesting that elements in the local inflammatory milieu may actually contribute to the persistence of skin inflammation. Previous, it was shown that autocrine regulation of IL-1, both IL-1α and IL-1β, is present in vitro [77, 78]. Therefore, a study was enforced to describe whether such autocrine regulation of the proinflammatory cytokine – TNFα – was present in keratinocytes. Indeed, it was found that stimulating keratinocytes with TNF-α in vitro led to an increase in

TNF-α mRNA expression [79]. This potential, interesting signaling pathway was critically dependent upon signaling through PKC-dependent pathways and involved increased gene transcription. Thus, it was shown that induction of the pro-inflammatory cytokine TNF-α, e.g., by skin irritants, could lead to induction of an autocrine signaling pathway locally in the skin, thereby substantiating the inflammatory reaction and as such contributing to the persistence of the clinical irritant skin reaction.

Core Message

■ Skin irritants can induce an inflammatory milieu, following which further amplification is possible. Today, data exist demonstrating autocrine regulation of both IL-1 and TNF-α in keratinocytes.

4.8 Hypothesis of the Immunological Events Leading to Irritant Contact Dermatitis

Following application of irritants to the skin, penetration of the stratum corneum is the primary event. During this, perturbation of the skin barrier occurs. This further facilitates the penetration of the skin by the irritant and other external agents. Following penetration of the stratum corneum, the irritant most likely induces the release of pre-formed IL-1α from the keratinocytes, and induces the synthesis of several other immunoregulatory keratinocyte-derived cytokines (Fig. 3). TNF-α in particular seems essential, because in a murine system injection of antibodies to TNF in vivo completely blocks the development of irritant reactions [61]. The mechanism of irritant-induced upregulation of TNF-α seems to involve increased transcription of the gene; however, irritant-induced stabilization of cytokine mRNA may also contribute [62]. Next, induction of cell adhesion molecules such as ICAM-1 on the keratinocytes and E-selectin on the endothelial cells facilitates the extravasation of inflammatory T lymphocytes to the skin. This process may be enforced by the release of the chemoattractant IL-8 by the keratinocytes [80]. During the first 24–72 h, an epidermal influx on non-Langerhans cell-derived antigen-presenting cells occurs. In addition, the number of epidermal Langerhans cells decreases and these cells possibly migrate towards the draining local lymph node. A cellular infiltrate comprised mainly of mononuclear cells, in particular CD4+ T lymphocytes, is then seen in the involved skin area. These cells are activated and they release inflammatory cytokines. In particular, increased levels of IFN-γ and IL-2 have been observed [41]. Ultimately, these events lead to the histological picture of acute irritant contact dermatitis.

The often-observed chronicity of irritant contact dermatitis is elusive. However, the irritant-induced inflammation may expose the immune system to immunogenic skin peptides that it does not normally see. The chronicity may therefore involve presentation of such self-peptides to the immune system resulting in the development of an autoimmune skin disease. Alternative, the irritant-induced TNF-α is regulated in an autocrine way and thereby involved in the maintenance of an inflammatory milieu locally in the skin. The resulting irritant contact dermatitis reaction may continue for years.

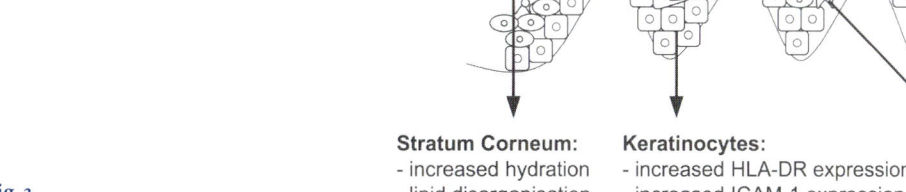

Fig. 3.
Epidermal changes following exposure to irritants

Suggested Reading

1. Piguet PF, Grau GE, Hauser C, Vassalli P (1991) Tumor necrosis factor is a critical mediator in hapten-induced irritant and contact hypersensitivity reactions. J Exp Med 173:673–679

This paper describe in detail the presence and significance of TNF-a in the contact irritant reaction as well as elicitation of the contact allergic reaction. Using the in situ hybridization technique, the authors directly demonstrate an important role of the keratinocyte in this induction, thus implicating the keratinocyte as an important player in the induction of the contact irritant reaction in skin.

References

1. Cua AB, Wilhelm KP, Maibach HI (1990) Frictional properties of human skin: Relation to age, sex and anatomical region, stratum corneum hydration and transepidermal water loss. Br J Dermatol 123:473–479
2. Berardesca E, Maibach HI (1988) Racial differences in sodium lauryl sulphate induced cutaneous irritation: black and white. Contact Dermatitis 18:65–70
3. Judge MR, Griffiths HA, Basketter DA, White IR, Rycroft RJ, McFadden JP (1996) Variation in response of human skin to irritant challenge. Contact Dermatitis 34:115–117
4. Frosch PJ, Kligman AM (1977) A method for appraising the stinging capacity of topically applied substances. J Soc Cosm Chem 28:197–209
5. Frosch P (1985) Hautirritation und empfindliche haut. Grosse, Berlin
6. Luger TA, stadler BM, Katz SI, Oppenheim JJ (1981) Epidermal cell (keratinocyte)-derived thymocyte-activating factor (ETAF). J Immunol 127:1493–1498
7. Sauder DN, Carter CS, Katz SI, Oppenheim JJ (1982) Epidermal cell production of thymocyte activating factor (ETAF). J Invest Dermatol 79:34–39
8. Lampert IA (1984) Expression of HLA-DR (ia like) antigen on epidermal keratinocytes in human dermatoses. Clin Exp Immunol 57:93–100
9. Volc-Platzer B, Steiner A, Radaszkiewicz T, Wolff K (1988) Recombinant gamma interferon and in vivo induction of HLA-DR antigens. Br J Dermatol 119:155–160
10. Dustin ML, Singer KH, Tuck DT, Springer TA (1988) Adhesion of T lymphoblasts to epidermal keratinocytes is regulated by interferon gamma and is mediated by intercellular adhesion molecule 1 (ICAM-1). J Exp Med 167:1323–1340
11. Norris P, Poston RN, Thomas DS, Thornhill M, Hawk J, Haskard DO (1991) The expression of endothelial leukocyte adhesion molecule-1 (ELAM-1), intercellular adhesion molecule-1 (ICAM-1), and vascular cell adhesion molecule-1 (VCAM-1) in experimental cutaneous inflammation: a comparison of ultraviolet B erythema and delayed hypersensitivity. J Invest Dermatol 96:763–770
12. Haraldsen G, Kvale D, Lien B, Farstad IN, Brandtzaeg P (1996) Cytokine-regulated expression of E-selektin, intercellular adhesion molecule-1 (ICAM-1), and vascular cell adhesion molecule-1 (VCAM-1) in human microvascular endothelial cells. J Immunol 156:2558–2565
13. Langerhans P (1868) Über die Nerven der menschlichen Haut. Virchows Arch (Pathol Anat) 44:325–337
14. Lore K, Sonerborg A, Spetz AL, Andersson U, Andersson J (1998) Erratum to "Immunocytochemical detection of cytokines and chemokines in Langerhans cells and in vitro derived dendritic cells". J Immunol Methods 218:173–187
15. Meunier L, Bata-Csorgo Z, Cooper KD (1995) In human dermis, ultraviolet radiation induces expansion of a $CD36^+$ $CD11b^+$ $CD1^-$ macrophage subset by infiltration and proliferation; $CD1^+$ Langerhans-like dendritic antigen-presenting cells are concomitantly depleted. J Invest Dermatol 105:782–788
16. Baadsgaard O, Fox DA, Cooper KD (1988) Human epidermal cells from ultraviolet light-exposed skin preferentially activate autoreactive $CD4^+2H4^+$ suppressor-inducer lymphocytes and $CD8^+$ suppressor/cytotoxic lymphocytes. J Immunol 140:1738–1744
17. Baadsgaard O, Salvo B, Manni A, Dass B, Fox DA, Cooper KD (1990) In vivo ultraviolet-exposed human epidermal cells activate T suppressor cell pathways that involve $CD4^+CD45RA^+$ suppressor-inducer T cells. J Immunol 145:2854–2861
18. Kang K, Gilliam AC, Chen G, Tootell E, Cooper KD (1998) In human skin, UVB initiates early induction of IL-10 over IL-12 preferentially in the expanding dermal monocytic/macrophagic population. J Invest Dermatol 111:31–38
19. Lisby S, Baadsgaard O, Cooper KD, Hansen ER, Mehregan D, Thomsen K, Vejlsgaard GL (1990) Phenotype, ultrastructure and function of $CD1^+DR^+$ epidermal cells that express CD36 (OKM5) in cutaneous T cell lymphoma. Scand J Immunol 32:111
20. Baadsgaard O, Lisby S, Avnstorp C, Clemmensen O, Vejlsgaard GL (1990) Antigen-presenting activity of non-Langerhans epidermal cells in contact hypersensitivity reactions. Scand J Immunol 32:217–224
21. Hansen ER, Baadsgaard O, Lisby S, Cooper KD, Thomsen K, Vejlsgaard GL (1990) Cutaneous T-cell lymphoma lesional epidermal cells activate autologous $CD4^+$ T lymphocytes: involvement of both $CD1^+OKM5^+$ and $CD1^+OKM5^-$ antigen-presenting cells. J Invest Dermatol 94:485–491
22. Lisby S, Baadsgaard O, Cooper KD, Vejlsgaard GL (1989) Decreased number and function of antigen-presenting cells in the skin following application of irritant agents: relevance for skin cancer? J Invest Dermatol 92:842–847
23. Mosmann TR, Cherwinski H, Bond MW, Giedlin MA, Coffman RL (1986) Two types of murine helper T cell clone. I. Definition according to profiles of lymphokine activities and secreted proteins. J Immunol 136:2348–2357
24. Kondo S, Kono T, Sauder DN, McKenzie RC (1993) IL-8 gene expression and production in human keratinocytes and their modulation by UVB. J Invest Dermatol 101:690–694
25. Pitzalis C, Cauli A, Pipitone N, Smith C, Barker J, Marchesoni A, Yanni G, Panayi GS (1996) Cutaneous lymphocyte antigen-positive T lymphocytes preferentially migrate to the skin but not to the joint in psoriatic arthritis. Arthritis Rheum 39:137–145
26. Santamaria LF, Perez Soler MT, Hauser C, Blaser K (1995) Allergen specificity and endothelial transmigration of T cells in allergic contact dermatitis and atopic dermatitis are associated with the cutaneous lymphocyte antigen. Int Arch Allergy Immunol 107:359–362
27. Santamaria Babi LF, Picker LJ, Perez Soler MT, Drzimalla K, Flohr P, Blaser K, Hauser C (1995) Circulating allergen-reactive T cells from patients with atopic dermatitis and allergic contact dermatitis express the skin-selective homing receptor, the cutaneous lymphocyte-associated antigen. J Exp Med 181:1935–1940
28. Brasch J, Burgard J, Sterry W (1992) Common pathogenetic pathways in allergic and irritant contact dermatitis. J Invest Dermatol 98:166–170

29. Scheynius A, Fischer T, Forsum U, Klareskog L (1984) Phenotypic characterization *in situ* of inflammatory cells in allergic and irritant contact dermatitis in man. Clin Exp Immunol 55:81–90

30. Lavrijsen APM (1997) Stratum corneum barrier in healthy and diseased skin. PhD Thesis, Leiden University, pp 26–38

31. Agner T, Serup J (1993) Time course of occlusive effects on skin evaluated by measurement of transepidermal water loss (TEWL). Including patch tests with sodium lauryl sulphate and water. Contact Dermatitis 28:6–9

32. De Fine Olivarius F, Agner T, Menné T (1993) Skin barrier function and dermal inflammation. An experimental study of transepidermal water loss after dermal tuberculin injection compared with SLS patch testing. Br J Dermatol 129:554–557

33. Lee JY, Effendy I, Maibach HI (1997) Acute irritant contact dermatitis: recovery time in man. Contact Dermatitis 36:285–290

34. Wilhelm KP, Cua AB, Wolf HH, Maibach HI (1993) Surfactant-induced stratum corneum hydration in vivo: prediction of the irritant potential of anionic surfactants. J Invest Dermatol 101:310–315

35. Fartasch M, Schnetz E, Diepgen TL (1998) Characterization of detergent-induced barrier alterations – effect of barrier cream on irritation. J Invest Dermatol 3:121–127

36. Fischer LB, Maibach HI (1975) Effect of some irritants on human epidermal mitosis. Contact Dermatitis 1:273–276

37. Wood LC, Jackson SM, Elias PM, Grunfeld C, Feingold KR (1992) Cutaneous barrier perturbation stimulates cytokine production in the epidermis of mice. J Clin Invest 90:482–487

38. Willis CM, Stephens CJM, Wilkinson JD (1989) Epidermal damage induced by irritants in man: a light and electron microscopic study. J Invest Dermatol 93:695–699

39. Willis CM, Young E, Brandon DR, Wilkinson JD (1986) Immunopathological and ultrastructural findings in human allergic and irritant contact dermatitis. Br J Dermatol 115:305–316

40. Avnstorp C, Ralfkiaer E, Jørgensen J, Wantzin GL (1987) Sequential immunophenotypic study of lymphoid infiltrate in allergic and irritant reactions. Contact Dermatitis 16:239–245

41. Hoefakker S, Caubo M, van't Erve EH, Roggeveen MJ, Boersma WJ, van Joost T, Notten WR, Claassen E (1995) In vivo cytokine profiles in allergic and irritant contact dermatitis. Contact Dermatitis 33:258–266

42. Jung K, Linse F, Pals ST, Heller R, Moths C, Neumann C (1997) Adhesion molecules in atopic dermatitis: patch tests elicited by house dust mite. Contact Dermatitis 37:163–172

43. De Vries IJ, Langeveld-Wildschut EG, van Reijsen FC, Bihari IC, bruijnzeel-Koomen CA, Thepen T (1997) Nonspecific T-cell homing during inflammation in topic dermatitis: expression of cutaneous lymphocyte-associated antigen and integrin alphaE beta7 on skin-infiltrating T cells. J Allergy Clin Immunol 100:694–701

44. Santamaria Babi LF, Moser R, Perez Soler MT, Picker LJ, Blaser K, Haser C (1995) Migration of skin-homing T cells across cytokine-activated human endothelial cell layers involves interaction of the cutaneous lymphocyte-associated antigen (CLA), the very late antigen-4 (VLA-4), and the lymphocyte function-associated antigen-1 (LFA-1). J Immunol 154:1543–1550

45. Van de Sandt JJ, Bos TA, Rutten AA (1995) Epidermal cell proliferation and terminal differentiation in skin organ culture after topical exposure to sodium dodecyl sulphate. In Vitro Cell Dev Biol Anim 31:761–766

46. Gawkrodger DJ, Carr MM, McVittie E, Guy K, Hunter JA (1987) Keratinocyte expression of MHC class II antigens in allergic sensitization and challenge reactions and in irritant contact dermatitis. J Invest Dermatol 88:11–16

47. Gatto H, Viac J, Charveron M, Schmitt D (1992) Study of immune-associated antigens (IL-1 and ICAM-1) in normal human keratinocytes treated with sodium lauryl sulphate. Arch Dermatol Res 284:186–188

48. Henseleit U, Steinbrink K, Goebeler M, Roth J, Vestweber D, Sorg C, Sunderkotter C (1996) E-selectin expression in experimental models of inflammation in mice. J Pathol 180:317–325

49. Mikulowska A, Falck B (1994) Distributional changes of Langerhans cells in human skin during irritant contact dermatitis. Arch Dermatol Res 286:429–433

50. Ranki A, Kanerva L, Forstrom L, Konttinen Y, Mustakallio KK (1983) T and B lymphocytes, macrophages and Langerhans´ cells during the course of contact allergic and irritant skin reactions in man. Acta Derm Venerol 63:376–383

51. Marks JG Jr, Zaino RJ, Bressler MF, Williams JV (1987) Changes in lymphocyte and Langerhans cell populations in allergic and irritant contact dermatitis. Int J Dermatol 26:354–357

52. Brand CU, Hunziker T, Braathen LR (1992) Studies on human skin lymph containing Langerhans cells from sodium lauryl sulphate contact dermatitis. J Invest Dermatol 99:109S–110S

53. Brand CU, Hunziker T, Limat A, Braathen LR (1993) Large increase of Langerhans cells in human skin lymph derived from irritant contact dermatitis. Br J Dermatol 128:184–188

54. Forsey RJ, Shahidullah H, Sands C, McVittie E, Aldridge RD, Hunter JA, Howie SE (1998) Epidermal Langerhans cell apoptosis is induced in vivo by nonanoic acid but not by sodium lauryl sulphate. Br J Dermatol 139:453–461

55. Haas J, Lipkow T, Mohamadzadeh M, Kolde G, Knop J (1992) Induction of inflammatory cytokines in murine keratinocytes upon *in vivo* stimulation with contact sensitizers and tolerizing analogues. Exp Dermatol 1:76–83

56. Kondo S, Pastore S, Shivji GM, McKenzie RC, Sauder DN (1994) Characterization of epidermal cytokine profiles in sensitization and elicitation phases of allergic contact dermatitis as well as irritant contact dermatitis in mouse skin. Lymphokine Cytokine Res 13:367–375

57. Hunziker T, Brand CU, Kapp A, Waelti ER, Braathen LR (1992) Increased levels of inflammatory cytokines in human skin lymph derived from sodium lauryl sulphate-induced contact dermatitis. Br J Dermatol 127:254–257

58. Holliday MR, Corsini E, Smith S, Basketter DA, Dearman RJ, Kimber I (1997) Differential induction of cutaneous TNF-α and IL-6 by topically applied chemicals. Am J Contact Dermatitis 8:158–164

59. Mohamadzadeh M, Muller M, Hultsch T, Enk A, Saloga J, Knop J (1994) Enhanced expression of IL-8 i normal human keratinocytes and human keratinocyte cell line HaCaT in vitro after stimulation with contact sensitizers, tolerogens and irritants. Exp Dermatol 3:298–303

60. Enk AH, Katz SI (1992) Early molecular events in the induction phase of contact sensitivity. Proc Natl Acad Sci USA 89:1398–1402

61. Piguet PF, Grau GE, Hauser C, Vassalli P (1991) Tumor necrosis factor is a critical mediator in hapten-induced irritant and contact hypersensitivity reactions. J Exp Med 173:673–679

62. Lisby S, Muller KM, Jongeneel CV, Saurat JH, Hauser C (1995) Nickel and skin irritants up-regulate tumor necro-

4

sis factor-alpha mRNA in keratinocytes by different but potentially synergistic mechanisms. Int Immunol 7: 343–352

63. Grängsjö A, Leijon-Kuligowski A, Torma H, Roomans GM, Lindberg M (1996) Different pathways in irritant contact eczema? Early differences in the epidermal element content and expression of cytokines after application of 2 different irritants. Contact Dermatitis 35:355–360

64. Wilmer JL, Burleson FG, Kayama F, Kanno J, Luster MI (1994) Cytokine induction in human epidermal keratinocytes exposed to contact irritants and its relation to chemical-induced inflammation in mouse skin. J Invest Dermatol 102:915–922

65. Zepter K, Haffner A, Soohoo LF, de Luca D, Tang HP, Fisher P, Chavinson J, Elmets CA (1997) Induction of biologically active IL-1 beta-converting enzyme and mature IL-1 beta in human keratinocytes by inflammatory and immunogic stimuli. J Immunol 159:6203–6208

66. Luger T (1991) The epidermis as a source of immunomodulating cytokines. Period Biol 93:97–104

67. Lee SV, Morhenn VB, Ilnicka M, Eugui EM, Allison AC (1991) Autocrine stimulation of interleukin-1 alpha and transforming growth factor alpha production in human keratinocytes and its antagonism by glucocorticoids. J Invest Dermatol 97:106–110

68. McKenzie RC, Sauder DN (1990) The role of keratinocyte cytokines in inflammation and immunity. J Invest Dermatol 95:105S–107S

69. Gearing AJH, Beckett P, Christodoulou M, Churchill M, Clements J, Davidson AH, Drummond AH, Galloway WA, Gilbert R, Gordon JL (1994) Processing of tumour necrosis factor-alpha precursor by metalloproteinases. Nature 370: 555–557

70. Trefzer U, Brockhaus M, Loetscher H, Parlow F, Kapp A, Schopf E, Krutmann J (1991) 55-kD tumor necrosis factor receptor is expressed by human keratinocytes and plays a pivotal role in regulation of human keratinocyte ICAM-1 expression. J Invest Dermatol 97:911–916

71. Groves RW, Allen MH, Ross EL, Barker JN, MacDonald DM (1995) Tumour necrosis factaor alpha is pro-inflammatory in normal human skin and modulates cutaneous adhesion molecule expression. Br J Dermatol 132:345–352

72. Detmar M, Orfanos CE (1990) Tumor necrosis factor-alpha inhibits cell proliferation and induces class II antigens and cell adhesion molecules in cultured normal human keratinocytes in vitro. Arch Dermatol Res 282:238–245

73. Yamazaki S, Yokozeki H, Satoh T, Katayama I, Nishioka K (1998) TNF-alpha, RANTES, and MCP-1 are major chemoattractants of murine Langerhans cells to the regional lymph nodes. Exp Dermatol 7:35–41

74. Wang B, Kondo S, Shivji GM, Fujisawa H, Mak TW, Sauder DN (1996) Tumour necrosis factor receptor II (p75) signalling is required for the migration of Langerhans' cells. Immunology 88:284–288

75. Corsini E, Terzoli A, Bruccoleri A, Marinovich M, Galli CL (1997) Induction of necrosis factor-α in vivo by a skin irritant. Tributyltin, through activation of transcription factors: its pharmacological modulation by anti-inflammatory drugs. J Invest Dermatol 108:892–896

76. Zuckerman SH, Evans GF, Guthrie L (1991) Transcriptional and post-transcriptional mechanisms involved in the differential expression of LPS-induced IL-1 and TNF mRNA. Immunology 73:460–465

77. Kamado K, Sato K (1994) Regulation of IL-1a expression in human karatinocytes. Lymphokine Cytokine Res 13:29–35

78. Warner SJC, Auger KR, Libby P (1987) Interleukin-1 induces interleukin-1. J Immunol 139:1911–1917

79. Lisby S, Hauser C (2002) Transcriptional regulation of tumor necrosis factor-α in keratinocytes mediated by interleukin-1β and tumor necrosis factor-α. Exp Dermatol 11: 592–598

80. Zachariae CO, Jinquan T, Nielsen V, Kaltoft K, Thestrup-Pedersen K (1992) Phenotypic determination of T-lymphocytes responding to chemotactic stimulation from fMLP, IL-8, human IL-10, and epidermal lymphocyte chemotactic factor. Arch Dermatol Res 284:333–338

Chapter 5

Immediate Contact Reactions

5

Arto Lahti, David Basketter

Contents

5.1 Introduction

Nonimmunologic contact urticaria (NICU) and other nonimmunologic immediate contact reactions (NIICRs) of the skin comprise a group of inflammatory reactions that appear within minutes to an hour after contact with the eliciting substance and usually disappear within a few hours. These reactions can also be called immediate-type irritancy. NIICRs can be caused by chemicals or proteins and occur without previous immunologic sensitization in most exposed individuals, and they are the most common type of immediate contact reaction [38].

In contrast to NICU, immunologic contact urticaria requires previous sensitization (not necessarily through the dermal route) to the offending agent, usually a protein. Subsequent contact with the material can then elicit the clinical symptoms, which are essentially indistinguishable from their nonimmunologic counterpart. However, in practice, from both a clinical and a mechanistic perspective, it can sometimes be difficult to be convinced whether one is dealing with an immunologic or a nonimmunologic (or a combination of both) type of urticaria.

5.2 Definitions, Concepts, and Symptoms

The symptoms of NIICRs are heterogeneous and the intensity of the reaction typically varies, depending on the concentration, the vehicle, the skin area exposed, the mode of exposure, and the substance itself [36]. A further important variable is the susceptibility of the exposed individual, which can vary widely [3]. Itching, tingling or burning accompanied by erythema are the weakest types of reactions. Sometimes only local sensations without any visible change in the skin are reported. The redness is usually follicular at first and then spreads to cover the whole application site. A local weal and flare suggest a contact urticarial reaction. Generalized urticaria after contact with NICU agents is a rare phenomenon but has been reported more often after contact with agents eliciting immunologic IgE-mediated contact urticaria. Repeated applications of NICU agents may cause eczematous reactions. Rapidly appearing microvesicles are frequently seen after contact with food products in protein contact dermatitis, which can be caused by nonimmunologic (irritant) or immunologic (allergic) mechanisms [21, 27]. In NICU reactions, the symptoms usually appear and remain in the contact area. In addition to local skin symptoms, other organs are occasionally involved, giving rise to conjunctivitis, rhinitis, an asthmatic attack, or anaphylactic shock [26]. This is called the contact urticaria syndrome and it mostly involves immunologic mechanisms [2, 59]. In some cases, NICU reactions

Table 1. Definitions and terms

Immediate contact reaction	Immunologic (allergic) or non-immunologic (irritant), urticarial or nonurticarial reactions. Does not define the appearance of the reaction
Contact urticaria	Allergic and nonallergic urticarial reactions
Immediate-type irritancy	Nonallergic urticarial or non-urticarial reactions
Protein contact dermatitis	Allergic or nonallergic eczematous immediate reactions caused by proteins or proteinaceous material
Contact urticaria syndrome	Local reactions in the skin and systemic symptoms in other organs, usually allergic

5

appear only on slightly compromised skin and can be part of the mechanism responsible for the maintenance of chronic eczemas.

The precise usage of the terms "immediate contact reaction," "contact urticaria," "immediate-type irritancy," "contact urticaria syndrome," "protein contact dermatitis," and "atopic contact dermatitis" varies considerably in the literature. Immediate contact reaction is the broadest concept, which covers both immunologic (allergic) and nonimmunologic (irritant) reactions, but does not say anything about the appearance of the reaction. Contact urticaria can be either allergic or irritant. The redness of skin appearing within tens of minutes after contact with the eliciting substance cannot be regarded as contact urticaria unless at least some people get urticarial reactions at the application site. Protein contact dermatitis is caused by proteins or proteinaceous materials, and it represents either allergic or irritant dermatitis, which has characteristic features of acute or chronic eczema [38]. Atopic contact dermatitis is a historical term and means an immediate-type (IgE-mediated) allergic contact reaction in an atopic person [20]. It is included in the concept of allergic protein contact dermatitis (Table 1).

5.3 Mechanisms and Clinical Aspects of Nonimmunologic Immediate Contact Reactions

5.3.1 Histamine

The mechanisms of NIICRs, similar to other irritant reactions, are not well understood. It was previously

assumed that substances eliciting NIICRs result in nonspecific histamine release from mast cells. However, it has been shown that H_1-antihistamines hydroxyzine, and terfenadine do not inhibit reactions to benzoic acid, cinnamic acid, cinnamic aldehyde (cinnamal), methyl nicotinate, or dimethylsulfoxide, although they inhibit reactions to histamine in prick tests [36, 37]. These results suggest that histamine is not the main mediator in NIICRs to these well-known contact urticants.

5.3.2 Skin Nerves

The role of skin nerves in NIICRs has been studied using capsaicin (trans-8-methyl-N-vanillyl-6-nonenamide), which is known to induce the release of bioactive peptides, such as substance P, from the axons of unmyelinated C-fibers of sensory nerves. Pretreatment of the skin with capsaicin inhibits erythema reactions in histamine prick tests [4], but does not inhibit either erythema or edema elicited by benzoic acid or methyl nicotinate [51]. This suggests that NIICRs to these model substances are not a type of neurogenic inflammation of the skin. Topical anesthesia inhibits erythema reactions to histamine, benzoic acid, and methyl nicotinate, but it is not known whether the inhibitory effect is due to the influence on the sensory nerves only, or whether the anesthetic also affects other cell types or regulatory mechanisms of immediate-type skin inflammation [51].

5.3.3 Ultraviolet Light

NIICRs to benzoic acid and methyl nicotinate can be inhibited by exposure to ultraviolet B and A light. The inhibition lasts for at least 2 weeks [50]. The reactions on nonirradiated skin sites also decrease, suggesting the possibility that UV irradiation may have "systemic effects" [49]. The mechanism of UV inhibition is not known, but it does not seem to be due to thickening of the stratum corneum, as has been speculated [18]. The inhibition of mast cell functions is one possible mechanism [10, 32].

5.3.4 Prostanoids

The NIICRs to benzoic acid, cinnamic acid, cinnamic aldehyde, methyl nicotinate, and diethyl fumarate can be inhibited by peroral acetylsalicylic acid and indometacin [42, 43] and by topical application of diclofenac or naproxen gels [29]. The duration of inhibition from a single dose of acetylsalicylic acid can be as long as 4 days [35]. The mechanism by which nonsteroidal anti-inflammatory drugs inhibit NIICRs in human skin has not been defined, but it is probably ascribable to the inhibition of prostaglandin (PG) metabolism.

New data provide evidence that PGD_2 is the primary mediator of contact urticarial reactions to benzoic acid, sorbic acid, and nicotinic acid esters. PGD_2 is dose-dependently released in human skin after application of these agents [63–65]. It is also known that intradermal injection of PGD_2 elicits erythema and weal formation in human skin. An interesting, but still unanswered, question in human skin is which types of cells are activated by these substances to release PGD_2. According to animal studies, good candidates are dermal macrophages and epidermal Langerhans cells [72, 84]. In rabbit skin, PGD_2 has been shown to be an intermediate in agonist-stimulated nitric oxide release, and the cutaneous vasodilatation can be inhibited by a nitric oxide synthase inhibitor [86]. This suggests that vasodilatation caused by PGD_2 is mediated by nitric oxide. Whether the mechanism is similar in human skin remains to be studied.

5.3.5 Molecular Structure

Molecular structure is important for the irritant properties of an NIICR agent. Pyridine carboxaldehyde (PCA) has three isomers: 2-, 3- and 4-PCA, depending on the position of the aldehyde group on the pyridine ring (Fig. 1). 3-PCA is a strong, and 2-PCA a weak, irritant in both human and animal skin (guinea pig ear swelling test). A slight change in the molecular structure of a chemical may substantially alter its capacity to produce NIICRs [24].

5.3.6 Agents Producing Nonimmunologic Immediate Contact Reactions

The best-studied substances producing NIICRs are benzoic acid, sorbic acid, cinnamic acid and aldehyde and nicotinic acid esters. Under optimal conditions, most individuals react with local erythema and/or edema to these substances within 45 min after application. Cinnamic aldehyde at a concentration of

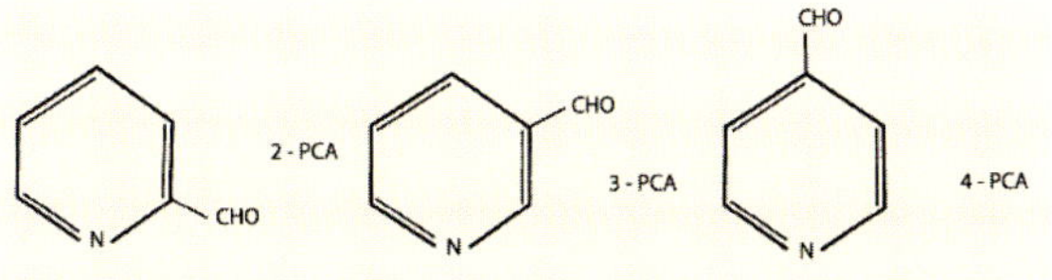

Fig. 1. Three isomers of pyridine carboxaldehyde (*PCA*)

Table 2. Agents producing immediate nonimmunologic contact reactions including contact urticaria

Animals
  Arthropods
  Caterpillars
  Corals
  Jellyfish
  Moths
  Sea anemones

Foods
  Cayenne pepper
  Fish
  Mustard
  Thyme

Fragrances and flavorings
  Balsam of Peru (*Myroxylon pereirae*)
  Benzaldehyde
  Cassis (cinnamon oil)
  Cinnamic acid
  Cinnamic aldehyde (cinnamal)

Medicaments
  Alcohols
  Benzocaine
  Camphor
  Cantharides
  Capsaicin
  Chloroform
  Dimethylsulfoxide
  Friar's balsam
  Iodine
  Methyl salicylate
  Methylene green
  Myrrh
  Nicotinic acid esters
  Resorcinol
  Tar extracts
  Tincture of benzoin
  Witch hazel

Metals
  Cobalt

Plants
  Chrysanthemum
  Nettles
  Seaweed

Preservatives and disinfectants
  Benzoic acid
  Chlorocresol
  Formaldehyde
  Sodium benzoate
  Sorbic acid

Miscellaneous
  Butyric acid
  Diethyl fumarate
  Histamine
  Pine oil
  Pyridine carboxaldehyde
  Sulfur
  Turpentine

5

0.01% may elicit erythema with a burning or stinging feeling in the skin. Some mouthwashes and chewing gums contain cinnamic aldehyde (cinnamal) at concentrations high enough to produce a pleasant tingling in the mouth and enhance the sale of the product. Higher concentrations may produce lip swelling. Some agents causing immediate irritant skin reactions are listed in Table 2.

5.3.7 Tests in Animal Skin

Animal test methods for determining NIICRs are needed to screen for putative agents and to clarify the mechanisms. At the moment, the guinea pig ear swelling test is the best animal test available for studying NIICRs [39, 40]. A positive reaction in the guinea pig ear lobe comprises erythema and edema. Quantification of the edema by measuring the change in ear thickness is an accurate, quick, and reproducible method. Similar to human skin, the swelling response in the guinea pig ear lobe depends on the concentration of the eliciting substance. The maximal response is a roughly 100% increase in ear thickness and it appears 40–50 min after the application, depending on the vehicle.

A decrease in reactivity to NIICR agents is noticed after reapplication on the following day [41]. This tachyphylaxis phenomenon is not specific to the substance that produces it, and reactivity to other agents also decreases. The length of the refractory period is 4 days for methyl nicotinate, 8 days for diethyl fumarate and cinnamic aldehyde, and 16 days for benzoic acid, cinnamic acid, and dimethylsulfoxide.

The guinea pig ear lobe resembles human skin in many respects, including the morphology of the reaction, the timing of the maximal response, the concentrations of the eliciting substances needed to produce the reaction, the tachyphylaxis phenomenon, and the lack of an inhibitory effect of antihistamines on the NIICRs.

5.3.8 Tests in Human Skin

Special tests for NIICRs are needed, because these reactions are not seen in ordinary tests for irritancy and contact allergy. The most frequently used tests are the open test and the chamber test.

5.3.8.1 Open Test

In the open test, 0.1 ml of the test substance is spread on a 3×3 cm area of the skin on the upper back, the extensor aspect of the upper arm, or the forearm. There are marked differences between skin sites in reactivity to NIICR substances. The face (especially the cheek), the antecubital space, the upper back, the upper arm, the volar forearm, the lower back, and the leg constitute a rough order of decreasing reactivity [18, 38, 52]. A 10-µl dose to a 1×1 cm area is often used if a greater number of substances are be tested at the same time. Petrolatum and water were the most often used vehicles 15 years ago [38], but it has been shown that the use of alcohol vehicles and the addition of propylene glycol to the vehicle enhance the sensitivity of the test to detect marginal immediate irritant reactions [44, 91]. The test is usually read at 20, 40, and 60 min in order to see the maximal response. In visual grading, scores for the erythema and edema components of the reaction (+ weak, ++ moderate, +++ strong) have been used [91], but objective measurement of erythema using chroma meters and laser Doppler flowmeters is strongly suggested [43, 45]. The test is usually performed on normal-looking skin, but it is sometimes useful to test suspected irritants on slightly or previously affected skin areas or on skin sites suggested by the patient's history. For example, if an immediate irritant reaction to a cosmetic cream has appeared on the face, one may see nothing if the test is performed on the back, but the reaction can be elicited by reapplication to the previously affected skin of the face. Repeated open tests on the same test site may be needed to detect weak immediate irritant reactions [25]. In a use test, the suspected product or substance is used in the same way as it was when the symptoms appeared.

5.3.8.2 Chamber Test

The chamber test is a routine method of patch testing for contact allergy, but it can also be used to study NIICRs. The test substances are applied in small aluminum chambers (Finn chamber, Epitest, Hyrylä, Finland) and fixed to the skin with porous acrylic tape. The occlusion time is 15 min and the test is read at 20, 40 and 60 min. Occlusion enhances percutaneous penetration and may increase the sensitivity of the test. The advantage of the chamber test is that a smaller skin area is needed than in the open test [22, 36].

5.3.8.3 Factors to be Considered in Skin Tests

The concentration of a NIICR agent needed in a skin test may be difficult to define, as it is in tests with classic, delayed-type irritants. Therefore, dilution series are recommended. They make it possible to determine the threshold irritant concentration for that particular patient and skin area. Examples of the concentrations often used in dilution series in alcohol vehicles are 250, 125, 62, 31 mM for benzoic acid and 50, 10, 2, and 0.5 mM for methyl nicotinate [37, 46].

It is known that oral and topical nonsteroidal anti-inflammatory drugs efficiently suppress NIICRs and may therefore cause false-negative results in testing [29, 43]. The minimum refractory period is 3 days [35]. Tanned skin has decreased reactivity to NIICR agents [18] and both UVB and UVA irradiation suppress these reactions for 2–3 weeks [49, 50]. Skin sites that are washed repeatedly may have a lowered threshold for immediate irritancy to NIICR agents [46]. The importance of the selection of the test site and the testing method has already been mentioned. These sources of false results should be kept in mind when tests for immediate irritancy are performed and the results of such tests are interpreted.

5.4 Mechanisms and Clinical Aspects of Immunologic Immediate Contact Reactions

The basic mechanisms involved are summarized in Fig. 2.

5.4.1 Induction

Immunologic contact urticaria is a type of immediate (type I) hypersensitivity reaction. In this manifestation of hypersensitivity, exposure to the offending agent, most commonly a protein but in some cases a chemical hapten, stimulates the production of IgE-class antibodies. These are manufactured by B lymphocytes and typically are highly specific to the protein or the hapten–protein complex, although cross-reactions do occur. Sensitization most commonly occurs via the respiratory or gastrointestinal tracts, but can also occur through the skin, as in the case of latex and some foods. The IgE antibodies produced bind to high-affinity Fc_ receptors (Fc_ R1) on the surface of mast cells and basophils, thereby sensitizing them [17].

The ability to mount an IgE response is dependent upon a subtype of helper T lymphocytes designated Th2 and the production of specific cytokines, notably interleukin-4 (IL-4) [15]. It is likely that those individuals whose physiology is biased towards this Th2 phenotype are more likely to develop an IgE response [71]. From this group, the factors determining who will display a contact urticarial reaction upon exposure are poorly understood, but will include the ease with which the agent penetrates skin, the fragility of their mast cells, and their tissue sensitivity to the inflammatory mediators released.

It is interesting to note in this respect that recent observations indicate that the processes associated

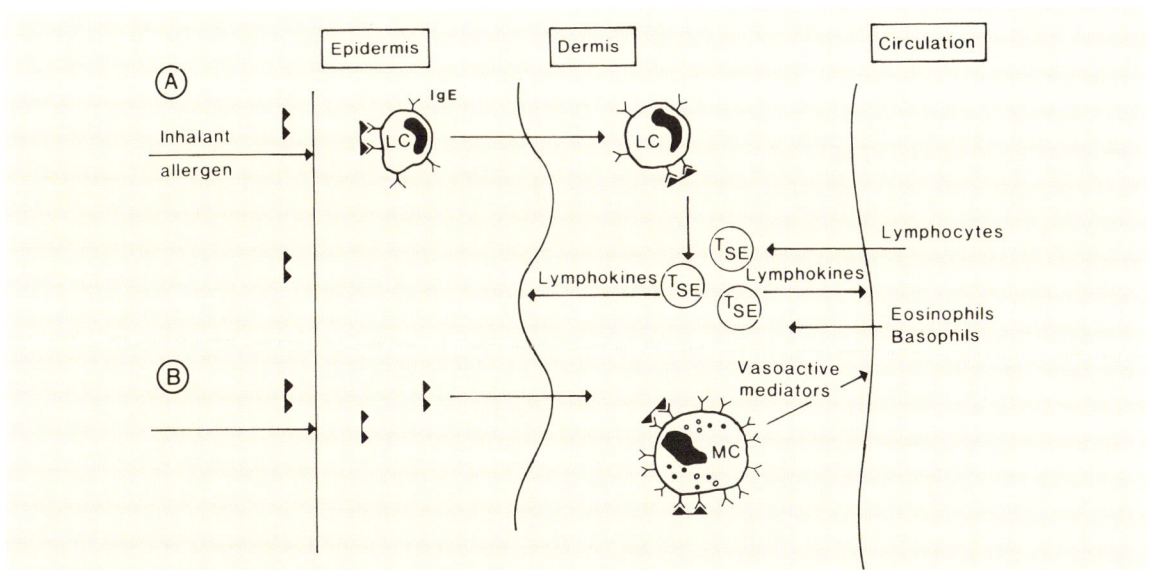

Fig. 2. Mechanisms by which protein allergens (pollen, mite, food, etc.) may produce delayed-type eczematous reactions (*A*) and immediate-type contact reactions (*B*) in patients with atopic dermatitis. (*LC* Langerhans cell, *MC* mononuclear cell, *T_{SE}* sensitized T lymphocyte)

with the induction of IgE sensitization can occur via skin contact [28, 57] and that Th2 responses may even be favored when there is stratum corneum damage [79]. This may of course have been an important factor in the epidemic of latex allergy – see below.

5.4.2 Elicitation

Following the induction of sensitization (a process for which the parameters are not well described), the clinical symptoms of immunologic contact urticaria are induced by direct skin contact with the antigen. Alternatively, inhalation of airborne protein or ingestion of food allergens may also lead to urticaria. This secondary exposure to the relevant urticant leads to binding of antigen to the IgE molecules on the surface of tissue mast cells and basophils. The consequent cross-linking of IgE causes an increase in intracellular calcium that triggers the release of both pre-formed and newly synthesized mediators. The most important of these mediators is the vasoactive amine histamine, the response to which can be blocked by pre-injection of compound 48/80 [48]. However, it is also likely that various leukotrienes, prostaglandins (PGD_2, PGE_2, PGI_2), platelet activating factor (PAF), and numerous other chemotactic and regulatory factors play a role [56, 75]. Furthermore, there is evidence, based on the use of the competitive inhibitor spantide, to suggest that the neuropeptide substance P, which is localized in peripheral sensory nerve endings, may be involved [85]. The importance of the role of nonhistamine mediators is reinforced by the relatively poor response of chronic idiopathic urticaria (caused by histamine-releasing autoantibodies to Fc_ R1) to antihistamine treatment [73].

Of significance from a clinical perspective is the fact that – in addition to the cutaneous manifestations of immunologic contact urticaria, which arise mainly from increased vascular permeability leading to erythematous and/or edematous swelling reactions in the dermis – other symptoms, such as rhinitis, conjunctivitis, asthma, and even anaphylaxis, may also be elicited in individuals who are highly sensitized or in whom a high degree of exposure occurs [17].

In addition to the clear role of histamine-releasing tissue mast cells in immunologic contact urticaria, a number of other cell types also possess functional IgE receptors and so, at least in some cases, may also participate in the responses observed. Langerhans cells have high-affinity (Fc_ R1) IgE receptors, at least in subjects with atopic dermatitis (reviewed in [6, 78]). However, Langerhans cell may express surface IgE receptors in response to the local inflammatory environment [34] and so it may be speculated that they might play a role in skin disorders other than atopic dermatitis. In addition to Langerhans cells, eosinophils [9], circulating lymphocytes (T and B) [92], platelets [30], and monocytes [60] also have Fc receptors for IgE, although not necessarily of high affinity. However, as with Langerhans cells, the role of these receptors in immunologic contact urticaria is largely unknown.

The typical symptoms of NIICRs have been described above (under Sect. 5.2, Definitions, Concepts, and Symptoms).

> **Core Message**
>
> ■ Immunologic and nonimmunologic contact reactions are morphologically indistinguishable.

5.4.3 Agents Producing Immunologic Immediate Contact Reactions

The commonest causes of immunologic contact urticaria are food proteins (via topical contact and oral ingestion), animal proteins, and natural rubber latex. However, the catalog of chemicals and proteins reported to have been implicated in immunologic contact urticaria is extensive (Table 3). In principle, it might be expected that any protein capable of generating formation of an IgE antibody response will also be capable of causing immunologic contact urticaria. Since, given appropriate exposure conditions, the majority of proteins can generate to some degree an IgE response (at least in a susceptible individual), the list in Table 3 is not particularly useful in identifying those proteins that are clinically most culpable, nor is it of much value in terms of clinical guidance or in risk assessment/management. Nevertheless, as mentioned above, certain materials either more commonly cause immunologic urticaria or, at least, are well recognized as such. These include foodstuffs (especially vegetables and shellfish), natural rubber latex, and proteins in the amniotic fluid of cows [31]. The relationship between food allergen ingestion and cutaneous symptoms, including urticaria, has been reviewed recently [89]. It is reported that acute urticaria is the most common food-induced adverse cutaneous reaction, occurring in approximately half of all patients with an IgE-mediated food allergy.

Table 3. Agents producing immediate immunologic contact reactions including contact urticaria

Animals and animal products
    Amnion fluid
    Blood
    Brucella abortus
    Bull terrier's seminal fluid
    Cercariae
    Cheyletus malaccensis
    Chironomidae, *Chironomus thummi thummi*
    Cockroach, *Blaberus giganteus*
    Dander
    Dermestes maculatus
    Gelatin
    Gut
    Hair
    Listrophorus gippus
    Liver
    Locust
    Mealworm, *Tenebrio molitor*
    Nereis diversicolor, worm
    Oyster
    Pine processionary caterpillar,
        Thaumetopoea pityocampa
        Placenta
        Saliva
        Serum
        Silk
        Spider mite, *Tetranychus urticae*
        Wool
Food
    Dairy
    Cheese
    Milk
Fruits
    Apple
    Apricot
    Banana
    Kiwi
    Litchi fruit, *Litchi chinensis*
    Mango
    Orange
    Peach
    Plum
Grains
    Buckwheat
    Maize
    Malt
    Rice
    Wheat
    Wheat bran
Nuts, seeds
    Peanut
    Sesame seed
    Sunflower seed
Meats
    Beef
    Chicken
    Lamb
    Liver
    Pork
    Roe deer, *Capreolus capreolus*
    Turkey

Table 3. Continued

Seafood
    Codfish
    Prawns
    Shrimp
Vegetables
    Asparagus, *Asparagus officinalis*
    Beans
    Cabbage
    Carrot
    Celery
    Chives
    Cucumber
    Endive
    Globe artichoke, *Cynara scolymus*
    Lettuce, *Lactuca sativa*
    Onion
    Paprika, *Capsicum annuum*
    Parsley
    Parsnip
    Potato
    Rutabaga (swede)
    Soybean
    Tomato
    Watermelon
Fragrances and flavorings
    Balsam of Peru (*Myroxylon pereirae*)
    Cinnamic aldehyde
    Menthol
    Vanillin
Medicaments
    Acetylsalicylic acid
    Albendazole
    Antibiotics
        Amoxicillin
        Ampicillin
        Bacitracin
        Cephalosporins
        Cefotiam dihydrochloride
        Cephalothin
        Chloramphenicol
        Cloxacillin
        Gentamicin
        Iodochlorhydroxyquin
        Mezlocillin
        Neomycin
        Nifuroxime
        Penicillin
        Rifamycin
        Streptomycin
        Virginiamycin
    Benzocaine
    Benzoyl peroxide
    Chlorothalonil
    Cisplatin
    Clobetasol-17-propionate
    Dinitrochlorobenzene
    Etofenamate
    Fumaric acid derivatives
    Ketoprofen
    Mechlorethamine
    Mexiletine
    Pentamidine

Table 3. Continued

      Phenothiazines
        Chlorpromazine
        Levomepromazine
        Promethazine
      Pyrazolones
        Aminophenazone
        Methimazole
        Propyl phenazone
      Sodium fluoride
      Tocopherol
Metals
    Aluminum
    Cobalt
    Copper
    Gold
    Iridium
    Mercury
    Nickel
    Palladium
    Platinum
    Rhodium
    Ruthenium
    Tin
    Zinc
Plants and plant products
    Abietic acid
    Aescin, *Aesculus hippocastanum*
    Algae
    Aster novi-belgii
    Beer
    Birch
    Bougainvillea
    Chamomile
    Campanula
    Castor bean
    Christmas cactus, *Schlumbergera*
    Chrysanthemum
    Cinchona
    Cnidoscolus angustidens
    Colophony
    Corn starch
    Cotoneaster
    Creeping fig, *Ficus pumila*
    Devils ivy, pothos, *Epipremnum aureum*
    Dianthus caryophyllus
    Dill
    Emetin
    Eucalyptus
    Fennel
    Gardenia, *Gardenia jasminoides*
    Garlic
    Gerbera
    Grevillea juniperina
    Gypsophila paniculata
    Hakea suaveolens
    Hawthorn, *Crataegus monogyna*
    Henna
    Hibiscus rosa-sinensis
    Hops, *Humulus lupulus*
    Latex rubber
    Lichens
    Lily, *Lilium longiflorum*
    Lime

5

Table 3. Continued

    Limonium tataricum
    Loligo japonica
    Lupin
    Madagascar jasmine, *Stephanotis floribunda*
    Mahogany
    Monstera deliciosa
    Mukali wood, *Aningeria robusta*
    Mulberry, *Morus alba*
    Mustard
    Obeche wood
    Papain
    Poppy flower, *Papaver rhoeas*
    Pelargonium
    Perfumes
    Phoenix canariensis
    Pickles
    Poinsettia, *Euphorbia pulcherrima*
    Pomegranate, *Punica granatum*
    Rice
    Rose
    Rouge
    Runner bean, *Phaseolus multiflorus*
    Semecarpus anacardium
    Shiitake mushroom
    Spathe, *Spathiphyllum*
    Spices
    Strawberry
    Teak
    Tobacco
    Tradescantia
    Tulip
    Verbena
    Weeping fig, *Ficus benjamina*
    Winged bean
Preservatives and disinfectants
    Benzoic acid
    Benzyl alcohol
    Butylated hydroxytoluene
    Chlorhexidine
    Chloramine
    Chlorocresol
    1,3-Diiodo-2-hydroxypropane
    Formaldehyde
    Gentian violet
    Hexanetriol
    p-Hydroxybenzoic acid
    Parabens
    2-Phenoxyethanol
    Phenylmercuric propionate
    o-Phenylphenate
    Polysorbates
    Polyvinylpyrrolidone
    Sodium hypochlorite
    Sorbitan monolaurate
    Tropicamide
Enzymes
    alpha-Amylase
    Cellulases
    Protease (detergent)
    Xylanases
Miscellaneous
    Acetyl acetone
    Acrylic monomer

Table 3. Continued

Alcohols (amyl-, butyl-, ethyl-, isopropyl)
Aliphatic polyamide
Ammonia
Ammonium persulfate
Aminothiazole
Aziridine
Basic Blue 99
Benzonitrile
Benzophenone
Carboxymethylcellulose
Chlorothalonil
Cu(II)-acetyl acetonate
Cresylglycidyl ether
Denatonium benzoate
Di(2-ethylhexyl) phthalate (DOP)
Diethyltoluamide
Diphenylmethane-4,4′-diisocyanate
Epoxy resin
Ethylenediamine dihydrochloride
Formaldehyde resin
Glyseryl thioglycolate
2-hydroxyethyl methacrylate
HATU
HBTU
Hexahydrophthalic anhydride
Lanolin alcohols
Lindane
Methyl ethyl ketone
Methylhexahydrophthalic anhydride
Monoamylamine
Naphtha
Naphthylacetic acid
Nylon
Oleylamide
Panthenol
Para-aminophenol
Para-methylaminophenol
Paraphenylenediamine
Patent Blue dye
Perlon
Petrolatum
Phenyl glycidyl ether
Phosphorus sesquisulfide
Phthalic anhydrides
Plastic
Polypropylene
Polyethylene gloves
Polyethylene glycol
Potassium ferricyanide
Potassium persulfate
Protein hydrolysates
Seminal fluid [76]
Sodium silicate
Sodium sulfide
Sorbitan sesquioleate
Sulfur dioxide
Terpinyl acetate
Textile finish
Vinyl pyridine
Xylene
Zinc diethyldithiocarbamate

Immediate allergic reactions to natural rubber latex (NRL) proteins have been recognized for about 20 years as an important medical and occupational health problem [80, 81] An expert group set up in 1999 by the European Commission wrote an opinion paper on NRL allergy (http://europa.eu.int/comm/food/fs/sc/scmp/out31en.pdf; European Commission – Opinion on natural rubber latex allergy; adopted by the Scientific Committee on Medical Products and Medical Devices on June 2000). Thirteen different NRL allergens (www.allergen.org) have been characterized at the molecular level, as reviewed recently [90]. Prevalence studies, based on skin prick testing, indicate that 2–17% of exposed health care workers are sensitized to NRL whereas the sensitization rate in the general population is less than 1% [58]. For the correct diagnosis of NRL allergy, the skin prick test and the measurement of NRL-specific IgE confirm the sensitization, but allergy diagnosis requires symptoms to be studied by a challenge or use test with NRL material. At the moment there is now standardized, sufficiently allergenic material available for the latex challenge test. Delayed-type reactions to NRL proteins have recently been studied and 1% (27/2738) was found to be patch-test positive to NRL, of which 19 (70%) were considered to be clinically relevant for eczematous skin conditions [77].

Results of recent animal studies indicate that cutaneous sensitization to NRL proteins eluting from latex gloves can, in addition to the production of high levels of NRL-specific IgE antibodies, also contribute the development of hand eczema (Fig. 3) [47, 55].

In the health care sector, change of all gloves from high-protein/powdered to low-protein/nonpowdered has had a beneficial effect but measuring the total

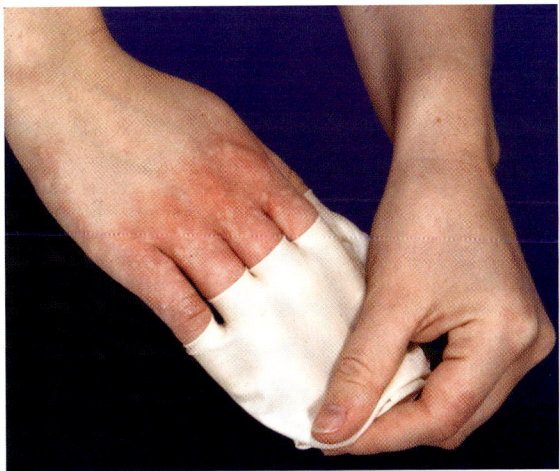

Fig. 3. Immunologic contact urticaria to natural rubber latex glove (Courtesy by Arto Lahti, University of Oulu, Department of Dermatology, Oulu, Finland)

protein cannot be deemed as a satisfactory regulatory measure to control allergen content in the future. Currently, one commercial test for measuring individual NRL allergens is available (FITkit; FIT Biotech, Tampere, Finland) and measurement of four main allergens in gloves and other rubber products is possible [68].

Allergen cross-reactions related to certain fruits and plant foods are known to be common in patients with NRL allergy. The molecular basis for a major part of these reactions seems to be in the structural similarity between the hevein domains in NRL and the ubiquitously occurring hevein-like class I endochitinases in various plants [12]. Although accumulating evidence suggests that the peak of the NRL allergy epidemic may have already passed in the health care sector, latex allergy remains an important disease entity with many unanswered questions.

The capacity of chemical haptens to provoke immunologic contact urticaria is not well studied, although a substantial number of chemicals have been implicated. However, it must be noted that the quality of the evidence to substantiate the argument that these chemical urticants have operated via an immune mechanism has not always been of the highest order. Reasons for this are discussed below.

5.4.4　Tests in Animals

Predictive models for the specific identification of materials capable of causing immunologic contact urticaria are not well developed. Animal models have been used (e.g., [62]), but the focus has been on mechanistic aspects rather than prediction. The guinea pig can be sensitized to foreign protein, as well as to a variety of chemicals that have been reported as immunologic contact urticants, e.g., cinnamic aldehyde (cinnamal). The process for the induction of sensitization may vary from techniques designed to examine the relative ability of proteins to behave as potential respiratory allergens (e.g., [7, 74]) to methods for the investigation of chemical respiratory sensitization (e.g., [8]) or even the evaluation of chemicals in skin sensitization tests, such as the guinea pig maximization test. In all of these procedures, once animals have been sensitized, intradermal challenge can be used to examine whether it is possible to elicit an immediate hypersensitivity response in the skin. This can readily be visualized if the animals have been given Evans blue dye (usually intracardially) prior to challenge. The reaction can be assessed some 20 min after the intradermal injection by measurement of the diameter and intensity of blueness. However, it might not be straightforward to relate this type of reaction to immunologic contact urticaria in humans; there are no data on the sensitivity/specificity of the predictions from such models, nor are there any data on the ability to elicit immediate skin reactions following epicutaneous rather than intradermal application. In addition to the guinea pig, the rabbit has also been shown to be capable of mounting immediate hypersensitivity reactions in skin, but use of this phenomenon as a model of immunologic contact urticaria is untried [70]. Whatever model is proposed, since it will be relatively easy to raise IgE antibodies, the key will be to find a way to determine the relevance of the predictions made.

The mouse has been proposed as a possible model of chemically induced immunologic contact urticaria. On the basis of work with trimellitic anhydride (a chemical capable of causing both immediate and delayed types of hypersensitivity) [11], an approach has been suggested that involves topical application of the test chemical to BALB/c strain mice, followed about 1 week later by epicutaneous challenge on the ear. The urticarial reaction is measured as ear swelling over a time course of 2 h [53, 54]. The only substance examined to date has been trimellitic anhydride, so clearly a large amount of work must still be done in order to demonstrate both the validity and the relevance of this potential model. Nevertheless, it can be argued that the approach is mechanistically based, fairly straightforward to conduct, and could perhaps prove of value in the future. It is interesting to speculate as to whether the model might work with proteins shown to produce immunologic contact urticaria, such as the hevein of latex (reviewed in [67]). The most likely problem of the approach would be poor specificity, with very many proteins demonstrating an ability to produce IgE responses.

Core Message

■ Reliable nonhuman predictive tests for either immunologic or nonimmunologic agents do not exist.

5.4.5　Tests in Humans

In contrast to animal studies, the only real purpose of human testing is to permit the diagnosis of disease. The typical clinical presentation of immunologic contact urticaria is essentially very similar to that of its nonimmunologic counterpart, although it is much more probable than for NICU that there may be some accompanying systemic organ involvement. However, there are a number of diagnostic test procedures that can be employed to identify the existence of an immunological mechanism. The main methods involve skin testing with the suspect substance and serological assays for specific IgE. In either situation, where a chemical hapten is the suspect material, it is then normally necessary to conjugate it to a protein prior to testing. Commonly, the protein selected is human serum albumin (HSA). However, the process of making a suitable hapten–protein complex should not be undertaken lightly; it may not be an easy process and insufficient attention to detail can easily result in false-negative data being obtained when the patient is assessed. Detailed guidance on the preparation of suitable hapten–protein conjugates has been published [5].

In theory, there is no reason why the tests for NIICR outlined above cannot also be applied to the investigation of immunologic contact urticaria. Simple open application of the suspect allergen may be sufficient [1]. However, the prick test approach developed for the identification of sensitization to protein respiratory allergens has been adopted as a means to detect the presence of immunologic contact urticaria when the epicutaneous tests are negative. It is used as a routine method by some dermatologists, being regarded as more reliable in terms of avoiding the risk of false-negative results. It should be noted that skin testing may carry a small risk of precipitating systemic reactions and thus low concentrations of putative allergen are employed. As with diagnostic patch testing for delayed allergic reactions, it is vital to ensure that the test conditions/concentrations do not lead to nonspecific reactions. If necessary, suitable testing of a control panel may be necessary.

As an adjunct to skin testing, or as an alternative where it is contraindicated (e.g., if the patient has experienced anaphylactic-type reactions in conjunction with the urticaria), serological assessment may be carried out. In this case, the serum sample is assayed for the presence of specific IgE antibodies directed against the suspect substances. Traditionally, IgE testing has been conducted using the radioallergosorbent test (RAST), although this has recently been replaced commercially by the UNICAP system. RAST methodology was originally described over 30 years ago [88] and has proven of value in the identification of many immunologic urticants, including natural rubber latex [83], and is useful for the assessment of potential cross-reactivity between allergens (e.g., [19]).

In recent years, the commercial RAST system (such as that available from Pharmacia) has been replaced by a number of alternatives, but all in essence follow the same principle, that of measuring antigen-specific IgE.

Core Message

■ Nonimmune agents can be identified by careful human testing.

Suggested Reading

Turjanmaa K, Alenius H, Mäkinen-Kiljunen S, Reunala T, Palosuo T (1996) Natural rubber latex allergy. Review. Allergy 51:593–602

References

1. Amin S, Maibach HI (1997) Immunologic contact urticaria definition. In: Amin S, Lahti A, Maibach HI (eds) Contact urticaria syndrome. CRC Press, Boca Raton, Fla., pp 11–26
2. Amin S, Lahti A, Maibach HI (1997) Contact urticaria syndrome. CRC Press, Boca Raton, Fla.
3. Basketter DA, Wilhelm K-P (1996) Studies on non-immune immediate contact reactions in an unselected population. Contact Dermatitis 35:237–240
4. Bernstein DI, Swift RM, Keyoumars S, Lorincz AL (1981) Inhibition of axon reflex vasodilatation by topically applied capsaicin. J Invest Dermatol 76:394–395
5. Bernstein JE, Zeiss CR (1989) Guidelines for preparation and characterization of chemical-protein conjugate antigens. Report of the subcommittee on preparation and characterization of low molecular weight antigens. J Allergy Clin Immunol 84:820–822
6. Bieber T (1996) Fc epsilon R1 on antigen presenting cells. Curr Opin Immunol 8:773–777
7. Blaikie L, Basketter DA and Morrow T (1995) Experience with a guinea pig model for the assessment of respiratory allergens. Hum Exp Toxicol 14:743
8. Dearman RJ, Basketter DA, Kimber I (1996) Characterisation of chemical allergens as a function of divergent cytokine secretion profiles induced in mice. Toxicol Appl Pharmacol 138:308–316
9. Capron M, Capron A, Dessaint J, Johansson S, Prin L (1981) Fc receptors for IgE on human and rat eosinophils. J Immunol 126:2087–2091
10. Czarnetzki BM, Rosenbach T, Kolde G, Frosch PJ (1985) Phototherapy of urticaria pigmentosa: clinical response and changes of cutaneous reactivity, histamine and chemotactic leukotrienes. Arch Dermatol Res 277:105–113
11. Dearman RJ, Mitchell JA, Basketter DA, Kimber I (1992) Differential ability of occupational chemical contact and respiratory allergens to cause immediate and delayed dermal hypersensitivity reactions in mice. Int Arch Allergy Toxicol 97:315–321
12. Dias-Perales A, Sanchez-Monge R, Blanco C et al (2002) What is the role of the hevein-like domain of fruit class I chitinases in their allergenic capacity? Clin Exp Allergy 32:448–454

5

13. Downard CD, Roberts LJ II, Morrow JD (1995) Topical benzoic acid induces the increased synthesis of prostaglandin D_2 in human skin in vivo. Clin Pharmacol Ther 57:441

14. Feczko PJ, Simms SM, Bakirci N (1989) Fatal hypersensitivity reaction during a barium enema. Am J Roentgenol 153:275–276

15. Finkelman FD, Katona IM, Urban JF Jr, Holmes J, Ohara T, Tung AS, Sample JG, Paul WE (1988) IL-4 is required to generate and sustain in vivo IgE responses. J Immunol 141:2335–2341

16. Garcia Ortiz JC, Moyano JC, Alvarez M, Bellido J (1998) Latex allergy in fruit-allergic patients. Allergy 53:532–536

17. Garssen J, Vandebriel RJ, Kimber I, van Loveren H (1996) Hypersensitivity reactions: definitions, basic mechanisms and localizations. In: Vos JG, Younes M, Smith E (eds) Allergic hypersensitivities induced by chemicals, recommendations for prevention. CRC Press, Boca Raton, Fla., pp 19–58

18. Gollhausen R, Kligman AM (1985) Human assay for identifying substances which induce non-allergic contact urticaria: the NICU-test. Contact Dermatitis 13:98–106

19. Halmepuro L, Lovestein H (1985) Immunological investigation of possible structural similarities between pollen antigens and antigens in apple, carrot and celery tuber. Allergy 40:264–272

20. Hannuksela M (1980) Atopic contact dermatitis. Contact Dermatitis 6:30

21. Hannuksela M (1986) Contact urticaria from foods. In: Roe DA (ed) Nutrition and the skin, vol 10. Liss, New York, pp 153–162

22. Hannuksela M (1995) Skin tests for immediate hypersensitivity. In: Rycroft RJG, Menné T, Frosch PJ (eds) Textbook of contact dermatitis. Springer, Berlin Heidelberg New York, pp 287–292

23. Hannuksela M, Lahti A (1977) Immediate reaction to fruits and vegetables. Contact Dermatitis 3:79–84

24. Hannuksela A, Lahti A, Hannuksela M (1989) Nonimmunologic immediate contact reactions to three isomers of pyridine carboxaldehyde. In: Frosch PJ, Dooms-Goossens A, Lachapelle J-M, Rycroft RJG, Scheper RJ (eds) Current topics in contact dermatitis. Springer, Berlin Heidelberg New York, pp 448–452

25. Hannuksela A, Niinimäki A, Hannuksela M (1993) Size of the test area does not affect the result of the repeated open application test. Contact Dermatitis 28:299–300

26. Harvell J, Bason M, Maibach H (1994) Contact urticaria and its mechanisms. Food Chem Toxicol 32:103–112

27. Hjorth N, Roed-Petersen J (1976) Occupational protein contact dermatitis in food handlers. Contact Dermatitis 2:28–42

28. Hsieh KY, Tsai CC, Wu CHH, Lin RH (2003) Epicutaneous exposure to protein antigen and food allergy. Clin Exp Allergy 33:1067–1075

29. Johansson J, Lahti A (1988) Topical non-steroidal anti-inflammatory drugs inhibit non-immunologic immediate contact reactions. Contact Dermatitis 19:161–165

30. Joseph M, Auriault C, Capron A, Vorng H, Viens P (1983) A new function for platelets: IgE dependent killing of schistosomes. Nature 303:810–812

31. Kalveram K-J, Kästner H, Frock G (1986) Detection of specific IgE antibodies in veterinarians suffering from contact urticaria. Z Hautkr 61:75–81

32. Kolde G, Frosch PJ, Czarnetzki BM (1984) Response of cutaneous mast cells to PUVA in patients with urticaria pigmentosa: histomorphometric, ultrastructural, and biochemical investigations. J Invest Dermatol 83:175–178

33. Köpman A, Hannuksela M (1983) Kumin aiheuttama kosketusurtikaria. Duodecim 99:221–224

34. Kraft S, Wessendorf JH, Hanau D, Bieber T (1998) Regulation of the high affinity receptor for IgE on human epidermal Langerhans cells. J Immunol 161:1000–1006

35. Kujala T, Lahti A (1989) Duration of inhibition of non-immunologic immediate contact reactions by acetylsalicylic acid. Contact Dermatitis 21:60–61

36. Lahti A (1980) Non-immunologic contact urticaria. Acta Derm Venereol 60:1–49

37. Lahti A (1987) Terfenadine (H1-antagonist) does not inhibit non-immunologic contact urticaria. Contact Dermatitis 16:220–223

38. Lahti A (1995) Immediate contact reactions. In: Rycroft RJG, Menné T, Frosch PJ (eds) Textbook of contact dermatitis. Springer, Berlin Heidelberg New York, pp 62–74

39. Lahti A, Maibach HI (1984) An animal model for nonimmunologic contact urticaria. Toxicol Appl Pharmacol 76:219–224

40. Lahti A, Maibach HI (1985a) Species specificity of nonimmunologic contact urticaria: guinea pig, rat and mouse. J Am Acad Dermatol 13:66

41. Lahti A, Maibach HI (1985b) Long refractory period after one application of nonimmunologic contact urticaria agents to the guinea pig ear. J Am Acad Dermatol 13:585–589

42. Lahti A, Oikarinen A, Viinikka L, Ylikorkala O, Hannuksela M (1983) Prostaglandins in contact urticaria induced by benzoic acid. Acta Derm Venereol 63:425–427

43. Lahti A, Väänänen A, Kokkonen E-L, Hannuksela M (1987) Acetylsalicylic acid inhibits non-immunologic contact urticaria. Contact Dermatitis 16:133–135

44. Lahti A, Kopola H, Harila A, Myllylä R, Hannuksela M (1993) Assessment of skin erythema by eye, laser Doppler flowmeter, spectroradiometer, two-channel erythema meter and Minolta chroma meter. Arch Dermatol Res 285:278–282

45. Lahti A, Poutiainen A-M, Hannuksela M (1993) Alcohol vehicles in tests for non-immunological immediate contact reactions. Contact Dermatitis 29:22–25

46. Lahti A, Pylvänen V, Hannuksela M (1995) Immediate irritant reactions to benzoic acid are enhanced in washed skin areas. Contact Dermatitis 33:177–182

47. Laouini D, Alenius H, Bryce P et al (2003) IL-10 is critical for Th2 responses in a murine model of allergic dermatitis. J Clin Invest 112:1058–1066

48. Larko O, Lindstedt G, Lundberg PA, Mobacken H (1983) Biochemical and clinical studies in a case of contact urticaria to potato. Contact Dermatitis 9:108–114

49. Larmi E (1989) Systemic effect of ultraviolet irradiation on nonimmunologic immediate contact reactions to benzoic acid and methyl nicotinate. Acta Derm Venereol 69:296–301

50. Larmi E, Lahti A, Hannuksela M (1988) Ultraviolet light inhibits nonimmunologic immediate contact reactions to benzoic acid. Arch Dermatol Res 280:420–423

51. Larmi E, Lahti A, Hannuksela M (1989a) Effects of capsaicin and topical anesthesia on nonimmunologic immediate contact reactions to benzoic acid and methyl nicotinate. In: Frosch PJ, Dooms-Goossens A, Lachapelle J-M, Rycroft RJG, Scheper RJ (eds) Current topics in contact dermatitis. Springer, Berlin Heidelberg New York, pp 441–447

52. Larmi E, Lahti A, Hannuksela M (1989b) Immediate contact reactions to benzoic acid and the sodium salt of pyrrolidone carboxylic acid. Comparison of various skin sites. Contact Dermatitis 20:38–40

53. Lauerma A, Maibach HI (1997) Model for immunologic contact urticaria. In: Amin S, Lahti A, Maibach HI (eds) Contact urticaria syndrome. CRC Press, Boca Raton, Fla., pp 27–32

54. Lauerma AI, Fenn B, Maibach HI (1997) Trimellitic anhydride sensitive mouse as an animal model for contact urticaria. J Appl Toxicol 17:357–360

55. Lehto M, Koivuluhta M, Wang G et al (2003) Epicutaneous natural rubber latex sensitization induces T helper 2-type dermatitis and strong prohevein-specific IgE response. J Invest Dermatol 120:633–640

56. Lewis RA, Austen KF (1981) Mediation of local homeostasis and inflammation by leukotrienes and other mast cell-dependent compounds. Nature 293:103

57. Li XM, Kleiner G, Huang CK, Lee S, Schofield B, Soter N, Sampson H (2001) Murine model of atopic dermatitis associated with food hepersensitivity. J Allerg Clin Immunol 107:693–702

58. Liss GM, Sussman GL (1999) Latex sensitization: occupational versus general population prevalence rates. Am J Ind Med 35:196–200

59. Maibach HI, Johnson HL (1975) Contact urticaria syndrome. Contact urticaria to diethyltoluamide (immediate-type hypersensitivity). Arch Dermatol 111:726–730

60. Melewicz F, Spiegelberg H (1980) Fc receptors for IgE on a subpopulation human peripheral blood monocytes. J Immunol 125:1026–1031

61. Mikkola JH, Alenius H, Kalkkinen N, Turjanmaa K, Palosuo T, Reunala T (1998) Hevein-like protein domains as a possible cause for allergen cross-reactivity between latex and banana. Allergy Clin Immunol 102:1005–1012

62. Moore KG, Dannenberg AM (1993) Immediate and delayed (late phase) dermal contact sensitivity reactions in guinea pigs. Int Arch Allergy Immunol 101:72–81

63. Morrow JD, Awad JA, Oates JA, Roberts LJ Jr (1992) Identification of skin as a major site of prostaglandin D_2 release following oral administration of niacin in humans. J Invest Dermatol 98:812

64. Morrow JD, Minton TA, Awad JA, Roberts LJ Jr (1994) Release of markedly increased quantities of prostaglandin D_2 from the skin in vivo in humans following the application of sorbic acid. Arch Dermatol 130:1408

65. Downard CD, Roberts LJ, Morrow JD (1995) Topical benzoic acid includes the increased biosynthesis of prostaglandin D2 in human skin in vivo. Clin Pharmacol Ther 57:441–445

66. Nutter AF (1979) Contact urticaria to rubber. Br J Dermatol 101:597–598

67. Palosuo T (1997) Latex allergens. Rev Fr Allerg Immunol Clin 37:1184–1187

68. Palosuo T, Alenius H, Turjanmaa K (2002) Quantitation of latex allergens. Methods 27:52–58

69. Pastorello EA, Ortolani C, Farioli L, Pravettoni V, Ispano M, Borga A, Bengtsson A, Incorvaia C, Berti C, Zanussi C (1994) Allergenic cross-reactivity among peach, apricot, plum, and cherry in patients with oral allergy syndrome: an in vivo and in vitro study. J Allergy Clin Immunol 94:699–707

70. Reijula KE, Kelly KJ, Kurup VP, Choi H, Bongard RD, Dawson CA, Fink JN (1994) Latex-included dermal and pulmonary hypersensitivity in rabbits. J Allergy Clin Immunol 94:891–902

71. Ricci M, Matucci A, Rossi O (1994) T cells, cytokines, IgE and allergic airways inflammation. J Invest Allergol Clin Immunol 4:214–220

72. Ruzicka T, Aubock J (1987) Arachinodic acid metabolism in guinea pig Langerhans cells: studies of cyclooxygenase and lipooxygenase pathways. J Immunol 138:539

73. Sabroe RA, Greaves MW (1997) The pathogenesis of chronic idiopathic urticaria. Arch Dermatol 133:1003–1008

74. Sarlo K, Fletcher ER, Gaines WG, Ritz HL (1997) Respiratory allergenicity of detergent enzymes in the guinea pig intratracheal test: association with sensitisaiton of occupationally exposed individuals. Fund Appl Toxicol 39:44–52

75. Schwartz LB, Austin KF (1984) Structure and function of the chemical mediators of mast cells. Prog Allergy 34:272

76. Shah A, Panjabi C (2004) Human seminal plasma allergy: a review of a rare phenomenon. Clin Exp Allergy 34(6):827–838

77. Sommer S, Wilkinson SM, Beck MH et al (2002) Type IV hypersensitivity reactions to natural rubber latex: results of a multicenter study. Br J Dermatol 146:114–117

78. Stingl G, Maurer D (1997) IgE mediated allergen presentation via Fc epsilon R1 on antigen presenting cells. Int Arch Allergy Immunol 113:24–29

79. Strid J, Hourihane J, Kimber I, Callard R, Strobel S (2004) Disruption of the stratum corneum allows potent epicutaneous immunization with protein antigens resulting in a dominant systemic Th2 response. Eur J Immunol 34:2100–2109

80. Turjanmaa K, Alenius H, Mäkinen-Kiljunen S et al (1996) Natural rubber latex allergy. Review. Allergy 51:593–602

81. Turjanmaa K, Alenius H, Reunala T, Palosuo T (2002) Recent developments in latex allergy. Curr Opin Clin Immunol 2:407–412

82. Turjanmaa K (1997) Contact urticaria from latex gloves. In: Amin S, Lahti A, Maibach HI (eds) Contact urticaria syndrome. CRC Press, Boca Raton, pp 173–188

83. Turjanmaa K, Reunala T, Räsänen L (1988) Comparison of diagnostic methods in latex surgical glove contact urticaria. Contact Dermatitis 20:360–364

84. Urade Y, Ujihara M, Hariguchi Y, Ikai K, Hayaishi O (1989) The major source of endogenous prostaglandin D_2 production is likely antigen-presenting cells: localization of glutathione-requiring PGD synthetase in histiocytes, dendritic and Kupffer cells in various rat tissues. J Immunol 143:2982

85. Wallengren J, Ekman R, Moller H (1986) Substance P and vasoactive intestinal peptide in bullous and inflammatory skin disease. Acta Derm Venereol 66:23–28

86. Wallengren J (1991) Substance P antagonist inhibits immediate and delayed type cutaneous hypersensitivity reactions. Br J Dermatol 124:324–328

87. Warren JB, Loi KR, Wilson AJ (1994) PGD_2 is an intermediate in agonist-induced nitric oxide release in rabbit skin microcirculation. Am J Physiol 226:1846

88. Wide L, Bennich H, Johansson SGO (1967) Diagnosis of allergy by an in vitro test for allergen antibodies. Lancet 2:1105–1108

89. Wuthrich B (1998) Food induced cutaneous adverse reactions. Allergy 53:131–13

90. Yeang HY (2004) Natural rubber allergens: new developments. Curr Opin Clin Immunol 4:99–10

91. Ylipieti S, Lahti A (1989) Effect of the vehicle on non-immunologic immediate contact reactions. Contact Dermatitis 21:105–106

92. Yodoi J, Iskizaka K (1979) Lymphocytes bearing Fc receptors for IgE. Presence of human and rat lymphocytes with Fc receptors. J Immunol 122:2577–2583

Chapter 6

Mechanisms of Phototoxic and Photoallergic Reactions

6

RENZ MANG, HELGER STEGE, JEAN KRUTMANN

Contents

6.1 Introduction

Solar radiation represents the most important environmental stress to which human beings are exposed. Within the spectrum of solar radiation reaching the Earth's surface, the ultraviolet (UV) and visible portions of electromagnetic radiation are of particular importance to human skin. According to different photochemical and photobiological reactions, the UV portion of the electromagnetic spectrum is divided into different regions: UVC (wavelength 200–290 nm), UVB (290–320 nm), UVA (320–400 nm), and visible light (400–800 nm) [1–3]. UV radiation is able penetrate the skin and blood. Its photon energy is sufficient to cause within the skin unimolecular and bimolecular chemical reactions.

The biological reactions resulting from the interaction of UV or visible radiation with human skin include physiological responses such as enhanced melanogenesis or thickening of the epidermal layers, and pathological reactions including photocarcinogenesis, photoaging, and the triggering of skin diseases characterized by an increased photosensitivity. In general, increased photosensitization is an abnormal reactivity of a biological substrate to, in principle, ineffective doses of UVA, UVB, and visible radiations. This can manifest as photodermatoses such as polymorphic light eruption or solar urticaria, as well as photoallergic and phototoxic reactions [4, 5].

For photosensitivity responses to occur, the relevant radiation must penetrate the tissue, be absorbed by biomolecules, and initiate chemical reactions in the tissue. The light-absorbing molecules are called *chromophores* or *photosensitizers*. In skin cells, the major UV-radiation-absorbing chromophores are nucleic acids, lipids, and proteins. Additionally other molecules such as porphyrins, vitamins or drugs are also able to absorb UV and visible radiation. In general, photosensitivity reactions result from the interaction of solar radiation with chromophores that are present constitutively in human skin or that have been topically or systemically applied [6]. Examples of endogenous molecules causing a photosensitivity reaction are porphyrins, whereas phytophotodermatitis is a prime example of an exogenous photosensitivity reaction. The combination of drugs and UV can produce both desired and undesired effects. Thus, PUVA-therapy (psoralen plus UVA radiation) has been long employed for the treatment of psoriasis, and porphyrins can be used therapeutically, i.e., in photodynamic therapy [7–9].

The present chapter focuses on the mechanisms underlying phototoxic and photoallergic reactions caused by exogenous chromophores, especially drugs.

6.2 Clinical Aspects of Photoallergic and Phototoxic Reactions

Phototoxicity is the result of direct cellular damage caused by an inflammatory nonimmunological mechanism, which is initiated by a phototoxic agent and subsequent irradiation. In contrast, photoallergic reactions represent delayed or cell-mediated or type IV hypersensitivity responses, which require the specific sensitization of a given human individual to a photoactivated drug. Differentiation of phototoxic

Table 1. Clinical and histological features that help to differentiate between types of photosensitivity (modified after [6])

	Phototoxicity	Photoallergy
Incidence	High	Low
Pathophysiology	Tissue injury	Delayed hypersensitivity response
Required dose of agent	Large	Low
Required dose of light	Large	Small
Onset after light exposure	Minutes to hours	24 h or more
Clinical appearance	Sunburn reaction	Eczematous
Reaction after a single contact	Yes	No
Localization	Only exposed area	Exposed area; may be spread
Pigmentation changes	Frequent	Unusual
Histology	Epidermal cell degeneration; dermal edema and vasodilatation; sparse dermal mononuclear infiltrate	Epidermal spongiosis and exocytosis of mononuclear cells, dermal mononuclear cell infiltrate

6

from photoallergic reactions is often difficult. This is due to the fact that most drugs are capable of causing both photoallergic and phototoxic reactions, and that the two types of photosensitivity reactions are very similar in their clinical and histological features. The following criteria can be used differentiate between these two types of photosensitivity (Table 1).

Phototoxic reactions develop in most individuals if they are exposed to sufficient amounts of light and the drug. They represent an unwanted pharmacolog- ical effect. Typically, reactions appear as an exagger- ated sunburn response (Figs. 1a, b, 2). Photoallergic reactions develop in only a minority of individuals exposed to the compound and light; its incidence is less than that of phototoxic skin reactions. The amount of drug required to elicit photoallergic reac- tions is considerably smaller than that required for phototoxic reactions. Moreover, photoallergic reac- tions are a delayed-type hypersensitivity; their onset is often delayed for as long as 24–72 h after exposure

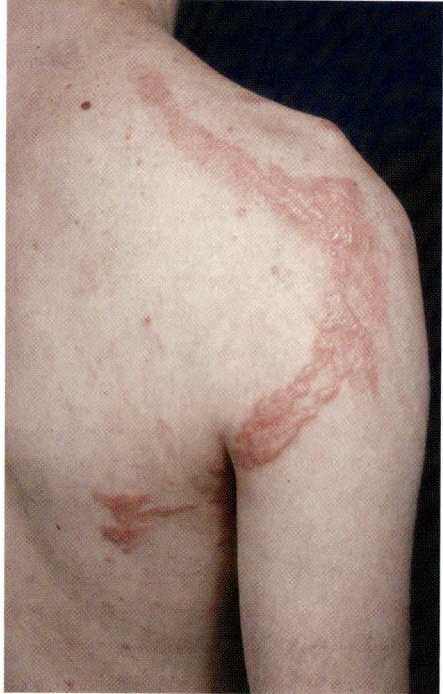
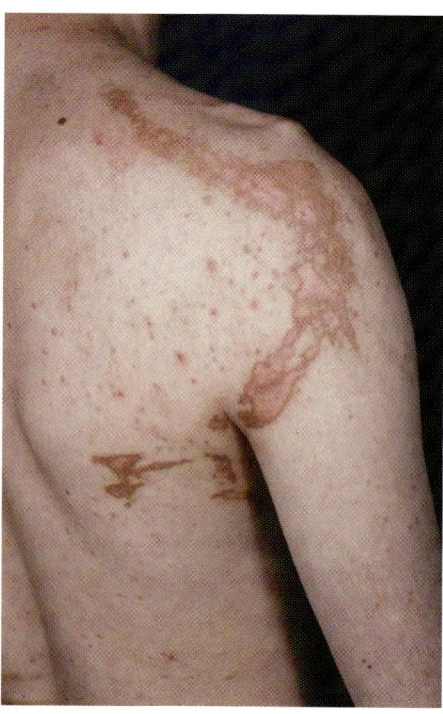

Fig. 1a, b. a Acute phototoxic dermatitis after contact to Cow parsnip (*Heracleum sphondylium*). b Hyperpigmentation 4 weeks later

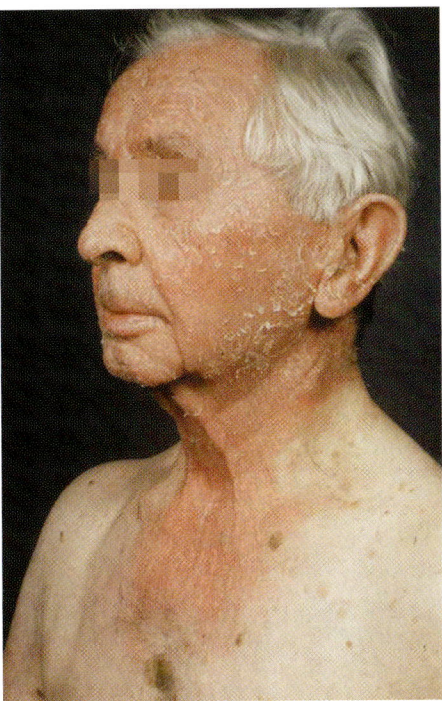

Fig. 2. Photoallergic dermatitis due to quinidine sulfate

to the drug and light. Although the clinical appearances of phototoxic and photoallergic reactions are similar, they result from photobiologic mechanisms that can be clearly differentiated [2–4, 10].

Core Message

■ Phototoxicity is the result of direct cellular damage caused by a nonimmunological inflammatory mechanism that results from the chemical or pharmacological structure of the used substances. In contrast, photoallergic reactions represent a cell-mediated hypersensitivity response, which requires the specific sensitization to a photoactivated drug.

6.3 Phototoxicity – General Mechanisms

In order for phototoxic reactions to occur they require photons to be absorbed by a molecule that is the chromophore or photosensitizer. The structural requirement of this molecule to induce photosensitization is its ability to absorb radiation. Typically these are wavelengths that penetrate the skin deeply (above 310 nm). This characteristic absorption spectrum is determined by the chemical structure of the molecule, in particular by the presence of single or double bonds or halogenated aromatic rings.

The absorbed photon promotes electrons within the molecule from a stable ground to an excited state, the so-called singlet or triplet state of the photosensitizer. Singlet and triplet states are higher-energy states that are defined by the spin state of the two electrons with the highest energies. When these two electrons have opposite spins, the electronic state is a singlet state; when they have the same spin, it is a triplet state. This excited singlet or triplet state is an unstable state and exists for only a very short time after photophysical formation. Typically, excited singlet states are stable for less than 10^{-10} s. Triplet states exist for a longer period and in tissues their lifetime is limited due to deactivation by oxygen (less than 10^{-6} s).

The excited states return to the ground state and the absorbed energy discharges by emission of radiation (fluorescence), heat or a chemical reaction producing a photoproduct. Complex processes are initiated by this photoproduct, which may then result in phototoxic reactions. It is important to keep in mind that not all drugs with the chemical features of a chromophore produce a photochemical reaction, because this also depends on variables such as drug absorption, metabolism, stability and solubility. In general, phototoxicity can be produced in all individuals given a high enough dose of a photosensitizer and light irradiation. The most common skin manifestation of a phototoxic reaction is an exaggerated sunburn reaction with or without edema, blisters and subsequent hyperpigmentation and desquamation in the exposed area. In other words phototoxicity represents an inflammatory reaction, which results from direct cellular damage produced by the photochemical reaction between a photosensitizer and the appropriate wavelength of radiation in the UV or visible range. In contrast to photoallergic reactions, phototoxic reactions can occur during the first exposure of a given individual to this chemical in combination with irradiation and do not require a previous sensitization phase [4, 10, 11] (Fig. 3).

From a photochemical point of view four pathways may be involved to exert phototoxic effects on a biological substrate. In general, these reactions can be further subdivided into oxygen-dependent photodynamic reactions and oxygen-independent nonphotodynamic reactions.

6

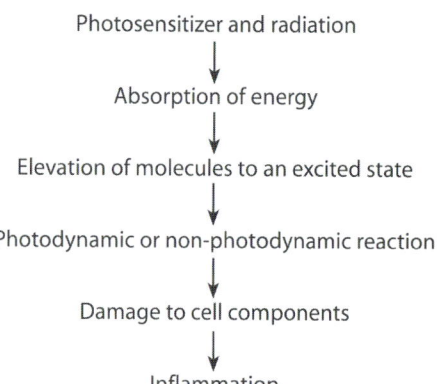

Photosensitizer and radiation

↓

Absorption of energy

↓

Elevation of molecules to an excited state

↓

Photodynamic or non-photodynamic reaction

↓

Damage to cell components

↓

Inflammation

Fig. 3. Pathomechanism of phototoxic reactions (modified after [6])

Photosensitizer + Photon → *Photosensitizer**

I. An energy transfer from the excited photosensitizer to the oxygen produces excited singlet oxygen, which can participate in lipid and/or protein oxidation or induce DNA damage.

$$Photosensitizer^* + O_2 \rightarrow Photosensitizer + {}^1O_2 \rightarrow {}^1O_2 + target$$

II. An electron or hydrogen transfer can lead to the formation of free radicals that directly attack biomolecules. In another pathway, interaction of these free radicals with ground-state oxygen can result in the generation of reactive oxygen species. These include superoxide anion, singlet oxygen, hydroxyl radicals, and hydrogen peroxide.

(I) *Photosensitizer** → *Photosensitizer•* → *Photosensitizer•* + target
(II) *Photosensitizer• + O_2* → *Photosensitizer O_2•* → *Photosensitizer O_2• + target*
(II) *Photosensitizer• + O_2* → *Photosensitizer^+ + O_2^{-•}* → H_2O_2 → OH• → OH• + target

Reactive oxygen intermediates generated through this process are then capable of damaging subcellular organelles, which in turn can lead to tissue injury and inflammation. Many photosensitization reactions may be explained on the basis of these reactions.

III. In contrast, the nonphotodynamic reaction is a direct reaction and leads to the generation of stable photoproducts independent of oxygen. A prime example of a nonphotodynamic type III reaction is a photosensitivity reaction induced by psoralens [11] (Fig. 3).

Photosensitizer* + target → Photosensitizer – target

IV. Finally, the photosensitizer can undergo decomposition so that the resulting photoproduct can act as either a toxin or a new photosensitizer (adapted by [12]).

Photosensitizer* → *Photosensitizer•* → *Photoproduct* → Photoproduct + target
↓ + *hv*
Photoproduct* → Photoproduct* + target

Core Message

■ There are direct and indirect photochemical mechanisms involved in phototoxicity.

The precise cellular target of phototoxic reactions depends on the physiochemical characteristics of the phototoxic agent. Topically applied agents are more likely to damage keratinocytes due to their higher concentration in the epidermis. Systemically applied drugs cause the greatest phototoxicity to components of the dermis, specifically mast cells and endothelial cells. At the cellular level several organelles may be damaged by the phototoxic reaction. A hydrophilic photosensitizer mainly damages the cell membranes, whereas lipophilic substances diffuse into the cell and have been shown to destroy components within the cell including lysosomes, mitochondria, and the nucleus [13, 14]. It should be noted that although effects on one organelle may predominate, most photosensitizers affect more than one structure. Damage to cells results in the release of soluble mediators that cause the inflammatory response. Among these mediators, eicosanoids, histamine, and complement have all been implicated in the generation of inflammatory responses induced by photosensitizers. Cytokines such as interleukin-1, interleukin-6, and tumor necrosis factor-α (TNF-alpha) which have been detected in UVB-induced erythema responses (sunburn reaction), may be involved in phototoxicity caused by drugs and chemicals; however, experimental evidence supporting this concept is lacking for most agents [15].

The specific wavelengths of light absorbed by a given phototoxic chemical depend on the physico-chemical characteristics of the phototoxic agent. As a general rule, in most instances, the wavelengths are within the UVA range. It is important to keep in mind, however, that a few agents such as sulfonamides, vinblastine, and fibric acid derivatives absorb in the UVB range, whereas porphyrins absorb energy from the long-wave UV and visible spectrum.

In general, phototoxic drugs pertain to different therapeutic classes, i.e., antibiotics, anti-diabetic drugs, antihistamines, cardiovascular drugs, diuretics, nonsteroidal anti-inflammatory drugs, psychiatric drugs, and others. These drugs appear in the literature as phototoxic either in vivo or in vitro. It is problematic that it is not possible to predict phototoxic potency [16, 17].

6.4 Some Examples of Specific Agents Capable of Causing Phototoxic Reactions

The following examples are given to illustrate the different mechanisms and factors that cause and influence phototoxic reactions.

6.4.1 Psoralens

Psoralens are heterocyclic, aromatic compounds derived from the condensation of a furan ring with a coumarin ring. Phototoxic reactions induced by psoralens constitute the major therapeutic principle of PUVA (psoralen plus UVA-radiation) therapy. For PUVA therapy, linear psoralens such as 8-methoxypsoralen, 5-methoxypsoralen, and trimethylpsoralen are mostly used in combination with UVA radiation (Fig. 4). PUVA therapy is a mainstay in the treatment of patients with psoriasis vulgaris, cutaneous T-cell lymphoma, and several other inflammatory skin diseases. Psoralens are able to produce photomodifications of various biomolecules. Unlike most other photosensitizing compounds, psoralens mediate their phototoxic effect for the most part through a non-oxygen-dependent photoreaction, although photodynamic reactions may additionally contribute. As opposed to other phototoxic agents, psoralens primarily target DNA. The interaction between psoralens and DNA occurs in two separate steps. In the first step the nonirradiated ground state of psoralen intercalates inside the nucleic acid duplex. In combination with UVA radiation the excited psoralen molecules then form monofunctional and bifunctional psoralen–DNA photoadducts (cross-links) with pyrimidine bases – mainly thymine, but also cytosine and uracil. This mechanism may explain the antiproliferative effects of psoralens. Psoralen-induced DNA damage is responsible for adverse effects such as increased mutagenicity and skin cancer [18].

Other important targets of psoralens are specific receptors, in particular the epidermal growth factor (EGF) receptor and this interaction could provide another basis to explain the antiproliferative effect of PUVA therapy in psoriasis [19]. There are, however, also effects on other cell membrane components [20]. It has been shown for example that psoralen–fatty acid adducts can activate a signaling transduction cascade leading to melanosynthesis in melanocytes. This effect may explain the beneficial effects of PUVA therapy in vitiligo patients [21] or the strong tanning following the treatment. More recently it has been noticed that PUVA therapy can induce programmed cell death (apoptosis) in skin infiltrating T-helper lymphocytes. Resulting depletion of skin-infiltrating T-cells from psoriatic skin is thought to be one of the major mechanisms by which PUVA therapy clears psoriasis. The precise mechanism by which PUVA induces T-helper-cell apoptosis remains to be elucidated [22].

In addition to PUVA therapy, psoralen-induced photosensitivity reactions may also cause unwanted reactions, as they are observed in phytophotodermatitis and berloque dermatitis such as hyperpigmentation of a bizarre configuration, blister formation, and erythema [23, 24].

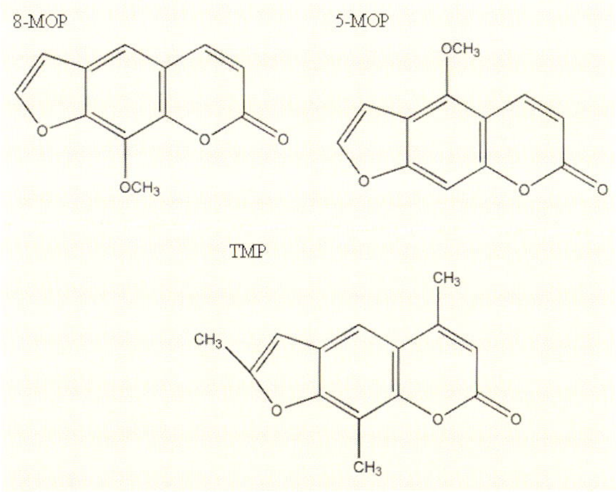

Fig. 4. Structure of 8-methoxypsoralen (*8-MOP*), 5-methoxypsoralen (*5-MOP*) and 4,5×,8-trimethylpsoralen (*TMP*)

6.4.2 Porphyrins

The phototoxicity of porphyrins and their derivatives is important for the pathogenesis of cutaneous symptoms of porphyrias and the therapeutic use of porphyrins in photodynamic therapy. The photoactivation of porphyrins results in the formation of singlet oxygen and thus represents a prime example of a type II reaction. The formation of singlet oxygen and of other free radicals then results in the production of peroxides, which can cause cell damage and cell death. It should be noted that the action spectrum of porphyrins does not lie within the UV range, but rather in the range of visible light (405 nm Soret band) [7, 8].

6.5 Fluoroquinolones

Quinolone antibiotics bearing fluorine substituent are commonly called fluoroquinolones (FQ). Chemically the parent compound is nalidixic acid. Some derivatives maintain the naphthyridinecarboxylic nucleus (enoxacin, trovafloxacin) but in others it is replaced by the quinolinecarboxylic acid (norfloxacin, lomefloxacin, sparfloxacin, clinafloxacin, ciprofloxacin). In both cases the nucleus is substituted with halogens in one or two positions. Phototoxicity induced by FQ appears to be related to structural features. 8-Halogenated FQ (i.e., lomefloxacin, clinafloxacin) provokes severe reactions in the skin in comparison with the low phototoxicity exhibited by 8-methoxy derivatives. Moreover, fluorine substituent on the 8-position of the quinoline ring of FQ also induces photoallergic responses. In general, the presence of an electron-donating substituent has been suggested to confer photostability to the halogenated substituent at the 8-position, reducing the phototoxicity. Although the exact mechanism of FQ photosensitization remains unclear, basically the following processes have been indicated to justify the FQ photoreactivity:

- An oxygen singlet is produced by the zwitterionic form resulting from dissociation of carboxylic acid and the simultaneous protonation of the piperazinyl group.
- The formation of reactive oxygen species including singlet oxygen, superoxide radical, hydroxyl radical, and hydrogen peroxide, although a mechanism based on these toxic agents does not appear to be correlated with the FQ photoreactivity.

- The photochemically induced dehalogenation generates a highly reactive carbene C-8, which reacts with some cell component.
- A combined process wherein the hemolytic defluorination leads to the formation of aryl radical which triggers attack of the cellular substrate, whereas the oxygen reactive species could operate in a secondary or a parallel process [12, 13, 25–28].

6.5.1 Nonsteroidal Anti-inflammatory Drugs

Nonsteroidal anti-inflammatory drugs (NSAIDs) frequently cause phototoxic reactions. The capacity of NSAIDs to cause an inflammatory skin reaction contrasts with their pharmacological capacity to inhibit inflammatory responses. NSAIDs are a chemically heterogeneous group of drugs. Basically, three subclasses may be considered: the carboxylic acids (salicylates, arylalkanoic acids and fenamates), pyrazoles, and oxicams. In any of these subclasses phototoxic and nonphototoxic molecules can be found.

It has been pointed out that their common use in clinical practice has led to multiple reports of photo-induced effects. The result is the existence of a number of mechanistic studies on this subject. There are numerous reports of phototoxic reactions resulting from the use of carprofen, ketoprofen, suprofen, tiaprofenic acid, and naproxen. Benoxaprofen was removed from the European market in 1982 because of a high frequency of phototoxic reactions. Photochemical studies have shown that NSAID phototoxicity is mainly mediated by reactive oxygen species and free radicals. This has been worked out mainly for naproxen. Diclofenac is lesser phototoxic than naproxen, for example. Nevertheless, this drug has received attention because of its wide use. The major photoproducts of diclofenac are carbazole derivates (compounds: 8ClCb and cb). In vitro assays performed with diclofenac and its photoproducts have shown phototoxicity only for 8ClCb, which has structural similarities to the phototoxic drug carprofen [1, 12, 29–31].

6.5.2 Amiodarone

Amiodarone – an anti-arrhythmic drug – often induces phototoxicity. As a clinical consequence a gray hyperpigmentation develops in the UV-exposed areas. Amiodarone and its metabolite desethylamiodarone are highly phototoxic and cause cell damage by injuring the cell membrane in an oxygen-dependent process. Because of the long half-time of amiodarone, this phototoxic reaction may persist for several months. The action spectrum of amiodarone-induced phototoxicity lies within the UVA range. This is surprising because in vitro studies have shown that the UVB range mediates the phototoxicity induced by amiodarone more efficiently than the UVA range. A possible explanation might be that the highest concentration of amiodarone in vivo was found in the dermis, which is reached preferentially by UVA, whereas the UVB portion of solar radiation is almost completely absorbed within the epidermis [32].

6.6 Photoallergic Reactions – General Mechanisms

Both phototoxic and photoallergic reactions require the presence of a chemical and radiation in the UV or visible range. Nevertheless, the mechanisms of action are completely different in both reactions. Photoallergic reactions are classic T-cell-mediated immune mechanisms (Gell and Coombs type IV reactions) and, as a consequence, patients do not have clinical manifestations upon first exposure, because sensitization to the photoallergic agent is an indispensable prerequisite. The photoallergic reaction can be produced by substances that are applied topically or systemically and, in contrast to phototoxic reactions, it does not depend on the concentration of the photosensitizer. The clinical features of photoallergic reactions closely resemble those of an eczematous reaction, as they are observed in contact dermatitis and usually occur 24–72 h after irradiation.

Agents that can cause photoallergic reactions include topical antimicrobials, fragrances, sunscreen ingredients, NSAIDs, psychiatric medications, and others. It is important to know that some of these substances might also have the potency to induce a common allergic contact dermatitis [6, 10, 32–35].

The steps involved in this photochemical reaction, which results in the formation of a complete antigen, are only poorly understood. From the mechanistic point of view, photoallergy involves covalent drug–protein photobinding (haptenization) leading to the formation of a complete photoantigen. This photoantigen may trigger a hypersensitivity reaction due to a cell-mediated immune response. In addition, the photosensitized modifications of proteins may also produce extensive structural changes associated with loss of biological function [6, 10].

For quinidine sulfate photoallergic reactions, the presence of serum components has been implicated in the pathogenesis of the photosensitivity reaction.

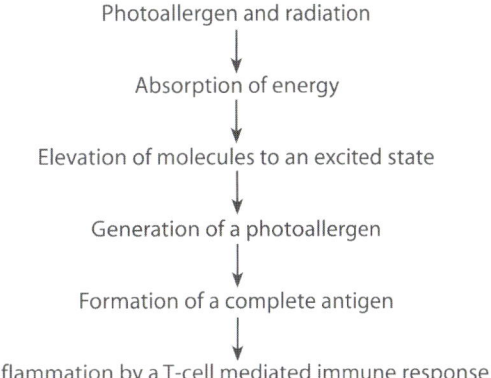

Fig. 5. Mechanism of a photoallergic reaction (modified after [6])

Accordingly, an eczematous reaction could be provoked after intradermal injection of the drug together with patient serum into previously UVA-irradiated skin, whereas injection of the drug alone in the absence of serum did not induce eczema. It has therefore been proposed that binding of the hapten quinidine sulfate to a potential carrier protein that is present in the serum may be of crucial importance in the pathogenesis of this particular type of photoallergic reaction [36].

In the past, most photoallergic reactions resulted from the topical use of soaps and deodorants containing halogenated salicylanilides and related compounds, whereas recently sunscreen ingredients have been found to be among the most frequent photoallergens. Systemic photoallergens include phenothiazines, chlorpromazine as well as NSAIDs. It should been noted that the same agents can also cause phototoxic reactions. For the majority of photoallergens the action spectrum lies within the UVA range. Exceptions are sulfonamides, benzodiazepines, diphenhydramine, isotretinoin, and thiazide diuretics, which produce photoallergic reactions upon exposure to UVB radiation [34] (Fig. 5).

References

1. Ferguson J (1999) Drug and chemical photosensitivity. In: Hawk JLM (ed) Photodermatology. Arnold, London pp 155–169
2. Krutmann J, Hönigsmann H, Elmets CA, Bergstresser PR (eds) (2000) Dermatological phototherapy and photodiagnostic methods. Springer, Berlin Heidelberg New York
3. Epstein JH (1989) Photomedicine. In: Smith KC (ed) The science of photobiology, 2nd edn. Plenum, New York, pp 155–192
4. Epstein JH (1983) Phototoxicity and photoallergy in man. J Am Acad Dermatol 8:141–147

6

5. Hölzle E, Plewig G, Lehmann P (1987) Photodermatoses – diagnostic procedures and their interpretation. Photodermatology 4:109–114
6. Gould JW, Mercurio MG, Elmets CA (1995) Cutaneous photosensitivity diseases induced by exogenous agents. J Am Acad Dermatol 33:551–573
7. Fritsch C, Goerz G, Ruzicka T (1998) Photodynamic therapy in dermatology. Arch Dermatol 134:207–214
8. Lim HW (1989) Mechanisms of phototoxicity in porphyria cutanea tarda and erythropoietic protoporphyria. Immunol Ser 46:671–685
9. Strauss GH, Bridges BA, Greaves M, Vella-Briffa D, Hall-Smith P, Price M (1980) Methoxypsoralen photochemotherapy. Lancet 122:1134–1135
10. Gonzalez E, Gonzalez S (1996) Drug photosensitivity, idiopathic photodermatoses, and sunscreens. J Am Acad Dermatol 35:871–885
11. Ljunggren B, Bjellerup M (1986) Systemic drug photosensitivity. Photodermatology 3:26–35
12. Quintero B, Miranda MA (2000) Mechanisms of photosensitization induced by drugs: a general survey. Ars Pharmadeutica 1:27–46
13. Quedraogo G, Morliere P, Santus R, Miranda, Castell JV (2000) Damage to mitochondria of cultured human skin fibroblasts photosensitized by fluoroquinolones. J Photochem Photobiol 58:20–25
14. Kochevar KE (1991) Phototoxicity mechanisms: chlorpromazine photosensitized damage to DNA and cell membranes. J Invest Dermatol 77:59–64
15. Terencio MC, Guillen I, Gomez-Lechon MJ, Miranda MA, Castell JV (1998) Release of inflammatory mediators (PGE2, IL-6) by fenofibric acid-photosensitized human keratinocytes and fibroblasts. Photochem Photobiol 68:331–336
16. Diffey BL, Farr PM, Adams SJ (1988) The action spectrum in quinine photosensitivity. Br J Dermatol 118:679–685
17. Diffey BL, Farr PM (1988) The action spectrum in drug induced photosensitivity. Photochem Photobiol 47:49–53
18. Dall'Acqua F, Vedaldi D, Bordin F, Rodighiero G (1979) New studies on the interaction between 8-methoxypsoralen and DNA in vitro. J Invest Dermatol 73:191–197
19. Laskin JD, Lee E, Laskin DL, Gallo MA (1986). Psoralens potentiate ultraviolet light-induced inhibition of epidermal growth factor binding. Proc Natl Acad Sci USA 83:8211–8215
20. Zarebska Z (1994) Cell membrane, a target for PUVA therapy. J Photochem Photobiol B 23:101–109
21. Anthony FA, Laboda HM, Costlow ME (1997) Psoralen-fatty acid adducts activate melanocyte protein kinase C: a proposed mechanism for melanogenesis induced by 8-methoxypsoralen and ultraviolet A light. Photodermatol Photoimmunol Photomed 13:9–16
22. Coven TR., Walters IB, Cardinale I, Krueger JG (1999) PUVA-induced lymphocyte apoptosis: mechanism of action in psoriasis. Photodermatol Photoimmunol Photomed 15:22–27
23. Pathak MA, Daniels F, Fitzpatrick TB (1962) The presently known distribution of furocomarins (psoralens) in plants. J Invest Dermatol 32:225–239
24. Kavli G, Volden G (1984) Phytophotodermatitis. Photodermatology 1:65–75
25. Dawe RS, Ibbotson SH, Sanderson JB, Thomson EM, Ferguson J (2003) A randomized controlled trial (volunteer study) of sitafloxacin, enoxacin, levofloxacin and sparfloxacin phototoxicity. Br J Dermatol 149:1232–1241
26. Kawada A, Hatanaka K, Gomi H, Matsuo I (1999) In vitro phototoxicity of new quinolones: production of active oxygen species and photosensitized lipid peroxidation. Photodermatol Photoimmunol Photomed 15:226–230
27. Neumann NJ, Holzle E, Lehmann P, Rosenbruch M, Klaucic A, Plewig G (1997) Photo hen's egg test: a model for phototoxicity. Br J Dermatol 136:326–330
28. Ferguson J, Johnson BE (1993) Clinical and laboratory studies of the photosensitizing potential of norfloxacin, a 4-quinolone broad-spectrum antibiotic. Br J Dermatol 128:285–295
29. Diffey BL, Daymond TJ, Fairgreaves H (1983) Phototoxic reactions to piroxicam, naproxen and tiaprofenic acid. Br J Rheumatol 22:239–242
30. Ljunggren B (1985) Propionic acid-derived nonsteroidal anti-inflammatory drugs and phototoxicity in vitro. Photodermatology 2:3–9
31. Stern RS (1983) Phototoxic-reactions to piroxicam and other non-steroidal anti-inflammatory agents. N Engl J Med 309:186–187
32. Ferguson J, Addo HA, Jones S, Johnson BE, Frain-Bell W (1985) A study of cutaneous photosensitivity induced by amiodarone. Br J Dermatol 113:537–549
33. Elmets CA (1986) Drug-induced photoallergy. Dermatol Clin 4:231–241
34. Emmett EA (1978) Drug photoallergy. Int J Dermatol 17:370–379
35. Horio T (1984) Photoallergic reaction. Classification and pathogenesis. Int J Dermatol 23:376–382
36. Schurer NY, Holzle E, Plewig G, Lehmann P (1992) Photosensitivity induced by quinidine sulfate: experimental reproduction of skin lesions. Photodermatol Photoimmunol Photomed 9:78–82

Part II

Pathology

II

Histopathological and Immuno-histopathological Features of Irritant and Allergic Contact Dermatitis

7

Jean-Marie Lachapelle, Liliane Marot

Contents

7.1 Introduction: General Considerations

Histopathological features of allergic and/or irritant contact dermatitis are not described in full detail in most textbooks of dermatology [1–3]. This is because they are not usually involved in the diagnostic procedures of both conditions. In most cases, contact dermatitis is suspected from anamnestic data and clinical signs [4]. Diagnosis is confirmed by patch testing and/or other tests, with additional information about the responsible agent(s). Nevertheless, in daily practice, contact dermatitis may be superimposed onto an underlying skin disease, the diagnosis of which is sometimes difficult.

In those circumstances, skin biopsy is highly recommended and considered an important tool of differential diagnosis.

Among such examples, the following can be quoted:

- Nummular dermatitis (eczema) versus parapsoriasis en plaques (benign type), psoriasis or *tinea incognito*.
- Seborrheic dermatitis versus lupus erythematosus or rosacea.
- Pompholyx versus pustular psoriasis, palmoplantar pustulosis or bullous pemphigoid.

When an eczematous reaction is involved, the histopathological clue in diagnosis is the presence of a spongiotic (spongiform) dermatitis, notwithstanding its origin: irritant, allergic or endogenous.

In each individual case, the histopathological picture is dependent on various parameters, which can play a confounding role, such as: (1) unknown duration of the disease; (2) lesions related to scratching; (3) infections; and (4) lichenification. Clinicians are sometimes advised to perform two biopsies instead of one, in order to focus on different stages of the disease.

A full description of histopathological signs of allergic and/or irritant contact dermatitis is better achieved by a careful study of positive allergic and/or irritant patch test reactions.

This approach has two advantages: (1) the histopathological signs reflect a practical situation, encountered daily at the patch test clinic; (2) a positive patch test reaction is a clear-cut, unmodified reaction – the direct consequence of the application of a substance on previously intact skin.

The only possible drawback to using patch test reactions is the role played by occlusion. This might be especially true for allergic reactions, and it is the reason for this description also being based upon open (unoccluded) reactions, the use of which is becoming commoner in many clinics.

This description will be a "freeze-frame photograph" of the situation at 48, 72 or 96 h; it does not take into account the chronology of events, starting at time 0 (with the application of the substance) and continuing for instance every 6 h – until 48 or 72 h. This dynamic view has been achieved in previous research studies [5].

It has to be emphasized that this description is useful when expressed in scientific (more than practical) terms, to improve our knowledge at the microscopic level. In this respect, patch testing has been used recently as a tool for evaluating the efficacy of topical drugs, such as pimecrolimus [6] or tacrolimus, [7] versus corticosteroids regarding the outcome of allergic positive patch test reactions to nickel sulfate in volunteers. The evaluation of results has been based on visual scoring and biometrical measurements using noninvasive technology, but not on the evaluation of histopathological parameters. Indeed, biopsy is considered an invasive procedure, rejected nowadays by most ethical committees.

A lot of information delivered in the next paragraphs comes from our own material, used in former studies, at a time when legal procedures were not as strictly codified as they are today.

Core Message

■ In clinical practice, when the diagnosis of allergic and/or irritant contact dermatitis is not clear-cut, skin biopsy is considered an important tool of differential diagnosis. In contrast, biopsies of positive patch tests are not recommended, except for scientific purposes.

7.2 Histopathological Features of Positive Allergic Patch Test Reactions

The histopathological picture of a positive allergic patch test reaction (read at 48 h) is a typical example of a spongiotic dermatitis [3]. Features are very similar in all cases.

7.2.1 Epidermal Changes

In the epidermis, spongiosis is an almost constant sign, resulting from the accumulation of fluid around individual keratinocytes (exoserosis) and the consequent stretching of intercellular desmosome complexes (or "prickles").

Spongiosis is focally or evenly distributed along the length of the epidermis; it is either limited to the lower layers or extends from the basal to the granular layer. In some but not all cases, it spares the cells of the sweat duct unit. Hair follicles are usually involved by the spongiotic process.

A more plentiful accumulation of fluid results in rupture of the intercellular prickles and the formation of vesicles. Thus, in allergic contact dermatitis, spongiotic vesiculation can be defined as an intraepidermal cavity with ragged walls and surrounding spongiosis. There is migration of inflammatory cells into the epidermis (exocytosis). These cells, mainly lymphocytes and occasionally polymorphonuclear neutrophils and eosinophils, accumulate in the spongiotic vesicles.

Some vesicles are rounded and tense; they are located in the stratum spinosum, whereas others are flat and located in the stratum corneum. They finally rupture at the surface of the epidermis and vertical channels of fluid discharge are occasionally seen on serial sections. These channels are sometimes colorfully described as "Devergie's eczematous wells." Intracellular edema of keratinocytes does occur, with accumulation of glycogen.

At the electron microscopic level, dissolution of interdesmosomal areas, or "microacantholysis," can be demonstrated; remaining desmosomes show tension and alignment of tonofilament bundles.

In photoallergic contact dermatitis, a biopsy of the photopatch test site, when positive, clearly shows transforming keratinocytes in sunburn cells.

7.2.2 Dermal Changes

Papillary blood capillaries are often congested and dilated; dilatation of lymphatic vessels is very conspicuous in some but not all cases. Dermal edema is prominent with deposits of acid mucopolysaccharides. A dense mononuclear cell infiltrate is usually present around blood vessels of the lower dermis, and even in the subcutaneous tissue. The cells of the infiltrate migrate from the perivascular spaces to the epidermis and are found throughout the dermal tissue, either isolated or grouped in small clumps.

It is not uncommon to see a dermal infiltration of inflammatory cells around and within hair sheaths and sebaceous ducts, which show some degree of spongiosis and cellular degeneration. This picture could be partly due to direct penetration of the allergens through the pilosebaceous unit.

The infiltrate is of the lymphohistiocytic type, composed almost exclusively of mononuclear cells, varying in form and size. The occurrence of an intimate contact between the cell surfaces of lymphocytes and the cell processes of macrophages was demonstrated many years ago at the ultrastructural

Fig. 1.
Allergic positive patch test reaction to balsam of Peru (*Myroxylon pereirae*) at 2 - days: spongiotic vesiculation in epidermis with exocytosis of mononuclear cells and dermal edema. Hematoxylin–eosin–saffron stain (×150)

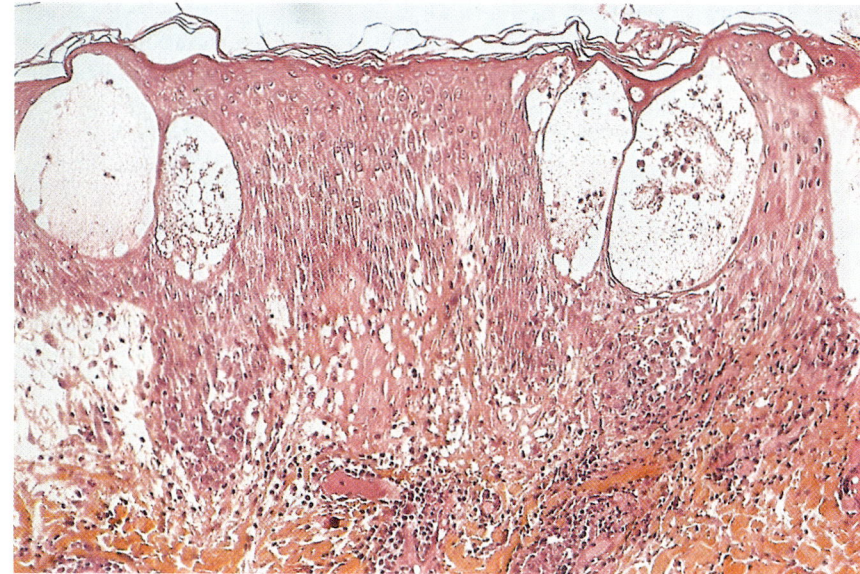

Fig. 2.
Allergic positive patch test reaction to wool wax alcohols (lanolin alcohol) at 2 - days: dense perivascular infiltrate of mononuclear cells. Hematoxylin–eosin–saffron stain (×250)

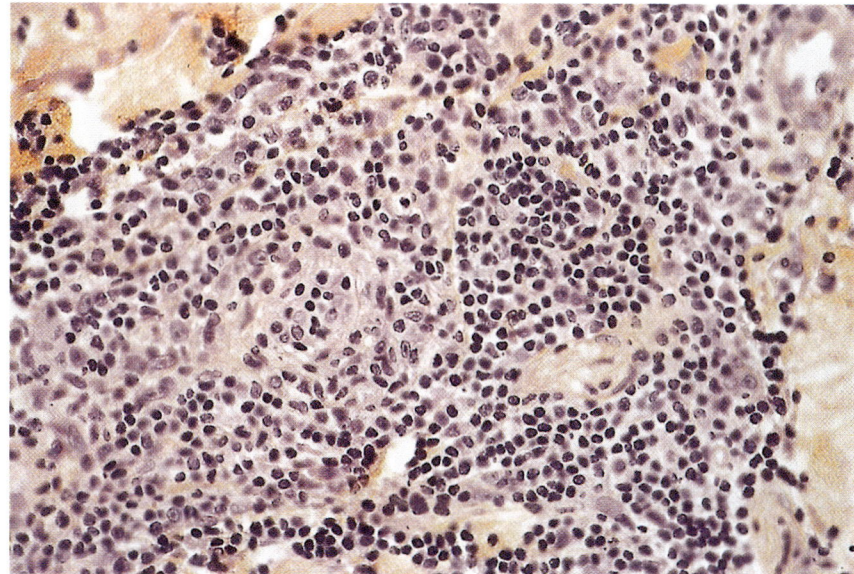

level. It was emphasized that, in delayed hypersensitivity, macrophages were thought to play an important role, together with lymphocytes. This view was later confirmed and broadened by the discovery of the role played by Langerhans cells.

Polymorphonuclear neutrophils are usually absent. Some eosinophils can be found in the edematous tissue of the upper dermis, migrating towards the epidermis.

The histopathological picture is very similar when the biopsy is taken 72 h or 96 h after application of the allergen. The dermal infiltrate around blood ves-sels is usually more pronounced. At this later stage, a few eosinophils can be observed very occasionally.

The role of the mast cell in allergic contact hypersensitivity remains controversial. Some studies showing histological evidence of mast cell degranulation suggest that early mast cell activation occurs [8].

In recent years, Hannuksela's repeated open application test (see Sect. 22.10.2) has become popular for confirming the clinical relevance of positive allergic patch test reactions [9]. We have taken biopsies from positive allergic open test reactions on the volar aspect of the forearm, or the cubital fossa, 48, 72, or 96 h after application of the allergen. In all cases, the histopathological picture was quite similar to that observed in positive allergic patch test reactions.

Two additional features can be observed occasionally:

- In some positive allergic patch test reactions, particularly to azo dyes, purpuric lesions are clinically present [10]: in those cases, there is an important extravasation of erythrocytes, mainly located around blood capillaries, but extending also to interstitial dermal tissue and invading epidermis (exocytosis).
- In some other positive allergic patch test reactions, e.g., to gold (more often at 96 h than 48 h), the infiltrate may be lymphomatoid and mimics pseudolymphoma [11]. It is dense, with a few mitotic figures, and subtle nuclear atypia. Rarely, the lymphoid cells may be very bizarre.

Core Message

- Histopathological features of positive allergic patch test reactions are typical of a spongiotic dermatitis, similar to that observed in different eczematous (exogenous or endogenous) reactions.

7.3 Histopathological Features of Positive Irritant Patch Test Reactions

The histopathological picture of positive allergic patch test reactions has been shown to be very similar ("monotonous and uniform") in most cases (see above). When irritants are applied – under occlusion – on the skin, a wide range of different lesions can be seen. This kaleidoscope of lesions concerns mainly epidermal alterations.

Various factors play a role in the formation of lesions: (1) the nature of the irritant agent, and consequently its mode of deleterious action on the cells, (2) the concentration of the irritant applied on the skin, (3) the ways of penetration of the skin, and (4) the individual reactivity of the skin to a well-defined irritant.

It is therefore possible that the same irritant chemical can produce different types of lesions in different patients, even when it is applied for the same duration and under the same conditions. There is no general rule in this respect.

7.3.1 Epidermal Changes

Various alterations of epidermal cells can be observed. In some cases, these alterations are limited to the superficial layers of the epidermis, the stratum granulosum and the upper part of the stratum spinosum; in others they extend to the dermo-epidermal junction, invading all layers of the epidermis. At first cells become karyopyknotic and lose their cytoplasmic staining properties on hematoxylin and eosin sections. These changes are known as "Bandmann's achromasia" [12]. When the irritation process becomes more severe, complete necrosis (or cytolysis) of epidermal cells occurs, leading to the formation of intra- or subepidermal vesicles and bullae. "Chemical acantholysis" of epidermal cells can be seen, mainly, but not exclusively, with certain irritants, such as cantharidin and trichloroethylene [13]. Polymorphonuclear neutrophils accumulate in the damaged epidermis, leading to the formation of subcorneal or intra-epidermal pustules.

In some cases, the formation of pustules is preferentially limited to the hair follicles. Follicular pustules are preferentially provoked by some irritants, such as croton oil ("croton oil effect"), or metal salts such as chromates, and those of mercury and nickel. Pustules due to metals are observed mainly, but not exclusively, in atopics. As already noted many years ago, some irritant reactions do not show any of the

Table 1. Epidermal lesions observed in relation to certain common irritants

Irritants	Epidermal lesions
Nonchlorinated organic solvents (i.e., alkanes, such as n-hexane; toluene; xylene; white spirit; turpentine, etc.)	Achromasia; superficial necrosis; karyopyknosis; very occasional acantholysis; subepidermal vesicles and/or bullae
Chlorinated organic solvents (i.e., trichloroethane; trichloroethylene; carbon tetrachloride; etc.)	Acantholysis ++; karyopyknosis; complete necrosis of epidermal cells; intraepidermal vesicles and/or bullae
Acids, alkalis, surfactants, detergents, aldehydes	Achromasia; superficial or complete necrosis of epidermal cells; subepidermal vesicles and/or bullae; no acantholysis

Fig. 3.
Irritant positive patch test reaction to croton oil at 2 - days: spongiotic vesiculation in epidermis with exocytosis of mononuclear cells. This picture is indistinguishable from an allergic reaction. Masson's trichrome blue stain (×150)

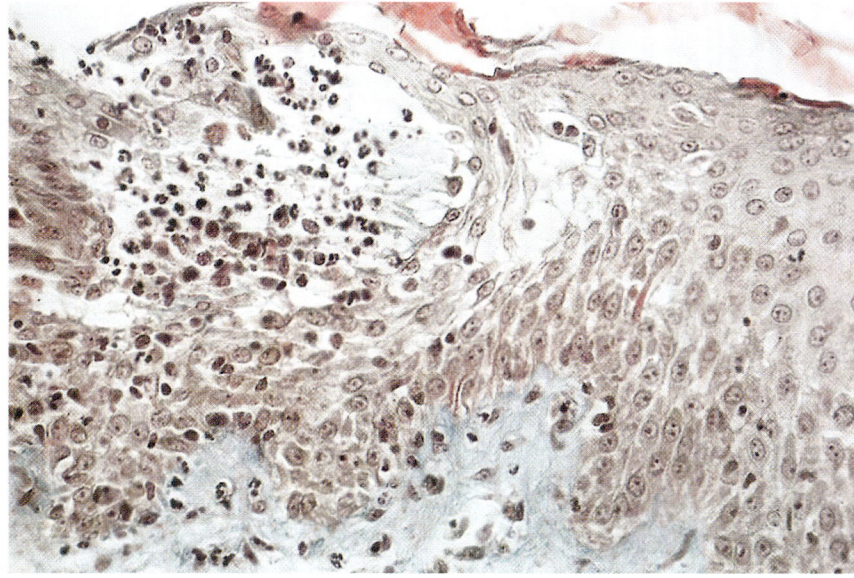

Fig. 4.
Irritant positive patch test reaction to trichloroethylene at 2 days: epidermal necrosis with acantholytic keratinocytes, exocytosis of inflammatory cells. Masson's trichrome blue stain (×150)

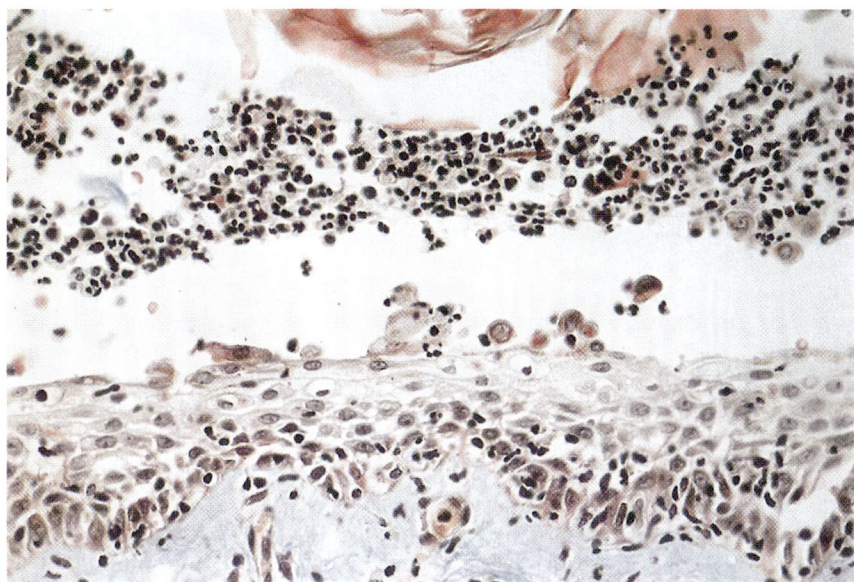

aforementioned histopathological signs; they are exclusively spongiotic (with or without vesicles).

Such observations can be made: (1) with weak irritants, (2) with strong irritants, applied on the skin at a low concentration, and (3) in the "excited" (or irritable) skin syndrome.

Examples of epidermal lesions classically observed with certain categories of irritants are given in Table 1.

Many years ago, ultrastructural studies threw some light on the mode of action of certain irritants, including croton oil, sodium hydroxide, and hydro-

chloric acid. More recently, Willis et al. [14, 15] completed an extensive study comparing the action of several categories of irritants, using semi-thin section technology. They noted in particular that various kinds of detergents damaged epidermal cells in different ways when applied at a low concentration. For instance, the major response to the anionic detergent sodium lauryl sulfate was parakeratosis, indicating increased epidermal cell turnover, whilst benzalkonium chloride, a cationic detergent, caused a different type of reaction – spongiosis and exocytosis with focal necrotic damage [16].

7

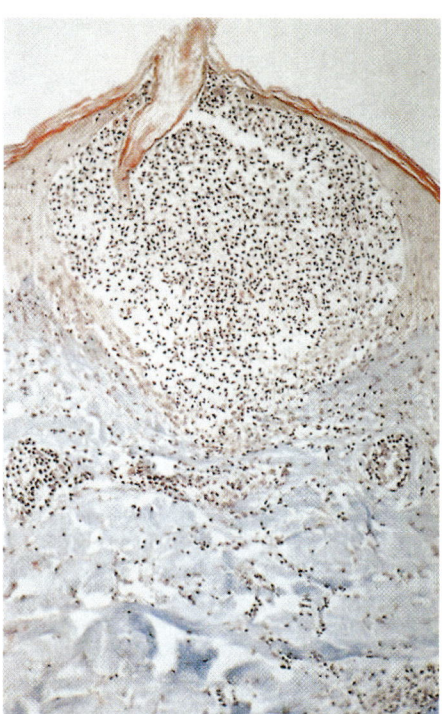

Fig. 5. Irritant positive patch test reaction to croton oil at 2 - days: a follicular pustule is filled with neutrophils and lymphoid cells. There is a perivascular infiltrate of mononuclear cells. Masson's trichrome blue stain (×75)

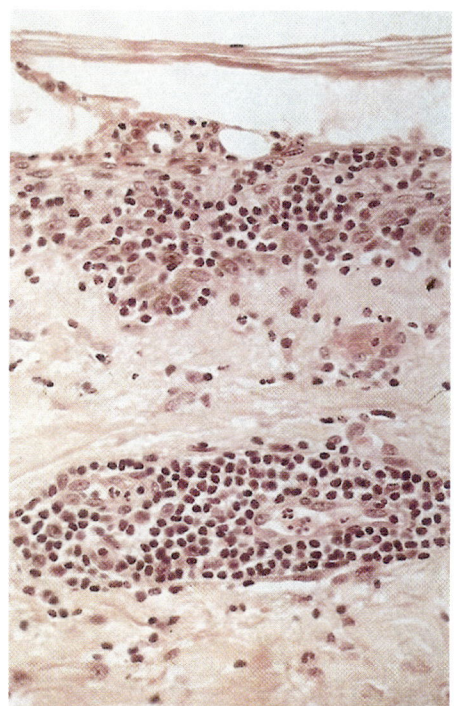

Fig. 6. Irritant positive patch test reaction to sodium lauryl sulfate at 2 days: the epidermis is partly necrotic with infiltration of mononuclear cells. There is a dermal perivascular infiltrate of mononuclear cells. Hematoxylin–eosin stain (×150)

Phototoxic reactions are characterized by the presence of eosinophilic necrotic keratinocytes ("sunburn cells").

7.3.2 Dermal Changes

Dermal changes are also related to the mechanisms involved in the mode of action of each individual irritant. Dermal edema is absent or slight. Blood capillaries and lymphatics are discretely dilated, but usually to a lesser extent than in positive allergic patch test reactions.

In some cases, there is an important inflammatory response distributed around the blood vessels of the upper and mid-dermis. It is either homogeneously mononuclear or mixed (polymorphonuclear neutrophils and lymphocytes/macrophages). Eosinophils are absent. In cases of severe irritation, it is usual to find pyknotic remnants of neutrophils in the upper part of the dermis.

> **Core Message**
>
> ■ Histopathological features of positive irritant patch test reactions are varied, according to the nature and/or concentration of irritant chemicals and to the individual reactivity of the skin. This "kaleidoscope" of lesions concerns mainly epidermal alterations.

7.4 Histopathological Criteria for Distinguishing Between Allergic and Irritant Patch Test Reactions in Humans

In the preceding paragraphs, the various histopathological signs encountered in allergic and irritant patch test reactions have been reviewed in detail [12, 17–20]. We must remember that this description re-

Table 2. Distinctive histopathological criteria between allergic and irritant patch test reactions in humans (modified from [8])

	Allergic reactions	Irritant reactions
Epidermis		
Spongiosis	+ to +++	+ or –
Exocytosis	+ to +++	+++
Vesicles	+ (spongiotic)	+ (rarely spongiotic)
Formation of bullae	Facultative (spongiotic)	Facultative (rarely spongiotic)
Pustules	–	+ or –
Necrosis of epidermal cells	–	+ to +++
Acantholysis of epidermal cells	–	+ or –
Distribution of the infiltrate in epidermis	Focal [21]	Diffuse [21]
Dermis		
Perivascular infiltrate	Mononuclear	Mononuclear or mixed (mononuclear + neutrophils)
Eosinophilic leucocytes	+ or –	–
Dilatation of lymphatic vessels	+ or –	–
Dilatation of blood capillaries	+ or –	+ or –
Edema	+ or –	Very unusual

fers to "typical" cases: irritant (without allergic component) or allergic (without irritant component). Comparative signs are presented in Table 2. These distinctive criteria are of limited value in practice for many reasons: (1) most criteria are present in irritant as well as in allergic positive patch test reactions; (2) other criteria are predominant either in irritant or in allergic reactions, but they lack specificity; (3) most allergens also have irritant properties. Even when allergens are patch tested at a concentration below the level of clinical irritancy to avoid "mixed" pictures, it is just possible that subclinically, at the microscopic level, they might show a mixed picture of irritation and allergy.

In practice, when a positive patch test reaction is clinically doubtful (irritant versus allergic), the help from a biopsy is minimal, due to the differential bias explained above.

Avnstorp et al. [21] conducted a semi-quantitative histopathological study of individual morphological parameters in allergic and irritant patch test reactions. Their conclusions were as follows: statistical analysis by correlation of 17 selected variables gives a diagnostic specificity of 87% and a sensitivity of 81% for allergic reactions. For irritant reactions, the specificity is 100% and the sensitivity 46%. By multiple regressive analysis, an index was calculated for the differentiation of allergic and irritant reactions. If this index were to be used in cases of allergic patch test reactions, all would also be reported as allergic reactions while half of the irritant reactions would be reported as allergic. Although this study has shed some light on the problem of the histopathological differentiation between allergic and irritant contact dermatitis, many difficulties remain in making such a differentiation [21].

When considering all these potential criteria of differential diagnosis, it is worth saying that spongiosis is in bulk a more consistent feature in allergic than in irritant reactions. Vestergaard et al. [22] have recently conducted a human study comparing allergic and irritant reactions. Biopsy samples were taken at a very early stage (6–8 h) after applying (1) an irritant (benzalkonium chloride) and (2) an allergen (that is colophony or quaternium-15) to individuals with known allergy to one of these allergens, selected because they rarely give rise to unspecific or irritant reactions. The significant finding was that focal spongiosis was present only in allergic reactions.

It is likely that the aggregation of monocytes/macrophages and proliferating T-cells, along with their chemical mediators, is responsible for the epidermal spongiosis in allergic contact dermatitis [23].

In conclusion, though conventional histopathology of positive patch test reactions can provide some useful information, it is of little help in separating allergic from irritant or mixed reactions. Drawing such a conclusion at the end of this section might appear to be negative, since a different view has prevailed for decades in so many European contact dermatitis clinics. Nevertheless, it is based on a careful review of the literature and a reappraisal of our own material. It coincides with the views of the basic scientists and must be considered by practicing dermatologists as reflecting reality.

7

Core Message

- Histopathological differential diagnosis between allergic and irritant patch test reactions is clearly explained in Table 2.

7.5 Comparative Immunohistochemical and Immunocytochemical Characteristics of Allergic and Irritant Patch Test Reactions in Humans

An explosion of knowledge concerning the mechanisms involved in contact dermatitis has been taking place over the past 10 years; the discovery of the key role played by the Langerhans cell and the ability to identify subpopulations of lymphocytes by the use of monoclonal antibodies must be considered as major advances. This has raised the question as to whether the use of new immunocytopathological techniques might help in distinguishing between irritant and allergic patch test reactions.

7.5.1 Epidermal Langerhans Cells in Irritant and Allergic Positive Patch Test Reactions

Semi-quantitative studies related to the number of Langerhans cells (LC; CD1 or T_6 dendritic cells) in the epidermis in positive irritant and allergic patch test reactions have been conducted. These studies have revealed a statistically significant decrease in LC 48 or 72 h after the application of various types of irritants: sodium lauryl sulfate, mercuric chloride, benzalkonium chloride, croton oil, or dithranol. There was also a significant reduction in dendritic length. These changes in density were unrelated to the intensity of the inflammatory response [24].

Similar studies in positive allergic patch test reactions show an early transitory increase in LC in the first few hours [25] following the application of allergens, though a similar response occurs at the sites of petrolatum application [25]. This phenomenon may therefore lack specificity. Later on, at 24, 48, or 72 h after application of the allergen, the number of LC is unchanged or decreases when compared with normal skin. It may also be reduced at the site of negative patch test reactions [26]. Current studies indicate that allergic and irritant patch test reactions cannot be differentiated reliably by counting LC, in spite of the small differences observed [27]. Moreover, lymphocyte/LC apposition is observed in both types of reaction [28, 29]. The presence of human leukocyte antigen (HLA) DR antigens on keratinocytes in allergic reactions may reflect an immunological response [30].

7.5.2 Cells of the Infiltrate in Irritant and Allergic Positive Patch Test Reactions: Immunophenotypic Studies

Early human studies showed little evidence of differential cytokine release between allergic and irritant contact dermatitis.

This strongly suggests that, although initiating events vary considerably, the cascade mechanisms responsible for the induction and release of regulating mediators are similar [31, 32]. Clearly, most, if not all, pro-inflammatory phenomena can be caused both by irritants and allergens. Therefore, they do not unambiguously discriminate between irritants and contact allergens [33].

In the various studies conducted so far, the composition of the infiltrates is similar in allergic and irritant reactions, and consists of T lymphocytes of helper/inducer types in association with T-cell accessory cells, that is, LC and HLA-DR-positive macrophages.

Probably, true differences between these types of compounds depend on whether or not allergen-specific T-cells become involved [33]. Thus, only after specific T-cell triggering might distinctive features be observed, e.g., local release of certain chemokines, such as CXCL10 (IP-10) and CXCL11 (I-TAC/IP9) [34].

The latter chemokines are produced by interferon-γ-activated keratinocytes and T lymphocytes [35].

Core Message

- New immunocytopathological techniques are of no real help in distinguishing between irritant and allergic patch test reactions, since there is little evidence of differential cytokine release.
  Clearly, most, if not all, of pro-inflammatory phenomena can be caused by both irritants and allergens. Therefore, they do not discriminate between irritants and contact allergens.

7.6 Conclusions

In spite of certain differences in the histopathological lesions observed in allergic and irritant patch test reactions, there is as yet no reliable diagnostic tool (either morphological or immunophenotypic) to "label" specifically each type of reaction.

References

1. Wilkinson SM, Beck MH (2004) Contact dermatitis: irritant. In: Burns DA, Breathnach SM, Cox N, Griffiths CE (eds) Rook's textbook of dermatology, 7th edn, Chap. 19. Blackwell Science, Oxford
2. Beck MH, Wilkinson SM (2004) Contact dermatitis: allergic. In: Burns DA, Breathnach SM, Cox N, Griffiths CE (eds) Rook's textbook of dermatology, 7th edn, Chap. 20. Blackwell Science, Oxford
3. Belsito DV (2003) Allergic contact dermatitis. In: Freedberg IM (ed) Fitzpatrick's dermatology in general medicine, 6th edn, Chap. 120. McGraw-Hill, New York, pp 1164–1180
4. Rietschel RL, Conde-Salazar L, Goossens A, Veien NK (1999) Atlas of contact dermatitis. Dunitz, London
5. Kerl H, Burg G, Braun-Falco O (1974) Quantitative and qualitative dynamics of the epidermal and cellular inflammatory reaction in primary toxic and allergic dinitrochlorobenzene contact dermatitis in guinea pigs. Arch Dermatol Forsch 249:207–226
6. Queille-Roussel C, Graeber M, Thurston M, Lachapelle JM, Decroix J, de Cuyper C, Ortonne JP (2000) SDZ ASM 981 is the first non-steroid that suppresses established nickel contact dermatitis elicited by allergen challenge. Contact Dermatitis 42:349–350
7. Alomar A, Puig L, Gallardo CM, Valenzuela N (2003) Topical tacrolimus 0.1% ointment (Protopic®) reverses nickel contact dermatitis elicited by allergen challenge to a similar degree to mometasone furoate 0.1% with greater suppression of late erythema. Contact Dermatitis 49:185–188
8. Angelini G, Vena GA, Filotico R, Tursi A (1990) Mast cell participation in allergic contact sensitivity. Contact Dermatitis 23:239
9. Hannuksela M, Salo H (1986) The repeated open application test (ROAT). Contact Dermatitis 14:221–227
10. Lazarov A, Cordoba M (2000) Purpuric contact dermatitis in patients with allergic reaction to textile dyes and resins. J Eur Acad Dermatol Venereol 14:101–105
11. Fleming C, Burden D, Fallowfield M et al (1997) Lymphomatoid contact reaction to gold earrings. Contact Dermatitis 37:298–299
12. Lachapelle JM (1973) Comparative histopathology of allergic and irritant patch test reactions in man. Current concepts and new prospects. Arch Belg Dermatol 28:83–92
13. Mahmoud G, Lachapelle JM (1985) Evaluation expérimentale de l'efficacité de crèmes barrière et de gels antisolvants dans la prévention de l'irritation cutanée provoquée par des solvants organiques. Cah Med Trav 22:163–168
14. Willis CM, Stephens CJM, Wilkinson JD (1989) Epidermal damage induced by irritants in man: a light and electron microscopic study. J Invest Dermatol 93:695–699
15. Willis CM, Stephens CJM, Wilkinson JD (1989) Preliminary findings on the patterns of epidermal damage induced by irritants in man. In: Frosch PJ, Dooms-Goossens A, Lachapelle JM, Rycroft RJ, Scheper RJ (eds) Current topics in contact dermatitis. Springer, Berlin Heidelberg New York, pp 42–45
16. Willis CM, Stephens CJM, Wilkinson JD (1993) Differential patterns of epidermal leukocyte infiltration in patch test reactions to structurally unrelated chemical irritants. J Invest Dermatol 101:364–370
17. Medenica M, Rostenberg A (1971) A comparative light and electron microscopic study of primary irritant contact dermatitis and allergic contact dermatitis. J Invest Dermatol 56:259–271
18. Lachapelle JM (1972) Comparative study of 3H-thymidine labelling of the dermal infiltrate of skin allergic and irritant patch test reactions in man. Br J Dermatol 87:460–465
19. Grosshans E, Lachapelle JM (1982) Comparative histo- and cytopathology of allergic and irritant patch test reactions in Man. In: Foussereau J, Benezra C, Maibach H (eds) Occupational contact dermatitis. Clinical and chemical aspects. Munksgaard, Copenhagen, pp 63–69
20. Nater JP, Hoedemaeker PHJ (1976) Histopathological differences between irritant and allergic patch test reactions in man. Contact Dermatitis 2:247–253
21. Avnstorp C, Balslev E, Thomsen HK (1989) The occurrence of different morphological parameters in allergic and irritant patch test reactions. In: Frosch PJ, Dooms-Goossens A, Lachapelle JM, Rycroft RJ, Scheper RJ (eds) Current topics in contact dermatitis. Springer, Berlin Heidelberg New York, pp 38–41
22. Vestergaard L, Clemmensen OJ, Sorensen FB, Andersen KE (1999) Histological distinction between early allergic and irritant patch test reactions: follicular spongiosis may be characteristic of early allergic contact dermatitis. Contact Dermatitis 41:207–210
23. Belsito DV (1999) The molecular basis of allergic contact dermatitis. In: Dyall-Smith D, Marks R (eds) Dermatology at the millennium. The Proceedings of the 19th World Congress of Dermatology. Parthenon, New York, pp 217–223
24. Ferguson J, Gibbs JH, Beck JS (1985) Lymphocyte subsets and Langerhans cells in allergic and irritant patch test reactions: histometric studies. Contact Dermatitis 13:166–174
25. Christensen OB, Daniels TE, Maibach HI (1986) Expression of OKT6 antigen by Langerhans cells in patch test reactions. Contact Dermatitis 14:26–31
26. Brasch J, Mielke V, Kÿnne N, Weber-Matthiesen V, Bruhn S, Sterry W (1990) Immigration of cells and composition of cell infiltrates in patch test reactions. Contact Dermatitis 23:238
27. Kanerva L, Ranki A, Lauharanta J (1984) Lymphocytes and Langerhans cells in patch tests. An immuno-histochemical and electron microscopic study. Contact Dermatitis 11:150–155
28. Willis CM, Young E, Brandon DR, Wilkinson JD (1986) Immunopathological and ultrastructural findings in human allergic and irritant contact dermatitis. Br J Dermatol 115:305–316
29. Illis CM, Wilkinson JD (1990) Changes in the morphology and density of epidermal Langerhans cells (CD1 + cells) in irritant contact dermatitis. Contact Dermatitis 23:239
30. Scheynius A, Fischer T (1986) Phenotypic difference between allergic and irritant patch test reactions in man. Contact Dermatitis 14:297–302
31. Hoeffaker S, Caubo M, Van't Erve EH (1995) In vivo cytokine profiles in allergic and irritant contact dermatitis. Contact Dermatitis 33:258–266

32. Ulfgren AK, Klareskog L, Lindberg M (2000) An immuno-histochemical analysis of cytokine expression in allergic and irritant contact dermatitis. Acta Derm Venereol (Stockh) 80:167–170
33. Rustemeyer T (2004) Immunological aspects of environmental and occupational contact allergies, Thela Thesis, Amsterdam
34. Flier J, Boorsma DM, Bruynzeel DP, van Beek PJ, Stoof TJ, Scheper RJ, Willemze R, Tensen CP (1999) The CXCR3 activating chemokines IP-10, MIG and IP-9 are expressed in allergic but not in irritant patch test reactions. J Invest Dermatol 113:574–578
35. Tensen CP, Flier J, van der Raaij-Helmer EM, Sampat-Sardjoepersad S, van den Schors RC, Leurs R, Scheper RJ, Boorsma DM, Willemze R (1999) Human IP-9: a keratinocyte derived high affinity CXC-chemokine ligand for the IP-10/Mig receptor (CXCR3). J Invest Dermatol 112:716–722

7

Ultrastructure of Irritant and Allergic Contact Dermatitis

CAROLYN M. WILLIS

Contents

8.1 Introduction

Electron microscopy has provided us with a valuable tool to investigate the cellular and subcellular effects of topical exposure to irritants and allergens, complementing histological examination at the light microscope level. Most reported data are based on the use of conventional preparative techniques, but developments such as post-fixation in ruthenium tetroxide to visualize intercellular lipids and the parallel examination of semi-thin and ultra-thin resin-embedded samples have enhanced our understanding of the cellular changes that take place. It is important to remember, however, that electron microscopy gives us only a snapshot of a minute fraction of a skin biopsy. Therefore, studies employing small sample numbers, with limited scrutiny of each specimen, should be viewed with a degree of caution. This is particularly true for irritant contact dermatitis investigations, where considerable inter-individual variation in the intensity of the response to chemicals occurs, and where the cellular damage inflicted is rarely uniform across the application site.

In the sections which follow, ultrastructural changes seen in skin exposed to irritants and allergens are described. With the exception of the last section, which deals specifically with a recent study of chronic chromate hand dermatitis, the data refer to the effects of acute exposure.

8.2 Ultrastructural Changes in the Epidermis

The stratified nature of the epidermis, and the presence of Langerhans cells and melanocytes in addition to keratinocytes, presents a wide variety of biochemical and immunological targets for topically applied irritants and allergens. Primary contact occurs at the outermost stratum corneum, which, depending on the chemical characteristics of the substance, may show ultrastructural evidence of damage. Diffusion into and penetration of the viable epidermal regions then take place. Again depending upon the chemical nature of the agent, as well as the severity of response and time of examination post-exposure, morphological indications of metabolic interruption may be seen.

8.2.1 Stratum Corneum

The outermost diffusion barrier of the skin, the stratum corneum, is a 20- to 30-cell-thick layer of flat, hexagonal, protein-rich corneocytes surrounded by intercellular lipids. Generally speaking, chemical irritants rather than allergens produce marked changes to its structure and behavior, as evidenced, biophysically, by increased transepidermal water loss. Recent ultrastructural studies utilizing ruthenium tetroxide as a post-fixative have greatly increased our understanding of the manner in which some irritant chemicals interact with this region of the epidermis and contribute to the development of irritant contact dermatitis (ICD). The application of low concentrations of the anionic surfactant sodium lauryl sulfate (SLS) to normal human skin was found by Fartasch to result not so much in an alteration of the existing lipid structure, but rather an alteration in the synthesis of new lipids [1]. Hence, disturbance of lamellar body lipid extrusion and transformation into lipid bilayers occurred, in the absence of any disruption to the intercellular lipid layers of the upper stratum corneum. By way of contrast, acetone produced a different pattern of change. Epidermal lipid lamellae displayed disruption and loss of cohesion throughout the stratum corneum – the transformed, more nonpolar, lamellar lipids showing greater disruption than the more polar lamellar body sheets [1]. A similar disruption of stratum corneum intercellular bilayers was also seen in human skin patch-tested with water alone [2], which would have the effect, as pointed out by the investigators, of enhancing skin permeability and susceptibility to irritants.

> ### Core Message
>
> ■ Chemical irritants generally have a greater impact than allergens on the ultrastructure of the stratum corneum.

8.2.2 Viable Keratinocytes

The greatest diversity of ultrastructural effects on viable keratinocytes within the epidermis is undoubtedly exerted by irritants, rather than by allergens.

While both induce varying degrees of spongiosis, clearly visible by both light and electron microscopy, chemical irritants also give rise to a heterogeneity of forms of intracellular damage that are time, dose and, in some cases, irritant dependent.

8.2.2.1 Irritant Contact Dermatitis

Two early studies provided some of the first evidence that irritants can damage the skin by different mechanisms. A comparison between the effects of an acid and an alkali on human epidermis found that sodium hydroxide dissolved the contents of horny cells and disrupted tonofilament–desmosome complexes, while hydrochloric acid did not [3]. Similarly, in a comparative study of two lipid solvents, the response to acetone, which was characterized by intracellular edema of keratinized cells and vacuolation of spinous cells, was conspicuously different to that to kerosene, in which the formation of large lacunae and cytolysis of spinous cells were seen [4]. In our own study, designed to systematically compare the morphological effects of six structurally unrelated irritants on normal human skin, electron microscopy also revealed significant differences in the nature of the cellular damage induced by different chemicals after 48 h of exposure [5]. Patch test reactions to SLS were characterized by parakeratotic cells in the upper epidermis, containing dense osmiophilic cytoplasm with numerous lipid droplets and vesicles, but an absence of keratohyalin granules (Figs. 1, 2). In contrast, the cationic detergent benzalkonium chlo-

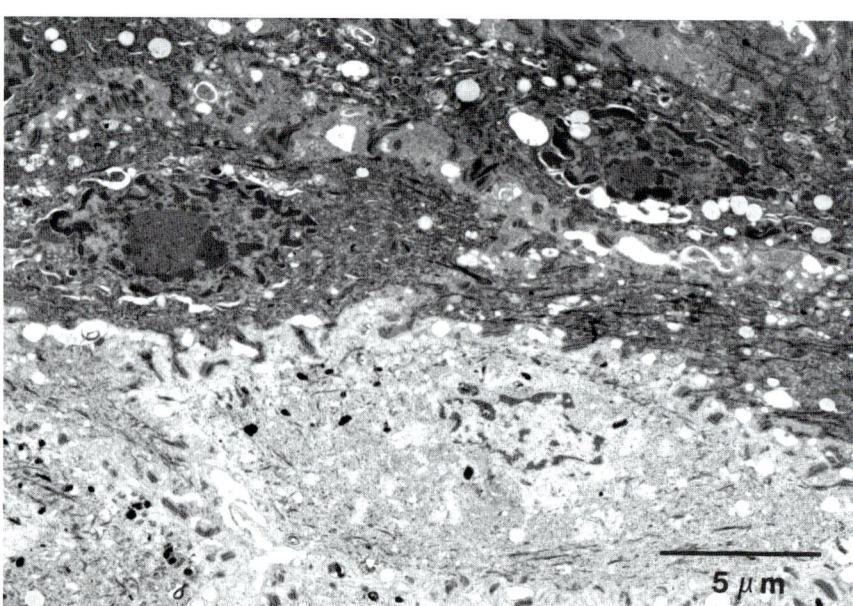

Fig. 1.
The interface between dark, osmiophilic, vesiculated, parakeratotic cells in the upper epidermis and paler cells of the stratum spinosum in a 48-h patch test reaction to sodium lauryl sulfate (*SLS*) (4%)

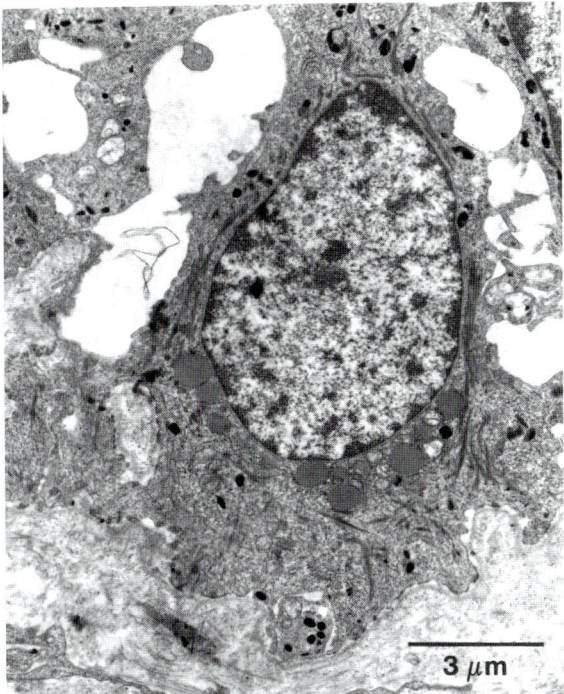

Fig. 2. Basal keratinocytes in a 48-h SLS (4%) patch test reaction, illustrating lipid droplet accumulation and prominent intracytoplasmic vesiculation

Table 1. Ultrastructural changes induced in the viable epidermis by acute exposure to selected irritants. Changes depend on the irritant, its concentration, and time

Irritant	Ultrastructural changes
Sodium lauryl sulfate	Spongiosis, vesiculation, nuclear/intra-cytoplasmic/mitochondrial vacuolation, lipid droplet accumulation, hydropic swelling, decreased desmosomes with aggregation of tonofilaments
Benzalkonium chloride	Nuclear/intracytoplasmic vacuolation, nuclear pyknosis, mitochondrial swelling, organelle disruption, hydropic swelling, spongiosis
Dithranol	Hydropic swelling, mitochondrial membrane disruption, spongiosis, intracytoplasmic vacuolation, dyskeratosis, apoptosis, colloid bodies
Croton oil	Marked spongiosis, intracytoplasmic vacuolation, pyknotic/enlarged nuclei
Nonanoic acid	Dyskeratosis, nuclear/intracytoplasmic vacuolation, vesiculation, lipid droplet accumulation, pyknotic nuclei
Acetone	Acantholysis, spongiosis, nuclear/intracytoplasmic edema and vacuolation
Sodium hydroxide	Disrupted tonofilament–desmosome complexes

Combined human and animal data [3–12]

ride produced distinct areas of necrosis (Fig. 3). Application of the 12-C-long chain fatty acid nonanoic acid resulted in the formation of tongues of dyskeratotic cells, largely composed of dense, wavy aggregates of osmiophilic keratin filaments associated with prominent intercellular desmosomes, and containing shrunken nuclei with condensed, marginated heterochromatin (Fig. 4). Exposure to dithranol produced different changes again, namely markedly enlarged upper epidermal keratinocytes, containing finely dispersed filaments and ribosomes, and, in keeping with previous findings [6, 7], disrupted mitochondria (Fig. 5).

The concept of ultrastructural changes being irritant-dependent was further supported by a recent study of the effects of a wide variety of irritant chemicals on the skin of hairless guinea pigs [8]. Although the skin changes described were not identical to those seen in human skin, partly perhaps as a result of concentration differences, it was clear, that again the nature of the epidermal damage elicited by SLS differed markedly from that of benzalkonium chloride.

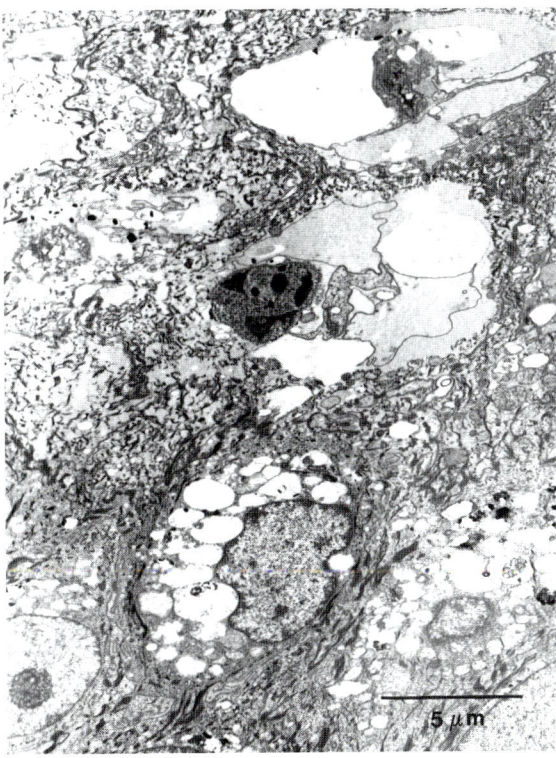

Fig. 3. An area of necrosis induced in the mid epidermis by 48-h patch testing with benzalkonium chloride (0.5%). Keratinocytes show extensive vacuolation, pyknotic nuclei, and disrupted organelles and membranes

Fig. 4.
Dyskeratotic upper epidermal cells, containing dense, wavy aggregates of osmiophilic keratin filaments, produced by 48-h patch testing with nonanoic acid (80%)

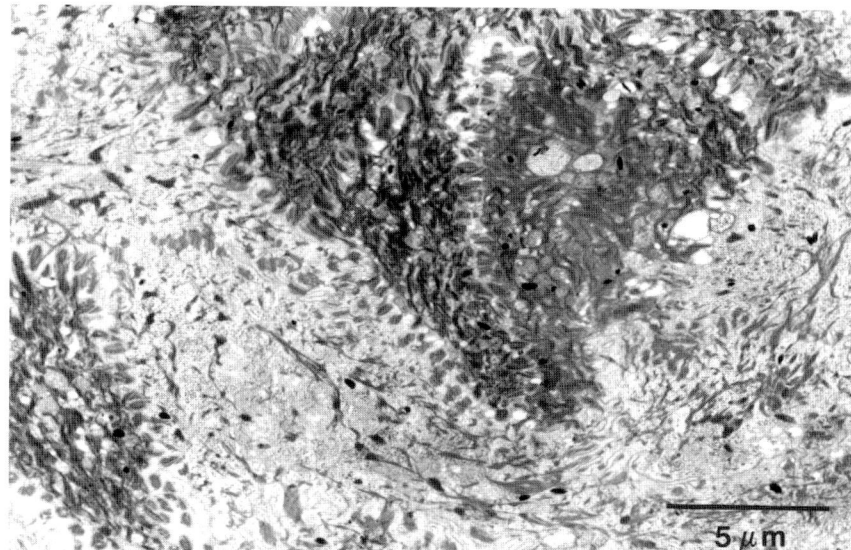

8

Fig. 5.
Enlarged upper epidermal keratinocyte, with cytoplasm containing finely dispersed filaments and ribosomes and perinuclearly clustered mitochondria, in a 48-h patch test reaction to dithranol (0.2%)

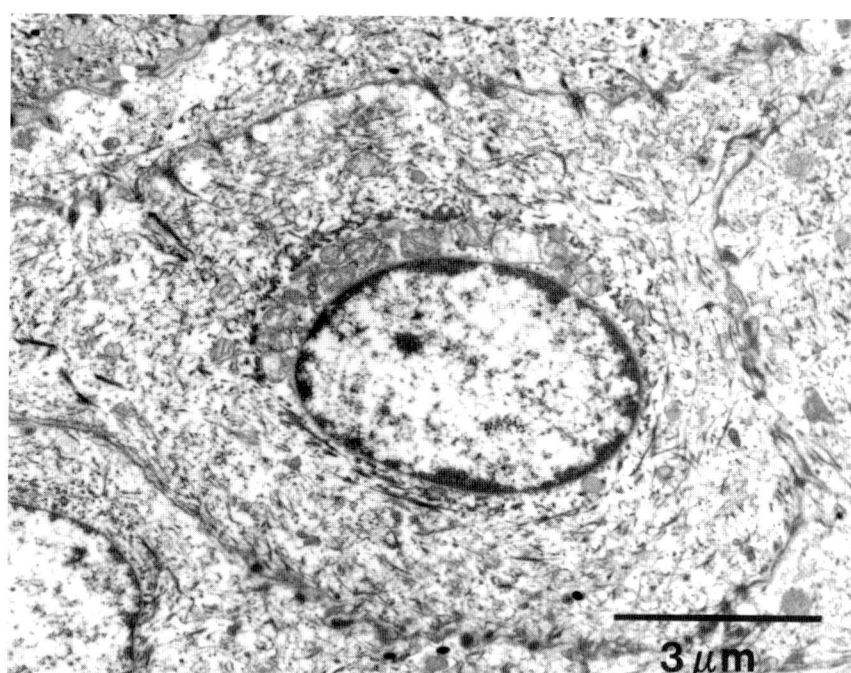

The ultrastructural changes to the viable cells in the epidermis variously described by investigators during the last three decades [3–10] (Table 1) are, in the main, indicative of autolysis or cytolysis, which would eventually lead to disintegration of the cell. In some cases, however, certain alterations, such as condensation of chromatin and cytosol, clumping of tonofilaments and budding of membrane-bound cell fragments, may be suggestive of another form of cell death, that of apoptosis. Often ultrastructurally indistinguishable from dyskeratotic cells in the early stages, apoptotic keratinocytes have been described in reactions to a number of well-studied irritants [11–13].

Core Message

- Structurally unrelated chemical irritants damage the skin by different mechanisms, which is reflected in the varying ultrastructural changes seen in the epidermis. These changes also depend on concentration, time, intensity of reaction, and species.

8.2.2.2 Allergic Contact Dermatitis

Intercellular edema or spongiosis, characterized by dilated intercellular spaces, stretched or absent tonofilament–desmosome complexes and the aggrega-

tion of tonofilaments into short bundles, is a consistent feature of the viable epidermal layers in allergic contact dermatitis (ACD) (Fig. 6), and one that is detectable in sensitized individuals by electron microscopy as early as 3 h after exposure to hapten [14]. Intracellular changes to keratinocytes, such as vacuolation and endoplasmic reticulum dilatation, also occur, but since the majority of allergens are also intrinsically irritant in nature, ascribing such changes with any degree of certainty to the process of sensitization itself is very difficult. Indeed, in a study of chromium reactions in humans and guinea pig, the authors concluded that keratinocyte intracellular reaction patterns were nonspecific and could not be distinguished from those of vehicle or occlusion alone [15].

Core Message

- The predominant ultrastructural change in the epidermis of acute allergic contact dermatitis lesions is spongiosis.

8.2.3 Langerhans Cells

Much of the ultrastructural data relating to Langerhans cell (LC) behavior in contact dermatitis focuses, not surprisingly, on ACD rather than ICD. Contradictory electron microscopy findings have emerged over

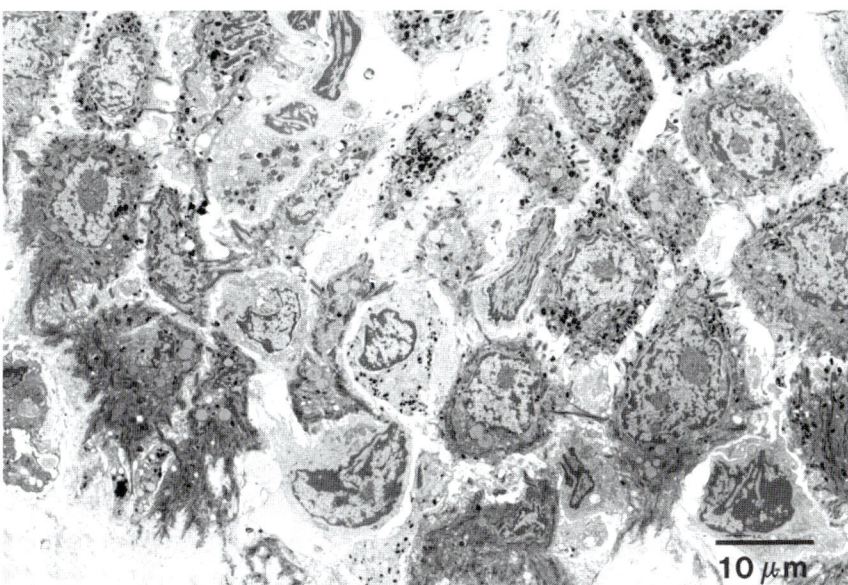

Fig. 6.
Low-power micrograph of the lower region of the epidermis of a 48-h patch test reaction to nickel sulfate (5%). Spongiosis and exocytosis are the predominant features

the years, however, stimulating debate on a number of issues, including whether overt cellular damage to LC is an inherent feature of allergic contact reactions, and the extent to which the changes seen are specific to ACD. Nevertheless, there is now no doubting the central role that this antigen-presenting, mononuclear cell occupies from an immunologic point of view [16]. As to whether LCs have a functional role in ICD also remains a matter of speculation, but, here, there is certainly a great deal of evidence of cellular damage to LC, most of which is likely to be nonspecific in origin.

8.2.3.1 Allergic Contact Dermatitis

As early as 1973, ultrastructural observations led to speculation that Langerhans cells might play a role in allergic contact reactions [17]. Close apposition to mononuclear cells was described as being an exclusive feature of ACD, and a variety of cellular changes suggestive of targeted physiological activity were seen. In the intervening years, numerous ultrastructural studies designed to elucidate the behavior of LC have been conducted, some of which are summarized in Table 2. From these, it would appear that there is early metabolic activation, as indicated by prominent rough endoplasmic reticulum and Golgi apparatus, during the early stages of induction and elicitation, followed later by degenerative changes, such as membrane disruption and condensation of nuclear chromatin (Fig. 7). In a rare ultrastructural study linking LC function and morphology more closely, Rizova et al. described an alteration in the pattern of endocytosis of major histocompatibility complex class II (HLA-DR) molecules specific to allergens. Sensitizer-treated LCs internalized HLA-DR preferentially in lysosomes collected near the nucleus, whereas irritant-treated and nontreated LCs internalized the molecules in prelysosomes located near the cell membrane [27].

8.2.3.2 Irritant Contact Dermatitis

Current immunological evidence does not support the concept of any specific functional activities for LC during the evolution of ICD, other than perhaps

Table 2. A summary of the major ultrastructural changes induced in Langerhans cells by selected chemical allergens. (*DNCB* Dinitrochlorobenzene, *DNFB* dinitrofluorobenzene)

Allergen(s)	Langerhans cell changes	Ref.
Various (human, 4–72 h)	Apposition to mononuclear cells. Prominent rough endoplasmic reticulum and Golgi complexes, glycogen accumulation, presence of polyribosomes, lysosome-like projections, ruffled cell membranes. Disruption to membranes	[17]
DNCB (guinea pig, 2–48 h)	Early cellular vacuolar and granular changes, with apposition to mononuclear cells. Later migration to/loss from the horny layer	[18]
Nickel, thiuram mix, epoxy resin, neomycin (man, 72 h)	Apposition to other cells, marked endocytosis with greatly increased cytoplasmic content of vesicles, the latter having trilaminar membranes and specific granules. Dark cytoplasmic vesicles (nickel). No evidence of cell damage	[19]
DNCB (guinea pig, 2 h to 14 days)	Early activation (6 h), with prominent rough endoplasmic reticulum and Golgi, and numerous lysosomes and vacuoles. After 12 h, cell damage, evidenced by disruption of cell membranes, etc.	[20]
Various (human, 3–168 h)	Increased metabolic activity in some cells, with distended endoplasmic reticulum, pronounced microtubules and increased numbers of Birbeck granules. Also occasional necrotic cells, with condensed chromatin and shrunken cytoplasm	[21]
Various (human, 3–72 h)	No morphological changes indicative of damage	[22]
Picryl chloride, DNFB (mouse, 1–96 h)	1–24 h, activation with enlargement of cell and nucleus and increase in mitochondria, Golgi and endoplasmic reticulum. After 48 h, degenerative changes	[23]
DNFB (induction) (guinea pig, 15 min to 24 h)	Activation from 15 min, with LC showing intense endocytotic activity – numerous coated vesicles and Birbeck granules	[24]
Various (human, 72 h)	Increased numbers of LC, increased synthesis and cell surface expression of HLA class II molecules	[25]
DNFB (mouse, 1–96 h)	During induction phase, cellular and endocytotic activation. Degenerative changes, including membrane rupture, cytoplasmic edema and irregular condensation of nuclear chromatin, in the late elicitation phase	[26]

Fig. 7.
Degenerative changes, including disrupted organelles and membranes, in a Langerhans cell within the epidermis of a 48-h patch test reaction to nickel sulfate (5%). Activated Langerhans cells were also present in the same biopsy sample

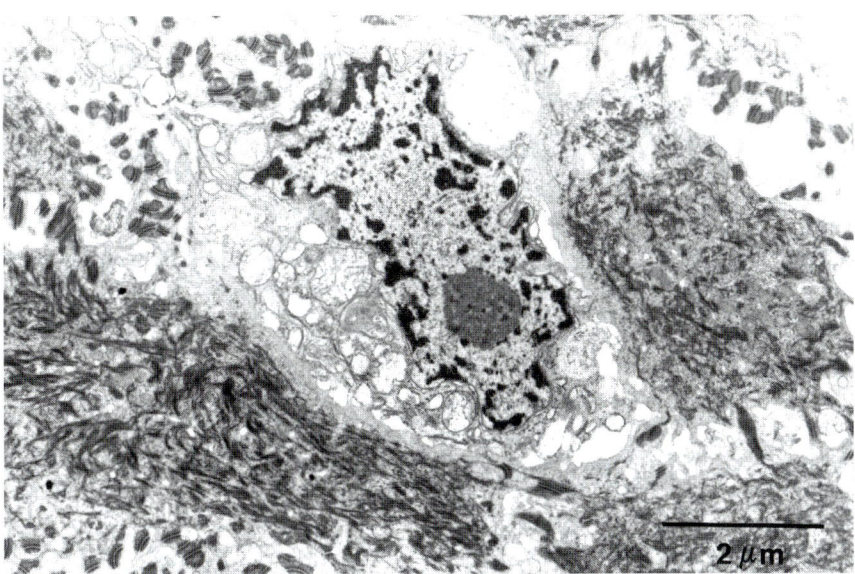

as a contributor to the milieu of inflammatory mediators, through their production and release of cytokines such as interleukin-1 (IL-1) [28]. Morphological evidence, however, certainly points to their participation in ICD, which, within the epidermis, shows variability with respect to time, severity of insult, and the chemical nature of the irritant applied [29]. Table 3 provides a summary of some of the ultrastructural studies in this area, which provide evidence for LC being both activated (Fig. 8) and in a state of degeneration during the evolution of ICD. Earlier beliefs that apposition of LC to mononuclear cells with-

Table 3. A summary of the predominant ultrastructural changes induced in Langerhans cells by acute exposure to selected chemical irritants. These are irritant-, dose-, time- and species-dependent. (*BC* Benzalkonium chloride, *CO* croton oil, *SLS* sodium lauryl sulfate)

Irritant(s)	Langerhans cell changes	Ref.
Mercuric chloride, soap, SLS (human, 24–48 h)	No apposition to mononuclear cells. Glycogen accumulation	[17]
Dithranol, nonanoic acid (human, 6–72 h)	Apposition to mononuclear cells. Ultrastructural evidence of both stimulation and degeneration	[30]
Dithranol (human, 24–48 h)	Fine structural changes in the mitochondria	[31]
BC (human, 3–168 h)	Evidence of both increased metabolic activity (distended endoplasmic reticulum and increased numbers of mitochondria and Birbeck granules) and necrosis (condensed chromatin and shrunken cytoplasm)	[21]
CO, BC, SLS (mice, 1–96 h)	Degenerative changes, with mitochondrial swelling and irregular cytoplasmic vacuolization, followed by membrane disruption and disorganization of the cellular components. With low concentration of CO, prior activation of LC, with increased numbers of mitochondria and enlargement of nuclei	[23]
Six irritants of varying chemical structure (human, 48 h)	Varying numbers of damaged cells displaying vesiculation, loss of integrity of organelles and membranes, condensed nuclear heterochromatin and lipid accumulation. Frequent activated LC, with numerous Birbeck granules in reactions to benzalkonium chloride	[29]

8

Fig. 8.
An activated Langerhans cell containing numerous Birbeck granules and widened rough endoplasmic reticulum, induced by patch testing with benzalkonium chloride (0.5%). Within the same biopsy sample, Langerhans cells displaying degenerative changes were also seen

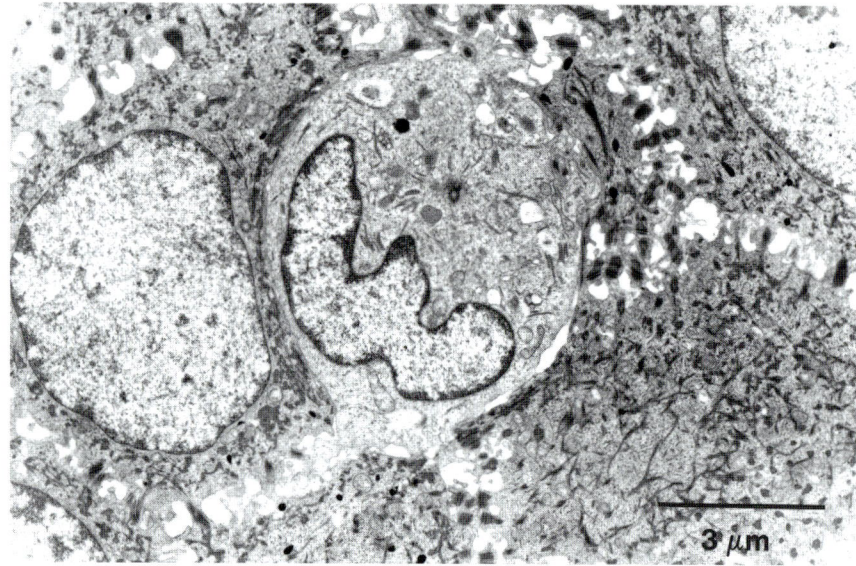

in the epidermis was unique to ACD [17] have now been set aside, following numerous reports of its occurrence also in ICD [31].

> **Core Message**
>
> ■ Langerhans cells within both allergic and irritant patch test reactions show ultrastructural evidence of both activation and degeneration.

8.3 Ultrastructural Changes in the Dermis

Commonly seen changes within the dermis of both ACD and ICD lesions include edema and capillary dilatation, with disruption and degeneration of collagen being an additional feature of some irritant reactions [32]. In their recent light- and electron-microscopic investigation of the effects of a range of chemical irritants on the skin of hairless guinea pigs, Sueki and Kligman [8] observed variations in the dermis that were, to a degree, irritant-dependent. Exposure to SLS and to organic solvents affected the dermis relatively little. In contrast, benzalkonium chloride and various urticariogens and comedogenic agents induced marked dilation of lymphatic vessels, as well as capillaries. Increased numbers of granules within dermal mast cells were also described for the latter irritants, although this was not quantified in any way.

An earlier light and electron microscopy study of hairless mice revealed that many irritant chemicals cause, in addition to the above changes, enlargement or hyperplasia of sebaceous glands, with basal cells displaying morphological signs of enhanced metabolic activity, such as increases in rough endoplasmic reticulum and sebum droplets [33]. Ultrastructural evidence has also led to the belief that platelets lining the dermal venular endothelium during irritant reactions contribute significantly to the pathogenesis of the overall response, at least in mice, being closely linked to the formation of edema [34].

> **Core Message**
>
> ■ Edema and capillary dilatation are commonly described ultrastructural features within the dermis of allergic and irritant patch test reactions.

8.4 Ultrastructural Changes in Chronic Contact Dermatitis

Little information is available regarding the ultrastructural changes associated with chronic contact dermatitis. This is largely because of the difficulty of accurately characterizing the disorder. Most clinical cases of chronic contact dermatitis are attributable to a complex admix of endogenously and exogenously derived provocation factors. Atopy often plays a role and even where sensitization to a relevant hapten is proven, the influence of concomitant irritant exposure is difficult to disentangle. However, recently, Shah and Palmer [35] attempted to document the variations in ultrastructural appearance of chronic occupational hand dermatitis linked to chromate allergy. Examination of a broad spectrum of clinical disease, in terms of intensity and duration, revealed cellular features within the epidermis common to other inflammatory dermatoses. These included marked spongiosis and intracellular vacuolation, particularly within the basal layers. However, the authors also described, for the first time in relation to chromate dermatitis, the presence of spindle-shaped granular cells, possibly mast cells, in the upper dermis, closely opposed to the dermo-epidermal junction.

Core Message

■ More studies of chronic contact dermatitis are required to appreciate more fully the ultrastructural changes which take place.

8.5 Summary

The past two or three decades have seen the publication of a wealth of information on the ultrastructural morphology of acute allergic and irritant contact dermatitis. Much still needs to be learnt, however, about the cellular features of the chronic forms of contact dermatitis. The introduction of modified tissue preparation techniques has greatly improved visualization of the stratum corneum and increased our understanding of the damage caused by topical exposure to chemicals. However, the continued paucity of studies utilizing correlative functional and morphological techniques still limits the extent to which purely electron microscopic findings can be meaningfully translated into pathophysiological events.

References

1. Fartasch M (1997) Ultrastructure of the epidermal barrier after irritation. Microsc Res Tech 37:193–199
2. Warner RR, Boissy YL, Lilly NA, Spears MJ, McKillop K, Marshall JL, Stone KJ (1999) Water disrupts stratum corneum lipid lamellae: damage is similar to surfactants. J Invest Dematol 113:960–966
3. Nagao S, Stroud JD, Hamada T, Pinkus H, Birmingham DJ (1972) The effect of sodium hydroxide and hydrochloric acid on human epidermis. Acta Derm Venereol (Stockh) 52:11–23
4. Lupulescu AP, Birmingham DJ, Pinkus H (1973) An electron microscopic study of human epidermis after acetone and kerosene administration. J Invest Dermatol 60:33–45
5. Willis CM, Stephens CJM, Wilkinson JD (1989) Epidermal damage induced by irritants in man. A light and electron microscopy study. J Invest Dermatol 93:695–700
6. Swanbeck G, Lundquist PG (1972) Ultrastructural changes of mitochondria in dithranol treated psoriatic epidermis. Acta Derm Venereol (Stockh) 52:94–98
7. Molière P, Dubertret L, Sa E, Melo MT, Salet C, Fosse M, Santus R (1985) The effect of anthralin (dithranol) on mitochondria. Br J Dermatol 112:509–515
8. Sueki H, Kligman AM (2003) Cutaneous toxicity of chemical irritants on hairless guinea pigs. J Dermatol 30:859–870
9. Metz J (1972) Elecktronenmikroskopische Untersuchungen an allergischen und toxischen Epicutantestreaktionen des Menschen. Arch Derm Forsch 245:125–146
10. Tovell PWA, Weaver AC, Hope J, Sprott WE (1974) The action of sodium lauryl sulphate on rat skin – an ultrastructural study. Br J Dermatol 90:501–506
11. Lindberg M, Forslind B, Wahlberg JE (1982) Reactions of epidermal keratinocytes in sensitized and non-sensitized guinea pigs after dichromate exposure: an electron microscopic study. Acta Derm Venereol (Stockh) 62:389–396
12. Kanerva L (1990) Electron microscopic observations of dyskeratosis, apoptosis, colloid bodies and fibrillar degeneration after skin irritation with dithranol. J Cutan Pathol 17:37–44
13. Forsey RJ, Shahidullah H, Sands C, McVittie E, Aldridge RD, Hunter JA, Howie SE (1998) Epidermal Langerhans cell apoptosis is induced in vivo by nonanoic acid but not by sodium lauryl sulphate. Br J Dermatol 139:453–461
14. Komura J, Ofuji S (1980) Ultrastructural studies of allergic contact dermatitis in man. Arch Dermatol Res 267:275–282
15. Forslind B, Wahlberg JE (1978) The morphology of chromium allergic skin reactions at electron microscopic resolution: studies in man and guinea pig. Acta Derm Venereol Suppl (Stockh) 79:43–51
16. Cumberbatch M, Dearman RJ, Griffiths CE, Kimber I (2003) Epidermal Langerhans cell migration and sensitisation to chemical allergens. APMIS 111:797–804
17. Silberberg I (1973) Apposition of mononuclear cells to Langerhans cells in contact allergic reactions. An ultrastructural study. Acta Derm Venereol (Stockh) 53:1–12
18. Hunziker N, Winkelman RK (1978) Langerhans cells in contact dermatitis of the guinea pig. Arch Dermatol 114:1309–1313
19. Falck B, Andersson A, Elofsson R, Sjöborg S (1981) New views on epidermis and its Langerhans cells in the normal state and in contact dermatitis. Acta Derm Venereol Suppl (Stockh) 99:3–27
20. Bian Z, Bing-He W (1985) Cytochemical and ultrastructural studies of the Langerhans cells. Int J Dermatol 24:653–659
21. Willis CM, Young E, Brandon DR, Wilkinson JD (1986) Immunopathological and ultrastructural findings in human allergic and irritant contact dermatitis. Br J Dermatol 115:305–316
22. Giannotti B, de Panfilis G, Manara GC (1986) Langerhans cells are not damaged in contact allergic reactions in humans. Am J Dermatopathol 8:220–226
23. Kolde G, Knop J (1987) Different cellular reaction patterns of epidermal Langerhans cells after application of contact sensitizing, toxic, and tolerogenic compounds. A comparative ultrastructural and morphometric time-course analysis. J Invest Dermatol 89:19–23

8

24. Hanau D, Fabre M, Schmitt DA (1989) ATPase and morphologic changes in Langerhans cells induced by epicutaneous application of a sensitizing dose of DNFB. J Invest Dermatol 92(5):689–694

25. Mommaas AM, Wijsman MC, Mulder AA, van Praag MC, Vermeer BJ, Koning F (1992) HLA class II expression on human epidermal Langerhans cells in situ: upregulation during elicitation of allergic contact dermatitis. Hum Immunol 34:99–106

26. Kolde G (1996) Turnover and kinetics of epidermal Langerhans cells and their dendritic precursor cells in experimental contact dermatitis. Arch Dermatol Res 288:197–202

27. Rizova H, Carayon P, Barbier A, Lacheretz F, Dubertret L, Michel L (1999) Contact allergens, but not irritants, alter receptor-mediated endocytosis by human epidermal Langerhans cells. Br J Dermatol 140:200–209

28. Kimber I (1999) Contact sensitisation mechanisms. In: Basketter DA (ed) Toxicology of contact dermatitis; allergy, irritancy and urticaria. Wiley, Chichester, chap 5

29. Willis CM, Stephens CJM, Wilkinson JD (1990) Differential effects of structurally-unrelated chemical irritants on the density and morphology of epidermal CD1a+ cells. J Invest Dermatol 95:711–716

30. Kanerva L, Ranki A, Mustakallio K, Lauharanta J (1983) Langerhans cell-mononuclear cell contacts are not specific for allergy in patch tests. Br J Dermatol 109 [Suppl 25]:64–67

31. Kanerva L, Ranki A, Lauharanta J (1984) Lymphocytes and Langerhans cells in patch tests. Contact Dermatitis 11:150–155

32. Willis CM (1995) The histopathology of irritant contact dermatitis. In: Van der Valk PGM, Maibach HI (eds) The irritant contact dermatitis syndrome. CRC, Boca Raton, Fla., pp 297–298

33. Lesnik RH, Kligman LH, Kligman AM (1992) Agents that cause enlargement of sebaceous glands in hairless mice. I. Topical substances. Arch Dermatol 284:100–105

34. Senaldi G, Piguet P-F (1997) Platelets play a role in the pathogenesis of the irritant reaction in mice. J Invest Dermatol 108:248–252

35. Shuh M, Palmer IR (2002) An ultrastructural study of chronic chromate hand dermatitis. Acta Derm Venereol (Stockh) 82:254–259

Chapter 9

Individual Predisposition to Irritant and Allergic Contact Dermatitis

9

Tove Agner, Torkil Menné

Contents

9.1 Introduction

Contact dermatitis is a skin disease that is either caused or exaggerated by environmental factors. However, development of contact dermatitis requires the combination of environmental factors and a susceptible host. While some individuals may develop contact dermatitis after only brief contact with irritants or allergens, other individuals may continue to remain unaffected even under extreme exogenous conditions. This chapter will focus on the susceptibility of the host to the development of irritant and/or allergic contact dermatitis.

9.2 Irritant Contact Dermatitis

Irritant contact dermatitis is a complex disease, with a multifactorial pathogenesis, to which individual as well as environmental factors contribute. Within the individual, the response to irritant stimuli depends on the skin barrier function, the inflammatory reactivity of the skin and – addressing chronic irritant contact dermatitis – its regeneration ability. Individual-related variables that influence these factors, and attempts to identify "sensitive skin," will be discussed in the following.

9.2.1 Can "Sensitive Skin" Be Identified?

9.2.1.1 Sensitive Skin

Exposed to the same exogenous conditions some individuals develop an irritant eczema while others do not. The group that develops eczema may be expected to have increased skin susceptibility or increased skin reactivity compared to the rest. Whether the concept of "sensitive skin" in fact exists has been debated. In his pioneering study of primary irritants, Björnberg found no correlation between the intensity evoked by 11 different primary irritants, and stated that the response to one particular irritant does not necessarily predict the response to another irritant [1]. This statement was supported by later studies [2, 3]. However, Frosch and Kligman [4] reported a statistically significant correlation between the skin response to particular irritants, and a group of individuals with sensitive skin could be identified by assessment of skin susceptibility to skin test with seven different irritants and assessment of minimal erythema dose (MED) [5]. For preselection of hyper-reactors, Frosch and Kligman [6] for practical reasons

9

used a 24-h forearm chamber exposure to 5% sodium lauryl sulfate (SLS).

The contradiction between reports that no correlation between irritant responses exists and that hyper-reactors can be identified may be specifically explained by choice of irritants, dose, test region, and test method. The different penetration abilities of particular irritants may account for discrepancies in the intensity of the evoked skin response. Use of high doses of irritants, eliciting severe reactions, may tend to equalize skin responses. Regional variation also exists [7].

9.2.1.2 Skin Irritancy Test

The identification of subjects with increased susceptibility to irritants would play an important role in the prevention of irritant contact dermatitis. Based on the original alkali test by Burckhardt [8], numerous pre-employment tests have been suggested [9–11]. However, reproducibility of the screening methods is low and the inter-individual variation high, and none of the tests has hitherto been found satisfactory for the purpose of pre-employment tests for sensitive skin.

9.2.1.3 Noninvasive Measuring Methods for Identification of Sensitive Skin

A number of noninvasive bioengineering methods have been used in an attempt to evaluate the biophysical properties of skin.

Experimental data, mainly based on SLS-induced skin irritation, indicate that measurement of baseline transepidermal water loss (TEWL) may be helpful for identification of sensitive skin. Tupker et al. [12] studied the role of baseline TEWL in skin susceptibility to weak irritants in healthy volunteers and found that barrier damage and inflammation evoked by the irritants were strongly related to baseline TEWL. In a group of 70 nonatopic healthy volunteers challenged with SLS, baseline TEWL was found to contribute significantly to a multiple regression analysis model using TEWL after exposure as the dependent variable [13], and, in the same study, subjects with high visual scores after SLS exposure had increased baseline TEWL compared with those who had low visual scores. Only a few studies have utilized individual baseline TEWL values for prediction of risk of irritant contact dermatitis. Repetitive measurements of baseline TEWL in workers in the metal industry in Singapore indicated that high TEWL values obtained

from the back of the hands may predict later development of irritant contact dermatitis [14]. This finding was supported by a recent study of apprentice hairdressers and apprentice nurses, reporting a trend toward a relationship between increased baseline TEWL and risk of hand dermatitis [15]. Findings were however not statistically significant. This indicates that baseline TEWL is only one of a number of factors influencing skin susceptibility, and the particular significance of this parameter may be overruled by other factors. Recently, the irritant threshold for an SLS patch test applied for 4 h was illustrated to correlate well with TEWL values obtained from SLS-irritated skin, indicating that the irritant threshold technique may be helpful in predicting the development of occupational contact dermatitis [16].

Attempts to identify sensitive skin have also been performed by other bioengineering methods. Measurements of skin hydration by electrical capacitance and electrical conductance measurements are generally considered of limited value as indicators of sensitive skin [17]. Measurement of skin color has been reported to be helpful in the evaluation of skin sensitivity to irritants [13, 18], but intermittent exposure to UV light may interfere with the accuracy of measurements. Biophysical properties such as pH values, skin lipids, and skin thickness as measured by ultrasound need further investigation with respect to their usefulness as indicators of sensitive skin [16]. Today, none of the bioengineering methods can by themselves identify sensitive skin. Further studies using varying experimental designs are necessary, and final conclusions depend on large-scale epidemiological studies.

9.2.2 Individual-Related Variation in Skin Susceptibility

9.2.2.1 Genetic Factors

Apart from the relationship between atopic dermatitis and development of irritant contact dermatitis, which is discussed below, the knowledge of influence of genetic factors is sparse, and systematic studies in this field are few. Holst and Möller studied the cutaneous sensitivity to benzalkonium chloride, SLS, and potash soap in twins [19]. Comparing the intra-pair reaction strength a higher degree of concordance was found among monozygotic than among dizygotic twins for one irritant, but not for all irritants tested. This indicates that a genetic predisposition to irritant susceptibility may be specific for each irritant (Table 1). In a recent questionnaire investigation in-

Table 1. Influence of individual related factors on skin reactivity to irritants and allergens

	Reactivity to irritants	Reactivity to allergens
Genetic factors	Yes	?
Sex	No	?
Age	Yes	?
Ethnic factors	?	?
Regional differences	Yes	Yes
Atopic dermatitis	Yes	?
Medication	Yes	Yes

cluding 6666 twins, hereditary risk factors were found to play a significant part in the development of hand eczema in the general population, when no extreme environmental exposure was present [20]. A subsample of the same twin material was studied with regard to contact allergy, atopic dermatitis and wet work, and the results indicated that a hitherto unrecognized genetic risk factor for hand eczema independent of atopic dermatitis and contact allergy is important for development of irritant contact dermatitis localized on the hands [21].

9.2.2.2 Sex

Hand eczema and contact dermatitis are known to occur more frequently in women than in men [22, 23]. This may, however, very well reflect differences in environmental hazards rather than endogenous differences between the sexes. Results from the above-mentioned twin study indicated that the high frequency of hand eczema in women in comparison with men was caused by environmental and not genetic factors [21].

Most experimental investigations have found no sex-relation in skin susceptibility [13, 24, 25].

Hormonal influence on skin reactivity in relation to the menstrual cycle has been discussed. Increased skin reactivity prior to and during the menstrual phase was initially reported by Halter in 1941 [26], and was supported by later casuistic reports [27, 28]. In an experimental study, skin reactivity to SLS was found to be significantly increased at day 1 in the menstrual cycle as compared to days 9–11 in non-menstruating women [29]. No cyclic variation in baseline TEWL has been reported. In experimental settings and in attempts of predictive patch testing, the influence of menstrual cycle on skin reactivity may be of some importance, but the clinical implication of the finding is uncertain.

9.2.2.3 Age

Increased susceptibility to irritants in childhood has been reported [30], as well as an increased susceptibility to SLS in young compared to elderly females [31]. Irritation, however, seemed to be more prolonged in the older group [32], indicating less skin reactivity but a prolonged healing period in older people. Barrier properties in aged skin (>80 years of age) were recently studied [33], and an abnormal barrier integrity and repair function as compared to young skin (20–30 years) was reported. These abnormalities were attributed to a deficiency in key stratum corneum lipids in old age.

9.2.2.4 Ethnic Factors

An inclination toward increased skin susceptibility to SLS in black and Hispanic skin was reported [34, 35], but a statistically significant difference was found only for particular concentrations of the irritant, and only when tested on pre-occluded skin. Decreased transcutaneous penetration was reported in black persons.

9.2.2.5 Regional Differences

Susceptibility to irritants differs between anatomical regions. In most studies skin susceptibility to irritants is ranked as extremities < back < forehead [36, 37]. Baseline TEWL with respect to anatomical sites can be ranked as back = abdomen = arm < dorsum of hand < forehead < palm [38]. However, a linear relationship between TEWL and skin reactivity to exogenous substances cannot be generalized, neither to all anatomical sites nor to every substance.

9.2.2.6 Atopy

The significance of a history of atopic dermatitis for the development of irritant hand eczema has been comprehensively demonstrated [21, 39, 40]. In experimental studies baseline TEWL has been reported to be increased in uninvolved skin in patients with atopic dermatitis [41–43], and patients with atopic dermatitis were reported to react more severely to irritants than healthy controls [43, 44]. The characteristic functional abnormalities as found in atopic dermatitis were not found in baseline conditions or after irritant exposure [45] in patients with respiratory atopy without atopic dermatitis.

9

9.2.2.7 Coincidental Diseases (Other Than Atopy)

In a recent study, the ability of individuals who perceive stinging to experience irritant reactions in the skin was examined. It was concluded that the ability to perceive stinging is not correlated to irritant susceptibility or other types of nonimmunological skin responses [46].

Hyper-reactive skin with an exaggerated response to irritants has been proven in patients with current active eczema [18, 23]. Hyporeactive skin with a decreased response to irritants was reported in patients with severe cancer [47].

9.2.2.8 Medication

Cortisol treatment is known to reduce skin responsiveness to irritants [48]. The influence of other drugs has not been thoroughly studied.

> **Core Message**
>
> ■ ICD is a complex disease, to which individual as well as environmental factors contribute.
> Atopic dermatitis (previous or current) is a major individual risk factor for development of ICD.

9.3 Allergic Contact Dermatitis

The development of contact allergy is dependent on individual susceptibility and exposure to potential allergens (Table 1).

9.3.1 Individual Predisposition to Contact Sensitization

9.3.1.1 Genetic Factors

Sulzberger and co-workers [49, 50] in human sensitization experiments with p-nitroso-dimethylaniline (NDMA) and 2,4-dinitrochlorobenzene (DNCB) established an individual variation in susceptibility to contact sensitization, and further showed that individuals who were highly susceptible to sensitization with one chemical showed little or no susceptibility to sensitization with other chemicals. More recent studies suggest that individual susceptibility occurs by a non-antigen-specific amplification of immune sensitization [51].

Twin studies on allergic contact sensitization are sparse. In a twin study of reactivity to DNCB and tuberculin no difference in concordance rate for dizygotic and monozygotic twins was reported [52]. Contradicting this, a study of nickel allergy in twins suggested that genetic influence over contact sensitization to nickel is likely [53]. In a recent Danish study including 630 female twins of whom 146 had a positive patch test to nickel, it was concluded that allergic nickel contact dermatitis is caused mainly by environmental factors and only to a lesser degree by genetic factors [54].

Numerous studies of the HLA genes in contact sensitization have not disclosed any consistent pattern [55]. The lack of association between the HLA genes and contact sensitization does not exclude the importance of genetic factors. Hitherto unknown HLA genes may be associated with allergic contact dermatitis, there may be heterogeneity in allergic contact dermatitis, and/or allergic contact dermatitis may not be associated or linked to the HLA region.

In conclusion, it seems that some individuals are more easily sensitized than others to common haptens due to their genetic background, but the total number of sensitized individuals in the population depends upon the degree of cutaneous exposure.

9.3.1.2 Sex

Women have higher immunoglobulin levels (IgM and IgG) than men, and stronger cell-mediated immune responses [56]. Both in animal studies and in humans, there is a preponderance of autoimmune disease in women compared to men.

Walker et al. [57], however, found that men are more susceptible to DNCB sensitization compared to women in a large well-controlled study. A similar study on patch sensitization to p-amino-diphenylamine and isopropyl-p-diphenylamine disclosed a significantly increased number of women sensitized as compared to men [58]. The authors suggest that women, through more frequent contact with para substances than men, may achieve subclinical sensitization. Rees et al. [59] report an increased reactivity to challenge with DNCB in DNCB-sensitized women compared to DNCB-sensitized men.

The main reason for female preponderance in clinical patch test studies is the high number of nickel- and cobalt-sensitive women. This is most likely a consequence of different exposure, with ear piercing the main risk factor for nickel allergy in women. A recent study of nickel allergy in men with pierced ears confirmed the role of ear piercing as a risk factor for nickel sensitization also in men, but the frequency of nickel allergy in men with pierced ears was lower than the frequency reported in women [60].

The influence of sex hormones on induction and elicitation of contact allergy is largely unknown. In a pilot study the response to DNCB was enhanced in women receiving oral contraceptive hormones [61] and a preliminary report indicates that the cutaneous reactivity to patch testing differs within the menstrual cycle [27]. The limited knowledge in this field is inconclusive, and deserves further systematic evaluation [62].

9.3.1.3 Age

The exposure pattern to environmental allergens differs between age groups. The most frequently recognized contact allergies in children are thiomersal, nickel, fragrance mix, and isothiazolinones [63] – and, in the United States, poison ivy and poison oak. Young people are more exposed to industrial and cosmetic chemicals than the elderly, who are more exposed to topical medicaments. The elderly may have one or more contact allergies reflecting exposure 30–40 years earlier, with the positive patch test being of historical interest only. Prevalence of contact allergy would be expected to increase with increasing age. In a recent study including 1501 8th-grade schoolchildren, as much as 15% were reported to have one or more positive patch tests [64]. In epidemiological studies of contact allergy, age is therefore an important confounder, which should be handled adequately, for example by stratification or multivariate analysis. Loss of sensitivity over the years – or reduction of the contact allergy to below a clinically relevant threshold – has been debated [65], and figures such as 20% to 50% have been suggested. However, these studies have not considered a possible overestimation of contact allergies in the primary studies due to excited skin syndrome.

9.3.1.4 Ethnic Factors

In an experimental study from 1966, black people were found to be less susceptible to contact sensitization with poison ivy and DNCB compared to white [66]. Newer data are not available.

9.3.1.5 Regional Differences

As mentioned above, exposure to allergens and ability of the allergens to penetrate the epidermis are essential factors for contact sensitization. These factors are influenced by regional variation. Sensitization is increased by traumatizing the skin, and skin exposed to irritants, for example on the hands, may often be traumatized. The barrier abilities of stratum corneum change from one region to another, as reflected by differences in TEWL values [38], and penetration abilities for different allergens may likewise change.

Occlusion promotes percutaneous penetration, and contributes to sensitization from topical medications in stasis dermatitis and perianal eczema.

Reactivity to diagnostic patch testing differs greatly according to anatomical site. Skin responsiveness is more pronounced on the back than on the arms and thighs, and only the upper back is recommended for routine diagnostic patch testing.

9.3.1.6 Atopy

Atopics downregulate Th1 cells, which explains their tendency to severe viral infections, particularly with herpes simplex [67]. Because of this Th1-cell downregulation, a decreased propensity to contact dermatitis is expected. Clinical studies addressing this problem are contradictory, but most find a decreased tendency to contact sensitization [68–71]. Some studies suggest that especially patients with severe atopic dermatitis have a decreased ability to develop contact allergies [72, 73]. In a population-based study no correlation, either positive or negative, was found between the presence of a positive patch test and IgE sensitivity [74]. Respiratory symptoms may also be of importance, and different subgroups of atopic patients with respect to contact sensitization may exist.

Another possible bias is the increased number of irritant patch test results in atopic patients, especially when testing metals, e.g., nickel, cobalt, and chromate [75]. Recent studies do, however, indicate that atopics seem to have an increased frequency of nickel sensitization [76]. Because of these uncertainties, patch test results should specify the number of patients included with atopy.

9.3.1.7 Coincidental Diseases (Other Than Atopy)

Patients with acute or debilitating diseases such as cancer (Hodgkin's disease and lymphoma) have impaired capacity for contact sensitization [47]. Patients with psoriasis are generally considered to have fewer contact allergies than others, but, due to the intensive treatment of psoriasis patients with topical agents, this impression may not be correct [77].

9.3.1.8 Medication

It is a general clinical experience that systemic prednisolone in a dose exceeding 15 mg/day may diminish or suppress allergic patch test reactions, as may topical corticoid treatment. Antihistamines and disodium cromoglycate do not seem to significantly influence the allergic contact dermatitis reaction. The influence of azathioprine and nonsteroidal anti-inflammatory drugs on the outcome of patch test reactions is unexplored.

Exposure to ultraviolet light, especially UVB [78, 79] and PUVA [80, 81], may reduce risk of sensitization and temporarily diminish the ability to elicit allergic reactions in sensitized individuals.

Suggested Reading

Björnberg A (1968) Skin reactions to primary irritants in patients with hand eczema. Isacson, Göteborg
Rystedt I (1985) Factors influencing the occurrence of hand eczema in adults with a history of atopic dermatitis in childhood. Contact Dermatitis 12:185–191
The thesis by Björnberg from 1968 was chosen as a classical reference, since the knowledge today about irritants and skin irritancy testing is still dependent on the results from this great work.

The epidemiological studies performed by Rystedt in the 1980s are still of current interest, and are the basis for the advice that we give today to atopic patients to prevent development of ICD.

References

1. Björnberg A (1968) Skin reactions to primary irritants in patients with hand eczema. Isacson, Göteborg
2. Coenraads PJ, Bleumik E, Nater JP (1975) Susceptibility to primary irritants. Contact Dermatitis 1:377–381
3. Wahlberg JE, Wrangsjö K, Hietasalo A (1985) Skin irritancy from nonanoic acid. Contact Dermatitis 13:266–269
4. Frosch PJ, Kligman AM (1982) Recognition of chemically vulnerable and delicate skin. In: Frost P, Horwitz S (eds) Principles of cosmetics for the dermatologist. Mosby, St Louis, Mo., pp 287–296
5. Frosch PJ, Wissing C (1982) Cutaneous sensitivity to ultraviolet light and chemical irritants. Arch Dermatol Res 272: 269–278
6. Frosch PJ, Kligman AM (1979) The soap chamber test. J Am Acad Dermatol 1:35–41
7. Flannigan SA, Smith RE, McGovern JP (1984) Intraregional variation between contact irritant patch test sites. Contact Dermatitis 10:123–124
8. Burkkhardt W (1947) Neure Untersuchungen bei die Alkali-empfindlichkeit der Haut. Dermatologica 94:73–96
9. Iliev D, Hinnen U, Elsner P (1997) Reproducibility of a non-invasive skin irritancy test in a cohort of metalworker trainees. Contact Dermatitis 36:101–103
10. Hinnen U, Elsner P, Burg G (1995) Assessment of skin irritancy by 2 short tests compared to acute irritation induced by sodium lauryl sulfate. Contact Dermatitis 33:236–239
11. Loffler H, Effendy I, Happle R (1996) The sodium lauryl sulfate test. A noninvasive functional evaluation of skin hypersensitivity. Hautarzt 47:832–838
12. Tupker RA, Coenraads PJ, Pinnagoda J, Nater JP (1989) Baseline transepidermal water loss (TEWL) as a prediction of susceptibility to sodium lauryl sulfate. Contact Dermatitis 20:265–269
13. Agner T (1992) Noninvasive measuring methods in the investigation of irritant patch test reactions. A study of patients with hand eczema, atopic dermatitis and controls. Acta Derm Venereol (Stockh) [Suppl] 177:44–46
14. Coenraads PJ, Lee J, Pinnagoda J (1986) Changes in water vapour loss from the skin of metal industry workers monitored during exposure to oils. Scand J Work Environ Health 12:494–498
15. Smit HA, van Rijssen A, Vandenbroucke JP, Coenraads PJ (1994) Susceptibility to and incidence of hand dermatitis in a cohort of apprentice hairdressers and nurses. Scand J Work Environ Health 20:113–121
16. Smith HR, Rowson M, Basketter DA, McFadden JP (2004) Intra-individual variation of irritant threshold and relationsship to transepidermal water loss measurement of skin irritation. Contact Dermatitis 51:26–29
17. Wilhelm KP, Maibach HI (1990) Factors predisposing to cutaneous irritation. Dermatol Clin 8:17–22
18. Agner T (1991) Skin susceptibility in uninvolved skin of hand eczema patients and healthy controls. Br J Dermatol 125:140–146
19. Holst R, Möller H (1975) One hundred twin pairs patch tested with primary irritants. Br J Dermatol 93:145–149
20. Bryld LE, Agner T, Kyvik KO, Brondsted L, Hindsberger C, Menné T (2000) Hand eczema in twins: a questionnaire investigation. Br J Dermatol 142:298–305
21. Bryld LE, Hindsberger C, Kyvik KO, Agner T, Menné T (2003) Risk factors influencing the development of hand eczema in a population-based twin sample. Br J Dermatol 149:1214–1220
22. Rystedt I (1985) Factors influencing the occurrence of hand eczema in adults with a history of atopic dermatitis in childhood. Contact Dermatitis 12:185–191
23. Meding B, Swanbeck G (1989) Epidemiology of different types of hand eczema in an industrial city. Acta Derm Venereol (Stockh) 69:227–233
24. Björnberg A (1975) Skin reactionsto primary irritants in men and women. Acta Derm Venereol (Stockh) 55:191–196
25. Tupker RA, Coenraads PJ, Pinnagoda J, Nater JP (1989) Baseline transepidermal water loss (TEWL) as a prediction of susceptibility to sodium lauryl sulfate. Contact Dermatitis 20:265–269
26. Halter K (1941) Zur Pathogenese des Ekzems. Arch Derm U Syph 181:593–719
27. Alexander S (1988) Patch testing and menstruation. Lancet i:751
28. Kemmet D (1989) Premenstrual exacerbation of atopic dermatitis. Br J Dermatol 120:715

29. Agner T, Damm P, Skouby SO (1991) Menstrual cycle and skin reactivity. J Am Acad Dermatol 24:566–570
30. Frosch JP (1985) Hautirritation und empfindliche Haut. Grosse, Berlin
31. Wilhelm KP, Cua AB, Maibach HI (1991) Skin aging. Effect on transepidermal water loss, stratum corneum hydration, skin surface pH, and casual sebum content. Arch Dermatol 127:1806–1809
32. Patil S, Maibach HI (1994) Effect of age and sex on the elicitation of irritant contact dermatitis. Contact Dermatitis 30:257–264
33. Ghadially R, Brown BE, Sequeira-Martin SM, Feingold KR, Elias PM (1995) The aged epidermal permeability barrier. Structural, functional, and lipid biochemical abnormalities in humans and a senescent murine model. J Clin Invest 95:2281–2290
34. Berardesca E, Maibach HI (1988) Racial differences in sodium lauryl sulfate induced cutaneous irritation: black and white. Contact Dermatitis 18:65–69
35. Berardesca E, Maibach HI (1988) Sodium lauryl sulfate induced cutaneous irritation. Comparison of white and Hispanic subjects. Contact Dermatitis 19:136–140
36. Frosch PJ, Kligman AM (1977) Rapid blister formation in human skin with ammonium hydroxide. Br J Dermatol 96:461–473
37. Frosch PJ, Duncan S, Kligman AM (1980) Cutaneous biometrics I. The response of human skin to dimethyl sulphoxide. Br J Dermatol 102:263–274
38. Pinnagoda J, Tupker R, Agner T, Serup J (1990) Guidelines for transepidermal water loss (TEWL) measurement. A report from the standardization group of the European Contact Dermatitis Society. Contact Dermatitis 22:164–178
39. Rystedt I (1985) Work-related hand eczema in atopics. Contact Dermatitis 12:164–171
40. Nilsson E, Bäck O (1986) The importance of anamnestic information of atopy, metal dermatitis and earlier hand eczema for the development of hand eczema in women in wet hospital work. Acta Derm Venereol (Stockh) 66:45–50
41. Werner Y, Lindberg M (1985) Transepidermal water loss in dry and clinically normal skin in patients with atopic dermatitis. Acta Derm Venereol (Stockh) 65:102–105
42. Tupker RA, Pinnagoda J, Coenraads PJ, Nater JP (1990) Susceptibility to irritants: role of barrier function, skin dryness and history of atopic dermatitis. Br J Dermatol 123:199–205
43. Agner T (1991) Susceptibility of atopic dermatitis patients to irritant dermatitis caused by sodium lauryl sulfate. Acta Derm Venereol (Stockh) 71:296–300
44. Van der Valk PGM, Vries MHK, Nater JP, Bleumink E, de Jong MCJM (1985) Eczematous reactions of the skin and barrier function as determined by water vapour loss. Clin Exp Dermatol 10:98–103
45. Seidenari S, Belletti B, Schiavi ME (1996) Skin reactivity to sodium lauryl sulfate in patients with respiratory atopy. J Am Acad Dermatol 35:47–52
46. Coverly J, Peters L, Whittle E, Basketter DA (1998) Susceptibility to stinging, nonimmunologic contact urticaria and acute skin irritation, is there a relationship? Contact Dermatitis 38:90–95
47. Johnson MW, Maibach HI, Salmon SE (1971) Skin reactivity in patients with cancer. N Engl J Med 284:1255–1256
48. Roper S, Jones HE (1982) A new look at conditioned hyper-irritability. J Am Acad Dermatol 7:643–650
49. Sulzberger MB, Rostenberg A (1939) Acquired specific hypersensitivity (allergy) to simple chemicals. J Immunol 36:17–27
50. Landsteiner K, Rostenberg A, Sulzberger MB (1939) Individual differences in susceptibility to eczematous sensitization with simple chemical substances. J Invest Dermatol 2:25–29
51. Moss C, Friedmann PS, Shuster S, Simpson JM (1985) Susceptibility and amplification of sensitivity in contact dermatitis. Clin Exp Immunol 61:232–241
52. Forsbeck M, Skog E, Ytterborn KH (1968) Delayed type of allergy and atopic disease among twins. Acta Derm Venereol (Stockh) 48:192–197
53. Menné T, Holm NV (1983) Nickel allergy in a female twin population. Int J Dermatol 22:22–28
54. Bryld LE, Hindsberger C, Kyvik KO, Agner T, Menné T (2004). Genetic factors in nickel allergy evaluated in a population based female twin sample. J Invest Dermatol 123:1025–1029
55. Menné T, Holm NV (1986) Genetic susceptibility in human allergic contact sensitization. Semin Dermatol 5:301–306
56. Ansar Ahmed S, Penhale WJ, Talal N (1985) Sex hormones, immune responses and autoimmune diseases. Am J Pathol 121:531–551
57. Walker FB, Smith PD, Maibach HI (1967) Genetic factors in human allergic contact dermatitis. Int Arch Allergy 32:453–462
58. Schønning L, Hjorth N (1969) Sex difference in capacity for sensitization. Contact Dermatitis 5:100
59. Rees Jl, Friedmann PS, Matthews JNS (1989) Sex differences in susceptibility to development of contact sensitization to DNCB. Br J Dermatol 120:371–374
60. Meijer C, Bredberg M, Fischer T, Widström L (1995) Ear piercing and nickel and cobalt sensitization, in 520 young Swedish men doing compulsory military service. Contact Dermatitis 32:147–149
61. Rea TH (1979) Quantitative enhancement of DNCB responsivity in women receiving oral contraceptives. Arch Dermatol 115:361–362
62. Modjtahedi BS, Modjtahedi SP, Maibach HI (2004) The sex of the individual as a factor in allergic contact dermatitis. Contact Dermatitis 50:53–59
63. Manzini BM, Ferdani G, Simonetti V, Donini M, Seidenari S (1998) Contact sensitization in children. Pediatr Dermatol 15:12–17
64. Mortz CG, Lauritsen JM, Bindslev-Jensen C, Andersen KE (2001) Prevalence of atopic dermatitis, asthma, allergic rhinitis, and hand and contact dermatitis in adolescents. The Odense adolescence cohort study on atopic diseases and dermatitis. Br J Dermatol 144:523–532
65. Valsecchi R, Rossi A, Bigardi A, Pigatto PD (1991) The loss of contact sensitization in man. Contact Dermatitis 24:183–186
66. Kligman AM (1966) The identification of contact allergens by human assay. II. Factors influencing the induction and measurements of allergic contact dermatitis. J Invest Dermatol 47:375–392
67. Bos JO, Wierenga EA, Smitt JHS, van der Heijden FL, Kaspenberg ML (1992) Immune dysregulation in atopic eczema. Arch Dermatol 128:1509–1512
68. Christoffersen J, Menné T, Tanghøj P, Andersen KE, Brandrup F, Kaaber K, Osmundsen PE, Thestrup-Pedersen K, Veien NK (1989) Clinical patch test data evaluated by multivariate analysis. Contact Dermatitis 5:291–300
69. Cronin E, Bandmann HJ, Calnan CD, Fregert S, Hjorth N, Magnusson B, Maibach HI, Malten K, Meneghini CL, Pirilä V, Wilkinson DS (1970) Contact dermatitis in the atopics. Acta Derm Venereol (Stockh) 50:1983–1987
70. Marghescu S (1985) Patch test reactions in atopic dermatitis. Acta Derm Venereol (Stockh) 114:113–116

71. De Groot AC (1990) The frequency of contact allergies in atopic patients with dermatitis. Contact Dermatitis 22: 273–277

72. Uehara M, Sawai T (1989) A longitudinal study of contact sensitivity in patients with atopic dermatitis. Arch Dermatol 125:366–368

73. Rystedt I (1985) Contact sensitivity in adults with atopic dermatitis in childhood. Contact Dermatitis 13:1–8

74. Nielsen NH, Menné T (1996) The relationship between IgE-mediated and cell-mediated hypersensitivities in an unselected Danish population: the Glostrup Allergy Study, Denmark. Br J Dermatol 134:669–672

75. Møller H, Svensson Å (1986) Metal sensitivity: positive history but negative test indicates atopy. Contact Dermatitis 14:57–60

76. Diepgen TL, Fartasc M, Hornstein OP (1989) Evaluation and relevance of atopic basic and minor features in patients with atopic dermatitis and in the general population. Acta Derm Venereol (Stockh) [Suppl] 144:50–54

77. Clark AR, Schwartz EF (1998) The incidence of allergic contact dermatitis in patients with psoriasis vulgaris. Am J Contact Dermat 9:96–99

78. Lauerma Al, Maibach HI; Granlaund H, Erkko P, Kartamaa M, Stubb S (1992) Inhibition of contact allergy reactions by topical FK506. Lancet 340:556

79. Cooper KD, Oberhelman L, Hamilton TA, Baadsgaard O, Terhune M, LeVee G, Anderson T, Koren H (1992) UV exposure reduces immunization rates and promotes tolerance to epicutaneous antigens in humans: relationship to dose, CD1a-DR+ epidermal macrophage induction, and Langerhans cell depletion. Proc Natl Acad Sci USA 15:89: 8497–8501

80. Skov L, Hansen H, Barker JN, Simon JC, Baadsgaard O (1997) Contrasting effects of ultraviolet-A and ultraviolet-B exposure on induction of contact sensitivity in human skin. Clin Exp Immunol 107:585–588

81. Thorvaldsen J, Volden G (1980) PUVA-induced diminution of contact allergic and irritant skin reactions. Clin Exp Dermatol 5:43–46

9

Chapter 10

Epidemiology

10

Pieter-Jan Coenraads, Thomas Diepgen, Wolfgang Uter,
Axel Schnuch, Olaf Gefeller

Contents

10.1 Basic Concepts of Population-based Epidemiology

Pieter-Jan Coenraads, Thomas Diepgen

10.1.1 Introduction

Contact dermatitis is a common disorder. Epidemiology is a tool to be used for appropriate summary measures to describe how common contact dermatitis is. Epidemiology is also used to analyze whether it is more common in specific groups, and which factors are associated with the occurrence of contact dermatitis (or its subtypes) in specific populations or subgroups. Typical questions are, for example, whether nickel allergy is more common in hairdressers, and whether this contact allergy enhances the risk of occupational contact dermatitis. A classic example is the occurrence of nickel allergy in Danish women [34]. Epidemiologic tools are also used to evaluate the results of interventions in specific populations [7].

10.1.2 Measures of Disease Frequency

Basic measures of disease frequency that are used in epidemiology are *incidence* and *prevalence*. The distinction is important: all too often in publications the term incidence is used, while prevalence is the appropriate term. For a meaningful analysis, both measures need a denominator: the number of persons in the population from which the cases arise, i.e., the source population.

The prevalence of contact dermatitis is the number of persons with contact dermatitis at a certain point in time (point prevalence) or during a certain (usually short) period of time (period prevalence). It is likely that the prevalence of contact dermatitis at one point in time is lower than a prevalence over a longer period because symptoms are not continuously present, as illustrated in a Danish study [38]. In

10

theory, the prevalence of contact dermatitis over a period of several years should be higher than the prevalence over a period of months. However, the difference may be small due to the fact that in many patients contact dermatitis is a condition with an unfavorable prognosis and a high rate of recurrence. In addition, the accuracy of recall will decrease with time, and it is conceivable that those persons who did not have symptoms recently will more often forget to report their earlier symptoms. The number of cases with a positive patch test in a large clinic, for example, suggests a prevalence, but is difficult to interpret: usually the source population from which the cases arise is not defined, nor is its size known.

The incidence of contact dermatitis refers to the number of new cases of contact dermatitis during a defined period in a specified population. The distinction with prevalence is important, because here an element of time (the transition from the healthy to the diseased state over time) is inserted. Commonly, the *incidence rate* is defined as the number of non-diseased persons who acquire contact dermatitis within a certain period of time, divided by the number of person-years for which the subjects in this population do not have contact dermatitis. Person-years are contributed only by those who are not ill at the beginning of the study. From the point in time at which a person acquires symptoms of contact dermatitis, he or she also no longer contributes to the total number of person-years in the denominator. The incidence rate is a summary measure that gives an indication of the force of transition to morbidity (such as contact allergy) over time.

This is different from the *cumulative incidence*. The cumulative incidence is the proportion of a fixed population that acquires contact dermatitis in a specific period of time. For example, suppose that workers in an epoxy-resin factory are patch tested and examined again after a few years. The number of new cases with epoxy allergy can only be determined at the end of this follow-up period; we do not know when they got their contact allergy. The proportion of new cases out of this fixed population of workers is a cumulative incidence. Cumulative incidences were used in a large follow-up study on work-related hand eczema in the automobile industry [19].

The difference between the two measures of incidence is small when the proportion of people that becomes ill in a specific period is small, but it can be sizeable when many people become ill in a short period of time. The incidence of contact dermatitis can be measured by periodic screening to detect all new cases in the study population over a certain period of time: this approach was used to study contact allergic sensitization in the Copenhagen region [40].

10.1.2.1 Source Population

The population in which the cases arise (source population) is the denominator of the measure of disease frequency (incidence or prevalence). A common feature of observational studies is the occurrence of nonresponders in the population that was invited to participate in the study. In many publications, the denominator refers to the responders only. Whether generalizations can be made to the source population as a whole depends on the extent to which the nonresponders were different in relevant characteristics from the source population. As a rule of thumb, response rates below 70% (some authors stipulate 80%) are prone to give spurious results.

> **Core Message**
>
> ■ Contact dermatitis is a common but a variable disease: symptoms accompanying the allergic state may vary in presentation or severity over time. Therefore the term prevalence should be used judiciously, restricted to defined populations and a defined point in time.

10.1.3 Observational Studies

The three most important types of observational study in the epidemiology of contact dermatitis are follow-up studies, case–control studies and cross-sectional studies. Important measures of association are the *relative risk*, the *rate ratio*, the *rate difference* and the *odds ratio*.

In follow-up studies, selection of subjects is based upon exposure to the factor of interest. Instead of exposure, the presence or absence of a risk factor (e.g., nickel allergy, or atopy) can also be chosen as the basis for comparison. For example, the relative risk of getting contact dermatitis in "wet" work (relative to dry work) can be studied in a follow-up study. This implies that a population of employees performing wet work and employees performing dry work is selected before the disease has developed and that they are followed over a certain period of time. The rate ratio (RR) is the incidence rate in persons exposed (to wet work) divided by the incidence rate among unexposed. This is a basic measure of association between exposure to wet work and contact dermatitis. Another measure of association is the rate difference (RD), being the difference between the incidence rates in exposed and unexposed subjects. It is also called attributable risk. A more elaborate application of this attributable risk has been used to study the impact of atopy on occupational contact dermatitis [14, 55].

In case–control studies, the subjects are selected according to their disease status. Information is collected on the past exposure of the persons with contact dermatitis (cases) and the nondiseased persons (controls). The odds of exposure among cases is compared to the odds of exposure among control persons (odds can be described as a proportion divided by 1 minus this proportion [$p/(1-p)$: this expression gives a certain mathematical advantage]. This can be expressed in an odds ratio (OR): when 38 cases with hand eczema (out of 97 cases) were exposed to a particular detergent and 59 were not exposed, the exposure odds are 38 : 59. When the exposure odds among 94 controls are 18 : 76, the odds ratio is the division of these two odds: the OR is 2.7.

A case–control study can be seen as a study among a defined population in which all diseased persons (for example those with hand eczema) and only a sample of the nondiseased persons are studied. This design is especially efficient in the study of a rare disease such as, for example, positive reactions to a very uncommon allergen. In this situation, the majority of the population does not have the disease, and it is not necessary to study all nondiseased persons. For reasons of interpretability, it is necessary to make an effort to select a population of controls in such a way that they reflect the exposure distribution among the nondiseased part of the source population from which the cases originated. Case–control studies can be based on incident cases or on prevalent cases. A study of incident cases includes as cases only those that develop the illness during a specified time period. In a case–control study of prevalent cases, existing cases of illness (e.g., persons with contact dermatitis, or persons with a specific allergy) at a point in time are selected. This approach has been chosen in population-wide study in Germany on the role of atopy [45]. Large registers of patch-test data may be good sources for case–control studies.

The choice of the right controls is essential in case–control studies; nonrepresentative controls will bias the results. This problem may easily arise from the inclusion of hospital-based controls, such as "other" dermatology patients.

In cross-sectional studies, a study population is selected regardless of exposure status or disease status (in contrast to case–control and follow-up studies). Usually, the information on exposure and disease in cross-sectional studies refers to the time of data collection. Thus, in cross-sectional studies on, for example contact dermatitis from cosmetic ingredients, it is not possible to draw conclusions with regard to the relationship between previous exposure to cosmetics and disease, because current exposure may be different from the exposure in the past that caused the disease. This problem is illustrated in a study that combines two prevalence investigations on contact sensitization with an 8-year interval [39].

In some situations the change of exposure status will be determined by the fact that the person has contact dermatitis. Persons who are susceptible to the development of eczematous symptoms are often aware of this, so they may change their habits (wear gloves or use medications) to suppress symptoms. In that case, when current exposure (as opposed to past exposure) is recorded in a case–control study or a cross-sectional study, the results will show that cases use gloves or medications more often than controls. Obviously the use of gloves is a result of being a case and not a cause. In many situations this type of distortion is less obvious. It is therefore preferable to record exposure with reference to the time prior to the first occurrence of eczematous symptoms. However, in practice it may be difficult to obtain reliable information on past exposure. In follow-up studies this poses less of a problem, because exposure is recorded before the symptoms of eczema become manifest.

10.1.3.1 Examples of Use and Misuse of Terms

Suppose a publication in which the authors state that "The incidence of nickel contact dermatitis at hospital X was 18/120 = 15%." They imply that, out of 120 patients seen, 18 were found to have this disease. In this common example the use of the term *incidence* is wrong and the term *prevalence* should be used.

If the authors had followed a group of 120 healthy nurses without contact dermatitis in their hospital over a certain time period, and at the end of that period had found 18 to have developed nickel dermatitis during that period, then they could use the term *cumulative incidence*.

The term "incidence rate" (often abbreviated to "incidence") could only be used if this group of 120 nurses was examined at the beginning of the study, to ascertain that nobody had nickel dermatitis, and if this group was continuously monitored during follow-up (e.g., 5 years). This design would yield exact information about the point in time at which anybody becomes diseased and would allow calculation of the number of person-months that each person contributes. A person no longer contributes after he or she becomes diseased. The number of months of follow-up until he or she shows dermatitis, or the total amount of months of follow-up (5×12 months) if no dermatitis appears, will be known at the end of the study. Suppose that the 18 persons who became diseased had a total of 300 months of follow-up without disease (e.g., 1 person 10 months until dermatitis appeared, another 14 months, etc.). The remaining 102 were followed for the total period of 5 years, contributing $102 \times 5 \times 12 = 6120$ months of follow-up. Thus, for the whole group, we have $300 + 6120 = 6420$ months of follow-up with a yield of 18 cases. This implies an incidence rate of $18/6420 = 0.0028$ cases per person-month of follow-up. If necessary, this can be converted to 0.034 cases per person-year of follow-up, and often this can be regarded as 0.034 cases per person-year exposure to nursing work.

Unfortunately, in contact dermatitis research, there are very few publications based on this more desirable design. The advantage of such a design is that it permits comparison with a different, unexposed group such as clerical staff [58], provided it is followed-up in the same way. The comparison can be expressed as a ratio of the two incidence rates, the rate ratio (RR), or as a difference between the two incidence rates, the rate difference (RD), which tells us about the association between exposure and dermatitis risk.

Suppose the incidence rate of dermatitis was 0.017 per person-year of follow-up in clerical staff, then the RR (sometimes called "relative risk") of $0.034/0.017 = 2$ would quickly tell us that the risk of developing dermatitis during nursing work is twice as high compared to low-risk clerical work. The RR and the RD are also amenable to further statistical elaboration, which could tell us more about, for example, the importance of soaps or gloves as specific exposure factors, or the role of nickel allergy.

10.1.4 Case Ascertainment

The case ascertainment refers to the methods used to let cases of contact dermatitis come to the attention of the investigator. It depends largely on the sources of data that are used, such as mortality statistics, morbidity statistics or observational studies. It may have major consequences for the magnitude of the disease frequency which one obtains. In morbidity statistics, case ascertainment usually involves registration of persons with eczema or dermatitis who fulfill additional criteria for registration, such as hospital admission or sickness leave. This restriction in the definition of a "case" will probably result in selec-

tive inclusion of the more severe cases, since a large proportion of individuals suffering from contact dermatitis do not come to medical attention.

Counting the number of persons with contact dermatitis in a population requires the explicit statement of diagnostic criteria to judge whether a person is considered to have contact dermatitis or not. In many publications, diagnostic criteria for the definition of contact dermatitis are not explicitly stated, and several authors reserve this term to denote allergic contact dermatitis. Since contact dermatitis refers to eczematous symptoms due to exposure of the skin to irritant or sensitizing agents, it can be considered as a subcategory of eczema. In some publications the terms "contact dermatitis" and "eczema" (especially of the hands) are used interchangeably, assuming that irritant or sensitizing agents play a role in the causation of eczema.

The ambiguity in diagnostic criteria also plays a role in the further distinction between allergic and irritant contact dermatitis. After further investigations (for example, patch testing) it is sometimes not certain whether the contact dermatitis is of allergic origin. In many instances, simultaneous exposure to irritant factors plays an essential part in the development of allergic contact dermatitis. Therefore, the distinction between allergic and irritant contact dermatitis should be interpreted with care in those publications where this distinction is made.

Nearly always, individuals are missed who might be sensitized to a specific allergen, while others are wrongly designated as cases of allergic contact dermatitis. In order to ascertain the validity of a used instrument, for example patch testing, the terms "sensitivity," "specificity," and "predictive value" are used. The sensitivity stands for the chance that cases with an allergic contact dermatitis (clinically relevant sensitization to a specific allergen) are correctly diagnosed, the specificity that the nonsensitized individuals are correctly diagnosed. Besides the sensitivity and specificity of the used instruments (e.g., patch testing) the positive predictive value (PPV) is an essential parameter. The PPV is the proportion of those individuals diagnosed by the used instrument (e.g., patch testing) who actually are sensitized. It should be kept in mind that the PPV is a function of the true prevalence of allergic sensitization in the population, of the sensitivity and of the specificity [16]. Thus, also from a statistical point of view, it is crucial to explore the patient's history carefully and exactly before performing patch testing: indiscriminate testing of many patients with a doubtful allergic origin of their skin problem (i.e., a low prevalence of true allergies) will lead to many cases of wrongly diagnosed contact dermatitis. In studies on contact allergy in the general population this issue is even more important than in a clinical setting because of the lower background prevalence. From a statistical point of view, an observed increase of the prevalence of contact allergy can theoretically be explained by a decrease of specificity over time because of an increased awareness of allergic diseases in the population (resulting in more false positives). In the interpretation of data on the occurrence of contact dermatitis it is important to distinguish between sensitization (i.e., a positive reaction in the patch-test reading) and the presence of allergic contact dermatitis ascribed to this sensitization. For example, a high rate of sensitization can be found in the population for some allergens, while a low frequency of allergic contact dermatitis due to these allergens was noticed (e.g., thiomersal, poison ivy).

Core Message

- Sensitivity and specificity of the used instruments are important. In epidemiological studies an overestimation of the true prevalence can result from low sensitivity/specificity.

In observational studies, active case ascertainment usually involves screening of the study population by clinical examination, by questionnaire or by a combination of both. However, the frequency of cases obtained by questionnaire may be quite different from those ascertained by clinical examination. Screening of the complete study population according to standardized criteria by one or more trained dermatologists is the most reliable and therefore preferred method. But it is generally not feasible, especially in large study populations: a questionnaire that can be self-administered by the whole study population is more cost-effective, but less valid.

Case Reports

- A study of occupational skin disease among California grape and tomato harvesters was prompted by reports of increased dermatitis amongst table grape growers [31]. The tomato harvesters were chosen as a comparison. To evaluate skin diseases, subjects were asked, "Have you had any type of skin rash or skin irritation within the last 3 months that has lasted 2 - days or more?" Fifty-two percent of grape

workers and 19% of tomato workers reported rashes lasting 2 days or more during the previous 3 months; a slightly greater difference was noted when the period in question was 1 year. No significant differences were seen between the two occupational groups, however, for prevalence of skin conditions on examination. One of the explanations raised by the authors was that rashes earlier in the growing season were reported in the questionnaire, while the symptoms had disappeared by the time of examination. Assuming that the investigators were blinded to the occupation of the workers, the authors also suggested the presence of information bias, in the sense that grape workers may have been more aware than tomato workers of dermatitis from harvest work. The questionnaire for evaluating current skin conditions detected only about one-third of the cases. This low sensitivity was attributed to differences in the understanding of skin changes between examiner and respondent. The authors stated that it might also relate to the observed skin conditions being of less than 2 days' duration; however, given the nature of those most common (acne and variants, folliculitis and eczematous dermatitis), this seems an unlikely explanation. The authors concluded that questionnaires may be insensitive for some dermatological conditions and active surveillance would improve case finding and the validity of incidence data.

The problems with questionnaires have been discussed in the context of studies on hand eczema [30, 48, 61]. But hand eczema does not always imply contact dermatitis, and certainly not always contact allergy. In the context of questionnaires, sensitivity, specificity, and PPV (as discussed above) have the same importance as in patch testing.

Given the practical limitations of a medical examination of large populations, some studies combine the validity of a clinical diagnosis with the easy applicability of a self-administered questionnaire.

In such a study, a set of three questions was developed, asking about symptoms of hand dermatitis, their duration, and whether these were recurrent [48]. The validity was evaluated among 109 nurses and compared with a medical diagnosis made by a dermatologist. A diagnosis of hand eczema, defined as "one or more symptoms, with a recurrent character, or lasting for more than 3 weeks" had a sensitivity of 100% and a specificity of 64%, resulting in a positive predictive value of 31%. This indicates that use of the questionnaire alone would result in a significant overestimation of the prevalence. Medical examination of only those who responded positively, to exclude false-positive cases, would, however, increase the specificity while maintaining the high sensitivity. It would reduce the screening effort by trained physicians. If the definition of hand eczema was based upon two or more symptoms with a recurrent character, or lasting for more than 3 weeks, the sensitivity remained high (80%) while the specificity increased to 89%, resulting in a PPV of 63%. When the same questionnaire, combined with a clinical examination, was applied to a different population (workers in a rubber factory), the results were quite different [61].

For current objective and past skin disorders on the face, a questionnaire was validated among employees who worked with visual display units [1]. Validation of a question on current skin symptoms has been applied in a study among farmers [51]. The use of the self-diagnosis term "hand-eczema" seems to be valid in questionnaire studies in Scandinavian countries [54]. Based on a combination of consensus and validation, an extensive set of questions has been developed for use in hand-eczema studies [53].

> ### Core Message
>
> ■ Very few dermatological questionnaires have been adequately validated. Response rates below 70% are likely to bias the results.

10.1.5 Incidence and Prevalence of Contact Dermatitis and Contact Sensitization

10.1.5.1 General Population

Morbidity statistics that provide information on the occurrence of skin diseases, and eczema or contact dermatitis specifically, are, for example, hospitalization records, case records from dermatology clinics, and data on sickness leave and occupational diseases. As mentioned before, it is likely that these statistics include mainly the more severe cases of skin disease.

There are several publications on the number and characteristics of patients visiting dermatology clin-

ics and/or patch testing units [46, 63]. However, no information on the incidence or prevalence of contact dermatitis can be derived from these publications, because information on the size of the source population from which the cases originated is usually lacking. It is difficult to interpret the distribution of occupations, age or sex in a patient population without knowing the distribution of these characteristics among the source population. Also, information on type and severity of skin disease in patient populations is difficult to interpret, because of selection mechanisms that play a role before a dermatology clinic is consulted. Within a population of clinic patients, systematic collection and registration of data can be the basis of a meaningful analysis, especially if it is on a transnational basis (ESSCA); guidelines for publication and analysis of such data have been published [59].

> ### Core Message
>
> ■ Publications based on data of patients visiting dermatology clinics and/or patch testing units have to be interpreted carefully since no information on population-based incidence or prevalence rates can be derived from those studies.

Publications that generate incidence-type data for the general population are scarce. A classic example is a retrospectively designed study among Danish women [34]. Data from incidence studies may support and direct strategies for prevention of contact allergy and allergic contact dermatitis. An example is the Copenhagen Allergy Study [40]: in 1990 a random sample of 567 persons of the 15- to 69-year-old population living in the western part of Copenhagen County, Denmark was patch tested in a cross-sectional study, and in 1998 a follow-up study was performed. In the follow-up study, 37 persons (12%) of the 313 patch-test-negative persons in 1990 had developed one or more positive patch tests (incident contact allergy). Twenty cases (6%) of incident nickel allergy and 25 cases (8%) of incident contact allergy to one or more haptens other than nickel were found. The data indicate that female sex, young age, and ear piercing (before 1990) were risk factors for developing nickel allergy. Contact sensitivity to one or more haptens was found in 16% and 19% in 1990 and 1998, respectively [39].

Information on the prevalence of hand eczema, contact sensitivity, and contact dermatitis in the general population can be obtained from cross-sectional

Table 1.1. Population-based studies on the prevalence of hand eczema, contact sensitization and contact dermatitis. (*E* Clinical examination, *I* interview, *Q* questionnaire)

Reference	Country	Target population	Method of case ascertainment	N	Outcome	Measures of prevalence	Rate (%)	Comment
Mortz et al. [37]	Denmark	12–16 years (children)	Q, I, E, patch test	1501	Hand eczema	Lifetime	9.2	Cross-sectional study of high quality
						1-year	7.3	
						Point	3.2	
					Contact sensitivity	Point	15.2	
					Allergic Contact Dermatitis	Point	0.7	
						Lifetime	7.2	
Nielsen et al. [39]	Denmark	15–41 years	Patch test in 1990	290	Contact sensitivity in 1990	Point in 1990	15.9	Small sample size, low participation rates (69% and 51%)
			Patch test in 1998	469	Contact sensitivity in 1998	Point in 1998	18.6	
Meding and Jarvholm [32]	Sweden	20–65 years	Q in 1983	16,708	Hand eczema in 1983	1-year in 1983	11.8	Response rate 83.5% in 1983
			Q in 1996	2218	Hand eczema in 1996	1-year in 1996	9.7	Response rate 73.9% in 1996
Schäfer et al. [45]	Germany	28–78 years	E, patch test	1141	Contact sensitivity	Point	40.0	Nested case–control study, biased target population (50% exhibited allergen-specific IgE antibodies to aeroallergens)

studies that were performed in recent years (Table 1.1). The aim of the Odense Adolescence Cohort Study was to assess prevalence measures of atopic dermatitis (AD), asthma, allergic rhinitis and hand and contact dermatitis in adolescents in Odense municipality, Denmark [37, 38]. This Odense study was carried out as a cross-sectional study among 1501 school children (age 12–16 years) and included questionnaire, interview, clinical examination, and patch testing. The lifetime prevalence of hand eczema based on the questionnaire was 9%, the 1-year period prevalence was 7.3%, and the point prevalence 3.2%, with a significant predominance in girls. The point prevalence of contact allergy was 15%; the most common contact allergens were nickel (8.6%) and fragrance mix (1.8%). Nickel allergy was clinically relevant in 69% and fragrance allergy in 29% of cases. A significant association was found between contact allergy and hand eczema while no association was

found between contact allergy and atopic dermatitis or inhalant allergy. The point prevalence of allergic contact dermatitis was 0.7% and the lifetime prevalence was 7%.

In two other cross-sectional studies the prevalence of hand eczema was compared between 1983 and 1996 in Swedish adults using the same questionnaire [32]. Random samples of 20,000 individuals from the population of Gothenburg, Sweden were drawn from the population register in 1983 and 1996. Data were collected with a postal questionnaire, which was identical in the two studies. The response rate was 83% in 1983 and 74% in 1996. The reported 1-year prevalence of hand eczema decreased from 12% in 1983 to 10% in 1996.

Within a population-based nested, case–control study in Germany patch tests were performed with 25 standard allergens in 1141 adults [45]. Additional information was obtained by a dermatological examination, a standardized interview, and blood analysis. At least one positive reaction was exhibited by 40% of the subjects, with reactions most frequently observed to fragrance mix (16%), nickel (13%), thimerosal (4.7%), and balsam of Peru (3.8%). Women were sensitized more often than men (50% versus 30%), and this was also significant for fragrance mix, nickel, turpentine, cobalt chloride, and thimerosal. Contact sensitization decreased with increasing degree of occupational training. Frequency estimates for the general adult population based on these findings were 28% for overall contact sensitization and 11% for fragrance mix, 10% for nickel, and 3.2% for thimerosal. In this study the sample was biased towards atopics because 50% of the subjects exhibited allergen-specific IgE antibodies to aeroallergens. The clinical relevance of the patch test reactions was not assessed. The high sensitization rate can also be explained by a high number of false-positive test results (see paragraph 3 of Sect. 10.1.4, "Case Ascertainment").

Previously other cross-sectional studies have been performed in the Netherlands [28, 49], Sweden [33], England [43], the United States [24], and Norway [26]. In all studies, a geographically defined population or a sample thereof was screened. In some of the studies all skin disorders were recorded, others focused on eczema or hand-eczema only. In most of the studies the term "eczema" included allergic contact dermatitis, irritant contact dermatitis, seborrheic eczema, nummular eczema, atopic eczema, dyshidrotic eczema, and unclassified eczema.

In the Netherlands, Norway and Sweden, the prevalence was higher among women, in London the prevalence was higher among men, while there was no difference between sexes in the United States. It is possible that the differences are obscured by differences in age distribution of the populations. The prevalence in women was especially high in the younger age groups.

In the United States, the prevalence of eczema seems to increase with age, while according to the publication from the Netherlands, Sweden and Norway, the prevalence seems to decrease slightly in the age groups above 50 years. The Dutch study [8] analyzed the relative contribution of age and occupation to the prevalence of hand eczema and found that the relationship with age disappeared after controlling for occupation. The same phenomenon was described in a population of Australian rubber and cement industry workers: the prevalence of dermatitis was relatively high in workers under 45 years, but the age effect also disappeared after controlling for job classification [60].

The major risk factor for contact dermatitis is considered to be exposure to irritant or sensitizing factors. This exposure is common during household activities and in certain occupations. This was evident in a study, using a validated questionnaire, which compared the general population with certain occupations, and which obtained a prevalence of 5% for men and almost 11% for women [49].

In conclusion, the prevalence studies strongly suggest that age and gender are not risk factors for contact dermatitis in themselves, but that these characteristics are associated with exposure in occupational and household activities. A review of the epidemiology of allergic contact sensitization, where similar phenomena were seen, concluded that the age-dependent immunological reactivity was less important than differences in exposure between age groups, and that differences in sensitization pattern between sexes seem to be caused by different exposures [35]. The dissimilarity was considered to be so obvious that patch test results were always given for men and women separately.

Core Message

■ Data from incidence studies may support and direct strategies for prevention of contact allergy and allergic contact dermatitis. Information on the prevalence of hand eczema, contact sensitivity, and contact dermatitis in the general population can be obtained from recent cross-sectional studies that demonstrate the high point and period prevalence in the general population, also in children and adolescents.

10.1.5.2 Incidence and Prevalence of Notified Occupational Contact Dermatitis

Occupational disease registries provide national incidence data based on the notification of occupational skin diseases and are available in many countries. Although the comparison of national data are hampered by differences across countries in reporting occupational diseases, the average incidence rate of registered occupational contact dermatitis in some countries lies around 0.5 to 1.9 cases per 1000 full-time workers per year [12, 22].

Most of the national registers combine all types of skin disease, while no distinction is made with regard to eczema or contact dermatitis. Skin diseases constitute up to 30% of all notified occupational diseases and it is estimated that eczema or contact dermatitis accounts for about 90% to 95% of all occupational skin diseases. Finland keeps also a register on occupational contact urticaria [25], and in Germany there is an additional register on occupational skin cancer [17]. Some of the occupational disease statistics give a breakdown by gender and occupation or branch of industry. Most national statistics do not provide information on the actual cause of contact dermatitis and predisposing factors.

National registries are usually incomplete as a result of underdiagnosis and underreporting of the disease. It has been estimated that the incidence of occupational skin diseases in the United States and Germany is being grossly underestimated [18, 56], the milder cases of skin disease not being registered at all. The extent of underreporting is likely to differ between countries, because each country has its own system of notification and its own criteria for compensation. In the United States, occupational disease statistics are collected annually from more than 170,000 private industries by the Bureau of Labor Statistics [2]. A detailed analysis has been made of the register of occupational diseases in Denmark [22]. In the United Kingdom the EPIDERM project in combination with OPRA (Occupational Physicians Reporting Activity) for recording occupational dermatoses requires dermatologists in a number of centers to report confirmed or suspected cases of occupational skin disease, including the occupation of the patient concerned [5]. It is a voluntary system, and operates on the principle of simplicity, ensuring compliance. The epidemiological limitations are well recognized, but the system corrects the virtual absence of meaningful official statistics in the UK. A population-based study of occupational skin diseases in North Bavaria and the Saarland, Germany, is one of the few that can claim completeness in terms of new cases (numerator) and size of the occupational population as denominator [3, 13].

In the United Kingdom the annual incidence of occupational contact dermatitis from dermatologist reports was 6.4 cases per 100,000 workers and 6.5 per 100,000 from reports by occupational physicians, an overall rate of 12.9 cases per 100,000 workers [36]. The highest incidence rates were seen in hairdressers [47]. Agents accounting for the highest number of allergic contact dermatitis cases were rubber, nickel, epoxies and other resins, aromatic amines, chromium and chromates, fragrances and cosmetics, and preservatives. Soaps, wet work, petroleum products, solvents, and cutting oils and coolants were the most frequently cited agents in cases of irritant dermatitis [36].

In Denmark the incidence is 17,700 cases on a workforce of about 2.6 million, i.e., about 0.8 per 1000 per year [22]. Out of 145 grouped exposure sources the 5 most frequently stated substances were detergents, water, metals, foodstuff, and rubber in notified occupational skin diseases in Denmark. These substances caused approximately half of the eczema cases. The most important irritant seems to be wet work.

In the Netherlands, a voluntary reporting system modeled more or less on the British EPIDERM project has been in operation since 2001. From the data generated by the pilot phase, based on a network of 25 dermatology practices distributed across the country as sentinel stations, an annual occupational skin disease incidence of 1.5 per 1000 employees could be estimated (Coenraads, unpublished report to Ministry of Social Affairs and Employment).

In Germany, occupational skin diseases excluding skin cancer are officially registered by the code "BK 5101," which is defined as "severe or recurrent skin diseases that force the discontinuation of any activity that causes or that could be causing the development, the worsening, or the recurrence of the skin disease.. In the year 2002 the industrial nonprofit insurance institutions reported 17,848 such skin disease cases. In Northern Bavaria, Germany, a detailed population-based prospective study was performed to classify all BK 5101 cases of occupational skin diseases [3, 11, 15, , 55]. From 1990 to 1999 in total of 5285 cases were recorded. In co-operation with the State Institute of Labour and Occupation the numbers of all persons employed in different occupations during the same time period were collected. Since the number of employees in the different occupations was known, a population-based study was performed to investigate incidences and demographic characteristics in specific occupational groups. The estimated overall incidence was 6.7 cases per 10,000 workers per year. The highest incidence per 1000 per year was in hairdressers (97), bakers (33), and florists (24). The induction period was very short: about 2 years in hairdressers, 3 years in the food industry, and about 4 years in health service and in metalworkers. Females had a considerable higher risk of developing occupational contact dermatitis than men. The incidence rate of contact dermatitis was highest between the age of 15 and 24 years. In about half of all cases a delayed-type sensitization with occupational relevance was detected. In Fig. 1.1 the incidence rates of irritant contact dermatitis (ICD) and allergic contact dermatitis (ACD) of employees of the 12 groups with the highest risk of an occupational skin disease are presented. The population-based register in Northern Bavaria, Germany, demonstrated a significant de-

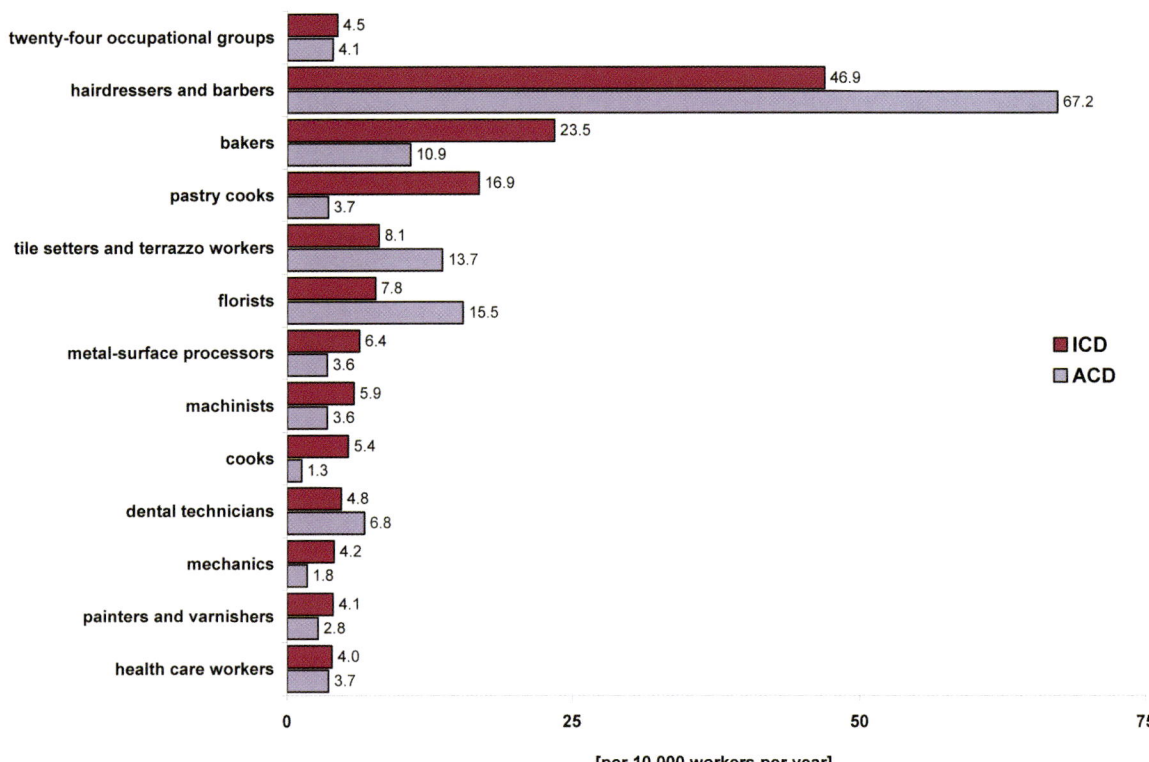

twenty-four occupational groups — 4.5 / 4.1
hairdressers and barbers — 46.9 / 67.2
bakers — 23.5 / 10.9
pastry cooks — 16.9 / 3.7
tile setters and terrazzo workers — 8.1 / 13.7
florists — 7.8 / 15.5
metal-surface processors — 6.4 / 3.6
machinists — 5.9 / 3.6
cooks — 5.4 / 1.3
dental technicians — 4.8 / 6.8
mechanics — 4.2 / 1.8
painters and varnishers — 4.1 / 2.8
health care workers — 4.0 / 3.7

■ ICD
□ ACD

[per 10,000 workers per year]

10

Fig. 1.1. Incidence rates (per 10,000 employees) of irritant contact dermatitis (*ICD*) and allergic contact dermatitis (*ACD*) in the 12 occupational groups with the highest risk for occupational skin diseases in North Bavaria (modified according to [15])

cline in incidence of occupational skin disease among hairdressers between 1990 and 1999 [13]. This supports a probable "intervention effect" by legislative and preventive measures that came into effect over the last decade for hairdressers. In contrast to this it could be demonstrated that potassium dichromate is still the most important allergen in the construction industry of Northern Bavaria; there was no significant decline during the 1990s [3]. This contrasts with the Scandinavian countries, where the prevalence of potassium dichromate sensitization declined following the reduction of chromate levels resulting from the addition of ferrous sulfate to cement. The impact of atopic skin diathesis on occupational contact dermatitis could be analyzed by using attributable risk figures; almost 22% of occupational skin disease cases may be ascribed to this endogenous risk factor [14].

Core Message

■ Skin diseases constitute up to 30% of all notified occupational diseases in most countries. National registries are usually incomplete as a result of underdiagnosis and underreporting of the disease.
The average incidence rate of registered occupational contact dermatitis is around 0.5 to 1.9 cases per 1000 full-time workers per year. The highest incidence rates are seen in hairdressers.

10.1.5.3 Incidence and Prevalence in Different Work Forces

Table 1.2 summarizes the results of two prospective cohort studies in working populations. In the prospective Audi cohort study 2078 apprentices were examined at the start of their apprenticeship and

Table 1.2. Prospective cohort studies on the incidence of work-related skin complaints [hand eczema (*HE*), contact sensitization, and contact dermatitis] in different professions. (*E* Clinical examination, *I* interview, *Q* questionnaire)

Reference	Country	Target population	Method of case ascertainment	N	Outcome	Measures of Incidence	Rate (%)	Comment
Funke et al. [19]	Germany	Apprentices in the car industry	Q, I, E	2078	HE in metal-workers (apprentices)	1-year	9.2	Prospective cohort study of high quality, Follow-up rate 98.2%
						3-years	15.3	
					HE in blue-collar apprentices	1-year	8.8	
						3-years	14.1	
					HE in white-collar apprentices	1-year	4.6	
						3-years	6.9	
Uter et al. [58]	Germany	Hair-dressing apprentices	Q, I, E	2352	HE at the first, second, and third examination during 3-year training	Point first year	12.9	Prospective cohort study of high quality, high initial response rate (91.5%) but 51.8% dropouts until final follow-up
						Point second year	23.5	
						Point third year	23.9	

systematically followed up over a 3-year period [19]. The main outcome variable was the incidences of work-related hand eczema in different apprenticeships. The 1-year cumulative incidences of hand eczema were 9.2% in metalworkers, 8.8% in other blue-collar workers, and 4.6% in white-collar apprentices. The 3-year cumulative incidences of hand eczema were 15% in metalworkers, 14% in other blue-collar workers, and almost 7% in white-collar apprentices. The incidence was not uniformly distributed over the 3-year period: within the first 6 months, a high rate of hand eczema occurred, which then declined and remained steady at a lower rate over the 2nd and the 3rd years.

In a prospective cohort study of 2352 hairdressing apprentices there were three examinations during their 3 years of vocational training [58]. The point prevalence of (mostly slight) irritant skin changes of the hands increased from 35% in the initial examination to almost 48% in the intermediate examination, and to 55% in the final examination. Given a more conservative definition of a case of "hand derma-

titis," these estimates were almost 13%, 24%, and 24%, respectively. Altogether, about 34 and 15 cases of "skin changes (any degree)" and "hand dermatitis," respectively, per 100 person-years were observed during the study period. The incidence rate decreased in the course of the study. However, the proportion of dropouts until final follow-up was almost 52%. This study demonstrates that apprentices with skin problems leave the work force more often than healthy apprentices.

During the 1980s and early 1990s several cross-sectional studies, mostly on hand eczema, were performed among specific occupational groups, for example in metal [10] and construction [9] workers, farmers [51], hospital workers [27], and painters [23]. Most of the recently published studies are also cross-sectional surveys (Table 1.3). A major problem in such studies is the healthy worker effect and the fact that a clear relationship between skin disease and work is difficult to assess retrospectively.

A postal questionnaire was mailed to 3500 Swedish dentists [62]. The response rate was 88%. Almost

Table 1.3. Cross-sectional studies on the prevalence of work-related skin complaints [hand eczema (*HE*), contact sensitization and contact dermatitis] in different professions. (*E* Clinical examination, *I* interview, *Q* questionnaire)

Reference	Country	Target population	Method of case ascertainment	N	Outcome	Measures of prevalence	Rate (%)	Comment
Wallenhammar et al. [62]	Sweden	Dentists	Q, E	3080	Hand eczema	1-year	14.9	Cross-sectional study based on a postal questionnaire, response rate 88%, subsequent patch testing of positive responders (158/191)
			Patch test	158				
Paulsen et al. [42]	Denmark	Gardeners and greenhouse workers	Q	1958	Occupational dermatitis	Lifetime	19.6	Cross-sectional study based on a postal questionnaire and subsequent patch testing of selected persons; response rate 84.6%
			Patch test	250				
Gruvberger et al. [20]	Sweden	Metalworkers	Q, E, patch test	163	Work-related contact dermatitis	Point ?	17.2	Cross-sectional study, selection bias, unclear measure of prevalence
Livesley et al. [30]	UK	Printing industry	Q, E	1189	Skin complaints	Lifetime	41.2	Cross-sectional study, response rate 62%
				1189	Current hand problem	Point	10.7	
Susitaival et al. [52]	California, USA	Veterinarians	Q	1416	Hand/forearm dermatitis	1-year	28	Response rate 73%
Leino et al. [29]	Finland	Hairdressers	I	355	Hand eczema	Lifetime	16.9	Response rate 71%, selection bias due to healthy worker effect
			E, patch test	130		Point	2.8	
Guo et al. [21]	Taiwan	Cement workers	I	1147	Work-related skin problems in males and females	1-year men	13.9	Response rate 68.2%, only 166/573 (29%) of randomly selected workers were patch tested
			E, patch test	166		1-year women	5.4	

15% (*n*=191) reported hand eczema during the previous year. They were invited to a clinical examination, including patch testing with a standard and a dental series: 158/191 (83%) dentists attended, and hand eczema diagnosis was confirmed in 94%, whereby 28% had allergic contact dermatitis. A cross-sectional study, based on a postal questionnaire and subsequent patch testing of selected persons, was carried out on almost 2000 gardeners in Denmark [42]. The lifetime prevalence of occupational dermatitis was almost 20%. Among 250 persons patch tested, the most frequently sensitizing occupational allergens were plants of the Compositae family and the fungicide captan. Allergic occupational contact dermatitis was suspected in 43/250 persons (17%). Irritant eczemas outnumbered allergic eczemas and both were mostly caused by plants.

In a metal working plant a questionnaire-based survey of occupational dermatoses was combined with clinical examination and patch testing [20]. According to the questionnaire, 214 out of 382 (56%) reported having or having had skin manifestations during the time of employment that were suspected to be work-related. Out of the 163 patch-tested metal workers, however, only 28 (17%) were found to have a work-related contact dermatitis: irritant contact dermatitis was diagnosed in 12/163, occupational allergic contact dermatitis in 10/163. In 66/163 (40%) metal workers it was impossible to determine the relationship between skin disease and work.

In the United Kingdom, a total of 1189 workers in the printing industry were investigated by a questionnaire [30]. A total of 490 respondents (41%) reported having a skin complaint at some time. Prevalence was highest in those working in printing compared to pre-press or finishing. The point prevalence was almost 11%. Clinical examination confirmed the high self-reported prevalence and also identified a substantial proportion of mild cases that were not reported. The overall prevalence of occupationally related skin complaints was estimated to be 40%.

A mailed questionnaire to a sample of California veterinarians showed that dermatoses during their career were reported by 46%, and hand and/or forearm dermatitis was reported more than once and during the past year by 22% of women and 10% of men [52]. Dermatitis related to work-related exacerbating factors was reported by 28%.

In Finland 355 out of a random sample of 500 female hairdressers were investigated by using a computer-aided telephone interview [29]. The telephone interview revealed a lifetime prevalence of almost 17% for hand dermatoses. Of the 189 reporting work-related skin and respiratory symptoms, 130 underwent a physical examination, lung function tests, prick and patch testing, and nasal and lung provocation tests. In the clinical investigations, the point prevalence was 2.8% for occupational dermatoses, 1.7% for occupational rhinitis, and 0.8% for occupational asthma. Ammonium persulfate caused 90% of the respiratory diseases and 27% of the hand dermatoses.

A study from Taiwan clearly demonstrates the difficulty of distinguishing between work-related and non-work-related skin problems and the difficulty of classifying severity [21]. A total of 1147 current regular cement workers were telephone-interviewed

about skin problems during the previous 12 months. The 1-year prevalence of skin problems in male workers was almost 22%; in female workers almost 13%. The 1-year prevalence of skin problems related to work or possibly related to work was lower: related to work in men, 11%; in women, 3%. Out of those with skin problems related or possibly related to work ($n = 116$) more than half reported that they had sought medical help, while about a quarter used non-prescription medicines. An average duration of 5 months of skin symptoms was reported during the previous 1 year. Only 13 workers (11%) took sick leave because of skin problems, with an average duration of 4.7 days. From those who were interviewed a random sample of 573 (50%) persons was selected, but only 166 were examined and patch tested with common contact allergens.

10.1.6 Special Considerations: Confounding, Atopy, Interactions, and Effect Modification

Contact dermatitis is a multifactorial disease: apart from exposure to irritating or sensitizing agents, there are many factors that may influence the development of contact dermatitis, such as weather conditions, humidity, psychological factors, and atopic constitution. These factors may act as confounders in studies if they are not properly controlled for, in either the design of the study or the analysis. Distortion of the study results, caused by confounding, occurs when an outside factor, for example history of atopic dermatitis, is associated with the exposure and also with the disease of interest.

For the ascertainment of atopic dermatitis, diagnostic criteria and scoring systems are available [4]. Evidence has accumulated that past or present atopic dermatitis is a risk factor for irritant contact dermatitis [6]. Earlier studies indicated that atopy was almost three times as high among patients with hand eczema as in the general population or a healthy control group. Later it appeared that atopic dermatitis was particularly associated with irritant contact dermatitis, not with contact allergy. The proportion of subjects with sporadic or continuous hand eczema was significantly greater in those with moderate and severe atopic dermatitis in childhood compared with those with respiratory allergy only, or a group without atopy. In a follow-up study of hospital workers, a history of atopic dermatitis increased the risk of developing hand eczema threefold [41]. Population-based studies in the food industry calculated a significantly greater risk of occupational contact dermatitis in employees with an atopic skin diathesis [14, 55].

Even if in epidemiological terms atopic dermatitis is an effect modifier, it can be argued that irritant contact dermatitis associated with atopy is primarily an exacerbation of underlying atopic dermatitis. Since atopic dermatitis is often associated with respiratory symptoms, respiratory atopy may appear as a risk factor. The same may apply to dry skin as an expression of atopic dermatitis.

The problem of contact dermatitis in a particular group of patients is easy to interpret when there is a straightforward cause–effect relationship; for example, hand eczema in a group of surgeons with a positive patch test to thiuram additives to their rubber gloves. However, the relevance of a positive patch test to very common allergens such as chromate or nickel may be difficult to assess in patients with a (contact) dermatitis that has a chronic relapsing course. As discussed above, there may be considerable (statistical) interaction between several exposure or risk factors of interest. Elucidation of such interactions may have consequences for preventive or other public-health strategies. To illustrate this point, in Table 1.4 an example is created from the data (modified for this purpose) generated in two Scandinavian follow-up studies on hand eczema and exposure to irritants [33, 44].

In Table 1.4, the relative risks of exposure to irritants on hand eczema are different according to the presence of a history of atopic dermatitis. There is an effect modification, meaning that the relative risks of exposure to irritants are not uniform (multiplicative) in the different levels of skin atopy: the risk of hand eczema in atopics is disproportionately increased by exposure to irritants.

The presence or absence of interactions between various factors operating on the risk of contact dermatitis have not yet been investigated in detail. One such example is the role of chromate allergy in foot eczema. As mentioned above, there are indications that such phenomena operate on nickel allergy: in the absence of signs of atopic dermatitis, the relative risk of a positive nickel patch test on the risk of hand eczema was only 1.7 in hairdressers and only 1.1 in nurses [50]. In a German study, nickel sensitivity was not associated with an elevated risk for hand eczema. Independent risk factors were: wet work, atopic skin, and exposure to permanent wave.

Suggested Reading

Menné T, Began O, Green A (1982) Nickel allergy and hand dermatitis in a stratified sample of the Danish female population: an epidemiological study including a statistic appendix. Acta Derm Venereol 62:35–41
In 1982 Menné et al. estimated the incidence of nickel allergy by asking a large stratified sample of the female general population about skin reactions to nickel and about hand eczema. Because they were able to obtain fairly reliable age-specific prevalence-rates, they were able to calculate incidence rates for developing nickel allergy. They were able to show a doubling of nickel allergy in all age groups. In the discussion of that publication, issues such as the relevance of a positive patch test and the question to what extent nickel allergy precedes or follows hand eczema are discussed (i.e., to what extent is nickel allergy a risk factor for hand eczema). It speculates on measures that forbid the use of nickel-releasing alloys; many years later this measure was implemented in Europe, following an earlier implementation of this regulation in Denmark.

References

1. Berg M, Axelson O (1990) Evaluation of a questionnaire for facial skin complaints related to work at visual display units. Contact Dermatitis 22:71–77
2. BLS: Bureau of Labor Statistics (2004) www.bls.gov/iff/home.htm
3. Bock M, Schmidt A, Bruckner T, Diepgen TL (2003) Occupational skin disease in the construction industry. Br J Dermatol 149:1165–1171
4. Charman C, Williams H (2000) Outcome measures of disease severity in atopic eczema. Arch Dermatol 136:763–769
5. Cherry N, Meyer JD, Adisesh A, Brooke R, Owen-Smith V, Swales C, Beck MH (2000) Surveillance of occupational skin disease: EPIDERM and OPRA. Br J Dermatol 142:1128–1134
6. Coenraads PJ, Diepgen TL (1998) Risk for hand eczema in employees with past or present atopic dermatitis. Int Arch Occup Environ Health 71:7–13
7. Coenraads PJ, Diepgen TL (2003) Problems with trials and intervention studies on barrier creams and emollients at the workplace. Int Arch Occup Environ Health 76:362–366
8. Coenraads PJ, Nater JP, van der Lende R (1983) Prevalence of eczema and other dermaloses of the hands and arms in the Netherlands. Association with age and occupation. Clin Exp Dermatol 8:495–503
9. Coenraads PJ, Nater JP, Jansen HA, Lantinga H (1984) Prevalence of eczema and other dermaloses of the hands and forearms in construction workers in the Netherlands. Clin Exp Dermatol 9:149–158
10. De Boer EM, van Ketel WG, Bruynzeel DP (1989) Dermatoses in metal workers. Contact Dermatitis 20:212–218

Table 1.4. Relative risks (modified) of contact dermatitis of the hands according to the level of atopic skin diathesis and exposure to irritants [6, 39, 51]

	No irritant exposure	Exposure to irritants
No atopy	1	1.5
Mild atopic dermatitis	2	4
Severe atopic dermatitis	4	12

10

11. Dickel H, Kuss O, Blesius CR, Schmidt A, Diepgen TL (2001) Occupational skin diseases in Nothern Bavaria between 1990 and 1999: a population based study. Br J Dermatol 145:453–462

12. Dickel H, Bruckner T, Berhard-Klimt C, Koch T, Scheidt R, Diepgen TL (2002) Surveillance scheme for occupational skin disease in the Saarland, FRG: first report from BKH-S. Contact Dermatitis 46:197–206

13. Dickel H, Kuss O, Schmidt A, Diepgen TL (2002) Impact of preventive strategies on trend of occupational skin disease in hairdressers: population-based register study. Br Med J 324:1422–1423

14. Dickel H, Bruckner TM, Schmidt A, Diepgen TL (2003) Impact of atopic skin diathesis on occupational skin disease incidence in a working population. J Invest Dermatol 121:37–40

15. Diepgen TL (2003) Occupational skin-disease data in Europe. Int Arch Occup Environ Health 76:331–338

16. Diepgen TL, Coenraads PJ (2000) The impact of sensitivity, specificity and positive predictive value of patch testing: the more you test, the more you get? Contact Dermatitis 42:315–317

17. Diepgen TL, Drexler H (2004) Skin cancer and occupational skin disease. Hautarzt 55:22–27

18. Diepgen TL, Schmidt A (2002) Werden Inzidenz und Prävalenz berufsbedingter Hauterkrankungen unterschätzt? Arbeitsmed Sozialmed Umweltmed 37:477–480

19. Funke U, Fartasch M, Diepgen TL (2001) Incidence of work-related hand eczema during apprenticeship: first results of a prospective cohort study in the car industry. Contact Dermatitis 44:166–172

20. Gruvberger B, Isaksson M, Frick M, Ponten A, Bruze M (2003) Occupational dermatoses in a metalworking plant. Contact Dermatitis 48:80–86

21. Guo YL, Wang BJ, Yeh KC, Wang JC, Kao HH, Wang MT, Shih HC, Chen CJ (1999) Dermatoses in cement workers in southern Taiwan. Contact Dermatitis 40:1–7

22. Halkier-Sorensen L (1996) Occupational skin diseases. Contact Dermatitis 35 [Suppl 1]:1–120

23. Hogberg M, Wahlberg JE (1980) Health screening for occupational dermatoses in housepainters. Contact Dermatitis 6:100–106

24. Johnson MLT, Roberts J (1978) Skin conditions and related need for medical care among persons 1–74 years. Vital Health Stat 11:1–72

25. Kanerva L, Toikkanen J, Jolanki R, Estlander T (1996) Statistical data on occupational contact urticaria. Contact Dermatitis 35:229–233

26. Kavli G, Forde OH (1984) Hand dermaloses in Tromso. Contact Dermatitis 10:174–177

27. Lammintausta K, Kalimo K, Aanton S (1982) Course of hand dermatitis in hospital workers. Contact Dermatitis 8:327–332

28. Lantinga H, Nater JP, Coenraads PJ (1984) Prevalence, incidence and course of ezema on the hands and forearms in a sample of thc general population. Contact Dermatitis 10:135–139

29. Leino T, Tammilehto L, Hytonen M, Sala E, Paakkulainen H, Kanerva L (1998) Occupational skin and respiratory diseases among hairdressers. Scand J Work Environ Health 24:398–406

30. Livesley EJ, Rushton L, English JS, Williams HC (2002) The prevalence of occupational dermatitis in the UK printing industry. Occup Environ Med 59:487–492

31. McCurdy SA, Wiggins P, Schenker MB, Munn S et al (1989) Assessing dermatitis in epidemiologic studies: occupational skin disease among California grape and tomato harvesters. Am J Industr Med 16:147–157

32. Meding B, Jarvholm B (2002) Hand eczema in Swedish adults – changes in prevalence between 1983 and 1996. J Invest Dermatol 118:719–723

33. Meding BE, Swanbeck G (1987) Prevalence of hand eczema in an industrial city. Br J Dermatol 16:627–634

34. Menné T, Bogan O, Green A (1982) Nickel allergy and hand dermatitis in a stratified sample of the Danish female population: an epidemiological study including a statistic appendix. Acta Derm Venereol 62:35–41

35. Menné T, Christoffersen J, Maibach HI (1987) Epidemiology of allergic contact sensitization. Monogr Allergy 21:132–161

36. Meyer JD, Chen Y, Holt DL, Beck MH, Cherry NM (2000) Occupational contact dermatitis in the UK: a surveillance report from EPIDERM and OPRA. Occup Med 50:265–273

37. Mortz CG, Lauritsen JM, Bindslev-Jensen C, Andersen KE (2001) Prevalence of atopic dermatitis, asthma, allergic rhinitis, and hand and contact dermatitis in adolescents. The Odense Adolescence Cohort Study on Atopic Diseases and Dermatitis. Br J Dermatol 144:523–532

38. Mortz CG, Lauritsen JM, Bindslev-Jensen C, Andersen KE (2002) Contact allergy and allergic contact dermatitis in adolescents: prevalence measures and associations. The Odense Adolescence Cohort Study on Atopic Diseases and Dermatitis (TOACS). Acta Derm Venereol 82:352–358

39. Nielsen NH, Linneberg A, Menné T, Madsen F, Frolund L, Dirksen A, Jorgensen T (2001) Allergic contact sensitization in an adult Danish population: two cross-sectional surveys eight years apart (the Copenhagen Allergy Study). Acta Derm Venereol 81:31–34

40. Nielsen NH, Linneberg A, Menné T, Madsen F, Frolund L, Dirksen A, Jorgensen T (2002) Incidence of allergic contact sensitization in Danish adults between 1990 and 1998; the Copenhagen Allergy Study, Denmark. Br J Dermatol 147:487–492

41. Nilsson GE, Mikaelsson B, Andersson S (1985) Atopy, occupation and domestic work as risk factors for hand eczema in hospital workers. Contact Dermatitis 13:216–223

42. Paulsen E, Sogaard J, Andersen KE (1997) Occupational dermatitis in Danish gardeners and greenhouse workers (I). Prevalence and possible risk factors. Contact Dermatitis 37:263–270

43. Rea JN, Newhouse ML, Halil T (1976) Skin diseases in Lambeth. A community study of prevalence and use of medical care. Br J Prev Soc Med 30:107–114

44. Rystedt I (1985) Hand eczema and long term prognosis in atopic dermatitis (thesis). Acta Derm Venereol [Suppl] 117:1–59

45. Schäfer T, Bohler E, Ruhdorfer S, Weigl L, Wessner D, Filipiak B, Wichmann HE, Ring J (2001) Epidemiology of contact allergy in adults. Allergy 56:192–196

46. Sertoli A, Francalanci S, Acciai MC, Gola M (1999) Epidemiological survey of contact dermatitis in Italy (1984–1993) by GIRDCA (Gruppo Italiano Ricerca Dermatiti da Contatto e Ambientali). Am J Contact Dermat 10:18–30

47. Shum KW, Meyer JD, Chen Y, Cherry N, Gawkrodger DJ (2003) Occupational contact dermatitis to nickel: experience of the British dermatologists (EPIDERM) and occupational physicians (OPRA) surveillance schemes. Occup Environ Med 60:954–957

48. Smit HA, Coenraads PJ, Lavrijsen APM, Nater JP (1992) Evaluation of a self-administered questionnaire on hand dermatitis. Contact Dermatitis 26:11–16

49. Smit HA, Burdorf A, Coenraads PJ (1993) The prevalence of hand dermatitis in different occupations. Int J Epidemiol 22:288–293

50. Smit HA, van Rijssen A, Vandenbroucke J, Coenraads PJ (1994) Individual susceptibility and the incidence of hand dermatitis in a cohort of apprentice hairdressers and nurses. Scand J Work Environ Health 20:113–121

51. Susitaival P, Husman L, Hollmen A, Horsmanheimo M (1995) Dermatoses determined in a population of farmers in a questionnaire-based clinical study including methodology validation. Scand J Work Environ Health 21:30–35

52. Susitaival P, Kirk J, Schenker MB (2001) Self-reported hand dermatitis in California veterinarians. Am J Contact Dermat 12:103–108

53. Susitaival P, Flyvholm MA, Meding B, Kanerva L, Lindberg M, Svensson A, Olafsson JH (2003) Nordic Occupational Skin Questionnaire (NOSQ-2002): a new tool for surveying occupational skin diseases and exposure. Contact Dermatitis 49:70–76

54. Svensson A, Lindberg M, Meding B, Sundberg K, Stenberg B (2002) Self-reported hand eczema: symptom-based reports do not increase the validity of diagnosis. Br J Dermatol 147:281–284

55. Tacke J, Schmidt A, Fartasch M, Diepgen TL (1995) Occupational contact dermatitis in bakers, confectioners and cooks. A population based study. Contact Dermatitis 33:112–118

56. Taylor JS (1988) Occupational disease statistics in perspective (editorial). Arch Dermatol 124:1557–1558

57. Thompson TR, Belsito DV (2002) Regional variation in prevalence and etiology of allergic contact dermatitis. Am J Contact Dermat 13:177–182

58. Uter W, Pfahlberg A, Gefeller O, Schwanitz HJ (1998) Prevalence and incidence of hand dermatitis in hairdressing apprentices: results of the POSH study. Prevention of occupational skin disease in hairdressers. Int Arch Occup Environ Health 71:487–492

59. Uter W, Schnuch A., Gefeller O (2004) European Surveillance System on Contact Allergies. Guidelines for the descriptive presentation and statistical analysis of contact allergy data. Contact Dermatitis 51(2)47–56

60. Varigos GA, Dunt DR (1981) Occupational dermatitis. An epidemiological study in the rubber and cement industries. Contact Dermatitis 7:105–110

61. Vermeulen R, Kromhout H, Bruynzeel DP, de Boer EM (2000) Ascertainment of hand dermatitis using a symptom-based questionnaire; applicability in an industrial population. Contact Dermatitis 42:202–206

62. Wallenhammar LM, Ortengren U, Andreasson H, Barregard L, Bjorkner B, Karlsson S, Wrangsjo K, Meding B (2000) Contact allergy and hand eczema in Swedish dentists. Contact Dermatitis 43:192–199

63. Wilkinson JD, Shaw S, Andersen KE, Brandao FM, Bruynzeel DP, Bruze M, Camarasa JM, Diepgen TL, Ducombs G, Frosch PJ, Goossens A, Lachapelle JM, Lahti A, Menné T, Seidenari S, Tosti A, Wahlberg JE (2002) Monitoring levels of preservative sensitivity in Europe. A 10-year overview (1991–2000). Contact Dermatitis 46:207–110

10.2 Statistical Methods in Clinical Epidemiology

Wolfgang Uter, Axel Schnuch, Olaf Gefeller

This text is based on a guidelines paper published in "*Contact Dermatitis*" 2004, **51**:47–56, on behalf of the ESCD working party "European Surveillance System on Contact Allergies (ESSCA)."

10.2.1 Introduction

Researchers will only be able to fully exploit the scientific potential of their study, and make this appreciable for the reader, if the design, the statistical analysis, and the presentation of its results have a sufficiently high standard. The present chapter aims at helping clinical researchers in the field of contact allergy (CA) to select those descriptive measures and statistical methods that are most appropriate for their problem. Its focus is on *clinical* epidemiology, i.e., *patient-based* research, thus supplementing the description of population-related studies and basic epidemiological concepts related to them, which are discussed in the preceding section (10.1 Basic Concepts of Population-based Epidemiology).

Many studies in the field of clinical epidemiology of contact dermatitis address CA by analyzing patch test data, and rather few clinical studies focus on other aspects of irritant or allergic contact dermatitis – excluding therapy studies, which will not be dealt with here (see textbooks such as [1]). Hence, we will pay particular attention to methods suitable for analyzing patch test data, describing, e.g., the profile of a certain allergen (e.g., pattern of reactions, probably under different test conditions, demographic variables of sensitized patients, spectrum of co-sensitization) or certain subpopulations (defined by sex, age, occupation, etc.) with their more or less characteristic spectrum of allergens. Due to the complexity of some research questions, however, the instruments included in this chapter might not suffice. Direct consultation with biostatisticians will always be advisable.

Type, extent, and severity of clinical dermatitis and patch test reactions, evaluated with the naked eye, remain the outcome of eminent importance in patient management and clinical CA research. This type of outcome, combined with information from the patient's history, such as occupation, possible sources of allergen exposure and the relevance of positive patch test reactions as factors potentially associated with the outcome, can be subject to statistical analysis. Hence, the present recommendations focus on such categorical outcomes. Instrument-based measurements, such as those for transepidermal water loss and other noninvasive techniques, microdialysates, digital image analysis, etc., have their own repertoire of statistical analysis methods, which would exceed the scope of this chapter, and are dealt with in other reviews or textbooks.

Core Message

■ Clinical (patch test) studies of contact allergy should not only be designed and performed adequately, but should also be analyzed and reported using appropriate descriptive and analytical statistics to achieve maximum scientific impact.

10.2.2 Outcome: the Patch Test Reaction

The grading of patch test reactions to allergens has been standardized largely on an international level [2], with partial refinement by national contact dermatitis groups, e.g., in central Europe [3]. With less well-known allergens in particular, not only should the number or percentage of positive reactions be given, but also the numbers of doubtful and irritant reactions, in order to obtain a complete view of the reaction profile of the allergen in question, tested (and read) as it has been in the particular study. If there should be uncertainty about the interpretation of reactions recorded as positive (erythema, infiltrate, possibly papules), these should be presented and analyzed separately from stronger positive reactions. Concerning supplementary test methods, useful suggestions for the scoring of repeated open application test (ROAT) results [4] and of reactions to occlusively tested sodium lauryl sulfate (SLS) [5] (which has recently been advocated as a useful supplement to allergen patch testing [6]), are available.

Supplementing the full description of the pattern of patch test reactions [doubtful, irritant, (weak/strong) positive], the following aggregating parameters have been suggested to give further information on the reaction profile of an allergen:

■ The reaction index (RI) [7]: (number of positive reactions – number of doubtful or irritant reactions) / (number of positive reactions + number of doubtful or irritant reactions). Val-

ues close to 1 indicate that the proportion of + to +++ reactions is much larger than the proportion of doubtful or irritant reactions; values close to –1, the opposite.
■ The positivity ratio (PR) [8], which is simply the proportion of positive reactions among all positive reactions (+ to +++). A value of >80% is considered indicative of a "problematic" allergen.
■ The time pattern in terms of the proportion of crescendo, plateau or decrescendo reactions, e.g., from D1 (day 1 of patch test) or D2 to D3 or D4. Comparisons between the types of time patterns have been found particularly useful in photopatch testing [9]. However, this kind of analysis may also prove interesting in the evaluation of conventional patch test results, as with problematic allergens [10] or different concentrations of a marginal irritant.

Although it can be argued that the RI and the PR provide redundant information already contained in a full description of the reaction profile, as above, they highlight specific aspects of the reaction profile characterizing a certain allergen preparation quantitatively "at a glance" and may thus be regarded as useful addition, e.g., when comparing different preparations of one allergen. Moreover, local patch test reading standards can easily be compared between centers in terms of quality control using these aggregate measures, preferably based on a set of well-established allergen preparations [11].

Core Message

■ A full description of the reaction profile, including the frequency of doubtful, irritant, and different grades of positive reactions, is recommended, in particular for allergens beyond the standard series.

10.2.3 Patient Selection

As a clear prerequisite for meaningful interpretation of research results in terms of CA frequency in a certain group of patients, the denominator must be described clearly in terms of:

10

■ The number of subjects included (if all persons are not tested with all allergens in a panel of allergens, the number tested must be stated for each allergen).
■ The period analyzed.
■ The way the allergen was patch tested. (Aimed testing versus testing consecutive patients, which has an evident impact on the prevalences of CA diagnosed. One example: CA to Disperse Blue 106/124 was diagnosed in up to 6.7% of patients patch tested with a special textile dyes series [12], whereas the prevalence was only 1.3% in consecutively tested patients [13]).
■ Important demographic characteristics which may have a profound impact on the observed spectrum of CA, e.g., according to the MOAHLFA index [14].

Clearly, the proportion of missing data for these items must be kept low by appropriate quality control of routine or study documentation [11].

The MOAHLFA index is an extension of the original MOHL [15] and the later MOAHL index [16], which lists the proportions of certain demographic variables, namely M for male sex, O for occupational causation of dermatitis, A for atopy, H for hand, L for leg, and F for face as affected site, and the last A for the proportion of patients aged 40 and above. Any of these factors may have a profound influence on the frequency of sensitization. For instance, a high proportion of patch test patients with lower leg dermatitis/varicose ulcers (the "L") will be associated with prevalences of neomycin sulfate and lanolin CA, to name but a few, well above the average [17]. A high proportion of occupational contact dermatitis cases (the "O") will evidently raise the frequency of positive reactions to epoxy resin, chromate, or other "occupational" allergens, depending on the spectrum of local industries. Hence, consideration of this basic demographic and clinical data will help to explain differing results from different centers [14]. Furthermore, consideration of the MOAHLFA index of the study group should put comparisons with other, dissimilar groups of patients into due perspective. With regard to the first "A," it should be mentioned that this stood for atopy in general in the MOAHL index, i.e., the presence of atopic eczema, allergic rhinoconjunctivitis or allergic bronchial asthma [16]. In contrast, in the MOAHLFA index as suggested, only atopic eczema is considered because, according to current evidence, there seems to be no reason to assume (1) an etiologically relevant association between CA and mucosal atopic symptoms and (2) a relevant impact

of the presence of these types of atopic symptoms on the indication for patch testing. Hence, the inclusion of mucosal atopic disease would render this "A" in the index less specific, while the proportion of patch-tested patients with underlying previous or current atopic eczema will have some impact on the spectrum of CA – due to either presumptive immunological abnormalities, or disease-specific exposures to topical medicaments, ointment base ingredients, etc., similar to leg dermatitis as the underlying condition.

In addition to a (standardized) description of the population characteristics as outline above, appropriate discussion of selection processes, as far as these are known, and their potential effect on CA frequencies or risk estimates should supplement the epidemiological interpretation of results. It is often a major criticism of patient-based studies (i.e., clinical epidemiology) that prevalences found in a particular group of patients are (mis-)interpreted by the authors as prevalences on a population level, which, expectedly, are usually much lower. Hence, prevalences should be put into the proper perspective by delineating the recruitment process for the study subjects, e.g., specialist versus general practitioner referral, and specialties of the center, such as medicolegal evaluation, dermatitis due to cosmetics or a strong background of phlebology, to mention but a few.

Core Message

■ The selection process until presentation in a patch test clinic and eventual inclusion as a patient in the study group, and the demographic and clinical characteristics of this group [namely the distribution of sex and age, occupational background and characteristic sites of dermatitis (MOAHLFA index)], can have a profound impact on the allergen spectrum and should thus be described in detail.

10.2.4 Proportions

Proportions (%) are a very common measure of an outcome of interest, such as the proportion of irritant, doubtful, and positive reactions to a certain allergen, or the frequency of selected population characteristics such as sex, occupation, atopy, etc., in the subset of patients testing positive or negative to a certain allergen. Primarily, such proportions are descriptive of the study population. In most cases, however, researchers want to communicate these results as typical or representative of other persons or patients sharing the characteristics defining their study group. Hence, the study group is regarded as a sample. This implies that the observed proportion is an estimate of the result that would theoretically be observed if all eligible persons in the target population were included in the study. Consequently, the precision of this estimate must be addressed by supplementing the point estimate (the observed proportion) with a confidence interval (CI), usually, but not necessarily, a 95% CI. Motivating the CI from a different perspective, it could be said that empirical results, such as an observed proportion, always carry an element of chance. Hence, it may well be that upon repetition of the study under the same conditions a slightly different proportion will be observed, especially if the sample was small (see below). The extremely useful concept of CI can be interpreted as follows: if 100 samples from a given target population were drawn, or 100 groups of patients sharing the same characteristics were assessed (or the study repeated 100 times), the observed proportion would, in 95 (90, 99) of these 100 samples or repetitions, lie within the limits indicated by the 95% (90%, 99%) CI.

Count data such as proportions often follow a binomial distribution; for more details see [18] or textbooks such as [19]. The binomial distribution, with increasing study sample size n, more and more resembles the well-known symmetrical, bell-shaped form of the normal distribution. Hence, a normal approximation to the binomial distribution can be used to calculate a CI according to Eq. 10.2.1 for large sample sizes. This formula exploits the fact that, given a normal distribution, the proportions of events within or beyond a certain span around the mean can be determined. Typically, a 5% error (α) is regarded as acceptable, i.e., that 2.5% of measurements may lie below, and 2.5% above the CI. Hence, the – symmetrical – 2.5% and 97.5% percentiles

$$\left(Z_{\frac{\alpha}{2}} \text{ for } \alpha = 0.05 \right)$$

of the standard normal distribution are of interest in determining the CI, i.e., –1.96 and +1.96 (as can be taken from statistical tabulations).

$$\text{CI}(\hat{p}) = Z_{\frac{\alpha}{2}} \cdot \text{SE}(\hat{p}) \quad \text{SE}(\hat{p}) = \sqrt{\frac{(\hat{p}(1-\hat{p}))}{n}} \quad (10.2.1)$$

where

$$Z_{\frac{\alpha}{2}} \text{ is the } 100\left(1 - \frac{\alpha}{2}\right)$$

percentile of the standard normal distribution, n is the total number of subjects, and $\hat{p}$ is the observed proportion (the estimate). The larger the study sample (n in Eq. 10.2.1), the smaller the standard error (SE in Eq. 10.2.1) will be, and hence the more precise the estimate, i.e., the narrower the CI. As an example: the point estimate 10% as 10 out of 100 is accompanied by a 95% CI of 4.1–15.9, while for 100 out of 1000, the corresponding CI is 8.1–11.9% according to Eq. 10.2.1. However, for small samples (e.g., $n<30$), the exact CI based directly on the binomial distribution is preferable, because the above normal approximation to the binomial distribution or other types of approximations do not hold. In summary, CIs provide an indispensable measure of the precision of observed proportions. Most statistical software packages offer the calculation of a CI to a proportion. However, if fewer than 100 cases are analyzed, the use of a percentage to describe proportions becomes questionable, and a sample size of less than 10 renders percentage meaningless.

Core Message

- Proportions, and other measures, should be supplemented with a confidence interval (CI) to quantify their precision; a 95% CI is commonly chosen. This may help to dispel overinterpretation of results, especially with very small samples.

10.2.5 Rates

While proportions quantify the frequency of a certain condition among those examined, rates are measures of the occurrence of events with reference to time, such as the heart rate (beats per minute) or cancer incidence rate (new cases per 100,000 persons per year). Thus, their unit contains an element of time. In the general field of epidemiology, incidence is the most important rate, see a detailed description and discussion in Sect. 10.1.

10.2.6 Statistical Testing of Proportions and Rates

Sometimes, the supplementation of CIs to proportions or rates will make formal statistical testing unnecessary. For instance, if CIs of proportions of different subgroups do not overlap, significant difference is already evident. For instance, 18.4% (95% CI: 15.7–21.0%) of hairdressers patch tested positively to ammonium persulfate, but only 4.4% (95% CI: 3.0–5.7%) of their clients [20], a significant difference. Moreover, the supplementation of CIs to proportions or other measures, for that matter, is being regarded as more informative and thus often even preferable to statistical testing [21]. If statistical tests for differences are performed, the following situations may arise:

- Comparison of the proportions observed in two (or more) independent groups of patients (e.g., those with a certain occupation versus those with other occupations, or males versus females). The statistical null hypothesis would be equality of proportions, or, in other words, that the two (or more) samples are derived from the same target population, with regard to the outcome. This hypothesis can be tested with the chi-square test, which examines the departure of observed n_{ij} from expected e_{ij} cell frequencies, summed up over each cell of the $k \times l$ contingency table, deriving a test statistic with a chi-squared distribution and $(k-1) \cdot (l-1)$ degrees of freedom.

$$X^2 = \sum_{i=1}^{k} \sum_{j=1}^{l} \frac{(n_{ij} - e_{ij})^2}{e_{ij}} \qquad (10.2.2)$$

Fisher's exact test (or its modified versions in the case of more than two groups) is an alternative preferable in cases of small samples, e.g., if any of the expected cell counts are less than 5. However, these tests **must not** be applied in dependent sample situations, i.e., if two factors are analyzed in one sample, which are primarily related, such as "left versus right" or "low versus high test concentration" comparisons of the same allergen (see Sect. 10.2.8 "Measures of Concordance" and [22]).

- A test for trend of proportions, e.g., over time. Although similar to the previous test problems in terms of the statistical null hypothesis of homogeneity, trend tests take the ordering of the (time) scale into account. One example of a trend test is the chi-squared test for trend [19]. Another possibility is the Cochran–Armitage trend test. For instance, the prevalence of nickel allergy remained largely stable in German patch test patients 1992 to 2001. However, a stratified analysis (see below) revealed a significant decline from 36.7% to 25.8% in the subgroup of female patients younger than 30 ($p < 0.0001$, Cochrane–Armitage trend test), coinciding with the EU nickel regulation [23].

However, if (1) more than one statistical test is performed and (2) statistical hypotheses testing is intended not just to be exploratory, but to be confirmative [i.e., aiming at empirically "proving" a scientific hypothesis within the framework of predefined α (and probably β) error], the well-known problem of "multiple testing" [19] arises, namely, spurious "significant" results. This should be counteracted by employing suitable α-adjustment techniques such as Bonferroni–Holm.

Core Message

- A CI is, in many situations, preferable to a p-value. For the statistical testing of differences of proportions (between disjunct subgroups of patients, across time), chi-square(d) tests are appropriate, but in cases of small samples Fisher's exact test is preferable.

10.2.7 Risk Estimates

The question of how much the frequency or likelihood of disease (or other conditions) is increased if a certain factor is present, relative to the frequency or likelihood if this factor is not present, is addressed by estimates of individual risk. These measures essentially comprise the – absolute or relative – risk difference, the relative risk (RR), the odds ratio (OR) and the prevalence ratio (PR). The interpretation of a difference in risk between exposed and unexposed heavily depends on the baseline risk of the disease and is thus uninformative if communicated alone.

For instance, a difference of 0.2% between the prevalence in exposed and unexposed is quite irrelevant if the disease is frequent (10, 20 or 30%), but important if the baseline prevalence is <1%. The RR, in contrast, is a quotient and thus quantifies the factor by which risk is increased in the exposed independent from baseline frequency. It is typically an incidence-based measure, namely the incidence found in those exposed divided by the incidence observed in the nonexposed, and can thus directly be estimated only in longitudinal (cohort) studies (see Sect. 10.1). In contrast, the OR and the PR, which are explained in this section, can be calculated in cross-sectional designs, to which clinical assessment of successive patients (who are seen just once during a certain study period) bears a similarity.

In the simplest, and often simplistic, case of a 2×2 contingency table (Table 2.1), cross-tabulating the dichotomized outcome with the dichotomized exposure variable, the prevalence ratio is easily calculated by dividing the proportion (prevalence) of the exposed study group by that of the nonexposed comparison group. The most common measure of risk, however, is the OR, by virtue of several advantages, which will not be discussed in depth here. In contrast to the prevalence ratio (and the RR), the OR is a quotient of two odds, see Table 2.1. With decreasing risk of a disease (which can be translated into decreasing prevalence here) p, the risk of that disease and its odds

$$p/(1-p)$$

become increasingly similar, because $1-p$ asymptotically approaches 1. Consequently, the quotients based on risk versus odds become more and more similar, i.e., the OR becomes a valid approximation of the RR when the "rare disease assumption" holds. There are no strict rules as to when a disease can be regarded rare enough; however, if the disease prevalence does not exceed 1%, the numerical discrepancy between

OR and RR is negligible. Asymptotic 95% CIs to the OR, based on an approximation of the normal distribution already introduced, can be calculated according to the following formula:

$$CI_{95\%}(\hat{OR}) = e^{(\ln \hat{OR} \pm Z_{\alpha/2} \cdot SE(\ln \hat{OR})} \qquad (10.2.3)$$

$$\hat{SE}(\ln \hat{OR}) = \sqrt{\frac{1}{a} + \frac{1}{b} + \frac{1}{c} + \frac{1}{d}}$$

Some statistical software packages offer the calculation of exact CIs, which are preferable especially in the case of small sample sizes.

However, while a valid method to estimate the precision of a crude (unadjusted) risk estimate is an important issue, the validity of the risk estimate itself may critically depend on other factors, the so-called confounders. As an example: the prevalence of nickel allergy has often been found to be very high in hairdressers, compared to other occupations (OR or PR well above 1), raising the suspicion that nickel is an occupational allergen. However, if the young age and predominantly female sex of hairdressers is taken into account – both factors strongly associated with nickel allergy via age- and sex-characteristic fashion habits – nickel CA appears only slightly more common, if at all. In this and similar situations, a multifactorial analysis or other techniques adjusting for such confounding effects must be employed (Fig. 2.1; see also section below).

Core Message

- The odds ratio (OR) or prevalence ratio (PR) is a suitable measure for the quantification of individual risk (e.g., of a certain CA) associated with certain exposure factors. It should be accompanied by a CI.

Table 2.1. Different risk estimates illustrated with a 2 × 2 contingency table. D represents disease, with $D=1$ being the diseased, and $D=0$ the healthy, E represents exposure (risk factor), with $E=1$ being the exposed, $E=0$ the nonexposed. (*OR* Odds ratio, *PR* prevalence ratio, *RR* relative risk)

	$D=1$	$D=0$		PR (RR)	OR
$E=1$	a	b	$n_{E=1}$	$\dfrac{a/n_{E=1}}{c/n_{E=0}}$	$\dfrac{a/(n_{E=1}-a)}{c/(n_{E=0}-c)} = \dfrac{a/b}{c/d}$
$E=0$	c	d	$n_{E=0}$		
	$n_{D=1}$	$n_{D=0}$	n_{Total}		

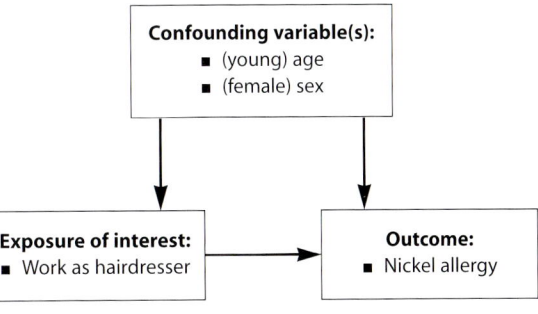

Fig. 2.1. Confounding: principle and an example (in *bullet list*)

10.2.8 Measures of Concordance

In CA research, the term concordance is colloquially used to describe simultaneous (concomitant) reactions to allergens, for which there may be several causes [24]. However, the concept of concordance in a stricter sense means agreement between ratings of two (or more) different observers, evaluating the same outcome in the same set of subjects. As such, it is a measure of the reliability (reproducibility) of a rating system under certain use conditions. Beyond this original application, the concept of concordance as outlined below can be applied to describe test reactions observed during synchronous patch testing in the following situations:

- Comparing test results obtained with different test methods, e.g., 24-h versus 48-h patch test application, large versus small test chambers [22], water versus ethanol as test vehicle, high versus low test concentration, or otherwise different preparations of the **same allergen**.
- Quantifying reproducibility upon synchronous duplicate patch testing of identical allergen preparations [25].
- Comparing test results with mixes and any of their individual constituents.
- Comparing test reactions to allergens which are structurally related, such as fragrances [26] or para-amino compounds [27].

The use of the concept of concordance to quantify agreement between test results is the only appropriate approach in the first two situations, and a useful additional measure in the other two situations. In this situation, the sole consideration of the percentage of concordant ratings (see Table 2.2) P_o,

$$P_o = \frac{n_{11} + n_{00}}{n}$$

as an intuitive measure, and other measures based directly on these proportions will give a misleading, overly optimistic impression of concordance, because by chance alone a certain proportion of ratings P_e will agree, with $\hat{p}$ being the probability of one positive rating, and $\hat{q}$ the probability of the other positive rating:

$$P_e = \hat{p} \cdot \hat{q} + (1 - \hat{p}) \cdot (1 - \hat{q})$$

Hence, only the agreement **beyond chance** should be considered.

A well-established measure of "chance-corrected" agreement for categorical data such as patch test results is Cohen's kappa [28], either as simple kappa for 2×2 contingency tables (Eq. 10.2.4), or as weighted kappa for larger, symmetrically structured tables of ordinal data.

$$\kappa = \frac{P_o - P_e}{1 - P_e} \tag{10.2.4}$$

The actual kappa value can be regarded as an estimate, and should thus be supplemented with CIs. Several interpretative scales of the kappa values have been suggested (e.g., [29]). In general, kappa values close to 0 indicate a (complete) lack of agreement beyond chance, and values close to 1 (almost) perfect agreement. As an example: upon synchronous duplicate patch testing with 48 h of exposure, kappa values between 0.85 (95% CI: 0.80–0.91) for nickel (5% pet.) and 0.50 (95% CI: 0.30–0.71) for formaldehyde (1% aqu.) have been found [25]. Considering this (very) good, but not perfect, agreement between identical allergens as an upper ceiling, concordance between different, but structurally related allergens is put into perspective: a kappa value of 0.64 (95% CI: 0.55–0.74) observed for the combination of p-phenylenediamine (PPD) and p-aminoazobenzene [30] appears to indicate more substantial agreement, if related to the kappa value 0.86 (95% CI: 0.79–0.92) for PPD alone [25] than if related to the theoretical upper bound of concordance, 1. However, the application of Cohen's kappa – or any other measure of concordance, for that matter – is not without pitfalls, e.g., similar kappa values may have an altogether different meaning in samples with very different prevalences of the outcome [31].

Core Message

- When quantifying concordance, i.e., the agreement between two related outcomes in a dependent sample, the sole consideration of observed agreement is misleading. Instead, Cohen's kappa coefficient, supplemented with CIs, should be used to describe "agreement beyond chance."

10.2.9 Statistical Testing in Dependent Samples

Concordance, as described above, is a concept suitable for describing agreement between two outcomes observed in one set of patients, i.e., in dependent samples. Sometimes, beyond description, statistical analysis of such paired sample results may be an issue. Examples for this include statistically testing for differences between:

- Test results obtained from the same patients with different concentrations, vehicles, exposure times, chamber sizes, etc. of an allergen.
- Responses to allergen or irritant challenge before and after some therapeutic intervention in the same patients.

In these and similar cases, it is not the concordant test results (using Table 2.2 for illustration purposes: n_{00} and n_{11}) that are informative, but the discordant test results (n_{01} and n_{10}); namely, the degree of asymmetry. If discordant results are essentially symmetrically distributed, it is reasonable to assume that they merely reflect chance variation, and not a systematic difference. If, however, more discordant results are observed in a particular area of the contingency table, this may indicate a systematic difference, such as "significantly more positive reactions with a higher test concentration" [32] or "borderline evidence for a higher detection rate of 5-chloro-2-methylisothiazol-3-one/2-methylisothiazol-3-one (MCI/MI) CA when using larger, compared with small, Finn Chambers" [22]. For 2×2 contingency tables (Table 2.2), McNemar's test, which is also available as an exact test based on the binomial distribution, is suitable to assess the null hypothesis of "no difference." In quadratic contingency tables larger than 2×2, the Bowker test or a generalized Cochran–Mantel–Haenszel test can be applied. For an extensive explanation, further examples, and a discussion of the application of this class of statistical tests, see [22].

Core Message

- In a dependent sample situation, i.e., when statistically testing (dis-)agreement of two related outcomes in one set of patients, tests for independent samples such as chi-squared or Fisher's exact test must not be used, but rather the McNemar, Bowker, or similar tests.

10.2.10 Assessment of Diagnostic Quality

The quality of a diagnostic test, and its statistical evaluation, is an issue in both population-based and clinical epidemiology. The preceding section (10.1) includes a comprehensive illustrative discussion of this issue. Hence, in this section, we will focus on a brief formal introduction, followed by those aspects that are important for patient-based studies.

Diagnostic tests are evaluated against a "gold standard" to examine their diagnostic properties. These include (for an explanation of abbreviations see Table 2.3):

- Sensitivity (the proportion of diseased testing positive: $a/n_{D=present}$).
- Specificity (the proportion of healthy persons testing negative, $d/n_{D=absent}$).
- The positive predictive value (the proportion of persons testing positive being actually diseased ($a/n_{T=pos}$).
- The negative predictive value (the proportion of persons testing negative being actually healthy ($d/n_{T=neg}$).

The "gold standard" generally is a method with high, proven validity. In the field of CA, there is not yet one ideal gold standard against which patch test results can be evaluated. For the time being, several "gold" standards – either combined or alternatively, namely "a positive history of intolerance (to the allergen in question)" [32], or the results of a provocative use test (PUT) or a repeated open application test (ROAT)

Table 2.2. A 2×2 contingency table illustrating a dependent sample situation with a left versus right comparison

Expected (random) concordance	Observed concordance		
	Right: positive	**Right: negative**	**Right: total**
Left: positive	n_{11} $n \cdot \hat{p} \cdot \hat{q}$	n_{10} $n \cdot \hat{p} \cdot (1-\hat{q})$	$n_{11}+n_{10}$ $n \cdot \hat{p}$
Left: negative	n_{01} $n \cdot (1-\hat{p}) \cdot \hat{q}$	n_{00} $n \cdot (1-\hat{p}) \cdot (1-\hat{q})$	$n_{01}+n_{00}$ $n \cdot (1-\hat{p})$
Left: total	$n_{11}+n_{01}$ $n \cdot \hat{q}$	$n_{10}+n_{00}$ $n \cdot (1-\hat{q})$	n

[33] – are employed to validate patch test results. Alas, the PUT or ROAT is cumbersome for doctor and patient, and thus possibly not used as often as is desirable.

When assessing the sensitivity, specificity, and other properties of allergen patch tests against the references mentioned, it should be kept in mind that these can only be as good as the "gold standard" chosen, which is as yet far from ideal, be it for reasons of feasibility. However, the concepts used for the assessment of diagnostic properties can also be applied successfully **within** the realm of patch testing itself, e.g., for the evaluation (1) of mixes against reactivity to their constituents (e.g., [34]) or (2) of single "marker allergens" against reactivity to allergens of which they are considered markers. Note that if constituents are tested only in the case of a positive reaction to the mix used for screening, just the PPV can be calculated, and not sensitivity and specificity, as the row "T = negative" is missing (Table 2.3).

Percentages such as sensitivity, specificity, and positive and negative predictive value should be supplemented with (95%) CIs, to address the issue of precision. Being proportions, these can be calculated as described above. When interpreting the positive and negative predictive value (PPV and NPV), their dependency not only on sensitivity (Sens) and specificity (Spec), but also on the prevalence P of disease (of CA, in this context) must be considered, which is illustrated in Sect. 10.1.

According to this, the PPV of a positive patch test result is (much) higher – hence, the proportion of false-positives (much) lower – in a typical clinical setting, where selected patients with suspected CA are patch tested and the a priori likelihood of CA is high, relative to patch testing in (subgroups of) the general population unselected for specific morbidity. This relationship seriously limits the value of patch test studies in the general population, at least concerning allergens that are not common. In contrast, in view of the relatively low prevalence of common CAs even in patch test patients (with, e.g., nickel sulfate rarely exceeding 20%), the NPV is not a problem, because it increases with decreasing prevalence.

Clearly, in individual cases the a priori likelihood of CA to a range of allergens is highly variable, if the history of the patient is carefully taken into account. If the patient's history is suggestive of a certain CA, a negative result, even with well-established test preparations such as nickel sulfate 5% pet. [35], should be challenged. The opposite, the evaluation of positive test reactions in the light of a possibly negative history, is the assessment of clinical relevance that will not be dealt with here.

Core Message

■ Patch testing even with optimum concentration and vehicle for a given allergen is, like most diagnostic tests, neither 100% sensitive nor 100% specific. Consequently, false-positive test results must be expected especially if the true CA prevalence is low, i.e., in population samples unselected for specific morbidity (suspected allergic contact dermatitis), compared to patch test patients.

10.2.11 Stratification and Standardization

In certain subgroups defined by age, sex, occupation or other characteristics, the outcome of interest (a specific CA) may occur with variable frequency. If these very differences in distribution are the main research interest, a stratified analysis, i.e., separate analyses for each subgroup, is usually performed and presented (for example [23, 36]). At the same time, stratification is one possible strategy of confounder control (Fig. 2.1), by performing separate analyses for each different level of the confounding factor, such as sex (male versus female) or age (≥40 versus <40 or 10-year age strata) or other factors. This will, however, lead to a multitude of stratum-specific prevalences, which may be hard to interpret as a whole. In this case, a unifying view may be achieved by suitably standardizing the prevalence by the confounders concerned.

Standardization is a well-established technique to increase comparability of descriptive study results, such as incidence and prevalence data. For instance, meaningful descriptive cancer epidemiology relies on age standardization, because: (1) the incidence of most cancers is strongly age-dependent, and (2) the age structure may differ between regions or vary across time, making valid comparisons (e.g., geo-

Table 2.3. Different measures of diagnostic performance illustrated with a 2×2 contingency table. [D Disease (according to "gold standard" criterion), T test to be evaluated]

	D=present	D=absent	
T=positive	a	b	$n_{T=pos}$
T=negative	c	d	$n_{T=neg}$
	$n_{D=present}$	$n_{D=absent}$	n_{Total}

graphical patterns or time trends) impossible. With this aim in mind, it has been introduced to clinical CA research [37]. There are essentially two methods of standardization: direct and indirect. To put it simply, indirect standardization involves calculating a quotient, in this context a "standardized morbidity ratio (SMR)," from the prevalence observed in the study sample P_{obs} and the expected prevalence P_{exp}. The expected prevalence P_{exp} is the weighted sum of the stratum-specific prevalences P_i^* in the reference population (the asterisk indicating that this quantity is not directly observable in the study and has to be "plugged in" using external information). The weights are the relative sizes of each stratum in the study group h_i (Eq. 10.2.5).

$$ \text{SMR} = \frac{P_{obs}}{P_{exp}} \qquad P_{exp} = \sum_i h_i \cdot P_i^* \qquad (10.2.5) $$

In contrast, direct standardization involves calculating a weighted sum P_{dir} of stratum-specific prevalences (of CA to a particular allergen) observed in the study group P_i, the stratum-specific weights being the relative sizes of each stratum in the reference population h_i^* (Eq. 10.2.6).

$$ P_{dir} = \sum_i h_i^* \cdot P_i \qquad (10.2.6) $$

The advantage of direct standardization is that the proportion – in terms of an "adjusted proportion" – is preserved as an intuitively accessible absolute measure of morbidity, whereas the SMR is a relative measure, similar to the relative risk (RR). The choice of the reference group for direct standardization is, in principle, arbitrary. The reference population can be self-defined [37], as long as the combined distribution of all relevant factors is known or defined. The effect of direct standardization is illustrated in a paper by Schnuch et al. [14]. Approximate CIs can be calculated to standardized proportions, based on the weighted sum of the variances per stratum (see formula 15–7, p 263 in [38]). For instance, a recent study compared the prevalence of CA between female hairdressers (median age 24) and female clients (median age 46); thanks to the restriction to the female sex, only age standardization was necessary. The unadjusted (crude) prevalence of fragrance mix CA was 9.4% and 9.6%, respectively. However, after age standardization, the proportions were 13.2% versus 9.0% [20]. This was a significant difference, which would have been missed if the differing age distribution had not been taken into account. Hence, age standardization (and additionally standardization for sex or other factors, if appropriate) is mandatory if: (1) the outcome (CA) of interest is associated with age (sex, …) and (2) subgroups to be compared differ with regard to age (sex, …). The process of direct age standardization is illustrated step-by-step in Table 2.4.

Table 2.4. Step-by-step illustration of the process of direct standardization, employing two age strata, based on published data [20]

Class	Age stratum	Step 1 N (%) in age stratum	Step 2 Prevalence (% pos.) P	Step 3 Standard weight w	Step 4 P · w	Step 5 Sum of P · w
Hairdressers	Age <40	633 (82.3%)	7.3	0.5	3.65	
	Age 40 +	136 (17.7%)	19.1	0.5	9.55	13.2
	Total:	769 (100%)	9.4	1.0		
Clients	Age <40	423 (38.4%)	6.4	0.5	3.2	
	Age 40 +	678 (61.6%)	11.6	0.5	5.8	9.0
	Total:	1101 (100%)	9.6	1.0		

Steps:
1. Divide the sample(s) into age strata, in this case, two. These strata are predefined by the choice of the standardization scheme (see step 3).
2. Determine the age stratum specific (CA) prevalences
3. Apply the weights to the stratum-specific prevalences; weights are defined to sum up to 1 (i.e., 100%). Here, the IVDK standard is applied (50% patients younger than 40, 50% 40 or above) [37]
4. Multiply each stratum-specific prevalence obtained in step 2 with the stratum specific weight
5. Add the weighted prevalences obtained in step 4 to derive the directly age-standardized prevalence for each of the subgroups, in this case female hairdressers and female clients, for an age-adjusted comparison

Core Message

■ Prevalences (of specific CA) may differ between subgroups defined, e.g., by age and sex, rendering stratified analysis a sensible approach. One unifying "adjusted prevalence" of the entire study group can be calculated using direct standardization, also allowing adjusted comparisons with other study populations possibly differing with regard to the confounding stratification variables such as age and sex.

10.2.12 Multifactorial Analysis

Many research questions will address one particular factor of interest, such as a certain occupation (compared to other occupations), or a certain year of patch testing versus another reference year, if changes over time are an issue. In this situation, other factors associated with both the factor of interest and the outcome, i.e., potential confounders, may distort this comparison (Fig. 2.1).

There are several ways of controlling for potential confounders:

■ Restriction: limiting analysis to a subset of persons who do not differ with regard to confounding variables, e.g., young females only, both in the study group and in the comparison group, in our "nickel and hairdressing" example. This, however, will impair generalizability of results and reduce the statistical power of the study due to the reduction in sample size.

■ Stratification: giving separate results for each subgroup defined by the (combined) confounding variable(s), see above. As adjusted overall risk estimate can be derived: the sum of all single stratum-specific estimates weighted by a weighting scheme, often reflecting the relative size of the stratum, given sufficient homogeneity across the strata.

■ Matching: by study design, the comparison group is made similar to the study group regarding the distribution of confounding variables, e.g., similar proportions of young and old, males and females (frequency matching), or by matching one or more controls to each single case with regard to confounding vari-

ables (individual matching). In the analysis of matched study data, the matching variables must be duly considered, which is an issue of multifactorial analysis beyond the scope of this chapter.

■ Standardization (if descriptive measures are concerned, see above).

■ Adjustment techniques in terms of multifactorial analysis. Multifactorial analysis plays an important role in the clinical epidemiology of CA (one of the first examples of its application was an analysis by the Danish Contact Dermatitis Group [39]).

Multifactorial analyses are often preferable because they offer the added value of being able to derive risk estimates for several factors of interest at the same time, which are mutually adjusted. Conceptually, this type of analysis is based on multiple linear regression analysis, which is an expansion of simple linear regression [19, 40]. In simple regression, a directional relationship between one independent factor X and one dependent outcome Y is postulated, estimated by fitting a regression line which optimally represents this relationship and quantified by a regression equation, which includes an intercept term α and a slope coefficient β:

$$Y = \alpha + \beta X \qquad (10.2.7)$$

Multiple linear regression analysis is a well-known means of analyzing the association between a metric response (outcome) variable and *several* – categorical or metric – explanatory (risk) factors. In this type of analysis, the β coefficient is an indicator of the strength of association between the outcome and the respective factor, adjusted for the impact of all other factors. This useful approach can be generalized to accommodate modeling of binary outcome or count data, such as the presence of a certain disease, or a positive reaction to a certain contact allergen (e.g., with logistic or Poisson regression analysis). Furthermore, dependent, e.g., longitudinal, data can be analyzed employing generalized estimating equations. A comprehensive discussion of all aspects of these complex statistical tools can be found in textbooks (e.g., [38, 41]) and exceeds the scope of this chapter. For applications to the field of CA research, see, e.g., [39, 42–44].

Core Message

■ Multifactorial analysis is a useful statistical tool to derive mutually adjusted risk estimates for a number of potential risk factors (for specific CA). For both the application and the interpretation of results, in-depth statistical knowledge or consultation with biostatisticians is required.

Case Report

■ Polidocanol is an antipruritic topical agent contained in some emollients, which are especially, but not exclusively, used for the adjuvant treatment of atopic eczema. The questions arose: (1) how common is contact allergy to polidocanol, and (2) do atopic eczema patients have a higher risk? A retrospective analysis of 1992–1999 data of the multicenter CA surveillance network IVDK (www.ivdk.org) yielded the following results: 6202 patients with suspected allergic contact dermatitis due to topical treatments were tested with 3.0% polidocanol in petrolatum, resulting in $n=111$ (1.79%, exact 95% CI: 1.47–2.15%) questionable, $n=30$ (0.48%, exact 95% CI: 0.33–0.69%) irritant, $n=110$ (1.77%, exact 95% CI: 1.46–2.13%) weak, and $n=21$ (0.34%, exact 95% CI: 0.21–0.52%) strong positive reactions, with an RI of –0.04 and a PR of 84% (exact 95% CI: 76.5–89.8%). Current or previous clinical relevance was documented for 53% of patients with positive reactions, based on probable or certain deterioration of pre-existing dermatitis by application of polidocanol-containing topicals; this proportion being independent from the strength of the positive reaction (p trend: 0.07, Cochrane–Armitage trend test). To elucidate the role of potential risk factors, namely age, sex, occupational cause of dermatitis and site of current dermatitis, (1) the distribution of these factors in different subgroups was assessed and (2) a logistic regression analysis with the outcome "polidocanol positive versus negative" was performed. Results showed that elderly patients (OR 3.78, 95% CI 2.01–7.93) were particular at risk. In contrast, atopic dermatitis was not a significant risk factor (OR 1.37, 95% CI 0.69–2.49).

■ **Comment:** The reaction profile of this allergen indicated that it is a somewhat difficult allergen to test. The overall proportion of positive reactions (2.11%, exact 95% CI: 1.77–2.50%), although patients were tested in an aimed manner, was quite low, relative to other allergens contained in topical preparations. Consideration of clinical relevance gave no indication for a substantial impact of possibly false-positive reactions on our analysis. After an analysis of the distribution of the "MOAHLFA factors" in positive versus negative patients gave a first impression on possible risk groups, a significant association between age (<40 versus 40+) and CA to polidocanol was found by a multifactorial analysis, while the risk in atopic eczema patients was only marginally elevated.

■ **Note:** The original study, including 3186 more patients tested with 0.5% polidocanol in water, gave slightly different results, namely yielding "leg dermatitis" as additional significant risk factor [43].

10.2.13 Conclusion

The recommendations given above are by no means an exhaustive review or cover all statistical methods potentially relevant to clinical research in the field of contact dermatitis, and CA in particular. However, according to our experience, they do address the most common problems and might thus be useful to researchers when preparing, performing and analyzing a study, and when eventually writing a manuscript.

References

1. Schwindt DA, Maibach HI (2000) Cutaneous biometrics. Kluwer Academic/Plenum, New York
2. Wahlberg JE (2001) Patch testing. In: Rycroft RJG, Menné T, Frosch PJ, Leppoittevin J-P (eds) Textbook of contact dermatitis. Springer, Berlin Heidelberg New York, pp 435–468
3. Schnuch A, Aberer W, Agathos M, Brasch J, Frosch PJ, Fuchs T, Richter G (2001) Leitlinien der Deutschen Dermatologischen Gesellschaft (DDG) zur Durchführung des Epikutantests mit Kontaktallergenen. Hautarzt 52:864–866
4. Johansen JD, Bruze M, Andersen KE, Frosch PJ, Dreier B, White IR, Rastogi S, Lepoittevin JP, Menné T (1998) The repeated open application test: suggestions for ascale of evaluation. Contact Dermatitis 39:95–96

10

5. Tupker RA, Willis C, Berardesca E, Lee CH, Fartasch M, Agner T, Serup J (1997) Guidelines on sodium lauryl sulfate (SLS) exposure tests. A report from the Standardization Group of the European Society of Contact Dermatitis. Contact Dermatitis 37:53–69

6. Geier J, Uter W, Pirker C, Frosch PJ (2003) Patch testing with the irritant sodium lauryl sulfate (SLS) is useful in interpreting weak reactions to contact allergens as allergic or irritant. Contact Dermatitis 48:99–107

7. Brasch J, Henseler T (1992) The reaction index: a parameter to assess the quality of patch test preparations. Contact Dermatitis 27:203–204

8. Geier J, Uter W, Lessmann H, Schnuch A (2003) The positivity ratio–another parameter to assess the diagnostic quality of apatch test preparation. Contact Dermatitis 48:280–282

9. Neumann NJ, Hölzle E, Lehmann P, Benedikter S, Tapernoux B, Plewig G (1994) Pattern analysis of photopatch test reactions. Photodermatol Photoimmunol Photomed 10:65–73

10. Brasch J, Geier J, Gefeller O (1996) Dynamic patterns of allergic patch test reactions to ten European standard allergens – an analysis of data recorded by the "Information Network of Departments of Dermatology (IVDK)". Contact Dermatitis 35:17–22

11. Uter W, Mackiewicz M, Schnuch A, Geier J (2005) Interne Qualitätssicherung von Epikutantest-Daten des multizentrischen Projektes "Informationsverbund Dermatologischer Kliniken" (IVDK). Dermatol Beruf Umwelt 53:107–114

12. Uter W, Geier J, Lessmann H, Hausen BM (2001) Contact allergy to Disperse Blue 106 and Disperse Blue 124 in German and Austrian patients, 1995 to 1999. Contact Dermatitis 44:173–177

13. Uter W, Geier J, Hausen BM (2003) Contact allergy to Disperse Blue 106/124 mix in consecutive German, Austrian and Swiss patients. Contact Dermatitis 48:286–287

14. Schnuch A, Geier J, Uter W, Frosch PJ, Lehmacher W, Aberer W, Agathos M, Arnold R, Fuchs T, Laubstein B, Lischka G, Pietrzyk P, Rakoski J, Richter G, Rueff F (1997) National rates and regional differences in sensitization to allergens of the standard series. Population adjusted frequencies of sensitization (PAFS) in 40,000 patients from a multicenter study (IVDK). Contact Dermatitis 37:200–209

15. Wilkinson JD, Hambly EM, Wilkinson DS (1980) Comparison of patch test results in two adjacent areas of England. II. Medicaments. Acta Derm Venereol 60:245–249

16. Andersen KE, Veien NK (1985) Biocide patch tests. Contact Dermatitis 12:99–103

17. Uter W, Ludwig A, Balda BR, Schnuch A, Pfahlberg A, Schäfer T, Wichmann HE, Ring J (2004) The prevalence of contact allergy differed between population-based and clinic-based data. J Clin Epidemiol 57:627–632

18. Uter W, Schnuch A, Gefeller O (2004) Guidelines for the descriptive presentation and statistical analysis of contact allergy data. Contact Dermatitis 51:47–56

19. Altman DG (1991) Practical statistics for medical research. Chapman and Hall, London

20. Uter W, Lessmann H, Geier J, Schnuch A (2003) Contact allergy to ingredients of hair cosmetics in female hairdressers and clients – an 8-year analysis of IVDK data. Contact Dermatitis 49:236–240

21. Gardner MJ, Altman DG (1986) Confidence intervals rather than Pvalues: estimation rather than hypothesis testing. Br Med J (Clin Res Ed) 292:746–750

22. Gefeller O, Pfahlberg A, Geier J, Brasch J, Uter W (1999) The association between size of test chamber and patch test reaction: a statistical reanalysis. Contact Dermatitis 40:14–18

23. Schnuch A, Uter W (2003) Decrease in nickel allergy in Germany and regulatory interventions. Contact Dermatitis 49:107–108

24. Benezra C, Maibach H (1984) True cross-sensitization, false cross-sensitization and otherwise. Contact Dermatitis 11:65–69

25. Uter W, Pfahlberg A, Brasch J (2002) Zur Reproduzierbarkeit der Epikutantestung – die Bewertung der Konkordanz bei synchroner Applikation. Allergologie 25:415–419

26. Schnuch A, Lessmann H, Geier J, Frosch PJ, Uter W (2004) Contact allergy to fragrances: frequencies of sensitization from 1996 to 2002. Results of the IVDK. Contact Dermatitis 50:65–76

27. Uter W, Lessmann H, Geier J, Becker D, Fuchs T, Richter G (2002) Die Epikutantestung mit "Parastoffen". Dermatol Beruf Umwelt 50:97–104

28. Fleiss JL (1981) Statistical methods for rates and proportions. Wiley, New York

29. Landis JR, Koch GG (1977) The measurement of observer agreement for categorical data. Biometrics 33:159–174

30. Uter W, Lessmann H, Geier J, Becker D, Fuchs T, Richter G (2002) The spectrum of allergic (cross-)sensitivity in clinical patch testing with "para amino" compounds. Allergy 57:319–322

31. Thompson WD, Walter SD (1988) A reappraisal of the kappa coefficient. J Clin Epidemiol 41:949–958

32. Frosch P, Pirker C, Rastogi SC, Andersen KE, Bruze M, Goossens A, White IR, Uter W, Menné T, Johansen JD (2005) Patch testing with a new fragrance mix detects additional patients sensitive to perfumes and missed by the current fragrance mix. Contact Dermatitis 52:207–215

33. Schnuch A, Kelterer D, Bauer A, Schuster C, Aberer W, Mahler V, Katzer K, Rakoski J, Jappe U, Krautheim A, Bircher A, Koch P, Worm M, Löffler H, Hillen U, Frosch PJ, Uter W (2005) Quantitative patch and repeated open application testing in Methyldibromo glutaronitrile sensitive-patients – results of the IVDK. Contact Dermatitis 52:197–206

34. Geier J, Gefeller O (1995) Sensitivity of patch tests with rubber mixes: results of the information network of departments of dermatology from 1990 to 1993. Am J Contact Derm 6:143–149

35. Dooms Goossens A, Naert C, Chrispeels MT, Degreef H (1980) Is a5% nickel sulphate patch test concentration adequate? Contact Dermatitis 6:232

36. Buckley DA, Rycroft RJ, White IR, McFadden JP (2003) The frequency of fragrance allergy in patch-tested patients increases with their age. Br J Dermatol 149:986–989

37. Schnuch A (1996) PAFS: population-adjusted frequency of sensitization. (I). Influence of sex and age. Contact Dermatitis 34:377–382

38. Rothman KJ, Greenland S (1998) Modern epidemiology. Lippincott/Raven, Philadelphia

39. Christophersen J, Menné T, Tanghoj P, Andersen KE, Brandrup F, Kaaber K, Osmundsen PE, Thestrup Pedersen K, Veien NK (1989) Clinical patch test data evaluated by multivariate analysis. Danish Contact Dermatitis Group. Contact Dermatitis 21:291–299

40. Matthews DE, Farewell VT (1996) Using and understanding medical statistics. Karger, Basel

41. Kleinbaum DG, Kupper LL, Morgenstern H (1982) Epidemiologic research. Van Nostrand Reinhold, New York

42. Nethercott JR, Holness DL, Adams RM et al (1994) Multivariate analysis of the effect of selected factors on the elicitation of patch test response to 28 common environmental contactants in North America. Am J Contact Derm 5: 13–18

43. Uter W, Geier J, Fuchs T (2000) Contact allergy to polidocanol, 1992 to 1999. J All Clin Immunol 106:1203–1204

44. Uter W, Schnuch A, Geier J, Pfahlberg A, Gefeller O (2001) Association between occupation and contact allergy to the fragrance mix: a multifactorial analysis of national surveillance data. Occup Environ Med 58:392–398

Part III

Dermatotoxicology

Chapter 11

Skin Penetration

11

Hans Schaefer, Thomas E. Redelmeier

Contents

tectable to all but the most sensitive techniques. Sampling the time-dependent changes in the concentration of a compound in individual compartments is thus technically challenging. Following application:

- Topical formulations may undergo radical changes in composition and structure.
- Xenobiotics are in general not evenly distributed on the skin surface.
- The effectiveness of the skin barrier often changes with time.
- The skin barrier is influenced by the type and progression of a disease.
- There is regional variation in the barrier properties of the skin.
- The viable tissues themselves respond to topical contact with xenobiotics in manners that may either enhance or retard percutaneous absorption.
- Drugs influence all of these processes in a more-or-less specific manner.

In view of these facts, the description of the kinetics of penetration after topical contact with a xenobiotic is a complex affair. A number of mathematical models have been developed to describe or define the relative importance of these processes in determining the bioavailability of compounds in a target tissue [1–6].

11.1 Introduction

Penetration of the skin is a key element in cutaneous reactions, be it to xenobiotics, to drugs, or to other compounds. The major difficulties in accurately describing percutaneous absorption are related to the size of the compartments. A topical application of a cream or ointment, for example, is routinely spread to a thickness corresponding to no greater than 10 µm.

The stratum corneum is also approximately 10 µm thick, whereas the viable epidermis, dermis, and to a greater extent the systemic compartment represent an effective large sink where absorbed substances undergo dilution to levels that often remain unde-

11.2 Diffusion

Any passage into and through the skin is governed by diffusion processes. In other words, active transport mechanisms play no role in penetration. Compounds that come into contact with the skin surface migrate down concentration gradients according to well-described laws governing diffusion of solutes in solutions and across membranes. For a more complete derivation of relevant equations, interested readers are referred to comprehensive reviews [7, 8].

11.2.1 Fick's Laws

Diffusion of uncharged compounds across a membrane or any homogeneous barrier is described by Fick's first and second laws. The first law states that the steady-state flux of a compound (J, mol/cm per second) per unit path length (δ, cm) is proportional to the concentration gradient (ΔC) and the diffusion coefficient (D, cm²/s):

$$J = -D(\Delta C/\Delta \delta) \qquad (11.1)$$

The negative sign indicates that the net flux is in the direction of the lower concentration. This equation holds for diffusion-mediated processes in isotropic solutions under steady-state conditions. Fick's second law predicts the flux of compounds under non-steady-state conditions. The solution to these equations depends upon defining appropriate boundary conditions [6–10]. However, regardless of whether diffusion occurs in a system under steady-state or non-steady-state conditions, the principal factors that determine the flux of a compound between two points in an isotropic medium are the concentration gradient, the path length, and the diffusion coefficient [11].

It is worthwhile pointing out that diffusion is a very effective transport mechanism over very short distances but not over long ones. The relationship between the time (Δt) it takes for a molecule to transverse a path length (x) and its diffusion coefficient is governed by:

$$\Delta t = x^2/2D \qquad (11.2)$$

For example, the diffusion coefficient for water in an aqueous solution is 2.5×10^{-5} cm²/s, suggesting that a water molecule would traverse a 10-µm path (the equivalent of the width of the stratum corneum) in 0.4 ms. However, since diffusion depends upon the square of the distance, longer pathlengths are not efficiently traversed: a 100-µm path would take 40 ms.

This explains why xenobiotics attain high concentrations in the upper layers of the skin, i.e., in the epidermis, while serum levels after cutaneous exposure remain low. The diffusional nature of percutaneous absorption also explains the exclusion of large molecules by the intact barrier: only a small number of such molecules per square centimeter can be brought into contact with the skin surface, which then encounter multilayers consisting of low-molecular-weight lipids with corresponding narrow intermolecular spaces (see below). As a rule of thumb, the passage of proteins and polymers >50,000 Da through the horny layer barrier becomes imperceptible.

Core Message

■ Penetration is based on passive diffusion. There is no mechanism of active transport through the horny layer barrier.

11.3 Three-Compartment Model

Although pharmacokinetic analysis of topical applications may require the description of a relatively large number of compartments, this discussion is confined to three compartments: the skin surface, the stratum corneum, and the viable tissue. In order to undergo percutaneous absorption, a compound must be released from its formulation, particulate state, solvent, etc., encounter the skin surface, penetrate the stratum corneum, diffuse through the viable epidermis into the dermis, and finally gain access to the systemic compartment through the vascular system. In addition, it may diffuse through the dermal and hypodermal layers to reach underlying muscular tissues. Within each compartment, the compound may diffuse down its concentration gradient, bind to specific compound, or be metabolized.

11.4 The Skin Surface

11.4.1 Surface Contact

The physical forms of contact with the skin surface, that is dust, powders, solutions, and formulations, all differ in their physicochemical properties, and, as discussed below, this influences the kinetics of release and/or absorption. However, the principal consideration is that topical contacts represent a physically small phenomenon, significantly limited by the amount of compound that is applied to the skin surface. When a patient applies, for example, a dermatologic preparation, the layer of a semisolid formulation covering the skin is very thin, corresponding to a volume of between 0.5 and 2 mg/cm². Thicker layers are felt as "undesirable" and consciously or subconsciously rubbed or spread to larger surfaces. This restricts the amount of compound that can effectively come into contact with the skin surface to approximately 0.5–2 µg/cm² for a 1% (wt/wt) topical formulation and other contact forms.

However, even after being rubbed in, material on the skin surface does not remain homogeneous over the time frame of penetration [15]. Topical applications undergo evaporation, such that even relatively nonvolatile substances such as water are rapidly lost [16, 17]. This phenomenon is readily recognized by patients as a cooling sensation. The evaporation results in rapid concentration of nonvolatile substances on the skin surface, which may result in the formation of supersaturated "solutions" or precipitation of active ingredients. Any material also mixes with skin-surface lipids and undergoes time-dependent changes in chemical composition, as their carrier undergoes absorption. Taken together, these considerations suggest that dramatic changes in the composition and structure of form occur following surface application, which determines the subsequent bioavailability.

An additional consideration is that topical contact does not result in an even distribution over the skin surface, but material will be deposited in crevices and appendages. This may result in a relative increase in absorption through appendages. This phenomenon may be accentuated in forms that contain particles or precipitates, since there is evidence that appropriately sized particles can rapidly penetrate along the shafts of hair follicles to a depth of up to 100–500 μm [18, 19]. Such deposits might be an important element in allergic reactions to airborne allergens such as house dust, pollen, etc.

11.5 The Skin Barrier

The primary compartment that limits the percutaneous absorption of compounds is the stratum corneum. This thin (10–20 μm) layer effectively surrounding the body represents a highly differentiated structure that determines the diffusion of compounds across the skin. The physical description of the stratum corneum has now been well documented [20], and it can be accurately characterized as 'bricks", i.e., cornified cells consisting of bundled, water-insoluble proteins, embedded in a "mortar" of intercellular lipid.

The general consensus today is that the stratum corneum is a highly organized, differentiated structure. In order to participate fully in forming an effective barrier to diffusion, the biogenesis of the corneocytes as well as the synthesis and processing of the intercellular lipid must proceed in an orderly manner. Recent evidence suggests that disruption in the kinetics of skin barrier formation by accelerating the division of the keratinocytes found in the underlying layers will lead to a disruption in the barrier properties of the skin [16, 17]. Thus the concept of dead or dying skin forming a passive barrier to diffusion is now replaced by a model of the stratum corneum as a highly differentiated structure that has unique properties particularly suited to its role in forming the skin barrier.

11.5.1 Corneocytes

Fully 85% of the stratum corneum is protein (as a percentage of dry mass), mostly associated with cornified cells, i.e., the corneocytes. These structures contain a core of keratins surrounded by an envelope made up of cross-linked proteins [21]. The keratins may account for up to 80% of the total dry mass of the corneocytes and thus represent the most important constituents. In addition to these fibrous proteins, the core contains low-molecular-weight polar compounds such as amino acids, urocanic and pyrrolidone carboxylic acid. These compounds play a role in maintaining the hydration properties of the stratum corneum.

11.5.2 Intercellular Lipid

Interspersed between corneocytes, the intercellular lipid is organized into sheets, which provide the primary barrier to diffusion across the stratum corneum [22]. This lipid is located in an extracellular domain and thus is not morphologically equivalent to a cellular membrane. The lipid accounts for approximately 15% of the dry weight of the stratum corneum or 20% of the volume. It is composed of roughly equimolar mixtures of ceramides, cholesterol, and long-chain free fatty acids. There is now substantial evidence that these lipids form structures [23, 24] wherein diffusion of the lipidic substances is more than 1,000-fold less than that found in cellular membranes [25, 26]. This material property of the intercellular lipid is particularly suited to play a role as a barrier to diffusion [20].

> ## Core Message
>
> ■ It is the complex structure of the thin stratum corneum that limits the penetration of compounds through the horny layer barrier.

11.5.3 Appendages

A variety of appendages penetrate the stratum corneum and epidermis, facilitating thermal control and providing a protective covering. Appendages are potential sites of discontinuity in the integrity of the skin barrier. Appendages account for 0.1% to 1% of the area of the skin and 0.01% to 0.1% of the total skin volume. It can be concluded that in order to significantly influence the flux of compounds across the skin, the diffusion coefficient has to be considerably higher than that across the intercellular lipid domains or corneocytes. For this reason, it is likely that "shunt" pathways are relatively more important for molecules exhibiting relatively slow rates of percutaneous absorption and are of primary importance during early stages after topical contact. There is unequivocal proof that solid material can enter the lower lumen of the hair follicle [27]. Follicular penetration was clearly demonstrated for titanium dioxide particles [28]. Thus one has to assume that any allergenic material associated with or presented as particles can take this route, thereby bypassing the horny layer barrier. The extent to which such a passage contributes to the allergic and irritant reaction to airborne xenobiotics (pollen allergens, etc.) and to bulky proteins in general merits further investigation.

> **Core Message**
>
> ■ Hair follicles present sites of imperfection in the skin protection afforded by the barrier function of the horny layer. They have to be taken into consideration as a port of entry for large molecules (proteins, etc.) as well as particles carrying adsorbed allergens.

11.5.4 Pathways Across the Stratum Corneum

The relevance of the intercellular lipid domain to permeation of compounds across the stratum corneum (Fig. 1) is inferred from the striking relationship between the hydrophobicity of compounds and their permeability coefficients across the skin [28, 29]. This suggests that the rate-limiting step for permeation includes a hydrophobic barrier, i.e., the intercellular lipid. The observation that small polar molecules such as urea exhibit higher permeability coefficients than expected on the basis of their partition coefficient between n-octanol and water has been interpreted to support the presence of polar and apolar pathways [29, 30]. However, alternative single-pathway models indicate that this observation can be accounted for by considering the influence of molecular volume on the relative diffusivity of compounds in membranes [30–32]. In addition, available evidence suggests that the only continuous domain within the stratum corneum is formed by the intercellular lipid space [32, 33]. This implies that compounds penetrating the stratum corneum must pass through intercellular lipid, although it does not exclude the possibility that compounds can also enter the inner lumen of corneocytes.

There are several studies that have directly visualized penetration pathways across the stratum corneum with electron microscopy. Osmium tetroxide vapor can be used to precipitate n-butanol that has penetrated the stratum corneum [32, 33]. Following a brief (5- or 60-s) exposure of murine or human stratum corneum, the alcohol was found enriched in the intercellular spaces (threefold), though significant levels were also found in the corneocytes. Using a different approach involving rapid freezing, water, ethanol, and cholesterol were also found preferentially concentrated in the intercellular lipid spaces [33, 34].

However, in most of these investigations there was also significant localization of compounds in the corneocytes, more prevalent in the upper layers (stratum disjunctum). Thus, corneocytes undergoing desquamation appear to be relatively permeable, even to rather bulky ions such as mercury. There is additional evidence that other compounds can and do penetrate the corneocytes. It is well established, for example, that occlusion or immersion of skin in a bath leads to swelling of the corneocytes, consistent with the entry of water. Other compounds have also been localized to corneocytes, including the binding of anionic surfactants to keratins. Low-molecular-weight moisturizers such as glycerol are likely to partition into the corneocytes and alter their water-binding capacity. Thus, the penetration of corneocytes cannot be excluded when considering percutaneous absorption pathways.

11.5.5 Inter- and Intra-individual Variation in Skin-Barrier Function

Finally, it is worthwhile considering the level of inter- and intra-individual variation in skin. The most ac-

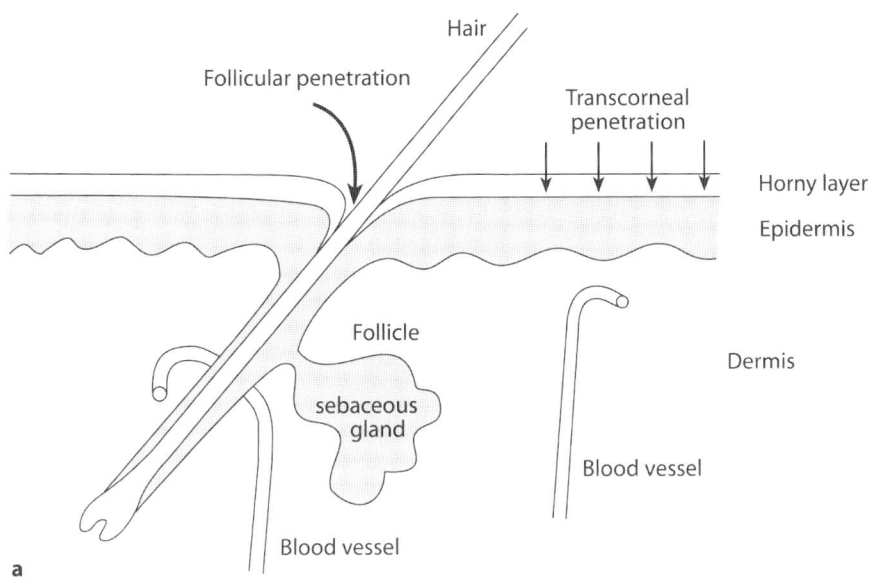

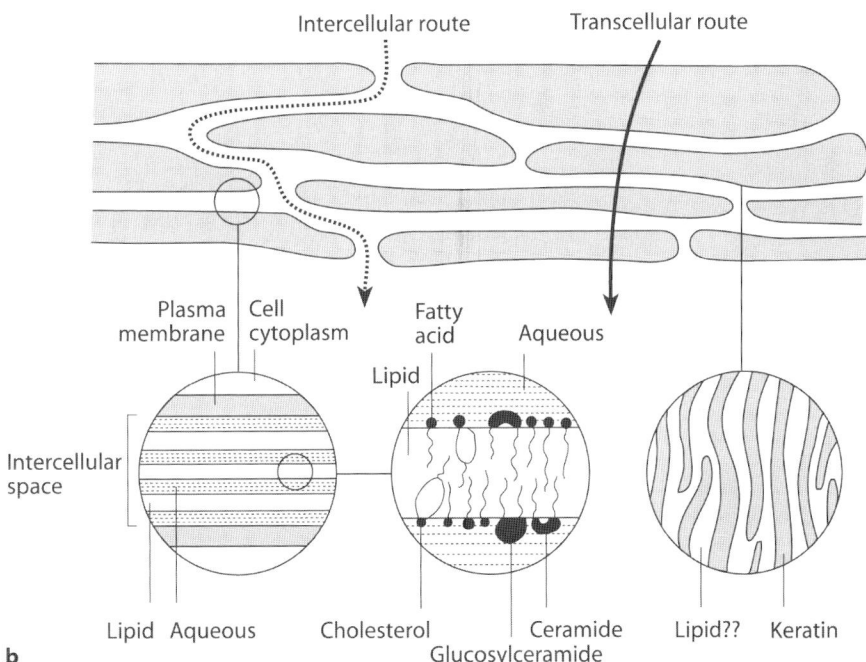

Fig. 1a, b. Model of penetration pathways. a Penetration occurs via appendages that exhibit a reduced barrier to diffusion but occupy a relatively small surface area. b Permeation through the stratum corneum (transcorneal permeation) may be considered to occur through the intercellular lipid domain or through the corneocytes (transcellular route). (From [20])

curate and reproducible method of measuring barrier activity is to follow transepidermal water loss (TEWL) [34–37]. The extent of within-individual variation in this parameter has been estimated to be 8% by site and 21% from day to day. The variations between individuals are reported to be somewhat larger, ranging from 35% to 48% [37, 38]. There appears to be no significant sex- or race-dependent differences in skin-barrier activity. The skin-barrier activity of premature infants (delivered more than 3 weeks premature) has been demonstrated to be markedly impaired, whereas skin-barrier function appears normal for full-term infants. There seems to be no significant alteration in skin-barrier activity as a function of age. Better-defined differences in skin barrier activity between different sites are observed; barrier function can be ranked as arm > abdomen > postauricular > forehead [34–37]. Undoubtedly contact sensitization and elicitation depend on threshold concentrations in the viable tissue, which however depend on quite a number of factors (surface concentration, size of contact area, antigenic potency of the allergen, number of exposures, effect of draining lymph node, vehicle, occlusion, eczematous conditions), as well as the degree and route of penetration [39, 40].

Core Message

■ Thresholds for sensitization and elicitation depend on many things including the degree of penetration by allergens: potency overrules penetration.

11

11.6 Viable Tissue

Although the primary barrier to percutaneous absorption lies within the stratum corneum (Fig. 2), diffusion within the viable tissue as well as metabolism and resorption will also influence the bioavailability of compounds in, and passage through, specific skin compartments. These processes are interrelated, and factors that increase the rate of one of these processes inevitably influence the others.

The passage of compounds from the stratum corneum into the viable epidermis results in a substantial dilution (Fig. 3). This reflects not only the relatively larger size of the epidermis as compared with the stratum corneum, but also the lower resistance to diffusion within viable tissues, corresponding approximately to that on an aqueous protein gel [37, 38]. Concentrations of 10^{-4}–10^{-6} M may be attained in the epidermis and dermis for substances that permeate readily (Fig. 3). Although the actual concentration gradient of a compound is influenced by both its physicochemical properties and the time of contact, the presence of a concentration gradient is visible at

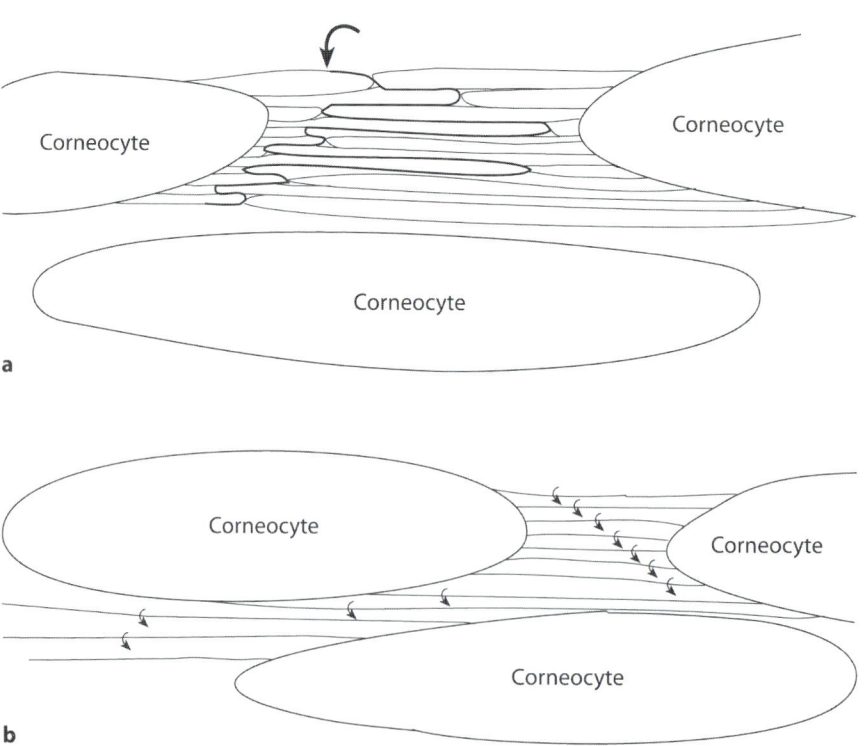

Fig. 2a, b. Schematic of possible penetration pathways through the intercellular lipid domain. **a** Diffusion of compounds may occur along lipid lamellae (*single line*), which occasionally penetrate the stratum corneum, or **b** diffusion occurs across the lamellae in a mechanism that is analogous to diffusion across lipid bilayers. **a** The pathway is indicated by a *heavy line*; **b** the pathway is denoted by an *arrow* to indicate translamellar diffusion and *lines* to denote lateral-lamellar diffusion. (From [20])

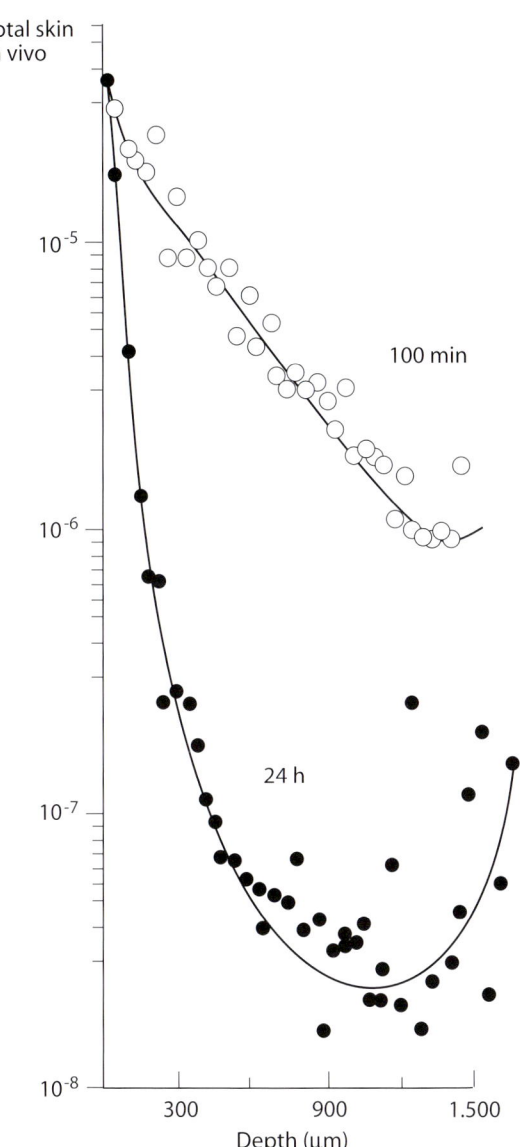

Fig. 3. Distribution of 8-methoxypsoralen (*8-MOP*) in the skin at the indicated time after application. At early time points, a steep nonlinear gradient is observed across the whole of the skin. At later periods, the concentration in the dermis has begun to level off. (From [20])

all times. In other words, strategies to enhance or decrease percutaneous absorption generally result in a relatively even increase or decrease in the concentration of compounds in all compartments.

11.6.1 Skin Metabolism

The skin contains a wide range of enzymatic activities, including phase-I oxidative, reductive, hydrolyt-

ic, and phase-II conjugative reactions as well as a full complement of metabolizing enzymes [38, 39, 41, 42]. Metabolic activity is a primary consideration in the design of prodrugs and may influence the bioavailability of drugs delivered via dermatologic or transdermal formulations.

Alterations in skin metabolism have been implicated in a range of diseases including hirsutism and acne, and they may be relevant to risk assessment of carcinogens. Metabolic processing of antigens by Langerhans cells is involved in the presentation of allergens to the immune system. Thus, metabolism in the skin compartments plays a significant role in determining the fate of a topically applied compound.

Significant cutaneous metabolism has been demonstrated for a wide variety of compounds of differing physicochemical properties, including the steroid hormones estrone, estradiol, and estriol as well as glucocorticoids, prostaglandins, retinoids, benzoyl peroxide, aldrin, anthralin, 5-fluorouracil, nitroglycerin, theophylline, and propranolol [38, 41]. It is convenient to classify metabolic reactions in terms of their cofactor dependence. Processes that require cofactors are likely to be energy-dependent and thus to be located within viable tissues. Among the best-studied examples are the interconversion of steroids (e.g., estrone and estradiol), and the oxidation of polycyclic aromatic hydrocarbons with mixed-function mono-oxygenases. Cinnamic aldehyde and cinnamic alcohol are known allergens, cinnamic aldehyde being the more potent sensitizer. It has been assumed that cinnamic alcohol is a "prohapten" that requires metabolic activation, presumably by oxidoreductase enzymes such as alcohol dehydrogenase or cytochrome P450 2E1, to the protein reactive cinnamaldehyde as hapten. In fact such bioconversion could be demonstrated in human skin [43]. In contrast, cofactor-independent processes involve catabolism and may be located outside of viable tissues, i.e., in the transition region between the stratum corneum and stratum granulosum. The best characterized of these involve hydrolytic reactions such as those described for nonspecific ester hydrolysis. Furthermore activation can take place outside the tissue: ethoxylated nonionic surfactants were shown to be susceptible to oxidation on air exposure and to form allergenic hydroxyaldehydes. More importantly irritant components present in the oxidation mixture facilitated the penetration [44].

Metabolic activity is found in: (1) skin-surface microorganisms, (2) appendages, (3) the stratum corneum, (4) the viable epidermis, and (5) the dermis. In considering the site of the most significant metabolism, one has to take into account the relevant enzymes and their specific activity as well as their capacity relative to the size of the compartment. Thus, though the level of many enzymes is highest in the epidermis, the relatively large size of the dermal compartment may play a significant role in determining the site of metabolism. A further consideration is that enzymes involved in cutaneous metabolism may be induced upon exposure to xenobiotics. This has been well described for various mixed-function mono-oxygenases [39, 42]. Finally, the quantitative extrapolation of results from animal models to humans is hazardous owing to the significant species differences in the metabolism of compounds.

However, despite the variety of skin-associated metabolic processes, the extent of metabolism is normally relatively modest, perhaps 2% to 5% of the absorbed compounds. Metabolism is limited not only by the relatively short period of time that a compound spends in the viable layers of the skin, but also by the overall level of enzyme activity. Thus, under many circumstances, the available enzymes are saturated by the level of compound undergoing percutaneous absorption [38, 41].

Core Message

- Pure compounds are not necessarily capable of eliciting allergic reactions: metabolism before and during penetration of the skin may activate compounds to potent allergens.

11.6.2 Resorption

Resorption, defined as the uptake of compounds by the cutaneous microvasculature, is directly related to the surface area of the exchanging capillaries as well as their blood flow. Total blood flow to the skin may vary up to 100-fold, a process primarily regulated by vascular shunts as well as by recruitment of new capillary beds [40, 41, 45, 46]. It has been estimated that, under resting conditions, only 40% of the blood flow passes via exchanging capillaries capable of acting as a sink for absorbed compounds. However, this value demonstrates considerable variation between body sites, individuals, and species [42, 47], and is influenced by disease states and environmental conditions. In particular, changes in temperature and humidity as well as the presence of vasoactive compounds may directly influence skin blood flow [43, 48].

11.6.3 The Influence of Pathologic Processes on Skin Barrier

It has been argued that the molecular weight of a compound must be under 500 Da to allow absorption through the skin [49]. This assumption is however based on a "macrophysiological" view of penetration kinetics, considering transcorneal diffusion to be the only route of entry into and through the skin. This view is contradicted by the very experience that proteins can be allergenic [39]. Two possible routes for protein penetration have to be taken into account: First, large molecules, and in fact particulate material, can enter deep into the lumen of hair follicles, as mentioned above [29]. Thereby they reach an area that is devoid of protection by a barrier [50], and which is surrounded by a dense population of immune-competent dendritic cells. Second, irritation is known to provoke barrier defects, thereby allowing proteins to enter into direct contact with the viable epidermis and its immune-competent Langerhans cells [20, 39, 44, 51, 52]. Environmental factors such as low humidity are suggested to increase the number of Langerhans cells as well as favor penetration by trinitrochlorobenzene [53]. Depending on the vehicle, occlusion may increase or decrease the response when testing the allergenic potency of parabens [54].

Reduced skin-barrier function is observed for a number of pathologic conditions including ichthyosis [44–46, 55–57], psoriasis [47, 48, 58, 59], atopic dermatitis [49, 50, 60, 61] and contact dermatitis [51, 62] (Tables 1 and 2). It is generally accepted that this can be attributed to structural alterations in the stratum corneum [20]. Structural deficiencies may arise from abrasion, from the extraction of lipids by solvents or strong detergents, by exposure to potent alkaline or acidic fluids and dusts, by the absence of an enzyme or structural protein in the underlying viable tissues, or they may be related to the improper formation of the stratum corneum resulting from an increase in keratinocyte proliferation [52, 63], as in the case of psoriasis. A consequence of poor barrier function is a further increase in penetration by xenobiotics, which

Table 1. Excretion of triamcinolone acetonide in the urine after topical application to normal and psoriatic skin

Skin area	Applied preparation	Excretion (%)	Time (h)
Uninvolved skin	0.1% cream	0.4	72
Psoriatic skin	0.1% cream	4.3	72
Healthy skin	0.1% cream	1.4	72

Table 2. Barrier function as measured by transepidermal water loss (*TEWL*) for normal, uninvolved, and involved psoriatic skin [20]. (*NS* Not significant)

Condition	TEWL (g/m² per h)	Student's *t* test
Healthy individual	4.3±1.2	NS
Uninvolved skin	6.3±1.8	n.a.
Psoriatic plaque	11.5±6.3	$p<0.05$
After scale removal	29.1±9.8	$p<0.05$
Fissured plaque	20.9±8.0	$p<0.05$

Student's *t* test is in comparison with uninvolved skin

may accentuate the problem. Thus in individuals predisposed to a defective barrier, a minor perturbation may become amplified as the skin attempts to compensate by increasing keratinocyte proliferation [52, 63]. As a rule of thumb in areas devoid of a functional horny layer, the penetration by a compound is increased by a factor of 3- to up to 15-fold. A further consideration is that the homeostatic mechanisms responsible for recovery of barrier activity after perturbation may be altered in some diseases or physiologic states. For example, whereas the skin of elderly people exhibits normal barrier function, the recovery of barrier activity after perturbation is markedly reduced [53, 64]. This kinetic basis for reduced barrier function may also account for inter-individual variation in barrier function and/or an apparently increased susceptibility of certain individuals to contact dermatitis [51, 62]. It follows that, on the one hand, in skin areas with pathologically disturbed barrier function the entrance of topical substances is accelerated and increased relative to the surrounding normal skin (targeting to the disease). On the other hand, once an irritant has overcome the barrier it facilitates its own penetration, thereby amplifying the damage [54, 65].

> ## Core Message
>
> - Any disturbance or disorder of the barrier function facilitates penetration by allergens. This is particularly true for eczematous conditions such as atopy, psoriasis, etc.

11.6.4 Allergens

Surprisingly little work has been published on penetration by allergens. Nickel penetrates through rubber gloves [55, 66]. However, its penetration of the skin is relatively minimal [56, 67] and depends on the vehicle [57, 68]. Occlusion enhances its penetration [58, 69]. Differences in higher penetration by squaric acid esters as compared to low penetration by squaric acid explain why the latter is a less-effective sensitizer in the sensitization therapy of alopecia areata [59, 70].

Pre-treatment with topical cyclosporin appears to provoke a perturbation of the horny layer barrier and thereby enhances penetration by allergens rather than inhibiting the allergic reaction by immunosuppression [60, 71].

One has to suppose that the elicitation of allergic reactions depends largely on the individual patient's barrier function, and thus on the influence of the site of elicitation, moisture, temperature, season, and environmental and endogenous factors on the penetration by the allergen in question.

Much more work is needed to address the prevention of elicitation by restricting allergen penetration: a hypothetical reduction of such penetration by a factor of three would lower the titer, and hence the frequency and severity of allergic reactions by a factor of three as well.

Several papers address the efficiency of barrier creams in reducing penetration by allergens and irritants [61–66, 72–77], demonstrating moderate to good protective capacity.

11.7 Vehicles

The influence of a carrier medium on percutaneous absorption of an incorporated substance is very complex [20]. It depends on the physicochemical interaction between a compound and its carrier as well as between the carrier and the skin surface. In very general terms the primary factor governing the passage of a compound is its own physicochemical property, that is its molecular size, polarity and lipophilicity: small nonpolar and moderately lipophilic substances penetrate best; highly polar water soluble compounds, least. The influence of classical vehicles on the passage of these two extremes is limited. The most prominent "vehicle effect" is reached either by pushing the concentration of a compound close to its solubility limits in a given carrier (thereby increasing its thermodynamic potential in favor of diffusion out of the vehicle and into the skin) or by disturbing the barrier function. However, the potential of so-called penetration enhancers is limited in practical terms, since the disturbance of the barrier function challenges the homeostatic equilibrium in the stratum corneum and provokes a counteraction in the sense of a strengthening of the barrier.

> ## Core Message
>
> ■ The carrier acts on the barrier – it can increase or decrease exposure to allergens.

11.8 Conclusions

The principal factors determining the kinetics of the diffusion into the skin of a xenobiotic are the physiochemical properties of the molecule. Hydrophobicity, molecular weight, and ionic charge determine the feasibility of transdermal delivery for any particular compound. Form of contact influences the kinetics largely from considerations of the thermodynamic activity of the compound. However, one should not exclude the impact of changes in the physical forms that occur following topical application. Evaporation, and changes in the structure of emulsion, dissolution in sebum, entry into the follicle, etc. may bring dramatic changes in the thermodynamic activity of the compound. Under some circumstances, this may lead to the retention of the drug on the skin surface.

The rate-limiting step for percutaneous absorption of most compounds is its penetration through the stratum corneum. There is substantial evidence that this is related to diffusion through a tortuous path around the corneocytes within the highly structured intercellular lipid, the constituents of which exhibit diffusional properties consistent with their role in the skin barrier. For skin diseases exhibiting reduced skin-barrier function, the absence of these critical structures may account for the decreased barrier activity. The progression of a disease and the inherent biological variability make predictions of percutaneous absorption for diseased skin inherently difficult. This contributes significantly to the challenges of developing topical applications of drugs as well as to that of barrier creams.

Processes occurring in viable tissues can have a significant though generally less-important influence on the bioavailability of compounds undergoing percutaneous absorption. It has been difficult to establish in vivo the level of skin-related metabolism of drugs undergoing percutaneous absorption.

References

1. Higuchi T (1960) Physical chemical analysis of percutaneous absorption process from creams and ointments. J Soc Cosmet Chem 11:85
2. Guy RH, Hadgraft J (1989) Mathematical models of percutaneous absorption. In: Bronaugh RL, Maibach HI (eds) Percutaneous absorption. Dekker, New York, p 13
3. Guy RH, Hadgraft J, Maibach AJ (1982) A pharmacokinetic model for percutaneous absorption. Int J Pharmaceut 11:119
4. Gupta SK et al (1993) Pharmokinetic and pharmodynamic modeling of transdermal products: in vivo methods, problems, and pitfalls. In: Shah VP, Maibach HI (eds) Topical drug bioavailability: bioequivalence and penetration. Plenum, New York, p 311
5. Kuboto K et al (1993) Percutaneous absorption: a single model. J Pharm Sci 82:450
6. Williams PL, Riviere JE (1995) A biophysically based dermatopharmokinetic compartment model for quantifying percutaneous penetration and absorption of topically applied agents. 1. Theory. J Pharm Sci 84:599
7. Jain MK (1980) In: Jain MK, Wagner RC (eds) Introduction to biological membranes. Wiley, Toronto, p 117
8. Gennis RB (1989) Biomembranes: molecular structure and function. Springer, Berlin Heidelberg New York
9. Barry BW (1983) Dermatological formulations: percutaneous absorption. Dekker, New York
10. Scheuplein RJ (1967) Mechanism of percutaneous absorption. II. Transient diffusion and the relative importance of various routes of skin penetration. J Invest Dermatol 45:334
11. Lieb WR, Stein WD (1986) Non-stokesian nature of transverse diffusion within human red blood cell membranes. J Membr Biol 92:111
12. Hatcher ME, Plachy WZ (1993) Dioxygen diffusion in the stratum corneum: an EPR study. Biochim Biophys Acta 1149:73
13. Packer KJ, Sellwood TC (1978) Proton magnetic resonance studies of hydrated stratum corneum, part 2. Self diffusion. J Chem Soc Faraday Trans 2:1592
14. Francoeur ML, Potts RO (1988) The perturbation of stratum corneum lipids affects the diffusive but not partitioning aspects of water vapor permeability. Pharm Res 5:S130
15. Brown S, Diffey BL (1986) The effect of applied thickness on sunscreen protection: in vivo and in vitro studies. Photochem Photobiol 44:509
16. Flynn GL (1993) General introduction and conceptual differentiation of topical and transdermal drug delivery systems. In: Shaw VP, Maibach HI (eds) Topical drug bioavailability: bioequivalence and penetration. Plenum, New York, p 369
17. Reifenrath WG (1995) Volatile substances. Cosmet Toil 110:85
18. Rolland A et al (1993) Site-specific drug delivery to pilosebaceous structures using polymeric microspheres. Pharm Res 10:1738
19. Rolland A (1993) Particulate carriers in dermal and transdermal drug delivery: myth or reality. In: Walters KA, Hadgraft J (eds) Pharmaceutical particulate carriers: therapeutic applications. Dekker, New York, p 1983
20. Schaefer H, Redelmeier TE (1996) Skin barrier principle of percutaneous absorption. Karger, Basel
21. Reichert U et al (1993) The cornified envelope: a key structure of terminally differentiating keratinocytes. In:

Darmon M, Blumenberg M (eds) The keratinocytes. Academic, San Diego, p 107

22. Elias PM, Menon GK (1991) Structural and lipid biochemical correlates of the epidermal permeability barrier. Adv Lipid Res 24:1

23. Madison KC et al (1987) Presence of intact intercellular lipid lamallae in the upper layers of the stratum corneum. J Invest Dermatol 88:714

24. Hou SYE et al (1991) Membranes structures in normal and essential fatty acid deficient stratum corneum: characterization by ruthenium tetroxide staining and x-ray diffraction. J Invest Dermatol 96:215

25. Bouwstra JA et al (1991) Structure of human stratum corneum by small-angle x-ray scattering. J Invest Dermatol 97:1005

26. Bouwstra JA et al (1992) Structure of human stratum corneum as a function of temperature and hydration: a wide angle x-ray diffraction study. Int J Pharm 84:205

27. Rolland A et al (1993) Site-specific drug delivery to pilosebaceous structures using polymeric microspheres. Pharm Res 10:1738

28. Lademann J et al (2001) Investigation of follicular penetration of topically applied substances. Skin Pharmacol Appl Skin Physiol 14:17–22

29. Flynn GL (1990) Physiochemical determinants of skin absorption. In: Gerrity TR, Henry CJ (eds) Principles of route-to-route extrapolation for risk assessment. Elsevier, New York, p 93

30. Tayar EL et al (1991) Percutaneous penetration of drugs: a quantitative structure-permeability relationship study. J Pharm Sci 80:744

31. Kastings GB et al (1987) Effect of lipid sollubility and molecular size on percutaneous absorption. In: Shroot B, Schaefer H (eds) Skin pharmakinetics, vol 1. Karger, Basel, p 138

32. Guy RH, Potts RO (1992) Structure-permeability relationships in percutaneous absorption. J Pharm Sci 81:603

33. Nemaniac MK, Elias PM (1980) In situ precipitation: a novel cytochemical technique for visualization of permeability pathways in mammalian stratum corneum. J Histol Cytochem 28:573

34. Squier CA, Lesch CA (1988) Penetration pathways of different compounds through epidermis and oral epithelial. J Oral Pathol 17:512

35. Pinnagoda J et al (1990) Guidelines for transepithelial water loss (TEWL) measurements. A report from the Standardization Group of the European Society of Contact Dermatitis. Contact Derm 22:164

36. Lavrijsen APM et al (1993) Barrier function parameters in various keratization disorders: transepithelial water loss and vascular response to hexyl nicotinate. Br J Dermatol 129:547

37. Rougier A, Lotte C (1993) Predictive approaches: I. The stripping technique. In: Shaw VP, Maibach HI (eds) Topical drug bioavailability: bioequivalence and penetration. Plenum, New York, p 163

38. Scheuplein RJ (1967) Mechanism of percutaneous absorption. II. Transient diffusion and the relative importance of various routes of skin penetration. J Invest Dermatol 45:33

39. Boukhman MP, Maibach HI (2001) Thresholds in contact sensitisation: immunologic mechanisms and experimental evidence in humans – an overview. Food Chem Tox 39:1125–1134

40. Berard F, Marty JP, Nicolas JF (2003) Allergen penetration through the skin. Eur J Dermatol 13:324–330

41. Kao J, Carver MP (1990) Cutaneous metabolism of xenobiotics. Drug Metab Rev 22:363

42. Mukhtar H, Khan WA (1989) Cutaneous cytochrome P-450. Drug Metab Rev 20:657

43. Smith CK, Moore CA, Elahi EN, Smart AT, Hotchkiss SA (2000) Human skin absorption and metabolism of the contact allergens, cinnamic aldehyde, and cinnamic alcohol. Toxical Appl Pharmacol 168:189–199

44. Bodin A, Li Ping Shao J, Nilsson LG, Karlberg AT (2001) Identification and allergenic activity of hydroxyaldehydes-a new type of oxidation product from an ethoxylated non-ionic surfactant. Contact Dermatitis 44:207–212

45. Ryan TJ (1983) Cutaneous circulation. In: Goldsmith LA (eds) Biochemistry and physiology of the skin, vol 2. Oxford University Press, New York, p 817

46. Riviere JE, Williams PL (1992) Pharmokinetic implication of changing blood flow in skin. J Pharm Sci 81:601

47. Monteiro-Riviere NA et al (1990) Interspecies and interregional analysis of the comparative histological thickness and laser Doppler blood flow measurements af five cutaneous sites in nine species. J Invest Dermatol 95:582

48. Riviere JE et al (1991) The effect of vasoactive drugs on transdermal lidocaine iontophoresis. J Pharm Sci 80:615

49. Bos JD, Meinardi MMHM (2000) The 500 Dalton rule for the skin penetration of chemical compounds and drugs. Exp Dermatol 9:165–169

50. Smith Pease CK, White IR, Basketter DA (2002) Skin as route of exposure to protein allergens. Clin Exp Dermatol 27:296–300

51. Zhai H, Maibach HI (2001) Skin occlusion and irritant and allergic contact dermatitis: an overview. Contact Dermatitis 44:201–206

52. Pedersen LK et al (2004) Augmentation of skin response by exposure to a combination of allergens and irritants – a review. Contact Dermatitis 50:265–273

53. Hosoi J et al (2000) Regulation of the cutaneous allergic reaction by humidity. Contact Dermatitis 42:81–84

54. Cross SE, Roberts MS (2000) The effect of occlusion on epidermal penetration of parabens from a commercial allergy test ointment, acetone and ethanol vehicles. J Invest Derm 115:914–918

55. Williams ML, Elias PM (1993) From basket weave to barrier: unifying concepts for the pathogenesis of the disorders of cornification. Arch Dermatol 129:626

56. Oestmann E et al (1993) Skin barrier function in healthy volunteers as assessed by transepidermal water loss and vascular response to hexyl nicotinate: intra- and interindividual variability. Br J Dermatol 128:130

57. Blichmann CW, Serup J (1989) Reproducibility and variability of transdermal water loss measurements. Acta Derm Venereol 67:206

58. Imokawa G et al (1991) Decreased levels of ceramides in stratum corneum of atopic dermatitis: an etiologic factor in atopic dry skin? J Invest Dermatol 96:523

59. Werner Y, Linberg M (1985) Transepidermal water loss in dry and clinically normal skin in patients with atopic dermatitis. Acta Derm Venereol 65:102

60. Takenouchi M, Suzuki H, Tagami H (1986) Hydration characteristics of pathological stratum corneum: evaluation of bound water. J Invest Dermatol 87:574–576

61. Werner Y, Linberg M (1985) Transepidermal water loss in dry and clinically normal skin in patients with atopic dermatitis. Acta Derma Venereol 65:102

62. Wilhelm KP et al (1991) Effect of sodium lauryl sulfate-induced skin irritation on in vivo percutaneous absorption of four drugs. J Invest Dermatol 97:927

63. Lavrijsen APM et al (1993) Barrier function parameters in various keratization disorders: transepithelial water loss and vascular response to hexyl nicotinate. Br J Dermatol 129:547

64. Lavrijsen APM et al (1995) Reduced skin barrier function parallels abnormal stratum corneum lipid organization in patients with lamellar ichtyosis. J Invest Dermatol 105:619
65. Fartasch M, Schnetz E, Diepgen TL (1998) Characterization of detergent-induced barrier alterations – effect of barrier cream on irritation. J Invest Dermatol 3:121–127
66. Wall LM (1980) Nickel penetration through rubber gloves. Contact Dermatitis 6:461–463
67. Kalimo K, Lammintausa K, Maki J, Teuho J, Jensen CT (1985) Nickel penetration in allergic individuals: bioavailability versus X-ray microanalysis detection. Contact Dermatitis 12:255–257
68. Fullerton A, Andersen JR, Hoelgaard A (1988) Permeation of nickel through human skin in vitro-effect of vehicles. Br J Dermatol 118:509–516
69. Fullerton A, Andersen JR, Hoelgaard A, Menne T (1986) Permeation of nickel salts through human skin in vitro. Contact Dermatitis 15:173–177
70. Sherertz EF, Sloan KB (1988) Percutaneous penetration of squaric acid and its esters in hairless mouse and human skin in vitro. Arch Dermatol Res 280:57–60
71. Surber C, Itin P, Buchner S, Maibach HI (1992) Effect of a new topical cyclosporin formulation on human allergic contact dermatitis. Contact Dermatitis 26:116–119
72. Loden M (1986) The effect of 4 barrier creams on the absorption of water, benzene, and formaldehyde into excised human skin. Contact Dermatitis 14:292–296
73. Boman A, Mellstrom G (1989) Percutaneous absorption of 3 organic solvents in the guinea pig. (III). Effect of barrier cream. Contact Dermatitis 21:134–140
74. Frosch PJ, Kurte A (1994) Efficacy of skin barrier creams (IV). The repetitive irritation test (RIT) with a set of 4 standard irritants. Contact Dermatitis 31:161–168
75. Zhai H, Maibach HI (1996) Effect of barrier creams: human skin in vivo. Contact Dermatitis 35:92–96
76. Zhai H, Maibach HI (1996) Percutaneous penetration (dermatopharmcokinetics) in evaluating barrier creams. Curr Prob Dermatol 25:193–205
77. Gawkrodger DJ, Healy J, Howe AM (1995) The prevention of nickel contact dermatitis. A review of the use of binding agents and barrier creams. Contact Dermatitis 32:257–265

11

Predictive Tests for Irritants and Allergens and Their Use in Quantitative Risk Assessment

DAVID BASKETTER, IAN KIMBER

Contents

12.1 Introduction

In this chapter, the main predictive methods, both animal and human, for the assessment of skin irritation and skin sensitization potential are described. The principles that they embody can be transcribed to the many variants that are also available (and which, for a variety of reasons, may be the preferred approach for some readers). A detailed discussion of these variants is beyond the scope of this article; rather the reader is encouraged to apply the basic principles outlined herein to consideration of all test methods. Whereas the panoply of assays available will serve in one way or another to identify irritation and sensitization hazards, it is in reality much more important to derive an estimation of the relative potency of the hazard presented, such that an appropriate risk assessment can be made and risk management measures applied. The second part of this chapter is therefore devoted to a consideration of the risk assessment approaches employed for chemicals known to have the capacity to irritate and/or to sensitize skin.

12.2 Definitions

Skin sensitization describes a state of heightened immunological reactivity for a particular chemical allergen, such that if this chemical allergen is encountered on the skin by a sensitized individual then a vigorous local immune response will be elicited resulting in cutaneous inflammation and the symptoms that are recognized clinically as allergic contact dermatitis. Skin irritation describes local damage or local trauma associated with the direct initiation of an inflammatory response and the symptoms characteristic of irritant contact dermatitis. Two important points should be made. First, that the properties of skin irritants and the potential to induce skin sensitization are not mutually exclusive. Indeed, many chemicals display both activities and these will, at appropriate concentrations, cause local inflammation at the site of first exposure, and initiate sensitization such that responses will be provoked following subsequent contact with lower concentrations of the material. The possession of both irritant and sensitizing properties by a chemical may have implications for the effectiveness with which skin sensitization is induced. Second, the morphological and histopathological characteristics of allergic contact dermatitis and irritant contact dermatitis are usually inseparable. Predictive tests identify irritant or sensitizing hazards (an intrinsic property) and these hazards may be scaled (e.g., by measuring relative potency). Risks to human health are then a function of the hazard, its relative potency, and the extent of skin exposure.

> ### Core Message
>
> - Impacts on human health depend on a combination of the sensitization and/or irritation hazard AND the conditions, duration, and extent of skin exposure.

12.3 Predictive Tests for Irritants

Human skin irritation is a more complex phenomenon than is sometimes recognized, especially by those who have devised simple tests for its assessment. The term "irritation" is deployed to embrace a broad range of skin effects, ranging (at least according to some) from immediate skin contact reactions (vide infra), through acute primary irritancy to traumiterative dermatitis that may well be chronic in nature [42]. Endpoints considered for these responses encompass both sensory and visible effects. However, for the purposes of this chapter, the focus has been restricted to acute and cumulative irritant reactions that produce symptoms of erythema, dryness, fissuring, and edema. Methods for the assessment of immediate skin contact reactions are covered in Chap. 5. It should be noted that in vitro methods have been validated only for the purposes of identification of corrosive substances (i.e., those that cause burns), and thus they are not considered here other than to direct the reader to appropriate references [8, 32, 54].

As mentioned above, it has become possible by a variety of means to identify, without the use of animals (or humans), those chemicals that may have a corrosive effect on skin [40]. In particular, two in vitro methods have been accepted formally as being validated for this purpose [21]. However, these methods generally do not extend to evaluation of lesser degrees of skin irritation. Animal methods for the prediction of acute and cumulative skin irritation potential were first described many years ago (reviewed in [46, 49]). Most infamous (notorious) amongst these is the rabbit skin irritation test devised by John Draize [17]. This method employs a single semi-occluded patch of undiluted chemical applied to shaved back skin (typically of three rabbits) for 4 h. Any resultant reactions are read, using a simple subjective scoring scheme, at 24 h, 48 h, and 72 h. The recovery from any induced skin irritation reaction may also be monitored. In essence, this test is now used to provide a first-pass assessment of the intrinsic acute skin irritation potential (i.e., hazard) of a chemical substance, so that basic risk management measures can be implemented. This is the situation for example with legislation in the European Union [18] that utilizes Draize test data effectively to compartmentalize chemicals into three basic categories – corrosive, irritant or unclassified. Such an approach has been largely ineffective in terms of prevention of clinical irritant contact dermatitis, since the rabbit is at best poorly predictive of human effects. Also the acute skin irritation potential measured is not an important clinical endpoint, and of course simple categorization hides important details/complexities and is simply no substitute for proper risk assessment. Furthermore, clinical skin irritation is more commonly associated with exposure to formulated products than with individual substances, and it is well known that the irritant activity of a formulation cannot be predicted by a simple summation of the irritant properties of the ingredients [29].

In order to derive more useful information, other animal models have been devised for the purpose of providing a better representation of the modalities of exposure that are encountered in practice. Typically, these methods involve both exaggeration and repetition of exposure, such as with the guinea pig immersion test, or repeated dosing in a modified rabbit test [42]. In addition, investigators have made recourse to relatively uncommon laboratory species (such as the Yucatan hairless micropig) in an attempt to obtain suitable predictive systems [23]. However, in most instances these methods have either failed to gain widespread acceptance, or have fallen out of favor. Rather than using animals, investigators have realized that it is more meaningful scientifically to conduct carefully controlled studies with human volunteers as these provide much more robust information on which to base safety assessments and risk management decisions. The generation of mild skin irritation effects in human volunteers is considered acceptable since such responses are both well tolerated and are reversible. The basic principles of these methods are discussed below.

Where human skin contact with a chemical is likely, or indeed intended, and given that the necessary ethical and safety requirements (reviewed in [51]) have been met, then carefully controlled studies in humans can yield by far the most useful information for the proper evaluation of skin irritation. Where the need is for basic regulatory classification, such as in the EU, a suitable approach, the human 4-h patch test, has been well described and validated [5]. However, the real value to be derived from human testing is where the protocol is able to mirror the pattern(s) of exposure that will occur in practice. In such studies, the chemical may be tested by itself, but it is very much more common that the chemical is tested as part of the final formulation in which it is to be used. Such an approach is not only of value for the testing of cosmetic products (e.g., [50]), but also for many other situations. For example, in clinical trials to examine the impact of formulation on irritancy of a pharmaceutical (e.g., [47]), or in the evaluation of potentially irritating surfactant-based household products [9], the use of carefully optimized methodologies permits the investigator to examine irritancy in what is essentially the in-use situation. Similarly, the approach can be adapted to permit the assessment of the irritancy of materials used in an occupational setting, such as cutting fluids [55]. Human volunteers may also be of particular value in the assessment of potential protective effects of products such as barrier creams (see e.g., [22]).

Typically, the process involved for human skin irritation studies will include the following steps:

- A scientific evaluation of the need for the investigation
- Identification of a suitable protocol
- Preparation of the safety dossier to support the proposed work
- Assessment of the study by an independent ethical review committee
- Initiation of the study by the recruitment of the participants who give fully informed written consent
- Progression of the study through the practical phase
- Formal reporting of the study

All of these elements are reviewed in detail elsewhere [50, 51].

Core Message

- Except where appropriate human testing can be conducted, skin irritation tests are only of limited value in the characterization of the potential effects associated with actual exposure of humans to irritants. In practice there is likely to be exposure to multiple sources of irritancy.

12.4 Predictive Tests for Allergens

A variety of methods is available for the identification of chemicals that have the potential to cause skin sensitization and allergic contact dermatitis. Historically, the guinea pig has been the species of choice for toxicological evaluations of skin sensitizing activity. Many guinea pig tests have been described, of which the guinea pig maximization test (GPMT [41]) and the occluded patch test [14] are the most widely used and most thoroughly characterized. Although guinea pig test methods vary with respect to detailed procedure, the principle is in most cases the same. Groups of animals are exposed by topical or intradermal exposure, or by a mixture of topical and intradermal exposure, to the test material. In some tests, adjuvant is also administered to enhance (maximize) immune responses provoked by the test material. Control guinea pigs receive the relevant vehicle alone, and where appropriate adjuvant treatments. Subsequent-

ly all animals (test and control) are exposed topically to the chemical (at the maximum concentration judged not to cause irritant effects) and the elicitation of cutaneous hypersensitivity reactions is determined as a function of challenge-induced erythema and/or edema. Sensitizing potential is judged on the basis of the frequency of specific reactions induced by challenge of treated animals. Detailed considerations of guinea pig test methods, including their conduct and interpretation, are available elsewhere [1, 10]. Suffice it to say here that the better-characterized guinea pig test methods have served toxicologists well, and if conducted and interpreted correctly provide an accurate indication of likely sensitization hazard.

Notwithstanding their proven utility, it must be recognized that guinea pig tests are not without limitations. Chief among these, in the context of this chapter, is the fact that such assays do not lend themselves to assessment of relative potency. Some attempts have been made to modify standard guinea pig methods for the purposes of deriving dose–response relationships [2], but these have met with only limited success. The difficulties are that it is not practicable in guinea pig assays to examine in detail multiple induction concentrations of the test chemical, and, even if this were to be done, then an endpoint that comprises a subjective assessment of the frequency of responses, rather than the vigor of responses, is not well suited to determination of the inherent potency of a sensitizing chemical.

In the last 15 years considerable progress has been made in characterizing the immunobiological processes that result in the induction of skin sensitization and the elicitation of allergic contact dermatitis. In parallel with this more sophisticated appreciation of the relevant cellular and molecular mechanisms, there have emerged opportunities to explore new approaches to skin sensitization testing. Attention has focused recently on the mouse and two alternative approaches to hazard identification have been developed using this species. One of these, the mouse ear swelling test (MEST [24]), is similar in principle to guinea pig methods insofar as activity is measured on the basis of reactions induced by challenge of previously treated mice. The other approach, the local lymph node assay (LLNA [34, 37, 39]), is predicated upon an alternative strategy in which activity is judged as a function of responses induced in mice during the induction, rather than elicitation, phase of contact sensitization. In this method skin sensitizers are identified as a function of their ability to provoke proliferative responses in draining lymph nodes following repeated topical exposure. In practice, skin sensitizing chemicals are defined as those which, at one or more test concentrations, induce a threefold or greater increase in lymph node cell proliferation compared with concurrent vehicle-treated controls. The LLNA has been the subject of extensive evaluations and the view currently is that the method provides a reliable and robust approach to the identification of sensitizing chemicals and as such represents a stand-alone alternative to guinea pig assays [4, 25, 45].

There is interest currently in the possibility that, in addition to providing a means for identifying hazard, the LLNA may be suitable also for measurement of relative potency as a first step in the risk assessment process [35]. The use of the LLNA for this purpose appears appropriate because the available evidence indicates that the vigor of induced proliferative responses by draining lymph node cells correlates closely with the extent to which skin sensitization will develop [36]. In practice, estimation of relative potency using the LLNA is based upon derivation by linear interpolation from dose–response curves of an EC3 value, this being defined as the effective concentration of chemical required to stimulate a 3-fold increase in lymph node cell proliferative activity compared with concurrent vehicle-treated controls [11], see Fig. 1. Experience to date indicates that the derivation in this way of an EC3 value provides a realistic, and apparently accurate and robust, measure of relative potency suitable for integration into the risk assessment process [11, 31, 52]. Further information on this aspect is given in Sect. 12.5.

The above methods are all in vivo tests. There has also been enthusiasm for the development of in vitro approaches to skin sensitization testing, but although some progress has been made in the context of hazard identification (reviewed in [38]), the iden-

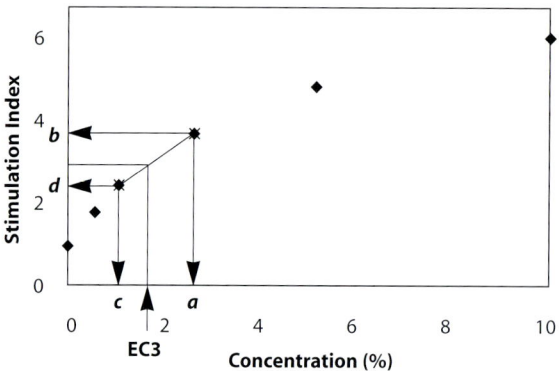

EC3 is calculated via: $c + \dfrac{(3-d) \times (a-c)}{(b-d)}$

Fig. 1. The derivation of the local lymph nose assay (*LLNA*) EC3 value

tification of chemical structural alerts, the derivation of (quantitative) structure–activity relationships, and methods based upon the in vitro assessment of cellular responses are not (yet) suitable for consideration of relative potency.

Core Message

■ Predictive tests for skin sensitization deliver information on the relative potency of individual sensitizing chemicals which is key to proper risk assessment. The optimal approach is to calculate the LLNA EC3 value and use this as an indicator of likely human potency.

12.5 Quantitative Risk Assessment

In toxicology, the initial evaluation involves the identification of intrinsic properties of chemicals/formulations, including skin irritation and sensitization hazards. However, this information, to be of any practical value, has to be placed in a real world context. Thus, where a hazard has been identified, it must be measured in terms of its potency and then judged in relation to the anticipated skin exposure that is likely to occur, both in normal use and in reasonably foreseeable misuse situations. These considerations form the topic of this section. Ultimately, where it is possible to make a fully quantitative risk assessment (a rare situation), then there will be a prediction of the number of cases of irritation and/or sensitization that are likely to arise.

For skin irritation, the opportunity to understand in detail the risk to humans does arise. Although quantitative measures of skin irritation potency are not readily available, as mentioned above, it is possible to undertake human studies that can provide a fairly accurate assessment of the risks presented. To achieve this, the participants in the study must comprise a representative sample of those who are likely to be exposed, and the skin exposure conditions in the study must approximate to those that are anticipated to occur in practice. In this way, the study will provide, in a microcosm, a picture of what is likely to happen in use.

An important consequence of the above is that it leads to the conclusion that simple patch testing, whether single or repeated, may not necessarily provide a fair representation of the skin irritancy of a test material that will be expressed in practice. For example, it has been shown that the rank order of ir-ritancy found under patch test conditions is not al-ways identical to that found under more realistic use conditions [30]. This comes as no great surprise, since cumulative irritancy is a function of both the intensity of each individual skin insult and the rate of recovery there from; this concept is based on that ex-pressed by Malten many years ago [43]. Furthermore, significant evidence of acute skin irritancy under 48-h patch test conditions on the arm has been shown to be of no relevance when a product was evaluated under exaggerated repeated open exposure condi-tions on the face, where it was essentially without ef-fect [7]. However, the practical experience of toxicol-ogists and safety evaluators is that appropriately de-signed human tests can be of great value in the pre-diction of skin irritancy in practice [6, 33, 46, 49].

For skin sensitization, it is not possible to conduct human testing in the same manner as for skin irrita-tion, not least for the obvious ethical reason that skin irritation is a reversible phenomenon, whereas the induction of skin sensitization represents an irrever-sible (health) change for the individual. In practice, it is necessary to use the predictive methods men-tioned in Sect. 12.4 to provide information on the rel-ative potency of the potential skin sensitizer. Typical-ly, this information on the newly identified skin sen-sitizer is then compared with that available for other skin sensitizers that are employed in similar expo-sure situations. In effect, the variables/unknowns as-sociated with the relationship between skin exposure to a sensitizer of known potency and the resultant likelihood of allergic contact dermatitis being elicit-ed are regarded as "constants" in the comparison of a known sensitizer in an existing use with a new sensi-tizer being used in the same situation. For example, the weak sensitizing potency of cocoamidopropyl betaine (CAPB) is well understood in terms of data from predictive models. In addition, the very limited

extent to which it causes clinical allergy through use in shampoos at levels up to approximately 10% is al-so quite well understood. Thus, were a novel material to be proposed for use in shampoos, CAPB could be employed as one potential benchmark for compari-son. Similarly, the much stronger sensitizing potency of (chloro)methylisothiazolinone is also well under-stood in predictive models and in humans; dose–re-sponse studies in mice, guinea pigs and humans exist [15, 53]. Furthermore, there are data on acceptable and unacceptable use concentrations and product types [16]. All of these data represent a valuable source of benchmark data for use in risk assessment.

Recently, a more quantitative approach to skin sensitization risk assessment has been promulgated. In essence, this is founded on the traditional toxicol-ogy approach of identifying a no effect level (NOEL) *in a predictive model* and then appropriate reduction of this NOEL to provide an indication *of human ex-posure limits* below which the adverse effect, in this case the induction of skin sensitization, should not occur. The approach indicates safe exposure levels for individual sensitizing chemicals under well-de-fined exposure conditions; exposure is expressed in dose per unit area and is calculated per diem. Com-prehensive details of this new approach have been delineated in a short series of publications [19, 20, 26]. Given the difficulties concerning the conduct of predictive human testing, this quantitative approach relies heavily on the direct prediction of NOELs from LLNA EC3 values. A number of publications now sup-port the validity of this relationship [12, 13, 26, 28, 48]. Quantitative risk assessment for skin sensitizing chemicals has been deployed to demonstrate the in-appropriately high level of exposure to a preserva-tive, methyldibromo glutaronitrile, providing an in-dependent demonstration of the utility of the ap-proach [56]. A generic overview of this new quantita-tive risk assessment strategy is outlined in Fig. 2.

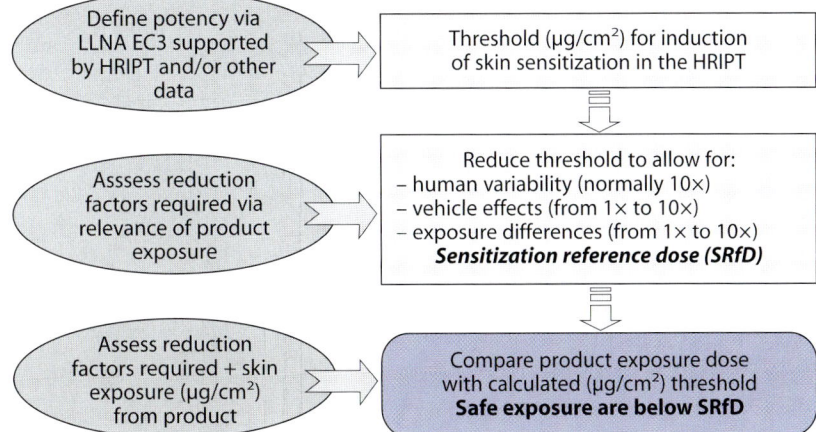

Fig. 2.
General approach to quanti-tative risk assessment for skin sensitization

Use of such a quantitative approach in defining human exposure limits for sensitizing chemicals relies heavily on both the accuracy and robustness of the measurement of potency in predictive models such as the LLNA. This aspect is mentioned in Sect. 12.4, but is also demonstrated by a comparison of potency categorizations in the LLNA compared to what is understood concerning potency in humans. The data in Table 1 display human potency categorizations based on EC3 results for 100 chemicals. It is important that these predictions are not only accurate, but also robust: such appears to be the case [3, 13]. As a further consequence, it is likely that data of this type will form the core sets of material against which in vitro alternatives ultimately will be validated [27].

12.6 Future Perspectives

In the context of skin irritation, there is a need to define in greater detail the elements of cutaneous inflammatory reactions that are a common feature of the irritant reactions provoked by diverse chemicals (which are likely to initiate irritancy via different mechanisms). This would in turn create new opportunities for the development of alternative test methods and also possibly provide a rational basis for the determination of relative potency. In addition, it is vital that this knowledge takes into account the fact that it is cumulative, rather than acute, irritancy which is of importance. With respect to translating hazard characterization into an accurate risk assessment, there is a need for an increased appreciation of the mechanistic basis for the polymorphic responses observed among exposed individuals.

Contact sensitization presents rather different challenges to those of skin irritation. Real progress is being made in development of approaches that allow robust and objective assessment of relative potency. In this regard, the utility of methods such as the LLNA need to be evaluated further and comparisons made between experimental estimates of skin sensitizing potential and what is known of allergenic activity among exposed human populations. This work also has implications for the future development of in vitro methods. To be of real value, in vitro methods must not only provide information on the presence (or absence) of sensitization hazard, they must in addition allow determination of the relative potency of an identified hazard. Only in this way can in vitro tests wholly replace the use of animal models for skin sensitization risk assessment.

Table 1. Prediction of human skin sensitization potency in the LLNA

Chemical	LLNA EC3 (%)	Human class
Oxazolone	0.01	Extreme
1,4-Benzoquinone	0.01	Extreme
1-Benzoylacetone	0.04	Extreme
Diphencyclopropenone	0.05	Extreme
N-Methyl-N-nitrosourea	0.05	Extreme
Methyl/chloromethyliso-thiazolinone	0.05	Extreme
2,4-Dinitrochlorobenzene	0.08	Extreme
Potassium dichromate	0.08	Extreme
Cyanuric chloride	0.09	Extreme
1,4-Dihydroquinone	0.11	Strong
Toluene diisocyanate	0.11	Strong
Chlorpromazine	0.14	Strong
Fluorescein isothiocyanate	0.14	Strong
Hexadecylmethane-sulfonate	0.14	Strong
Maleic anhydride	0.16	Strong
p-Phenylenediamine	0.16	Extreme
Dimethyl sulfate	0.19	Strong
Benzoyl bromide	0.20	Strong
Dodecylthiosulfonate	0.20	Strong
Glutaraldehyde	0.20	Strong
β-Propriolactone	0.20	Strong
Trimellitic anhydride	0.22	Strong
Benzoyl chloride	0.23	Strong
Benzoyl peroxide	0.30	Strong
Lauryl gallate	0.30	Strong
5-Methyl iso-eugenol	0.30	Strong
Propyl gallate	0.32	Strong
Phthalic anhydride	0.36	Strong
Chloramine-T	0.40	Strong
Formaldehyde	0.40	Strong
Methylisothiazolinone	0.40	Strong
2-Nitro-4-phenylene-diamine	0.40	Strong
2-Aminophenol	0.50	Strong
Glyoxal	0.60	Strong
Hexahydrophthalic anhydride	0.84	Strong
Iso-eugenol	1.3	Moderate
Methyldibromo glutaronitrile	1.3	Moderate
1-Phenyl-1,2-propanedione	1.3	Moderate
2-Hydroxyethyl acrylate	1.4	Moderate
Vinyl pyridine	1.6	Moderate
2-Mercaptobenzothiazole	1.7	Moderate
Cinnamic aldehyde (cinnamal)	2.0	Moderate

12

Table 1. Continued

Chemical	LLNA EC3 (%)	Human class
2-Amino-6-chloro-4-nitrophenol	2.2	Moderate
3-dimethylamino-propylamine	2.2	Moderate
Trans-2-decanal	2.5	Moderate
Zinc dimethyldithio-carbamate	2.7	Moderate
Phenylacetaldehyde	3.0	Moderate
3-Aminophenol	3.2	Moderate
Diethyl sulfate	3.3	Moderate
3-Methylisoeugenol	3.6	Moderate
3-Propylidenephthalide	3.7	Moderate
Benzylidene acetone	3.7	Moderate
1-Bromopentadecance	5.1	Moderate
Dipentamethylenethiuram disulfide	5.2	Moderate
Tetramethylthiuram disulfide	5.2	Moderate
3,4-Dihydrocoumarin	5.6	Moderate
Diethylmaleate	5.8	Moderate
4-Chloroaniline	6.5	Moderate
Dihydroeugenol	6.8	Moderate
1-(*p*-Methoxyphenyl)-1-penten-3-one	9.3	Moderate
Camphorquinone	10	Weak
Hexylcinnamal	11	Moderate
Citral	13	Weak
Eugenol	13	Weak
p-Methylhydrocinnamal	14	Weak
Abietic acid	15	Weak
Mercaptobenzimidazole	15	Weak
p-tert-Butyl-α-methyl hydrocinnamal	19	Weak
Hydroxycitronellal	20	Weak
Phenyl benzoate	20	Moderate
Dipentamethylene-thiuramtetrasulfide	21	Weak
Cyclamen aldehyde	22	Weak
Benzocaine	22	Weak
5-Methyl-2,3-hexanedione	26	Weak
Ethyleneglycol dimethacrylate	28	Weak
Ethyl acrylate	29	Weak
Linalool	30	Weak
Penicillin G	30	Weak
Butylglycidylether	31	Weak
3-Methyleugenol	32	Weak
Isopropyl myristate	44	Weak
2-Ethyl butyraldehyde	60	Weak

Table 1. Continued

Chemical	LLNA EC3 (%)	Human class
Limonene	69	Weak
Aniline	89	Weak
Acetanisole	Non-sensitizing	Not classified
1-Bromobutane	Non-sensitizing	Not classified
Chlorobenzene	Non-sensitizing	Not classified
Dextran	Non-sensitizing	Not classified
Diethylphthalate	Non-sensitizing	Not classified
Glycerol	Non-sensitizing	Not classified
Hexane	Non-sensitizing	Not classified
4-Hydroxybenzoic acid	Non-sensitizing	Not classified
2-Hydroxypropyl methacrylate	Non-sensitizing	Not classified
Isopropanol	Non-sensitizing	Not classified
Lactic acid	Non-sensitizing	Not classified
6-Methyl coumarin	Non-sensitizing	Not classified
Methyl salicylate	Non-sensitizing	Not classified
Octanoic acid	Non-sensitizing	Not classified
Resorcinol	Non-sensitizing	Not classified
Tween 80	Non-sensitizing	Not classified

LLNA EC3 value derived as indicated in Fig. 1. Human class assignment based on order of magnitude EC3 groups

Core Message

■ In vitro tests for the identification of skin irritants and skin sensitizers are not yet available. However, opportunities have been identified and are the subject of active investigation currently.

References

1. Andersen KE, Maibach HI (1985) Contact allergy predictive tests in guinea pigs. Karger, Basel (Current problems in dermatology, vol 14)
2. Andersen KE, Volund A, Frankild S (1995) The guinea pig maximization test with a multiple dose design. Acta Derm Venereol 75:463–469
3. Basketter DA, Cadby P (2004) Reproducible prediction of contact allergenic potency using the local lymph node assay. Contact Dermatitis 50:15–17
4. Basketter DA, Gerberick GF, Kimber I, Loveless SE (1996) The local lymph node assay: a viable alternative to currently accepted skin sensitisation tests. Food Chem Toxicol 34:985–997
5. Basketter DA, Chamberlain M, Griffiths HA, York M (1997a) The classification of skin irritants by human patch test. Food Chemical Toxicol 35:845–852

6. Basketter DA, Reynolds FS, York M (1997b) Predictive testing in contact dermatitis – irritant dermatitis. In: Goh CL, Koh D (eds) Clinics in dermatology – contact dermatitis, vol 15. Elsevier, Amsterdam, pp 637–644

7. Basketter DA, Gilpin GR, Kuhn M, Lawrence RS, Reynolds FS, Whittle E (1998) Patch tests versus use tests in skin irritation risk assessment. Contact Dermatitis 39:252–256

8. Basketter DA, Gerberick GF, Kimber I, Willis C (1999a) The toxicology of contact dermatitis, chap 3. Wiley, Chichester, pp 39–56

9. Basketter DA, Gerberick GF, Kimber I, Willis C (1999b) The toxicology of contact dermatitis, chap 4. Wiley, Chichester, pp 57–72

10. Basketter DA, Gerberick GF, Kimber I, Willis CM (1999c) Toxicology of contact dermatitis. Allergy, irritancy and urticaria. Wiley, Chichester

11. Basketter DA, Lea LJ, Dickens A, Briggs D, Pate I, Dearman RJ, Kimber I (1999d) A comparison of statistical approaches to derivation of EC3 values from local lymph node assay dose responses. J Appl Toxicol 19:261–266

12. Basketter DA, Blaikie L, Dearman RJ, Kimber I, Ryan CA, Gerberick GF, Harvey P, Evans P, White IR, Rycroft RJG (2000) Use of the local lymph node assay for the estimation of relative contact allergenic potency. Contact Dermatitis 42:344–348

13. Basketter DA, Pease Smith CK, Patlewicz GY (2003) Contact allergy: the local lymph node assay for the prediction of hazard and risk. Clin Exp Dermatol 28:218–221

14. Buehler EV (1965) Delayed contact hypersensitivity in the guinea pig. Arch Dermatol 91:171–177

15. Chan PD, Baldwin RC, Parson RD, Moss JN, Sterotelli R, Smith JM, Hayes AW (1983) Kathon biocide: manifestation of delayed contact dermatitis in guinea pigs is dependent on the concentration for induction and challenge. J Invest Dermatol 81:409–411

16. De Groot AC (1990) Methylisothiazolinone/methylchloroisothiazolinone (Kathon CG) allergy: an updated review. Am J Contact Dermatitis 1:151–156

17. Draize JH, Woodard G, Calvery HO (1944) Methods for the study of irritation and toxicity of substances applied topically to the skin and mucous membranes. J Pharmacol Exp Ther 82:377–390

18. EC (1992) Annex to Commission Directive 92/69/EEC of 31 July 1992 adapting to technical progress for the seventeenth time Council Directive 67/548/EEC on the approximation of laws, regulations and administrative provisions relating to the classification, packaging and labelling of dangerous substances. Official J Eur Commun L383A:35

19. Felter SP, Robinson MK, Basketter DA, Gerberick GF (2002) A review of the scientific basis for default uncertainty factors for use in quantitative risk assessment of the induction of allergic contact dermatitis. Contact Dermatitis 47:257–266

20. Felter SP, Ryan CA, Basketter DA, Gerberick GF (2003) Application of the risk assessment paradigm to the induction of allergic contact dermatitis. Regul Toxicol Pharmacol 37:1–10

21. Fentem JH, Archer GEB, Balls M, Botham PA, Curren RD, Earl LK, Esdaile DJ, Holzhutter H-G, Liebsch M (1998) The ECVAM international validation study on in vitro tests for skin corrosivity. 2. Results and evaluation by the Management Team. Toxicol In Vitro 12:483–524

22. Frosch PJ, Kurte A, Pilz B (1993) Efficacy of skin barrier creams. III. The repetitive irritation test (RIT) in humans. Contact Dermatitis 29:113–118

23. Gabard B, Treffel P, Charton-Picard F, Eloy R (1995) Irritant reactions on hairless micropig skin: a model for testing barrier creams? Karger, Basel, pp 275–287 (Current problems in dermatology, vol 23)

24. Gad SC, Dunn BJ, Dobbs DW, Reilly C, Walsh RD (1986) Development and validation of an alternative dermal sensitisation test: the mouse ear swelling test (MEST). Toxicol Appl Pharmacol 84:93–114

25. Gerberick GF, Ryan CA, Kimber I, Dearman RJ, Lea LJ, Basketter DA (1999) Local lymph node assay: validation assessment for regulatory purposes. Am J Cont Derm 11(1):3–18

26. Gerberick GF, Robinson MK, Felter S, White I, Basketter DA. (2001) Understanding fragrance allergy using an exposure-based risk assessment approach. Contact Dermatitis 45:333–340

27. Gerberick GF, Ryan CA, Kern PS, Dearman RJ, Kimber I, Patlewicz GY, Basketter DA (2004) A chemical dataset for the evaluation of alternative approaches to skin sensitization testing. Contact Dermatitis 50:274–288

28. Griem P, Goebel C, Scheffler H (2003) Proposal for a risk assessment methodology for skin sensitization based on sensitization potency data. Regul Toxicol Pharmacol 38:269–290

29. Hall-Manning TJ, Holland GH, Basketter DA, Barratt MD (1995) Skin irritation potential of mixed surfactant systems in a human 4 hour covered patch test. Allergologie 18:465

30. Hannuksela A, Hannuksela M (1995) Irritant effects of a detergent in wash and chamber tests. Contact Dermatitis 32:163–166

31. Hilton J, Dearman RJ, Harvey P, Evans P, Basketter DA, Kimber I (1998) Estimation of relative skin sensitising potency using the local lymph node assay: a comparison of formaldehyde with glutaraldehyde. Am J Contact Derm 9:29–33

32. Holland G, York M, Basketter DA (1995) Irritants – corrosive materials, oxidising/reducing agents, acids and alkalis, concentrated salt solutions etc. In: Maibach HI, Coenraads PJ (eds) Irritant contact dermatitis syndrome. CRC Press, Boca Raton, pp 55–64

33. Jenkins HL, Adams MG (1989) Progressive evaluation of skin irritancy of cosmetics using human volunteers. Int J Cosmet Sci 11:141–149

34. Kimber I, Basketter DA (1992) The murine local lymph node assay: a commentary on collaborative studies and new directions. Food Chem Toxic 30:165–169

35. Kimber I, Basketter DA (1997) Contact sensitisation: a new approach to risk assessment. Hum Ecol Risk Assess 3:385–395

36. Kimber I, Dearman RJ (1991) Investigation of lymph node cell proliferation as a possible immunological correlate of contact sensitizing potential. Food Chem Toxic 29:125–129

37. Kimber I, Dearman RJ, Scholes EW, Basketter DA (1994) The local lymph node assay: developments and applications. Toxicology 93:13–31

38. Kimber I, Pichowski JP, Betts CJ, Cumberbatch M, Basketter DA, Dearman RJ (2001) Alternative approaches to the identification and charactersiation of chemical allergens. Toxicol In Vitro 15:307–331

39. Kimber I, Dearman RJ, Basketter DA, Ryan CA, Gerberick GF (2002) The local lymph node assay: past, present and future. Contact Derm 47:315–328

40. Lewis RW, Basketter DA (1995) Transcutaneous electrical resistance: application in predicting skin corrosives. In: Elsner P, Maibach HI (eds) Irritant dermatitis: new clinical and experimental aspects. Karger, Basel, pp 243–255

41. Magnusson B, Kligman AM (1970) Allergic contact dermatitis in the Guinea pig. Thomas, Springfield, IL

12

42. Maibach HI, Coenraads PJ (1995) The irritant contact dermatitis syndrome. CRC Press, Boca Raton
43. Malten KE (1981) Thoughts on irritant contact dermatitis. Contact Dermatitis 7:238–247
44. Marzulli FN, Maibach HI (1975) The rabbit as a model for evaluating skin irritants: a comparison of results obtained on animals and man using repeated skin exposures. Food Cosmet Toxicol 13:533–540
45. NIH publication no 99–4494 (1999) The murine local lymph node assay: a test method for assessing the allergic contact dermatitis potential of chemical compounds
46. Patil SM, Patrick E, Maibach HI (1996) Animal, human, and in vitro test methods for predicting skin irritation. In: Marzulli FN, Maibach HI (eds) Dermatotoxicology. Taylor and Francis, Washington, DC, pp 411–436
47. Prins M, Swinkels OQ, Kolkman EG, Wuis EW, Hekster YA, van der Valk PG (1998) Skin irritation by dithranol cream. A blind study to assess the role of the cream formulation. Acta Derm Venereol 78:262–265
48. Schneider K, Akkan Z (2004) Quantitative relationship between the local lymph node assay and human skin sensitization assays. Regul Toxicol Pharmacol 39:245–255
49. Simion FA (1995) In vivo models to predict skin irritation. In: Van der Valk PGM, Maibach HI (eds) The irritant contact dermatitis syndrome. CRC Press, Boca Raton, pp 329–334
50. Walker AP, Basketter DA, Baverel M, Diembeck W, Matthies W, Mougin D, Paye M, Rothlisburger R, Dupuis J (1996) Test guideline for assessment of skin compatibility of cosmetic finished products in man. Food Chem Toxicol 34:551–560
51. Walker AP, Basketter DA, Baverel M, Diembeck W, Matthies W, Mougin D, Paye M, Rothlisburger R, Dupuis J (1997) Test guidelines for assessment of skin tolerance of potentially irritant cosmetic ingredients in man. Food Chem Toxicol 35:1099–1106
52. Warbrick EV, Dearman RJ, Lea LJ, Basketter DA, Kimber I (1999) Local lymph node assay responses to paraphenylenediamine: intra- and inter-laboratory evaluations. J Appl Toxicol 19:255–260
53. Weaver JE, Carding CW, Maibach HI (1985) Dose response assessments of Kathon biocide. I. Diagnostic use and diagnostic threshold patch testing with sensitised humans. Contact Dermatitis 12:141–145
54. Welss T, Basketter DA, Schroder KR (2004) In vitro skin irritation: facts and future. State of the art review of mechanisms and models. Toxicol In Vitro 18:231–243
55. Wigger-Alberti W, Hinnen U, Elsner P (1997) Predictive testing of metalworking fluids: a comparison of 2 cumulative human irritation models and correlation with epidemiological data. Contact Dermatitis 36:14–20
56. Zachariae C, Rastogi S, Devantier C, Menne T, Johansen JD (2003) Methyldibromo glutaronitrile: clinical experience and exposure-based risk assessment. Contact Dermatitis 48:150–154

Chapter 13

Allergic Contact Dermatitis in Humans – Experimental and Quantitative Aspects

Jeanne Duus Johansen, Peter J. Frosch, Torkil Menné

Contents

13.2 Individual Variation

The degree of contact allergy can be graded either according to the patch test outcome (+ to +++) or by serial dilution [2, 3] (Fig. 1). There is a correlation between the two grading systems, such that individuals with a +++ reaction generally react to a lower patch test concentration than those with only a + reaction [4]. The degree of contact allergy is an important individual risk factor for development of allergic contact dermatitis. In a study of 101 patients with contact allergy to 5-chloro-2-methylisothiazol-3-one (MCI) and 2-methylisothiazol-3-one (MI), a significantly greater number of patients had a positive use test to emollients preserved with 15 ppm MCI/MI

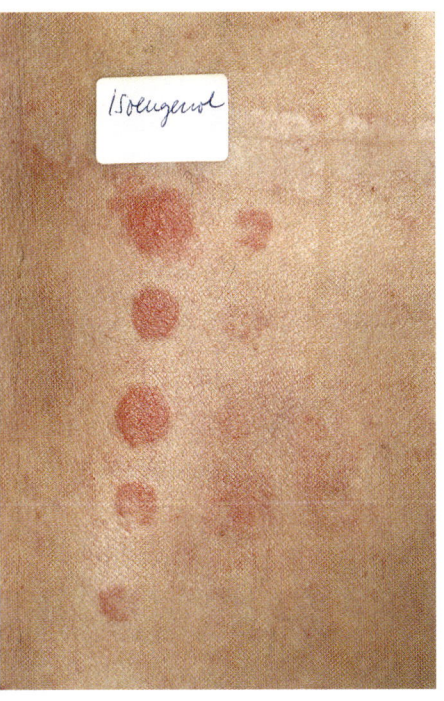

Fig. 1. Result of patch testing with a serial dilution of isoeugenol (2% to 0.008% in ethanol). The patient was highly sensitive and still showed a papular reaction at 0.125% (*upper right*)

13.1 Introduction

Allergic contact dermatitis is a common and potentially disabling disease. The clinical definition of the disease is based on the history of the patient, clinical examination, patch testing, and a detailed, often repeated exposure assessment.

The literature on evaluation and standardization of the diagnostic patch test is extensive [1]. Less effort has been focused on experimental elicitation of the disease allergic contact dermatitis. Such studies are essential for confirmation of the diagnosis allergic contact dermatitis in the clinical situation, and serve as an important guideline for establishing estimates of the exposure concentrations that are safe with respect to elicitation of contact allergy in sensitized individuals.

The present chapter reviews methods for experimental allergic contact dermatitis in humans, and the most important individual and exposure-related variables for the elicitation of allergic contact dermatitis.

among those reacting with a positive patch test to 25 ppm than among those only reacting with a positive patch test to 100 ppm [5]. Similarly, it has been shown that the degree of contact allergy is an important risk factor for perfume dermatitis in fragrance-sensitive individuals [6].

Frosch et al. [7] have demonstrated that patients with a strong patch test reaction to the fragrance mix (++ or +++) have a positive history of fragrance sensitivity to a much higher degree than those with a weak (+) or doubtful (?+) reaction (Table 1).

Rudzki et al. [8] have clearly illustrated that the numbers of patients with shoe dermatitis among chromate-sensitive individuals are greatest in those with a high degree of contact allergy.

An important observation in relation to the tendency to persistent regional dermatitis, e.g., hand eczema, is the study by Hindsen et al. [9], who illustrated that nickel dermatitis is followed by long-lasting local hyper-reactivity to nickel but not to other allergens or irritants. Recently similar results were obtained in a study of patients sensitized to methyldibromo glutaronitrile [10]. In the case of multiple contact allergies, as is frequently seen in patients with fragrance contact allergy, synergistic effects may result in an unpredictable propensity to react to perfumed products [11].

Core Message

■ The degree of contact allergy is an important individual risk factor for development of allergic contact dermatitis. Local specific hyper-reactivity to an allergen at a previously exposed skin site may persist for a long time.

13.3 Exposure-related Factors

The amount of allergen per skin surface area is the key factor that determines the risk of induction [12–14] and the same may apply for elicitation. As illustrated in Table 2 the exposures to MCI/MI from different sources, calculated as $\mu g/cm^2$, parallel the risk of elicitation of allergic contact dermatitis from different product types. Elicitation of allergic contact dermatitis occurs in approximately 50% of MCI/MI-sensitive individuals when exposed to leave-on product preserved with 15 ppm MCI/MI, while elicitation with a shampoo preserved with the same amount is relatively uncommon [15].

Elicitation depends not only on exposure concentration but also on the duration of exposure. Increasing the duration of exposure to 1% p-phenylene-diamine (PPD) gave a proportionate increase in the number of reactors among PPD-sensitized individuals. The same effect could be obtained by increasing the PPD exposure concentration [16]. A cumulative effect of exposures has been demonstrated, so that repeating exposures cause elicitation in more individuals [16, 17]. Using low concentrations of allergen means that more exposures are required to elicit a reaction than for higher concentrations, as demonstrated with the fragrance ingredient isoeugenol [17]. Repeated open exposure on the lower forearm to a solution containing 0.05% isoeugenol produced reactions in 42% of sensitized individuals within a 4-week period and in 67% at exposure to 0.2% isoeugenol. The median time until reaction was 15 days for the low and 7 days for the high concentration [17]. This and other experiments indicate that the accumulated total dose is a major determinant of the elicitation response [16, 18, 19]. Jensen et al. showed that the effect of applying a 0.04% solution of methyldibromo glutaronitrile once a day in a use test had an almost equal capability of provoking allergic contact dermatitis as application of 0.01% four times a day [18].

The matrix may influence the elicitation capacity of an allergen and the addition of irritants such as

Table 1. Intensity of patch test reactions to the fragrance mix and/or constituents in relation to history (*IR* Irritative reactions)

Fragrance history	?+/IR	+	++	+++	Total
Positive	13	14	39	16	82
Negative	52	25	26	0	103
Doubtful	5	14	18	2	39
Total	70	53	83	18	224

Table 2. Degree of MCI/MI exposure from different sources (the much lower exposure with the shampoo results from the wash-off effect)

Source	MCI/MI exposure ($\mu g/cm^2$)
Diagnostic patch test 100 ppm	3
Lotion preserved with 15 ppm	6×10^{-2}
Shampoo preserved with 15 ppm	8.7×10^{-4}

detergents has been shown to increase the clinical response to an allergen by a factor of 4–6 [20–22].

Skin regions differ in sensitivity. The upper arm has been shown to be more sensitive than the forehead and ventral aspect of the lower arm in use tests [23], the axilla more sensitive than the outer aspect of the upper arm [24], and recently it has been shown that the neck and face are more sensitive than the outer aspect of the upper arm [25].

Core Message

■ Exposure-related factors that influence the risk of elicitation are allergen concentration (dose), duration and frequency of exposure, matrix, presence of irritants, and region of application.

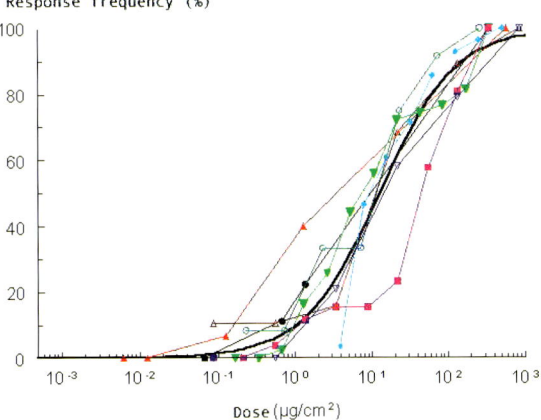

Fig. 2. Dose–response curves based on patch test data from eight studies of nickel allergy. The data are analyzed by logistic regression. The *black curve* represents the weighed adjusted average curve from all the studies [35]

13.4 Experimental Human Models

13.4.1 Serial Dilution Patch Test

A dilution series of a relevant allergen usually in ethanol, petrolatum or water is the most used method for quantification of the elicitation response. The test is performed on the upper back similar to standard testing just with one allergen at different concentrations. The dilution steps depend on the allergen and the purpose of investigation, but usually steps of two, three or ten are used, with a span of concentrations covering a factor 100–10,000. Thresholds are determined either as the minimal elicitation concentration (MEC) or as the maximum no effect level (NOEL).

There is a considerable inter-individual variation in reactivity to an allergen, but also an intra-individual variation over time as shown for nickel-allergic patients [26]. Compiling results for groups of nickel-allergic patients, however, gives a fairly constant dose–response curve also over time [26]. At low allergen levels the clinical response will be less pronounced: typically the reactions will become papular (Fig. 1). From a biological point of view the assessment of thresholds should take these weaker responses into consideration and not rely just on diagnostic patch test criteria [27].

Serial dilution patch tests have been used to determine the optimal patch test concentration for a substance [28, 29], as a predictor of chronic disease [30], or to obtain data of thresholds relevant for groups of sensitized individuals to be used in risk assessments

and prevention [31, 32]. Overviews of published dose–response data for individual allergens have been produced [15, 33, 34]; further such data have been subjected to a kind of meta-analysis combining results from several studies into a single dose–response curve (Fig. 2), which again may be used in risk assessments [27, 35]. One of the results of such data analysis is that the variation between studies is limited considering that they were performed in different geographical regions and time periods. A further standardization suggested is to implement dose–response elicitation data in risk assessment routinely [35, 36], and to systematically and prospectively assess the relationship between thresholds obtained by serial dilution patch tests and repeated open applications tests [35].

13.4.2 The Repeated Open Application Test

Different names have been used for the repeated open application of allergens to contact-sensitized individuals, such as the usage test, provocative use test, and open patch test. The name ROAT (repeated open application test) was coined by Hannuksela and Salo [37] and has since been the generally accepted term for this procedure. The test consists of an open exposure, often with a finished product or with a well-defined vehicle containing the defined allergen at a nonirritant concentration. A 5×5-cm^2 skin area on the forearm or upper arm close to the antecubital fossa is used. Application in the antecubital fossa should be avoided because the degree of natural occlusion is unpredictable. The vehicle used in the ROAT may be a finished product or patch test vehicles such as petrolatum or alcohol. Twice a day application is recommended for practical reasons. Most ROAT studies have used an application time of 1–2 weeks. One week is undoubtedly too short, depending on the reactivity of individual patients and the hapten exposure concentration [17, 38]. In newer studies applications of emollients with relevant preservatives have been made on the neck and face, which have been shown to be more sensitive than the upper arm [25, 39]. Clinical tests need to take the region of application into consideration, and testing should preferably be done simulating normal exposure as closely as possible in order to avoid false-negative results.

Itching may be the first symptom in the allergic contact dermatitis reactions elicited. In a double-blind ROAT study of cinnamal, some individuals registered itching at the site of specific allergen exposure before any visible skin signs [38]; however, nonimmunologic contact urticaria may alternatively have caused these symptoms [38]. Further studies, which systematically focus on this point, are necessary. The morphology of the positive ROAT has given important information as to the early clinical signs of the allergic contact dermatitis reaction. The first objective sign in allergic contact dermatitis may be a follicular papular eruption, as seen from low concentrations of allergens in serial dilution patch testing (Fig. 1). The follicular morphology of the allergic contact dermatitis reaction is not generally recognized in textbooks, but nevertheless may be the first clinical symptoms in a ROAT with a specific allergen. The explanation for this morphology is the increased accumulation and absorption of allergens through the follicles and sweat duct orifices [40, 41]. More rarely, uniform redness is the primary symptom. Continued exposure leads to infiltration and eventually vesicle formation. There are no generally accepted guidelines for evaluation of the ROAT. The terminology used for diagnostic patch test reading is less suitable, as early allergic reactions will be disregarded. Further, an experimental ROAT will usually be terminated before strong positive reactions comparable to ++ or +++ patch test reactions have developed. As the ROAT is usually done with nonirritant allergen concentrations and the response compared to a vehicle-treated controlled area, both the follicular reaction pattern and noninfiltrated redness represent allergic reactions and should be scored as such, in contrast to reading the occluded patch test. Johansen et al. [42] have proposed a semi-quantitative reading scale for the ROAT (Tables 3–7). This system is based mainly on the experience obtained with perfume ingredient testing and needs broader evaluation.

Noninvasive so-called bioengineering methods are useful in the quantification of the experimental irritant response, but because of the heterogeneous and often follicular pattern of the early allergic contact dermatitis reaction, such methods are less suitable in evaluation of the ROAT [43].

Table 3. Reading use tests: involved area application

	Percentage of application area involved (%)				
	90–100	50–89	25–49	1–24	0
Score	4	3	2	1	0

Table 4. Reading use test: erythema

	Involvement			Strength		
	Homo-geneous	Spotty	None	Strong	Medium	Weak
Score	2	1	0	3	2	1

Table 5. Reading use test: papules/infiltration

	Papules/infiltration				
	Homogeneous infiltration	Many (>25)	Some (10–15)	Few (<10)	None
Score	4	3	2	1	0

Table 6. Reading use test: vesicles

	Vesicles				
	Confluent	Many (>25)	Some (10–25)	Few (<10)	None
Score	4	3	2	1	0

Table 7. Overall clinical impression of the use test reaction

Strong	Moderate	Weak	Doubtful	Negative
Positive	Positive	Positive		

Core Message

■ ROATs should be continued for at least 14 days if negative. The neck and face are more sensitive than the upper arm to allergen exposure in sensitized individuals.

13.4.3 The Axillary Exposure Test

Allergens related to deodorants and textiles are relevant to the axillary region. Published research has focused on formaldehyde and fragrances. Industry has long experience of irritancy testing in the development of deodorants and antiperspirants. It is recognized that this particular skin area is problematic in relation to product development, as this moist and occluded skin area has a propensity to irritant reactions. When performing axillary allergen exposure studies, it is therefore always necessary to include both sensitized and nonsensitized individuals to control for irritancy.

The early morphology of the positive reactions is similar to that seen in the ROAT, with papulofollicular elements being a common feature. Studies including formaldehyde and fragrances have demonstrated lower concentration thresholds in the axillae, as compared to the skin of the upper arm and back [44, 45]. Exposure studies with standard deodorants containing cinnamal or hydroxycitronellal in increasing concentration illustrate a dose–response relationship in patients sensitive to the substance in question [45, 46]. This type of study, combined with product analysis, clearly demonstrates the relevance of fragrance allergy in relation to deodorants. Further, it is an important step in the risk assessment process for the continued improvement of product safety [45, 46].

13.4.4 The Shampoo Test

Shampoos are widely used cosmetic products with few side-effects. Reports of allergic contact dermatitis from shampoos are mainly case-based. Shampoos can cause dermatitis of the scalp, face, and neck. Cases simulating seborrheic dermatitis have been reported. The rarity of allergic contact dermatitis from shampoos is probably explained by the small degree of exposure (Table 2), because of allergen dilution.

In controlled exposure studies with an MCI/MI-containing shampoo including MCI/MI-sensitive individuals, Frosch et al. [47] identified cases with elicitation of exudative scalp dermatitis, facial dermatitis, and flare of hand eczema. Even if such cases are rarely reported [15], the outcome of the shampoo use test alerts the clinician to consider this possibility in the case of contact dermatitis of the scalp, face, neck, and retroauricular regions.

13.4.5 The Liquid Soap Test

Liquid soaps are a well-known cause of irritant contact dermatitis, especially at the workplace. Allergic contact dermatitis from allergens in liquid soaps is rarely documented, possibly due to the lack of adequate methods of investigation. However, a new method of testing liquid soaps has been developed [48] following clinical evidence that these types of products were involved in many cases of contact allergy to methyldibromo glutaronitrile [49–51].

Testing is performed on two identical areas of 5 cm × 10 cm at the fore arms. In a blinded and randomized fashion, a soap containing the allergen in question, in this case methyldibromo glutaronitrile, is applied on one arm and an identical placebo product without the allergen on the other arm. The test site is moistened with water and two drops of soap applied. The test area is washed with the soap by moving a small water-soaked nylon sponge back and forward over the area 10 times. The soap is left for a maximum of 30 s before the skin sites are rinsed with running water and dried [48]. Applications are made twice daily for up to 4 weeks. Using this protocol it was demonstrated that 37% (7/19) of sensitized individuals gave a reaction to a liquid soap containing methyldibromo glutaronitrile in the currently permitted concentration [48]. This was an important part of the chain of evidence that liquid soaps with methyldibromo glutaronitrile cause allergic contact dermatitis, and it also provided a new model for testing liquid soaps. The model was optimized recently, as it will often be relevant to test products with less potent allergens. In the suggested design, the skin of the lower part of each arm was pretreated with the allergen in question by patch testing with a concentration range of the allergen using 12-mm Finn chambers [10]. One month later a use test was performed with a liquid soap containing the allergen on one arm and an identical soap without the allergen on the other arm. An increased reactivity was shown on the areas that had been pretreated with the allergen (methyldibromo glutaronitrile), while pre-irritated skin gave no augmented response to allergen exposure; furthermore, a control group was negative [10]. It is a design that may prove useful in assessing the risk of exposure to allergens in liquid soaps. Testing of more allergens is needed for further validation.

Core Message

- New models for testing allergens in liquid soaps have been developed for the purpose of risk assessment.

13.4.6 The Finger Immersion Test/ Experimental Hand Eczema

Hand eczema is a common disease and may lead to sick leave and permanent disability. The diagnosis of allergic contact dermatitis on the hands is based upon the outcome of patch testing and qualitative exposure assessment. In some cases this procedure is straightforward, as for example with rubber gloves. There is solid evidence that the rubber chemicals, thiurams and mercaptobenzothiazole in the standard patch test series are present in rubber gloves, and are leached out during use in amounts sufficient to elicit allergic contact dermatitis [52–54]. But in many cases, when the diagnosis allergic hand dermatitis is established, e.g., from metals, preservatives, and naturally occurring substances, the evidence is circumstantial because experimental disease models combined with quantitative exposure assessment are not developed.

There have been attempts in the past to establish such models. Hjorth and Roed Petersen [55] made provocation studies of the fingers of chefs and sandwich makers using fresh food. Christensen and Möller [56] established vesicular nickel hand eczema as part of systemic contact dermatitis.

Allenby and Basketter [57] introduced the finger immersion model. They intended to investigate whether trace amounts of nickel (0.1–1 ppm), present in some consumer products, were able to elicit allergic hand eczema. Four nickel-sensitive individuals, without previous or present hand eczema, had their thumbs immersed in a solution containing nickel (0.1–1 ppm) and sodium dodecyl sulfate (0.1–0.3%) twice daily for 10 min over 21 days. None of the volunteers developed an eczematous response. Accumulation of nickel in the fingernails was used as an objective exposure parameter (Table 8). Recently, Nielsen et al. [58] made a double-blind placebo-controlled finger immersion study, including 35 nickel-sensitive individuals with low-grade hand eczema (redness and scaling, but no vesicles) over 2 weeks. Finger exposure for 10 min daily to first 10 ppm and later 100 ppm nickel elicited a statistically significant flare of vesicular hand eczema in nickel-exposed patients,

Table 8. Nickel in nails reflecting exposure

Type of exposure	Nickel µg/g (mean)	Reference
Occupational exposure		
None (controls)	1.19	[60]
Moderate	29.20	[60]
Heavy	123.00	[60]
Experimental exposure		
Baseline	1.58	[59]
Immersion of finger in 0.1–1 ppm nickel twice a day for 21 days[a]	7.80	[57]
Immersion of finger in 10 ppm nickel once a day for 1 week	5.50	[59]
Immersion of finger in 100 ppm nickel once a day for 1 week	12.00	[59]

[a] Four observations

as compared to vehicle-exposed patients. As objective response parameters, the number of vesicles was counted and the blood flow measured by laser Doppler. The nickel concentrations in nails (Table 8) and skin as a consequence of experimental nickel exposure were measured [59]. Combination of the knowledge from this experimental study and the quantification of nickel exposure in different industries [60] might give a more solid basis for the diagnosis of occupational hand eczema caused by nickel allergy in the future. Similar pilot studies have been done with chromate and cobalt [61]. Also perfume ingredients, e.g., hydroxycitronellal and Lyral®, have been tested in similar protocols with exposure concentrations equal to diluted and undiluted dish washing liquid [62]. In contrast to the studies of nickel, chromate and cobalt, no significant difference could be found between active exposure and placebo, possibly due to the use of less potent allergens, which under normal exposure conditions would be in combination with irritants.

13.5 The Comparative Approach

Formaldehyde has been studied in different human models. Table 9 compares the concentration threshold for reactivity to formaldehyde in formaldehyde-sensitive patients in different experimental exposure tests. It is important to notice that some of the results are based on one or few patients. Notwithstanding this, the variation in concentration thresholds depending on exposure site and exposure condition is

Table 9. Concentration threshold for reactivity to formaldehyde in formaldehyde-sensitive patients in different experimental exposure tests

Method	Threshold (ppm)	Reference
Repeated (1-week) exposure on normal skin	300 ppm	[4]
Repeated axillary exposure	150 ppm	[44]
Finn chamber patch test	150 ppm	[72]
Repeated patch testing in the same area	30 ppm	[19]
Hand eczema skin immersion (40 min) 1 patient	0.2 ppm	[63]

challenging. Horsfall [63] found a positive exposure test with 0.2 ppm formaldehyde in a patient with allergic formaldehyde dermatitis on the hands. If this observation can be confirmed, it is important for our understanding of formaldehyde hand dermatitis. When making the final risk assessment, the wide variation in elicitation concentration threshold, as illustrated for formaldehyde in Table 9, needs to be considered. Similar comparative data are not yet present for other allergens.

13.6 Elicitation Data Used in Prevention and Regulations

Experimental clinical exposure studies may form the basis for regulation of allergen exposure in the future. This has been the case in the regulation of nickel released from metal items designed to be in direct and prolonged skin contact. This question is relatively simple, as exposure to metal items such as jewelry, claps, buttons etc. is comparable to that in the patch test, and the evaluation can therefore be based on this technology. A number of studies have uniformly shown that metal items releasing less than 0.5 $\mu g/cm^2$ nickel per week elicit an allergic reaction in only a few nickel-sensitive individuals [64]. This observation was the basis for the regulation of nickel exposure in Denmark and later in the EU [65]. Future studies may illustrate that the measurement of nickel in the skin, released from such items, will be a more reliable parameter than nickel released from the items in artificial sweat. Studies of nickel in nails, as shown in Table 8, measured in different industrial settings and during experimental nickel exposure, illustrate that it is possible to quantify nickel exposure, even though the variation is not insignificant [57, 59, 60]. Based on nickel nail concentrations, the expo-

sure used in the experimental studies that provoked a flare of dermatitis is comparable to a moderate industrial nickel exposure. Data now exist supporting the view that nickel regulation has been an effective tool of prevention and caused a decrease in the numbers of nickel-sensitized individuals in the young part of the female population [66, 67].

Exposure to chemicals from rubber gloves is analogous to nickel exposure from metal items designed to be in direct and prolonged contact with the skin. It has been shown that the amount of rubber chemicals released from rubber gloves, under the influence of synthetic sweat, is comparable to the amount of rubber chemical necessary to elicit a positive patch test [52, 53]. Such data explain why a positive patch test to thiurams is frequently relevant to exposure to rubber gloves.

Experimental exposure studies with important perfume chemicals have been made, with concentrations based on the outcome of chemical analysis of perfumed products and fine fragrances [68, 69]. In this way, it has been substantiated that the concentrations of perfume chemicals in cosmetic products and fine fragrances not infrequently exceed those that may elicit allergic contact dermatitis in sensitized individuals. Studies of thresholds for fragrance allergens such as Lyral® [31] and the main allergens in oak moss abs., chloroatranol [32], have formed the basis for risk assessments and recommendations for safer use concentrations for these substances.

In patients with contact allergy to more than one perfumed ingredient, combined exposure to both may lead to a synergistic eliciting effect [6]. This illustrates that a detailed knowledge of environmental exposure to well-defined allergens is needed for the performance of meaningful experimental exposure studies. The development of chemical methods in recent years to quantify exposure to metals, preservatives [70], plastics, fragrances, and rubber chemicals has facilitated the conduct of clinically relevant experimental exposure studies in specifically sensitized individuals. However, much is still to be learnt in this area, as the main allergens from many naturally occurring sources remain unknown, e.g., perfume ingredients such as ylang ylang oil [71].

Core Message

- Elicitation data derived from dose–response studies have been used for preventive actions with success.

13.7 Comments

Studies on experimental allergic contact dermatitis in humans have in several cases formed part of the basis for regulations of specific contact allergens – and with success. A further integration in the legislative process is desired, as the relevant end-point of prevention, allergic contact dermatitis in humans, is the subject of these investigations. However, to implement data from quantitative elicitation studies more systematically, some methodological aspects need further consideration and standardization. The studies need careful planning and highly motivated volunteers to obtain the necessary compliance. By combining such studies with measurements of allergen concentrations, e.g., in skin and nails, a powerful instrument for evidence-based diagnosis of allergic contact dermatitis can be established in the future. Finally, such studies are an important part of the risk assessment for chemicals that come into contact with the skin, from either consumer products or occupational exposures.

References

1. Wahlberg JE (2000) Patch testing. In: Rycroft RJG, Menné T, Frosch PJ, Lepoittevin J-P (eds) Textbook of contact dermatitis, 3rd edn. Springer, Berlin Heidelberg New York
2. Andersen KE, Liden C, Hansen J, Volund A (1993) Dose-response testing with nickel sulphate using the TRUE test in nickel-sensitive individuals. Multiple nickel sulphate patch-test reactions do not cause an "angry back". Br J Dermatol 129:50–56
3. Menné T, Calvin G (1993) Concentration threshold of non-occluded nickel exposure in nickel-sensitive individuals and controls with and without surfactant. Contact Dermatitis 29:180–184
4. Flyvholm MA, Hall BM, Agner T, Tiedemann E, Greenhill P, Vanderveken W, Freeberg FE, Menné T (1997) Threshold for occluded formaldehyde patch test in formaldehyde-sensitive patients. Relationship to repeated open application test with a product containing formaldehyde releaser. Contact Dermatitis 36:26–33
5. Menné T (1991) Relationship between use test and threshold patch test concentration in patients sensitive to 5-chloro-2-methyl-4-isothiazolin-3-one and 2- methyl-4-isothiazolin-3-one (MCI/MI). Contact Dermatitis 24:375
6. Johansen JD, Andersen KE, Menné T (1996) Quantitative aspects of isoeugenol contact allergy assessed by use and patch tests. Contact Dermatitis 34:414–418
7. Frosch PJ, Pilz B, Burrows D, Camarasa JG, Lachapelle JM, Lahti A, Menné T, Wilkinson JD (1995) Testing with fragrance mix. Is the addition of sorbitan sesquioleate to the constituents useful? Contact Dermatitis 32:266–272
8. Rudzki E, Rebandel P, Karas Z (1997) Patch testing with lower concentrations of chromate and nickel. Contact Dermatitis 37:46
9. Hindsen M, Bruze M (1998) The significance of previous contact dermatitis for elicitation of contact allergy to nickel. Acta Derm Venereol 78:367–370
10. Jensen CD, Johansen JD, Menné T, Andersen KE (2005) Increased retest activity by both patch and use test with methyldibromo glutaronitrile in sensitized individuals. Acta Derm Venereol (in press)
11. Johansen JD, Skov L, Volund A, Andersen K, Menné T (1998) Allergens in combination have a synergistic effect on the elicitation response: a study of fragrance-sensitized individuals. Br J Dermatol 139:264–270
12. Kligman AM (1966) The identification of contact allergens by human assay. 3. The maximization test: a procedure for screening and rating contact sensitizers. J Invest Dermatol 47:393–409
13. Rees JL, Friedmann PS, Matthews JN (1990) The influence of area of application on sensitization by dinitrochlorobenzene. Br J Dermatol 122:29–31
14. Upadhye MR, Maibach HI (1992) Influence of area of application of allergen on sensitization in contact dermatitis. Contact Dermatitis 27:281–286
15. Fewings J, Menné T (1999) An update of the risk assessment for methylchloroisothiazolinone/methylisothiazolinone (MCI/MI) with focus on rinse-off products. Contact Dermatitis 41:1–13
16. Hextall JM, Alagaratnam NJ, Glendinning AK, Holloway DB, Blaikie L, Basketter DA, McFadden JP (2002) Dose–time relationship for elicitation of contact allergy to para-phenylenediamine. Contact Dermatitis 47:96–99
17. Andersen KE, Johansen JD, Bruze M, Frosch PJ, Goossens A, Lepoittevin JP, Rastogi S, White I, Menné T (2001) The time-dose-response relationship for elicitation of contact dermatitis in isoeugenol allergic individuals. Toxicol Appl Pharmacol 170:166–171
18. Jensen CD, Johansen JD, Menné T, Andersen KE (2005) Methyldibromo glutaronitrile contact allergy: effect of single versus repeated daily exposures. Contact Dermatitis 52:88–92
19. Jordan WPJ, Sherman WT, King SE (1979) Threshold responses in formaldehyde-sensitive subjects. J Am Acad Dermatol 1:44–48
20. Heydorn S, Andersen KE, Johansen JD, Menné T (2003) A stronger patch test reaction to the allergen hydroxycitronellal and the irritant sodium lauryl sulfate. Contact Dermatitis 49:133–139
21. Pedersen LK, Haslund P, Johansen JD, Held E, Volund A, Agner T (2004) Influence of a detergent on skin response to methyldibromo glutaronitrile in sensitized individuals. Contact Dermatitis 50:1–5
22. Agner T, Johansen JD, Overgaard L, Volund A, Basketter D, Menné T (2002). Combined effects of irritants and allergens. Synergistic effects of nickel and sodium lauryl sulfate – in nickel sensitized individuals (1991). Contact Dermatitis 47:21–26
23. Hannuksela M (1991) Sensitivity of various skin sites in the repeated open application test. Am J Contact Dermat 2:102–104
24. Johansen JD, Rastogi SC, Bruze M, Andersen KE, Frosch PJ, Dreier B, Lepoittevin JP, White IR, Menné T (1998). Deodorants: a clinical provocation study in fragrance-sensitive individuals. Contact Dermatitis 39:161–165.
25. Zachariae C, Hall B, Cottin M, Andersen KE, Menné T (2004). Formaldehyde allergy – clinically relevant threshold reactions. Contact Dermatitis (abstract) 50:136
26. Hindsen M. Bruze M, Christensen OB (1999) Individual variation in nickel patch test reactivity. Am J Contact Dermat 10:62–67
27. Hansen MB, Johansen JD, Menné T (2003) Chromium allergy: significanse of both Cr(III) and Cr(VI). Contact Dermatitis 49:206–212

13

28. Frosch PJ, Pirker C, Rastogi SC, Andersen KE, Bruze M, Svedman C, Goossens A, White IR, Uter W, Giménez Arnau E, Lepoittevin JP, Menné T, Johansen JD (2005) Patch testing with a new fragrance mix detects additional patients sensitive to perfumes and missed by the current fragrance mix. Contact Dermatitis 52:207–215

29. Gruvberger B, Andersen KE, Brandao FM, Bruynzeel DP, Bruze M, Frosch PJ, Goosens A, Lathi A, Lindberg M, Menné T, Orton D, Seidinari S (2005). Patch testing with methyldibromo glutaronitrile, a multicentre study with the EECDRG. Contact Dermatitis 52:14–18

30. Mortz CG, Lauritzen JM, Bindslev-Jensen C, Andersen KE (2002) Nickel sensitization in adolescents and association with ear piercing, use of braces and hand eczema. The Odense Adolescence Cohort Study on Atopic Diseases and Dermatitis (TOACS). Acta Derm Venereol 82:352–358

31. Johansen JD, Frosch PJ, Svedman C, Andersen KE, Bruze M, Pirker C, Menné T (2003) Hydroxyisohexyl 3-cyclohexene carboxaldehyde – known as Lyral: quantitative aspects and risk assessment of an important fragrance allergen. Contact Dermatitis 48:310–316

32. Johansen JD, Andersen KE, Svedman C, Bruze M, Bernard G, Giminez-Arnau E, Rastogi SC, Lepoittevin JP, Menné T (2003) Chloroatranol an extremely potent allergen hidden in perfumes – a dose-response elicitation study. Contact Dermatitis 49:180–184

33. Boukhman MP, Maibach HI (2001) Thresholds in contact sensitization: immunologic mechanisms and experimental evidence in humans – an overview. Food Chem Toxicol 39:1125–1134

34. Trattner A, Johansen JD, Menné T (1998) Formaldehyde concentration in diagnostic patch testing: comparison of 1% with 2%. Contact Dermatitis 38:9–13

35. Fischer LA, Menné T, Johansen JD (2005) Experimental nickel elicitation thresholds – a review focusing on occluded nickel exposure. Contact Dermatitis 52:57–64

36. Villarama CD, Maibach HI (2004) Correlations of patch test reactivity and the repeated open application test (ROAT)/provocative use test (PUT). Food Chem Toxicol 42:1719–1725

37. Hannuksela M, Salo H (1986) The repeated open application test (ROAT). Contact Dermatitis 14:221–227

38. Johansen JD, Andersen KE, Rastogi SC, Menné T (1996) Threshold responses in cinnamic-aldehyde-sensitive subjects: results and methodological aspects. Contact Dermatitis 34:165–171

39. Pedersen LK, Agner T, Held E, Johansen JD (2004) Methyldibromo glutaronitrile in leave-on products elicits contact allergy at low concentration. Br J Dermatol 151:817–822

40. Rolland A, Wagner N, Chatelus A, Shroot B, Schaefer H (1993) Site-specific drug delivery to pilosebaceous structures using polymeric microspheres. Pharm Res 10:1738–1744

41. Vestergaard L, Clemmensen OJ, Sorensen FB, Andersen KE (1999) Histological distinction between early allergic and irritant patch test reactions: follicular spongiosis may be characteristic of early allergic contact dermatitis. Contact Dermatitis 41:207–210

42. Johansen JD, Bruze M, Andersen KE, Frosch PJ, Dreier B, White IR, Rastogi S, Lepoittevin JP, Menné T (1998) The repeated open application test: suggestions for a scale of evaluation. Contact Dermatitis 39:95–96

43. Held E, Lorentzen H, Agner T, Menné T (1998) Comparison between visual score and erythema index (DermaSpectrometer) in evaluation of allergic patch tests. Skin Res Technol 4:188–191

44. Maibach HI (1983) Formaldehyde: effects on animal and human skin. In: Gibson JE (ed) Formaldehyde toxicity. Hemisphere, Washington DC, pp 166–174

45. Bruze M, Johansen JD, Andersen KE, Frosch PJ, Lepoittevin JP, Rastogi S, Wakelin S, White IR, Menné T (2003) Deodorants: an experimental provocation study with cinnamic aldehyde. J Am Acad Dermatol 48:194–200

46. Svedman C, Bruze M, Johansen JD, Andersen KE, Goossens A, Frosch PJ, Lepoittevin JP, Rastogi S, White IR, Menné T (2003) Deodorants: an experimental provocation study with hydroxycitronellal. Contact Dermatitis 48:217–223

47. Frosch PJ, Lahti A, Hannuksela M, Andersen KE, Wilkinson JD, Shaw S, Lachapelle JM (1995) Chloromethylisothiazolone/methylisothiazolone (CMI/MI) use test with a shampoo on patch-test-positive subjects. Results of a multicentre double-blind crossover trial. Contact Dermatitis 32:210–217

48. Jensen CD, Johansen JD, Menné T, Andersen KE (2004) Methyldibromo glutaronitrile in rinse-off products causes allergic contact dermatitis: an experimental study. Br J Dermatol 150:90–95

49. Zachariae C, Rastogi S, Devantier Jensen C, Menné T, Johansen JD (2003). Methyldibromo glutaronitrile: clinical experience and exposure-based risk assessment. Contact Dermatitis 48:150–154

50. Zachariae C, Johansen JD, Rastogi SC, Menné T (2005) Allergic contact dermatitis from methyldibromo glutaronitrile – clinical cases from 2003. Contact Dermatitis 52:6–8

51. Johansen JD, Veien NK, Laurberg G, Kaaber K, Thormann J, Lauritzen M, Avnstorp C (2005) Contact allergy to methyldibromo glutaronitrile – data from a front line network. Contact Dermatitis 52:138–141

52. Knudsen BB, Larsen E, Egsgaard H, Menné T (1993) Release of thiurams and carbamates from rubber gloves. Contact Dermatitis 28:63–69

53. Knudsen BB, Menné T (1996) Elicitation thresholds for thiuram mix using petrolatum and ethanol/sweat as vehicles. Contact Dermatitis 34:410–413

54. Hansson C, Bergendorff O, Ezzelarab M, Sterner O (1997) Extraction of mercaptobenzothiazole compounds from rubber products. Contact Dermatitis 36:195–200

55. Hjorth N, Roed-Petersen J (1976) Occupational protein contact dermatitis in food handlers. Contact Dermatitis 2:28–42

56. Christensen OB, Moller H (1975) External and internal exposure to the antigen in the hand eczema of nickel allergy. Contact Dermatitis 1:136–141

57. Allenby CF, Basketter DA (1994) The effect of repeated open exposure to low levels of nickel on compromised hand skin of nickel-allergic subjects. Contact Dermatitis 30:135–138

58. Nielsen NH, Menné T, Kristiansen J, Christensen JM, Borg L, Poulsen LK (1999) Effects of repeated skin exposures to low nickel concentrations – a model for allergic contact dermatitis to nickel on the hands. Br J Dermatol 141:676–682

59. Kristiansen J, Christensen JM, Henriksen T, Nielsen NH, Menné T (1999) Determination of nickel in fingernails and forearm skin (stratum corneum). Anal Chim Acta 403:265–272

60. Peters K, Gammelgaard B, Menné T (1991) Nickel concentrations in fingernails as a measure of occupational exposure to nickel. Contact Dermatitis 25:237–241

61. Nielsen NH, Kristiansen J, Borg L, Christensen JM, Poulsen LK, Menné T (2000) Repeated exposures to cobalt and

chromate on the hands of patients with hand eczema and the specific metal contact allergy. Contact Dermatitis 43: 212–215

62. Heydorn S, Menné T, Andersen KE, Bruze M, Svedman C, Basketter D, Johansen JD (2003). The fragrance hand immersion study – an experimental model simulating exposure for allergic contact dermatitis on the hands. Contact Dermatitis 48:324–330

63. Horsfall FL (1934) Formaldehyde hypersensitiveness. An experimental study. J Immunol 27:569–581

64. Menné T (1994) Quantitative aspects of nickel dermatitis. Sensitization and eliciting threshold concentrations. Sci Total Environ 148:275–281

65. Liden C, Menné T, Burrows D (1996) Nickel-containing alloys and platings and their ability to cause dermatitis. Br J Dermatol 134:193–198

66. Schnuch A, Uter W (2003) Decrease in nickel allergy in Germany and regulatory interventions. Contact Dermatitis 49:107–108

67. Jensen CS, Lisby S, Baadsgaard O, Volund A, Menné T (2002) Decrease in nickel sensitization in a Dansih school-girl population with ears pierced after implementation of a nickel-exposure regulation. Br J Dermatol 146:636–642

68. Rastogi SC, Lepoittevin JP, Johansen JD, Frosch PJ, Menné T, Bruze M, Dreier B, Andersen KE, White IR (1998) Fragrances and other materials in deodorants: search for potentially sensitizing molecules using combined GC-MS and structure activity relationship (SAR) analysis. Contact Dermatitis 39:293–303

69. Johansen JD, Rastogi SC, Menné T (1996) Contact allergy to popular perfumes; assessed by patch test, use test and chemical analysis. Br J Dermatol 135:419–422

70. Gruvberger B (1997) Methylisothiazolinones. Diagnosis and prevention of allergic contact dermatitis. Acta Derm Venereol [Suppl] (Stockh) 200:1–42

71. Frosch PJ, Johansen JD, Menné T, Pirker C, Rastogi SC, Andersen KE, Bruze M, Goossens A, Lepoittevin JP, White IR (2002) Further important sensitizers in patients sensitive to fragrances. II. Reactivity to essential oils. Contact Dermatitis 47:279–287

72. Fischer T, Andersen K, Bengtsson U, Frosch P, Gunnarsson Y, Kreilgard B, Menné T, Shaw S, Svensson L, Wilkinson J (1995) Clinical standardization of the TRUE Test formal-dehyde patch. Curr Probl Dermatol 22:24–30

13

Part IV

Clinical Features

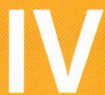

Chapter 14

General Aspects

14

Niels K. Veien

Contents

14.1 Introduction

A diagnosis of contact dermatitis requires the careful consideration of many variables, including patient history, physical examination, and various types of skin testing. A thorough knowledge of the clinical features of the skin's reactions to various contactants is important in making a correct diagnosis of contact dermatitis.

While an eczematous reaction is the most commonly encountered adverse reaction to contactants, other clinical manifestations may also be seen. These include erosions, ulcerations, urticaria, erythema multiforme, purpura, lichenoid eruptions, exanthems, erythroderma, allergic contact granuloma, lymphocytoma, sarcoidal reactions, toxic epidermal necrolysis, pigmented contact dermatitis, and photosensitive reactions [1–3]. Generalized symptoms have also been described in association with contact sensitivity, as documented by challenge experiments [4, 5], and contact urticaria may become anaphylactoid [6] and life-threatening [7].

The emphasis in this chapter will be on eczemas as a manifestation of contact dermatitis. Other clinical manifestations will be described in detail in Chap. 21 – and hand eczema, in particular, in Chap. 19.

14.2 The Medical History of the Patient

14.2.1 History of Hereditary Diseases

The family and personal history of a patient with contact dermatitis should be taken in detail, especially with regard to atopy. Patients who have suffered from severe atopic dermatitis in childhood are likely to experience irritant contact dermatitis later in life, particularly on the hands [8]. A history of contact urticaria, in particular on the lips and hands, due to uncooked food items is common among atopics [8]. Contact urticaria due to animal dander may aggravate atopic dermatitis of the arms and the periorbital area. It can be useful to note the results of prick tests carried out; for example, in previous attempts to discover the cause of respiratory allergy. A positive prick test to house dust mites, animal dander or pollen may correlate with the results of an atopic patch test and may be relevant as an aggravating factor in atopic dermatitis [9, 10].

Patients with recurrent vesicular hand eczema are often atopic [11], and Schwanitz [12] coined the term "*das atopische Palmoplantareksem*" after a study of the literature and having seen 58 patients with recurrent vesicular hand eczema. Edman, however [13], found no statistical correlation between atopy and this type of hand dermatitis. Details concerning the relationship between atopy and contact sensitization are given in Sect. 14.3.5.5 Atopy.

It is unusual for a patient to have a family history of contact dermatitis. Although hereditary factors were seen to have some significance among twins with nickel allergy, these were found to be less important than environmental factors [14].

A family history of psoriasis is important as it may be difficult to distinguish psoriasis from contact dermatitis and seborrheic dermatitis. This is particularly true on the scalp, the face, the anogenital area, and the hands. Köbner reactions on the hands of psoriasis patients can mimic irritant or allergic contact dermatitis [15]. Likewise, Köbner reactions on the hands may show a striking resemblance to hyperkeratotic hand eczema. Both psoriasis and hyperkeratotic hand eczema can be aggravated by physical trauma from, for example, the handles of tools.

14.2.2 General Medical History

Malnutrition may cause eczematous lesions in, for example, alcohol dependency [16] or in patients with acrodermatitis enteropathica or metabolic disorders such as phenylketonuria. In order to make a diagnosis of systemically induced dermatitis it is necessary to take a complete history of drug intake. Cutaneous sensitization to a drug may give rise to symmetrical dermatitis when the same drug, or a chemically related drug, is taken orally or injected [17] (see Chaps. 16 and 35). Drug intake can also play a significant role in a number of photodermatoses.

Obesity is an important factor in the development of intertriginous dermatoses and mechanical contact dermatitis due to friction; the latter may be seen, for example, on the inner surfaces of the thighs of obese children.

Psychiatric disorders can lead to contact dermatitis caused by the compulsive clutching of keys containing nickel (Fig. 1) or mechanical dermatitis caused by the compulsive rubbing of the skin (Fig. 2).

Core Message

■ Both family and medical history are important when making a diagnosis of contact dermatitis. Rashes seen in metabolic diseases and in obese persons may mimic contact dermatitis. Contact urticaria and irritant contact dermatitis are common in persons with current or previous atopic dermatitis.

Fig. 1.
Allergic contact dermatitis in a nickel-sensitive psychiatric patient who clutched nickel-containing keys all day

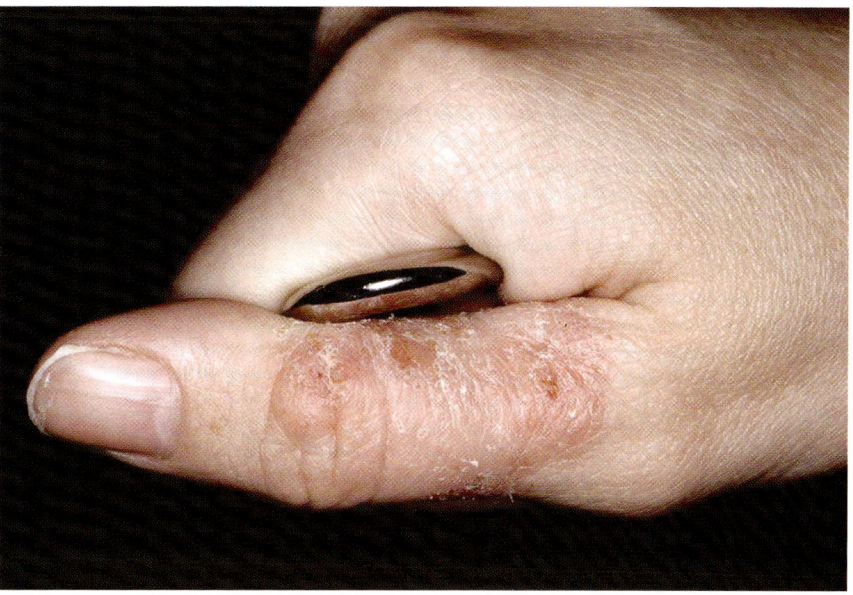

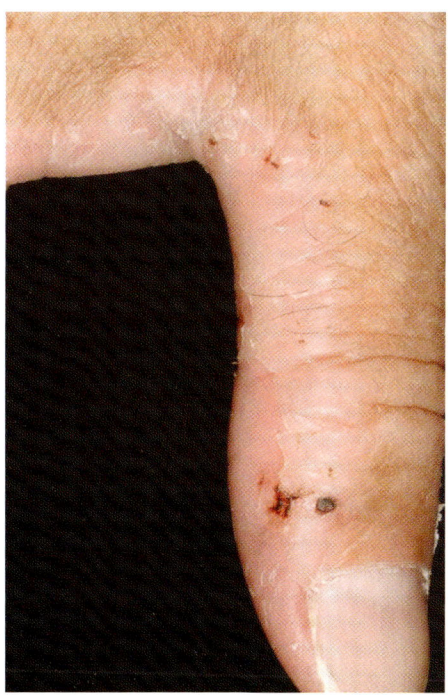

Fig. 2. Factitious dermatitis from compulsory rubbing of the skin of the fingers. Note the sharp delineation from normal skin

14.2.3 History of Previous Dermatitis

A firm history of previous allergic contact dermatitis from, for example, nickel, fragrances or topical medicaments would be reason to suspect inadvertent contact with the same haptens if an otherwise unexplained eruption of contact dermatitis occurs. A history of axillary intolerance to spray deodorants is a good indication of fragrance allergy [18]. Further details on the relationship between the history of nickel allergy and atopy are given in Sect. 14.3.5.5 Atopy.

A history of previous dermatitis near leg ulcers should lead to a suspicion of topical medicaments as the cause of current or possible future eruptions of dermatitis in this area or elsewhere. A history of dermatitis where adhesive tape has been applied should lead the physician to search for possible colophony sensitivity. It should be mentioned, however, that most modern adhesive tapes contain no colophony, as the adhesive substance is now usually an acrylate.

14.2.4 Time of Onset

For long-standing contact dermatitis, the exact time of onset is usually ill-defined and is not useful in establishing the final diagnosis. The cause of contact dermatitis with recent abrupt onset may be established by taking a careful history of contactants during the days immediately preceding the onset of dermatitis. The history should include occupational exposures and exposures during leisure time and while working in the home or doing hobbies, as well as any changes in clothing or cosmetics, including soaps and detergents. Topical remedies used for the treatment of the dermatitis, both prescription and over-the-counter products, should be recorded, as well as any recent changes in systemic drug therapy.

14.2.5 History of Aggravating Factors

For chronic contact dermatitis, the history should include information about contactants in relation to aggravation of the dermatitis rather than to its onset. Two types of flares of chronic dermatoses should be considered: eruptions that appear suddenly and without warning, and eruptions that show seasonal variation. Seasonal variations may help to establish the type of dermatitis and possibly also the specific cause, a point that is illustrated in Fig. 3.

The sudden aggravation of chronic dermatitis or recurrences at short intervals may help to establish the cause of the dermatitis or, if this is not possible, those factors which aggravate it. Recurrent vesicular eczema of the hands provides a typical example of how such help can be obtained. Although a definite cause for this type of dermatitis is rarely determined, a number of factors may cause the eruption of a crop of vesicles. The time elapsing between exposure to aggravating factors and the eruption of vesicles is 1–3 days, and with proper instruction a patient is often able to recall exposures that occurred up to 3 days prior to the onset of dermatitis and thus identify aggravating factors.

There are certain fundamental types of dermatitis such as atopic dermatitis, seborrheic dermatitis, allergic contact dermatitis, and irritant contact dermatitis. Possible aggravating factors include contact allergens, contact irritants (chemical, physical), contact urticaria, extreme variations in temperature, low or high humidity, ingestion of certain foods, smoking, psychological stress, sweating, drug intake, sun exposure, and infections (local and systemic) – dermatophytes and yeasts, bacteria, herpes simplex virus [19, 20].

When discussing sun exposure with the patient, it should be stressed that the offending ultraviolet irradiation may penetrate window glass, both in the home and in an automobile, as well as thin clothing. It should also be stressed that aggravation during out-

14

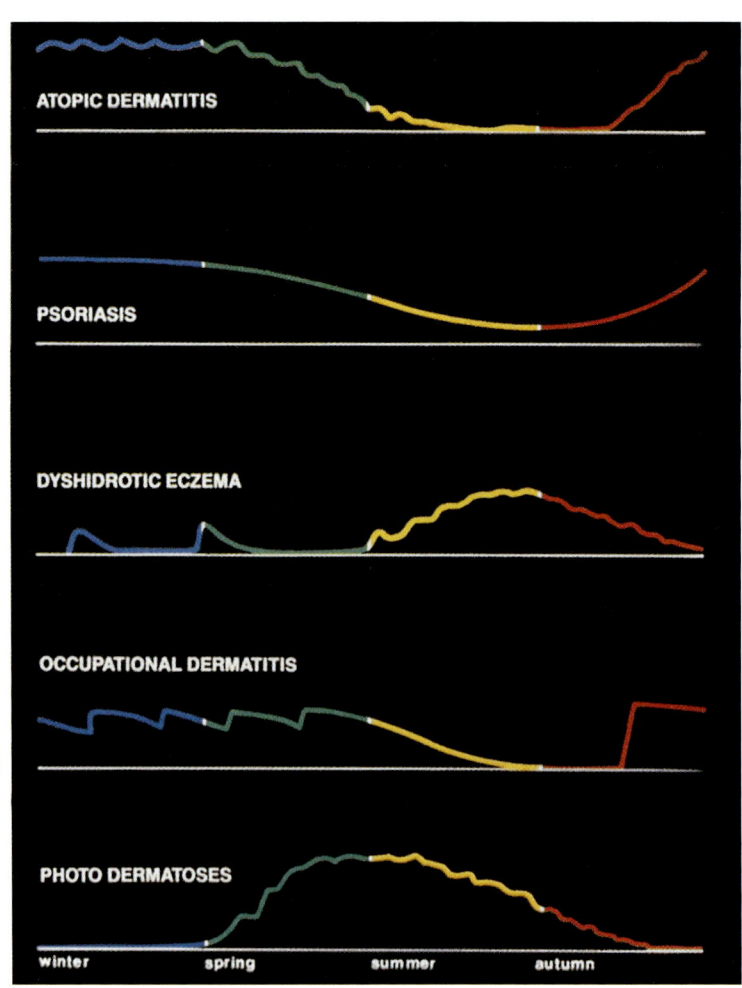

Fig. 3a–e.
Seasonal variation in dermatitis.
a *Atopic dermatitis*: fluctuates, severely pruritic, improves during the summer months. **b** *Psoriasis*: no pruritus, slow or no fluctuations, improves during the summer months. **c** *Dyshidrotic eczema*: eruptive throughout the year, often especially active during the summer months. **d** *Occupational dermatitis*: slow improvement seen over several consecutive days away from the workplace, fades during long periods of vacation, typically during the summer months; prompt recurrence upon resumption of work. **e** *Photodermatoses*: sudden onset during the spring, fluctuates during the summer months, fades during late summer; there is increased sun tolerance as pigmentation and epidermal thickness increase during the summer months

door activities is not necessarily related to the sun. Dermatitis in areas of the body normally exposed to the sun can also be caused by airborne irritants and allergens in dust particles, aerosols, pollen, and other plant material [21]. Seasonal variations in patch test results due to dry weather have been seen [22], and sun exposure may suppress immune reactions [23].

Core Message

■ It is difficult for patients with persistent dermatitis to designate a precise time of onset. However, patients with chronic dermatitis may have either seasonal flares or sudden unexplained flares of dermatitis. Patients should be instructed to make a note of circumstances related to sudden aggravation of their dermatitis.

14.2.6 Course of the Dermatitis

In dealing with chronic dermatoses it is important to record treatment response as well as response to the elimination of suspected causative substances. Some endogenous dermatoses, such as seborrheic dermatitis, are easily suppressed by means of topical treatment, but recurrence is common. Contact dermatitis usually requires intensive treatment and recurs after discontinuation of therapy if the causative substance is not removed.

While allergic contact dermatitis usually recurs relatively quickly after re-exposure to the causative agent, irritant contact dermatitis tends to recur more slowly [24]. This difference can be useful in making the diagnosis.

The response to vacation periods and sick leave is of particular importance when occupational contact dermatitis is suspected. The result of re-exposure to the suspected causative agent is equally important.

14.2.7 Types of Symptoms

Pruritus is the fundamental symptom of irritant and allergic contact dermatitis, and in sensitized persons it usually occurs during the first day of further contact with the offending item. The intensity of symptoms varies greatly and depends on the type of dermatitis and also on various individual factors. Some persons with irritant contact dermatitis have practically no symptoms, while some adults with atopic dermatitis suffer so much from itching that it is difficult for them to sleep and to carry out everyday tasks.

Subtle symptoms of insidious onset include the stinging sensation felt in some cosmetic reactions in which there is no visible physical symptom. Stinging can be caused by a number of substances and is elicited on very sensitive skin. This symptom does not necessarily represent irritancy in general [25]. Pain and burning, rather than itching, are frequent in phototoxic dermatitis such as that caused by giant hogweed. A burning sensation is also common in herpes simplex and in herpes zoster. If it proves difficult to differentiate between the diagnosis of contact dermatitis and other dermatoses, a detailed description of the symptoms can be helpful.

Symptoms of contact urticaria are often noticed seconds to minutes after contact with the causative substance. Characteristically, the symptoms include stinging and smarting in addition to pruritus. Such symptoms are often caused by uncooked foods touching the perioral area or the hands, or animal dander on exposed skin. In many patients, the symptoms fade quickly if the causative substance is rinsed off.

Mayonnaise preserved with sorbic acid caused an epidemic of perioral contact urticaria in a group of kindergarten children. The careful histories that were taken proved to be the most important tool in arriving at the correct diagnosis [26].

Patients who suffer from hay fever in the birch pollen season often have a history of contact urticaria of the oral mucosa caused by hazelnuts and apples due to antigens common to all three [27]. Birch pollen and grass may cause cellular immune reactions and contact dermatitis with an airborne pattern [28, 29]. An association has also been found between birch pollen allergy and reactions to apple, carrot, pear and cherry and between grass pollen and tomato and certain types of melon [30, 31]. A careful history is, therefore, very important in the diagnostic work-up of patients with stomatitis and contact urticaria.

Core Message

■ Pruritus is the hallmark symptom of contact dermatitis. The intensity is variable and stinging may be more common than pruritus in cosmetic contact dermatitis. Phototoxic dermatitis is characterized by burning and smarting rather than pruritus. Contact urticaria is characterized by pruritus, burning or smarting seconds to minutes after contact with the offending substance.

14.3 Clinical Features of Eczematous Reactions

14.3.1 Acute and Recurrent Dermatitis

Spongiosis of the epidermis is one of the histological hallmarks of acute eczematous reactions. Clinically, confluence of spongiosis can lead to vesicles and even bullae [32] (see Chap. 7).

Macroscopically, the vesicular response is associated with acute and recurrent contact dermatitis and is best visualized on the palms (Figs. 4, 5), the sides of the fingers (Fig. 6), around the fingernails (Fig. 7) and on the soles of the feet. Vesicular erup-tions on the palms and soles often occur simultane-ously [33]. Vesicular palmar eruptions are not specif-ic to eczema, as discussed in Sect. 14.6, Differential Diagnosis.

Vesicular eruptions at other than the above-men-tioned sites are uncommon. Acute dermatitis usually presents with papules, although occasionally with vesicles (Fig. 8) or even bullae (Fig. 9). The vesicular or bullous reaction may be seen in allergic as well as in irritant reactions and cannot be used to distin-guish between these two types of dermatitis. Bullous contact dermatitis may be seen after the application of a typical irritant, cantharidin, in the treatment of warts (Fig. 10).

14

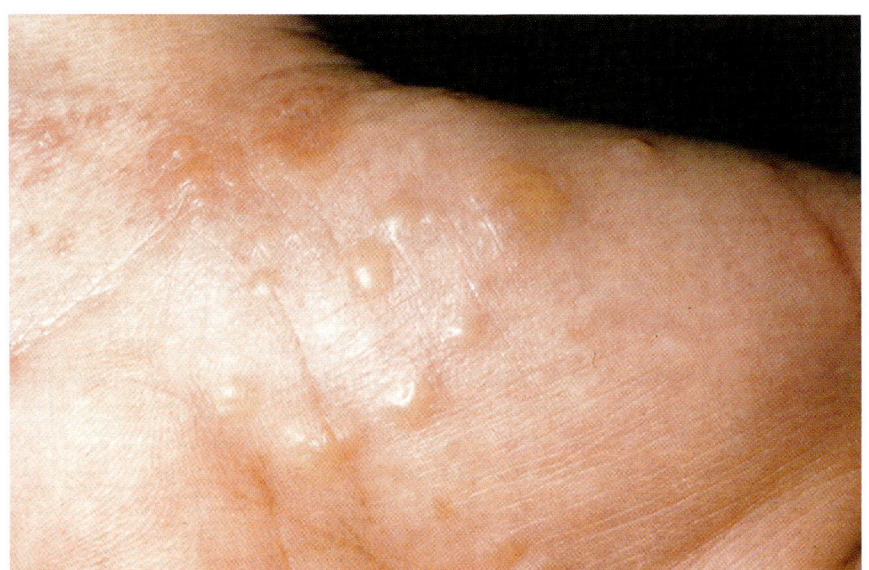

Fig. 4.
Confluent vesicles on the palm

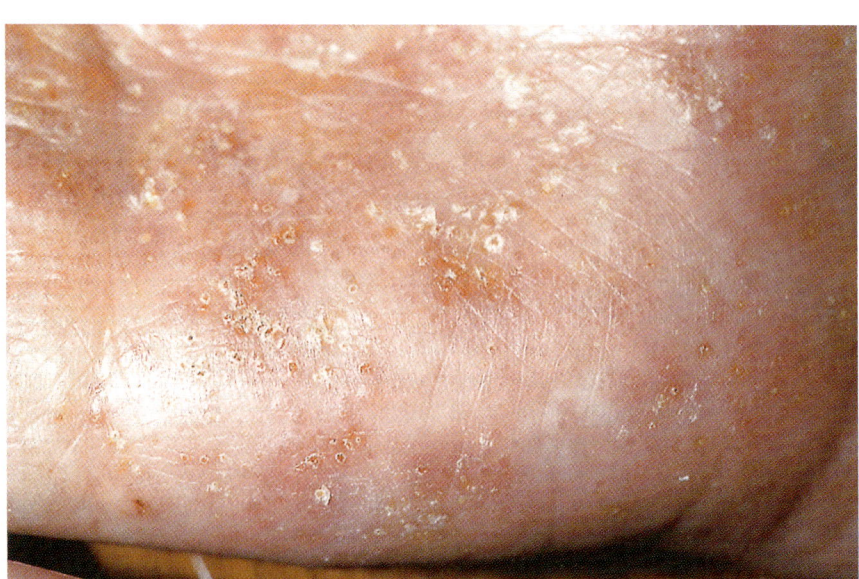

Fig. 5.
Deep-seated vesicles on the palm

Fig. 6.
Vesicles with inflammation on the sides of the fingers

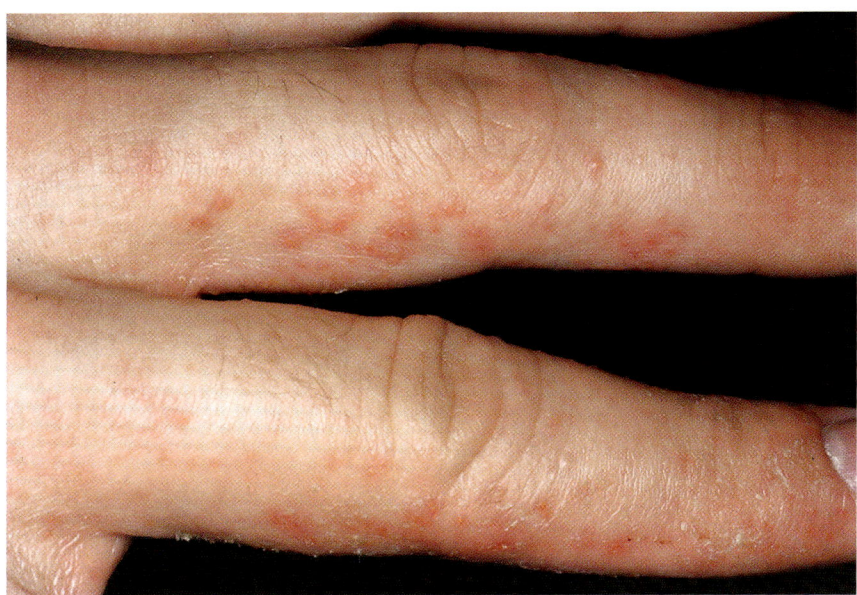

Fig. 7.
Periungual vesicles

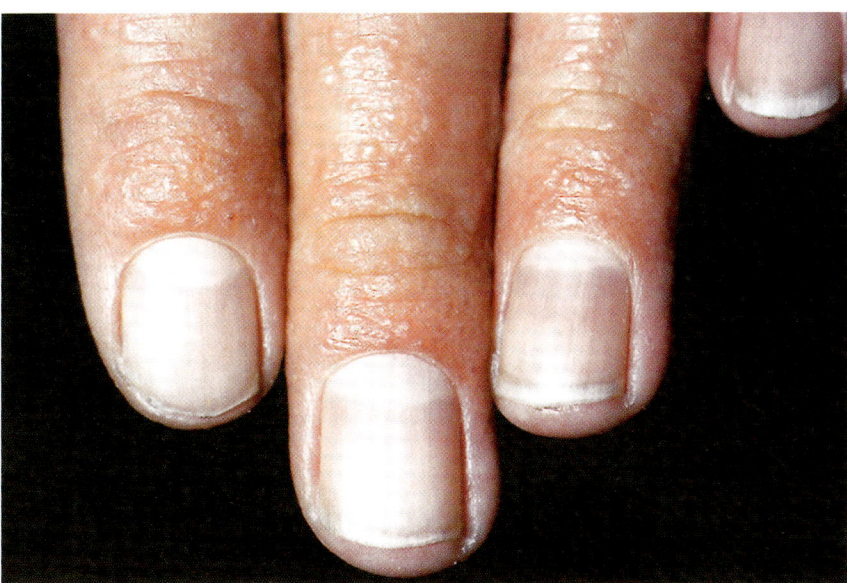

The onset of an eczematous reaction can be more subtle. On the dorsa of the hands, the initial symptoms may be "chapping" (Fig. 11) [24]. Irritants may subsequently cause the chapping to progress to frank eczema. The environmental temperature and humidity are of significance for the development of dermatitis from low-grade irritants [34–37].

It is difficult to distinguish between allergic and irritant contact dermatitis. A distinction can sometimes be made at the site of "experimental" contact dermatitis, for example a patch test site. Minimal itching occurs when a primary irritant is placed on the skin and subsequently occluded, and erythema and slight infiltration will be strictly limited to the area of the patch. Strong irritants may produce bullous or pustular reactions (Fig. 12), but these will also be limited to the occluded area. Similar occlusive testing with a substance to which the patient has a cellular immune reaction tends to give a markedly pruritic, infiltrated, papular or vesicular reaction which extends beyond the rim of the occluding disc (Fig. 13).

One possible explanation for this difference in the periphery of the test area is that it is necessary to have a higher concentration of the offending substance to elicit an irritant reaction than to elicit an al-

Fig. 8.
Vesicular dermatitis on the dorsum of the hand

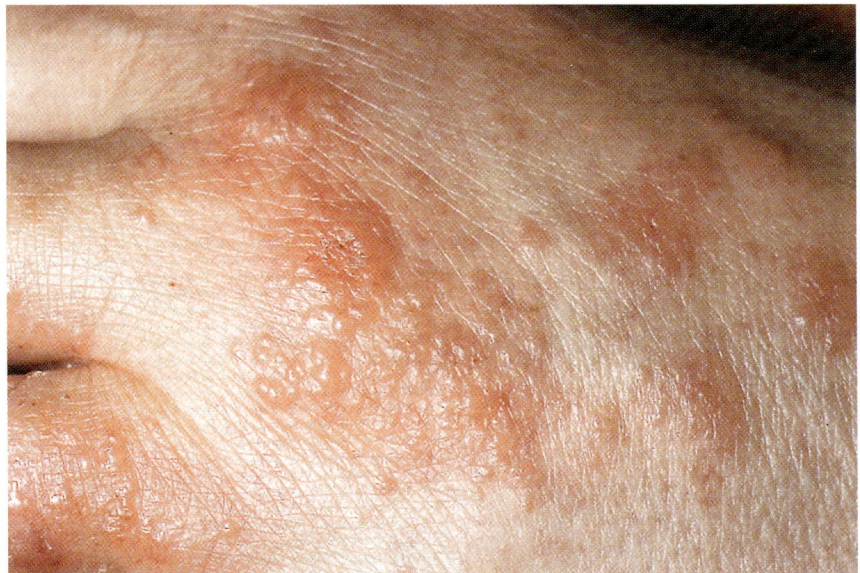

Fig. 9.
Bullous dermatitis

14

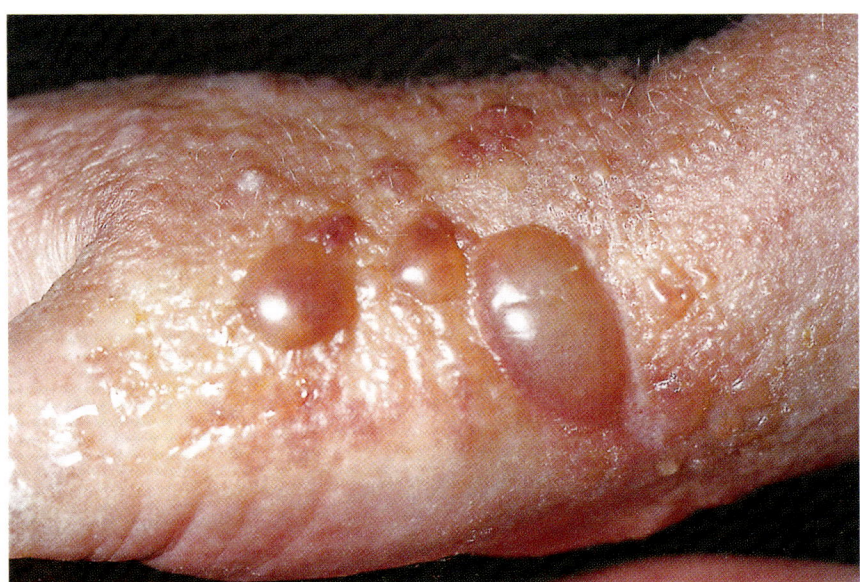

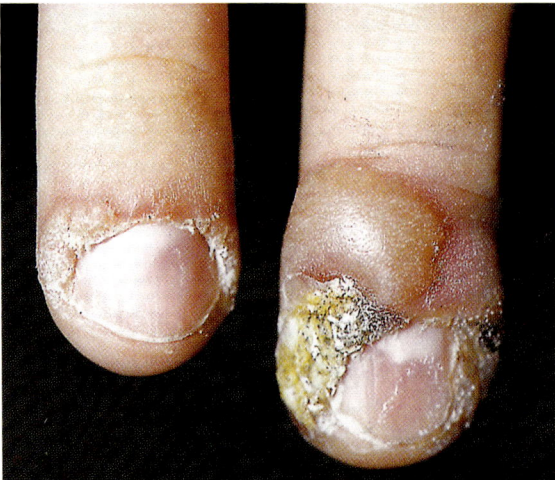

Fig. 10.
Bullous periungual dermatitis caused by cantharidin

Fig. 11.
"Chapping" on the dorsum
of the hand

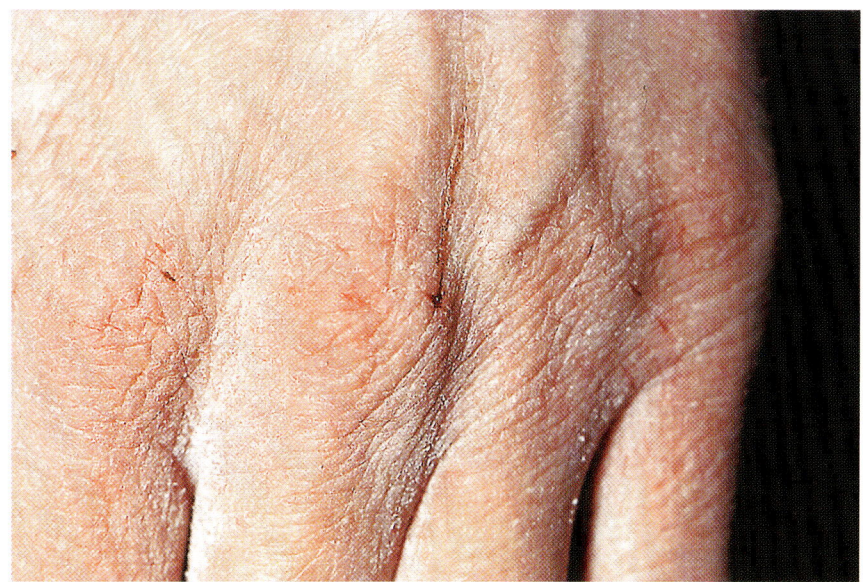

Fig. 12.
A bullous irritant patch test
reaction to a varnish

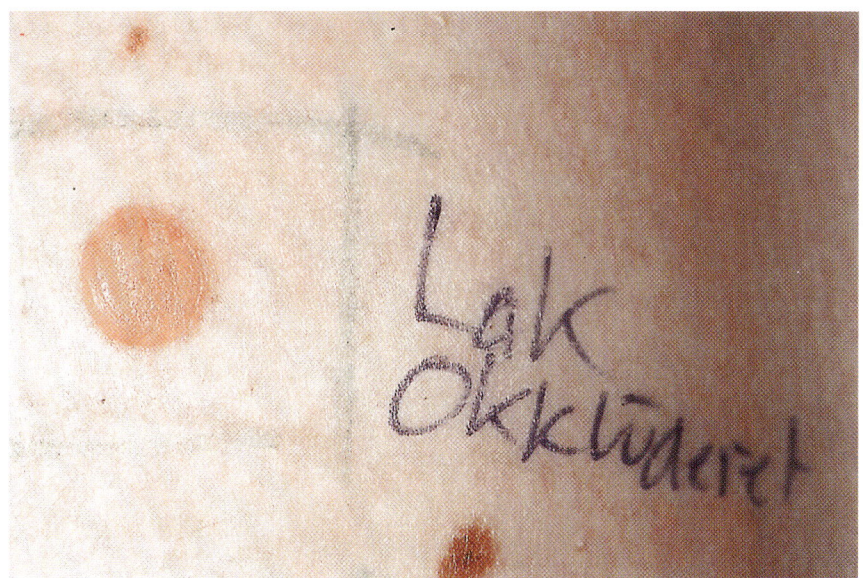

Fig. 13.
A vesicular allergic patch test
reaction to nickel

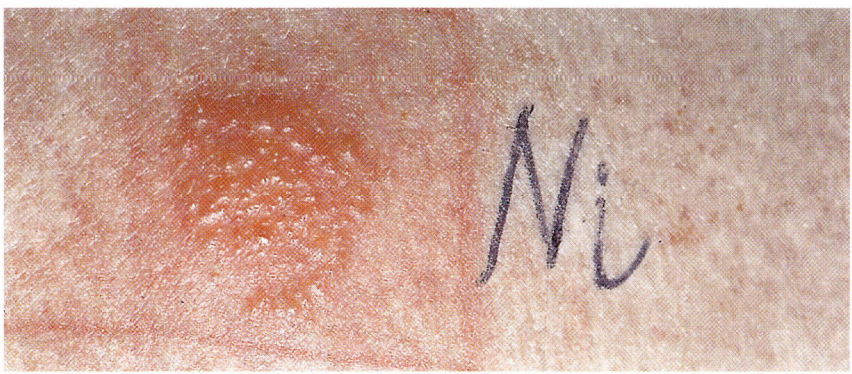

Fig. 14.
Recurrent vesicular hand
eczema mimicking chronic
hand eczema. Note vesicles
at the periphery of the involved area

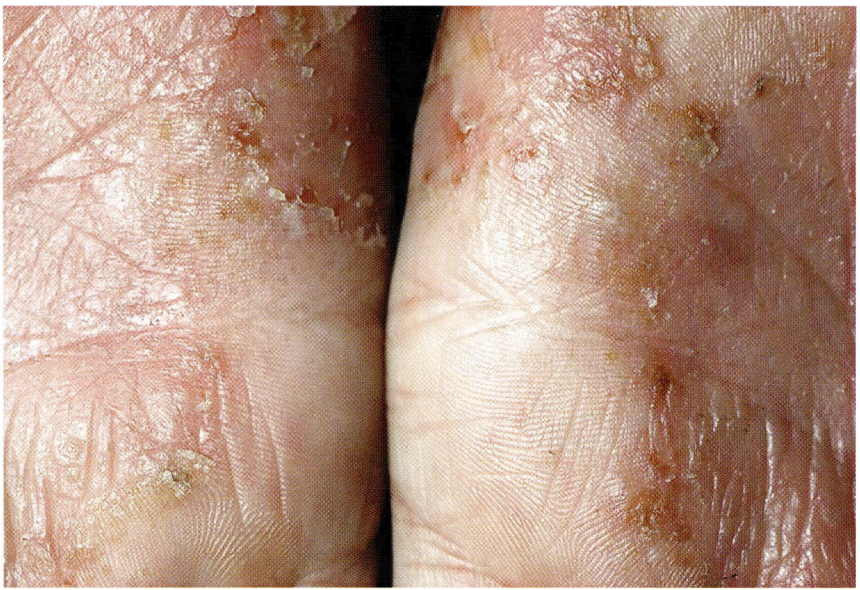

lergic reaction. The concentration of the substance used for a patch test will ordinarily be quite low outside the occluded area and will thus be less than the amount necessary to elicit an irritant reaction, even though an allergic reaction may still occur. The recruitment of specifically sensitized cells and the ensuing release of nonspecific cytokines facilitate the allergic response outside the area of direct contact.

The vesicular response is often seen as recurrent vesicular dermatitis of the palms and soles. If frequent acute eruptions occur, this type of eruption tends to take on the appearance of a chronic eczematous reaction. Careful inspection will often reveal a purely vesicular reaction, particularly at the periphery of the area of skin involved (Fig. 14).

14.3.2 Chronic Dermatitis

If contact with an offending item persists, chronic dermatitis may eventually develop. The characteristic features of chronic dermatitis are pruritus, lichenification, erythema, scaling, fissures and excoriations

14

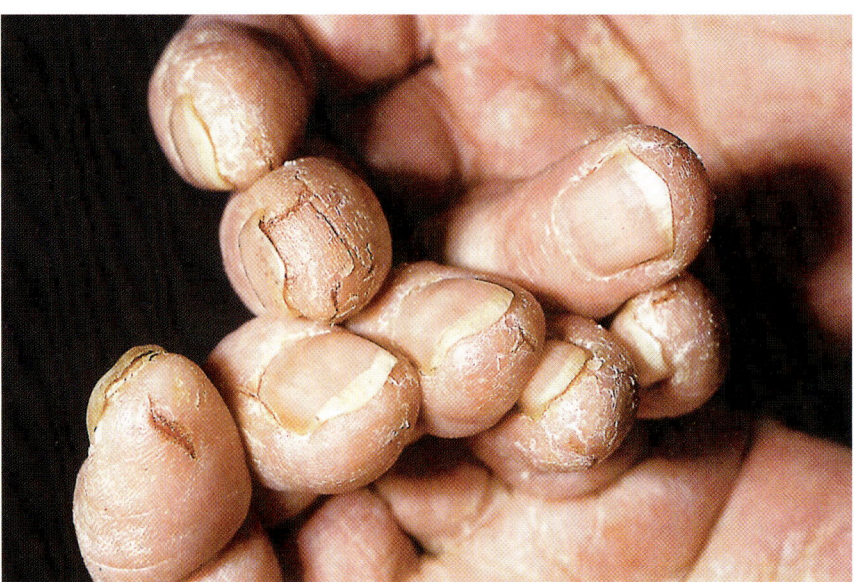

Fig. 15.
Chronic hand eczema with
fissures

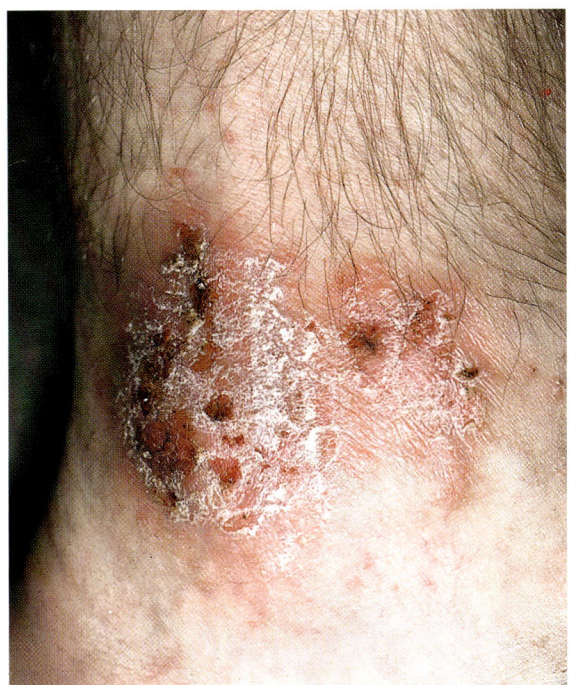

Fig. 16. Lichen simplex chronicus of the ankle

(Fig. 15). Histologically, spongiosis becomes less pronounced, and psoriasiform features supervene. The clinical correlate to this histological transition is lichen simplex chronicus (neurodermatitis) (Fig. 16).

14.3.3 Nummular (Discoid) Eczema

The term "nummular" (or "discoid") eczema is based on the morphology or coin shape of the lesions (Fig. 54). This type of dermatitis may be of endogenous origin and can be confused with contact dermatitis from soluble oils, irritant dermatitis from depilatory cream [38–40] or with psoriasis.

14.3.4 Secondarily Infected Dermatitis

When, as in chronic dermatitis, the epidermal barrier is no longer intact, secondary infection can develop at the site of the dermatitis. In fact, chronic dermatitis is often the result of cumulative insults by irritants, microorganisms, and allergens to which the patient has become sensitized. Frank bacterial infection of contact dermatitis is common (Fig. 17), and the possibility of pathogenic bacteria being present should therefore be considered before initiating treatment of chronic contact dermatitis.

Secondary infection should be distinguished from pustular irritant contact dermatitis caused by, for example, croton oil [41] or fluorouracil [42] and from palmo-plantar pustulosis, which typically exhibits pustules of uniform size as opposed to the varying size of the pustules in infected dermatitis (Fig. 18).

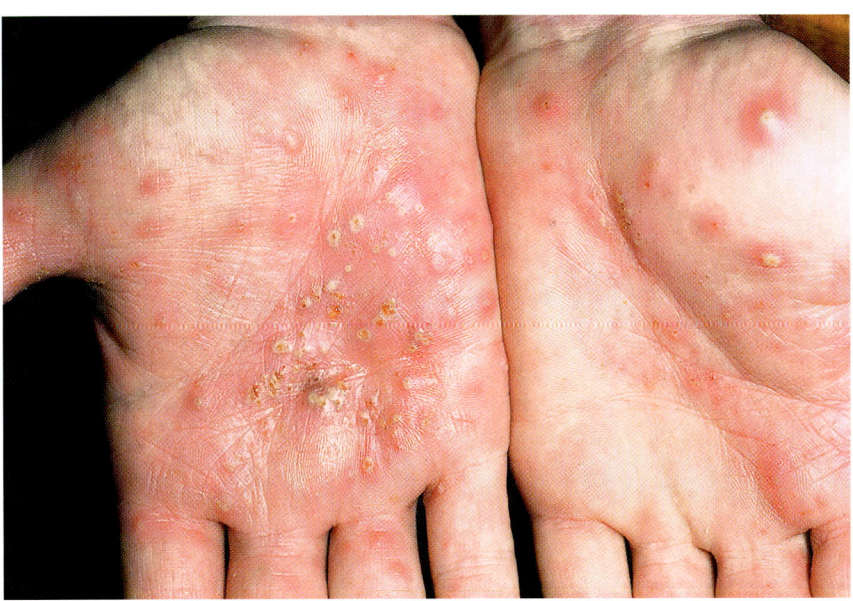

Fig. 17.
Hand eczema with secondary bacterial infection

Fig. 18.
Palmo-plantar pustulosis
with uniform pustules and
brown, dried-up lesions

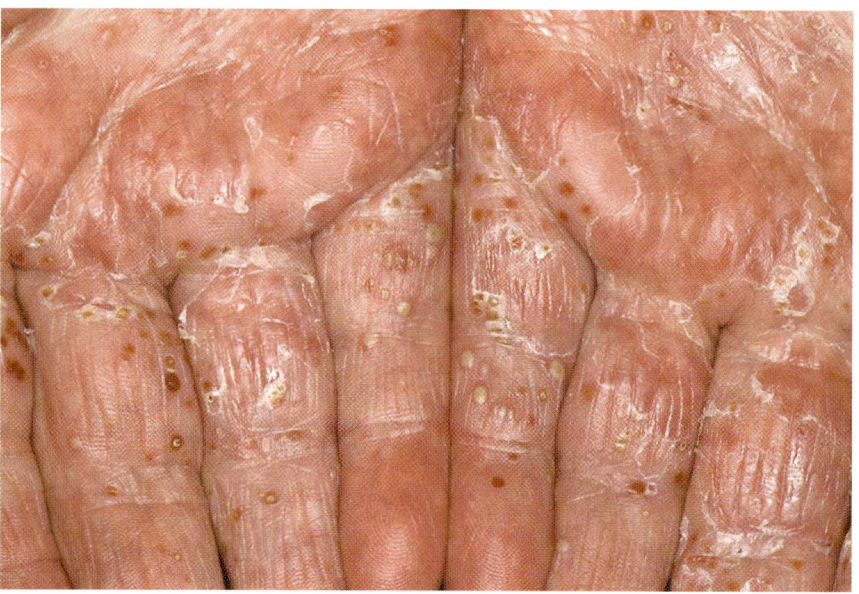

14.3.5 Clinical Features of Contact Dermatitis in Specific Groups of Persons

The clinical features of contact dermatitis may vary among specific groups of persons.

14.3.5.1 Gender

Allergic contact dermatitis is more common among women than among men. This is probably due more to exposure pattern than to gender [43]. Hand eczema is also more common among women than among men [44].

14.3.5.2 Children

Children have been thought to develop allergic contact dermatitis less often than adults. However, Weston and Weston [45] reviewed the literature and concluded that allergic contact dermatitis was common in children and that the clinical pattern of the dermatitis provided an important clue to the specific diagnosis. The pattern of sensitization is similar to that of adults [46, 47].

Paraphenylene diamine used in so-called temporary henna tattoos is a commonly described cause of allergic contact dermatitis in children [48]. See Case Report 2 at the end of the chapter.

Epidemics of irritant contact dermatitis caused by caterpillars are particularly common among children. See Sect. 14.4.2.3 Caterpillar Dermatitis and Irritant Dermatitis from Plants and Animals.

Core Message

■ Children appear to develop contact dermatitis with the same frequency as adults. Babies may be an exception. The exposure pattern in children may be different from that of adults.

14.3.5.3 Elderly Persons

Elderly persons frequently develop allergic contact dermatitis from substances in topical medicaments, fragrances and balsam of Peru [49–50]. Inflammatory reactions are subtler in elderly persons [51], and their contact dermatitis therefore often has a scaly appearance and is less vesicular than in younger individuals. Dry skin in combination with low humidity may in older persons cause a peculiar cracked "*eczema craquelée*", with inflammatory dermatitis and superficial breaks in the skin surface (Fig. 19).

14

Fig. 19.
Eczema craquelée on the
lower leg

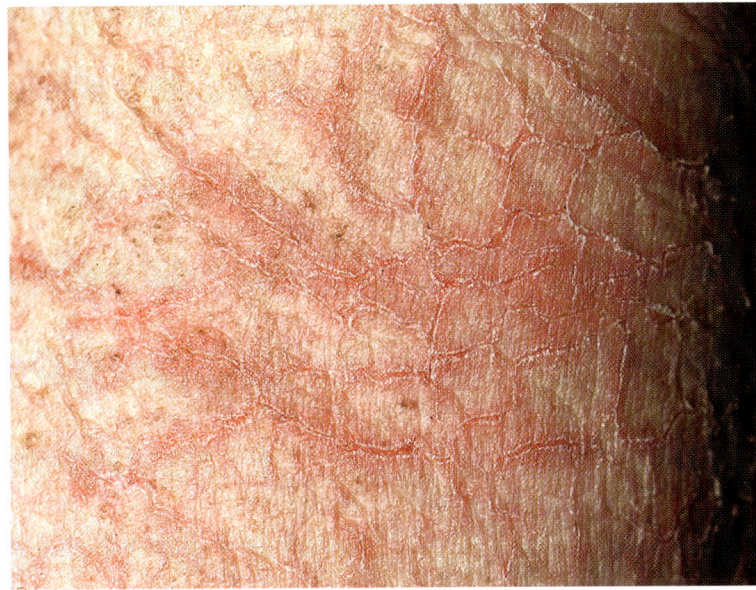

Core Message

■ Elderly persons often develop allergic
contact dermatitis from medicaments,
fragrances and balsam of Peru as well as
low humidity dermatitis such as eczema
craquelée.

14.3.5.4 Ethnicity

Black individuals and others with dark skin tend to
develop hyperpigmentation and infiltration, particularly in chronic contact dermatitis, to a greater degree than those with light-colored skin (Fig. 20).
Contact dermatitis in dark-skinned persons frequently has the appearance of lichen simplex chronicus. The frequency of contact dermatitis or sensitive
skin is probably unrelated to ethnicity [52–55]. Irritant contact dermatitis may be more common among

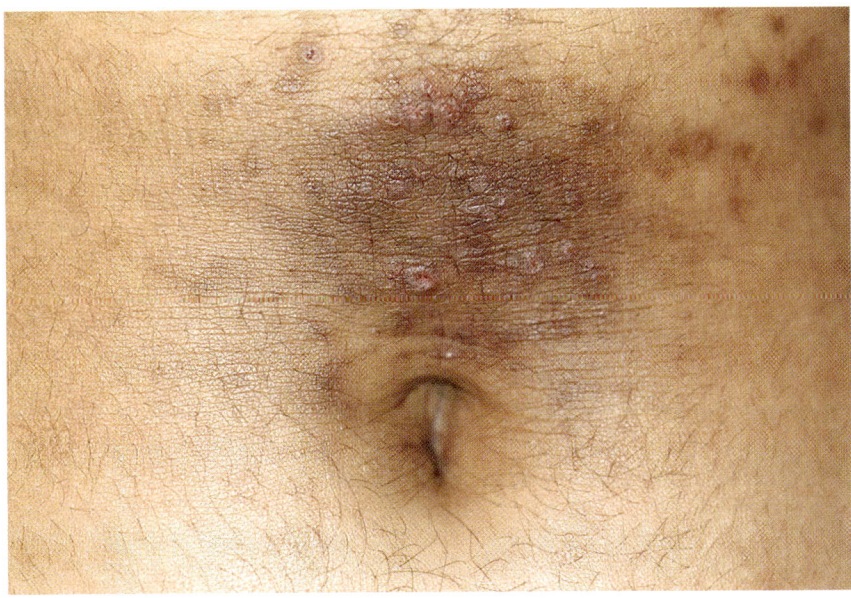

Fig. 20.
Post-inflammatory hyper-
pigmentation following allergic nickel contact dermatitis

persons of Asian descent than among Caucasians [56].

14.3.5.5 Atopy

Patients with atopic dermatitis who develop allergic contact dermatitis from a given substance often react with both aggravation of their atopic dermatitis and a pattern of allergic contact dermatitis. There is some question as to the exact relationship between atopy and contact sensitization. It has been suggested that atopics become contact sensitized less often than nonatopics [57]. Of a group of 130 adults who had moderate atopic dermatitis in childhood, 23% had positive patch tests to one or more allergens in a standard series, whereas 17% of 159 adults who had severe atopic dermatitis in childhood had similar positive patch tests [58]. The results of this and another study [59] support the theory that atopics experience fewer delayed-type sensitizations.

Christophersen et al. [60] carried out a multivariate statistical analysis of various parameters in 2166 patch-tested patients and found that nickel allergy was significantly less common among atopics than among nonatopics. This difference could not be demonstrated for other common contact allergens. Since nickel is a ubiquitous environmental allergen, atopics and nonatopics are equally exposed to this allergen.

Negative nickel patch tests in patients with a history of nickel allergy have been linked to atopy [61], but no agreement has as yet been reached on the relevancy of such findings [62].

Irritant hand eczema is common among children with atopic dermatitis [63].

Core Message

■ While contact allergy is probably slightly less common in atopic persons than in nonatopic persons, irritant hand eczema is more common in persons with atopy. Ethnicity does not appear to play a role in contact allergy, but the exposure pattern may vary among races.

14.4 Identifying the Cause of Contact Dermatitis from the Clinical Pattern

It is often difficult to trace the substance which has caused the skin to react to contact, particularly if the patient has chronic lesions. Reactions to substances that are not a part of everyday life, such as dinitrochlorobenzene or infrequently used topical drugs, usually present little diagnostic difficulty, while the source of reactions to ubiquitous allergens such as nickel and fragrances may be much more difficult to trace. Certain patterns of skin disease can, however, point in the direction of particular groups of substances, or even towards one specific causative substance.

14.4.1 Clinical Patterns Indicating General Causes of Contact Dermatitis

14.4.1.1 Contact Pattern

In the most obvious cases, an eczematous reaction is seen at the exact site of contact with the offending item. This type of reaction is frequently recognized by the patient and will commonly not be brought to the attention of a physician.

A typical example of contact-pattern dermatitis is allergic nickel contact dermatitis (Fig. 21). Historically, the most characteristic nickel contact sites have changed with changes in women's fashions. While, in the 1930s, most of Bonnevie's [64] patients had dermatitis at the site of contact with nickel-plated stocking suspender clasps, later the metal hooks on brassieres became a common offender. In the 1970s, sites of contact with metal buttons and studs in blue jeans became the most common sites of nickel dermatitis. At present, the earlobes, particularly if the patient has pierced ears [65], and sites of contact with nickel-plated watchbands and clasps are the most common primary sites of nickel dermatitis. Euro coins caused nickel dermatitis on the fingers of a taxi driver [66]. Gawkrodger et al. [67] examined 134 patients with positive patch tests to nickel and found the following prevalence of sites: palm 49%, dorsum of the hands 39%, wrist 22%, face 20%, arm 16%, neck 14%, and periorbital area 12%.

A study carried out in Singapore showed the most common sites to be the wrist, the ears, and the waist [68]. The contact pattern of nickel dermatitis is also dependent on cultural tradition and on the groups of patients studied, as well as on climatic factors. For example, sweating caused by high temperatures increases the release of nickel from nickel-plated items [69]. Nickel is also released by plasma, a fact that may explain the high rate of nickel sensitization after ear piercing [70].

In 1969, Kanan [71] described the typical site of nickel dermatitis among males in Kuwait as the sites of contact with metal studs in undergarments. Fisher

Fig. 21.
Allergic nickel contact dermatitis

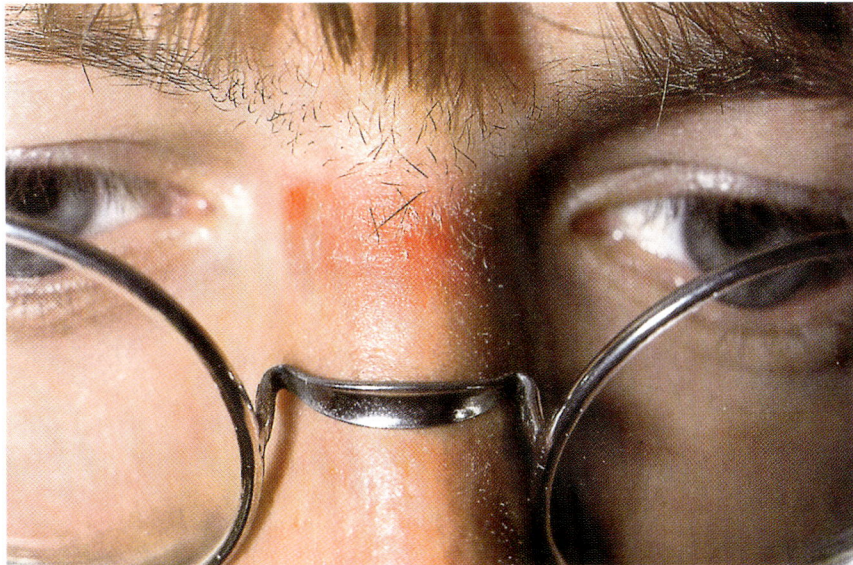

[72] noted that the most common sites of nickel dermatitis in males were under blue jeans' buttons and under watchbands.

Unusual sites of nickel contact dermatitis seen by the author include a small eczematous patch at the entry site of a venepuncture needle and a patch of eczema caused by the small nickel-plated part of a rubber stopper used to make a prosthesis airtight. Nickel dermatitis has also developed at sites of Dermojet injection [73], sites of the closure of surgical wounds with skin clips [74], and in tattoos, possibly due to contamination with nickel in red tattoo pigment [75].

Irritant contact dermatitis occurring under objects that occlude the skin, such as the metal case of a watch or a plastic watchstrap, may mimic nickel dermatitis. Repeated licking of the lips may cause irritant contact dermatitis induced by humidity and irritants in saliva. Such dermatitis is seen in areas that can be reached by the tongue (Fig. 22). Compulsive washing of the hands may cause irritant dermatitis on the dorsum of the hands and part of the forearms (Fig. 23). An older woman developed peculiar irritant dermatitis on her back due to compulsive washing with soap (Fig. 24).

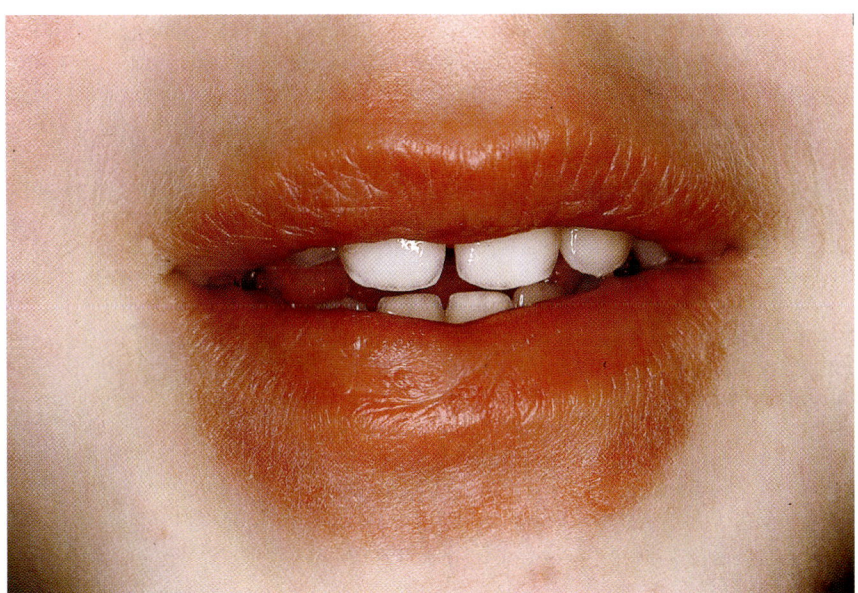

Fig. 22.
Irritant contact dermatitis with sharp demarcation caused by lip licking

14

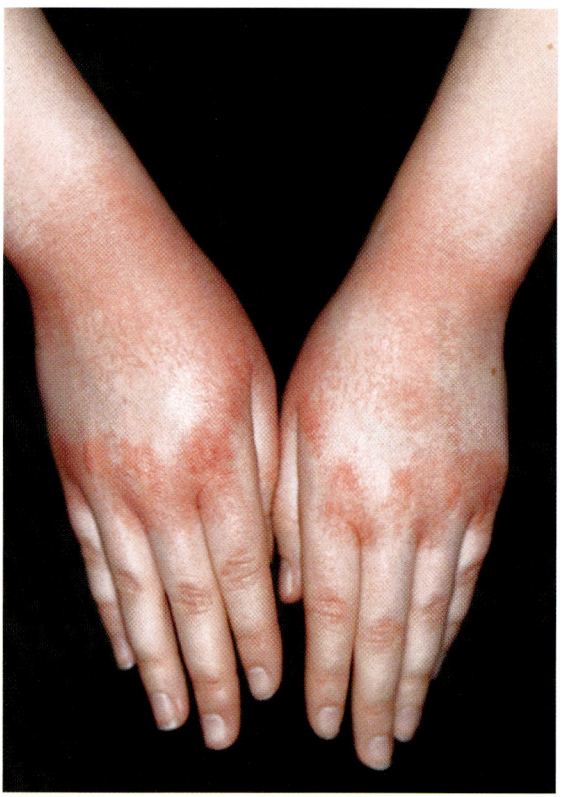

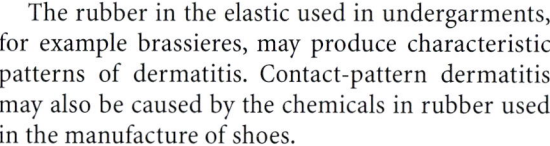

Fig. 23. Irritant contact dermatitis in a young girl caused by compulsive hand washing

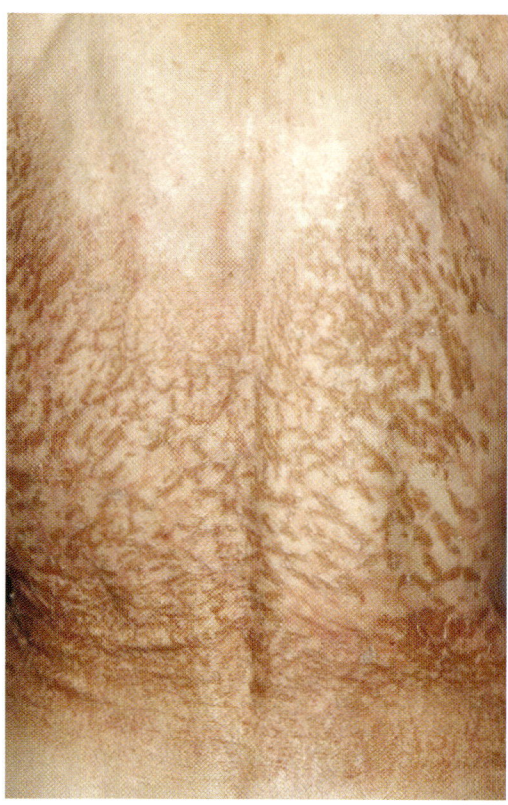

Fig. 24. Severe irritant contact dermatitis. This woman's husband washed her back 3 times a day with soap because he thought her itching was due to an infestation

The rubber in the elastic used in undergarments, for example brassieres, may produce characteristic patterns of dermatitis. Contact-pattern dermatitis may also be caused by the chemicals in rubber used in the manufacture of shoes.

Topical medicaments may also produce eczematous contact-pattern reactions, and these often have a biphasic course. Improvement initially seen following the use of a certain medicament applied to relieve an existing problem may be followed by aggravation in the area of application.

If a contact allergen – typically a topical drug – repeatedly applied to the legs of a sensitized person results in severe dermatitis, this will tend to spread in an id-like manner to the arms and possibly to the entire body. This pattern of spread is also seen in patients with severe stasis dermatitis, and it has been suggested that this is caused by cell-mediated autoimmunity [76, 77].

Since dermatitis caused by topical medicaments is most common in occluded areas and at sites where the skin is particularly delicate, this cause should be suspected if there is aggravation of existing dermatitis of the anogenital area, the lower leg, the ear or the eyelids [78–80].

Treatment with caustic agents may produce ulcerations at the sites of application. Severe reactions may follow the erroneous use of topical wart remedies applied to nevi on parts of the body that are normally occluded.

The computer mouse is suggested as the cause of contact dermatitis in the form of both allergic contact dermatitis [81] and occlusive dermatitis with negative patch tests (Fig. 25).

Certain contact allergens can produce contact-pattern dermatitis that does not appear at the actual site of contact. Nail polish is such an allergen, and typical sites of allergic contact dermatitis caused by nail polish are the eyelids, neck and genitalia, rather than the skin around the fingernails [82].

Core Message

■ The contact pattern of contact dermatitis depends on fashion and local traditions. Some contact allergens cause dermatitis at distant sites – eyelid dermatitis may, for example, be caused by nail polish.

Fig. 25.
Irritant or sweat retention dermatitis on the palmar side of the fingers of the right hand caused by prolonged contact with a computer mouse

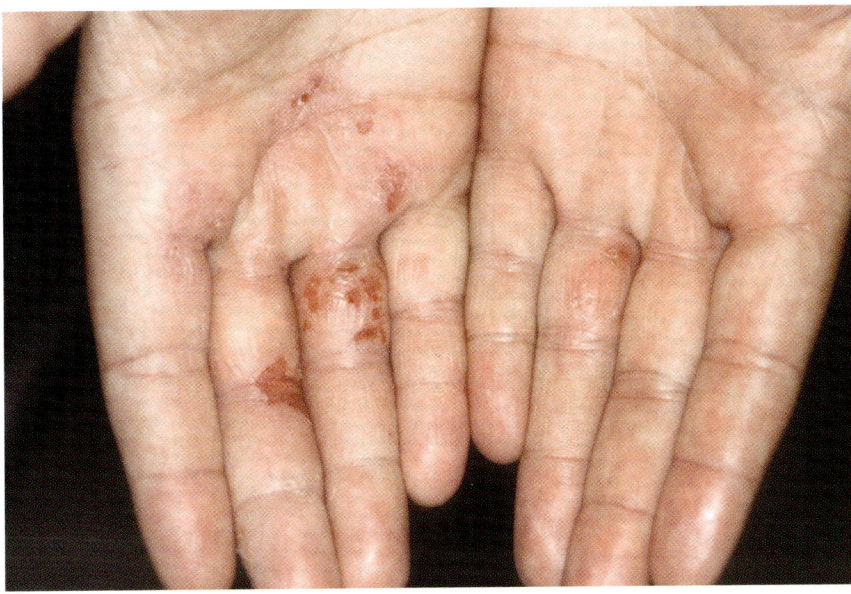

14.4.1.2 Streaked Dermatitis in Exposed Areas

Dermatitis may appear in streaks if it has been caused by liquids allowed to run down the skin. Caustic substances such as those used by farmers to clean milking equipment can cause such reactions.

Dermatitis caused by plant juices or the toxin from jellyfish such as the Portuguese man-of-war often appears in a bizarre streaked pattern [83]. Dermatitis caused by juices from Umbelliferae is often phototoxic. Upon resolution, a streaked bullous dermatitis can be followed by marked hyperpigmentation, which may last for many months (Figs. 26, 27).

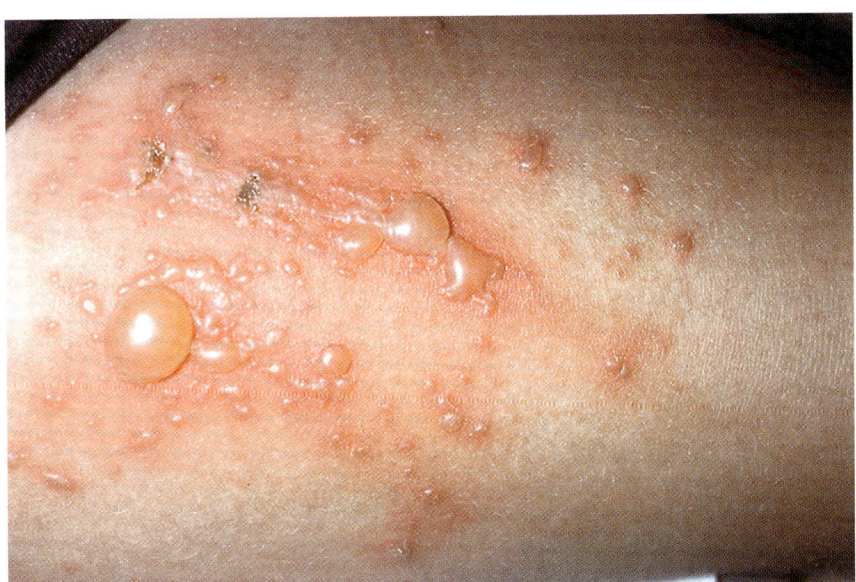

Fig. 26.
Phototoxic dermatitis caused by giant hogweed

Fig. 27.
Post-inflammatory hyper-pigmentation following resolution of phototoxic dermatitis caused by giant hogweed

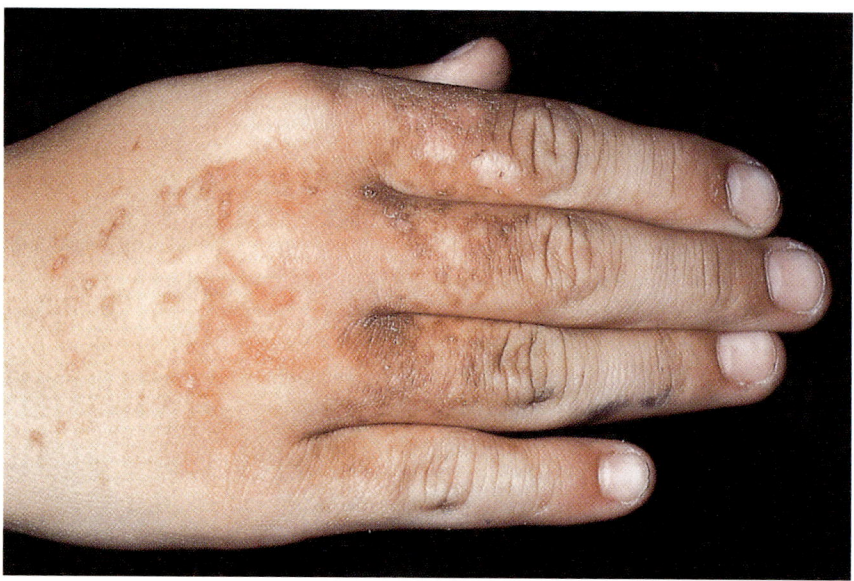

14.4.1.3 Airborne Contact Dermatitis

Airborne contact dermatitis may be caused by such substances as:

- Fibrous materials such as glass fiber, rock wool and grain dust, which give rise to mechanical dermatitis [84].
- Wood and cement dust, which cause irritant reactions [85]. Wood may also sensitize.
- Dust containing particles from plants such as *Parthenium hysterophorus*, ragweed or certain types of wood or medicaments to which the patient has delayed-type sensitivity [86–89].
- Aerosols of mineral oils that cause irritant reactions.

Huygens and Goossens have reviewed the causes of airborne contact dermatitis [90].

Particles of medicaments in dust, from for example pigsties, can cause dermatitis if the patient has contact allergy to the medicament in question. Airborne contact dermatitis appears on areas of the skin where the dust or fibers can be trapped, for example on the eyelids, neck (under a shirt collar), forearms (under cuffs) or lower legs (inside trouser legs) [21, 91]. Chronic airborne contact dermatitis tends to mimic photocontact dermatitis [92]. A combination of these two forms of dermatitis may also be seen.

Dermatitis from wood dust and dust from plant particles often leads to lichenified dermatitis at the sites of contact. The handling of large amounts of carbonless copy paper and laser printed paper can cause irritation of the mucous membranes of the nose and eyes and pruritus on exposed skin. In one study an increased level of plasma histamine was documented after exposure to carbonless copy paper [93].

Various cutaneous symptoms, including pruritus and paresthesia, have been described after long-term exposure to computer screens, but few patients exhibit diagnostic skin lesions [94, 95].

Core Message

- Airborne contact dermatitis can mimic photo contact dermatitis. Airborne contact dermatitis may be seen on exposed skin and at sites where dust is trapped under a shirt collar, shirt cuffs or trouser legs.

14.4.1.4 Mechanical Dermatitis

Friction can cause both hyperkeratosis and dermatitis. Acute lesions may appear as actual abrasions of the skin (Fig. 28), while chronic mechanical dermatitis is often more subtle and therefore more difficult to diagnose. Mechanical trauma is particularly important as an occupational disorder. Many different aspects of this type of dermatitis were detailed at a conference on the cutaneous effects of repeated mechanical trauma to the skin [96]. Most computer-related occupational dermatoses are mechanical [97, 98].

14

Fig. 28.
Abrasion caused by contact with rough fibers in a sack made of jute

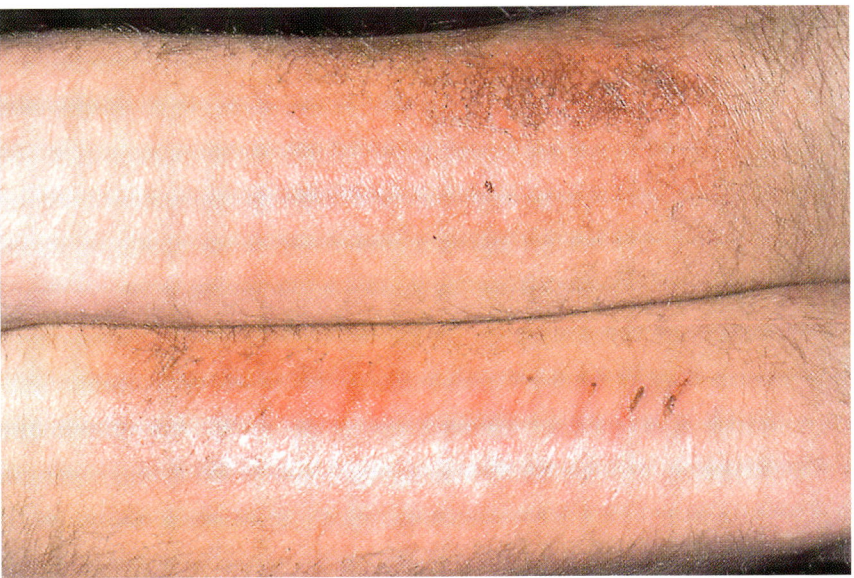

The handling of large quantities of paper, for example computer printouts, may eventually lead to hyperkeratosis on the involved fingers. Eczematous dermatitis may develop after long-term, often subconscious, manipulation of the skin (Fig. 29). Some popular sports activities have given rise to new dermatological entities caused by physical trauma. These include "rower's rump", "jogger's nipples", "black heel" [99–101], "canyoning hand" [102], and "baseball pitcher's friction dermatitis" [103].

Mechanical dermatitis on the inner aspects of the thighs may mimic intertrigo. The treatment given to HIV-positive patients may cause "buffalo hump," and mechanical dermatitis may be seen on the hump [104]. Bizarre patterns of dermatitis and purpura may result from curious cultural habits, such as coin rubbing. Unusual patterns of skin lesions can also be seen in the victims of physical or electrical torture. Cellular phone chargers caused ulcerations at the site of contact in two persons who slept on the chargers [105].

> ### Core Message
>
> ■ Mechanical contact dermatitis is a consequence of repeated physical trauma at the site of contact. Characteristic patterns of mechanical contact dermatitis are seen among participants in certain sports.

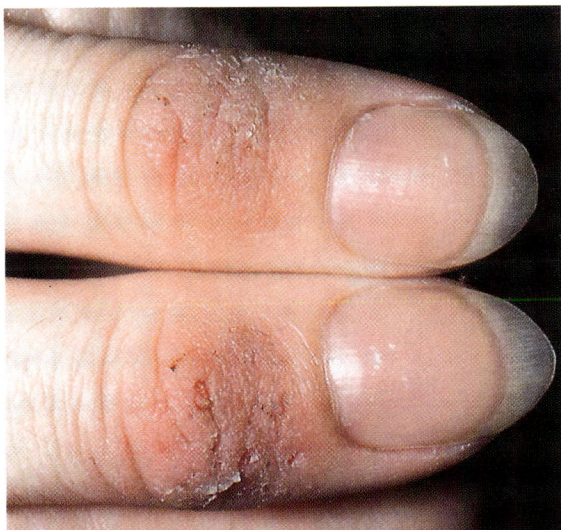

Fig. 29. Mechanical contact dermatitis caused by manipulation of the skin

14.4.1.5 Hyperkeratotic Eczema

Symmetrical, hyperkeratotic plaques on the central parts of the palms and/or soles represent an entity that is clinically distinct from other types of eczema, because no vesicles are seen. At the onset of an eruption, this dermatitis is often pruritic, while pruritus is uncommon in chronic lesions (Fig. 30). Although this type of eczema is distinct from psoriasis histologically, clinically it is difficult to distinguish from psoriasis [106]. The etiology is unknown. The condition is most common in middle-aged men, is very

Fig. 30.
Hyperkeratotic palmar eczema

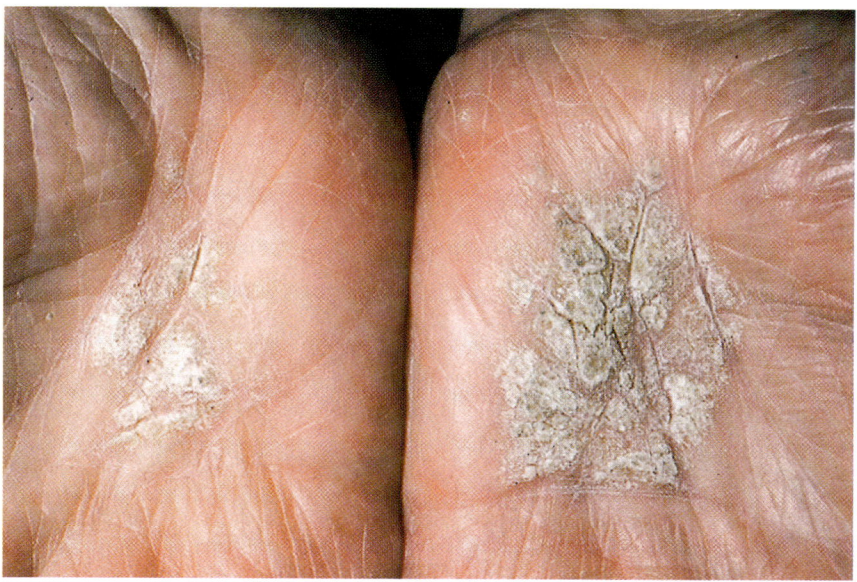

persistent, and is aggravated by mechanical trauma. Oral acitretin has been shown to be an effective treatment [107].

14.4.1.6 Ring Dermatitis

Dermatitis which occurs under tight-fitting jewelry, such as finger rings, can be due to allergic reactions to constituents of the jewelry. Ring finger dermatitis is significantly more common in patients who are patch test positive to gold sodium thiosulfate than in patients who do not have this contact allergy [108]. If a ring is made of relatively pure gold or of plastic, this type of eczema is most commonly due to sweat retention and the accumulation under the ring of occluded irritants from detergents (Fig. 31).

14.4.1.7 Follicular Reactions

Folliculitis or an acneiform appearance may develop following cutaneous contact with or the absorption of certain polyhalogenated aromatic hydrocarbons, such as dioxin, or following skin contact with crude oil or its derivatives. Exposed areas of the body are most commonly involved due to direct contact or to aerosols (Fig. 32), but chloracne caused by the inhala-

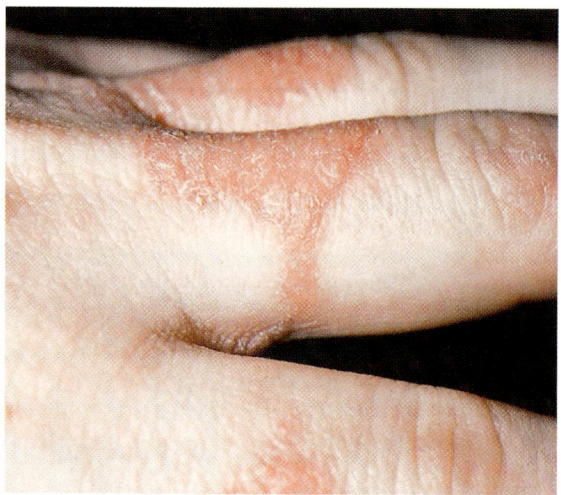

Fig. 31. Irritant contact dermatitis under a finger ring

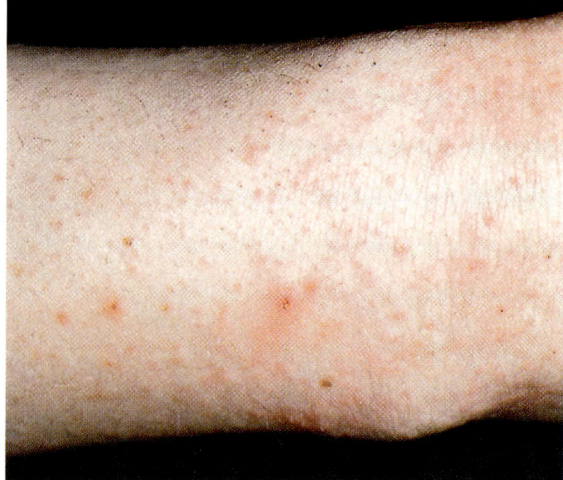

Fig. 32. Folliculitis caused by oil

14

tion of chlorinated compounds can appear on parts of the body that are normally covered, and oil folliculitis may occur on the thighs if a patient has worn trousers that have become soaked in oil. Pomade acne of the forehead caused by oils applied to the hair is usually found only on the forehead and the temples, while cosmetic acne is most often distributed over the entire face [109].

Allergic contact dermatitis may appear as a pustular dermatosis. Pustular reactions have been described in allergic contact dermatitis caused by mercaptobenzothiazoles [110]. A galvanizer was seen to have occupational contact folliculitis [111]. Pustular patch test reactions, interpreted as nonallergic, were seen in 2% of 853 persons tested with sodium tungstate. The reactions were often reproducible [112].

Core Message

- Follicular or pustular reactions are commonly due to irritant reactions to mineral oils or certain pesticides. Pustular reactions are rarely an expression of allergic contact dermatitis.

14.4.1.8 Connubial and Consort Dermatitis

Contact with rubber condoms can cause genital eczema in women. Allergic contact urticaria may occur following contact with semen, and such contact can also cause systemic symptoms and even anaphylactic reactions [113, 114]. Males can develop dermatitis of the penis after contact with contraceptive cream. Connubial dermatitis is not confined solely to the genitals, as witnessed by the fact that some women develop allergic contact dermatitis on the face after contact with a partner's aftershave lotion or other cosmetic preparations used by the sexual partner [115, 116].

14.4.1.9 Recurrent Vesicular Hand and/or Foot Dermatitis

This common pruritic dermatosis occurs as eruptions of crops of vesicles on the palms, the sides of fingers, the central part of the soles or the sides of the toes (Figs. 4–8). There may be little or no inflammation. The eruptions heal with subsequent scaling, but repeated frequent eruptions may lead to chronic hand and/or foot eczema. Recurrent vesicular der-

matitis is a nonspecific clinical reaction pattern which may be caused by external agents, but it is commonly considered to be an example of an endogenous dermatosis [33, 117] (see Chap. 16). There is a statistical correlation between vesicular eruptions on the hands and tinea pedis [118].

Core Message

- Recurrent vesicular hand dermatitis is an eruptive, pruritic, vesicular, nonspecific reaction pattern on palmar or plantar skin. This pattern is seen in both contact dermatitis and in endogenous dermatitis.

14.4.1.10 Fingertip Eczema (Pulpitis)

Contact dermatitis of the fingertips, particularly on the thumb and the index and middle fingers of the nondominant hand, is a common ailment among chefs due to their repeated contact with irritants or allergens found in plants such as garlic (Fig. 33). Dental technicians and dentists can also develop fingertip eczema on the same three digits – but on the dominant hand – due to contact with the acrylic substances used to make dental prostheses and plastic dental fillings [119, 120].

Pulpitis can also present as mechanical contact dermatitis in persons who handle large amounts of paper and cardboard.

Some children develop pulpitis on all 10 digits. Clinically, shiny erythema, possibly with fissures, is seen. Although some children with this condition

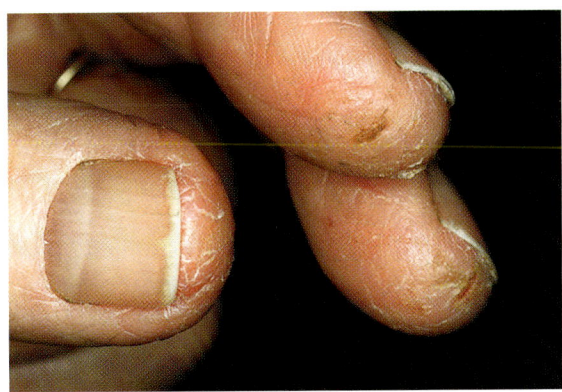

Fig. 33. Pulpitis caused by the handling of garlic on the thumb, index and middle fingers of the nondominant hand of a garlic-sensitive woman

have a history of atopic dermatitis, the etiology is unknown.

14.4.1.11 Eczema Nails

A characteristic pattern of transverse grooves and ridges may be seen in the nail plates of patients with eczema on the dorsal aspects of the fingers. There is usually also involvement or disappearance of the nail

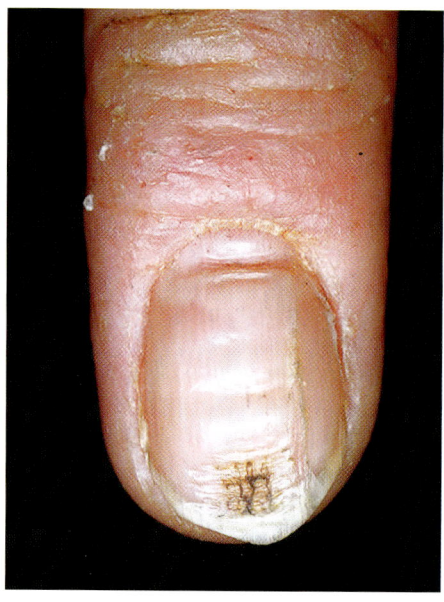

Fig. 34. Transverse ridges and grooves in the nail plate of a patient with eczema on the dorsal aspects of the fingers

cuticle. The number of grooves on the nail often corresponds to the number of episodes of flare of the eczema (Fig. 34). Subungual vesicular dermatitis under the periphery of the nail plate is less common [121]. This pattern of subungual dermatitis has been seen, however, following work with anaerobic acrylic sealants [122]. Allergic contact dermatitis from formaldehyde-based hardening resins in nail polish and acrylates used to build up artificial nails can cause severe nail damage, including irreversible nail dystrophy [123, 124].

14.4.1.12 Papular and Nodular Excoriated Lesions

Most reported cases of delayed hypersensitivity to aluminum have occurred following deposition in the dermis or subcutis of vaccines used for childhood immunizations or following hyposensitization procedures. Persistent, pruritic, excoriated, deeply infiltrated lesions at injection sites are characteristic (Figs. 35, 36) [125–128]. Histologically, histiocytic infiltrates are characteristic, but other features may be present [129]. Intolerance to antiperspirants that contain aluminum salts has been described, but such cases appear to be rare [130].

Infiltrated papular lesions have also been seen at the sites of injection of zinc-bound insulin. The patients in question had zinc hypersensitivity, as demonstrated by intracutaneous testing and lymphocyte transformation studies [131]. There have been no further reports of such cases. A similar morphology of contact sensitization is seen if tattoo pigment causes

14

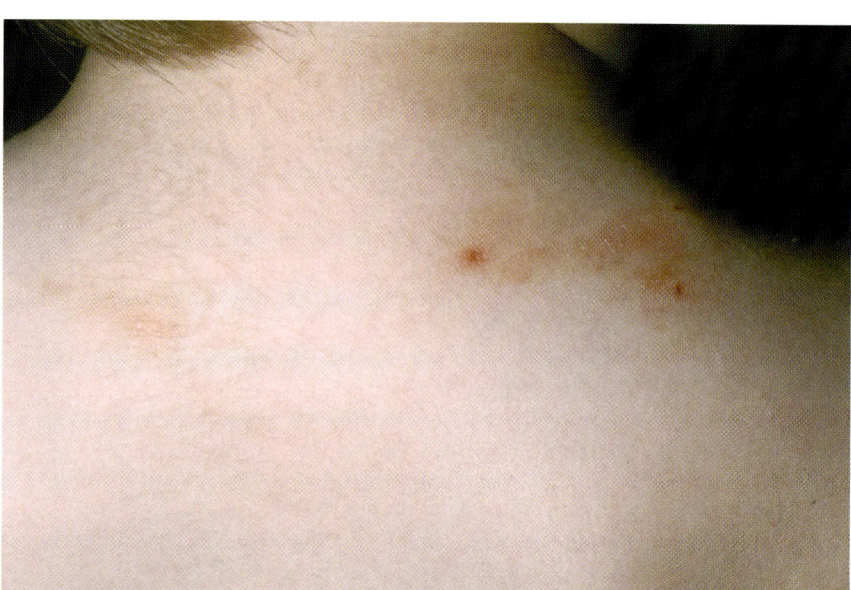

Fig. 35.
Persistent, pruritic infiltrates following childhood immunizations in an aluminum-sensitive child

Fig. 36.
Papular, nodular, and excoriated lesions in an aluminum-sensitive person following hyposensitization with a vaccine containing aluminum

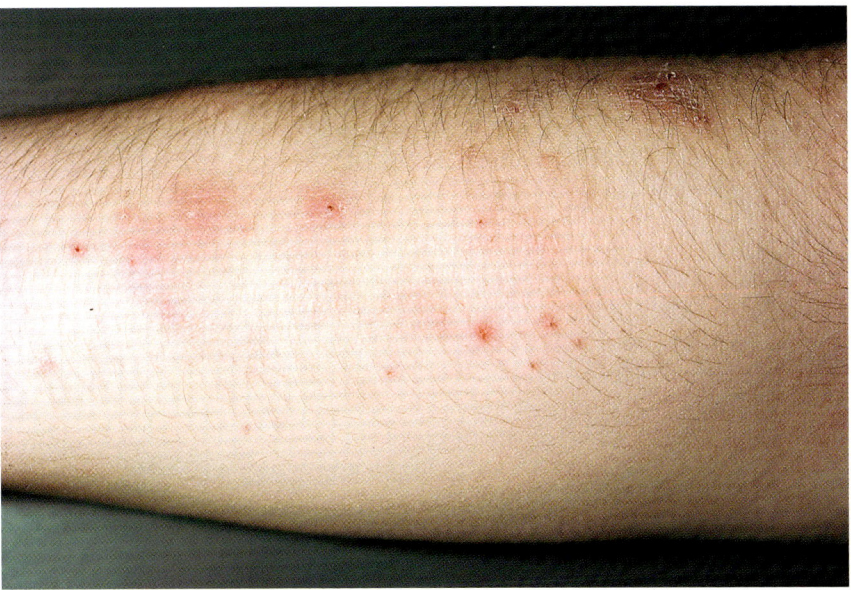

sensitization. Chromium, cobalt, and mercury salts used to be common sensitizing tattoo pigments [132]. Modern tattoo pigments, however, rarely sensitize. See also Sect. 14.5.7 Contact Stomatitis.

penetrate eczematous skin, but the same allergens cannot usually penetrate intact skin [137] (see Chap. 5).

Core Message

- Pruritic, papular, excoriated infiltrates at the sites of childhood immunizations or hyposensitization injections may be due to contact allergy to aluminum – otherwise a rare sensitizer.

14.4.1.13 Contact Urticaria of the Hands and Lips

Contact urticaria should be suspected if dermatitis or intermittent urticaria is seen on the lips and/or the hands, particularly if an itching or a burning sensation has arisen seconds to minutes after contact with uncooked food items or with latex gloves (Fig. 37). Anaphylactic reactions may also occur. The symptoms on the hands sometimes disappear when the hands are rinsed; in some cases hand eczema develops or, more commonly, an existing hand eczema is aggravated [133–135]. This problem is particularly common among atopics. A skin application food test (SAFT) has been developed to diagnose this type of dermatitis in children [136]. Allergens in foods may

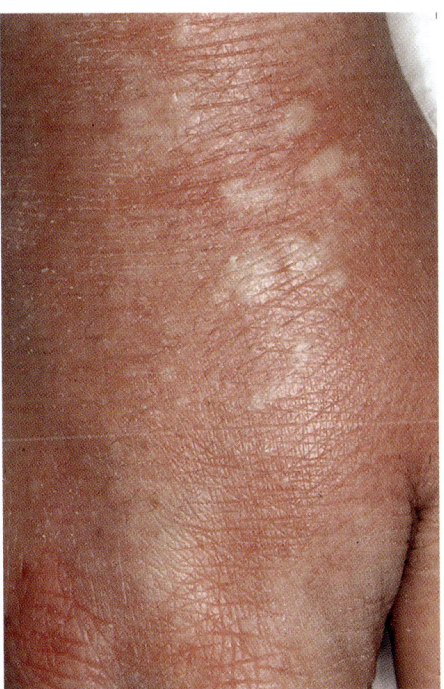

Fig. 37. Contact urticaria due to latex seen after a few minutes of challenge with, or exposure to, latex gloves

14.4.1.14 Clinical Patterns of Systemically Induced Contact Dermatitis

If a substance to which a person has developed cellular immunity due to contact with the skin is subsequently ingested or otherwise absorbed, a variety of cutaneous reactions may occur (see Chap. 16) [138, 139]. Vesiculation of the hands, for example, may be seen in patients who have not previously experienced this reaction pattern. A patient who suffers from recurrent vesicular hand eczema may experience a flare of dermatitis after experimental oral challenge with the substance to which he or she is sensitive. One nickel-sensitive patient developed palmar vesicles and small bullae a few days after beginning a weight-reducing diet that called for the ingestion of vegetables rich in nickel. Nickel-sensitive patients may have dermal lesions with evidence of vasculitis, which can be reproduced by placebo-controlled oral challenge [140]. A keratotic eruption of the elbows has been described as accompanying a systemically induced dermatitis [141]. See Chapter 16.

So-called secondary eruptions were noted by Calnan [142] when he described the clinical features of large groups of nickel-allergic patients. These secondary eruptions consisted of erythematous flares in skin folds such as the antecubital fossae and on the sides of the neck, the eyelids, and the inner thighs. Widespread edematous erythema in the skin folds of the anogenital area has been termed the "baboon syndrome" [143], and edematous lesions of this type have also been observed in nickel-sensitive patients following oral challenge with nickel [144].

Sensitization from the topical application of drugs is common. If a drug to which a patient is sensitized is taken orally, a variety of reactions can be seen, ranging from recurrence of the dermatitis in its original site and reactivation of a patch test site, to widespread dermatitis. Such widespread dermatitis may be accompanied by fever and toxic epidermal necrolysis, which may be life-threatening [17, 145, 146]. Toxicoderma and fever have also been seen in gold-sensitive patients after the intramuscular injection of gold preparations [4].

Fixed drug eruption is a distinct nummular eruption occurring repeatedly in the same location after the ingestion of the drug in question [147]. It may be, but is not necessarily, associated with topical sensitivity to the drug. In one study, a fixed eruption could be reproduced in 18 of 24 patients after topical application of the drug. The study showed topical sensitivity to phenazones to be especially common [148].

Core Message

■ The systemic administration of a hapten in contact sensitized persons can lead to a variety of symptoms such as flare-up of the current dermatitis or previous sites of contact dermatitis or previous patch test sites. Vesicular eruptions on the hands, flexural dermatitis, or widespread rashes or the "baboon syndrome" may be seen.

14.4.2 Characteristic Clinical Patterns of Dermatitis Associated with Specific Substances or Types of Application

14.4.2.1 Cement Ulcerations

Caustic reactions and acute irritant contact dermatitis at the site of prolonged contact with wet cement are sometimes seen under the tops of socks or on other parts of the lower leg that are normally occluded. The alkalinity of the cement and prolonged skin contact with wet cement are the most likely causes of this dermatitis [149–151] (Fig. 38).

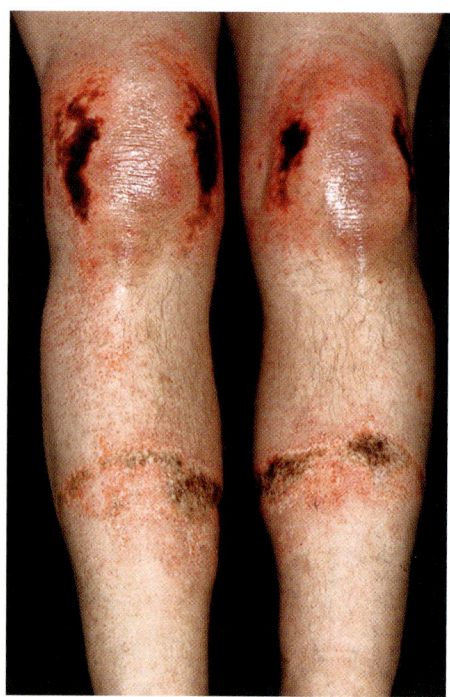

Fig. 38. Caustic reaction caused by cement

14.4.2.2 Pigmented Contact Dermatitis

Optical brighteners were originally described by Osmundsen and Alani [152] as the cause of severely pruritic, purpuric, allergic contact dermatitis which caused little or no discernible change in the epidermis. In Japan, pigmented contact dermatitis is relatively common [153]. A resin commonly used in the dyeing of cotton fabrics (Naphthol AS) can cause pigmented allergic contact dermatitis that is typically seen on the neck and upper arms [154] (see Chap. 18).

14.4.2.3 Caterpillar Dermatitis and Irritant Dermatitis from Plants and Animals

Spicules hidden among the hairs of certain caterpillars contain a toxin which can cause persistent pruritic vesicles or papules at sites of contact with the skin. This is a characteristic clinical finding among children who have played with these caterpillars [155, 156] (Fig. 39). Sun-worshippers may come in contact with this toxin on beaches where large numbers of such species of caterpillars have wandered in procession [157]. Occupational immunologic contact urticaria has also been described [158]. Similar toxic substances are found in sea urchins and sea anemones and in various plants such as those of the *Dieffenbachia* species and in *Agave tequilana* [159]. Mechanical injuries from thorns and similar projections on plants or fish may mimic this dermatosis.

> **Core Message**
>
> - Long-lasting, pruritic, papular, and vesicular eruptions may result from contact with spicules from certain caterpillars. Children who play with caterpillars have eruptions on the hands, while forestry workers may have more widespread eruptions.

14.4.2.4 Head and Neck Dermatitis

Adults with atopic dermatitis and persistent pruritic dermatitis of the face, the sides of the neck and the shoulders may have immediate-type sensitivity to the saprophytic fungus *Pityrosporum ovale* [160, 161].

14.4.2.5 Dermatitis from Transcutaneous Delivery Systems

Eczematous lesions as well as general cutaneous reactions and systemic symptoms sometimes occur where transcutaneous drug delivery systems have been applied [162, 163]. Generally speaking, such reactions are rare. Continuous percutaneous drug delivery systems are used for such drugs as clonidine, nitroglycerin, scopolamine, estradiol, nicotine, and testosterone [164, 165]. Studies of why the drugs applied in this manner sometimes cause cutaneous re-

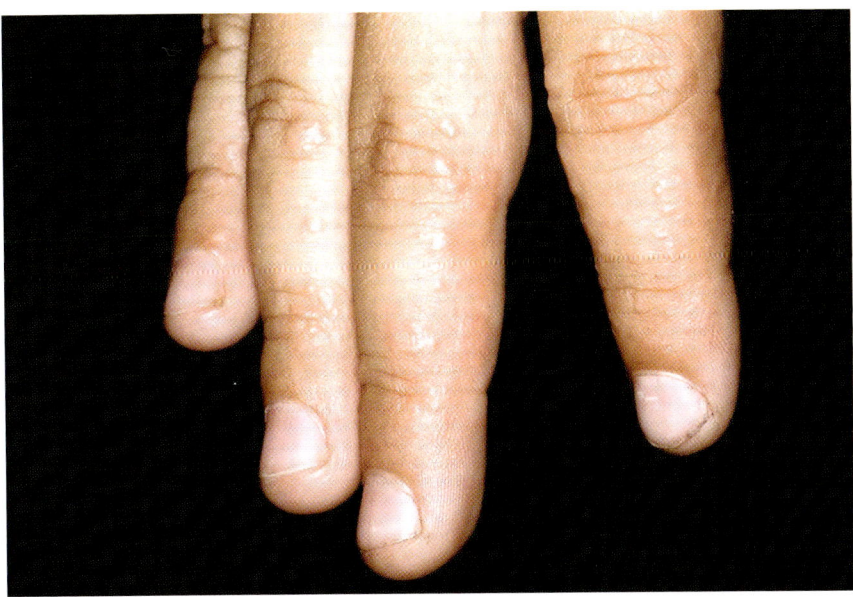

Fig. 39.
Persistent papules and vesicles on the fingers of a child who played with a caterpillar

actions have revealed that a limited number of patients have allergic contact dermatitis from the active drug or from ingredients in the delivery system itself [166–168]. Oral ingestion of the drugs in question has been seen to produce widespread dermatitis in a few patients [164].

14.4.2.6 Berloque Dermatitis

The application of perfumes on the sides of the neck may give rise to a phototoxic reaction with edematous dermatitis and subsequent pigmentation at the exact sites of application of the perfume [169].

14.4.2.7 Stomatitis due to Mercury or Gold Allergy

Grayish streaks, erythema or erosions on the oral mucous membranes at sites of contact with amalgam dental fillings indicate irritant or allergic contact stomatitis from the mercury in the amalgam fillings or from the gold on capped teeth (Fig. 40). There has been some controversy as to the use of amalgam dental fillings containing mercury. This entity is discussed in detail in Sect. 14.6 Differential Diagnosis.

14.5 Regional Contact Dermatitis

The diagnosis of contact dermatitis is facilitated by a thorough knowledge of substances which characteristically cause dermatitis of specific areas of the skin.

Computer analyses of the relationship between eczema sites and contact allergens have shown statistically significant correlations between, for example, nickel and cobalt and various sites on the fingers and palms, and between lanolin and the lower legs. Sensitivity to the fragrance mix was shown to correlate with dermatitis of the axillae, sensitivity to balsam of Peru with dermatitis of the face and the lower legs, and sensitivity to neomycin and "caine" mix with dermatitis of the lower leg [170]. Other examples of substances that cause dermatitis in specific areas of the body are presented in the following sections.

14.5.1 Dermatitis of the Scalp

Allergic contact dermatitis of the scalp itself is surprisingly rare in view of the fact that the level of percutaneous absorption through skin of the scalp is high compared with other areas of the body. While sensitization to leave-on products such as pomades and minoxidil does occur, dermatitis is more commonly seen on adjacent areas such as the ears, forehead and sides of the neck than on the scalp itself [171–174] (Fig. 41).

Contact sensitizers applied to the scalp, such as thioglycolates in permanent wave solutions or dyes used to color the hair, more frequently cause hand eczema in the persons who apply the substances than contact dermatitis in the person to whom they are applied [175]. Fifty-five patients who had their hair dyed had rather severe reactions on the face or scalp. All those patch tested reacted to paraphenylene diamine [176].

14

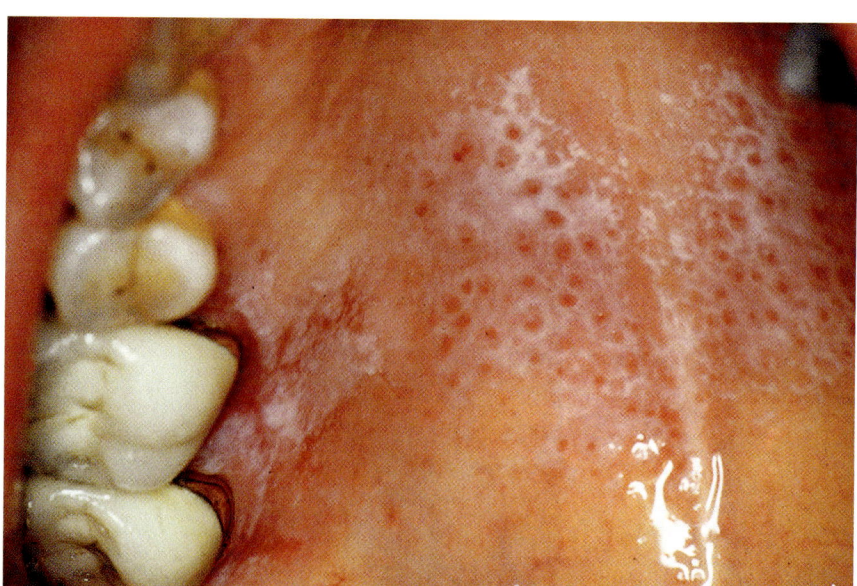

Fig. 40.
Oral lichenoid lesions in a gold-sensitive person (courtesy of P.J. Frosch)

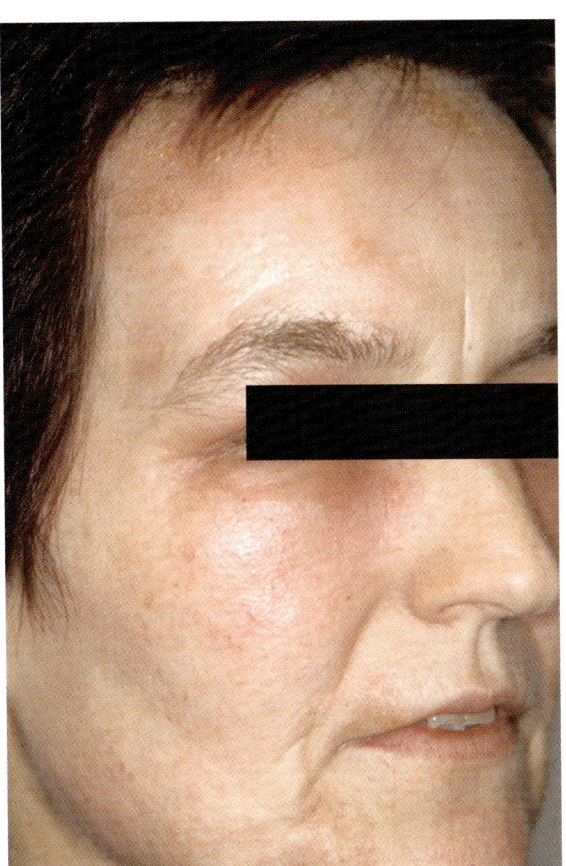

Fig. 41. A woman developed edematous facial dermatitis and dermatitis of the neck after having her hair dyed. She had a positive patch test to paraphenylene diamine

Contact dermatitis of the scalp may be followed by telogen effluvium [177].

Nickel in hairpins and decorative items of nickel used near the scalp may cause dermatitis at the sites of contact.

Rinse-off products such as shampoos may cause allergic contact dermatitis of the scalp due to surfactants, preservatives or fragrances, but such reactions are rare in view of the amounts used [178–183]. Patients who have previously become sensitized to preservatives may react to similar compounds in shampoos and other hair-care products. Methyl dibromo-glutaranitril is an example of a preservative that commonly sensitizes. Bovine collagen in hair conditioners can cause contact urticaria of the scalp and face [184]. Medicated shampoos, for example those containing tar, may cause irritant contact dermatitis of the scalp or aggravation of the seborrheic dermatitis or psoriasis they were intended to improve.

Microorganisms such as *Pityrosporum ovale* may aggravate existing diseases of the scalp, and seborrheic dermatitis of the scalp has been seen to improve following treatment with ketoconazole shampoo [185, 186]. Bacterial infection may aggravate atopic dermatitis of the scalp and cause folliculitis as well as exudative dermatitis.

Discoloration of the hair due to external contactants may be caused by the copper salts found in swimming pool water (green color), dithranol (anthralin) preparations used on the scalp (reddish color) or hydroxyquinoline preparations (brownish-yellow color). Irritant dermatitis may be seen after bleaching the hair (Fig. 42).

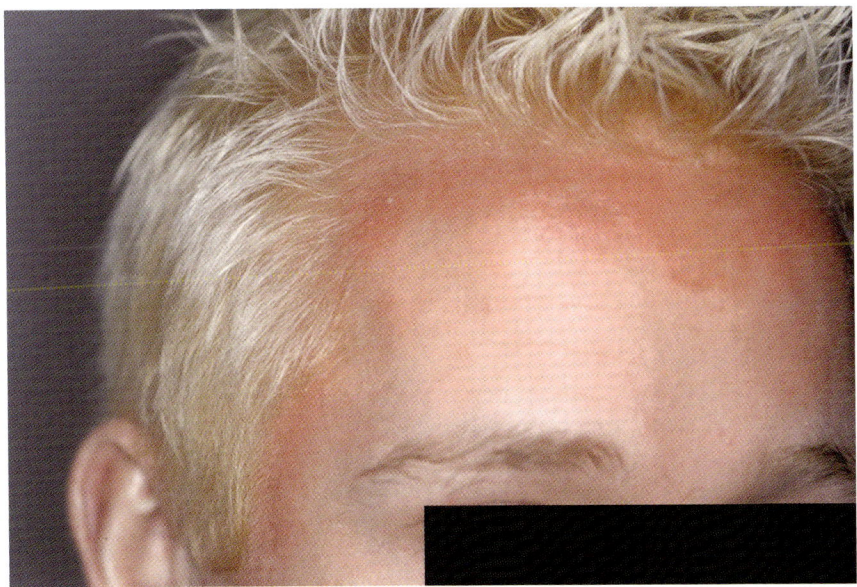

Fig. 42.
A young man developed irritant contact dermatitis of the frontal and temporal regions after lightening his hair

Core Message

■ Contact dermatitis caused by irritants or contact allergens applied to the scalp commonly occurs on the forehead, the ears, and the neck. Hair dyes and permanent wave solutions are more often the cause than rinse-off products.

14.5.2 Dermatitis of the Face and Neck

The face and neck, like the backs of the hands, are the areas of the body most heavily exposed to the sun. These areas are, therefore, the prime targets for photocontact dermatitis. Common causes of photosensitive dermatoses were reviewed by Fotiades et al. [187]. Olaquindox used in pig feed has been seen to cause photoallergic contact dermatitis [188]. In typical cases, the symptoms of this photodermatosis are burning, stinging, and itching. There is a sharp delineation along the collar and no dermatitis under the chin or behind the earlobes. Less typical cases may include symptoms similar to the above but with little to be seen on physical examination. The pigmentation seen following some types of phototoxic contact dermatitis is caused by furocoumarins, and such pigmentation is in itself almost diagnostic.

Photocontact dermatitis following contact with tar products appears where drops of wood preservatives, for example, have fallen on the skin. Hyperpigmentation is more commonly seen after photocontact dermatitis caused by furocoumarins than by tar.

Photocontact dermatitis that remains undiagnosed, or that is caused by substances which are difficult to avoid, may eventually become what is known as chronic actinic dermatitis or the actinic reticuloid syndrome [189–191]. The etiology of this entity is not clear, and airborne contact dermatitis may be a causative factor. Even when the substance causing this dermatitis has been removed, some patients remain permanently light sensitive.

The face and neck are also typical sites of airborne contact dermatitis, which in its early phases may be distinguished from photocontact dermatitis by the presence of dermatitis in submental areas and behind the ears. Airborne contact dermatitis is commonly most intense where dust is trapped under the shirt collar, while light-induced dermatitis is seen only above the collar. An airborne pattern of dermatitis may be caused by plants, in particular plants of the Compositae family [192–195] (Fig. 43), or among farm workers from fodder and cow dander [196, 197].

A typical mechanical dermatitis in this area is the classic fiddler's neck, caused by long-term contact with the chin rest on a violin [198].

Allergic contact dermatitis of the neck is commonly caused by nickel in jewelry, but jewelry made of exotic woods can also be the cause [199]. Plastics rarely cause dermatitis on the neck. Nurses in intensive-care units who wear a stethoscope for many hours a day may develop nickel dermatitis on the sides of the neck.

In a study by Hausen and Oestmann [200], 50% of 64 flower vendors with contact dermatitis caused by plants had dermatitis of the face. The most common causative plants were chrysanthemums, tulips and alstroemeria, while daffodils and primulas were rarely the cause.

Facial dermatitis is commonly caused by cosmetics. Of 119 patients with cosmetic dermatitis, 63% had involvement of the face, while 26% had involvement of the hands and arms [201]. Of 13,216 patients with contact dermatitis seen by members of the North American Contact Dermatitis Group over a 5-year period, 713 had dermatitis caused by cosmetics. Interestingly, in most cases, neither patient nor physician had suspected cosmetics as the cause of the contact dermatitis on the basis of the clinical features, and diagnoses were not made until the results of patch testing were known. Of the patients, 81% had dermatitis that could be described as allergic contact dermatitis; irritation accounted for the reactions of 16% of the patients, and phototoxic and photoallergic reactions each accounted for less than 1% of the reactions. Fragrances, preservatives, hair-coloring agents, and permanent wave solutions accounted for most of the cases of allergic contact dermatitis seen in this study [202]. Eight men developed dermatitis of the beard area due to *para*-phenylenediamine in dyes for the beard [203].

In an investigation of positive patch tests to preservatives, Jacobs et al. [204] found that the face was the most commonly involved site for relevant reactions to the preservatives quaternium-15, 2-bromo-2-nitropropane-1,3-diol, imidazolidinyl urea and diazolidinyl urea. Over time the relative frequency of allergy to quaternium-15 has decreased. Allergy to methyl dibromoglutaronitrile is, on the other hand, increasing in frequency [205].

The use of soap containing chromium is a rare cause of pigmented contact dermatitis of the face [206]. Depigmentation may also be seen following the use of cosmetic products such as toothpaste containing cinnamic aldehyde (cinnamal) [207] and the use of incense [208].

Ammonium persulfate used to bleach hair is a peculiar substance in that it may produce symptoms in

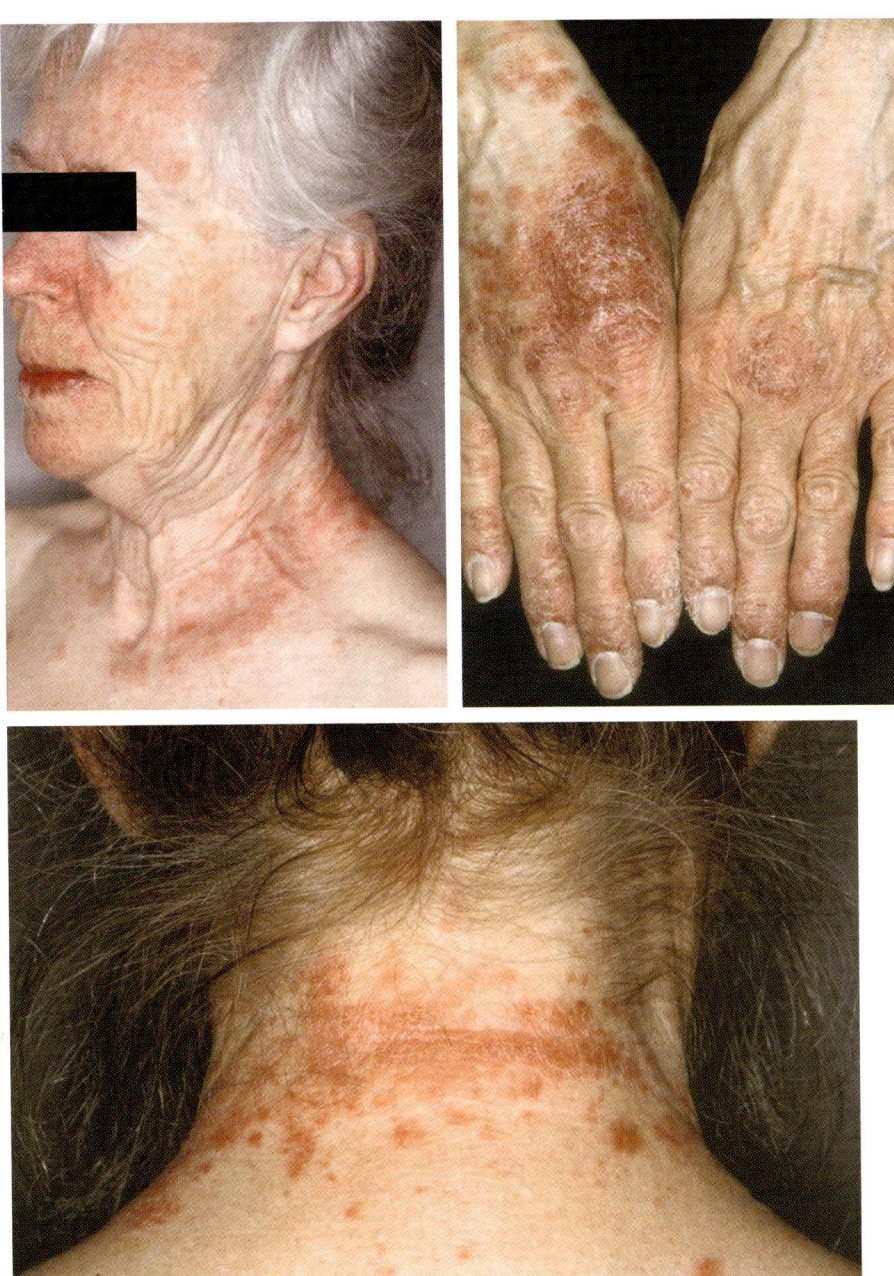

Fig. 43a–c. A woman sensitive to sesquiterpene lactone developed airborne contact dermatitis of the face (a), neck (b), and dorsal aspects of the hands (c)

both the hairdresser and the customer, following contact with either the solution used to treat the hair or its airborne particles. The substance can cause histamine release, leading to severe respiratory symptoms and urticaria. It may also produce irritant contact dermatitis and allergic reactions, which may be either immediate-type or delayed-type [209] (Fig. 42).

Cosmetic acne presenting as discrete poral occlusion is common. An acneiform folliculitis of the fore-

head known as pomade acne is occasionally seen after the long-term use of oily hair-care products [109]. A transient stinging sensation on the face, with no apparent dermatitis, following the application of cosmetic preparations is common [25]. The stinging sensation may in some cases be due to contact urticaria. Individuals with fair, freckled skin are probably more likely than others to develop irritation from cosmetics. A questionnaire study of 90 student nurses revealed contact dermatitis from cosmetics in 29, while 25 others had rhinitis caused by cosmetic preparations [210]. Sunscreen preparations may produce allergic as well as photoallergic contact dermatitis at the sites of application.

Facial dermatitis can also be caused by allergens and irritants in face masks (surgical masks, scuba-diving masks, and masks worn to filter out dust or used to supply fresh air while working with dangerous substances) [211]. The contact pattern of the dermatitis characteristically follows the outline of the mask worn (Fig. 44). Nickel dermatitis, as illustrated in Fig. 21, is usually located at the site of specific contact with, for example, metal spectacle frames. The earlobe sign is a term used to describe facial dermatitis caused by substances applied to the face and neck with one hand. While there is dermatitis on the earlobe on the contralateral side of the hand used for application, the earlobe on the ipsilateral side is not involved [212].

Particular attention should be paid to three specific locations on the face and neck, as discussed below.

> ### Core Message
>
> ■ Photocontact dermatitis, airborne contact dermatitis, and cosmetic contact dermatitis are commonly seen on the face. Sesquiterpene lactones from plants, fragrances, and preservatives in cosmetics are common causes. Methyl dibromoglutaronitrile is a common contact allergen in cosmetics.

14.5.2.1 The Lips

On the lips, dermatitis may be caused by cosmetics and foods that make contact with the lips. Contact urticaria is commonly the cause when contact with certain foods results in cheilitis. The characteristic symptoms include stinging, burning, tingling, and itching of the lips seconds to minutes after contact with the offending item [213]. Similar symptoms may occur on the oral mucosa. Compositae plants such as lettuce may cause cheilitis in patients sensitive to sesquiterpene lactones [214].

Common causes of allergic contact cheilitis were reviewed by Ophaswongse and Maibach [215], and by Strauss and Orton [216]. Series of patients sensitive to volatile oils in toothpastes, to metals and to ingredients in lipsticks have also been reported [217–221].

14.5.2.2 The Eyes and Eyelids

The skin of the eyelid is very thin and delicate. It is covered by a coat of water-fast make-up by a large proportion of the female population, and the cosmetic products used for this purpose are often based on oils considered to be irritants.

Many people rub the eyelids frequently, and substances otherwise found on the hands are thereby transported to the eyelids. The classical site of allergic contact dermatitis caused by nail varnish is the face and, in particular, the eyelids [222]. The eyelids are also common sites of airborne and systemic contact dermatitis. It is therefore not surprising that eye-

14

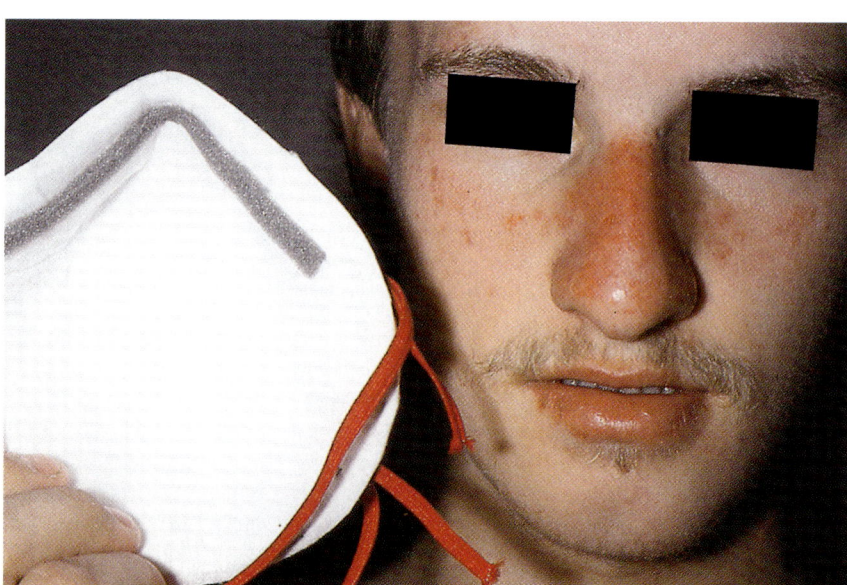

Fig. 44.
Allergic contact dermatitis due to formaldehyde in a protective mask

Fig. 45.
Eyelid eczema

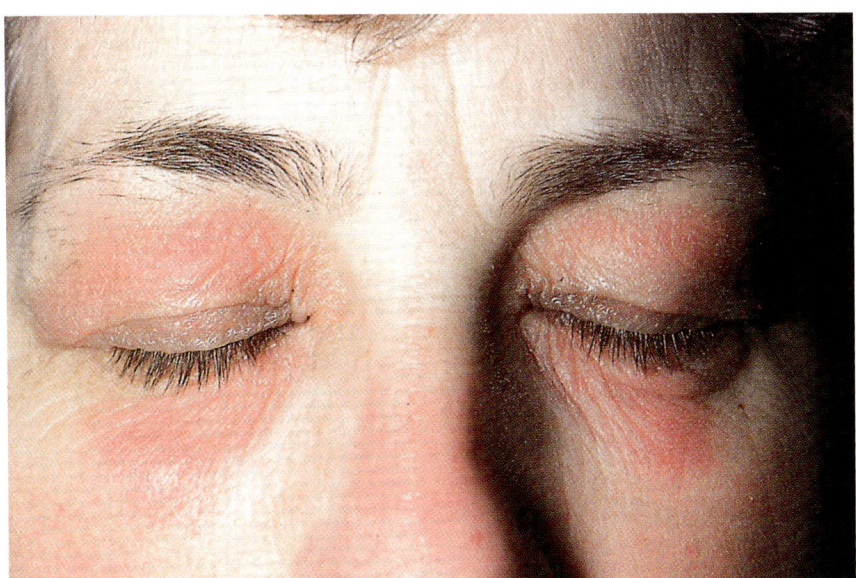

lid dermatitis is common and that it can have a multitude of causes [58, 223–226] (Fig. 45). Guin [227] found that 151 of 203 patients with eyelid dermatitis had allergic contact dermatitis. Forty-six had protein contact dermatitis, 23 had atopic dermatitis and 18 had seborrheic dermatitis or psoriasis. Ayala et al. [228] found that 50% of 447 patients with eyelid dermatitis had allergic contact dermatitis, most commonly caused by nickel, perfume, and cobalt; 21% had irritant contact dermatitis, 14% atopic dermatitis and 6% seborrheic dermatitis. The very loosely bound subcutis of the eyelid makes marked edema a characteristic feature of eyelid dermatitis.

Eyelid dermatitis has been used as a model for various enhanced patch test techniques such as patch testing on tape-stripped skin and patch testing on scarified skin. These techniques have been recommended for the detection of weak sensitizers such as eye medications used for prolonged periods of time [229].

Atopic persons frequently have fissured dermatitis of the upper eyelids, probably due to mechanical irritation from rubbing the eyes and from airborne irritants such as fibers from carpets, animal hair, and other sources. In patients sensitized to house dust mites and animal dander, contact urticaria on the eyelids may also be caused by these allergens.

Nickel dermatitis of the eyelids may be due to nickel in eyelid make-up or to the systemic administration of nickel, as evidenced by the flares seen after oral challenge with nickel. Shellac in mascara caused allergic contact dermatitis of the eyelids in six patients [230].

Topical ophthalmic products and preparations used in the care of contact lenses can cause contact dermatitis of the eyelids [231, 232]. Irritant contact conjunctivitis has been seen after the use of acrylic monomers found in printing inks [233], and after contact with calcium oxalate crystals from plants of the genus *Dieffenbachia* [234].

Core Message

- Irritant eyelid dermatitis is common in atopic persons. Irritants include eyelid make-up, dust, and irritants brought to the eyelid from the hands. Contact allergens include perfume and topical medicaments. Eyelid dermatitis may also be a manifestation of systemic contact dermatitis.

14.5.2.3 The Ear

There are three common causes of dermatitis of the ear. One of these is seborrheic dermatitis, often seen in conjunction with dermatitis of the scalp and face. This condition frequently recurs after periods of quiescence and may require long-term or intermittent treatment. Such treatment may result in sensitization and allergic contact dermatitis from topical medicaments [78–80].

A second major cause of dermatitis of the ear is objects or medicaments put into the ear. In a study involving a large number/series of patients, neomycin, framycetin and gentamicin were the most common sensitizers [235]. Corticosteroids have also caused external otitis [236]. Hairpins containing nickel used to relieve itching in the ear canal may cause allergic contact dermatitis. Matches containing chromate or phosphorus sesquisulfide may likewise cause allergic contact dermatitis of the external ear. Hearing aids rarely produce allergic contact dermatitis [237, 238] but can cause dermatitis as a result of occlusion, particularly in patients with seborrheic dermatitis.

The third type of dermatitis commonly found on the ear is earlobe dermatitis caused by nickel sensitization. In fact, today's most commonly described cause of nickel sensitization is earrings worn in pierced ears [65, 239]. There is sometimes a discrepancy between a history of dermatitis at sites which have been in contact with cheap jewelry and patch test results, which may be negative in spite of the repeated appearance of a rash after such jewelry is worn. One explanation for this discrepancy could be that nickel sensitization has not actually occurred and that the dermatitis is caused by irritancy or is some other nonimmunological reaction. Other possibilities are that sensitization has taken place, but that the patch test results were false negative [240]. Gold sensitization is statistically associated with ear piercing [241], and granulomatous dermatitis of the earlobe in a gold-sensitive person has been described [242]. Nickel-plated spectacle frames may cause dermatitis at the site of contact on the ear and nose, while dermatitis from plastic frames is rare [243].

Eight patients who had dermatitis on the ears had relevant positive patch tests to potassium dichromate. This substance was found in the casing of their cell phones [244].

Core Message

- The ears are classic sites of allergic contact dermatitis from medicaments used to treat external otitis as well as nickel dermatitis from cheap jewelry.

14.5.3 Dermatitis of the Trunk

The principal sensitizers causing dermatitis of the trunk are

- Nickel in brassiere straps, zippers and buttons.
- Rubber in the elastic of undergarments and other clothing (rubber items may cause contact urticaria as well as allergic contact dermatitis).
- Fragrances used in soaps, skin-care products, and detergents.
- Formaldehyde and other textile resins and dyes.

Textile fiber dermatitis is usually most pronounced at sites of intense contact with the fibers and at typical sweat retention sites such as the axillary folds, the sides of the neck, the waist, the inner aspects of the thighs, and the gluteal folds [245, 246]. In addition to the fibers themselves, the chemicals used to dye or improve the appearance of textiles may also cause dermatitis at the above-mentioned sites [247]. Of 6203 consecutively patch tested patients, 263 reacted to at least one azo dye used to dye textiles. Common sites of dermatitis were the neck and axillae [248]. This was also the case in 16 patients sensitized to various azo dyes [249]. Forty-nine patients with positive patch tests to textile dyes had dermatitis at various sites, including the hands, trunk, face, and feet [250]. Of 437 patients sensitive to azo dyes, most had dermatitis in areas in contact with clothing [251]. The incidence of textile dermatitis caused by the release of formaldehyde has decreased recently due to a reduction in the release of formaldehyde from fabrics [252].

New, unwashed, permanent-press sheets caused moderately pruritic burning papules of the helices and lobes of the ears, the cheeks and the sides of the neck in 25 patients. An irritant reaction to textile resins was thought to have caused the dermatitis [253]. Irritant contact dermatitis may be caused by detergents that have not been thoroughly rinsed out of clothing after washing. Children with atopic dermatitis are particularly susceptible to irritation from detergent residues.

Mechanical dermatitis caused by rough woolen fibers and various artificial fibers is common, particularly among atopics, who may also suffer from sweat retention dermatitis on the trunk. The pressure exerted by tight-fitting items of clothing such as girdles, brassieres, and belts can lead to dermatitis and hyperpigmentation. Similar dermatitis may be seen from safety shoes, particularly in atopics, and from face masks in pilots and firemen.

One distinct type of mechanical dermatitis of the upper back is a patch of excoriated dermatitis seen at the site of a label in a blouse. This condition is very common among patients with atopic dermatitis, but it also occurs in adults with no history of atopic dermatitis. The label causing the dermatitis is often

14

made of stiff artificial fibers, which cause pruritus in atopic patients and others with sensitive skin [254].

Another distinct type of clothing dermatitis is seen in patients who wear undergarments that have been machine washed together with textiles containing glass fiber, for example curtains, or work clothes contaminated with rock wool or glass fiber. The fibers bound in the undergarments may cause an intensely pruritic mechanical dermatitis at the sites of contact.

Rare causes of dermatitis of the trunk include contact with the electrode jelly used for electrocardiograms, rubber in electrodes used for electrocardiograms [255], tattoo pigment used for coloring the nipple after breast reconstruction following breast cancer [256], and transcutaneous drug delivery systems and ostomy bags (see Sect. 14.5.3.3 Stoma Dermatitis). Brassiere paddings with propylene glycol caused allergic contact dermatitis on one patient [257].

Dermatitis under swimwear may be "'seabather's eruption," a very pruritic papular dermatitis probably caused by the larvae of the sea anemone (*Edwardsiella lineata*) [258].

A papular dermatitis of the trunk of persons who bathed in hot sulfur springs was probably irritant contact dermatitis caused by sulfur or the acidity of the baths [259].

Core Message

■ Textile dermatitis and other types of clothing dermatitis are usually seen on the trunk, particularly in areas of skin in intense contact with the item of clothing in question. Allergic contact dermatitis from detergents is rare. Mechanical contact dermatitis from rough fibers, especially labels in clothing, is common.

14.5.3.1 The Axillary Region

There are certain types of dermatitis which are peculiar to the axillary region.

In view of the extensive use of antiperspirant products containing aluminum, aluminum allergy is rare. Aluminum sensitization has been seen largely as a consequence of the injection of vaccines precipitated with aluminum hydroxide, while dermatitis elicited by aluminum in antiperspirants is uncommon.

Of 20 patients with cosmetic dermatitis, 5 had axillary dermatitis due to the perfume in their deodorants or antiperspirants [260]. A history of axillary rash after the use of deodorant spray correlated well with fragrance allergy [18]. A similar correlation was seen between a history of a rash from scented products and fragrance allergy [261]. Fragrance dermatitis caused by deodorants and antiperspirants is characteristically seen in the entire axillary region. Dermatitis due to textile resins, on the other hand, is most intense in axillary folds and often does not affect the central area of the axilla. Dermatitis of the axillary folds caused by friction between clothes and the skin is common in patients with atopic dermatitis. It is possible that in the past the diagnosis of perfume dermatitis was obscured by the fact that a corticosteroid preparation used to suppress axillary eczema once contained perfume [262].

A form of contact dermatitis commonly seen in both the axillary and the genital area is caused by irritant reactions to chemical depilatory agents or various mechanical means of hair removal. Shaving off the pubic hair may cause pseudofolliculitis when regrowth occurs.

Core Message

■ A rash in the axillae after the use of deodorant sprays correlates well with fragrance allergy. Textile dermatitis is usually most intense in the axillary fold rather than in the central part of the axillae.

14.5.3.2 The Anogenital Region

The anogenital area is a common site of contact dermatitis [263]. This is due, among other things, to the fact that allergens and irritants can easily penetrate the delicate skin of this normally occluded area.

Age plays an important role in the development of anogenital contact dermatitis, as witnessed by the irritant contact dermatitis caused by urine and feces during the first years of life and also in the elderly incontinent [264]. In the elderly, mechanical pressure from sitting in a fixed position can cause characteristic, striated dermatitis on the sacral area ("grandfather's disease") (Fig. 46). Diapers may cause mechanical dermatitis as well as irritant contact dermatitis, but they rarely cause allergic contact dermatitis. In baby girls, dermatitis at the top of the vulval folds is

Fig. 46.
Pressure-induced, mechanical contact dermatitis with a peculiar linear pattern ("Grandfather's disease")

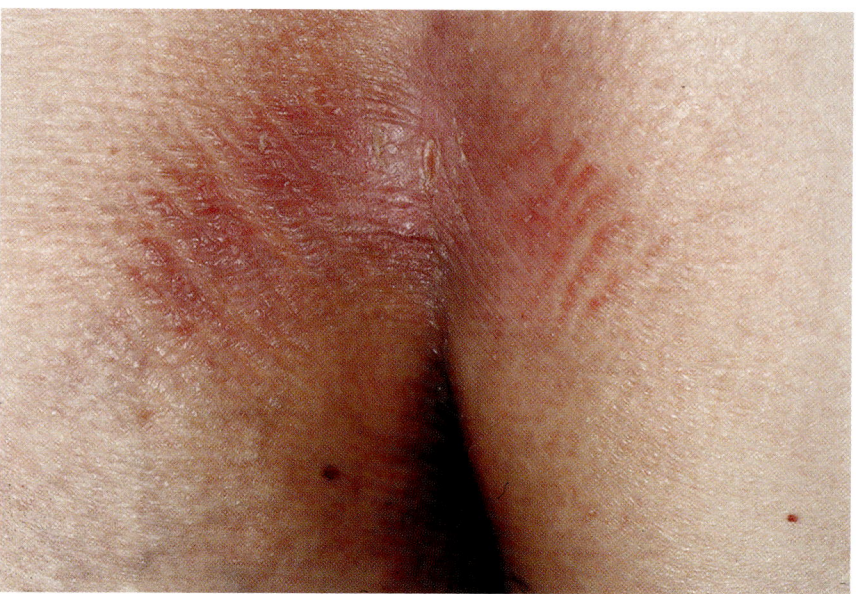

often considered to be evidence of dermatitis caused by diapers (W pattern) (Fig. 47), while dermatitis that is most intense in the vulval creases is more likely to be caused by microorganisms. "Lucky Luke" diaper dermatitis is an irritant diaper dermatitis [265].

Mothers tend to exchange disposable paper diapers for old-fashioned cloth diapers when diaper rash appears. This change is unnecessary and is, in fact, potentially harmful. A 26-week double-blind study of various diaper types used for infants with atopic dermatitis showed that the use of disposable diapers gave rise to diaper dermatitis less often than the use of conventional cloth diapers [266].

Among sexually active individuals, connubial dermatitis may occur in the vulval area and on the penis and scrotum, or even the face [267]. One characteristic of this dermatitis is that its activity fluctuates with the sexual activity of the patient. If connubial dermatitis in the male can be relieved by the use of a condom, this suggests that it is caused by substances applied to the vulva or vagina. Such substances include spermicidal creams, jellies or suppositories, the fragrances in creams and cleansing agents, and the rubber in diaphragms. Microorganisms in the vagina such as *Candida albicans* commonly cause transient balanitis in the male.

14

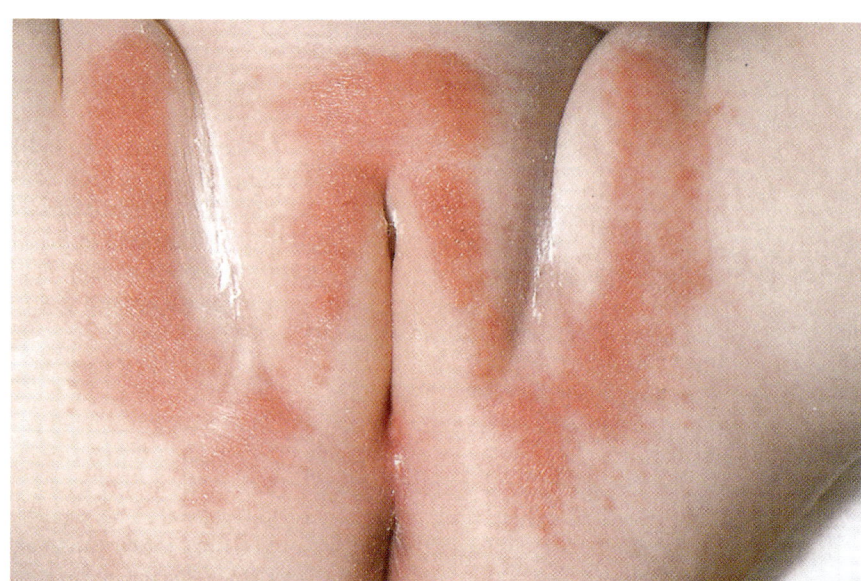

Fig. 47.
Irritant diaper dermatitis ("W-dermatitis")

Vulvitis is less frequently relieved by the use of a condom. Females have been observed to suffer from contact urticaria caused by semen. This is an important entity, as anaphylactoid reactions have occurred [113, 268]. Allergic contact dermatitis from semen has also been described [269].

Pruritus vulvae may be associated with allergic contact dermatitis [270–272], while vulval vestibulitis has not been associated with relevant contact allergy [273]. A history of atopy and seborrheic dermatitis are important endogenous causes of vulvar dermatitis [274].

Other dermatological problems associated with sexual activity include traumatic lesions such as fissures, erosions or even ulcers caused by the friction of intense sexual activity, lack of lubrication or bizarre habits. In both sexes a mechanical Köbner phenomenon may cause eruptions or aggravation of psoriasis lesions on the genitals. Lichen planus is common on the penis, and the Köbner phenomenon may delay clearing of this disease. Lichen simplex chronicus of the vulva may remain active due to sexual activity. A particular problem in males is sclerosing lymphangitis of the penile lymph vessels. This condition is commonly considered to be traumatic.

In addition to problems related to sexual activity, dermatitis on the genitals may be caused by substances normally found on the hands, which have been transferred to the genitals. In males this type of dermatitis may present as allergic contact dermatitis caused, for example, by sawdust or preservatives in paints [86]. Females may develop irritant or allergic contact dermatitis of the vulva or perianal area following contact with nail polish or colophony in sanitary pads [275, 276].

Widespread pruritus and dermatitis with features similar to those of systemically induced contact dermatitis appeared following the introduction of intrauterine contraceptive devices made of copper [277]. Sensitivity to copper is unusual, and this may not be the sole explanation of these symptoms.

Another curious eruption in the anogenital and bikini area is the "baboon syndrome" described in Chap. 16.

Allergic and/or irritant contact dermatitis in the anogenital area is often caused by the topical application of various medicaments. A wide range of compounds can cause such reactions, including antifungal agents used to combat dermatophyte infections and candidiasis, as well as hemorrhoid remedies and agents used to relieve anogenital pruritus. Some of the sensitizing agents commonly used in this area of the body are benzocaine, neomycin, the hydroxyquinolines and bufexamac [78–80, 270–272, 278]. Recy-cled paper used for toilet paper may contain up to 5–10 mg nickel per kg [279].

Ingested irritants and sensitizers may cause pruritus and contact dermatitis in the perianal region. The mechanism here may be the deposition of the suspected substance on perianal skin. In some situations, however, systemically induced contact dermatitis or other systemic mechanisms may be to blame, as in the case of coffee drinker's rash [280]. The anal pruritus seen after oral challenge with nickel or Balsam of Peru may be due to unabsorbed substances in the feces present in higher concentrations than those normally experienced [139].

Core Message

■ In infants and incontinent adults, the anogenital region is exposed to irritants. Irritant dermatitis may also result from intense cleansing of the area. Allergic contact dermatitis from topical medicaments is common in the perianal region.

14.5.3.3 Stoma Dermatitis

Excretions from a stoma may cause dermatitis when irritant substances come into contact with skin which is not suited for such contact. Incorrectly attached ostomy bags may be responsible. Leakage from ileostomies is potentially the most irritating, as the feces are rather liquid and may contain enzymes and other irritants that would normally be degraded during passage through the colon and rectum [281, 282]. The materials used for the stoma appliances themselves, or their adhesive surfaces, are today so well researched and carefully selected that they rarely cause sensitization or irritation [283]. An important exception was noted by Beck et al. [284], who discovered low-molecular-weight epoxy resin in a type of ostomy bag which sensitized six patients. A similar patient was described by Mann et al. [285].

Dermatological problems in connection with the use of ostomy bags may also be due to sweat retention in the area of the stoma or under the bag itself if this makes direct contact with the skin [286]. Rothstein [287] has provided a detailed review of the problems associated with stoma care and their management.

Core Message

■ Stoma dermatitis is more commonly
   due to ill-fitting ostomy bags with leakage
   of intestinal content or to sweat retention
   than to allergic contact dermatitis.

14.5.4 Dermatitis of the Legs

Dermatitis of the thighs may be clinically characterized by patches of eczema at sites where pockets make contact with the skin. Persons who normally carry nickel-plated items, "strike-anywhere" matches containing phosphorus sesquisulfide, or matches with heads containing chromium in their pockets may suffer from dermatitis of the thighs. Follicular dermatitis on the anterior aspects of the thighs is a typical consequence of wearing trousers that have become soaked with splashing cutting oil or caked with oil rubbed off the hands.

Thirty-three patients developed allergic contact dermatitis to a modified colophonium derivative in an epilating agent used on the legs [288].

The dermatitis occasionally seen on the stump of a femur amputee has several possible causes. Among the most common are friction and pressure exerted on specific skin areas due to an ill-fitting prosthesis or insufficient tissue under the distal tip of the femur bone. In such situations there may also be trophic disturbance of the skin overlying the bone. Irritant contact dermatitis and dermatitis due to sweat retention under the prosthesis may also occur, even when it fits well [289].

Allergic contact dermatitis may be caused by materials in the prostheses themselves or by substances used under them [290, 291].

Dermatitis at the site of, or in close proximity to, varicose veins is an early indication of stasis dermatitis (Fig. 48). This type of dermatitis tends to become chronic, and eventually the pattern of dermatitis becomes less characteristic (Fig. 49). Trophic disturbance, often aggravated by the edema of the lower leg typical of patients with varicose veins, is probably an etiological factor. Patients with stasis dermatitis may develop venous leg ulcers.

The chronicity of leg ulcers and stasis dermatitis, in combination with the occlusive bandages applied to afflicted legs, makes this area a rival to the anogenital region as the most common site of allergic contact dermatitis caused by topical medicaments [292–294]. Unless a short course of treatment can be anticipated, the selection of agents for the topical treatment of stasis dermatitis should be made with emphasis on substances that rarely sensitize.

Of 1,270 patients with leg ulcers, 106 patients had positive patch tests to colophonium and/or ester gum resin. Had ester gum resin not been used for testing, the diagnosis of 47 patients would not have been based on a relevant positive patch test [295].

Stocking dermatitis is seen in those areas with the most intense contact with stockings or socks [248, 249, 296]. Rubber dermatitis due to the elastic in

14

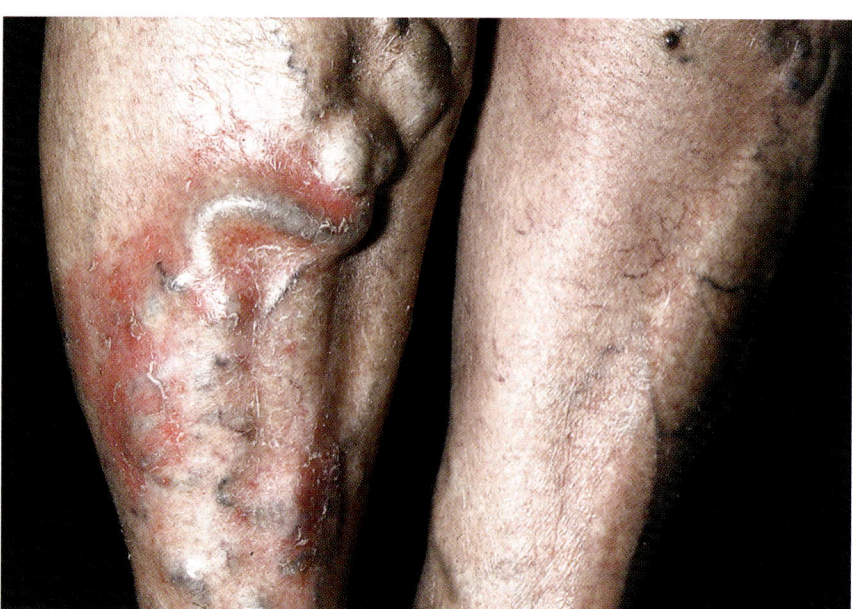

Fig. 48.
Early stasis dermatitis

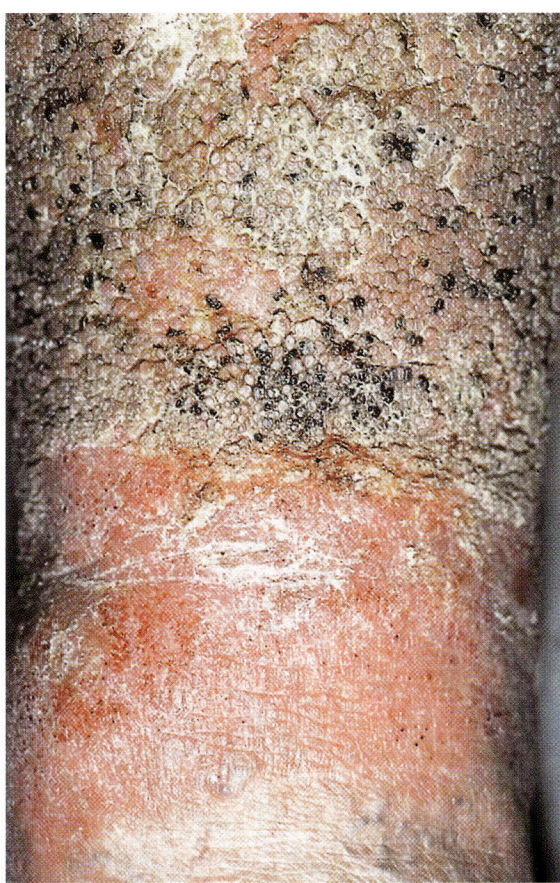

Fig. 49. Chronic stasis dermatitis

14.5.5 Dermatitis of the Feet

Dermatitis of the feet presents with specific characteristic clinical patterns at, for example, the points of shoe contact, primarily on the dorsal aspects of the feet and toes and on the sides of the feet. This dermatitis rarely appears on the sides of the toes or in the plantar flexure creases of the toes. Rubber chemicals, in particular mercaptobenzothiazole, glues such as *p-tert*-butylphenolformaldehyde, and chromates, are commonly the cause of allergic footwear dermatitis [298–302]. Seventeen men who wore the same type of socks at work developed foot dermatitis caused by basic red 46 in the socks [303]. Frictional dermatitis on the dorsal aspects of the toes, usually on the big toes, may be seen in children with atopic dermatitis.

One type of dermatitis which is specific to children is juvenile plantar dermatosis. Although the etiology of this dermatitis is unknown, friction and pressure probably play significant roles in the pathogenesis, as illustrated in Fig. 50 [304–306]. In this patient the dermatitis appeared only on the weight-bearing aspects of the soles. There are two character-

men's socks occurs in a limited area of the lower legs, while nylon stocking dermatitis may appear on the medial aspects of the thighs as well as in the popliteal fossae and on the feet. Shoe dermatitis may mimic stocking dermatitis on the feet, and mercaptobenzothiazole leached from shoes has been shown to accumulate in socks [297]. Children with atopic dermatitis often develop irritant contact dermatitis from synthetic fibers in tights (panty hose), wool in leggings or rubber chemicals in the shin protectors used by football players. Obese children, in particular, may also develop friction dermatitis on the medial aspects of the thighs.

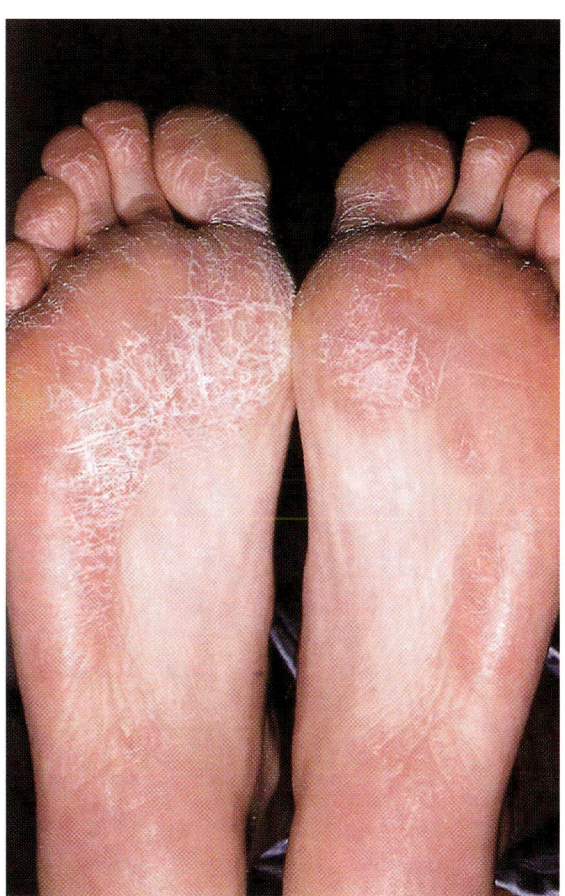

Fig. 50. Juvenile plantar dermatosis in pressure areas on the soles

Core Message

■ The lower leg is a prime site of allergic contact dermatitis from topical medicaments, particularly in leg ulcer patients. Textile dermatitis may be seen under socks and on the thighs. Detergents and mineral oils in work clothes may cause irritant dermatitis.

istic morphologies of plantar dermatoses in addition to juvenile plantar dermatitis. These are recurrent, pruritic, vesicular plantar dermatitis and hyperkeratotic eczema.

14.5.5.1 Recurrent, Pruritic, Vesicular, Plantar Dermatitis

This dermatitis consists of crops of vesicles in the central part of the sole and sometimes also on the sides of the toes. If frequent eruptions occur, this dermatitis may appear to be a chronic eczematous condition. This plantar eruption is less common than an eruption of similar morphology that appears on the hands. It is not usually possible to identify the etiology of the dermatitis, although it has been reproduced by oral challenge with metal salts in some patients with positive patch tests to the same substances, and even in some patch-test-negative patients [33].

14.5.5.2 Hyperkeratotic Plantar Eczema

Hyperkeratotic eczema consists of well-demarcated plaques of hyperkeratosis, often with painful fissures (Fig. 51). It is commonly associated with similar lesions on the palms. For further details, see Sect. 14.4.1.5 Hyperkeratotic Eczema.

> **Core Message**
>
> ■ Allergic contact dermatitis on the feet may be due to dichromates in leather, to rubber chemicals in shoes, or to dyes in socks.

14.5.6 Dermatitis of the Arms

There are two main sites of dermatitis of the arms. One is the antecubital fossa, which is a typical site of sweat retention dermatitis, atopic dermatitis, and secondary nickel dermatitis. The other is the forearm, to which hand dermatitis frequently spreads. Eczema of the forearm with no involvement of the hands can be seen in occupational eczema caused by dust, detergents, isocyanate lacquer [307], and the juices of meat and fish. Isothiazolinones caused allergic contact dermatitis of the forearms of one patient (Fig. 52).

Tattoos are commonly placed on the upper arm. Modern tattoo pigments rarely sensitize. Patchy Red 904A and DC 99060 each caused allergic contact dermatitis in one tattooed person [308, 309].

14

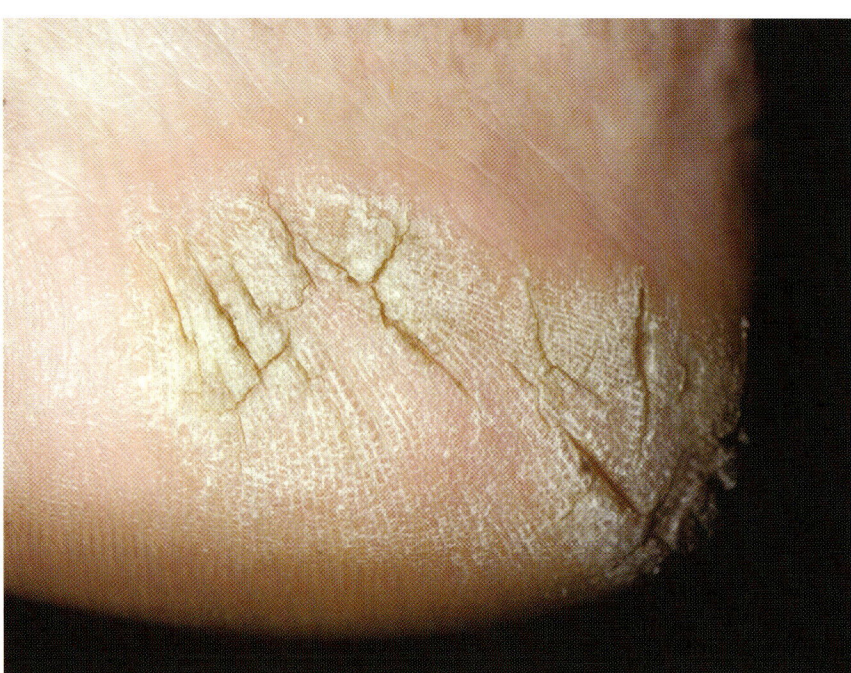

Fig. 51.
Fissured, hyperkeratotic eczema on a heel

Fig. 52.
Allergic contact dermatitis
on the arms caused by the
preservative MCI/MI
(5-chloro-2-methylisothiazol-
3-one/2-methylisothiazol-3-
one or Kathon CG) in an
emollient

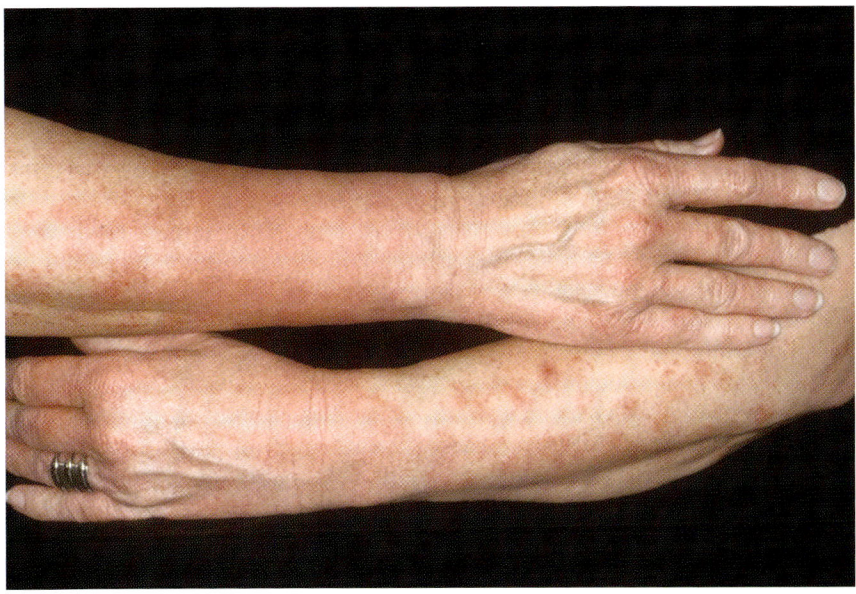

14.5.7 Contact Stomatitis

The metals and plastics used in dentistry may cause
allergic contact stomatitis. Erythema, lichen planus-
like lesions and erosion and ulceration of the oral
mucosa have been linked to mercury allergy elicited
by mercury in amalgam dental fillings and to gold
[310–318]. Grayish streaks on the buccal mucosa at
the sites of contact with amalgam dental fillings in
patients who have positive patch tests to mercury
salts certainly suggest a causative relationship
(Fig. 53). The relationship is less clear if the oral lesions are not directly in contact with metals in the
mouth [319, 320].

Of a group of 67 patients with atrophic-erosive
oral lichen planus, 17% had positive patch tests to
mercury compounds, compared with 8% of a reference group [321]. In another group of 29 patients with
similar symptoms, 18 patients (62%) had contact allergy to mercury compared with 3.2% of a control
group. For three of the patients, the symptoms disappeared after removal of all amalgam dental fillings

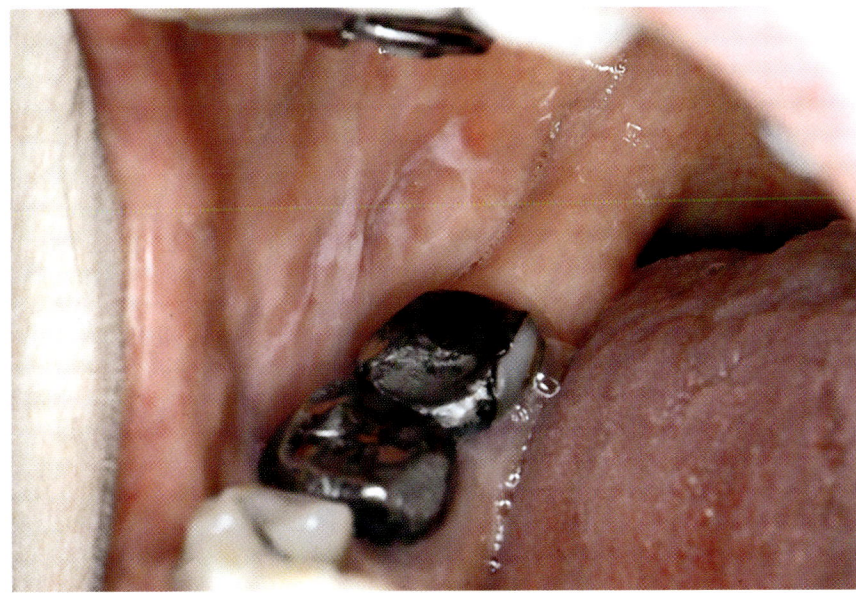

Fig. 53.
Lichen planus-like stomatitis
adjacent to amalgam dental
fillings in a mercury-sensitive person

[322]. Sensitization to mercury and systemic toxicity of amalgam dental restorations are subjects still open to discussion [323].

It has been suggested that dental braces made of steel and containing nickel, cobalt and/or chromium are sometimes responsible for systemic contact dermatitis [324, 325]. In view of the common use of dental plates and their intense contact with the oral mucosa, sensitization to such plates is rare [326]. Dental technicians who manufacture the uncured dental plates may, however, become sensitized to the acrylic materials they handle.

Flavorings added to toothpaste may also cause contact stomatitis. Common causes of contact stomatitis and cheilitis have been reviewed by Fisher [327] and Chan and Mowad [328]. Foodstuffs rarely cause allergic contact stomatitis, but contact urticaria of the oral mucosa caused by foods is common. Sonnex et al. [329] described a patient with contact stomatitis from coffee. The term "oral allergy syndrome" has been proposed to describe immediate-type reactions which include irritation of the oral mucosa shortly after the ingestion of certain foods [30, 31]. Cross-sensitivity between pollen and food allergens may precipitate such symptoms. The burning mouth syndrome is a poorly understood entity, which may be caused by a number of factors including systemic diseases, psychological stress and, occasionally, contact sensitivity [330].

Core Message

■ Lichen planus-like grayish streaks on the buccal mucosa adjacent to dental fillings can be caused by mercury or gold in the fillings. Stomatitis from acrylates in dental prostheses is rare.

14.5.8 Dermatitis Caused by Items Within the Body

Implanted items such as pacemakers have been blamed for widespread pruritic dermatitis and for eczema and bullous eruptions on the skin overlying them. The etiology of such dermatitis is uncertain, but traces of metals, and in some cases epoxy resin, released from the case of the pacemaker have been suggested as a cause of these rare reactions [331, 332]. Copper intrauterine devices have been blamed for similar types of dermatitis [277], as have metal orthodontic braces [324].

Nickel wiring left in the tissues following surgery may give rise to dermatitis of the skin overlying these tissues or to vesicular hand eczema. Such dermatitis has also been seen in sensitized individuals whose fractures have been set with metal plates and screws, and in a patient who had shrapnel fragments left in the tissues [333].

Artificial hip joints are now primarily of the metal-to-plastic type and rarely give rise to allergic reactions [333].

Widespread dermatitis and vesicular hand eczema have been seen in patients who have swallowed coins containing nickel. The dermatitis faded when the coins were removed [334].

The tattoo pigments used today rarely lead to sensitization, but one study described a granulomatous reaction in a tattoo caused by aluminum [335], and Patchy Red 904A caused allergic contact dermatitis in one patient [308].

Metals in the oral cavity are dealt with in Sect. 14.5.7 Contact Stomatitis.

14.6 Differential Diagnosis

Two main groups of diseases should be considered in the differential diagnosis when dealing with possible contact dermatitis, namely:

■ Other types of eczema.
■ Noneczematous dermatoses which have clinical features similar to those of contact dermatitis.

Atopic dermatitis may have a number of features in common with contact dermatitis, and contact dermatitis is commonly superimposed on atopic dermatitis. One example of this is "head and neck dermatitis" which has already been described as a contact urticaria reaction caused by *Pityrosporum ovale*.

Lichen simplex chronicus (neurodermatitis) and nummular eczemas are morphological terms used to describe eczema which may be endogenous, the nummular eczema often with superimposed bacterial infection (Fig. 54). Lichen simplex chronicus may be mechanically aggravated by, for example, rubbing a foot on the eczematous plaque. (Figs. 55) [38]. The patch testing of 48 patients with discoid eczema gave 16 relevant reactions, but this was not reproduced by other studies [336]. There is some evidence of a connection between discoid eczema and alcohol dependence.

Seborrheic dermatitis is usually so characteristic that it presents no diagnostic difficulty but, when there is facial and anogenital involvement, seborrhe-

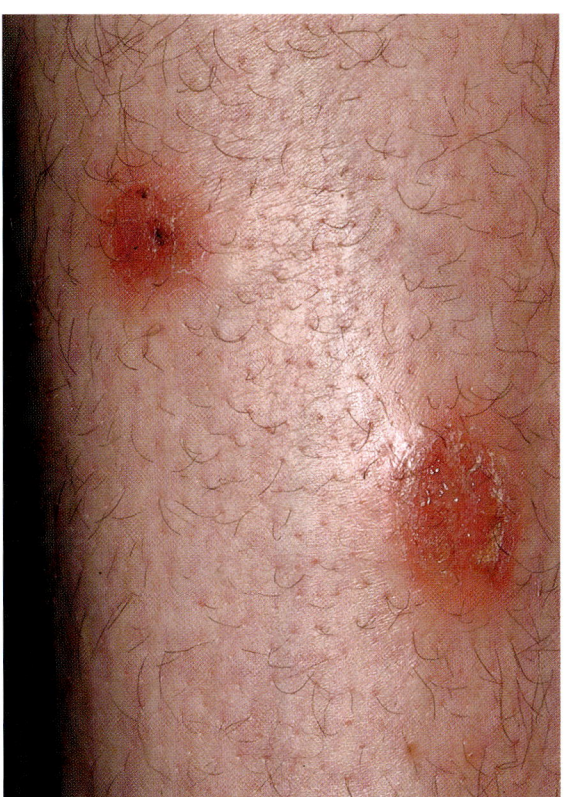

Fig. 54. Nummular eczema on the lower leg

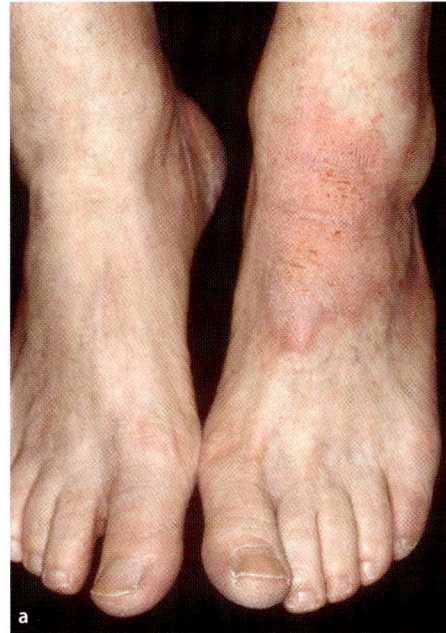

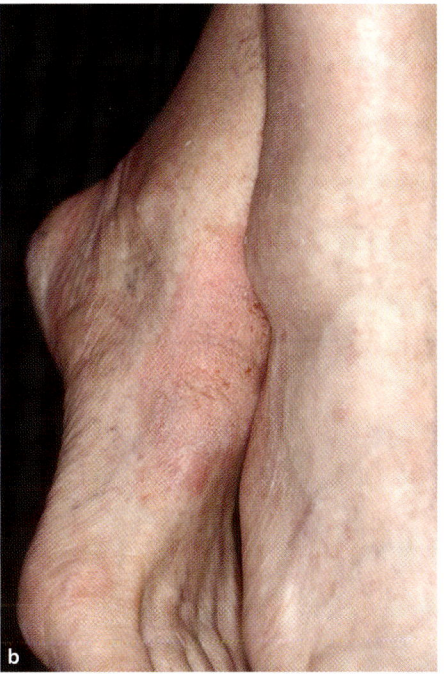

Fig. 55a, b. Lichen simplex chronicus of the left ankle (a) maintained by rubbing the right heel against the area of dermatitis (b)

ic dermatitis can be difficult to distinguish from contact dermatitis and from psoriasis. The term sebopsoriasis has been coined to describe dermatitis with features of both psoriasis and seborrheic dermatitis [337, 338]. Low-humidity dermatoses may have clinical features similar to those of seborrheic dermatitis of the face [36] and may also mimic lichen simplex chronicus of the lower leg [339]. Eczematous eruptions associated with rare metabolic diseases such as acrodermatitis enteropathica, other zinc deficiency syndromes or phenylketonuria may also mimic contact dermatitis.

Pityriasis alba may be mistaken for contact dermatitis, but is morphologically characteristic with dry patches of eczema on the cheeks and/or upper arms followed by post-inflammatory hypopigmentation (Fig. 56). Asteatotic eczema is seen mainly in elderly persons due to xerosis of the skin. Hailey–Hailey disease, as well as intertrigo, may mimic contact dermatitis and acrodermatitis continua. Acrodermatitis continua Hallopeau and palmoplantar pustulosis may have clinical features similar to those of contact dermatitis.

Most cases of psoriasis and hyperkeratotic eczema are easily recognized as distinct entities, but psoria-

sis on the hands may be difficult to distinguish from contact dermatitis (Fig. 57). Köbner-induced psoriasis at the site of nickel contact in a nickel-sensitive person is another difficult differential diagnosis. Occasionally, patients with psoriasis may have relevant positive patch tests [340, 341].

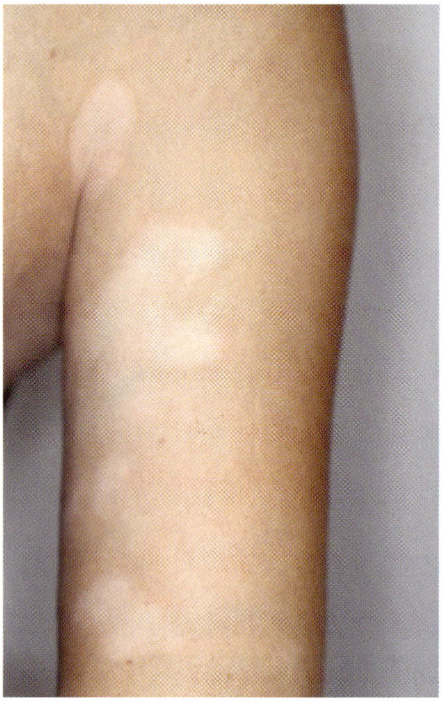

Fig. 56. Pityriasis alba of the upper arm with central post-inflammatory hypopigmentation and discrete dermatitis at the periphery of the lesions

Collagenoses such as lupus erythematosus of the palms may have eczematous features similar to those of contact dermatitis.

It calls for a high degree of suspicion to make a correct diagnosis of Norwegian scabies, which, clinically, can mimic contact dermatitis.

Another important differential diagnosis is dermatophytosis, particularly when there is involvement of the feet or when *Trichophyton rubrum* has infected the skin of the hands (Fig. 58). The diagnostic problems increase if the dermatophytosis has been treated with topical steroids. Dermatophytids on the fingers resulting from plantar dermatophytosis are clinically indistinguishable from vesicles associated with other causes, such as systemic contact dermatitis [117]. This supports the view that a vesicular eruption on the fingers is a nonspecific reaction pattern that may have a number of different causes. Examples are lichen planus [342], cutaneous T-cell lymphoma [343] and bullous pemphigoid (Fig. 59). Palmar lichen planus can also have a striking resemblance to hand eczema (Fig. 60).

Dysplasias such as actinic keratoses and in situ tumors such as Bowen's disease may mimic contact dermatitis (Fig. 61).

A diagnosis of contact dermatitis cannot be made by means of histological examination of a biopsy specimen. Nonetheless, a biopsy may be a useful tool in making this diagnosis, as it will enable the exclusion of a number of the above-mentioned diseases that have specific histological features.

Core Message

■ Contact dermatitis may be mimicked by other types of dermatitis such as seborrheic dermatitis, atopic dermatitis, and nummular dermatitis. Tinea, particularly in the face or perianal regions, is an important differential diagnosis together with Bowen's disease, in particular on the fingers.

14

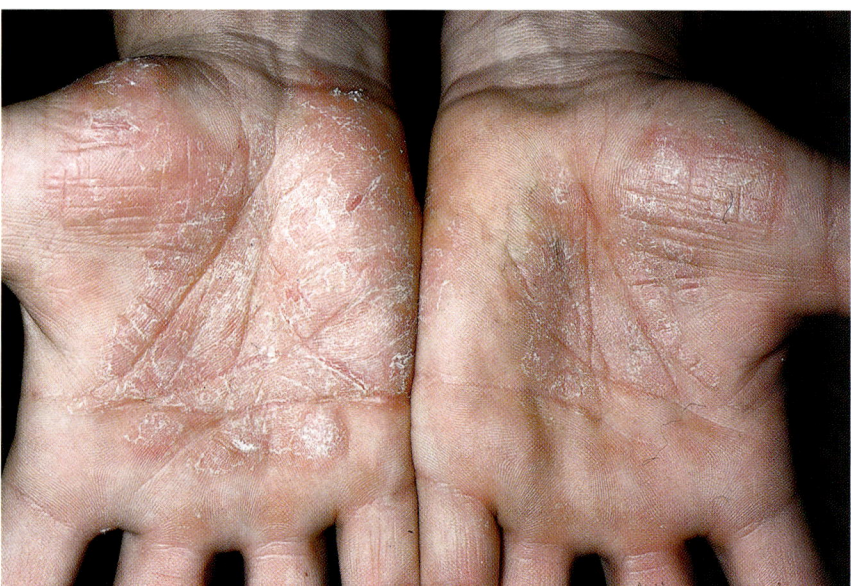

Fig. 57.
Psoriasis on the hands

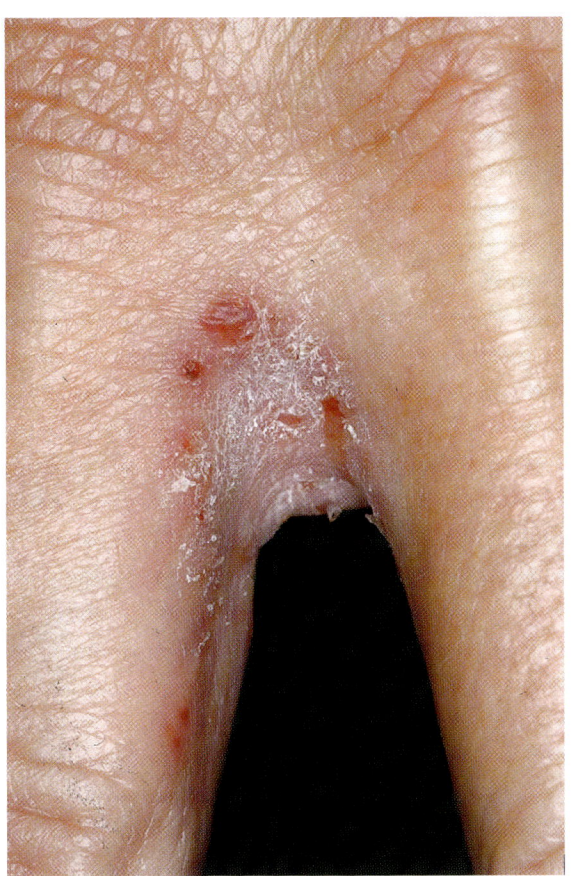

Fig. 58. Dermatophyte infection on a finger web

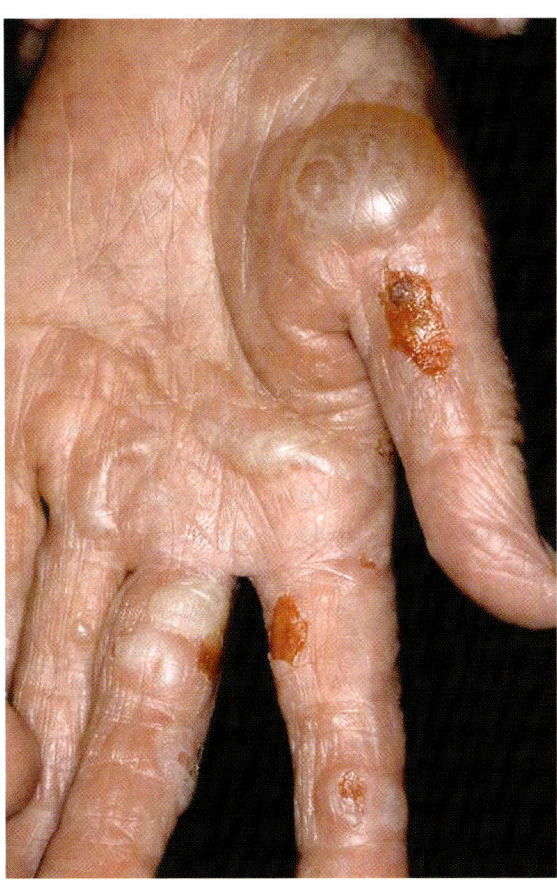

Fig. 59. Bullous pemphigoid presenting with vesicular and bullous lesions on the hands

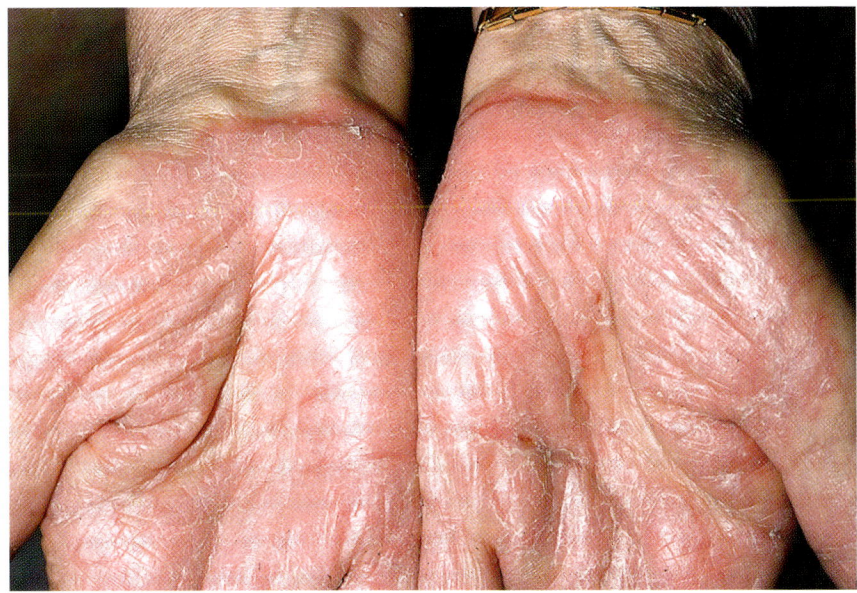

Fig. 60.
Lichen planus of the palms

Fig. 61.
Bowen's disease on a finger

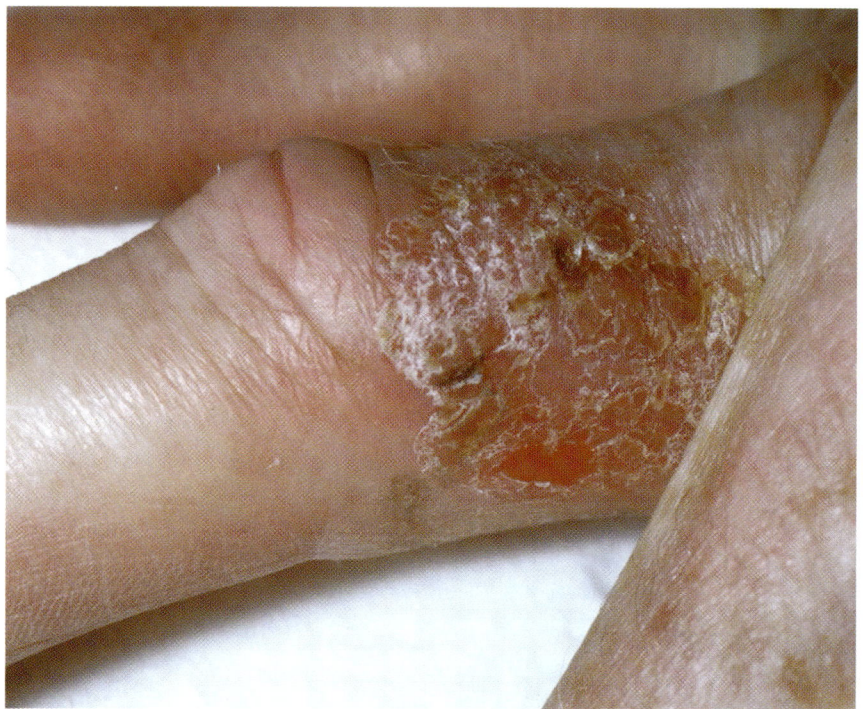

14.7 Case Reports

Case Reports

■ **1.** A 47-year-old woman had worked as a flower vendor in a supermarket for 15 years. She was seen because she had developed dermatitis on her hands and forearms, particularly on the right side (Fig. 62).

Patch testing with the European Standard Series showed a ++ reaction to primin. While discussing the relevance of this test, she remembered that a different type of primula had been introduced in the store where she worked.

She brought a plant to our clinic, and we identified it as *Primula obconica* (Fig. 63). A close-up of a leaf of this plant shows the spicules that contain primin (Fig. 64).

■ **Comment:** Most positive patch tests to primin are seen in older women, and the reaction is most often of past relevance. A low-allergenic *Primula obconica* has been developed, and contact allergy to primin should become a thing of the past.

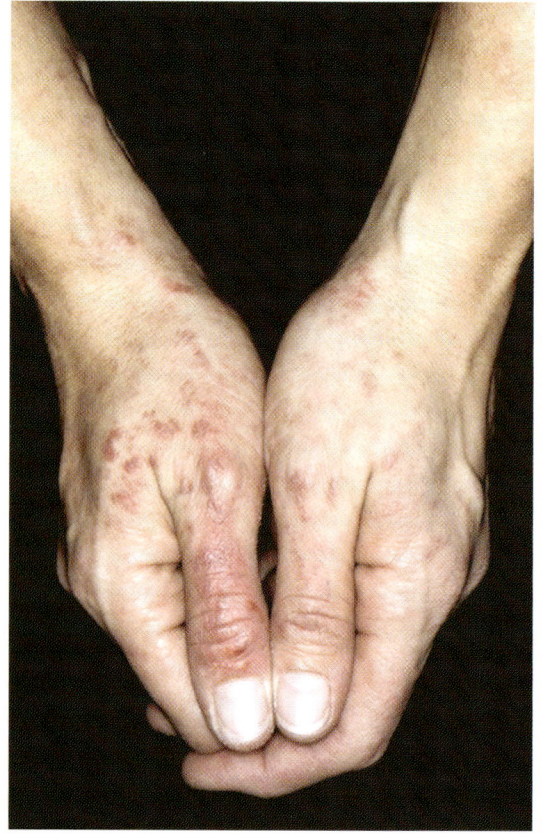

Fig. 62. Allergic contact dermatitis caused by *Primula obconica,* mostly on the right hand

14

Fig. 63.
Primula obconica

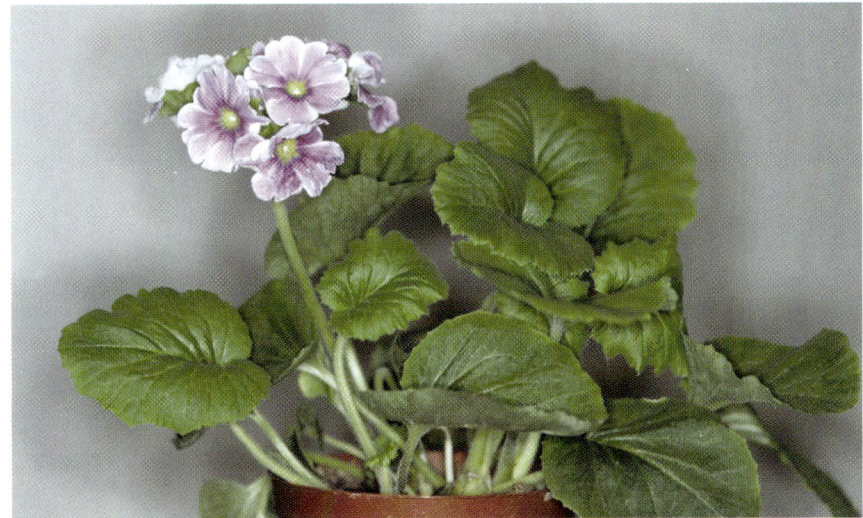

Fig. 64.
Tiny spicules on a leaf of
Primula obconica

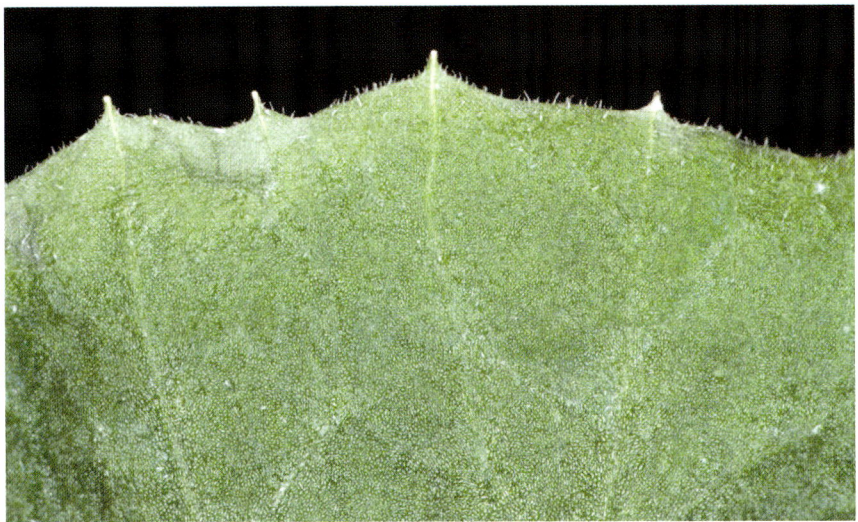

■ **2.** A family of four had a 1-week vacation in Turkey. After their return, 5-year-old twin sons developed intense dermatitis at the sites of temporary tattoos they had made during the holiday (Figs. 65, 66). Both the boys had positive patch tests to para-phenylene diamine. One of the boys subsequently developed an id-like eruption on the trunk (Fig. 67a). Curiously, the eruption was seen on areas of the skin that had not been exposed to the sun (Fig. 67b). The eruption became so intense that a short course of systemic steroid was necessary to suppress the symptoms.

■ **Comment:** It is well known that the colors used to make temporary so-called henna tattoos often contain paraphenylene diamine. In this case, twins became sensitized to paraphenylene diamine, and one of them developed a widespread id-like eruption.

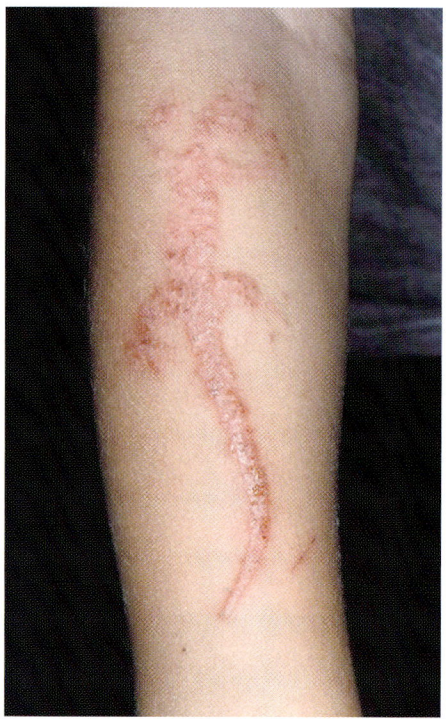

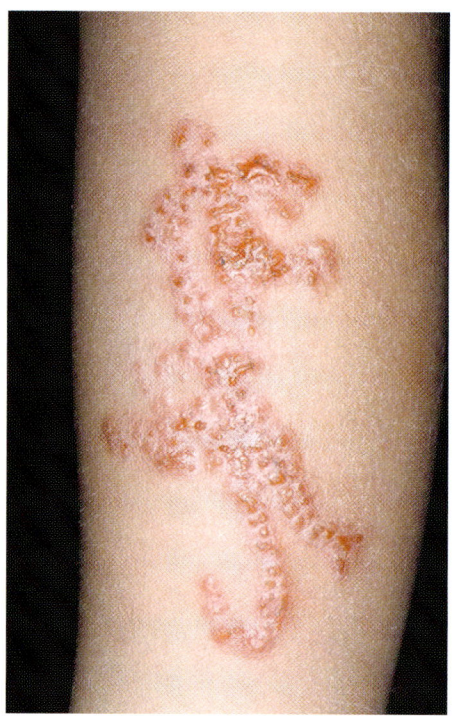

Fig. 65. Allergic contact dermatitis on the forearm of one of 5-year-old twin boys after a temporary, black "Henna" tattoo

Fig. 66. Allergic contact dermatitis on the forearm of the other twin

14

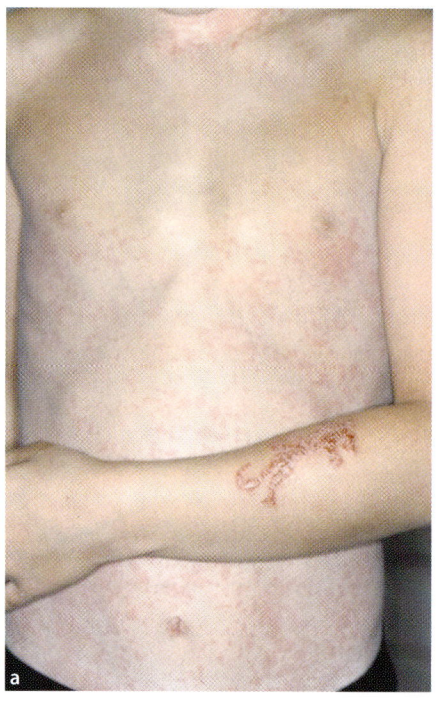

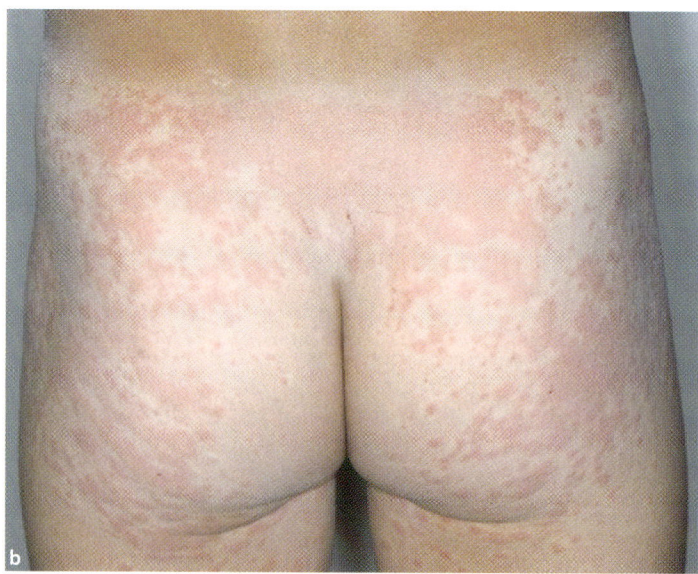

Fig. 67a, b. The twin in Fig. 66 developed an id-like eruption on the trunk (a). The eruption was most predominant on skin that was not exposed to the sun (b)

References

1. Armstrong DKB, Walsh MY, Dawson JF (1997) Granulomatous contact dermatitis due to gold earrings. Br J Dermatol 136:776–778
2. Evans AV, Banerjee P, McFadden JP, Calonje E (2003) Lymphomatoid contact dermatitis to para-tertyl-butyl phenol resin. Clin Exp Dermatol 28:272–273
3. Blum R, Baum HP, Ponnighaus M, Kowalzick L (2003) Sarcoidal allergic contact dermatitis due to palladium following ear piercing (in German). Hautarzt 54:160–162
4. Möller H, Ohlsson K, Linder C, Björkner B, Bruze M (1998) Cytokines and acute phase reactants during flareup of contact allergy to gold. Am J Contact Dermat 9:15–22
5. Möller H, Björkner B, Bruze M (1996) Clinical reactions to systemic provocation with gold sodium thiomalate in patients with contact allergy to gold. Br J Dermatol 135:423–427
6. Fisher AA (1987) Contact urticaria and anaphylactoid reaction due to corn starch surgical glove powder. Contact Dermatitis 16:224–235
7. Van der Meeren HLM, van Erp PEJ (1986) Life-threatening contact urticaria from glove powder. Contact Dermatitis 14:190–191
8. Rystedt I (1985) Hand eczema and long-term prognosis in atopic dermatitis (dissertation). Department of Occupational Dermatology, National Board of Occupational Safety and Health and Karolinska Hospital, Karolinska Institute, Stockholm
9. Darsow U, Vieluf D, Ring J (1999) Evaluating the relevance of aeroallergen sensitization in atopic eczema with the atopy patch test: a randomized, double-blind multicenter study. J Am Acad Dermatol 40:187–193
10. Tan BB, Weald D, Strickland I, Friedmann PS (1996) Double-blind controlled trial of effect of housedust-mite allergen avoidance on atopic dermatitis. Lancet 347:15–18
11. Thelin I, Agrup G (1985) Pompholyx – a one year series. Acta Derm Venereol (Stockh) 65:214–217
12. Schwanitz HJ (1986) Das Atopische Palmoplantarekzem. Springer, Berlin Heidelberg New York
13. Edman B (1988) Palmar eczema: a pathogenetic role for acetylsalicylic acid, contraceptives and smoking? Acta Derm Venereol (Stockh) 68:402–407
14. Menné T (1983) Nickel allergy. Dissertation, University of Copenhagen
15. Ancona A, Fernandez-Diez J, Bellamy C (1986) Occupationally induced psoriasis. Derm Beruf Umwelt 34:71–73
16. Rothenborg HW, Andersen HB (1993) Alcohol and skin disorders. J Eur Acad Dermatol Venereol 2:113–120
17. Menné T, Veien N, Sjølin K-E, Maibach HI (1994) Systemic contact dermatitis. Am J Contact Dermat 5:1–12
18. Johansen JD, Andersen TF, Kjoller M, Veien, N, Avnstorp C, Andersen KE, Menné T (1998) Identification of risk products for fragrance contact allergy: a case-referent study based on patients' histories. Am J Contact Dermat 9:80–86
19. Linneberg A, Nielsen NH, Menné T, Madsen F, Jørgensen T (2003) Smoking might be a risk factor for contact allergy. J Allergy Clin Imunol 111:980–984
20. Niemeier V, Nippesen M, Kupfer J, Schill WB, Gieler U (2002) Psychological factors associated with hand dermatoses: which subgroup needs additional psychological care? Br J Dermatol 146:1031–1037
21. Dooms-Goosens AE, Debusschere KM, Gevers DM et al (1986) Contact dermatitis caused by airborne agents. J Am Acad Dermatol 15:1–11
22. Uter W, Geier J, Land M, Pfahlberg A, Gefeller O, Schnuch A (2001) Another look at seasonal variation in patch test results. A mulifactorial analysis of surveillance data of the IVDK. Contact Dermatitis 44:146–152
23. Veien NK, Hattel T, Laurberg G (1992) Is patch testing a less accurate tool during the summer months? Am J Contact Dermat 3:35–36
24. Malten KE (1981) Thoughts on irritant contact dermatitis. Contact Dermatitis 7:238–247
25. Frosch PJ, Kligman AM (1977) A method for appraising the stinging capacity of topically applied substances. J Soc Cosmet Chem 28:197–209
26. Clemmensen O, Hjorth N (1982) Perioral contact urticaria from sorbic acid and benzoic acid in a salad dressing. Contact Dermatitis 8:1–6
27. Andersen KE, Løwenstein H (1978) An investigation of the possible immunological relationship between allergen extracts from birch pollen, hazelnut, potato and apple. Contact Dermatitis 4:73–79
28. Murphy GM, Rycroft RJG (1989) Allergic contact dermatitis from silver birch pollen. In: Frosch PJ, Dooms-Goosens A, Lachapelle J-M, Rycroft RJG, Scheper RJ (eds) Current topics in contact dermatitis. Springer, Berlin Heidelberg New York, pp 146–148
29. Koh D, Goh CL, Tan HTW, Ng SK, Wong WK (1997) Allergic contact dermatitis from grasses. Contact Dermatitis 37:32–34
30. Amlot PL, Kemeny DM, Zachary C, Parkes P, Lessor MH (1987) Oral allergy syndrome (OAS): symptoms of IgE-mediated hypersensitivity to foods. Clin Allergy 17:33–42
31. Ortolani C, Ispano M, Pastorello E, Bigi A, Ansaloni R (1988) The oral allergy syndrome. Ann Allergy 61:47–52
32. Ackerman AB (1978) Histological diagnosis of inflammatory skin diseases. Lea and Febiger, Philadelphia, Pa., p 863
33. Veien NK, Menné T (2000) Acute and recurrent vesicular hand dermatitis (pompholyx). In: Menné T, Maibach HI (eds) Hand eczema, 2nd edn. CRC, Boca Raton, Fla., pp 147–164
34. Frosch PJ (1989) Irritant contact dermatitis. In: Frosch PJ, Dooms-Goosens A, Lachapelle J-M, Rycroft RJG, Scheper RJ (eds) Current topics in contact dermatitis. Springer, Berlin Heidelberg New York, pp 385–403
35. Rothenborg HW, Menné T, Sjølin K-E (1977) Temperature dependent primary irritant dermatitis from lemon perfume. Contact Dermatitis 3:37–48
36. Rycroft RJG (1985) Low humidity and microtrauma. Am J Ind Med 8:371–373
37. Rycroft RJG (1987) Low-humidity occupational dermatoses. In: Gardner AW (ed) Current approaches to occupational health, 3rd edn. Wright, Bristol, pp 1–13
38. Hellgren L, Mobacken H (1969) Nummular eczema – clinical and statistical data. Acta Derm Venereol (Stockh) 49:189–196
39. Rycroft RJG (1981) Soluble oil dermatitis. Clin Exp Dermatol 6:229–234
40. Le Coz C-J (2002) Contact nummular (discoid) eczema from depilating cream. Contact Dermatitis 46:111–112
41. Torinuki W, Tagami H (1987) Pustular irritant dermatitis due to croton oil. Acta Derm Venereol (Stockh) 68:257–260

42. Sevadjian CM (1985) Pustular contact hypersensitivity to fluorouracil with rosacealike sequelae. Arch Dermatol 121:240–242

43. Modjtahedi BS, Modjtahedi SP, Maibach HI (2004) The sex of the individual as a factor in allergic contact dermatitis. Contact Dermatitis 50:53–59

44. Meding B (1990) Epidemiology of hand eczema in an industrial city (dissertation). Acta Derm Venereol [Suppl] (Stockh) 153:1–43

45. Weston WL, Weston JA (1984) Allergic contact dermatitis in children. Am J Dis Child 138:932–936

46. Romaguera C, Vilaplana J (1998) Contact dermatitis in children: 6 years experience (1992–1997). Contact Dermatitis 39:277–280

47. Brasch J, Geier J (1997) Patch test results in schoolchildren. Contact Dermatitis 37:286–293

48. Wolf R, Wolf D, Matz H, Orion E (2003) Cutaneous reactions to temporary tattoos. Dermatol Online J 9:3

49. Wantke F, Hemmer W, Jarisch R, Gotz M (1996) Patch test reactions in children, adults and the elderly. A comparative study in patients with suspected allergic contact dermatitis. Contact Dermatitis 34:316–319

50. Uter W, Geier J, Pfahlberg A, Effendy I (2002) The spectrum of contact allergy in elderly patients with and without lower leg dermatitis. Dermatology 204:266–272

51. Nedorost ST, Stevens SR (2001) Diagnosis and treatment of allergic skin disorders in the elderly. Drugs Aging 18:827–835

52. Berardesca E, Maibach HI (1988) Contact dermatitis in blacks. Dermatol Clin 6:363–368

53. Jourdain R, De Lacharrière O, Bastien P, Maibach HI (2002) Ethnic variations in self-perceived sensitive skin: epidemiological survey. Contact Dermatitis 46:162–169

54. Deleo VA, Taylor SC, Belsito DV, Fowler JF Jr, Fransway AF, Maibach HI, Marks JG Jr, Mathias CG, Nethercott JR, Pratt MD, Reitschel RR, Sherertz EF, Storrs FJ, Taylor JS (2002) The effect of race and ethnicity on patch test results. J Am Acad Dermatol 46:S107–S112

55. Modjtahedi SP, Maibach HI (2002) Ethnicity as a possible endogenous factor in irritant contact dermatitis: comparing the irritant response among Caucasians, blacks, and Asians. Contact Dermatitis 47:272–278

56. Robinson MK (2002) Population differences in acute skin irritation responses. Race, sex, age, sensitive skin and repeat subject comparisons. Contact Dermatitis 46:86–93

57. Jones HE, Lewis CW, McMarlin SL (1973) Allergic contact sensitivity in atopic patients. Arch Dermatol 107:217–222

58. Rystedt I (1985) Contact sensitivity in adults with atopic dermatitis in childhood. Contact Dermatitis 12:1–8

59. Svensson A, Möller H (1986) Eyelid dermatitis: the role of atopy and contact dermatitis. Contact Dermatitis 15:178–182

60. Christophersen J, Menné T, Tanghøj P, Andersen KE, Brandrup F, Kaaber K, Osmundsen PE, Thestrup-Pedersen K, Veien NK (1989) Clinical patch test data evaluated by multivariate analysis. Contact Dermatitis 21:291–299

61. Möller H, Svensson A (1986) Metal sensitivity: positive history but negative test indicates atopy. Contact Dermatitis 14:57–60

62. Todd DJ, Burrows D, Stanford CF (1989) Atopy in subjects with a history of nickel allergy but negative patch tests. Contact Dermatitis 21:129–133

63. Dotterud LK, Falk ES (1995) Contact allergy in relation to hand eczema and atopic diseases in north Norwegian schoolchildren. Acta Paediatr 84:402–406

64. Bonnevie P (1939) Aethiologie und Pathogenese der Eczemkrankheiten (Dissertation) Nyt Nordisk, Copenhagen

65. Larsson-Stymne B, Widström L (1985) Ear piercing – a cause of nickel allergy in schoolgirls? Contact Dermatitis 13:289–293

66. Sánchez-Pérez J, Ruís-Genao, García del Río I, García Diez A (2003) Taxi driver's occupational allergic contact dermatitis from nickel in euro coins. Contact Dermatitis 48:340–341

67. Gawkrodger DJ, Vestey JP, Wong W-K, Buxton PK (1986) Contact clinic survey of nickel-sensitive subjects. Contact Dermatitis 14:165–169

68. Moorthy TT, Tan GH (1986) Nickel sensitivity in Singapore. Int J Dermatol 25:307–309

69. Hemingway JD, Molokhia MM (1987) The dissolution of metallic nickel in artificial sweat. Contact Dermatitis 16:99–105

70. Emmett EA, Risby TH, Jiang L, Ng Sk, Feinman S (1988) Allergic contact dermatitis to nickel: bioavailability from consumer products and provocation threshold. J Am Acad Dermatol 19:314–322

71. Kanan MW (1969) Contact dermatitis in Kuwait. J Kuwait Med Assoc 3:129–144

72. Fisher AA (1985) Nickel dermatitis in men. Cutis 35:424–426

73. De Corres LF, Garrastazu MT, Soloeta R, Escayol P (1982) Nickel contact dermatitis in a blood bank. Contact Dermatitis 8:32–37

74. Oakley AMM, Ive FA, Car MM (1987) Skin clips are contraindicated when there is nickel allergy. J R Soc Med 80:290–291

75. Corazza M, Zampio MR, Montanari A, Pagnoni A, Virgili A (2002) Lichenoid reaction from a permanent red tatto: has nickel a possible aetiologic role? Contact Dermatitis 46:114–115

76. Kasteler JS, Petersen MJ, Vance JE, Zone JJ (1992) Circulating activated T lymphocytes in autoeczematization. Arch Dermatol 128:795–798

77. Cunningham MJ, Zone JJ, Petersen MJ, Green JA (1986) Circulating activated (DR-positive) T lymphocytes in a patient with autoeczematization. J Am Acad Dermatol 14:1039–1041

78. Andersen KE, Maibach HI (1983) Drugs used topically. In: De Weck AL, Bundgaard H (eds) Allergic reactions to drugs. Springer, Berlin Heidelberg New York, pp 313–377

79. Wilkinson JD, Hambly EM, Wilkinson DS (1980) Comparison of patch test results in two adjacent areas of England. II. Medicaments. Acta Derm Venereol (Stockh) 60:245–249

80. Edman B, Möller H (1986) Medicament contact allergy. Derm Beruf Umwelt 34:139–143

81. Goossens A, Blondeel S, Zimerson E (2002) Resorcinol monobenzoate: a potential sensitizer in a computer mouse. Contact Dermatitis 47:235

82. Avnstorp C, Hamann K (1981) Neglelakeksem. Ugeskr Laeger 143:2504–2505

83. Burnett JW, Calton GJ (1987) Jellyfish envenomation syndromes updated. Ann Emerg Med 16:1000–1005

84. Hogan DJ, Dosman JA, Li KYR et al (1986) Questionnaire survey of pruritus and rash in grain elevator workers. Contact Dermatitis 14:170–175

85. Lachapelle JM (1986) Industrial airborne irritant or allergic contact dermatitis. Contact Dermatitis 14:137–145

14

86. Beck MH, Hausen BM, Dave VK (1984) Allergic contact dermatitis from *Machaerium scleroxylum* Tul. (Pao ferro) in a joinery shop. Clin Exp Dermatol 9:159–166

87. Ippen H, Wereta-Kubek M, Rose U (1986) Haut- und Schleimhautreaktionen durch Zimmerpflanzen der Gattung Dieffenbachia. Dermatosen 34:93–101

88. Hausen BM (1982) Häufigkeit und Bedeutung toxischer und allergischer Kontaktdermatitiden duch *Machaerium scleroxylum* Tul. (Pao ferro), einem Ersatzholz für Palisander (*Dalbergia nigra* All.). Hautarzt 33:321–328

89. Møller NE, Nielsen B, von Würden K (1986) Contact dermatitis to semisynthetic penicillins in factory workers. Contact Dermatitis 14:307–311

90. Huygens S, Goossens A (2001) An update on airborne contact dermatitis. Contact Dermatitis 44:1–6

91. Karlberg AT, Gafvert E, Meding B, Stenberg B (1996) Airborne contact dermatitis from unexpected exposure to rosin (colophony). Rosin sources revealed with chemical analyses. Contact Dermatitis 35:272–278

92. Hjorth N, Roed-Petersen J, Thomsen K (1976) Airborne contact dermatitis from Compositae oleoresins simulating photodermatitis. Br J Dermatol 95:613–619

93. LaMarte FP, Merchant JA, Casale TB (1988) Acute systemic reactions to carbonless copy paper associated with histamine release. J Am Med Assoc 260:242–243

94. Berg M (1988) Skin problems in workers using visual display terminals. Contact Dermatitis 19:335–341

95. Berg M, Lonne-Rahm SB, Fischer T (1998) Patients with visual display unit-related facial symptoms are stingers. Acta Derm Venereol (Stockh) 78:44–45

96. Kligman AM, Klemme JC, Susten AS (eds) (1985) The chronic effects of repeated mechanical trauma to the skin. Am J Ind Med 8:253–513

97. Wintzen M, Van Zuuren EJ (2003) Computer-related skin diseases. Contact Dermatitis 48:241–243

98. García-Morales I, García Bravo B, Camacho Martínez F (2003) Occupational contact dermatitis caused by a personal-computer mouse mat. Contact Dermatitis 49:172

99. Powell FC (1994) Sports dermatology. J Eur Acad Dermatol Venereol 3:1–15

100. Tomecki KJ, Mikesell JF (1987) Rower's rump. J Am Acad Dermatol 16:890–891

101. Kanerva L (1998) Knuckle pads from boxing. Eur J Dermatol 8:359–361

102. Descamps V, Peuchal X (2002) 'Canyoning hand': a new recreational hand dermatitis. Contact Dermatitis 47:363–364

103. Inue S, Yamamoto S, Ikegami R, Ozawa K, Itami S, Yoshikawa K (2002) Baseball pitcher's friction dermatitis. Contact Dermatitis 47:176–177

104. Sullivan JR, Rachlis A, Phillips E (2003) 'Buffalo-hump' dermatitis: a hat trick of antiretroviral side-effects. Contact Dermatitis 48:169–170

105. Kato A, Shoji A, Aoki N (2003) Very-low-voltage electrical injuries caused by cellular-phone chargers. Contact Dermatitis 49:168–169

106. Hersle K, Mobacken H (1982) Hyperkeratotic dermatitis of the palms. Br J Dermatol 107:195–202

107. Thestrup-Pedersen K, Andersen KE, Menné T, Veien NK (2001) Treatment of hyperkeratotic dermatitis of the palms (eczema keratoticum) with oral acitretin. A single-blind, placebo-controlled study. Acta Derm Venereol (Stockh) 81:353–355

108. Sabroe RA, Sharp LA, Peachey RDG (1996) Contact allergy to gold sodium thiosulfate. Contact Dermatitis 34:345–348

109. Plewig G, Fulton JE, Kligman AM (1970) Pomade acne. Arch Dermatol 101:580–584

110. Pecegueiro M, Brandao M (1984) Contact plantar pustulosis. Contact Dermatitis 11:126–127

111. Andersen KE, Sjølin KE, Solgard P (1989) Actuce irritant contact folliculitis in a galvanizer. In: Frosch PJ, Dooms-Goossens A, Lachapelle J-M, Rycroft RJG, Scheper RJ (eds) Current topics in contact dermatitis. Springer, Berlin Heidelberg New York, pp 417–418

112. Rystedt I, Fischer T, Lagerholm B (1983) Patch testing with sodium tungstate. Contact Dermatitis 9:69–73

113. Freeman S (1986) Woman allergic to husband's sweat and semen. Contact Dermatitis 14:110–112

114. Poskitt BL, Wojnarowska FT, Shaw S (1995) Semen contact urticaria. J R Soc Med 88:108P–109P

115. Held JL, Ruszkowski AM, Deleo VA (1988) Consort contact dermatitis due to oak moss. Arch Dermatol 124:261–262

116. Bernedo N, Audicana MT, Uriel O, Velasco M, Gastaminza G, Fernández E, Muñoz D (2004) Allergic contact dermatitis from cosmetics applied by the patient's girlfriend. Contact Dermatitis 50:252–253

117. Veien NK, Hattel T, Laurberg G (1994) Plantar *Trichophyton rubrum* infections may cause dermatophytids on the hands. Acta Derm Venereol (Stockh) 74:403–404

118. Bryld LE, Agner T, Menné T (2003) Relation between vesicular eruptions on the hands and tinea pedis, atopic dermatitis and nickel allergy. Acta Derm Venereol (Stockh) 83:186–188

119. Rustemeyer T, Frosch PJ (1996) Occupational skin diseases in dental laboratory technicians. (I). Clinical picture and causative factors. Contact Dermatitis 34:125–133

120. Delaney TZ, Donnelly AM (1996) Garlic dermatitis. Australas J Dermatol 37:109–110

121. Rycroft FJG, Baran R (1984) Occupational abnormalities and contact dermatitis. In: Baran R et al (eds) Diseases of the nails. Blackwell, London, pp 267–287

122. Mathias CGT, Maibach HI (1984) Allergic contact dermatitis from anaerobic acrylic sealants. Arch Dermatol 120:1202–1205

123. Cronin E (1982) "New" allergens of clinical importance. Semin Dermatol 1:33–41

124. Foti C, Cassano N, Conserva A, Vena GA (2003) Irritant paronychia with onychodystrophy caused by cyanoacrylate nail glue. Contact Dermatitis 49:274–275

125. Veien NK, Hattel T, Justesen O, Nørholm A (1986) Aluminium allergy. Contact Dermatitis 15:295–297

126. Kaaber K, Nielsen AO, Veien NK (1992) Vaccination granulomas and aluminium allergy: course and prognostic factors. Contact Dermatitis 26:304–306

127. Lopez S, Pelaez A, Navarro LA, Montesinos E, Morales C, Carda C (1994) Aluminium allergy in patients hyposensitized with aluminium-precipitated antigen extracts. Contact Dermatitis 31:37–40

128. Bergfors E, Trollfors B, Inerot A (2003) Unexpectedly high incidence of persistent itching odules and delayed hypersensitivity to aluminium in children after the use of adsorbed vaccines from a single manufacturer. Vaccine 22:64–69 (Erratum in: Vaccine 22:1586, 2004)

129. Culora GA, Ramsay AD, Theaker JM (1996) Aluminium and injection site reactions. J Clin Pathol 49:844–847

130. Fischer T, Rystedt I (1982) A case of contact sensitivity to aluminium. Contact Dermatitis 8:343

131. Feinglos MN, Jegasothy BV (1979) "Insulin" allergy due to zinc. Lancet 1:122–124

132. Cronin E (1980) Contact dermatitis. Churchill Livingstone, Edinburgh

133. Hjorth N, Roed-Petersen J (1976) Occupational protein contact dermatitis in food handlers. Contact Dermatitis 2:28–42

134. Chan EF, Mowad C (1998) Contact dermatitis to foods and spices. Am J Contact Dermatol 9:71–79

135. Kanerva L, Toikkanen J, Jolanki R, Estlander T (1996) Statistical data on occupational contact urticaria. Contact Dermatitis 35:229–233

136. Oranje AP, van Gysel D, Mulder PG, Dieges PH (1994) Food-induced contact urticaria syndrome (CUS) in atopic dermatitis: reproducibility of repeated and duplicate testing with a skin provocation test, the skin application food test (SAFT). Contact Dermatitis 31:314–318

137. Iliev D, Wuthrich B (1998) Occupational protein contact dermatitis with type I allergy to different kinds of meat and vegetables. Int Arch Occup Environ Health 71:289–292

138. Menné T, Veien N, Sjølin K-E, Maibach HI (1994) Systemic contact dermatitis. Am J Contact Dermat 5:1–12

139. Veien NK (1989) Systemically induced eczema in adults. Acta Derm Venereol (Stockh) [Suppl] 147:1–58 (Dissertation, University of Copenhagen)

140. Veien NK, Krogdahl A (1989) Is nickel vasculitis a clinical entity? In: Frosch PJ, Dooms-Goossens A, Lachapelle J-M, Rycroft RJG, Scheper RJ (eds) Current topics in contact dermatitis. Springer, Berlin Heidelberg New York, pp 172–177

141. Kaaber K, Sjølin KE, Menné T (1983) Elbow eruptions in nickel and chromate dermatitis. Contact Dermatitis 9:213–216

142. Calnan CD (1956) Nickel dermatitis. Br J Dermatol 68:229–236

143. Andersen KE, Hjorth N, Menné T (1984) The baboon syndrome: systemically-induced allergic contact dermatitis. Contact Dermatitis 10:97–100

144. Christensen OB (1981) Nickel allergy and hand eczema in females. Dissertation, University of Lund, Malmö

145. Lechner T, Grytzmann B, Bäurle G (1987) Hämatogenes allergisches Kontaktekzem nach oraler Gabe von Nystatin. Mykosen 30:143–146

146. Bernard P, Rayol J, Bonnafoux A et al (1988) Toxidermies apres prise orale de pristinamycine. Ann Dermatol Venereol 115:63–66

147. Sehgal VN, Gangwani OP (1987) Fixed drug eruption. Int J Dermatol 26:67–74

148. Alanko K, Stubb S, Reitamo S (1987) Topical provocation of fixed drug eruption. Br J Dermatol 116:561–567

149. Rycroft RJG (1980) Acute ulcerative contact dermatitis from Portland cement. Br J Dermatol 102:487–489

150. Rycroft RJG (1980) Acute ulcerative contact dermatitis from ready mixed cement. Clin Exp Dermatol 5:245–247

151. Koch P (1996) Brulures, necroses et ulcerations cutanees dues au ciment, au beton premixe et a la chaux. Huit cas. Ann Dermatol Venereol 123:832–836

152. Osmundsen PE, Alani MD (1971) Contact allergy to an optical whitener, "CRY", in washing powders. Br J Dermatol 85:61–66

153. Valsecchi R, de Landro A, Pansera B, Cainelli T (1995) Pigmented contact dermatitis. Contact Dermatitis 33:70–71

154. Hayakawa R, Matsunaga K, Kojima S, Kaniwa M, Nakamura A (1985) Naphthol AS as a cause of pigmented contact dermatitis. Contact Dermatitis 13:20–25

155. Dunlop K, Freeman S (1997) Caterpillar dermatitis. Australas J Dermatol 38:193–195

156. Balit CR, Geary MJ, Russell RC, Isbister GK (2004) Clinical effects of exposure to the White-stemmed gum moth (Chelepteryx collesi). Emerg Med Australas 16:74–81

157. Maier, Spiegel W, Kinaciyan T, Krehan H, Cabaj A, Schopf A, Honigsmann H (2003) The oak processionary caterpillar as the cause of an epidemic airborne disease: survey and analysis. Br J Dermatol 149:990–997

158. Vega J, Vega JM, Moneo I, Armentia A, Caballero ML, Miranda A (2004) Occupational immunologic contact urticaria from pine processionary caterpillar (Thaumetopoea pityocampa): experience in 30 cases. Contact Dermatitis 50:60–64

159. Salinas ML, Ogura T, Soffchi L (2001) Irritant contact dermatitis caused by needle-like calcium oxalate crystals, raphides, in Agave tequilana among workers in tequila distilleries and agave plantations. Contact Dermatitis 44:94–96

160. Waersted A, Hjorth N (1985) Pityrosporum orbiculare – a pathogenic factor in atopic dermatitis of the face, scalp and neck? Acta Derm Venereol (Stockh) [Suppl] 114:146–148

161. Kieffer M, Bergbrant IM, Faergemann J et al (1990) Immune reactions to Pityrosporum ovale in adult patients with atopic dermatitis and seborrhoeic dermatitis. J Am Acad Dermatol 29:739–742

162. Maibach HI (1987) Oral substitution in patients sensitized by transdermal clonidine treatment. Contact Dermatitis 16:1–8

163. Harai Z, Sommer I, Knobel B (1987) Multifocal contact dermatitis to nitroderm TTS 5 with extensive postinflammatory hypermelanosis. Dermatologica 174:249–252

164. Holdiness MR (1989) A review of contact dermatitis associated with transdermal therapeutic systems. Contact Dermatitis 20:3–9

165. Carmichael AJ (1994) Skin sensitivity and transdermal drug delivery. A review of the problem. Drug Saf 10:151–159

166. Weickel R, Frosch PJ (1986) Kontaktallergie auf Glyceroltrinitrat (Nitroderm TTS). Hautarzt 37:511–512

167. Wilson DE, Kaidbey K, Boike SC, Jorkasky DK (1998) Use of topical corticosteroid pretreatment to reduce the incidence and severity of skin reactions associated with testosterone transdermal therapy. Clin Ther 20:299–306

168. Jordan WP Jr (1997) Allergy and topical irritation associated with transdermal testosterone administration: a comparison of scrotal and nonscrotal transdermal systems. Am J Contact Dermatol 8:108–113

169. Zaynoun ST, Aftimos BA, Tenekjian KK, Kurban AK (1981) Berloque dermatitis – a continuing cosmetic problem. Contact Dermatitis 7:111–116

170. Edman B (1985) Sites of contact dermatitis in relationship to particular allergens. Contact Dermatitis 13:129–135

171. Näher H, Frosch PJ (1987) Contact dermatitis to thioxolone. Contact Dermatitis 17:250–251

172. Tosti A, Guerra L, Bardazzi F (1991) Contact dermatitis caused by topical minoxidil: case reports and review of the literature. Am J Contact Dermatol 2:56–59

173. Ebner H, Müller E (1995) Allergic contact dermatitis from minoxidil. Contact Dermatitis 32:316

174. Friedman ES, Friedman PM, Coen DE, Washenik K (2002) Allergic contact dermatitis to topical minoxidil solution: etiology and treatment. J Am Acad Dermatol 46:309–312

175. Storrs FJ (1984) Permanent wave contact dermatitis: contact allergy to glyceryl monothioglycolate. J Am Acad Dermatol 11:74–85

14

176. Søsted H, Agner T, Andersen KE, Menné T (2002) 55 cases of allergic reactions to hair dye: a descriptive, consumer complaint-based study. Contact Dermatitis 47:299–303

177. Tosti A, Piraccini BM, van Neste DJ (2001) Telogen effluvium after allergic contact dermatitis of the scalp. Arch Dermatol 137:187–190

178. Andersen KE, Roed-Petersen J, Kamp P (1984) Contact allergy related to TEA-PEG-3 cocamide sulfate and cocamidopropyl betaine in a shampoo. Contact Dermatitis 11:192–193

179. Pérez RG, Aguirre A, Ratón JA, Eizaguirre X, Díaz-Pérez JL (1995) Positive patch tests to zinc pyrithione. Contact Dermatitis 32:118–119

180. Brand R, Delaney TA (1998) Allergic contact dermatitis to cocamidopropylbetaine in hair shampoo. Australs J Dermatol 39:121–122

181. Nielsen NH, Menné T (1997) Allergic contact dermatitis caused by zinc pyrithione associated with pustular psoriasis. Am J Contact Dermatol 8:170–171

182. Fowler JF, Fowler LM, Hunter JE (1997) Allergy to cocamidopropyl betaine may be due to amidoamine: a patch test and product use test study. Contact Dermatitis 37:276–281

183. Fowler JF Jr, Zug KM, Taylor JS, Storrs, FJ, Sherertz EA, Sasseville DA, Rietschel RL, Pratt MD, Mathias CGT, Marks JG, Mailbach HI, Fransway AF, Deleo VA, Belsito DV (2004) Allergy to cocamidopropyl betaine and amidoamine in North America. Dermatitis 15:5–6

184. Pasche-Koo F, Claeys M, Hauser C (1996) Contact urticaria with systemic symptoms caused by bovine collagen in a hair conditioner. Am J Contact Dermat 7:56–58

185. Dobrev H, Zissova L (1997) Effect of ketoconazole 2% shampoo on scalp sebum level in patients with seborrhoeic dermatitis. Acta Derm Venereol (Stockh) 77:132–134

186. Peter RU, Richarz-Barthauer U (1995) Successful treatment and prophylaxis of scalp seborrhoeic dermatitis and dandruff with 2% ketoconazole shampoo: results of a multicentre, double-blind, placebo-controlled trial. Br J Dermatol 132:441–445

187. Fotiades J, Soter NA, Lim HW (1995) Results of evaluation of 203 patients for photosensitivity in a 7.3-year period. J Am Acad Dermatol 33:597–602

188. Schauder S, Schroder W, Geier J (1996) Olaquindox-induced airborne photoallergic contact dermatitis followed by transient or persistent light reactions in 15 pig breeders. Contact Dermatitis 35:344–354

189. Frain-Bell W, Lakshmipathi T, Rogers J, Willock J (1974) The syndrome of chronic photosensitivity dermatitis and actinic reticuloid. Br J Dermatol 91:617–634

190. Russell SC, Dawe RS, Collins P, Man I, Ferguson J (1998) The photosensitivity dermatitis and actinic reticuloid syndrome (chronic actinic dermatitis) occurring in seven young atopic dermatitis patients. Br J Dermatol 138:496–501

191. Healy E, Rogers S (1995) Phtosensitivity dermatitis/actinic reticuloid syndrome in an Irish population: a review and some unusual features. Acta Derm Venereol (Stockh) 75:72–74

192. Goulden V, Wilkinson SM (1998) Patch testing for Compositae allergy. Br J Dermatol 138:1018–1021

193. Machet L, Vaillant L, Callens A, Demasure M, Barruet K, Lorette G (1993) Allergic contact dermatitis from sunflower (*Helianthus annuus*) with cross-sensitivity to arnica. Contact Dermatitis 28:184–200

194. Hausen BM (1996) A 6-year experience with compositae mix. Am J Contact Dermatol 7:94–99

195. Paulsen E, Søgaard J, Andersen KE (1998) Occupational dermatitis in Danish gardeners and greenhouse workers (III). Compositae-related symptoms. Contact Dermatitis 38:140–146

196. Mahajan VK, Sharma VK, Kaur I, Chakrabarti (1996) Contact dermatitis in agricultural workers: rôle of common crops, fodder and weeds. Contact Dermatitis 35:373–374

197. Mahler V, Diepgen TL, Heese A, Peters K-P (1998) Protein contact dermatitis due to cow dander. Contact Dermatitis 38:47–48

198. Moreno JC, Gata IM, Garcia-Bravo B, Camacho FM (1997) Fiddler's neck. Am J Contact Dermatol 8:39–42

199. Hausen BM (1997) Allergic contact dermatitis from a wooden necklace. Am J Contact Dermatol 8:185–187

200. Hausen BM, Oestmann G (1988) Untersuchungen über die Häufigkeit berufsbedingter allergischer Hauterkrankungen auf einem Blumengrossmarkt. Dermatosen 36:117–124

201. De Groot AC, Bruynzeel DP, Bos JD et al (1988) The allergens in cosmetics. Arch Dermatol 124:1525–1529

202. Adams RM, Maibach HI (1985) A five-year study of cosmetic reactions. J Am Acad Dermatol 13:1062–1069

203. Hsu TS, Davis MD, el-Azhary R, Corbett JF, Gibson LE (2001) Beard dermatitis due to para-phenylenediamine use in Arabic men. J Am Acad Dermatol 44:867–869

204. Jacobs M-C, White IR, Rycroft RJG, Taub N (1995) Patch testing with preservatives at St John's from 1982 to 1993. Contact Dermatitis 33:247–254

205. Wilkinson JD, Shaw S, Andersen KE, Brandao FM, Buynzeel DP, Bruze M, Camarasa JM, Diepgen TL, Ducombs G, Frosch PJ, Goossens A, Lachapelle JM, Lahti A, Menné T, Seidenari S, Tosti A, Wahlberg JE (2002) Monitoring levels of preservative sensitivity in Europe. A 10-year overview (1991–2000). Contact Dermatitis 46:207–210. Comment in: Contact Dermatitis 46:189–190, 2002

206. Mathias CGT (1982) Pigmented cosmetic dermatitis from contact allergy to a toilet soap containing chromium. Contact Dermatitis 8:29–31

207. Mathias CGT, Maibach HI, Conant MA (1980) Perioral leukoderma simulating vitiligo from use of a toothpaste containing cinnamic aldehyde. Arch Dermatol 116:1172–1173

208. Hayakawa R, Matsunaga K, Arima Y (1987) Depigmented contact dermatitis due to incense. Contact Dermatitis 16:272–274

209. Fisher AA, Dooms-Goossens A (1976) Persulfate hair bleach reactions. Arch Dermatol 112:1407–1409

210. Guin JD, Berry VK (1980) Perfume sensitivity in adult females. J Am Acad Dermatol 3:299–302

211. Brandrup F, Hansen NS, Schultz K (1987) Ansigtseksem fremkaldt af gummi i åndedraetsvaern. Ugeskr Laeger 149:968

212. Rotstein E, Rotstein H (1997) The ear-lobe sign: a helpful sign in facial contact dermatitis. Australas J Dermatol 38:215–216

213. Hannuksela M, Lahti A (1977) Immediate reactions to fruits and vegetables. Contact Dermatitis 3:79–84

214. Paulsen E (1996) Compositae-dermatitis på Fyn (dissertation), Odense University, Odense

215. Ophaswongse S, Maibach HI (1995) Allergic contact cheilitis. Contact Dermatitis 33:365–370

216. Strauss RM, Orton DI (2003) Allergic contact cheilitis in the United Kingdom: a retrospective study. Am J Contact Dermatol 14:75–77

217. Downs AMR, Lear JT, Sansom JE (1998) Contact sensitivity in patients with oral symptoms. Contact Dermatitis 39:258–259

218. Goldsmith PC, White IR, Rycroft FJG, McFadden JP (1995) Probable active sensitization to tixocortol pivalate. Contact Dermatitis 33:429–430

219. Serra-Baldrich E, Puig LL, Arnau AG, Camarasa JG (1995) Lipstick allergic contact dermatitis from gallates. Contact Dermatitis 32:359–372

220. Niinimäki A (1995) Spice allergy. Acta Univ Oul D 357 (dissertation), University of Oulu

221. Francalanci S, Sertoli A, Giorgini S, Pigatto P, Santucci B, Valsecchi R (2000) Multicentre study of allergic contact cheilitis from toothpastes. Contact Dermatitis 43:216–222

222. Liden C, Berg M, Farm G, Wrangsjo K (1993) Nail varnish allergy with far-reaching consequences. Br J Dermatol 128:57–62

223. Ockenfels HM, Seemann U, Goos M (1997) Contact allergy in patients with periorbital eczema: an analysis of allergens. Data recorded by the Information Network of the Departments of Dermatology. Dermatology 195:119–124

224. Shah M, Lewis FM, Gawkrodger DJ (1996) Facial dermatitis and eyelid dermatitis: a comparison of patch test results and final diagnoses. Contact Dermatitis 34:140–141

225. Karlberg AT, Gafvert E, Meding B, Stenberg B (1996) Airborne contact dermatitis from unexpected exposure to rosin (colophony). Rosin sources revealed with chemical analyses. Contact Dermatitis 35:272–278

226. Herbst RA, Uter W, Pirker C, Geier J, Frosch PJ (2004) Allergic and non-allergic periorbital dermatitis: patch test results of the Information Network of the Departments of Dermatology during a 5-year period. Contact Dermatitis 51:13–19

227. Guin JD (2002) Eyelid dermatitis: experience in 203 cases. J Am Acad Dermatol 47:755–765

228. Ayala F, Fabbrocini G, Bacchilega R, Berardesca E, Caraffini S, Corazza M, Flori ML, Francalanci S, Guarrera M, Lisi P, Santucci B, Schena D, Suppa F, Valsecchi R, Vincenzi C, Balato N (2003) Eyelid dermatitis: an evaluation of 447 patients. Am J Contact Dermatol 14:69–74

229. Frosch PJ, Weickel R, Schmitt T, Krastel H (1988) Nebenwirkungen von opthalmologischen Externa. Z Hautkr 63:126–136

230. Le Coz C-J, Leclere J-M, Arnoult E, Raison-Peyron N, Pons-Guiraud A, Vigan M (2002) Allergic contact dermatitis from shellac in mascara. Contact Dermatitis 46:149–152

231. Grundmann H, Wozniak K-D, Tost M (1981) Zum allergischen Kontakteksem im Lid- und Augenbereich. Folia Ophthalmol 6:258–261

232. Valsecchi R, Imberti G, Martino D, Cainelli T (1992) Eyelid dermatitis: an evaluation of 150 patients. Contact Dermatitis 27:143–147

233. Nethercott JR (1978) Skin problems associated with multifunctional acrylic monomers in ultraviolet curing inks. Br J Dermatol 98:541–551

234. Ottosen C-O, Irgens-Møller L (1984) Øjenskader kan skyldes stueplanten *Dieffenbachia*. Ugeskr Laeger 146:3927–3928

235. Millard TP, Orton DI (2004) Changing patterns of contact allergy in chronic inflammatory ear disease. Contact Dermatitis 50:83–86

236. Wilkonson SM, Bech MH (1993) Hypesensitivity to topical corticosteroids in otitis externa. J Laryngol Otol 107:597–599

237. Lear JT, Sandhu G, English JSC (1998) Hearing aid dermatitis: a study in 20 consecutive patients. Contact Dermatitis 38:212–238

238. Sood A, Taylor JS (2004) Allergic contact dermatitis from hearing aid materials. Dermatitis 15:48–50

239. Nielsen NH, Menné T (1993) Nickel sensitization and ear piercing in an unselected Danish population. Glostrup Allergy Study. Contact Dermatitis 29:16–21

240. Kieffer M (1979) Nickel sensitivity: relationship between history and patch test reaction. Contact Dermatitis 5:398–401

241. Nakada T, Iijima M, Nakayama H, Maibach HI (1997) Role of ear piercing in metal allergic contact dermatitis. Contact Dermatitis 36:233–236

242. Armstrong DK, Walsh MY, Dawson JG (1997) Granulomatous contact dermatitis due to gold earrings. Br J Dermatol 136:776–778

243. Carlsen L, Andersen KE, Egsgaard H (1986) Triphenyl phosphate allergy from spectacle frames. Contact Dermatitis 15:274–277

244. Seishima M, Yama Z, Oda M (2003) Cellular phone dermatitis with chormate allergy. Dermatology 207:48–50

245. Hatch KL, Maibach HI (1985) Textile fiber dermatitis. Contact Dermatitis 12:1–11

246. Hatch KL, Maibach HI (1986) Textile chemical finish dermatitis. Contact Dermatitis 14:1–13

247. Fowler JF Jr, Skinner SM, Belsito DV (1992) Allergic contact dermatitis from formaldehyde resins in permanent press clothing: an underdiagnosed cause of generalized dermatitis. J Am Acad Dermatol 27:962–968

248. Seidenari S, Mantovani L, Manzini BM, Pignatti M (1997) Cross-sensitizations between azo dyes and para-amino compound. A study of 236 azo-dye-sensitive subjects. Contact Dermatitis 36:91–96

249. Seidenari S, Manzini BM, Schiavi ME, Motolese A (1995) Prevalence of contact allergy to non-disperse azo dyes for natural fibers: a study in 1814 consecutive patients. Contact Dermatitis 33:118–122

250. Giusti F, Seidenari S (2003) Textile dyes sensitization: a study of 49 patients allergic til disperse dye alone. Contact Dermatitis 48:54–55

251. Seidenari S, Giusti F, Massone F, Mantovani L (2002) Sensitization to disperse dyes in a patch test population over a five-year period. Am J Contact Dermat 13:101–107

252. Scheman AJ, Carroll PA, Brown KH, Osburn AH (1998) Formaldehyde-related textile allergy: an update. Contact Dermatitis 38:332–336

253. Tegner E (1985) Sheet dermatitis Acta Derm Venereol (Stockh) 65:254–257

254. Veien NK, Hattel T, Laurberg G (1992) Can 'label dermatitis' become 'creeping neurotic excoriations'? Contact Dermatitis 27:272–273

255. Corazza M, Maranini C, La Malfa W, Virgili A (1998) Unusual suction-like contact dermatitis due to ECG electrodes. Acta Derm Venereol (Stockh) 78:145–159

256. Goossens A, Verhamme B (2002) Contact allergy to permanent colorants used for tattooing a nipple after breast reconstruction. Contact Dermatitis 47:250

257. Lamb SR, Ardley HE, Wilkinson SM (2003) Contact allergy to propylene glycol in brassiere padding inserts. Contact Dermatitis 48:224–225

258. Freudenthal AR, Joseph PR (1993) Seabather's eruption. N Engl J Med 329:542–544

259. Sun C-C, Sue M-S (1995) Sulfur spring dermatitis. Contact Dermatitis 32:31–34

260. Larsen WG (1977) Perfume dermatitis. Arch Dermatol 113:623–626

261. Johansen JD, Andersen TF, Veien N, Avnstorp C, Andersen KE, Menné T (1997) Patch testing with markers of fragrance contact allergy. Do clinical tests correspond to

14

patients' self-reported problems? Acta Derm Venereol (Stockh) 77:149–153

262. Larsen WG (1979) Allergic contact dermatitis to the perfume in Mycolog cream. J Am Acad Dermatol 1:131–133

263. Bauer A, Geier J, Elsner P (2000) Allergic contact dermatitis in patients with anogenital complaints. J Reprod Med 45:649–654

264. Longhi F, Carlucci G, Bellucci R, di Girolamo R, Palumbo G, Amerio P (1992) Diaper dermatitis: a study of contributing factors. Contact Dermatitis 26:248–252

265. Di Landro A, Greco V, Valsecchi R (2002) 'Lucky Luke' contact dermatitis from diapers with negative patch tests. Contact Dermatitis 46:48–49

266. Seymour JL, Keswick BH, Haifin JM, Jordan WP, Milligan MC (1989) Clinical effects of diaper types on the skin of normal infacts and infants with atopic dermatitis. J Am Acad Dermatol 17:988–997

267. De Groot AC, Frosch PJ (1997) Adverse reactions to fragrances. A clinical review. Contact Dermatitis 36:57–86

268. Poskitt BL, Wojnarowska FT, Shaw S (1995) Semen contact urticaria. J R Soc Med 88:108P–109P

269. Guillet G, Dagregorio G (2004) Seminal fluid as a missed allergen in vulvar allergic contact dermatitis. Contact Dermatitis 50:318–319

270. Lewis FM, Shah M, Gawkrodger DJ (1997) Contact sensitivity in pruritus vulvae: patch test results and clinical outcome. Am J Contact Dermat 8:137–140

271. Kanerva L, Estlander T (1995) Occupational allergic contact dermatitis associated with curious pubic nickel dermatitis from minimal exposure. Contact Dermatitis 32:309–310

272. Marren P, Wojnarowska F, Powell S (1992) Allergic contact dermatitis and vulvar dermatoses. Br J Dermatol 126:52–56

273. Nunns D, Ferguson J, Beck M, Mandal D (1997) Is patch testing necessary in vulval vestibulitis? Contact Dermatitis 37:87–89

274. Crone AM, Stewart EJ, Wojnarowska F, Powell SM (2000) Aetiological factors in vulvar dermatitis. J Eur Acad Dermatol Venereol 14:181–186

275. Lazarov A (1999) Perianal contact dermatitis caused by nail lacquer allergy. Am J Contact Dermat 10:43–44

276. Lauerma AI (2001) Simultaneous immediate and delayed hypersensitivity to chlorhexidine digluconate. Contact Dermatitis 44:59–60

277. Romaguera C, Grimalt F (1981) Contact dermatitis from a copper-containing intrauterine contraceptive device. Contact Dermatitis 7:163–164

278. Frosch PJ, Raulin C (1987) Kontaktallergie auf Bufexamac. Hautarzt 38:331–334

279. Blecher P, Korting HC (1992) Irritative und allergologische Aspekte der Verwendung Altpapier-haltiger Hygienepapiere im Analbereich. Dermatosen 40:30–34

280. Veien NK, Hattel T, Justesen O, Nørholm A (1987) Dermatoses in coffee drinkers. Cutis 40:421–422

281. Ratliff CR, Conovan AM (2001) Frequency of peristomal complications. Ostomy Wound Manage 47:26–29

282. Lyon CC, Smith AJ, Griffiths CE, Beck MH (2000) The spectrum of skin disorders in abdominal stoma patients. Br J Dermatol 143:1248–1260

283. Heskel NS (1987) Allergic contact dermatitis from stomaadhesive paste. Contact Dermatitis 16:119–121

284. Beck MH, Burrows D, Fregert S, Mendelsohn S (1985) Allergic contact dermatitis to epoxy resin in ostomy bags. Br J Surg 72:202–203

285. Mann RJ, Stewart E, Peachey RDG (1983) Sensitivity to urostomy pouch plastic. Contact Dermatitis 9:80–81

286. Fisher AA (1995) Contact dermatitis, 4th edn. Lea and Febiger, Philadelphia, Pa., pp 418–423

287. Rothstein MS (1986) Dermatologic considerations of stoma care. J Am Acad Dermatol 15:411–432

288. Goossens A, Armingaud P, Avenel-Audran M, Begon-Bagdassarian I, Constandt L, Giordano-Labadie F, Girardin P, Coz CJLE, Milpied-Homsi B, Nootens C, Pecquet C, Tennstedt D, Vanhecke E (2002) An epidemic of allergic contact dermatitis due to epilating products. Contact Dermatitis 46:67–70

289. Fisher AA (1995) Contact dermatitis, 4th edn. Lea and Febiger, Philadelphia, Pa., pp 426–429

290. van Ketel WG (1977) Allergic contact dermatitis of amputation stumps. Contact Dermatitis 3:50–61

291. Komamura H, Foi T, Inui S, Yoshikawa K (1997) A case of contact dermatitis due to impurities of cetyl alcohol. Contact Dermatitis 36:44–46

292. Wilkinson SM (1994) Hypersensitivity to topical corticosteroids. Clin Exp Dermatol 19:1–11

293. Tavadia S, Bianchi J, Dawe RS, Mcevoy M, Wiggins E, Hamill E, Urcelay M, Strong AMM, Douglas WS (2003) Allergic contact dermatitis in venous leg ulcer patients. Contact Dermatitis 48:261–265

294. Machet L, Couhe C, Perrinaud A, Hoarau C, Lorette G, Vaillant L (2004) A high prevalence of sensitization still persists in leg ulcer patients: a retrospective series of 106 patients tested between 2001 and 2002 and a meta-analysis of 1975–2003 data. Br J Dermatol 150:929–935

295. Salim A, Shaw S (2001) Recommendation to include ester gum resin when patch testing patients with leg ulcers. Contact Dermatitis 44:34–60

296. Hausen BM, Schulz (1984) Strumpffarben-Allergie. Dtsch Med Wochenschr 109:1469–1475

297. Rietschel RL (1984) Role of socks in shoe dermatitis. Arch Dermatol 120:398

298. Roul S, Ducombs G, Leaute-Labreze C, Labbe L, Taïeb A (1996) Footwear contact dermatitis in children. Contact Dermatitis 35:334–336

299. Freeman S (1997) Shoe dermatitis. Contact Dermatitis 36:247–249

300. Cockayne SE, Shah M, Messenger AG, Gawkrodger DJ (1998) Foot dermatitis in children: causative allergens and follow-up. Contact Dermatitis 38:203–206

301. Saha M, Srinivas CR, Shenoy SD, Balachandran C, Acharya S (1993) Footwear dermatitis. Contact Dermatitis 28:260–264

302. Trattner A, Farchi Y, David M (2003) Shoe contact dermatitis in Israel. Am J Contact Dermat 14:12–14

303. Opie J, Lee A, Frowen K, Fewings J, Nixon R (2004) Foot dermatitis caused by the textile dye Basic Red 46 in acrylic blend socks. Contact Dermatitis 49:297–303

304. Möller H (1972) Atopic winter feet in children. Acta Derm Venereol (Stockh) 52:401–405

305. Jones SK, English JSC, Forsyth A, mackie RM (1987) Juvenile plantar dermatosis: an 8-year follow-up of 102 patients. Clin Exp Dermatol 12:5–7

306. Ashton RE, Griffiths WAD (1986) Juvenile plantar dermatosis: atopiy or footwear? Clin Exp Dermatol 11:529–534

307. Frick M, Isaksson M, Björkner B, Hindsén M, Pontén A, Bruze M (2003) Occupational allergic contact dermatitis in a company manufacturing boards coated with isocyanate lacquer. Contact Dermatitis 48:255–260

308. Bhardwaj SS, Brodell RT, Taylor JS (2003) Red tattoo reactions. Contact Dermatitis 48:236–237

309. Greve B, Chytry R, Raulin C (2003) Contact dermatitis from red tattoo pigment (quinacridone) with secondary spread. Contact Dermatitis 49:265–266

310. Ahlgren C, Ahnlide I, Björkner B, Bruze M, Liedholm R, Möller H, Nilner K (2002) Contact allergy to gold is correlated to dental gold. Acta Derm Venereol 82:41–44

311. Crissey JT (1965) Stomatitis, dermatitis, and denture materials. Arch Dermatol 92:45–48

312. Koutis D, Freeman S (2001) Allergic contact stomatitis caused by acrylic monomer in a denture. Aust J Dermatol 42203–206

313. Tosti A, Piraccini BM, Peluso AM (1997) Contact and irritant stomatitis. Semin Cutan Med Surg 16:314–319

314. Koch P (1998) Orale lichenoide Läsionen. Auslösung durch exogene Faktoren? Dermatosen 46:196–201

315. Von Mayenburg J, Frosch PJ, Fuchs T, Aberer W, Bäurle G, Brehler R, Busch R, Gaber G, Hensel O, Koch P, Peters K-P, Rakoski J, Rueff F, Szliska C (1996) Mercury and amalgam sensitivity. Possible clinical manifestations and sources of contact sensitization. Dermatosen 44:213–221

316. Räsänen L, Kalimo K, Laine J, Vainio O, Kotiranta J, Pesola I (1996) Contact allergy to gold in dental patients. Br J Dermatol 134:673–677

317. Bruze M, Edman B, Björkner B, Möller H (1994) Clinical relevance of contact allergy to gold sodium thiosulfate. J Am Acad Dermatol 31:579–583

318. Wong L, Freeman S (2003) Oral lichenoid lesions (OLL) and mercury in amalgam fillings. Contact Dermatitis 48:74–79

319. Östman P-O, Anneroth G, Skoglund A (1996) Amalgam-associated oral lichenoid reactions. Clinical and histologic changes after removal of amalgam fillings. Oral Surg Oral Med Oral Pathol Oral Radiol Endod 81:459–465

320. Laine J, Kalimo K, Happonen R-P (1997) Contact allergy to dental restorative materials in patients with oral lichenoid lesions. Contact Dermatitis 36:141–146

321. Mobacken H, Hersle K, Sloberg K, Thilander H (1984) Oral lichen planus: hypersensitivity to dental restoration material. Contact Dermatitis 10:11–15

322. Finne K, Göransson K, Winckler L (1982) Oral lichen planus and contact allergy to mercury. Int J Oral Surg 11:236–239

323. Burrows D (1989) Mischievous metals – chromate, cobalt, nickel and mercury. Clin Exp Dermatol 14:266–272

324. Veien NK, Borchorst E, Hattel T, Laurberg G (1994) Stomatitis or systemically-induced contact dermatitis from metal wire in orthodontic materials. Contact Dermatitis 30:210–213

325. Pigatto PD, Guzzi G (2004) Systemic contact dermatitis from nickel associated with orthodontic appliances. Contact Dermatitis 50:100–101

326. Hensten-Pettersen (1989) Nickel allergy and dental treatment procedures. In: Maibach HI, Menné T (eds) Nickel and the skin: immunology and toxicology. CRC, Boca Raton, Fla., pp 195–205

327. Fisher AA (1987) Reactions of the mucous membrane to contactants. Clin Dermatol 5:123–136

328. Chan EF, Mowad C (1998) Contact dermatitis to foods and spices. Am J Contact Dermat 9:71–79

329. Sonnex TS, Dawber RPR, Ryan TJ (1981) Mucosal contact dermatitis due to instant coffee. Contact Dermatitis 7:298–300

330. Guerra L, Vincenzi C, Peluso AM, Tosti A (1993) Role of contact sensitizers in the burning mouth syndrome. Am J Contact Dermat 4:154–157

331. Peters MS, Schroeter AL, Van Hale VM, Braodbent JC (1984) Pacemaker contact sensitivity. Contact Dermatitis 11:214–218

332. Romaguera C, Grimalt F (1981) Pacemaker dermatitis. Contact Dermatitis 7:333

333. Wilkinson JD (1989) Nickel allergy and orthopedic prostheses. In: Maibach HI, Menné T (eds) Nickel and the skin: immunology and toxicology. CRC, Boca Raton, Fla., pp 187–193

334. Lacroix J, Morin CL, Collin P-P (1979) Nickel dermatitis from a foreign body in the stomach. J Pediatr 95:428–429

335. McFadden N, Lyberg T, Hensten-Pettersen A (1989) Aluminium-induced granulomas in a tattoo. J Am Acad Dermatol 20:903–908

336. Fleming C, Parry E, Forsyth A, Kemmett D (1997) Patch testing in discoid eczema. Contact Dermatitis 36:261–264

337. Janniger CK, Schwartz RA (1995) Seborrhoeic dermatitis. Am Fam Physician 52:149–155, 159–160

338. Kerl H, Pachinger W (1979) Psoriasis: odd varieties in the adult. Acta Derm Venereol (Stockh) [Suppl] 87:90–94

339. Veien NK, Hattel T, Laurberg G (1997) Low-humidity dermatosis from car heaters. Contact Dermatitis 37:138

340. Clark AR, Sherertz EF (1998) The incidence of allergic contact dermatitis in patients with psoriasis vulgaris. Am J Contact Dermat 9:96–99

341. Heule F, Tahapary GJM, Bello CR, van Joost Th (1998) Delayed-type hypersensitivity to contact allergens in psoriasis. A clinical evaluation. Contact Dermatitis 38:78–82

342. Feuerman EJ, Ingber A, David M, Weissman-Katzenelson V (1982) Lichen ruber planus beginning as a dyshidrosiform eruption. Cutis 30:401–404

343. Jakob T, Tiemann M, Kuwert C, Abeck D, Mensing H, Ring J (1996) Dyshidrotic cutaneous T-cell lymphoma. J Am Acad Dermatol 34:295–297

14

Chapter 15

Clinical Aspects of Irritant Contact Dermatitis

15

PETER J. FROSCH, SWEN MALTE JOHN

Contents

multifactorial disease in most cases. Toxic chemicals (irritants) are the major cause, but mechanical, thermal, and climatic effects are important contributory cofactors. The clinical spectrum of irritant contact dermatitis is much wider than that of allergic contact dermatitis and ranges from slight scaling of the stratum corneum, through redness, whealing, and deep caustic burns, to an eczematous condition indistinguishable from allergic contact dermatitis. Acute forms of irritant contact dermatitis may be painful and may be associated with sensations such as burning, stinging or itching. Individual susceptibility to irritants is extremely variable.

Core Message

■ Irritant contact dermatitis is caused by chemicals which damage skin structures in a direct nonallergic way. The clinical picture is extremely variable and ranges from chemical burns to chronic irritant forms, often indistinguishable from allergic contact dermatitis.

15.2 Clinical Pictures

The morphology of cutaneous irritation varies widely and depends on the type and intensity of the irritant(s). Based on clinical criteria we may distinguish the following types:

■ Chemical burns
■ Irritant reactions
■ Acute irritant contact dermatitis
■ Chronic irritant contact dermatitis (cumulative insult dermatitis).

Folliculitis, acneiform eruptions, miliaria, pigmentary alterations, alopecia, contact urticaria and gran-

15.1 Definition

Irritant contact dermatitis may be defined as a nonallergic inflammatory reaction of the skin to an external agent. The acute type comprises two forms, the irritant reaction and acute irritant contact dermatitis, and usually has only a single cause. In contrast, the chronic form, cumulative insult dermatitis, is a

Table 1. Clinical effects of chemical irritants (adapted from [1])

Ulcerations	Strong acids (chromic, hydrofluoric, nitric, hydrochloric, sulfuric) Strong alkalis (especially calcium oxide, calcium hydroxide, sodium hydroxide, sodium metasilicate, sodium silicate, potassium cyanide, trisodium phosphate) Salts (arsenic trioxide, dichromates) Solvents (acrylonitrile, carbon disulfide) Gases (ethylene oxide, acrylonitrile)
Folliculitis and acneiform lesions	Arsenic trioxide Fiberglass (Fig. 1) Oils and greases Tar Asphalt Chlorinated naphthalenes Polyhalogenated biphenyls
Miliaria	Occlusive clothing and dressing Adhesive tape Aluminum chloride
Hyperpigmentation	Any irritant (especially phototoxic agents such as psoralens, tar, asphalt) Metals (inorganic arsenic, silver, gold, bismuth, mercury)
Hypopigmentation	*p-tert*-Amylphenol *p-tert*-Butylphenol Hydroquinone Monobenzyl ether of hydroquinone *p-tert*-Catechol 3-Hydroxyanisole 1-*tert*-Butyl-3, 4-catechol
Alopecia	Borax Chloroprene dimers
Urticaria	Chemicals (dimethylsulfoxide) Cosmetics (sorbic acid) Animals Foods Plants Textiles Woods
Granulomas	Silica Beryllium Talc

15

ulomatous reactions may result from irritancy to chemicals (Table 1, Fig. 1), but in the following only the first four types, clinically the most important, will be discussed in detail.

15.2.1 Chemical Burns

Highly alkaline or acid materials can cause severe tissue damage even after short skin contact. Painful erythema develops at exposed sites, usually within minutes, and is followed by vesiculation and formation of necrotic eschars (Figs. 2–7). Occasionally, intense whealing can be observed in the erythematous phase due to toxic degranulation of mast cells

(Fig. 7). The shape of lesions is bizarre and "artificial" in most cases and does not follow the usual pattern of known dermatoses. This is an important hallmark in differentiating accidental and self-inflicted lesions from genuine skin disease (Figs. 8, 9). In accidents the clothing may cause a sharp border due to its protective effect (e.g., explosion of liquids in containers).

Strong acids and alkalis are the major causes of chemical burns (Fig. 10). The halogenated acids are particularly dangerous because they may lead to deep continuous tissue destruction even after short skin contact (Fig. 2). Holes in protective gloves may result in serious injuries with scar formation. Caustic chemicals are also often trapped by clothing and footwear, resulting in deep ulceration down to the

Fig. 1.
Glass fiber dermatitis. Severe itchy small papules on the forearms of a teacher who isolated his roof with glass wool from a do-it-yourself store without any protection

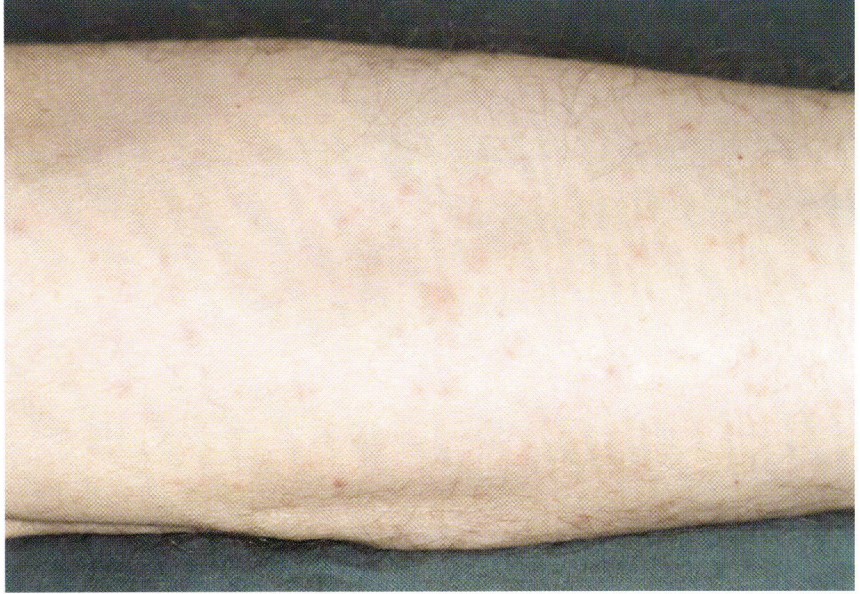

Fig. 2a, b.
Severe chemical burn caused by bromoacetic acid.
a Immediate effect.
b After 21 days there is still erythema, edema, and deep necrotic lesions

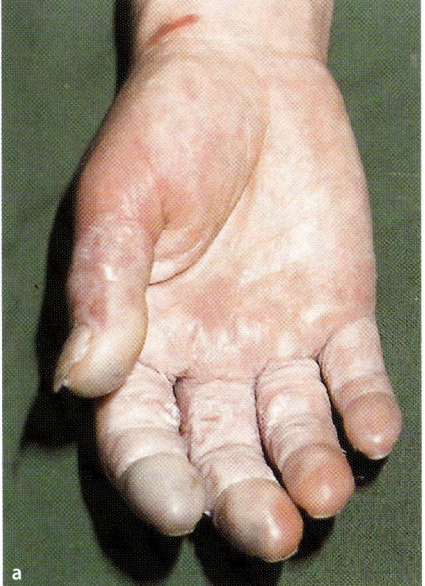
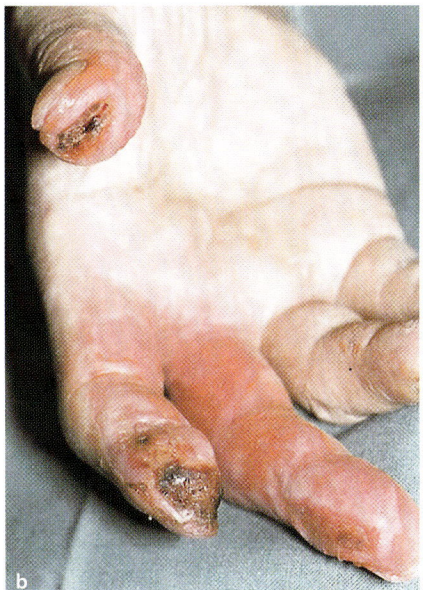

subcutaneous tissue, whereas other, open, areas are less severely affected because of the possibility of rapid removal (Figs. 3, 4).

It is important to realize that a number of other chemicals, including dusts and solids, may also cause severe necrotic lesions after prolonged skin contact, particularly under occlusion (cement, amine hardeners, etc.). If the concentration of the irritant is low or contact time short, multiple lesions can develop (Fig. 11).

Core Message

■ Chemical burns result from strong acids or alkalis. Halogenated acids are particularly dangerous. Severe tissue damage may result after short contact only. Typical is the initial painful whitening and edema of the skin, followed by deep necrosis and scarring.

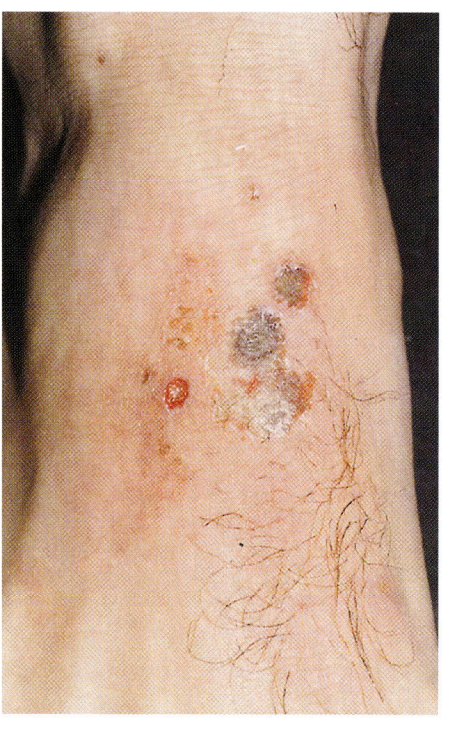

Fig. 3. Sharply demarcated ulcerative lesions on the dorsum of a chemistry student's foot caused by sodium hydroxide

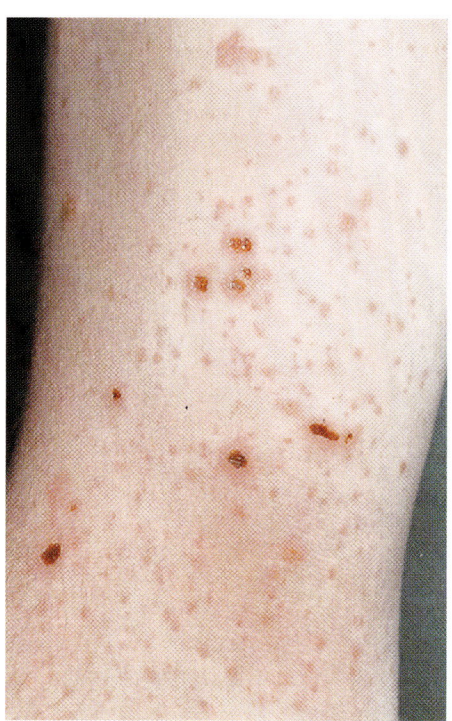

Fig. 4. Multiple follicular papules and necrotic lesions on the arm of a factory worker caused by sodium hydroxide trapped in the clothes after explosion of a container

15

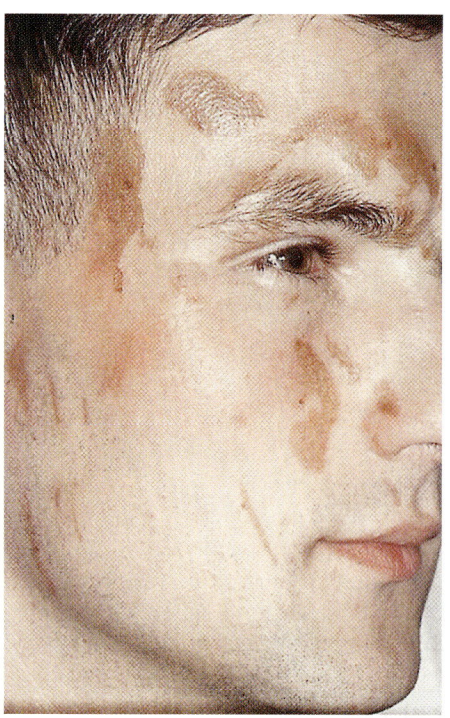

Fig. 5. Brown-yellow staining and superficial epidermal damage induced by splashes of nitric acid. Note the streaky pattern

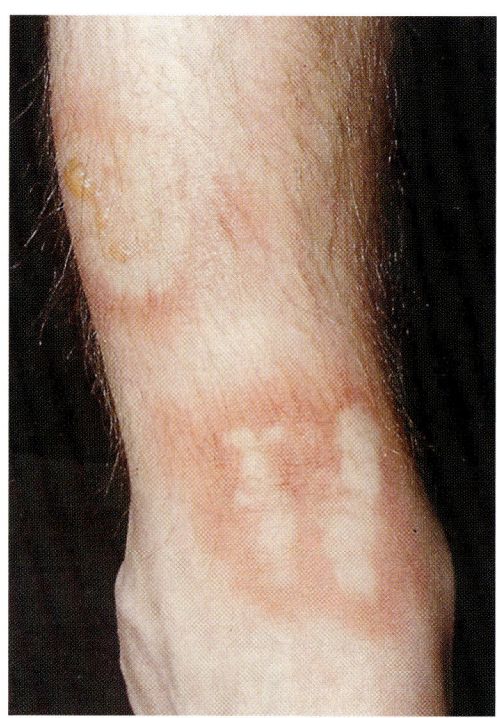

Fig. 6. Erythema and blistering on the lower leg caused by undiluted isothiazolinone (Kathon WT) trapped in the rubber boot of a machinist adding the biocide to cutting oil

Fig. 7.
Urticarial plaques 20 min after contact with concentrated phenol (explosion of a container)

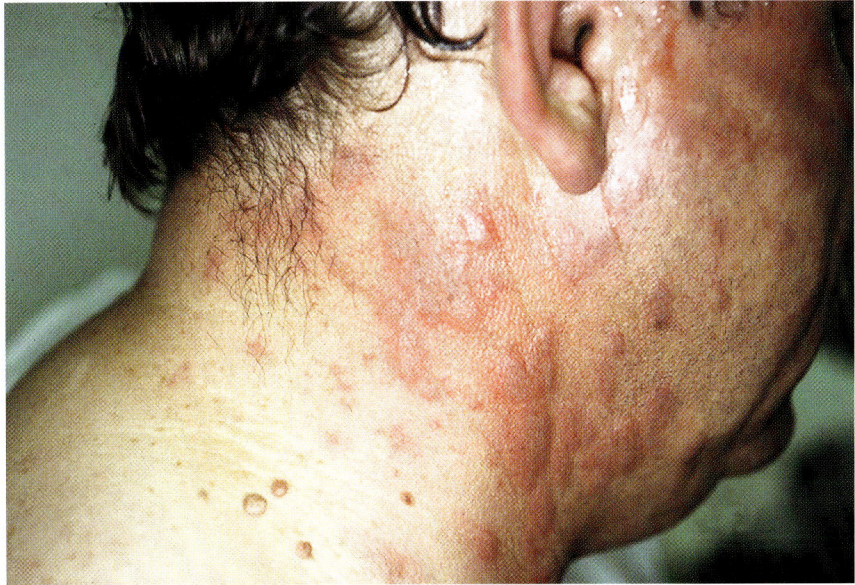

Fig. 8.
Acute chemical burn with sharply demarcated erythema and superficial erosions due to a concentrated acid (most likely hydrochloric acid); pH in the lesion was 1.2, in the adjacent areas 5.4. This artifactual dermatitis was seen in a car mechanic who claimed for legal compensation

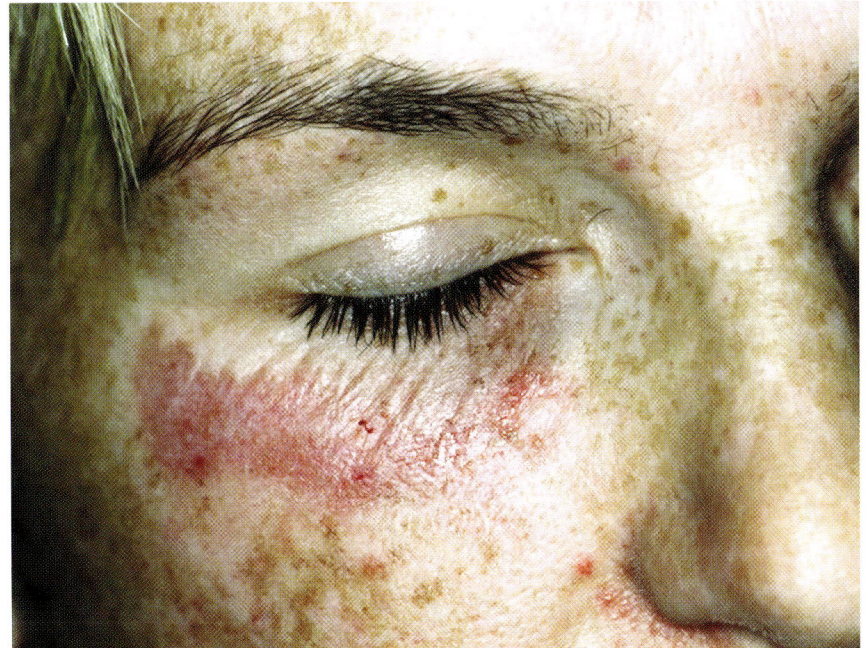

15.2.2 Irritant Reactions

Irritants may produce cutaneous reactions that do not meet the clinical definition of a "dermatitis." In English-speaking countries the term "dermatitis" is held to be synonymous with "eczema" by most authors, though this can be disputed. The diagnosis "acute irritant reaction" is thus increasingly used if the clinical picture is monomorphic rather than polymorphic and characterized by one or more of the following signs: scaling (including the initial stage of "dryness"), redness (starting with faint follicular spots, up to dusky red areas with hemorrhages), vesicles (blisters), pustules, and erosions (follicular and planar). Severe cutaneous damage reaching down to dermal structures should be termed a "chemical burn" (German: *Verätzung*, French: *cautérisation*). In practice some overlap will exist which may result in a

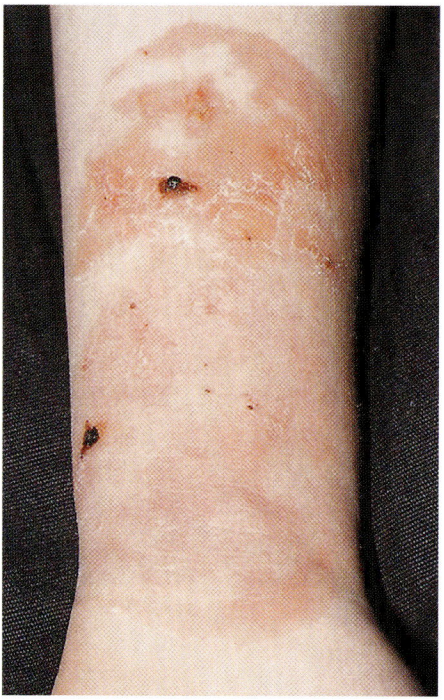

Fig. 9. Artefactual dermatitis with erythema, scaling and crusting in a psychotic patient caused by rubbing in a harsh floor cleanser. Typical of an artifact is the sharp demarcation

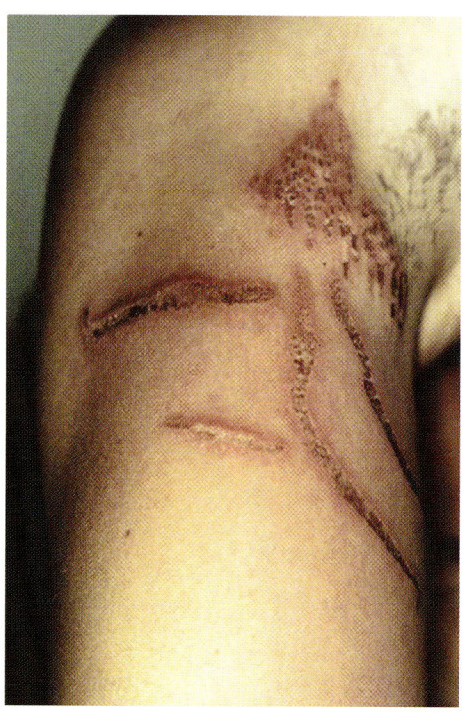

Fig. 10. Deep ulcerations with scar formation after contact with a jellyfish when bathing in the Mediterranean Sea

15

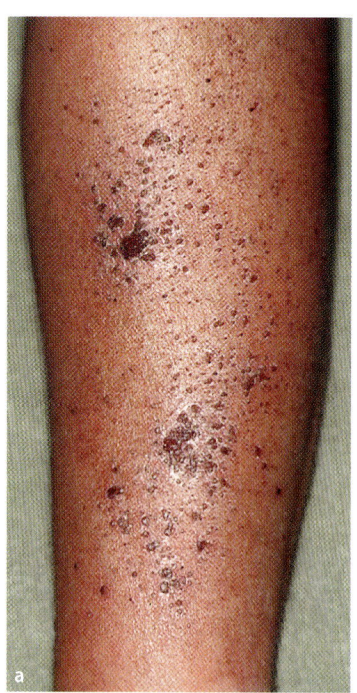

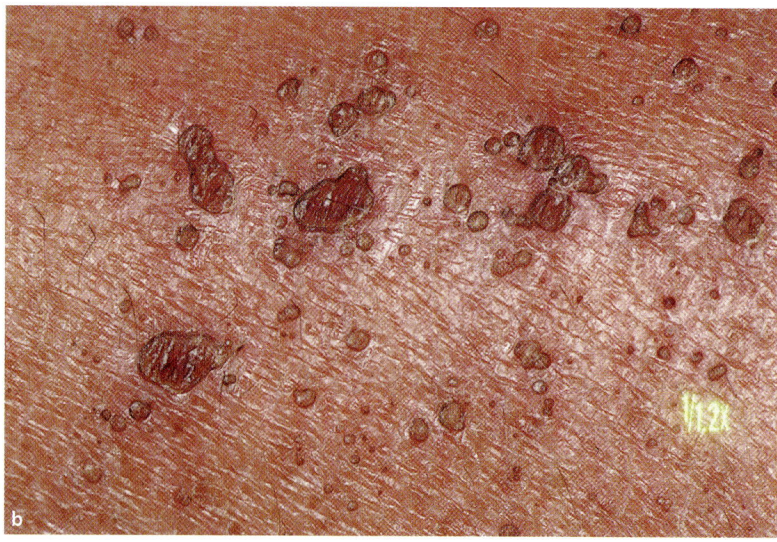

Fig. 11 a, b. Multiple small chemical burns due to cement dust on the arms of a mason. The lesions appeared when freshly set plaster was roughened with a sharp instrument

variable clinical picture, particularly when the course over time is followed (Table 6).

Chemicals which can cause irritant reactions are listed in Table 2, and typical clinical effects are shown in Figs. 12 and 13. The substances are mainly "mild irritants," i.e., ones that do not cause a severe skin reaction on short contact (<1 h). The resulting skin lesion may vary with the type of exposure, body region, and individual susceptibility (Fig. 14).

Core Message

- An irritant reaction is monomorphous (erythema, wheals, papules, pustules) and often experimentally induced.

Table 2. Common irritants which are important causes of occupational dermatitis (adapted from [36, 66, 188])

Water and its additives	(Salts and oxides of calcium, magnesium, and iron)
Skin cleansers	Soaps, detergents, "waterless cleansers," and additives (sand, silica)
Industrial cleaning agents	Detergents, surface-active agents, sulfonated oils, wetting agents, emulsifiers, enzymes
Alkalis	Soap, soda, ammonia, potassium and sodium hydroxides, cement, lime, sodium silicate, trisodium phosphate, and various amines
Acids	Severe irritancy (caustic): sulfuric, hydrochloric, nitric, chromic, and hydrofluoric acids
	Moderate irritancy: acetic, oxalic, and salicylic acids
Oils	Cutting oils with various additives (water, emulsifiers, antioxidants, anticorrosive agents, preservatives, dyes and perfumes)
	Lubricating and spindle oils
Organic solvents	White spirit, benzene, toluene, trichloroethylene, perchloroethylene, methylene chloride, chlorobenzene
	Methanol, ethanol, isopropanol, propylene glycol
	Ethyl acetate, acetone, methyl ethyl ketone, ethylene glycol monomethyl ether, nitroethane, turpentine, carbon disulfide
	Thinners (mixtures of alcohols, ketones, and toluene)
Oxidizing agents	Hydrogen peroxide, benzoyl peroxide, cyclohexanone peroxide, sodium hypochlorite
Reducing agents	Phenols, hydrazines, aldehydes, thioglycolates
Plants	Citrus peel and juice, flower bulbs, garlic, onion, pineapple, pelargonium, iris, cucumbers, buttercups, asparagus, mustard, barley, chicory, corn
	Various plants of the spurge family (Euphorbiaceae), Brassicaceae family (Cruciferae) and Ranunculaceae family (for further details see [61])
Animal products	Pancreatic enzymes, bodily secretions
Miscellaneous irritants	Alkyl tin compounds and penta-, tetra-, and trichlorophenols (wood preservatives)
	Bromine (in gasoline, agricultural chemicals, paper industry, flame retardant)
	Methylchloroisothiazolinone and methylisothiazolinone (irritant at high concentrations during production or misuse)
	Components of plastic processing (formaldehyde, phenol, cresol, styrene, di-isocyanates, acrylic monomers, diallyl phthalate, aliphatic and aromatic amines, epichlorohydrin)
	Metal polishes
	Fertilizers
	Propionic acid (preservative in animal feed)
	Rust-preventive products
	Paint removers (alkyl bromide)
	Acrolein, crotonaldehyde, ethylene oxide, mercuric salts, zinc chloride, chlorine

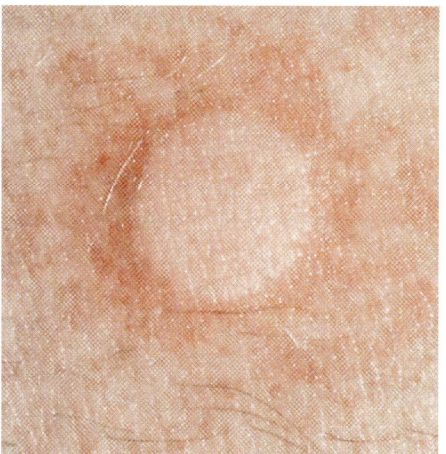

Fig. 12. Marked whealing induced by application of undiluted dimethylsulfoxide (*DMSO*) in a cup for 5 min

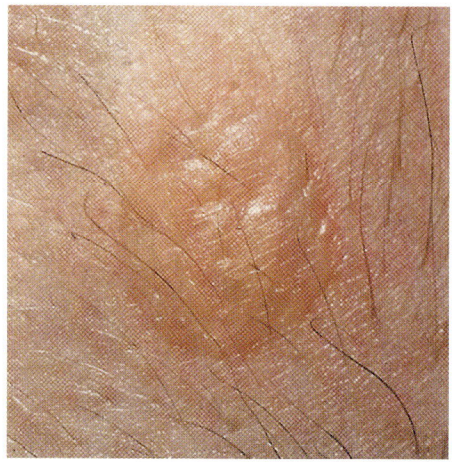

Fig. 13. Superficial blister after the application of 0.1% cantharidin in acetone for 24 h

Fig. 14.
Regional variation in cutaneous reactivity to the irritant dimethylsulfoxide (*DMSO*). The whealing response is most intense in the facial region and least on the palms of the hands (*AF* Antecubital fossa, *B* upper back, *FH* forehead, *L* lower leg, *W* wrist)

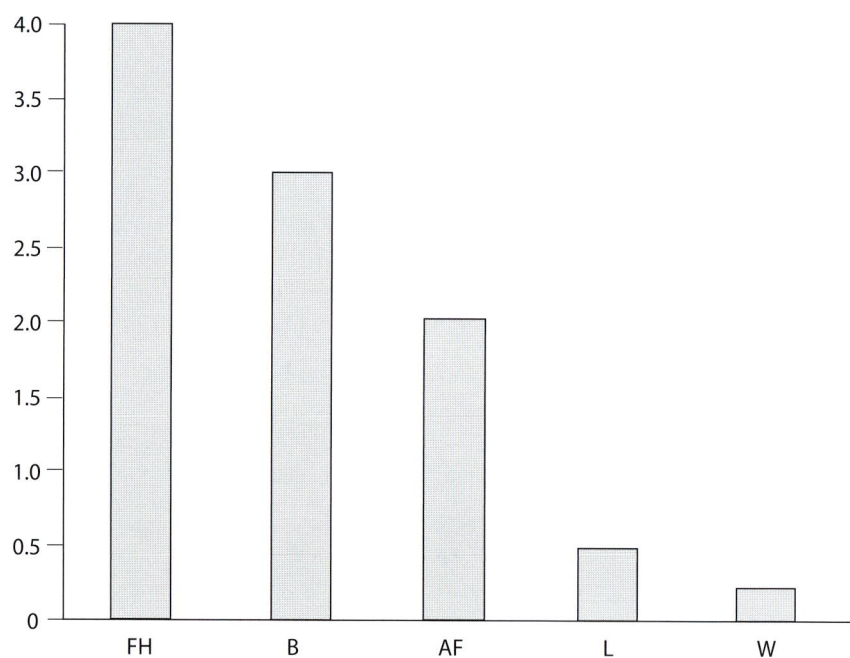

15

15.2.3 Acute Irritant Contact Dermatitis

The clinical appearance of acute irritant contact dermatitis is very variable and it may even be indistinguishable from the allergic type. There are numerous reports in the literature of even experienced dermatologists being misled into an initial assumption of allergic contact dermatitis, which later, after a careful work-up, turned out to be "only irritation." (Fig. 15).

Most instructive is the report by Malten et al. [145] on hexanediol diacrylate. A UV-cured paint used in a door factory contained hexanediol diacrylate, which caused an epidemic of papular and burning, rather than itching, dermatitis among the workers. Retrospectively, it is clear that the irritant contact dermatitis did not show the typical polymorphic picture of contact allergy, with the synchronous presence of macules, papules, and vesicles. These lesions developed one after another over the course of a few days (metachronic polymorphism). Malten et al. used the term "delayed irritation" for this type of cutaneous irritancy. In the meantime it has also been reported

Table 3. Substances causing delayed irritancy. The peak of intensity may show a crescendo pattern more typical of contact allergens

Benzalkonium chloride
Benzoyl peroxide
Bis (2-chloroethyl) sulfide
Bromine
Butanediol diacrylate
Calcipotriol
Dichlor (2-chlorovinyl) arsine
Diclofenac
Dithranol
Epichlorhydrin
Ethylene oxide
Hexanediol diacrylate
Nonanoic acid
Octyl gallate
Podophyllin
Propane sulfone
Propylene glycol
Sodium lauryl sulfate
Tetraethylene glycol diacrylate
Tretinoin

with other diacrylates [158] and various other substances [143].

Delayed irritation may be more common than so far generally thought. Further substances causing it are listed in Table 3. Irritant patch test reactions to benzalkonium chloride may be papular and increase in intensity with time [20, 30, 35]. On the normal skin surrounding psoriatic plaques, dithranol causes redness and edema, which may become very severe on the legs with venous stasis.

Calcipotriol frequently causes delayed irritation after several applications. Although redness and edema dominate, papules and vesicles may develop and mimic contact allergy. The latter has been verified only in rare cases, requiring patch testing with serial dilutions, repeated open application and, if possible, repeat of those procedures at a later stage [79]. Diclofenac gel is now widely used for the treatment of solar keratoses. In patients with sensitive skin a severe irritant dermatitis may develop within a few days, clinically indistinguishable from allergic contact dermatitis (Fig. 16).

Recently, a series of cases with chemical burns due to bromide was reported [120]. Small vesicles and bullae, or erythematous patches followed by hyperpigmentation, developed 2–5 days after exposure to bromine in the face and neck region of workers exposed to bromine vapors or liquids [120]. Bromine is used for gasoline additives, agricultural chemicals, flame retardants, dyes, photographic and pharmaceutical chemicals, bleaching of pulp and paper, etc.

The model irritants sodium lauryl sulfate (SLS) and nonanoic acid have been used in many patch test studies as a "positive control." Using detailed visual scoring, and particularly with bioengineering methods (transepidermal water loss, skin blood flow, skin surface contour), it can be demonstrated that the intensity of reaction may increase over time (48 h versus 96 h), at least within a certain low concentration range [4, 176]. Furthermore, data from right to left comparisons showed good reproducibility. The traditional view in patch testing that reactions that fade

Fig. 15.
Acute irritant contact dermatitis with acneiform features in a patient with severe acne vulgaris. Initially thought to be caused by the prescribed topical medications (benzoyl peroxide washing solution, clindamycin gel) it turned out to be due to an epilating wax, which the patient applied once weekly

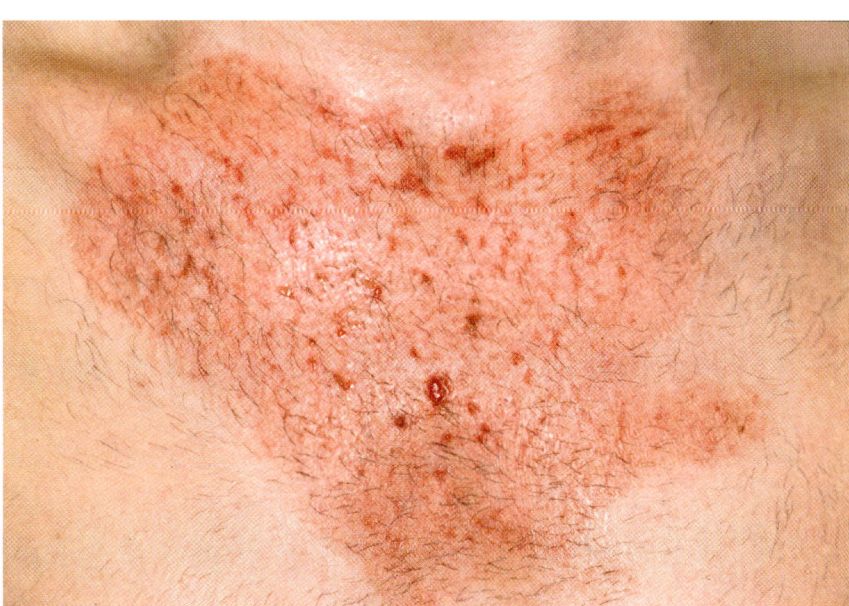

Fig. 16.
Acute irritant contact dermatitis on the forehead 1 -
week after the application of
diclofenac gel (twice daily)
for the treatment of actinic
keratoses. The patient had
skin type I and very sensitive
skin all his life. Patch testing
with diclofenac gel as well as
a repetitive open application
test on the forearm for 1 -
week was negative

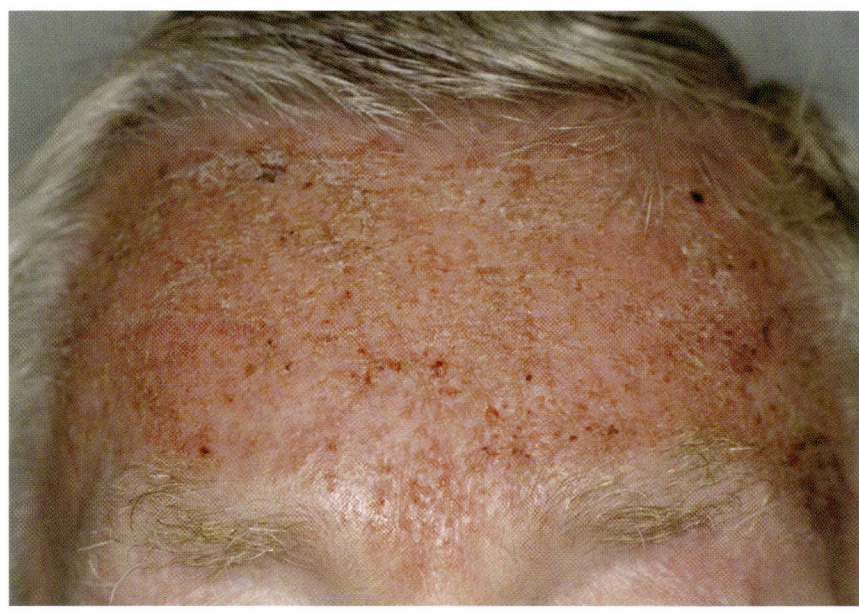

after 48 h are necessarily irritant, rather than allergic, has to be discarded.

Irritation due to tretinoin develops usually after a few days and is characterized by mild to fiery redness, followed by large flakes of stratum corneum. The dermatitis is burning rather than itching. The skin becomes sensitive to touch and to water (Fig. 17).

Acute irritant contact dermatitis includes other well-known entities such as irritation from adhesive tapes (Fig. 18), diaper dermatitis [10], perianal der-

15

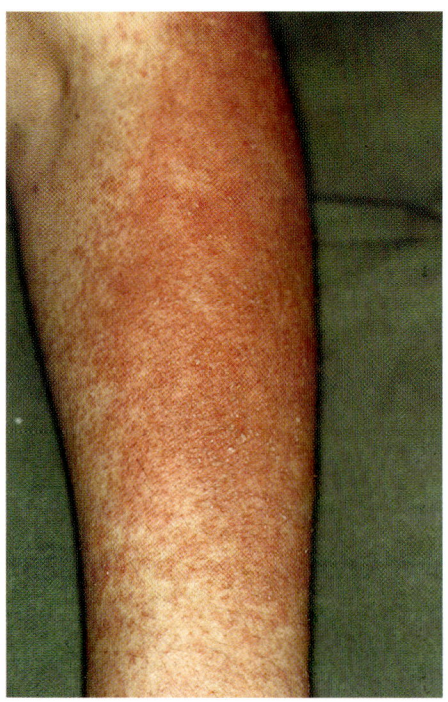

Fig. 17. Acute irritant contact dermatitis with erythema, papules, and scaling after 2 weeks of application of a cream containing tretinoin and urea for follicular hyperkeratosis. Patch testing was negative

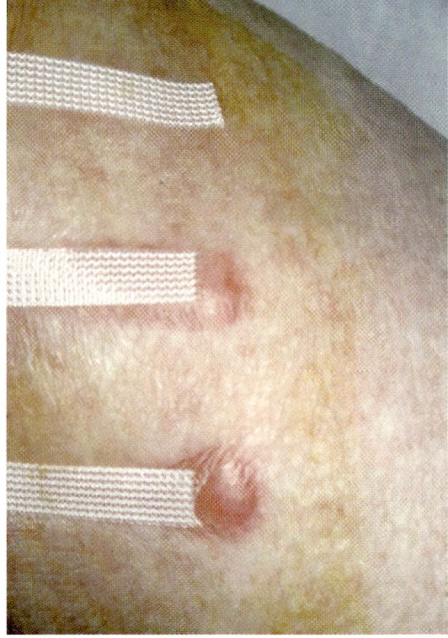

Fig. 18. Bullous lesions caused by tension along tape strips for the closure of a surgical wound. There was no dermatitis; patch testing with the tape was negative

Fig. 19.
Airborne irritant contact
dermatitis with slight erythema and scaling caused by
irritating stone dust (lime
and chalk)

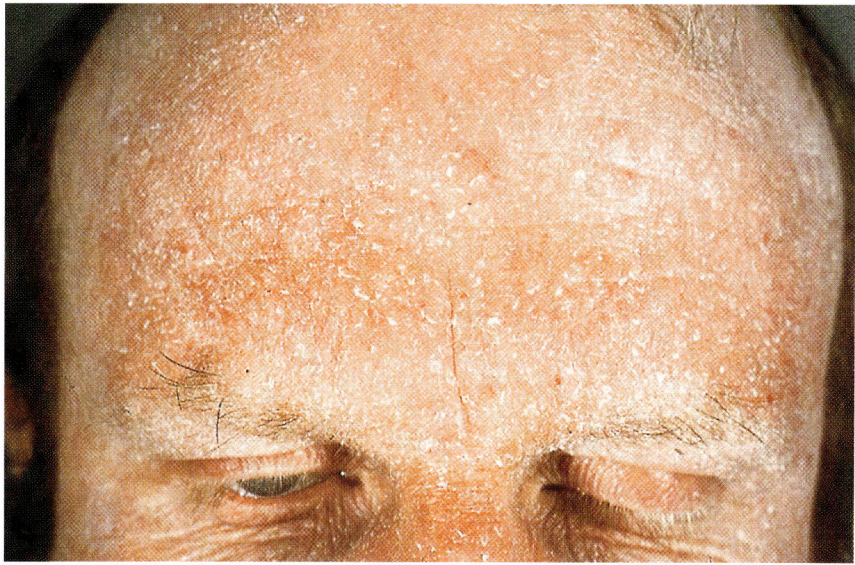

Table 4. Dermatoses where irritants play a major role in the
pathogenesis. Depending on individual susceptibility and intensity of exposure to the irritant(s), the dermatitis may be
more acute or more chronic

Hand eczema
Cosmetic dermatitis
Eyelid eczema
Reactions to therapeutics
Tape irritation
Diaper dermatitis
Perianal and stoma dermatitis
Asteatotic eczema
"Status eczematicus"
Juvenile plantar dermatosis
Photoirritation
Plant dermatitis
Reactions to wool and textiles
Contact urticaria
Subjective irritation ("stinging")
Airborne irritant contact dermatitis

ments this may provoke a severe spreading dermatitis, even with vulvodynia [144]. It has also been described in patients taking danthron laxatives, converted in the colon to the well-known irritant dithranol.

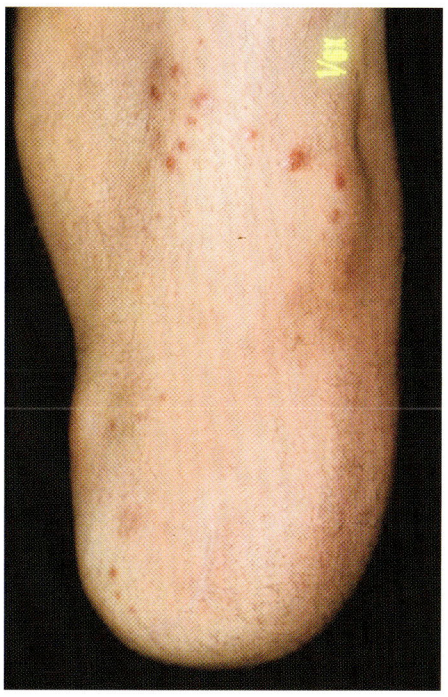

Fig. 20. Acneiform lesions and erythema on an amputated leg
due to occlusion of the prosthesis. Extensive patch testing was
negative

matitis, and airborne irritant contact dermatitis due
to dusts and vapors (Table 4, Fig. 19). A long list of
airborne irritants that caused a dermatitis, which initially was often thought to be allergic, has been compiled and recently updated (Table 5) [52, 102].

Cosmetics are not infrequently the cause of mild
irritant contact dermatitis on the face, particularly
the eyelids, where contact allergy has to be excluded
by appropriate patch and use testing.

Reaction to prostheses of the limbs (Fig. 20) or
hearing aids are often not allergic but irritant. Perianal dermatitis is primarily due to fecal enzymes, but
in patients taking pancreatic enzymes as supple-

Table 5. Causes of airborne contact dermatitis. Listed are reports on allergic contact dermatitis, irritant contact dermatitis, photoallergic reactions, contact urticaria, contact allergy syndrome, erythema-multiforme-like eruption, pigmented contact dermatitis and various eruptions (adapted from [52, 102, 128])

1. Plants, natural resins, and wood allergens	*Acacia melanoxylon* (Australian blackwood)
	Alstroemeria (tulipalin A)
	Anethole
	Apuleia leiocarpa wood (Brazilian wood)
	Atranorin (metabolite of oak moss)[a]
	Bowdichia nitida (sucupira, South-American wood)
	Champignon mushroom
	Citrus fruits (lemon essential oils)
	Coleus plant[a]
	Colophonium[a] and pine dust
	Compositae (Asteraceae)
	Dalbergia latifolia Roxb. (East-Indian rosewood)
	Dendranthema morifolium
	Entandrophragma cylindricum
	Essential oils[a]
	Fraxinus americanus (a domestic wood)
	Frullania (liverwort)
	Garlic
	Helianthus annuus (sunflower)
	Iroko (*Chlorophora excelsa*, West-African hard wood)
	Lichens
	Machaerium acutiforium (Bolivian rosewood, a tropical wood)
	Machaerium scleroxylon (Santos rosewood. pao ferro)
	Panthenium hyserophorus
	Primula obconica
	Soybean
	Tea tree oil[a]
	Tropical woods (e.g., framire)
	Wild plants (*Anthemis nobilis*, *Sisymbrium officinale*)
2. Plastics, rubbers, glues	Acrylates
	Aziridine derivates
	Benzoyl peroxide
	Diaminodiphenylmethane
	Dibutylthiourea
	Epoxy acrylates
	Epoxy resin (and amines)[a]
	Formaldehyde and formaldehyde resins isocyanates (diphenylmethane-4, 4′-diisocyanate)
	Isophoronediamine
	Triglycidyl isocyanurate
	Unsaturated polyester resin
3. Metals	Arsenic salts
	Chromate (potassium dichromate)
	Cobalt
	Gold
	Mercury
	Nickel

15

Table 5. Continued.

4. Industrial and pharmaceutical chemicals	Albendazole(antihelminthic agent)
	2-Aminophenyldisulfide
	2-Aminothiophenol
	Apomorphine[a]
	Benzalkonium chloride
	Bis-(aminopropyl)-laurylamine
	Budesonide[a]
	Cacodylic acid
	Cefazolin
	Chloroacetamide
	Chlorprothixene
	Color developers
	Didecyldimethylammonium chloride
	Difencyprone
	Di-isopropyl carbodi-imide
	DOPPI
	Ethylenediamine
	FADCP
	Famotidine and intermediates
	Hydroxylammonium chloride
	Isoflurane
	Isothiazolinones
	Metaproterenol
	Methyl red (dye)
	Nicergoline
	Ortho-chlorobenzylidenemalonitrile
	Paracetamol
	Phosphorus sesquisulfide
	Phthalocyanine pigments
	Propacetamol
	Pyritinol (and pyritinol hydrochloride)
5. Pesticides and animal feed additives	Carbamates (fungicides)
	Cobalt (animal feed additive)
	Dyrene
	Ethoxyquin (antioxidant in animal feed)
	Olaquindox
	Oxytetracycline hydrochloride (animal feed antibiotic)
	Penicillin (animal feed antibiotic)
	Pyrethrum
	Spiramycin (animal feed antibiotic) tetrachloroacetophenone (insecticide)
	Tylosin (animal feed antibiotic)
6. Miscellaneous	Cigarettes and matches
	Tyrophagus putrescentiae
	Pig epithelia
	Penicillium[a]
	Cladosporium[a]

[a] Non-occupational

Various irritants have been tested under experimental conditions and it has been shown that a wide range of lesions can be produced by varying the dose and mode of exposure (Table 6).

The reaction's intensity depends on numerous exogenous and endogenous factors. Under experimental conditions a full range of lesions may be produced with the same irritant by varying its dose. In this table, the most typical skin changes are given as observed frequently after more or less "normal" exposure. Most irritants can produce severe bullous reactions if applied under occlusion at high concentration for 24 h. For further details, see [30, 72, 107, 220–222, 240]. The irritant potential of water after repetitive short contact or long continuous exposure has been underestimated in the past [204]. Recently Warner et al. have shown by ultrastructural studies that water directly disrupts stratum corneum lipid lamellar bilayers even after a 4-h occlusion phase [225]. Effects are similar to those induced by surfactants [224].

15.2.4 Chronic Irritant Contact Dermatitis

Other terms synonymous with chronic irritant contact dermatitis include "cumulative insult dermatitis," "traumiterative dermatitis," and "wear and tear dermatitis" (German: *Abnutzungsdermatose, chronisch degeneratives Ekzem*). Although never clearly defined, this diagnosis applies to an eczematous condition that persists for a considerable time period (minimum 6 weeks) and for which careful diagnostic investigation has failed to demonstrate an allergic cause. Taking a detailed history usually reveals the dermatitis to be caused by repetitive contact with water, detergents, organic solvents, irritant foods or other known mild to moderate irritants.

The prime localization is on the hands ("housewives' eczema"). In a fully developed case, redness, infiltration and scaling with fissuring are seen all over the hands (Fig. 21). The dermatitis includes the fingers, initially starting in the webs, but spreading later to the sides and backs of the hands and finally including the palmar aspect. This is frequently observed in hairdressers [80] (Fig. 22a–c). The volar aspect of the wrist is usually unaffected, in contrast to allergic or

15

Table 6. Materials causing irritant reactions on human skin

Irritant	Cutaneous reaction
Water	Dryness, erythema, scaling, wrinkling ("immersion foot")
Detergents (anionic), soaps	Dryness erythema scaling, fissuring, (rarely vesicles)
Tretinoin, benzoyl peroxide dithranol, calcipotriol, diclofenac	Dryness, erythema, scaling
Benzalkonium chloride (and other cationic detergents)	Erythema, pustules (rarely delayed reactions) with papules
Dimethylsulfoxide	Erythema, whealing (strong)
Methyl nicotinate	Erythema, whealing (weak)
Capsaicin	Erythema, vesiculation
Sodium hydroxide	Erythema, erosions (follicular initially)
Lactic acid	Erythema, whealing
Nonanoic acid	Erythema, scaling
Croton oil	Erythema, pustules, purulent bullae
Kerosene	As croton oil
Cantharidin	Erythema, bullae
Metal salts (mercury chloride, cobalt chloride, nickel sulfate, potassium dichromate)ae	Erythema, pustules, purulent bull
Formic acid	Erythema, superficial blistering (removal of stratum corneum)
Xylene	Dryness, erythema
Toluene	Dryness, erythema, purpura

Fig. 21a, b.
Chronic irritant contact dermatitis (cumulative insult dermatitis).
a Housewife's eczema due to wet work and a number of irritants.
b Close-up view of the thumb

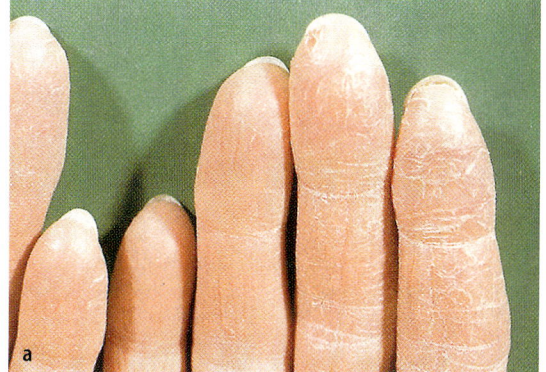
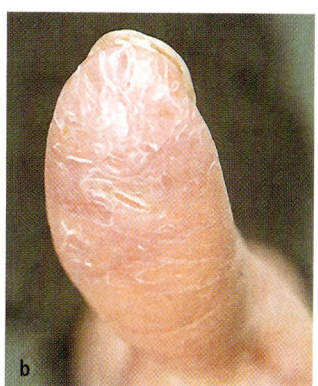

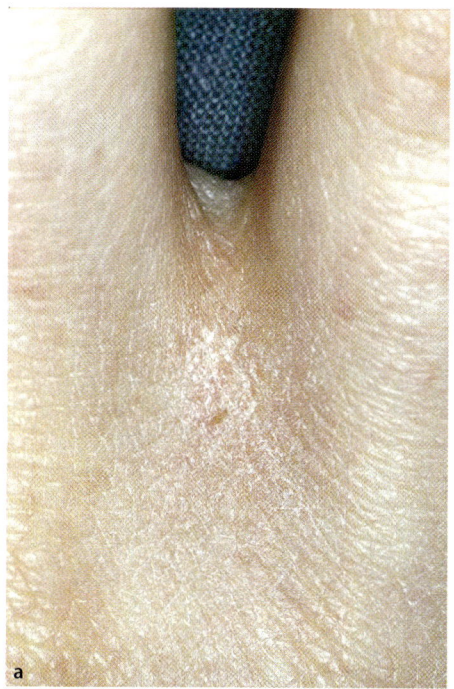
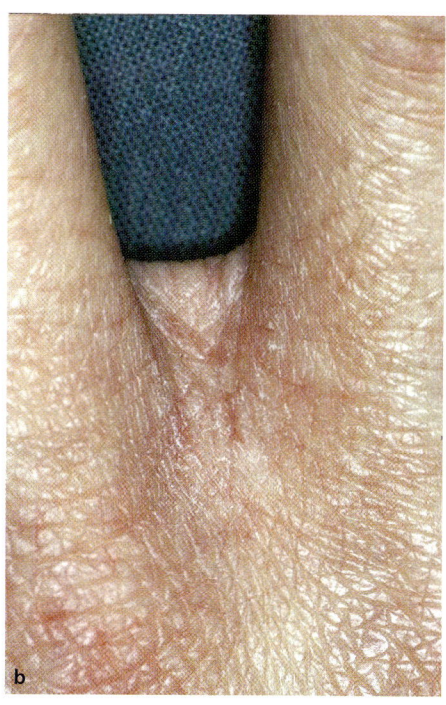

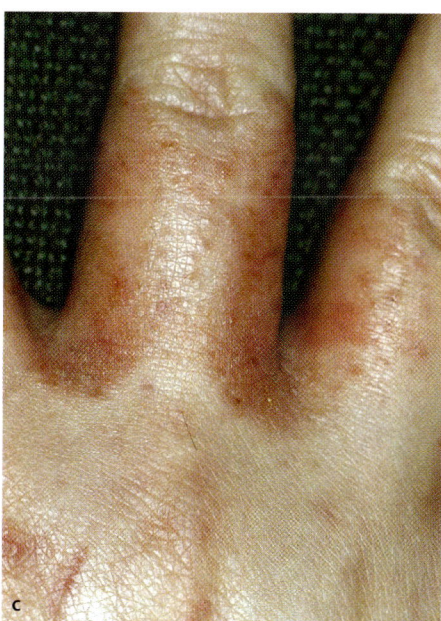

Fig. 22a–c.
Characteristic sequence of events in the development of irritant hand dermatitis due to unprotected wet work in the hairdressing trade (17-year-old female apprentice): initial mild interdigital scaling (**a**), gradual onset of erythema, lichenification, superficial fissures (**b**), marked erythema, vesicles, deep fissures and erosions (**c**)

Fig. 23.
Chronic irritant contact dermatitis of the nummular type on the back of the hand of a housewife

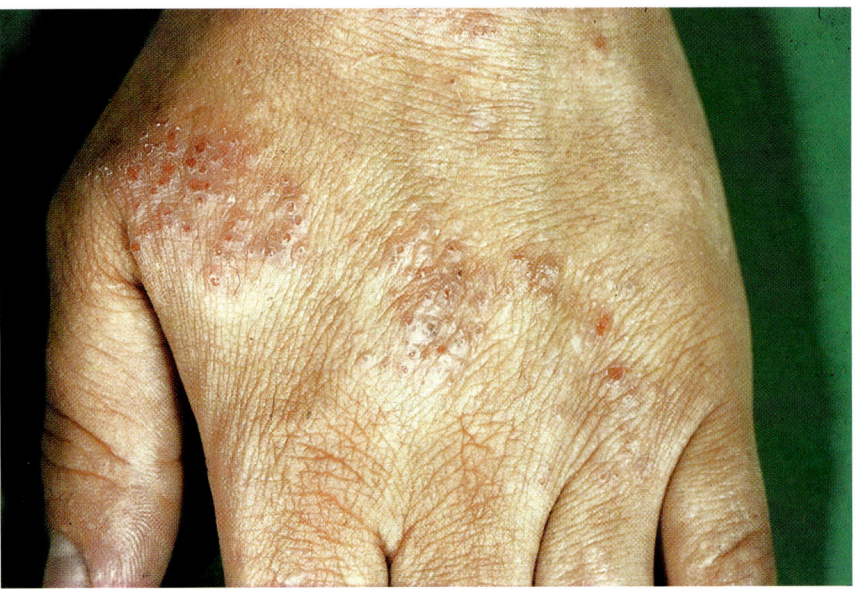

atopic hand eczema. Occasionally, there is a nummular pattern on the backs of the hands (Fig. 23). If there is extensive occupational contact with moderate irritants (organic solvents, detergents), the dermatitis may be limited to those fingers with most exposure. Friction is a further contributing factor and plays an important part in determining the localization of the dermatitis [90, 151, 152]. Hyperkeratosis of the fingertips was observed in nearly half of the shoemakers in the sole-cutting department as a reaction to the continuous trauma of working with leather [147].

The hallmark of chronic irritant contact dermatitis may be the absence of vesicles and the predominance of dryness and chapping, and a number of studies on hand eczema have confirmed that vesiculation is less frequent in the irritant type than in allergic and atopic types [22, 23, 127, 150]. However, the diagnosis is often complicated by so-called hybrids, where there is a combination of irritancy and contact allergy, or of irritancy and atopy, or even all three [150, 179]. For further information see Chap. 19 and a recent monograph on hand eczema [154].

Dermatitis due to metalworking fluids is irritant in most cases and shows a variable morphological pattern (Fig. 24). Some workers exhibit only dryness and scaling of the hands, whereas others develop an

15

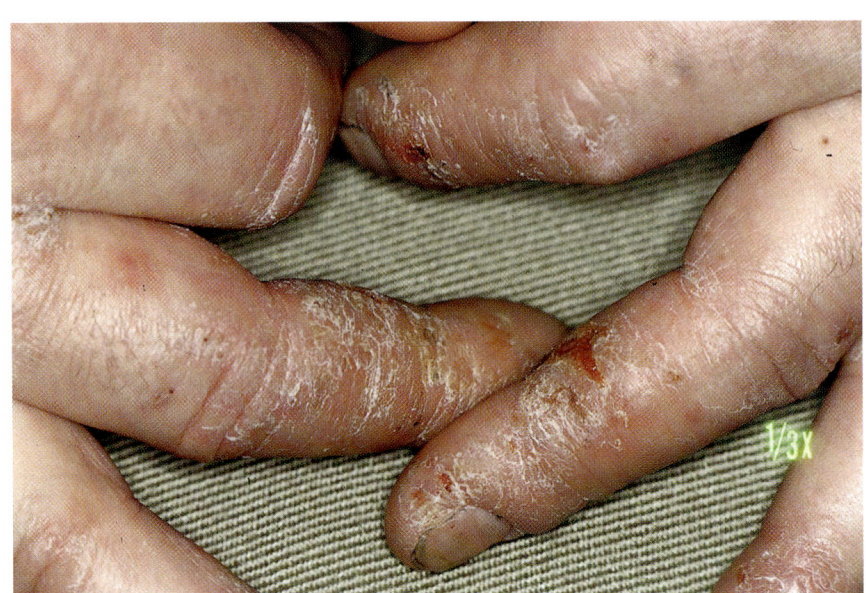

Fig. 24.
Chronic irritant contact dermatitis on the fingers from metalworking fluids in a metalworker polishing small objects

Table 7. High-risk occupations for chronic irritant (cumulative insult) contact dermatitis (adapted from [48])

Baker
Butcher
Canner
Caterer
Cleaner
Cook
Construction worker
Dental assistant or technician
Fisherman
Florist
Hairdresser
Health care worker
Horticulture and nursery gardening
Machinist
Masseur
Mechanic
Metalworker (surface processor)
Motor mechanic
Nurse (hospitals and nursing homes for elderly)
Painter
Pastry cook
Printer
Shoemaker
Tile setter and terrazzo worker

itchy nummular type of dermatitis spreading to the forearms and sometimes other exposed body regions. The correct diagnosis can often only be made after careful patch testing and re-exposure to the work environment [46].

In atopic hand eczema, irritant factors often play a major role in the pathogenesis. It is sometimes a matter of definition whether these cases are diagnosed primarily as atopic or irritant contact dermatitis.

High-risk occupations for chronic irritant contact dermatitis are listed in Table 7, and the major irritants in various occupations are summarized Table 8.

Core Message

■ Chronic irritant contact dermatitis is most frequently localized on the hands. Usually several chemical irritants are involved and cumulate together with climatic and mechanical factors to low-grade damage over months. Redness, scaling, and fissures on the back of the hands, between fingers or on the most exposed parts of the hands are prominent clinical signs. Lack of itching and slow aggravation after resuming work are typical. However, the diagnosis is often difficult, requires careful patch testing and a follow up. Furthermore, combined forms with a contact allergy may exist.

Case Reports

■ A 28-year old teacher developed a mild dermatitis on the back of both hands, on the finger webs, and on the finger tips of the right hand. There were slight redness, scaling, and fissures on the right thumb and index finger. The dermatitis started about 4 months after she gave birth to her first child. For 10 years she had slight rhinitis in early spring but had never suffered from atopic eczema. Skin testing revealed positive prick test to birch and hazelnut pollens. Patch testing with the standard series, vehicle/emulsifier series, preservatives and corticosteroid series showed a 2+ reaction to thiomersal and a doubtful reaction to thiuram mix (day 3 reading). In order to determine the clinical relevance of these reactions she reported upon focused questioning to have had several vaccinations without adverse effects. After the hand dermatitis had started she frequently wore rubber gloves during housework; occasionally she noticed slight itching, particularly when using them for more than 1 h.

Diagnosis: Chronic irritant contact dermatitis of hands. Allergic rhinitis. Contact allergy to thiomersal and possibly to thiuram mix.

Treatment and course: The patient was advised to avoid harsh detergents and long exposures to water and other known irritants (information leaflet for hand eczema). Bland emollients without fragrance were to be applied several times daily. She was told that she probably had a rubber allergy and should therefore use vinyl gloves. The thiomersal sensitization was of no current relevance but could become important in the future (eye make up, eye drops).

Comment: If the contact allergy to thiuram were certain, a combined form of hand eczema would exist in this case (irritant and contact allergic). The use of fragrance-free skin care products was recommended prophylactically to prevent further sensitizations common in patients with chronic hand eczema.

Table 8. List of irritants in various occupations (based on [1, 36, 42, 66])

Occupation	Irritants
Agricultural workers	Pesticides, artificial fertilizers, disinfectants and cleansers for milking utensils, petrol, diesel oil, plants, animal secretions
Artists	Solvents used for cleansing and degreasing, soaps and detergents, paint removers
Bakers and pastry makers	Soaps and detergents, oven cleaners, fruit juices, acetic, ascorbic and lactic acid, enzymes
Bartenders	Wet work, soaps and detergents, fruit juices, alcohol
Bathing attendants	Wet work, soaps and detergents, free or combined chlorine/bromine
Bookbinders	Glue, solvents
Building workers	Cement, chalk, hydrochloric and hydrofluoric acids, wood preservatives, glues
Butchers	Soaps and detergents, wet work, spices, meat, entrails
Canning and food industry workers	Soaps and detergents, wet work, brine, syrup, vegetables and vegetable juices, fruit and fruit juices, fish, meat, crustaceans
Carpenters, cabinet makers	French polish, solvents, glues, cleansers, wood preservatives
Chemical and pharmaceutical industry workers	Soaps and detergents, wet work, solvents, numerous other irritants that industry are specific for each work-place
Cleaners	Wet work, detergents, solvents
Coal and other miners	Oil, grease, cement, powdered limestone
Cooks, catering industry	Soaps and detergents, wet work, vegetable and fruit juices, spices, fish, meat, crustaceans, dressing, vinegar
Dentists and dental technicians	Soaps and detergents, wet work, soldering, fluxes, adhesives, acrylic monomers, solvents
Dyers	Solvents, oxidizing and reducing agents, hypochlorite, hair removers
Electricians, electronics industry	Soldering flux, metal cleaners, epoxy resin hardeners
Fishermen	Wet work, oils, petrol fish, crustaceans, entrails
Floor layers	Detergents, solvents, cement, adhesives
Florists, gardeners, plant growers	Manure, fertilizers, pesticides, irritating plants and plant parts
Foundry workers	Cleansers, oils, phenol-formaldehyde and other resins
Hairdressers and barbers	Soap, wet work, shampoos, permanent wave liquids, bleaching agents
Histology technicians	Solvents, formaldehyde
Hospital workers	Soaps and detergents, wet work, hand creams, disinfectants, quaternary ammonium compounds
Housework	Soaps and detergents, wet work, cleaners, polishes, food
Jewelers	Acids and alkalis for metal cleaning, polishes, soldering fluxes, rust removers, adhesives
Laundry workers	Detergents, wet work, bleaches, solvents, stain removers
Masons	Cement, chalk, acids
Mechanics	Detergents, hand cleansers, degreasers, lubricants, oils, cooling system fluids, battery acid, soldering flux, petrol, diesel oil
Metalworkers	Hand cleansers, cutting and drilling oils, solvents
Office workers	Ammonia from photocopy paper, carbonless copy paper
Painters	Solvents, emulsion paints, paint removers, organic tin compounds, hand cleanser
Photographers	Alkalis, acids, solvents, oxidizing and reducing agents
Plastics industry workers	Solvents, acids, oxidizing agents, styrene, di-isocyanates, acrylic monomers, phenols, formaldehyde, diallyl phthalate, ingredients in epoxy resin systems
Plating industry workers	Acids, alkalis, solvents, detergents
Plumbers	Wet work, hand cleansers, oils, soldering flux
Printers	Solvents, hand cleansers, acrylates in radiation-curing printing lacquers and inks
Radio and television repairers	Organic solvents, metal cleansers, soldering fluxes
Roofers	Tar, pitch, asphalt, solvents, hand cleansers
Rubber workers	Talc, zinc stearate, solvents
Shoemakers	Solvents, polishes, adhesives, rough leather
Shop assistants	Detergents, vegetables, fruit, fish, meat
Tanners	Wet work, acids, alkalis, oxidizing and reducing agents, solvents, proteolytic enzymes
Textile workers	Solvents, bleaching agents, detergents
Veterinarians	Soaps and detergents, hypochlorite, cresol, entrails, animal secretions
Welders	Oils, metal cleansers, degreasing agents
Woodworkers	Detergents, solvents, oils, wood preservatives

15

15.2.5 Special Forms of Irritation

15.2.5.1 Climatic Factors

Low outdoor temperatures and low humidity may cause dryness and scaling on the hands and face, and later on also on other body regions. Erythema is usually absent but may be prominent in more severe conditions with fissures or nummular eczema-like lesions ("eczema craquelée"). Living or working in overheated dry rooms will further aggravate the process, which has also been termed "low-humidity dermatosis" [186]. Office workers and outdoor occupations of various types are predisposed. Atopics are more easily affected than nonatopics. In a retrospective analysis of 29,000 patients who attended a contact dermatitis clinic in London, a diagnosis of physical irritant contact dermatitis was made in 1.15% of all patients. The most common cause was low humidity due to air-conditioning, which caused dermatitis of face and neck in office workers due to drying out of the skin [156].

Meteorological factors (dry and cold weather) can contribute to the pathogenesis of irritant hand dermatitis in wet work professions [209]. Some authors found increased irritability to standard irritants such as SLS, even of skin not directly exposed to weather conditions during the winter season in bioengineering studies [2, 15, 141]. Thus, it is no surprise that there is also a seasonal variation in allergy patch test results: the likelihood of weak, i.e., "false-positive" reactions is increased. This will particularly be the case for those allergens that are also marginal irritants [34, 86, 211–213].

Thermal injury can be very subtle and lead to an itchy eczematous plaque on the lower legs of car drivers in the winter ("car heater dermatitis", Fig. 25, [218].

15.2.5.2 Aggravation of Endogenous Dermatoses by Friction and Occlusion

Shoes, helmets, and other garments or carried equipment can lead to circumscribed lesions that may mimic allergic contact dermatitis. This is primarily seen in patients with a past or present atopic dermatitis or psoriasis (*Köbner phenomenon*) [155]. Typical cases are shown in Figs. 26–28. Friction, heat, and occlusion are triggering factors for manifestation of the endogenous disease in previously nonaffected regions. The sharp demarcation often suggests an allergic contact dermatitis, which must always be excluded by adequate testing. On the hand, psoriasis can be due to contact allergy to rubber gloves [101] but may also result solely from irritation, particularly in hospital personnel wearing gloves frequently [84, 175]. Several studies have shown that gloves impair skin barrier function and can further damage primarily irritated skin [175, 243]. A recent review summarizes the effects of occlusion on irritant and allergic contact dermatitis [250]: barrier function is decreased; the effect of irritants and contact allergens is increased, particularly on compromised skin; hydrocolloid patches that absorb water can decrease the irritant reaction caused by the occlusive agent itself;

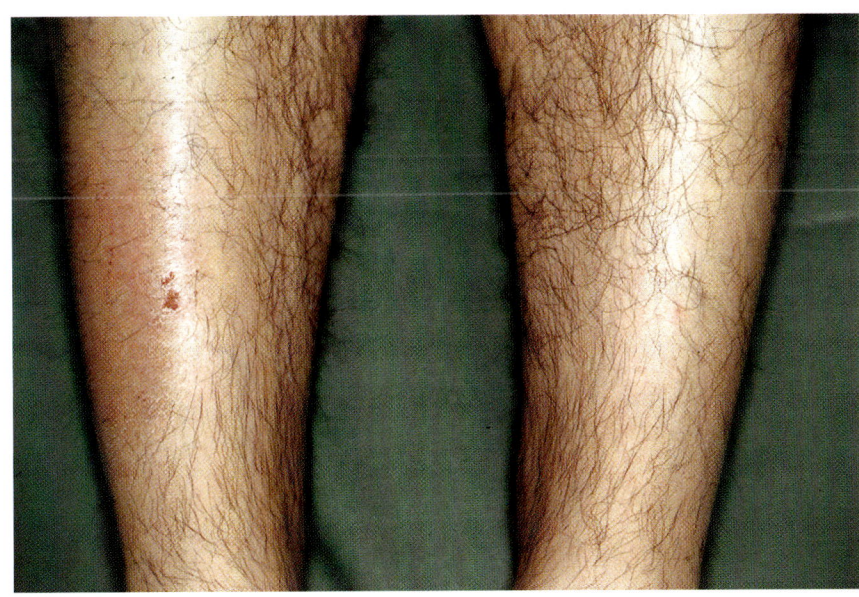

Fig. 25.
Car heater dermatitis in a salesman due to frequent long car driving. The hot air stream came from the center of the car and induced redness and scaling only on the directly exposed right leg

Fig. 26.
Psoriatic lesions on the forehead due to a tightly fitting
safety helmet. Patch testing
was negative – the patient
had only minor psoriatic lesions on the extremities

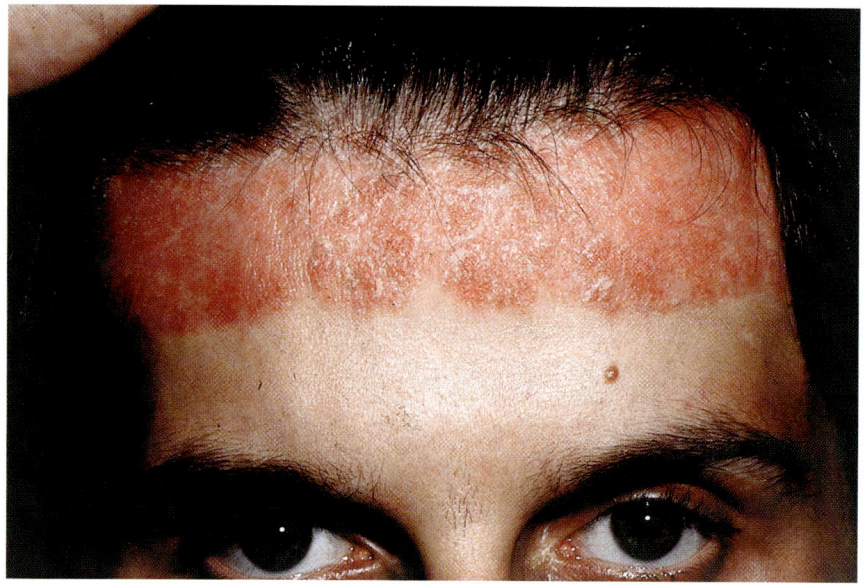

Fig. 27.
Nonallergic frictional dermatitis from safety boots in
a coal miner with mild atopic dermatitis on the neck and
flexures. Hyperhidrosis visible between the toes was
certainly a cofactor in this
case

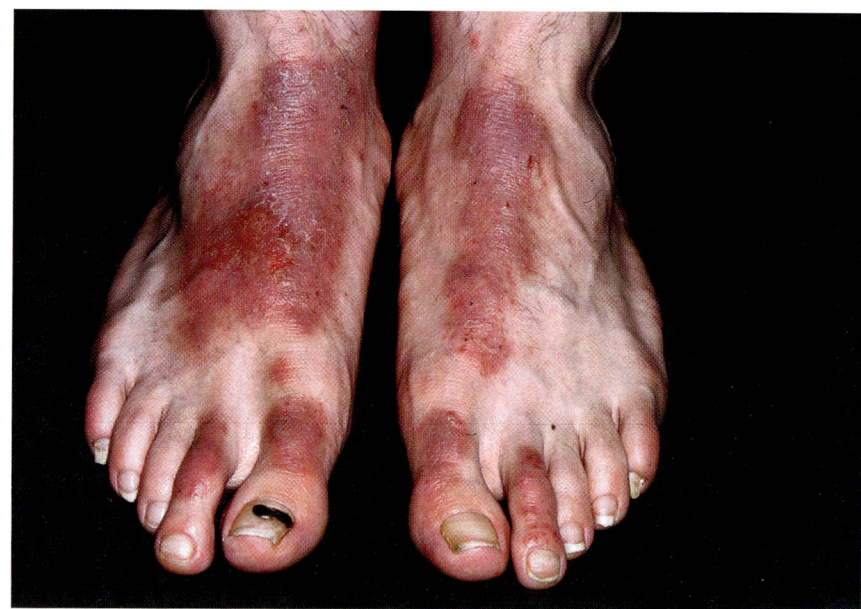

15

and occlusion does not significantly delay barrier repair in humans. The ubiquitous usage of the computer mouse has led to reports of low-grade frictional irritant dermatitis and formation of calluses [117, 203].
Contact allergy to plastic materials present in the
mouse or in the pad has also been observed [37]. In
view of the high numbers of users worldwide these
side-effects are apparently very rare.

15.3 Epidemiology

Hard data on the incidence of irritant contact dermatitis are still very limited. In many studies on contact
dermatitis no clear distinction is made between irritant and allergic types. The source population is also
often either ill-defined or highly selected (patients
attending a contact dermatitis clinic, for example),
and cases of slight cutaneous irritation where medical attention is not sought are therefore missed. Recent data are presented and discussed in detail in
Chap. 10. Some studies are, however, worthy of note
in this context.

Fig. 28.
Psoriasis, Köbner effect by stainless steel watch on left wrist. Note small adjacent psoriatic plaque. Patch test was negative

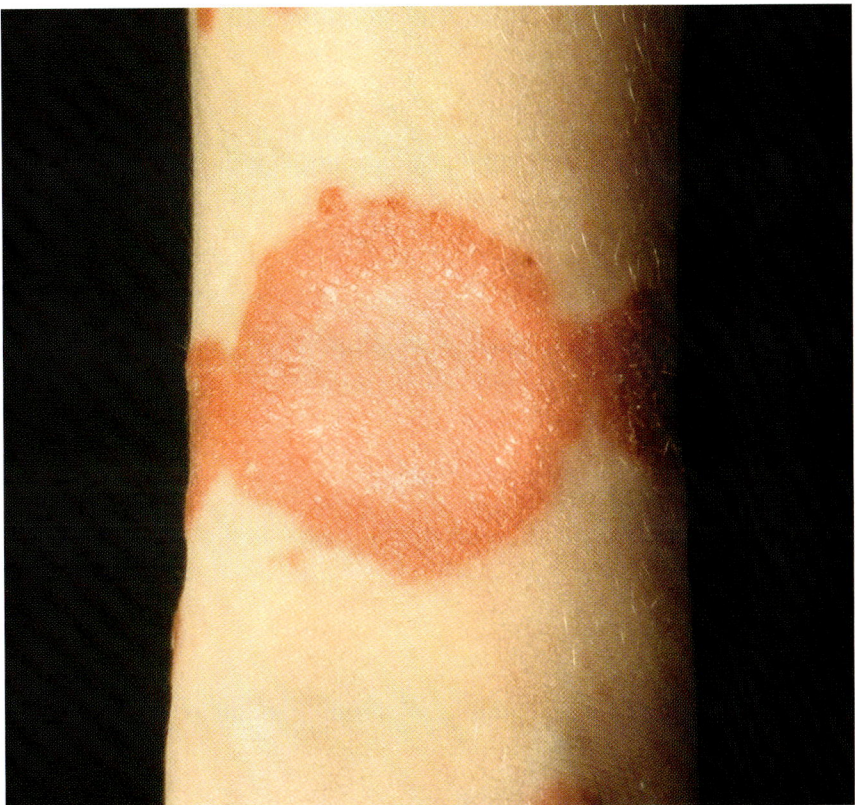

In Denmark, the compensation paid for occupational skin diseases was analyzed by Halkier-Sørensen [95]. Skin diseases represented 36% of all compensated cases and were closely followed by musculoskeletal disorders. For irritant eczema (59%) a total of DKr 102,671,567 was paid in comparison to allergic eczema (41%), DKr 71,147,070.

In a large multicenter prospective study on reactions caused by cosmetics, Eiermann et al. [55] found irritancy to account for 16% of 487 cases of contact dermatitis due to cosmetics. Over a time period of 40 months, approximately 179 800 patients were seen by 11 dermatologists and 8,093 patients were tested for contact dermatitis. In all, 487 cases (6%) were caused by cosmetics, the majority of them (407) being due to contact allergy. The authors pointed out that during the course of the study irritation was more frequently diagnosed once the physicians had been mentally "sensitized" to this type of reaction. When the adverse effects of 253 cosmetics and toiletries as reported to the Swedish Medical Products Agency were analyzed, 90% were eczematous reactions. Of these, 70% were classified as allergic and 30% as irritant [29]. The number of reports for the years of 1989–1994 appears to be small and can be explained by underreporting.

In Heidelberg, Germany, a retrospective study of 190 cases of hand dermatitis revealed the following distribution of diagnoses: atopic dermatitis 40%, chronic irritant contact dermatitis 27%, allergic contact dermatitis 23%, and various other diseases 10% [127]. The 50 patients with chronic irritant hand dermatitis (without clinical or laboratory signs of atopy) came from typical high-risk occupations: housework, nursing, hairdressing, and cleaning.

Bäurle and co-workers [22, 23] studied 683 patients with hand eczema in Erlangen, Germany. They considered 24.2% to suffer from chronic irritant contact dermatitis, 15.8% from allergic contact dermatitis and 38.5% from atopic hand dermatitis.

Meding [150] made an extensive study of hand eczema in Gothenburg, an industrial city in southern Sweden. When a questionnaire was sent out to 20,000 inhabitants, the point prevalence of hand eczema was determined to be 5.4% (1-year period prevalence 11%). Females outnumbered males by 2:1. The distribution of the three main diagnoses in her panel of 1,585 patients who were investigated further was: 35% irritant contact dermatitis, 22% atopic hand dermatitis, and 19% allergic contact dermatitis. The author pointed out that, due to careful clinical examination, a considerable number of mild cases of irritant contact dermatitis were recognized, hence the relatively high figure for irritant contact dermatitis. In this study, the most harmful exposures turned out to be to "unspecified chemicals," water, detergents, dust, and dry dirt. For irritant contact dermatitis of the hand, a significantly higher period prevalence was found in people doing service work (15.4%; even higher in hairdressers), medical and nursing work and administrative work (11.8%). The lowest prevalence was found in female computer operators (3.2%).

For dental personnel in Finland, exact figures on the incidence rates per 10,000 workers were published recently [116]. The incidence rates for irritant contact dermatitis as reported in the years 1982–1994 varied between 11 and 21 per 10,000, while there was a sharp increase in the rate of allergic cases (26 to 79 respectively) due to the extensive use of acrylates. Detergents, wet and dirty work, plastic chemicals, and antimicrobials were considered to be the major irritants. In a German study on 55 dental technicians suffering from moderate to severe occupational dermatitis, allergic contact dermatitis was diagnosed in 63.6% and irritant contact dermatitis in 23.6% [185].

Paulsen [165] studied 253 gardeners in Odense (Denmark) and found irritant occupational contact dermatitis in 59%. Plants were the most commonly involved irritants (Compositae, Primulaceae, Araceae, Euphorbiaceae, Eraliaceae, Geraniaceae), but pesticides and rubber gloves must also be considered.

Based on the clinical criteria used by dermatologists, slight chronic irritant contact dermatitis of the hands may affect nearly 100% of exposed persons in certain occupations, such as food processing, fishing, hairdressing, construction, or veterinary medicine. In the metal industry at least 50% of dermatoses due to cutting oils are of the irritant type (see Chap. 39). Most workers do not seek medical attention because the effect is not serious and is accepted as "normal" in that occupation.

The most accurate figures on incidence of irritant and allergic contact dermatitis as a cause of occupational disease have been generated in Northern Bavaria (Germany) by Diepgen's group [48–50]. The data are based on all workers' compensation claims reported to the register of occupational skin diseases in the years from 1990 to 1999. Incidence rates were calculated for 24 occupational groups using the known number of insured employees in those professions. Of 5,285 patients an occupational skin disease was diagnosed in 59% after careful diagnostic procedures including extensive patch testing. This amounted to an incidence rate of 4.5 patients per 10,000 workers for irritant contact dermatitis and 4.1 patients for 10,000 workers for allergic contact der-

matitis. The highest incidence of irritant contact dermatitis rates were found in hairdressers (46.9 per 10,000 workers per year), bakers (23.5 per 10,000 workers per year), and pastry cooks (16.9 per 10,000 workers per year); at the same time irritant contact dermatitis was the main diagnosis of occupational skin disease in pastry cooks (76%), cooks (69%), food processing industry workers and butchers (63%), mechanics (60%), and locksmiths and automobile mechanics (59%). The results of a questionnaire showed frequent skin contact with detergents (52%), disinfectants (24%), and acidic and alkaline chemicals (24%) in the workplace.

In a patch test clinic of Kansas City (Kansas, USA) a retrospective analysis between 1994 and 1999 was performed [125]. Of 437 patients who underwent patch testing, 25% had occupational skin disease. Allergic contact dermatitis was diagnosed in 60% of the patients and irritant contact dermatitis in only 34%. Healthcare professionals, machinists, and construction workers accounted for nearly half of all patients with occupational skin disease. Nickel sulfate, glutaraldehyde, and thiuram mix were the most common allergens. The authors emphasize the importance of patch testing and particularly an extension of the very limited number of materials officially available in the USA in order not to miss cases of occupational contact allergy. Thus, as other authors have pointed out, the investigator's knowledge of allergens and irritants at the workplace and the quality of allergological work up, including the patient's own materials which might reveal the decisive allergen, are of utmost importance, and influence the ratio of irritant contact dermatitis to allergic contact dermatitis [47, 49, 78, 87, 111, 125, 153, 214].

Core Message

- In general, irritant contact dermatitis is more frequent than allergic contact dermatitis. High-risk professions are nursing work, hair dressing, food processing, construction work, and handling of plants. Water, detergents, dust, and dry dirt are the most common causes. Water-soluble cutting oils are the major culprit for occupational dermatitis in the metal industry. Figures on prevalence are extremely variable due to differences in the spectrum of irritants, working conditions, and protective measures. Furthermore, the observed frequency depends on the type of population studied and the quality of diagnostic work up.

15

15.4 Pathogenesis

A number of factors have now been identified as being involved in the pathogenesis of irritant contact dermatitis, particularly of the chronic cumulative type [64, 85, 122, 134, 146, 178]. These can be divided into exogenous and endogenous factors (Table 9).

15.4.1 Exogenous Factors

Table 9 lists the numerous exogenous factors influencing the irritant response. These include the type of chemical, the mode of exposure, and the body site, but the most important are the inherent toxicity of the chemical for human skin and its penetration.

Agner et al. [3] have studied the penetration of human skin by sodium lauryl sulfate (SLS) using an in vitro model. Different formulations of SLS applied to the skin for 24 h (aqueous solution and gels) were studied, but irrespective of the vehicle used permeation of SLS into the recipient phase was poor. Results were compared to in vivo patch testing in 12 subjects. Approximately 70% of SLS applied in aqueous solution was released from the patch test system. Release from gels was poorer. Good agreement was found between the in vivo results and the in vitro model. No correlation was found between the amount of SLS left in the filter disc and the strength of the clinical reaction in vivo.

Apart from strong acids and alkalis, it is not possible to predict the irritant potential of a chemical on the basis of its molecular structure as, to a certain extent, can be done for contact allergens (Chaps. 3 and 12). The pH is not strictly correlated with irritancy, as studies with detergents, alkaline soaps and α-hydroxy acids have shown [67, 69, 215, 216]. However, in a study with 12 basic compounds a positive correlation was found between increasing dissociation constant (pKa) and skin irritation capacity on human volunteers, measured either visually or by reflectance spectroscopy [157]. Compounds with low pKa induced vasoconstriction whereas high values generated vasodilation. Disruption of barrier was minimal with these irritants except mecamylamine.

Prediction of the irritation potential is even more difficult if one deals with formulated products containing many and sometimes ill-defined chemicals. Instructive is the report of Fischer and Bjarnason [63] on an epidemic outbreak of skin symptoms after a new class of diesel oil ("green diesel") had been marketed in Sweden. Initially thought to be a problem of contact allergy related to the added dyes, it turned out to be irritant contact dermatitis. The new "lighter" diesel oils are considered to be "friendlier" to the environment due to a lower concentration of aromatic compounds and low sulfur content. But these features caused more cutaneous irritation than the old types with high sulfur levels and a high degree of aromatic compounds, as careful studies on human volunteers including the use of laser Doppler perfusion imaging revealed. Paradoxically, the authors conclude, "what is good for the environment is not always good for the skin."

The intensity of the resulting irritation depends greatly on the body region. The face and the postauricular and genital regions are particularly sensitive skin areas, a major reason being a reduced barrier and the abundance of "holes" in the skin (sweat ducts and hair follicles) [62]. Figure 14 shows the large regional variation in reactivity to the solvent dimethylsulfoxide (DMSO), which causes toxic degranulation of mast cells [70]. Cua et al. [43] studied the reactivity to SLS in ten body regions: the thigh had the highest sensitivity and the palm the lowest.

Important but frequently unrecognized cofactors of irritant reactions are mechanical, thermal and climatic influences. Rough sheets have produced facial dermatitis in babies, and rough tabletops and paper have aggravated hand dermatitis in post-office workers [45, 151]. In a cohort of 111 office apprentices, the point prevalence of irritant or atopic eczema of the

Table 9. Exogenous and endogenous factors influencing the irritant response of human skin

Exogenous factors	Endogenous factors
Type of irritant (chemical structure, pH)	Individual susceptibility to irritant(s)
Amount of irritant penetrating (solubility, time of application)	Primary hyperirritable ("sensitive") skin
Body site	Atopy (particularly atopic dermatitis)
Body temperature	Inability to develop hardening
Mechanical factors (pressure, friction, abrasion)	Secondary hyperirritability (status eczematicus)
Climatic conditions (temperature, humidity, wind speed)	Racial factors
	Age
	Sensitivity to UV light

hands was 18.9% in the initial and 25% in the final examination after 3 years [208]. Handling of paper, particularly carbonless copy paper, and low relative humidity were considered to be the major causative factors, in agreement with other reports [1, 187].

In an epidemiological study on 246 shoemakers in 5 different factories, the prevalence of occupational contact dermatitis was found to be 14.6%: 8.1% irritant contact dermatitis and 6.5% allergic contact dermatitis. Solvents, adhesives, varnishes, and mechanical forces were considered to be the major irritants [147].

One detergent caused an epidemic in hospital kitchen workers, mainly because it was used at too high a temperature [183]. The influence of temperature of two different detergents was studied in a hand/forearm immersion test [39].

Cold windy climates produce drying of the skin due to the reduced capacity of the stratum corneum to retain water at lower temperatures. The condition is aggravated by frequent bathing or showering and the use of soaps and detergent bars. An eczema-like picture is seen in elderly persons. In a wash study, hard water with a higher content of calcium was found to be more irritating than soft water [226]. The type of water also had an influence on soap deposition to the skin. On the other hand, in hot humid climates sweating and friction may induce a clothing dermatitis, which seems to be a contact allergy. Elevated plaques with a sharp margin followed by scaling, fissures and hyperpigmentation, associated with various types of garment closely apposed to the skin, were observed in a series of Indian patients [173]. Most patients reported mild burning or stinging and some had developed the condition several times only in the hot summer months.

15.4.2 Endogenous Factors

Relevant endogenous factors include atopy and skin sensitivity. A number of studies from Scandinavia, such as those by Nilsson et al. [161], Rystedt [189] and Lammintausta and Kalimo [130], have confirmed the supposition of experienced clinicians that previous or current atopic dermatitis is a risk factor for the development of hand eczema in occupations involving wet work. Further confirmation came from a large study of 1,600 hand eczema patients in Erlangen, Germany [22, 23], and one in Osnabrueck, Germany [207]. It is important to point out that, on the basis of these studies, persons with a history of hay fever and/or bronchial asthma do not show a markedly increased risk of developing hand eczema in comparison to nonatopic controls. However, in Meding's study [150] there was a statistically significant but weak correlation between hand eczema and atopic mucosal symptoms.

Persons with atopic dermatitis in childhood often have dry skin for the rest of their lives. Histologically, dry skin shows some similarities to subclinical eczema. Clinically, overt irritation may therefore be precipitated more easily by a number of irritant factors.

Using SLS patch testing for 24 h and measuring transepidermal water loss, Löffler and Effendy [139] found enhanced skin susceptibility only in individuals with active dermatitis. Subjects with a history of past atopic dermatitis or rhinoconjunctivitis/asthma were not more sensitive. However, this experimental design might not reliably predict the actual conditions in most occupations, where there is repetitive low-dose irritancy over a long time.

If clinical signs of an atopic skin diathesis are carefully evaluated this can be of help in estimating the risk of occupational irritant contact dermatitis. In a study on bakers and confectioners in Germany, a significant correlation was found between a high score (>10 points on the Erlangen atopy score) and the development of hand dermatitis [21]. Other studies of high-risk professions have not corroborated such a correlation; recent reviews summarize the complexity of this issue [83, 206]. Differences in methodology account in part for the discrepancies in results.

15.4.3 Sensitive (Hyperirritable) Skin

Individuals with sensitive, hyperirritable skin do exist. This may be due to a genetic predisposition, independent of atopy. Racial differences in cutaneous irritability have been well documented [70, 72, 227, 228]. Blacks in general have less irritable skin than whites of northern (Celtic) extraction. In recent studies this view has been challenged. Using noninvasive techniques such as transepidermal water loss (TEWL) measurements a higher susceptibility to SLS has been found in blacks compared to whites [25]. Similarly a greater sensitivity to SLS was reported in Hispanic skin than in white skin [26].

It has been shown that subjects with light skin complexions (types 1 and 2) not only have high UVB sensitivity but also skin that is hyperirritable to chemicals in general [71]. Hyperirritable skin can also develop secondarily during the course of hand or leg eczema. Status eczematicus and "angry back syndrome" fall into this category. There is evidence that secondary (acquired) hyperirritability in a subgroup of patients may persist even months and years after a previous eczema has healed [109, 110].

In a recent study on human volunteers it was demonstrated that previous chronic irritant contact dermatitis sites to SLS showed hyper-reactivity compared to normal skin even after the tenth week post-induction [38].

The cause of hyperirritable skin is still unknown. There is good evidence so far that a thin and/or permeable stratum corneum plays a key role. Based on Fick's law of penetration, the thickness of the stratum corneum influences the flux of the penetrating chemical. Weigand et al. [228] have shown that the stratum corneum of blacks has more cell layers on average than that of whites. This group also found that the buoyant density of black stratum corneum was higher, which may indicate a more compact barrier. Marks' group was able to demonstrate a relationship between the minimal irritancy dose for dithranol and the mean corneocyte surface area: the smaller the corneocyte area, the lower the irritancy threshold [96]. They also found a positive correlation between the minimal blistering time with ammonium hydroxide and the skin surface contour. This was also true for other irritants.

Regional variations in irritability are related to differences in keratinization and to the density of transepidermal shunts allowing penetration (sweat ducts, hair follicles). The intercellular lipids of the stratum corneum play an important part in the barrier function of the skin, as has been shown by a number of investigators [53, 56, 57, 133, 230]. Based on recent reports, it seems that the ceramides and glycosylceramides may be the key elements in storage of water in the stratum corneum. In animals fed a diet free of essential fatty acids, administering linoleic acid either topically or systemically has been shown to improve the stratum corneum barrier [57]. There is also some clinical evidence that this may have an effect in humans, but therapeutic trials with linoleic acid or ceramide-containing medicaments in atopic eczema and dry skin have not been encouraging [11].

Ceramides in the stratum corneum are also considered to be important in the regulation of the skin barrier. Inverse correlations were found between baseline ceramide 6I and the 24-h erythema score for SLS 3%, between ceramide 1 and 24-h TEWL, and between ceramide 6II and 72-h TEWL for SLS 3% [51]. These findings suggest that low levels of ceramides may determine a proclivity to SLS-induced irritation.

Individuals with hyperirritable skin are also more reactive when tested on scarified or stripped skin, i.e., after removal of the stratum corneum, the major rate-limiting factor for penetration [239]. This is also the basis for the assumption that these individuals may release more inflammatory mediators or may be more reactive to them in comparison to normal or hyporeactive skin [71, 88].

Recently, using noninvasive bioengineering methods, it has been possible to demonstrate that female skin is more reactive to the anionic detergent SLS in the premenstrual phase than in the remainder of the menstrual cycle [5]. In general, however, females do not seem to have more sensitive skin than males [30, 131]. Rather, it is assumed that females are exposed more frequently to potential irritants than males (household products, cosmetics) and are therefore more prone to develop irritant contact dermatitis, of both acute and chronic types. Accordingly, in a recent large multicenter study in 5,971 individuals male sex was a weak but significant risk factor for a clinically positive reaction to 0.25% and 0.5% SLS [213].

Cutaneous irritability is influenced by age. There is now increasing evidence that, for several compounds, percutaneous penetration in the old age group is less than in the young one [182, 184]. In one study, susceptibility to detergents was found to increase with age, whereas the pustulogenic effect of croton oil decreased [40]. The same group found no difference with the irritants thymoquinone and croton aldehyde. In another study with SLS, the old age group showed significantly less reactivity than young adults [43]. This was quantified by visual scoring and measurements of TEWL. TEWL in the elderly is usually lower than in the young, which might be related to the latter group having a better stratum corneum barrier against water [238]. Grove et al. [91] studied different irritants in young and old cohorts. With ammonium hydroxide, blistering occurred more rapidly in older persons. Histamine, DMSO, 48/80, chloroform, methanol, lactic acid, and ethyl nicotinate induced stronger (visual) reactions in the younger cohort (Fig. 29). A comparison of cumulative irritation (7.5% SLS on 5 days consecutively, open application) revealed delayed and decreased reaction of older compared to younger skin and recovery appeared to be prolonged [194]. Further details on population differences regarding skin structure, physiology, and susceptibility to irritants are given in recent reviews [27, 100, 181, 202]. See also Chap. 28.

The phenomenon of "hardening" has been little studied, despite its common occurrence in many occupations [245]. The skin becomes slightly erythematous and hyperkeratotic from daily contact with a mild irritant, and high concentrations of the irritant can then be tolerated. If the hardening stimulus stops, the skin shows desquamation and reactivity returns to its previous level. Hardening can be induced by SLS. It seems to be an irritant-specific phenomenon because reactivity to other irritants may even be increased [149].

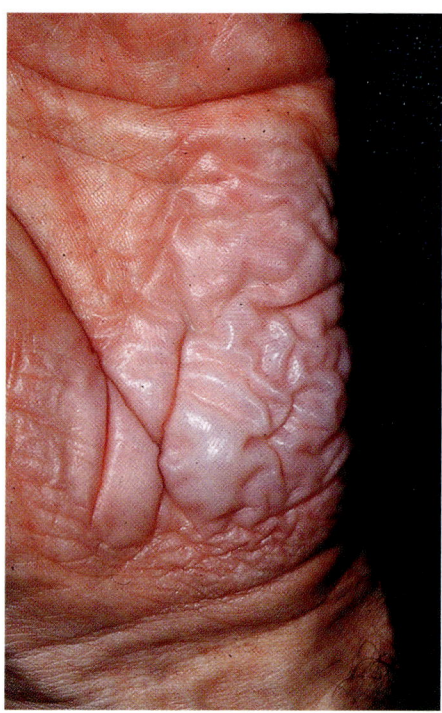

Fig. 29. Intensive swelling of the stratum corneum and edema caused by undiluted DMSO applied for 12 h under a dressing. DMSO was used as an "antidote" after the patient had accidentally pricked himself with the needle of a syringe containing a cytostatic drug [170]

15

> ### Core Message
>
> ■ Individuals with primary (endogenous) sensitive skin react to many but not all irritants more strongly compared to individuals with "tough" skin. So far, no single test can identify these persons or predict their reactivity to a certain (new) irritant.

15.5 Diagnostic Tests and Experimental Irritant Contact Dermatitis

The diagnostic tests used to quantify a patient's susceptibility to irritants are [4, 15, 68, 71, 72, 222]:

■ Alkali resistance (sodium hydroxide)
■ Ammonium hydroxide
■ Dimethylsulfoxide

■ Threshold response to various irritants (sodium lauryl sulfate, nonanoic acid, benzalkonium chloride, kerosene, croton oil, anthralin)
■ Lactic acid stinging
■ Minimal erythema dose of UVB light
■ Measurement of TEWL.

None is really so simple and reliable that it can be used clinically on a large scale, and the diagnostic value of the older tests such as Burckhardt's alkali resistance test has been overestimated, particularly in regard to their capacity to distinguish between allergic and irritant eczema.

Recently, a quick NaOH-challenge as a routine irritant patch test in occupational dermatology [Swift Modified Alkali Resistance Test (SMART)] was suggested [110]. The test comprises a 0.5 M NaOH-challenge for only 2 × 10 min with intermediate biophysical measurements (TEWL) and a clinical assessment. It also incorporates a 0.9% NaCl-control. This test has recently been validated in two cohorts of 1,111 individuals with former occupational dermatoses (now healed). Performed on the volar forearm, it was helpful to detect constitutional risks, namely atopic skin. It showed an almost fivefold increased chance of a positive reaction in the forearm in atopics, and a threefold increased chance on the back of the hand [109]. Comparing skin reactivity to SMART on the forearm and the back of the hand simultaneously (Differential Irritation Test, DIT), the study confirmed that in general the back of the hand is relatively robust, even in skin-sensitive individuals. However, there is a minority of ca. 10% of patients who formerly suffered from hand eczema where the normal hierarchy of skin sensitivity to NaOH is absent, and an isolated reactivity of the back of the hand occurs. The authors claim that this a priori paradoxical constellation – which is not to be found in healthy controls – provides strong evidence for a persistent acquired hyperirritability after previous eczema. Some patients with healed irritant contact dermatitis complain of experiencing ongoing increased skin sensitivity. However, in many of these cases the clinician cannot identify any skin impairment. The DIT is an approach to objectify the phenomenon of subclinical secondary cutaneous hyper-reactivity.

The results confirm that there may be pertinent options associated with epicutaneous NaOH-challenges [28, 123, 237]. An interesting aspect as to why NaOH may be a candidate for a predictive patch test in occupational dermatology is that the major cause of occupational dermatoses – "wet work" – alkalinizes the skin (dilution and exhausting of buffer-systems [92]). This occupational hazard may be mimicked by the test. The vital importance of a physiological, **acidic** pH for barrier homeostasis, especially for the formation of the lamellar lipid bilayer system, was recently demonstrated [93].

Nevertheless, the topic of predictive testing remains controversial. The diagnostic methods listed, however, are very useful in determining threshold responses to various irritants. Subjects with increased reactivity to one or more irritants can be identified and various influences such as the effect of repeated UVB exposure, the cumulative effects of mild irritants, or the protective effects of "barrier" creams can be quantified. Using these techniques, Frosch [72] demonstrated that in a normal population with healthy skin the proportion of subjects with hyperirritable skin was 14%; 25% were regarded as "hypoirritable" and 61% as "normal." The distinction between the three groups was made by use of cluster analysis, a statistical method that can compare and validate a number of criteria in one subject. Although some individuals seem to have hyperirritable skin per se, one finds that the correlation between some irritants is rather weak if a large number of irritants of very different chemical structure are used. In one study, we found a good correlation between the responses to sodium hydroxide, ammonium hydroxide and water-soluble irritants, but a very weak and insignificant one between SLS and lipid-soluble irritants such as croton oil and kerosene [71]. As early as 1968, Björnberg showed that one might not necessarily be able to predict the reactivity to one irritant on the basis of reactivity to another irritant [30].

Recently, the model irritant SLS has been studied extensively [98, 139, 148]. Concentrations vary from 0.5% to 2.5% usually applied with small or large Finn chambers for 24 h. Then most Caucasian subjects will develop an erythema of different intensity. Reactions are rarely severe and, even if a blistering reaction does occur, healing is swift and rarely followed by pigmentary changes. Basketter's group [18, 148, 180] has developed a 4-h test with large Hill Top chambers (25 mm diameter, 0.1 ml). With a concentration gradient of 0.1% to 20%, the threshold of erythema is determined, rather than a visual grading of intensity. Using this technique, they could not find any significant differences in a population of six different skin types (typing according to complexion and UVB sensitivity). Neither did they find differences between atopics and nonatopics. This suggests that short-term relatively high dosing of an irritant such as SLS cannot detect subtle differences in the susceptibility to cumulative insults over a longer period of time. On the other hand, this test is of value in providing a positive control for studies with other irritants for comparative reasons. According to an EU guideline, the irritancy potential of new chemicals must be assessed, avoiding animal tests whenever possible [13–15, 17, 54, 112, 246]. For predictive testing of irritants and quantitative risk assessment see also Sect. 12.3 of this book and a recent monograph [19].

The measurement of the baseline TEWL may be a useful indicator of reactivity to irritants. After 3-weeks of treatment with SLS, TEWL showed significant linear correlation with pretreatment TEWL values [236]. This supported an earlier study [171]. However, when a single 24-h occlusive SLS application was employed, no correlation was found [235].

15.6 Action of Irritants and Inflammatory Mediators

In contrast to contact allergy, the basic inflammatory mechanisms of irritants have been less studied, but recently new pathogenetic concepts began to emerge [58, 206, 242]. As irritants are very diverse in chemical structure, pH, penetration, and other features, they are generally assumed to have very different modes of action in the skin. However, some basic initial mechanisms seem to be fairly common to the early events in the elicitation of acute and chronic irritant contact dermatitis, e.g., the release of the pro-inflammatory mediators interleukin-1 (IL-1) and tumor necrosis factor alpha (TNF-α) following any kind of barrier perturbation, regardless of whether chemically or mechanically induced. Furthermore, for SLS-induced irritation, the role of heat-shock proteins [33] and oxidative stress [241] has recently been demonstrated. The body of evidence is growing, to enable skin irritation research to move on from the descriptive level to assessment of the underlying cascade of pathogenetic events, which seem to be pivotally influenced by multiple genetic polymorphisms. These recent findings may provide the crucial key to explaining the as yet enigmatic great inter-individual variability in irritant susceptibility, including the enhanced irritant response in atopics [206].

The reader is referred to Chaps. 4 and 8 of this volume, recent reviews, and some pertinent original publications [12, 19, 44, 70, 74, 103, 126, 135, 137, 159, 162, 164, 172, 177, 179, 199, 217, 223, 236].

15.7 Quantification of the Irritant Response (Bioengineering Techniques)

A very worthwhile approach in the study of cutaneous toxicity is the use of noninvasive methods to quantify the irritant response. This rapidly expanding research area is reviewed in Chap. 28. Many groups are now using evaporimeters to measure TEWL [171, 215], and laser flowmeters can quantify blood flow using the Doppler principle [31, 160, 161, 220]. Both techniques are quite sensitive and measurements can be made in minutes without damaging the skin or requiring a biopsy.

Limitations of these instruments have been demonstrated: very high rates of TEWL, as well as very intense hyperemia due to venous stasis may be evaluated inaccurately by these instruments [2]. Despite this, they are very useful in attempts to measure objectively the degree of skin damage, and have been successfully used to measure the toxic effects of surfactants and organic solvents, singly or in combination ("tandem application" [65, 119, 232, 233]). Recently, several groups assessed the protective function of barrier creams [59, 75, 76, 190–192, 201].

The quantification of increased cutaneous irritability has proven to be helpful for the interpretation of weak or query reactions to contact allergens as allergic or irritant; that is why recent recommendations were made to include SLS 0.25% and 0.5% – applied for 24 or 48 h on the back – in routine allergy patch testing [34, 86, 140, 213].

Lammintausta et al. [132] have shown that subjects with increased susceptibility to stinging have more vulnerable skin than those with no increased susceptibility to stinging. After applying various irritants they found a greater increase in blood flow and TEWL in "stingers" than in "non-stingers." These differences in cutaneous reactivity were not detected on clinical examination. This supports the view that the measurement of skin functions is worthwhile and should be promoted in future studies, even though recent studies could not corroborate marked differences in cutaneous irritability between stingers and nonstingers (see below).

Studying the dose–response relationship for SLS in humans, Agner and Serup [4] found measurement of TEWL to be the method best suited overall for quantification of patch test results, whereas colorimetry was found to be the least sensitive of the methods tested. Wilhelm et al. [234] quantified the cutaneous response to six concentrations of SLS using visual scores, skin color reflectance, TEWL and laser Doppler flow (LDF) measurements. All noninvasive techniques were more sensitive than the human eye in detecting irritation by the lowest concentration of SLS (0.125%). TEWL showed the highest discriminating power and the best correlation with visual scores. Change in total color (ΔE^*) correlated better than redness (Δa^*) to the SLS dose applied and to visual score, whereas Δa^* correlated better with TEWL and with LDF than ΔE^*.

Ultrasound A-mode scanning was found to be a promising method for quantification of the inflammatory response, being consistently more sensitive than measurement of skin color. Wahlberg has successfully used the LDF technique in assessing the irritant response to organic solvents [221], and van der Valk and coworkers [215, 216] have used evaporimetry in a series of studies quantifying the irritant potential of various detergents. Pinnagoda et al. [171] have described a repetitive exposure test for 3 weeks on human forearm skin using SLS. Baseline TEWL before exposure to the irritant correlated with the resulting cumulative irritancy caused by the detergent. The authors concluded that baseline TEWL might be a valuable predictor of cutaneous irritability.

The topic, however, remains controversial [206]. Unlike some laboratory studies, in a number of recent field studies of high-risk professions, such as hairdressers [108, 197, 198], metal workers [28] and nurses [197], it could not be proven that baseline TEWL and other baseline bioengineering parameters are relevant predictors of occupational dermatitis, and even pre-employment irritation tests were not or only poorly predictive [28, 198]. At the workplace there are many complex, interacting factors apart from pre-employment barrier function that influence the likelihood of the development of occupational skin disease. Obviously, one factor of particular importance is the individual motivation to employ skin protection measures. As could be shown for hairdressers' apprentices, even atopics could reduce their risks of suffering an occupational dermatosis by 50% if they continuously used skin protection [210].

Core Message

■ Today, the measurement of transepidermal water loss (TEWL) is the most frequently used procedure for quantifying impaired function of the stratum corneum. Clinically invisible subtle damage, e.g., by detergents, is reliably detected by an increase in TEWL.

15.8 Therapy and Prevention

The reader is referred to Chap. 44, which provides many details on this important subject.

In the acute stage of irritant contact dermatitis, topical corticosteroids are indicated. If there is deep tissue destruction or signs of bacterial infection, systemic corticosteroids and antimicrobial agents should be administered. Long-term administration of potent corticosteroids is dangerous because of the risk of atrophy and impairment of the stratum corneum [73]. The anti-inflammatory effect of corticosteroids against various irritants is weak or nonexistent. The effect depends on the potency of the corticosteroid and mode of application (before or after the irritant, single or repetitive application, topical, or systemic administration). This explains the discrepant results reported in the literature [8, 136, 174].

Recent studies have revealed that even short-term glucocorticoid treatment – down to 3 days of clobetasol – compromises both barrier permeability and stratum corneum integrity [118, 124].

Dental laboratory technicians are frequently affected by occupational skin disease due to multiple irritants and allergens [168, 185]. In a controlled clinical trial two popular commercial barrier creams and two moisturizers containing urea and beeswax respectively were evaluated in a total of 192 technicians [81]. Every technician used one barrier cream (several applications during work) and one moisturizer applied at home at least once daily for 4 weeks each with a wash-out period of 2 weeks in between. The sequence barrier cream – moisturizer, and vice versa, was randomized in two single, blind cross-over designs for both combinations. The skin condition was evaluated on a clinical score by a dermatologist at regular intervals and TEWL was measured on the back of the hand and on the forearm. Both moisturizers were assessed as "good" or "very good" in 77–98% and superior to both barrier creams (58–67% respectively). Regarding TEWL, both moisturizers proved to be significantly more effective than the barrier creams. The acceptance of the products was high. The results demonstrate the high value of skin care after work.

In a controlled study on 39 nurses a prevention model was evaluated and compared to regular work [113]. In the prevention model the use of hand alcohol instead of soap and water in disinfection procedures when the hands were not visibly dirty was followed; furthermore, the use of gloves in wet activities such as patient washing to prevent the hands from becoming wet and visibly dirty was mandatory. After 3 weeks the prevention model was found to be beneficial and less damaging to the stratum corneum as assessed by measurements of TEWL even though the time of occlusion by wearing gloves more frequently had increased.

In all cases of chronic irritant contact dermatitis a systematic approach on a wide front must be undertaken. Potential irritants in the work and home environments must be identified and, whenever possible, eliminated (replacement by other less irritant substances, reduction of exposure, use of protective gloves, etc.). Skin cleansing should be as mild as possible (liquid detergents based on alkylether sulfates or sulfosuccinate esters, avoiding organic solvents and hard brushes or other abrasives). Several methods have been described recently for irritancy ranking of detergents. The one-time patch test provides orienting data that must be compared to the results of immersion or wash tests, which better simulate the in-use situation [60, 166, 205, 231]. Corneosurfametry involves superficial biopsy of the stratum corneum with cyanoacrylate, exposure to detergents, and measuring the absorbed toluidine/fuchsin dye by colorimetry. Harsh surfactants considerably increase the staining of the corneocytes. With this technique detergents can be evaluated regarding mildness [88, 169]. Furthermore, subjects with self-perceived sensitive skin showed an increased reactivity in this assay when compared to individuals with normal skin who had not experienced any adverse reaction to detergents, wool or rough textile objects in the past. This suggests that these sensitive subjects could have a weakened resistance of their stratum corneum to surfactants.

Interestingly, the application of ionized water (mineral water, CO_2-enriched water) seems to be beneficial in the treatment of irritant contact dermatitis and may accelerate barrier recovery [32, 247].

Regular application of bland emollients to counteract desiccation should be encouraged. Several groups have shown in elegant experiments that the application of skin moisturizers improves repair mechanisms [94, 138]. Forearm immersion in SLS and measurement of TEWL seems to be the most discriminating procedure [97, 98]. For further information there are helpful reviews [99, 248]. The use of barrier creams remains controversial. Few well-controlled clinical studies have been conducted (for review [75, 89]). In a model called the repetitive irritation test (RIT), designed for guinea pigs as well as for human volunteers, Frosch and co-workers [76, 77] were able to demonstrate large differences in efficacy among commercial products. While some were quite effective in suppressing the irritation of SLS, sodium hydroxide and lactic acid, others were not, or even aggravated the irritation. In a similar model, Zhai et al. [249] found several commercial formulations effective against irritation by SLS – although to a variable degree – but all failed against a mixture of ammonium hydroxide and urea. A modified version of the RIT was recently evaluated in a multicenter study showing remarkable differences in various dermatological emollients. Interlaboratory differences were present but the ranking of the formulations stayed the same [192].

The value of phototherapy for chronic cases of eczema has been well established. Results with portable UVB lamps permitting home treatment for hand eczema are encouraging [24, 196].

If all measures fail, the diagnosis of an irritant contact dermatitis must be re-evaluated: atopy may be the dominant cause or contact allergy (e.g., to preservatives, fragrances or corticosteroids) may be preventing recovery. Recent studies have shown synergistic effects of irritants and allergens [7, 167]. The realistic combined exposure of irritants and allergens at the workplace can lead to augmentation of the cutaneous response. Mechanisms for a changed response involve immunological effects and enhanced penetration. Low levels of sensitization may thus become clinically relevant. As chronic contact dermatitis is commonly a multifactorial disease, psychological factors and lack of compliance by the patient must also be kept in mind. Recently, the value of "eczema schools" has been substantiated [6, 229]. If patients in high-risk occupations are trained in detail as how to avoid irritant and allergic factors in their job, the prognosis improves considerably [82, 106, 115, 193, 208]. This special education must start early with apprentices before dangerous habits are established [114, 210].

> ## Core Message
>
> ■ The most important therapeutic approach in the treatment of irritant contact dermatitis is the identification of causative chemicals and climatic as well as mechanical factors. Mild forms may be sufficiently controlled by regular use of emollients/moisturizers. Severe relapsing forms require corticosteroids, UV treatment, and the attendance at "eczema schools." In such cases it is not rare for the causative activity to be completely abandoned, particularly if the patient's compliance is low.

15.9 Neurosensory Irritation ("Stinging")

While the subjective hallmark of allergic cutaneous reactions is often an unbearable pruritus, many irritants cause painful sensations described as burning, stinging or smarting. We may distinguish two types of reactions regarding the time course: (1) immediate-type stinging, and (2) delayed-type stinging.

15.9.1 Immediate-Type Stinging

A few chemicals cause painful sensations within seconds of contact with normal intact skin. Best known is a mixture of chloroform and methanol (1:1). Depending on the body region and, to some extent, on individual susceptibility, a sharp pain develops within a few seconds or a few minutes of exposure. This phenomenon has been used for assessment of the cutaneous barrier, which mainly resides in the stratum corneum [72, 121]. On the volar forearm of healthy white subjects, discomfort is experienced after an average exposure time of 47 s (range 13–102 s). The irritant mixture is applied in abundant quantity in a small plastic cup (8 mm diameter). Regional differences in sensitivity can easily be documented (mastoid region – upper back – forearm – palmar region; in order of decreasing sensitivity). Once they have started, subjective reactions to chloroform:methanol increase in intensity within seconds to such an extent that the irritant must be removed in order to avoid torturing the subject. The pain abates quickly, with some individual differences. In most cases only faint erythema is visible for a short duration. Rarely, superficial necrosis of the epidermis is seen in "tough" subjects who endure the pain for a longer exposure of several minutes.

Undiluted ethanol (95%) causes a short-lasting sharp stinging sensation in most individuals in sensitive skin regions (face and neck, genital area). If the skin has slight abrasions, e.g., due to shaving, this phenomenon is experienced by everybody. The immediate type of stinging can also be observed with strong caustic chemicals, primarily acids in irritant concentrations. Typical of these agents is that severe cutaneous damage is nearly always associated with the subjective reaction. The latter is the warning signal of imminent somatic destruction if exposure is continued.

15.9.2 Delayed-Type Stinging

When a sunscreen containing amyldimethyl-*p*-aminobenzoic acid (ADP, Padimate) was marketed on a wide scale in Florida, many users experienced disagreeable stinging or burning after application. The discomfort usually occurred 1 or 2 min after application and intensified over the next 5–10 min.

Attempts to remove the sunscreen by washing brought no relief. The pain slowly abated over the next half hour. Objective signs of irritation did not develop. The condition was primarily experienced on the face after sweating and contact with salt water [163].

This is a typical example of the phenomenon of delayed-type stinging, which can be induced by a number of substances. Frosch and Kligman [67] were the first to study this systematically on human skin. The key observation was that this type of discomfort is not experienced by everybody but only by certain "stingers." A panel of subjects can be screened for stingers by the application of 5% aqueous lactic acid to the nasolabial fold after induction of profuse sweating in a sauna. Stinging is scored on an intensity scale of 0–3 (severe) at 10 s, 2.5 min, 5 min, and 8 min. A subject is regarded a stinger if he or she complains of severe (3+) discomfort between 2.5 and 8 min.

Table 10. Agents causing subjective reactions of the skin in the form of stinging or burning (from [67])

Stinging type	Agent	Concentration
Immediate-type stinging	Chloroform	50% Ethanol
	Methanol	100%
	Ethanol (primarily on abraded skin)	100%
	Strong acids	
	Hydrochloric acid	1% Water
	Trichloracetic acid	5% Water
	Weak acids	
	Ascorbic, acetic, citric and sorbic acids	5% Water
	Retinoic acid	0.05% Ethanol
Delayed-type stinging		
Slight stinging	Benzene	1% Ethanol
	Phenol	1% Ethanol
	Salicylic acid	5% Ethanol
	Resorcinol	5% Water
	Phosphoric acid	1% Water
	Aluminum chloride	30% Water
	Zirconium hydroxychloride	30% Water
Moderate stinging	Sodium carbonate	15% Water
	Trisodium phosphate	5% Water
	Propylene glycol	100%
	Propylene carbonate	100%
	Propylene glycol diacetate	100%
	Dimethylacetamide	100%
	Dimethylformamide	100%
	Dimethylsulfoxide	100%
	Diethyltoluamide (Deet)	50% Ethanol
	Dimethyl phthalate	50% Ethanol
	Benzoyl peroxide	5% Grease-free washable lotion base
Severe stinging	Crude coal tar	5% Dimethylformamide
	Lactic acid	5% Water
	Phosphoric acid	3.3% Water
	Hydrochloric acid	1.2% Water
	Sodium hydroxide	1.3% Water
	Amyldimethyl-*p*-aminobenzoic acid (Escalol 506)	5% Ethanol
	2-Ethoxyethyl-p-methoxy-cinnamate (Giv-Tan FR)	2% Ethanol

The *immediate type of stinging* develops after short exposure (seconds or minutes) and abates quickly after removal of the irritant. The *delayed type of stinging* builds up over a certain time period, does not disappear quickly after removal of the causative agent, and is experienced only by predisposed individuals ("stingers")

In the *stinging assay* the material to be evaluated is applied to the cheek of preselected sensitive subjects after intensive sweating has been induced. The stinging score of a material is the mean score of three readings taken at 2.5, 5.0, and 8.0 min. Substances with average scores falling between 0.4 and 1.0 are arbitrarily regarded as having "slight" stinging potential, the range 1.1–2.0 signifies "moderate" stinging, and the range 2.1–3.0 indicates "severe" stinging. The immediate, and in most cases transient, type of stinging is identified by questioning the subject 10 s after application of the material. Thus, the subjective tolerance of a cosmetic or topical drug can be evaluated under exaggerated test conditions on subjects with increased sensitivity.

Although a very subjective and seemingly unreliable method, this stinging assay has stood the test of time and proven valuable in screening various agents for subjective discomfort. The existence of the stinging phenomenon was, however, frequently disputed because signs of objective irritation are missing and there is no method of validation. In Table 10 are listed several substances with which this phenomenon has been observed for years. Among them are the sunscreens ADP and 2-ethoxyethyl-pimethoxycinnamate, the insect repellent *N*, *N*-diethyltoluamide, the solvent propylene glycol (undiluted), and dermatological therapeutics such as salicylic acid, aluminum chloride, benzoyl peroxide, and crude coal tar. The intensity of stinging depends on the concentration of the agent and its vehicle. For further details the reader is referred to the original publication and to a review [67, 200].

Based on extensive experience with this test, Soschin and Kligman [200] found the classification of a substance to be more reliable if the cumulative score in a 12-member panel is used:

- ■ <10: Insignificant stinging potential in normal use.
- ■ 11-24: Modest stinging potential, creating a problem for persons with sensitive skin.
- ■ >25: Definite stinging potential, certain to be "troublesome."

These authors confirmed that stingers have a higher susceptibility to a number of diverse chemical irritants and have a history of "sensitive" skin due to reactions to toiletries and cosmetics. Stingers also usually suffer from generalized dry skin in winter time, and persons with a past history of atopic dermatitis of the face usually sting severely.

The eye area is the most sensitive portion of the entire face. Certain eye-shadows may pass the sting-ing test on the nasolabial fold but produce subjective discomfort upon regular use. Therefore, eye cosmetics should be tested in this region to assure optimal compatibility.

15.9.3 Pathogenesis of Stinging and Influencing Factors

The pathogenesis of the stinging phenomenon remains uncertain, although it clearly involves excitation of sensory nerve endings. The fact that these are more abundant around hair follicles may explain why the stinging threshold is lowest on the face, particularly on the cheek and nasolabial fold. Sweating and increase in body temperature might further enhance penetration of the sting-inducing agent.

Initially, it was thought that stingers were primarily females with a fair complexion and very sensitive (hyperirritable) skin. Further experience on larger panels of subjects failed to confirm this in regard to the fair complexion: dark-skinned individuals can be stingers, too. However, Lammintausta et al. provided evidence that hyperirritability is associated with the stinging phenomenon [132]. The repeated application of the anionic detergent SLS to the skin of the upper back damaged the stratum corneum barrier in stingers more than in nonstingers. This was quantified by visual scoring and measurements of TEWL. Furthermore, in the facial region of stingers lactic acid produced an increase in blood flow recognized by the laser Doppler technique but not with the naked eye. Subjects who did not experience stinging with lactic acid showed less or no change in blood flow.

Issachar et al. [105] measured the blood flow induced by methyl nicotinate, applying a computer-assisted Doppler perfusion image technique. Significant differences were found between stingers and nonstingers. Reactors to lactic acid also showed an increased response to methyl nicotinate as early as 5 min after application, and for 30 min afterwards, though the duration of inflammation in these two groups was the same. This suggests an increased penetration of (water-soluble) substances and a higher vascular reactivity in subjects who are susceptible to neurosensory irritation.

However, when irritant reactions are assessed only visually without the use of bioengineering equipment, the differences in reactivity between stingers and nonstingers were very small or nonexistent. This is the conclusion of a series of experiments conducted by Basketter and coworkers [41]. For DMSO, methyl nicotinate, and cinnamic aldehyde, there was no difference in the response of stingers and nonstingers. In contrast, for benzoic acid and *trans*-cinnamic acid, both the mean intensity of erythema and its spread were greater in the panelists graded as stingers. It was confirmed that a high reactivity to one urticant was not predictive of high reactivity to the other urticants [16]. There was no significant difference in reactivity of males and females.

Measurement of the pH on the face revealed no difference before but after the application of lactic acid. Stingers showed a sharp decrease and a slight, but persistent over 30 min, increase in pH [104]. Nonstingers had a similar pattern but the pH values remained lower and it took longer to regain the values before lactic acid application. This finding may be explained by differences in penetration and neutralization of the acid on the skin surface.

Seidenari et al. [195] studied 26 Caucasian women with sensitive skin by their own assessment and with high scores in the lactic acid stinging test. Furthermore a wash test with a harsh soap was undertaken. Several baseline biophysical parameters were used: TEWL, capacitance, pH, sebum, and skin color measurements. The skin of sensitive subjects was described as less subtle, less hydrated and more erythematous and telangiectatic with respect to the skin of normal subjects. A trend towards an increase in TEWL, pH, and colorimetric a^* values, and a decrease in capacitance, sebum, and colorimetric L^* values was observable. However, significances were only present for capacitance and a^* values.

Wu et al. recently reported similar findings in 50 healthy Chinese volunteers, who underwent a modified lactic acid stinging test with 3% and 5% aqueous solutions of lactic acid and biophysical measurements (TEWL, capacitance). Again, there was only a trend but no statistically significant association between lactic acid stinging test score and TEWL increase [244].

Blacks develop stinging less frequently than whites. This is Frosch and Kligman's experience as well as that of Weigand and Mershon [227] when evaluating the tear gas *o*-chlorobenzylidene malononitrile.

It is a common clinical observation that skin care products and topical medicaments frequently cause stinging sensations in patients with atopic dermatitis. This symptom often worsens during stress. In a recent Swedish study of 25 patients with atopic dermatitis various neuroimmune mechanisms were studied [142]. In the 16 patients who developed stinging to lactic acid the following differences compared to the 9 nonstingers were found: in stingers the papillary dermis had an increased number of mast cells, vasoactive intestinal polypeptide-positive fibers, and a tendency to a higher number of substance P-posi-

tive nerve fibers, but a decrease of calcitonin gene-related peptide fibers. The stingers had a tendency to lower salivary cortisol. Finally, there is now evidence that the stinging phenomenon is linked to neuroimmunological mechanisms and that chronic stress may be an aggravating factor.

A set of experiments has elucidated further factors influencing delayed-type stinging [67]. They can be summarized as follows:

- Stinging is markedly reduced after inhibition of sweating.
- Prior damage to the skin increases stinging (sunburn, tape stripping, chemical irritation by detergents).
- The intensity of stinging is dose-dependent with regard to concentration and frequency of application.
- The vehicle plays an important role (solutions in ethanol or propylene glycol are more effective than fatty ointments).
- There are marked regional differences: the intensity of stinging decreases in the order nasolabial fold >cheek >chin >retroauricular region >forehead; scalp, back, and arm are virtually unreactive in respect of stinging.

The correlation of stinging with irritancy is inconsistent. With the α-hydroxy acids a positive correlation was found (pyruvic >glycolic >tartaric >lactic acid) [67]. pH did not account for the differences in either stinging or irritancy. Laden [129] also found that acids of the same pH could have quite different stinging capacities. The esters of *p*-aminobenzoic acid are examples of divergent action with regard to irritancy and stinging. A stinging ester such as ADP was found to be nonirritating on scarified skin, while an irritating one (glyceryl-*p*-aminobenzoic acid) was nonstinging.

Strong irritants (undiluted kerosene, benzalkonium chloride) may cause severe blistering reactions if applied under occlusion for 24 h, and yet they do not induce delayed- or immediate-type stinging.

In summary, our knowledge about the stinging phenomenon is still very limited [219]. Stinging undoubtedly exists and causes considerable discomfort in susceptible persons. They may as a result discontinue the use of a cosmetic or a medicament prescribed by a dermatologist.

Core Message

■ The immediate type of stinging (e.g., as induced by alcohol) develops after exposure
and abates quickly within seconds or minutes. The delayed type of stinging builds up
over a certain time, does not disappear after removal of the causative agent, occurs
frequently in the face when sweating, and
is experienced primarily by predisposed
individuals ("stingers"). These individuals
can be identified by a positive response to
5% lactic acid. They are often fair-skinned,
have a history of "sensitive" or "dry" skin
and reveal an atopic background. Neuroimmunological mechanisms are probably involved.

Suggested Reading

1. Björnberg A (1968) Skin reactions to primary irritants in
patients with hand eczema. Isacsons, Göteborg
The first careful prospective hand eczema study: 100 patients with active hand eczema, 50 patients with hand eczema healed for at least 3 months, 20 patients with active
hand eczema and eczematous lesions elsewhere on the
body, and 100 healthy control persons were investigated
with a series of irritants applied open or under occlusion
(NaOH, sodium lauryl sulfate, benzalkonium chloride, hydrochloric acid, croton oil, mercury bichloride, phenol, tri-
chloracetic acid, etc.). Patients with atopic and dyshidrotic
eczema were excluded. The main conclusions were as follows. A constitutional increase in skin reactivity to primary
irritants was not present in patients with hand eczema. A
general increase in skin reactivity to primary irritants was
found in patients with an active eczematous process ("status eczematicus"). The alkali tests were judged to be of no
value in the diagnosis of "alkali eczema" and "occupational
eczema." It is not possible to predict the intensity of skin reaction to one irritant by knowing the strength of a reaction
to another irritant.
These observations still hold true after many years. The use
of one or several irritants as a pre-employment test to
judge a predisposition to eczema has no scientific basis.
2. Frosch PJ, Kligman AM (1977) A method for appraising the
stinging capacity of topically applied substances. J Soc Cosmet Chem 28 : 197–209
Subjective discomfort such as smarting or prolonged stinging known for decades was studied in a systematic way for
the first time. The phenomenon does not occur in everybody but is frequent in so-called stingers. These individuals
are identified by the application of 5% lactic acid to the
cheek after induction of profuse sweating in a sauna. Stinging is scored on a 0 to 3+ scale at various intervals up to
8 min. Numerous substances causing delayed-type of stinging have been identified (propylene glycol, diethyltoluamide, benzoyl peroxide, coal tar, amyldimethyl-*p*-amino-

benzoic acid, etc.). There is no correlation between the
stinging capacity of a material and its irritancy.
Most cosmetics are now routinely tested for stinging in volunteers before marketing. Various modifications of the
original stinging assay have been described in order to increase its reliability.

References

1. Adams RM (1999) Occupational skin disease, 3rd edn.
Saunders, Philadelphia
2. Agner T, Serup J (1989) Seasonal variation of skin resistance to irritants. Br J Dermatol 121 : 323–328
3. Agner T, Fullerton A, Broby-Johnson U, Batsberg W
(1990) Irritant patch testing: penetration of sodium lauryl
sulphate into human skin. Skin Pharmacol 3 : 213–217
4. Agner T, Serup J (1990) Sodium lauryl sulphate for irritant patch testing – a dose-response study using bioengineering methods for determination of skin irritation.
J Invest Dermatol 95 : 543–547
5. Agner T, Damm P, Skouby SO (1991) Menstrual cycle and
skin reactivity. J Am Acad Dermatol 24 : 566–570
6. Agner T, Held E (2002) Skin protection programmes.
Contact Dermatitis 46 : 253–256
7. Agner T, Johansen JD, Overgaard L, Volund A, Basketter D,
Menné T (2002) Combined effects of irritants and allergens. Contact Dermatitis 47 : 21–26
8. Anveden I, Kindberg M, Andersen KE, Bruze M, Isaksson
M, Lidén C, Sommerlund M, Wahlberg JE, Wilkinson JD,
Willis CM (2004) Oral prednisone suppresses allergic but
not irritant patch test reactions in individuals hypersensitive to nickel. Contact Dermatitis 50 : 298–303
9. Aramaki J, Effendy I, Happle R, Kawana S, Löffler C,
Löffler H (2001) Which bioengineering assay is appropriate for irritant patch testing with sodium lauryl sulfate?
Contact Dermatitis 45 : 286–290
10. Atherton DJ (2004) A review of the pathophysiology, prevention and treatment of irritant diaper dermatitis. Curr
Med Res Opin 20 : 645–649
11. Bamford JTM, Gibson RW, Renier CM (1985) Atopic eczema unresponsive to evening primrose oil (linoleic and
gammalinolenic acids). J Am Acad Dermatol 13 : 959–965
12. Barr RM, Brain SC, Camp RD, Cilliers J, Greaves MW, Mal-
let Al, Misch K (1984) Levels of arachidonic acid and its
metabolites in the skin in human allergic and irritant
contact dermatitis. Br J Dermatol 111 : 23–28
13. Basketter DA, Whittle E, Chamberlain M (1994) Identification of irritation and corrosion hazards to skin: an alternative strategy to animal testing. Food Chem Toxicol
32 : 539–542
14. Basketter DA, Whittle E, Griffiths HA, York M (1994) The
identification and classification of skin irritation hazard
by human patch test. Food Chem Toxicol 32 : 769–775
15. Basketter DA, Griffiths HA, Wang XM, Wilhelm KP,
McFadden J (1996) Individual, ethnic and seasonal variability in irritant susceptibility of skin: the implications
for a predictive human patch test. Contact Dermatitis 35 :
208–213
16. Basketter DA, Wilhelm KP (1996) Studies on non-immune
contact reactions in an unselected population. Contact
Dermatitis 35 : 237–240
17. Basketter DA, Chamberlain M, Griffiths HA, York M
(1997) The classification of skin irritants by human patch
test. Food Chem Toxicol 35 : 845–852

15

18. Basketter DA, Miettinen J, Lahti A (1998) Acute irritant reactivity to sodium lauryl sulfate in atopics and non-atopics. Contact Dermatitis 38:253–256

19. Basketter D, Gerberick F, Kimber I, Willis C (1999) Toxicology of contact dermatitis. Wiley, Chichester

20. Basketter DA, Marriott M, Gilmour NJ, White IR (2004) Strong irritants masquerading as skin allergens: the case of benzalkonium chloride. Contact Dermatitis 50:213–217

21. Bauer A, Bartsch R, Stadeler M, Schneider W, Grieshaber R, Wollina U, Gebhardt M (1998) Development of occupational skin diseases during vocational training in baker and confectioner apprentices: a follow-up study. Contact Dermatitis 39:307–311

22. Bäurle G, Hornstein OP, Diepgen TL (1985) Professionelle Handekzeme und Atopie. Dermatosen 33:161–165

23. Bäurle G (1986) Handekzeme. Studie zum Einfluß von konstitutionellen und Umweltfaktoren auf die Genese. Schattauer, Stuttgart

24. Bayerl C, Garbea A, Peiler D, Rzany B, Allgäuer T, Kleesz P, Jung EG, Frosch PJ (1999) Pilotstudie zur Therapie des beruflich bedingten Handekzems mit einer neuen tragbaren UVB-Bestrahlungseinheit. Aktuel Dermatol 25:302–305

25. Berardesca E, Maibach HI (1988) Racial differences in sodium lauryl sulphate induced cutaneous irritation: black and white. Contact Dermatitis 18:65–70

26. Berardesca E, Maibach HI (1988) Sodium-lauryl-sulphate-induced cutaneous irritation: comparison of white and hispanic subjects. Contact Dermatitis 19:136–140

27. Berardesca E, Maibach HI (2003) Ethnic skin: overview of structure and function. J Am Acad Dermatol 48 [Suppl]:S139–S142

28. Berndt U, Hinnen U, Iliev D, Elsner P (1999) Is occupational irritant contact dermatitis predictable by cutaneous bioengineering methods? Results of the Swiss metalworkers' eczema study (PROMETES). Dermatology 198:351–354

29. Berne B, Boström Å, Grahnén AF, Tammela M (1996) Adverse effects of cosmetics and toiletries reported to the Swedish Medical Products Agency 1989–1994. Contact Dermatitis 34:359–362

30. Björnberg A (1968) Skin reactions to primary irritants in patients with hand eczema. Isacsons, Göteborg

31. Blanken R, van der Valk PGM, Nater JP (1986) Laser-Doppler flowmetry in the investigation of irritant compounds on human skin. Dermatosen 34:5–9

32. Bock M, Schürer NY, Schwanitz HJ (2004) Effects of CO_2-enriched water on barrier recovery. Arch Derm Res 296:163–168

33. Boxman IL, Hensbergen PJ, van der Schors RC, Bruynzeel DP, Tensen CP, Ponec M (2002) Proteomic analysis of skin irritation reveals the induction of HSP27 by sodium lauryl sulphate in human skin. Br J Dermatol 146:777–785

34. Brasch J, Schnuch A, Geier J, Aberer W, Uter W (2004) Iodopropynylbutyl carbamate 0.2% is suggested for patch testing of patients with eczema possibly related to preservatives. Br J Dermatol 151:608–615

35. Bruynzeel DP, van Ketel WG, Scheper RJ, von Blomberg-van der Feier BME (1982) Delayed time course of irritation by sodium lauryl sulfate: observations on threshold reactions. Contact Dermatitis 8:236–239

36. Bruze M, Emmett EA (1990) Occupational exposures to irritants. In: Jackson EM, Goldner R (eds) Irritant contact dermatitis. Dekker, New York, pp 81–106

37. Capon F, Cambie MP, Clinard F, Bernardeau K, Kalis B (1996) Occupational contact dermatitis caused by computer mice. Contact Dermatitis 35:57–58

38. Choi JM, Lee JY, Cho BK (2000) Chronic irritant contact dermatitis: recovery time in man. Contact Dermatitis 42:264–269

39. Clarys P, Manou I, Barel AO (1997) Influence of temperature on irritation in the hand/forearm immersion test. Contact Dermatitis 36:240–243

40. Coenraads PJ, Bleumink E, Nater JP (1975) Susceptibility to primary irritants. Age dependance and relation of contact allergic reactions. Contact Dermatitis 1:177–181

41. Coverly J, Peters L, Whittle E, Basketter DA (1998) Susceptibility to skin stinging, non-immunologic contact urticaria and acute skin irritation; is there a relationship? Contact Dermatitis 38:90–95

42. Cronin E (1980) Contact dermatitis. Churchill Livingston, Edinburgh

43. Cua AB, Wilhelm KP, Maibach HI (1990) Cutaneous sodium lauryl sulfate irritation potential: age and regional variability. Br J Dermatol 123:607–613

44. Cumberbatch M, Dearman RJ, Groves RW, Antanopoulos C, Kimber I (2002) Differential regulation of epidermal Langerhans cell migration by interleukins (IL)-1alpha and IL-1beta during irritant and allergen-induced cutaneous immune responses. Toxicol Appl Pharmacol 182:126–135

45. Dahlquist I, Fregert S (1979) Skin irritation in newborns. Contact Dermatitis 5:336

46. De Boer EM, van Keitel WG, Bruynzeel DP (1989) Dermatoses in metal workers. I. Irritant contact dermatitis. Contact Dermatitis 20:212–218

47. Dickel H, Kuss O, Blesius CR, Schmidt A, Diepgen TL (2001) Occupational skin diseases in Northern Bavaria between 1990 and 1999: a population-based study. Br J Dermatol 145:453–462

48. Dickel H, Kuss O, Schmidt A, Kretz J, Diepgen TL (2002) Importance of irritant contact dermatitis in occupational skin disease. Am J Clin Dermatol 3:283–289

49. Dickel H, John SM (2003) Ratio of irritant contact dermatitis in occupational skin disease. J Am Acad Dermatol 49:361–362

50. Diepgen TL (2003) Occupational skin disease data in Europe. Int Arch Occup Environ Health 76:331–338

51. Di Nardo A, Sugino K, Wertz P, Ademola J, Maibach HI (1996) Sodium lauryl sulfate (SLS) induced irritant contact dermatitis: a correlation study between ceramides and in vivo parameters of irritation. Contact Dermatitis 35:86–91

52. Dooms-Goossens AE, Debusschere KM, Gevers DM, Dupre KM, Degreef HJ, Loncke JP, Snaauwaert JE (1986) Contact dermatitis caused by airborne agents. J Am Acad Dermatol 15:1–10

53. Downing DT, Stewart ME, Wertz PW, Colton SW, Abraham W, Strauss JS (1987) Skin lipids: an update. J Invest Dermatol 88:2s–62

54. EC Annex to Commission Directive 92/69/EEC of 31 July 1992 adapting to technical progress for the seventh time Council Directive 67/548/EEC on the approximation of laws, regulations and administrative provisions relating to the classification, packaging and labelling of dangerous substances. Official J Eur Commun L383A:35 (1992)

55. Eiermann HJ, Larsen W, Maibach HI, Taylor JS (1982) Prospective study of cosmetic reactions: 1977–1980. J Am Acad Dermatol 6:909–917

56. Elias PM, Brown BE, Zoboh VA (1980) The permeability barrier in essential fatty acid deficiency: evidence for a direct role for linoleic acid in barrier function. J Invest Dermatol 74:230–233

15

57. Elias PM (1985) The essential fatty acid deficient rodent: evidence for a direct role for intercellular lipid in barrier function. In: Maibach HI, Lowe N (eds) Models in dermatology, vol 1. Karger, Basel, pp 272–285

58. Elias PM, Wood LC, Feingold KR (1999) Epidermal pathogenesis of inflammatory dermatoses. Am J Contact Dermat 10:119–126

59. Elsner P, Wigger-Alberti W (2003) Skin-conditioning products in occupational dermatology. Int Arch Occup Environ Health 76:351–354

60. English JSC, Ratcliffe J, Williams HC (1999) Irritancy of industrial hand cleansers tested by repeated open application on human skin. Contact Dermatitis 40:84–88

61. Epstein WL (1990) House and garden plants. In: Jackson EM, Goldner R (eds) Irritant contact dermatitis. Dekker, New York, pp 127–165

62. Feldman RJ, Maibach HI (1967) Regional variations in percutaneous absorption of 14 C cortisol in man. J Invest Dermatol 48:181–185

63. Fischer T, Bjarnason B (1996) Sensitizing and irritant properties of 3 environmental classes of diesel oil and their indicator dyes. Contact Dermatitis 34:309–315

64. Fleming MG, Bergfeld WF (1990) The etiology of irritant contact dermatitis. In: Jackson EM, Goldner R (eds) Irritant contact dermatitis. Dekker, New York, pp 41–66

65. Fluhr JW, Bankova L, Fuchs S, Kelterer D, Schliemann-Willers S, Norgauer J, Kleesz P, Grieshaber R, Elsner P (2004) Fruit acids and sodium hydroxide in the food industry and their combined effect with sodium lauryl sulphate: controlled in vivo tandem irritation study. Br J Dermatol 151:1039–1048

66. Fregert S (1981) Manual of contact dermatitis, 2nd edn. Munksgaard, Copenhagen

67. Frosch PJ, Kligman AM (1977) A method for appraising the stinging capacity of topically applied substances. J Soc Cosmet Chem 28:197–209

68. Frosch PJ, Kligman AM (1977) Rapid blister formation in human skin with ammonium hydroxide. Br J Dermatol 96:461–473

69. Frosch PJ, Kligman AM (1979) The soap chamber test: a new method for assessing the irritancy of soaps. J Am Acad Dermatol 1:35–41

70. Frosch PJ, Duncan S, Kligman AM (1980) Cutaneous biometrics 1: the DMSO test. Br J Dermatol 102:263–274

71. Frosch PJ, Wissing C (1982) Cutaneous sensitivity to ultraviolet light and chemical irritants. Arch Dermatol Res 272:269–278

72. Frosch PJ (1985) Hautirritation und empfindliche Haut. Grosse, Berlin

73. Frosch PJ (1985) Human models for quantification of corticosteroid adverse effects. In: Maibach HI, Lowe NJ (eds) Models in dermatology, vol 2. Karger, Basel, pp 5–15

74. Frosch PJ, Czarnetzki BM (1987) Surfactants cause in vitro chemotaxis and chemokinesis of human neutrophils. J Invest Dermatol 88:52s–55s

75. Frosch PJ, Kurte A, Pilz B (1993) Biophysical techniques for the evaluation of skin protective creams In: Frosch PJ, Kligman AM (eds) Noninvasive methods for the quantification of skin functions. Springer, Berlin Heidelberg New York, pp 214–222

76. Frosch PJ, Kurte A (1994) Efficacy of skin barrier creams. IV. The repetitive irritation test (RIT) with a set of four standard irritants. Contact Dermatitis 31:161–168

77. Frosch PJ, Pilz B (1994) Hautschutz für Friseure – die Wirksamkeit von zwei Hautschutzprodukten gegenüber Detergentien im repetitiven Irritationstest. Dermatosen 42:199–202

78. Frosch PJ, Pilz B, Peiler D, Dreier B, Rabenhorst S (1997) Die Epikutantestung mit patienten- eigenen Produkten. In: Plewig G, Przybilla B (eds) Fortschritte der praktischen Dermatologie und Venerologie. Springer, Berlin Heidelberg New York, pp 166–181

79. Frosch PJ, Rustemeyer T (1999) Contact allergy to calcipotriol does exist. Contact Dermatitis 40:66–71

80. Frosch PJ, Rustemeyer T (2000) Hairdresser's eczema. In: Menné T, Maibach HI (eds) Hand eczema, 2nd edn. CRC Press, Boca Raton, pp 195–207

81. Frosch PJ, Peiler D, Grunert V (2003) Wirksamkeit von Hautschutzprodukten im Vergleich zu Hautpflegeprodukten bei Zahntechnikern – eine kontrollierte Feldstudie. JDDG 1:547–557

82. Funke U, Diepgen T, Fartasch M (1996) Risk-group-related prevention of hand eczema at the workplace. Curr Probl Dermatol 25:123–132

83. Gallacher G, Maibach HI (1998) Is atopic dermatitis a predisposing factor for experimental acute irritant contact dermatitis? Contact Dermatitis 38:1–4

84. Gawkrodger DJ, Lloyd MH, Hunter JAA (1986) Occupational skin disease in hospital cleaning and kitchen workers. Contact Dermatitis 15:132–135

85. Gehse M, Kändler-Stürmer P, Gloor M (1987) Über die Bedeutung der Irritabilität der Haut für die Entstehung des berufsbedingten allergischen Kontaktekzems. Dermatol Monatsschr 173:400–404

86. Geier J, Uter W, Pirker C, Frosch PJ (2003) Patch testing with the irritant sodium lauryl sulfate (SLS) is useful in interpreting weak reactions to contact allergens as allergic or irritant. Contact Dermatitis 48:99–107

87. Geier J, Uter W, Lessmann H, Frosch PJ (2004) Patch testing with metal-working fluids from the patient's workplace. Contact Dermatitis 51:172–179

88. Goffin V, Piérard-Franchimont C, Piérard G (1996) Sensitive skin and stratum corneum reactivity to household cleaning products. Contact Dermatitis 34:81–85

89. Goh CL, Gan SL (1994) Efficacies of a barrier cream and an afterwork emollient cream against cutting fluid dermatitis in metal workers. A prospective study. Contact Dermatitis 31:176–180

90. Gollhausen R, Kligman AM (1985) Effects of pressure on contact dermatitis. Am J Ind Med 8:323–328

91. Grove GL, Duncan S, Kligman AM (1982) Effect of ageing on the blistering of human skin with ammonium hydroxide. Br J Dermatol 107:393–400

92. Grunewald AM, Gloor M, Gehring W, Kleesz P (1995) Damage to the skin by repetitive washing. Contact Dermatitis 32:225–232

93. Hachem J, Crumrine D, Fluhr J (2003) pH directly regulates epidermal permeability barrier homeostasis, and stratum corneum integrity/cohesion. J Invest Dermatol 121:345–353

94. Halkier-Sørensen L, Thestrup-Pedersen K (1993) The efficacy of a moisturizer (Locobase) among cleaners and kitchen assistants during everyday exposure to water and detergents. Contact Dermatitis 29:1–6

95. Halkier-Sørensen L (1998) Occupational skin disease: reliability and utility of the data in the various registers; the course from notification to compensation and the costs. Contact Dermatitis 39:71–78

96. Hamami I, Marks R (1988) Structural determinants of the response of the skin to chemical irritants. Contact Dermatitis 18:71–75

97. Hannuksela A, Hannuksela M (1996) Irritant effects of a detergent in wash, chamber and repeated open application tests. Contact Dermatitis 34:134–137

98. Held E, Agner T (1999) Comparison between 2 test models in evaluating the effect of a moisturizer on irritated human skin. Contact Dermatitis 40:261–268

99. Held E (2002) Prevention of irritant skin reactions in relation to wet work. Thesis, University of Copenhagen

100. Hicks SP, Swindells KJ, Middelkamp-Hup MA, Sifakis MA, Gonzalez E, Gonzalez S (2003) Confocal histopathology of irritant contact dermatitis in vivo and the impact of skin color (black vs white). J Am Acad Dermatol 48:727–734

101. Hill VA, Ostlere LS (1998) Psoriasis of the hands köbnerizing in contact dermatitis. Contact Dermatitis 39:194

102. Huygens S, Goossens A (2001) An update on airborne contact dermatitis. Contact Dermatitis 44:1–6

103. Imokawa G, Mishima Y (1981) Cumulative effect of surfactants on cutaneous horny layers. Contact Dermatitis 7:65–71

104. Issachar N, Gall Y, Borell MT, Poelman MC (1997) pH measurements during lactic acid stinging test in normal and sensitive skin. Contact Dermatitis 36:152–155

105. Issachar N, Gall Y, Borrel MT, Poelman MC (1998) Correlation between percutaneous penetration of methyl nicotinate and sensitive skin, using laser Doppler imaging. Contact Dermatitis 39:182–186

106. Itschner L, Hinnen U, Elsner P (1996) Prevention of hand eczema in the metal-working industry. Risk awareness and behaviour of metal worker apprentices. Dermatology 193:226–229

107. Jackson EM, Goldner R (eds) (1990) Irritant contact dermatitis. Dekker, New York

108. John SM, Uter W, Schwanitz HJ (2000) Relevance of multiparametric skin bioengineering in a prospectively-followed cohort of junior hairdressers. Contact Derm 43:161–168

109. John S, Uter W (2005) Meteorological influence on NaOH irritation varies with body site. Arch Derm Res 296:320–326

110. John SM (2005) Functional skin testing: the SMART-procedures. In: Chew A-L, Maibach HI (eds) Handbook of irritant dermatitis. Springer, Berlin Heidelberg New York (in press)

111. Jolanki R, Estlander T, Alanko K, Kanerva L (2000) Patch testing with a patient's own material handled at work. In: Kanerva L, Elsner P, Wahlberg JE, Maibach HI (eds) Handbook of occupational dermatology, vol 47. Springer, Berlin Heidelberg New York, pp 375–383

112. Judge MR, Griffiths HA, Basketter DA, White IR, Rycroft RJG, McFadden JP (1996) Variation in response of human skin to irritant challenge. Contact Dermatitis 34:115–117

113. Jungbauer FHW, van der Harst JJ, Groothoff JW, Coenraads PJ (2004) Skin protection in nursing work: promoting the use of gloves and hand alcohol. Contact Dermatitis 51:135–140

114. Jungbauer FHW, van der Vleuten P, Groothoff JW, Coenraads PJ (2004) Irritant hand dermatitis: severity of disease, occupational exposure to skin irritants and preventive measures 5 years after initial diagnosis. Contact Dermatitis 50:245–251

115. Kalimo K, Kautiainen H, Niskanen T, Niemi L (1999) "Eczema school" to improve compliance in an occupational dermatology clinic. Contact Dermatitis 41:315–319

116. Kanerva L, Lahtinen A, Toikkanen J, Forss H, Estlander T, Susitaival P, Jolanki R (1999) Increase in occupational skin diseases of dental personnel. Contact Dermatitis 40:104–108

117. Kanerva L, Estlander T, Jolanki R (2000) Occupational contact dermatitis caused by personal-computer mouse. Contact Dermatitis 43:362–363

118. Kao JS, Fluhr JW, Man M-Q, Fowler AJ, Hachem J-P, Crumrine D, Ahn SK, Brown BE, Elias PM, Feingold KR (2003) Short-term glucocorticoid treatment compromises both permeability barrier homeostasis and stratum corneum integrity: inhibition of epidermal lipid synthesis accounts for functional abnormalities. J Invest Dermatol 120:456–464

119. Kappes UP, Goritz N, Wigger-Alberti W, Heinemann C, Elsner P (2001) Tandem application of sodium lauryl sulfate and n-propanol does not lead to enhancement of cumulative skin irritation. Acta Derm Venereol (Stockh) 81:403–405

120. Kim IH, Seo SH (1999) Occupational chemical burns caused by bromine. Contact Dermatitis 41:43

121. Klaschka F (1979) Arbeitsphysiologie der Hornschicht in Grundzügen. In: Marchionini A (ed) Jadassohns Handbuch der Haut- und Geschlechtskrankheiten. Ergänzungswerk, vol 1, part 4A. Springer, Berlin Heidelberg New York, pp 153–261

122. Kligman AM (1979) Cutaneous toxicity: an overview from the underside. Curr Probl Dermatol 7:1–25

123. Kolbe L, Kligman AM, Stoudemayer T (1998) The sodium hydroxide erosion assay: a revision of the alkali resistance test. Arch Derm Res 290:382–387

124. Kolbe L, Kligman AM, Schreiner V, Stoudemayer T (2001) Corticosteroid-induced atrophy and barrier impairment measured by non-invasive methods in human skin. Skin Res Technol 7:73–77

125. Kucenic MJ, Belsito DV (2003) Occupational allergic contact dermatitis is more prevalent than irritant contact dermatitis: a 5-year study. J Am Acad Dermatol 49:360–361, authors' reply 362

126. Kucharekova M, Hornix M, Ashikaga T et al (2003) The effect of the PDE-4 inhibitor (cipamfylline) in two human models of irritant contact dermatitis. Arch Dermatol Res 295:29–32

127. Kühner-Piplack B (1987) Klinik und Differentialdiagnose des Handekzems. Eine retrospektive Studie am Krankengut der Universitäts-Hautklinik Heidelberg 1982–1985. Thesis, Ruprecht-Karls-University, Heidelberg

128. Lachapelle JM, Mahmoud G, Vanherle R (1984) Anhydrite dermatitis in coal miners. Contact Dermatitis 11:188–189

129. Laden K (1973) Studies on irritancy and stinging potential. J Soc Cosmet Chem 24:385–393

130. Lammintausta K, Kalimo K (1981) Atopy and hand dermatitis in hospital wet work. Contact Dermatitis 7:301–308

131. Lammintausta K, Maibach HI (1987) Irritant reactivity in males and females. Contact Dermatitis 17:276–280

132. Lammintausta K, Maibach HI, Wilson D (1988) Mechanisms of subjective (sensory) irritation. Dermatosen 36:45–49

133. Landmann L (1985) Permeabilitätsbarriere der Epidermis. Grosse, Berlin (Grosse Scripta 9)

134. Landman G, Farmer ER, Hood AF (1990) The pathophysiology of irritant contact dermatitis In: Jackson EM, Goldner R (eds) Irritant contact dermatitis. Dekker, New York, pp 67–77

135. Larsen CG, Ternowitz T, Larsen EG, Thestrup-Pedersen K (1989) ETAF/interleukin 1 and epidermal lymphocyte chemotactic factor in epidermis overlying an irritant patch test. Contact Dermatitis 20:335–340

136. Levin C, Zhai H, Bashir S, Chew AL, Anigbogu A, Stern R, Maibach H (2001) Efficacy of corticosteroids in acute experimental irritant contact dermatitis? Skin Res Technol 7:214–218

137. Li LF, Fiedler VC, Kumar R (1998) Down-regulation of protein kinase C isoforms in irritant contact dermatitis. Contact Dermatitis 38:319–324

138. Lodén M (1997) Barrier recovery and influence of irritant stimuli in skin treated with a moisturizing cream. Contact Dermatitis 36:256–260

139. Löffler H, Effendy I (1999) Skin susceptibility of atopic individuals. Contact Dermatitis 40:239–242

140. Löffler H, Pirker C, Aramaki J, Frosch PJ, Happle R, Effendy I (2001) Evaluation of skin susceptibility to irritancy by routine patch testing with sodium lauryl sulfate. Eur J Dermatol 11:416–419

141. Löffler H, Happle R (2003) Influence of climatic conditions on the irritant patch test with sodium lauryl sulphate. Acta Derm Venereol (Stockh) 83:338–341

142. Lonne-Rahm S, Berg M, Mrin P, Nordlind K (2004) Atopic dermatitis, stinging, and effects of chronic stress: a pathocausal study. J Am Acad Dermatol 51:899–905

143. Lovell CR, Rycroft RCG, Williams DMJ, Hamlin J (1985) Contact dermatitis from the irritancy (immediate and delayed) and allergenicity of hydroxypropyl acrylate. Contact Dermatitis 12:117–118

144. Lyon CC, Yell J, Beck MH (1998) Irritant contact dermatitis from pancreatin exacerbating vulvodynia. Contact Dermatitis 38:362

145. Malten KE, den Arend JACJ, Wiggers RE (1979) Delayed irritation: hexanediol diacrylate and butanediol diacrylate. Contact Dermatitis 5:178–184

146. Malten KE (1981) Thoughts on irritant contact dermatitis. Contact Dermatitis 7:238–247

147. Mancuso G, Reggiani M, Berdondini RM (1996) Occupational dermatitis in shoemakers. Contact Dermatitis 34:17–22

148. McFadden JPP, Wakelin SH, Basketter DA (1998) Acute irritation thresholds in subjects with Type I-Type VI skin. Contact Dermatitis 38:147–149

149. McOsker DE, Beck LW (1967) Characteristics of accomodated (hardened) skin. J Invest Dermatol 48:372–383

150. Meding B (1990) Epidemiology of hand eczema in an industrial city. Acta Derm Venerol (Stockh) [Suppl] 153:1–43

151. Menné T (1983) Frictional dermatitis in post-office workers. Contact Dermatitis 9:172–173

152. Menné T, Hjorth N (1985) Frictional contact dermatitis. Am J Ind Med 8:401–402

153. Menné T, Dooms-Goossens A, Wahlberg JE, White IR, Shaw S (1992) How large a proportion of contact sensitivities are diagnosed with the European Standard series? Contact Dermatitis 26:201–202

154. Menné T, Maibach HI (eds) (2000) Hand eczema, 2nd edn. CRC, Boca Raton, Fla.

155. Moroni P, Cazzaniga R, Pierini F, Panella V, Zerboni R (1988) Occupational contact psoriasis. Dermatosen 36:163–164

156. Morris-Johns R, Robertson SJ, Ross JS et al (2002) Dermatitis caused by physical irritants. Br J Dermatol 147:270–275

157. Nangia A, Andersen PH, Berner B, Maibach HI (1996) High dissociation constants (pKA) of basic permeants are associated with in vivo skin irritation in man. Contact Dermatitis 34:237–242

158. Nethercott JR, Gupta S, Rosen C, Enders LJ, Pilger CW (1984) Tetraethylene glycol diacrylate. A cause of delayed cutaneous irritant reaction and allergic contact dermatitis. J Occup Med 26:513–516

159. Nickoloff BJ (1988) The role of gamma interferon in cutaneous trafficking of lymphocytes with emphasis on molecular and cellular adhesion events. Arch Dermatol 124:1835–1843

160. Nilsson GE, Otto U, Wahlberg JE (1982) Assessment of skin irritancy in man by laser Doppler flowmetry. Contact Dermatitis 8:401–406

161. Nilsson E, Mikaelsson B, Andersson S (1985) Atopy, occupation and domestic work as risk factors for hand eczema in hospital workers. Contact Dermatitis 13:216–223

162. Oxholm AM, Oxholm P, Avnstorp C, Bendtzen K (1991) Keratinocyte-expression of interleukin-6 but not of tumour necrosis factor-alpha is increased in the allergic and the irritant patch test reaction. Acta Derm Venereol (Stockh) 71:93–98

163. Parrish JA, Pathak MA, Fitzpatrick TB (1975) Facial irritation due to sunscreen products (letter to the editor). Arch Dermatol 111:525

164. Patrick E, Burkhalter A, Maibach HI (1987) Recent investigations of mechanisms of chemically induced skin irritation in laboratory mice. J Invest Dermatol 88:24s–31s

165. Paulsen E (1998) Occupational dermatitis in Danish gardeners and greenhouse workers (II.) Etiological factors. Contact Dermatitis 38:14–19

166. Paye M, Gomes G, Zerweck CR, Piérard GD, Grove GL (1999) A hand immersion test under laboratory-controlled usage conditions: the need for sensitive and controlled assessment methods. Contact Dermatitis 40:133–138

167. Pedersen LK, Johansen JD, Held E, Agner T (2004) Augmentation of skin response by exposure to a combination of allergens and irritants – a review. Contact Dermatitis 50:265–273

168. Peiler D, Rustemeyer T, Pflug B, Frosch PJ (2000) Allergic contact dermatitis in dental laboratory technicians. II. Major allergens and their clinical relevance. Dermatosen 48:48–54

169. Piérard GE, Goffin V, Herrmanns-Lê T, Arrese JE, Piérard-Franchimont C (1995) Surfactant induced dermatitis. A comparison of corneosurfametry with predicitve testing on human and reconstructed skin. J Am Acad Dermatol 33:462–469

170. Pilz B, Löffler T, Frosch PJ (1994) Toxische Dermatitis durch Dimethylsulfoxid (DMSO) als Antidot gegen Epirubicin. Dermatosen 42:204–209

171. Pinnagoda J, Tupker RA, Coenraads PJ, Nater JP (1989) Prediction of susceptibility to an irritant response by transepidermal water loss. Contact Dermatitis 20:341–346

172. Prottey C (1978) The molecular basis of skin irritation. In: Breuer MM (ed) Cosmetic science, vol 1. Academic, London, pp 275–349

173. Ramam M, Khaitan BK, Singh MK, Gupta SD (1998) Frictional sweat dermatitis. Contact Dermatitis 38:49

174. Ramsing DW, Agner T(1995) Efficacy of topical corticosteroids on irritant skin reactions. Contact Dermatitis 32:293–297

175. Ramsing DW, Agner T (1996) Effect of glove occlusion on human skin (II). Long-term experimental exposure. Contact Dermatitis 34:258–262

176. Reiche L, Willis C, Wilkinson J, Shaw S, de Lacharièrre O (1998) Clinical morphology of sodium lauryl sulfate (SLS) and nonanoic acid (NAA) irritant patch test reactions at 48 h and 96 h in 152 subjects. Contact Dermatitis 39:240–243

177. Reilly DM, Green MR (1999) Eicosanoid and cytokine levels in acute skin irritation in response to tape stripping and capsaicin. Acta Derm Venereol (Stockh) 79:187–190

15

178. Rietschel RL (1989) Persistent maleic acid irritant dermatitis in the guinea pig. In: Frosch PJ, Dooms-Goossens A, Lachapelle JM, Rycroft RJG, Scheper RJ (eds) Current topics in contact dermatitis. Springer, Berlin Heidelberg New York, pp 429–434

179. Rietschel RL (1990) Diagnosing irritant contact dermatitis. In: Jackson EM, Goldner R (eds) Irritant contact dermatitis. Dekker, New York, pp 167–171

180. Robinson MK, Perkins MA, Basketter DA (1998) Application of a 4-h human patch test method for comparative and investigative assessment of skin irritation. Contact Dermatitis 38:194–202

181. Robinson MK (1999) Population differences in skin structure and physiology and the susceptibility to irritant and allergic contact dermatitis: implications for skin safety testing and risk assessment. Contact Dermatitis 41:65–79

182. Roskos KV, Maibach HI, Guy RH (1989) The effect of aging on percutaneous absorption in man. J Pharmacokinet Biopharm 17:617–630

183. Rothenborg HW, Menné T, Sjolin KE (1977) Temperature dependent primary irritant dermatitis from lemon perfume. Contact Dermatitis 3:37–48

184. Rougier A, Lotte C, Corcuff P, Maibach HI (1988) Relationship between skin permeability and corneocyte size according to anatomic site, age, and sex in man. J Soc Cosmet Chem 39:15–26

185. Rustemeyer T, Frosch PJ (1996) Occupational skin diseases in dental laboratory technicians. I. Clinical picture and causative factors. Contact Dermatitis 34:125–133

186. Rycroft RJG, Smith WD (1980) Low humidity occupational dermatoses. Contact Dermatitis 6:488–492

187. Rycroft RJG (1986) Occupational dermatoses among office personnel. Occup Med State Art Rev 1:323–328

188. Rycroft RJG (1998) The principal irritants and sensitizers. In: Rook A, Wilkinson DS, Ebling FJG, Champion RH, Burton JL, Burns DA, Breathnach SM (eds) Textbook of dermatology, 6th edn. Blackwell, Oxford, pp 821–860

189. Rystedt I (1985) Atopic background in patients with occupational hand eczema. Contact Dermatitis 12:247–254

190. Schliemann-Willers S, Wigger-Alberti W, Elsner P (2001) Efficacy of a new class of perfluoropolyethers in the prevention of irritant contact dermatitis. Acta Derm Venereol (Stockh) 81:392–394

191. Schliemann-Willers S, Wigger-Alberti W, Kleesz P, Grieshaber R, Elsner P (2002) Natural vegetable fats in the prevention of irritant contact dermatitis. Contact Dermatitis 46:6–12

192. Schnetz E, Diepgen TL, Elsner P, Frosch PJ, Klotz AJ, Kresken J, Kuss O, Merk H, Schwanitz HJ, Wigger-Alberti W, Fartasch M (2000) Multi-centre study for the development of an in vivo model to evaluate the influence of topical formulations on irritation. Contact Dermatitis 42:336–343

193. Schwanitz HJ, Uter W, Wulfhorst B (eds) (1996) Neue Wege zur Prävention – Paradigma Friseurekzem. Rasch, Osnabrück

194. Schwindt DA, Wilhelm KP, Miller DL, Maibach HI (1998) Cumulative irritation in older and younger skin: a comparison. Acta Derm Venereol (Stockh) 78:279–283

195. Seidenari S, Francomano M, Mantovani L (1998) Baseline biophysical parameters in subjects with sensitive skin. Contact Dermatitis 38:311–315

196. Sjövall P, Christensen OB (1994) Treatment of chronic hand eczema with UV-B Handylux in the clinic and at home. Contact Dermatitis 31:5–8

197. Smit HA, van Rijssen A, Vandenbrouke JP, Coenrads PJ (1994) Susceptibility to and incidence of hand dermatitis in a cohort of apprentice hairdressers and nurses. Scand J Work Environ Health 20:113–121

198. Smith HR, Armstrong DK, Holloway D, Whittam L, Basketter DA, McFadden JP (2002) Skin irritation thresholds in hairdressers: implications for the development of hand dermatitis. Br J Dermatol 146:849–852

199. Smith HR, Basketter DA, McFadden JP (2002) Irritant dermatitis, irritancy and its role in allergic contact dermatitis. Exp Dermatol 27:138–146

200. Soschin D, Kligman AM (1982) Adverse subjective reactions. In: Kligman AM, Leyden JJ (eds) Safety and efficacy of topical drugs and cosmetics. Grune and Stratton, New York, pp 377–388

201. Spoo J, Wigger-Alberti W, Berndt U, Fischer T, Elsner P (2002) Skin cleansers: three test protocols for the assessment of irritancy ranking. Acta Derm Venereol (Stockh) 82:13–17

202. Swindells K, Burnett N, Ruis-Diaz F, Gonzalez E, Mihm MC, Gonzalez S (2004) Reflectance confocal microscopy may differentiate acute allergic and irritant contact dermatitis in vivo. J Am Acad Dermatol 50:220–228

203. Tanaka M, Fujimoto A, Kobayashi S et al (2001) Keyboard wrist pad. Contact Dermatitis 44:253–254

204. Tsai TF, Maibach HI (1999) How irritant is water? An overview. Contact Dermatitis 41:311–314

205. Tupker RA, Bunte EE, Fidler V, Wiechers JW, Coenraads PJ (1999) Irritancy ranking of anionic detergents using one-time occlusive, repeated occlusive and repeated open tests. Contact Dermatitis 40:316–322

206. Tupker R (2003) Prediction of irritancy in the human skin irritancy model and occupational setting. Contact Derm 49:61–69

207. Uter W, Pfahlberg A, Gefeller O, Schwanitz HJ (1998) Risk factors for hand dermatitis in hairdressing apprentices. Dermatosen 46:151–158

208. Uter W, Pfahlberg A, Gefeller O, Schwanitz HJ (1998) Hand eczema in a prospectively-followed cohort of office-workers. Contact Dermatitis 38:83–89

209. Uter W, Gefeller O, Schwanitz HJ (1998) An epidemiological study of the influence of season (cold and dry air) on the occurrence of irritant skin changes of the hands. Br J Dermatol 138:266–272

210. Uter W (1999) Epidemiologie und Prävention von Handekzemen in Feuchtberufen am Beispiel des Friseurhandwerks. Universitätsverlag Rasch, Osnabrück

211. Uter W, Geier J, Land M, Pfahlberg A, Gefeller O, Schnuch A (2001) Another look at seasonal variation in patch test results. A multifactorial analysis of surveillance data of the IVDK. Information Network of Departments of Dermatology. Contact Dermatitis 44:146–152

212. Uter W, Hegewald J, Pfahlberg A, Pirker C, Frosch PJ, Gefeller O (2003) The association between ambient air conditions (temperature and absolute humidity), irritant sodium lauryl sulfate patch test reactions and patch test reactivity to standard allergens. Contact Dermatitis 49:97–102

213. Uter W, Geier J, Becker D, Brasch J, Löffler H (2004) The MOAHLFA index of irritant sodium lauryl sulfate reactions: first results of a multicentre study on routine sodium lauryl sulfate patch testing. Contact Dermatitis 51:259–262

214. Uter W, Balzer C, Geier J, Schnuch A, Frosch PJ (2005) Ergebnisse der Epikutantestung mit patienteneigenen Parfums, Deos und Rasierwässern. Dermatol Beruf Umwelt 53:25–36

215. Van der Valk PGM, Crijns MC, Nater JP, Bleumink E (1984) Skin irritancy of commercially available soap and deter-

gent bars as measured by water vapour loss. Dermatosen 32:87–90

216. Van der Valk PGM, Nater JP, Bleumink E (1984) Skin irritancy of surfactants as assessed by water vapor loss measurements. J Invest Dermatol 82:291–293

217. Van der Valk PGM, Maibach HI (eds) (1996) The irritant contact dermatitis syndrome. CRC Press, Boca Raton

218. Veien NK, Hattel T, Laurberg G (1997) Low-humidity dermatosis from car heaters. Contact Dermatitis 37:138

219. Villarama C, Maibach HI (2005) Sensitive skin and transepidermal water loss. In: Fluhr J, Elsner P, Berardesca E, Maibach HI (eds) Bioengineering and the skin. CRC Press, Boca Raton, pp 135–141

220. Wahlberg JE (1984) Skin irritancy from alkaline solutions assessed by laser Doppler flowmetry. Contact Dermatitis 10:111

221. Wahlberg JE (1989) Assessment of erythema: a comparison between the naked eye and laser Doppler flowmetry. In: Frosch PJ, Dooms-Goossens A, Lachapelle JM, Rycroft RJG, Scheper RJ (eds) Current topics in contact dermatitis. Springer, Berlin Heidelberg New York, pp 549–553

222. Wahlberg JE, Lindberg M (2003) Nonanoic acid – an experimental irritant. Contact Dermatitis 49:117–123

223. Wallengren J, Larsson B (2001) Nitric oxide participates in prick test and irritant patch test reactions in human skin. Arch Derm Res 293:121–125

224. Warner RR, Boissy YL, Lilly NA, Spears MJ, McKillop K, Marshall JL, Stone KJ (1999) Water disrupts stratum corneum lipid lamellae: damage is similar to surfactants. J Invest Dermatol 113:960–966

225. Warner RR, Stone KJ, Boissy YL (2003) Hydration disrupts human stratum corneum ultrastructure. J Invest Dermatol 120:275–284

226. Warren R, Ertel KD, Bartolo RG, Levine MJ, Bryant PB, Wong LF (1996) The influence of hard water (calcium) and surfactants on irritant contact dermatitis. Contact Dermatitis 35:337–343

227. Weigand DA, Mershon MM (1970) The cutaneous irritant reaction to agent o- chlorobenzylidene malononitrile (CS). II. Quantitation and racial influence in human subjects. Edgewood Arsenal Technique no 4332

228. Weigand DA, Haygood C, Gaylor JR (1974) Cell layers and density of negro and caucasian stratum corneum. J Invest Dermatol 62:563–568

229. Weisshaar E, Radulescu M, Bock M et al (2005) Hautschutzseminare zur sekundären Individualprävention bei Beschäftigten in Gesundheitsberufen: erste Ergebnisse nach über 2-jähriger Durchführung. JDDG 3:33–38

230. Wertz PW, Miethke MC, Long SA, Strauss JS, Downing DT (1985) The composition of the ceramides from human stratum corneum and from comedones. J Invest Dermatol 84:410–412

231. Wigger-Alberti W, Fischer T, Greif C, Maddern P, Elsner P (1999) Effects of various grit-containing cleansers on skin barrier function. Contact Dermatitis 41:136–140

232. Wigger-Alberti W, Krebs A, Elsner P (2000) Experimental irritant contact dermatitis due to cumulative epicutaneous exposure to sodium lauryl sulphate and toluene: single and concurrent application. Br J Dermatol 143:551–556

233. Wigger-Alberti W, Spoo J, Schliemann-Willers S, Klotz A, Elsner P (2002) The tandem repeated irritation test: a new method to assess prevention of irritant combination damage to the skin. Acta Derm Venereol (Stockh) 82:94–97

234. Wilhelm KP, Surber C, Maibach HI (1989) Quantification of sodium lauryl sulfate irritant dermatitis in man: comparison of four techniques: skin color reflectance, transepidermal water loss, laser Doppler flow measurement and visual scores. Arch Dermatol Res 281:293–295

235. Wilhelm KP, Maibach HI (1990) Susceptibility to SLS-induced irritant dermatitis: relation to skin pH, TEWL, sebum concentration, and stratum corneum turnover time. J Am Acad Dermatol 23:122–124

236. Wilhelm KP, Saunders JC, Maibach HI (1990) Increased stratum corneum turnover induced by subclinical irritant dermatitis. Br J Dermatol 122:793–798

237. Wilhelm KP, Pasche F, Surber C, Maibach HI (1990) Sodium hydroxide- induced subclinical irritation. A test for evaluating stratum corneum barrier function. Acta Derm Venereol (Stockh) 70:463–367

238. Wilhelm KP, Maibach HI (1993) The effect of aging on the barrier function of human skin evaluated by in vivo transepidermal water loss measurement. In: Frosch PJ, Kligman AM (eds) Noninvasive methods for the quantification of skin functions. Springer, Berlin, Heidelberg New York, pp 181–189

239. Willers P (1984) Die Bedeutung der Hornschicht für die Irritabilität der Haut. Thesis, Westfälische Wilhelms University, Münster

240. Willis CM, Stephens CJM, Wilkinson JD (1988) Experimentally-induced irritant contact dermatitis. Contact Dermatitis 18:20–24

241. Willis CM, Britton LE, Reiche L, Wilkinson JD (2001) Reduced levels of glutathione S-transferases in patch test reactions to dithranol and sodium lauryl sulphate as demonstrated by quantitative immunocytochemistry: evidence for oxidative stress in acute irritant contact dermatitis. Eur J Dermatol 11:99–104

242. Willis CM (2002) Variability in responsiveness to irritants: thoughts on possible underlying mechanisms. Contact Dermatitis 47:267–271

243. Wrangsjö K, Osterman K, van Hage-Hamsten M (1994) Glove-related skin symptoms among operating theatre and dental care unit personnel. Contact Dermatitis 30:102–107

244. Wu Y, Wang X, Zhou Y, Tan Y, Chen D, Chen Y, Ye M (2003) Correlation between stinging, TEWL and capacitance. Skin Res Technol 9:90–93

245. Wulfhorst B (2000) Skin hardening in occupational dermatology. In: Kanerva L, Elsner P, Wahlberg J, Maibach H (eds) Handbook of occupational dermatology. Springer, Berlin, Heidelberg, New York, pp 115–121

246. York M, Griffiths HA, Whittle E, Basketter DA (1996) Evaluation of human patch test for the identification and classification of skin irritation potential. Contact Dermatitis 34:204–212

247. Yoshizawa Y, Kitamura K, Kawana S, Maibach HI (2003) Water, salts and skin barrier of normal skin. Skin Res Technol 9:31–33

248. Zhai H, Maibach HI (1998) Moisturizers in preventing irritant contact dermatitis: an overview. Contact Dermatitis 38:241–244

249. Zhai H, Willard P, Maibach HI (1999) Putative skin-protective formulations in preventing and/or inhibiting experimentally-produced irritant and allergic contact dermatitis. Contact Dermatitis 41:190–192

250. Zhai H, Maibach HI (2001) Skin occlusion and irritant and allergic contact dermatitis: an overview. Contact Dermatitis 44:201–206

15

Chapter 16

Systemic Contact Dermatitis

16

Niels K. Veien, Torkil Menné

Contents

16.1 Introduction

Systemic contact dermatitis may occur in persons with contact sensitivity when these persons are exposed to the hapten orally, transcutaneously, intravenously or by inhalation. The entity can present with clinically characteristic features or be clinically indistinguishable from other types of contact dermatitis. Contact sensitization to ubiquitous haptens is common. In a Danish population-based study, 15.2% reacted to one or more of the haptens in the European standard patch test series [1]. Many of these haptens can be presented to the immune system by a systemic route. The total number of individuals at risk of developing systemic contact dermatitis is therefore large.

The first description of systemic contact dermatitis can probably be ascribed to the pioneering British dermatologist, Thomas Bateman [2]. His description of the mercury dermatitis called eczema rubrum is similar to what we today describe as the "baboon syndrome": "Eczema rubrum is preceded by a sense of stiffness, burning, heat and itching in the part where it commences, most frequently the upper and inner surface of the thighs and about the scrotum in men, but sometimes it appears first in the groin, axillae or in the bends of the arms, on the wrists and hands or on the neck."

In the 20th century, the systemic spread of nickel dermatitis to areas other than the sites of contact was described by Schittenhelm and Stockinger in Kiel in 1925 [3]. After patch testing nickel-sensitive workers with nickel sulfate, they observed dermatitis and flares in former areas of contact dermatitis even when there was no current contact with nickel items in these areas. The literature on systemic contact dermatitis is now comprehensive. Reviews include Cronin [4], Fisher [5], Menné et al. [6] and Veien et al. [7].

Core Message

■ Systemic contact dermatitis may occur after the systemic administration of a hapten in persons with contact sensitivity to the hapten. Systemic contact dermatitis may be indistinguishable from other types of contact dermatitis.

16.2 Clinical Features

The clinical features of systemic contact dermatitis are summarized in Table 1.

A causal relationship between systemic administration of the hapten and these clinical manifestations is most easily documented in persons sensitized to medicaments. For such persons, the exposure to the hapten can be controlled. This is less feasible for persons sensitized to, for example, ubiquitous metals.

Flare-up reactions at former sites of dermatitis or previously positive patch test sites raise a suspicion of systemic contact dermatitis [8–10]. A flare at a

Table 1. Clinical aspects of systemic contact dermatitis

Dermatitis in areas of previous exposure	Flare-up of previous dermatitis
	Flare-up of previously positive patch test sites
Dermatitis on previously unaffected skin	Vesicular hand eczema
	Flexural dermatitis
	Baboon syndrome
	Maculopapular rash (toxicoderma)
	Vasculitis-like lesions
General symptoms	Headache
	Malaise
	Arthralgia
	Diarrhea and vomiting
	Fever

previously positive patch test site following ingestion of the hapten is a fascinating and specific sign of systemic contact dermatitis. Such reactions may be caused by medicaments and are also sometimes seen in experimental oral provocation studies. This symptom is hapten specific and can be seen years after the original patch testing [11, 12].

Vesicular hand eczema (Fig. 1) [13] is a pruritic eruption on the palms, volar aspects and sides of the fingers, around the nails and occasionally on the plantar aspects of the feet with deep-seated vesicles and sparse or no erythema. If the periungual area is involved, transverse ridging of the fingernails can be a consequence. Vesicular hand eczema is a common disease, often with unknown etiology. It may have the appearance of chronic hand eczema if frequent vesicular eruptions occur, and the dermatitis does not clear completely between eruptions. Crops of vesicles may be seen at the periphery of an area of dermatitis. This type of hand eczema may be a symptom of systemic contact dermatitis.

A flare-up of dermatitis in the elbow and the knee flexures is a common symptom of systemic contact dermatitis. Such flares are difficult to distinguish from the early lesions of atopic dermatitis [14].

The "baboon syndrome" (Fig. 2) [15] is a characteristic, although rare, clinical manifestation of systemic contact dermatitis. It is a well-demarcated eruption on the buttocks, in the genital area and in a V-shape on the inner thighs, of a color ranging from dark-violet to pink. It may occupy the whole area or only part of it. Nakayama et al. [16] described the same clinical features as mercury exanthema. In mercury-sensitive patients, the baboon syndrome may also be seen in connection with acute generalized exanthematous pustulosis [17].

A nonspecific, maculopapular rash (toxicoderma) is often seen in systemic contact dermatitis. General symptoms such as headache and malaise are rarely seen in sensitized individuals following oral provocation with gold and medicaments. In patients sensitive to neomycin [8] and chromate [18], oral provocation with the hapten can cause nausea, vomiting, and diarrhea. A few patients have complained of arthralgia. Systemic administration of gold to gold-sensitized individuals has led to toxicoderma and slight fever [19, 20]. Malaise, leukocytosis, and pyrexia have also been seen in patients with systemic contact dermatitis from mercury [21].

16

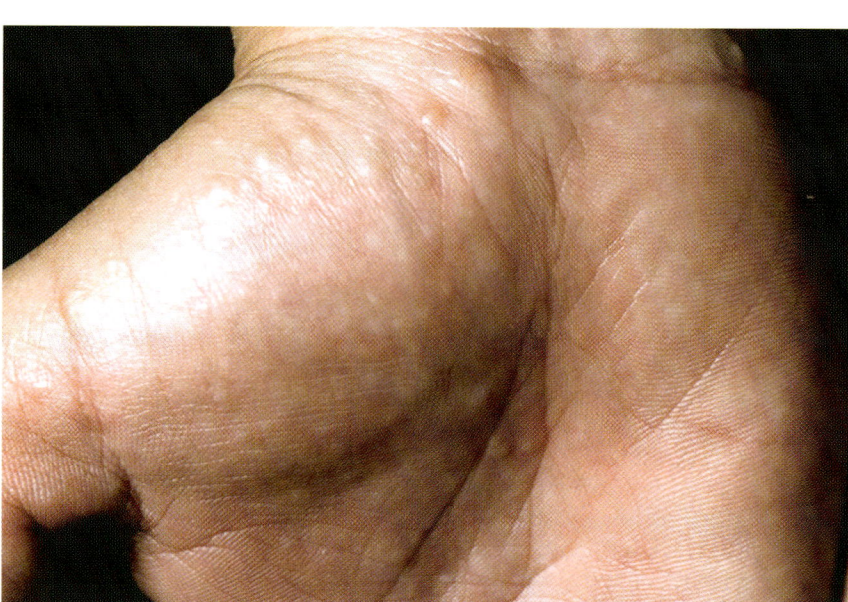

Fig. 1.
Vesicular eruption in the thenar region after oral challenge with 4 mg nickel

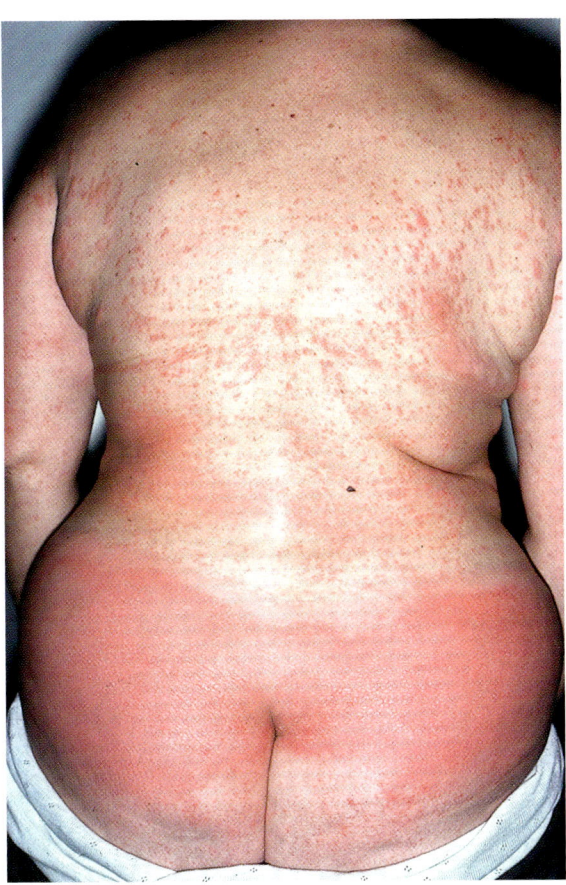

Fig. 2. Baboon syndrome in a patient sensitive to balsam of Peru after the use of suppositories that contained balsam of Peru

---

Core Message

■ The clinical features of systemic contact dermatitis include flare-up of previous dermatitis or previously positive patch test sites, vesicular palmar and/or plantar dermatitis, flexural dermatitis, and the baboon syndrome.

16.3 Mechanism

Based on human and animal experiments, it appears that both the humoral and the cellular immune systems are activated in systemic contact dermatitis. The histopathology of flare-up reactions is similar to that seen in ordinary contact dermatitis, while the accumulation of neutrophils in the baboon syndrome

---

suggests that circulating immune complexes play a role [7].

Flares at sites of previous dermatitis or previously positive patch test sites are probably caused by specifically sensitized T-cells, either resting at the site or homing to the area after specific hapten exposure [12, 22, 23]. A reduction of CD_4+ cells, CD_4+ CD45Ro+ and CD_8+ cells was seen in the peripheral blood of nickel-sensitive women after oral challenge with nickel. The oral challenge induced maturation of naive T-cells into memory cells. Memory cells were seen particularly in the intestinal mucosa [24].

A reduction of the number of CLA+ CD_{45}Ro+ CD_3+ and CLA+ CD_{45}Ro+ CD_8+ but not CLA+ CD_{45}Ro+ CD_4+ cells was seen in the peripheral blood of nickel-sensitive patients after oral challenge with nickel [25].

CD_4+ T-cell clones reacted to cobalt but not to nickel in a patient following the removal of a cobalt-containing metal joint prosthesis [26].

Flexural eczema, vesicular hand eczema, the baboon syndrome, and toxicoderma may be caused by nonspecific cytokine release [27]. Möller et al. [19] recorded a significant increase of cytokines such as IL-ra, interferon-γ (IFN-γ), tumor necrosis factor α (TNF-α), type-1 TNFα receptor (TNF-R1), IL-6 and acute phase reactants during systemic contact reactions to gold. In a patient with systemic contact dermatitis from prednisolone, elevated serum values of the IL-5, IL-6, and IL-10 were seen [28].

Antigen-specific tolerance to nickel has been demonstrated in guinea pigs [29]. Flares of dermatitis are frequently seen in clinical hyposensitization experiments when the hapten is given orally. Of 20 *Parthenium*-sensitive patients, 6 had to stop oral hyposensitization therapy due to aggravation of their dermatitis [30].

Core Message

■ The mechanism of systemic contact dermatitis includes both specifically sensitized T-cells and nonspecific cytokine release. The latter could explain nonspecific symptoms such as flexural dermatitis and the baboon syndrome.

16.4 Medicaments

Most diagnosed cases of systemic contact dermatitis have occurred as a consequence of systemic exposure to medicaments in specifically contact-sensitized individuals. Such cases were common in the early era of the use of antibiotics, when drugs such as streptomycin and penicillin were given both topically and systemically.

Medicaments known to cause systemic contact dermatitis are summarized in Chap. 35 and elsewhere [7]. Many case reports are available, and while the list illustrates the wide range of possibilities, it is not complete. Any drug is probably capable of causing systemic contact dermatitis if cutaneous sensitization precedes systemic exposure. In this context, it should be kept in mind, as it is not uncommon that a drug reaction can be diagnosed later by patch testing (Chap. 35).

Table 2 shows how contact sensitization to medicaments may result in systemic contact dermatitis. Contact sensitization is most commonly caused by the use of topical antibiotics in the treatment of leg ulcers, but the less common exposures outlined in Table 2 should be kept in mind. In a controlled study, Isaksson [31] showed that some budesonide-sensitive patients react to the inhalation of budesonide. Inhalation of budesonide caused angioedema in one contact-sensitized person [32]. Occupational exposure to drugs is seen in the pharmaceutical industry as well as among health care professionals such as nurses, who administer tablets or give injections. Among those with occupational contact with medicaments, veterinarians have a high frequency of contact allergy to medicaments. Systemic contact dermatitis can be caused by the cross-reactivity of certain medicaments. Corticosteroids can cause anaphylactoid-like reactions [33].

16

Table 2. Routes of sensitization to medicaments

Use as a topical medicament (particularly in leg ulcer patients)
Leaking of the medicament to the epidermis from various sites of intravenous injection
Occupational exposure
Eye drops
Suppositories
Intravesical installation
Injection of medicaments, middle ear, surgical wounds and intraperitoneal injection
Cross-reactivity

Core Message

■ Drugs used both topically and systemically may cause systemic contact dermatitis either as a flare-up of dermatitis in previous areas of dermatitis or as a widespread rash.

16.5 Metals

16.5.1 Nickel

Schittenhelm and Stockinger [3] observed the spread of nickel dermatitis after cutaneous exposure to nickel. Many patients with severe suspender dermatitis in the 1950s and 1960s had widespread dermatitis, with vesicular hand eczema and flexural dermatitis similar to that seen in systemic contact dermatitis [34, 35]. Systemic exposure from the absorption of nickel in the area of the dermatitis was thought to explain the clinical picture. Recently, it has been documented that avoidance of prolonged skin contact

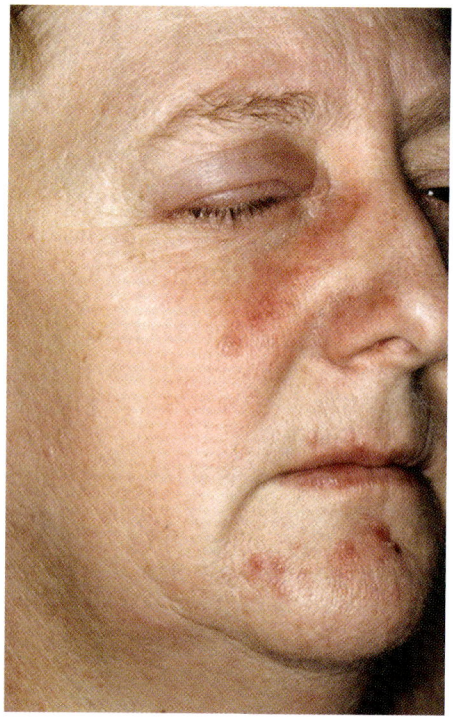

Fig. 3. Edematous eruption of the eyelid and dermatitis where spectacle frames touched the facial skin after oral challenge with 2.5 mg nickel

with nickel-releasing alloys results in a statistically significant decrease in the frequency of hand eczema in nickel-sensitive individuals [36]. It has also been shown that following the adoption in Denmark of a regulation prohibiting the use of nickel in clothing or jewelry, a previously identified statistical association between nickel sensitivity and hand eczema no longer exists [37].

The study of orally provoked flare-ups of nickel dermatitis was pioneered by Christensen and Möller [9], followed up by Kaaber et al. [38, 39], and Veien et al. [40]. In a double-blind study, Christensen and Möller [9] provoked 12 nickel-sensitive individuals with an oral dose of 5.6 mg nickel. Of the 12 patients, 9 reacted with systemic contact dermatitis after an average of 8 h. These patients had the symptoms listed in Table 1, in particular, vesicular hand eczema (Fig. 1). The results of this study have been repeated and confirmed by several authors [6, 12]. The evidence for immunological specificity includes flare-up reactions at previous nickel contact sites, for example under metal spectacle frames (Fig. 3). Such a reaction was seen under previous sites of suspender nickel dermatitis in a woman who had not used garter belts containing nickel for over 30 years (Fig. 4). Vasculitis-like lesions may also be seen (Fig. 5).

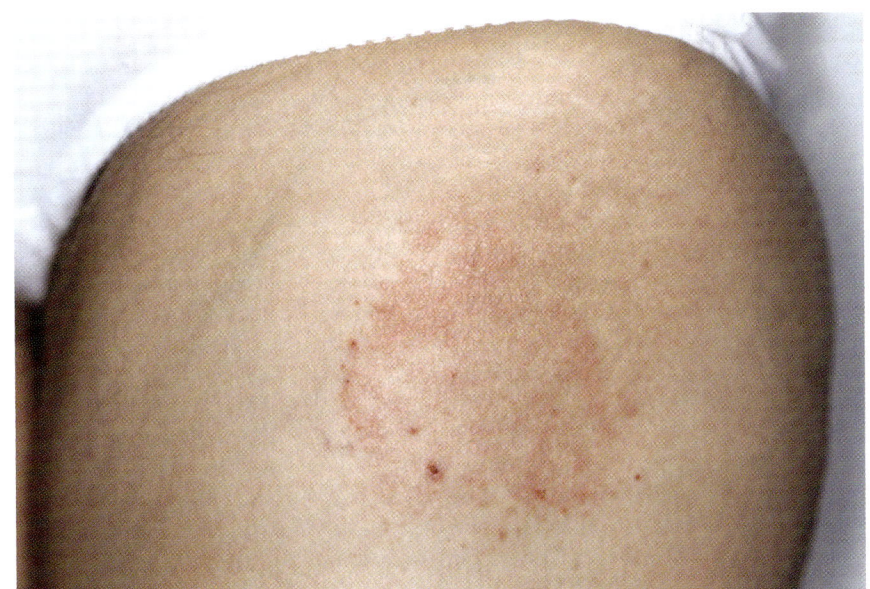

Fig. 4.
A plaque of dermatitis on the upper thigh in a 64-year-old woman after oral challenge with 2.5 mg nickel. As a young girl she had suspender dermatitis on the thighs from nickel in garter belts. She had not worn a garter belt for 30 years

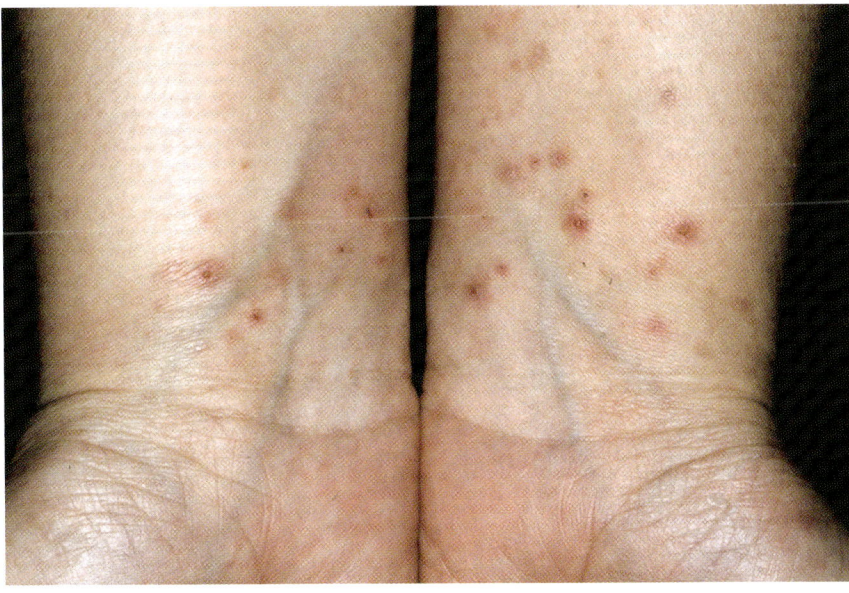

Fig. 5.
Following a placebo-controlled challenge with 2.5 mg nickel, this nickel-sensitive patient developed discrete, very pruritic, vasculitis-like lesions on the forearms and thighs

The above-mentioned studies illustrate that few patients react to a dose of less than 0.5 mg nickel given as a single oral dose, while the majority of patients react to a dose of 5 mg or more. Dose responsiveness in nickel-sensitive patients has been demonstrated in two studies in which 0.3–4 mg and 1 or 3 mg nickel, respectively, was used for oral challenge [41, 42]. Systemic nickel dermatitis has been seen following accidental intravenous exposure to micrograms of nickel [43–45]. Nickel released from dental braces [46–48] and from older types of orthopedic prostheses can cause systemic nickel dermatitis and/or loosening of the prostheses [49, 50].

The daily ingestion of nickel from food varies from 150 to 500 µg and depends both on the type of food and the production environment of the individual foodstuff. Foods with high nickel content include whole-grain flour, oats, soybeans, legumes, shellfish, nuts, licorice, and chocolate [51]. Nickel may be leached from cooking utensils [52]. The amount of nickel absorbed depends upon the concurrent intake of other foodstuffs such as proteins and alcohol. Chelating medicaments can interfere with nickel absorption and metabolism and in that way provoke systemic contact dermatitis. This has been well described for disulfiram (Fig. 6) [39].

Dietary intervention is indicated for nickel-sensitive patients with vesicular hand eczema or more widespread systemic contact dermatitis, if the elimination of nonoccupational as well as occupational nickel exposure does not improve or clear the dermatitis. Dietary restriction following the guidelines by Veien et al. [53] should be followed for 1–2 months, and the outcome at that time should determine whether dietary restriction should be continued. Clinical studies suggest that approximately one-quarter of selected patients benefit from prolonged dietary treatment [54, 55].

Core Message

- A flare-up of dermatitis at a previously positive patch test site or widespread eruptions may be seen after placebo-controlled oral challenge with nickel.

16.5.2 Chromium and Cobalt

Cobalt and chromium salts can provoke systemic contact dermatitis [6, 56]. Dose–response studies with chromium suggest that a range from 0.05 mg to 14.2 mg potassium dichromate given as a single oral dose is appropriate. Chromium picolinate given as a nutritional supplement caused systemic contact dermatitis in one person [57]. Only one study has been made of cobalt-sensitive individuals. Four of six cobalt-sensitive patients with vesicular hand eczema had a flare of the dermatitis after placebo-controlled oral challenge with 1 mg cobalt given as 4.75 mg cobalt chloride [58]. The removal of chromium- and cobalt-releasing dental braces or dietary restrictions may help individual patients.

16

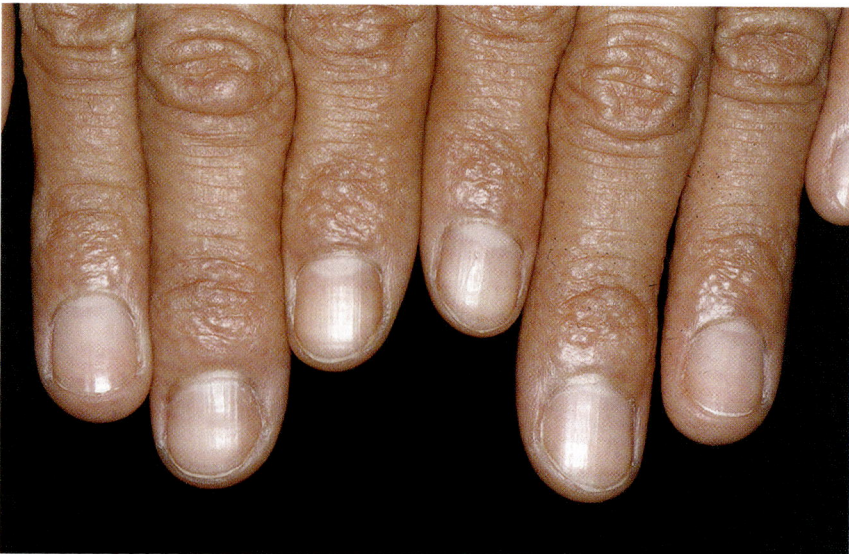

Fig. 6.
Symmetrical vesicular dermatitis of the periungual area in a nickel-sensitive person a few days after beginning treatment for alcohol dependence with disulfiram

16.5.3 Gold

Following the introduction of routine testing with gold sodium thiosulfate, a frequency of up to 10% positive reactions has been seen among consecutively patch-tested patients. Systemic contact dermatitis from gold in patients with rheumatoid arthritis treated with gold salts is probably common, as indicated by both clinical and experimental experience [59–62].

16.5.4 Mercury

Widespread eruptions, erythema-multiforme-like eruptions, and the baboon syndrome have been described in mercury-sensitive patients exposed to systemic mercury. Exposure can be from the vapors released from a broken thermometer, from homeopathic drugs or the drilling of amalgam dental fillings [21, 63–66].

> **Core Message**
>
> ■ Mercury-sensitive persons exposed to mercury vapors from a broken thermometer may develop baboon syndrome.

16.6 Other Contact Allergens

Most clinical and experimental studies of systemic contact dermatitis deal with either metals or medicaments, but important anecdotal evidence suggests that systemic contact dermatitis may be caused by certain plants, spices, and preservatives [67].

In a study of 42 patients with systemic contact dermatitis from *Rhus*, it was suggested that a toxic rather than an immunological reaction caused the symptoms. No information about patch test results was provided [68].

Kligman [69] attempted to hyposensitize persons with *Rhus* dermatitis by giving increasing oral doses of the allergen. Half of the moderately to severely sensitive patients developed either pruritus or a rash; 10% of the patients experienced flares of their dermatitis at sites of previously healed contact dermatitis. Flare-ups of vesicular hand eczema and erythema multiforme were rare. Perianal pruritus occurred in 10% of the highly sensitive individuals. Severe systemic contact dermatitis has been described in *Rhus*-sensitive patients who had eaten cashew nuts

[70]. This reaction was explained by an allergen in cashew nut shells that cross-reacts with urushiols in poison ivy [71].

The oral hyposensitization of 20 patients sensitive to *Parthenium hysterophorus* resulted in such severe flares in 6 of them that hyposensitization had to be stopped. Fourteen other patients successfully completed the hyposensitization procedure [72].

Systemic contact dermatitis has been seen in patients sensitive to balsam of Peru (*Myroxylon pereirae*) which contains naturally occurring flavors. Hjorth [73] observed systemic contact dermatitis in balsam-of-Peru-sensitive patients who had eaten flavored ice cream and orange marmalade. Veien et al. [74] challenged 17 patients sensitive to balsam of Peru with an oral dose of 1 g balsam of Peru. Ten patients reacted to balsam of Peru and one to a placebo (Fig. 7).

Of 102 patients sensitive to balsam of Peru, 8 reacted to coniferous benzoate and benzyl alcohol. All 8 had systemic contact dermatitis. Three had hand eczema, and three had widespread dermatitis [75].

In other studies, reduction of the dietary intake of balsams has been shown to improve the dermatitis of more than half of selected patients who were sensitive to balsam of Peru [76–78].

> **Core Message**
>
> ■ Patients with contact sensitivity to balsam of Peru may develop systemic contact dermatitis from spices and other flavorings. Open studies indicate that diet treatment may be helpful.

Members of the Compositae family of plants commonly cause allergic contact dermatitis. Systemic contact dermatitis in this group of patients is easily overlooked [79]. Sesquiterpene lactones are found in food and herbal remedies containing laurel, chamomile, and goldenrod [80–83]. One of four patients with contact allergy to lettuce had a flare of vesicular hand dermatitis after oral challenge with lettuce, and one of ten reacted to feverfew [79].

> **Core Message**
>
> ■ Herbal remedies such as laurel, chamomile, and goldenrod contain sesquiterpene lactones and may cause systemic contact dermatitis in sensitized persons.

Fig. 7.
Facial dermatitis in a baker sensitive to balsam of Peru after oral challenge with 1 g balsam of Peru

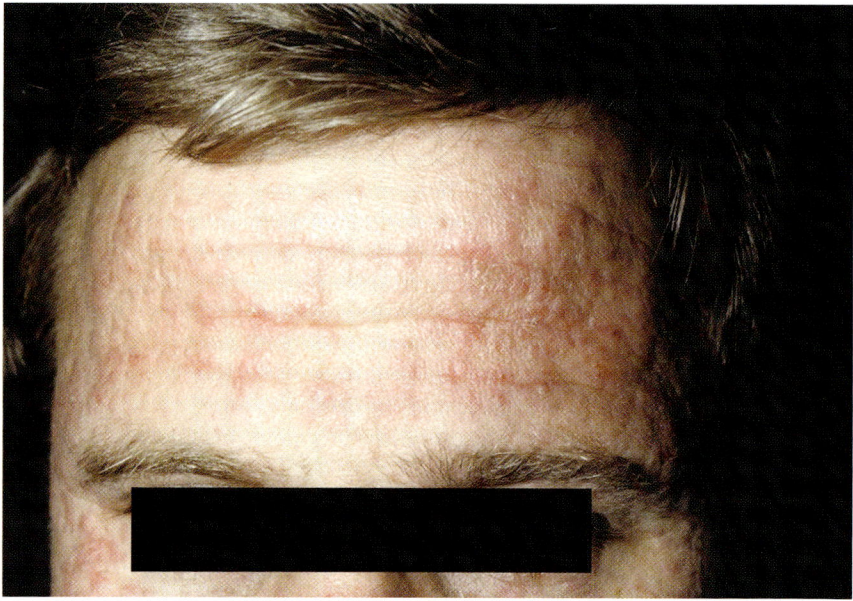

Garlic tablets caused a flare of vesicular hand eczema in a 58-year-old man with a positive patch test to garlic. A double-blind oral challenge was positive, and the dermatitis resolved when the garlic tablets were discontinued [84]. Periorbital and flexural dermatitis were seen in another garlic-sensitive person after the ingestion of garlic [85].

The antioxidant butylated hydroxyanisole (BHA), used both in cosmetics and in foods, can cause systemic contact dermatitis [86] as can the preservative sorbic acid [87–89].

Systemically aggravated contact dermatitis has been caused by aluminum in toothpaste in children sensitized to aluminum in vaccines [90].

16.7 Risk-Assessment-Oriented Studies

While the risk of systemic contact dermatitis from drugs can be assessed, it is more difficult to carry out similar studies on ubiquitous contact allergens such as metals and naturally occurring flavors. In spite of intensive research on the significance of orally ingested nickel in nickel-sensitive individuals, we are unable to give firm advice concerning the oral dose that would represent a risk for the wide range of nickel-sensitive individuals. Many variables, such as the route of administration, bioavailability, individual sensitivity to nickel, interaction with naturally occurring amino acids, and interaction with medicaments, must be considered. A number of as yet unknown factors could influence nickel metabolism. Furthermore, immunological reactivity to nickel can change with time [12] and can be influenced by sex hormones and the development of tolerance. It is important to recognize that this area of research is extremely complex and that much well-controlled research is still needed.

Core Message

- Systemic contact dermatitis in nickel-sensitive patients is complex. Reactions may vary with individual sensitivity to nickel, with bioavailability, with interaction with other food items or medicaments. Reactions may also be influenced by sex hormones and the development of tolerance.

Well-controlled oral challenge studies can be carried out with medicaments in sensitized individuals. The beta-adrenergic blocking agent alprenolol is a potent contact sensitizer. Ekenvall and Forsbeck [91] identified 14 workers employed in the pharmaceutical industry who were contact sensitized to this compound. Oral challenge with a therapeutic dose (100 mg) led to a flare-up in one worker who developed pruritus and widespread dermatitis.

The preservative Merthiolate (thimerosal) is widely used in sera and vaccines. Förström et al. [92] investigated 45 thimerosal contact-sensitive persons to evaluate the risk of a single therapeutic dose of 0.5 ml of a 0.01% Merthiolate solution given subcutaneously. Only 1 of the 45 patients developed a systemic contact dermatitis reaction. Aberer [93] did not observe any reactions in a similar study involving 12 patients.

Maibach [94] studied a group of patients who had discontinued the use of transdermal clonidine because of dermatitis. Of 52 patients with positive patch tests to clonidine, 29 were challenged orally with a therapeutic dose of the substance. Only one patient reacted with a flare-up at the site of the original dermatitis.

Propylene glycol is used as a vehicle in topical medications and cosmetics and as a food additive. Propylene glycol is both a sensitizer and an irritant. Hannuksela and Förström [95] challenged ten contact-sensitized individuals with 2–15 ml propylene glycol. Eight reacted with exanthema 3–16 h after the ingestion.

The overall impression of these studies is that systemic contact dermatitis in patients sensitized to a particular medicament is rare when the same patients are exposed to a therapeutic systemic dose of the medicament. Gold may constitute an exception to this general impression.

Core Message

- Although systemic contact dermatitis to medicaments given in therapeutic doses is probably rare in relation to the number of patients treated, there are many case reports of such reactions.

16.8 Diagnosis

Systemic contact dermatitis can occur in patients who are contact sensitized to a particular hapten if these patients are then systemically exposed to the same hapten or to breakdown products such as formaldehyde, a breakdown of aspartame [96].

The number of persons who will actually react to systemic exposure depends on the dose administered. In the case of nickel, whether a patient reacts to systemic exposure may also depend on the strength of the patch test reaction and the time that has elapsed since patch testing [42].

According to the available literature, particularly from experimental nickel challenge studies and challenge studies with medicaments, a relatively high dose of the hapten is needed to produce systemic contact dermatitis. The number of patients with

systemic contact dermatitis seen in clinical practice is low compared to the number of patients with allergic and irritant contact dermatitis [97]. In spite of the fact that systemic contact dermatitis is relatively rare, it is important to identify this type of reaction to provide optimal management of the individual patient. The diagnosis rests on the history of the patient, patch testing, and oral challenge and elimination studies. Severe reactions are unusual. Anaphylactic reactions following the administration of corticosteroids have been described [33].

16.9 Case Reports

Case Report 1

- A 37-year-old woman had had severe anogenital dermatitis for 3 years (Fig. 8). She had previously been treated by her gynecologist who had found no explanation for the dermatitis.

  The result of various topical treatments was unsatisfactory. Patch testing showed a ++ reaction to nickel. She had no memory of rashes under cheap jewelry or other nickel items.

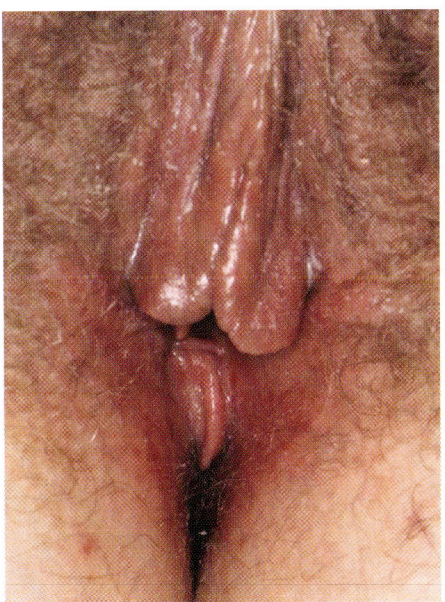

Fig. 8. Edematous anogenital dermatitis in a nickel-sensitive patient prior to initiation of a low-nickel diet

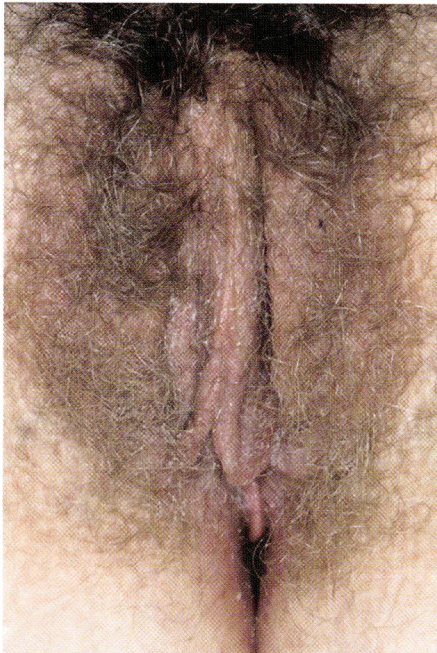

Fig. 9. The same patient as in Fig. 8 after 2 months on a low-nickel diet

Placebo-controlled oral challenge with 2.5 mg nickel produced a severe flare of her anogenital dermatitis after 2 days. The flare lasted more than a week. She was instructed to follow a low-nickel diet, and after 2 months the dermatitis was quiescent (Fig. 9).

Two years later the woman was seen again. The current problem was very pruritic perianal dermatitis. She was again advised to reduce the nickel intake in food, and after 2 months, the dermatitis had practically cleared. She admitted that on both occasions she had eaten lots of chocolate, known to contain significant amounts of nickel.

Case Report 2

■ A 43-year-old woman was seen because of an acute eruption of vesicular hand eczema (Fig. 10). She was known to have nickel allergy, and the eruption had occurred after 1 week on a weight-reducing diet. Many of the foods included in this diet were high in nickel content. She was instructed in how to avoid food items with a high content of nickel, and the dermatitis faded (Fig. 11).

16

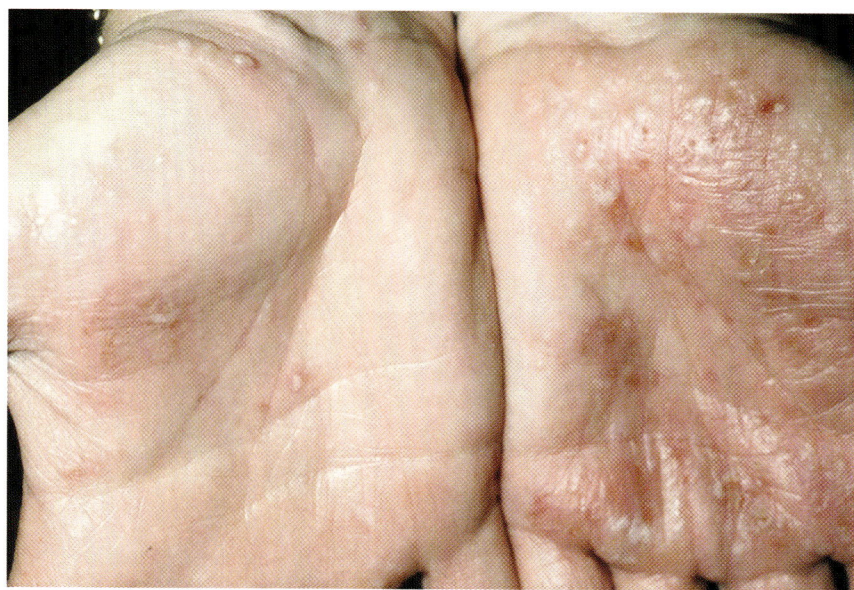

Fig. 10.
An acute eruption of vesicular hand eczema after a weight-reducing diet that included foods with a high nickel content

Fig. 11.
The same patient as in
Fig. 10. The dermatitis faded
after she was instructed to
follow a low-nickel diet

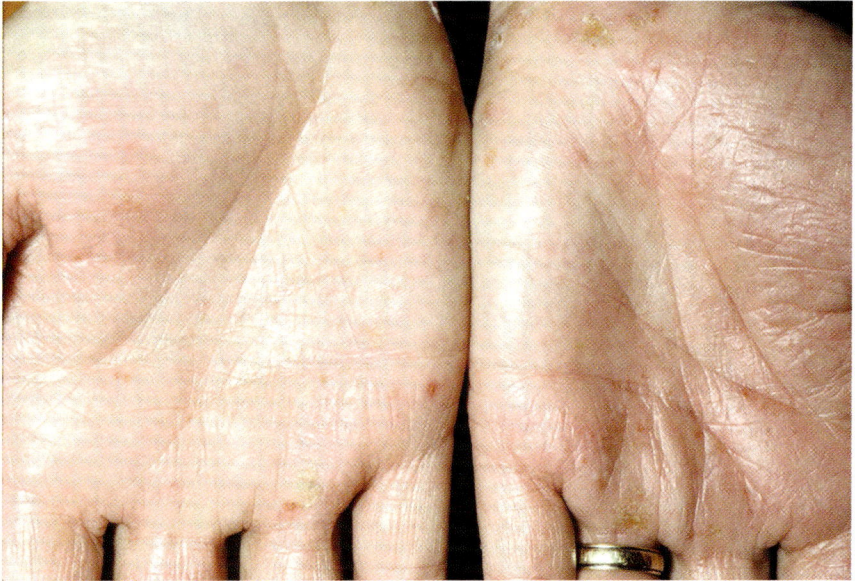

References

1. Nielsen NH, Menné T (1992) Allergic contact sensitization in an unselected Danish population. Acta Derm Venereol (Stockh) 72:456–460
2. Shelley WB, Crissey JT (1970) Thomas Bateman. In: Shelley WB, Crissey JT (eds) Classics in clinical dermatology. Thomas, Illinois, p 22
3. Schittenhelm A, Stockinger W (1925) Über die Idiosynkrasie gegen Nickel (Nickel-krätze) und ihre Beziehung zur Anaphylaxie. Z Ges Exp Med 45:58–74
4. Cronin E (1980) Reactions to the systemic absorption of contact allergens. Contact dermatitis. Churchill Livingstone, London, pp 26–29
5. Fisher AA (1986) Systemic contact-type dermatitis. Contact dermatitis. Lea and Febiger, Philadelphia, Pa., pp 119–131
6. Menné T, Veien NK, Sjølin K-E, Maibach HI (1994) Systemic contact dermatitis. Am J Cont Dermat 5:1–12
7. Veien NK, Menné T, Maibach HI (2004) Systemic contact dermatitis. In: Zhai H, Maibach HI (eds) Dermatotoxicology, 6th edn. CRC, Boca Raton, Fla., pp 285–320
8. Ekelund A-G, Möller H (1969) Oral provocation in eczematous contact allergy to neomycin and hydroxyquinolines. Acta Derm Venereol (Stockh) 49:422–426
9. Christensen OB, Möller H (1975) External and internal exposure to the antigen in the hand eczema of nickel allergy. Contact Dermatitis 1:136–141
10. Menné T, Weisman K (1984) Hämatogenes Kontakteksem nach oraler Gabe von Neomycin. Hautarzt 35:319–320
11. Christensen OB, Lindström C, Löfberg H, Möller H (1981) Micromorphology and specificity of orally induced flare-up reactions in nickel-sensitive patients. Acta Derm Venereol (Stockh) 61:505–510
12. Hindsén M (1998) Clinical and experimental studies in nickel allergy. Dissertation, Malmö
13. Veien NK, Menné T (2000) Acute and recurrent vesicular hand dermatitis (pompholyx). In: Menné T, Maibach HI (eds) Hand eczema, 2nd edn. CRC, Boca Raton, Fla., pp 147–165
14. Wintzen M, Donker AS, van Zuuren EJ (2003) Recalcitrant atopic dermatitis due to allergy to Compositae. Contact Dermatitis 48:87–88
15. Andersen KE, Hjorth N, Menné T (1984) The baboon syndrome: systemically induced allergic contact dermatitis. Contact Dermatitis 10:97–101
16. Nakayama H, Niki F, Shono M, Hada S (1983) Mercury exanthem. Contact Dermatitis 9:411–417
17. Lerch M, Bircher AJ (2004) Systemically induced allergic exanthem from mercury. Contact Dermatitis 50:349–353
18. Kaaber K, Veien NK (1977) The significance of chromate ingestion in patients allergic to chromate. Acta Derm Venereol (Stockh) 57:321–323
19. Möller H, Ohlsson K, Linder C, Björkner B, Bruze M (1998) Cytokines and acute phase reactants during flare-up of contact allergy to gold. Am J Contact Dermat 9:15–22
20. Möller H, Gjörkner B, Bruze M et al (1999) Laser Doppler perfusion imaging for the documentation of flare-up in contact allergy to cold. Contact Dermatitis 41:131
21. Vena GA, Foti C, Grandolfo M, Angelini G (1994) Mercury exanthem. Contact Dermatitis 31:214–216
22. Scheper RJ, von Blomberg M, Boerrigter GH, Bruynzeel D, van Dinther A, Vos A (1983) Induction of local memory in the skin. Role of local T cell retention. Clin Exp Immunol 51:141–151
23. Yamashita N, Natsuaki M, Sagamis (1989) Flare-up reactions on murine contact hypersensitivity. I. Description of an experimental model: rechallenge system. Immunology 67:365–369
24. Di Gioacchino M, Boscolo P, Cavallucci E, Verna N, di Stefano F, di Sciascio M, Masci S, Andreassi M, Sabbioni E, Angelucci D, Conti P (2000) Lymphocyte subset changes in blood and gastrointestinal mucosa after oral nickel challenge in nickel-sensitized women. Contact Dermatitis 43:206–211
25. Jensen CS, Lisby S, Larsen JK, Veien NK, Menné T (2004) Characterization of lymphocyte subpopulations and cytokine profiles in peripheral blood of nickel-sensitive individuals with systemic contact dermatitis after oral nickel exposure. Contact Dermatitis 50:31–38

16

26. Thomssen H, Hoffmann B, Schank M, Hohler T, Thabe H, Meyer zum Buschenfelde KH, Marker-Hermann E (2001) Cobalt-specific T lymphocytes in synovial tissue after an allergic reaction to a cobalt alloy joint prosthesis. J Rheumatol 28:1121–1128

27. Möller H, Ohlsson K, Linder C, Björkner B, Bruze M (1999) The flare-up reactions after systemic provocation in contact allergy to nickel and gold. Contact Dermatitis 40: 200–204

28. Yawalka N, Hari Y, Helbling A, von Gregerz S, Kappeler A, Braathen LR, Pichler WJ (1998) Elevated serum levels of interleukins 5,6 and 10 in a patient with drug-induced exanthem caused by systemic corticosteroids. J Am Acad Dermatol 39:790–793

29. Van Hoogstraten IMW, Boden D, von Blomberg ME, Kraal G, Scheper RJ (1992) Persistent immune tolerance to nickel and chromium by oral administration prior to cutaneous sensitization. J Invest Dermatol 99:607–611

30. Hamilton TK, Zug KA (1998) Systemic contact dermatitis to raw cashew nuts in a pesto sauce. Am J Contact Dermat 9:51–54

31. Isaksson M (2000) Clinical and experimental studies in corticosteroid contact allergy (Dissertation). Malmö, Sweden, Department of Dermatology, University Hospital

32. Pirker C, Misic A, Frosch PJ (2003) Angioedema and dysphagia caused by contact allergy to inhaled budesonide. Contact Dermatitis 49:77–79

33. Vidal C, Tomé S, Fernándex-Redondo V, Tato F (1994) Systemic allergic reactions to corticosteroids. Contact Dermatitis 31:273–274

34. Calnan CD (1956) Nickel dermatitis. Br J Dermatol 68: 229–236

35. Marcussen PV (1957) Spread of nickel dermatitis. Dermatologica 115:596–607

36. Kalimo K, Lammintausta K, Jalava J, Niskanen T (1997) Is it possible to improve the prognosis in nickel contact dermatitis? Contact Dermatitis 37:121–124

37. Nielsen NN, Linneberg A, Menné T, Madsen F, Frolund L, Dirksen A, Jørgensen T (2002) The association between contact allergy and hand eczema in 2 cross-sectional surveys 8 years apart. Contact Dermatitis 47:71–77

38. Kaaber K, Veien NK, Tjell JC (1978) Low nickel diet in the treatment of patients with chronic nickel dermatitis. Br J Dermatol 98:197–201

39. Kaaber K, Menné T, Tjell JC, Veien N (1979) Antabuse treatment of nickel dermatitis. Chelation – a new principle in the treatment of nickel dermatitis. Contact Dermatitis 5: 221–228

40. Veien NK, Hattel T, Justesen O, Nørholm A (1987) Oral challenge with nickel and cobalt in patients with positive patch tests to nickel and/or cobalt. Acta Derm Venereol (Stockh) 67:321–325

41. Jensen CS, Menné T, Lisby S, Kristiansen J, Veien NK (2003) Experimental systemic contact dermatitis from nickel: a dose-response study. Contact Dermatitis 49:124–132

42. Hindsen M, Bruze M, Christensen OB (2001) Flare-up reactions after oral challenge with nickel in relation to challenge dose and intensity and time of previous patch test reactions. J Am Acad Dermatol 44:616–623

43. Stoddard JC (1960) Nickel sensitivity as a cause of infusious reaction. Lancet 2:741–742

44. Smeenk G, Teunissen PC (1977) Allergische reacties op nikkel uit infusietoedieningssystemen. Ned Tijdschr Geneeskd 121:4–9

45. Olerud JE, Lee MY, Ulvelli DA, Goble GJ, Babb AL (1984) Presumptive nickel dermatitis from hemodialysis. Arch Dermatol 120:1066–1068

46. Veien NK, Borchorst E, Hattel T, Laurberg G (1994) Stomatitis or systemically induced contact dermatitis from metal wire in orthodontic materials: Contact Dermatitis 30: 210–213

47. Kerosuo H, Kanerva L (1997) Systemic contact dermatitis caused by nickel in a stainless steel orthodontic appliance. Contact Dermatitis 36:112–113

48. Mancuso G, Berdondini RM (2002) Eyelid dermatitis and conjunctivitis as sole manifestations of allergy to nickel in an orthodontic appliance. Contact Dermatitis 46:245

49. Wilkinson JD (1989) Nickel allergy and orthopaedic prostheses. In: Maibach HI and Menné T (eds) Nickel and the skin immunology and toxicology. CRC, Boca Raton, Fla., pp 188–193

50. Antony FC, Dudley W, Field R, Holden CA (2003) Metal allergy resurfaces in failed hip endoprostheses. Contact Dermatitis 48:49–50

51. Veien NK, Menné T (1990) Nickel contact allergy and a nickel-restricted diet. Semin Dermatol 9:197–205

52. Berg T, Petersen A, Pedersen GA, Petersen J, Madsen C (2000) The release of nickel and other trace elements from electric kettles and coffee machines. Food Addit Contam 17:189–196

53. Veien NK, Hattel T, Laurberg G (1993) Low nickel diet: an open, prospective trial. J Am Acad Dermatol 29:1002–1007

54. Veien NK, Hattel T, Justesen O, Nørholm A (1985) Dietary treatment of nickel dermatitis. Acta Derm Venereol (Stockh) 65:138–142

55. Antico A, Soana R (1999) Chronic allergic-like dermatopathies in nickel-sensitive patients. Results of dietary restrictions and challenge with nickel salts. Allergy Asthma Proc 20:235–242

56. Veien NK, Hattel T, Laurberg G (1994) Chromate-allergic patients challenged orally with potassium dichromate. Contact Dermatitis 31:137–139

57. Fowler JF Jr (2000) Systemic contact dermatitis caused by oral chromium picolinate. Cutis 65:116

58. Veien NK, Hattel T, Laurberg G (1995) Placebo-controlled oral challenge with cobalt in patients with positive patch test to cobalt. Contact Dermatitis 33:54–55

59. Wichs IP, Wong D, McCullagh RB, Fleming A (1988) Contact allergy to gold after systemic administration of gold for rheumatoid arthritis. Ann Reum Dis 47:421–422

60. Möller H, Björkner B, Bruze M (1996) Clinical reactions to provocation with gold sodium thiomalate in patients with contact allergy to gold. Br J Dermatol 135:423–427

61. Möller H. Larsson Å, Björkner B, Bruze M, Hagstam Å (1996) Flare up of contact allergy sites in a gold-treated rheumatic patient. Acta Derm Venereol (Stockh) 76:55–58

62. Möller H, Svensson Å, Björkner B, Bruze M, Lindroth Y, Marthorpe R, Theander J (1997) Contact allergy to gold and gold therapy in patients with rheumatoid arthritis. Acta Derm Venerol (Stockh) 77:370–373

63. Nakayama H, Shono M, Hada S (1984) Mercury exanthem. J Am Acad Dermatol 11:137–139

64. Audicana M, Bernedo N, Gonzalex I, Munoz D, Fernandez E, Gastaminza G (2001) An unusual case of baboon syndrome due to mercury present in a homeopathic medicine. Contact Dermatitis 45:185

65. Adachi A, Horikawa T, Takashima T et al (2000) Mercury-induced nummular dermatitis. J Am Acad Dermatol 43: 383–385

66. Zimmer J, Grange F, Straub P et al (1997) Erytheme meruriel apres exposition accidentelle a des vapeurs de mercure. Ann Med Interne Paris 148:317–320

67. Veien NK (1997) The role of ingested food in systemic allergic contact dermatitis. Clin Dermatol 15:547–555

68. Oh S-H, Haw C-R, Lee M-H (2003) Clincial and immunologic features of systemic contact dermatitis from ingestion of *Rhus* (*Toxicodendron*). Contact Dermatitis 48: 251–254

69. Kligman AM (1958) Hyposensitization against rhus dermatitis. Arch Dermatol 78: 47–72, 93

70. Ratner JH, Spencer SK, Grainge JM (1974) Cashew nut dermatitis. Arch Dermatol 110: 921–923

71. Kligman AM (1958) Cashew nut shell oil for hyposensitization against rhus dermatitis. Arch Dermatol 78: 359–363

72. Handa S, Sahoo B, Sharma VK (2001) Oral hyposensitization in patients with contact dermatitis from *Parthenium hysterophorus*. Contact Dermatitis 44: 279–282

73. Hjorth N (1965) Allergy to balsams. Spectrum Int 7: 97–101

74. Veien NK, Hattel T, Justesen O, Nørholm N (1985) Oral challenge with balsam of Peru. Contact Dermatitis 12: 104–107

75. Hausen BM (2001) Rauchen, Süssigkeiten, Perubalsam – ein Circulus vitiosus? Aktuel Dermatol 27: 136–143

76. Veien NK, Hattel T, Laurberg G (1996) Can oral challenge with balsam of Peru predict possible benefit from a low-balsam diet? Am J Contact Dermat 7: 84–87

77. Salam TN, Fowler JF Jr (2001) Balsam-related systemic contact dermatitis. J Am Acad Dermatol 45: 377–381

78. Pfutzner W, Thomas P, Niedermeier A, Pfeiffer C, Sander C, Przybilla B (2003) Systemic contact dermatitis elicited by oral intake of balsam of Peru. Acta Derm Venereol (Stockh) 83: 294–295

79. Oliwiecki S, Beck MH, Hausen BM (1991) Compositae dermatitis aggravated by eating lettuce. Contact Dermatitis 24: 318–319

80. Dooms-Goossens A, Bubelloy R, Degreef H (1990) Contact and systemic contact-type dermatitis to spices. Dermatol Clin 8: 89–93

81. Rodríguez-Serna M, Sánchez-Motilla MM, Ramón R, Aliaga A (1998) allergic and systemic contact dermatitis from *Matricaria chamomilla* tea. Contact Dermatitis 39: 192–193

82. Schatzle M, Agathos M, Breit R (1998) Allergic contact dermatitis from goldenrod (*Herba solidaginis*) after systemic administration. Contact Dermatitis 39: 271–272

83. Rycroft RJG (2003) Recurrent facial dermatitis from chomomile tea. Contact Dermatitis 48: 229

84. Barden AD, Wilkinson SM, Bech MH, Chalmers RJG (1994) Garlic induced systemic contact dermatitis. Contact Dermatitis 30: 299–300

85. Pereira F, Hatia M, Cardoso J (2002) Systemic contact dermatitis from diallyl disulfide. Contact Dermatitis 46: 124

86. Roed-Petersen J, Hjorth N (1976) Contact dermatitis from antioxidants. Br J Dermatol 94: 233–241

87. Gierdano: Labadil F, Pech-Ormieres C, Bazex J (1996) Systemic contact dermatitis from sorbic acid. Contact Dermatitis 34: 61–62

88. Raison-Peyron N, Meynadier JM, Meynadier J (2000) Sorbic acid: an unusual cause of systemic contact dermatitis in an infant. Contact Dermatitis 43: 247–248

89. Dejobert Y, Delaporte E, Piette F, Thomas P (2001) Vesicular eczema and systemic contact dermatitis from sorbic acid. Contact Dermatitis 45: 291

90. Veien NK, Hattel T, Laurberg G (1993) Systemically aggravated contact dermatitis caused by aluminium in tooth paste. Contact Dermatitis 28: 199–200

91. Ekenvall L, Forsbeck M (1978) Contact eczema produced by a beta-adrenergic blocking agent (alprenolol). Contact Dermatitis 4: 190–194

92. Förström L, Hannuksela M, Kousa M, Lehmuskallio E (1980) Merthiolate hypersensitivity and vaccines. Contact Dermatitis 6: 241–245

93. Aberer W (1991) Vaccinations despite thiomersal sensitivity. Contact Dermatitis 24: 6–10

94. Maibach HI (1987) Oral substitution in patients sensitized by transdermal clonidine treatment. Contact Dermatitis 16: 1–9

95. Hannuksela M, Förström L (1978) Reactions to peroral propylene glycol. Contact Dermatitis 4: 41–45

96. Hill AM, Belsito DV (2003) Systemic contact dermatitis of the eyelids caused by formaldehyde derived from aspartame? Contact Dermatitis 49: 258–259

97. Veien NK, Hattel T, Justensen O, Nørholm A (1987) Diagnostic procedures for eczema patients. Contact Dermatitis 17: 35–40

Chapter 17

Phototoxic and Photoallergic Reactions

17

Roy A. Palmer, Ian R. White

Contents

17.1 Introduction

An exogenous substance may cause photosensitivity by phototoxic or photoallergic mechanisms, or by inducing a dermatosis which is exacerbated by exposure to ultraviolet (UV) radiation (Table 1). Phototoxicity is commoner than photoallergy, and is distinguished from it by the lack of an immunological basis. The characteristics of these two reaction patterns are shown in Table 2. However, it must be recognized that all attempts to classify substances causing these reactions are partly arbitrary; in particular, many agents are capable of producing photosensitivity by multiple and unique mechanisms, with corresponding differences in clinical presentation.

Phototoxicity may be due to systemically administered agents (usually drugs), or contact with substances (most commonly plants). Photoallergy is almost always due to topically applied substances (including sunscreens).

Mechanisms of phototoxicity and photoallergy are discussed in greater detail in Chap. 6. With regard to photoallergy, its predisposing factors and prevalence, individual photoallergens and the investigation of suspected photoallergy are described in the chapter on photopatch testing (Chap. 27).

17.2 Mechanisms of Photosensitization

Molecules that absorb photons are called chromophores. The chemical structure of a chromophore determines the wavelengths of radiation that it absorbs (its "absorption spectrum"). UVB is radiation of wavelength 280–315 nm, UVA is 315–400 nm, and wavelengths above this are visible light. Only a few chromophores, for example eosin, absorb light in the visible spectrum. Most phototoxicity and photoallergy is caused by UVA rather than UVB for several reasons: (1) most photosensitizers absorb UVA more than UVB; (2) there is much more UVA than UVB in sunlight; (3) sunburn occurs with small doses of UVB and so creates an upper limit to the dose of UVB that can be tolerated; and (4) more UVA penetrates to the dermis (particularly relevant to systemically administered photosensitizers). The latter is one reason why *in vitro* absorption spectra may differ from *in vivo* action spectra [1] (the action spectrum is the ability of different wavelengths of radiation to cause an effect).

17.2.1 Mechanisms of Phototoxicity

When a chromophore absorbs a photon, the energy promotes electrons within the molecule into an excited state. These return to the ground state by giving out radiation (for example, fluorescence) or heat, or by causing a chemical reaction. Products of the latter

Table 1. Mechanisms and clinical manifestations of photosensitivity caused by exogenous substances (adapted from Ferguson [18])

Mechanism	Clinical manifestations	Examples of topical agents	Examples of systemic agents
Phototoxicity	Immediate-onset erythema. Prickling, burning, edema or urticaria. May show delayed erythema or hyperpigmentation	Coal tar, anthraquinone-based dyes	Benoxaprofen, amiodarone, chlorpromazine
	Delayed-onset erythema (at 12–24 h; = exaggerated sunburn)		Fluoroquinolones, tetracyclines, thiazides, quinine, amiodarone, chlorpromazine retinoids
	Late-onset erythema (24–120 h), may develop blisters, hyperpigmentation	Psoralens	Psoralens
	Pseudoporphyria		Frusemide, amiodarone, tetracyclines
	Photoonycholysis		Tetracyclines, psoralens
	Telangiectasia		Calcium-channel blockers
Photoallergy	Eczema	Sunscreens, Musk ambrette	Rare/controversial
Induction of photo-sensitive dermatosis	Lupus erythematosus		Hydralazine
	Lichenoid reaction		Thiazides
	Melasma		Oral contraceptive pill
	Pellagra		Hydantoin

Table 2. Comparison between phototoxic and photoallergic reactions (adapted from [37])

	Phototoxic	Photoallergic
Occurs in all individuals with sufficient dose	Yes	No
Incidence after exposure	High	Low
Required concentration of photosensitizing agent	High	Low
Required dose of ultraviolet	High	Low
Reaction possible after single exposure	Yes	No
Ultraviolet action spectrum	Same as absorption spectrum	Broader than absorption spectrum
Commonest appearance	Erythema	Eczema
Limited to exposed area	Yes	May spread
Flare-up reactions	No	Possible
Cross-reactions	No	Possible

17

are called photoproducts and the reactions generating them can be divided into three types:

- Type I   Transfer of an electron leads to the formation of free radicals. These free radicals react with oxygen thereby generating reactive oxygen species.

- Type II   Energy transfer leads directly to the formation of reactive oxygen species.

- Type III   Energy transfer leads directly to the formation of stable phototoxic products.

As can be seen from the above, types I and II are dependent on oxygen; they are sometimes called "photodynamic reactions" and the reactive oxygen species they produce cause damage to cells. They are more common than type III reactions. An individual phototoxic substance usually causes phototoxicity by multiple molecular pathways. Systemically administered phototoxic agents tend to cause most damage to endothelial cells and mast cells, and topically applied ones to keratinocytes. The cellular location of damage tends to be inside the cell in the case of lipophilic sensitizers, and hydrophilic ones tend to damage cell membranes (Chap. 6).

17.2.1.1 Examples

Furocoumarins (Psoralens)

These are unusual among photosensitizing substances in several respects: they operate predominantly through a type III mechanism, they target DNA, and some of the processes involved are reasonably well understood. They form complexes between adjacent base pairs in DNA, and then on UVA irradiation a covalent bond is formed between the furocoumarin and a pyrimidine base (particularly thymine) on the DNA. This process is an example of cycloaddition and it yields a monoadduct with a furocoumarin molecule linked to one DNA strand. If there is now further absorption of UVA, a similar reaction can take place with a pyrimidine base on the opposite strand of DNA, a process of bifunctional cycloaddition which results in interstrand cross-linking [2]. The mechanism of erythema production from furocoumarin phototoxicity is not fully clear, but there is a correlation between the ability of a psoralen to cross-link strands of DNA with the production of an erythematous response [3]. 4,6,4´-Trimethylangelicin, a psoralen that forms monoadducts only, is far less phototoxic than 8-methoxypsoralen, which engages in bifunctional cycloaddition [4]. However, the erythema from furocoumarin phototoxicity may also be related to membrane damage caused by photodynamic processes [5].

Dyes

The absorption of visible light and UVA by dyes such as acridine orange causes generation of singlet oxygen which results in tissue damage, particularly to membranes [6].

Nonsteroidal Anti-inflammatory Drugs (NSAIDs)

These produce photoproducts which generate free radicals [7, 8].

Amiodarone

After exposure to UV, amiodarone loses iodine (deiodination) and there is aryl radical formation. This aryl radical is able to take hydrogen from chemical donors such as linoleic acid. A dienyl radical is formed, which can then produce a peroxy radical causing lipid peroxidation. This reaction may be the reason for the deposition of lipofuscin in the skin associated with amiodarone phototoxicity [9].

17.2.2 Mechanisms of Photoallergy

A stable photoproduct is generated by a photochemical reaction as described above. In photoallergy, that photoproduct acts as a hapten or a complete antigen to generate a type-IV hypersensitivity reaction. This hypersensitivity is essentially the same as that underlying allergic contact dermatitis; in the sensitization phase Langerhans cells migrate to lymph nodes and present antigens to T-lymphocytes. In the elicitation phase these T-cells meet the antigen in the skin and react to it. The histology and morphology of a photoallergic contact reaction are similar to those of an ordinary allergic contact reaction and, on immunohistological examination, $CD4^+$ lymphocytes are present in the infiltrate [10]. Both the sensitization and elicitation phases of the reaction require the generation of the allergen by ultraviolet radiation.

Many compounds that can cause photoallergy are halogenated aromatic hydrocarbons [11]. One chemical that has been studied is tetrachlorosalicylanilide, which used to be a common photoallergen until it was withdrawn. UV causes it to undergo photochemical dechlorination, generating free radicals that react with albumin; albumin modified in this way may be antigenic [11].

The action spectrum of photoallergy is usually in the UVA range. Exceptions to this, in which both UVA and UVB have been incriminated, include NSAIDS [12] and diphenhydramine hydrochloride [13].

Some agents, for example phenothiazines, are capable of producing both phototoxicity and photoallergy.

17.3 General Features of Photosensitive Eruptions

Phototoxicity and photoallergy due to topically applied substances have a distribution corresponding to the overlap of the application of the substance and UV exposure. Photosensitivity due to systemic administration of a phototoxic substance tends to have a distinctive distribution identical to that of chronic actinic dermatitis. It involves the face (especially the forehead, cheeks, chin, and helices of ears), upper chest, sides and back of the neck, and dorsal aspects of the forearms and hands. The skin proximal to the second and third fingers is more affected than that proximal to the fourth and fifth, and the proximal phalanges are affected but not the middle or distal ones. There may be well-demarcated cut-offs at the edges of clothing, such as on the V-of-the-chest and beyond the sleeves. Shaded areas of exposed skin, such as upper eyelids, behind the ears, under the chin, skin creases and finger-web spaces, are typically spared. This may help distinction from airborne allergic contact dermatitis.

However, this classic distribution is not always obviously present, reasons for which include the penetration of thin loose-weave clothing by UVA, and the spread of photoallergic (but not phototoxic) reactions to include unexposed skin. Asymmetrical exposure to UV (for example, due to car travel) may cause an asymmetrical rash.

When attempting to determine if a patient is photosensitive it is very helpful if the patient has noticed that their condition deteriorates with sun exposure. Patients sensitive to UVA are less likely to observe this than those sensitive to UVB. This is because UVA shows less seasonal variation and penetrates cloud, windows, and thin loose-weaved clothing. Therefore, exacerbations related to discrete episodes of intense sun exposure, which are more easily recognized by patients, do not dominate the clinical picture. Also, the shorter the latent period between exposure and deterioration the easier it is for the patient to make the association.

17.4 Phototoxicity

Some of the systemic and topical agents reported to cause phototoxic reactions are listed in Tables 3 and 4. The incidence of phototoxicity with each drug varies greatly between reports. The commonest types of phototoxicity seen by dermatologists are phototoxicity due to psoralen-UVA (PUVA) therapy and to other orally administered drugs, and phytophototoxic dermatitis.

Phototoxicity will theoretically occur in all individuals exposed to a high enough dose of both the phototoxic substance and UV. However, in practice it frequently seems to be idiosyncratic, for reasons that are not entirely clear. Differences in drug metabolism between individuals (which may be genetic) may predispose some people. Fair-skinned individuals who report high sunburn sensitivity (Fitzpatrick skin-types I and II) may be more susceptible. This is certainly the case with PUVA therapy, and may be due not only to the fact that a lower dose of UV is required to cause erythema in these people, but also to possible differences in the shape of the dose-response curve and duration of erythema.

Investigation of contact phototoxic reactions by photopatch testing is not usually indicated; these reactions are difficult to interpret because all individuals will theoretically react given enough sensitizer and the cutaneous absorption of that sensitizer is difficult to reliably calibrate. Instead, the diagnosis comes from the history and examination. In the case of systemic phototoxic reactions, irradiation with a broad-band source or monochromatic irradiation, on and off the suspected drug, will establish to what degree the minimum phototoxic dose (on the drug, evaluated at an appropriate time interval after UV, which depends on the suspected photosensitizer) is lower than the minimum erythema dose (off the drug).

Phototoxicity usually resolves quickly after ceasing exposure to the photosensitizer. If there are strong reasons not to stop a systemic drug that is causing phototoxicity, changing the time of administration from the morning to the evening may help [14], as may reducing the dose, because phototoxicity is, by its nature, dose-dependent. Amiodarone and its major metabolite can persist in the skin for months after stopping it so that phototoxicity can be prolonged. During the development of new drugs that are chemically related to known photosensitizers, it is essential to test for phototoxicity before they are marketed. A variety of *in vitro* methods exist, and *in vivo* testing is performed which allows the calculation of a "phototoxicity index" [15].

The increased carcinogenic risk in patients who have had many oral PUVA treatments is well recognized, and the possibility exists that other photosensitizing drugs may also promote photocarcinogenesis. It has been shown in mice that fluoroquinolones can do this, but it is probably of no significance for humans who usually take only short courses [16]. The significance is uncertain for patients with cystic fibrosis who take long courses of high-dose fluoroquinolones and have a high incidence of phototoxicity [17].

17.4.1 Clinical Features of Phototoxicity

These vary depending on the photosensitizing agent. The complexity and variability of the processes involved defy the construction of a perfect classification. The following attempt is summarized in Table 1 (adapted from Ferguson [18]).

17.4.1.1 Immediate-onset Erythema

During UVA exposure patients develop a prickling or burning sensation with erythema, which becomes edematous or urticarial if severe. This is similar to the features of erythropoietic protoporphyria. In addition, there may be associated subsequent hyperpigmentation.

Tar

Workers exposed to coal tar, or derivatives such as creosote, may develop tar "smarts." The reaction consists of burning and smarting of the exposed skin and this is often associated with erythema that leads to hyperpigmentation. The phenomenon occurs in the summer months and is related to the degree of UVA exposure. The reactions may be caused by volatile fumes as well as by direct contact.

Amiodarone

Approximately 50% of patients develop an immediate prickling or burning sensation with erythema [19]. This immediate erythema settles but may re-emerge 24 h later [20]. It is dose-related. The minimum erythema dose is reduced over the range 335–460 nm. A minority of patients get a slate grey pigmentation due to the deposition of an amiodarone metabolite complex in the skin. Amiodarone and its major metabolite can persist in the skin for months after stopping administration, so that the symptoms of acute phototoxicity can be prolonged for months, and the pigmentation for years.

Chlorpromazine

This can produce immediate erythema and discomfort. In addition, a slate-grey pigmentation may occur, as with amiodarone.

17.4.1.2 Delayed-onset Erythema

This has a time-course similar to that of sunburn (peak erythema at 12–24 h) and if severe may look like "exaggerated sunburn." Tetracyclines, retinoids, thiazides, and quinine may produce this response. Among the tetracyclines, the order of likelihood of provoking phototoxicity is: demeclocycline (syn. demethylchlorotetracycline) >doxycycline>others.

17.4.1.3 Late-onset Erythema

This is caused by psoralens, and is characterized by erythema maximal at 72–96 h after UVA exposure, which may be followed by hyperpigmentation lasting months or even years. If the dose is low and the exposures are repeated only hyperpigmentation develops.

Phytophototoxic Contact Dermatitis

This is caused by topical contact with psoralens from plants, followed by UVA exposure. Many common plants contain psoralens and examples are listed in Table 5. The compounds are lipid soluble and penetrate the epidermis readily, and this is enhanced by high humidity. There are a variety of manifestations possible depending on the manner in which exposure occurs. For example, strimmers (weed whackers) deliver a buckshot of weeds creating irregular, nonlinear red macules ("strimmer dermatitis"). Topical contact with lime juice is a famous culprit. If walking through long weeds, bizarre linear angular red streaks can develop at the site of contact, which may become bullous. This may be confused with "pseudophytophototoxic dermatitis" (caused by an irritant contact dermatitis in response to compounds in, for example, buttercups), and allergic contact dermatitis (for example to poison ivy, common in the USA).

Berloque Dermatitis

This was caused by the inclusion in some perfumes of bergamot oil, which contains "bergapten" (5-methoxypsoralen). The reaction occurred where the perfume had been applied; the term "berloque" refers to the drop-like shape of the patches. It is now rare due to the prohibition of psoralens from cosmetic products; if bergamot oil is used it must be psoralen-free.

17.4.1.4 Pseudoporphyria, Photoonycholysis, and Telangiectasia

Some phototoxic drugs are capable of producing pseudoporphyria, characterized by skin fragility, blistering and milia formation after minor trauma, features also seen in porphyria cutanea tarda and variegate porphyria. A similar picture may develop in patients with chronic renal failure on dialysis, and in frequent users of sunbeds; the mechanisms of these are not clear. Photoonycholysis occurs via a phototoxic mechanism. Exposed-site telangiectasia is a rare side-effect of calcium channel blockers, usually occurs without a history of acute phototoxicity, and resolves over many months. It is believed the vasculature is the phototoxic target [15].

17.5 Photoallergy

Photoallergy is a type-IV hypersensitivity reaction to an antigen generated by the interaction of sunlight with a topically applied substance. Its predisposing factors and prevalence, individual photoallergens, and the investigation of suspected photoallergy by photopatch testing are described in Chap. 27. Currently, the commonest photoallergens in the western world are sunscreens. Some photoallergens are also contact allergens, and some also cause phototoxic reactions.

17.5.1 Clinical Features of Photoallergy

Photoallergy nearly always manifests as eczema, and has histological features identical to allergic contact dermatitis. It may be acute, subacute or chronic, and a spectrum of reactions is therefore possible including erythema, bullae, and lichenification. There may be spread onto unexposed sites and the eruption can become widespread but the exposed areas tend to remain the most severe. The latent period between exposure and appearance/deterioration of eczema depends on the severity of the reaction, but is usually 2–48 h later.

The differential diagnosis of photoallergic contact dermatitis includes the following.

17.5.1.1 Phototoxicity

Many photoallergens also have phototoxic potential. Clinically, it may be difficult to differentiate between phototoxic and photoallergic contact reactions. Table 2 lists features that may help in the differentiation. Typical phototoxicity has the appearance of sunburn (which may be severe); however, in practice the distinction can be difficult, and repeat episodes of phototoxicity can cause a dermatitis clinically and histologically [15]. The presence of sunburn-type erythema alone probably indicates a toxic reaction, which may be confirmed on histological examination. Many case reports allocating the type of photosensitivity reaction to a particular compound do so on insecure grounds; there has been a tendency to falsely ascribe a photoallergic basis to phototoxic reactions.

Table 3. Systemic agents causing phototoxicity

Antibiotics	Fluoroquinolones
	Nalidixic acid
	Sulphonamides, e.g., sulphamethoxazole
	Tetracyclines, e.g., tetracycline, oxytetracycline, doxycycline, chlortetracycline, demethylchlortetracycline
Anticancer agents	Dacarbazine
	Fluorouracil
	Vinblastine
Cardiovascular agents	Amiodarone
	Frusemide
	Quinidine
	Thiazide diuretics, e.g., chlorothiazide, hydrochlorothiazide, cyclopenthiazide
Psychoactive agents	Phenothiazines, e.g., chlorpromazine, phenothiazine
	Tricyclic antidepressants, e.g., protriptyline, clomipramine, dothiepin, imipramine, maprotiline
Therapeutic agents	Psoralens
	Porphyrins
Miscellaneous	Antimalarials; chloroquine, hydroxychloroquine
	Griseofulvin
	Nonsteroidal anti-inflammatory drugs, e.g., azapropazone, benoxaprofen, piroxicam, tiaprofenic acid
	Quinine
	Retinoids, e.g., acitretin, isotretinoin
	Sulphonylureas

Table 4. Some topical agents causing phototoxicity

Dyes	Eosin, acridine orange, acriflavin
Psoralens	Present in plants (see Table 5), essential oils, used therapeutically
Biocides	Fenticlor Halogenated salicylanilides
Sunscreens	2-Ethoxyethyl-*p*-methoxycinnamate Isoamyl-*p*-N, N′-dimethylamino-benzoate
Miscellaneous	Balsam of Peru Buclosamide Coal tar and derivatives Cadmium sulfide Chlorpromazine Porphyrins

17.5.1.2 Allergic Contact Dermatitis

It may also be difficult to differentiate between photoallergy and allergic contact dermatitis (ACD). Many photoallergens can also cause ACD. Sunscreens can cause ACD and because they are typically applied at times of sun exposure it is usually clinically impossible to differentiate photoallergy from ACD to sunscreens. A chronic eczema on the exposed areas is usually not due to photosensitivity but is the result of airborne ACD. Airborne ACD characteristically involves the upper eyelids and extends below the chin and behind the ears, but does not always do so.

Table 5. Examples of plants containing psoralens (from [21])

Family name	Source	Common
Moraceae	*Ficus carica*	Fig
Rutaceae	*Citrus aurantifolia*	Sweet lime
	Citrus bergamia	Bergamot orange
	Citrus limon	Lemon
	Ruta graveolens	Rue
Umbelliferae	*Heracleum mantegazzianum*	Giant hogweed
	Pastinaca sativa	Parsnip
	Apium graveolens	Celery
	Daucus carota	Carrot

Causes of airborne ACD include colophony, fragrances, and phosphorus sesquisulfide, but the most common cause worldwide is Compositae (Asteraceae). Exposure to Compositae allergens is increased in summer. Patch testing with leaves or flowers of Compositae will not always detect Compositae dermatitis, because of ranges in the amount of the allergens in species and seasonal variation. Occlusive patch tests performed with some commercially available oleoresin extracts have caused false-positive irritant reactions. Open tests with these oleoresins may give false-negative results in Compositae-sensitive subjects. The development of a sesquiterpene lactone mix by Ducombs and Benezra [21] gave reliability in the detection of Compositae sensitivity. This mix consists of a 0.1% dilution of an equal mixture of alantolactone, costunolide, and dehydrocostuslactone. The latter two substances are the more important allergens in the mix. This mixture is not irritating, and active sensitization is rare at this concentration. As an alternative to this mix, 1% costus oil may detect the majority of Compositae-sensitive individuals, but the oil contains a variable amount of allergen and may be sensitizing. A Compositae mix developed by Hausen [22] contains the oleoresins of five Compositae species. Compositae are contact allergens; there is no convincing evidence that Compositae are significant photoallergens [23].

A further source of diagnostic confusion is that ACD can be photoexacerbated, in the same way that, for example, atopic eczema can be in some patients. This has been reported with a number of allergens, for example tosylamide/formaldehyde resin [24], but rather than being specific to particular allergens this may reflect a general tendency among particular individuals. There is experimental evidence for this in mice and humans, which is discussed in Chap. 27 in relation to photoaugmentation of photopatch test reactions.

17.5.1.3 Photodermatoses

Chronic actinic dermatitis (CAD) is discussed below. Polymorphic light eruption (PLE) is rarely, if ever, truly eczematous but may cause diagnostic confusion particularly because approximately 15% of patients report that it is exacerbated by sunscreens [25]. Theoretically this may occur if the sunscreen is more effective at filtering UVB than UVA, and UVA is provoking the eruption and UVB is helping to prevent it by causing immunosuppression. Patients who develop PLE for the first time while using a sunscreen often wrongly believe they are allergic to it.

17.5.2 Prognosis of Photoallergy

The duration of photoallergy after stopping the application of a topical sensitizer is variable, typically between a few days [26] and several weeks [27]. Ketoprofen may persist in the epidermis for at least 17 days [28].

For decades it has been reported that occasionally after withdrawal of a topical photoallergen a tendency to dermatitis from sun exposure can persist for years, and this is termed "persistent light reactivity" (PLR) or, if the duration is shorter, sometimes "recurrent transient light reactions." It has been postulated that the drug results in allergic sensitization to endogenous allergens. There is claimed experimental support for such a mechanism [29], whereby tetrachlorosalicylanilide causes oxidation of histidine with modification of albumin into a weak allergen. Further irradiation with UVB, in the absence of the initial photosensitizer, may produce enough oxidized antigenic protein to elicit a cell-mediated immune response at all skin sites. Many agents have been implicated including musk ambrette, ketoprofen, and halogenated phenols (e.g., fenticlor). However, the existence of PLR as a discrete entity is controversial. Many argue that the evidence for a causative role for topical photoallergens in the generation of a prolonged state of endogenous photosensitivity is weak and prefer to regard such patients as having developed chronic actinic dermatitis (CAD) without preceding topical photoallergy [15, 23]. They challenge the basis on which the diagnosis of contact photoallergy was made, usually believing that the reaction was a phototoxic one, or turn causality in the opposite direction and regard such patients as having CAD which has predisposed to the development of contact photoallergy.

17.5.3 Photoallergy due to Systemically Administered Drugs

Photosensitivity with an eczematous morphology that is claimed to be due to a systemic agent has been reported many times. Substances reported to cause photoallergy in this way include sulphonamides, sulphonylurea derivatives, chlorothiazides, quinine, quinidine, and piroxicam [30]. Some of these reports support the diagnosis with positive photopatch tests but the systemic agents reported to cause photoallergy are generally also known to cause phototoxicity, and therefore photopatch tests in such reports may have been misinterpreted (see Chap. 27). Experimen-

tally, it has been claimed that the intraperitoneal injection of chlorpromazine or sulphanilamide in mice, with UV irradiation to the skin, causes photosensitivity that can be transferred with lymph node cells [31]. In a suspected case, it is possible to dilute the drug, preferably to several concentrations, and photopatch test the patient; other subjects should also be tested in this way to investigate possible phototoxicity. However, metabolites may be the relevant photosensitizers so this procedure might lead to false-negative results. Therefore systemic photochallenge, giving twice the normal dose of the suspected agent with irradiation of the skin before and at intervals after ingestion, has been advocated [32].

17.6 Chronic Actinic Dermatitis (CAD)

Synonyms: photosensitivity dermatitis, actinic reticuloid [33].

This condition will be discussed here because of its photosensitive nature, the high prevalence among sufferers of concomitant allergic contact dermatitis (ACD) to airborne allergens, and the relatively high prevalence of CAD among patients with photoallergy.

CAD is uncommon, typically affects patients over 60 years of age with a male:female ratio of approximately 6:1, affects all races, and is commoner in temperate climes. It sometimes occurs on the background of endogenous nonphotosensitive eczema. Patients frequently have ACD, particularly to Compositae, colophony and fragrances, which may precede the development of CAD. Many patients are keen gardeners who have therefore had considerable exposure to these allergens and sunshine. The occurrence of CAD among atopic eczema patients aged 30–50 years is increasingly being recognized [34]. The pathogenesis is not completely understood but may involve a type-IV hypersensitivity response to a UV-induced autoantigen [35].

It presents as a persistent patchy or confluent eczematous eruption, which is often lichenified and may show very infiltrated pseudo-lymphomatous papules or plaques. It typically has a photosensitive distribution and worsens in summer and after episodes of sun exposure. However, the condition is often perennial and patients are often unaware of the role of sun exposure. Also, the condition may only patchily affect exposed sites, and may progress to covered areas and occasionally erythroderma.

On monochromator phototesting, there are usually abnormal reactions to UVA and UVB wavelengths, and sometimes also to visible light [35, 36]. Testing with broad-band sources provokes the eruption. Patch testing is vital to detect ACD. Histology is not usually helpful in making the diagnosis, but when examined shows a chronic eczema and, in severe long-standing cases, pseudo-lymphomatous changes.

Treatment comprises avoidance of sun exposure by changes in behavior, use of tight-weave long sleeves/trousers and a hat, and the application of broad-spectrum high-factor sunscreens of low allergenic potential. Patients should be advised how to avoid any relevant allergens. Topical steroids and emollients are useful. If these measures are inadequate, oral immunosuppressive therapy with ciclosporin, azathioprine or mycophenolate mofetil may be required. Prolonged low-dose PUVA or TL-01 treatment is sometimes effective. With avoidance of sunshine and relevant airborne allergens, many patients notice a gradual reduction in their photosensitivity over a few years [36].

References

1. Diffey BL, Farr PM (1988) The action spectrum in drug induced photosensitivity. Photochem Photobiol 47:49–53
2. Hearst JE, Isaacs ST, Kanne D, Rapoport H, Straub K (1984) The reaction of the psoralens with deoxyribonucleic acid. Q Rev Biophys 17:1–44
3. Vedaldi D, Dall'Acqua F, Gennaro A, Rodighiero G (1983) Photosensitized effects of furocoumarins: the possible role of singlet oxygen. Z Naturforsch 38c:866–869
4. Takashima A, Yamamoto K, Mizuno N (1989) Photobiological activities of a newly synthesized 4,6,4'-trimethylangelicin on human skin. Photomed Photobiol 11:155–162
5. Kochevar IE (1987) Mechanism of drug photosensitization. Photochem Photobiol 45:891–895
6. Moan J, Pettersen EO, Christensen T (1979) The mechanism of photodynamic inactivation of human cells in vitro in the presence of haematoporphyrin. Br J Cancer 39:398–407
7. Ljunggren B, Bjellerup M (1986) Systemic drug phototoxicity. Photodermatology 3:26–35
8. Moore DE, Chappins PP (1988) A comparative study of the photochemistry of the non-steroidal anti-inflammatory drugs, naproxen, benoxaprophen and indomethacin. Photochem Photobiol 47:173–180
9. Li ASW, Chignell CF (1987) Spectroscopic studies of cutaneous photosensitizing agents. IX. A spin trapping study of the photolysis of amiodarone and desethylemiodarone. Photochem Photobiol 45:191–197
10. Takashima A, Yamamoto K, Kimura S, Takakuwa Y, Mizuno N (1991) Allergic contact and photocontact dermatitis due to psoralens in patients with psoriasis treated with topical PUVA. Br J Dermatol 124:37–42
11. Epling GA, Wells JL, Ung Chan Yoon (1988) Photochemical transformations in salicylanilide photoallergy. Photochem Photobiol 47:167–171
12. Adamski H, Benkalfate L, Delaval Y, Ollivier I, le Jean S, Toubel G, le Hir-Garreau I, Chevrant-Breton J (1998) Photodermatitis from non-steroidal anti-inflammatory drugs. Contact Dermatitis 38:171–174
13. Yamada S, Tanaka M, Kawahara Y, Inada M, Ohata Y (1998) Photoallergic contact dermatitis due to diphenhydramine hydrochloride. Contact Dermatitis 38:282
14. Lowe NJ, Fakouhi TD, Stern RS, Bourget T, Roniker B, Swabb EA (1994) Photoreactions with a fluoroquinolone antimicrobial: evening versus morning dosing. Clin Pharmacol Ther 56:587–591
15. Ferguson J (2002) Photosensitivity due to drugs. Photodermatol Photoimmunol Photomed 18:262–269
16. Urbach F (1997) Ultraviolet radiation and skin cancer of humans. J Photochem Photobiol B 40:3–7
17. Burdge DR, Nakielna EM, Rabin HR (1995) Photosensitivity associated with ciprofloxacin use in adult patients with cystic fibrosis. Antimicrob Agents Chemother 39:793
18. Ferguson J (1999) Drug and chemical photosensitivity. In: Hawk JLM (ed) Photodermatology, chap 12. Arnold, London
19. Chalmers RJ, Muston HL, Srinivas V, Bennett DH (1982) High incidence of amiodarone-induced photosensitivity in North-west England. Br Med J (Clin Res Ed) 285:341
20. Ferguson J, Addo HA, Jones S, Johnson BE, Frain Bell W (1985) A Study of cutaneous photosensitivity induced by amiodarone. Br J Dermatol 113:537–549
21. Benezra C, Ducombs G, Sell Y Foussereau J (1985) Plant contact dermatitis. Mosby, London, p 11
22. Hausen BM (1996) A 6-year experience with compositae mix. Am J Contact Dermatitis 7:94–99
23. British Photodermatology Group (1997) Photopatch testing–methods and indications. Br J Dermatol 136:371–376
24. Vilaplana J, Romaguera C (2000) Contact dermatitis from tosylamide/formaldehyde resin with photosensitivity. Contact Dermatitis 42:311–312
25. Palmer RA, van de Pas CB, Campalani E, Walker SL, Young AR, Hawk JL (2004) A simple method to assess severity of polymorphic light eruption. Br J Dermatol 151:645–652
26. Buckley DA, Wayte J, O'Sullivan D, Murphy GM (1995) Duration of response to UVA irradiation after application of a known photoallergen. Contact Dermatitis 33:138–139
27. Durieu C, Marguery MC, Giordano-Labadie F, Journe F, Loche F, Bazex J (2001) Photoaggravated contact allergy and contact photoallergy caused by ketoprofen: 19 cases. Ann Derm Venereol (Stockh) 128:1020–1024
28. Sugiura M, Hayakawa R, Kato Y, Sugiura K, Ueda H (2000) 4 cases of photocontact dermatitis due to ketoprofen. Contact Dermatitis 43:16–19
29. Kochevar IE, Harber LC (1977) Photoreactions of 3,3',4',5-tetrachlorosalicylanilide with proteins. J Invest Dermatol 68:151–156
30. Isaksson M, Bruze M (1997) Photopatch testing. Clin Dermatol 15:615–618
31. Giudici PA, Maguire HC (1985) Experimental photoallergy to systemic drugs. J Invest Dermatol 85:207–210
32. Holzle E (2001) The photopatch test. In: Krutmann J, Honigsmann H, Elmets CA, Bergstresser PR (eds) Dermatological phototherapy and photodiagnostic methods, chap 17. Springer, Berlin Heidelberg New York
33. Norris PG, Hawk JLM (1990) Chronic actinic dermatitis: a unifying concept. Arch Dermatol 126:376–378
34. Russell SC, Dawe RS, Collins P, Man I, Ferguson J (1998) The photosensitivity dermatitis and actinic reticuloid syndrome (chronic actinic dermatitis) occurring in seven young atopic dermatitis patients. Br J Dermatol 138:496–501
35. Hawk JL (2004) Chronic actinic dermatitis. Photodermatol Photoimmunol Photomed 20:312–314
36. Dawe RS, Ferguson J (2003) Diagnosis and treatment of chronic actinic dermatitis. Dermatol Ther 16:45–51
37. Maurer T (1983) Contact and photocontact allergens. Dekker, New York, p 132

Chapter 18

Pigmented Contact Dermatitis and Chemical Depigmentation

18

Hideo Nakayama

Contents

18.1 Hyperpigmentation Associated with Contact Dermatitis

18.1.1 Classification

Hyperpigmentation associated with contact dermatitis is classified into three categories: (1) hyperpigmentation due to incontinentia pigmenti histologica; (2) hyperpigmentation due to an increase in melanin in the basal layer cells of the epidermis, i.e., basal melanosis; and (3) hyperpigmentation due to slight hemorrhage around the vessels of the upper dermis, resulting in an accumulation of hemosiderin, such as in Majocchi–Schamberg dermatitis.

It is easy to understand that when the grade of contact dermatitis is more severe, or its duration longer, the secondary hyperpigmentation following dermatitis is more prominent. However, the first type mentioned above, incontinentia pigmenti histologica, often occurs without showing any positive manifestations of dermatitis such as marked erythema, vesiculation, swelling, papules, rough skin or scaling. Therefore, patients may complain only of a pigmentary disorder, even though the disease is entirely the result of allergic contact dermatitis. Hyperpigmentation caused by incontinentia pigmenti histologica has often been called a lichenoid reaction, since the presence of basal liquefaction degeneration, the accumulation of melanin pigment, and the mononuclear cell infiltrate in the upper dermis are very similar to the histopathological manifestations of lichen planus. However, compared with typical lichen planus, hyperkeratosis is usually milder, hypergranulosis and saw-tooth-shape acanthosis are lacking, hyaline bodies are hardly seen, and the band-like massive infiltration with lymphocytes and histiocytes is lacking.

A lichenoid reaction is considered to be a scaled-down type-IV allergic reaction of the lichen planus type, based on positive patch test reactions in patients and negative reactions in controls, as in ordinary allergic contact dermatitis.

An increase in melanin pigment in keratinocytes is noted after allergic contact dermatitis, presumably caused by hyperfunction of melanocytes, but the same phenomenon is also seen with irritant contact dermatitis. When sodium lauryl sulfate, a typical skin irritant, was repeatedly applied on the forearms of Caucasians, the number of epidermal melanocytes was observed to almost double, suggesting hyperplasia, hypertrophy, and increased function [1].

The pathological processes involved in the third form of hyperpigmentation with contact dermatitis, purpuric dermatitis, have not yet been clarified. Shiitake mushroom, very commonly eaten in Asia, has been known to produce a transient urticarial dermatitis with severe itching, which results in a purpuric scratch effect, when insufficiently cooked. This is thought to be due to toxic substances in the mushroom unstable to heat, and the pigmentation due to purpura is not caused by hypersensitivity [2]. As with other forms of dermatitis, accompanying capillary fragility results in purpura. Some cases are associat-

ed with contact hypersensitivity to rubber components or textile finishes, but in many cases the causes
are not known.

18.1.2 Pigmented Contact Dermatitis

18.1.2.1 History and Causative Agents

Core Message

■ Pigmented contact dermatitis on the
covered area cannot be cured by the
application of corticosteroid ointments,
even though it is a result of contact

allergens from textiles, soaps or washing
powders for textiles. Successive contact
with small amounts of allergens destroys
basal layer cells of the epidermis, resulting
in melanin accumulation in the upper
dermis for a long time. Treatment entails
finding out the contact allergens, and
avoiding them for a long time.

Pigmented contact dermatitis was first reported by
Osmundsen in Denmark in 1969. In 8 months he had
120 patients, 7 of whom showed a pronounced and
bizarre hyperpigmentation. In 4 of these 7 cases contact dermatitis preceded the hyperpigmentation,

Table 1. The main contact sensitizers producing secondary hyperpigmentation

Name	Chemical structure	Purpose	Patch test concentration and base
Tinopal CH3566	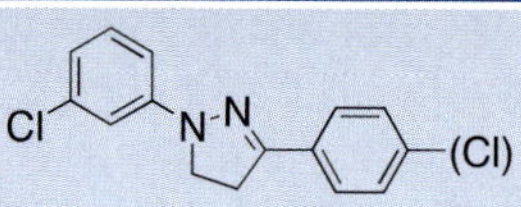	Optical whitener in washing powder	1% pet.
Naphthol AS	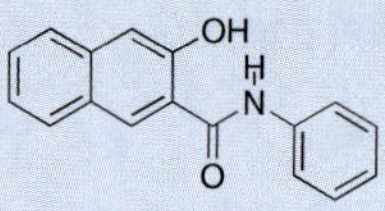	Dye for textile	1% pet.
Benzyl salicylate	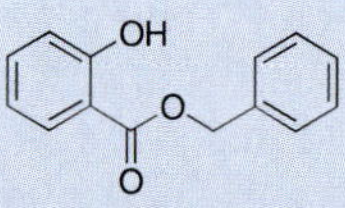	Fragrance	5–1% pet.
Hydroxycitronellal	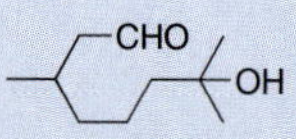	Fragrance	5–1% pet.
D &C Red 3 and brilliant lake red R	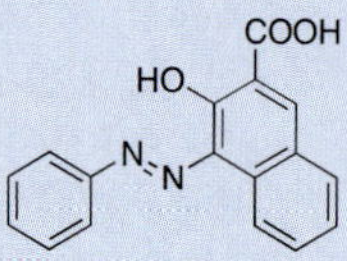	Pigment for cosmetics	1% pet.
Phenyl-azo-2-naphthol (PAN)	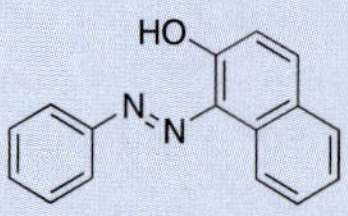	Impurity	0.1% pet.
D & C Yellow 11	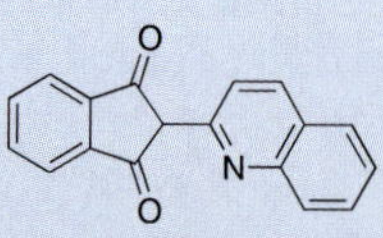	Pigment for cosmetics	0.1% pet.
Ylang-ylang oil	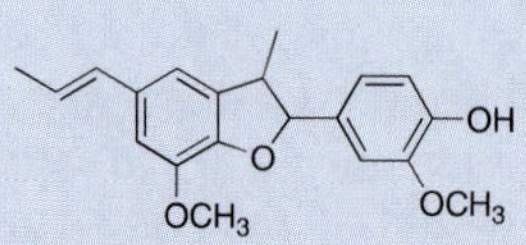 dehydrodiisoeugenol	Fragrance, incense	5% pet.

18

Table 1. Continued

Name	Chemical structure	Purpose	Patch test concentration and base
Jasmine absolute	Main sensitizer not yet identified	Fragrance	10–5% pet.
Synthetic sandalwood	Main sensitizer not yet identified	Fragrance	10% pet.
Cinnamic alcohol		Fragrance	1% pet.
Musk ambrette		Fragrance, incense	5% pet.
Biocheck 60		Pesticide for textiles	0.2% aq.
PPP-HB		Textile finish	5% eth.
Impurity of commercial CI Blue 19 (Brilliant Blue)	Main sensitizers not yet identified	Dye	5% eth.
Mercury compounds	Hg^{2+}	Bactericides	0.1–0.05% aq. or pet. (not with aluminum chamber)
Nickel (sulfate)	Ni^{2+}	Metal product	5% aq. or pet.
Chromate (K dichromate)	Cr^{6+}	Leather, soap	0.5% aq. or pet.

while the other 3 did not notice any signs of dermatitis such as itching or erythema before the pigmentation appeared [3, 4].

Hyperpigmentation, with or without dermatitis, was located mostly in covered areas, such as the chest, back, waist, arms, neck, and thighs. After a patient wanted to conceal the pigmentation by wearing long sleeves and a high-neck sweater, which she washed with a washing powder every day, the hyperpigmentation extended from the neck and axillae to all over the neck, chest, and arms. The hyperpigmentation was brown, slate-colored, grayish-brown, reddish-brown, bluish-brown, etc., according to the case, and often had a reticulate pattern. The histopathology of the pigmentation showed incontinentia pigmenti histologica.

Patch tests with the standard series current at that time gave no information as to the causative allergens. However, Osmundsen noticed that the patients had used washing powders that contained a new op-tical whitener, Tinopal or CH3566 (Table 1). This was one of numerous optical whiteners which became available at that time to make textiles "whiter than white." Patch tests with CH3566 1% pet. finally explained the pigmentary disorder, as they showed strong positive reactions in the patients and negative results in the controls. The pigmentation was persistent, but the dermatitis that often preceded hyperpigmentation was observed to disappear following the elimination of washing powders that contained CH3566. Fortunately, the identification of the causative chemical was made rapidly, and the widespread usage of CH3566 was avoided in time.

Pigmented contact dermatitis is rare in Caucasians but not uncommon in Mongoloids. The next pigmented contact dermatitis was reported by Ancona-Alayón et al. in Mexico [5]. Among 53 workers handling azo dyes in a textile factory, 12 developed a spotted hyperpigmentation without pruritus, and 18 suffered from hyperpigmentation to a lesser extent.

This new occupational skin disorder appeared 4 months after the introduction of a new dyeing process of azo-coupling on textiles, and most of the patients had contact with azo dyes on weaving machines. Hyperpigmentation varied from a bizarre dark pigmentation to a streaky milder pigmentation of the neck, arms, face, and, in exceptional cases, covered areas.

Histopathological examination of the pigmentary disorder showed spongiosis, irregular acanthosis, edema of the dermis, pericapillary lymphocytic infiltration, basal liquefaction degeneration, and incontinentia pigmenti histologica. Melanocyte proliferation at the affected sites was also noted.

Patch tests showed that 24 of the 53 workers were positive to Naphthol AS 5% in water, while the other 29, as well as 10 controls, were negative to Naphthol AS. The dermatoses disappeared after the dyeing process was changed so that the workers did not directly touch Naphthol AS, an azo dye coupling agent.

In the early 1980s, pigmented contact dermatitis due to Naphthol AS appeared in central Japan, but this time it was not occupational. A textile factory manufacturing flannel nightwear, a traditional Japanese garment called *yukata*, economized on water for washing the products after the process of azo-coupling using Naphthol AS. This modification of production resulted in the appearance of pigmented contact dermatitis of the covered areas of skin of people living in the districts where the products were distributed and worn. Kawachi et al. [6] and Hayakawa et al. [7] reported such cases, and the hyperpigmentation was mainly located on the back and neck. The factory was said to have improved the washing process and the materials quickly, but the presence of such cases indicates that whenever the textile industry uses Naphthol AS, and at the same time economizes on water for washing the products, there must be a risk of producing pigmented contact dermatitis of the covered areas. According to Hayakawa et al. [7] the amount of Naphthol AS detected in the patients' nightwear was 4,900–8,700 ppm, a considerable amount. A case due to Naphthol AS in a pillow case was later reported [8].

In 1984, the city of Tokyo decided to investigate new textile finishes which seemed to have produced contact dermatitis of the covered skin areas, including pigmented contact dermatitis (Fig. 1). Based on information about the textile finishes which actually came into contact with the patients' skin or were very commonly used, 115 chemicals were finally chosen and patch tested. The test materials included 50 dyes of all colors, 13 whiteners, 5 fungicides, 32 resin components, 13 softening agents, and 15 other miscellaneous textile finishes which were widely used at that

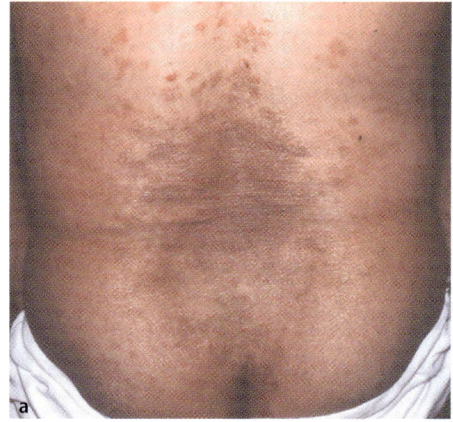

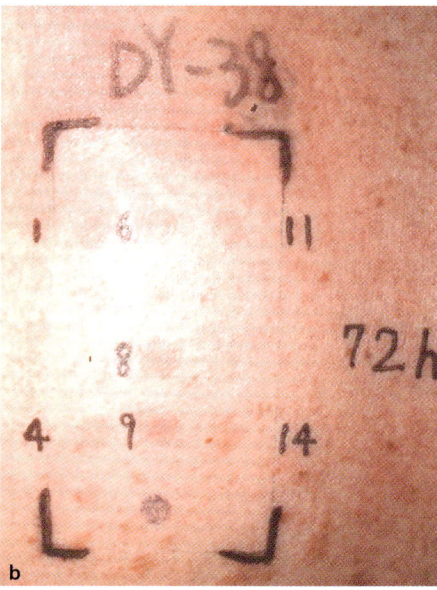

Fig. 1a, b. Pigmented contact dermatitis (a) in a 67-year-old man who was sensitized by several textile finishes, including commercial grade red and brown dyes and fungicides (b)

time by the textile industry in Japan. They were chosen from approximately 1,200 textile finishes, either imported or produced in Japan. They were checked as to solubility in water, ethanol, acetone, etc., diluted to 5% (except bactericides, fungicides, and other pesticides for textiles which were diluted to 1%), and then applied to dry paper discs 8 mm in diameter, to make dry allergen-containing discs named "instant patch test allergens." They were peeled off silicon-treated covering paper before use.

The results obtained from five hospitals in and around Tokyo revealed that several new contact sensitizers were responsible for producing textile dermatitis and secondary hyperpigmentation. These textile finishes included Biochek 60, a very toxic fungicide which seemed also to have acted as a sensitizer, a phosphite polymer of pentaerythritol and hydrogenated bisphenol A (PPP-HB), impurities in a dye CI Blue 19 (or Brilliant Blue R), and mercury compounds [9].

The research on these 115 chemicals was performed in the 5 hospitals on 80–101 persons, among whom 51–62 were patients suffering from textile contact dermatitis, and the rest, 29–39, were controls with atopic dermatitis and dermatitis due to causes other than textiles. Among those with textile contact dermatitis, 27–33 had pigmented contact dermatitis. Such cases had been deliberately chosen for patch testing because the investigators hoped to find out the causative contact sensitizers producing such hyperpigmentation. Of these pigmented contact dermatitis patients, 9 showed positive reactions suggestive of an allergy to Biochek 60, and 1 to several textile finishes. The results were rather disappointing, but they did show that it is not easy to discover the contact sensitizers producing pigmented contact dermatitis from contact with textile finishes. The discoveries of CH3566 and Naphthol AS can be regarded as having been important and valuable. Pigmented contact dermatitis due to blue dyes, Blue 106 and 124 was reported by Kovacevic et al. in 2001 [10].

Besides the above-mentioned textile finishes, rubber components can also produce dermatitis resulting in hyperpigmentation, mainly around the waist. Sometimes in such cases the pigmentation is not due to incontinentia pigmenti histologica but to purpura (see Sect. 18.1.4, Purpuric Dermatitis). Thus far, only cases of pigmented contact dermatitis in which causative allergens were found have been reported. Causes other than contact sensitivity have not yet been well investigated, except for friction melanosis which is described in Sect. 18.1.2.2, Differential Diagnosis.

18.1.2.2 Differential Diagnosis

Differential diagnosis of pigmented contact dermatitis due to washing powder or textile components includes Addison's disease, friction melanosis, amyloidosis cutis, drug eruption, atopic dermatitis with pigmentation and dermatitis and secondary hyperpigmentation due to dental metal sensitivity (dental metal eruption).

Friction melanosis was frequently seen in Japan in the 1970s and 1980s, the disease consisting of dark brown or black hyperpigmentation unaccompanied by dermatitis or itching [11]. Friction melanosis occurred predominantly on the skin over or along bones, such as the clavicles, ribs, scapulae, spine, knees, and elbows. The color and distribution of friction melanosis sometimes leads to confusion with

pigmented contact dermatitis. The disease, however, is produced by patients vigorously rubbing the skin with a hard nylon towel or nylon brush every day when bathing. Patch testing with various contact allergens failed to demonstrate allergens that seemed to be correlated with the disease. It was Tanigaki et al. [12] in 1983 who pointed out the causative association of rubbing with a nylon towel or brush, and the disease has gradually decreased since this hazard has become known to the public.

The use of nylon towels or brushes for washing the skin should therefore be checked before the diagnosis of pigmented contact dermatitis due to textiles is made. If the dark hyperpigmentation of the skin over bones gradually fades and disappears after use of nylon towels or brushes is discontinued and patients change their mode of washing to a milder technique, the diagnosis of friction melanosis should be considered. Curiously, the histopathology of friction melanosis shows incontinentia pigmenti histologica, which is a characteristic feature of pigmented contact dermatitis. However, liquefaction degeneration of basal layer cells of the epidermis is not present [11].

Another skin disorder to be distinguished is skin amyloidosis, especially lichen amyloidosus or papular amyloidosis. It is possible that a small amount of amyloid, which can be demonstrated by Dylon staining, is found in lichenoid tissue reactions, probably because amyloid in the upper dermis is considered to be derived from degenerate epidermal cells produced by epidermal inflammation. Special staining with Congo red or thioflavine T and electron-microscopic study of the skin specimen are also helpful in the differential diagnosis.

18.1.2.3 Prevention and Treatment

It is essential to avoid the use of textiles and washing powders containing strong contact sensitizers, in order to prevent contact dermatitis and pigmented contact dermatitis of the skin areas that come into contact with the fabric and washing powders or softening agents that remain on them even after rinsing. There are, however, many textile finishes available today, with more than 1,200 commercial finishes being sold to the textile industry, and unfortunately their components are mainly secret. The purity of dyes is, in general, very low and some of the many impurities are allergenic. For example, the very commonly used CI Blue 19 (or Brilliant Blue R) turned out to be allergenic and caused some patch-test-positive cases of pigmented contact dermatitis in 1985 [9]. Purified CI Blue 19, in contrast, never produced positive patch test reactions at the same 5% concentration.

The experiences accumulated in the past show that, when entirely new textile finishes are introduced to the textile industry, the minimum safety evaluation tests such as LD50, Ames test, and skin irritation test should be performed, and their sensitization potential should be investigated by a research team including dermatologists. Strong contact sensitizers can be detected by several experimental procedures using animals. Although animal experiments are now the subject of ethical scrutiny in connection with such investigations, they remain indicated if the irritability and allergenicity of textile finishes are to be adequately investigated.

The textile industry should cooperate with dermatologists when pigmented contact dermatitis has once occurred, by immediately informing them of the components of the chemical finishes of the textile suspected to have caused the disease, and a precise study of impurities and quality control in the factory should also be performed. Shortening of the washing process should be strictly refrained, otherwise surplus dyes, their impurities, and other chemical finishes may remain and produce a problem.

When a causative allergen is discovered, the solution of pigmented contact dermatitis is not difficult [4, 5, 7]. However, when causative allergens are not identified, the solution of the pigmentary disorder is usually very difficult. In 1985, in Japan, a new strategy for the treatment of both recurrent textile dermatitis and pigmented contact dermatitis was introduced. Based on the research project for finding out contact sensitizers and irritants in textiles [9], underwear with only four or five kinds of textile finishes which showed no evidence of positive reactions in patients with contact dermatitis, pigmented contact dermatitis, atopic dermatitis, and healthy controls was put into mass production and became available. This is a measure to prevent the patients coming into contact with the responsible allergen in ordinary underwear again, and keeps the patients out of range of the responsible allergens.

Such allergen-free underwear for patients is called allergen-controlled wearing apparel (ACW) and has successfully counteracted pigmented contact dermatitis. The idea was inspired by the success of allergen-controlled cosmetics in 1970, which is discussed later (see Sect. 18.1.3, Pigmented Cosmetic Dermatitis). It is not surprising that persistent secondary hyperpigmentation disappears only very slowly when the causative contact allergens are completely eliminated from the patient's environment for a long period, as the hyperpigmentation is considered to be brought about by frequent and repeated contact with a very small amount of contact sensitizer in the textile or washing material. Patients were requested to use allergen-free soaps and allergen-eliminated washing

materials for their clothing at the same time, so that their skin was not contaminated by the responsible allergens in ordinary soaps and washing materials. Matsuo et al. reported several cases in which this treatment was successful [13, 14].

Even though cases are very rare, pigmented contact dermatitis can also occur following systemic contact dermatitis. In a 50-year-old man, for example, recurrent and persistent dermatitis accompanied diffuse secondary hyperpigmentation. The use of corticosteroid ointments, oral antihistamines, and allergen-free soaps did not improve the condition at all. A patch test with nickel sulfate 5% aq. showed a strong positive reaction, with a focal flare of most of the original skin lesion. This implied not only that the patient was sensitive to nickel, but also that only a few hundred parts per million of nickel ions absorbed from the patch test site into the bloodstream were enough to provoke an allergic reaction over a wide area of the site of the original skin lesions. This observation led to a search for a source of nickel ions in the patient, and five nickel alloys were subsequently found in the patient's oral cavity. He agreed to eliminate these nickel crowns, as they turned out to have been acting as cathodes, attracting an electric current of 1–3 mA at 100–200 mV. According to Faraday's law of electrolysis, cations elute from the cathode in proportion to the amount of electric current passing into the cathode.

The complete elimination of nickel-containing alloys from his oral cavity and their substitution with gold alloys, which did not contain any nickel at all, resulted in complete cure of the dermatitis and secondary hyperpigmentation in 3 months, and there has never been any recrudescence of the disease. The patient's pigmented contact dermatitis had been kept going for a long period by metal allergens continuously supplied from his own oral cavity [15].

18.1.3 Pigmented Cosmetic Dermatitis

18.1.3.1 Signs

Core Message

■ Pigmented cosmetic dermatitis is caused by the same mechanism as pigmented contact dermatitis of the covered area; however, the causative allergens are quite different, and they are a number of cosmetic allergens. Patch test of cosmetic series allergens is recommended, and continual and exclusive usage of allergen-controlled cosmetics and soaps cures the disease.

The most commonly seen hyperpigmentation due to contact dermatitis in the history of dermatology must be the pigmented cosmetic dermatitis which affected the faces of Oriental women [16]. Innumerable patients with this pigmentary disorder presented in the 1960s and 1970s in Japan, and similar patients were also seen in Korea, India, Taiwan, China, and the USA.

The signs of pigmented cosmetic dermatitis are diffuse or reticular, black or dark brown hyperpigmentation of the face, which cannot be cured by the use of corticosteroid ointments or the continuous ingestion of vitamin C. The border of pigmented cosmetic dermatitis is not sharp, as in lichen planus or melasma, and it is not spot-like as in nevus of Ota tardus bilateralis.

Slight dermatitis is occasionally seen with hyperpigmentation, or dermatitis may precede hyperpigmentation. In contrast to Addison's disease, pigmented cosmetic dermatitis does not show any systemic symptoms such as weakness, fatigue, and emaciation. Laboratory findings such as full blood count, liver function tests, daily urinary excretion of 17-ketosteroid and 17-hydroxy corticosteroid, and serum immunoglobulins and electrolytes are normal in the majority of patients with pigmented cosmetic dermatitis [16].

Histopathological examination of pigmented cosmetic dermatitis shows basal liquefaction degeneration of the epidermis and incontinentia pigmenti histologica. The epidermis maybe mildly acanthotic, however it is sometimes atrophic, presumably the effect of frequently applied corticosteroid ointments for the treatment of itchy dermatitis of the face. Cellular infiltrates of lymphocytes and histiocytes are seen perivascularly, as are often seen in ordinary allergic contact dermatitis (Fig. 2).

In some cases, the dark brown or black hyperpigmentation is also seen on skin other than on the face. The neck, chest, and back can be involved and, in a few exceptional cases, hyperpigmentation may extend to the whole body. In these cases, the allergens cinnamic alcohol and its derivatives sensitize the patients first to cosmetics and then provoke allergic reactions to soaps, domestic fabric softeners, and food, all of which sometimes contain cinnamic derivatives. The ingestion of 1 g cinnamon sugar from a cup of tea in a supermarket was enough to provoke a mild focal flare of dermatitis at the sites of diffuse reticular black hyperpigmentation of the whole body in one reported case [17]. When one of the common potent sensitizers producing pigmented cosmetic dermatitis, D & C Red 31 (Japanese name R-219), was discovered, a focal flare of dermatitis at the site of facial hyperpigmentation was occasionally noted by patch testing 5% R-219 in petrolatum. These findings show that the allergen could provoke the dermatitis not only by contact with the skin surface but also from within the skin, by allergens transported via blood vessels, just as allergic contact dermatitis can be provoked by the administration of small amounts of nickel or drugs.

18.1.3.2 Causative Allergens

The term "pigmented cosmetic dermatitis" was introduced in 1973 for what had previously been known

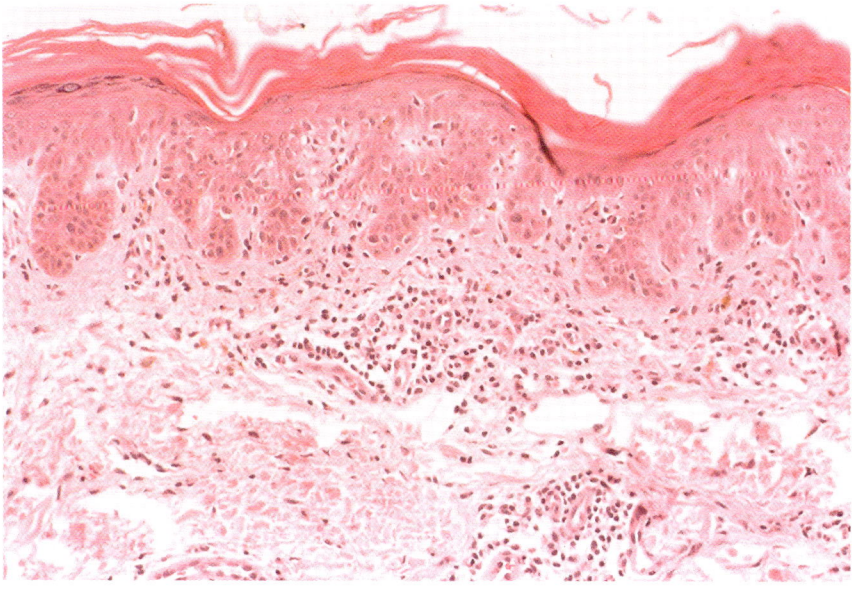

Fig. 2.
Histopathology of a typical lichenoid reaction, with incontinentia pigmenti histologica of pigmented cosmetic dermatitis. The epidermis shows mild acanthosis, and occasional liquefaction degeneration in the basal layer of the epidermis has dropped melanin pigments into the upper dermis. Note that the cellular infiltration in the upper dermis is not as dense as in lichen planus

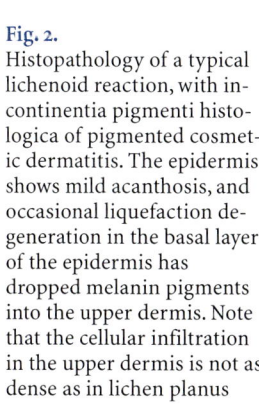

as melanosis faciei feminae when the mechanism (type IV allergy), most of the causative allergens, and successful treatment with allergen control for this miserable pigmentary disorder were clarified for the first time [18, 19]. The name was adopted by modifying Osmundsen's designation pigmented contact dermatitis, for the disease caused by CH3566 on the trunk.

Historically, the first description of the disease goes back to 1948, when Japanese dermatologists encountered this peculiar pigmentary disorder for the first time, and were greatly embarrassed as to diagnosis. Bibliographical surveys showed that Riehl's melanosis, described in 1917 [20], seemed probable, because World War II had ended just 3 years before the investigation. Subsequently, the disease was erroneously called Riehl's melanosis for almost 30 years in Asian countries. Riehl's melanosis, however, was a dark brown hyperpigmentation observed during World War I in Caucasian men, women and children, when food was extremely scarce and the patients had to eat decayed corn and weed crops instead of the normal food of peacetime. Besides hyperpigmentation of the face, ears and scalp, there were nodules and, histopathologically, dense cellular infiltration was present in the dermis. Cosmetics could be excluded as a cause, because it was during World War I, and it was not possible for all these people, especially the men and children, to have used cosmetics before they had the disease. Riehl could not discover the true cause of this pigmentary disorder, but suspected the role of the abnormal wartime diet [20]. Riehl's melanosis disappeared when World War I ended, when people obtained normal food again, to reappear for a short period in France during the German occupation in World War II, when food again became scarce.

Consequently, Riehl's melanosis, a wartime melanosis having no relationship to cosmetic allergy, should not be confused with pigmented cosmetic dermatitis, which involved many Asian women in peacetime for many years. In 1950, Minami and Noma [21] designated the disease melanosis faciei feminae, and recognized the disease as a new entity. The causation was not known for many years. However, Japanese dermatologists gradually became aware of the role of cosmetics in this hyperpigmentation. First, it occurred only on those women, and very exceptionally men, who used cosmetics and, secondly, even though the bizarre brown hyperpigmentation was so conspicuous, the presence of slight, recurrent, or preceding dermatitis was observed. The problem for the dermatologists at that time was that the components of cosmetics were completely secret, and the kinds of cosmetic ingredients were too many (more

than 1,000) for their allergenicity to be evaluated.

Finally, in 1969, a research project was set up to identify the causative allergens from 477 cosmetic ingredients by patch and photopatch testing. It was a new idea, because melanosis faciei feminae had been regarded as a metabolic disorder rather than a type of contact dermatitis. This was 7 years before Finn chambers became available; therefore, small patch test plasters of 10 × 2 cm with six discs 7 mm in diameter (Miniplaster) were put into production to enable 48–96 samples to be patch tested at one time on the backs of volunteer control subjects and patients. Many cosmetic ingredients, adjusted to nonirritant concentrations with the cooperation of 30–40 volunteers, were subsequently patch and photopatch tested in the patients. Results for each ingredient were obtained from 172–348 patients, including 79–121 with melanosis faciei feminae. Statistical evaluation brought to light a number of newly discovered contact sensitizers amongst the cosmetic ingredients, mainly fragrance materials and pigments, including jasmine absolute, ylang-ylang oil, cananga oil, benzyl salicylate, hydroxycitronellal, sandalwood oil, artificial sandalwood, geraniol, geranium oil, D & C Red 31, and Yellow No. 11 [16, 18, 19, 22].

18.1.3.3 Treatment

The above-mentioned research project at the same time included a plan to produce soaps (acylglutamate) and cosmetics for the patients from whom the causative allergens had been completely eliminated, as even those who suffered from severe and bizarre hyperpigmentation usually could not accept abandoning their use of cosmetics to remove this pigmentary disorder. Patch testing with a series of 30 standard cosmetic ingredients to find the allergens causing the disease [23], followed by the exclusive use of soaps and cosmetics that were completely allergenfree for such patients, designated the allergen control system, produced dramatic effects. Around 1970, most textbooks of dermatology in Japan said that melanosis faciei feminae was very difficult to cure and that the causation was unknown. However, after allergen control was introduced, the disease became completely curable. Table 2 shows the effect of allergen control in 165 cases reported to the American Academy of Dermatology in 1977, and also the longterm follow-up results of allergen control obtained by Watanabe after 3–11 years (mean, 5 years). In 50 cases of pigmented cosmetic dermatitis cured by allergen control (i.e., patch test with 30 cosmetic series patch test allergens [25] followed by the exclusive use of allergen-free soaps and cosmetics, Acseine® in Ja-

Table 2. Effect of allergen-controlled cosmetics on pigmented cosmetic dermatitis patients

	Nakayama et al. [22]	Watanabe [24]
Total	165	53
Complete cure	52	40
Almost complete cure	21	0
Remarkable improvement	51	13
Improvement	22	0
Not effective	19	0
Follow-up	3 months to 5 years	3–11 years (mean 5 years)

pan and Hong Kong), there were, on average, 2.5 allergens for each patient. It usually required 1–2 years for a patient to regain normal nonhyperpigmented facial skin (Fig. 3). Contamination with ordinary soaps and cosmetics was the most influential and decisive factor inhibiting therapy, because such ordinary daily necessities contained the allergens that were producing the disease. The patients were therefore requested to visit the dermatologist once a month to be checked for improvement, and were persuaded every time to avoid such contamination, including products used in beauty parlors [16, 24].

In 1979, Kozuka [25] discovered a new contact sensitizer, phenylazo-2-naphthol (PAN), as an impurity

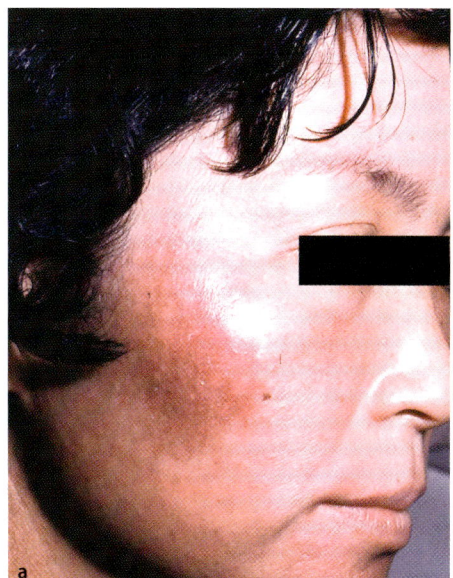
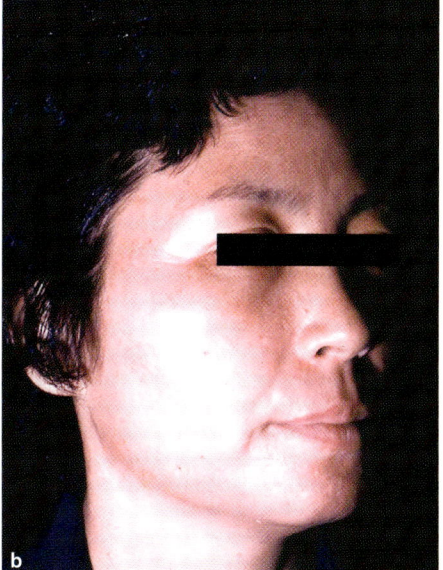
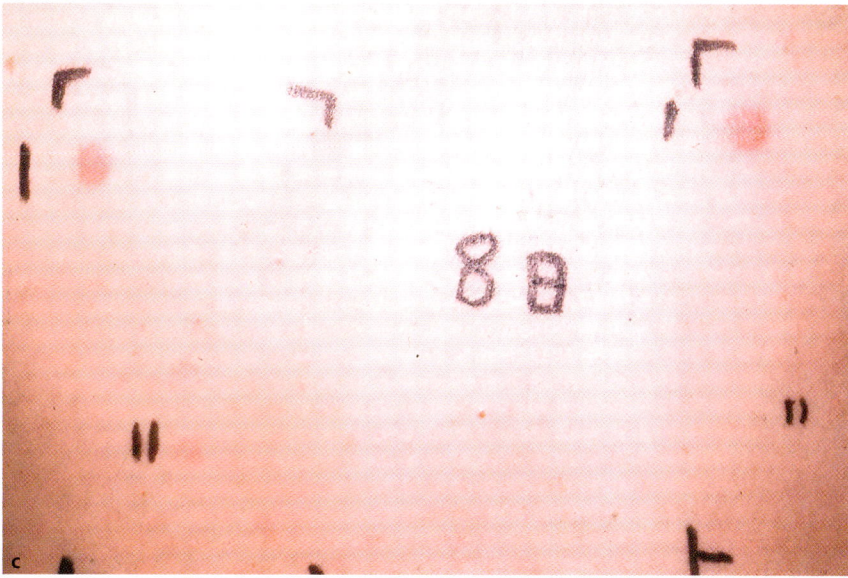

Fig. 3a–c.
Pigmented cosmetic dermatitis in a 43-year-old woman, caused by contact hypersensitivity to jasmine absolute (a). Jasmine absolute 10% in petrolatum produced reactions (site 1) which were still positive even on the eighth day of the patch test (b). The exclusive use of soaps and cosmetics that did not contain common and rare cosmetic sensitizers cleared the persistent dermatitis with pigmentation completely after 1 year and 8 months of use (c)

in commercial supplies of D & C Red 31. Its sensitizing ability and ability to produce secondary hyperpigmentation were as great as those of Yellow No. 11, and therefore many industries began to eliminate or considerably decrease the amount of PAN and Yellow No. 11 in their products. The legal partial restriction of Red No. 31 and Yellow No. 11 by the Japanese government and the voluntary restriction by cosmetic companies of the use of allergenic fragrances, bactericides, and pigments resulted in a remarkable decrease in pigmented cosmetic dermatitis after 1980. One of the reasons for the proposal to change the name from "melanosis faciei feminae" to "pigmented cosmetic dermatitis" [18] was that the latter name makes it easier for the patients to understand the causation of the disease and, at the same time, for industry to recognize the danger of cosmetics in producing such disastrous pigmentary disorders through contact sensitization. The disease was still present in the 1990s [26, 27], and it is necessary for

dermatologists to recognize the importance of cosmetic allergens in producing hyperpigmentation.

18.1.4 Purpuric Dermatitis

In 1886 Majocchi described purpura annularis telangiectodes and, 4 years later, Schamberg described a progressive pigmentary dermatitis which is now well known as Schamberg's disease. The pigmentation in this dermatitis is due to the intradermal accumulation of hemosiderin, the predominant sites being the legs and thighs. Later, Gougerot and Blum described a similar dermatosis as pigmented purpuric lichenoid dermatitis.

The disease was rare but most often occurred in middle-aged or elderly men. However, when a similar disease occurred in many British soldiers during World War II, especially in those who sweated freely or experienced friction when wearing khaki shirts or

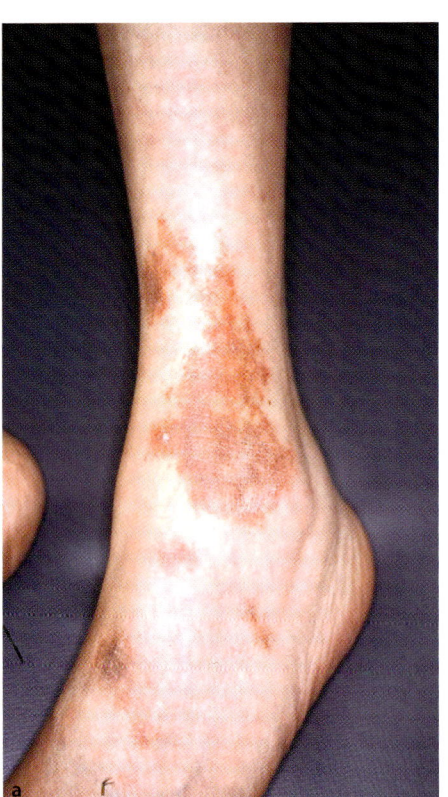
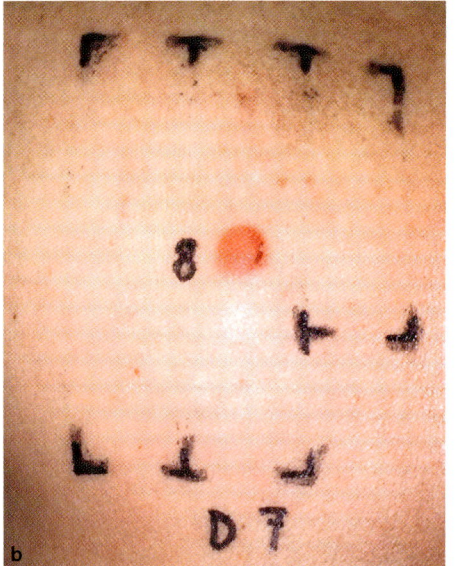

Fig. 4a, b. Reticular brown hyperpigmentation of pigmented purpuric lichenoid dermatitis on an 80-year-old male (**a**). Biopsy showed marked hemorrhage around capillaries of the upper dermis, along with the cellular infiltrates composed of lymphocytes and histiocytes. Patch test revealed strong contact hypersensitivity to paratertiarybutyl phenolformaldehyde resin at 1% petrolatum (**b**). It had been (H) positive from D2 to D14 and confirmative patch test was again strongly positive.

Exposure to the contact allergen was considered to have been from the textile finishes of his socks. The exclusive usage of well-washed white cotton socks gradually improved the dermatitis. Complete blood count (CBC) and liver function test results were normal. This case indicates the importance of patch test of textile finishes if possible, for the treatment of this pigmentary disorder woolen socks, with severe pruritus, dermatitis and pigmentation due to purpura, dermatologists became aware that some textile finishes must have been responsible for the disease [28, 29]. Patch tests and use tests revealed that a blend of vegetable oils and oleic acid seemed to have been responsible.

In 1968, Batschvarov and Minkov [30] reported that rubber components such as *N*-phenyl-*N´*-isopropyl-*p*-phenylenediamine (IPPD), *N*-phenyl-β-naphthylamine (PNA), 2-mercaptobenzothiazole (MBT) and dibenzothiazole disulfide (DBD), i.e., derivatives of *p*-phenylenediamine, naphthylamine, and benzothiazoles, were the allergens responsible for a purpuric dermatitis around the waist underneath the elastic of underwear. A similar pigmented dermatitis was recognized in the shoulders, breasts, groins, and thighs. The capillary resistance (Rumpel-Leede) test was positive in all 23 cases studied. Similar test results were obtained in a smaller proportion of patients with the khaki dermatitis mentioned above. In Bulgaria, over 600 patients were recorded, and the necessity for dermatologists to investigate contact allergens in textiles to solve the problem of purpuric dermatitis of covered areas of skin was stressed [30]. A dye, blue 85, was reported as a causation in 1988 [31]. A case due to a textile finish of socks is demonstrated (Fig. 4).

18.1.5 "Dirty Neck" of Atopic Eczema

Core Message

■ Today, there is much evidence that house dust mites are one of the most important causations of severe atopic dermatitis. Suffering from this dermatitis for many years often leads to reticular dark brown hyperpigmentation of the neck, i.e., the dirty neck. Using the patch test and RAST to identify exacerbating factors and then actively removing them is recommended, as is measuring mite fauna levels in patients' homes.

Atopic dermatitis has been increasing in incidence in many countries, and approximately 1.7–2% of moderate or severe atopic dermatitis patients suffer from reticular dark brown or dark purple pigmentation of the neck. It has been called "dirty neck" [32, 33]. Atopic dermatitis is a multifactorial disease with increased serum IgE in 70–80% of moderate or severe

cases, and also shows an aspect of contact hypersensitivity to house dust mites [34–36], metals [37], and other environmental substances.

The elevation of serum IgE in patients with moderate or severe atopic dermatitis up to 2,000 or even to 20,000 IU/ml is peculiar, since with bronchial asthma, rhinitis, conjunctivitis, and urticaria, only rarely does the level of IgE exceed 1,000 IU/ml [38]. However, it is certain that some 20–30% of moderate or severe atopic dermatitis patients do not show any rise in serum IgE levels; therefore, one explanation for this controversy is that atopic dermatitis has two aspects of immunity for the production of eczema: first, IgE-mediated allergy resulting in spongiosis [39], and, second, cell-mediated allergic contact dermatitis [40, 41].

So-called dirty neck is, histologically, a moderate dermatitis composed of slight acanthosis, lymphocyte and histiocyte infiltration around the vessels in the upper dermis, and incontinentia pigmenti histologica. The reticular pattern of "dirty neck" resembles macular amyloidosis; however, amyloid is usually negative according to Congo red stain, and only a small amount of amyloid was detected by electron microscopy [32]. The pigmentation and configuration are also similar to pigmented cosmetic dermatitis morphologically; however, the most commonly detected contact allergens with severe atopic dermatitis including "dirty neck" were not previously described cosmetic allergens, but frequently house dust mite components [34, 35]. Today, a test to demonstrate mite contact hypersensitivity is possible using a commercially sold patch test reagent Dermatophagoides Mix® (Chemotechnique, Sweden) in a Finn chamber. House dust mite proteins such as Der 1 to 7 have been known as sensitizers, and recently α-acaridial, a component of a house dust mite *Tyrophagus putrescentiae*, turned out to be a primary sensitizer [42]. Active sensitization was observed by the patch test of α-acaridial at 5–0.5% in petrolatum, and the positive reactions were maintained for 1–11 months. It is amazing that such a strong contact sensitizer is present in house dust mites.

The treatment of "dirty neck" is not easy. When the mite fauna were investigated by a new methylene blue agar method in the homes of atopic dermatitis patients, and environmental improvements were made to decrease the mite numbers to fewer than 20/m² at 20 second aspiration using a 320-W cleaner, 88% of severe atopic dermatitis patients showed considerable improvement in their severe dermatitis when they were followed up for 1–2 years [43]. The statistically significant effect of house dust mite elimination with controls in atopic dermatitis was also reported by Tan et al. [44]. The "dirty neck," however,

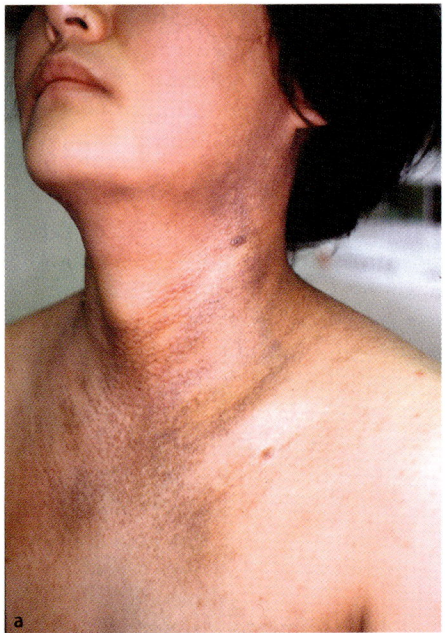
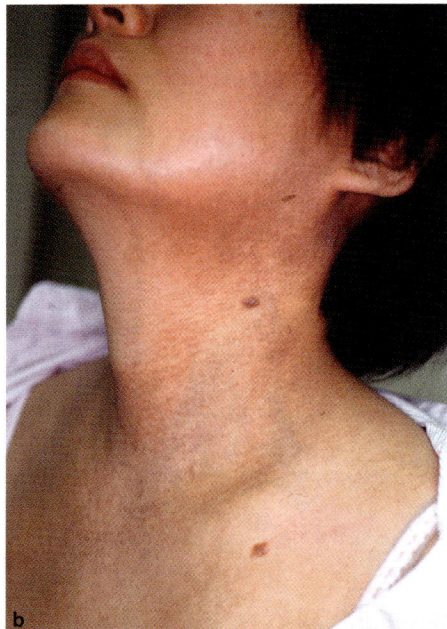

Fig. 5a, b. A severe case of atopic dermatitis of a 28-year-old woman had resulted in "dirty neck" for almost 10 years (**a**). The generalized severe eczema could not be sufficiently controlled by corticosteroid ointments; therefore, among her multiple allergens, mite and metal were selected for elimination to obtain improvement. First, mite fauna was investigated in her home followed by environmental improvement to efficiently decrease *Dermatophagoides*. Second, she was hypersensitive to stannic (tin) derivatives; therefore, dental metals containing stannic were all eliminated and replaced by other metals to which she was not hypersensitive. Tacrolimus ointment has been used as an antisymptomatic treatment recently. Generalized severe eczema disappeared after the above-mentioned allergen elimination, then "dirty neck" slowly disappeared in 4 years, as the last symptom of this case (**b**)

was difficult to cure even with this method, and it can be regarded as the last symptom to improve for atopic dermatitis (Fig. 5).

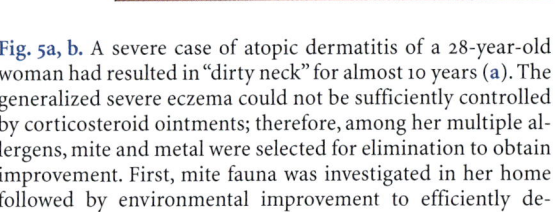

18.2 Depigmentation from Contact with Chemicals

18.2.1 Mechanism of Leukoderma due to Chemicals

There are at least three kinds of mechanism producing leukoderma from contact with chemicals:

- Leukoderma due to selective destruction of melanocytes
- Leukomelanoderma or photoleukomelanoderma due to pigment blockade
- Hypopigmentation due to reduction of melanin synthesis

Allergic contact dermatitis and irritant contact dermatitis can both produce a secondary leukoderma which is almost impossible to differentiate from idiopathic vitiligo. The incidence is low, except for certain phenol derivatives and catechols, which produce a much higher incidence in workers who frequently come into contact with them (Table 3).

Monobenzyl ether of hydroquinone (MBEH) has been known to be a cause of occupational vitiligo since the 1930s [45], the main source of contact having been rubber, in which it is used as an antioxidant to prevent degeneration. The use of MBEH in the rubber industry today is rare, as it had a long history of causing occupational leukoderma by destroying melanocytes. Instead, MBEH came to be used as a bleaching agent for melanotic skin, being used to treat diseases such as melasma and solar lentigo and by dark-skinned people for cosmetic purposes. However, as its toxic effect on melanocytes was too strong, the treatment often resulted in a mottled pattern of leukoderma (confetti-like depigmentation), which was worse than simple hyperpigmentation, and produced problems [46].

Historically, the next chemical to produce leukoderma by contact was 4-*tert*-butylcatechol (PTBC), known since the 1970s [47, 48]. Approximately half of

18

the 75 workers in a tappet assembly plant in the United States were reported to have various grades of leukoderma from daily occupational contact with PTBC. Four severe cases reported in 1970 by Gellin et al. [47] initially had itchy erythematous reactions at the sites of contact, then developed sharply outlined or confluent leukoderma on the face, scalp, hands, fingers, forearms, etc. The patients were all Caucasians.

Patch tests revealed that 0.1% PTBC in acetone produced positive reactions in three of these four cases, one of whom later developed leukoderma at the site of the patch test. However, an exposure test with 1% PTBC in the assembly oil, carried out with occlusion of the forearms in six volunteers, failed to produce leukoderma artificially. Animal tests revealed that PTBC was an irritant, producing erythema and necrosis in albino rabbits, and a bleaching test with 10% PTBC in black guinea pigs resulted in depigmentation of the black skin, both macroscopically and histologically, from the loss of pigment in the epidermis and hair follicles.

At almost the same time, at the beginning of the 1970s, occupational contact leukoderma due to *p-tert*-butylphenol (PTBP) began to be recognized. The incidence of vitiligo vulgaris in the general population was considered to be less than 1%. Therefore, the presence of several cases of vitiligo, located mainly on exposed areas of skin, in the same factory of 20–30 workers alerted dermatologists to the fact that the depigmentation was an occupational dermatosis [49]. PTBP is contained in cobblers' glues, shoes cemented with rubber glues, resins, industrial oils, paints, adhesives, bactericides, plasticizers for cellulose acetate, and printing inks [49–52].

The changes produced by PTBP are similar to those caused by *p-tert*-butylcatechol, and can occur with or without sensitization. Kahn [50] and Romaguera et al. [53] reported patients who were apparently sensitized to PTBP with positive reactions on a closed patch test with 1% PTBP.

Hydroquinone is an excellent depigmenting agent for clinical treatment of various pigmentations [54]. However, it may rarely produce leukoderma that is similar to vitiligo vulgaris [55,56]. The mechanism of the hypopigmentation caused by hydroquinone is thought to be decreased formation of melanosomes and destruction of the membranous organelles in the melanocytes, thus causing degeneration of melanocytes [57].

These historically accumulated cases of contact leukoderma caused by phenol derivatives indicate that selective toxicity of these chemicals to melanocytes is the main cause of leukoderma, judging from the degeneration of melanocytes, the irritation often noted, and the fact that sensitization is not always demonstrated.

Table 3. Chemicals producing leukoderma or hypopigmentation on contact

Another hazard of using hydroquinone as a bleaching agent is ochronosis, especially when it is used at high concentrations (e.g., 3.5–7.5%) [58]. Ochronosis means "yellow disease," and black Africans suffer from hyperpigmentation of the face due to the degeneration of elastic fibers caused by this topical agent [59]. Therefore, the use of hydroquinone as a bleaching agent by blacks should be advised carefully, and high concentrations are not recommended.

18.2.2 Contact Leukoderma Caused Mainly by Contact Sensitization

Very rarely, allergic contact dermatitis produces a secondary depigmentation similar to vitiligo. A gardener was reported to have developed secondary leukoderma after allergic contact dermatitis due to *Alstroemeria* [60], and when squaric acid dibutylester was used for immunotherapy in a 26-year-old male with alopecia areata, depigmentation over the whole scalp was reported after repeated contact dermatitis produced by nine courses of treatment. Regrowth of hair was also noted [61]. A herbicide, Carbyne R, and cerium oxide have also been reported to produce contact hypersensitivity and secondary leukoderma [62, 63].

References

1. Papa CM, Kligman AM (1965) The behavior of melanocytes in inflammation. J Invest Dermatol 45:465–474
2. Nakamura T (1977) Toxicoderma caused by "Shiitake", lentinus edodos (in Japanese). Rinsho-Hifuka 31:65–68
3. Osmundsen PE (1969) Contact dermatitis due to an optical whitener in washing powders. Br J Dermatol 81:799–803
4. Osmundsen PE (1970) Pigmented contact dermatitis. Br J Dermatol 83:296–301
5. Ancona-Alayón A, Escobar-Márques R, González-Mendoza A et al (1976) Occupational pigmented contact dermatitis from Naphthol AS. Contact Dermatitis 2:129–134
6. Kawachi S, Kawashima T, Akiyama J et al (1985) Pigmented contact dermatitis due to dyes from nightgown (in Japanese). Hifuka No Rinsho 27:91–92, 181–187
7. Hayakawa R, Matsunaga K, Kojima S et al (1985) Naphthol AS as a cause of pigmented contact dermatitis. Contact Dermatitis 13:20–25
8. Osawa J, Takekawa K, Onuma S, Kitamura K, Ikezawa Z (1997) Pigmented contact dermatitis due to Naphthol AS in a pillow case. Contact Dermatitis 37:37–38
9. Nakayama H, Suzuki A (1985) Investigation of skin disturbances caused by the chemicals contained in daily necessities, part 1. On the ability of textile finishes to produce dermatitis (in Japanese). Tokyo-To Living Division Report 1–27
10. Kovacevic Z, Kränke B (2001) Pigmented purpuric contact dermatitis from Disperse Blue 106 and 124 dyes. J Am Acad Dermatol 45:456–458
11. Takayama N, Suzuki T, Sakurai Y et al (1984) Friction melanosis (in Japanese). Nishinihon Hifuka (West Japan Dermatol) 46:1340–1345
12. Tanigaki T, Hata S, Kitano M et al (1983) On peculiar melanosis occuring on the trunk and extremities (in Japanese). Rinsho Hifuka 37:347–351
13. Matsuo S, Nakayama H, Suzuki A (1989) Successful treatment with allergen controlled wearing apparel of textile dermatitis patients (in Japanese). Hifu 31 [Suppl 6]:178–185
14. Nakayama H (1989) Allergen control, an indispensable treatment for allergic contact dermatitis. Dermat Clin 8:197–204
15. Nakayama H (1987) Dental metal and allergy (in Japanese). Jpn J Dent Assoc 40:893–903
16. Nakayama H, Matsuo S, Hayakawa K et al (1984) Pigmented cosmetic dermatitis. Int J Dermatol 23:299–305
17. Matsuo S, Nakayama H (1984) A case of pigmented dermatitis induced by cinnamic derivatives (in Japanese). Hifu 26:573–579
18. Nakayama H (1974) Perfume allergy and cosmetic dermatitis (in Japanese). Jpn J Dermatol 84:659–667
19. Nakayama H, Hanaoka H, Ohshiro A (1974) Allergen controlled system. Kanehara Shuppan, Tokyo, pp 1–42
20. Von Riehl G (1917) Über eine eigenartige Melanose. Wien Klin Wochenschr 30:780–781
21. Minami S, Noma Y (1950) Melanosis faciei feminae (in Japanese). Dermatol Urol 12:73–77
22. Nakayama H, Harada R, Toda M (1981) Pigmented cosmetic dermatitis. Int J Dermatol 15:673–675
23. Nakayama H (1983) Cosmetic series patch test allergens, types 19 to 20 (in Japanese, with English abstract). Fragrance Journal Publications, Tokyo, pp 1–121
24. Watanabe N (1989) Long term follow-up of allergen control system on patients with cosmetic dermatitis (in Japanese). Nishinihon Hifuka 51:113–130
25. Kozuka T, Tashiro M, Sano S et al (1979) Brilliant Lake Red R as a cause of pigmented contact dermatitis. Contact Dermatitis 5:294–304
26. Gonçalo S, Sil J, Gonçalo M, Polares Batista A (1991) Pigmented photoallergic contact dermatitis from musk ambrette. Contact Dermatitis 24:229–231
27. Trattner A, Hodak E, David M (1999) Screening Patch tests for pigmented contact dermatitis in Israel. Contact Dermatitis 40:155–157
28. Greenwood K (1960) Dermatitis with capillary fragility. Arch Dermatol 81:947–952
29. Twiston Davies JH, Neish Barker A (1944) Textile dermatitis. Br J Dermatol 56:33–43
30. Batschvarov B, Minkov DM (1968) Dermatitis and purpura from rubber in clothing. Trans St John's Hosp Dermatol Soc 54:178–182
31. Van der Veen, JPW, Neering H, DeHaan P et al (1988) Pigmented purpuric clothing dermatitis due to Disperse Blue 85. Contact Dermatitis 19:222–223
32. Humphreys F, Spencer J, McLaren K, Tidman MJ (1996) An histological and ultrastructural study of the dirty neck appearance in atopic eczema. Clin Exp Dermatol 21:17–19
33. Manabe T, Inagaki Y, Nakagawa S et al (1987) Ripple pigmentation of the neck in atopic dermatitis. Am J Dermatopathol 9:301–307
34. Nakayama H (1995) The role of the house dust mite in atopic eczema. Practical contact dermatitis. McGraw-Hill, New York, pp 623–630
35. Vincenti C, Trevisi P, Guerra L, Lorenzi S, Tosti A (1994) Patch testing with whole dust mite bodies in atopic dermatitis. Am J Contact Dermatitis 5:213–215

18

36. Sakurai M (1996) Results of patch tests with mite components in atopic dermatitis patients (in Japanese with English abstract). Allergy 45:398–408
37. Shanon J (1965) Pseudoatopic dermatitis, contact dermatitis due to chrome sensitivity simulating atopic dermatitis. Dermatologica 131:118–190
38. Okudaira H (1997) Atopic diseases and house dust mite allergens (in Japanese with English abstract). Hifu 39 [Suppl 19]:45–51
39. Bruynzeel-Koomen, C VanWichen DF, Toonstra J et al (1986) The presence of IgE molecules on epidermal Langerhans cells in patients with atopic dermatitis. Arch Dermatol Res 278:199–205
40. Imayama S, Hashizume T, Miyahara H et al (1992) Combination of patch test and IgE for dust mite antigens differences 130 patients with atopic dermatitis into four groups. J Am Acad Dermatol 27:531–538
41. Rawle FC, Mitchell EB, Platts-Mills TAE (1984) T cell responses to major allergen from the house dust mite Dermatophagoides pteronyssinus antigen P1: comparison of patients with asthma, atopic dermatitis, and perennial rhinitis. J Immunol 44:195–201
42. Nakayama H, Kumei A (2003) House dust mite – an important causation of atopic dermatitis. SP World 31:13–20
43. Kumei A (1995) Investigation of mites in the house of atopic dermatitis (AD) patients, and clinical improvements by mite elimination (in Japanese with English abstract). Allergy 44:116–127
44. Tan BB, Weald D, Strickland I, Friedmann PS (1996) Double-blind controlled trial of effect of housedust-mite allergen avoidance on atopic dermatitis. Lancet 347:15–18
45. Oliver EA, Schwartz L, Warren LH (1939) Occupational leukoderma: preliminary report. J Am Med Assoc 113:927–928
46. Yoshida Y, Usuba M (1958) Monobenzyl ether of hydroquinone leukomelanodermia (in Japanese). Rinsho Hifuka Hinyokika 12:333–338
47. Gellin GA, Possik PA, Davis IH (1970) Occupational depigmentation due to 4-tertiarybutyl catechol (TBC). J Occup Med 12:386–389
48. Gellin GA, Maibach HI, Mislazek MH, Ring M (1979) Detection of environmental depigmenting substances. Contact Dermatitis 5:201–213
49. Malten KE, Sutter E, Hara I, Nakajima T (1971) Occupational vitiligo due to paratertiary butylphenol and homologues. Trans St John's Hosp Dermatol Soc 57:115–134
50. Kahn G (1970) Depigmentation caused by phenolic detergent germicides. Arch Dermatol 102:177–187
51. Malten KE (1967) Contact sensitization caused by p-tert-butylphenol and certain phenolformaldehyde-containing glues. Dermatologica 135:54–59
52. Malten KE (1975) Paratertiary butylphenol depigmentation in a consumer. Contact Dermatitis 1:180–192
52. Romaguera C, Grimalt F (1981) Occupational leukoderma and contact dermatitis from paratertiary-butylphenol. Contact Dermatitis 7:159–160
54. Arndt KA, Fitzpatrick TB (1965) Topical use of hydroquinone as a depigmenting agent. J Am Med Assoc 194:965–967
55. Frenk E, Loi-Zedda P (1980) Occupational depigmentation due to a hydroquinone-containing photographic developer. Contact Dermatitis 6:238–239
56. Kersey P, Stevenson CJ (1981) Vitiligo and occupational exposure to hydroquinone from servicing self-photographing machines. Contact Dermatitis 7:285–287
57. Jimbow K, Obata H, Pathak M, Fitzpatrick TB (1974) Mechanism of depigmentation by hydroquinone. J Invest Dermatol 62:436–449
58. Findlay GH (1982) Ochronosis following skin bleaching with hydroquinone. J Am Acad Dermatol 6:1092–1093
59. Hoshaw RA, Zimmerman KG, Menter A (1985) Ochronosis-like pigmentation from hydroquinone bleaching creams in American Blacks. Arch Dermatol 121:105–108
60. Björkner BE (1982) Contact allergy and depigmentation from alstromeria. Contact Dermatitis 8:178–184
61. Valsecchi R, Cainelli T (1984) Depigmentation from squaric acid dibutyl ester. Contact Dermatitis 10:108
62. Brancaccio RR, Chamales MH (1977) Contact dermatitis and depigmentation produced by the herbicide carbyne. Contact Dermatitis 3:108–109
63. Rapaport MJ (1982) Depigmentation with cerium oxide. Contact Dermatitis 8:282–283

Hand Eczema

19

Tove Agner

Contents

Hand eczema is a common disease in the general population, and one the most frequent diagnoses in dermatology. It affects occupational as well as private aspects of life, and the severity varies from mild and transient to severe and chronic disease. Being a disease that affects mainly young people, and often interfering with their professional career, the disease is a burden not only to the patient but also to society.

Development of hand eczema is in most cases influenced by multiple factors, involving exogenous as well as endogenous aspects. An exact diagnosis is necessary to correctly advise the patient about treatment and prevention of the eczema. Unfortunately many cases of hand eczema take a chronic course. The best way to avoid this seems to be early diagnoses and effective treatment in the initial phase.

19.1 Epidemiology

19.1.1 Frequency

The occurrence of hand eczema depends on basal characteristics such as age, sex, atopy, and occupation in the population that are investigated. In a Swedish study the self-reported 1-year prevalence of hand eczema in the general population was 11.8% in 1983 and had decreased to 9.7% in 1996 [36, 39]. The crude incidence rate of self-reported hand eczema in individuals aged 20–65 years was recently reported to be 5.5 cases per 1,000 person-years [40]. The incidence of hand eczema is high among young people. In school children the 1-year prevalence of hand eczema was reported to be 7.3% for children aged 12–16 years and 10.0% for children aged 16–19 years [50, 82]. Early onset of hand eczema is frequent, and in around one-third of cases onset of hand eczema occurs before the age of 20 [40].

19.1.2 Risk Factors

Hand eczema may often take a chronic course with a tendency to frequent relapses. A history of earlier hand eczema is a major indication of vulnerable skin, predisposing the individual to the development of hand eczema. Even short episodes of eczema may predict a tendency to future disease, and the most important risk factor for development of hand eczema seems to be previous episodes of hand eczema earlier in life [56]. Atopic dermatitis is another major predictive factor, and considerably increased risk for development of hand eczema in persons with previous or current atopic dermatitis is well established. In a population study a history of childhood eczema was found to be more important for development of hand eczema compared to other risk factors such as female sex and occupational exposure [41]. The prevalence of hand eczema in adults reporting moderate and severe atopic dermatitis in childhood was 25% and 41%, respectively [62], and a long-term follow-up study confirmed that more than 40% of patients attending the Karolinska Hospital in Stockholm for atopic dermatitis in childhood had developed hand eczema when re-examined 25 years later [63, 64]. In a recent population-based survey including 15,000 people, 42% of those who reported childhood eczema stated positively that they had had hand eczema at some time [44]. The importance of mucosal atopy for development of hand eczema is not fully agreed, but it is a significantly less essential risk factor than atopic dermatitis [23, 40, 57, 62]. Although the frequency of atopic dermatitis had been on the increase, the prevalence of hand eczema slightly decreased between 1983 and 1996 in Swedish adults (from 11.8 to 9.7 [39]). The decrease in prevalence of hand eczema could be an effect of an increased focus on preventive measures for occupational diseases recently.

Hand eczema occurs more frequently in females than in males [6, 12, 36, 41], the female:male ratio being 1.8:1 [40]. Females are traditionally more exposed to wet work than males, and many jobs involving extensive wet work, e.g., hairdressing, health care work, catering and cleaning, are usually female jobs. Generally, females report more hand washings per day than males [40, 44], and they may often have more exposure to domestic skin irritants, including cooking and child caring. No sex-related difference in skin susceptibility to irritants has been reported from experimental studies [2]. In a recent population-based twin study, female sex was confirmed to be a risk factor for development of hand eczema, but when covariates such as nickel allergy and wet work were included in the analysis the effect of gender was no longer statistically significant [7]. This clearly indicates that the high frequency of hand eczema in females compared to males is caused by different exposures.

Recent findings indicate that the increased risk for adult women to develop hand eczema is present in the age group 20–29 years only, in which group the incidence rate is doubled as compared to males, while no increased risk for women is present beyond the age of 30 [40]. An increased amount of wet work in young females most likely explains this pattern [40]. However, female preponderance among hand eczema patients in school pupils has been reported, probably due to increased frequency of atopic dermatitis and nickel allergy among females in the study population [50].

Contact allergy and especially nickel allergy is generally accepted to be a risk factor for development of hand eczema [7, 8, 51]. The interaction between nickel allergy and hand eczema was analyzed by Menné et al. [49], who found it to be "both ways": compared with non-nickel-sensitive females, those who had become nickel sensitized ran an increased risk of developing hand eczema, and those who had developed hand eczema first ran an increased risk of later developing nickel allergy [49]. This association has been confirmed in more recent studies [8, 44, 50]. In two cross-sectional studies examining the prevalence of hand eczema and contact allergy of the general population in Copenhagen, performed before and after nickel exposure regulation in Denmark, the first study in 1990 found a significant association between nickel allergy and a history of hand eczema in women, while the second study in 1998 could not find this association [54]. This is probably due to diminished exposure to nickel after nickel legislation was introduced [14], and is an interesting example of how regulations and legislation as preventive measures may diminish the risk of contact allergy and subsequently hand eczema.

19.1.3 Validity of Self-reported Hand Eczema

Much information about occurrence and risk factors for hand eczema is based on questionnaires asking either risk groups or the general population about clinical signs of previous and present hand eczema. Naturally, this way of obtaining information is not as precise as an objective assessment by a dermatologist. The validity of self-reported hand eczema depends on the type of population investigated, and has been evaluated in several studies. It is generally agreed that the self-reported prevalence of hand eczema underestimates the true prevalence [38]. A simple question as "do you have hand eczema?" had higher sensitivity and specificity than more complex symptom-based questions, since it is difficult for individuals to identify skin signs compatible with the clinical diagnosis of hand eczema [73]. Standardized questions for occupational hand eczema have been developed, providing more standardized data [72].

19.2 Etiology and Morphology

Core Message

■ A precise diagnosis is necessary for optimal treatment and prevention.

The most common etiology for hand eczema is irritant contact dermatitis (35%), followed by atopic hand eczema (22%), and allergic contact dermatitis (19%), while endogenous forms other than atopic hand eczema such as pompholyx and hyperkeratotic eczema only constitute a minor group [36].

It is important to realize that the etiology of hand eczema cannot be determined from the clinical manifestations, and that different etiological diagnoses cannot be distinguished by clinical pattern [28, 35]. Although a clinical presentation with numerous vesicles may indicate an allergic contact dermatitis, and a chronic, scaly appearance may lead to a suspicion of irritant contact dermatitis, these clinical signs may in some cases be misleading, and omission of a full diagnostic program cannot be justified.

Core Message

- Morphology may not be related to etiology.

19.2.1 Allergic Contact Dermatitis

Core Message

- Patients with hand eczema lasting for more than 1 month should be patch tested.

A positive patch test with relevance to the current hand eczema may be expected to occur in less than one-third of all cases of hand eczema. Contact sensitization may be the primary cause of hand eczema, or may be a complication of irritant or atopic hand eczema. The number of positive patch tests has been reported to correlate with the duration of hand eczema, indicating that long-standing hand eczema may often be complicated by sensitization [30]. The most common contact allergies in patients with hand eczema are nickel, cobalt, fragrance-mix, balsam of Peru, and colophony [36]. Contact sensitivity, especially to nickel but also to other allergens, is generally considered to be a risk factor for development of hand eczema [30, 49, 50], and the risk increases with increasing strength of contact allergy [7, 8]. The importance of metal allergy for flare-up of hand eczema was underlined in experimental studies of hand eczema in patients with metal allergy. Exposure to even very low doses of the metal caused a flare-up in the sensitized patients, but not in controls [52, 53].

Recent papers also indicate that fragrance allergy can be a common and relevant problem in patients with hand eczema, since perfumes are often present in consumer products to which the hand are exposed [22]. Formaldehyde allergy was found to be of significance for patients with hand eczema. Of 117 women sensitized to formaldehyde, 52% had hand eczema, and the dominating exposure source was domestically used cleaning products [13]. More recently, allergy to methyldibromo glutaronitrile was frequently found to be relevant in patients with hand eczema [83].

19.2.2 Irritant Contact Dermatitis

Irritant contact dermatitis is the most common cause of hand eczema. In an epidemiological population-based study irritant factors were found to play either a primary or an additional role in 73% of all cases of hand eczema [31]. The most common exposure causing irritant contact dermatitis on the hands is wet work, at the working place or at home. Young women are at special risk of this type of hand eczema, since this group has an increased frequency of occupational exposure to wet work, and at the same time has a significant domestic exposure.

Having children below 4 years of age in the family and lacking a dishwashing machine have both been demonstrated to be separate and significant risk factors for hand eczema [57]. The level of pre-existing skin irritation and barrier disruption is important for the skin's susceptibility to further irritation. Detergents have a significant ability to harm the barrier function of the skin, which can be quantified as increased transepidermal water loss. This explains why wet work is, in the majority of cases, a complicating factor, since the disturbed barrier function leads to increased penetration by irritants, allergens, and bacteria. The combined effects of irritants and allergens may change the threshold value for elicitation of allergic contact dermatitis, either by immunological effects or by enhanced penetration by allergen [58]. Elicitation thresholds for allergens may be considerably influenced by simultaneous exposure.

In a population-based twin study, hereditary risk factors were found to play a significant part in the development of hand eczema in the general population, when no extreme environmental exposure exists [6]. This hereditary risk factor could only partly be explained by atopic dermatitis or contact allergy, and a separate genetic risk factor, independent of atopic dermatitis and contact allergy, is suggested to be of importance for development of irritant contact dermatitis of the hands [7].

19.2.3 Contact Urticaria

Contact urticaria on the hands may, in a chronic phase, imitate eczema, meaning that this entity cannot be recognized from just the clinical examination. Skin prick tests or RAST tests are necessary to identify contact urticaria, which on the hands is most often found after occupational exposure to latex gloves or food. Contact urticaria on the hands has an increased frequency in atopics.

19.2.4 Atopic Dermatitis

Persons with atopic dermatitis have a significantly increased risk for development of hand eczema when exposed to irritants at work or at home [10]. Preventive measures are taken to inform young people with atopic dermatitis to avoid professions including wet or dirty work or food handling. Hand eczema in atopics often takes a chronic course, and a change of job seems to improve the prognosis less for atopics than for others [63]. Cellular immunity in atopics is decreased, and allergic contact dermatitis seems to occur in a smaller number of patients with past or present atopic disease than in nonatopics [65]. Positive patch tests, often related to topical treatments, are however sometimes found in atopics, and patch tests should be performed as in other patients with hand eczema.

19.2.5 Endogenous Forms

19.2.5.1 Acute and Recurrent Vesicular Hand Eczema (Pompholyx)

Pompholyx is a clinical manifestation of hand eczema with an uncertain etiology [48]. Preceded by itching, a vesicular eruption occurs on the palmar aspects of fingers and hands, interdigitally and sometimes in the periungual area. Infections and allergic contact dermatitis should be excluded. A relationship with atopic dermatitis, to tinea pedis, and to nickel allergy has been suspected. In a recent study an association with tinea pedis was statistically confirmed, while no association with atopy or nickel allergy could be established [8].

19.2.5.2 Hyperkeratotic Eczema

Hyperkeratotic dermatitis of the palms is a clinically characteristic entity which occurs mainly in men above the age of 40. Hyperkeratosis is present symmetrically in the palms, and fissures are common, while vesicles are not found. It may, however, be preceded by an initial vesicular stage. Although hard manual labor may be a risk factor for hyperkeratotic hand eczema, no such thing can be identified in the majority of cases [21, 46]. The differential diagnosis to psoriasis may sometimes be difficult, but widespread lesions are not found in hyperkeratotic ecze-

Table 1. Diagnosis of hand eczema

Medical history questions:
    Previous episodes of hand eczema
    Atopic dermatitis (previous or current)
    Psoriasis

Exposures
    Domestic
    Occupational
    Leisure time

Clinical examination
    Assessment of severity
    Assessment of morphology
        Localization
        Extension
        Hyperkeratotic
        Pompholyx

Patch testing
    Should be performed in all patients with hand eczema lasting for more than 1 month
    In case of positive patch test reactions
        Present relevance? (exposure assessment)
        Past relevance?
        Unknown relevance?

Based on the examination above one of the following diagnoses should be reached
    Irritant contact dermatitis
        Occupational
        Nonoccupational
    Allergic contact dermatitis (or allergic contact urticaria)
        Occupational
        Nonoccupational
    Atopic dermatitis
    Endogenous dermatitis (other than atopic)

Several etiological factors may often be included in the diagnosis, e.g., irritant contact dermatitis and atopic dermatitis, or allergic contact dermatitis and irritant contact dermatitis

19

Table 2. Treatment and prevention of hand eczema

Allergen and irritant avoidance

   Exposure assessment

   Substitution of products causing irritation (domestic and occupational)

   Substitution of products causing elicitation of allergy (domestic and occupational)

   Personal protection

   Avoidance of wet work

   Avoidance of dirty work and mechanical irritation of the skin of the hands

Information

   Skin protection program

   Expectations – what can be done and what is the prognosis

   Notification of possible occupational cases

Treatment

   Basic treatment (skin care program and moisturizers)

   Topical therapy (topical steroids being the most frequently used treatment)

   Systemic therapy (limited to severe cases)

   Physical therapy (UVB, PVVA)

ma. Also in the case of clinically typical hyperkeratotic hand eczema, patch testing should be performed, since the clinical pattern may sometimes be misleading, or a complicating contact allergy may be identified (Tables 1, 2).

19.3 Occupational Hand Eczema

Skin diseases constitute up to 30% of all occupational diseases. The most common work-related dermatosis is contact dermatitis, for which the annual incidence is reported to be 12.9 per 100,000 workers [9, 19].

Core Message

■ Hand eczema is one of the most commonly recognized occupational diseases, and also one of the most expensive in worker's compensation.

Occupational contact dermatitis is most often located on the hands. The true incidence of occupational hand eczema varies from one region to another, depending on industrialization and workplaces in the region. Legal aspects regarding occupational hand eczema and worker's compensation influence the frequency at which cases are reported to the authorities, and the true number of cases may very well be much higher than the reported and/or recognized number. The cost to society is high, including worker's compensation, sick leave, retraining, and costs to health services. In addition to being a burden to the individual, the disease is expensive for society since it most often affects young people and is a predictor of long-term sick leave and unemployment [32].

Occupational hand eczema is more often due to irritant than to allergic contact dermatitis [17, 68]. Frequent, harmful occupational exposures were reported to be unspecified chemicals, water and detergents, dust and dry dirt [42]. In a recent Danish study the highest numbers of occupational hand eczema were found among health care workers [68]. A large number of hand eczema cases was reported among cleaners and in people with wet work in hospitals [30, 42]. High numbers were also reported among factory workers, cleaners, kitchen workers/cooks, and hairdressers. The highest relative risk of eczema per employee was found for bakers [68]. Bakers were reported to have a threefold increased risk of hand eczema as compared to the background population, due to exposure to dough and wet work [45]. A high relative risk was also reported for hairdressers, dental surgery assistants, and kitchen workers/cooks. Common for occupations with high risk of occupational hand eczema is exposure to wet work, which has also been identified as a risk factor for development for hand eczema. Many female-dominated occupations involve extensive wet work (healthcare workers, hairdressers, catering). Focus on prevention of hand eczema within this area would be a benefit for the workers as well as for society, due to a reduction in economic costs.

Also metal workers have an increased risk for development of hand eczema. In a prospective study the 3-year cumulative incidence of hand eczema in metal workers was 15.3% as compared to 6.9% in "white collar-workers" [16]. A study of metal worker trainees found that, apart from atopic dermatitis, other major risk factors for development of hand eczema were mechanical factors as well as chemical irritants, and insufficient amount of recovery time [5]. Frequent causes of occupational allergic contact dermatitis are allergy to metals, rubber, biocides, and fragrances.

Cases of occupational hand eczema should be reported to the authorities as work-related disease. For further information on legal aspects of occupational contact dermatitis within different countries see Chap. 45.

19.4 Prognosis

Hand eczema is a long-lasting disease. A mean duration of 11.6 years was reported [36], 12.0 and 9.9 years for allergic and irritant contact dermatitis, respectively, while atopic hand eczema was reported to have a duration of 16.3 years. Another study reported 41% of cases to be healed when re-examined after 3 years [30]. Hand eczema may often lead to sick leave, and the mean total sick leave time for hand eczema patients was reported to be 4 weeks per year [43]. In a cohort of patients with occupational hand eczema, sick leave for more than 5 weeks per year owing to the eczema was reported by 19.9%. It is generally agreed that frequent and long-lasting sick leave is often related to atopic hand eczema. Earlier studies have reported a higher degree of severity in patients with allergic contact dermatitis as compared to irritant contact dermatitis on the hands, as measured by symptom duration, sick leave, and extent of involvement [1, 15, 43, 47]. New data, however, indicate that this has changed. A recent study reports occupational irritant contact dermatitis to be more strongly associated with severe hand eczema than allergic contact dermatitis [25], and in a recent Danish study on occupational hand eczema a substantially greater severity among those with occupational irritant contact dermatitis was found [69]. This alteration in risk factors for severity is probably explained by recent regulation of exposure to allergens such as nickel and chromate, which has reduced the risk for allergic contact dermatitis. Having a food-related occupation appears to be associated with an increased risk of job loss [69].

It is generally assumed that a long delay before diagnosis and treatment of hand eczema leads to a poor prognosis, although there are no substantial data available to support this hypothesis.

Considering the severe consequences of having hand eczema, it is evident that prevention of the disease should be promoted.

19.5 Treatment

Three important steps in the treatment of hand eczema are:

- ▪ To ensure that the patient understands the precise diagnosis (e.g., allergic or toxic contact dermatitis) and its consequences
- ▪ To teach the patient good skin care habits
- ▪ To initiate an effective medical treatment (topical, systemic, or physical thereapy/therapies).

Understanding the diagnosis improves the prognosis for the patient [3, 24], and is necessary to ensure compliance. Making the patient understand the importance of avoiding skin contact with allergens in the case of allergic contact dermatitis may be a time-consuming procedure, and several consultations may often be necessary. The message that the patient needs to understand is often quite complex, and it is a challenge for the dermatologist to keep the information as simple and as practical as possible. Independent of the diagnosis the patient should be instructed in good skin care habits. Written information and videos may be helpful. Reports on eczema schools for patients with hand eczema are few, and more experience is needed [27] (Table 3).

An extremely important aspect of the treatment of hand eczema is use of moisturizers. Topically applied lipids improve skin barrier function, and the effect of the moisturizer corresponds to the amount of lipids in the product [18]. Recently it was investigated whether moisturizers containing skin-related lipids were more effective than petrolatum-based creams in patients with chronic hand eczema, and advantage of the skin-related lipids for treatment of contact dermatitis could not be demonstrated [29]. Since use of moisturizers may sometimes be neglected or looked upon as being "not important" by the patients, it is necessary for the dermatologist to underline the significance of moisturizers, and help the patient to select an effective and acceptable one. Males seem to be less familiar than females with the use of moisturizers, and the importance of moisturizers should be emphasized to this group in particular.

Table 3. Skin protection program based on evidence from clinical and experimental studies

Wash your hands in lukewarm water. Rinse and dry your hands thoroughly after washing
Use gloves when starting wet-work tasks
Protective gloves should be used when necessary but for as short a time as possible
Protective gloves should be intact and clean and dry inside
When protective gloves are used for more than 10 min, cotton gloves should be worn underneath
Hand wash may be substituted by use of disinfectant when the hands are not wet a visibly contaminated
Do not wear finger rings at work
Apply moisturizers on your hands during the working day or after work
Select a lipid-rich and fragrance-free moisturizer
Moisturizers should be applied all over the hands including the fingerwebs, fingertips, and back of the hand
Take care also when doing housework, use protective gloves for dishwashing, and warm gloves when going outside in winter

19

Topical corticosteroids are still the core treatment for hand eczema [78], and their use is reported in 51% of patients with hand eczema [43]. However, few studies are available on the efficacy and side-effects when used as a long-term treatment. Nine weeks of treatment with mometasone furoate was reported to clear 80% of cases, and maintenance therapy 3 times weekly for 36 weeks did not cause any significant side-effects [79]. However, the chronicity of the disease increases the risk of side-effects due to long-term treatment with topical corticosteroids. Use of topical steroids under occlusion for short periods, e..g., 1 h a day for a few weeks, may be helpful for hyperkeratotic eczema, but increases the risk of side-effects considerably. When the eczema continues in spite of treatment the possibility of contact allergy to topical corticosteroids should be considered.

Tacrolimus or pimecrolimus may be suitable treatments for some types of hand eczema, but more experience with these preparations is needed [66, 75, 76].

In severe cases systemic treatment with immunosuppressants such as cyclosporine, azathioprine or methotrexate may sometimes be necessary, but randomized controlled trials on these treatments for hand eczema are not available. Acitretin is an effective treatment for keratotic hand eczema [77]. Botulinum toxin has been used in the treatment of pompholyx [74]. Physical treatment with PUVA therapy or UVB may be considered, and UVA-1 treatment was recently advocated for pompholyx [59]. Grenz rays have traditionally been used particularly for treatment of hyperkeratotic hand eczema [33], although nowadays it has been widely replaced by newer treatments because of its potential carcinogenic side-effects.

To compare the efficacy of different medical treatments for hand eczema randomized controlled trials are needed. In clinical trials the evaluation should comprise objective assessment of the eczema as well as self-assessment by the patients. Instruments for self-assessment are available either as a VAS-score or as health-related quality of life [80], and a scoring systems for standardized objective evaluation has been proposed [20, 84].

19.6 Prevention

Since hand eczema is a disease that may often become chronic, is a burden for the patient, and is a great cost to society, prevention is obviously an attractive alternative. Prevention should aim mainly at exposure, but knowledge about endogenous risk factors should also be taken into account.

19.6.1 Regulation of Threshold Values for Allergens

Exposure of the skin to allergens in sufficiently high concentrations to cause sensitization is decisive in the development of allergic contact dermatitis on the hands. Regulation of allergen exposure, by either legislation on threshold values or regulation of precautions in the handling of allergenic products, reduces allergen exposure and subsequently reduces the frequency of allergic contact dermatitis. One example of this is nickel exposure regulation, of which a positive effect has been documented [54]; other examples are regulation of chromate in cement, and recently prohibition of the preservative methyldibromo glutaronitrile in cosmetics.

19.6.2 Identification of Risk Groups

Previous or current atopic dermatitis is, as already mentioned, a significant endogenous risk factor for development of hand eczema, and counseling about avoiding wet and dirty occupations should be given to atopics as early as in childhood. A separate genetic risk factor, independent of atopic dermatitis, has recently been suggested to be important in the development of irritant contact dermatitis of the hands [7], but further studies are needed to confirm this hypothesis.

Exposure to wet work is a special risk factor for development of hand eczema, and to achieve the optimal effect of preventive efforts the focus for prevention should aim at reducing wet exposure.

19.6.3 Skin Protection

Protection of the hands is essential for the prevention of hand eczema and is a fundamental aspect in its treatment. The effects of protective measures, such as use of moisturizers and gloves, have mostly been documented in laboratory studies with experimentally damaged skin [11]. An intervention program for people working in wet occupations has been developed, based on results from experimental studies, and its effectiveness was documented in an intervention study [19].

Use of gloves in wet work has generally been recommended and accepted as an important preventive measure. Compliance with this recommendation is good in some but far from all jobs [81]. Although the protective effect of gloves should not be doubted, gloves may sometimes be the cause of hand eczema. Protective gloves may cause irritant contact dermatitis or allergic contact dermatitis due to contact sensitization to rubber additives, or they may cause contact urticaria due to immediate natural rubber latex allergy [60, 61, 71]. The diagnostic work to be done when suspecting glove-related dermatitis includes exposure assessment (how many hours a day), as well as a patch test for rubber additives and a skin prick test or RAST test for latex.

19.7 Quality of Life

Not surprisingly, hand eczema has been demonstrated to have a negative impact on quality of life, and females seem to report a higher degree of discomfort than males [37]. Also psychological factors may have a significant impact on the disease, although this area needs further studies [55]. Subjects diagnosed by patch testing more than 36 months after disease onset seem to have worse quality of life scores than those diagnosed earlier, and hand eczema and generalized eczema seem to be equally detrimental to quality of life [26, 67].

19.8 Differential Diagnosis

In most cases of hand eczema the diagnosis does not provide any difficulties, but there are some pitfalls that should be avoided. A diagnosis often to be mistaken for hand eczema is dermatomycosis, which should always be suspected when hand eczema is limited to one hand. Psoriasis is more difficult to differentiate from hand eczema, but sharply demarcated extension of the lesions should raise the suspicion. Scabies in the hand and porphyria cutanea tarda may also sometimes mimic hand eczema, the latter being localized to the dorsal side of the hands [70].

References

1. Adiesh A, Meyer JD, Cherry NM (2002) Prognosis and work absence due to occupational contact dermatitis. Contact Dermatitis 46:273–279
2. Agner T (1992) Noninvasive measuring methods for the investigation of irritant patch test reactions. A study of patients with hand eczema, atopic dermatitis and controls. Acta Derm Venereol Suppl (Stockh) 1731–26
3. Agner T, Flyvholm MA, Menné T (1999) Formaldehyde allergy: a follow-up study. Am J Contact Dermat 10:12–17
4. Berndt U, Hinnen U, Iliev D, Elsner P (1999) Role of the atopy score and of single atopic features as risk factors for the development of hand eczema in trainee metal workers. Br J Dermatol 140:922–924
5. Berndt U, Hinnen U, Iliev D, Elsner P (2000) Hand eczema in metalworker trainees – an analysis of risk factors. Contact Dermatitis 43:327–332
6. Bryld LE, Agner T, Kyvik KO, Brøndsted L, Hindsberger C, Menné T (2000) Hand eczema in twins: a questionnaire investigation. Br J Dermatol 142:298–305
7. Bryld LE, Hindsberger C, Kyvik KO, Agner T, Menné T (2003a) Risk factors influencing the development of hand eczema in a population-based twin sample. Br J Dermatol 149:1214–1220
8. Bryld LE, Agner T, Menné T (2003b) Relation between vesicular eruptions on the hands and tinea pedis, atopic dermatitis and nickel allergy. Acta Derm Venereol (Stockh) 83:186–188
9. Cherry N, Meyer JD, Adisesh A (2000) Surveillance of occupational skin disease: EPIDERM and OPRA. Br J Dermatol 142:1128–1134
10. Coenraads PJ, Diepgen TL (1998) Risk for hand eczema in employees with past or present atopic dermatitis. Int Arch Occup Environ Health 71:7–13
11. Coenraads P, Diepgen TL (2003) Problems with trials and intervention studies on barrier creams and emollients at the workplace. Int Arch Occup Environ Health 76:362–366
12. Coenraads PJ, Nater JP, van der Lende R (1983) Prevalence of eczema and other dermatoses of the hands and arms in the Netherlands. Association with age and occupation. Clin Exp Dermatol 8:495–503
13. Cronin E (1991) Formaldehyde is a significant allergen in women with hand eczema. Contact Dermatitis 25:276–282
14. Danish Ministry of the Environment (1989) Statutory order no 472, 27 June 1989
15. Fregert S (1975) Occupational dermatitis in a 10-year material. Contact Dermatitis 1:96–107
16. Funke U, Fartasch M, Diepgen TL (2001) Incidence of work-related hand eczema during apprenticeship: first results of a prospective cohort study in the car industry. Contact Dermatitis 44:166–172
17. Halkier-Sorensen L (1996) Occupational skin diseases. Contact Dermatitis 35:1–120
18. Held E, Agner T (2001) Effect of moisturizers on skin susceptibility to irritants. Acta Derm Venereol (Stockh) 81:104–107
19. Held E, Mygind K, Wolff C, Gyntelberg F, Agner T (2002) Prevention of work-related skin problems: an intervention study in wet work employees. Occup Environ Med 59:556–561
20. Held E, Skoet R, Johansen JD, Agner T (2005) The hand eczema severity index (HECSI): a scoring system for clinical assessment of hand eczema. A study of inter- and intraobserver reliability. Br J Dermatol 152(2)302–307
21. Hersle K, Mobacken H (1982) Hyperkeratotic dermatitis of the palms. Br J Dermatol 107:195
22. Heydorn S, Johansen JD, Andersen KE, Bruze M, Svedman C, White I, Basketter DA, Menné T (2003) Fragrance allergy in patients with hand eczema. Contact Dermatitis 48:317–323
23. Holm JO, Veierod MB (1994) An epidemiological study of hand eczema. II. Prevalence of atopic diathesis in hairdressers, compared with a control group of teachers. Acta Derm Venereol (Stockh) [Suppl] 187:12–14
24. Holness DL, Nethercott JR (1991) Is a worker's understanding of their diagnosis an important determinant of outcome in occupational contact dermatitis? Contact Dermatitis 25:296–301
25. Jungbauer FH, van der Vleuten P, Groothoff JW, Coenraads PJ (2004) Irritant hand dermatitis: severity of disease, occupational exposure to skin irritants and preventive measures 5 years of initial diagnosis. Contact Dermatitis 50:245–251

19

26. Kadyk DL, McCarter K, Achen F, Belsito DV (2003) Quality of life in patients with allergic contact dermatitis. J Am Acad Dermatol 49:1037–1048

27. Kalimo K, Kautiainen H, Niskanen T, Niemi L (1999) Eczema school to improve compliance in an accupational dermatology clinic. Contact Dermatitis 41:315–319

28. Kang YC, Lee S, Ahn SK, Choi EH (2002) Clinical manifestations of hand eczema compared by etiological classification and irritation reactivity to SLS. J Dermatol 29:477–483

29. Kucharekova M, van de Kerkhof PC, van der Valk PG (2003) A randomized comparison of an emollient containing skinrelated lipids with a petrolatum-based emollient as adjunct in the treatment of chronic hand eczema. Contact Dermatitis 48:293–299

30. Lammintausta K, Kalimo K, Havu VK (1982) Occurrence of contact allergy and hand eczema in hospital wet work. Contact Dermatitis 8:84–90

31. Lantinga H, Nater JP, Coenraads PJ (1984) Prevalence, incidence and course of eczema on the hands and forearms in a sample of the general population. Contact Dermatitis 10:135–139

32. Leino-Arjas P, Liira J, Mutanen P (1999) Predictors and consequences of unemployment among construction workers: prospective cohort study. BMJ 4:600–605

33. Lindelof B, Wrangsjo K, Lidén S (1987) A double-blind study of Grenz ray therapy in chronic eczema of the hands. Br J Dermatol 117:77–80

34. Ling TC, Coulson IH (2002) What do trainee hairdressers know about hand dermatitis? Contact Dermatitis 47:227–231

35. Magina S, Barros MA, Ferreira JA, Mesquita-Guimaraes J (2003) Atopy, nickel sensitivity, occupation, and clinical patterns in different types of hand eczema. Am J Contact Dermat 14:63–68

36. Meding B (1990) Epidemiology of hand eczema in an industrial city. Acta DermVenereol (Stockh) [Suppl] 153:1–43

37. Meding B (2000) Differences between the sexes with regard to work-related skin disease. Contact Dermatitis 43:65–71

38. Meding B, Barregard L (2001) Validity of self-reports of hand eczema. Contact Dermatitis 45:99–103

39. Meding B, Järvholm B (2002) Hand eczema in Swedish adults: changes in prevalence between 1983 and 1996. J Invest Dermatol 118:719–723

40. Meding B, Jarvholm B (2004) Incidence of hand eczema – a polulation-based retrospective study. J Invest Dermatol 122:873–877

41. Meding B, Swanbeck G (1990a) Predictive factors for hand eczema. Contact Dermatitis 23:154–161

42. Meding B, Swanbeck G (1990b) Occupational hand eczema in an industrial city. Contact Dermatitis 22:13–22

43. Meding B, Swanbeck G (1990c) Consequences of having hand eczema. Contact Dermatitis 23(1)6–14

44. Meding B, Lidén C, Berglind N (2001) Self-diagnosed dermatitis in adults – results from a population survey in Stockholm. Contact Dermatitis 45:341–345

45. Meding B, Wrangsjo K, Brisman J, Jarvholm B (2003) Hand eczema in 45 bakers – a clinical study. Contact Dermatitis 48:7–11

47. Menné T, Bachmann E (1979) Permanent disability from skin diseases. A study of 564 patients registered over a 6 year period. Derm Beruf Umwelt 27:37–42

46. Menné T (1994) Hyperkeratotic dermatitis of the palms. In: Menné T, Maibach HI (eds) Hand eczema. CRC, Boca Raton, Fla.

48. Menné T, Hjorth N (1985) Pompholyx: dyshidrotic eczema. Semin Dermatol 2:5

49. Menné T, Borgan Ø, Green A (1982) Nickel allergy and hand dermatitis in a stratified sample of the Danish female population: an epidemiological study including a statistic appendix. Acta Derm Venereol (Stockh) 62:35–41

50. Mortz CG, Lauritsen JM, Bindslev-Jensen C, Andersen KE (2001) Prevalence of atopic dermatitis, asthma, allergic rhinitis, and hand and contact dermatitis in adolescents. The Odense adolescence cohort study on atopic diseases and dermatitis. Br J Dermatol 144:523–532

51. Mortz CG, Lauritsen JM, Bindslev-Jensen C, Andersen KE (2002) Contact allergy and allergic contact dermatitis in adolescents: prevalence measures and associations. The Odense Adolescent Cohort Study on Atopic Diseases and Dermatitis. Acta Derm Venereol (Stockh) 82:352–358

52. Nielsen NH, Menné T, Kristiansen J, Christensen JM, Borg L, Poulsen LK (1999) Effects of repeated skin exposure to low nickel concentrations: a model for allergic contact dermatitis to nickel on the hands. Br J Dermatol 141:676–682

53. Nielsen NH, Kristiansen J, Borg L, Christensen JM, Poulsen LK, Menné T (2000) Repeated exposures to cobalt or chromateon the hands of the patients with hand eczema and contact allergy to that metal. Contact Dermatitis 43:212–215

54. Nielsen NH, Linneberg A, Menné T, Madsen F, Frolund L, Dirksen A, Jørgensen T (2002) The association between contact allergy and hand eczema in two cross-sectional surveys 8 years apart. Contact Dermatitis 47:71–77

55. Niemeier V, Nippesen M, Kupfer J, Schill WB, Gieler U (2002; Psychological factors associated with hand dermatoses: which subgroups needs additionally care? Br J Dermatol 146:1031–1037

56. Nilsson E, Back O (1986) The importance of anamnestic information of atopy, metal dermatitis and earlier hand eczema for development of hand dermatitis in women in wet hospital work. Acta Derm Venereol (Stockh) 66:45–50

57. Nilsson E, Mikaelsson B, Andersson S (1985) Atopy, occupation and domestic work as risk factors for hand eczema in hospital workers. Contact Dermatitis 13:216–233

58. Pedersen LK, Johansen JD, Held E, Agner T (2004) Augmentation of skin response by exposure to a combination of allergens and irritants – a review. Contact Dermatitis 50:265–273

59. Polderman MC, Govaert JC, le Cessie S, Pavel S (2003) A double-blind placebo-controlled trial of UVA-1 in the treatment of dyshidrotic eczema. Clin Exp Dermatol 28:584–587

60. Ramsing DW, Agner T (1996a) Effect of glove occlusion on human skin. (I). short-term experimental exposure. Contact Dermatitis 34:1–5

61. Ramsing DW, Agner T (1996b) Effect of glove occlusion on human skin (II). Long-term experimental exposure. Contact Dermatitis 34:258–262

62. Rystedt I (1985a) Long term follow-up in atopic dermatitis. Acta Derm Venereol [Suppl] (Stockh) 114:117–120

63. Rystedt I (1985b) Work-related hand eczema in atopics. Contact Dermatitis 12:164–171

64. Rysted I (1985c) Hand eczema in patients with a history of atopic manifestations in childhood. Acta Derm Venereol (Stockh) 65:305–312

65. Rystedt I (1985d) Atopic background in patients with occupational hand eczema. Contact Dermatitis 12:247–254

66. Schnopp C, Remling R, Mohrenschlager M, Weigl L, Ring J, Abeck D (2002) Topical tacrolimus (FK506) and mometa-

sone furoate in treatment of dyshidrotic palmar eczema: a randomized, observer-blinded trial. J Am Acad Dermatol 46:73–77

67. Skoet R, Zachariae R, Agner T (2003) Contact dermatitis and quality of life: a structured review of the literature. Br J Dermatol 149:452–456

68. Skoet R, Olsen J, Mathiesen B, Iversen L, Johansen JD, Agner T (2004) A survey of occupational hand eczema in Denmark. Contact Dermatitis 51(4)159–166

69. Skoet R, Rothman KJ, Olsen J, Mathiesen B, Iversen L, Johansen JD, Agner T (2005) Effect of diagnoses and sub-diagnoses on severity, sick leave and loss of job in a population of occupational hand eczema patients. Br J Dermatol (in press)

70. Sommer S, Wilkinson SM (2004) Porphyria cutanea tarda-masquerading as chronic hand eczema. Acta Derm Venereol (Stockh) 84:170–171

71. Strauss RM, Gawkrodger DJ (2001) Occupational contact dermatitis in nurses with hand eczema. Contact Dermatitis 44:293–296

72. Susitaival P, Flyvholm MA, Meding B, Kanerva L, Lindberg M, Svensson A, Olafsson JH (2003) Nordic Occupational Skin Questionnaire (NOSQ-2002): a new tool for surveying occupational skin diseases and exposures. Contact Dermatitis 49:70–76

73. Svensson A, Lindberg M, Meding B, Sundberg K, Stenberg B (2002) Self-reported hand eczema: symptom-based reports do not increase the validity of diagnosis. Br J Dermatol 147:281–284

74. Swartling C, Naver H, Lindberg M, Anveden I (2002) Treatment of dyshidrotic hand dermatitis with intradermal botulinum toxin. J Am Acad Dermatol 47:667–671

75. Thaci D, Steinmeyer K, Ebelin M, Scott G, Kaufmann R (2003) Occlusive treatment of chronic hand dermatitis with pimecrolimus cream 1% results in low systemic exposure, is well tolerated, safe and effective. Dermatology 207:37–42

76. Thelmo MC, Lang W, Brooke E, Osborne BE, McCarty MA, Jorizzo JL, Fleischer A Jr (2003) An open-label pilot study to evaluate the safety and efficacy of topically applied tacrolimus ointment for the treatment of hand and/or foot eczema. J Dermatolog Treat 14:136–140

77. Thestrup-Pedersen K, Andersen KE, Menné T, Veien NK (2001) Treatment of hyperkeratotic dermatitis of the palms (eczema keratoticum) with oral acitretin. A single-blind placebo-controlled study. Acta Derm Venereol (Stockh) 81:353–355

78. Veien NK, Menné T (2003) Treatment of hand eczema. Skin Therapy Lett 8:4–7

79. Veien NK, Olholm Larsen P, Thestrup-Pedersen K, Schou G (1999) Long-term, intermittent treatment of chronic hand eczema with mometasone furoate. Br J Dermatol 140:882–886

80. Wallenhammar LM, NyfjallM, Lindberg M, Meding B (2004) Health-related quality of life and hand eczema – a comparison of two instruments, including factor analysis. J Invest Dermatol 122:1381–1389

81. Wrangsjo K, Wallenhammar LM, Ortengren U, Barregard L, Andreasson H, Bjorkner B, Karlsson S, Meding B (2001) Protective gloves in Swedish dentistry: use and side effects. Br J Dermatol 145:32–37

82. Yngveson M, Svensson Å, Isacsson Å (1998) Prevalence of self-reported hand dermatosis in upper secondary school pupils. Acta Derm Venereol (Stockh) 78:371–374

83. Zachariae C, Rastogi S, Devantier C, Menné T, Johansen J (2003) Methyldibromo glutaronitrile: clinical experience and exposure based risk assessment. Contact Dermatitis 48:150–154

84. Coenraads PJ, Van Der Walle H, Thestrup-Pedersen K, Ruzicka T, Dreno B, De La Loge C, Viala M, Querner S, Brown T, Zultak M (2005) Construction and validation of a photografic guide for assessing severity of chronic hand dermatitis. Br J Dermatol 152:296–301

19

Chapter 20

Protein Contact Dermatitis

20

Matti Hannuksela

Contents

20.1 Definition

The term protein contact dermatitis (PCD) was introduced by Niels Hjorth and Jytte Roed-Petersen in 1976 [1]. They suggested PCD to be a further category of occupational contact dermatitis in addition to irritant and allergic contact dermatitis. Patients with PCD may show positive patch or skin prick or scratch test reactions, or a combination of both, or all skin tests may remain negative. Only those with a positive scratch but negative patch test result were considered to belong to this new category of contact dermatitis. Later on, the term PCD was widened to include cases of type IV contact allergies to proteins. The most usual causes of PCD are foodstuffs and animal danders, and other animal products such as meat, milk, feces, and urine. Clinically, PCD is indistinguishable from other types of contact dermatitis. The dermatitis begins often as fingertip dermatitis.

Core Message

■ Protein contact dermatitis is caused by proteins. The clinical picture is indistinguishable from that of other types of contact dermatitis. The patients may show positive immediate or delayed reactions in skin prick, scratch or patch tests, or the skin tests may remain negative.

20.2 Clinical Features

The first sign of PCD is often eczematous dermatitis in the tips of the fingers that are in touch with the causative foodstuff, animal or some other proteinaceous item. Hjorth and Roed-Petersen were not the first to describe the phenomenon. The entity was well known in the 1930s and 1940s especially among people working in dairy farming [2]. Wheal and flare reactions (i.e., immunologic contact urticaria) resulting in eczematous dermatitis are also seen. Dermatitis is usually sharply restricted to the contact area, and eczematids are seen only rarely. Eczema heals usually rapidly when the causative agent is avoided. It seems obvious that chronic forms of dermatitis do not occur, or at least such cases are rare.

Core Message

■ Protein contact dermatitis is usually restricted sharply to the area involved. It may begin directly as eczema, or the first sign is contact urticaria resulting in eczematous dermatitis.

20.3 Causes of PCD

The list of causes of occupational contact urticaria and PCD in Finland in 2002 included animal danders and other material of animal origin (50 out of the total of 108 cases), various cereals (27 cases), natural rubber latex (9 cases), trees and other plants (8 cases), foodstuffs (4 cases), and miscellaneous causes (10 cases) [3]. The total number of occupational skin diseases in 2002 was 965, 11.2% of which were 108 cases of contact urticaria and PCD.

The most common and most important causes of PCD are listed in Table 1, cow dander being probably one of the most frequent.

Table 1. Causes of protein contact dermatitis

Animals
  Dander
  Saliva, milk, blood, urine, feces
  Meat, internal organs such as liver and gut
  Amnion fluid
  Skin

Fishes and crustaceans
  Mackerel, eel, codfish, plaice, herring, salmon, cuttlefish
  Shrimps, lobsters, crabs
  Pearl oysters

Plants and plant products
  Lettuce, chicory salad, spinach
  Onion, chives
  Cucumber, melon
  Potato, tomato, paprika
  Carrot, parsley, horseradish
  Asparagus
  Fruits
  Spices
  Weeds, grasses
  Verbena
  Natural rubber latex

Insects, mites and spiders
  Cockroach
  Storage mites
  House dust mites
  Silk
  Maggots (*Calliphora vomitoria*), chironomids (nonbiting midgets)
  Spiders

Other causes
  Cellulolytic enzymes
  Pollens
  Malassezia furfur
  Molds
  Mushrooms (e.g., *Lentinus edodes, Pleurotus ostreatus*)

A current hand dermatosis was reported by 10.7% of 5266 female and by 4.2% of 5581 male farmers in Finland [4]. Most dermatoses were eczemas. A total of 138 farmers with self-reported hand dermatosis were subjected to further investigation. Skin prick and patch tests were both made in 106 farmers. Cow dander elicited positive reactions in 41 (39%) of them, cow dander thus being the most common cause of their hand dermatitis.

Natural rubber latex (NRL) is a well-known cause of contact urticaria. It produces also PCD without signs of urticaria [5, 6].

> **Core Message**
>
> ■ The list of causes of PCD is long, including mostly animal and plant allergens. The allergenic proteins remain poorly identified.

20.4 Mechanisms of PCD

Irritation may be the commonest pathogenetic mechanism leading to eczematous dermatitis caused by foodstuffs (Table 2) [7]. Many housewives and other food handlers have found that tomato and paprika in particular irritate the skin. Spices, on the other hand, are capable of producing both immunologic and nonimmunologic contact urticaria and PCD. Immediate contact dermatitis appears as tiny eczematous vesicles, and the process may result in dermatitis within days. Erythema multiforme is possible from, e.g., NRL [8] but the mechanism remains unclear. Reaction between immunoglobulin E (IgE) and high-affinity IgE receptors on Langerhans cells is probably the main mechanism resulting in eczema but the classical delayed-type allergy mechanism is also possible.

Table 2. Possible mechanisms of protein contact dermatitis (*PCD*) and contact urticaria (CU)

Type of PCD	Mechanism and mediators
Irritation	Mechanism is unknown
Nonimmunologic CU	Mostly unknown. Prostaglandins deal often with the reaction
Immunologic CU	1. IgE on mast cells. Histamine and other mediators are released
	2. IgG on mast cells (?)
	3. Unknown
Eczematous dermatitis	1. Classical delayed allergy
	2. IgE on Langerhans cells
	3. Prolonged or repeated CU
Erythema multiforme	IgE-mediated?

20

Core Message

■ Several immunologic and nonimmunologic mechanisms may lead to dermatitis known as PCD. Specific IgE is obviously crucial in most reactions.

20.5 Atopic Dermatitis – a Special Type of PCD?

Type I and IV hypersensitivities to house dust mites (*Dermatophagoides pteronyssinus* and *D. farinae*) and their role in atopic dermatitis (AD) have been a matter of major interest since the 1980s [9]. In AD, positive patch test (PT) reactions to purified house dust mite allergens in petrolatum are seen more often than positive skin prick test (SPT) reactions, and interestingly also in patients with only respiratory symptoms [10]. Recent findings suggest that the IgE molecule has a key role, at least as an amplifier, in the atopy PT reaction [9]. Other contact allergens, the role of which in the pathogenesis of AD has been studied during the past two decades, include, e.g., pollens and *Malassezia furfur* [11–13].

Delayed allergy to *Malassezia furfur* seems to play role in the type of AD known as head and shoulders [12], but the role of the house dust mite remains controversial [14–17]. In some studies, the amount of dust mite allergens in the bed does not seem to show any correlation with the extent and severity of the patients' dermatitis [16, 17]. Airborne allergens such as pollens may worsen AD but the route of allergen exposure is the airways rather than the skin.

Core Message

■ House dust mites, pollens and *Malassezia* allergens elicit often positive reaction in PTs in AD patients. *Malassezia* allergy probably plays role in the head and shoulders AD but the significance of mite allergens is a controversial matter. Airborne allergens such as pollens are less likely to worsen AD by direct skin contact.

20.6 Diagnostic Tests in PCD

Ordinary SPTs, prick-prick test, scratch test, 20-min PTs, 24- to 72-h PTs, open PT, and use test comprise the arsenal of skin tests needed in PCD (see Chaps. 22, 23, and 26). Measuring the amount of specific IgE in serum [radioallergosorbent test (RAST) and RAST inhibition and others], basophil degranulation test (histamine release), and Western blot are also sometimes utilized. The significance of positive test results should be decided on clinical grounds separately in every case.

SPT is intended for standardized, commercial allergens. The scratch test is more suitable for nonstandardized allergens. Fresh fruits and vegetables are usually tested with the prick-prick method. The scratch-chamber test is seldom used because of its low specificity [18].

The 20-min PT is rarely used. Hjorth and Roed-Petersen [1] found only six positive responses in 20-min PTs in 33 kitchen workers, while a 48-h PT was positive 21 times. The 20-min PT did not add any further information to SPT, scratch test, and 48-h PT. Susitaival et al. [19] made 20-min PTs with cow dander and found positive results in patients with negative results in SPT and 24-h PT.

Only a few protein allergens for PTs are standardized. Most often the suspected materials are tested as such. As to the vehicle, petrolatum seems to be more suitable than other vehicles.

Studies comparing various occlusion times are few. Holm et al. [9] found the 74-h PT to be more sensitive than 24-h and 48-h PTs when testing house dust mite allergens, but the clinical relevance of the tests with longer occlusion times remains unresolved.

Open PT means simply placing the suspected material on the skin or rubbing it gently. Previously diseased skin is more prone to react than healthy skin. Hjorth and Roed-Petersen [1] reported three cases showing dyshidrotic (eczema) vesicles in 20 min from fish or shellfish. Tomato caused vesicular reaction in 20 min in one patient, and potato and carrot a delayed vesicular reaction in rub tests in a study on food handler dermatitis by Niinimäki [20].

Core Message

■ Immediate reactivity to proteins in PCD can usually be verified in scratch tests or prick tests. The 20-min PT may produce some extra information. Open PT or rub test on previously diseased skin may show a 20-min or delayed eczematous or vesicular reaction without contact urticaria. RAST and other tests for specific IgE in the serum are sometimes helpful.

20.7 Treatment of PCD

PCD shows no tendency to become chronic. Avoiding the causative material usually leads to rapid healing of the eruption. In severe cases, corticosteroid creams or ointments speed up the healing process.

References

1. Hjorth N, Roed-Petersen J (1976) Occupational protein contact dermatitis in food handlers. Contact Dermatitis 2: 28–42
2. Epstein S (1948) Milker's eczema. J Allergy 19:333–341
3. Riihimäki H, Kurppa K, Karjalainen A, Aalto L, Jolanki R, Keskinen H, Mäkinen I, Saalo A (2003) Ammattitaudit (Occupational diseases) 2002. Työterveyslaitos, Helsinki, pp 68–70
4. Susitaival P, Husman L, Horsmanheimo M, Notkola V, Husman K. (1994) Prevalence of hand dermatoses among Finnish farmers. Scand J Work Environ Health 20:206–212
5. Sommer S, Wilkinson SM, Beck MH, English JS, Gawkrodger DJ, Green C (2002) Type IV hypersensitivity to natural rubber latex: results of a multicentre study. Br J Dermatol 146:114–117
6. Kanerva L (2000) Occupational protein contact dermatitis and paronychia from natural rubber latex. J Eur Acad Dermatol Venereol 14:504–506
7. Hannuksela M (1997) Immediate and delayed type protein contact dermatitis. In: Amin S, Lahti A, Maibach HI (eds) Contact urticaria syndrome. CRC, Boca Raton, Fla., pp 279–287
8. Bourrain J-L, Woodward C, Dumas V, Caperan D, Beani J-C, Amblard P (1996) Natural rubber latex contact dermatitis with features of erythema multiforme. Contact Dermatitis 35:55–56
9. Holm L, Matuseviciene G, Scheynius A, Tengvall Linder M (2004) Atopy patch test with house dust mite allergen – an IgE-mediated reaction? Allergy 59:874–882
10. Fuiano N, Incorvaia C (2003) Comparison of skin prick test and atopy patch test with dust mite extracts in patients with respiratory symptoms or atopic eczema dermatitis syndrome. Allergy 58:828
11. Reitamo S, Visa K, Kähönen K, Käyhkö K, Stubb S, Salo OP (1986) Eczematous reactions in atopic patients caused by epicutaneous testing with inhalant allergens. Br J Dermatol 114:303–309
12. Johansson C, Sandström MH, Bartosik J, Särnhult T, Christiansen J, Zargari A, Bäck O, Wahlgren CF, Faergemann J, Scheynius A, Tengvall Linder M (2003) Atopy patch test reactions to *Malassezia* allergens differentiate subgroups of atopic dermatitis patients. Br J Dermatol 148:479–488
13. De Groot AC, Young E (1989) The role of contact allergy to aeroallergens in atopic dermatitis. Contact Dermatitis 21:209–214
14. Shah D, Hales J, Cooper D, Camp R (2002) Recognition of pathogenically relevant house dust mite hypersensitivity in adults with atopic dermatitis: a new approach? J Allergy Clin Immunol 109:1012–1018
15. Beltrani VS (2003) The role of house dust mites and other aeroallergens in atopic dermatitis. Clin Dermatol 21:177–182
16. Gutgesell C, Heise S, Seubert S, Domhof S, Brunner E, Neumann C (2001) Double-blind placebo-controlled house dust mite control measures in adult patients with atopic dermatitis. Br J Dermatol 145:70–74
17. Koopman LP, Strien RT, Kerkhof M, Wijga A, Smit HA, de Jongste JC, Gerritsen J, Aalberse RC, Brunekreef B, Neijens HJ (2002) Plecabo-controlled trial of house dust mite-impermeable mattress covers: effect on symptoms in early childhood. Am J Respir Crit Care Med 166:307–313
18. Osterballe M, Scheller R, Stahl Skov P, Andersen KE, Bindslev-Jensen C (2003) Diagnostic value of scratch-chamber test, skin prick test, histamine release and specific IgE in birch-allergic patients with oral allergy syndrome to apple. Allergy 58:950–953
19. Susitaival P, Husman L, Hollmén A, Horsmanheimo M, Husman K, Hannuksela M (1995) Hand eczema in Finnish farmers. A questionnaire-based clinical study. Contact Dermatitis 32:150–155
20. Niinimäki A (1987) Scratch-chamber tests in food handler dermatitis. Contact Dermatitis 16:11–20

20

Chapter 21

Noneczematous Contact Reactions 21

ANTHONY GOON, CHEE-LEOK GOH

Contents

21.1 Introduction

Cutaneous contact reactions may present as noneczematous eruptions. Several noneczematous eruptions resulting from contact reactions have been described. The exact mechanisms of these eruptions are unknown. It is important for the clinician to recognize these noneczematous contact reactions, as often the cause can be confirmed by simple patch testing and unnecessary investigations into systemic diseases can be avoided. Contact reactions manifesting as noneczematous eruptions include the following:

- Erythema multiforme-like eruption (urticarial papular and plaque eruption)
- Pigmented purpuric eruption
- Lichen planus-like or lichenoid eruption
- Bullous eruption
- Papular and nodular eruption
- Granulomatous eruption
- Pustular eruption
- Erythematous and exfoliative eruption
- Scleroderma-like eruption
- Pigmented contact dermatitis
- Lymphomatoid contact dermatitis
- Vascular occlusive contact dermatitis

21.2 Erythema Multiforme-like Reaction (Urticarial Papular and Plaque Eruptions)

This is an important contact reaction, as it is often mistaken for erythema multiforme from various systemic causes. Several contact allergens including metals, topical medicaments, woods, and industrial chemicals have been reported to cause "erythema multiforme-like" eruptions (see Table 1). In these reports the allergic nature of the reactions can be confirmed by positive patch test reactions. These eruptions have been described as "target-like," "erythematovesicular," and "urticarial" by different authors. In Asian countries such reactions have been reported to be due to contact allergy to proflavine and trinitrotoluene.

21.2.1 Clinical Features

The characteristic presentation is usually an urticarial eruption about 1–14 days after an episode of aller-

Table 1. Reported causes of UPPE

Woods and plants
   Dalbergia nigra (Brazilian rosewood)
   Machaerium scleroxylon (pao ferro)
   Eucalyptus saligna (gum)
   Toxicodendron radicans (poison ivy)
   Primula obconica
   Artemisia vulgaris (common mugwort)

Topical medicaments
   Ethylenediamine
   Sulfanilamide
   Pyrrolnitrin
   Furazolidone
   Sulfonamide
   Nifuroxime
   Promethazine
   Scopolamine
   Balsam of Peru
   Hydrobromide
   p-Phenylenediamine
   Clioquinol (Vioform)
   Mafenide acetate
   Diaminodiphenylmethane
   Proflavine
   Mefenesin
   Vitamin E
   Econazole
   Diphencyprone
   Nitrogen mustard
   Nitroglycerin
   Tea tree oil

Metals and chemicals
   Nickel
   Cobalt
   9-Bromofluorene precursors
   Phenylsulfone derivatives
   Epoxy resin
   p-Chlorobenzene sulfonylglycolic acid
   Nitrile
   Formaldehyde
   Trichloroethylene
   Trinitrotoluene
   Dimethoate
   Eumulgin L
   Bisphenol A
   Costus resinoid

gic contact dermatitis. The primary site may be eczematous but becomes urticarial within a few days. This will be followed by erythematous urticarial papular and/or plaque eruptions (Fig. 1) around the primary contact site. The eruption often also appears at distant sites. This lasts longer than the primary ec-zematous lesion and tends to persist after the clearance of the initial dermatitis. The lesions are usually pruritic.

21.2.2 Patch Test

Contact allergy to the allergens can be confirmed by a positive patch test. The patch test reactions are eczematous and often vesicular or bullous, but may occasionally be urticarial.

21.2.3 Histology

The histology of these lesions does not show the classical changes of erythema multiforme. The epidermis is either normal or shows mild spongiosis with upper dermal edema and a mild perivascular lymphohistiocytic infiltrate. Vacuolar degeneration of the basal cells is rarely present. There is no epidermal necrosis or interface infiltration, as are present in erythema multiforme (Fig. 2).

21.2.4 Differentiation from Classical Erythema Multiforme

Besides the occasional target-like lesions, the morphology, clinical course, and history of erythema-multiforme-like eruptions of contact allergy are not characteristic of classical erythema multiforme. Lesions of erythema multiforme tend to have an acral distribution, appear in crops and are almost all target-like. The term "urticarial papular and plaque eruption" (UPPE) of contact allergy was suggested to describe such an eruption [1]. UPPE will be used synonymously with erythema-multiforme-like eruption in the rest of this chapter.

The exact mechanism of UPPE is unknown. The eruption appears to represent an allergic immune complex reaction. The allergens are probably absorbed percutaneously, causing an allergic contact dermatitis with concurrent immune complex reaction.

21.2.5 Causes

Allergens reported to cause erythema multiforme-like eruptions include: (1) woods and plants, (2) topical medications, and (3) chemicals. Table 1 lists the known causes of UPPE.

21

Fig. 1.
Erythema-multiforme-like eruption from contact allergy to trinitrotoluene. Note urticular papular and plaque eruption (*UPPE*)

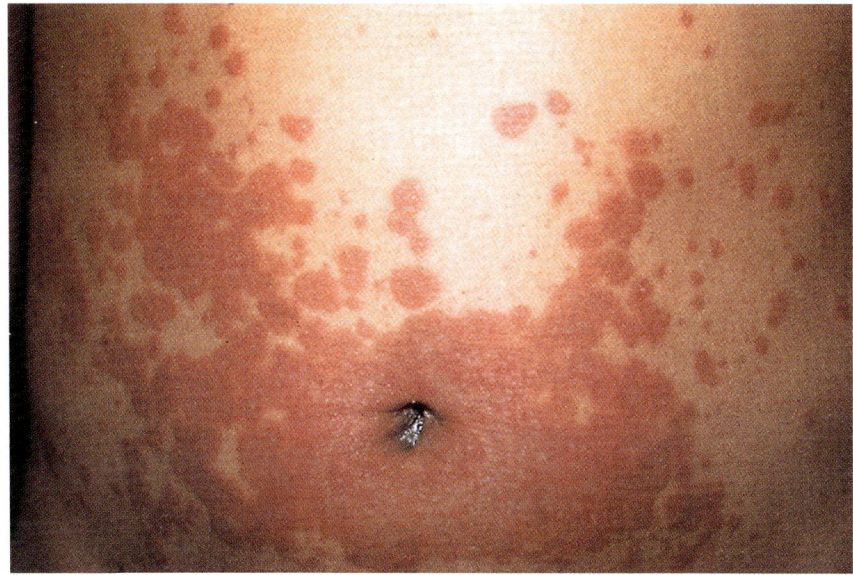

Fig. 2.
Histology of a UPPE lesion from the patient in Fig. 1. Mild upper dermal edema and lymphohistiocytic infiltrates with normal epidermis. Note absence of changes typical of erythema multiforme

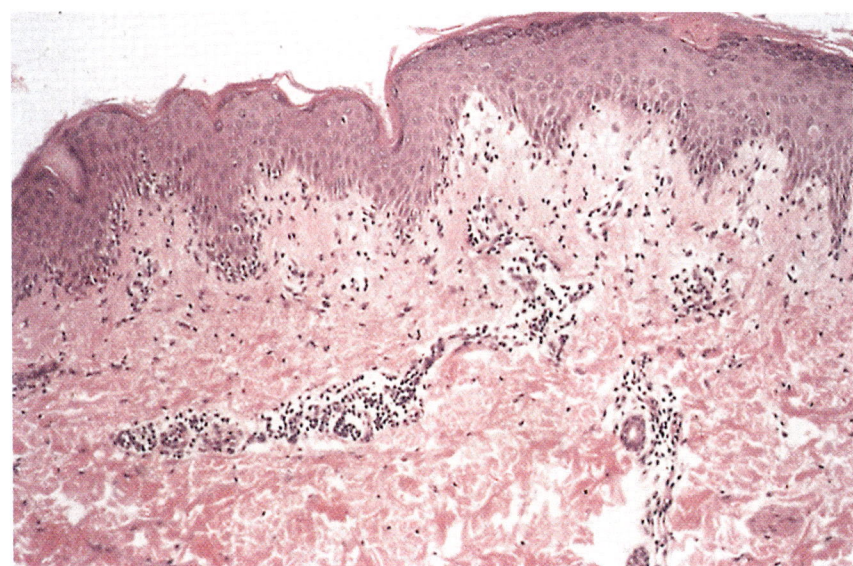

21.2.5.1 Woods and Plants

Tropical woods, including Brazilian rosewood (*Dalbergia nigra*), pao ferro (*Machaerium scleroxylon*), and *Eucalyptus saligna* have been reported to cause occupational UPPE in three carpenters [2]. The allergen in pao ferro is *R*-3,4-dimethoxy-dalbergione. Patients wearing wooden bracelets [3] and pendants [4] made from *Dalbergia nigra* and hobbyists handling pao ferro wood [5] have been reported to develop UPPE. The specific chemical antigen in Brazilian rosewood is the quinone *R*-4-methoxy-dalbergione. The antigen in pao ferro is *R*-3,4-dimethoxy-dalber-

gione [6]. Plants reported to cause UPPE include poison ivy (*Toxicodendron radicans*) [7, 8], primula (*Primula obconica*) [9], mugwort (*Artemisia vulgaris*) [10] and Compositae weeds [11].

21.2.5.2 Topical Medicaments

Ethylenediamine [12, 13], pyrrolnitrin, sulfonamide, promethazine, balsam of Peru, diaminodiphenylmethane and clioquinol (Vioform) have been reported as the contact allergens responsible for such eruptions. Some of the patients reported had vasculitic or purpuric lesions. Other implicated medicaments include a cream containing mafenide acetate [14], mephenesin [15, 16] (Fig. 3), econazole [17], vitamin E [18], nitroglycerin patches [19], tea tree oil [20], and topical nitrogen mustard. In Asia, proflavin [21] has been reported to cause purpuric contact dermatitis and UPPE when applied to abrasions.

UPPE due to diphencyprone was also described in a patient who received the sensitizer as immunotherapy for plane warts on the face [22].

Medicaments that are applied to mucosae are rapidly absorbed systemically and may enhance the skin and systemic sensitization process. UPPE occurred in a patient who applied sulfanilamide cream for vulvovaginitis; she had a positive patch test reaction to the sulfanilamide cream and also developed UPPE after ingesting sulfanilamide [23]. UPPE was also described in contact allergy to furazolidone- and nifuroxime-containing suppositories in another patient. A flare-up of the eruption developed when she was patch tested to the suppository. UPPE was also reported from contact allergy to eyedrops. Two case reports of Stevens–Johnson syndrome from contact allergy to sulfonamide-containing eyedrops were de-

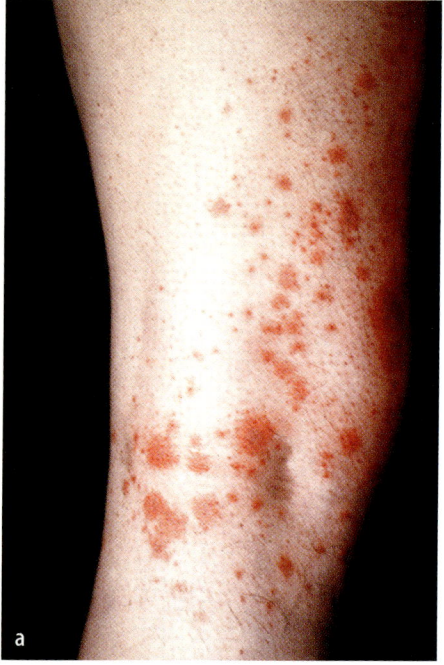

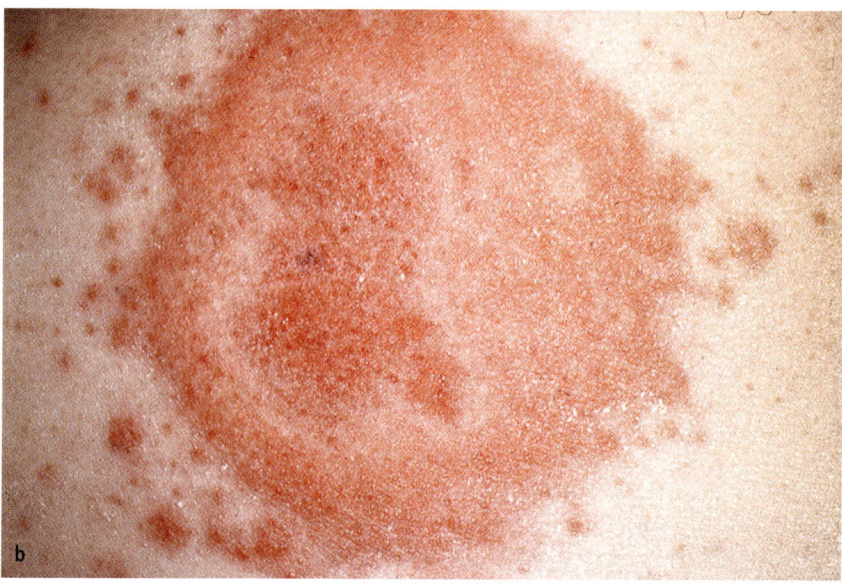

Fig. 3a, b.
Erythema-multiforme-like lesions on the leg after use of an ointment containing mephenesin (**a**). The patch test with the active ingredient was strongly positive (**b**) (courtesy of P.J. Frosch)

21

scribed [24, 25]. Another patient developed UPPE from scopolamine hydrobromide eyedrops; his eruption recurred on rechallenge to the eyedrops [26].

21.2.5.3 Metals and Chemicals

Metals

UPPE may be a manifestation of contact allergy to some metals and industrial chemicals. Calnan first described UPPE in the secondary spread of nickel dermatitis [27]. Cook reported UPPE in a 13-year-old girl following allergic contact dermatitis from nickel and cobalt in the metal studs of her jeans [28]. A similar eruption was reported in a garment worker who developed nickel dermatitis on her hands from nickel-plated scissors; she had a vesiculopapular patch test reacting to nickel salt and during patch testing her hand dermatitis and UPPE reappeared [29]. UPPE in a patient with nickel dermatitis due to a metallic necklace was also reported [30].

Noneczematous urticarioid dermatitis involving the axillae from contact allergy to Eumulgin L (cetearyl alcohol) in deodorant has been reported. Patch test to the emulsifier was strongly positive [31].

Laboratory Chemicals

UPPE from laboratory chemicals was first described by Cavendish in 1940 in a student who developed recurrent eruptions after 9-bromofluorene exposure. During patch testing, one of the control patients became sensitized to the chemical and developed UPPE 13 days after the patch test [32]. Powell also reported a student with a similar eruption due to 9-bromofluorene and, similarly, one control patient became sensitized to the chemical [33]. De Feo also described how, out of 250 chemistry students, 24 developed localized acute contact eczema followed by generalized UPPE, while synthesizing 9-bromofluorene in the laboratory. They had positive patch tests to the chemical [34]. Roed-Petersen reported a chemistry student who developed UPPE on the exposed skin from a phenyl sulfone derivative that he was synthesizing. He had a strong positive reaction to the compound [35].

Industrial Chemicals

Several industrial chemicals have been suspected to cause UPPE. Nethercott et al. reported UPPE in four workers handling printed circuit boards. Liver involvement was documented in three of the workers. Two of the workers had a positive reaction to formaldehyde and formaldehyde was implicated as the cause of the eruptions [36]. Phoon et al. described five workers who developed UPPE and Stevens–Johnson syndrome after exposure to trichloroethylene in an electronics factory. Three workers had hepatitis and one died of hepatic failure. A patch test to trichloroethylene on one worker was negative. The eruption was suspected to be due to a hypersensitivity reaction to trichloroethylene from percutaneous and/or transrespiratory absorption of trichloroethylene [37].

UPPE was also reported in a worker with allergic contact dermatitis from trinitrotoluene; the patient had a strong eczematous patch test reaction to trinitrotoluene [38]. It was recently reported to occur in a warehouseman allergic to dimethoate, an organophosphorous insecticide and acaricide [39]. Other industrial chemicals include epoxy resin and *para*-chlorobenzene sulfonylglycolic acid nitrile.

Others

More recently, there have been reports of UPPE due to paraphenylenediamine in henna tattoos [40], rubber gloves [41], cutting oil [42], and costus resinoid [43].

> ### Core Message
>
> ■ A persistent erythema multiforme-like reaction may occur after an episode of allergic contact dermatitis from woods and plants, medicaments, metals, and chemicals. The histology of these lesions does not show the classical changes of epidermal necrosis or interface infiltration that are present in erythema multiforme.

21.3 Pigmented Purpuric Eruption

Contact allergy may present as a purpuric eruption. The eruption is usually asymptomatic, macular and purpuric, with or without preceding itch or erythema (Fig. 4). The purpuric eruption then becomes brownish and fades away. The exact mechanism of the reaction is unknown.

Allergic contact dermatitis in response to isopropyl-*N*-phenyl-*p*-phenylenediamine (IPPD) in rubber clothing [44], rubber boots [45], rubber diving suits, elasticized shorts, rubberized support bandages [46] and rubberized brassieres [47] has been reported, manifest as contact purpuric eruptions.

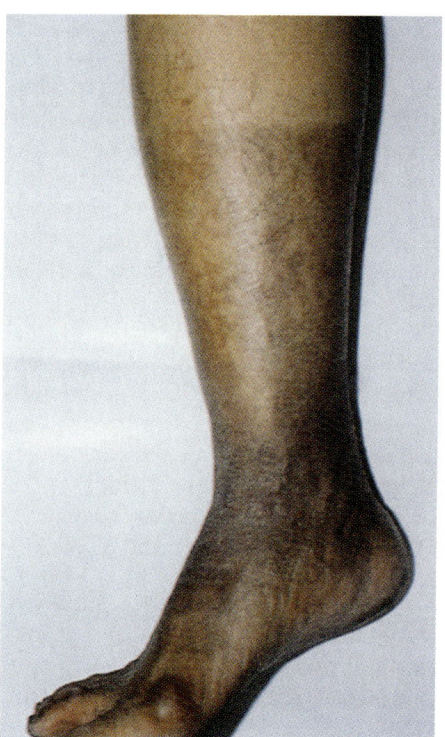

Fig. 4. Pigmented purpuric dermatitis from isopropyl-*N*-phenyl-p-phenylenediamine (*IPPD*) in rubber boots

Allergic contact dermatitis from paraphenylene-diamine after handling black hats [48] has been reported to be associated with a purpuric eruption. Raw wool was also reported to cause a contact purpuric eruption [49].

Contact allergy to balsam of Peru [50] and proflavine [21] in medicaments, and the azo dye Disperse Blue 85 [51] in naval uniforms may also manifest as a purpuric eruption. More recently, contact allergy to the azo dyes Disperse Blue 106 and Disperse Blue 124 [52] has been reported to cause progressive pigmented purpura.

An acute nonpruritic eruption with focal purpura from contact allergy to 5% benzoyl peroxide in acne gel has been reported. Patch tests with benzoyl peroxide in petrolatum and the acne gel containing benzoyl peroxide produced similar reactions. Alterations of the capillary endothelium included obliteration of the lumina with perivascular mononuclear cell infiltrates, with no epidermal alterations in the histology [53].

Emla cream, a topical anesthetic, has been reported to cause toxic purpuric contact reactions [54, 55]. Four patients were reported to develop toxic purpuric reaction 30 min after Emla application before the treatment of molluscum contagiosum. Patch tests

with Emla and its individual ingredients were negative. The authors concluded that the purpuric reaction was not of an allergic nature. Possibly, it was caused by a toxic effect on the capillary endothelium [54].

The sap of *Agave americana*, a popular ornamental plant, has been reported to cause purpuric irritant contact dermatitis [56].

Core Message

■ Contact reactions from black rubber, dyes, and medicaments may present usually as asymptomatic macular purpuric eruptions that become brownish and fade away. These may be allergic, toxic or irritant in nature.

21.4 Lichen Planus-like or Lichenoid Eruption

Lichenoid eruptions mimicking lichen planus may be a manifestation of allergic contact dermatitis to some color developers. The eruptions present as

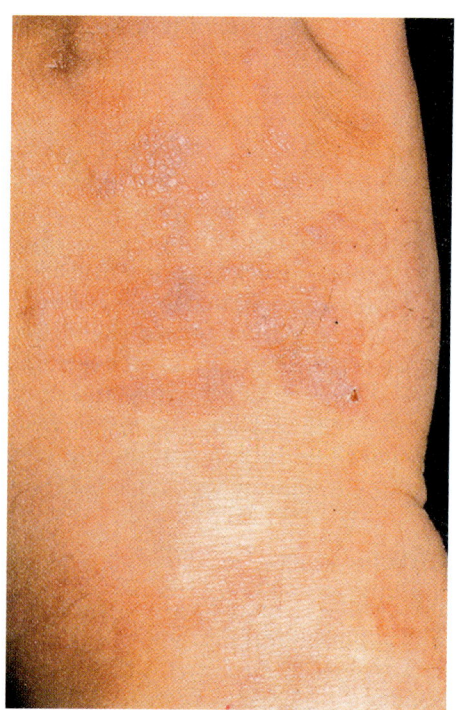

Fig. 5. Lichenoid eruption on the back of the hand from color developer (CD 4) (courtesy of P.J. Frosch)

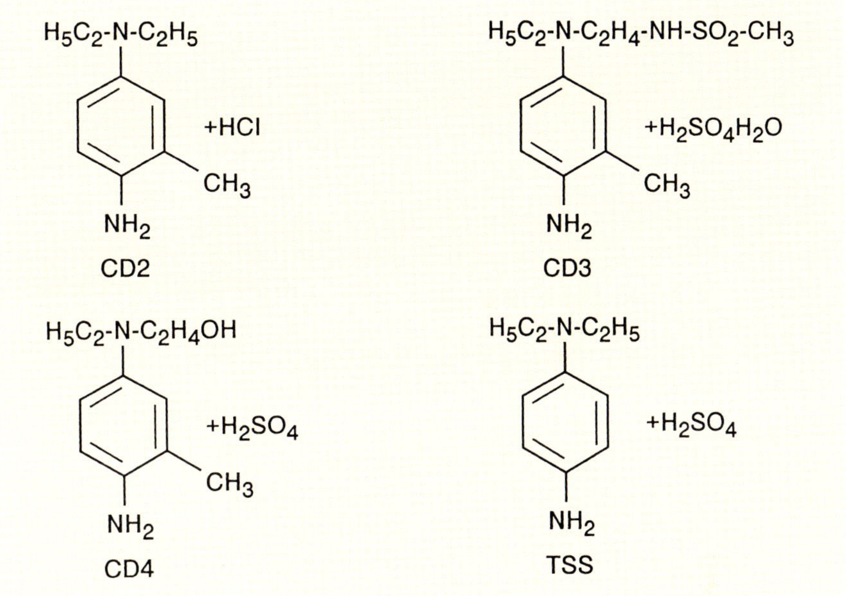

Fig. 6.
Contact sensitizing color developers

itchy dusky or violaceous papules or plaques on areas of skin exposed to the allergen (Fig. 5). The hands and forearms are commonly affected sites. Unlike idiopathic lichen planus, the skin lesions clear within a few weeks upon cessation of contact with the causative allergen.

Several color developers have been reported to cause such eruptions (Fig. 6). Kodak CD2 (4-*N*, *N*-diethyl-2 methylphenylenediamine monohydrochloride), Kodak CD3 [4-(*N*-ethyl-*N*-2-methanesulphonylaminoethyl)-2-methyl-phenylenediamine sesquisulfate monohydrate], Agfa TSS (4-amino-*N*-diethylaniline sulfate), Ilford MI 210 [*N*-ethyl-*N*(5-hydroxyamyl) *p*-phenylenediamine hydrogen sulfate] and Kodak CD4 [2-amino-5-*N*-ethyl-*N*-(β-hydroxyethyl)-aminotoluene sulfate] are reported allergens [57]. Mandel reported that 9 out of 11 workers with contact allergy to color developer showed lichen-planus-like eruptions [58], but Fry reported a lower rate of 7 out of 20 patients, the remainder presenting with eczematous reactions [59].

21.4.1 Histology

The histology of lichen-planus-like eruptions from color developers may show features compatible with lichen planus or a nonspecific chronic superficial perivascular dermatitis. Some reports indicate that the histology in the majority of patients shows changes compatible with lichen planus [60–63], but others indicate that a nonspecific chronic dermatitis change is more common [55, 58]. In Fry's report, out of seven patients with lichenoid lesions biopsied, one showed changes of eczema, two showed lichenoid dermatitis, and two showed lichen planus changes [58].

21.4.2 Mechanism

There is controversy about the etiology of the lichen-planus-like eruption from color developers. Lichenoid eruptions may be due to direct contact with the chemicals on the skin producing allergic contact dermatitis, but may also represent eruptions resulting from systemic absorption of the allergen [59, 61]. A combination of both mechanisms may be responsible.

Other allergens reported to cause lichenoid eruptions include metallic copper [63] and mercury [64] from dental amalgam. These patients presented with lichen-planus-like lesions on the buccal mucosa. Both had positive patch test reactions to the respective allergen. Nickel salts were also reported to cause lichenoid dermatitis [65, 66]. Lembo et al. reported a chronic lichenoid eruption in a schoolboy from aminoglycoside-containing creams. Biopsy showed a band-like mononuclear upper dermal infiltrate. Patch tests showed a lichenoid reaction to neomycin [67]. A lichenoid reaction has also been reported to epoxy resin [68].

Other contact allergens more recently reported to cause lichenoid eruptions include *para*-substituted amino compounds in temporary henna tattoos [69] and *Parthenium hysterophorus* [70].

Core Message

■ Lichenoid eruptions clinically and histologically resembling lichen planus may be due to allergic contact dermatitis from color developers, metals, aminoglycosides, epoxy resin, and other agents.

21.5 Bullous Eruption

Contact allergy to cinnamon produced bullous eruptions in a female in Singapore after she used cinnamon powder to treat scars on her lower limbs [71]. The morphology and histology of the eruption resembled bullous pemphigoid. However, direct immunofluorescence studies were negative. Patch test showed a strong positive reaction to the cinnamon powder, cinnamic aldehyde and cinnamic alcohol. Her eruption was attributed to the latter allergens present in the cinnamon powder. The exact mechanism of the cell-mediated hypersensitivity reaction is unknown.

Contact allergy to nickel and its oral ingestion has also been reported to cause dyshidrosiform pemphigoid [72].

Bullous irritant reactions may also occur upon application of cantharidin, a vesicant produced by beetles in the order Coleoptera [73], which has a long history in both folk and traditional medicine.

Core Message

■ Bullous contact allergic reactions have been reported from cinnamon and nickel while bullous contact irritant reactions may be due to vesicants from Coleoptera beetles.

21.6 Nodular and Papular Eruption

Contact allergy to gold is known to cause chronic papular and nodular skin eruptions. Such eruptions tend to be on the earlobes of sensitized individuals after the wearing of pierced-type gold earrings. The eruptions characteristically persist for months after the patients have avoided contact with metallic gold [74–79]. Patch test reactions to gold and gold salts in these patients are usually strongly positive. In some patients, the positive reactions to gold salts tend to be indurated and persist for months. Occasionally the patch test may evoke an infiltrative lymphoblastic reaction, which persists for months [75, 79–81]. The histology of these eruptions or its patch test reaction usually shows a dense lymphomonocytic infiltrate mimicking mycosis fungoides, but mycosis fungoides cells are absent. The cellular infiltrate consists mainly of suppressor/cytotoxic T-cells [80]. Dental amalgam allergy was reported to cause a nodular eruption mimicking oral carcinoma [82].

Core Message

■ Chronic papular and nodular skin eruptions due to gold may sometimes last for months. A nodular eruption due to dental amalgam allergy may mimic oral carcinoma.

21.7 Granulomatous Eruption

Skin injury from zirconium, silica, magnesium, and beryllium may cause granulomas. Some reactions are usually due to a delayed-type allergic reaction that can be confirmed by patch testing while others are nonallergic reactions.

Zirconium granuloma was first reported to be a manifestation of allergic contact dermatitis from zirconium compounds in deodorants [83–85]. Clinically, the granulomatous eruptions appear 4–6 weeks after applying the zirconium compounds and are usually confined to the area of application, e.g., the axillae. Eczema is usually present but pruritus is minimal. Patients with the eruptions have associated positive patch test reactions to zirconium compounds. The histology shows epithelioid cells and may be indistinguishable from sarcoidosis. Allergic granulomatous eruptions were also reported in sensitized patients who use zirconium compounds to treat *Rhus* dermatitis [86–89].

Cutaneous granulomas may also occur following immunization with vaccines containing aluminum hydroxide, such patients having positive patch tests to aluminum chloride and/or aluminum Finn chambers. In 1 series of 21 children, the granulomas of 11 improved with time [90].

Chromium and mercurial pigments in tattoos can produce allergic granulomatous reactions. Mercury (red cinnabar, mercury sulfide-red pigment), chromium (chromium oxide powder-green pigment), cobalt (cobaltous aluminate-blue pigment) and cadmium (cadmium sulfide-yellow pigment) are known causative agents [91]. An unknown substance in purple tattoo pigment has also been reported to cause a granulomatous reaction [92, 93]. Granulomatous reactions may be preceded by or associated with eczematous reactions (Fig. 7). The lesions are usually nonpruritic. Histology shows typical granulomas. These patients usually have positive patch test reactions to the respective metallic salts.

A young woman developed persistent nodules at sites of ear piercing with gold earrings and patch testing demonstrated a positive allergic response to gold sodium thiosulfate. Histological examination of the nodules demonstrated a prominent sarcoidal-type granulomatous tissue reaction. This is in contrast to previous reports of lymphocytoma-cutis-type histology and was associated with the occurrence of epithelioid granulomata at the site of a strongly positive and long-lasting patch test reaction [94].

Contact orofacial granulomatosis has been reported to be caused by delayed hypersensitivity to gold and mercury [95]. Sarcoidal allergic contact dermatitis due to palladium following ear piercing and ex-

udative granulomatous reactions to hyaluronic acid (Hylaform) have also been reported [96].

21.8 Pustular Eruption

Metallic salts, e.g., nickel, copper, arsenic, and mercury salts, have been reported to cause transient sterile pustular reactions [97]. These reactions have also been reported following contact allergy to black rubber [98]. The significance of such pustular reactions remains speculative. Stone and Johnson explained that such reactions may represent an enhanced reaction of prior inflammation rather than an irritant or allergic reaction [99]. Atopics are predisposed to such reactions [100]. Wahlberg and Maibach believe that such reactions are usually irritant in nature but may also be a manifestation of allergic reactions [101].

Allergic contact dermatitis from a nitrofurazone-containing cream manifested as a pustular eruption [102]. Subcorneal pustular eruption may also be a manifestation of allergy to trichloroethylene [103].

21.9 Erythematous and Exfoliative Eruption

Some industrial chemicals, e.g., trichloroethylene and methyl bromide, appear to cause characteristic localized or generalized erythema with or without a papulo-vesicular eruption followed by exfoliation. The skin lesions usually take several weeks to clear. In most cases, the skin reaction was believed to be a toxic or allergic reaction from percutaneous or mucosal absorption of the chemicals. The allergic mechanism may be confirmed in some cases by a positive patch test reaction to trichloroethylene and trichloroethanol (its metabolite).

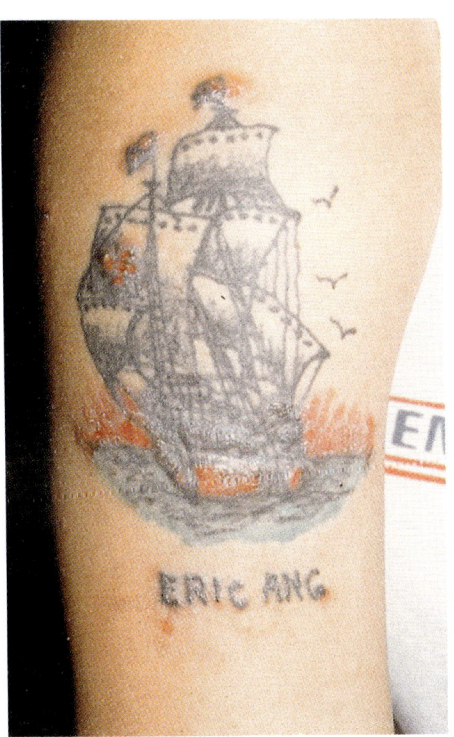

Fig. 7. Allergic granulomatous reaction from mercury pigment (red) and cobalt pigment (blue). Note overlying eczematous reactions

21.9.1 Trichloroethylene

Generalized erythema followed by exfoliation resulting from exposure to trichloroethylene was first described by Schwartz et al. [104] and later by Bauer and Rabens [105]. The reaction was believed to be due to a systemic sensitization to trichloroethylene.

Conde-Salazar et al. reported a patient who developed a generalized erythema and subcorneal pustular eruption from a cutaneous hypersensitivity reaction to trichloroethylene [103]. The allergic reaction was confirmed by a positive erythematous scaly patch test reaction to 5% trichloroethylene. The patient also reacted systemically to a cutaneous challenge test made by exposing his leg to an environment saturated with trichloroethylene. Nakayama et al. [106] also described generalized erythema and exfoliation with mucous membrane ulceration in a patient from cutaneous exposure to trichloroethylene. The patient had positive patch test reactions to trichloroethylene and trichloroethanol (a metabolite of trichloroethylene) [106]. The patient's skin eruption continued to appear after cessation of exposure to trichloroethylene. The prolonged duration of the eruption was believed to be due to the slow release of accumulated trichloroethylene and its metabolites in the patient's fatty tissue.

Cutaneous reaction to inhaled trichloroethylene can also cause a characteristic skin eruption consisting of localized erythematous xerotic plaques which become parched and fissured [107].

21.9.2 Methyl Bromide

Exposure to methyl bromide was described as causing sharply demarcated erythema with vesiculation in six fumigators [108]. Plasma bromide levels in these patients after exposure strongly suggested percutaneous absorption of methyl bromide. The lesions were more prominent on skin that was relatively moist or subject to mechanical pressure, such as the axillae, groins, and abdomen. Histologically, the early skin lesions showed keratinocytes, necrosis, severe upper dermal edema and bullae, and diffuse dermal neutrophilic infiltration. The skin eruptions were believed to be due to the direct toxic effect of methyl bromide as an alkylating agent.

Core Message

- Localized or generalized erythema with or without a papulo-vesicular eruption followed by exfoliation may be due to a toxic or allergic reaction from percutaneous or mucosal absorption of chemicals. This reaction may persist for weeks.

21.10 Scleroderma-like Eruption

Solvents have been reported as predisposing or eliciting factors in some patients with scleroderma-like eruptions [109, 110]. The pathogenic mechanism is unknown. Solvents implicated include aromatic hydrocarbon solvents, such as benzene, toluene and white spirit, and aliphatic hydrocarbons, such as naphtha, *n*-hexane and hexachloroethane. Unlike chlorinated hydrocarbons, these hydrocarbons do not produce multisystem disease resembling vinyl chloride disease. The associated scleroderma and morphea-like sclerosis is usually limited to the skin of the hands and feet, where direct contact took place, but occasionally may be widespread.

In 1972, Texier et al. [111] reported atrophic sclerodermoid patches following phytonadione injections. Intradermal testing with phytonadione gave positive results in 50% of patients. The clinical findings are indistinguishable from those of morphea [112–114]. Histology shows dense sclerosis of the reticular dermis and subcutaneous fat and a lymphocytic inflammatory infiltrate. The pathogenesis is unknown. A possible immune mechanism has been suggested. Pang et al. reported a cutaneous reaction to intradermal phytomenadione challenge in a patient with sclerodermoid plaques that had persisted more than 10 years after subcutaneous phytomenadione injections. Positive intradermal test produced a persistent erythematous indurated plaque at the test site for more than 5 months, suggesting a marked cutaneous hypersensitivity to the drug. Serial biopsies of the test site showed transition from spongiotic eczematous features initially to inflammatory morphea-like histology over a 5-month period [115].

21

Core Message

■ Aromatic and aliphatic hydrocarbons may be associated with scleroderma-like eruptions but do not produce multisystem disease. The sclerosis is usually limited to the sites of contact but may occasionally be widespread.

21.11 Pigmented Contact Dermatitis

Pigmented contact dermatitis is a characteristic allergic contact dermatitis reaction manifesting as macular pigmentation on sites of contact. Patients often observe brownish to gray pigmentation on the face after using cosmetics containing azo-dyes (as contaminants) [116] or fragrances [117]. Optical whiteners have been reported to cause similar reactions. Characteristically, female patients present with patchy macular pigmentation mimicking melasma. Patients may experience slight erythema and itch before the onset of pigmentation. Unlike melasma, the pigmentation clears upon avoidance of the causative allergen. The allergic nature of the skin lesion can be confirmed by patch testing with the incriminated allergens.

An outbreak of pigmented contact dermatitis was reported in Japan in the 1970s [118]. Fragrances and Sudan I (an impurity in Brilliant Lake Red) were the causative allergens. In Asian countries, pigmented contact dermatitis from fragrances in cosmetics and Sudan I have also been reported. The source of these contact allergens is usually cosmetics that are produced by small-time cosmetic manufacturers where there is little product quality control. Another common cause of pigmented contact dermatitis is seen in Hindu women who present with pigmentation on their mid-forehead due to allergens (usually Sudan I) in the red dye applied to their forehead for cultural reasons [119].

More recently reported causes of pigmented contact dermatitis include ricinoleic acid in lipsticks causing pigmented contact cheilitis [120], topical minoxidil [121] and para-tertiary butylphenol formaldehyde resin used as an adhesive in a watch strap [122].

Chapter 18 is devoted to pigmented contact dermatitis, where it is covered in greater detail.

21.12 Lymphomatoid Contact Dermatitis

Lymphomatoid contact dermatitis refers to the relatively little-known phenomenon of allergic contact dermatitis producing histological features suggestive of cutaneous T-cell lymphoma. The skin lesions are mainly localized to areas in contact with the allergen and resolve with avoidance. This condition was first reported in 1976 by Orbaneja et al. [123] and 13 cases have been reported to date. The histology is characterized by a superficial band-like T-cell infiltrate, which resembles early-stage mycosis fungoides. The density of infiltrate exceeds that seen in allergic contact dermatitis, and atypical lymphocytes are present. This reaction has been reported to be caused by nickel [124], gold [125], isopropyl-diphenylenediamine [126], cobalt naphthenate [127], ethylenediamine dihydrochloride [128], *para*-phenylenediamine [129] and *para*-tertyl-butyl phenol resin [130].

A second type of lymphomatoid contact dermatitis had been reported by Ecker and Winkelmann in 1981 [131], where patients had erythroderma resembling actinic reticuloid associated with positive patch test findings. However, most other authors contended that this latter group does not fit into the original description of lymphomatoid contact dermatitis.

Core Message

■ Allergic contact dermatitis producing histological features suggestive of cutaneous T-cell lymphoma can occur in areas in contact with various chemical allergens. The skin lesions will resolve with avoidance.

21.13 Vascular-Occlusive Contact Dermatitis

A 75-year-old man presented with purpuric papulonecrotic lesions on his back 2 days after applying a spray containing the nonsteroidal anti-inflammatory drug fepradinol [132]. Patch tests showed strong positive reactions to the spray as well as fepradinol 0.1, 1 and 2% eth., while 30 controls tested negative to fepradinol at the same concentrations. The histology of his lesions showed a thrombotic vasculopathy with epidermal necrosis without related leukocytoclastic vasculitis. This is the first reported case of vascular-occlusive contact dermatitis.

References

1. Goh CL (1989) Urticarial papular and plaque eruption. A manifestation of allergic contact dermatitis. Int J Dermatol 28:172–176
2. Holst R, Kirby J, Magnusson B (1976) Sensitization to tropical woods giving erythema multiforme-like eruptions. Contact Dermatitis 2:295–296
3. Fisher AA (1986) Erythema multiforme-like eruptions due to exotic woods and ordinary plants, part I. Cutis 37:101–104
4. Fisher AA, Bikowski J (1981) Allergic contact dermatitis due to wooden cross made of *Dalbergia nigra*. Contact Dermatitis 7:45–46
5. Irvine C, Reynolds A, Finlay AY (1988) erythema multiforme-like reaction to "rosewood." Contact Dermatitis 19:24–25
6. Hausen BM (1981) Woods injurious to human health. De Gruyter, Berlin, p 59
7. Mallory SB, Miller OF, Tyler WB (1982) Toxicodendron radicans dermatitis with black lacquer deposit on the skin. J Am Acad Dermatol 6:363–368
8. Schwartz RS, Downham TF (1981) Erythema multiforme associated with Rhus contact dermatitis. Contact Dermatitis 27:85–86
9. Hjorth N (1966) Primula dermatitis. Trans St John's Hosp Derm Soc 52:207–219
10. Kurz G, Rapaport MJ (1979) External/internal allergy to plants (Artemesia). Contact Dermatitis 5:407–408
11. Jovanovic M, Mimica-Dukic N, Poljacki M, Boza P (2003) Erythema multiforme due to contact with weeds: a recurrence after patch testing. Contact Dermatitis 48:17–25
12. Fisher AA (1986) Erythema multiforme-like eruptions due to topical medications, part II. Cutis 37:158–161
13. Meneghini CL, Angelini G (1981) Secondary polymorphic eruptions in allergic contact dermatitis. Dermatologica 163:63–70
14. Yaffe H, Dressler DP (1969) Topical application of mafenide acetate. Its association with erythema multiforme and cutaneous reactions. Arch Dermatol 100:277–281
15. Degreef H, Conamie A, van Derheyden D et al (1984) Mephenesin contact dermatitis with erythema multiforme-like features. Contact Dermatitis 10:220–223
16. Schulze-Dirks A, Frosch PJ (1993) Kontaktallergie auf Mephenesin. Hautarzt 44:403–406
17. Valsecchi R, Foiadelli L, Cainelli T (1982) Contact dermatitis from econazole. Contact Dermatitis 8:422
18. Saperstein H, Rapaport M, Rietschel RL (1984) Topical vitamin E as a cause of erythema multiforme-like eruptions. Arch Dermatol 120:906 908
19. Silvestre JF, Betlloch I, Guijarro J, Albares MP, Vergara G (2001) Erythema-multiforme-like eruption on the application site of a nitroglycerin patch, followed by widespread erythema multiforme. Contact Dermatitis 45:299–300
20. Khanna M, Qasem K, Sasseville D (2000) Allergic contact dermatitis to tea tree oil with erythema multiforme-like id reaction. Am J Contact Dermatitis 11:238–242
21. Goh CL (1987) Erythema multiforme-like and purpuric eruption due to contact allergy to proflavine. Contact Dermatitis 17:53–54
22. Puig L, Alegre M, Cuatrecasas M, de Moragas JM (1994) Erythema multiforme-like reaction following diphencyprone treatment of plane warts. Int J Dermatol 33:201–203
23. Goette DK, Odom RB (1980) Vaginal medications as a cause for varied widespread dermatitides. Cutis 26:406–409
24. Gottschalk HR, Stone OJ (1976) Stevens-Johnson syndrome. Arch Dermatol 113:235–236
25. Rubin Z (1977) Ophthalmic sulfonamide-induced Stevens-Johnson syndrome. Arch Dermatol 113:235–236
26. Guill MA, Goette DK, Knight CG et al (1979) Erythema multiforme and urticaria. Eruptions induced by chemically-related ophthalmic anticholinergic agents. Arch Dermatol 115:742–743
27. Calnan CD (1956) Nickel dermatitis. Br J Dermatol 68:229–232
28. Cook LJ (1982) Associated nickel and cobalt contact dermatitis presenting as erythema multiforme. Contact Dermatitis 8:280–281
29. Friedman SF, Parry HO (1985) Erythema multiforme associated with contact dermatitis. Contact Dermatitis 12:21–23
30. Fisher AA (1986) Erythema multiforme-like eruptions due to topical miscellaneous compounds, part III. Cutis 37:262–264
31. Corazza M, Lombardi AR, Virgili A (1997) Non-eczematous urticarioid allergic contact dermatitis due to Eumulgin L in a deodorant. Contact Dermatitis 36:159–160
32. Cavendish A (1968) A case of dermatitis from 9. bromofluorene and a peculiar reaction to a patch test. Br J Dermatol 52:155–164
33. Powell EW (1968) Skin reactions to 9-bromofluorene. Br J Dermatol 80:491–496
34. De Feo CP (1966) Erythema multiforme bullosum caused by 9-bromofluorene. Arch Dermatol 94:545–551
35. Roed-Petersen J (1975) Erythema multiforme as an expression of contact dermatitis. Contact Dermatitis 1:270–271
36. Nethercott JR, Albers J, Gurguis S et al (1982) Erythema multiforme exudativum linked to the manufacture of printed circuit boards. Contact Dermatitis 3:314–322
37. Phoon WH, Chan MOY, Rajan VS et al (1984) Stevens-Johnson syndrome associated with occupational exposure to trichloroethylene. Contact Dermatitis 10:270–276
38. Goh CL (1988) Erythema multiforme-like eruption due to trinitrotoluene allergy. Int J Dermatol 27:650–651
39. Schena D, Barba A (1992) Erythema-multiforme-like contact dermatitis from dimethoate. Contact Dermatitis 27:116–117
40. Jappe U, Hausen BM, Petzoldt D (2001) Erythema-multiforme-like eruption and depigmentation following allergic contact dermatitis from a paint-on henna tattoo, due to para-phenylenediamine contact hypersensitivity. Contact Dermatitis 45:249–50
41. Lu CY, Sun CC (2001) Localized erythema-multiforme-like contact dermatitis from rubber gloves. Contact Dermatitis 45:311–2
42. Hata M, Tokura Y, Takigawa M (2001) Erythema multiforme-like eruption associated with contact dermatitis to cutting oil. Eur J Dermatol 11:247–248
43. Le Coz CJ, Lepoittevin JP (2001) Occupational erythema-multiforme-like dermatitis from sensitization to costus resinoid, followed by flare-up and systemic contact dermatitis from beta-cyclocostunolide in a chemistry student. Contact Dermatitis 44:310–311
44. Batchvaros B, Minkow DM (1968) Dermatitis and purpura from rubber in clothing. Trans St John's Hosp Derm Soc 54:73–78
45. Calnan CD, Peachey RDG (1971) Allergic contact purpura. Clin Allergy 1:287–290

21

46. Fisher AA (1974) Allergic petechial and purpuric rubber dermatitis. The PPPP syndrome. Cutis 14:25–27
47. Romaguera C, Grimalt F (1977) PPPP syndrome. Contact Dermatitis 3:103
48. Shmunes E (1978) Purpuric allergic contact dermatitis to paraphenylenediamine. Contact Dermatitis 4:225–229
49. Agarwal K (1982) Contact allergic purpura to wool dust. Contact Dermatitis 8:281–282
50. Bruynzeel DP, van den Hoogenband HM, Koedijk F (1984) Purpuric vasculitis-like eruption in a patient sensitive to balsam of Peru. Contact Dermatitis 11:207–209
51. Van der Veen JPW, Neering H, de Haan P, Bruynzeel (1988) Pigmented purpuric clothing dermatitis due to Disperse Blue 85. Contact Dermatitis 19:222–223
52. Calobrisi SD, Drolet BA, Esterly NB (1998) Petechial eruption after the application of EMLA cream. Pediatrics 101:471–473
53. Van Joost T, van Ulsen J, Vuzevski VD, Naafs B, Tank BA (1990) Purpuric contact dermatitis to benzoyl peroxide. J Am Acad Dermatol 22:359–361
54. De Waard van der Spek FB, Oranje AP (1997) Purpura caused by Emla is of toxic origin. Contact Dermatitis 36:11–13
55. Komericki P, Aberer W, Arbab E, Kovacevic Z, Kranke B (2001) Pigmented purpuric contact dermatitis from Disperse Blue 106 and 124 dyes. J Am Acad Dermatol 45:456–458
56. Cherpelis BS, Fenske NA (2000) Purpuric irritant contact dermatitis induced by Agave americana. Cutis 66:287–288
57. Goh CL, Kwok SF, Rajan VS (1984) Cross sensitivity in Colour developers. Contact Dermatitis 10:280–285
58. Mendel EH (1960) Lichen planus-like eruption caused by a colourfilm developer. Arch Dermatol 70:516–519
59. Fry L (1965) Skin disease from colour developers. Br J Dermatol 77:456–461
60. Buckley WR (1958) Lichenoid eruptions following contact dermatitis. Arch Dermatol 78:454–457
61. Canizares O (1959) Lichen planus-like eruption caused by colour developer. Arch Dermatol 80:81–86
62. Hyman AB, Berger RA (1959) Lichenoid eruption due to colour developer. Arch Dermatol 80:243–244
63. Frykholm KO, Frithiof L, Fernstorm AI et al (1969) Allergy to copper derived from dental alloys as a possible cause of oral lesions of lichen planus. Acta Derm Venereol (Stockh) 49:268–269
64. Bircher AJ, von Schultheiss A, Henning G (1993) Oral lichenoid lesions and mercury sensitivity. Contact Dermatitis 29:275–276
65. Lombardi F, Campolmi P, Sertoli A (1983) Lichenoid dermatitis caused by nickel salts? Contact Dermatitis 9:520–521
66. Meneghine CL (1971) Lichenoid contact dermatitis. Contact Dermatitis Newslett 9:194
67. Lembo G, Balato N, Patruno C, Pini D, Ayala F (1987) Lichenoid contact dermatitis due to aminoglycoside antibiotics. Contact Dermatitis 17:122–123
68. Lichter M, Drury D Remlinger K (1992) Lichenoid dermatitis caused by epoxy resin. Contact Dermatitis 26:275
69. Schultz E, Mahler V (2002). Prolonged lichenoid reaction and cross-sensitivity to para-substituted amino-compounds due to temporary henna tattoo. Int J Dermatol 41:301–303
70. Verma KK, Sirka CS, Ramam M, Sharma VK (2002) Parthenium dermatitis presenting as photosensitive lichenoid eruption. A new clinical variant. Contact Dermatitis 46:286–289
71. Goh CL, Ng SK (1988) Bullous contact allergy from cinnamon. Dermatosen 36:186–187
72. Atakan N, Tuzun J, Karaduman A (1993) Dyshidrosiform pemphigoid induced by nickel in the diet. Contact Dermatitis 29:388–391
73. You DO, Kang JD, Youn NH, Park SD (2003) Bullous contact dermatitis caused by self-applied crushed Paederus fuscipes for the treatment of vitiligo. Cutis 72:385–388
74. Shelley WB, Epstein E (1963) Contact-sensitivity to gold as a chronic papular eruption. Arch Dermatol 87:388–391
75. Monti M, Berti E, Cavicchini S, Sala F (1983) Unusual cutaneous reaction after gold chloride patch test. Contact Dermatitis 9:150–151
76. Petros H, Macmillan AL (1973) Allergic contact sensitivity to gold with unusual features. Br J Dermatol 88:505–508
77. Young E (1974) contact hypersensitivity to metallic gold. Dermatologica 149:294–298
78. Fisher AA (1974) Metallic gold: the cause of persistent allergic "dermal" contact dermatitis. Cutis 14:177–180
79. Iwatsuki K, Tagami H, Moriguchi T, Yamada M (1982) Lymphoadenoid structure induced by gold hypersensitivity. Arch Dermatol 118:608–611
80. Iwatsuki K, Yamada M, Takigawa M, Inoue K, Matsumoto K (1987) Benign lymphoplasia of the earlobes induced by gold earrings: immunohistologic study on the cellular infiltrates. J Am Acad Dermatol 16:83–88
81. Fleming C Burden D, Fallowfield M, Lever R (1997) Lymphomatoid contact reaction to gold earrings. Contact Dermatitis 37:298–299
82. Zenarola P, Lomuto M, Bisceglia M (1993) Hypertrophic amalgam dermatitis of the tongue simulating carcinoma. Contact Dermatitis 29:157–158
83. Rubin L (1956) Granulomas of axillae caused by deodorants. JAMA 162:953–955
84. Sheard G (1957) Granulomatous reactions due to deodorant sticks. JAMA 164:1085–1087
85. Shelley WB, Hurley HJ (1958) Allergic origin of zirconium deodorant granuloma. Br J Dermatol 70:75–101
86. Williams RM, Skipworth GB (1959) Zirconium granulomas of glabrous skin following treatment of rhus dermatitis. Arch Dermatol 80:273–276
87. Epstein WL, Allen JR (1964) Granulomatous hypersensitivity after use of zirconium-containing poison oak lotions. JAMA 190:162–163
88. Baler GR (1965) Granulomas from topical zirconium in poison ivy dermatitis. Arch Dermatol 91:145–148
89. LoPresti PJ, Hambrick GW (1965) Zirconium granuloma following treatment of rhus dermatitis. Arch Dermatol 92:188–189
90. Kaaber K, Nielsen AO, Veien NK (1992) Vaccination granulomas and aluminium allergy: course and prognostic factors. Contact Dermatitis 26:304–306
91. Levy J, Sewell M, Goldstein N (1979) A short history of tattooing. J Derm Surg Oncol 5:851–853
92. Nguyen LQ, Allen HB (1974) Reactions to manganese and cadmium in tatoos. Cutis 23:71–72
93. Schwartz RA, Mathias CGT, Miller CH, Rojas-Corona R, Lamber WC (1987) Granulomatous reaction to purple tattoo pigment. Contact Dermatitis 16:198–202
94. Armstrong DK, Walsh MY, Dawson JF (1997) Granulomatous contact dermatitis due to gold earrings. Br J Dermatol 136:776–778
95. Lazarov A, Kidron D, Tulchinsky Z, Minkow B (2003) Contact orofacial granulomatosis caused by delayed hypersensitivity to gold and mercury. J Am Acad Dermatol 49:1117–1120

96. Raulin C, Greve B, Hartschuh W, Soegding K (2000) Exudative granulomatous reaction to hyaluronic acid (Hylaform). Contact Dermatitis 43:178–179

97. Fisher AA, Chargrin L, Fleischmayer R et al (1959) Pustular patch test reactions. Arch Dermatol 80:742–752

98. Schoel VJ, Frosch PJ (1990) Allergisches Kontaktekzem durch Gummiinhaltsstoffe unter dem Bild einer Pustulosis palmaris. Dermatosen 38:178–180

99. Stone OJ, Johnson DA (1967) Pustular patch test-experimentally induced. Arch Dermatol 95:618–619

100. Hjorth N (1977) Diagnostic patch testing. In: Marzulli F, Maibach HI (eds) Dermatoxicology and pharmacology. Wiley, New York, p 344

101. Wahlberg JE, Maibach HI (1981) Sterile cutaneous pustules – a manifestation of primary irritancy? J Invest Dermatol 76:381–383

102. Burkhart CG (1981) Pustular allergic contact dermatitis: a distinct clinical and pathological entity. Cutis 27:630–638

103. Conde-Salazar L, Guimaraens D, Romero LV, Yus ES (1983) Subcorneal pustular eruption and erythema from occupational exposure to trichloroethylene. Contact Dermatitis 9:235–237

104. Schwartz L, Tulipan L, Birmingham A (1947) Occupational diseases of the skin, 3rd edn. Lea and Febiger, Philadelphia, p 771

105. Bauer M, Rabens SF (1977) Trichloroethylene toxicity. Int J Dermatol 16:113–116

106. Nakayama H, Bobayashi M, Takahashi M, Ageishi Y, Takano T (1988) Generalized eruption with severe liver dysfunction associated with occupational exposure to trichloroethylene. Contact Dermatitis 19:48–51

107. Goh CL, Ng SK (1988) A cutaneous manifestation of trichloroethylene toxicity. Contact Dermatitis 18:59–60

108. Hezemans-Boer M, Toonstra J, Meulenbelt J, Zwaveling JH, Sangster B, van Vloten WA (1988) Skin lesions due to exposure to methyl bromide. Arch Dermatol 124:917–921

109. Walder BK (1983) Do solvents cause scleroderma? Int J Dermatol 22:157–158

110. Yamakage A, Ishikawa H (1982) Generalized morphea-like scleroderma occurring in people exposed to organic solvents. Dermatologica 165:186–193

111. Texier L, Gautheir Y, Gauthier O et al (1972) Hypodermite sclerodermiforme lombo-fessiere induite par des injections de vitamine K1 et de Fer 300. Bull Soc Fr Dermatol Syphil 79:499–500

112. Rommel A, Saurat JH (1982) Hypodermite fessiere sclerodermiforme et injections de vitamine K1 a la naissance. Ann Pediatr 29:64–66

113. Janin-Mercier A, Mosser C, Bourges M (1985) Subcutaneous sclerosis with fasciitis and eosinophilia after phytoadione injections. Arch Dermtol 121:1421–1423

114. Pujol RM, Puig L, Moreno A, Perez M, de Moragas JM (1989) Pseudoscleroderma secondary to phytonadione (Vitamin K1) injections. Cutis 43:365–368

115. Pang BK, Munro V, Kossard S (1996) Pseudoscleroderma secondary to phytomenadione (vitamin K1) injections: Texier's disease. Aust J Dermatol 37:44–47

116. Kozuka T, Tashiro M, Sano S, Fujimoto K, Nakamura Y, Hashimoto S, Nakaminami G (1979) Brilliant Lake Red R as a cause of pigmented contact dermatitis. Contact Dermatitis 5:297–304

117. Ippen H, Tesche S (1971) Freund's pigmented photodermatitis. ("Berloque-dermatitis","eau de cologne-pigmentation"). Hautarzt 22:535–536

118. Sugai T, Takahashi Y, Takagi T (1977) Pigmented cosmetic dermatitis and coal tar dyes. Contact Dermatitis 3:249–256

119. Kozuka I, Goh CL, Doi T, Yioshikawa K (1988) Sudan I as a cause of pigmented contact dermatitis in "kumkum" (an Indian cosmetic). Ann Acad Med Singapore 17:492–494

120. Leow YH, Tan SH, Ng SK (2003) Pigmented contact cheilitis from ricinoleic acid in lipsticks. Contact Dermatitis 49:48–49

121. Trattner A, David M (2002) Pigmented contact dermatitis from topical minoxidil 5%. Contact Dermatitis 46:246

122. Ozkaya-Bayazit E, Buyukbabani N (2001) Non-eczematous pigmented interface dermatitis from para-tertiary-butylphenol-formaldehyde resin in a watchstrap adhesive. Contact Dermatitis 44:45–46

123. Orbaneja JG, Diez LI, Lozano JL, Salazar LC (1976) Lymphomatoid contact dermatitis: a syndrome produced by epicutaneous hypersensitivity with clinical features and a histopathologic picture similar to that of mycosis fungoides. Contact Dermatitis 2:139–143

124. Danese P, Bertazzoni MG (1995) Lymphomatoid contact dermatitis due to nickel. Contact Dermatitis 33:268–269

125. Fleming C, Burden D, Fallowfield M, Lever R (1997) Lymphomatoid contact reaction to gold earrings. Contact Dermatitis 37:298–299

126. Marliere V, Beylot-Barry M, Doutre MS, Furioli M, Vergier B, Dubus P, Merlio JP, Beylot C (1998) Lymphomatoid contact dermatitis caused by isopropyl-diphenylenediamine: two cases. J Allergy Clin Immunol 102:152–153

127. Schena D, Rosina P, Chieregato C, Colombari R (1995) Lymphomatoid-like contact dermatitis from cobalt naphthenate. Contact Dermatitis 33:197–198

128. Wall LM (1982) Lymphomatoid contact dermatitis due to ethylenediamine dihydrochloride. Contact Dermatitis 8:51–54

129. Calzavara-Pinton P, Capezzera R, Zane C, Brezzi A, Pasolini G, Ubiali A, Facchetti F (2002) Lymphomatoid allergic contact dermatitis from para-phenylenediamine. Contact Dermatitis 47:173–174

130. Evans AV, Banerjee P, McFadden JP, Calonje E (2003) Lymphomatoid contact dermatitis to para-tertyl-butyl phenol resin. Clin Exp Dermatol 28:272–273

131. Ecker RI, Winkelmann RK (1981) Lymphomatoid contact dermatitis. Contact Dermatitis 7:84–93

132. Santos-Briz A, Antunez P, Munoz E, Moran M, Fernandez E, Unamuno P (2004) Vascular-occlusive contact dermatitis from fepradinol. Contact Dermatitis 50:44–46

21

Part V

Diagnostic Tests

V

Chapter 22

Patch Testing

22

Jan E. Wahlberg, Magnus Lindberg

Contents

22.1 Introduction

22.1.1 The Purpose of Patch Testing

Patch testing is a well-established method of diagnosing contact allergy– a delayed type of hypersensitivity (type IV reaction). Patients with a history and clinical picture of contact dermatitis are re-exposed to the suspected allergens under controlled conditions to verify the diagnosis. Also testing patients with hand (dyshidrotic, hyperkeratotic), arm, face or leg eczema (stasis dermatitis), testing of other types of eczema (atopic, seborrheic dermatitis, nummular eczema), including patients with chronic psoriasis, vulval disorders or drug reactions (Chap. 24), is sometimes indicated, especially when they are recalcitrant to prescribed treatment and the dermatologist suspects contact allergy to prescribed topical medicaments and their vehicles.

Apart from its use to confirm a suspected allergic contact dermatitis, the patch test procedure can also be used before recommending alternative medicaments, skin care products, cosmetics, gloves, etc. in a particular patient. If the patient does not react to the alternatives tested, it is unlikely that he or she will react to the products in ordinary use.

Early classic publications on patch testing are reviewed in Chap. 1. More recent, often quoted, guidelines are presented by Malten et al. [1], Fregert [2] and Bandmann and Wohn [3].

Several studies (e.g. [4–6]) have shown that detailed patch testing is beneficial for patients and improve their quality of life (QoL). However, it has also been claimed that random patch testing with a standard series should be discouraged due to low pretest probability [7].

When performing patch testing it has to be remembered that the patch test is a biological provocation test and as such the outcome is dependent on multiple factors including the test system and test material, the biological/functional status of the tested person, and the responsible dermatologist. Most of theses aspects will be discussed in this chapter.

> ### Core Message
>
> - Indications for patch testing:
>   - Cases of contact dermatitis
>   - Other types of eczema and dermatoses, where a superimposed contact allergy is suspected, particularly if recurrent and nonresponsive to treatment
>   - Suspected contact allergy to topical medicaments and their vehicles
>   - "Predictive testing" of alternative products such as gloves, skin care products, medicaments

22.1.2 Standardization

The first patch tests according to present principles were carried out in 1895 [8], but were preceded by some preliminary experiments [9] (see Chap. 1). During the last few decades much effort has been put into standardization of allergens, vehicles, concentrations, patch test materials, tapes, and the scoring of test reactions, and the method today is considered accurate and reliable. A series of papers has demonstrated good reproducibility of patch test results [10–18]. Standardization has facilitated comparisons of contact allergy frequency in and between clinics, geographical areas, and areas with various degrees of industrialization but some questions still remain, especially concerning the reading and scoring of test reactions. This will be discussed in detail below.

22.1.3 Bioavailability

To obtain optimal bioavailability of a hapten one can influence the following five variables:

- Intrinsic penetration capacity
- Concentration, dose
- Vehicle
- Occlusivity of patch test system and tape
- Exposure time

Since it is desirable to remove all test strips at the same time – usually at day 2 (48 h) – four factors remain and can be varied and optimized by the manufacturers of patch test materials and allergen preparations and by the dermatologist responsible for the testing. The penetration capacity can depend upon the salts used; for example, there is a big difference between the penetration of nickel achieved by nickel sulfate and nickel chloride [19]. The higher penetration of nickel from the chloride is probably explained by the partition skin/vehicle of the salts, when applied in the same vehicle in equimolar concentration and under occlusion.

22.2 Test Systems

One can distinguish two test systems: the original one, where the allergens, patches, and tapes are supplied separately, and the modern ready-to-use system, where only a covering material has to be removed before the test is applied.

22.2.1 Original System (Allergen–Patch–Tape)

22.2.1.1 Patches

Some of the patch test units available are depicted in Fig. 1. In Finn chamber (Epitest, Finland) the test area is circular and in van der Bend (van der Bend, Netherlands) and IQ chambers (Chemotechnique Diagnostic, Sweden) they are square. The latter is claimed to facilitate distinguishing allergic from irritant reactions, since an irritant reaction tends to look square, while an allergic reaction tends to look round [1]. Based on a comparative study with ordinary (8 mm) and large (12 mm) Finn chambers, it was found that the larger chambers may be useful for detection of weak sensitization to some contact allergens [20–22]. However, the larger chambers are usually recommended for experimental studies when testing for irritancy.

22.2.1.2 Allergens

The standard patch test allergens sold by Chemotechnique Diagnostics [21] and Trolab Hermal [23], for example, can, according to the suppliers' product catalogues, be considered chemically defined and pure. However, the dermatologist responsible for

patch testing is recommended repeatedly to request the manufacturers to provide results of chemical analyses.

The test preparations are presented in plastic syringes or bottles of inert material to prevent degradation or other chemical changes due to air, humidity, and light. The suppliers' recommendations on storage must be followed in order to minimize these risks. It is suspected that several of the contact allergies reported earlier were due to impurities or degradation products [24]. It has not been possible to confirm the allergenic potential of some claimed "allergens."

22.2.1.3 Vehicles

Each allergen almost certainly has its own optimal vehicle; it is improbable that just one vehicle (e.g., petrolatum) could be optimal for all allergens. White petrolatum is the most widely used vehicle, but its general reliability can be questioned. It gives good occlusion, keeps the allergens stable and is inexpensive. On the other hand, it can retain the allergen (see Sect. 22.5.6.1, Common Causes), irritate the skin, and even give rise to allergic skin reactions [25]. Liquid vehicles such as water and solvents (acetone, ethanol, methyl ethyl ketone) are recommended since they facilitate penetration of the skin, but they also have some drawbacks. Solvents may evaporate, which does not favor exact dosing, and most test solutions must be freshly prepared. Liquid vehicles are used mainly when testing chemicals and products brought by patients (see Sect. 22.13, Tests with Unknown Substances), and in research projects.

In the present standard series water is used for formaldehyde and for 5-chloro-2-methylisothiazol-3-one plus 2-methylisothiazol-3-one (MCI/MI). By using buffer solutions for acid and alkaline products,

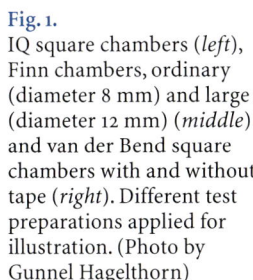

Fig. 1.
IQ square chambers (*left*), Finn chambers, ordinary (diameter 8 mm) and large (diameter 12 mm) (*middle*) and van der Bend square chambers with and without tape (*right*). Different test preparations applied for illustration. (Photo by Gunnel Hagelthorn)

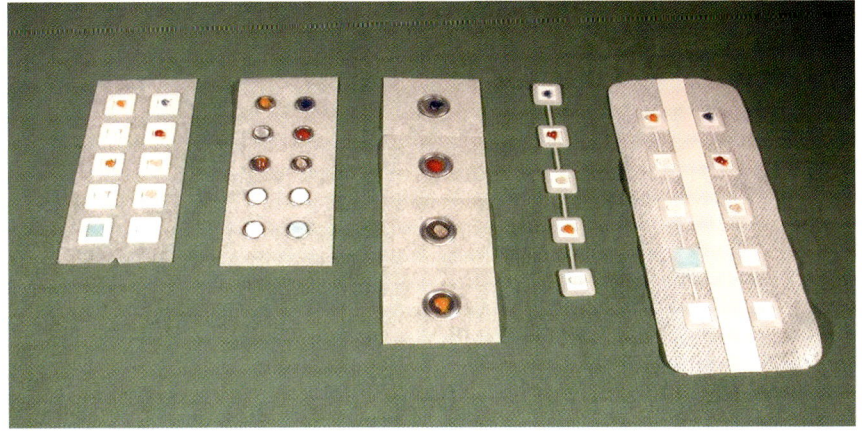

the test concentration can be raised [26]. A filter paper must be used for liquid allergen preparations when using Finn chambers. Modern vehicles are hydrophilic gels (cellulose derivatives), used for example in the TRUE test (Mekos Laboratories, Denmark) [27].

When using more sophisticated vehicles containing salicylic acid, anionic detergents, solvents and others than those mentioned above (e.g., dimethylsulfoxide, DMSO), alkalis, etc. to increase penetration (see Sect. 22.1.3, Bioavailability), an extra patch with the vehicle, as is, must be applied to exclude the possibility that the vehicle is irritant. Since the number of test sites is limited, these vehicles cannot be recommended for routine use. However, they might be valuable where the standard preparation has given a negative reaction but the clinical impression of an allergic contact dermatitis remains.

Core Message

■ White petrolatum is used as the vehicle in the majority of patch test preparations. However, in cases of unexpected, negative patch test results alternative vehicles have to be considered.

22.2.1.4 Concentrations

In textbooks on contact dermatitis and patch testing, and in suppliers' catalogues, the concentration of an allergen is given as a percentage. In one catalogue [19] molality (M) is given together with percentage (weight/weight) and in the TRUE Test concentration is given in milligrams or micrograms per square centimeter. The traditional method of presenting concentrations as a percentage is simple and probably practical, but has been questioned [28, 29], as we do not know if this means weight/weight, volume/volume, volume/weight or weight/volume. Especially when comparing substances and in research projects, it is the dose, the number of molecules delivered, that is of interest [30]. The concentration of Ni ions is 20.9% in nickel sulfate ($NiSO_4 \cdot 7H_2O$) compared to 24.7% in nickel chloride ($NiCl_2 \cdot 6H_2O$) [31]. Thus in comparative studies with these salts it is essential to use the same molality [32].

Core Message

■ Test concentrations should preferably be expressed as weight per area, e.g., milligrams or micrograms per square centimeter (mg/cm^2, $\mu g/cm^2$).

22.2.1.5 Tapes

Previously, most tapes were based on colophony and could cause severe and lasting reactions in patients for whom such a sensitivity was not anticipated.

By introducing modern acrylate-based adhesive tapes, for example Scanpor (Norgeplaster, Alpharma, Norway), the problem has almost been eliminated. Finn chambers on Scanpor tape are commercially available. In cases where loosening can be anticipated (oily or hairy skin, sweating, high humidity), some reinforcing tapes are recommended. Methods for studies on conformability and irritancy of tapes have been published [33, 34].

22.2.1.6 Application of Test Preparations to the Patches

Commercial test preparations – allergens in petrolatum and kept in syringes – are applied directly into the test chambers, or onto the filter paper discs of the other patches (Fig. 2a) and a small amount, "a snake" (approx. 5 mm long) [23], of the mixture is applied across the diameter of the disc. The orifice of the syringe is adjusted to facilitate this.

Liquid test preparations are preferably applied via a digital pipette with disposable plastic tips to allow exact dosing (15 μl calculated for ordinary Finn chambers) (Fig. 2b).

22.2.1.7 Some Practical Suggestions

Storage

The allergens should be kept in a cool, dark place (refrigerator) to minimize degradation. Those diluted in liquids (water, solvents) should be kept in dark bottles. Allergens should be renewed according to their expiry dates.

22

Fig. 2a–e. Patch testing. **a, b** Application of allergens to test patches (**a** allergen in petrolatum, **b** allergen in liquid test preparation using digital pipette with disposable tip). **c** Application of patch tests on the upper back. **d** Marking the test area. **e** Test applied to the upper back. (Photo by Gunnel Hagelthorn)

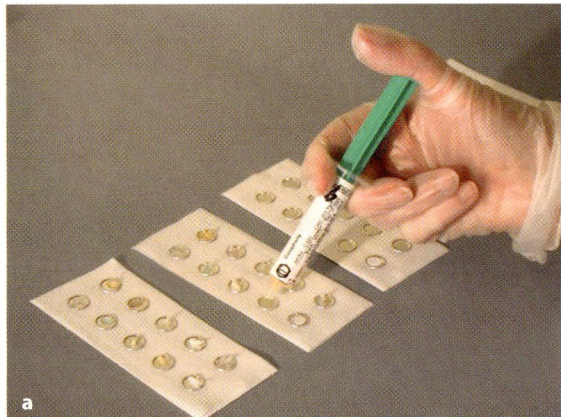

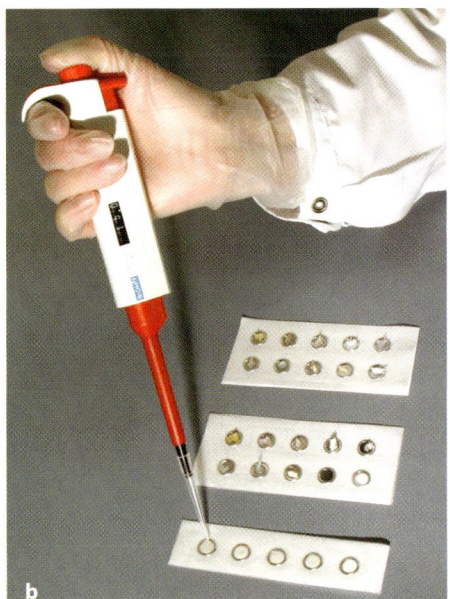

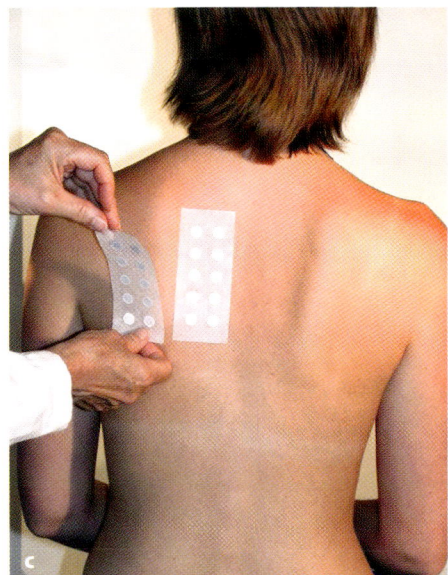

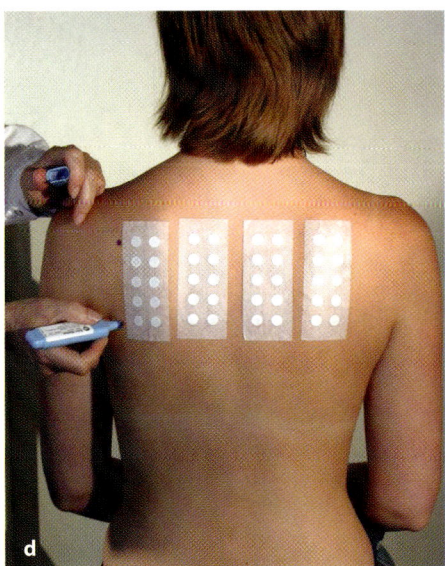

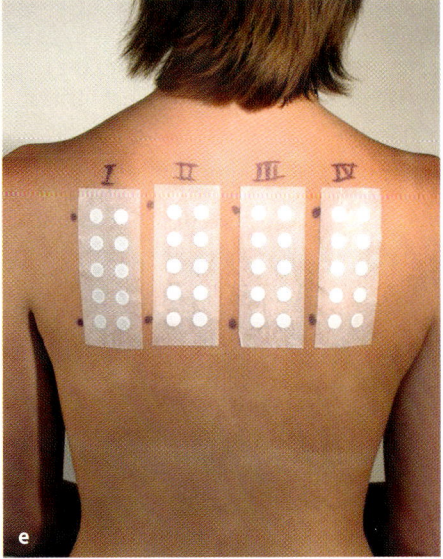

Sequence of Allergens

Adjust the sequence of the allergens so that those frequently causing strong, cross or concomitant reactions are not adjacent. In a study [35] using the TRUE Test system it was found that positive tests to nickel did not intensify reactions to dichromate (distance 1, 3, and 7 cm between the patches) while another [36] concluded that substances with a tendency to cross-reaction or co-sensitizing substances should be tested distant from one another, thus preventing the occurrence of false-positive results. The order given in the catalogues [21, 23] can usually be followed.

Testing in Pregnancy

We usually do not test pregnant women. There are no indications that the minute amounts of allergens absorbed in patch testing could influence the fetus, but in cases of miscarriage or deformity it is natural to blame several things, including medical investigations.

Test Sites

The preferred site is the upper back. For a small number of allergens, for example at retesting, the outer aspect of the upper arm is also acceptable. False-negative test results can be obtained when testing on the lower back or on the volar forearms (see Sect. 22.5.6.1, Common Causes).

Removal of Hair

On hairy areas of the back it is difficult to get acceptable skin contact, and for this reason clipping is recommended. However, a combination of clipping, petrolatum, and tapes sometimes contributes to the irritation seen, which makes reading somewhat difficult.

Degreasing of Test Site

In cases of oily skin, gentle treatment with ethanol or other mild solvents is recommended. The solvent must evaporate before the test strips are applied.

Application of Test Strips

Test strips should be applied from below with mild pressure to remove air pouches, followed by some moderate strokes with the back of the hand to improve adhesion [37] (Fig. 2c).

Skin Markers

Several solutions, inks or marking pens are available [2, 21, 23, 37, 38] Fig. 2d, e). If test strips with constant distance between the discs are used, only two marks are needed.

Positive Control

To exclude hyporeactivity, an impaired inflammatory response, and the possibility that the test patches do not adhere properly, sodium lauryl sulfate and nonanoic acid have been suggested as positive controls [39–42].

Instructions

We have found it valuable to inform our patients as to the aim of the test; about avoidance of showers, wetting the test site, irradiation, and excessive exercise; and about symptoms such as itch, loosening of patches, and late reactions. Examples of such written instructions and guidelines for patients are available [1, 38].

Reading

The light should be good (side lighting may be of help) and adjustable. A magnifying lamp or lens is often helpful. To facilitate reading, most test systems have a special reading plate with punched-out holes corresponding to the test sites.

22.2.2 Ready-to-use Systems

In the ready-to-use patch test system, all necessary material is prepared in advance and the dermatologist, nurse or technician only has to remove the covering material, apply the test strips and mark. In the TRUE Test system (Mekos Laboratories, Denmark) [27] the allergens are incorporated in hydrophilic gels and the patches are 9 mm by 9 mm (Fig. 3). At present, this system is commercially available for the standard series.

Some comparative studies have been carried out with TRUE Test versus Finn chambers [43–47], demonstrating good concordance. The accuracy, reliability, simplicity, and costs of the ready-to-use system must be balanced by the costs, including personnel, of the original systems [see Sect. 22.2.1, Original System (Allergen–Patch–Tape)].

22

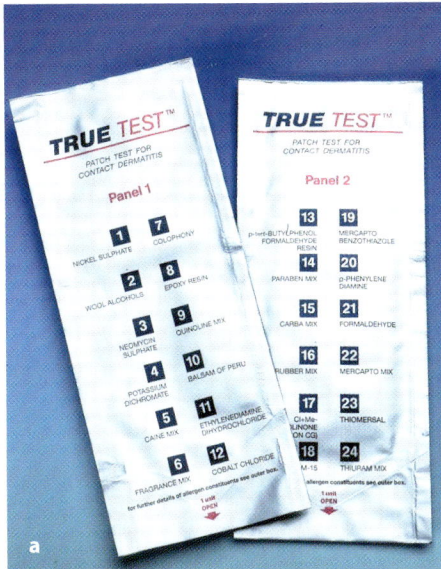

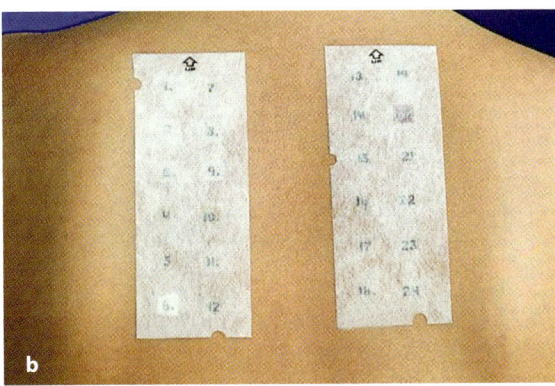

Fig. 3a, b. TRUE Test ready-to-use system. **a** Tests delivered in ready-to-use packages; **b** tests applied to the upper back. Note the square patches. Courtesy by Mekos Laboratories, Denmark.

22.3 Allergens

22.3.1 Numbers

There are 3,700 chemicals described that can cause allergic contact dermatitis [48], and data on new ones are published every year. In de Groot's first book [49], 2,800 allergens were reviewed, indicating that 900 additional substances were identified as sensitizers between 1986 and 1994. The new ones are identified when carrying out predictive testing and when examining and testing patients with contact dermatitis.

22.3.2 Suppliers

The catalogs from the suppliers (e.g., Chemotechnique Diagnostics [21] and Trolab, Hermal [23]) contain lists of approximately 350–400 test preparations in alphabetical order, allergens in the European and International standard series, tables of mixes, and lists of screening series. The catalogs also contain information on the occurrence of allergens and cross-reactivity, as well as some service items such as test sheets, guides to patch testing, skin markers, questionnaires, and advice to patients.

22.3.3 Screening Series

To evaluate the significance of special exposures – mainly occupational – a number of screening series are available (Table 1). They are compiled from the experience gathered at departments of occupational dermatology, and from the literature [50, 51]. Newly defined allergens are added regularly and these series can be considered to cover the present exposure situation.

However, the allergens are pure chemicals and, if the original offending agent was an impurity, a metabolite, a degradation product etc., the cause will be missed. A supplementary test with the patient's own working materials should be done in those cases where the test with the screening series was negative but the suspicion of allergic contact dermatitis remains. A matter of dispute is the ethical question: "should a patient be tested with a number of well-known contact allergens to which he or she has never been exposed?" Is there a risk of patch test sensitization? (see Sect. 22.8, Complications).

22.3.4 Variations Concerning Concentration and Vehicle

Slight differences in recommendations on concentrations and vehicles can be found in catalogs [21, 23] and textbooks on contact dermatitis and patch testing [2, 38, 52–54]. There are thus no ultimate test preparations that are optimal in all clinics or geographical areas. Patch and tape occlusion, humidity, temperature and other climatic factors (see also below Sect. 22.7.4, Irradiation), local experience, and tradition can motivate deviations from these recommendations. Test concentrations for children are presented in Chap. 43. However, the test preparations offered in catalogs are based on tests of several thousands of patients and must be considered very useful

Table 1. Examples of commercially available screening series and number of allergens in each series (*n*)

Chemotechnique [19]	*n*	Trolab Hermal [21]	*n*
Bakery	19	Antioxidants	6
Corticosteroids	8	Bakery allergens	14
Cosmetics	48	Cosmetics	13
Dental	30	Cutting oils (current)	26
Epoxy	9	Cutting oils (historical)	13
Fragrance	24	Dental materials	20
Hairdressing	26	Disinfectants	6
Isocyanate	6	Hairdressing	8
Medicaments	13	Industrial biocides	15
(Meth)acrylate:		Medicaments I Antibiotics	9
Adhesives, dental and other	15	Medicaments II Antiseptics, antimycotics	5
Nails – artificial	13	Medicaments III Miscellaneous	5
Printing	24	Medicaments IV Local anesthetics	5
Oil and cooling fluid	35	Medicaments V Corticosteroids	8
Photographic chemicals	16	Medicaments VI Ophthalmics	5
Plant	13	Metal compounds	7
Plastic and glues	25	Perfumes, flavors	24
Rubber additives	25	Photoallergens	17
Scandinavian photopatch	20	Photographic chemicals	16
Shoe	22	Plants	8
Sunscreen	10	Plastic, glues	30
Textile colors and finish	32	Preservatives	20
Various allergens	59	Shoe allergens	9
		Rubber chemicals	17
		Sunscreen agents	9
		Textile and leather dyes	13
		Vehicles, emulsifiers	8
		Miscellaneous	5

guidelines when setting up and running a patch test clinic.

22.4 Standard Series

The present European standard series contains 25 items, but 6 of them are *mixes*, so in fact at least 24 additional allergens are applied. Balsam of Peru, colophony, and lanolin are examples of natural mixes, where much effort has been spent identifying the allergens [55–58]. The basic idea of using mixes instead of single allergens is to save time and space. Also, the patients are tested with a number of closely related substances, among others rubber chemicals. The screening capacity of the standard series is thereby greatly increased. However, the value of these mixes is sometimes questioned [59]. It is difficult to find an optimal concentration for each allergen in a common vehicle (usually petrolatum) and to determine whether the allergens metabolize or interact to potentiate or decrease reactivity [60, 61].

At our clinic we use the mixes for screening purposes, positive cases being retested with the ingredients. Not unusually, these tests are negative and we then have to ask ourselves whether the initial reaction was an expression of irritancy and/or whether the ingredients have interacted. The opposite has also been noticed. The patient may be negative to a particular mix, but react when retested with its ingredients.

The advantages and disadvantages of using a standard series of patch tests were recently discussed by Lachapelle and Maibach [62]. They pointed out that it can be considered a limited technical tool, representing one of the pieces of a puzzle, to be combined with other means of diagnosis, and that it also compensates for anamnestic failures. The allergens of the standard series are presented in detail in Chap. 29 and the test concentrations in Chap. 49.

22.4.1 Deciding What to Include in the Standard Series

The original standard series was based on the experience of the members of the International Contact Dermatitis Research Group and mirrored the findings and current situation in different parts of Europe and the United States. The series is evaluated regularly by national and international contact dermatitis groups. Each test clinic is recommended to

22

compile its patch test results yearly. If the frequency of positive reactions to a particular allergen is less than 1%, its presence in a standard series can be questioned and it should probably be replaced by another compound. In these ways, the standard series continually changes in composition and in the total number of substances included.

The new allergens introduced are often preservatives. 5-Chloro-2-methylisothiazol-3-one (MCI) plus 2-methylisothiazol-3-one (MI) can be mentioned as a typical example. The first cases were observed in Southern Sweden in 1980 [63] and isothiazolinone then became an almost universal allergen, with local epidemics in Finland, the Netherlands, Italy, and Switzerland [64]. It was included in the Swedish standard series in 1985 and in the European standard series in 1988 [65].

A scheme [66] for identification of new contact allergens includes:

- **Clinical**
  - Positive patch test reaction to a product
  - Test with ingredients of the product
  - Serial dilution test to define a threshold of sensitivity
  - Control tests for irritancy
  - Cross-reactivity – equimolar concentrations
  - Use tests – repeated open application test (ROAT), provocative use test (PUT)
- **Experimental**
  - Structural formula
  - Chemical analyses – test material, product, purity, stability
  - Animal testing – allergenic potency, cross-reactivity pattern

The choice of patch test concentrations is initially decided by the dermatologist studying a suspected allergen in an index case of contact dermatitis. Most allergens are tested in the concentration range 0.01–10% and by analogy with similar chemicals the dermatologist will probably start within this range and then continue with a serial dilution test (Table 2). The threshold of sensitivity defined must be checked for irritancy by tests in controls [66]. If these control tests are negative, information on the case and on the test preparation, where allergen, concentration, and vehicle are stated, will be published as scientific reports and also disseminated to suppliers of patch test allergens. An instructive example of the procedure of defining a new allergen – the preservative iodopropynyl butylcarbamate – was recently presented [67, 68]. The issue is further discussed in Sect. 22.13.3, Test or Not?.

Table 2. Results of a serial dilution test with nickel sulfate in a patient who previously reacted to 5.0% (+++)

Dilution step (%)		Score
1.	1.0	+++
2.	0.3	++
3.	0.1	+
4.	0.03	+
5.	0.01	A few papules
6.	0.003	?
7.	0.001	–
8.	0.0003	–

Nowadays, following local epidemics, conference reports, and communications in scientific journals, several patch test clinics may choose to include a newly identified allergen in their standard series to investigate the frequency in their geographical area. If the initial reports can be confirmed and the allergen is diffused in many and various products, it is then recommended for inclusion in the standard series [69].

At a joint meeting of the International and European Environmental and Contact Dermatitis Research Groups [65], it was recommended to include MCI/MI and at the same meeting some other changes in the tray were made: carba mix (three rubber chemicals) was removed and replaced by another rubber chemical (mercaptobenzothiazole); p-phenylenediamine hydrochloride was replaced by the corresponding free base and the concentration was raised from 0.5% to 1.0%. In 1995 [70] the introduction of the sesquiterpene lactone mix in the standard series, replacement of ingredients in the PPD black rubber mix and the quinolone mix by single components, and the dropping of ethylenediamine dihydrochloride and a p-hydroxybenzoate from the paraben mix took place. More recently budesonide and tixocortolpivalate were recommended for inclusion in the European standard series [71]. A comparison of the European standard series with the North American and Japanese series shows some differences in composition, concentrations, and vehicles [70, 72]. An extended international standard series was suggested [72]. The groups' official recommendations for changes can be read by all interested parties, which also gives opportunities for questions and discussion.

22.5 Reading and Evaluation of Patch Tests

The diagnosis allergic contact dermatitis is based on patch testing and quantitative and qualitative exposure assessment. The frequency of patch testing in national health care systems varies considerably around the world. In Denmark with a population of 5 million, approximately 25,000 new patients are patch tested yearly. Patch testing is a medical technology that has developed over the last 100 years and is now of major significance in the evaluation and classification of dermatitis. In cases of allergic contact dermatitis a clear outcome of the patch test can be obtained in most cases with a significant impact on clinical diagnosis and prognosis. Difficulties in discriminating weak allergic and irritant reactions will undoubtedly occur. Such gray zones need to be handled by supplementary tests such as dose–response, serial dilution, and ROATs and in the final conclusion related to the clinical history. Reading of patch tests is based on morphological criteria only. Reading of a patch test, as with all other tests in medicine, is a question of strictly following objective criteria. The interpretation of test results and the relevance depend on a global evaluation including the history of the patient, clinical observations, and exposure assessment.

22.5.1 Reading – When and How

The reading should be done by the dermatologist him- or herself, after adequate training.

22.5.1.1 Exposure Time

Most authors advocate an exposure time of 48 h. A few comparisons of 1-day (24 h) and 2-day (48-h) allergen exposure show some reactions positive only at day 1 (24 h) and some positive only at day 2 (48 h) [73]. A 1-day exposure would reduce the number of questionable reactions [74]. No definite conclusions can be drawn from the studies published so far [75].

It would be convenient for the patient, and probably for the dermatologist, if the exposure time could be reduced with retained accuracy. Preliminary studies with exposure to $NiSO_4$ for 5 h [76], to $K_2Cr_2O_7$ for 6 h and 48 h [77], and *para*-phenylenediamine (PPDA) for 15, 30, and 120 min [78] demonstrated that some patients will react at these brief exposures, but also showed great variability. To achieve reduced exposure time while retaining accuracy, the penetration capacity of the hapten must be increased, among other things by using higher concentrations or doses, more efficacious vehicles and optimal occlusion (see Sect. 22.1.3, Bioavailability). Working out these parameters for all existing allergens, however, would be an overwhelming task.

22.5.1.2 Reading When?

Wherever possible, it was strongly recommended that two readings be carried out, the first after removal of the patches (usually day 2) and the second 2–5 days later [79]. In a study, paired readings on days 4 and 7 were found to be more reliable than those on days 2 and 4 [80]. The readings must be related to the exposure times (see Sect. 22.5.1.1, Exposure Time) and if the patches are applied for only 1 day, readings should be at days 1 and 3.

If they are removed at the dermatologist's clinic or office, it is possible to check that they have adhered properly and that the marking is adequate. However, this procedure must be balanced by the great(er) value of later readings for the patients (see below). One should wait at least 15–30 min after the removal, since the combination of allergen, vehicle, patches, and tape causes a transient increase in skin blood flow, a sign of irritation [81]. At later readings it is possible to record which reactions have turned negative and which reactions have become apparent and/or increased (crescendo) or decreased (decrescendo) in intensity. From studies with repeated readings it is obvious that the same patch test preparation can produce lost as well as found reactions [82, 83]. Neomycin, corticosteroids, and gold are often-quoted examples of allergens with late appearance ("slow" allergens) while others (fragrance mix, Balsam of Peru) are classified as "early" allergens. When readings were carried out on days 2, 3, and 7, 3% and 8.2% respectively of the reactions first appeared on day 7 [84, 85]. However, some of the positive late reactions proved negative when retested [84]. Long-lasting reactions persisting weeks or months after the initial readings are increasingly attended [86]. However, the clinical significance is not yet settled.

A reaction positive on day 2 and a negative one on day 4 has been suggested to indicate irritancy. There are some examples where such a pattern has been found to be clinically relevant, but the frequency is not known. To contribute to the confusion, a few substances are known to cause "delayed irritancy" [1].

22.5.1.3 Compromise

Multiple readings are thus highly justified and the importance of readings beyond day 2 is stressed [87]. If practical or geographical circumstances permit only one reading, the present accepted compromise is at day 3 (72 h), i.e., 24 h after removal of the patches. However in recent papers [88, 89] it was stated that a single reading on day 4 would have been most useful. Patients are instructed to report any late reactions.

Table 3. Multiple readings – options and recommendations

Option	No. of visits	Day 0 Application	Day 2 Removal, reading	Day 3/4 Reading	Day 5/7 Reading	Comment
1	2	×	×			Not recommended
2	3	×	×	×		Recommended
3	3	×		×	×	Recommended
4	4	×	×	×	×	Highly recommended

Options and recommendations concerning multiple readings are presented in Table 3. Options 2–4 enable discrimination between crescendo and decrescendo reactions. When comparing options 2 and 3 – both with three visits – we slightly prefer option 3 since it gives an opportunity to do a late reading (day 5/7).

The value of repeated readings must be balanced by the discomfort, costs, and practical problems (e.g., travel) the repeated visits will cause the patients. However, it is our firm belief that repeated readings will increase the accuracy of our only method of establishing contact allergy.

Core Message

■ Late-appearing positive patch test reactions can appear for most allergens and are common for some. These reactions are missed if only early readings are carried out. Multiple readings are thus encouraged and if one wants to restrict the number of visits to three we consider that a reading at day 5/7 is more valuable than at day 2 – just after the removal of the patches.

Table 4. Recording of patch test reactions according to the International Contact Dermatitis Research Group (ICDRG) [36]

?+	Doubtful reaction; faint erythema only
+	Weak positive reaction; erythema, infiltration, possibly papules
++	Strong positive reaction; erythema, infiltration, papules, vesicles
+++	Extreme positive reaction; intense erythema and infiltration and coalescing vesicles
–	Negative reaction
IR	Irritant reactions of different types
NT	Not tested

22.5.2 Recording of Test Reactions

The common method of recording patch test reactions, recommended by the International Contact Dermatitis Research Group [2], is presented in Table 4. These recommendations are followed worldwide and are referred to in most scientific reports. Typical examples are shown in Fig. 4.

However, this recording system is somewhat simplified and not all types of reaction fit this outline. While experienced patch testers rarely disagree concerning the reading of the obvious irritant (IR), ++ and +++ reactions, the reading of the +? and + reactions and some of the IR may cause difficulties.

For documentation of patch test results it is recommended that forms are used with space for additional notes on the morphological appearance of the test reactions. It should be mentioned that some investigators record any changes from normal skin and others might ignore a very weak follicular reaction and record it as negative. Especially when repeated readings are taken, or lesser-known or new substances have been applied, it is essential to follow the appearance and disappearance of the various components of the reactions. Pictures can be of value for documentation, but can rarely replace our traditional aids: inspection and palpation. Instruction and supervision by an experienced patch tester is recommended for the *novice*. Each test site should be inspected and palpated and daily readings in selected cases would enable her/him to follow the dynamics of test reactions.

22.5.3 Interpretation of Reactions at Test Sites

A reaction at a test site merely indicates some kind of change compared to adjacent, nontested skin: it is not synonymous with "allergic" or "relevant"! Some important and somewhat controversial issues on the interpretation of patch test reactions will now be discussed.

Fig. 4a–d. Allergic patch test reactions (all day 3) of increasing intensity. **a** + Reaction to nickel sulfate; **b** still a + reaction to *para*-phenylenediamine (*PPDA*); **c** ++ reaction to PPDA; **d** +++ reaction to PPDA. (Courtesy of P.J. Frosch)

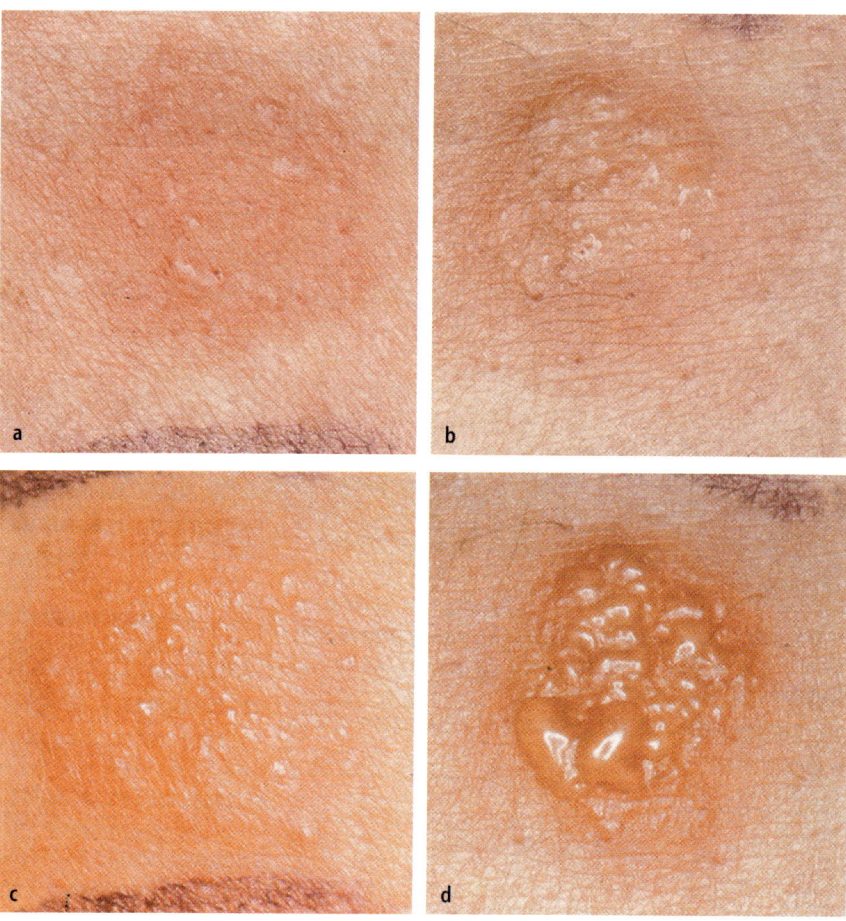

Core Message

■ Patch test reactions should be recorded according to the scheme presented in Table 4.
Repeated readings would enable the reader – especially when under training – to follow the appearance and disappearance of various components of a reaction.
A reaction at a test site merely indicates some kind of change compared to adjacent, nontested skin: it is not synonymous with "allergic" or "relevant."

22.5.3.1 Discrimination Between Allergic and Irritant Reactions

To distinguish allergic (Fig. 4) reactions from irritant (Fig. 5) reactions on morphological grounds alone is difficult. Irritant reactions (IR) are said [1, 37, 52] to be characterized by: fine wrinkling ("silk paper"), erythema, and papules in follicular distribution, petechiae, pustules, bullae and necrosis and with minimal infiltration. Typical examples are shown in Fig. 5. Extension beyond the defined area exposed to the allergen is used to discriminate between allergic and irritant reactions [1]. Fisher [38] frankly states: "There is no morphological way of distinguishing a weak irritant patch test from a weak allergic test." Examples are benzalkonium chloride and MCI/MC, where there has been some discussion concerning the somewhat peculiar features of the test reactions.

In Table 2 the results from a serial dilution test with nickel sulfate are shown. At dilution step 5 (0.01%), a few papules have been recorded and in this case we know that the reaction is relevant and that this patient is highly sensitive. However, if "a few papules" are noticed in another patient, where only *one* concentration of an allergen has been applied, the interpretation is much more difficult. Usually, we have to repeat the test and probably raise the concentration and/or carry out a serial dilution test.

22

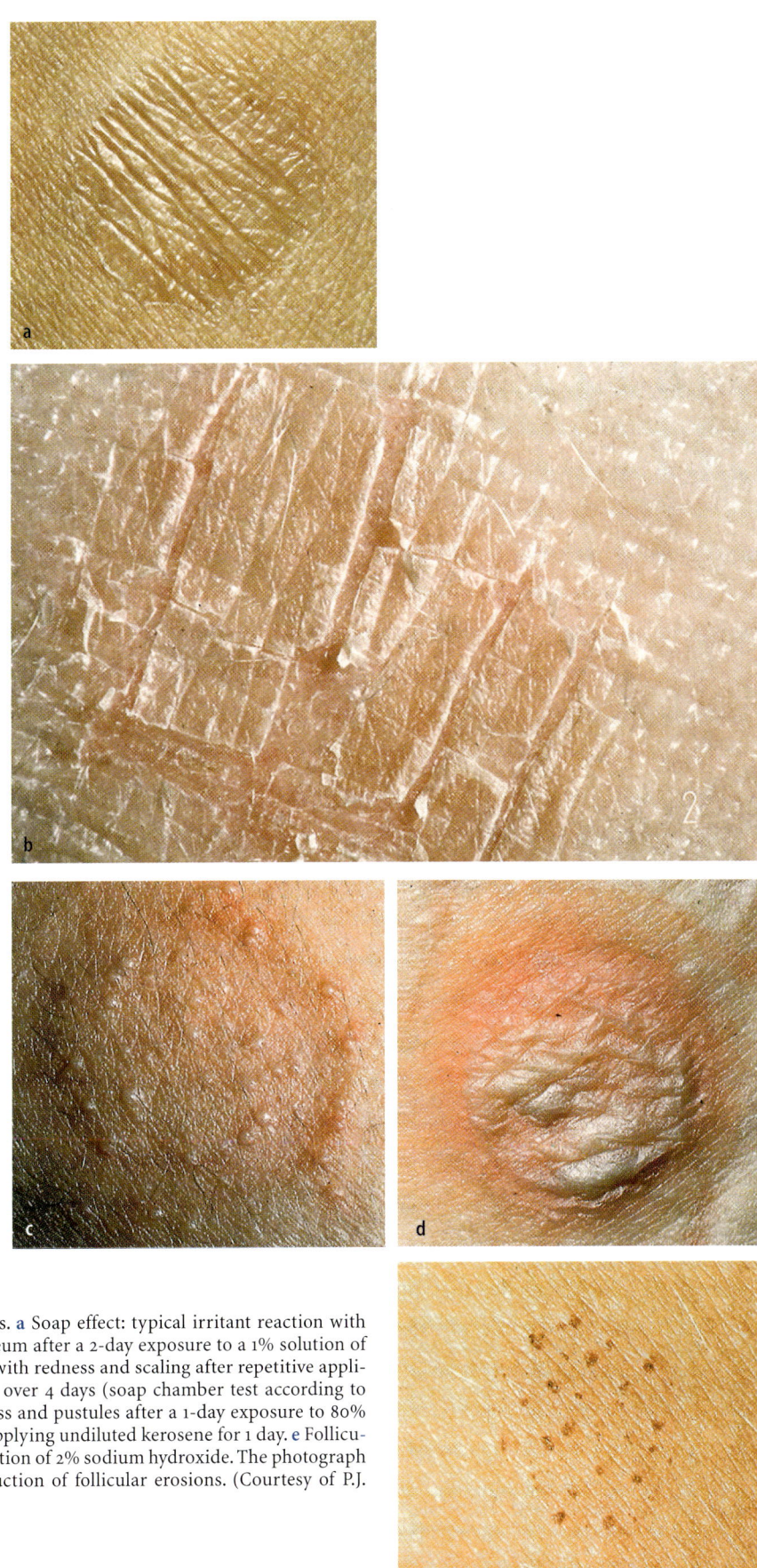

Fig. 5a–e. a, b Irritant reactions. **a** Soap effect: typical irritant reaction with glistening of the stratum corneum after a 2-day exposure to a 1% solution of toilet soap. **b** Irritant reaction with redness and scaling after repetitive application of an 8% soap solution over 4 days (soap chamber test according to Frosch and Kligman). **c** Redness and pustules after a 1-day exposure to 80% croton oil. **d** Full blister after applying undiluted kerosene for 1 day. **e** Follicular crusts after a 15-min application of 2% sodium hydroxide. The photograph was taken 1 day after the induction of follicular erosions. (Courtesy of P.J. Frosch)

22.5.3.2 Ring-Shaped Test Reactions

The somewhat peculiar ring-shaped test reactions (the "edge effect"), observed with – among other allergens – formaldehyde and MCI/MC in liquid vehicles, are in most cases an expression of contact allergy [90]. A special type can be seen with corticosteroids where the margins of the positive test are red, whereas the central area is whitish.

22.5.3.3 Ultrastructure

For distinguishing between allergic and irritant patch test reactions, traditional light or electronic microscopy has been of minimal help (see Chap. 8). Studies with monoclonal antibodies (e.g., [91]) and newer molecular techniques have not yet provided methods for clinical use to separate the two types of patch test reactions.

22.5.3.4 Doubtful and One Plus Reactions

When vesicles are present there is rarely any discussion of the allergic nature of the reaction, but the presence or absence of papules is more controversial [62, 92]. However, observed +? and + reactions may cause difficulties. As can be seen from Table 4, "possibly papules" is included in the + reaction. This expression can be interpreted in different ways: to be classified as a one plus (+) reaction – is erythema plus infiltration enough? What about erythema and papules, but no infiltration? According to Cronin [52], + is a palpable erythema. Historically the reading criteria for +? and + have not developed in parallel in all geographical areas. These differences in the interpretation of the objective skin changes explain some of the differences seen between departments and geographical areas.

When such a weak reaction (+? or +) has been obtained we recommend – as discussed in Sect. 22.5.3.1, Discrimination Between Allergic and Irritant Reactions – repeating the test, increasing the concentration by a factor of 5 or 10, and carrying out serial dilution (Table 2) and Use tests (see below).

Consensus on the denomination and interpretation of doubtful and weak reactions would be of great value and would facilitate comparisons between clinics and geographical areas.

Core Message

- Doubtful (+?) and weak test reactions (+) are hard to interpret. In those cases repeating the test, increasing the test concentration, serial dilution tests or Use tests are recommended.

22.5.3.5 Cross-Sensitivity

In cross-sensitivity, contact allergy caused by a primary allergen is combined with allergy to other chemically closely related substances. In those patients who have become sensitized to one substance, an allergic contact dermatitis can be provoked or worsened by several other related substances. A patient positive to *para*-phenylendiamine not only reacts to the dye itself, but also to immunochemically related substances that have an amino group in the *para* position, e.g., azo compounds, local anesthetics, and sulfonamides. When studying cross-reactivity it is essential to use pure test compounds [24].

22.5.4 Relevance

Evaluating the relevance of a reaction is the most difficult and intricate part of the patch test procedure, and is a challenge to both dermatologist and patient. The dermatologist's skill, experience, and curiosity are crucial factors.

For standard allergens, detailed lists are available that present the occurrence of each in the environment. The patient and the dermatologist should study the lists together, in order to judge the relevance of a positive patch test reaction, in relation to the exposure, site, course, and relapses of the patient's current dermatitis. A positive test reaction can also be explained by a previous, unrelated episode of contact dermatitis (past relevance).

Sometimes, the relevance of a positive reaction remains unexplained ("unexplained positive") until the patient brings a package or bottle where the allergen in question is named on the label. In other cases, chemical analyses demonstrate the presence of the allergen, or the manufacturer finally – after many inquiries – admits that the offending substance is present in the product. Methods for increasing the accuracy of the relevance of positive patch test reactions were recently presented [59, 93]. See also below, Sect. 22.10, Use Tests.

22

In cosmetics, skin care products, detergents, paints, cutting fluids, glues, etc., it is common that new ingredients are added or replace previous ones, but the product keeps its original trade name. Alternatively, well-known allergens are included in new products but with other fields of application than the original. To discover the cause of the patient's dermatitis the dermatologist must sometimes be obstinately determined!

The relative importance of different exogenous and endogenous factors to a given case of dermatitis might be hard to evaluate.

> ### Core Message
>
> ■ Evaluating the relevance of positive test reactions is the most difficult and intricate part of the test procedure and in this process the dermatologist's skill, experience, and curiosity are crucial factors. Clinical examination, repeated checking of history and exposure, Use tests, chemical analyses, and work-site visits ("the patient's chemical environment") can be of great help.

22.5.5 False-Positive Test Reactions

A false-positive reaction is a positive patch test reaction in the absence of contact allergy [94]. The most common causes can be summarized as follows:

1. Too high a test concentration for that particular patient
2. Impure or contaminated test preparation
3. The vehicle is irritant (especially solvents and sometimes petrolatum)
4. Excess of test preparation applied
5. The test substance, usually as crystals, is unevenly dispersed in the vehicle
6. Influence from adjacent test reactions (see above "Sequence of Allergens")
7. Current or recent dermatitis at test site
8. Current dermatitis at distant skin sites
9. Pressure effects of tapes, mechanical irritation of solid test materials, furniture and garments (brassiere)
10. Adhesive tape reactions
11. The patch itself has caused the reactions
12. Artifacts

Some are self-evident and can be predicted and monitored by the dermatologist carrying out patch testing, while others cannot.

22.5.5.1 The Compromise (Item 1)

While the current recommendations on allergen concentrations in relation to vehicle, patch, and tapes are based on long experience, they are nevertheless a compromise! The general problem is that if you lower the concentration to avoid irritancy you will also lose some cases that will be of special occupational and medicolegal importance. Well-known examples are dichromate, formaldehyde, tars, fragrance-mix and, previously, carba mix. It is probably better to have a (weak) false-positive reaction than a false-negative reaction because at least with a potentially false-positive reaction one is *alerted* to the possibility of allergy, which one can then confirm or deny, whereas with a false-negative reaction one is never alerted at all and may altogether miss a true allergy. Therefore, most dermatologists seem to prefer the higher concentrations of these marginal irritants, even though they know that nonspecific reactions from them are not uncommon.

> ### Core Message
>
> ■ Current recommendations on allergen concentrations in relation to vehicles, patches, and tapes are based on long experience but are nonetheless a compromise. If you lower the concentration to avoid irritancy you will also lose some cases. It is probably better to have a weak false-positive reaction than a false-negative reaction because the dermatologist is then alerted.

22.5.5.2 Excited-Skin Syndrome – "Angry Back" (Items 7 and 8)

Patients with current eczema may show cutaneous hyperirritability which can cause problems in patch testing. In the excited-skin syndrome, the presence of a strong positive reaction will influence the reactivity at adjacent test sites. When more than one site shows a reaction, this phenomenon must be considered, and retesting of the items one at a time is the usual recommendation (Fig. 6). Thanks to Björnberg's [95]

Fig. 6. Patients with multiple sensitizations do exist. This leg ulcer patient was allergic to numerous allergens. The strong reactions have been reproduced and were clinically relevant (wool wax alcohols, propylene glycol, parabens, *para*-phenylenediamine, MCI/MI, imidazolidinyl urea, thimerosal, thiuram mix, triamcinolone acetonide, amcinonide, and bufexamac). (Courtesy of P.J. Frosch)

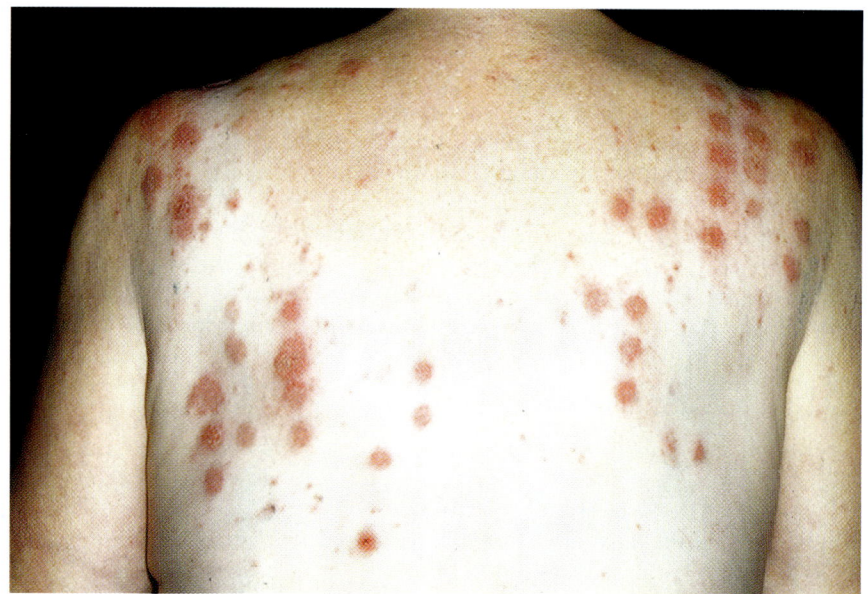

important observations, we have always avoided patch testing a patient with current eczema and labile skin, and the excited-skin syndrome is seldom seen in our latitudes [96]. There is extensive literature on this syndrome [97, 98].

22.5.5.3 The Patch (Item 11)

After receiving intradermal allergen extracts due to pollen allergy, a few patients will develop sensitivity to aluminum. They will then react to an Al-test as well as to Finn chambers. Mercury-containing test preparations can react with aluminum, but nowadays plastic-coated Finn chambers are available.

22.5.5.4 Artifacts (Item 12)

Sometimes strong, necrotic reactions are seen and an artifact is suspected. In medicolegal cases, control patches (empty or containing water or petrolatum) are recommended for application simultaneously and in random order.

22.5.6 False-Negative Test Reactions

22.5.6.1 Common Causes

A false-negative reaction is a negative patch test reaction in the presence of contact allergy [94]. The most common causes can be summarized as follows:

1. Insufficient penetration of the allergen
   a. Too low a test concentration for that particular patient
   b. The test substance is not released from the vehicle or retained by the filter paper
   c. Insufficient amount (dose) of test preparation applied; patch test concentration lower than declared [99]
   d. Insufficient occlusion
   e. Duration of contact too brief – the test strip has fallen off or slipped
   f. The test was not applied to the recommended site – the upper back
2. Failure to perform delayed readings; e.g., neomycin and corticosteroids are known to give delayed reactions (see Table 3)
3. The test site has been treated with corticosteroids or irradiated with UV or Grenz rays
4. Systemic treatment with corticosteroids or immunomodulators
5. Allergen is not in active form, insufficiently oxidized (oil of turpentine, rosin compounds, D-limonene) or degraded
6. Compound allergy

Some of them are self-evident and can be predicted and monitored by the dermatologist, while others cannot. Examples of the latter category may arise in the following situations: when testing has been carried out in a refractory or "anergic" phase [97]; when the test does not reproduce the clinical exposure to reach the critical elicitation level (multiple applica-

22

tions), where some adjuvant factors are present (sweating, friction, pressure, damaged skin); or penetration at the test site (see Sect. 22.1.3, Bioavailability) is lower than that of clinical exposure (eyelids, axillae). A stripped skin technique is recommended in the last case, where the test sites are stripped with tape before application of test preparations.

The differential diagnoses photoallergy and contact urticaria should also be considered. Skin hyporeactivity in relation to patch testing was recently reviewed [100] and it was pointed out that the failure to elicit a response might be due to a faulty immune response, a defective inflammatory response or both. The defective inflammatory response can be evaluated by using a positive control, such as the irritant sodium lauryl sulfate [41] or nonanoic acid [39].

22.5.6.2 Compound Allergy (Item 6)

The term "compound allergy" is used to describe the condition in patients who are patch test positive to formulated products, usually cosmetic creams or topical medicaments, but are test negative to all the ingredients tested individually [101]. This phenomenon can sometimes be explained by irritancy of the original formulation, but in some cases it has been demonstrated that reactivity was due to combination of the ingredients to form reaction products [102, 103]. Another reason might be that the ingredients were patch tested at the usage concentrations, which are too low for many allergens (e.g., MCI/MI, neomycin). Pseudo-compound allergy, due to faulty patch testing technique, is likely to be commoner than true compound allergy. In recent publications [104, 105], several proven or possible compound allergens were listed. The formation of allergenic reaction products can take place within the product ("chemical allergenic reactions") but probably also metabolically in the skin ("biological allergenic reactions") [104]. The topic remains the subject of continuing debate [106, 107]. False-positive and false-negative reactions have recently been reviewed [59].

22.6 Ethnic and Climatic Considerations

Problems and recommendations when patch testing at different climatic environments and in oriental and black populations were recently reviewed [62].

22.7 Effect of Medicaments and Irradiation on Patch Tests

22.7.1 Corticosteroids

Treatment of test sites with topical corticosteroids [108] can give rise to false-negative reactions (see Sect. 22.5.6.1, Common Causes).

Testing a patient on oral corticosteroids always creates uncertainty. The problem was studied 25–30 years ago [109–111] by comparing the intensity of test reactions before and during treatment with corticosteroids (20–40 mg prednisone). Diminution and disappearance of test reactions were noted in several cases, but not regularly. These findings have been interpreted as allowing us to test patients on oral doses equivalent to 20 mg of prednisone without missing any important allergies. However, the test reactions studied were strong (+++), and fairly weak (+) and questionable reactions were not evaluated. In a recent study [112] patch testing with serial dilution tests with nickel, it was found that the total number of positive nickel patch tests decreased significantly when the patients were on 20 mg prednisone compared to on placebo. The threshold concentration to elicit a patch test reaction increased and the overall degree of reactivity to nickel shifted toward weaker reactions. In clinical practice we prefer to defer testing until the patient's dermatitis has cleared. When testing a patient with labile skin there is also the risk of excited-skin syndrome [97]. In selected cases where one or two allergens are strongly suspected, we choose to test for these only, even if the patient is on oral corticosteroids. However, when the dermatitis has cleared, we repeat the test with the whole series to relieve our uncertainty.

22.7.2 Antihistamines

In one study [110], the antihistamine Incidal did not influence reactivity, while in another [113] a decrease in intensity was seen in 6 out of 17 patients after cinnarizine had been administered for 1 week. Oral loratadine was found to reduce patch test reactions; evaluated clinically and echographically [114]. These results also give the dermatologist a feeling of uncertainty, and we prefer either to discontinue antihistamine treatment during testing or to defer testing. However, this contraindication is not universally accepted [115].

22.7.3 Immunomodulators

Topical cyclosporine inhibits test reactions in humans and in animal models [116–118]. As yet there is no comparison of test reactions in allergic patients before and during treatment with orally or parenterally administered cytostatic agents.

22.7.4 Irradiation

It has been shown that irradiation with UVB [119] and Grenz rays [120, 121] reduced the number of Langerhans cells and the intensity of patch test reactions in humans. Repeated suberythema doses of UVB depressed reactivity even at sites shielded during the exposures. This indicates a systemic effect of UVB [119]. Experiments to clarify the mechanism behind these observations have been carried out on experimental animals, but their relevance to humans is not finally settled [122, 123].

22.7.5 Seasonal Variations

Seasonal variations in patch test reactivity is not fully explored. In Israel negative patch test reactivity was found among 55% in winter and 70% in summer among tested patients [124]. In a German study [125] formaldehyde exhibited a distinct increase in questionable or irritant as well as weak-positive reactions associated with dry, cold weather. In a more recent German study [126] it was concluded that ambient temperature and humidity and sodium lauryl sulfate reactivity independently contribute information on individual irritability at the time of patch testing. We recommend avoidance of patch testing on severely tanned persons and that a minimum of 4 weeks after heavy sun exposure should be allowed before testing. At our clinic we refrain from testing during July and August.

22.8 Complications

Reported complications of patch testing are listed below. However, most can be predicted and avoided:

1. Patch test sensitization
2. Irritant reactions from nonstandard allergens or products, brought by the patient
3. Flare of previous or existing dermatitis due to percutaneous absorption of the allergen
4. Subjective complaints
5. Depigmentation, e.g., phenols
6. Pigmentation, sometimes after sunlight exposure of test sites
7. Scars, keloids
8. Granulomas from beryllium, zirconium
9. Anaphylactoid reactions or shock from, e.g., neomycin, bacitracin (regarding penicillin, see below)
10. Infections (bacteria, virus)

22.8.1 Patch Test Sensitization (Item 1)

By definition, a negative patch test reaction followed by a flare-up after 10–20 days, and then a positive reaction after 3 days at retesting, means that sensitization was induced by the patch test procedure. There is a small risk of active sensitization from the standard series and common examples are *para*-phenylenediamine, primula extracts and, in recent years, isothiazolinone [63], acrylates [127], and a bleach accelerator (PBA-1) [128]. The risk, however, is an extremely low one when the testing is carried out according to internationally accepted guidelines.

It must be emphasized that the overall risk–benefit equation of patch testing patients is much in favor of the benefit.

22.8.2 Subjective Complaints (Item 4)

Subjective complaints, e.g., fever, fatigue, indisposition, vomiting, headache, dizziness, were more often reported on the day of test application compared to the day of reading, however with one exception – itch on the back [129]. This itch can mainly be related to positive patch test reactions and irritation from adhesive tapes. However, 10–15% of patients with positive test reactions, but without itch, reported complaints such as tiredness, feeling unwell, headache, shakiness, and light-headedness [130]. Of patients without complaints on the day of application 36% later reported complaints other than itch [131].

22.8.3 Penicillin (Item 9)

Penicillin can give rise to anaphylactoid reactions or shock and is therefore not recommended for routine patch testing (see also Chap. 40). To minimize the risk, which is essential also from a medicolegal point of view, we recommend radioallergosorbent tests, an oral provocation test with half or one tablet of penicillin, and an open test prior to the closed patch test.

22

22.9 Open Tests

22.9.1 Open Test

"Open test" and "Use test" (see Sect. 22.10, Use Tests) are sometimes used as synonyms and no clear-cut definitions seem to exist. Open testing usually means that a product, as is or dissolved in water or some solvent (e.g., ethanol, acetone, ether), is dropped onto the skin and allowed to spread freely. No occlusion is used.

An open test is recommended as the first step when testing poorly defined or unknown substances or products, such as those brought by the patient (paints, glues, oils, detergents, cleansing agents based on solvents, etc.). The test site should be checked at regular intervals during the first 30–60 min after application, especially when the history indicates immediate reactions or contact urticaria (see Chap. 26). A second reading should be done at 3–4 days.

The usual test site is the volar forearm, but this is less reactive than the back or the upper arms. A negative open test can be explained by insufficient penetration, but indicates that one dares to go on with an occlusive patch test.

22.9.2 Semi-open Test

This method was introduced by Goossens [132] and is mainly used for products – brought by the patients – with suspected irritant properties due to solvents or emulsifiers, e.g., detergents, shampoos, paints, resins, varnishes, glues, waxes, cooling fluids, pharmaceuticals, and cosmetics. The product (solution or suspension) is applied with a cotton swab as is in a small amount (about 15 μL) to an area of 2 × 2 cm. After complete drying it is covered with acrylate tape for 2 days. The site is checked for contact urticaria and at days 2 and 4 for signs of contact eczema.

22.10 Use Tests

22.10.1 Purpose

The original (provocative) use (or usage) tests (PUT) were intended to mimic the actual use situation (repeated open applications) of a formulated product such as a cosmetic, a shampoo, an oil or a topical medicament. A positive result supported the suspicion that the product had caused the patient's dermatitis. The primary goal was not to clarify the nature (allergic or irritant) of the dermatitis – just to reproduce it!

Nowadays these tests are increasingly used to evaluate the clinical significance of ingredient(s) of a formulated product previously found reactive by ordinary patch testing. The concentration of the particular ingredient can be so low that one may wonder whether the positive patch test reaction can explain the patient's dermatitis.

22.10.2 Repeated Open Application Test

The repeated open application test (ROAT) in a standardized form was introduced by Hannuksela and Salo [133]. Test substances, either commercial products, as is, or special test substances (e.g., patch test allergen) are applied twice daily for 7 days to the outer aspect of the upper arm, antecubital fossa or back skin (scapular area). The size of the test area is not crucial: a positive result may appear on a 1 cm × 1 cm area 1–2 days later than on a larger area. The amount of test substance should be approx. 0.1 ml to a 5 cm × 5 cm area and 0.5 ml to a 10 cm × 10 cm area [134, 135].

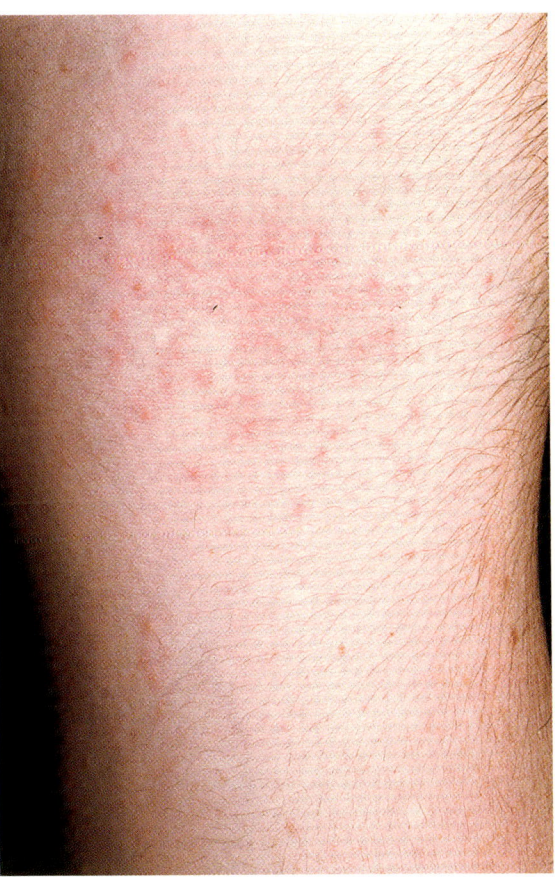

Fig. 7. A positive ROAT on the third day in a patient allergic to iso-eugenol. (Courtesy of P.J. Frosch)

A positive response – eczematous dermatitis – usually appears on days 2–4 (Fig. 7), but it is recommended to extend the applications beyond 7 days in order not to miss late-appearing reactions [136–138]. A refined scheme for scoring of ROAT reactions has recently been presented [139]. The patient is told to stop the application of the test substance(s) when he or she notices a reaction [133].

If a ROAT is carried out with a formulated product, the observed reaction may be due to allergy to an ingredient, but irritancy from other ingredients cannot be excluded. At our clinic we therefore use two coded samples – one containing the allergen and one without it. We instruct the patient to apply one product to the left arm and the other to the right arm, according to a special protocol where the treatments and any observed reaction can be noted. If there is a reaction only at the test site where the allergen-containing product has been applied, we consider the initial patch test reaction relevant. On the other hand, we interpret reactions of the same intensity on both arms as an expression of irritancy.

The value of ROAT has been verified in cases with positive, negative or questionable reactions at initial patch testing [136, 137, 140–142] and in animal studies [138], and it was pointed out that Use testing has significant potential in refinement of the evidence-based diagnosis of clinical relevance [143].

22.11 Noninvasive Techniques

To reduce the well-known interindividual variation when scoring patch test reactions, several attempts have been made to introduce objective bioengineering techniques for assessment. Erythema and skin color can be assessed by laser Doppler flowmetry (LDF), skin reflectance and colorimeters, and edema with calipers, ultrasound and electrical impedance. The advantages and limitations of these methods have been reviewed [144]. These sophisticated techniques cannot replace visual assessment and palpation of test sites by the dermatologist, but are valuable in research work [145]. The topic is further reviewed in Chap. 28.

A significant correlation between visual scoring of patch test reactions and LDF values was claimed by Staberg et al. [146]. The method discriminated between negative and positive reactions, but failed to quantify strong positive reactions. However, in a recent guideline from the standardization group of the European Society of Contact Dermatitis it was stated that laser Doppler perfusion imaging does not directly distinguish between allergic and irritant patch test reactions [147].

It has also been shown that the combination of allergen, vehicle, patch, and tape will cause a transient increase in skin blood flow, even in healthy subjects [80]. An increase was noticed for 1–2 days after removal of the patches, without causing any visual changes. Skin blood flow must be increased three to four times before the naked eye can detect an erythema [148].

22.12 Quality Control of Test Materials

22.12.1 Identification and Purity

As pointed out above (see Sect. 22.2.1.2, Allergens), the dermatologist is recommended to obtain protocols of chemical analyses and data on purity from suppliers of test preparations. Some dermatologists have the laboratory facilities to check the information presented, but most just have to accept it. Especially when "new" allergens are detected, in cases of unexpected multiple reactivity or suspected cross-reactivity, detailed information on purity, chemical identification, and stability of the allergen is indispensable [24]. Some mixes, such as fragrance mix, contain emulsifiers (sorbitan sesquioleate) and a correct retest with ingredients of a mix should thus include the individual fragrances as well as the emulsifier.

22.12.2 Test Preparations Under the Microscope

Light microscope examination (magnification ×100–400) of commercial test preparations with petrolatum as vehicle is usually disappointing. Crystals [149–151] or globules [152] of different size are seen and one wonders how this influences the bioavailability of the allergen. However, in one comparative study no difference in reactivity was found [153].

In the TRUE Test, the allergens are incorporated in hydrophilic gels and are evenly distributed [27].

22.12.3 Fresh Samples

In cases of unexpected negative test reactions, the items listed in Sect. 22.5.6.1, Common Causes should be considered. If the case remains unsolved, it is suggested that a fresh sample of the allergen be purchased from a different supplier.

22.12.4 Adhesive Tapes

A significant development in tape quality has taken place [33, 154] (see also above Sect. 22.2.1.5, Tapes).

22.13 Tests with Unknown Substances

22.13.1 Warning!

A word of warning: totally unknown substances or products should never be applied to human skin! Scarring, necrosis, keloids, pigmentation, depigmentation, systemic effects following percutaneous absorption, and any other complications listed earlier can appear and the dermatologist may be accused of malpractice.

22.13.2 Strategy

When patients bring suspected products or materials from their (work) environment we recommend that adequate product safety data sheets, lists of ingredients, etc. are requested from the manufacturer so that a general impression of the product, ingredients, concentrations, intended use, etc. can be formed. There are usually one or two ingredients that are of interest as suspected allergens, while the rest are well-known substances of proven innocuousness for which detailed information is available. For substances or products where skin contact is unintentional and the dermatitis is a result of misuse or accident, detailed information from the manufacturer is required before any tests are initiated.

22.13.3 Test or Not?

The next step is to look for the suspected allergens. If they are available from suppliers of patch test allergens [21, 23], one can rely on the choice of vehicle and concentration. If one suspects that impurities or contaminants have caused the dermatitis, this can only be discovered via samples of the ingredient from the manufacturer.

If it is an entirely new substance, where no data on toxicity, etc. are available, the patient and dermatologist have to decide how to find an optimal test concentration and vehicle, and to discuss the risk of complications. To minimize the risk, one can start with an open test and, if this is negative, continue with occlusive patch testing. Most allergens are tested in the concentration range 0.01–10% and we usually start with the lowest and raise the concentration when the preceding test is negative. A very practical method is to apply 0.01% and 0.1% for 1 day in a region where the patient can easily remove the patch her- or himself (upper back or upper arm). If severe stinging or burning occurs, he or she should be instructed to remove it immediately. If the test is negative, the concentration can be raised to 1%. Occasionally, the likely irritant or sensitization potential of a chemical may be such that starting with concentrations of 0.001% and 0.01% is advisable, increasing to 0.1% if negative. An alternative is to start with a higher concentration, but with reduced exposure time (5 h) [76]; but this procedure is not sufficiently standardized.

If the test is positive in the patient, one has to demonstrate in unexposed controls that the actual test preparation is nonirritant [66]. Otherwise the observed reaction in the particular patient does not prove allergenicity. It is important to check the pH of products before testing.

When testing products brought by the patient, it is essential to use samples from the actual batch to which the patient has been exposed, but also when testing, for example, cutting fluids, unused products must be tested for comparison. When testing with dilutions, one runs the risk of overlooking true allergens by using over-diluted materials. See also Chap. 50.

22.13.4 Solid Products and Extracts

When a solid product is suspected (textiles, rubber, plants, wood, paper etc.), these can usually be applied as is. Rycroft [94] recommends that the material be tested as wafer-thin, regular-sided, smooth sheets (e.g., rubber) or as finely divided particulates (e.g., woods). A transient so-called pressure effect is sometimes seen when testing with solids. Plants and woods and their extracts constitute special problems, due to variations in the quantity of allergens produced and their availability on the surface. Extracts for testing can be obtained by placing the product or sample in water, synthetic sweat, ethanol, acetone or ether, and heating to 40–50°C. False reactions to nonstandardized patch tests have been reviewed by Rycroft [94]. Patch testing with thin-layer chromatograms has been found valuable for products such as textiles, plastics, food, plants, perfumes, drugs, and grease [155].

22.13.5 Cosmetics and Similar Products

For most products with intended use on normal or damaged skin (cosmetics, skin care products, soap, shampoos, detergents, topical medicaments, etc.), detailed predictive testing and clinical and consumer trials have been performed. The results can usually be obtained from the manufacturer. For this category of products, open tests and Use tests probably give more information than an occlusive patch test on the pathogenesis of the patient's dermatitis. Suggestions on concentrations and vehicles can be found in textbooks [38, 52].

22.14 The Future

This chapter concludes with the following list of hopes and needs for the future:

- Diversified vehicles to obtain optimal bio-availability of allergens
- Statements in suppliers' catalogs on the purity and stability of individual allergens
- Decrease of test exposure times (24 h or less) with retained accuracy
- Consensus on the reading, scoring, interpretation, and relevance of weak test reactions
- Objective assessment of test reactions
- Further standardization of Use tests
- Irritancy from test preparations – refinement of predictive methods
- Systemic treatment with immunomodulators and antihistamines– influence on patch test reactivity
- Influence on patch test reactivity due to seasonal variation, latitude, temperature, and humidity.

References

1. Malten KE, Nater JP, van Ketel WG (1976) Patch testing guidelines. Dekker and van de Vegt, Nijmegen
2. Fregert S (1981) Manual of contact dermatitis, 2nd edn. Munksgaard, Copenhagen
3. Bandmann HJ, Dohn W (1967) Die Epicutantestung. Bergmann, Munich
4. Rajagopalan R, Anderson R (1997) Impact of patch testing on Dermatology-specific quality of life in patients with allergic contact dermatitis. Am J Contact Dermat 8: 215–221
5. Thomson KF, Wilkinson SM, Sommer S, Pollock B (2002) Eczema: quality of life by body site and the effect of patch testing. Br J Dermatol 146: 627–630
6. Woo PN, Hay IC, Ormerod AS (2003) An audit of the value of patch testing and its effect on quality of life. Contact Dermatitis 48: 244–247
7. Van der Valk PGM, Devos SA, Coenraads P-J (2003) Evidence-based diagnosis in patch testing. Contact Dermatitis 48: 121–125
8. Jadassohn J (1896) Zur Kenntnis der medikamentösen Dermatosen, Verhandlungen der Deutschen Dermatologischen Gesellschaft. Fünfter Congress, Raz, 1895. Braunmuller, Vienna, p 106
9. Foussereau J (1984) History of epicutaneous testing: the blotting-paper and other methods. Contact Dermatitis 11: 219–223
10. Fischer TI, Hansen J, Kreilgård B, Maibach HI (1989) The science of patch test standardization. Immunol Allergy Clin North Am 9: 417–443
11. Belsito DV, Storrs FJ, Taylor JS, Marks JG Jr, Adams RM, Rietschel RL, Jordan WP, Emmett EA (1992) Reproducibility of patch tests: a United States multi-centre study. Am J Contact Dermat 3: 193–200
12. Breit R, Agathos M (1992) Qualitätskontrolle der Epikutantestung – Reproduzierbarkeit im Rechts-Links-Vergleich. Hautarzt 43: 417–421
13. Bousema MT, Geursen AM, van Joost T (1991) High reproducibility of patch tests. J Am Acad Dermatol 24: 322–323
14. Lachapelle JM, Antoine JL (1989) Problems raised by the simultaneous reproducibility of positive allergic patch test reactions in man. J Am Acad Dermatol 21: 850–854
15. Macháčková J, Seda O (1991) Reproducibility of patch tests. J Am Acad Dermatol 25: 732–733
16. Lindelöf B (1990) A left versus right side comparative study of Finn Chamber™ patch tests in 220 consecutive patients. Contact Dermat 22: 288–289
17. Stransky L, Krasteva M (1992) A left versus right side comparative study of Finn Chamber patch tests in consecutive patients with contact sensitization. Dermatosen 40: 158–159
18. Brasch J, Henseler T, Aberer W, Bäuerle G, Frosch PJ, Fuchs T, Fünfstück V, Kaiser G, Lischka GG, Pilz B, Sauer C, Schaller J, Scheuer B, Szliska C (1994) Reproducibility of patch tests. A multicenter study of synchronous left-versus right-sided patch tests by the German Contact Dermatitis Research Group. J Am Acad Dermatol 31: 584–591
19. Fullerton A, Rud Andersen J, Hoelgaard A, Menné T (1986) Permeation of nickel salts through human skin in vitro. Contact Dermatitis 15: 173–177
20. Brasch J, Szliska C, Grabbe J (1997) More positive patch test reactions with larger test chambers? Contact Dermatitis 37: 118–120
21. Chemotechnique Diagnostics (2003) Patch test products. Catalogue. Malmö, Sweden
22. Gefeller O, Phahlberg A, Geier J, Brasch J, Uter W (1999) The association between size of test chamber and patch test reaction: a statistical reanalysis. Contact Dermatitis 40: 14–18
23. Trolab Hermal (2003) Patch test allergens. Trolab, Hermal, Reinbek, Germany
24. Fregert S (1985) Publication of allergens. Contact Dermatitis 12: 123–124
25. Dooms-Goossens A, Degreff H (1983) Contact allergy to petrolatums I. Sensitizing capacity of different brands of yellow and white petrolatums. Contact Dermatitis 9: 175–185
26. Bruze M (1984) Use of buffer solutions for patch testing. Contact Dermatitis 10: 267–269

27. Fischer T, Maibach H (1989) Easier patch testing with TRUE test. J Am Acad Dermatol 20:447–453
28. Magnusson B, Blohm S-G, Fregert S, Hjorth N, Høvding G, Pirilä V, Skog E (1966) Routine patch testing II. Acta Derm Venereol (Stockh) 46:153–158
29. Benezra C, Andanson J, Chabeau C, Ducombs G, Foussereau J, Lachapelle JM, Lacroix M, Martin P (1978) Concentrations of patch test allergens: are we comparing the same things? Contact Dermatitis 4:103–105
30. Bruze M (1986) Sensitizing capacity of 2-methylol phenol, 4-methylol phenol and 2,4,6-trimethylol phenol in the Guinea Pig. Contact Dermatitis 14:32–38
31. Wall LM, Calnan CD (1980) Occupational nickel dermatitis in the electroforming industry. Contact Dermatitis 6:414–420
32. Wahlberg JE (1996) Nickel: the search for alternative, optimal and non-irritant patch test preparations. Assessments based on laser Doppler flowmetry. Skin Res Technol 2:
33. Tokumura F, Ohyama K, Fujisawa H, Matsuda T, Kitazaki Y (1997) Conformability and irritancy of adhesive tapes on the skin. Contact Dermatitis 37:173–178
34. Fischer T, Dahlén Å, Bjkarnason B (1999) Influence of patch-test application tape on reactions to sodium lauryl sulphate. Contact Dermatitis 40:32–37
35. Brasch J, Kreilgård B, Henseler T, Aberer W, Fuchs T, Pfluger R, Hoeck U, Gefeller O (2000) Positive nickel patch tests do not intensify positive reactions to adjacent patch tests with dichromate. Contact Dermatitis 43:144–149
36. Duarte I, Lazzarini R, Buense R (2002) Interference of the position of substances in an epicutaneous patch test battery with the occurrence of false-positive results. Am J Contact Dermat 13:125–132
37. Fischer T, Maibach HI (1986) Patch testing in allergic contact dermatitis: an update. Semin Dermatol 5:214–224
38. Fisher AA (1986) Contact Dermatitis, 3rd edn. Lea and Febiger, Philadelphia
39. Wahlberg JE, Maibach HI (1980) Nonanoic acid irritation – a positive control at routine patch testing? Contact Dermatitis 6:128–130
40. Wahlberg JE, Wrangsjö K, Hietasalo A (1985) Skin irritancy from nonanoic acid. Contact Dermatitis 13:266–269
41. Geier J, Uter W, Pirker C, Frosch PJ (2003) Patch testing with the irritant sodium lauryl sulphate (SLS) is useful in interpreting weak reactions to contact allergens as allergic or irritant. Contact Dermatitis 48:99–107
42. Wahlberg JE, Lindberg M (2003) Nonanoic acid – an experimental irritant. Contact Dermatitis 49:117–123
43. Gollhausen R, Przybilla B, Ring J (1989) Reproducibility of patch test results: comparison of True test and Finn Chamber test. In: Frosch PJ, Dooms-Goossens A, Lachapelle JM, Rycroft RJ, Scheper RJ (eds) Current topics in contact dermatitis. Springer, Berlin Heidelberg New York, pp 524–529
44. Lachapelle J-M, Bruynzeel DP, Ducombs G, Hannuksela M, Ring J, White IR, Wilkinson J, Fischer T, Billberg K (1988) European multicenter study of the True test™. Contact Dermatitis 19:91–97
45. Ruhnek-Forsbeck M, Fischer T, Meding B, Pettersson L, Stenberg B, Strand A, Sundberg K, Svensson L, Wahlberg JE, Widström L, Wrangsjö K, Billberg K (1988) Comparative multi-center study with True test™ and Finn Chamber® patch test methods in eight Swedish hospitals. Acta Derm Venereol (Stockh) 68:123–128
46. Stenberg B, Billberg K, Fischer T, Nordin L, Pettersson L, Ruhnek-Forsbeck M, Sundberg K, Swanbeck G, Svensson L, Wahlberg JE, Widström L, Wrangsjö K (1989) Swedish multicenter study with True test, panel 2. In: Frosch PJ, Dooms-Goossens A, Lachapelle JM, Rycroft RJ, Scheper RJ (eds) Current topics in contact dermatitis. Springer, Berlin Heidelberg New York, pp 518–523
47. Wilkinson JD, Bruynzeel DP, Ducombs G, Frosch PJ, Gunnarsson Y, Hannuksela M, Ring J, Shaw S, White IR (1990) European multicenter study of TRUE test, panel 2. Contact Dermatitis 22:218–225
48. de Groot AC (1994) Patch testing. Test concentrations and vehicles for 3700 chemicals, 2nd edn. Elsevier, Amsterdam
49. De Groot AC (1986) Patch testing. Test concentrations and vehicles for 2800 allergens. Elsevier, Amsterdam
50. Cronin E (1986) Some practical supplementary trays for special occupations. Semin Dermatol 5:243–248
51. Kanerva L, Elsner P, Wahlberg JE, Maibach HI (2000) Handbook of occupational dermatology. Springer, Berlin Heidelberg New York
52. Cronin E (1980) Contact dermatitis. Churchill Livingstone, London
53. Adams RM (1990) Occupational skin disease, 2nd edn. Saunders, Philadelphia
54. Foussereau J, Benezra C, Maibach HI (1982) Occupational contact dermatitis. Clinical and chemical aspects. Munksgaard, Copenhagen
55. Hjorth N (1961) Eczematous allergy to balsams. Allied perfumes and flavouring agents. Munksgaard, Copenhagen
56. Takano S, Yamanaka M, Okamoto K, Saito F (1983) Allergens of lanolin: parts I and II. J Soc Cosmet Chem 34:99–125
57. Fregert S, Dahlquist I, Trulsson L (1984) An attempt to isolate and identify allergens in lanolin. Contacts Dermatitis 10:16–19
58. Karlberg A-T (1988) Contact allergy to colophony. Chemical identifications of allergens, sensitization experiments and clinical experiences. Thesis, Karolinska Institute, Stockholm, Sweden
59. Alé SI, Maibach HI (2002) Scientific basis of patch testing. Dermatol Beruf Umwelt 50:43–50, 91–96, 131–133
60. Hansson C, Agrup G (1993) Stability of the mercaptobenzothiazole compounds. Contact Dermatitis 28:29–34
61. Bergendorff O, Hansson C (2001) Stability of thiuram disulfides in patch test preparations and formation of asymmetric disulfides. Contact Dermatitis 45:151–157
62. Lachapelle J-M, Maibach HI (2003) Patch testing, prick testing. A practical guide. Springer, Berlin Heidelberg New York
63. Björkner B, Bruze M, Dahlquist I, Fregert S, Gruvberger B, Persson K (1986) Contact allergy to the preservative Kathon® CG. Contact Dermatitis 14:85–90
64. de Groot AC (1988) Adverse reactions to cosmetics. Thesis, Rijksuniversiteit Groningen, the Netherlands
65. Andersen KE, Burrows D, Cronin, Dooms-Goossens A, Rycroft RJG, White IR (1988) Recommended changes to standard series. Contact Dermatitis 19:389–390
66. Wahlberg JE (1998) Identification of new allergens and non-irritant patch test preparations. Contact Dermatitis 39:155–156
67. Bryld LE, Agner T, Rastogi SC, Menné T (1997) Idopropynyl butylcarbamate: a new contact allergen. Contact Dermatitis 36:156–158
68. Schnuch A, Geijer J, Brasch J, Uter W (2002) The preservative iodopropynyl butylcarbamate: frequence of allergic reactions and diagnostic considerations. Contact Dermatitis 46:153–156

69. Bruze M, Condé-Salazar L, Goossens A, Kanerva L, White I (1999) Thoughts on sensitizers in a standard patch test series. Contact Dermatitis 41: 241–250

70. Bruynzeel DP, Andersen KE, Camarasa JG, Lachapelle J-M, Menné T, White IR (1995) The European standard series. Contact Dermatitis 33:145–148

71. Isaksson M, Brandao FM, Bruze M, Goossens A (2000) Recommendation to include budesonide and tixocortol pivalate in the European standard series. Contact Dermatitis 43:41–42

72. Lachapelle J-M, Ale SI, Freeman S, Frosch PJ, Goh CL, Hannuksela M, Hayakawa R, Maibach HI, Wahlberg JE (1997) Proposal for a revised international standard series of patch tests. Contact Dermatitis 36:121–123

73. Kalimo K, Lammintausta K (1984) 24 and 48 h allergen exposure in patch testing. Comparative study with 11 common contact allergens and NiCl₂. Contact Dermatitis 10:25–29

74. Brasch J, Geier J, Henseler T (1995) Evaluation of patch test results by use of the reaction index. An analysis data recorded by the Information Network of Departments of Dermatology (IVDK). Contact Dermatitis 33: 375–380

75. Manuskiatti W, Maibach HI (1996) 1- versus 2- and 3-day diagnostic patch testing. Contact Dermatitis 35:197–200

76. Bruze M (1988) Patch testing with nickel sulphate under occlusion for five hours. Acta Derm Venereol (Stockh) 68: 361–364

77. Kosann MK, Brancaccio RR, Shupack JL, Franks AG Jr, Cohen DE (1998) Six-hour versus 48-hour patch testing with varying concentrations of potassium dichromate. Am J Contact Dermat 9:92–95

78. McFadden JP, Wakelin SH, Holloway DB, Basketter DA (1998) The effect of patch duration on the elicitation of para-phenylenediamine contact allergy. Contact Dermatitis 39:79–81

79. Rietschel R, Adams RM, Maibach HI, Storrs FJ, Rosenthal LE (1988) The case for patch test readings beyond day 2. J Am Acad Dermatol 18:42–45

80. MacFarlane AW, Curley RK, Graham RM, Lewis-Jones MS, King CM (1989) Delayed patch test reactions at days 7 and 9. Contact Dermatitis 20:127–132

81. Wahlberg JE, Wahlberg ENG (1987) Quantification of skin blood flow at patch test sites. Contact Dermatitis 17: 229–233

82. Geier J, Gefeller O, Wiechmann K, Fuchs T (1999) Patch test reactions at D4, D5 and D6. Contact Dermatitis 40:119–126

83. Dickel H, Taylor JS, Evey P, Merk HF (2000) Delayed readings of a standard screening patch test tray: frequency of "lost", "found", and "persistent" reactions. Am J Contact Dermatitis 11:213–217

84. Saino M, Rivara P, Guarrera M (1995) Reading patch tests on day 7. Contact Dermatitis 32:312

85. Jonker MJ, Bruynzel DP (2000) The outcome of an additional patch-test reading on days 6 or 7. Contact Dermatitis 42:330–335

86. Bygum A, Andersen KE (1998) Persistent reactions after patch testing with TRUE Test™ panels 1 and 2. Contact Dermatitis 38:218–220

87. Uter WJC, Geier J, Schnuch A (1996) Good clinical practice in patch testing: readings beyond day 2 are necessary: a confirmatory analysis. Am J Contact Dermat 7:231–237

88. Shehade SA, Beck MH, Hiller VF (1991) Epidemiological survey of standard series patch test results and observations on day 2 and day 4 readings. Contact Dermatitis 24: 119–122

89. Todd DJ, Handley J, Metwali M, Allen GE, Burrows D (1996) Day 4 is better than day 3 for a single patch test reading. Contact Dermatitis 34:402–404

90. Lachapelle JM, Tennstedt D, Fyad A, Masmoudi ML, Nouaigui H (1988) Ring-shaped positive allergic patch test reactions to allergens in liquid vehicles. Contact Dermatitis 18:234–236

91. Scheynius A, Fischer T (1986) Phenotypic difference between allergic and irritant patch test reactions in man. Contact Dermatitis 14:297–302

92. Bruze M, Isaksson M, Edman B, Björkner B, Fregert S, Möller H (1995) A study on expert reading of patch test reactions: inter-individual accordance. Contact Dermatitis 32:331–337

93. Lachapelle J-M (1997) A proposed relevance scoring system for positive allergic patch test reactions: practical implications and limitations. Contact Dermatitis 36:39–43

94. Rycroft RJG (1986) False reactions to nonstandard patch tests. Semin Dermatol 5:225–230

95. Björnberg A (1968) Skin reactions to primary irritants in patients with hand eczema. An investigation with matched controls. Thesis, Sahlgrenska Sjukhuset, Gothenburg, Sweden

96. Andersen KE, Lidén C, Hansen J, Vølund Å (1993) Dose-response testing with nickel sulphate using the TRUE test in nickel-sensitive individuals. Multiple nickel sulphate patch-test reactions do not cause an 'angry back'. Br J Dermatol 129:50–56

97. Bruynzeel DP, Maibach HI (1990) Excited skin syndrom and the hyporeactive state: current status. In: Menné T, Maibach HI (eds) Exogenous dermatoses: environmental dermatitis. CRC, Boca Raton, Fla., pp 141–150

98. Cockayne SE, Gawkrodger DJ (2000) Angry back syndrome is often due to marginal irritants: a study of 17 cases seen over 4 years. Contact Dermatitis 43:280–282

99. Kanerva L, Estlander T, Jolanki R, Alanko K (2000) False-negative patch test reactions due to a lower concentration of patch test substance than declared. Contact Dermatitis 42:289–291

100. Koehler AM, Maibach HI (2000) Skin hyporeactivity in relation to patch testing. Contact Dermatitis 42:1–4

101. Kelett JK, King CM, Beck MH (1986) Compound allergy to medicaments. Contact Dermatitis 14:45–48

102. Aldridge RD, Main RA (1984) Contact dermatitis due to a combined miconazole nitrate/hydrocortisone cream. Contact Dermatitis 10:58–60

103. Smeenk G, Kerckhoffs HPM, Schreurs PHM (1987) Contact allergy to a reaction product in Hirudoid® cream: an example of compound allergy. Br J Dermatol 116:223–231

104. Bashir SJ, Maibach HI (1997) Compound allergy. An overview. Contact Dermatitis 36:179–183

105. Bashir SJ, Kanervaq L, Jolanki R, Maibach HI (2000) Occupational and non-occupational compound allergy. In: Kanerva L, Elsner P, Wahlberg JE, Maibach HI (eds) Handbook of occupational dermatology. Springer, Berlin Heidelberg New York, pp 351–355

106. McLelland J, Shuster S, Matthews JNS (1991) "Irritants" increase the response to an allergen in allergic contact dermatitis. Arch Dermatol 127:1016–1019

107. McLelland J, Shuster S (1990) Contact dermatitis with negative patch tests. Br J Dermatol 122:623–630

108. Sukanto H, Nater JP, Bleumink E (1981) Influence of topically applied corticosteroids on patch test reactions. Contact Dermatitis 7:180–185

109. O'Quinn SE, Isbell KH (1969) Influence of oral prednisone on eczematous patch test reactions. Arch Dermatol 99:380–389

110. Feuerman E, Levy A (1972) A study of the effect of prednisone and an antihistamine on patch test reactions. Br J Dermatol 86:68–71

111. Condie MW, Adams RM (1973) Influence of oral prednisone on patch-test reactions to Rhus antigen. Arch Dermatol 107:540–543

112. Anveden I, Lindberg M, Andersen KE, Bruze M, Isaksson M, Lidén C, Sommerlund M, Wahlberg J, Wilkinson J, Willis C (2004) Oral prednisone suppresses allergic but not irritant patch test reactions in individuals hypersensitive to nickel. Contact Dermatitis 50:298–303

113. Lembo G, Presti ML, Balato N, Ayala F, Santoianni P (1985) Influence of cinnarizine on patch test reactions. Contact Dermatitis 13:341–343

114. Motolese A, Ferdani G, Manzini BM, Seidenari S (1995) Echographic evaluation of patch test inhibition by oral antihistamine. Contact Dermatitis 32:251

115. Elston D, Licata A, Rudner E, Trotter K (2000) Pitfalls in patch testing. Am J Contact Dermat 11:184–188

116. Aldridge RD, Sewell HF, King G, Thomson AW (1986) Topical cyclosporin A in nickel contact hypersensitivity: results of a preliminary clinical and immunohistochemical investigation. Clin Exp Immunol 66:582–589

117. Nakagawa S, Oka D, Jinno Y, Takei Y, Bang D, Ueki H (1988) Topical application of cyclosporine on guinea pig allergic contact dermatitis. Arch Dermatol 124:907–910

118. Biren CA, Barr RJ, Ganderup GS, Lemus LL, McCullough JL (1989) Topical cyclosporine: effects on allergic contact dermatitis in guinea pigs. Contact Dermatitis 20:10–16

119. Sjövall P (1988) Ultraviolet radiation and allergic contact dermatitis. An experimental and clinical study. Thesis, University of Lund, Sweden

120. Lindelöf B, Lidén S, Lagerholm B (1985) The effect of grenz rays on the expression of allergic contact dermatitis in man. Scand J Immunol 21:463–469

121. Ek L, Lindelöf B, Lidén S (1989) The duration of Grenz ray-induced suppression of allergic contact dermatitis and its correlation with the density of Langerhans cells in human epidermis. Clin Exp Dermatol 14:206–209

122. Cruz PD (1996) Effects of UV light on the immune system: answer to five basic questions. Am J Contact Dermatitis 7:47–52

123. Tie C, Golomb C, Taylor JR, Strelein JW (1995) Suppressive and enhancing effects of Ultraviolet B radiation on expression of contact hypersensitivity in man. J Invest Dermatol 104:18–22

124. Ingber A, Sasson A, David M (1998) The seasonal influence on patch test reactions is significant in Israel. Contact Dermatitis 39:318–319

125. Uter W, Geier J, Land M, Phahlberg A, Gefeller O, Schnauch A (2001) Another look at seasonal variation in patch test results. Contact Dermatitis 44:146–152

126. Uter W, Hegewald J, Phahlberg A, Pirker C, Frosch PJ, Gefeller O (2003) The association between ambient air conditions (temperature and absolute humidity), irritant sodium lauryl sulphate patch test reactions and patch test reactivity to standard allergens. Contact Dermatitis 49:97–102

127. Kanerva L, Estlander T, Jolanki R (1988) Sensitization to patch test acrylates. Contact Dermatitis 18:10–15

128. Lidén C, Boman A, Hagelthorn G (1982) Flare-up reactions from a chemical used in the film industry. Contact Dermatitis 8:136–137

129. Inerot A, Möller H (2000) Symptoms and signs reported during patch testing. Am J Contact Dermatitis 11:49–52

130. Kunkeler L, Bikkers SCE, Bezemer PD, Bruynzeel DP (2000) (Un)usual effects of patch testing? Br J Dermatol 143:582–586

131. Kamphof WG, Kunkeler L, Bikkers SCE, Bezemer PD, Bruynzeel DP (2003) Patch-test-induced subjective complaints. Dermatology 207:28–32

132. Dooms-Goossens A (1995) Patch testing without a kit. In: Guyin JD (ed) Practical contact dermatitis. McGraw-Hill, New York, pp 63–74

133. Hannuksela M, Salo H (1986) The repeated open application test (ROAT). Contact Dermatitis 14:221–227

134. Hannuksela M (1991) Sensitivity of various skin sites in the repeated open application test. Am J Contact Dermat 2:102–104

135. Hannuksela A, Niinimäki A, Hannuksela M (1993) Size of the test area does not affect the result of the repeated open application test. Contact Dermatitis 28:299–300

136. Johansen JD, Andersen KE, Rastogi SC, Menné T (1996) Threshold responses in cinnamic-aldehyde-sensitive subjects: results and methodological aspects. Contact Dermatitis 34:165–171

137. Johansen JD, Andersen KE, Menné T (1996) Quantitiative aspects of isoeugenol contact allergy assessed by use and patch tests. Contact Dermatitis 34:414–418

138. Wahlberg JE, Färm G, Lidén C (1997) Quantification and specificity of the repeated open application test (ROAT). Acta Derm Venereol (Stockh) 77:420–424

139. Johansen JD, Bruze M, Andersen KE, Frosch PJ, Dreier B, White IR, Rastogi S, Lepoittevin JP, Menné T (1997) The repeated open application test: suggestions for a scale of evaluation. Contact Dermatitis 39:95–96

140. Flyvholm M-A, Hall BM, Agner T, Tiedemann E, Greenhill P, Vanderveken W, Freeberg FE, Menné T (1997) Threshold for occluded formaldehyde patch test in formaldehyde-sensitive patients. Contact Dermatitis 36:26–33

141. Tupker RA, Schuur J, Coenraads PJ (1997) Irritancy of antiseptics tested by repeated open exposures on the human skin, evaluated by non-invasive methods. Contact Dermatitis 37:213–217

142. Färm G (1998) Repeated open application tests (ROAT) in patients allergic to colophony – evaluated visually and with bioengineering techniques. Acta Derm Venereol (Stockh) 78:130–135

143. Nakada T, Hostynek JJ, Maibach HI (2000) Use tests: ROAT (repeated open application test) / PUT (provocative use test): an overview. Contact Dermatitis 43:1–3

144. Berardesca E, Maibach HI (1988) Bioengineering and the patch test. Contact Dermatitis 18:3–9

145. Bjarnason B, Flosadottir E, Fischer T (1999) Objective non-invasive assessment of patch tests with the laser Doppler perfusion scanning technique. Contact Dermatitis 40:251–260

146. Staberg B, Klemp P, Serup J (1984) Patch test responses evaluated by cutaneous blood flow measurements. Arch Dermatol 120:741–743

147. Fullerton A, Stucker M, Wilhelm K-P, Wårdell K, Anderson C, Fischer T, Nilsson GE, Serup J (2002) Guidelines for visualization of cutaneous blood flow by laser Doppler perfusion imaging. Contact Dermatitis 46:129–140

148. Wahlberg JE (1989) Assessment of erythema: a comparison between the naked eye and laser Doppler flowmetry. In: Frosch PJ, Dooms-Goossens A, Lachapelle JM, Rycroft RJ, Scheper RJ (eds) Current topics in contact dermatitis. Springer, Berlin Heidelberg New York, pp 549–553

149. Wahlberg JE (1971) Vehicle role of petrolatum. Acta Derm Venereol (Stockh) 51:129–134

150. Vanneste D, Martin P, Lachapelle JM (1980) Comparative study of the density of particles in suspension for patch testing. Contact Dermatitis 6:197–203
151. Fischer T, Maibach HI (1984) Patch test allergens in petrolatum: a reappraisal. Contact Dermatitis 11:224–228
152. Mellström GA, Sommar K, Wahlberg JE (1992) Patch test preparations of metallic mercury under the microscope. Contact Dermatitis 26:64–65
153. Karlberg A-T, Lidén C (1988) Comparison of colophony patch test preparations. Contact Dermatitis 18:158–165
154. Magnusson B, Hersle K (1966) Patch test methods. III. Influence of adhesive tape on test response. Acta Derm Venereol (Stockh) 46:275–278
155. Bruze M, Frick M, Persson L (2003) Patch testing with thin-layer chromatograms. Contact Dermatitis 48:278–279

22

Chapter 23

Atopy Patch Testing with Aeroallergens and Food Proteins

23

Ulf Darsow, Johannes Ring

Contents

23.1 Introduction

An epicutaneous patch test with allergens known to elicit IgE-mediated reactions and the evaluation of eczematous skin lesions after 24 h to 72 h is called the atopy patch test (APT) [1]. This test was developed as a diagnostic tool for characterizing patients with aeroallergen-triggered atopic eczema (AE, atopic dermatitis), a chronic inflammatory skin disease. AE is characterized by a combination of clinical features, including pruritus and a typically age-related distribution and skin morphology [2, 3]. Patients with AE often have elevated serum levels of immunoglobulin E (IgE), often directed against aeroallergens (e.g., house dust mites) and food allergens. These allergens produce flares in some patients with AE, but not in all sensitized individuals [4]. Also, aeroallergen avoidance, especially with regard to house dust mites, can result in marked improvement of skin lesions [5]. Among the allergens found to be relevant in AE, aeroallergens and food allergens (in children) are the most important. Therapeutic consequences of the diagnosis of allergy are based upon avoidance strategies, thus, the relevance of (often multiple) IgE-mediated sensitizations in patients with AE for the skin disease has to be evaluated. In spite of these clinical aspects, the role of allergy in eliciting and maintaining the eczematous skin lesions was controversial [6], partially due to a lack of specificity of the classic tests for IgE-mediated hypersensitivity, skin prick test, and measurement of specific serum IgE.

Mite allergen in the epidermis of patients with AE under natural conditions [7], as well as in APT sites [8, 9], has been demonstrated in proximity to Langerhans cells. Langerhans cells in the skin express IgE receptors of three different classes [10–12]. In addition, a Birbeck-granule-negative, non-Langerhans-cell population with an even higher IgE receptor expression than the Langerhans cell, the so-called inflammatory dendritic epidermal cells (IDEC) [13], has recently been demonstrated in freshly induced APT lesions, a phenomenon which occurred in both "intrinsic" and "extrinsic" patients [14]. This might explain the IgE-associated activation of allergen-specific T-cells, leading finally to eczematous skin lesions in the APT (Fig. 1) [15, 16]. According to the results of Langeveld-Wildschut et al., the positive APT reaction requires the presence of epidermal IgE$^+$ CD1a$^+$ cells [17]. From APT biopsies, allergen-specific T-cells have been cloned [16]. These T-cells showed a characteristic TH2 (T helper cell subpopulation) secretion pattern initially, whereas, after 48 h, a TH1 pattern was predominant. This same pattern is also found in chronic lesions of AE.

Core Message

■ The atopy patch test (APT), an epicutaneous patch test with allergens known to elicit IgE-mediated reactions, and the evaluation of eczematous skin lesions after 24 h to 72 h, was developed as a diagnostic tool for characterizing patients with aeroallergen-triggered atopic eczema (AE, atopic dermatitis). Positive APT reactions are associated with allergen-specific T-cell responses.

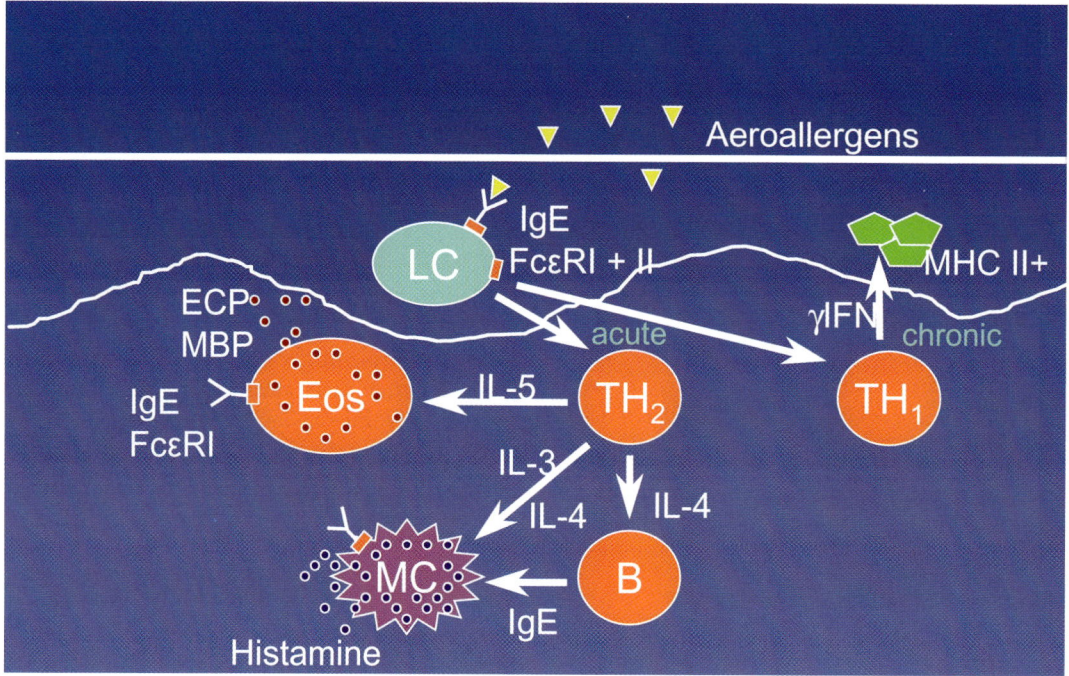

Fig. 1. Proposed pathophysiology of aeroallergen-triggered atopic eczema (AE, atopic dermatitis). (*LC* Langerhans cell, *FcεR* IgE receptor, *Eos* eosinophil granulocyte, *TH* T-cell populations, *B* B-cell, *MC* mast cell)

Early studies describing experimental patch testing with aeroallergens were published in 1937 by Rostenberg and Sulzberger [18] and in 1982 by Mitchell et al. [19]; the methods and results since have shown wide variations. Potentially irritating procedures such as skin abrasion [8, 20], tape stripping [21, 22], and sodium lauryl sulfate (SLS) application [9] were used to enhance allergen penetration. No clear-cut correlations to the skin prick test or specific IgE measurements could be obtained, and the sensitivity and specificity of experimental APT with regard to clinical history remained unclear. For better standardization, we performed APT on non-lesional, non-abraded, untreated skin during remission [1, 23]. The results were compared for vehicle and dose of allergen in the preparations used. It was shown that healthy controls and patients with respiratory atopy without a history of eczema do not react in the APT [23], or with a lower frequency and intensity of APT reactions to whole-body mite extract compared to patients with AE [24]. The sensitivity and specificity of different diagnostic procedures were calculated [25].

23.2 APT Methods

Table 1 summarizes the methods for APT resulting from methodological studies [14, 25–27]: APT with significant correlations to clinical parameters like allergen-specific IgE or the patient's history are today

Table 1. Atopy patch test (*APT*) methods resulting from methodological studies [25–27]

Allergen-specific individual history, eczema pattern, and routine diagnosis skin prick test and specific IgE
Patients in remission phase of eczema
Atopy patch test:
Lyophilized aeroallergens (house dust mites, cat dander, grass and birch pollen)
Allergen doses: 5,000–7,000 PNU/g or 200 IR/g
Vehicle: petrolatum, large Finn chambers
Application for 48 h on clinically uninvolved, *unpretreated* back skin (no tape stripping)
Evaluation after 48 h and 72 h according to ICDRG guidelines or ETFAD key[a]

[a] (see Table 5)

performed with a very similar technique to conventional patch tests for the diagnosis of classical contact allergy. Exclusion criteria (use of antihistamines, systemic and in loco topical steroids: 1 week, UV radiation 3 weeks, acute eczema flare) and the possibility of contact urticaria should be considered. Epicutaneous tests with lyophilized allergens, e.g., from house dust mites (*Dermatophagoides pteronyssinus, D. pter.*), cat dander, and grass pollen, are performed with a petrolatum vehicle (including a vehicle control). Patients should be in a state of remission of their eczema, the patch test is applied in large Finn chambers for 48 h on their back on non-abraded and uninvolved skin. Any potentially irritating methods of skin barrier disruption, like tape stripping of the skin, should be avoided. In several studies, non-atopic volunteers and patients suffering from allergic rhinoconjunctivitis only presented negative APT reactions with the methods described in Table 1. The reproducibility of different APT methods is high if the test is performed on the back (Table 2). Allergens in petrolatum elicited twice as many APT reactions as allergens in a hydrophilic vehicle [23]. High-allergen specific IgE in serum is not a prerequisite for a positive APT, but patients with *D.-pter.*-positive APT showed in 62% of patients a corresponding positive skin prick test and in 77% of cases a corresponding elevated specific IgE. In other allergens, the concordance was even higher. Allergen concentrations of 500, 3,000, 5,000, and 10,000 PNU (protein nitrogen units)/g in petrolatum were comparatively used in 57 patients [26]. It was shown that the percentage of patients with clear-cut positive reactions was significantly higher in patients with eczematous skin lesions in air-exposed areas (69%) compared to patients without this predictive pattern (39%; p=0.02).

Table 2. Intra-individual reproducibility of different APT models. Reproducibility of positive APT reactions at different time points

Patch test	n	Time (months)	Reproducibility
APT petrolatum[a] D. pter., grass and birch pollen, no tape stripping	20	6–12	18
APT petrolatum[b] D. pter., cat dander, grass and birch pollen, no tape stripping	16	12–24	15
APT aqueous[c] D. pter., 10 × tape stripping	5	6	5

[a,b] Own data; [c]from [17]

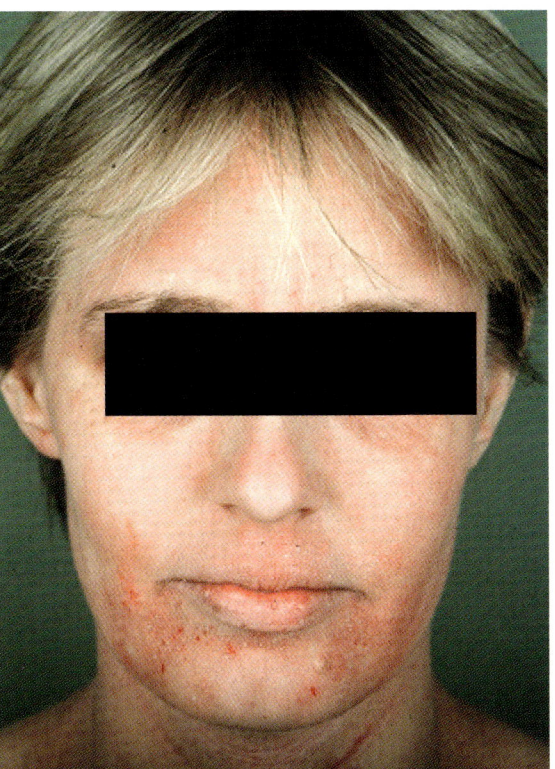

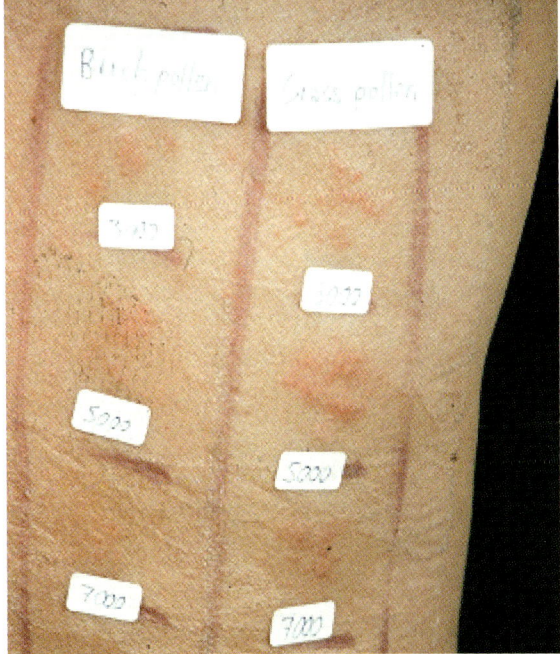

Fig. 2. Case report
- 25 y., atopic eczema for 18 years
- Repeated eczema flares in spring and summer
- Lesion in free skin areas
- SPT/sIgE: mult. positive to aero-allergens incl. grass- and birch pollen
- APT: +++ to grass- and birch pollen
- Standard patch test negative

23

Table 3. Summary of principal study results for aeroallergen APT [14, 25–27]

Controls: no positive reaction (non-atopic/rhinoconjunctivitis only)
Vehicle: petrolatum better than hydrogel
Allergen concentration >1,000 PNU/g: 7,000 PNU/g gave "optimal results" in adults
Biologically standardized allergens: 200 IR/g
Atopic eczema (AE) in uncovered skin areas:
Associated with higher frequency of positive APT
Seasonal eczema flares: positive grass pollen APT
APT correlates with clinical history

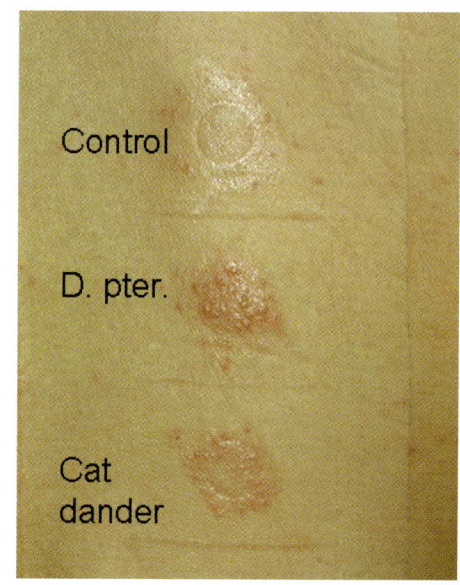

Fig. 3. APT reactions to different allergens after removal of Finn chambers after 48 h. Clear-cut eczematous appearance with infiltration and spreading papules, partially with a follicular pattern. Control: petrolatum

A case of a patient is given with Fig. 2. In the first group, the maximum reactivity was nearly reached with 5,000 PNU/g. The data from a randomized, double-blind multicenter trial, involving 253 adult patients and 30 children with AE, were used to calculate a suitable APT allergen dosage [25, 28]. Adults were tested with four concentrations; 3,000 to 10,000 PNU/g of *D. pter.*, cat dander, grass pollen, and (in two study centers only; $n=88$) with birch and mugwort pollen. A dose response for APT could be obtained by McNemar statistics, comparing with only questionable, only erythematous, or irritative reactions. The optimal allergen doses were in the range of 5,000 PNU/g to 7,000 PNU/g. For children, lower allergen concentrations seem possible [28]. Simultaneously tested, the allergen doses of 7,000 PNU/g and 200 IR/g (biological unit; Index réactif) of the most important aeroallergens in Europe showed comparable concordance with the patient's history, suggest-

ing clinical relevance in another study in 50 patients with AE. An example of a positive APT reaction to a biologically standardized allergen preparation is shown in Fig. 3. The clinical outcome of the methods studied is summarized in Table 3.

The standardization of aeroallergen APT is currently more advanced than food patch testing. In Europe, the efforts are coordinated by the European Task Force on Atopic Dermatitis (ETFAD), a sister society of the European Academy of Dermatology and Venereology (EADV). A recent ETFAD study in six

Table 4. Positive test results and patient's history of allergen-associated eczema flare. Frequency of positive APT reactions is lower than positive IgE-mediated sensitizations. Patient's allergen-specific history of eczema flares after allergen exposure was obtained prospectively. $n=314$, 24% children ≤10 years old. (*APT* Atopy patch test ≥+, *Hx-concordance* allergen-specific concordance of APT result and clinical history, *sIgE* specific IgE ≥0.35 kU/l, *SPT* skin prick test ≥3 mm.) Data from [29]

	SPT (%)	sIgE (%)	APT (%)	History (%)	Hx-concordance (%)
Aeroallergens					
D. pter.	56	56	39	34	57
Birch pollen	49	53	17	20	61
Grass pollen	57	59	15	31	64
Cat dander	44	46	10	30	62
Food allergens					
Egg white	25	19	11	7	77
Wheat flour	16	38	10	3	78
Celery	20	30	9	1	79

European Countries (n=314) showed again that house dust mites (*D. pter.*) most often elicited positive APT reactions, followed by pollen allergens (Table 4) [29]. This study also investigated food extract preparations in petrolatum. To date, food APT are performed with unstandardized fresh food preparations, with conflicting results.

23.3 Evaluation of APT Reactions

Usually, APT reactions are read after 48 h and 72 h. In patients with contact urticaria, a wheal-and-flare reaction may be seen after 30 min. Most reactions are visible and palpable at 48 h, sometimes with decrescendo to 72 h. After tape stripping followed by allergen application, there are more early reactions visible. Clear-cut positive reactions should be distinguished from negative or questionable reactions, understanding the fact that only reactions showing papules or at least some degree of infiltration were correlated with clinical relevance. Consensus meetings of most groups performing APT for clinical use in Europe were held in Munich in 1997 and 1998, and a consensus APT reading key for describing the intensity of APT reactions was developed and published [30]. Following its use in a multicenter trial in six European countries, in 2003, the ETFAD proposed a simplified version, as given in Table 5. However, clinically meaningful APT results were also obtained with the International Contact Dermatitis Research Group (ICDRG) key for conventional patch testing [23, 25].

> **Core Message**
>
> ■ APT result is graded according to ETFAD or ICDRG guidelines.

Table 5. ETFAD key for the grading of positive APT reactions (modified from [30]). (*ETFAD* European Task Force on Atopic Dermatitis)

–	Negative
?	Only erythema, questionable
+	Erythema, infiltration
++	Erythema, few papules
+++	Erythema, many or spreading papules
++++	Erythema, vesicles

23.4 Predictors, Sensitivity, and Specificity of APT

As long as no "gold standard" of provocation for aeroallergen allergy in AE exists, the history of allergen-specific exacerbation is used as a parameter for clinical relevance. A previous study compared the outcome of the APT with a seasonal history of "summer eruption" of AE in 79 patients [27]. Significantly higher frequencies of positive grass pollen APT reactions (with two methods used) occurred in patients with a corresponding history of exacerbation of skin lesions during the grass pollen season of the previous year (75% with positive APT). Patients without this history showed significantly lower APT reactivity (16% with positive APT; $p<0.001$).

> **Core Message**
>
> ■ The APT specificity exceeded the specificity of the classic tests of IgE-mediated hypersensitivity, which was 0.33 for the skin prick test and radioallergosorbent test (RAST). On the other hand, the sensitivity of the classical methods was higher (0.92 for RAST and 1.0 for the skin prick test, Table 6).

In two multicenter studies with up to five aeroallergens, the predictors of a positive APT reaction were investigated (Table 7) [25, 29]. The sensitivity and specificity of the APT in these studies are also shown in Table 6. It has to be kept in mind that, at least for non-seasonal aeroallergens, the history may be unreliable, thus, limiting the precision of such calculations like in Table 6. For most allergens, a significant association of APT and specific IgE could be demonstrated.

Problems such as irrelevant positive or spreading APT reactions may occur in patients undergoing APT during an eczema flare, or if methods of abrasion of the stratum corneum are used. The issue of pharmacological influence on APT still holds many unanswered questions. As the standardization of the high-molecular-weight allergens has some specific problems, a commercial provider of test substances with reproducible quality and major allergen content is desirable. However, to date, such allergen preparations are not easily available. Even more problems with allergen standardization are known for food APT.

23

Table 6. Sensitivity and specificity of different test procedures with regard to clinical history: the APT shows a higher specificity than classical tests for IgE-mediated hypersensitivity with regard to the allergen-specific history. Studies used different allergen standardizations. Data from [25, 27, 29]

Test	Sensitivity (%)[a]	Specificity (%)[a]
Different grass pollen preparations, n=79		
Skin prick	100	33
sIgE	92	33
APT	75	84
European multicenter study, n=314, four allergens		
Skin prick	68–80	50–71
sIgE	72–84	52–69
APT	14–45	64–91
German multicenter study, n=253, three allergens		
Skin prick	69–82	44–53
sIgE	65–94	42–64
APT	42–56	69–92

[a] Depending on the allergen, with regard to a clinical history with eczema flares in pollen season or after direct contact with the allergen

Table 7. Logistic regression model: predictors of a positive APT reaction (from [25]); highest significance at the top of table

Positive reactions are associated with:
Increased specific serum IgE
Positive skin prick test reaction
Allergen-specific corresponding history
Increased total IgE
Long eczema duration
Rhinoconjunctivitis (grass pollen)

23.5 APT with Food Proteins

The APT with foods is still an experimental method, but the available standardized food challenge protocols allowed the evaluation of the clinical relevance of food APT reactions to a certain degree. Often, native foods, such as hen's eggs, wheat flour, cow's milk, or soy products, were applied in 12-mm aluminum test chambers for 24 h or 48 h on the patient's skin. Majamaa et al. [31] investigated 142 children under 2 years old with suspected cow's milk allergy. In 50% of the cases, the oral provocation test was positive (22 immediate-type reactions). Of these patients, 26% had an increased corresponding specific IgE, 14% a positive skin prick test, and 44% a positive APT with cow's milk. In this age group, most positive APT reactions were seen without corresponding pos-

Table 8. Can APT with food replace oral provocation tests? A combination of positive APT with elevated specific serum IgE ($\geq$0.35 kU/l for milk, $\geq$17.5 kU/l for eggs) resulted in 94–100% positive predictive value in this study by Roehr et al. [35]. (*APT* Native APT, *SPT* skin prick test, *sIgE* specific IgE)

Test	Sensitivity (%)			Specificity (%)		
	SPT	sIgE	APT	SPT	sIgE	APT
Cow's milk	78	84	47	69	38	96
Hen's eggs	89	96	57	57	36	93
Wheat flour	67	67	89	53	47	94
Soy	50	75	75	90	52	86

n=98 children (median 13 months) with AE and suspected food allergy, oral provocation test: 95 (55%) positive

itive skin prick test results. Further investigations by Isolauri and Turjanmaa [32] showed an association between the clinical pattern of the reaction and the result of the skin prick test and APT. They also suggested to perform the skin prick test and APT simultaneously to increase the precision of diagnosis. In the investigated group of children (aged 2–36 months) with AE, the skin prick test with cow's milk was positive in 67% of cases with *immediate-type* reactions in the oral challenge, mostly accompanied by negative APT. On the other hand, a positive APT was seen in 89% of cases with *delayed eczematous* reaction, whereas, in these cases, the skin prick test was mostly negative.

An association of positive APT (with native preparations of cow's milk, hen's eggs, wheat flour, and soy) with eczema flares following oral provocation was described by Niggemann et al. [33, 34]. Roehr et al. [35] calculated, for the APT with these native foods, a sensitivity of 47–89% and a specificity of 86–96% with regard to the result of the oral provocation. The positive predictive value of the diagnostic method could be increased to 94– 100% when positive skin prick tests, elevated specific IgE, and a positive APT were combined for these calculations (Table 8). However, a practical problem for such combinations is discordant test results. Our own investigations in a multicenter study in six European countries using an APT with food preparations in petrolatum [29] showed a concordance of APT result and clinical history of 77% (hen's eggs), 78% (wheat flour), and 79% (celery). The specificity of this APT was 91% with regard to a predictive clinical history but the sensitivity was only 30– 33% (n=314).

Core Message

■ Different results of different study groups are obvious, especially for the sensitivity of unstandardized food APT. Further clinical studies for the standardization and patient group selection for food APT are necessary.

23.6 APT and "Intrinsic Type" Atopic Eczema

A sensitization detected by APT, which is supposedly T-cell-mediated, may be even more relevant for the clinical course of AE than the demonstration of an IgE-mediated sensitization. Interestingly, 7% of the tested patients who would be labeled as "intrinsic type" of AE, according to Schmid-Grendelmeier et al.'s definition [36], show a sensitization in the APT. A similar finding of positive APT reactions in subjects without sIgE to *Dermatophagoides* was described by Seidenari et al. [37] and Manzini et al. [38]. Also, recently, 8 out of 12 "intrinsic" AE patients were reported to react to a partially purified whole-mite APT preparation [39]. Similar results have been obtained by APT with *Malassezia sympodialis* antigens [40]. House-dust-mite-specific antibodies of the IgG4 subtype, as well as a rapid influx of IDEC in the APT lesions, has recently been reported in two otherwise "intrinsic" AE patients [41]. However, the mechanism of these "intrinsic" APT reactions remains hypothetical to date, but a T-cell-mediated mechanism without IgE involvement seems probable.

Core Message

■ With regard to the recently proposed novel nomenclature for allergy by the European Academy of Allergy and Clinical Immunology (EAACI) [42], these cases may be diagnosed as "non-IgE-associated (nonatopic) eczema" or "T-cell-mediated eczema."

23.7 Outlook

The APT with aeroallergens may provide an important diagnostic tool, as has been shown in two patient subgroups. In patients with an air-exposed eczema distribution pattern, positive APT reactions occurred at lower allergen doses compared with other patients with AE. Patients with an aeroallergen-specific history had significantly more positive APT reactions.

Core Message

■ The lower sensitivity but higher specificity of the APT compared to the skin prick test or RAST favors the notion that the classical tests may have some value as screening tests; specificity may be added by the APT. The APT does not replace the classical methods of diagnosis of IgE-mediated allergy.

Questions remain open concerning the clinical relevance of positive APT results in patients with a negative history and discordant negative skin prick tests or RAST, since no gold standard exists for the provocation of eczematous skin lesions in aeroallergen-triggered AE. These questions may only be answered by controlled studies using specific provocation and elimination procedures in patients with positive and negative APT results. However, this does not argue against the clinical use by allergists at the present time, since one has to keep in mind that, in many classical contact allergens, the standardization and evaluation efforts have been less systematic. Still, these allergens are used for routine diagnosis in patch test clinics. Appropriate allergen-specific avoidance strategies are recommended in patients showing positive APT reactions. The diagnostic validity of APT in routine diagnosis of aeroallergen-triggered AE is investigated in further controlled studies.

Suggested Reading

Tanaka Y, Tanaka M, Anan S, Yoshida H (1989) Immunohistochemical studies on dust mite antigen in positive reaction site of patch test. Acta Derm Venereol Suppl (Stockh) 144:93–96
Eczematous reactions could be induced by patch testing with mite antigens in patients with atopic eczema (AE). Using an immuno-double-labeling technique, the authors demonstrated that many mite-antigen-bearing Langerhans cells are visible in the epidermis in the early stage of the atopy patch testing (APT) reaction. Twenty-four hours later, these cells were observed only in the deep dermis. Immuno-electron microscopically, it was found that the mite antigens were trapped by macrophages, which were in contact with lymphocytes. Many IgE-positive dendritic cells bearing mite antigens were seen in positive APT sites.
One of the first and most often cited studies suggesting IgE-mediated contact hypersensitivity to mite antigens in

23

the pathogenesis of AE. These observations still hold true and are also discussed with regard to the allergen specificity of APT reactions, which was later corroborated by other investigators.

References

1. Ring J, Kunz B, Bieber T, Vieluf D, Przybilla B (1989) The "atopy patch test" with aeroallergens in atopic eczema. J Allergy Clin Immunol 82:195
2. Rajka G (1989) Essential aspects of atopic dermatitis. Springer, Berlin Heidelberg New York
3. Ruzicka T, Ring J, Przybilla B (eds) (1991) Handbook of atopic eczema. Springer, Berlin Heidelberg New York
4. Tupker R, DeMonchy J, Coenraads P, Homan A, van der Meer J (1996) Induction of atopic dermatitis by inhalation of house dust mite. J Allergy Clin Immunol 97:1064–1070
5. Tan B, Weald D, Strickland I, Friedman P (1996) Double-blind controlled trial of effect of housedust-mite allergen avoidance on atopic dermatitis. Lancet 347:15–18
6. Oosting AJ, de Bruin-Weller MS, Terreehorst I, Tempels-Pavlica Z, Aalberse RC, de Monchy JG, van Wijk RG, Bruijnzeel-Koomen CA (2002) Effect of mattress encasings on atopic dermatitis outcome measures in a double-blind, placebo-controlled study: the Dutch mite avoidance study. J Allergy Clin Immunol 110:500–506
7. Maeda K, Yamamoto K, Tanaka Y, Anan S, Yoshida H (1992) House dust mite (HDM) antigen in naturally occurring lesions of atopic dermatitis (AD): the relationship between HDM antigen in the skin and HDM antigen-specific IgE antibody. J Derm Sci 3:73–77
8. Gondo A, Saeki N, Tokuda Y (1986) Challenge reactions in atopic dermatitis after percutaneous entry of mite antigen. Br J Dermatol 115:485–493
9. Tanaka Y, Anan S, Yoshida H (1990) Immunohistochemical studies in mite antigen-induced patch test sites in atopic dermatitis. J Derm Sci 1:361–368
10. Bieber T, Rieger A, Neuchrist C, Prinz JC, Rieber EP, Boltz-Nitulescu G, Scheiner O, Kraft D, Ring J, Stingl G (1989) Induction of FCeR2/CD23 on human epidermal Langerhans' cells by human recombinant IL4 and IFN. J Exp Med 170:309–314
11. Bieber T, de la Salle H, Wollenberg A, Hakimi J, Chizzonite R, Ring J, Hanau D, de la Salle C (1992) Human epidermal Langerhans cells express the high affinity receptor for immunoglobulin E (Fc epsilon RI). J Exp Med 175:1285–1290
12. Wollenberg A, de la Salle H, Hanau D, Liu FT, Bieber T (1993) Human Keratinocytes release the endogenous beta-galactoside-binding soluble lectin immunoglobulin E (IgE-binding protein) which binds to Langerhans cells where it modulates their binding capacity for IgE glycoforms. J Exp Med 178:777–785
13. Wollenberg A, Kraft S, Hanau D, Bieber T (1996) Immunomorphological and ultrastructural characterization of Langerhans cells and a novel, inflammatory dendritic epidermal cell (IDEC) population in lesional skin of atopic eczema. J Invest Dermatol 106:446–453
14. Kerschenlohr K, Decard S, Przybilla B, Wollenberg A (2003) Atopy patch test reactions show a rapid influx of inflammatory dendritic epidermal cells in patients with extrinsic atopic dermatitis and patients with intrinsic atopic dermatitis. J Allergy Clin Immunol 111:869–874
15. van Reijsen FC, Bruijnzeel-Koomen CAFM, Kalthoff FS (1992) Skin-derived aeroallergen-specific T-cell clones of Th2 phenotype in patients with atopic dermatitis. J Allergy Clin Immunol 90:184–193
16. Sager N, Feldmann A, Schilling G, Kreitsch P, Neumann C (1992) House dust mite-specific T cells in the skin of subjects with atopic dermatitis: frequency and lymphokine profile in the allergen patch test. J Allergy Clin Immunol 89:801–810
17. Langeveld-Wildschut EG, Bruijnzeel PLB, Mudde GC, Versluis C, van Leperen-van Dijk AG, Bihari IC, Knol EF, Thepen T, Bruijnzeel-Koomen CAFM, van Reijsen F (2000) Clinical and immunologic variables in skin of patients with atopic eczema and either positive or negative atopy patch test reactions. J Allergy Clin Immunol 105:1008–1016
18. Rostenberg A, Sulzberger MD (1937) Some results of patch tests. Arch Dermatol 35:433–454
19. Mitchell E, Chapman M, Pope F, Crow J, Jouhal S, Platts-Mills T (1982) Basophils in allergen-induced patch test sites in atopic dermatitis. Lancet 1:127–130
20. Norris P, Schofield O, Camp R (1988) A study of the role of house dust mite in atopic dermatitis. Br J Dermatol 118:435–440
21. van Voorst Vader PC, Lier JG, Woest TE, Coenraads PJ, Nater JP (1991) Patch tests with house dust mite antigens in atopic dermatitis patients: methodological problems. Acta Derm Venereol (Stockh) 71:301–305
22. Bruijnzeel-Koomen C, van Wichen D, Spry C, Venge P, Bruijnzeel P (1988) Active participation of eosinophils in patch test reactions to inhalant allergens in patients with atopic dermatitis. Br J Dermatol 118:229–238
23. Darsow U, Vieluf D, Ring J (1995) Atopy patch test with different vehicles and allergen concentrations: an approach to standardization. J Allergy Clin Immunol 95:677–684
24. Seidenari S, Giusti F, Pellacani G, Bertoni L (2003) Frequency and intensity of responses to mite patch tests are lower in nonatopic subjects with respect to patients with atopic dermatitis. Allergy 58:426–429
25. Darsow U, Vieluf D, Ring J, Atopy Patch Test Study Group (1999) Evaluating the relevance of aeroallergen sensitization in atopic eczema with the atopy patch test: a randomized, double-blind multicenter study. J Am Acad Dermatol 40:187–193
26. Darsow U, Vieluf D, Ring J (1996) The atopy patch test: an increased rate of reactivity in patients who have an air-exposed pattern of atopic eczema. Br J Dermatol 135:182–186
27. Darsow U, Behrendt H, Ring J (1997) Gramineae pollen as trigger factors of atopic eczema – evaluation of diagnostic measures using the atopy patch test. Br J Dermatol 137:201–207
28. Darsow U, Vieluf D, Berg B, Berger J, Busse A, Czech W, Heese A, Heidelbach U, Peters KP, Przybilla B, Richter G, Rueff F, Werfel T, Wistokat-Wülfing A, Ring J (1999) Dose response study of atopy patch test in children with atopic eczema. Pediatr Asthma Allergy Immunol 13:115–122
29. Darsow U, Laifaoui J, Bolhaar S, Bruijnzeel-Koomen CAFM, Breuer K, Wulf A, Werfel T, Brönnimann M, Braathen LR, Dangoisse C, Blondeel A, Song M, Didierlaurent A, André C, Drzimalla K, Simon D, Disch R, Borelli S, Elst L, Devilliers A, Oranje AP, de Raeve L, Reiser K, Wollenberg A, Przybilla B, Roul S, Taieb A, Seidenari S, Wüthrich B, Ring J (2004) Atopy patch test with aeroallergens and food allergens in petrolatum: a European multicenter study. Allergy 59:1318–1325
30. Darsow U, Ring J (2000) Airborne and dietary allergens in atopic eczema: a comprehensive review of diagnostic tests. Clin Exp Dermatol 25:544–551

31. Majamaa H, Moisio P, Holm K, Kautiainen H, Turjanmaa K (1999) Cow's milk allergy: diagnostic accuracy of skin prick and patch tests and specific IgE. Allergy 54:346–351

32. Isolauri E, Turjanmaa K (1996) Combined skin prick and patch testing enhances identification of food allergy in infants with atopic dermatitis. J Allergy Clin Immunol 97: 9–15

33. Niggemann B, Reibel S, Wahn U (2000) The atopy patch test (APT) – a useful tool for the diagnosis of food allergy in children with atopic dermatitis. Allergy 55:281–285

34. Niggemann B, Reibel S, Roehr CC, Felger D, Ziegert M, Sommerfeld C, Wahn U (2001) Predictors of positive food challenge outcome in non-IgE-mediated reactions to food in children with atopic dermatitis. J Allergy Clin Immunol 108:1053–1058

35. Roehr CC, Reibel S, Ziegert M, Sommerfeld C, Wahn U, Niggemann B (2001) Atopy patch tests, together with determination of specific IgE levels, reduce the need for oral food challenges in children with atopic dermatitis. J Allergy Clin Immunol 107:548–553

36. Schmid-Grendelmeier P, Simon D, Simon HU, Akdis CA, Wüthrich B (2001) Epidemiology, clinical features, and immunology of the "intrinsic" (non-IgE-mediated) type of atopic dermatitis (constitutional dermatitis). Allergy 56: 841–849

37. Seidenari S, Manzini BM, Danese P, Giannetti A (1992) Positive patch tests to whole mite culture and purified mite extracts in patients with atopic dermatitis, asthma, and rhinitis. Ann Allergy 69:201–206

38. Manzini BM, Motolese A, Donini M, Seidenari S (1995) Contact allergy to Dermatophagoides in atopic dermatitis patients and healthy subjects. Contact Dermatitis 33: 243–246

39. Ingordo V, D'Andria G, D'Andria C, Tortora A (2002) Results of atopy patch tests with house dust mites in adults with "intrinsic" and "extrinsic" atopic dermatitis. J Eur Acad Derm Venereol 16:450–454

40. Johansson C, Sandstrom MH, Bartosik J, Sarnhult T, Christiansen J, Zargari A, Back O, Wahlgren CF, Faergemann J, Scheynius A, Tengvall Linder M (2003) Atopy patch test reactions to Malassezia allergens differentiate subgroups of atopic dermatitis patients. Br J Dermatol 148:479–488

41. Kerschenlohr K, Decard S, Darsow U, Ollert M, Wollenberg A (2003) Clinical and immunologic reactivity to aeroallergens in "intrinsic" atopic dermatitis patients. J Allergy Clin Immunol 111:195–197

42. Johansson SGO, Bieber T, Dahl R, Friedmann PS, Lanier BQ, Lockey RF, Motala C, Ortega Martell JA, Platts-Mills TAE, Ring J, Thien F, van Cauwenberge P, Williams HC (2004) Revised nomenclature for allergy for global use: report of the Nomenclature Review Committee of the World Allergy Organization, October 2003. J Allergy Clin Immunol 113:832–836

Chapter 24

Patch Testing in Adverse Drug Reactions

24

Derk P. Bruynzeel, Margarida Gonçalo

Contents

> ## Core Message
>
> - A drug eruption is an adverse skin reaction caused by a drug used in normal doses and presents a wide variety of cutaneous reactions.

24.1 Introduction

A drug eruption is an adverse skin reaction caused by a drug used in normal doses. Systemic exposure to drugs can lead to a wide variety of cutaneous reactions, ranging from erythema, maculopapular eruptions (the most frequent reaction pattern), acrovesicular dermatitis, localized fixed drug eruptions, to toxic epidermal necrolysis and from urticaria to anaphylaxis (Figs. 1, 2). The incidence of these eruptions is not exactly known; 2%–5% of inpatients experience such a reaction and it is a frequent cause of consultation in dermatology [1–3]. Topically applied drugs may cause contact dermatitis reactions. Topical sensitization and subsequent systemic exposure may induce dermatological patterns similar to drug eruptions or patterns more typical of a systemic contact dermatitis, like the "baboon syndrome" (Chap. 16). It is clear that, in these situations, patch testing can be of great help as a diagnostic tool [4].

In patients with drug eruptions without previous contact sensitization, patch testing seems less logical, but is still a strong possibility, as systemic exposure of drugs may also lead to T-cell sensitization and to delayed type IV hypersensitivity reactions [5–8]. The value of patch testing in adverse drug reactions has not always been appreciated, but there is growing interest in this field. Positive test results can be very helpful, mainly as a complementary tool in drug imputation, but also for studying cross-reactions and understanding pathomechanisms involved in drug eruptions [9].

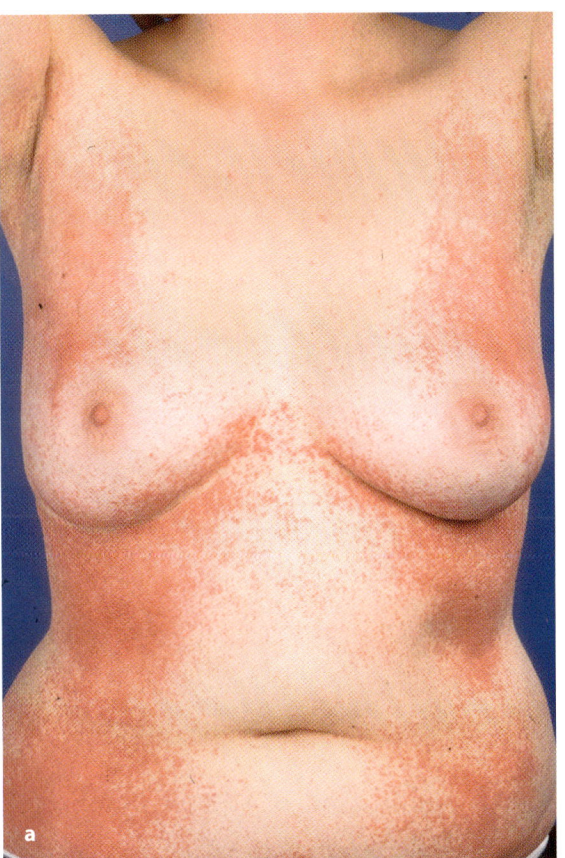

Fig. 1a–c. Acute generalized exanthematous pustular eruption (AGEP) due to phenobarbital (**a**). The detail shows numerous vesicles (**b**). The patch test with phenobarbital was clearly positive with vesicles and few pustules on day 2 (**c**)

24

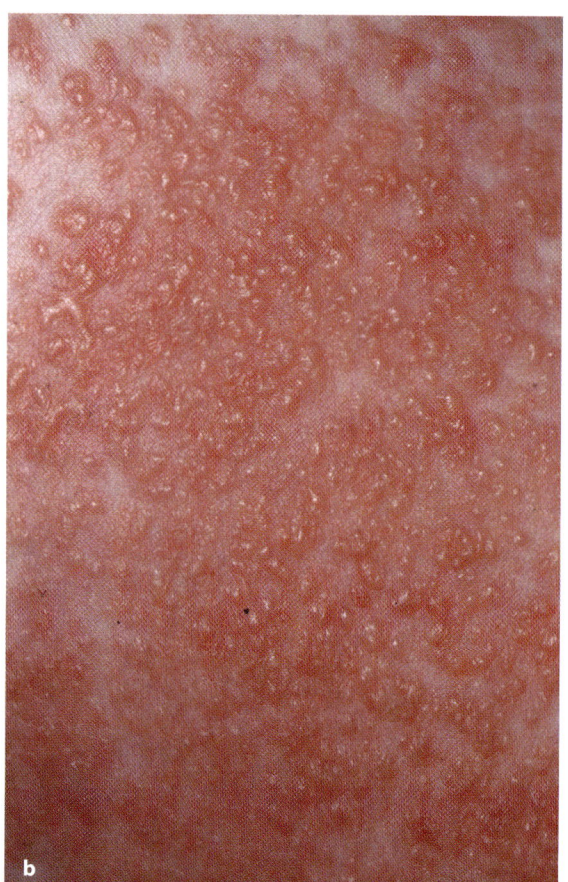

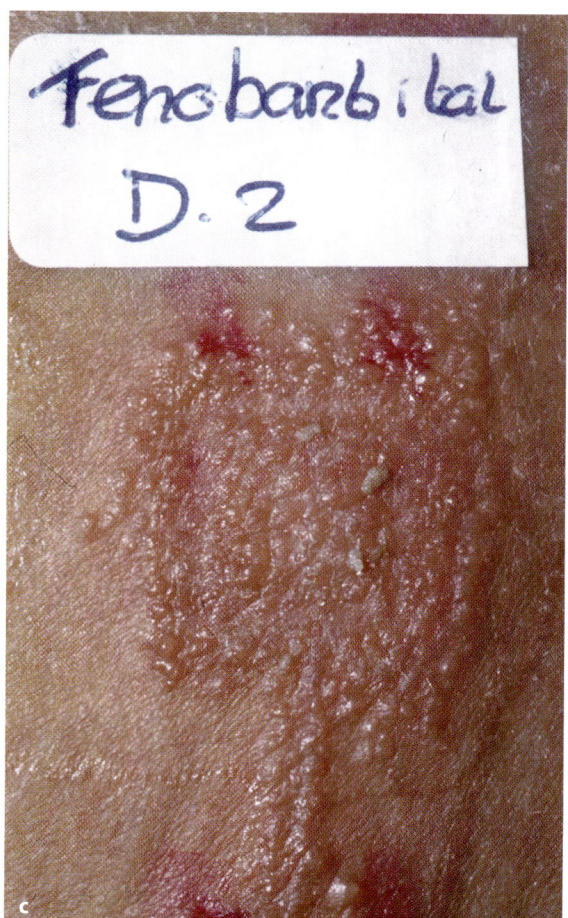

Fig. 1b, c.

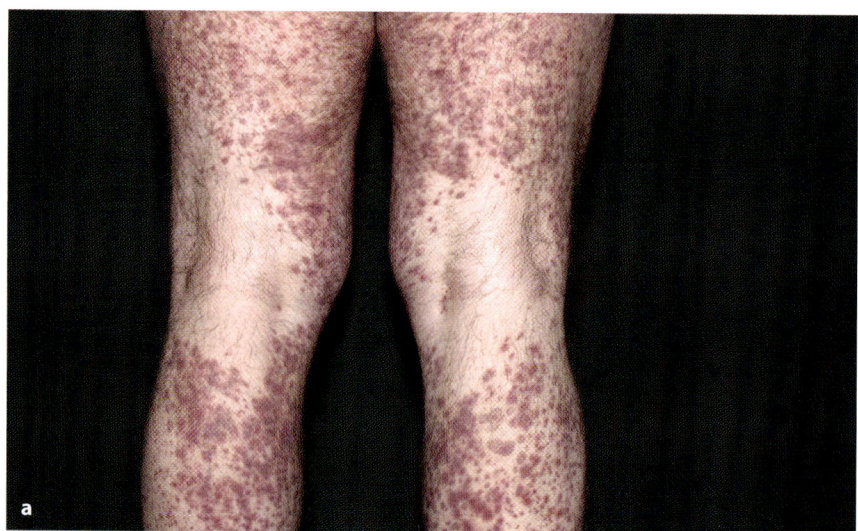

Fig. 2a–c.
Erythema multiforme-like drug eruption due to tetrazepam (a). Close up shows target lesions (b). Patch test with tetrazepam was positive both at 1% and 10% (c) (courtesy of PJ Frosch [89])

Fig. 2b, c.
Erythema multiforme-like
drug eruption due to tetrazepam (a). Close up shows
target lesions (b). Patch test
with tetrazepam was positive
both at 1% and 10% (c) (courtesy of PJ Frosch [89])

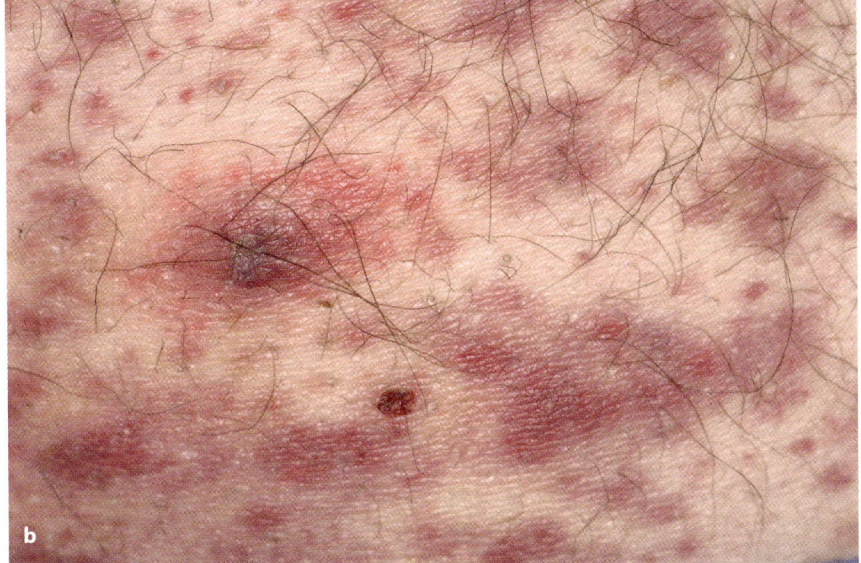

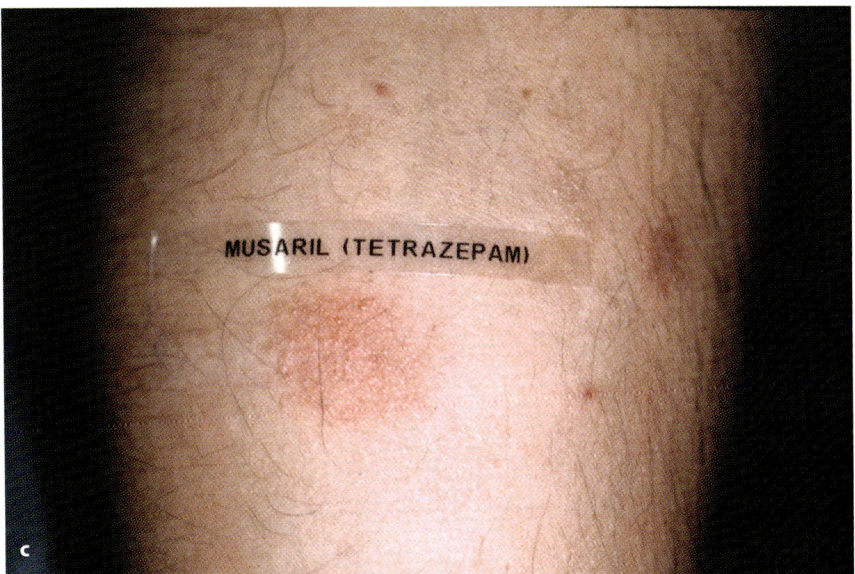

24.2 Pathomechanisms

Most adverse drug reactions are probably not allergic at all, but are caused by pharmacological properties of the drug, special sensitivity of the patient, or events such as accumulation and interactions. Usual-ly it is not possible to decide from the clinical picture which mechanism is involved. The pseudo-allergic (anaphylactoid) reaction, observed with acetylsali-cylic acid and other nonsteroidal anti-inflammatory drugs, is an example of a nonimmunological reaction mimicking a true (type I) allergic reaction due to nonspecific release of large amounts of histamine

and other mediators of inflammation [10]. Allergic drug reactions can be classified according to the im-munological reaction types of Gell and Coombs (Chap. 2), but often, it is not one isolated immunolog-ical mechanism that is responsible for the event: combinations of type I and IV reactivity exist [11]. Delayed type IV hypersensitivity involving drug (or drug metabolite) specific T-cells have been docu-mented in several patterns of drug eruptions. In ma-culopapular exanthema, specific T-cells were isolated from the skin and blood during the acute episode and, later, from positive patch tests [12]. Specific T-cells have been documented in other patterns of drug eruptions, where the different clinical aspects of the

24

eruption depend on the preferential activity of the T-cell: IL-5 production with eosinophil recruitment and activation in the drug hypersensitivity syndrome (DHS) or drug reaction eosinophilia and systemic symptoms (DRESS), production of the chemokine CXCL8 (IL-8) with preferential neutrophil recruitment in acute generalized exanthematic pustulosis (AGEP) or a T-cell cytotoxic activity in exanthems, bullous lesions, Stevens–Johnson syndrome (SJS) and toxic epidermal necrolysis [6, 12–16]. Fixed drug eruptions are also typical T-cell-mediated reactions, with a special localization pattern and a very particular retention of drug-specific T-cells in lesional areas, which induces lesional reactivation shortly after drug exposure, both after drug intake or topical application as a patch or open test [13, 17]. Delayed type hypersensitivity is also involved in some photosensitive drug reactions, mainly in those with an eczematous pattern [18, 19].

Therefore, this makes patch testing suitable in several drug eruptions other than dermatitis. Nevertheless, sometimes it is not the drug itself but a systemic metabolite that is the hapten responsible for the adverse reaction. This may be a cause of false-negative test results if the test is performed with the drug itself and not with the metabolite, which is usually not known or not available. Although skin metabolism is quite efficient, some drugs are not metabolized by skin cells [7].

Core Message

■ A wide variety of clinically different adverse eruptions may be T-cell-mediated.

24.3 Patch Test Indications

The diagnosis of a drug eruption and the imputation of the culprit drug are performed mainly on clinical grounds, based on chronological and semiological criteria: the clinico-evolutive pattern of the eruption, its chronological relation with the initiation and suspension of the drug, and data on a previous drug reaction (accidental rechallenge) [20]. No single test can replace a good characterization of these parameters. Even in cases where very accurate data is available, which, most often, is not the case, and especially if the patient is on multiple drugs, the imputability index for a single drug is very low. Drug reintroduction would be the more definitive test for confirming the culprit drug, but it does not always reproduce the

skin reaction and it is often contraindicated due to the risk of inducing a severe drug reaction, as in toxic epidermal necrolysis or in the hypersensitivity syndrome. Therefore, complementary clinical and laboratory investigations can then be performed in order to try to confirm, and seldom to exclude, an imputable drug.

Patch testing with drugs is simple to perform and is a relatively safe method of investigation. The risk of reactivation of the drug eruption is very low. Serious immediate reactions evoked by patch testing are rare [21–25], the risk is considerably lower compared with intracutaneous (i.c.) tests. Thus, the patch test is a good test to start with. If patch tests are negative, prick or scratch, i.c. tests, and a provocation test, performed sequentially in a hospital setting, may be the next steps [9].

Patch testing in the study of drug eruptions has been performed for many years, but not as a systematic investigation. Therefore, controlled studies with large numbers of patients with well characterized patterns of drug eruptions induced by different drugs are still lacking. Nevertheless, there are many reports showing that positive patch tests are found relatively often in cases of eczematous eruptions, maculopapular and delayed urticarial rashes, and AGEP (Table 1). Nevertheless, the frequency of positive tests ranges from 7.5% to 43%, depending on the selection of patients, the pattern of drug eruption, and the drugs involved [26, 27]. Positive patch tests with carbamazepine, tetrazepam, synergistins, and aminopenicillins are observed in more than 50% of the cases with delayed reactions [9, 28–37]. Fixed drug erup-

Table 1. Patch test results in patients with a possible adverse drug eruption, classified according to the type of eruption (adapted from [26] and [27])

Eruption	Number of positives/patients (%)	
	Osawa et al. [26] (*n*=197)	Barbaud et al. [27] (*n*=72)
Maculopapular	10/72 (14)	16/27 (59)
Erythroderma	8/15 (53)	5/7 (71)
Eczematous	9/17 (53)	3/9 (33)
Erythema multiforme (EM)	6/29 (21)	
Lichenoid	2/11 (18)	
Photosensitivity		4/4[a] (100)
Fixed eruptions	2/6 (33)	0/3
Urticaria/angioedema		2/18 (11)
Miscellaneous	15/47 (32)	1/6[b] (17)
Total	62/197 (31)	31/72 (43)

[a] Photopatch test. [b] Positive test in AGEP

tions are unique, T-cell-mediated eruptions, so we can expect to find positive tests on the residual lesions in a high percentage of cases [12, 17]. Alanko [38] found as many as 26 out of 30 cases (87%) [17, 39]. In photosensitive eruptions, when it is not a clearly phototoxic reaction, photopatch tests can be rewarding [18, 40]. Examples of drugs reported to give positive patch test reactions are shown in Tables 2–5.

Core Message

■ Positive patch tests are found especially in eczematous and maculopapular eruptions, fixed eruptions, and, sometimes, in urticarial and photosensitive eruptions.

Table 2. Examples of drugs reported to elicit positive photopatch test reactions in patients with photosensitive adverse drug eruptions. The test concentrations and vehicles are those mentioned by the authors. The UVA test dose was usually 5 J/cm² but ranged from 4.5 J/cm² to 15.5 J/cm². (*acet.* Acetone, *aq.* water, *pet.* petrolatum)

Drug	Test concentration, vehicle	Reference
Actarit[a]	1% pet.	[56, 57]
Althiazide[b]	10% pet./aq.	[58]
Amitriptyline[a]	5% pet.	[59]
Carbamazepine	0.01% pet.	[60]
Clomipramine[a]	0.1% pet.	[61]
Chloroquine sulfate	–	[62]
Chlorpromazine[a]	1% aq., pet.	[57]
Doxycycline[a]	10% pet.	[63]
Flutamide[a]	1–20% acet., pet.	[64, 65]
Griseofulvin	1% pet.	[66]
Hydrochlorothiazide[a]	1–10% pet.	[67]
Lomefloxacin[a]	1–10% pet.	[40, 67, 68]
NSAIDs[a]	1–10% pet.	[18, 69]
Ampiroxicam[a]	1% pet.	[70]
Ketoprofen[a]	1% pet.	[47, 176]
Piroxicam[a]	1% pet.	[18, 19, 71–74]
Tiaprofenic acid	1% pet.	[47]
Promethazine[a]	0.1–1% pet.	[57]
Pyridoxine HCl	–	[75]
Pyritinol	20% pet.	[76]
Quinidine	0.1% aq.	[77]
Quinine	0.1% aq.	[77]
4-Quinolines[a]	10% pet.	[78]
Simvastatin[a]	10% pet.	[79, 80]
Tetrazepam[a]	10% pet.	[81]
Thioridazine	1% pet.	[57]
Triflusal[a] (HTB[c])	1% pet.	[82]

[a] Tests in controls reported.
[b] Positive tests with UVB, not with UVA.
[c] *HTB* 2-hydroxy-4-trifluoro-methyl benzoic acid, a triflusal metabolite

Table 3. Examples of drugs reported to elicit positive patch test reactions in patients with adverse drug eruptions. The test concentrations and vehicles are those mentioned by the authors. (*alc.* Alcohol, *aq.* water, *eth.* ethanol, *pet.* petrolatum)

Drug	Test concentration, vehicle	Reference
Aminoglycosides	20% pet.	[26]
Anesthetics, local	0.5–2% aq.	[83]
Atenolol[a]	10% pet.	[84]
β-Lactam antibiotics[a]	1–20%, pet.	[11, 28, 41, 45, 85–87]
Benzodiazepines[a]	1% aq., 5–10% pet.	[30–33, 88, 89]
Bucillamine[a]	1% pet.	[90]
Carbamazepine[a]	0.1–10% pet.	[26, 34–36, 60]
Carbenicillin	5% aq.	[91]
Captopril[a]	0.1–3% pet.	[26, 92]
Celecoxib[a]	10% pet	[93]
Cephalosporins	5–20% aq., pet.	[11, 26, 41, 94–96]
Cimetidine[a]	1% aq.	[97]
Clindamycin phosphate	1–20% pet., aq.	[98, 99]
Codeine phosphate	0.05% aq.	[100]
Dihydroquinidine[a]	pulverized tablet	[101]
Diltiazem[a]	1% pet., saline	[102, 103]
Ephedrine HCl[a]	5% aq.	[104]
Erythromycin base[a]	as is –2.5% pet.	[101, 105]
Gold sodium thiomalate	5% pet.	[26]
Heparins	as is	[106– 109]
Hydromorphone[a]	2% aq.	[110]
Metoprolol[a]	10% pet.	[84]
Nifuroxazide[a]	10% pet.; 1–0.001% aq.	[111, 112]
Nystatin	30,000 IU/g PEG	[113]
Oxprenolol	10% pet.	[84]
Oxyphenbutazone[a]	1–5% pet.	[114, 115]
Penicillin G[a]	100,000 units/ml aq.	[11, 42, 85, 91, 116]
Penicillins[a]	1–20% pet.	[26, 28, 45]
Phenazone[a]	5% pet.	[117]
Phenobarbital	1–20% pet.	[26]
Phenylbutazone	1–5% pet.	[114, 115, 118]
Phytotherapeutics:		
Herba solidaginis extr.	as is; 1:10	[119]
Piroxicam[a]	1–10% pet.	[26]
Piperazine	1% aq.	[114]
Pravastatin	pulverized tablet	[120]
Pristinamycin	1–10% aq., pet.	[29]
Propranolol[a]	10% pet.	[84]
Propicillin	20% pet.	[121]
Pyrazinamide	1–10% alc.	[122]
Ranitidine[a]	1% pet.	[123]
Sertraline[a]	5–10% pet., eth.	[124]
Sodium valproate	1–5% pet.	[26]
Spiramycin[a]	5% pet.	[102]
Stepronin[a]	18% sol.	[125]
Sulfamethoxazole[a]	as is	[43]
Sulfonamide[a]	10% pet.	[102]
Tiopronin	0.3–5% pet.	[26, 126]
Tobramycin	5% aq.	[98]
Virginiamycin[a]	0.5% pet.	[102]
Vitamin K[a]	0.1% pet.	[127]
Zinc acexamate[a]	5% aq.	[128]

[a] Tests in controls reported

24

Table 4. Examples of drugs reported to elicit positive epicut-aneous tests in fixed-drug eruptions, using an open or occlu-sive technique. The test concentrations and vehicles are those mentioned by the authors. (*alc.* Alcohol, *aq.* water, *DMSO* dim-ethylsulfoxide, *pet.* petrolatum)

Drug	Test concentration, vehicle	Reference
Acyclovir	5% pet.	[129]
Aminophylline	10% pet.	[130]
Amlexanox	50% pet.	[131]
Apronal	5% pet.	[130]
Barbiturates	10% pet., alc.	[38, 130]
Carbamazepine	10% pet., alc.	[38]
Chlormezanone	10% pet., alc.	[38, 130]
Citiolone	10% DMSO	[132]
Ciprofloxacin	10% pet.	[133]
Clarithromycin	10% aq.	[134]
Dipyrone	10% pet.	[130]
Doxycycline	10% pet., alc.	[38, 130]
Ethenzamide	20% pet.	[135]
Ibuprofen	10% pet.	[130]
Mefenamic acid	10% pet.	[130]
Metronidazole	50% pet	[136]
Nimesulide	1–10% pet.	[17, 137]
Ofloxacin	20% pet.	[138]
Phenazone derivatives	10% pet., alc.	[38, 130]
Piroxicam	1–10% pet.	[17, 139]
Promethazine	10% pet.	[130]
Sulfasalazine	10% pet.	[140]
Sulfonamides	10% pet., alc.	[38]
Trimethoprim	10% pet., alc.	[38, 39]
Tenoxicam	1–10% pet	[17]

Table 5. Examples of drugs and chemically related materials which may, after contact sensitization, elicit systemic contact dermatitis when used systemically [4, 175]

Drug	Reference
Amantadine	[141]
Aminophylline	[142]
Clonidine	[143]
Corticosteroids	[144–148]
Erythromycin	[105]
Estradiol	[46]
Ethylenediamine	[142, 149]
Ephedrine HCl	[104]
5-Fluorouracil	[150]
Gentamycin	[151]
Gold salts	[152, 153]
Heparins	[154]
Hydroxyquinolines	[155, 156]
Hydroxyzine	[149, 157]
Imidazoles	[46, 158, 159]
Lignocaine, local anesthetics	[83, 160–162]
Mitomycin C	[163–165]
Neomycin	[156]
Netilmycin	[151]
NSAIDs:	
Arylpropionic acid derivatives	[47]
Arylalcanoic acid derivatives	[166, 167]
Pyrazolone derivatives	[168, 169]
Nystatin	[170]
Pantothenic acid (vitamin B5)	[171]
Penicillins	[4]
Sorbic acid	[172]
Sulfonamides	[4]
Synergistins	[173]
Tetraethylthiuram disulfide	[4]
Thimerosal	[174]

24.4 Technique and Test Materials

It can take weeks before skin reactivity is measurable by patch testing. Thus, it is advisable to wait several weeks after the rash has gone to perform the patch tests. How long exactly is not known, but 6 weeks is usually advised [9, 41, 42].

Patch testing is performed in the generally accept-ed way on the back, as in contact dermatitis [9]. In particular cases, such as in fixed eruptions, reactivity occurs only in skin areas where the skin reaction has occurred [43, 44]. The application time is usually 2 days, but, occasionally, it can be convenient to re-move tests at D1 [45]. Readings are performed at D2 and at D3 or D4, according to the International Con-tact Dermatitis Research Group (ICDRG) guidelines.

In fixed eruptions, the test materials are applied on an inactive, residual lesion, usually for one day, with occlusion as in patch testing. The residual pig-mentation is a useful marker to indicate the area to apply the tests. Readings are performed at D1 and D2 or at D3, if previously negative [17]. Another test is applied on normal skin on the back and serves as a negative control. Alanko [38] prefers an open test, as, sometimes, positive reactions are seen only in the first 24 h, which makes observations necessary dur-ing the first 24-h period. A reaction is regarded as positive when clear erythema is visible for at least 6 h, but often, we can observe an eczematous or bul-lous reaction, sometimes mimicking the fixed drug eruption [17].

In drug photosensitivity, photoepicutaneous patch tests can be performed as in photoallergic con-tact dermatitis, using mainly UVA irradiation, at a dose of 5 J/cm² [18].

There is not much knowledge available about the ideal test concentrations of drugs. Concentrations found in textbooks are often based on experiences with contact dermatitis patients. Sometimes, these concentrations seem to be too low in cases of drug eruptions. Recommended concentrations are usually between 1% and 20% of the pure chemical, but we need to know the safe ranges of test concentrations, for which, larger studies with patients and controls are needed. For example, carbamazepine, hydrochlorothiazide, propranolol, sulfamethoxazole, and trimethoprim did not evoke reactions when tested at 20% in petrolatum in 200 volunteers [1]. In patients with delayed exanthematous eruptions due to carbamazepine, ampicillin, and amoxicillin patch-test concentrations of 1% and 5% are sufficient, as all patients reacting at 20% also reacted at 1% or 5% pet [28, 45]. In cases of very severe drug eruptions, it is advisable to start with lower concentrations to prevent reactivation of the eruption [9].

If the pure drug is not available, which is often the case, the test can be done with the drug as such, in powdered form or in solutions for oral, i.v., or i.m. use. The amount of active drug in a tablet varies, but is approximately 20% (w/w). Serial dilutions can be helpful. Petrolatum and water are the most frequently used vehicles, but ethanol and dimethylsulfoxide (DMSO) can be more adequate for certain drugs [46]. A pharmacist can give advice on a suitable vehicle for maximum penetration and bioavailability.

Whenever possible, chemically related compounds or other drugs of the same pharmacological group are tested in order to obtain information on possible cross-reactivity. Sometimes, the pattern of cross-reactivity may be very informative for the patient and the doctor. In this way, cross-reactivity was demonstrated between: amoxicillin and ampicillin [28]; in more than half of the cases between pristinamycin and virginiamycin [29]; in systemic photosensitivity for the arylpropionic nonsteroidal anti-inflammatory drugs (NSAIDs), ketoprofen and tiaprofenic acid, and the hypolipemiant agent fenofibrate [47]. There is cross-reactivity between piroxicam and tenoxicam in fixed drug eruptions, whereas tenoxicam is safe in piroxicam photosensitive patients, as shown by photopatch testing and drug challenge [17, 19].

When tests are done with pure chemicals, it can also be worthwhile to perform tests with the filler materials and the original drug preparation. In principle, reactions to the "inert" filler substances and additives are possible, but in practice, they are rare [48–51]. Occasionally, they are the cause of false positive reactions (irritation, low pH), and induce nonrelevant positive patch test reactions in previously contact-sensitized patients [51]. Testing with pure drugs or with low concentrations of the commercial products seldom gives false positive reactions. Nevertheless, a positive reaction with a non-standardized drug concentration needs to be checked in at least 20 controls.

Although rarely encountered, anaphylactic reactions can occur due to topical application of drugs, e.g., penicillins, neomycin, or bacitracin [21–23]. For safety reasons, it is practical to observe the patient for approximately half an hour after application of the test material. Another adverse patch test effect is sensitization by patch testing; this is rarely seen, even with penicillins [52].

False-negative reactions can be expected, either because the responsible hapten is a drug metabolite that is not formed in the skin, because the vehicle or the concentration is not adequate, or because, as occurs in viral infections, the drug eruption is due to other concomitant factors that may enhance individual hypersensitivity [37, 53].

Core Message

■ Patch tests are best performed not earlier than 6 weeks after disappearance of the rash.

24.5 Relevance and Consequences

The tests should be interpreted very carefully. A positive test has to be checked with the controls to exclude false-positive reactions. Although ethical problems may arise over the use of controls, we can perform control tests on individuals who take the drug but who developed a drug eruption from a different drug. A true positive test can be regarded as a sign of immunological reactivity of the patient and should be taken seriously if compatible with the history. Re-administration of the drug should be avoided as it can again elicit an adverse reaction, which might be even more severe.

A negative test result far from excludes hypersensitivity or an adverse drug reaction. The test method might not be adequate due to another pathomechanism, the bioavailability of the test material might have been insufficient, the wrong drug may have been tested, history and drug records can be surprisingly inaccurate, the right drug may have been tested but the allergen could be a metabolite, and so on. Thus, a negative test result does not allow a definitive conclusion.

24

If necessary, other tests have to be performed, such as prick, scratch, and intradermal tests or even a challenge (provocation) test [54]. The provocation test is regarded as the gold standard, but occasionally also gives false negatives [55]. In vitro tests for IgE (RAST) exist for some drugs, as well as lymphocyte proliferation/activation tests. However, these tests are rarely available and not performed on a routine basis.

In conclusion, although many suspected patients have negative patch test reactions, it remains worthwhile to perform the tests on individual patients.

They can confirm a clinical imputability and avoid any eventual drug reintroduction with more severe consequences and, in very particular cases, can give important information on other cross-reacting drugs.

Core Message

■ It is worthwhile to perform patch tests on individual patients with a suspected drug eruption.

References

1. Bruynzeel DP, Maibach HI (1997) Patch testing in systemic drug eruptions. Clin Dermatol 15:479–484
2. Roujeau JC (1997) Drug-induced skin reactions. In: Grobb JJ, Stern RS, Mac Kie RM, Weinstock WA (eds) Epidemiology, causes and prevention of skin diseases. Blackwell, Oxford, UK
3. Bigby M (2001) Rates of cutaneous reactions to drugs. Arch Dermatol 137:765–770
4. Menné T, Maibach HI (1966) Systemic contact-type dermatitis. In: Marzulli FN, Maibach HI (eds) Dermatoxicology, 5th edn. Taylor and Francis, Washington, DC, pp 161–175
5. Pichler WJ, Schnyder B, Zanni MP, Hari Y, von Greyerz S (1998) Role of T cells in drug allergies. Allergy 53:225–232
6. Pichler W (2003) Delayed drug hypersensitivity reactions. Ann Intern Med 139:683–693
7. Griem P, Wulferink M, Sachs B, González JB, Gleichmann E (1998) Allergic and autoimmune reactions to xenobiotics: how do they arise? Immunol Today 19:133–141
8. Hari Y, Fruitig-Schnyder K, Hurni M, Yawalker N, Zanni MP, Schnyder B, Kappeler A, von Greyerz S, Braathen LR, Pichler WJ (2001) T cell involvement in cutaneous drug eruptions. Clin Exp Allergy 31:1398–1408
9. Barbaud A, Gonçalo M, Bruynzeel D, Bircher A (2001) Guidelines for performing skin tests with drugs in the investigation of cutaneous adverse drug reactions. Contact Dermatitis 45:321–328
10. Kallós P, Kallós L (1980) Histamine and some other mediators of pseudo-allergic reactions. In: Dukor P, Kallós P, Schlumberger HD, West GB, (eds) PAR. Pseudo-allergic reactions, vol 1: genetic aspects and anaphylactoid reactions. Karger, Basel, Switzerland, pp 28–55
11. Bruynzeel DP, von Blomberg-van der Flier M, Scheper RJ, van Ketel WG, de Haan P (1985) Allergy for penicillin and the relevance of epicutaneous tests. Dermatologica 171:429–434
12. Yawalker N, Hari Y, Frutig K, Egli F, Wendland T, Braathen LR, Pichler WJ (2000) T cells isolated from positive epicutaneous test reactions to amoxicillin and ceftriaxone are drug specific and cytotoxic. J Invest Dermatol 115:647–652
13. Barbaud A (2002) Tests cutanés dans l'investigation des toxidermies: de la physiopathologie aux résultats des investigations. Thérapie 57:258–262
14. Kuechler PC, Britschgi M, Schmid S, Hari Y, Grabscheid B, Pichler WJ (2004) Cytotoxic mechanisms in different forms of T-cell-mediated drug allergies. Allergy 59:613–622
15. Britschgi M, Pichler WJ (2002) Acute generalized exanthematous pustulosis, a clue to neutrophil-mediated inflammatory processes orchestrated by T cells. Curr Opin Allergy Clin Immunol 2:325–331
16. Choquet-Kastylevsky G, Intrator L, Chenal C, Bocquet H, Revuz J, Roujeau JC (1998) Increased levels of interleukin 5 are associated with the generation of eosinophilia in drug-induced hypersensitivity syndrome. Br J Dermatol 139:1026–1032
17. Gonçalo M, Oliveira HS, Fernandes B, Robalo-Cordeiro M, Figueiredo A (2002) Topical provocation in fixed drug eruption from nonsteroidal anti-inflammatory drugs. Exogenous Dermatol 1:81–86
18. Gonçalo M (1998) Exploration dans les photo-allergies médicamenteuses. In: Groupe d'Etudes et de Recherches en Dermato-Allergologie (GERDA) (eds) Progrès en dermato-allergologie. John Libbey Eurotext, Nancy, France, pp 67–74
19. Gonçalo M, Figueiredo A, Tavares P, Fontes Ribeiro CA, Teixeira F, Poiares Baptista A (1992) Photosensitivity to piroxicam: absence of cross reaction with tenoxicam. Contact Dermatitis 27:287–290
20. Moore N, Paux G, Begaud B, Biour M, Loupi E, Boismare F, Royer RJ (1985) Adverse drug reaction monitoring: doing it the French way. Lancet 2:1056–1058
21. Pietzcker F, Kuner V (1975) Anaphylaxie nach epicutanem Ampicillin-Test. Z Hautkr 50:437–440
22. Maucher OM (1972) Anaphylaktische Reaktionen beim Epicutantest. Hautarzt 23:139–140
23. Shechter JF, Wilkinson RD, dei Carpio J (1984) Anaphylaxis following the use of bacitracin ointment. Report of a case and review of the literature. Arch Dermatol 120:909–911
24. Jonker MJ, Bruynzeel DP (2003) Anaphylactic reaction elicited by patch testing with diclofenac. Contact Dermatitis 49:114–115
25. Mashiah J (2003) A systemic reaction to patch testing for the evaluation of acute generalized exanthematous pustulosis. Arch Dermatol 139:1181–1183
26. Osawa J, Naito S, Aihara M, Kitamura K, Ikezawa Z, Nakajima H (1990) Evaluation of skin test reactions in patients with non-immediate type drug eruptions. J Dermatol 17:235–239
27. Barbaud A, Reichert-Penetrat S, Tréchot P, Jaquin-Petit M-A, Ehlinger A, Noirez V, Faure GC, Schmutz J-L, Béné M-C (1998) The use of skin testing in the investigation of cutaneous adverse drug reactions. Br J Dermatol 139:49–58

28. Gonçalo M, Fernandes B, Oliveira HS, Figueiredo A (2000) Epicutaneous patch testing in drug eruptions. Contact Dermatitis 42:22

29. Barbaud A, Tréchot P, Weber-Muller F, Ulrich G, Coomun N, Schmutz J-L (2004) Drug skin tests in cutaneous adverse drug reactions to pristinamycin: 29 cases with a study of cross-reactions between synergistins. Contact Dermatitis 50:22–26

30. Camarasa JG, Serra-Baldrich E (1990) Tetrazepam allergy detected by patch test. Contact Dermatitis 22:246

31. Reichert C, Gall H (1998) Type-IV-Allergie auf Tetrazepam. Dermatosen 46:75–78

32. Ortega NR, Barranco P, López Serrano C, Romualdo L, Mora C (1996) Delayed cell-mediated hypersensitivity to tetrazepam. Contact Dermatitis 34:139

33. Ortiz-Frutos FJ, Alonso J, Hergueta JP, Quintana I, Iglesias L (1995) Tetrazepam: an allergen with several clinical expressions. Contact Dermatitis 33:63–65

34. Alanko K (1993) Patch testing in cutaneous reactions caused by carbamazepine. Contact Dermatitis 29:254–257

35. Camarasa JG (1985) Patch test diagnosis of exfoliative dermatitis due to carbamazepine. Contact Dermatitis 12:49

36. Puig L, Nadal C, Fernández-Figueras M-T, Alomar A (1996) Carbamazepine-induced drug rashes: diagnostic value of patch tests depends on clinico-pathologic presentation. Contact Dermatitis 34:435–437

37. Renn CN, Straff W, Dorfmüller A, Al-Masoudi T, Merk HF, Sachs B (2002) Amoxicillin-induced exanthema in young adults with infectious mononucleosis: demonstration of drug-specific lymphocyte reactivity. Brit J Dermatol 147:1166–1170

38. Alanko K (1994) Topical provocation of fixed drug eruption. A study of 30 patients. Contact Dermatitis 31:25–27

39. Ozkaya-Bayazit E, Güngôr H (1997) Trimethoprim-induced fixed drug eruption: positive topical provocation on previously involved and uninvolved skin. Contact Dermatitis 39:87–88

40. Oliveira HS, Gonçalo M, Figueiredo A (2000) Photosensitivity to lomefloxacin. A clinical and photobiological study. Photodermatol Photoimmunol Photomedic 16:116–120

41. Bruynzeel DP, van Ketel WG (1989) Patch testing in drug eruptions. Semin Dermatol 8:196–203

42. Fellner MJ (1968) An immunologic study of selected penicillin reactions involving the skin. Arch Dermatol 96:503–519

43. Klein CE, Trautmann A, Zillikens D, Bröcker EB (1995) Patch testing in an unusual case of toxic epidermal necrolysis. Contact Dermatitis 33:448–449

44. Barbaud A, Tréchot P, Reichert-Pénétrat S, Granel F, Schmutz JL (2001) The usefulness of patch testing on the previously most severely affected site in a cutaneous adverse drug reaction to tetrazepam. Contact Dermatitis 44:259–260

45. Torres M-J, Sanchez-Sabaté E, Alvarez J, Mayorga C, Fernández J, Padial A, Cornejo-Garcia J-A, Bellón T, Blanca M (2004) Skin test evaluation in nonimmediate allergic reactions to penicillins. Allergy 59:219–234

46. Gonçalo M, Oliveira S, Monteiro C, Clerins I, Figueiredo A (1999) Allergic and systemic contact dermatitis from estradiol. Contact Dermatitis 40:58–59

47. Le Coz CJ, Bottlaender A, Scrivener J-N, Santinelli F, Cribier BJ, Heid E, Grosshans EM (1998) Photocontact dermatitis from ketoprofen and tiaprofenic acid: cross-reactivity study in 12 consecutive patients. Contact Dermatitis 38:245–252

48. Shmunes E (1984) Allergic dermatitis to benzyl alcohol in an injectable solution. Arch Dermatol 120:1200–1201

49. Schäfer T, Enders F, Przybilla B (1995) Sensitization to thimerosal and previous vaccination. Contact Dermatitis 32:114–116

50. Verecken P. Birringer C, Knitelius A-C, Herbaut D, Germaux M-A (1998) Sensitization to benzyl alcohol: a possible cause of "corticosteroid allergy". Contact Dermatitis 38:106

51. Barbaud A, Tréchot P, Reichert-Penetrat S, Commun N, Schmutz JL (2001) Relevance of skin tests with drugs in investigating cutaneous adverse drug reactions. Contact Dermatitis 45:265–268

52. van Ketel WG (1975) Patch testing in penicillin allergy. Contact Dermatitis 1:253–254

53. Vieira R, Gonçalo M, Figueiredo A (2004) Patch testing with allopurinol and oxypurinol in drug eruptions. Contact Dermatitis 50:156

54. Hannuksela M (1998) Skin testing in drug hypersensitivity. In: Kauppinen K, Alanko K, Hannuksela M, Maibach H (eds) Skin reactions to drugs. CRC, Boca Raton, Fla., pp 81–95

55. Alanko K, Kauppinen K (1998) Diagnosis of drug eruptions: clinical evaluation and drug challenge. In: Kauppinen K, Alanko K, Hannuksela M, Maibach H (eds) Skin reactions to drugs. CRC, Boca Raton, Fla., pp 75–79

56. Kawada A, Hiruma M, Miura Y, Noguchi H, Akiyama M, Ishibashi A (1997) Photosensitivity due to actarit. Contact Dermatitis 36:175–176

57. Suhonen R (1976) Thioridazine photosensitivity. Contact Dermatitis 2:179

58. Schwarze HP, Albes B, Marguery MC, Loche F, Bazex J (1998) Evaluation of drug-induced photosensitivity by UVB photopatch testing. Contact Dermatitis 39:200

59. Sandra A, Srinivas CR, Deshpande SC (1998) Photopatch test reaction to amitriptyline. Contact Dermatitis 39:208–209

60. Terni T, Tagami H (1989) Eczematous drug eruption from carbamazepine: coexistence of contact and photocontact sensitivity. Contact Dermatitis 20:260–264

61. Ljunggren B, Bos G (1991) A case of photosensitivity and contact allergy to systemic tricyclic drugs, with unusual features. Contact Dermatitis 24:259–265

62. van Weelden H, Bolling HH, Baart de la Faille H, van der Leun JC (1982) Photosensitivity caused by chloroquine. Arch Dermatol 118:290

63. Tanaka N, Kawada A, Ohnishi Y, Hiruma M, Tajima S, Akiyama M, Ishibashi A (1997) Photosensitivity due to doxycycline hydrochloride with an unusual flare. Contact Dermatitis 37:93–94

64. Vilaplana J, Romaguera C, Azón A, Lecha M (1998) Flutamide photosensitivity – residual vitiliginous lesions. Contact Dermatitis 38:68–70

65. Martín-Lázaro J, Buján JG, Arrondo AP, Lozano JR, Galindo EC, Capdevila EF (2004) Is photopatch testing useful in the investigation of photosensitivity due to flutamide? Contact Dermatitis 50:325–326

66. Kojima T, Hasegawa T, Ishida H, Fujita M, Okamoto S (1988) Griseofulvin-induced photodermatitis – report of six cases. J Dermatol 15:76–82

67. Gonçalo M, Barros MA, Azenha A, Basto S, Figueiredo A (1996) The importance of photopatch testing in patients with photosensitive drug eruptions. In: Jadassohn Centenary Congress abstract book. European Society of Contact Dermatitis (ESCD), London, p 15

24

68. Kurumajin Y, Shono M (1992) Scarified photopatch testing in lomefloxacin photosensitivity. Contact Dermatitis 26:5–10

69. Przybilla B, Ring J, Scwab U, Galosi A, Dom M, Braun-Falco O (1987) Photosensibilisierende Eigenschaften nichtsteroidaler Antirheumatika im Photopatch- Test. Hautarzt 38:18–25

70. Kurumaji Y (1996) Ampiroxicam-induced photosensitivity. Contact Dermatitis 34:298–299

71. Vasconcelos C, Magina S, Quirino P, Barros MA, Mesquita-Guimarães J (1997) Cutaneous drug reactions to piroxicam. Contact Dermatitis 39:145

72. Varela P, Amorim I, Massa A, Sanches M, Silva E (1998) Piroxicam-beta-cyclodextrin and photosensitivity reactions. Contact Dermatitis 38:229

73. Youn JL, Lee HG, Yeo UC, Lee YS (1993) Piroxicam photosensitivity associated with vesicular hand dermatitis. Clin Exp Dermatol 18:52–54

74. Figueiredo A, Fontes Reibeiro CA, Gonçalo S, Caldeira HM, Poiares-Baptista A, Teixeiro F (1987) Piroxicam-induced photosensitivity. Contact Dermatitis 17:73–79

75. Morimoto K. Kawada A, Hiruma M, Ishibashi A (1996) Photosensitivity from pyridoxine hydrochloride (vitamin B6). J Am Acad Dermatol 35:304–305

76. Ishibashi A, Hirano K. Nishiyama Y (1973) Photosensitive dermatitis due to pyritinol. Arch Dermatol 107:427–428

77. Ljunggren B, Hindesen M, Isaksson (1992) Systemic quinine photosensitivity with photoepicutaneous cross-reactivity to quinidine. Contact Dermatitis 26:1–4

78. Kimura M, Kawada A (1998) Photosensitivity induced by lomefloxacin with cross-photosensitivity to ciprofloxacin and fleroxacin. Contact Dermatitis 38:180

79. Morimoto K, Kawada A, Hiruma M, Ishibashi A, Banda H (1995) Photosensitivity to simvastatin with an unusual response to photopatch and photo tests. Contact Dermatitis 33:274

80. Rodriguez Granados MT, De La Torre C, Cruces MJ, Pifteiro G (1998) Chronic actinic dermatitis due to simvastatin. Contact Dermatitis 38:294–295

81. Quiftones D, Sanchez I, Garcia-Abujeta JL, Fernandez L, Rodriguez F, Martil-Gil D, Jerez J (1998) Photodermatitis from tetrazepam. Contact Dermatitis 39:84

82. Serrano G, Aliaga A, Planells I (1987) Photosensitivity associated with triflusal (Disgren). Photodermatology 4:103–105

83. Ruzicka T, Gerstmeier M, Przybilla B, Ring J (1987) Allergy to local anesthetics: comparison of patch test with prick and intradermal test results. J Am Acad Dermatol 16:1202–1208

84. van Joost T, Sillevis Smitt JH (1981) Skin reactions to propranolol and cross-sensitivity to beta-adrenoreceptor blocking agents. Arch Dermatol 117:600–601

85. Romano A, Di Fonso M, Pietrantonio F, Pocobelli D, Giannarini L, Dei Bono A, Fabrizi G, Venuti A (1993) Repeated patch testing in delayed hypersensitivity to beta-lactam antibiotics. Contact Dermatitis 28:190

86. Lisi P, Lapomarda V, Stingeni L, Assalve D, Handel K, Caraffini S, Agostinelli D (1997) Skin tests in the diagnosis of eruptions caused by betalactams. Contact Dermatitis 37:151–154

87. Moreno-Ancillo A, Dominguez-Noche C, Gil-Adrados AC, Cosmes PM (2003) Near-fatal delayed hypersensitivity reaction to cloxacillin. Contact Dermatitis 49:44–49

88. Kämpgen E, Bürger T, Bröcker E-V, Klein E (1995) Cross-reactive type IV hypersensitivity reactions to benzodiazepines revealed by patch testing. Contact Dermatitis 33:356–357

89. Pirker C, Misic A, Brinkmeier T, Frosch PJ (2002) Tetrazepam drug sensitivity – usefulness of the patch test. Contact Dermatitis 47:135–138

90. Kimura M, Kawada A (1998) Drug eruption due to bucillamine. Contact Dermatitis 39:98–99

91. Prieto López C, Gamboa PM, Zugazaga Prieto M, Fernández Martínez JC, Miguel de la Villa F, Antépara Ercoreca I (1990) Study of various immunological parameters in the diagnosis of allergy to penicillin G and its derivatives. Allergol Immunpathol 18:141–148

92. Smit AJ, Van der Laan S, De Monchy J, Kallenberg CGM, Donker AJM (1984) Cutaneous reactions to captopril. Predictive value of skin tests. Clin Allergy 14:413–419

93. Alonso JC, Ortega JD, Gonzalo MJ (2004) Cutaneous reaction to oral celecoxib with positive patch test. Contact Dermatitis 50:48–49

94. Galindo Bonilla PA, Garcia Rodríguez R, Feo Brito F, Garrido Martin JA, Fernández Martinez F (1994) Patch testing for allergy to beta-lactam antibiotics. Contact Dermatitis 31:319–320

95. Romano A, Pietrantonio F, di Fonso M, Venuti A (1992) Delayed hypersensitivity to cefuroxime. Contact Dermatitis 27:270–271

96. Filipe P, Silva R, Almeida S, Guerra Rodrigo F (1996) Occupational allergic contact dermatitis from cephalosporins. Contact Dermatitis 34:226

97. Peters K (1986) Delayed hypersensitivity to oral cimetidine. Contact Dermatitis 15:190–191

98. Mufioz D, dei Pozo MD, Audícana M, Fernández E, Fernandez de Corres L (1996) Erythema-multiforme-like eruption from antibiotics of 3 different groups. Contact Dermatitis 34:227–228; 20:72–73

99. Lammintausta K, Tokola R, Kalimo K (2002) Cutaneous adverse reactions to clindamycin: results of skin tests and oral exposure. Br J Dermatol 146:643–648

100. de Groot AC, Conemans I (1986) Allergic urticarial rash from oral codeine. Contact Dermatitis 14:209–214

101. Moreau A, Dompmartin A (1995) Drug-induced acute generalized exanthematous pustulosis with positive patch tests. Int J Dermatol 34:263–266

102. Wolkenstein P, Chosidow O, Fléchet M-L, Robbiola O, Paul M, Dumé L, Revuz J, Roujeau J-C (1996) Patch testing in severe cutaneous adverse drug reactions, including Stevens-Johnson syndrome and toxic epidermal necrolysis. Contact Dermatitis 35:234–236

103. Wakelin SH, James MP (1995) Diltiazem-induced acute generalised exanthematous pustulosis. Clin Exp Dermatol 20:341–344

104. Audicana M, Urrutia I, Echechipia S, Mufioz D, Fernandez de Corres L (1991) Sensitization to ephedrine in oral anti-catarrhal drugs. Contact Dermatitis 24:223

105. Fernadez Redondo V, Casas L, Taboada M, Toribio J (1994) Systemic contact dermatitis from erythromycin. Contact Dermatitis 30:43–44

106. Bircher AJ (1993) Allergische Reaktionen vom Spättyp auf Heparine. Allergologie 16:268–274

107. Bircher AJ, Flückiger R, Buchner SA (1990) Eczematous infiltrated plaques to subcutaneous heparin: a type IV allergic reaction. Br J Dermatol 123:507–514

108. Boehncke W-H, Weber L, Gall H (1996) Tolerance to intravenous administration of heparin and heparinoid in a patient with delayed-type hypersensitivity to heparins and heparinoids. Contact Dermatitis 35:73–75

109. Koch P, Hindi S, Landwehr D (1996) Delayed allergic skin reactions due to subcutaneous heparin-calcium, enoxaparin-sodium, pentosan polysulfate and acute skin lesions from systemic sodium-heparin. Contact Dermatitis 34:156–158

110. De Cuyper C, Goeteyn M (1992) Systemic contact dermatitis from subcutaneous hydromorphone. Contact Dermatitis 27:220–223
111. Machet L, Jan V, Machet MC, Lorette G, Vaillan L (1997) Acute generalized exanthematous pustulosis induced by nifuroxazide. Contact Dermatitis 36:308–309
112. Kiec-Swierczynska M, Krecisz B (1998) Occupational contact allergy to nifuroxazide simulating prurigo nodularis. Contact Dermatitis 39:93–94
113. Quirce S, Farra F, Lázaro M, Gómez MI, Sánchez Cano M (1991) Generalized dermatitis due to oral nystatin. Contact Dermatitis 25:197–198
114. Fernández de Corres L, Bernaola G, Lobera T, Leanizbarrutia I, Mufioz D (1986) Allergy from pyrazolone derivatives. Contact Dermatitis 14:249–250
115. Valsecchi R, Tornaghi A, Falgheri G, Rossi A, Cainelli T (1983) Drug reaction from oxyphenbutazone. Contact Dermatitis 9:419
116. Haneke EG, Körner E, Haneke E (1980) Klinische Bedeutung positiver Penicillinreaktione. Dtsch Med Wochenschr 105:635–639
117. Landwehr AJ, van Ketel WG (1982) Delayed-type allergy to phenazone in a patient with erythema multiforme. Contact Dermatitis 8:283–284
118. Vooys RC, van Ketel WG (1977) Allergic drug eruption from pyrazolone compounds. Contact Dermatitis 3:57–58
119. Schätzle M, Agathos M, Breit R (1998) Allergic contact dermatitis from goldenrod (Herba solidaginis) after systemic administration. Contact Dermatitis 39:271–272
120. De Boer EM, Bruynzeel DP (1994) Allergy to pravastatin. Contact Dermatitis 30:238
121. Gebhardt M, Lustig A, Bocker T, Wollina U (1995) Acute generalized exanthematous pustulosis (AGEP): manifestation of drug allergy to propicillin. Contact Dermatitis 33:204–205
122. Goday I, Aguirre A, Díaz-Pérez JL (1990) A positive patch test in a pyrazinamide drug eruption. Contact Dermatitis 22:181–182
123. Juste S, Blanco J, Garcés M, Rodriguez G (1992) Allergic dermatitis due to oral ranitidine. Contact Dermatitis 27:339–340
124. Fernandes B, Brites M, Gonçalo M, Figueiredo A (2000) Maculopapular eruption from sertraline with positive patch tests. Contact Dermatitis 42:287
125. Romano A, Pietrantonio F, di Fonso M, Pocobelli D, Venuti A (1993) Delayed hypersensitivity to stepronin: a case report. Contact Dermatitis 29:166
126. Romano A, Pietrantonio F, di Fonso M, Venuti A, Fabrizi G (1995) Contact allergy to tiopronin: a case report. Contact Dermatitis 33:269
127. Bruynzeel I, Hebeda CL, Folkers E, Bruynzeel DP (1995) Cutaneous hypersensitivity reactions to vitamin K: 2 case reports and a review of the literature. Contact Dermatitis 32:78–82
128. Galindo PA, Garrido IA, Gómez E, Borja J, Feo F, Encinas C, García R (1998) Zinc acexamate allergy. Contact Dermatitis 38:301–302
129. Montoro J, Basomba A (1997) Fixed drug eruption due to acyclovir. Contact Dermatitis 36:225
130. Lee AY (1998) Topical provocation in 31 cases of fixed drug eruption: change of causative drugs in 10 years. Contact Dermatitis 38:258–260
131. Sugiura M, Hayakawa R, Osada T (1998) Fixed drug eruption due to amlexanox. Contact Dermatitis 38:65–67
132. Gonzales Delgado P, Florido Lopez F, Saenz de San Pedro B (1995) Fixed drug eruption due to citiolone. Contact Dermatitis 33:352
133. Rodriguez-Morales A, Alonso Llamazares A, Palacios Benito R, Martinez Cocera C (2001) Fixed drug eruption from quinolones with a positive lesional patch test to ciprofloxacin. Contact Dermatitis 44:255
134. Rosina P, Chieregato C, Schena D (1998) Fixed drug eruption from clarithromycin. Contact Dermatitis 38:105
135. Kawada A, Hiruma M, Noguchi H, Akagi A, Ishibashi A, Marshall I (1996) Fixed drug eruption induced by ethenzamide. Contact Dermatitis 34:369–370
136. Gastaminez G, Anda M, Audicana MT, Fernandez E, Munoz D (2001) Fixed-drug eruption due to metronidazole with positive topical provocation. Contact Dermatitis 44:36
137. Cordeiro MR, Gonçalo M, Fernandes B, Oliveira HS, Figueiredo A (2000) Positive lesional patch tests in fixed drug eruptions from nimesulide. Contact Dermatitis 43:307
138. Kawada A, Hiruma M, Noguchi H, Banba K, Ishibashi A, Banba H, Marshall J (1996) Fixed drug eruption induced by ofloxacin. Contact Dermatitis 34:427
139. Oliveira HS, Gonçalo M, Reis JP, Figueiredo A (1999) Fixed drug eruption to piroxicam. Positive patch tests with cross-sensitivity to tenoxicam. J Dermatol Treatment 10:209–212
140. Kawada A, Kobayashi T, Noguchi H, Hiruma M, Ishibashi A, Marshall 1 (1996) Fixed drug eruption induced by sulfasalazine. Contact Dermatitis 34:155–156
141. van Ketel WG (1988) Systemic contact-type dermatitis by derivatives of adamantane? Derm Beruf Umwelt 36:23–24
142. van den Berg WHHW, van Ketel WG (1983) Contactallergie voor ethyleendiamine. Ned Tijdschr Geneeskd 127:1801–1802
143. Maibach HI (1987) Oral substitution in patients sensitized by transdermal clonidine treatment. Contact Dermatitis 16:1–8
144. Stingeni L, Caraffini S, Assolve D, Lapomarda V, Lisi P (1996) Erythema-multiforme-like contact dermatitis from budesonide. Contact Dermatitis 34:154–155
145. Isaksson M, Persson L-M (1998) Contact allergy to hydrocortisone and systemic contact dermatitis from prednisolone with tolerance of betamethasone. Am J Contact Dermatitis 9:136–138
146. McKenna DB, Murphy GM (1998) Contact allergy to topical corticosteroids and systemic allergy to prednisolone. Contact Dermatitis 38:121–122
147. Valsecchi R, Reseghetti P, Leghissa P, Cologni L, Cortinovis R (1998) Erythema-multiforme-like lesions from triamcinolone acetonide. Contact Dermatitis 38:362–363
148. Whitmore SE (1995) Delayed systemic allergic reactions to corticosteroids. Contact Dermatitis 32:193–198
149. Ash S, Scheman AJ (1997) Systemic contact dermatitis to hydroxyzine. Am J Contact Dermatitis 8:2–5
150. Nadal C, Pujol RM, Randazzo E, Alomar A (1996) Systemic contact dermatitis from 5-fluorouracil. Contact Dermatitis 35:124–125
151. Grob JJ, Mege JL, Follana J, Legre R, Andrac L, Bonerandi JJ (1990) Skin necrosis after injection of aminosides. Dermatologica 180:258–262
152. Möller H, Ohlsson K, Linder C, Björkner B, Bruze M (1998) Cytokines and acute phase reactants during flare-up of contact allergy to gold. Am J Contact Dermat 9:15–22
153. Fleming C, Porter D, MacKie R (1998) Absence of gold sodium thiosulfate contact hypersensitivity in rheumatoid arthritis. Contact Dermatitis 38:55–56

24

154. Krasovec M, Kämmerer R, Spertini F, Frenk E (1995) Contact dermatitis from heparin gel following sensitization by subcutaneous heparin administration. Contact Dermatitis 33:135–136

155. Silvestre JF, Alfonso R, Moragón M, Ramón R, Botella R (1997) Systemic contact dermatitis due to norfloxacin with a positive patch test to quinoline mix. Contact Dermatitis 39:83

156. Ekelund A-G, Möller H (1969) Oral provocation in eczematous contact allergy to neomycin and hydroxy-quinolines. Arch Derm Venereol (Stockh) 49:422–426

157. Michel M, Dompmartin A, Louvet S, Szczurko C, Castel B, Leroy D (1997) Skin reactions to hydroxyzine. Contact Dermatitis 36:147–149

158. Fernández L, Maquiera E, Rodríguez F, Picans I, Duque S (1996) Systemic contact dermatitis from miconazole. Contact Dermatitis 34:217

159. Van Dijke CPH, Veerman FR, Haverkamp HCH (1983) Anaphylactic reactions to ketoconazole. Br Med J 287:1673

160. Curley RK, Macfarlane AW, Kong CM (1986) Contact sensitivity to the amide anesthetics lidocaine, prilocaine, and mepivacaine. Case report and review of the literature. Arch Dermatol 122:924–926

161. Downs AMR, Lear JT, Wallington TB, Sanson JE (1998) Contact sensitivity and systemic reaction to pseudoephedrine and lignocaine. Contact Dermatitis 39:33

162. Marques C, Faria E, Machado A, Gonçalo M, Gonçalo S (1995) Allergic contact dermatitis and systemic contact dermatitis from cinchocaine. Contact Dermatitis 33:443

163. Christensen OB (1990) Two cases of delayed hypersensitivity to mitomycin C following intravesicular chemotherapy of superficial bladder cancer. Contact Dermatitis 23:263

164. de Groot AC, Conemans JM (1991) Systemic allergic contact dermatitis from intravesical instillation of the antitumor antibiotic mitomycin C. Contact Dermatitis 24:201–209

165. Echechipía S, Alvarez MJ, García BE, Olaguíbel JM, Rodriguez A, Lizaso MT, Acero S, Tabar AI (1995) Generalized dermatitis due to mitomycin C patch test. Contact Dermatitis 33:432

166. Barbaud A, Tréchot P, Aublet-Cuvelier A, Reichert-Penetrat S, Schmutz J-L (1998) Bufexamac and diclofenac: frequency of contact sensitization and absence of cross-reactions. Contact Dermatitis 39:272–273

167. Dooms-Goossens A, Dooms M, van Lint L, Degreef H (1979) Skin sensitizing properties of arylalcanoic acids and their analogues. Contact Dermatitis 5:324–328

168. Kerre S, Busschots A, Dooms-Goossens A (1995) Erythema-multiforme-like contact dermatitis due to phenylbutazone. Contact Dermatitis 33:213–214

169. Walchner M, Rueff F, Przybilla B (1997) Delayed-type hypersensitivity to mofebutazone underlying a severe drug reaction. Contact Dermatitis 36:54–55

170. Lechner T, Grytzmann B, Bäurle G (1987) Hämatogenes allergisches Kontaktekzem nach oraler Gabe von Nystatin. (Hematogenous allergic contact dermatitis after oral administration of nystatin) Mykosen 30:143–146

171. Hemmer W, Bracun R, Wolf-Abdolvahab S, Focke M, Götz M, Jarisch R (1997) Maintenance of hand eczema by oral pantothenic acid in a patient sensitized to dexpanthenol. Contact Dermatitis 37:51

172. Giordano-Labadie F, Pech-Ormieres C, Bazex J (1996) Systemic contact dermatitis from sorbic acid. Contact Dermatitis 34:61–62

173. Michel M, Dompmartin A, Szczurko C, Castel B, Moreau A, Leroy D (1996) Eczematous-like drug eruption induced by synergistins. Contact Dermatitis 34:86–87

174. Zenerola P, Gimma A, Lomuto M (1995) Systemic contact dermatitis from thimerosal. Contact Dermatitis 32:107–108

175. Fisher AA (1966) Systemic eczematous "contact-type" dermatitis medicamentosa. Ann Allergy 24:406–420

176. Hom HM, Humphreys F, Aldridge RD (1998) Contact dermatitis and prolonged photosensitivity induced by ketoprofen and associated with sensitivity to benzophenone-3. Contact Dermatitis 38:353–354

Chapter 25

Allergens Exposure Assessment

25

Birgitta Gruvberger, Magnus Bruze, Sigfrid Fregert, Carola Lidén

Contents

25.1 Spot Tests and Chemical Analyses

Birgitta Gruvberger, Magnus Bruze, Sigfrid Fregert

25.1.1 Introduction

Many allergens are widely used in both environmental and occupational products. In many cases, it is difficult to know all the ingredients of a product, since most products are not sufficiently labeled. To diagnose and prevent allergic contact dermatitis, the demonstration of allergens in products from the patient's environment is important. Chemical analysis of a product can make it possible to demonstrate the presence or absence of known allergens. Simple spot tests or documented analytical methods, such as thin-layer chromatography (TLC), high-performance liquid chromatography (HPLC), gas chromatography (GC), atomic absorption spectrophotometry (AAS), and inductively coupled plasma–mass spectrometry (ICP–MS) can be used. Moreover, with chemical methods, the purity of a substance can be checked and new allergens can be isolated and identified. Advanced methods such as mass spectrometry (MS), nuclear magnetic resonance spectroscopy (NMR), and infrared spectrophotometry (IR) are often required to identify isolated allergens.

In this chapter, some principal chemical methods and some examples of chemical methods for dermatological applications are described.

25.1.2 pH Measurement

Acidic and, particularly, alkaline products play a significant role in the development of irritant contact dermatitis and in chemical skin burns [1]. It is important to determine the degree of acidity or alkalinity in a product suspected of causing skin problems in order to avoid false-positive diagnoses of allergic contact dermatitis.

25

pH determinations are relevant only in water-based products/solutions. A universal pH paper is usually satisfactory for clinical work. A few drops of the solution/emulsion to be investigated are applied on the pH paper. The resulting color is compared with the color scale on the package of the pH paper. pH paper moistened with water can be applied to solid subjects to demonstrate residual acidic or alkaline solution on the object. For accurate determination of the pH in a solution, a pH meter is necessary.

25.1.3 Spot Tests

Spot tests can be used to demonstrate both inorganic and organic compounds [2, 3]. A specific reagent may react with a specific substance to give a specific color and, thus, indicate the occurrence of the specific substance. However, other substances can disturb the chemical reaction and the specific color can be difficult to identify. A discolored sample can contain the investigated substance. To confirm its presence and quantify the substance, more sophisticated methods are required.

To demonstrate nickel ions released from metal objects, a spot test is commonly used.

25.1.4 Thin-Layer Chromatography

Chromatography is a general term applied to a variety of separation techniques based upon the sample partitioning between a moving phase, which can be a gas or a liquid, and a stationary phase, which may be either liquid or solid.

In thin-layer chromatography (TLC), the stationary phase consists of an inert absorbent, e.g., silica gel. The stationary phase covers the surface of a glass plate. The moving phase constitutes an eluting solvent. The sample to be analyzed is dissolved in a low-boiling solvent and a small amount is applied near the bottom of the plate. The plate is placed in a closed vessel containing a small amount of the eluting solvent. The eluent is drawn up to the top of the plate owing to the capillary forces. Substances with high affinity to the stationary phase will move slower than substances with a low affinity. When the eluent has almost reached the top of the plate, the plate is removed from the glass vessel and dried. To detect the spots on the plate, they must be made visible. UV-absorbing substances can be detected by irradiating the plate with a UV lamp. Some substances may react with various reagents applied to the plates, giving visible compounds. The R_F value for a substance is the ratio between the distance traveled by the substance and the distance traveled by the eluent. To investigate whether a sample contains a specific substance (reference), the reference is applied beside the sample on the plate. If the sample contains a substance with the same R_F value as the reference, it will indicate that the substance and the reference may be identical. However, more chromatographic methods are required to confirm this.

25.1.5 Gas Chromatography

A gas chromatograph consists of an injector, a column, and a detector. In gas chromatography (GC), the mobile phase constitutes a carrier gas, e.g., nitrogen or helium, and the stationary phase is a nonvolatile liquid on a solid support or on the walls of the column. The most common supports are inert porous materials. The sample, dissolved in an organic solvent, is injected into the column and heated. The components evaporate and the gas carries the components through the column. Depending on the molecular weight of the components, and the polar interactions between them and the stationary phase, they will be retarded. Detectors with different sensitivity for specific compounds are available on the market. A flame ionization detector (FID) is a common device that detects most organic components passing through the column. The organic compounds are readily pyrolyzed when introduced into a hydrogen–air flame, and ions are produced in the process. The signals are recorded as peaks on a chromatogram.

To identify substances in a sample, it is often necessary to use several columns with different stationary phases that give the substances different retention times. GC combined with a mass spectrometer often makes it possible to identify unknown substances.

25.1.6 High-Performance Liquid Chromatography

In high-performance liquid chromatography (HPLC), the eluent is pumped through the column under high pressure in a closed system. In an isocratic system, the composition of the mobile phase is the same throughout the analysis. In a gradient system, at least two pumps are used, delivering varying amounts of different eluents. In this manner, the composition of the mobile phase can be changed during the analysis. The sample, dissolved in the mobile phase, is injected into the HPLC setup. The components of the sample pass through the column to the detector at different speeds. The most common detector is a UV detector. A refractive index (RI) detector can be used to detect components that do not absorb UV radiation. In some cases, derivatization can be used by adding a UV-absorbing substance, which will react with the component, to give a new component detectable by UV. The signals from the detector are registered as a chromatogram. A variety of columns of both nonpolar and polar types are available on the market. Columns containing polar groups are used in straight-phase HPLC and columns with nonpolar groups are used in reversed-phase HPLC.

The HPLC technique can be employed for both analytical and preparative purposes. In preparative HPLC, larger amounts of a sample can be injected, and fractions containing various components can be separated and collected for further analyses and/or patch testing.

25.1.7 Atomic Absorption Spectrophotometry

Atomic absorption spectrophotometry (AAS) is one of the most common methods to identify and quantify small amounts of metals in both organic and inorganic materials. The method relies on the absorption of light by atoms. The atoms can absorb light, but only at certain wavelengths corresponding to the energy requirements of the particular atoms. The successful operation of an atomic absorption spectrophotometer lies in generating a supply of free, uncombined atoms in the ground state and exposing this atom population to light at the characteristic absorption wavelength. The atomization process consists of heating a solution to a temperature that is sufficient to dissociate the compound. The thermal energy required can be supplied by a flame (air–acetylene) or by a flameless technique (graphite furnace). For quantitative measurements, the sample must be compared with standard solutions of known concentrations.

25.1.8 UV–Vis Spectrophotometry

With an ultraviolet–visible (UV–Vis) spectrophotometer, substances that absorb light in the ultraviolet and visible regions can be detected. The substance is dissolved in a solvent with a low UV absorption and is placed in the light beam in the spectrophotometer. The absorbance is plotted as a function of the wavelengths. An absorption curve often includes both maximum/maxima and minimum/minima. Many substances have characteristic absorption curves in the UV–Vis region, and this information can be useful to identify substances.

A UV detector is the most commonly used in HPLC.

25.1.9 Infrared Spectrophotometry

Infrared (IR) spectrophotometry is used especially to identify organic substances. Nearly all molecules containing covalent bonds will show some degree of selective absorption in the (IR) region. Various functional groups in a molecule give specific patterns of peaks in an IR spectrum, which can be used to identify, for example, amino groups, carbonyl groups, and nitro groups. Transparent samples, such as plastic films, can be analyzed without processing. Other samples can be mixed with potassium bromide and pressed into a tablet. The IR spectra can be compared with the reference spectra.

25.1.10 Mass Spectrometry

Mass spectrometry (MS) is used especially to determine the molecular weights and structures of organic substances. Pure substances can be analyzed directly, while components in products have to be separated before analysis. GC is often combined with MS (GC–MS). The gas flow containing separated components is introduced directly into the mass spectrometer. In MS, ions are generated by collision of rapidly moving electrons with the molecules of the gas. The ions are separated in an electromagnetic field according to their mass-to-charge ratio. The result of the analysis is demonstrated in a mass spectrum, showing the relative intensities of the ions formed. Fragmentation of a substance into smaller ions is very common. This fragmentation pattern is unique for each compound and gives valuable information about its chemical structure.

25.1.11 Inductively Coupled Plasma–Mass Spectrometry

Inductively coupled plasma–mass spectrometry (ICP–MS) is a technique where the inductively couple plasma (ICP) is used as the ion source for a mass spectrometry (MS). The ions are separated according to their mass and charge, and are measured individually. The major attractiveness of ICP–MS is its exceptional sensitivity combined with high analysis speed. For most elements, ICP–MS offers detection limits which are better than those of graphite furnace AAS.

25

25.1.12 Nuclear Magnetic Resonance Spectroscopy

Using nuclear magnetic resonance spectroscopy (NMR) together with MS and/or IR analysis, it is often possible to elucidate the molecular structures of unknown substances.

The NMR technique is based on the absorption of energy by the sample to be analyzed. The sample is placed in a strong magnetic field that will affect atoms within the sample. The nucleus can absorb energy from an additionally applied radio pulse when the frequency of the pulse matches that of the oscillating nucleus. The absorption is recorded by the instrumentation.

The atom most commonly studied is hydrogen (^{1}H-NMR). An NMR spectrum consists of absorption peaks from which information on functional groups and the relative number of hydrogen atoms can be retrieved. Other atoms that can be studied are carbon 13, fluorine 19, and phosphorus 31.

Many reports have been published concerning chemical methods for detecting various allergens. In Table 1.1, the methods applying to allergens in the European standard test series are shown. The chemical methods for identifying and/or quantifying miscellaneous sensitizers are shown in Table 1.2.

Table 1.1. Literature references of chemical methods for allergens in the European standard series. (*AAS* Atomic absorption spectrophotometry, *GC* gas chromatography, *HPLC* high-performance liquid chromatography, *ICP–MS* inductively coupled plasma––mass spectrometry, *TLC* Thin-layer chromatograph, *UV–Vis* ultraviolet–visible spectrophotometry)

Allergen	Spot test	TLC	HPLC	GC	AAS/ICP–MS	UV–Vis
Potassium dichromate					[4–14]	[11, 15]
4-phenylenediamine base			[16]			
Thiuram mix			[17]	[18]		
Neomycin sulfate						
Cobalt chloride					[6, 8, 12–14, 19]	
Benzocaine		[20–22]	[21, 22]			
Nickel sulfate	[23–26]				[13, 14, 25, 27–31]	
Quinoline mix						
Colophony			[32–34, 38]	[32, 34–37]		
Parabens			[39–41]			
N-Isopropyl-N-phenyl-4-phenylenediamine			[42]	[42]		
Wool wax alcohols						
Mercapto mix		[44]	[43–45]	[44, 45]		
Epoxy resin		[46–48]	[47–50]			
Balsam of Peru			[51]			
4-*tert*-Butylphenol formaldehyde resin			[45, 52]			
Mercaptobenzothiazole		[44, 45]	[44, 45]	[44, 45]		
Formaldehyde	[53–58]		[56, 59–63]			[55]
Fragrance mix				[64, 65]		
Sesquiterpene lactone mix						
Quaternium 15			[66] and Kreilgård, personal communication 1996			
Primin						
Methylchloroisothiazolinone/methylisothiazolinone			[67, 68]			
Budesonide			[69]			
Tixocortol-21-pivalate			[69]			
Methyldibromo glutaronitrile			[66, 70, 71]			

Table 1.2. Literature references of chemical methods for miscellaneous sensitizers. (*AAS*, atomic absorption spectrophotometry, *GC* gas chromatography, *HPLC* high-performance liquid chromatography, *TLC* Thin-layer chromatography, *UV–Vis* ultraviolet–visible spectrophotometry)

Sensitizer	Spot test	TLC	HPLC	GC	AAS	UV–Vis
Various acrylates				[72]		
Allyl glycidyl ether			[73]			
p-aminobenzoic acid		[20, 21]	[21, 22]			
Amyl p-dimethylaminobenzoate			[21, 22]			
Atranorin	[74]	[74]				
Bithionol		[20]				
2-bromo-2-nitropropane-1,3-diol			[66, 75, 76]			
Buclosamide		[20]				
Cadmium chloride					[77]	
Chlorhexidine acetate		[20]				
Chlorhexidine gluconate		[20]				
Chlorpromazine hydrochloride		[20]				
Diazolidinyl urea			[66, 78]			
Dichlorophene		[20]				
Diethylthiourea		[79]	[79]			
Diglycidylether of bisphenol F			[80]			
Dimethyloldimethylhydantoin			[66, 81]			
Diphenhydramine chloride		[20]				
Diphenylmethane-4,4'-diisocyanate			[82]			
Diphenylthiourea		[83]	[83, 84]			
Ethyl 4-bis(hydroxypropyl)aminobenzoate		[21]	[21, 22]			
Ethylene thiourea		[83, 85]	[85]			
2-ethylhexyl p-dimethylaminobenzoate		[21]	[21, 22]			
Fentichlor		[20]				
Various fragrances				[86–88]		
Glyceryl p-aminobenzoate		[21]	[21, 22]			
Hexachlorophene		[20]				
Hydrocortisone-17-butyrate			[69]			
Imidazolidinyl urea			[41, 66]			
d-limonene				[89, 90]		
6-Methylcoumarin		[20]				
Moskene		[91]	[91]			
Musk ambrette		[91]	[91, 92]			
Musk ketone		[91]	[91]			
Musk tibetine		[91]	[91]			
Musk xylene		[91]	[91]			
Phenol formaldehyde resin			[93]			
Phenylisothiocyanate			[84]			
Promethazine hydrochloride		[20]				
Tetrachlorosalicylanilide		[20]				
Thiourea		[20]				
Tinuvin P			[94–96]	[94]		
Tribromosalicylanilide		[20]				
Trichlorocarbanilide		[20]				
Triclosan		[20]				
Zinc dibutyldithiocarbamate		[97]	[97]			
Zinc dimethyldithiocarbamate		[97]	[97]			
Zinc ethylphenyldithiocarbamate		[97]	[97]			

25

25.1.13 Common Chemical Methods Used by Dermatologists

25.1.13.1 Detection of Nickel Ions Released from Metal Objects

Nickel is most commonly detected by using the dimethylglyoxime test [23]. A few drops each of dimethylglyoxime 1% in ethanol and ammonia 10% in water are applied to a cotton-tipped applicator, which is rubbed against the metal object to be investigated. Dimethylglyoxime reacts with nickel ions in the presence of ammonia, giving a pink–red salt (Fig. 1.1). Coins known to contain nickel can be used to test the reagent and to observe the pink–red color.

The sensitivity of the test can be enhanced by pretreatment of the surface of the object with a solution of artificial sweat and by heating. This test is proposed by the European Committee for Standardization [24].

The method is very simple and can be used, for example, by dermatologists and nickel-allergic individuals to detect nickel release from various metal objects.

25.1.13.2 Detection of Hexavalent Chromium (Chromate)

The chromium spot test is valid only for hexavalent chromium. *Sym*-diphenylcarbazide reacts with chromate and dichromate ions in the presence of sulfuric acid, giving a red–violet color. *Reagents*: I. *Sym*-diphenylcarbazide 1% w/v in ethanol (must be prepared immediately before the investigation). II. Sulfuric acid 1 mol/l. *Reference*: Solutions of potassium chromate 2.0, 1.0, 0.5, and 0.25 µg chromate/ml.

Chromate on the Surface of a Solid Object

A few drops each of reagents I and II are applied to a cotton swab. The cotton swab is, thereafter, rubbed against the surface of the object for 1 min. If chromate is present, a red–violet color appears.

Chromate in Solutions

To a sample of approximately 10 ml, a few drops each of reagents I and II are added. If chromate is present, a red–violet color appears (Fig. 1.2).

Chromate in Powders Insoluble in Water (e.g., Cement)

Five grams of cement is mixed with 10 ml of water for some minutes. The mixture is then filtered and the filtrate is handled as for chromate in solutions. Iron ions can interfere with the reagent and give discolored solutions.

25.1.13.3 Detection of Epoxy Resin Based on Bisphenol A

The most common epoxy resin of the bisphenol A type is diglycidyl ether of bisphenol A resin (DGEBA-R). This epoxy resin contains oligomers of various molecular weights (e.g., 340, 624, 908, 1,024). Since DGEBA with a molecular weight of 340 is a strong sensitizer, a chemical method to detect the sensitizer in various types of products is important. There is a simple TLC method to demonstrate the oligomers [46].

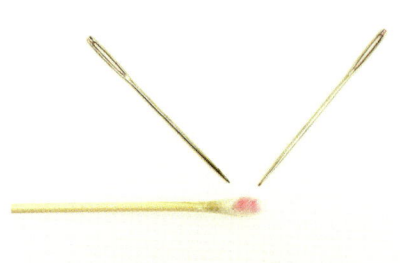

Fig. 1.1. Detection of nickel ions released from sewing needles. A few drops each of dimethylglyoxime 1% in ethanol and ammonia 10% in water were applied to the cotton-tipped applicator, which was rubbed against the needles. The pink–red color of the cotton indicates the presence of nickel ions

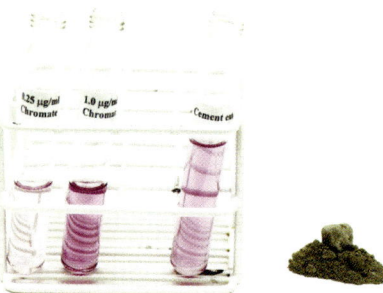
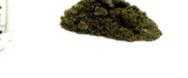

Fig. 1.2. Detection of chromate in cement. A few drops of the reagents were added to the reference solutions and to the cement extract. The red–violet color of the extract indicates the presence of chromate in the investigated cement

Demonstration of epoxy resin of bisphenol A type (Fig. 1.3a) requires the following:

- Materials: TLC plates (silica gel 60, F 254). Eluent: chloroform/acetonitrile 90/10 (v/v). Spray reagents: sulfuric acid 1 mol/l. Anisaldehyde in methanol 2.5% (v/v). Standard: 1% (w/v) epoxy resin of bisphenol A type in acetone containing low-mol.-wt. (340, 624, 908, etc.) oligomers. Extraction solution: acetone/methanol (90/10 v/v) or ethanol.
- Procedure: The sample to be investigated is dissolved in the extraction solution. Solid samples are extracted at room temperature or in an ultrasonic bath. The required extraction time is dependent on the amount of low-molecular epoxy resin in the sample. The extract is evaporated to a volume of a few milliliters before being applied to the plate. The standard solution, 2–5 µl (20–50 µg), is deposited with a capillary pipette on a TLC plate. A similar volume of the sample is applied beside the standard. Since the concentration of the epoxy resin in the sample is often unknown, it is advisable to apply double and triple amounts of the sample on the same plate. The plate is eluted in a tank lined with filter paper saturated with the eluent. The plate is air-dried and sprayed with sulfuric acid until it is just moist, and then sprayed lightly with anisaldehyde. After being heated in an oven at 100°C for 10 min, the oligomers are visible as violet spots with oligomer 340 at the top, followed by 624 (Fig. 1.3b). If the sample contains unhardened low-molecular epoxy resin, the oligomers 340, 624, and 908 can be identified with the same R_F values as the oligomers in the standard.

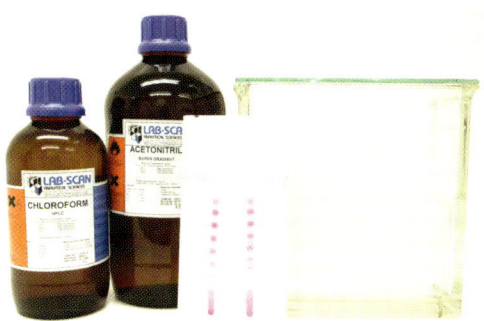

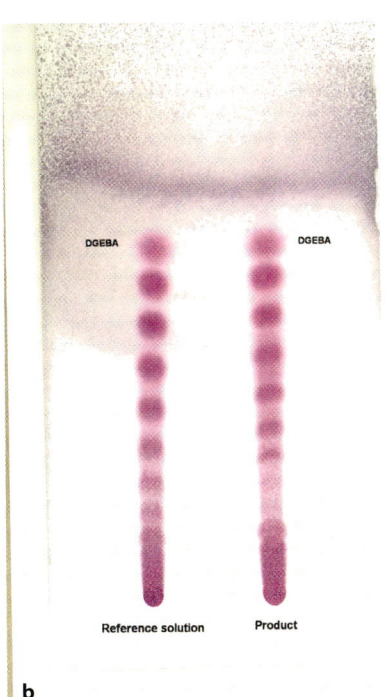

Fig. 1.3a, b. TLC analysis of epoxy resin based on bisphenol A. a Small amounts of the reference solution and the extract of the product to be investigated were applied on the plate before eluting in a tank. After spraying with the reagents and heating in an oven, the oligomers are visible as violet spots. b Product containing diglycidyl ether of bisphenol A (DGEBA)

Fillers and pigments in the sample can disturb the analysis. In such cases, special treatment of the sample may be required.

25.1.13.4 Detection of Formaldehyde

Formaldehyde is a gas that dissolves easily in water-based products. Small amounts may be released from many preservatives, and many water-based products may, thus, contain formaldehyde. Two simple methods are frequently used to identify formaldehyde in various types of products.

Chromotropic Acid Method

- **Reagent.** Forty milligrams of chromotropic acid is dissolved in 10 ml of concentrated sulfuric acid (freshly prepared). Standard solutions: a concentrated water solution of formaldehyde (35%) is diluted to 100 µg/ml and refrigerated (stock solution). Standard solutions containing 2.5, 10, 20, and 40 µg formaldehyde/ml are prepared. The standard solutions should be refrigerated and freshly prepared every week.

25

Approximately 0.5 g of the sample is placed in a 25-ml glass jar with a ground-glass stopper. Then 1 ml of each standard solution and 1 ml water (blank) is placed in separate glass jars. Then, 0.5 ml of the reagent is added to small glass tubes and then placed individually in the glass jars containing the sample, the standards, and the blank, respectively. The jars are kept in the dark and observed after 1 and 2 days. A violet reagent indicates the presence of formaldehyde (Fig. 1.4).

This method is based on a chemical reaction of chromotropic acid and free formaldehyde evaporated from the sample/standards [54]. However, other aldehydes and ketones can also react with chromotropic acid, giving colors that can interfere with the violet reagent.

With the chromotropic acid method, a rough estimation of the concentration of formaldehyde can be obtained by comparing the intensity of the sample color with those of the standards.

Acetylacetone Method

■ **Reagent.** Fifteen g ammonium acetate, 0.2 ml acetylacetone, and 0.3 ml glacial acetic acid are dissolved in water to 100 ml. The solution should be refrigerated and freshly prepared every week.

■ **Standard Solutions.** From the stock solution of formaldehyde (100 µg/ml), standards containing 2.5, 10, 20, and 40 µg formaldehyde/ml are prepared. The standard solutions should be refrigerated and freshly prepared every week.

Approximately 0.5 g of the sample is placed in a glass jar with a ground-glass stopper. Ointments and other fat products should be emulsified with a few drops of formaldehyde-free emulsifier, such as Triton X-100. One ml of each standard solution and 1 ml water (blank) is added to separate glass jars. To each glass jar, 2.5 ml of the reagent solution is added and the jar is then shaken. The jars are heated at 60°C for 10 min. A yellow mixture indicates the presence of formaldehyde. If the concentration of formaldehyde is high, the yellow will already appear before heating. The intensity of the yellow can be compared with that of the standards to estimate the content of formaldehyde in the sample.

If the sample to be analyzed is colored, an extraction procedure with 1-butanol can be performed, as described by Fregert et al. [55]. Quantification of the content can be performed using a UV–Vis spectrophotometer [55].

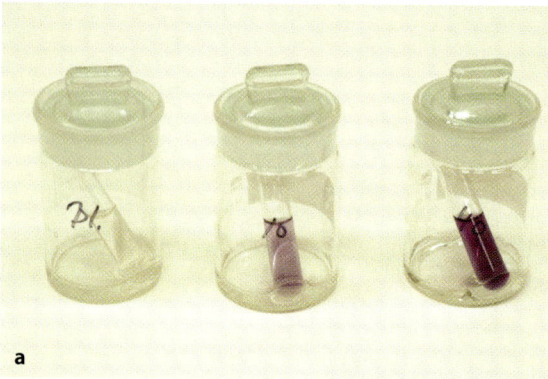

a

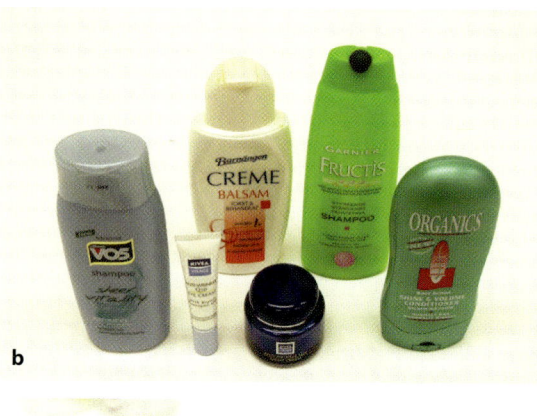

b

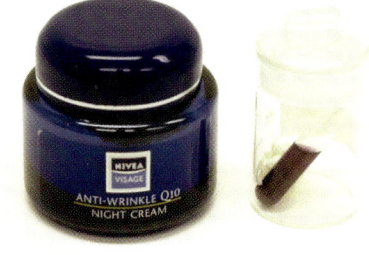

c

Fig. 1.4a–c. Detection of formaldehyde with the chromotropic acid method. Violet color of the reagent indicates the presence of formaldehyde. **a** One blank and two standard solutions of formaldehyde. **b** Products to be analyzed. **c** A leave-on product containing formaldehyde

25.1.14 Summary

To diagnose and prevent allergic contact dermatitis, it is important to demonstrate allergens in products from the patient's environment. With various chemical methods, it is possible to demonstrate the presence or absence of known allergens in products and to isolate and identify new allergens. However, chemical methods have limitations, and false-positive as well as false-negative results can be obtained, especially when simple methods are used.

References

1. Bruze M, Fregert S, Gruvberger B (2000) Chemical skin burns. In: Menné T, Maibach HI (eds) Hand eczema, 2nd edn. CRC, Boca Raton, Fla., pp 117–127
2. Feigl F, Anger V (1972) Spot tests in inorganic analysis, 6th edn. Elsevier, Amsterdam, The Netherlands
3. Feigl F, Anger V (1966) Spot tests in organic analysis, 7th edn. Elsevier, Amsterdam, The Netherlands
4. Adams RM, Fregert S, Gruvberger B, Maibach HI (1976) Water solubility of zinc chromate primer paints used as antirust agents. Contact Dermatitis 6:357–358
5. Bruze M, Gruvberger B, Hradil E (1990) Chromate sensitization and elicitation from cement with iron sulfate. Acta Derm Venereol (Stockh) 70:160–162
6. Fregert S, Gruvberger B (1972) Chemical properties of cement. Berufsdermatosen 20:238–248
7. Fregert S, Gruvberger B (1973) Factors decreasing the content of water-soluble chromate in cement. Acta Derm Venereol (Stockh) 53:267–270
8. Fregert S, Gruvberger B, Heijer A (1972) Sensitization to chromium and cobalt in processing of sulphate pulp. Acta Derm Venereol (Stockh) 52:221–224
9. Ingber A, Gammelgaard B, David M (1998) Detergents and bleaches are sources of chromium contact dermatitis in Israel. Contact Dermatitis 38:101–104
10. Lachapelle JM, Lauwerys R, Tennstedt D, Andanson J, Benezra C, Chabeau G, Ducombs G, Foussereau J, Lacroix M, Martin P (1980) Eau de Javel and prevention of chromate allergy in France. Contact Dermatitis 6:107–110
11. Nygren O, Wahlberg JE (1998) Speciation of chromium in tanned leather gloves and relapse of chromium allergy from tanned leather samples. Analyst 123:935–937
12. Spruit D, Malten KE (1975) Occupational cobalt and chromium dermatitis in an offset printing factory. Dermatologica 151:34–42
13. Tandon R, Aarts B (1993) Chromium, nickel and cobalt contents of some Australian cements. Contact Dermatitis 28:201–205
14. Wahlberg JE, Lindstedt G, Einarsson Ö (1977) Chromium, cobalt and nickel in Swedish cement, detergents, mould and cutting oils. Berufsdermatosen 25:220–228
15. Wass U, Wahlberg JE (1991) Chromated steel and contact allergy. Recommendation concerning a "threshold limit value" for the release of hexavalent chromium. Contact Dermatitis 24:114–118
16. Lind M-L, Boman A, Surakka J, Sollenberg J, Meding B (2004) A method for assessing occupational dermal exposure to permanent hair dyes. Ann Occup Hyg 48:533–539
17. Bergendorff O, Hansson C (2001) Stability of thiuram disulfides in patch test preparations and formation of asymmetric disulfides. Contact Dermatitis 45:151–157
18. Knudsen BB, Larsen E, Egsgaard H, Menné T (1993) Release of thiurams and carbamates from rubber gloves. Contact Dermatitis 28.63–69
19. Fregert S, Gruvberger B (1978) Solubility of cobalt in cement. Contact Dermatitis 4:14–18
20. Bruze M, Fregert S (1983) Studies on purity and stability of photopatch test substances. Contact Dermatitis 9:33–39
21. Bruze M, Fregert S, Gruvberger B (1984) Occurrence of para-aminobenzoic acid and benzocaine as contaminants in sunscreen agents of para-aminobenzoic acid type. Photodermatology 1:277–285
22. Bruze M, Gruvberger B, Thulin I (1990) PABA, benzocaine, and other PABA esters in sunscreens and after-sun products. Photodermatol Photoimmunol Photomed 7:106–108
23. Rietschel RL, Fowler JF Jr (eds) (1995) Fisher's contact dermatitis, 4th edn. Williams and Wilkins, Baltimore, Maryland, pp 857–857
24. European Committee for Standardisation (CEN) (2002) Screening tests for nickel release from alloys and coatings in items that come into direct and prolonged contact with the skin. CR 12471
25. Lidén C, Röndell E, Skare L, Nalbanti A (1998) Nickel release from tools on the Swedish market. Contact Dermatitis 39:127–131
26. Lidén C, Johnsson S (2001) Nickel on the Swedish market before the Nickel Directive. Contact Dermatitis 44:7–12
27. European Committee for Standardization (CEN) (1998) Reference test method for release of nickel from products intended to come into direct and prolonged contact with the skin. EN 1811
28. Andersen KE, Nielsen GD, Flyvholm M-A, Fregert S, Gruvberger B (1983) Nickel in tap water. Contact Dermatitis 9:140–143
29. Bang Pedersen N, Fregert S, Brodelius P, Gruvberger B (1974) Release of nickel from silver coins. Acta Derm Venereol (Stockh) 54:231–234
30. Fischer T, Fregert S, Gruvberger B, Rystedt I (1984) Contact sensitivity to nickel in white gold. Contact Dermatitis 10:23–24
31. Fischer T, Fregert S, Gruvberger B, Rystedt I (1984) Nickel release from ear piercing kits and earrings. Contact Dermatitis 10:39–41
32. Bergh M, Menné T, Karlberg A-T (1994) Colophony in paper-based surgical clothing. Contact Dermatitis 31:332–333
33. Ehrin E, Karlberg A-T (1990) Detection of rosin (colophony) components in technical products using an HPLC technique. Contact Dermatitis 23:359–366
34. Karlberg A-T, Gäfvert E, Meding B, Stenberg B (1996) Airborne contact dermatitis from unexpected exposure to rosin (colophony). Rosin sources revealed with chemical analyses. Contact Dermatitis 35:272–278
35. Karlberg A-T, Magnusson K (1996) Rosin components identified in diapers. Contact Dermatitis 34:176–180
36. Karlberg A-T, Gäfvert E, Lidén C (1995) Environmentally friendly paper may increase risk of hand eczema in rosin-sensitive persons. J Am Acad Dermatol 33:427–432
37. Meding B, Åhman M, Karlberg A-T (1996) Skin symptoms and contact allergy in woodwork teachers. Contact Dermatitis 34:185–190

25

38. Sadhra S, Gray CN, Foulds IS (1997) High-performance liquid chromatography of unmodified rosin and its applications in contact dermatology. J Chromatogr B Biomed Sci Appl 700:101–110

39. Rastogi SC, Schouten A, de Kruijf N, Weijland JW (1995) Contents of methyl-, ethyl-, propyl-, butyl-, and benzylparaben in cosmetic products. Contact Dermatitis 32:28–30

40. Seventh Commission Directive 96/45/EC of 2 July 1996 relating to methods of analysis necessary for checking the composition of cosmetics products

41. Sottofattori E, Anzaldi M, Balbi A, Tonello G (1998) Simultaneous HPLC determination of multiple components in a commercial cosmetic cream. J Pharm Biomed Anal 18:213–217

42. Kaniwa MA, Isama K, Nakamura A, Kantoh H, Itoh M, Ichikawa M, Hayakawa R (1994) Identification of causative chemicals of allergic contact dermatitis using a combination of patch testing in patients and chemical analysis. Application to cases from industrial rubber products. Contact Dermatitis 30:20–25

43. Hansson C, Bergendorff O, Ezzelarab M, Sterner O (1997) Extraction of mercaptobenzothiazole compounds from rubber products. Contact Dermatitis 36:195–200

44. Kaniwa M-A, Momma J, Ikarashi Y, Kojima S, Nakamura A, Nakaji Y, Kurokawa Y, Kantoh H, Itoh M (1992) A method for identifying causative chemicals of allergic contact dermatitis using a combination of chemical analysis and patch testing in patients and animal groups: application to a case of rubber boot dermatitis. Contact Dermatitis 27:166–173

45. Kaniwa M-A, Isama K, Nakamura A, Kantoh H, Itoh M, Miyoshi K, Saito S, Shono M (1994) Identification of causative chemicals of allergic contact dermatitis using a combination of patch testing in patients and chemical analysis. Application to cases from rubber footwear. Contact Dermatitis 30:26–34

46. Fregert S, Trulsson L (1978) Simple methods for demonstration of epoxy resins of bisphenol A type. Contact Dermatitis 4:69–72

47. Fregert S, Meding B, Trulsson L (1984) Demonstration of epoxy resin in stoma pouch plastic. Contact Dermatitis 10:106

48. Jenkinson HA, Burrows D (1987) Pitfalls in the demonstration of epoxy resins. Contact Dermatitis 16:226–227

49. Hansson C (1994) Determination of monomers in epoxy resin hardened at elevated temperature. Contact Dermatitis 31:333–334

50. Le Coz CJ, Coninx D, van Rengen A, Al Aboubi S, Ducombs G, Benz MH, Boursier S, Av Audran M, Verret JL, Erikstam U, Bruze M, Goossens A (1999) An epidemic of occupational contact dermatitis from an immersion oil for microscopy in laboratory personnel. Contact Dermatitis 40:77–83

51. Oxholm A, Heidenheim M, Larsen E, Batsberg W, Menné T (1990) Extraction and patch testing of methylcinnamate, a newly recognized fraction of balsam of Peru. Am J Contact Dermat 1:43–46

52. Avenel-Audran M, Goossens A, Zimerson E, Bruze M (2003) Contact dermatitis from electrocardiograph-monitoring electrodes: role of p-tert-butylphenol-formaldehyde resin. Contact Dermatitis 48:108–111

53. Blohm G (1959) Formaldehyde contact dermatitis. Acta Derm Venereol (Stockh) 39:450–453

54. Dahlquist I, Fregert S, Gruvberger B (1980) Reliability of the chromotropic acid method for qualitative formaldehyde determination. Contact Dermatitis 6:357–358

55. Fregert S, Dahlquist I, Gruvberger B (1984) A simple method for the detection of formaldehyde. Contact Dermatitis 10:132–134

56. Gryllaki-Berger M, Mugny C, Perrenoud D, Pannatier A, Frenk E (1992) A comparative study of formaldehyde detection using chromotropic acid, acetylacetone and HPLC in cosmetics and household cleaning products. Contact Dermatitis 26:149–154

57. Sheretz EF (1992) Clothing dermatitis: practical aspects for the clinician. Am J Contact Dermat 3:55–64

58. Stonecipher MR, Sherertz EF (1993) Office detection of formaldehyde in fabric: assessment of methods and update on frequency. Am J Contact Dermat 4:172–174

59. Benassi CA, Semenzato A, Bettero A (1989) High-performance liquid chromatographic determination of free formaldehyde in cosmetics. J Chromatogr 464:387–393

60. Bergendorff O, Ezzelarab M, Wallengren J, Hansson C (1994) Airborne contact dermatitis from formaldehyde released from heated plastic polymers. Am J Contact Dermat 5:223–225

61. Flyvholm M-A, Hall BM, Agner T, Tiedemann E, Greenhill P, Vanderveken W, Freeberg FE, Menné T (1997) Threshold for occluded formaldehyde patch test in formaldehyde-sensitive patients. Contact Dermatitis 36:26–33

62. Karlberg A-T, Skare L, Lindberg I, Nyhammar E (1998) A method for quantification of formaldehyde in the presence of formaldehyde donors in skin-care products. Contact Dermatitis 38:20–28

63. Second Commission Directive 82/434/EEC, Annex IV, Identification and determination of free formaldehyde

64. Rastogi SC (1995) Analysis of fragrances in cosmetics by gas chromatography-mass spectrometry. J High Resol Chromatogr 18:653–658

65. Rastogi SC, Johansen JD, Menné T (1996) Natural ingredients based cosmetics. Content of selected fragrance sensitizers. Contact Dermatitis 34:423–426

66. Gruvberger B, Bruze M, Tammela M (1998) Preservatives in moisturizers on the Swedish market. Acta Derm Venererol (Stockh) 78:52–56

67. Gruvberger B, Persson K, Björkner B, Bruze M, Dahlquist I, Fregert S (1986) Demonstration of Kathon CG in some commercial products. Contact Dermatitis 15:24–27

68. Rastogi SC (1990) Kathon CG and cosmetic products. Contact Dermatitis 22:155–160

69. Isaksson M, Gruvberger B, Persson L, Bruze M (2000) Stability of corticosteroid patch test preparations. Contact Dermatitis 42:144–148

70. Rastogi SC, Johansen SS (1995) Comparison of high-performance liquid chromatographic methods for the determination of 1,2-dibromo-2,4-dicyanobutane in cosmetic products. J Chromatogr A 692:53–57

71. Rastogi SC, Zachariae C, Johansen JD, Devantier C, Menne T (2004) Determination of methyldibromoglutaronitrile in cosmetic products by high-performance liquid chromatography with electrochemical detection. Method validation. J Chromatogr 26:315–317

72. Henriks-Eckerman M-L, Kanerva L (1997) Gas chromatographic and mass spectrometric purity analysis of acrylates and methacrylates used as patch test substances. Am J Contact Dermat 8:20–23

73. Dooms-Goossens A, Bruze M, Buysse L, Fregert S, Gruvberger B, Stals H (1995) Contact allergy to allyl glycidyl ether present as an impurity in 3-glycidyloxypropyltrimethoxysilane, a fixing additive in silicone and polyurethane resins. Contact Dermatitis 33:17–19

74. Dahlquist I, Fregert S (1980) Contact allergy to atranorin in lichens and perfumes. Contact Dermatitis 6:111–119

75. Guthrie WG (1984) Analysis of bronopol in water-based lotion. Provisional HPLC method. Boots Company PLC, Nottingham, UK

76. Wang H, Provan GJ, Helliwell K (2002) Determination of bronopol and its degradation products by HPLC. J Pharm Biomed Anal 29:387–392

77. Wahlberg JE (1977) Routine patch testing with cadmium chloride. Contact Dermatitis 3:293–296

78. Williams RO 3rd, Mahaguna V, Sriwongjanya M (1997) Determination of diazolidinyl urea in a topical cream by high-performance liquid chromatography. J Chromatogr B Biomed Sci Appl 29:303–306

79. Kerre S, Devos L, Verhoeve L, Bruze M, Gruvberger B, Dooms-Goossens A (1996) Contact allergy to diethylthiourea in a wet suit. Contact Dermatitis 35:176–178

80. Pontén A, Zimerson E, Sörensen Ö, Bruze M (2004) Chemical analysis of monomers in epoxy resins based on bisphenols F and A. Contact Dermatitis 50:289–297

81. Schouten A, Vermeulen M (1994) Methods of determination for preservatives mentioned in the EC Council directive regarding cosmetic products. 115. The determination of dimethyloldimethylhydantoin (DMDMH) in cosmetic products. TNO Nutr Food Res Rep V 94.608

82. Frick M, Zimerson E, Karlsson D, Marand Å, Skarping G, Isaksson M, Bruze M (2004) Poor correlation between stated and found concentrations of diphenylmethane-4,4′-diisocyanate (4,4′-MDI) in petrolatum patch test preparations. Contact Dermatitis 51:73–78

83. Meding B, Baum H, Bruze M, Roupe G, Trulsson L (1990) Allergic contact dermatitis from diphenylthiourea in Vulkan heat retainers. Contact Dermatitis 22:8–12

84. Fregert S, Trulsson L, Zimerson E (1982) Contact allergic reactions to diphenylthiourea and phenylisothiocyanate in PVC adhesive tape. Contact Dermatitis 8:38–42

85. Bruze M, Fregert S (1983) Allergic contact dermatitis from ethylene thiourea. Contact Dermatitis 9:208–212

86. Rastogi SC, Johansen JD, Frosch P, Menné T, Bruze M, Lepoittevin JP, Dreier B, Andersen KE, White IR (1998) Deodorants on the European market: quantitative chemical analysis of 21 fragrances. Contact Dermatitis 38:29–35

87. Rastogi SC, Lepoittevin J-P, Johansen JD, Frosch PJ, Menné T, Bruze M, Dreier B, Andersen KE, White IR (1998) Fragrances and other materials in deodorants: search for potentially sensitizing molecules using combined GC-MS and structure activity relationship (SAR) analysis. Contact Dermatitis 39:293–303

88. Gimenez-Arnau A, Gimenez-Arnau E, Serra-Baldrich E, Lepoittevin JP, Camarasa JG (2002) Principles and methodology for identification of fragrance allergens in consumer products. Contact Dermatitis 47:345–352

89. Karlberg AT, Dooms-Goossens A (1997) Contact allergy to oxidized d-limonene among dermatitis patients. Contact Dermatitis 36:201–206

90. Karlberg AT, Magnusson K, Nilsson U (1992) Air oxidation of d-limonene (the citrus solvent) creates potent allergens. Contact Dermatitis 26:332–340

91. Bruze M, Edman B, Niklasson B, Möller H (1985) Thin layer chromatography and high pressure liquid chromatography of musk ambrette and other nitromusk compounds including photopatch studies. Photodermatology 2:295–302

92. Bruze M, Gruvberger B (1985) Contact allergy to photoproducts of musk ambrette. Photodermatology 2:310–314

93. Bruze M, Persson L, Trulsson L, Zimerson E (1986) Demonstration of contact sensitizers in resins and products based on phenol-formaldehyde. Contact Dermatitis 14:146–154

94. Arisu K, Hayakawa R, Ogino Y, Matsunaga K, Kaniwa M-A (1992) Tinuvin P in a spandex tape as a cause of clothing dermatitis. Contact Dermatitis 26:311–316

95. Björkner B, Niklasson B (1997) Contact allergy to the UV absorber Tinuvin P in a dental restorative material. Am J Contact Dermat 8:6–7

96. Niklasson B, Björkner B (1989) Contact allergy to the UV-absorber Tinuvin P in plastics. Contact Dermatitis 21:330–334

97. Kaniwa M-A, Isama K, Nakamura A, Kantoh H, Hosono K, Itoh M, Shibata K, Usuda T, Asahi K, Osada T, Matsunaga K, Ueda H (1994) Identification of causative chemicals of allergic contact dermatitis using a combination of patch testing in patients and chemical analysis. Application to cases from rubber gloves. Contact Dermatitis 31:65–71

25.2 Skin Exposure Assessment

CAROLA LIDÉN

25.2.1 Introduction

Contact allergens, skin irritants, and other hazardous substances can come into contact with the skin, but there is little experience on how to measure the dose deposited on the skin. Solid materials, solutions, vapors, gases, and particles may contaminate the skin by direct contact, indirect contact, or airborne exposure. Exposure may be intended or unintended, voluntarily or accidental, known or unknown, visible, or invisible, etc.

Occupational hygiene has traditionally been concerned mainly with exposure by inhalation. Skin exposure to pesticides and some organic solvents has been an exception, due to the importance of skin absorption for their toxic effects (see Chap. 42: Pesticides). During recent years, there has been increasing attention to exposure by dermal contact; however, it is still mainly focused on exposure causing systemic effects, rather than dermatitis and other local effects. The EC Dermal Exposure Network (DEN) and the EU RISKOFDERM projects have made large efforts to increase knowledge in the area. A review over dermal exposure data in EU workplaces is given in [19]. The hands were found to be the most contaminated parts of the body, which is no surprise to experts in occupational dermatology and contact dermatitis.

A conceptual model of the process leading to uptake via the dermal route has been postulated [22]. The model describes uptake as a result of the transport of mass between the source, air, surface contaminant, outer and inner clothing contaminant layer, and the skin contaminant layer. A method for structured, semi-quantitative dermal exposure assessment (DREAM) has been developed [25]. The meth-

25

od consists of an inventory and an evaluation part. It can be used in occupational hygiene and in epidemiological studies. A European Standardisation project (CEN/TC 137) is developing a technical report for guidance on a strategy for the evaluation of dermal exposure in workplaces [8].

25.2.2 Techniques for Assessment of Skin Exposure

A brief review is given of techniques which may be useful in the assessment of skin exposure to contact allergens, skin irritants, and other skin hazardous substances.

25.2.2.1 Fluorescent Tracer Technique

The fluorescent tracer technique has often been used for the assessment of skin exposure to pesticides [1, 2, 7, 9] (See Chap. 42, Pesticides). The technique has also been applied for the assessment of skin exposure to dental acrylates (Fig. 2.1) [3] and paint [5, 21].

In brief, a fluorescent tracer is dissolved or mixed in the preparation of interest, e.g., a pesticide. Different fluorescent tracers have been used (e.g., Uvitex OB, Tinopal CBS-X, Calcofluor, and riboflavin). Some of them are used as laundry whitener. After the work process has been carried out, the body surface, clothes, gloves, and possibly the surrounding surfaces and equipment are illuminated with UV light in a darkened room, preferably under standardized conditions. The contaminated areas are, thus, visualized. A video camera, together with a computer program for image analysis, may be used for the recording and

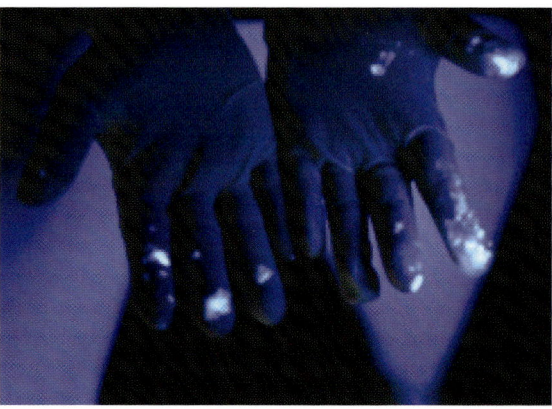

Fig. 2.1. Contamination of protective gloves with dental acrylates, visualized by the fluorescence tracer technique (courtesy of A. Boman).

analysis of the area and intensity of contamination. Documentation and evaluation may also be performed in a less sophisticated manner, depending on conditions, resources, and needs of the investigation.

The fluorescent tracer technique may be used for qualitative or quantitative assessment of skin exposure [6]. As the contamination is visualized, the method may be used, and have a great impact on training workers, to minimize contamination of skin and surfaces. Other applications may be to identify sources of contamination, to improve risk assessment, and to follow-up intervention. A comparison was made between the assessment of skin exposure by the fluorescent tracer technique and by using a rinsing method. Good agreement was found between the methods [21].

25.2.2.2 Removal Techniques

Among the most frequently used methods for sampling chemicals deposited on the skin are removal techniques, e.g., different washing methods and tape stripping.

Washing, Rinsing, and Wiping

Different washing techniques have been much used in studies of skin exposure to pesticides, as reviewed in [4]. The methods may be used also for skin irritants and contact allergens. Recent studies have been carried out to study the deposition of permanent hair dyes on the hands of hairdressers and the contamination of surfaces [12, 13]. Sampling was carried out by bag rinsing. The hands were shaken in plastic bags containing a borate buffer in 10% ethanol, before and after work. The hands of more than 50% of the hairdressers studied were contaminated by the permanent hair dyes analyzed (Tables 2.1 and 2.2). Studies have also been carried out to study the deposition of nickel, chromium, and cobalt on the hands of cashiers, locksmiths, and office employees (Lidén, to be published). Sampling was performed by wipe-washing defined areas on the hands with a weak acid before and after working for one or two h. It was shown that the sampling method was efficient and that the skin is contaminated by the metals in normal work situations (Tables 2.1 and 2.2).

When sampling by washing, rinsing, or wiping, it is essential to consider the choice of materials used (soap, solvent, wipe, plastic bag, etc.). They may interfere with skin absorption or chemical analysis. Sampling efficiency and sampling strategy are important factors for the outcome. By washing and rinsing, the chemicals deposited on large areas may be

Table 2.1. Method development for skin exposure assessment – some examples. (*AAS* Atomic absorption spectrophotometry, *GC* gas chromatography, *GC–MS* gas chromatography with mass spectrometry, *HPLC* high-performance liquid chromatography, *ICP–MS* inductively coupled plasma–mass spectrometry)

Substance	Sampling	Analytical method	Result	Ref.
Multifunctional acrylates	Tape stripping	GC	The first tape strip removed 94% of tripropylene glycol diacrylate (TPGDA) and 89% of UV resin	[16]
Jet fuel (naphthalene)	Tape stripping	GC–MS	The first two tape strips removed 70% of the applied dose	[15]
Permanent hair dyes	Bag rinsing	HPLC	Sampling efficiency 70–90%	[12]
Nickel	Tape stripping	ICP–MS	Adsorption studied by 20 strips	[10]
Nickel	Tape stripping	AAS	Baseline: 1–3 ng/tape sample	[11]
Nickel	Nail clipping	AAS	Baseline: 1.58 µg/g	[11]
Nickel, chromium, cobalt	Wipe-wash	ICP–MS	Sampling efficiency 93–100%	–[a]
Particles	Vacuuming	Light microscopy, X-ray fluorescence (XRF)	Sampling efficiency 95–100%	[14]
Particles	Tape stripping	Light microscopy, XRF	The first two strips removed 99.8%	[14]

[a] Lidén, to be published

Table 2.2. Examples of skin exposure assessment by different technique in the occupational setting. (*AAS* atomic absorption spectrophotometry, *GC* gas chromatography, *HPLC* high-performance liquid chromatography, *ICP–MS* inductively coupled plasma–mass spectrometry)

Exposure	Sampling	Analytical method	Dose on skin (mean value); (number of subjects or samples)	Ref.
Metalworking fluid	Whole-body oversuits, sampling gloves	HPLC, inductively coupled plasma–atomic emission spectrometry (ICP–AES)	Boron in suit: 62 µg/cm^2 per h (n=31) In gloves: 2,900 µg/cm^2 per h (n=7)	[20]
Electroplating fluid	Whole-body oversuits, sampling gloves	Portable X-ray fluorescence (PXRF)	Ni, Cr, Cu, and Zn in suit: 37 µg/cm^2 per h (n=26) In gloves: 190 µg/cm^2 per h (n=25)	[20]
Permanent hair dyes in hairdressers	Bag rinsing	HPLC	Paraphenylenediamine (PPD): 22–939 nmol/hand (n=33) Exposure by dye application, cutting newly dyed hair, or from background exposure	[13]
UV-curable acrylates in the furniture industry	Tape stripping	GC	TPGDA: 30.4 µg or 10 cm^2/work shift (n=36)	[24]
Workers exposed to nickel	Nail clipping	AAS	Moderate exposure (n=83): 29.2 µg/g Heavy exposure (n=51): 123 µg/g	[18]
Nickel in different occupations (2 h work)	Wipe washing	ICP–MS	Cashiers (n=7): 0.3 µg/cm^2 Locksmiths (n=3): 0.9 µg/cm^2 Office workers (n=4): 0.03 µg/cm^2	–[a]

[a] Lidén, to be published

sampled. By wipe-washing, the mass per area unit, e.g., µg/cm², may be calculated, which is of high relevance when considering contact allergy.

Tape Stripping

Tape stripping, by stripping up to 20 times, is often used in dermatology for studies of different processes in the stratum corneum. Tape stripping has been applied also for sampling in the assessment of skin exposure to acrylates, jet fuel, nickel, and particles (Tables 2.1 and 2.2) [11, 14–16, 24]. Stripping up to 3 times may also be done. Tape stripping, by several strippings, has been used for studies of how nickel is adsorbed in the skin (Table 2.1) [10]. Such an application may be referred to as biomonitoring. Different types of tape have been used, depending on the substance of interest and the analytical procedure used.

Nail Clippings

Analysis of nickel in fingernails has been developed as a method suggested for the assessment of occupational skin exposure to nickel (Tables 2.1 and 2.2) [11, 18]. It was shown that the level of nickel in fingernails increased significantly when low doses of nickel nitrate solution were applied to the fingers. (See Chap. 32, Metals)

Vacuuming

Vacuuming may be used for sampling particles deposited on skin. A suction sampler was constructed for this purpose and it was used in method development in an exposure chamber (Table 2.1) [14]. Comparisons were made with results from tape stripping and patch sampling, confirming good agreement. The suction sampler allows for dust sampling from large areas of skin. The technique will be further developed and applied in work place studies.

25.2.2.3 Surrogate Skin Sampling

In skin exposure assessment, the concept of surrogate skin is used as a medium used to collect chemicals deposited on the sampler, as a surrogate for the skin surface. The technique has been much used in the assessment of skin exposure to pesticides ([17], review in [23]).

Whole-body oversuits, gloves, and patches applied in different locations on the body are used as samplers. They may be made of cotton or other fabric, filter paper, aluminum foil or other material. After exposure, the substance is extracted and analyzed; oversuits may be sectioned before analysis. Skin ex-

posure to metal working fluids and electroplating fluid was studied by the use of oversuits and sampling gloves worn inside protective gloves (Table 2.2) [20].

A patch sampler with a sampling surface of tape was developed for the assessment of skin exposure to particles. The patch sampler was used for wheat flour, corn starch, and wood dust. The analysis was carried out by different methods. The results were compared with sampling by tape stripping and vacuuming (Table 2.1) [14].

25.2.2.4 Biomonitoring

Common biomonitoring has little use in the assessment of skin exposure to contact allergens and skin irritants. Tape stripping and microdialysis may, however, in the future be used more for this purpose.

25.2.3 Analytical Methods

See Sect. 25.1, Tables 2.1 and 2.2, and the publications referred to above for a broad range of analytical methods suitable for contact allergens.

25.2.4 Application of Results

There is a great need for further development and application of methods for the assessment of skin exposure to contact allergens, skin irritants, and other skin-hazardous substances. The application of solid methods for skin exposure assessment will increase the understanding of skin contamination, the dose–effect relationship, and the possibilities for prevention. The results may be used in risk assessment, in setting occupational dermal exposure limits, and in follow-up after intervention by exposure control. Skin exposure assessment may, in the future, be applied in the evaluation of patients with contact dermatitis.

Core Message

- Assessment of skin exposure to contact allergens, skin irritants, and other skin-hazardous substances is a new research area. It will help us to understand better skin contamination, the dose–effect relationship, and conditions for the prevention of dermatitis.

References

1. Aragón A, Blanco L, López L, Lidén C, Nise G, Wesseling C (2004) Reliability of a visual scoring system with fluorescent tracers to assess dermal pesticide exposure. Ann Occup Hyg 48:601–606

2. Blanco LE, Aragón A, Lundberg I, Lidén C, Wesseling C, Nise G (2005) Determinants of dermal exposure among Nicaraguan subsistence farmers during pesticide applications with backpack sprayers. Ann Occup Hyg 49:17–24

3. Boman A, Sandborgh-Englund G, Andreasson H, Johnsson S, Lidén C (2002) Hand contamination and protection during dental work. In: Proceedings of the international conference on occupational and environmental exposures of skin to chemicals: science and policy. Crystal City Hilton, Washington, DC 8–11 September 2002

4. Brouwer DH, Boeniger MF, van Hemmen J (2000) Hand wash and manual skin wipes. Ann Occup Hyg 44:501–510

5. Brouwer DH, Lansink CM, Cherrie JW, van Hemmen JJ (2000) Assessment of dermal exposure during airless spray painting using a quantitative visualisation technique. Ann Occup Hyg 44:543–549

6. Cherrie JW, Brouwer DH, Roff M, Vermeulen R, Kromhout H (2000) Use of qualitative and quantitative fluorescence techniques to assess dermal exposure. Ann Occup Hyg 44:519–522

7. Cohen Hubal EA, Suggs JC, Nishioka MG, Ivancic WA (2005) Characterizing residue transfer efficiencies using a fluorescent imaging technique. J Expo Anal Environ Epidemiol 15:261–270

8. European Committee for Standardisation (CEN) (working document) (2005) Workplace exposure – strategy for the evaluation of dermal exposure. CEN/TC 137 prCEN/TR 137027

9. Fenske RA (1988) Visual scoring system for fluorescent tracer evaluation of dermal exposure to pesticides. Bull Environ Contam Toxicol 41:727–736

10. Hostýnek JJ, Dreher F, Nakada T, Schwindt D, Anigbogu A, Maibach HI (2001) Human stratum corneum adsorption of nickel salts. Investigation of depth profiles by tape stripping in vivo. Acta Derm Venereol Suppl (Stockh) 212:11–18

11. Kristiansen J, Molin Christensen J, Henriksen T, Nielsen NH, Menné T (2000) Determination of nickel in fingernails and forearm skin (stratum corneum). Anal Chim Acta 403:265–272

12. Lind M-L, Boman A, Surakka J, Sollenberg J, Meding B (2004) A method for assessing occupational dermal exposure to permanent hair dyes. Ann Occup Hyg 48:533–539

13. Lind M-L, Boman A, Sollenberg J, Johnsson S, Hagelthorn G, Meding B (2004) A method for assessing occupational dermal exposure to permanent hair dyes. Ann Occup Hyg 48:533–539

14. Lundgren L, Lidén C, Skare L, Sundström G (2003) Stripping, vacuuming and surrogate skin – measurement of dust on skin. In: Selected abstracts of the 1st world congress on work-related and environmental allergy (1st WOREAL), Helsinki, Finland, 9–12 July 2003. Exog Dermatol 2:90

15. Mattorano DA, Kupper LL, Nylander-French LA (2004) Estimating dermal exposure to jet fuel (naphthalene) using adhesive tape strip samples. Ann Occup Hyg 48:139–146

16. Nylander-French LA (2000) A tape-stripping method for measuring dermal exposure to multifunctional acrylates. Ann Occup Hyg 44:645–651

17. OECD (1997) Guidance document for the conduct of studies of occupational exposure to pesticides during agricultural application. Environment, health and safety publications series on testing and assessment, no 9

18. Peters K, Gammelgaard B, Menné T (1991) Nickel concentrations in fingernails as a measure of occupational exposure to nickel. Contact Dermatitis 25:237–241

19. Rajan-Sithamparanadarajah R, Roff M, Delgado P, Eriksson K, Fransman W, Gijsbers JHJ, Hughson G, Mäkinen M, van Hemmen JJ (2004) Patterns of dermal exposure to hazardous substances in European Union workplaces. Ann Occup Hyg 48:285–297

20. Roff M, Bagon DA, Chambers H, Dilworth EM, Warren N (2004) Dermal exposure to electroplating fluids and metalworking fluids in the UK. Ann Occup Hyg 48:209–217

21. Roff M, Wheeler J, Baldwin P (2001) Comparison of fluorescence and rinsing methods for assessing dermal exposure. Appl Occup Environ Hyg 16:319–322

22. Schneider T, Vermeulen R, Brouwer DH, Cherrie JW, Kromhout H, Fogh CL (1999) Conceptual model for assessment of dermal exposure. Occup Environ Med 56:765–773

23. Soutar A, Semple S, Aitken RJ, Robertson A (2000) Use of patches and whole body sampling for the assessment of dermal exposure. Ann Occup Hyg 44:511–518

24. Surakka J, Lindh T, Rosén G, Fischer T (2000) Workers' dermal exposure to UV-curable acrylates in the furniture and parquet industry. Ann Occup Hyg 44:635–644

25. Van Wendel-de-Joode B, Brouwer DH, Vermeulen R, van Hemmen JJ, Heederik D, Kromhout H (2003) DREAM: a method for semi-quantitative dermal exposure assessment. Ann Occup Hyg 47:71–87

Chapter 26

Skin Tests for Immediate Hypersensitivity

26

Matti Hannuksela

Contents

26.1 Introduction

Immediate contact reactions comprise both immunologic (allergic) and nonimmunologic (non-allergic) reactions. Itching, burning, and tingling are the most usual subjective symptoms. Mild reactions appear as redness only, but in stronger reactions, contact urticaria or eczematous dermatitis can be seen.

Skin tests are usually reliable in detecting immediate allergies. Medication, such as acetylsalicylic acid and other prostaglandin inhibitors, and ultraviolet radiation readily abolish nonimmunological reactivity. They have less influence on allergic reactions. This chapter deals with the most usual and most useful skin tests, discussing their advantages and disadvantages (Table 1).

26.2 Skin Prick Test

The skin prick test (SPT) is usually the most convenient and reliable method for detecting clinically significant, immunoglobulin E (IgE)-mediated allergy. Large numbers of standardized allergens are available commercially. Self-made test material can also be used.

Drops of SPT allergen solutions are applied to the skin of the back or lower arm, 3–5 cm apart, and pierced with a special prick test lancet. Histamine dihydrochloride, 10 mg/ml, is used as a positive control and the base solution as a negative control. After piercing the skin, the drops are wiped off with a soft tissue. After 15–20 min, the diameters or areas of the wheals are measured. Redness around the weal is usually not taken into consideration. The result is usually expressed as the mean of the longest diameter of the weal and the longest diameter perpendicular to it. Reactions larger than 3 mm and at least half the size of that produced by histamine are regarded as positive [1–3]. Reactions at least the size of that by histamine are usually clinically relevant. Those smaller than half the size of the histamine reaction are usually not significant.

In a cheaper modification of the ordinary SPT, the lancet is first dipped in the allergen solution and, im-

Table 1. Skin tests for immediate hypersensitivity reactions

Test	Remarks
Skin prick test (SPT)	For immediate allergy. Especially for standardized allergen solutions
Prick-by-prick	For testing with fresh foods
Scratch test	For immunoglobulin E (IgE)-mediated immediate allergy. Non-standardized allergens
Scratch-chamber test	May be less sensitive than scratch test
Open application test	For both immunologic and nonimmunologic reactions
	Previously affected skin reacts more readily than healthy skin
Skin application food test	Resembles chamber test. An alternative to open application test
Rub test	Another modification of the open application test

mediately after that, the skin is pricked [4]. No statistical difference has been noticed in the size of the wheals.

Another modification of the SPT is the prick-by-prick method used especially for testing with fresh foodstuffs [5, 6]. A piece of food is pricked with the lancet, immediately after which, the skin is pricked with the same lancet. The results are grouped as mentioned above.

> ## Core Message
>
> ■ The skin prick test is the standard skin test method for detecting immediate allergies. Commercial standardized allergens are recommended. Skin from the back and the arm are the preferable test sites. The result is read after 15–20 min. Reactions greater than 3 mm and at least the size of histamine dihydrochloride, 10 mg/ml, are usually clinically significant. Reactions smaller than half of that from histamine are considered negative.

26.3 Scratch Test

This previously common method for detecting immediate allergy is still used when only non-standardized allergens are available. In SPT with, e.g., fresh meat, poultry, flours, spices, fruits, and vegetables, skin infection and other untoward effects are more likely than in a scratch test. Scratches approximately 5-mm long are made with a blood lancet or venipuncture needle on arm or back skin 3–5 cm apart, and bleeding is avoided. Allergen solutions are applied to the scratches for 5–10 min, after which, they can be wiped off with a soft tissue. Powdered allergens are mixed with a drop of physiological saline or 0.1 N sodium hydroxide. Histamine dihydrochloride, 10 mg/ml, is the positive and saline or 0.1 N sodium hydroxide is the negative control. The results are read 15–20 min after application. Only the longest diameter of the weal perpendicular to the scratch is measured. Reactions equal to or greater than that from histamine are usually clinically significant. Spices like cinnamon and mustard also produce nonimmunologic contact urticaria reactions, often indistinguishable from true allergic reactions. The significance of such reactions should be interpreted with caution.

26.4 Scratch-Chamber Test

In this test, the scratch with the allergen is covered with an 8-mm, or, preferably, a 12-mm Finn chamber (Epitest, Helsinki, Finland). This method has been used when fruits, vegetables, and other fresh foods have been tested [7]. The control substances and reading are the same as for the scratch test. In a study on apple allergy, the sensitivity of the scratch-chamber test has been found to be inferior to that of SPT [8].

> ## Core Message
>
> ■ The scratch test and its modification, the scratch-chamber test, are suitable for testing with non-standardized materials, such as meat, flours, fruits, vegetables, and spices. Covering the scratch with an epicutaneous test chamber may decrease the sensitivity or specificity of the scratch test.

26.5 Chamber Test

In addition to the SPT, scratch test, and scratch-chamber test, the chamber test has been used in the diagnosis of immediate contact allergy. There might be two types of immediate allergy: that detected by the SPT, and that found by an occluded epicutaneous test (chamber test) [9, 10]. There seems to be three kinds of patients: those reacting to SPT only, those reacting to the chamber test only, and those reacting to both [9].

The test material is put into an ordinary patch test chamber (e.g., Finn chamber), moistened with physiological saline when needed, and applied to the back or upper arm for 15–20 min. The test is read some minutes after the removal of the test chamber. A weal-and-flare reaction is regarded as positive, and erythema without edema as unlikely to be positive. One should keep in mind that materials such as cinnamon and mustard elicit readily nonimmunologic contact urticaria reactions. When testing materials of unknown irritancy, an appropriate number of control cases should also be tested.

26.6 Open Application Test

This test is also known as the contact urticaria test, open patch test, and provocative test. It can be used for both immunologic (allergic) and nonimmunologic reactions. Immunologic reactions appear on the arms as readily as on the back skin. Nonimmunologic reactions, on the other hand, appear less readily on the ventral aspects of lower arms, while the back skin and the outer aspects of the upper arms are equally sensitive [11]. Allergic reactions are usually more readily produced on previously affected skin than on normal-looking, healthy skin [12]. Cosmetic creams may produce positive reactions on the cheek while the back skin shows no response.

Liquids, creams, and ointments are tested by spreading 0.1 ml of the test substance to an area of about 3 × 3 cm in size on the upper back or the outer aspect of the upper arm [13]. When testing a greater number of substances at the same time, 10-μl aliquots are applied to 1 × 1-cm areas. After 15–60 min, the test materials are gently wiped off with a soft paper towel or tissue. Dry test materials, such as latex gloves and carbonless copy paper, are applied directly to the skin moistened with two or three drops of water for better contact. Powders should be mixed with a proper vehicle. Petrolatum and water were the most popular vehicles some decades ago, but alcohol vehicles with propylene glycol may enhance the reactivity [14, 15].

The test is usually read at 20, 40, and 60 min. When testing previously unknown substances, it is advisable to follow the result for 6–8 h at 1–2-h intervals. Nonimmunologic reactions tend to appear more slowly than allergic ones. The time of maximal reactivity depends on the substance itself and on the vehicle used [14].

In visual grading, redness and edema are usually assessed separately (+ weak, ++ moderate, +++ strong). However, objective measurements are preferred. Erythema can be measured, e.g., with chromameter or with laser Doppler flowmeter.

Core Message

■ The open application test, also known as the contact urticaria test, open patch test, and provocative test, is usually done on the upper back skin or on the outer aspects of the upper arms. Allergic reactions also appear as readily on the lower arms. Aliquots of 0.1 ml are spread onto 3 × 3-cm areas. When testing a greater number of substances, 10-μl aliquots are applied to 1 × 1-cm areas. Allergic reactions usually appear usually within 15–20 min, but may last several hours.

26.7 Rub Test

In the rub test, the suspected substance is gently rubbed into slightly affected or healthy skin [7]. Rubbing may enhance the reactivity compared to the open application test.

In the skin application food test (SAFT), 0.8 ml of liquid food or a solid piece of food is placed on a 4-cm² gauze and fixed onto the back skin with acrylic tape [16]. The test can also be performed by using patch test chambers (e.g., van der Bend or large Finn chambers). The results are followed up every 10 min, the maximal occlusion time being 30 min. The test results are highly reproducible.

Core Message

■ The rub test and the skin application food test (SAFT) are modifications of the open application and chamber tests. The results are followed up for 30–40 min. The tests are used especially in cases of suspected food contact allergy.

26.8 Factors Suppressing Immediate Skin Test Reactivity

H_1 antihistamines suppress histamine-mediated skin test reactions for 1–4 days, astemizole for at least 3–4 weeks.

Over 10 mg of prednisone and equivalent doses of other glucocorticosteroids suppress allergic reactions to the extent that the result may not be relevant. Non-steroidal anti-inflammatory drugs abolish the nonimmunologic reactivity for at least 3 days, but have no or little effect on allergic reactions.

Both ultraviolet A (UVA) and ultraviolet B (UVB) exposure weakens the skin reactivity for 2–3 weeks to substances producing nonimmunologic immediate reactions. On the other hand, UV usually shows no effect on the size of immediate allergic contact reactions.

26.9 Control Tests

When testing with non-standardized allergens, control tests ought to be performed to detect false-positive and non-relevant test results. It is advocated to use at least (20–)50 atopic control persons when testing substances causing IgE-mediated allergy.

References

1. Basomba A, Sastre A, Pelaez A, Romar A, Campos A, Garcia-Villalmanzo A (1985) Standardization of the prick test. A comparative study of three methods. Allergy 40: 395–399
2. Malling H-J (1985) Reproducibility of skin sensitivity using a quantitative skin prick test. Allergy 40:400–404
3. Taudorf E, Malling H-J, Laursen LC, Lanner A, Weeke B (1985) Reproducibility of histamine skin prick test. Allergy 40:344–349
4. Zawodniak A, Kupczyk M, Gorski P, Kuna P (2003) Comparison of standard and modified SPT method. Allergy 58 :257–259
5. Dreborg S, Foucard T (1983) Allergy to apple, carrot and potato in children with birch pollen allergy. Allergy 38: 167–172
6. Rancé F, Juchet A, Brémont F, Dutau G (1997) Correlations between skin prick tests using commercial extracts and fresh foods, specific IgE, and food challenges. Allergy 52: 1031–1035
7. Niinimäki A (1987) Scratch-chamber tests in food handler dermatitis. Contact Dermatitis 16:11–20
8. Osterballe M, Scheller R, Stahl Skov P, Andersen KE, Bindslev-Jensen C (2003) Diagnostic value of scratch-chamber test, skin prick test, histamine release and specific IgE in birch-allergic patients with oral allergy syndrome to apple. Allergy 58:950–953
9. Susitaival P, Husman K, Husman L, Hollmén A, Horsmanheimo M, Hannuksela M, Notkola V (1994) Hand dermatoses in dairy farmers. In: McDuffie HH, Dosman JA, Semchuk KM, Olenchock SA, Senthilselvan A (eds) Human sustainability in agriculture: health, safety, environment. Lewis, Chelsea, Missouri
10. Morren M-A, Janssens V, Dooms-Goossens A, van Hoeyveld E, Cornelis A, De Wolf-Peeters C, Heremans A (1993) a-amylase, a flour additive: an important cause of protein contact dermatitis in bakers. J Am Acad Dermatol 29: 723–728
11. Lahti A (1980) Non-immunologic contact urticaria. Acta Derm Venereol Suppl (Stockh) 91:1–49
12. Tosti A, Guerra L (1988) Protein contact dermatitis in food handlers. Contact Dermatitis 19:149–150
13. Lahti A (1997) Nonimmunologic contact urticaria. In: Amin S, Lahti A, Maibach HI (eds) Contact urticaria syndrome. CRC Press, Boca Raton, Florida, pp 5–10
14. Ylipieti S, Lahti A (1989) Effects of the vehicle on non-immunologic immediate contact reactions. Contact Dermatitis 21:105–106
15. Lahti A, Poutiainen A-M, Hannuksela M (1993) Alcohol vehicles in tests for non-immunological immediate contact reactions. Contact Dermatitis 29:22–25
16. Oranje AP, Van Gysel D, Mulder PGH, Dieges PH (1994) Food-induced contact urticaria syndrome (CUS) in atopic dermatitis patients: reproducibility of repeated and duplicate testing with a skin provocation test, the skin application food test (SAFT). Contact Dermatitis 31:314–318

26

Chapter 27

Photopatch Testing

27

Roy A. Palmer, Ian R. White

Contents

27.1 Introduction

Photopatch testing (PhPT) is primarily used to diagnose photoallergy to topical agents. Mechanisms of photoallergy are discussed in Chap. 6, and clinical features of photoallergy are covered in Chap. 17. In a research context, PhPT can be used to evaluate the phototoxic potential of substances, but it is not useful for the diagnosis of suspected phototoxic reactions.

Photoallergy is the result of a type-IV hypersensitivity reaction to a photoproduct or photoactivated chemical. It is rare, and is less common than phototoxicity. The allergens responsible have changed over the past four decades; currently, in the Western world, the most frequent culprits are sunscreens, but even these compounds have a low potential for photosensitization [1]. The rarity of photoallergy is one

of the reasons that PhPT has remained, arguably, an imprecise investigation. The interaction of two agents (a topical chemical and ultraviolet) creates a complexity and potential variability that hinders accuracy and reproducibility. The subject has suffered from straddling two subspecialities; namely, contact dermatitis and photodermatology, and variations in the methodology of PhPT have hindered the comparison of data from different studies. Nevertheless, PhPT has a vital role in distinguishing patients with photoallergy, airborne allergic contact dermatitis, and photodermatoses.

There are reported to be 49 known PhPT centers in Europe; the 34 who responded to a survey [2] each conducted only an average of 16 photopatch tests per year, and only two centers conducted more than 50. There is a lack of standardization in the methodology of PhPT, with wide variations in the agents used, test concentrations, and interpretation of reactions. This is partly because evidence to recommend any particular approach has not been available. Groups from Scandinavia [3, 4], Germany, Austria and Switzerland [5], Italy [6], and Britain [7] have made separate and differing attempts at standardization of the technique. Recently, the European Taskforce for Photopatch Testing has produced a consensus methodology [2]. This development was long overdue, and is a major step forwards. It ensures an appropriate degree of standardization, while recognizing that some variation between centers will always exist as a necessity, due to regional variations in allergen exposure and logistical factors.

27.2 Prevalence and Factors Predisposing to Photoallergy

Although it has not been investigated, the prevalence of photoallergy in the general population is likely to be extremely small. Patients diagnosed with photoallergy usually have an underlying photodermatosis [1, 8–10]. This may be explained by the original indication for referral to the investigating unit, the frequent

27

use of sunscreens in photosensitive patients, and the application of sunscreens on inflamed skin (thereby, increasing penetration). It is also possible that such patients are intrinsically prone to sensitization, which is suggested in chronic actinic dermatitis (CAD) by the very high prevalence of contact allergy in that condition.

Until 10 years ago, most reports of PhPT series suggested that 7–20% of patients tested had at least one photoallergic reaction [9, 11–13]. Many of these studies used substances that are now either obsolete or likely to give phototoxic reactions that may be misinterpreted as photoallergic. Studies in the past decade using series consisting predominantly of sunscreen allergens have tended to show lower rates of 2.3–10% [1, 8, 14, 15]. The largest of these studies reviewed the results of 2,715 patients who underwent PhPT between 1983 and 1998 [1]. It found that 2.3% of patients had at least one photoallergic reaction; the average number of positive reactions among these photoallergic patients was 1.3.

27.3 Contact Photoallergens

27.3.1 A Historical Perspective

Only a small number of substances have been responsible for causing the majority of cases of photoallergy. When substances are recognized as photoallergens, they tend to be withdrawn, so the list of currently relevant allergens is constantly changing. The problem of topical photoallergy was first identified in 1961 by Wilkinson in regard to tetrachlorosalicylanilide [16], which belongs to the family of halogenated salicylanilides. These substances, and also the chlorinated phenols (fentichlor and bithionol), were used as antibacterial agents in soaps and other products. They caused an epidemic of photosensitivity until they were removed from the European environment in the 1970s, although extremely rare cases seemed to develop "persistent light reactivity" (see Chap. 17). Wilkinson described the sparing of skin behind the lower part of the ears in photosensitive individuals with facial eczema; his name is now immortalized in the term "Wilkinson's triangle."

Musk ambrette was used extensively, and in high concentrations (up to 4%), as a fragrance enhancer in toiletries and aftershaves. It was also found in other products, such as soaps, hair sprays, furniture polish, and fruit-flavored edibles, including yoghurts and sweets. In 1978, it was identified as a photoallergen by Larsen [17]; it is also a simple contact allergen. It became an increasing menace, typically causing local-

ized eczema corresponding to the application of aftershave, or a more widespread dermatitis, resembling chronic actinic dermatitis [18]. Following recommendations from the International Fragrance Association, the concentrations were reduced and the incidence of new cases fell dramatically. It is now prohibited from Europe and most other major markets. However, it is still widely available in some Asian countries and large quantities are exported from China.

In the West, photoallergy is now rare and legislation requires the evaluation of substances before they are marketed. The stringent guidelines for such evaluations now ensure that it is unlikely for significant photoallergens to become widely available ever again.

27.3.2 UV Filters

Over the last 20 years, there has been a dramatic increase in the use of sunscreens, driven by a desire to avoid skin cancer and photoaging. In addition, ultraviolet (UV) filters are sometimes included in cosmetics to increase the shelf life of the product by preventing photodegradation [19], and to increase the shelf-life of the user by preventing photoaging. As a result, there has been an increase in the incidence of photoallergy to these agents but, again, once the major culprits were identified (for example, isopropyl dibenzoylmethane [20]), they were removed from the marketplace. Although currently, sunscreens are the most frequent photoallergens [8], they, nevertheless, have a low potential for photoallergenicity, and they also have an excuse; their job is to absorb UV radiation.

There has been an increasing recognition of the role of UVA in photoaging and photocarcinogenesis and, therefore, an increasing drive to provide protection against it, in addition to UVB. UV filters can be divided into organic and physical agents. The physical agents zinc oxide and titanium dioxide, when in pigment form, predominantly reflect (but not absorb) UV, so do not undergo photochemical reactions and, therefore, do not cause sensitization. They tend to have a white appearance because they also reflect visible light, which is an undesirable characteristic that has been reduced by the use of *microfine* titanium dioxide. This substance predominantly absorbs UV and is usually used in high concentrations; there is no percutaneous absorption so sensitization does not occur [21, 22]. Organic agents absorb ultraviolet radiation (UVR) by undergoing a chemical transformation, which gives them the potential to be photoallergenic. They can be grouped as follows:

- *Benzophenones*; absorb UVB and some UVA.
- *PABA and its esters*; mostly absorb UVB. They have become less frequently used.
- *Cinnamates*; have largely replaced para-aminobenzoic acid (PABA) and its esters as UVB absorbers. Ethylhexyl methoxycinnamate (octyl methoxycinnamate) is commonly used, but is a very rare photoallergen.
- *Dibenzoylmethanes*; mostly absorbs UVA.
- *Camphor derivatives*.

In the PhPT study of 2,715 patients referred to earlier, 65% of photoallergic reactions were to sunscreens, particularly benzophenone-3 and benzophenone-10 [1]. In addition, 2% of patients had an ordinary contact allergic reaction to the PhPT series, most commonly to UV filters, again, particularly benzophenone-3 and benzophenone-10.

UV filters can cause an acute reaction with clinical features identical to those of an ordinary allergic contact dermatitis. However, because they are usually applied before exposure to sunlight, it is often difficult to make a diagnosis on the basis of the history alone; reactions to them may be misinterpreted as an idiopathic photodermatosis, and people using sunscreens to treat idiopathic photodermatoses may acquire an allergy to them that exacerbates the pre-existing condition.

27.3.3 Other Photoallergens

Chlorpromazine can induce photoallergic (and phototoxic) reactions in, for example, healthcare workers handling tablets [23]. In the PhPT study of 2,715 patients, 12% of photoallergic responses were to promethazine and 7% to chlorpromazine; the authors recognized that these reactions may have been phototoxic and wrongly diagnosed [1]. Photoallergy due to topical non-steroidal anti-inflammatory drugs (NSAIDs) has been reported many times over the last decade, particularly from mainland Europe, where they are used frequently [24–27]. There is no convincing evidence that Compositae, lichens, and wood mixes are significant photoallergens, except, possibly, in extremely rare cases [7, 28]. They can cause airborne allergic contact dermatitis and patients with chronic actinic dermatitis often have positive patch tests to Compositae.

Many other contact photoallergens have been described [29] (Table 1), but most are unconfirmed and some of the reports are probably erroneous, attributing photoallergy to cases of phototoxicity. Cross-reactions between chemically related substances have been reported [30], such as between ketoprofen with benzophenone-3, which share a benzophenone moiety [31].

27.4 General Considerations for Photopatch Testing

The major indication for PhPT is the investigation of eczema affecting UV-exposed sites. Some patients will give a history of using potentially photoallergenic preparations and exacerbations following sun exposure. Individuals having PhPTs should also be phototested and patch-tested with a "standard series" that includes allergens that may mimic photosensitivity (such as Compositae), a "facial series," and their own skin-care products. Patch tests can be performed at the same time as PhPTs. Although published evidence is lacking, false-negative results may be caused by immunosuppressive therapy (topical and systemic) and antihistamines. Therefore, when possible, these should be stopped prior to PhPT, perhaps 1 week beforehand for topical steroids [7] or 2 weeks for systemic immunosuppressants [2].

As regards to the choice of substances for PhPT, those which frequently cause phototoxic reactions should generally be avoided. There cannot be a "standard light series" for all countries because of geographical variations in exposure. A working party of the British Photodermatology Group suggested a routine list of photoallergens for Britain, and the European Taskforce for Photopatch Testing have recently published their recommendations (Table 2) [2, 7]. These will need to be continually reviewed to reflect research and changes in the use of products. Very little information exists regarding the optimal concentration of agents for PhPT. Patients' own products should be tested when appropriate, and other agents listed in Table 2 when indicated, such as thiourea (used as an antioxidant in photocopy paper [32]). Photoallergy to *systemic* agents, and the difficulties of using PhPT to diagnose it, is discussed in Chap. 17.

27.5 Source and Dose of UVA

UVA is more relevant than UVB or visible light to photoallergy for reasons discussed in Chap. 17. Fluorescent UVA lamps of the kind used for psoralen-UVA (PUVA) therapy are preferred [2], since they are cheap, easily available, and have an output which is broad across the UVA region. Also, their irradiance is relatively high and uniform across a large irradiated site, and the different types of these tubes have similar spectra, allowing comparison between centers.

27

Table 1. Examples of topical agents reported to cause (but not necessarily confirmed as causing) photoallergy. Others are listed in Table 2 [1, 29]

Sunscreens
　Benzophenone-10
　Digalloyl trioleate
　Dimethoxane
　2-ethoxyethyl-*p*-methoxycinnamate
　Glyceryl *p*-aminobenzoate
　4-isopropyldibenzoylmethane
　Amyl dimethyl PABA

Halogenated antimicrobials
　Bis(2-hydroxy-5-chlorophenyl) sulfide (fentichlor)
　5-bromo-4′-chlorosalicylanilide
　Buclosamide
　Chlorhexidine
　Chloro-2-phenylphenol
　4,5-Dibromosalicylanilide
　Hexachlorophene
　Tetrachlorosalicylanilide (TCSA)
　2,2′-thiobis(4,6-dichlorophenol) (bithionol)
　Tribromosalicylanilide
　Trichlorocarbanilide
　Triclosan

Fragrance ingredients
　6-Methyl coumarin
　Musk ambrette
　Musk xylol

Others
　Brilliant lake red R (DC-R31)
　Permanent orange (DC-017)
　Benzocaine
　Benzydamine
　Chlorpromazine
　Chlorprothixene
　NSAIDs, e.g., tiaprofenic acid, ibuproxam
　Promethazine
　Quinine sulfate
　Thiourea, dimethylthiourea
　Zinc pyrithione

---

cm^2 [7]). Also, the dose needs to be low enough not to cause, in association with the topical substance, a clinically irrelevant phototoxic response. The latter have been mostly studied with promethazine. Reactions to this are more likely to be phototoxic than photoallergic. With a 5 J/cm^2 dose, reactions to promethazine only occur in 1.8% of patients, but with a dose of 10 J/cm^2, they occur in 34–45% [7]. There is no evidence that clinically important reactions are missed by 5-J/cm^2 and revealed by 10-J/cm^2 doses. Although doses of 1 J/cm^2 or even lower *can* elicit photoallergic reactions [18, 33], the yield of positive reactions decreases below 5 J/cm^2 [34]. Therefore, although more research is required, a dose of 5 J/cm^2 has been recommended and gradually seems to be becoming standard [2, 7, 9, 11, 13, 18, 33]. This may be increased for dark-skinned subjects.

If patients who are very sensitive to UVA are exposed to 5 J/cm^2 of UVA, they may have severe reactions. Therefore, the dose may be reduced to 2.5 J/cm^2 (or lower) in patients with suspected chronic actinic dermatitis and/or a history of severe photosensitivity [1]. It is helpful if the results of standard phototests are known before the administration of UVA in the PhPT, because this identifies UVA-sensitive patients. In these patients, the UVA MED can be determined using the same UVA source as that to be used for PhPT; a suitable dose for PhPT may be 50% of their UVA MED [33]. Such patients have an increased risk of photoexacerbated reactions (irritant and allergic) [2, 35], which are of uncertain relevance and may be falsely interpreted as indicating photoallergy. Ideally, the UVA MED should be tested in all patients prior to PhPT, but this is not essential.

27.6　Allergen Application and Reading of Reactions

Testing should be conducted on skin that has been clinically normal for the preceding two weeks [2]. Patients should be advised of the possible risks of sensitization and strong reactions, preferably with an information sheet. The mid-upper back skin is used, avoiding the paravertebral groove. Two identical sets of allergens are applied as parallel series on either side of the back using conventional patch-test techniques. Two days later, both are discarded and the sites are examined for reactions, which are recorded using the standard scoring system. One set of sites is shielded while the other is irradiated with UVA. A reading immediately after irradiation (up to 20 min later) is sometimes performed, and detects immediate phototoxic urticarial reactions that may occur with, for example, benzophenone-3 [36]. In sunny

Whole-body units can be used with appropriate shielding, or, more conveniently, small-area units (of the kind used for hand/foot PUVA) can be mounted on a wall. The irradiance of the latter varies with the distance from the lamps, so the gap should be maintained at 15 cm from the front panel; then, a change of ±5 cm causes a change in dose of ±12% [7]. The UVA output may fluctuate over weeks to months, so the apparatus must be regularly calibrated.

The dose of UVA has traditionally been 5–15 J/cm^2. The dose needs to be low enough not to cause sunburn; in white subjects, the UVA minimum erythema dose (MED) of unacclimatized upper-back skin is about 15–20 J/cm^2 (95% confidence interval; 8–40 $J/$

Table 2. Photopatch testing: choice of photoallergens [2, 7]. This table lists the photoallergens suggested by two working groups for routine inclusion in photopatch series. (*BPG*, British Photodermatology Group [7], *ETPT*, European Taskforce for Photopatch Testing [2].) All agents are available through Hermal (Trolab) or Chemotechnique Diagnostics, except those marked with *, which need to be prepared "in-house"

		BPG (%)	ETPT (%)
Control	Petrolatum	100	100
UV filters	PABA	5 or 10	10
	Ethylhexyl dimethyl PABA	2 or 10	10
	Ethylhexyl methoxycinnamate (Parsol MCX[b])	2 or 10	10
	Benzophenone-3 (Oxybenzone[a])	2 or 10	10
	Butyl methoxydibenzoylmethane (Parsol 1789[b], Avobenzone[a])	2 or 10	10
	4-Methylbenzylidene camphor (Mexoryl SD[b])	–	10
	Benzophenone-4	–	10
	Isoamyl p-methoxycinnamate	–	10
	Phenylbenzimidazole sulfonic acid	–	10
NSAIDs	Naproxen	–	5*
	Ibuprofen	–	5*
	Diclofenac	–	1*
	Ketoprofen	–	2.5*
Other	Musk ambrette	1 or 5	–
	Patients' own products	As appropriate	As appropriate

The first name in the list is the International Nomenclature of Cosmetic Ingredients (*INCI*) name, which must be used for ingredient labeling purposes in Europe.
[a] International Nonproprietary Names (INN names)
[b] Trade name

climates, all sites should then be covered with opaque material. Two days later, the sites are examined again.

Some variations on this scheme are used with no published evidence to favor one over the others. In the most common variant, the sites are occluded with allergen for only 1 day (protocol 2 in Table 3). This decreased occlusion time does not seem to reduce the sensitivity of the test and it does permit, within a

Monday–Friday protocol, a reading 3 days after irradiation. At this time, photoallergic reactions may be more obvious and more easily distinguished from phototoxic reactions by the "crescendo" pattern (see below). A later reading after 1 week has also been proposed [37]. The relevance of the result should be determined.

The penetration of PhPT allergens can be increased by "scarifying" the skin or tape-stripping

Table 3. Commonly used photopatch test protocols

Protocol	Day						
	0	1	2	3	4	5	6
1	Application of allergens		Irradiate with 5 J/cm² UVA; immediate reading		Reading	[a]	[a]
2	Application of allergens	Irradiate with 5 J/cm² UVA; immediate reading		Reading	[a]	[a]	[a]

[a] Desirable but not essential reading

[38], or using a prick method [39], but these techniques are now rarely used.

27.7 Interpretation of Results

If there is a reaction to the UVA alone, then the patient is UVA-sensitive and the PhPT results should usually be disregarded; if necessary, the test may be repeated with a lower dose of UVA.

Assuming this has not occurred, there are seven possible reactions to PhPT:

- *Negative*
- *Photoallergic*
- *Phototoxic*
- *Irritant* (unlikely to be clinically relevant):
- *Photo-augmented irritant* (unlikely to be clinically relevant)
- *Photo-suppressed irritant* (unlikely to be clinically relevant)
- *Allergic*:
- *Photo-augmented allergic*
- *Photo-suppressed allergic*

No reaction at the unirradiated site but a reaction at the irradiated site signifies photoallergy. Equal reactions at both sites are interpreted as "ordinary" allergy. Allergic and photoallergic reactions, when strongly positive, are usually easy to interpret. However, diagnostic difficulties arise with weaker reactions and two particular issues have to be considered.

27.7.1 Photoallergy vs Phototoxicity

The tendency of the agent in question to give phototoxic reactions at the concentration and UVA dose being used should be known. Weak reactions tend to be phototoxic and strong ones photoallergic. A peak of the reaction within the first 24 h ("decrescendo") tends to indicate phototoxicity, whereas a reaction that becomes stronger after 24 h ("crescendo") tends to indicate photoallergy [5, 40]. However, these criteria often fail to distinguish the nature of reactions. When they were used in an analysis of 1,500 patients with 2,859 positive reactions, 28% of reactions were phototoxic, 4% were photoallergic, and 27% of reactions had a reaction pattern that did not fit into the typical patterns of either phototoxicity or photoallergy [40]. In addition, 29% were classified as allergic reactions (erythematous or palpable immediately after removal of the patches; the possibility of subsequent exacerbation or suppression of these reactions

by UV was not examined) and 12% as immediate, short-lived, non-specific reactions. The agents making up the 27% of reactions not fitting the typical patterns of either phototoxicity or photoallergy were, particularly, NSAIDs, phenothiazines, and disinfectants, and were thought to mostly have phototoxic mechanisms.

One method to distinguish photoallergy from phototoxicity is to carry out a serial dilution of the suspected photoallergen and also vary the dose of irradiation, for example, using a series from 10–50% of the UVA MED [7]. A positive response at a very low concentration and/or a very low UV dose points to photoallergy rather than phototoxicity. It is helpful to test controls negatively to exclude phototoxicity. Histology may be helpful to distinguish phototoxic reactions from photoallergic ones.

27.7.2 The Possibility of Photo-augmentation or Photo-suppression of Simple Allergic and Irritant Reactions

It is well known that UV has a profound suppressive effect on the *sensitization* phase of contact hypersensitivity (in one model, 93% suppression from one exposure to a dose of UV equal to double the minimum erythema dose [41]). However, in this context, we are concerned with the effect of one exposure to UVA on the *elicitation* phase and, here, the picture is more complicated. Murine studies show that UV may actually augment the elicitation phase [42–44], and this also seems to occur in a considerable proportion of people [45–47]. The effect may be age-dependent, with older individuals being less likely to undergo photo-suppression [46]. Photo-augmentation of irritant reactions has also been shown to occur [47].

Therefore, reactions where both sites are positive but the irradiated site is only slightly stronger should be interpreted with caution. It is, of course, possible that such reactions indicate that contact allergy is co-existing with photoallergy, but this may be rare in comparison to the phenomenon of photo-augmentation of simple contact reactions. Furthermore, weakly positive reactions at an irradiated site with negative reactions at the unirradiated site could be due to photo-augmentation of an otherwise subclinical contact allergy.

27.8 Summary

So, from all of the above discussion, there are four factors that can lead to a false diagnosis of photoallergy: (1) phototoxicity; (2) photo-augmentation of irritant responses; (3) photo-augmentation of allergic responses; and (4) technical error. With these issues in mind, the results of PhPT can be interpreted.

References

1. Darvay A, White IR, Rycroft RJ, Jones AB, Hawk JL, McFadden JP (2001) Photoallergic contact dermatitis is uncommon. Br J Dermatol 145:597–601
2. Bruynzeel DP, Ferguson J, Andersen K, Goncalo M, English J, Goossens A, Holzle E, Ibbotson SH, Lecha M, Lehmann P, Leonard F, Moseley H, Pigatto P, Tanew A; European Taskforce for Photopatch Testing (2004) Photopatch testing: a consensus methodology for Europe. J Eur Acad Dermatol Venereol 18:679–682
3. Wennersten G, Thune P, Brodthagen H, Jansen C, Rystedt I (1984) The Scandinavian multicenter photopatch study. Preliminary results. Contact Dermatitis 10:305–309
4. Jansen CT, Wennersten G, Rystedt I, Thune P, Brodthagen H (1982) The Scandinavian standard photopatch test procedure. Contact Dermatitis 8:155–158
5. Neumann NJ, Holzle E, Plewig G, Schwarz T, Panizzon RG, Breit R, Ruzicka T, Lehmann P (2000) Photopatch testing: the 12-year experience of the German, Austrian, and Swiss photopatch test group. J Am Acad Dermatol 42:183–192
6. Pigatto PD, Legori A, Bigardi AS, Guarrera M, Tosti A, Santucci B, Monfrecola G, Schena D (1996) Gruppo Italiano Ricerca Dermatiti da Contatto ed Ambientali Italian Multicenter Study of Allergic Contact Photodermatitis: epidemiological aspects. Am J Contact Dermat 7:158–163
7. British Photodermatology Group (1997) Photopatch testing: methods and indications. Br J Dermatol 136:371–376
8. Bell HK, Rhodes LE (2000) Photopatch testing in photosensitive patients. Br J Dermatol 142:589–590
9. Thune P, Jansen C, Wennersten G, Rystedt I, Brodthagen H, McFadden N (1988) The Scandinavian multicenter photopatch study 1980–1985: final report. Photodermatology 5:261–269
10. Bilsland D, Ferguson J (1993) Contact allergy to sunscreen chemicals in photosensitivity dermatitis/actinic reticuloid syndrome (PD/AR) and polymorphic light eruption (PLE). Contact Dermatitis 29:70–73
11. DeLeo VA, Suarez SM, Maso MJ (1992) Photoallergic contact dermatitis. Results of photopatch testing in New York, 1985 to 1990. Arch Dermatol 128:1513–1518
12. Fotiades J, Soter NA, Lim HW (1995) Results of evaluation of 203 patients for photosensitivity in a 7.3-year period. J Am Acad Dermatol 33:597–602
13. Holzle E, Neumann N, Hausen B, Przybilla B, Schauder S, Honigsmann H, Bircher A, Plewig G (1991) Photopatch testing: the 5-year experience of the German, Austrian, and Swiss Photopatch Test Group. J Am Acad Dermatol 25:59–68
14. Bryden AM, Ibbotson SH, Ferguson J (on behalf of the UK Multicentre Photopatch Group) (2003) Photopatch testing: results of the U.K. multicentre photopatch study. Br J Dermatol 149(Suppl 64):3 (abstract)
15. Berne B, Ros AM (1998) 7 years experience of photopatch testing with sunscreen allergens in Sweden. Contact Dermatitis 38:61–64
16. Wilkinson DS (1961) Photodermatitis due to tetrachlorsalicylanilide. Br J Dermatol 73:213–219
17. Larsen W (1978) Photoallergy to musk ambrette found in an aftershave lotion. Presented at the American Academy of Dermatology meeting, San Francisco, California, December 1978
18. Cronin E (1984) Photosensitivity to musk ambrette. Contact Dermatitis 11:88–92
19. English JSC, White IR, Cronin E (1987) Sensitivity to sunscreens. Contact Dermatitis 17:159–162
20. Schauder S, Ippen H (1997) Contact and photocontact sensitivity to sunscreens. Review of a 15-year experience and of the literature. Contact Dermatitis 37:221–232
21. Ang P, Ng SK, Goh CL (1998) Sunscreen allergy in Singapore. Am J Contact Dermat 9:42–44
22. Dromgoole SH, Maibach HI (1990) Sunscreening agent intolerance: contact and photocontact sensitization and contact urticaria. J Am Acad Dermatol 22:1068–1078
23. Horio T (1975) Chlorpromazine photoallergy. Coexistence of immediate and delayed type. Arch Dermatol 111:1469–1471
24. Durieu C, Marguery MC, Giordano-Labadie F, Journe F, Loche F, Bazex J (2001) Photoaggravated contact allergy and contact photoallergy caused by ketoprofen: 19 cases. Ann Dermatol Venereol 128:1020–1024
25. Adamski H, Benkalfate L, Delaval Y, Ollivier I, le Jean S, Toubel G, le Hir-Garreau I, Chevrant-Breton J (1998) Photodermatitis from non-steroidal anti-inflammatory drugs. Contact Dermatitis 38:171–174
26. Durbize E, Vigan M, Puzenat E, Girardin P, Adessi B, Desprez PH, Humbert PH, Laurent R, Aubin F (2003) Spectrum of cross-photosensitization in 18 consecutive patients with contact photoallergy to ketoprofen: associated photoallergies to non-benzophenone-containing molecules. Contact Dermatitis 48:144–149
27. Matthieu L, Meuleman L, Van Hecke E, Blondeel A, Dezfoulian B, Constandt L, Goossens A (2004) Contact and photocontact allergy to ketoprofen. The Belgian experience. Contact Dermatitis 50:238–241
28. Lovell CR (1993) Plants and the skin, 1st edn. Blackwell Scientific Publications, Oxford, UK
29. De Groot AC, Weyland JW, Nater JP (1994) Unwanted effects of cosmetics and drugs used in dermatology, 3rd edn. Elsevier, Amsterdam, The Netherlands, pp 136–154
30. Goossens A (2004) Photoallergic contact dermatitis. Photodermatol Photoimmunol Photomed 20:121–125
31. Bosca F, Miranda MA, Carganico G, Mauleon D (1994) Photochemical and photobiological properties of ketoprofen associated with the benzophenone chromophore. Photochem Photobiol 60:96–101
32. Dooms-Goossens A, Chrispeels MT, De Veylden H, Roelandts R, Willems L, Degreef H (1987) Contact and photocontact sensitivity problems associated with thiourea and its derivatives: a review of the literature and case reports. Br J Dermatol 116:573–579
33. Duguid C, O'Sullivan D, Murphy GM (1993) Determination of threshold UV-A elicitation dose in photopatch testing. Contact Dermatitis 29:192–194
34. Hasan T, Jansen CT (1996) Photopatch test reactivity: effect of photoallergen concentration and UVA dosaging. Contact Dermatitis 34:383–386
35. Addo HA, Sharma SC, Ferguson J, Johnson BE, Frain-Bell W (1985) A study of compositae plant extract reactions in photosensitivity dermatitis. Photodermatology 2:68–79

36. Collins P, Ferguson J (1994) Photoallergic contact dermatitis to oxybenzone. Br J Dermatol 131:124–129

37. DeLeo V, Gonzalez E, Kim J, Lim H (2000) Phototesting and photopatch testing: when to do it and when not to do it. Am J Contact Dermat 11:57–61

38. Hölzle E, Plewig G, Lehmann P (1987) Photodermatoses – diagnostic procedures and their interpretation. Photodermatology 4:109–114

39. Bourrain JL, Paillet C, Woodward C, Beani JC, Amblard P (1997) Diagnosis of photosensitivity to flupenthixol by photoprick testing. Photodermatol Photoimmunol Photomed 13:159–161

40. Neumann NJ, Holzle E, Lehmann P, Benedikter S, Tapernoux B, Plewig G (1994) Pattern analysis of photopatch test reactions. Photodermatol Photoimmunol Photomed 10:65–73

41. Kelly DA, Young AR, McGregor JM, Seed PT, Potten CS, Walker SL (2000) Sensitivity to sunburn is associated with susceptibility to ultraviolet radiation-induced suppression of cutaneous cell-mediated immunity. J Exp Med 191:561–566

42. Polla L, Margolis R, Goulston C, Parrish JA, Granstein RD (1986) Enhancement of the elicitation phase of the murine contact hypersensitivity response by prior exposure to local ultraviolet radiation. J Invest Dermatol 86:13–17

43. Yoshikawa T, Kurimoto I, Streilein JW (1992) Tumour necrosis factor-alpha mediates ultraviolet light B-enhanced expression of contact hypersensitivity. Immunology 76:264–271

44. Grabbe S, Steinbrink K, Steinert M, Luger TA, Schwarz T (1995) Removal of the majority of epidermal Langerhans cells by topical or systemic steroid application enhances the effector phase of murine contact hypersensitivity. J Immunol 155:4207–4217

45. Tie C, Golomb C, Taylor JR, Streilein JW (1995) Suppressive and enhancing effects of ultraviolet B radiation on expression of contact hypersensitivity in man. J Invest Dermatol 104:18–22

46. Palmer RA, Hawk JLM, Young AR, Walker SL (2005) The effect of solar-simulated radiation on the elicitation phase of contact hypersensitivity does not differ between controls and patients with polymorphic light eruption. J Invest Dermatol 124:1308–1312

47. Beattie PE, Traynor NJ, Woods JA, Dawe RS, Ferguson J, Ibbotson SH (2004) Can a positive photopatch test be elicited by subclinical irritancy or allergy plus suberythemal UV exposure? Contact Dermatitis 51:235–240

27

Chapter 28

Noninvasive Techniques for Quantification of Contact Dermatitis

28

Jørgen Serup

Contents

28.1 Introduction

History and clinical examination are the main tools of clinical dermatologists. Inspection of the skin is rapid, and the lateral extension and severity of a dermatitis are easily assessed. The disadvantage is that this method is, essentially, subjective. As a research tool, it is open to bias and is, thus, difficult to use. With punch biopsy and microscopy, detailed information about the layers of the skin and their involvement with dermatitis is obtained; however, a punch usually represents only a very small fraction of diseased skin, and processing and staining are a kind of desirable artifact. The result still has a subjective element, which is related to the pathologist's examination.

Information and knowledge are not simply a matter of high magnification and fine detail. In the dermatological armamentarium, there is an area between clinical evaluation and sophisticated technique, where noninvasive bioengineering techniques may be relevant. Bioengineering techniques offer: (1) noninvasiveness and in vivo information, with instant results; (2) objective assessment (quantitation or imaging as a basis for computerized analysis); (3) choice of body region and site of examination, with only a few limitations, depending on technique; and (4) the same site can be studied by different techniques, and follow-up examinations can be performed to study the spontaneous course and effect of treatment, without interfering with the subject being studied.

28.2 Prerequisites and Planning of Study by Noninvasive Techniques

Various devices for the noninvasive evaluation of the skin have become available. It is straightforward to put a probe on the skin and to get a reading on a digital display. Generally, variation and inconclusiveness are more likely to be attributable to the way in which devices are used, rather than to inaccuracy of the equipment. Before a study based on bioengineering methods is conducted, the essentials of the method need to be known, and a number of questions must be asked. These include the following:

- What information is expected?
- What is the most relevant variable to be measured, and which variables serve for description, comparison, support, or exclusion?
- What is the expected time course of variables, and when should measurements be performed?
- Are variables expected to develop linearly or not?
- What are the ranges of variables in relation to the expected phenomenon or structure being studied, including interindividual and intraindividual variation and dependence of anatomical site, sex, and age?
- What function or structure is actually being tested?
- What is the measuring area, and, if small, should more recordings be taken and averaged to overcome local site variation?

28

- Are recordings with the equipment reproducible, and is the accuracy acceptable relative to variables being measured and their expected range?
- What are the measuring standards and calibration procedures?
- Are there environmental standards and calibration procedures?
- Are there environmental influences, including season, and a need for special laboratory room facilities?
- Is preconditioning of the individual necessary before testing?
- What precludes measurements from being performed?
- Has the researcher or technician both the training and sufficient practical experience to conduct the study?

As in any other research field, the results depend essentially on the ratio between signal and noise, where noise means sources of variation, some predictable, others unknown. At the moment, the success of studies based on noninvasive techniques depends mainly on the training of the researcher and appropriate planning, with an emphasis on proper control of predictable sources of variation.

28.3 Review of Noninvasive Techniques Relevant to the Study of Contact Dermatitis

The essentials of skin structure and function as a basis for bioengineering studies were reviewed in the past by Frosch and Kligman [1] and more recently by Goldsmith [2] and Serup and Jemec [3]. Various monographs about bioengineering methods and their technical principles and applications have appeared [3–7]. Previously, bioengineering and the patch test were summarized [8].

Several noninvasive techniques were used in the past to study contact dermatitis, often prototypes or laboratory equipment. Some techniques, such as polysulfide rubber replica, are simple and can be used directly, while others are complicated, and validation, multiplication, and commercialization are needed before they can attract general interest. This introduction deals mainly with techniques that are available and which can be practiced in a variety of laboratories.

28.3.1 Changes in the Skin Surface

A change of color and skin surface are central to the visual assessment of contact dermatitis. The color of the skin, including erythema, can be measured by two different principles: (1) spectrophotometric scanning, using wavelengths of 400–800 nm and measurements of absorbency and reflectance; and (2) tristimulus analysis of reflected flash light. Spectrophotometric scanning has proven to be of little practical use because the broad melanin absorption band overlaps with the hemoglobin band, and because nonspecific optical phenomena of the skin, related to scaling and scattering, influence recordings significantly.

However, devices that measure the hemoglobin band specifically and express erythema as an index of hemoglobin relative to melanin have appeared; if they are of technically high precision, these devices are useful [9].

The alinear perception of color by the human eye and brain is in the range 400–800 nm, with the most sensitive range of detection being between 500 nm and 600 nm, corresponding to the color of blood and, therefore, redness. Equipment based on tristimulus analysis of reflected light and the Commission International d'Eclairage (CIE) takes this alinearity of the eye into account and expresses any color in a three-dimensional system (Fig. 1), with green–red ($a\star$), yellow–blue ($b\star$), and L axes, where $L\star$ expresses brightness [10]. In erythema, $a\star$ increases, $L\star$ decreases, and $b\star$ is unaltered [11]. Tristimulus devices are convenient and rapid to operate.

The contour of the skin surface, with scales, papules, vesicles, etc., can be studied by clinical photography and by various replica techniques. The main difficulty of close-up photography is that the flashgun light, after scattering within the skin, is reflected back to the camera lens from different layers of the skin with different microstructures and under different angles from the same structure. Skin surface pictures become much sharper if the surface is coated and transmission and scattering are eliminated. If immersion oil is applied and the optical effects of the surface are thus eliminated, dermal structures, such as blood vessels, may be seen. Reflections from the surface may also be avoided by using polarized light. In clinical photography, the film and copy process are also subject to variation between batches, with significant influences on the photograph [12]. Today, digital photography is taking over. This allows sophisticated image analysis of color and surface structures of clinical relevance. Using polysulfide rubber imprint material, 30° incident light, and a stereomi-

Fig. 1.
The Commission International d'Eclairage (*CIE*) color system, which is essentially constructed to substitute for the human eye, taking the alinearity of color perception into account. Each color has its position in a three-dimensional coordinate system, with two horizontal axes for color and a vertical axis for brightness

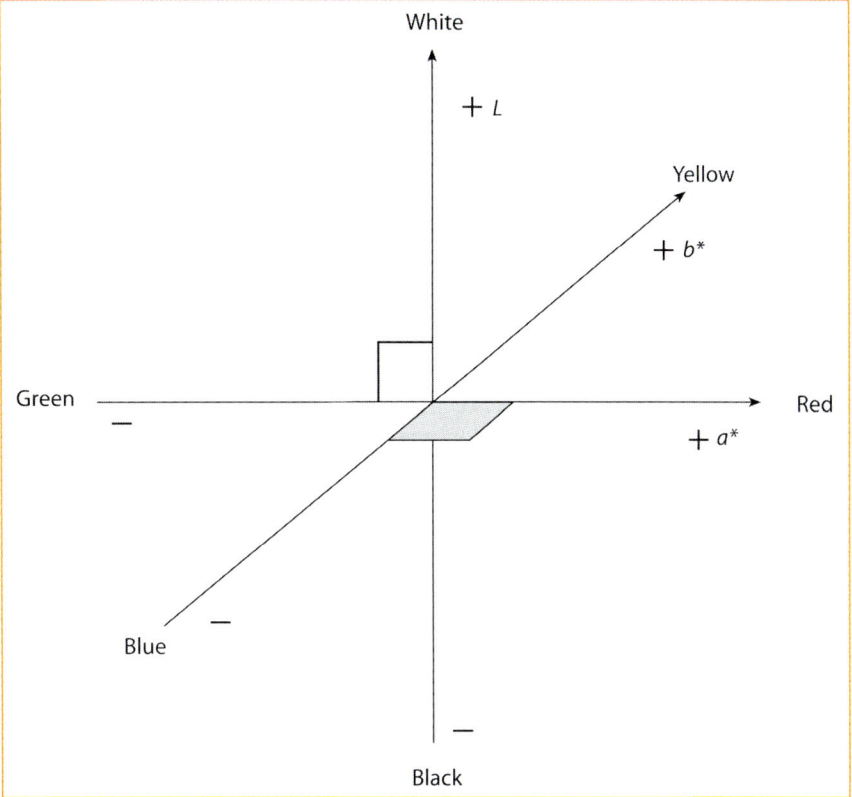

croscope surface, the finer details are clearly illustrated, since the flexible rubber material is not transparent. Replicas are cheap and simple and can be stored and evaluated blind and in batches under routine laboratory conditions. Replicas can also be used as a basis for advanced quantification by the stylus method and by computerized image analysis [13]. A tape method, representing a development of the sticky slide technique for harvesting stratum corneum material, is commonly employed. This is useful for quantitative evaluation of the scaling and hyperkeratosis of dermatitis [14].

28.3.2 Epidermal Hydration and Water Barrier Function

Although invisibly, the water barrier of the skin is very often damaged in dermatitis, with consequences for the biology of the epidermis and the clinical manifestations. Hydration of the skin surface can be measured by electrical methods [15, 16]. The construction of the detector and the technical specifications determine the layer of the epidermis that is measured. The contour of the skin and the size and shape of the detector determine the electrical contact and influence the results. If the detector is small,

more measurements need to be taken and averaged to minimize local site variation. The conductance measurer described by Tagami [16] measures very superficially, and the Corneometer of Courage and Khazaka, based on electrical capacitance, is able to measure more deeply in the epidermis [17, 18]. The compartment of the epidermis that is able to bind water is only small, and diffusional equilibrium between stratum corneum and ambient air takes place quickly, i.e., within 10 min [19]. Following occlusion, the biology of the epidermis changes, and equilibrium with ambient air takes longer, i.e., after 24 h of occlusion, 30 min or longer. Thus, when skin surface hydration is being measured, the skin should be uncovered for a predetermined period before the recordings. The temperature and humidity of the laboratory also need to be kept within certain limits.

The parameter of transepidermal water loss (TEWL) expresses diffusional water loss through the skin and is of major importance in irritant reactions to detergents. Various closed-chamber methods have been used in the past; however, these were cumbersome and interfered with the spontaneous TEWL parameter. The method of open-chamber water vapor evaporation and gradient estimation, as described by Nilsson [20] and Spencer [21], is widely used. The water vapor pressure gradient is measured with sensors

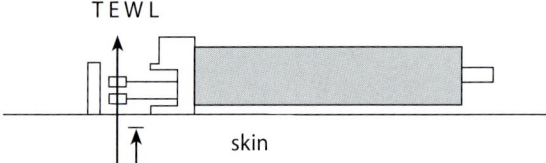

Fig. 2. Open-chamber probe for the measurement of the TEWL. Pairs of sensors (hygrosensors coupled with thermistors) mounted in the chamber at different levels above the skin for the determination of the humidity gradient in the chamber, representing the flux of water out of the skin, or the TEWL

28

(Fig. 2) at two different levels above the skin, and then the TEWL is calculated [20, 21]. Proper preconditioning and good control of the measuring conditions is essential for accurate recordings. Sources of variation were reviewed and guidelines were given by the standardization group of the European Society of Contact Dermatitis (ESCD) [22]. The water barrier of the skin does not resemble a filter or membrane within the skin, but, instead, a gradient across the skin, including a 10-mm layer of ambient air. Thus, the environment is part of the water barrier, and changes in temperature and humidity influence the passage of water out of the skin, and also the skin surface's hydration. Eccrine sweating is, in most body regions, less important, except after physical activity, when it has the capacity to increase manifoldly. Environmental changes related to the seasons also need to be considered [23].

28.3.3 Parameters of Inflammation

Vasodilatation and edema formation are the essential features of inflammation. Blood flow has been extensively studied, while edema formation has been comparatively overlooked.

The use of the skin surface's temperature as a measure of inflammatory activity is more or less obsolete in contact dermatitis. In normal skin, the temperature varies within narrow limits. In dermatitis, vasodilatation tends to increase the temperature towards the core temperature, but evaporation, crusting, and scaling tend to decrease the temperature. Skin surface temperature can be measured by contact methods, including cholesteric crystal sheets, and by infrared nontouch methods. The main application of contact thermography in contact dermatitis is to image lateral temperature gradients, which may give detailed information about inflammation and crusting of patch test reactions [7, 24, 25].

The *vasodilatation* of inflammation and the increase in blood flow is often measured by laser Dop-

pler flowmetry [6]. A variety of equipment is available. The tone of the cutaneous vasculature is normally in a relatively contracted condition, and it may be difficult to monitor vasoconstriction, such as blanching, due to corticosteroids. A 30-fold increase in flow may be seen in dermatitis; however, in advanced inflammation, the edema may compress vessels, and the degree of inflammatory activity may be underestimated. As compared with other methods, laser Doppler flowmetry is both sensitive and discriminative. Recently, laser Doppler scanners have been developed. With this method, the mapping of, for example, the hyperperfusion of a patch reaction is possible (Fig. 3). Site variation in patch test reactions is major. With the scanner, the average hyperperfusion is easily calculated. The vasculature and its tone are in a state of dynamic balance, and factors such as mental stress and noise instantly influence the flow. Thus, both preconditioning and measuring conditions need to be considered.

Measurement of the *edema* of inflammatory reactions may be carried out with skin-fold calipers and with high-frequency ultrasound (Fig. 4). Calipers inevitably compress the edema, and it is unclear what layer of the skin is being included in the fold and measured. With ultrasound, high frequency and broad bandwidth are needed. Transducers of 20 MHz have provided a good compromise between the needs of resolution and depth of the viewing field. With A-mode scanners, the thickness of dermatitis skin can be measured and the increase in thickness representing the edema formation calculated [26]. With B-mode and C-mode scanners, cross-sectional imaging of the skin is possible [27]. In vivo distances, areas, volume, and structure analysis are possible

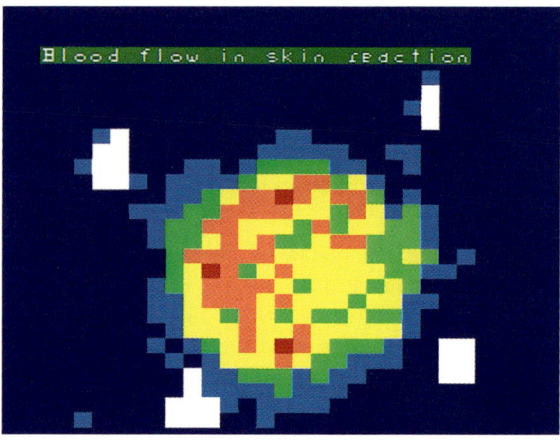

Fig. 3. Laser Doppler scanning. Irritant reaction to sodium lauryl sulfate (*SLS*). *Red* is high perfusion, *blue* is low. *White pixels* represent markings made on the skin with black ink

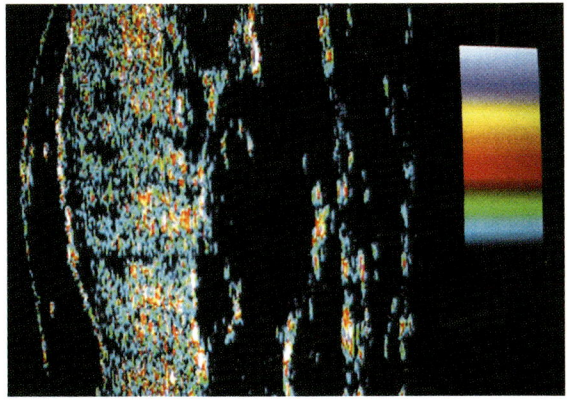

Fig. 4. High-frequency B-mode scanning of a 2+ allergic reaction to nickel, obtained with Dermascan C. A plastic membrane from the probe chamber is seen over the skin. Underneath the epidermis, an echolucent band of edema formation appears, with projections along the hair follicles and sebaceous glands. *White* and *blue* represent strong ultrasound reflections, *yellow* and *red* moderate, and *green* weak reflections. Subcutaneous fat is minimally echogenic and is shown in *black*, as is the coupling medium between the ultrasound transducer and the skin surface with the plastic membrane

with the use of computerized analysis. Ultrasound shows that inflammatory edema develops mainly in the papillary dermis, where it propagates and results in an echolucent band, which can be measured and followed during the different stages of the inflammatory process (Fig. 4). Education and training are needed in order to perform ultrasound examination, as in any other specialty. Generally, methods assessing static features, such as structure and dimension, are less vulnerable to measuring conditions and are easier to standardize compared to methods based on functions.

28.4 Allergic Contact Dermatitis

Erythema, edema, papules, and vesicles are the well known manifestations of acute allergic contact dermatitis that are read in diagnostic patch testing. Using noninvasive techniques, the same manifestations can be quantified. In strong reactions, bullae, erosions, and crusts may appear. Once elicited, it is held that the cascade of events follows essentially the same course. In the chronic stage, hyperkeratosis and scaling are often prominent. Unlike the situation in irritant contact dermatitis, allergic reactions have been relatively seldom studied by noninvasive techniques in the past.

Study of the skin surface contour by polysulfide rubber replica shows that counts of papules and vesicles correlate with clinical readings, and doubtful reactions may be divided into those with sporadic papules and those without, but with an impression from the margin of the test chamber instead [28].

Studies of skin color and allergic contact dermatitis have not appeared. It is likely that weak and moderate reactions can be ranked, but in strong reactions, changes of the physical character of the skin surface are likely to influence the optical properties and create variation.

Epidermal hydration and TEWL depend very much on the clinical state of the dermatitis. In chronic dermatitis with scaling, the conductance is decreased, due to a reduced water-binding capacity, in contrast to TEWL, which is increased [29]. The value of conductance measurements seems to lie not in the grading of early-stage dermatitis, but in the assessment of chronic stages and documentation of healing. Decreased conductance and increased TEWL are very common in long-lasting dermatitis, irrespective of its origin. Nevertheless, increased TEWL is not a primary event in allergic reactions; rather, the water barrier becomes progressively damaged during the first few days, as inflammation develops [30].

The surface temperature of acute allergic reactions is increased; however, if vesicles and bullae leaving crusts appear, the temperature pattern of the surface may be irregular, with decreased temperature corresponding to the crusts [24, 25, 31]. Increased temperature may persist for a period after visible changes have disappeared [7].

Allergic reactions to nickel show increased blood flow as measured by laser Doppler flowmetry, and positive, doubtful, and negative reactions can be distinguished [32]. However, the positive reactions may be difficult to rank. Probably, the inflammatory response has an initial stage dominated by vasodilation and a more advanced stage dominated by edema formation, which compresses the vasculature. Allergic patch test reactions and irritant reactions to sodium lauryl sulfate (SLS) show an increase of blood flow at the same level [33].

Ultrasound measurement of skin thickness and the edema of allergic patch test reactions show progressive thickening of the skin as the clinical reaction increases [26, 27, 34]. With ultrasound, strong reactions can also be graded. The edema formation of allergic reactions is more severe as compared with irritant reactions after SLS, matched with respect to the strength of the reactions clinically [26]. With ultrasound B-mode scanning, an echolucent band is seen in the papillary dermis immediately underneath the epidermis, representing more advanced edema and swelling of the outer dermis (Fig. 4) [27]. It is a general feature that the inflammation of contact dermatitis involves mainly the papillary dermis, which is more easily distended than the reticular dermis under the influence of the pressure of edema. Such changes cannot be evaluated by routine histology, since histological processing is highly intrusive to tissue water, which is extracted and replaced by lipophilic media prior to embedding in paraffin.

28.5 Irritant Contact Dermatitis

Irritant contact dermatitis is not a uniform disease entity; each irritant exerts its particular noxious effects on the skin, and each occupation has its special set of risk substances and mode of physical contact [35]. Obviously, this creates diversity in the manifestations of irritancy and the way in which it is best assessed. Moreover, reactions are dependent on age, body region, menstrual phase, skin complexion, and skin type, including sensitivity to sunlight, etc. Thus, control of a great number of variables is a prerequisite.

A number of substances and test procedures were evaluated in the past by Björnberg [36] and more recently by Frosch [37]. Monographs on irritant contact dermatitis and TEWL have been published by van der Valk [38], Pinnagoda [39], and Tupker [40]. Irritancy and laser Doppler flowmetry was studied by de Boer [41], and Agner has studied irritancy by various methods, including replica, thermography, TEWL, laser Doppler flowmetry, colorimetry, high-frequency ultrasound, and conductance [42].

The change in color in the direction of redness as elicited by the irritant SLS is characterized by an increase in a^*, a minor decrease in L^*, and unchanged b^*, as measured according to the CIE system [11]. Colorimeters based on the CIE system and tristimulus color analysis are especially suited to a busy routine and for situations in which preconditioning is difficult. Colorimetry appears accurate for the distinction of positive reactions from negative reactions; however, colorimetry is less precise for a more differentiated ranking of redness, depending on the irritant being studied [42, 43]. A major reason why the grading of redness can be difficult is that the vasodilatation of inflammation, as mentioned above, does not run linearly, but fades out as the edema progresses. Moreover, microanatomical changes in the skin surface of strong reactions influence the optical properties of the skin nonspecifically, with consequences for the measurement of color. In chronic dermatitis, hyperkeratosis and scaling may influence colorimeter measurements.

The skin surface contour changes depending on the irritant and the time of examination, as demonstrated by studies with polysulfide rubber replica [44]. Sodium lauryl sulphate (SLS) has become the preferred experimental irritant. Some irritants induce a papular pattern; others, a nonpapular pattern. Propanol, which is used as a vehicle for nonanoic acid, is itself irritant and changes the skin relief.

The skin surface hydration of irritant contact dermatitis is the result of damage to the cutaneous water barrier induced by the irritant on the one hand, resulting in increased water vapor pressure in and over the stratum corneum, and, by the formation of crusts, hyperkeratosis and scales on the other, resulting in reduced water-binding capacity and decreased stratum corneum hydration. Already in the acute stage of dermatitis, most irritants exert a noxious effect, with a decrease of electrical conductance and capacitance, depending on the specific irritant and its ability to coagulate the skin surface, while increased hydration is found only in some individuals and mainly from the detergent SLS [18]. In chronic-stage contact dermatitis, the electrical measurements are decreased almost without exception [29]. Due to the variable structure and pathophysiology of acute irritant reactions, electrical methods have not been found to be very useful for the grading of irritancy [43].

Measurement of the TEWL and damage to the water barrier have proven to be important for the characterization of irritant effects on skin elicited by detergents [38–40, 42]. Studies using mainly SLS as a model detergent have demonstrated that the TEWL measurement is more accurate than other methods, such as laser Doppler flowmetry, colorimetry, and ultrasound, for the grading of this irritant [39, 40, 42, 43, 45]. Impairment of the water barrier and increase of the TEWL are found not only in the acute stage of dermatitis, but also in chronic stages, with hyperkeratosis and scaling [29]. The difficulty with TEWL is that a number of prerequisites with respect to preconditioning and laboratory conditions need to be fulfilled for measurements to be accurate, as described by the standardization group [21]. It must be stressed again that different irritants act differently on the skin, and experiences obtained with detergents cannot be uncritically extended to any other substance [35, 44, 45]. The use of TEWL to detect sensitive skin and predict the occupational risk of irritant contact dermatitis is described below.

Skin-surface temperature, as mentioned above, is not an accurate measure of the inflammatory activity of irritant contact dermatitis. However, thermographic imaging of skin-surface temperature gradients demonstrates that some reactions to irritants are cold, due to the formation of a temperature-insulating crusting, while others are warm [24, 25, 31]. Different skin-surface temperature patterns appear during the course of irritant reactions, and such patterns may be followed using thermographic methods and compared with allergic reactions.

Laser Doppler flowmetry has been used extensively for the evaluation of irritant contact dermatitis [41, 42, 46]. Experiments with SLS and laser Doppler flowmetry have demonstrated a dose–response relationship [41–43, 45, 46], and the method has proven to be valuable for the quantification of irritant reactions and their inflammatory component. In the evaluation of reactions elicited by SLS, laser Doppler flowmetry with monochannel equipment is less accurate than TEWL and ultrasound measurements [43, 45]. However, with modern laser scanners, the precision is substantially improved (Fig. 3). As noted above, the edema of strong reactions may compress the vasculature and influence the flow. Also, changes in the skin surface, such as vesicles, bullae, crusts, hyperkeratosis, and scaling, may influence the optics of the skin and the laser signal. Using probes covering a small surface area only, averaging of three or more recordings is necessary to overcome local site variation in the cutaneous blood supply. The laser Doppler method registers the total blood flow, and recordings are easily influenced by the measuring conditions, such as talking, breathing, noise, and mental stress. Thus, preconditioning and laboratory conditions need to be carefully controlled.

28.5.1 Edema

High-frequency (20 MHz) ultrasound measurement of skin thickening and edema formation has been used in numerous studies of SLS irritant reactions [26, 27, 42, 43, 45], and a dose–response relationship has been demonstrated. For the evaluation of SLS reactions in which damage of the water barrier is prominent, ultrasound has a level of accuracy in between those of TEWL and laser Doppler flowmetry [43, 45]. In types of reactions with less pronounced damage to the water barrier, ultrasound is probably more accurate. The cross-sectional ultrasound image of contact dermatitis has been relatively seldom studied to date. However, inflammatory edema of the skin does not expand it in a uniform way. Edema extends mainly in the more soft and pliable papillary dermis, and an echolucent band is seen by ultrasound [27]. Ultrasound has the advantage in that structure is studied, and preconditioning and laboratory conditions are, therefore, not critical. Its disadvantage is that training in this special technique is necessary.

28.5.2 Sensitive Skin and Hyperirritable Skin

During his or her lifetime, almost every person experiences a dermatitis on some occasion, and skin sensitivity represents a spectrum of reactivity. On the basis of reactivity to SLS, Frosch and Kligman defined a group of people who suffer more constantly from irritant contact dermatitis [47]. A skin type with high basal TEWL reacts more strongly to SLS, and this may be used to predict occupational risk [39, 40, 42, 48], although prognostic and epidemiological studies gave no convincing confirmation of this. Sensitive skin was also found to be more sensitive to light; more fair, with a higher L^* and lower b^* according to colorimetry, and thinner, according to ultrasound. These findings may indicate a more profound structural and functional inferiority of sensitive skin, including deviations in both the epidermis and the dermis [42, 49]. However, skin sensitivity is not simply a constant, but it also changes with age, menstrual cycle, season of the year, etc. – factors which interfere and overlap, and which may occasionally create the preconditions for an irritant contact dermatitis to appear [23, 50]. All of these variables need be taken into account whenever skin sensitivity is evaluated by noninvasive techniques, and when the determination of risk factors or dynamic testing by provocation with a standard noxious agent, such as SLS, are performed.

Patients with active hand dermatitis and young patients with atopic dermatitis have hyperirritable skin and react more strongly to SLS, while reactivity in chronic or healed eczema and in adult atopy and hand dermatitis is normal [51–53]. Thus, whenever groups of patients are studied by noninvasive techniques, they need to be clearly defined clinically. Extensive guidelines on provocative and sensibility testing with SLS were published by the standardization group of the ESCD [54].

28.6 Urticarial Wheals

Wheals or hives are very dynamic lesions with rapid changes during the initial 30 min when a triple response develops (Fig. 5). Thus, in the measurement of wheals, the timing of the recordings needs to be precise and relevant.

Laser Doppler flowmetry of wheals shows an increase of blood flow in both the center and the flare of the weal. The edema formation interferes with the vasculature, and measurements in the flare are more suitable for the distinction of the strength of the re-

Fig. 5.
Histamine wheal followed for 30 min with laser Doppler flowmetry (center and perilesional flare), ultrasound measurement of wheal thickness, and measurement of mean diameter

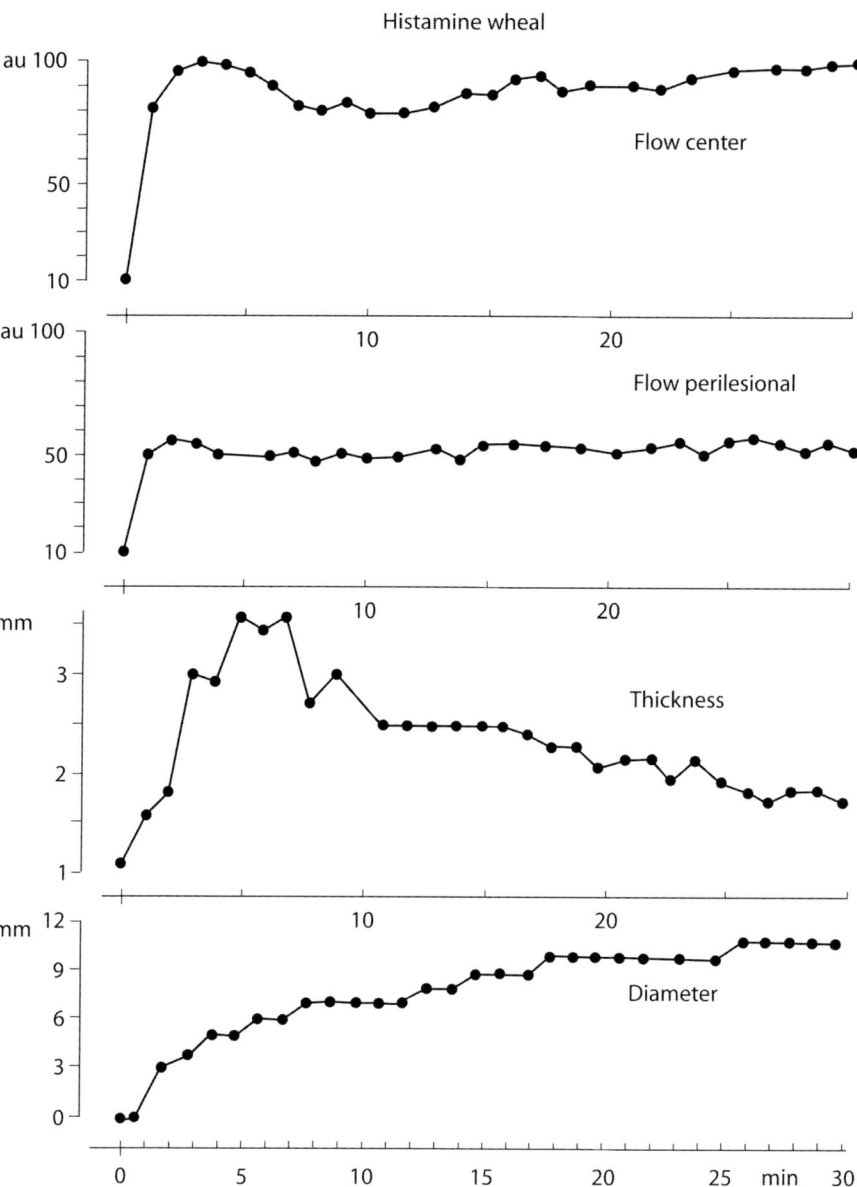

action after different concentrations of histamine [55, 56].

Ultrasound examination of histamine wheals shows that the wheal is initially globoid, and, at a diameter of about 5 mm, it extends laterally in the skin and becomes more flat [27, 57]. With ultrasound, the thickness and volume of wheals can be measured. Ultrasound cross-sectional imaging shows that the edema of wheal reactions propagates mainly laterally in the skin of the papillary dermis, which is more easily distended [27]. At the same time, this explains the formation of pseudopodia. Van Neste developed the noninvasive measurement of wheal reactions into a

useful method for the quantification of the effect of antihistamines [56, 58–60].

Wheal reactions to dimethylsulfoxide have been studied by TEWL, conductance, ultrasound skin thickness, and laser Doppler measurements, and all the methods were concluded to be suitable for the quantification of responses, except for laser Doppler flowmetry, this being due to the influence of edema on the vasculature [61].

References

1. Frosch PJ, Kligman AM (eds) (1993) Noninvasive methods for the quantification of skin functions. Springer, Berlin Heidelberg New York

2. Goldsmith LA (ed) (1983) Biochemistry and physiology of the skin. Oxford University Press, New York

3. Serup J, Jemec G (eds) (1995) Handbook of non-invasive methods and the skin. CRC, Boca Raton, Fla.

4. Agache P, Humbert P (eds) (2004) Measuring the skin. Springer, Berlin Heidelberg New York

5. Berardesca E, Elsner P, Wilhelm K-P, Maibach HI (eds) (1995) Bioengineering of the skin: methods and instrumentation. CRC, Boca Raton, Fla.

6. Wilhelm K-P, Elsner P, Berardesca E, Maibach HI (eds) (1997) Bioengineering of the skin: skin surface imaging and analysis. CRC, Boca Raton, Fla.

7. Elsner P, Barel AO, Berardesca E, Gabard B, Serup J (eds) (1998) Skin bioengineering techniques and applications in dermatology and cosmetology. Karger, Basel, Switzerland

8. Berardesca E, Maibach HI (1988) Bioengineering and the patch test. Contact Dermatitis 18:3–9

9. Diffey BL, Oliver RJ, Farr PM (1984) A portable instrument for quantifying erythema induced by ultraviolet radiation. Br J Dermatol 111:663–672

10. Robertson AR (1977) The CIE 1976 color difference formulas. Color Res Appl 2:7–11

11. Serup J, Agner T (1990) Colorimetric quantification of erythema – a comparison of two colorimeters (Lange Micro Color and Minolta Chroma Meter CR-200) with a clinical scoring scheme and laser-Doppler flowmetry. Clin Exp Dermatol 15:267–272

12. Slue WE (1989) Photographic cures for dermatologic disorders. Arch Dermatol 125:960–962

13. Grove GL, Grove MJ (1989) Objective methods for assessing skin surface topography noninvasively. In: Leveque J-L (ed) Cutaneous investigation in health and disease. Dekker, New York

14. Serup J, Winther A, Blichmann C (1989) A simple method for the study of scale pattern and effects of a moisturizer: qualitative and quantitative evaluation by D-Square tape compared with parameters of epidermal hydration. Clin Exp Dermatol 14:277–282

15. Leveque J-L, de Rigal J (1983) Impedance methods for studying skin moisturization. J Soc Cosmet Chem 34:419–428

16. Tagami H (1989) Impedance measurement for evaluation of the hydration state of the skin surface. In: Leveque J-L (ed) Cutaneous investigation in health and disease. Dekker, New York, pp 79–111

17. Blichmann C, Serup J (1988) Assessment of skin moisture. Measurement of electrical conductance, capacitance and transepidermal water loss. Acta Derm Venereol (Stockh) 68:284–290

18. Agner T, Serup J (1988) Comparison of two electrical methods for measurement of skin hydration. An experimental study on irritant patch test reactions. Bioeng Skin 4:263–269

19. Stender IM, Blichmann C, Serup J (1990) Effects of oil and water baths on the hydration state of the epidermis. Clin Exp Dermatol 15:206–209

20. Nilsson GE (1977) Measurement of water exchange through skin. Med Biol Eng Comput 15:209–218

21. Spencer TS (1990) Transepidermal water loss: methods and applications. In: Rietschel RL, Spencer TS (eds) Methods for cutaneous investigation. Dekker, New York, pp 191–217

22. Pinnagoda J, Tupker RA, Agner T, Serup J (1990) Guidelines for transepidermal water loss (TEWL) measurement. A report from the standardization group of the European Society of Contact Dermatitis. Contact Dermatitis 22:164–178

23. Agner T, Serup J (1989) Seasonal variation of skin resistance to irritants. Br J Dermatol 121:323–328

24. Agner T, Serup J (1988) Contact thermography for assessment of skin damage due to experimental irritants. Acta Derm Venereol (Stockh) 68:192–195

25. Baillie AJ, Biagioni PA, Forsyth A, Garioch JJ, McPherson D (1990) Thermographic assessment of patch-test responses. Br J Dermatol 122:351–360

26. Serup J, Staberg B (1987) Ultrasound for assessment of allergic and irritant patch test reactions. Contact Dermatitis 17:80–84

27. Serup J (1992) Ten years' experience with high-frequency ultrasound examination of the skin: development and refinement of technique and equipment. In: Altmeyer P, Hoffman K (eds) Ultrasound in dermatology. Springer, Berlin Heidelberg New York, pp 41–54

28. Peters K, Serup J (1987) Papulo-vesicular count for the rating of allergic patch test reactions. A simple technique based on polysulfide rubber replica. Acta Derm Venereol (Stockh) 67:491–495

29. Blichmann C, Serup J (1987) Hydration studies on scaly hand eczema. Contact Dermatitis 16:155–159

30. Serup J, Staberg B (1987) Differentiation of allergic and irritant reactions by transepidermal water loss. Contact Dermatitis 16:129–132

31. Serup J (1987) Contact thermography – towards the Sherlock Holmes magnifying glass for solving allergic and irritant patch test reactions? Contact Dermatitis 17:61–62

32. Staberg B, Serup J (1984) Patch test responses evaluated by cutaneous blood flow measurements. Arch Dermatol 120:741–743

33. Staberg B, Serup J (1988) Allergic and irritant skin reactions evaluated by laser Doppler flowmetry. Contact Dermatitis 18:40–45

34. Serup J, Staberg B, Klemp P (1984) Quantification of cutaneous oedema in patch test reactions by measurement of skin thickness with high-frequency pulsed ultrasound. Contact Dermatitis 10:88–93

35. Willis CM, Stephens CJM, Wilkinson JD (1989) Epidermal damage induced by irritants in man. A light and electron microscopy study. J Invest Dermatol 93:695–700

36. Bjørnberg A (1968) Skin reactions to primary irritants in patients with hand eczema. An investigation with matched controls. Thesis, Oscar Isacson, Göteborg, Sweden

37. Frosch P (1985) Hautirritation und empfindliche Haut. Grosse, Berlin, Germany

38. van der Valk PGM (1983) Water vapour loss measurements on human skin. Thesis, State University Hospital, Gröningen, the Netherlands

39. Pinnagoda J (1990) Transepidermal water loss. Its role in the assessment of susceptibility to the development of irritant contact dermatitis. Thesis, State University Hospital, Gröningen, the Netherlands

40. Tupker RA (1990) The influence of detergents on the human skin. A study on factors determining the individual susceptibility assessed by transepidermal water loss. Thesis, State University Hospital, Gröningen, the Netherlands

41. De Boer EM (1989) Occupational dermatitis by metalworking fluids. An epidemiological study and an investigation on skin irritation using laser Doppler flowmetry. Thesis, Vrije University, Amsterdam, the Netherlands

28

42. Agner T (1991) Noninvasive measuring methods for the investigation of irritant contact dermatitis. Thesis, University of Copenhagen, Denmark

43. Agner T, Serup J (1990) Sodium lauryl sulphate for irritant patch testing. A dose response study using bioengineering methods for determination of skin irritation. J Invest Dermatol 95:543–547

44. Agner T, Serup J (1987) Skin reactions to irritants assessed by polysulfide rubber replica. Contact Dermatitis 17: 205–211

45. Agner T, Serup J (1990) Individual and instrumental variations in irritant patch-test reactions – clinical evaluation and quantification by bioengineering methods. Clin Exp Dermatol 15:29–33

46. Bircher AJ, Guy RH, Maibach HI (1990) Laser-Doppler blood flowmetry. Skin pharmacology and dermatology. In: Shepherd AP, Öberg PÅ (eds) Laser-Doppler blood flowmetry. Kluwer, Boston, Mass., pp 141–174

47. Frosch PJ, Kligman AM (1982) Recognition of chemically vulnerable and delicate skin. In: Frost PH, Horwith SN (eds) Principles of cosmetics for the dermatologist. Mosby, St Louis, Mo., pp 287–296

48. Murahata RI, Crowe DM, Roheim JR (1986) The use of transepidermal water loss to measure and predict the irritation response to surfactants. Int J Cosmet Sci 8:225–231

49. Frosch P, Wissing C (1982) Cutaneous sensitivity to ultraviolet light and chemical irritants. Arch Dermatol Res 272: 269–278

50. Agner T, Damm P, Skouby SO (1991) Menstrual cycle and skin reactivity. J Am Acad Dermatol 24:566–570

51. Werner Y, Lindberg M (1985) Transepidermal water loss in dry and clinically normal skin in patients with atopic dermatitis. Arch Dermatol Res 65:102–105

52. Agner T (1991) Skin susceptibility in uninvolved skin of hand eczema patients and healthy controls. Br J Dermatol 125:140–146

53. Agner T (1990) Susceptibility to sodium lauryl sulphate in patients with atopic dermatitis and controls. Acta Derm Venereol (Stockh) 71:296–300

54. Tupker RA, Willis C, Berardesca E, Lee CH, Fartasch M, Agner T, Serup J (1997) Guidelines on sodium lauryl sulfate (SLS) exposure tests. A report from the Standardization Group of the European Society of Contact Dermatitis. Contact Dermatitis 37:53–69

55. Serup J, Staberg B (1985) Quantification of weal reactions with laser Doppler flowmetry. Comparative blood flow measurements of the oedematous centre and the perilesional flare of skin-prick histamine weals. Allergy 40: 233–237

56. Van Neste D (1991) Skin response to histamine: reproducibility study of the dry skin prick test method and of the evaluation of microvascular changes with laser Doppler flowmetry. Acta Derm Venereol (Stockh) 71:25–28

57. Serup J (1984) Diameter, thickness, area, and volume of skin-prick histamine weals. Allergy 39:359–364

58. Van Neste D, Ghys L, Antoine JL, Rihoux JP (1989) Pharmacological modulation by cetirizine and atropine of the histamine- and methacholine-induced wheals and flares in human skin. Skin Pharmacol 2:93–102

59. Van Neste D (1990) Skin response to histamine dry skin prick test: influence of duration of the skin prick on clinical parameters and on skin blood flow monitoring. J Dermatol Sci 1:435–439

60. Leroy T, Tasset C, Valentin B, Van Neste D (1998) Comparison of the effects of cetirizine and ebastine on the skin response to histamine iontophoresis monitored with laser Doppler flowmetry. Dermatology 197:146–151

61. Agner T, Serup J (1989) Quantification of the DMSO response, a test for assessment of sensitive skin. Clin Exp Dermatol 14:214–217

Part VI

Allergic Contact Dermatitis Related to Specific Exposures

VI

Chapter 29

Allergens from the Standard Series   29

Klaus E. Andersen, Ian R. White, An Goossens

Contents

29.1 Introduction

The distinction between allergic and irritant contact dermatitis is based on a patient's history and clinical features, in combination with diagnostic patch testing. This test procedure is indicated in the investigation of long-standing cases of contact dermatitis and should also be used to exclude contact allergy as a complicating factor in stubborn cases of other eczematous diseases, such as atopic dermatitis, stasis eczema, seborrheic dermatitis, and vesicular hand eczema. A patch test is the cutaneous application of a small amount of the suspected allergen in a suitable concentration and vehicle. The test site, usually the back, is covered with an occlusive dressing for 2 days. The skin condition, vehicle and concentration, volume of the test substance, size of the test chamber, test site, application time, and the number of readings influence the result, and frequent errors are possible [1–4] (see Chap. 2). The proper performance and interpretation of this bioassay require considerable training and experience.

Patch testing is routinely performed by applying a standard series of the most frequently occurring contact allergens and those contact allergens that may be missed without routine screening. The choice of test concentration is based on patch test experience such that there is a minimum number of irritant reactions and a maximum of clinically explicable allergic positive reactions. Test concentrations are generally expressed in percentages. This can be misleading, since the molecular weight of allergens can be very different. A better way of expressing concentration would be both the percentage and molality (m=number of moles per 1,000 g of solvent or vehicle) [5].

An experienced contact dermatologist will be able to guess correctly the clinically relevant contact allergen in some patients, based on the history and the clinical appearance of the eczema. This guess is more likely to be correct for common allergens, such as nickel (50–80%), and less likely to be correct for less common allergens (<10%) [6,7]. This failure to guess correctly explains the general acceptance of the use of a standard series in the evaluation of all patients suspected of having a contact dermatitis.

Supplementary tests with working materials properly diluted, and extra allergens selected on the basis of patient history and known exposures, are often required in order to determine the nature of the patient's suspected contact dermatitis. The standard series detects approximately 75–80% of all contact allergies [8].

The European standard series is dynamic and subject to continual modification depending on population exposures and prevalence of contact allergy [9, 10] (Table 1). Among the major patch test material companies, Hermal and Chemotechnique supply with

Table 1. The current European standard patch test series from Trolab Hermal and Chemotechnique, and the contact allergens available from TRUE Test Panel 1 and Panel 2. The patch test concentrations are shown. (*aq.* water, *pet.* petrolatum)

	Trolab Hermal[a]	Chemotechnique[a]	TRUE Test[b]
Potassium dichromate	0.5% pet.	–	23 µg/cm^2
Neomycin sulfate	20% pet.	–	230 µg/cm^2
Thiuram mix	1% pet.	–	25 µg/cm^2
p-phenylenediamine free base	1% pet.	–	90 µg/cm^2
Cobalt chloride	1% pet.	–	20 µg/cm^2
Benzocaine	5% pet.	–	–
Formaldehyde	1% aq.	–	180 µg/cm^2
Colophony (colophonium)	20% pet.	–	850 µg/cm^2
Clioquinol	5% pet.	–	–
Balsam of Peru (*Myroxylon pereirae*)	25% pet.	–	800 µg/cm^2
N-Isopropyl-*N'*-phenyl-paraphenylenediamine (IPPD)	0.1% pet.	–	–
Wool alcohols (lanolin alcohol)	30% pet.	–	1,000 µg/cm^2
Mercapto mix	1% pet.	2% pet.	75 µg/cm^2
Epoxy resin	1% pet.	–	50 µg/cm^2
Paraben mix	16% pet.	–	1,000 µg/cm^2
para-Tertiary-butylphenol-formaldehyde resin (PTBP resin)	1% pet.	–	40 µg/cm^2
Fragrance mix	8% pet.	–	430 µg/cm^2
Quaternium-15	1% pet.	–	100 µg/cm^2
Nickel sulfate	5% pet.	–	200 µg/cm^2
Cl+Me-isothiazolinone[c]	0.01% aq.	–	4 µg/cm^2
Mercaptobenzothiazole	2% pet.	–	75 µg/cm^2
Primin	0.01% pet.	–	–
Sesquiterpene lactone mix	0.1% pet.	–	–
Budesonide	–	0.01% pet.	–
Tixocortol pivalate	–	0.1% pet.	–
Hydroxyisohexyl-3-cyclohexene carboxaldehyde (Lyral)	5% pet.	–	–
Caine mix	–	–	630 µg/cm^2
Quinoline mix	–	6% pet.	190 µg/cm^2
Black rubber mix	–	–	75 µg/cm^2
Carba mix	–	–	250 µg/cm^2
Thimerosal	–	–	8 µg/cm^2
Ethylenediamine	–	–	50 µg/cm^2

[a] Hermal and Chemotechnique offer more than these allergens
[b] TRUE allergens for a Panel 3 are under development
[c] Methylchloroisothiazolinone/methylisothiazolinone

some modifications the European standard series, as recommended by the European Environmental and Contact Dermatitis Research Group (EECDRG), and Mekos supplies TRUE Test Panel 1 and Panel 2, which, in the collection and preparation of the allergens, differ from the European standard series on several positions, as seen in Table 1. The standard series can be extended to include allergens of local importance to specific departments. The frequency of allergic contact sensitization to the allergens of the standard series varies from study to study, depending on the composition of the study population. Comparison of the frequencies in different populations is only valid when the results are standardized with respect to confounding factors, such as age, sex, presence of atopy, presence of diseased skin, and occupational exposure – the MOAHLFA index, indicating the frequency of occurrence of males, occupational dermatitis, atopy, hand dermatitis, leg ulcers or stasis dermatitis, facial dermatitis, and age above 40 years [11, 12]. Moreover, when evaluating multicenter patch test studies, the patch test application time, the amount of the allergens applied on the chambers, the reading time, and the reading scale should be taken into account as well [13].

References

1. Wahlberg JE, Elsner P, Kanerva L, Maibach HI (2003) Management of positive patch test reactions. Springer, Berlin Heidelberg New York
2. Rietschel RL, Fowler JF (2001) Fisher's contact dermatitis, 5th edn. Lippincott Williams and Wilkins, Philadelphia, Pa.
3. Kanerva L, Elsner P, Wahlberg JE, Maibach HI (2000) Handbook of occupational dermatology. Springer, Berlin Heidelberg New York
4. Brasch J, Szlinka C, Grabbe J (1997) More positive patch test reactions with larger test chambers? Contact Dermatitis 37:118–120
5. Benezra C, Andanson J, Chabeau C, Ducombs G, Foussereau J, Lachapelle JM, Lacroix M, Martin P (1978) Concentrations of patch test allergens: are we comparing the same things? Contact Dermatitis 4:103–105
6. Cronin E (1972) Clinical prediction of patch test results. Trans St John's Hosp Dermatol Soc 58:153–162
7. Podmore P, Burrows D, Bingham EA (1984) Prediction of patch test results. Contact Dermatitis 11:283–284
8. Menné T, Dooms Goossens A, Wahlberg JE, White IR, Shaw S (1992) How large a proportion of contact sensitivities are diagnosed with the European standard series? Contact Dermatitis 26:201–202
9. Bruynzeel DP, Andersen KE, Camarasa JG, Lachapelle J-M, Menné T, White IR (1995) The European standard series. European Environmental and Contact Dermatitis Research Group (EECDRG). Contact Dermatitis 33:145–148
10. Isaksson M, Brandao FM, Bruze M, Goossens A (2000) Recommendation to include budesonide and tixocortol pivalate in the European standard series. Contact Dermatitis 43:41–42
11. Christophersen J, Menné T, Tanghoj P, Andersen KE, Brandrup F, Kaaber K, Osmundsen PE, Thestrup-Pedersen K, Veien NK (1989) Clinical patch test data evaluated by multivariate analysis. Danish Contact Dermatitis Group. Contact Dermatitis 21:291–299
12. Wilkinson JD, Hambly EM, Wilkinson DS (1980) Comparison of patch test results in two adjacent areas of England. II. Medicaments. Acta Derm Venereol (Stockh) 60:245–249
13. Andersen KE (1998) Multicentre patch test studies: are they worth the effort. Contact Dermatitis 38:222–223

29.2 Nickel

Nickel is a metal which is used in a large number of alloys and chemical compounds. Only iron, chromium, and lead are produced in larger amounts. Nickel is ubiquitous in the environment and constitutes about 0.008% of the Earth's crust. Humans are constantly exposed, though in variable amounts [1]. Nickel is the most common contact allergen in children and adults [2, 3]. Metallic nickel (only after corrosion), as well as nickel salts, gives rise to contact allergy. The corrosiveness of sweat, saliva, and other body fluids to nickel and nickel alloys is of primary importance [4].

Nickel is the most common allergen in the standard series and the most common cause of allergic contact dermatitis, particularly in women. The frequency of nickel allergy in women is 3–10 times higher than in men [2, 5]. This gender difference is traditionally explained by increased exposure in women, due to direct skin contact with nickel-releasing metal, such as in jewelry, wristwatches, and clothing accessories. Wet work at home and exposure in certain occupational groups with a majority of women, such as hairdressers, cleaners, and food service workers, are also associated with the increased frequency of nickel allergy in women [6,7]. The incidence of nickel allergy in women has increased until the most recent decade, and has reached a plateau of around 15–20%, depending on the source of reference [3, 5, 8]. The most common cause of sensitization is thought to be ear piercing [2, 9], even in men [10]. The clinical pattern of nickel dermatitis is described in the classic paper of Calnan and Wells [11]. The primary sites of dermatitis develop as a result of direct skin contact with nickel-releasing metal. The secondary sites are unrelated to direct skin contact. A systemic contact dermatitis may develop in particularly sensitive patients through oral intake through foods. The systemic contact dermatitis is symmetrical and often includes the neck and face, eyelids, elbow flexures and forearms, hands, inner thighs, anogenital region, and may be generalized [12]. Flare-up reactions of previous nickel patch test sites may oc-

29

cur. The systemic allergic nickel dermatitis is hapten-specific and with a clear dose–response relationship. Immunological investigations in nickel-sensitive individuals whose dermatitis flared after oral nickel provocation showed that CD8+ "memory" CLA+ T lymphocytes and T lymphocytes with a type 2 cytokine profile are involved in the development of systemic nickel dermatitis [13]. The doses used experimentally have been much larger than the normal daily dietary nickel intake, which varies between 0.1 mg to 0.5 mg nickel, and the induction of systemic nickel dermatitis from daily dietary nickel intake remains controversial [14–17]. However, nickel-sensitive patients with vesicular hand eczema worsened after an oral challenge with nickel in water and with a diet naturally high in nickel [18]. Nickel absorption and retention in the body is highly dependent on food intake and fasting, but nickel toxicokinetics is the same in nickel-allergic women and age-matched controls [19].

The relationship between nickel allergy and hand eczema is controversial as well. It is evident that allergic dermatitis of the hands occurs as a result of contact with solubilized nickel and takes place more rapidly if the patient has preexisting irritant hand eczema [20]. Hand eczema is more common in nickel-sensitized women than in the general population [21, 22]. However, a Swedish study in men [10] did not reveal a higher frequency of hand eczema among metal-sensitive subjects, nor in individuals with pierced ears, compared to a nonsensitized group, and recent Danish studies have shown contradictory results. Mortz et al. [2] found a significant association between hand eczema and nickel allergy in a population of unselected adolescents, and Bryld et al. found the same in a population-based twin sample [23, 24]. However, when the analysis was limited to twins with vesicular hand eczema, there was no association [23].

Other conundrums about nickel allergy remain unresolved; for instance, does nickel allergy render a person, even with normal skin, more vulnerable to irritant contact dermatitis? It would appear that it can [25], but atopic dermatitis is the major risk factor to the development of hand eczema [24, 26, 27]. A survey of 368 nickel-sensitive subjects attempted to determine the overall importance of nickel as an occupational allergen and it was found in about 23% of the cases to function as a secondary occupational allergen, in conjunction with other factors [6].

The incidence of allergy in men, even in those with earrings, is lower than in females; the cause not being clear. Some experimental studies claim that women are more easily sensitized than men [28]. A more likely explanation for the fewer nickel-allergic men may be less exposure from wet work and less skin contact with nickel-releasing jewelry.

Certainly, in nickel allergy, one can see patterns of dermatitis which are unusual for contact dermatitis; for instance, on the palmar aspects of the fingers and the adjacent palm. This can sometimes be explained by local contact. It is to be expected that a solid such as metal will produce a different distribution of dermatitis compared to liquids and detergents. However, intensive handling of nickel coins in a controlled experiment did not provoke allergic contact hand eczema in nickel-sensitive individuals [29].

There is no method of desensitization, but it is possible to produce immune tolerance in animals fed nickel prior to attempted sensitization, and this has been confirmed in humans. Adolescents who have dental braces (causing ingestion of nickel) prior to ear piercing develop much less nickel allergy [2, 30]. This is clearly not a practical method of solving the problem. Oral administration of nickel sulfate 5.0 mg once a week for 6 weeks in nickel-allergic patients lowered the degree of contact allergy significantly, as measured by the patch test reactions before and after nickel administration [31].

There is little doubt that metal plates on bones can initiate a dermatitis, which occurs particularly over the areas of the plate [32, 33], but it is now well accepted that nickel allergy is not a contraindication to a metal hip of stainless steel or vitallium type. There is no convincing evidence that these sensitize or exacerbate a preexisting dermatitis, or lead to rejection of the hip [34].

Nickel allergy was claimed not to increase the risk of developing other allergies [35, 36]. However, nickel allergy is often associated with reactivity to other metals. This seems, in most cases, to be caused by multiple exposure and sensitization and not to cross reactivity [37] and may simply be due to the fact that these metals are commonly associated. It is difficult to obtain pure compounds and most of these metals are contaminated with another. On the other hand, Moss et al. [38] suggested that the acquisition of sensitivity to one allergen might predispose to the acquisition of another unrelated sensitivity – based on a statistical analysis of patch test data from 2,200 consecutive patients and experimental sensitization using dinitrochlorobenzene (DNCB). Further, guinea pigs sensitized to nickel were found to be more easily sensitized to cobalt [39], and it has been shown that lymphocytes with monoclonal sensitivity to nickel will react to palladium and copper, but not with cobalt [40]. Nickel is an intriguing contact allergen, and some cases of nickel patch test reactivity may be unspecific, as nickel, in analogy to superantigens, may directly link to the T cell receptor (TCR) and major histocompatibility complex (MHC) in a peptide-independent manner. However, nickel requires human histocompatibility leukocyte antigen (HLA) determined TCR amino acids [41].

The dimethylglyoxime (DMG) test, which is used to detect nickel release from metal surfaces, is accurate to about 10 ppm (0.001%=2.1 µg Ni/g) and is a good routine test to eliminate metals as a source of nickel which may be causing allergy. However, metals containing lower amounts can still produce an exacerbation of nickel dermatitis, and, therefore, the dimethylglyoxime test cannot be relied upon absolutely to rule out a piece of metal as the cause of a patient's dermatitis [42, 43]. The release of nickel from stainless steel is minimal and is directly correlated with its sulfur content, since sulfur affects corrosion resistance, and, hence, also the release of nickel [44]. Experimental studies have shown that nickel-sensitive patients rarely react following repeated exposures to levels below 10 ppm nickel [45]. The EU nickel directive aimed at the prevention of nickel allergy covers metal items in direct contact with skin, piercing materials, and requirements on resistance to wear (Council Directive 94/27/EC, OJ No. L 188 of 22.7.94). The nickel release threshold is 0.5 µg/cm² per week, and a European standard for testing nickel release from articles intended to come in prolonged and direct skin contact has been adopted.

The nickel directive seems to be effective, as a significant decrease in the frequency of nickel allergy in Denmark is reported in the age group 0–18 years [46], and in Germany in patients below 31 years of age [47].

The standard patch test concentration of nickel sulfate is in Europe 5% pet. or 200 µg/cm² in the TRUE test. In the USA, 2.5% pet. is recommended. Follicular and irritant reactions may occur and complicate clinical interpretation. A problem in patch testing is that, depending on the questioning procedure, 15–50% of those who give a clear history of reaction to metal jewelry, which strongly suggests nickel allergy, do not react [16, 48]. The reason for this is not clear. It does not appear to be due to a fault in the test reagent, or method of testing, as other salts, for instance, nickel chloride, or intradermal (ID) testing will increase the positive yield by a very small amount [49]. Nickel contact allergy seems not to be associated with atopic dermatitis [50, 51]. Positive nickel sulfate patch tests are, in general, very reproducible [52, 53]. However, the individual variation in nickel patch test threshold reactivity from test session to test session with a dilution series among nickel-sensitive patients may vary considerably [54].

References

1. Grandjean P, Nielsen GD, Andersen O (1989) Human nickel exposure and chemobiokinetics. In: Maibach HI, Menne T (eds) Nickel and the skin: immunology and toxicology. CRC, Boca Raton, Fla., pp 9–34
2. Mortz CG, Lauritsen JM, Bindslev-Jensen C, Andersen KE (2002) Nickel sensitization in adolescents and association with ear piercing, use of dental braces and hand eczema. The Odense Adolescence Cohort Study on Atopic Diseases and Dermatitis (TOACS). Acta Derm Venereol (Stockh) 82:359–364
3. Nielsen NH, Linneberg A, Menne T, Madsen F, Frolund L, Dirksen A, Jorgensen T (2001) Allergic contact sensitization in an adult Danish population: two cross-sectional surveys eight years apart (the Copenhagen Allergy Study). Acta Derm Venereol 81:31–34
4. Morgan LG, Flint GN (1989) Nickel alloys and coatings: release of nickel. In: Maibach HI, Menne T (eds) Nickel and the skin: immunology and toxicology. CRC, Boca Raton, Fla., pp 45–54
5. Schnuch A, Geier J, Uter W, Frosch PJ, Lehmacher W, Aberer W, Agathos M, Arnold R, Fuchs T, Laubstein B, Lischka G, Pietrzyk PM, Rakoski J, Richter G, Rueff F (1997) National rates and regional differences in sensitization to allergens of the standard series. Population-adjusted frequencies of sensitization (PAFS) in 40,000 patients from a multicenter study (IVDK). Contact Dermatitis 37:200–209
6. Shah M, Lewis FM, Gawkrodger DJ (1998) Nickel as an occupational allergen. A survey of 368 nickel-sensitive subjects. Arch Dermatol 134:1231–1236
7. Shum KW, Meyer JD, Chen Y, Cherry N, Gawkrodger DJ (2003) Occupational contact dermatitis to nickel: experience of the British dermatologists (EPIDERM) and occupational physicians (OPRA) surveillance schemes. Occup Environ Med 60:954–957
8. Marks JG Jr, Belsito DV, DeLeo VA, Fowler JF Jr, Fransway AF, Maibach HI, Mathias CG, Pratt MD, Rietschel RL, Sherertz EF, Storrs FJ, Taylor JS; North American Contact Dermatitis Group (2003) North American Contact Dermatitis Group patch-test results, 1998 to 2000. Am J Contact Dermat 14:59–62
9. Larsson-Stymne B, Widström L (1985) Ear piercing – a cause of nickel allergy in schoolgirls? Contact Dermatitis 13:289–293
10. Meijer C, Bredberg M, Fischer T, Widstrom L (1995) Ear piercing, and nickel and cobalt sensitization, in 520 young Swedish men doing compulsory military service. Contact Dermatitis 32:147–149
11. Calnan CD, Wells GC (1956) Suspender dermatitis and nickel sensitivity. Br Med J (4978):1265–1268
12. Andersen KE, Hjorth N, Menne T (1984) The baboon syndrome: systemically-induced allergic contact dermatitis. Contact Dermatitis 10:97–100
13. Jensen CS, Lisby S, Larsen JK, Veien NK, Menne T (2004) Characterization of lymphocyte subpopulations and cytokine profiles in peripheral blood of nickel-sensitive individuals with systemic contact dermatitis after oral nickel exposure. Contact Dermatitis 50:31–38
14. Jensen CS, Menne T, Lisby S, Kristiansen J, Veien NK (2003) Experimental systemic contact dermatitis from nickel: a dose-response study. Contact Dermatitis 49:124–132
15. Veien N (1989) Systemically induced eczema in adults. Acta Derm Venereol Suppl (Stockh) 147:1–58

29

16. Burrows D (1989) The Prosser White oration 1988. Mischievous metals – chromate, cobalt, nickel and mercury. Clin Exp Dermatol 14:266–272
17. Santucci B, Manna F, Cristaudo A, Cannistraci C, Capparella MR, Picardo M (1990) Serum concentrations in nickel-sensitive patients after prolonged oral administration. Contact Dermatitis 22:253–256
18. Nielsen GD, Jepsen LV, Jorgensen PJ, Grandjean P, Brandrup F (1990) Nickel-sensitive patients with vesicular hand eczema: oral challenge with a diet naturally high in nickel. Br J Dermatol 122:299–308
19. Nielsen GD, Soderberg U, Jorgensen PJ, Templeton DM, Rasmussen SN, Andersen KE, Grandjean P (1999) Absorption and retention of nickel from drinking water in relation to food intake and nickel sensitivity. Toxicol Appl Pharmacol 154:67–75
20. Wilkinson DS, Wilkinson JD (1989) Nickel allergy and hand eczema. In: Maibach HI, Menne T (eds) Nickel and the skin: immunology and toxicology. CRC, Boca Raton, Fla., pp 133–163
21. Menne T, Holm NV (1983) Hand eczema in nickel-sensitive female twins. Genetic predisposition and environmental factors. Contact Dermatitis 9:289–296
22. Menne T, Borgan O, Green A (1982) Nickel allergy and hand dermatitis in a stratified sample of the Danish female population: an epidemiological study including a statistic appendix. Acta Derm Venereol (Stockh) 62:35–41
23. Bryld LE, Agner T, Menne T (2003) Relation between vesicular eruptions on the hands and tinea pedis, atopic dermatitis and nickel allergy. Acta Derm Venereol (Stockh) 83:186–188
24. Bryld LE, Hindsberger C, Kyvik KO, Agner T, Menne T (2003) Risk factors influencing the development of hand eczema in a population-based twin sample. Br J Dermatol 149:1214–1220
25. van der Burg CK, Bruynzeel DP, Vreeburg KJ, von Blomberg BM, Scheper RJ (1986) Hand eczema in hairdressers and nurses: a prospective study. I. Evaluation of atopy and nickel hypersensitivity at the start of apprenticeship. Contact Dermatitis 14:275–279
26. Nilsson EJ, Knutsson A (1995) Atopic dermatitis, nickel sensitivity and xerosis as risk factors for hand eczema in women. Contact Dermatitis 33:401–406
27. Mortz CG, Lauritsen JM, Bindslev-Jensen C, Andersen KE (2001) Prevalence of atopic dermatitis, asthma, allergic rhinitis, and hand and contact dermatitis in adolescents. The Odense Adolescence Cohort Study on Atopic Diseases and Dermatitis. Br J Dermatol 144:523–532
28. Rees JL, Friedmann PS, Matthews JN (1989) Sex differences in susceptibility to development of contact hypersensitivity to dinitrochlorobenzene (DNCB). Br J Dermatol 120:371–374
29. Zhai H, Chew AL, Bashir SJ, Reagan KE, Hostynek JJ, Maibach HI (2003) Provocative use test of nickel coins in nickel-sensitized subjects and controls. Br J Dermatol 149:311–317
30. Van Hoogstraten IM, Andersen KE, von Blomberg BM, Boden D, Bruynzeel DP, Burrows D, Camarasa JG, Dooms-Goossens A, Kraal G, Lahti A (1991) Reduced frequency of nickel allergy upon oral nickel contact at an early age. Clin Exp Immunol 85:441–445
31. Sjovall P, Christensen OB, Moller H (1987) Oral hyposensitization in nickel allergy. J Am Acad Dermatol 17:774–778
32. Thomas RH, Rademaker M, Goddard NJ, Munro DD (1987) Severe eczema of the hands due to an orthopaedic plate made of Vitallium. Br Med J Clin Res Ed 294:106–107
33. Wilkinson JD (1989) Nickel allergy and orthopedic prosthesis. In: Maibach HI, Menne T (eds) Nickel and the skin: immunology and toxicology. CRC, Boca Raton, Fla., pp 187–193
34. Gawkrodger DJ (2003) Metal sensitivities and orthopaedic implants revisited: the potential for metal allergy with the new metal-on-metal joint prostheses. Br J Dermatol 148:1089–1093
35. Lammintausta K, Kalimo K (1987) Do positive nickel reactions increase nonspecific patch test reactivity? Contact Dermatitis 16:160–163
36. Paramsothy Y, Collins M, Smith AG (1988) Contact dermatitis in patients with leg ulcers. The prevalence of late positive reactions and evidence against systemic ampliative allergy. Contact Dermatitis 18:30–36
37. Liden C, Wahlberg JE (1994) Cross-reactivity to metal compounds studied in guinea pigs induced with chromate or cobalt. Acta Derm Venereol (Stockh) 74:341–343
38. Moss C, Friedmann PS, Shuster S, Simpson JM (1985) Susceptibility and amplification of sensitivity in contact dermatitis. Clin Exp Immunol 61:232–241
39. Lammintausta K, Pitkanen OP, Kalimo K, Jansen CT (1985) Interrelationship of nickel and cobalt contact sensitization. Contact Dermatitis 13:148–152
40. Moulon C, Vollmer J, Weltzien HU (1995) Characterization of processing requirements and metal cross-reactivities in T cell clones from patients with allergic contact dermatitis to nickel. Eur J Immunol 25:3308–3315
41. Gamerdinger K, Moulon C, Karp DR, Van Bergen J, Koning F, Wild D, Pflugfelder U, Weltzien HU (2003) A new type of metal recognition by human T cells: contact residues for peptide-independent bridging of T cell receptor and major histocompatibility complex by nickel. J Exp Med 197:1345–1353
42. Menne T, Brandup F, Thestrup-Pedersen K, Veien NK, Andersen JR, Yding F, Valeur G (1987) Patch test reactivity to nickel alloys. Contact Dermatitis 16:255–259
43. Kanerva L, Sipilainen-Malm T, Estlander T, Zitting A, Jolanki R, Tarvainen K (1994) Nickel release from metals, and a case of allergic contact dermatitis from stainless steel. Contact Dermatitis 31:299–303
44. Haudrechy P, Mantout B, Frappaz A, Rousseau D, Chabeau G, Faure M, Claudy A (1997) Nickel release from stainless steels. Contact Dermatitis 37:113–117
45. Basketter DA, Angelini G, Ingber A, Kern PS, Menne T (2003) Nickel, chromium and cobalt in consumer products: revisiting safe levels in the new millennium. Contact Dermatitis 49:1–7
46. Johansen JD, Menne T, Christophersen J, Kaaber K, Veien N (2000) Changes in the pattern of sensitization to common contact allergens in Denmark between 1985–1986 and 1997–1998, with a special view to the effect of preventive strategies. Br J Dermatol 142:490–495
47. Schnuch A, Geier J, Lessmann H, Uter W (2003) (Decrease in nickel sensitization in young patients–successful intervention through nickel exposure regulation? Results of IVDK, 1992–2001). Hautarzt 54:626–632
48. Kieffer M (1979) Nickel sensitivity: relationship between history and patch test reaction. Contact Dermatitis 5:398–401
49. Moller H, Svensson A (1986) Metal sensitivity: positive history but negative test indicates atopy. Contact Dermatitis 14:57–60
50. Uter W, Pfahlberg A, Gefeller O, Geier J, Schnuch A (2003) Risk factors for contact allergy to nickel – results of a multifactorial analysis. Contact Dermatitis 48:33–38

51. Mortz CG, Lauritsen JM, Bindslev-Jensen C, Andersen KE (2002) Contact allergy and allergic contact dermatitis in adolescents: prevalence measures and associations. The Odense Adolescence Cohort Study on Atopic Diseases and Dermatitis (TOACS). Acta Derm Venereol (Stockh) 82: 352–358

52. Memon AA, Friedmann PS (1996) Studies on the reproducibility of allergic contact dermatitis. Br J Dermatol 134: 208–214

53. Andersen KE, Liden C, Hansen J, Volund A (1993) Dose-response testing with nickel sulfate using the TRUE test in nickel-sensitive individuals. Multiple nickel sulfate patch-test reactions do not cause an 'angry back'. Br J Dermatol 129:50–56

54. Hindsen M, Bruze M, Christensen OB (1999) Individual variation in nickel patch test reactivity. Am J Contact Dermat 10:62–67

29.3 Chromium

It is probably more accurate to use the term "chromate," because chromium is unique in that the metal itself does not sensitize, but, rather, its salts. Both hexavalent ($Cr_2O_7^-$) and trivalent (Cr^{3+}) chromate may cause allergic contact dermatitis. Trivalent chromate is poorly soluble and penetrates the skin poorly, binding with proteins on the surface skin, whilst hexavalent chromate is easily soluble and penetrates skin easily but binds poorly with proteins. It is thought that hexavalent chromate penetrates the skin and is then reduced enzymatically to trivalent chromate, which combines with protein as the hapten. Using standard patch test techniques, Fregert and Rorsman [1] showed that, if the concentration of trivalent chromate is high enough, and the exposure time sufficiently prolonged, positive patch tests will also result. However, the evidence would suggest that, at a cellular level, the body develops an allergy to both hexavalent and trivalent chromate [2, 3]. Recent clinical dose–response patch test experiments using volunteer chromate allergic patients showed that the calculated minimal elicitation threshold (MET) giving a positive patch test reaction in 10% of the patients was 0.18 µg/cm² (6 ppm.) for Cr(III) and 0.03 µg/cm² (1 ppm) for Cr(VI) [4]. The frequency of patch test positives to chromate on routine patch testing varies considerably from region to region. In Denmark, about 2% of consecutively tested eczema patients have chromate allergy [5], much less than in neighboring countries such as Germany and England, where the frequency of chromate allergy ranges from 3.1% to 10.5% [6, 7]. Where higher rates are reported, some irritant reactions may be included. It is difficult to compare these results unless the patient materials are examined for confounding factors, such as age, sex, atopy, occupational dermatitis, site of dermatitis, etc. Cement has been considered as the main cause of chromate allergy. All authorities agree that cement dermatitis is decreasing in incidence and increasing evidence indicates that this may be partly due to the introduction of ferrous sulfate in cement in some countries in order to reduce the levels of hexavalent chromium [8–11]. However, the decline in cement dermatitis may also result from other factors, such as automation and prefabrication processes in the construction industry [12, 13]. A remarkable observation is the fact that chromate allergy was common among construction workers employed at the Channel Tunnel project, in which normal cement was used [14]. In contrast, only a few workers developed cement dermatitis during the construction of the Great Belt tunnel and bridge in Denmark, a project of a comparable size [5]. In Denmark, legislation has, since 1981, regulated the concentration of hexavalent chromate in ready-to-use cement, and, since 2003, a similar legislation has been adopted in the EU, making it illegal to sell cement and cement products containing more than 2 ppm hexavalent chromium. Recent epidemiological investigations support this legislation, since chromate sensitization among construction workers in Northern Bavaria, Germany was still common throughout the 1990s, without the declining frequency seen in Scandinavian countries, where the addition of ferrous sulfate to cement had been used since the 1980s [15]. Chromate allergy is more common in male than in female eczema patients, due to the occupational exposure in male-dominated occupations, such as building and machine industry [6]. This has changed in Denmark since introduction of the legislation limiting the content of hexavalent chromate in cement. Now, chromate allergy is more common in female patients, probably caused by chromate tanned leather in gloves and shoes [16].

There are many causes of chromate allergy other than cement, including chrome tanned leather, anti-rust paint, timber preservatives, the wood pulp industry, ash either from burnt wood in general or matches with chromate in the match head, coolants and machine oils, galvanizing, defatting solvents, brine added to yeast residues, welding, the dye industry (due to either a dye, a reducing agent, or a mordant), printing, glues, foundry sand, boiler linings, television work (ammonium bichromate to produce cross-linking of light-sensitive polyvinyl alcohol), magnetic tapes (chromium dioxide), solutions used to facilitate tire fitting, chromium plating, hardeners and resins in the aircraft industry, preservatives used in milk testing, bleaches, and detergents. An extensive list of possible sources of contact allergy is in Table 2. Of these sources, many are rare and one-off contacts. The commonest sources of chromate aller-

Table 2. Industrial exposure to chromium is possible during contact with the following compounds or work procedures (from [17])

Analytic standards reagents
Anticorrosion agents
Batteries
Catalysts (for hydrogenation, oxidation, and polymerization)
Ceramics
Corrosion inhibitors
Chromate surface treatments
Drilling muds
Electroplating and anodizing agents
Engraving
Explosives
Fire retardants
Magnetic tapes
Milk preservatives
Paints and varnishes
Paper
Photography
Roofing
Surgical sutures
Tanning leather
Textile mordants and dyes
Television screens
Textile mordants and dyes
Wood preservatives

29

gy by far still remains cement, followed by welding, chrome tanning, leather, pigments, and chrome plating. The relevance of a positive chromate patch test may be difficult to ascertain. More detailed information can be obtained in references [3] and [17]. Allergic chromate dermatitis is often widespread and persistent, and may appear in a nummular eczema pattern [18]. However, if the patient carefully aims to avoid contact with chromate-containing products, the chromate dermatitis often clears [19]. A change of occupation may be beneficial in some cases, but it does not ensure the healing of the dermatitis. Substitution for the chromate-containing products is often possible for leather gloves, shoes, and printing material, among others. The occasionally seen persistent nature of chromate dermatitis is not clear. It may be due to chromate remaining in the skin for a long time, or it may require minute quantities of chromate to flare up a contact allergy, and minute quantities of an amount similar to that in cement are found in many everyday objects, such as paper, soil, ash, etc. Recent clinical experimental exposure studies in volunteer patients have revealed that the vast majority of sensitized individuals fail to react to levels of chromate below 10 ppm under realistic exposure conditions [20, 21]. It has been suggested that dermatitis can be aggravated in those allergic to chromate by oral ingestion, but this remains unproven and has not received the attention that the same theory has received in nickel allergy [22].

Chromium is an essential element in the body, especially for glucose metabolism.

Potassium dichromate 0.5% pet. is the standard dilution for testing. However, this percentage can produce an irritant reaction, which may explain the wide difference in dichromate allergy reported throughout the world. It has been suggested that 0.25% would be more accurate, but while this produces fewer reactions, it does miss some true dichromate allergies [23]; the same applies to a dilution of 0.375% [24]. The patch test concentration in the TRUE Test system is 23 $\mu g/cm^2$. The closeness of irritant concentration to that to detect contact allergy is a problem in assessing the true incidence of chromate allergy and in diagnosing individual patients.

References

1. Fregert S, Rorsman H (1964) Allergy to trivalent chromium. Arch Dermatol 90:4–6
2. Burrows D (1984) The dichromate problem. Int J Dermatol 23:215–220
3. Burrows D (1983) Chromium: metabolism and toxicity. CRC, Boca Raton, Fla.
4. Hansen MB, Johansen JD, Menne T (2003) Chromium allergy: significance of both Cr(III) and Cr(VI). Contact Dermatitis 49:206–212
5. Zachariae CO, Agner T, Menne T (1996) Chromium allergy in consecutive patients in a country where ferrous sulfate has been added to cement since 1981. Contact Dermatitis 35:83–85
6. Schnuch A, Geier J, Uter W, Frosch PJ, Lehmacher W, Aberer W, Agathos M, Arnold R, Fuchs T, Laubstein B, Lischka G, Pietrzyk PM, Rakoski J, Richter G, Rueff F (1997) National rates and regional differences in sensitization to allergens of the standard series. Population-adjusted frequencies of sensitization (PAFS) in 40,000 patients from a multicenter study (IVDK). Contact Dermatitis 37:200–209
7. Olsavszky R, Rycroft RJ, White IR, McFadden JP (1998) Contact sensitivity to chromate: comparison at a London contact dermatitis clinic over a 10-year period. Contact Dermatitis 38:329–331
8. Avnstorp C (1989) Prevalence of cement eczema in Denmark before and since addition of ferrous sulfate to Danish cement. Acta Derm Venereol (Stockh) 69:151–155
9. Avnstorp C (1989) Follow-up of workers from the prefabricated concrete industry after the addition of ferrous sulphate to Danish cement. Contact Dermatitis 20:365–371
10. Roto P, Sainio H, Reunala T, Laippala P (1996) Addition of ferrous sulfate to cement and risk of chromium dermatitis among construction workers. Contact Dermatitis 34:43–50
11. Turk K, Rietschel RL (1993) Effect of processing cement to concrete on hexavalent chromium levels. Contact Dermatitis 28:209–211
12. Goh CL, Gan SL (1996) Change in cement manufacturing process, a cause for decline in chromate allergy? Contact Dermatitis 34:51–54

13. Wong SS, Chan MT, Gan SL, Ng SK, Goh CL (1998) Occupational chromate allergy in Singapore: a study of 87 patients and a review from 1983 to 1995. Am J Contact Dermat 9:1–5

14. Irvine C, Pugh CE, Hansen EJ, Rycroft RJ (1994) Cement dermatitis in underground workers during construction of the Channel Tunnel. Occup Med Oxf 44:17–23

15. Bock M, Schmidt A, Bruckner T, Diepgen TL (2003) Occupational skin disease in the construction industry. Br J Dermatol 149:1165–1171

16. Johansen JD, Menne T, Christophersen J, Kaaber K, Veien N (2000) Changes in the pattern of sensitization to common contact allergens in Denmark between 1985–1986 and 1997–1998, with a special view to the effect of preventive strategies. Br J Dermatol 142:490–495

17. Burrows D, Adams RM, Flint GN (1999) Metals. In: Adams RM (ed) Occupational skin disease, 3rd edn. Saunders, Philadelphia, Pa., pp 395–433

18. Thormann J, Jespersen NB, Joensen HD (1979) Persistence of contact allergy to chromium. Contact Dermatitis 5:261–264

19. Lips R, Rast H, Elsner P (1996) Outcome of job change in patients with occupational chromate dermatitis. Contact Dermatitis 34:268–271

20. Fowler JFJ, Kauffman CL, Marks JG Jr, Proctor DM, Fredrick MM, Otani JM, Finley BL, Paustenbach DJ, Nethercott JR (1999) An environmental hazard assessment of low-level dermal exposure to hexavalent chromium in solution among chromium-sensitized volunteers. J Occup Environ Med 41:150–160

21. Basketter DA, Angelini G, Ingber A, Kern PS, Menne T (2003) Nickel, chromium and cobalt in consumer products: revisiting safe levels in the new millennium. Contact Dermatitis 49:1–7

22. Kaaber K, Veien N (1977) The significance of chromate ingestion in patients allergic to chromate. Acta Derm Venereol (Stockh) 57:321–323

23. Andersen KE, Burrows D, Cronin E, Dooms Goossens A, Rycroft RJ, White IR (1988) Recommended changes to standard series. Contact Dermatitis 19:389–390

24. Burrows D, Andersen KE, Camarasa JG, Dooms-Goossens A, Ducombs G, Lachapelle JM, Menne T, Rycroft RJ, Wahlberg JE, White IR, et al (1989) Trial of 0.5% versus 0.375% potassium dichromate. European Environmental and Contact Dermatitis Research Group (EECDRG). Contact Dermatitis 21:351

29.4 Cobalt

Today, more than 75% of the world's production of cobalt is used in the manufacture of alloys. It is also an integral and necessary component of vitamin B12. Meats, fruits, vegetables, and cereals are major sources of vitamin B12, and, thus, of cobalt [1].

A positive patch test to cobalt often occurs in association with a positive test to nickel or chromate, more particularly, nickel, although the pattern may be different in males and in females [2, 3]. However, cobalt allergy without nickel allergy may occur in about 30% of the cases [4]. The association between nickel and cobalt allergy is explained by the metals being commonly present in alloys and products so that considerable contact with nickel means a corre-

spondingly high contact with cobalt, and, hence, a corresponding possibility of sensitization to both [5]. Experimental studies in guinea pigs have shown that concomitant nickel and cobalt patch test reactivity is due to multiple sensitizations rather than cross reactivity [6]. However, a positive test to cobalt occurs 20 times more frequently in those allergic to nickel than in those not allergic, and a person with a +++ nickel positive patch test is 50 times more likely to have +++ positive cobalt reaction [7]. Rystedt and Fischer [8] reported 7% positive patch tests in 4,034 eczema patients, and of these, 50 were isolated cobalt reactions.

Cases of allergy have been reported due to contact with nonmetal sources, such as cobalt naphthenate and oleate used as dryers for varnishes, paints, and printing inks, or as a contact catalyst in polyester resin systems, an oxidizing agent in automobile exhaust controls, in electroplating, and in the rubber tire industry. Exposure and allergy has also occurred to cobalt in wet alkaline clay in pottery and china plants; the latter may be due to porcelain dyes. Cobalt is often added to animal feeds and dermatitis has been described due to it. Cobalt and chromate are still prominent allergens in construction workers in Germany [9], though the cobalt content in cement is low. Cobalt chloride was the third most frequently occurring contact allergen among construction workers with occupational eczema, after chromate and epoxy resin [10]. It is often difficult to identify the source of a single positive cobalt patch test; that is, one with a negative nickel test. However, most of these patients are probably allergic to jewelry, as with nickel.

The importance of cobalt exposure for maintaining allergic hand dermatitis in sensitized individuals is questionable, as patients who immersed a finger in a cobalt salt solution containing 200 mg/l for 10 min daily for 2 weeks failed to develop a flare of hand eczema [11]. Cobalt chloride 1% pet. is the standard dilution for patch testing, and the concentration in the TRUE Test is 20 $\mu g/cm^2$. Cobalt reactions may appear late [12], and cobalt may also be an irritant, giving rise to false-positive reactions of a spotty nature ("poral") associated with a toxic effect on the eccrine acrosyringium [13].

References

1. Basketter DA, Angelini G, Ingber A, Kern PS, Menne T (2003) Nickel, chromium and cobalt in consumer products: revisiting safe levels in the new millennium. Contact Dermatitis 49:1–7

2. Schafer T, Bohler E, Ruhdorfer S, Weigl L, Wessner D, Filipiak B, Wichmann HE, Ring J (2001) Epidemiology of contact allergy in adults. Allergy 56:1192–1196

29

3. Kanerva L, Jolanki R, Estlander T, Alanko K, Savela A (2000) Incidence rates of occupational allergic contact dermatitis caused by metals. Am J Contact Dermat 11: 155–160

4. Edman B (1985) Sites of contact dermatitis in relationship to particular allergens. Contact Dermatitis 13:129–135

5. Basketter DA, Briatico-Vangosa G, Kaestner W, Lally C, Bontinck WJ (1993) Nickel, cobalt and chromium in consumer products: a role in allergic contact dermatitis? Contact Dermatitis 28:15–25

6. Wahlberg JE, Liden C (2000) Cross-reactivity patterns of cobalt and nickel studied with repeated open applications (ROATS) to the skin of guinea pigs. Am J Contact Dermat 11:42–48

7. van Joost T, van Everdingen JJ (1982) Sensitization to cobalt associated with nickel allergy: clinical and statistical studies. Acta Derm Venereol (Stockh) 62:525–529

8. Rystedt I, Fischer T (1983) Relationship between nickel and cobalt sensitization in hard metal workers. Contact Dermatitis 9:195–200

9. Uter W, Ruhl R, Pfahlberg A, Geier J, Schnuch A, Gefeller O (2004) Contact allergy in construction workers: results of a multifactorial analysis. Ann Occup Hyg 48:21–27

10. Bock M, Schmidt A, Bruckner T, Diepgen TL (2003) Occupational skin disease in the construction industry. Br J Dermatol 149:1165–1171

11. Nielsen NH, Kristiansen J, Borg L, Christensen JM, Poulsen LK, Menne T (2000) Repeated exposures to cobalt or chromate on the hands of patients with hand eczema and contact allergy to that metal. Contact Dermatitis 43:212–215

12. Geier J, Gefeller O, Wiechmann K, Fuchs T (1999) Patch test reactions at D4, D5 and D6. Contact Dermatitis 40: 119–126

13. Storrs FJ, White CR Jr (2000) False-positive "poral" cobalt patch test reactions reside in the eccrine acrosyringium. Cutis 65:49–53

29.5 Fragrance Mix

Fragrance and flavor substances are organic compounds with characteristic, usually pleasant, odors [1]. They are ubiquitous and are used in perfumes and perfumed products and are found not only in cosmetics, but also in detergents, fabric softeners, and other household products where fragrance may be used to mask unpleasant odors from raw materials. Flavors are used in foods, beverages, and dental products. Common clinical features of fragrance contact dermatitis are (Fig. 1a, b):

- Axillary dermatitis
- Dermatitis of the face and neck
- Well-circumscribed patches in areas where perfumes are dabbed on (wrists, behind the ears) and (aggravation of) hand eczema

Depending on the degree of sensitivity, the severity of dermatitis may range from mild to severe with dissemination. Airborne and connubial contact dermatitis occurs. There is a possible association between fragrance allergy and hand eczema [2].

Other less frequent adverse reactions to fragrances are: photocontact dermatitis, contact urticaria, irritation, and pigmentary disorders [3, 4].

Evaluation of perfume allergy may be difficult. A complete perfume compound consists of from 10 to more than 300 basic components, selected from about 3,000 materials (http://pharmacos.eudra.org/ F3/cosmetic/cosm_inci_index.htm), which can be divided into the following [1, 3, 4]:

- Natural products isolated from various parts of plants, e.g., blossoms, buds, fruit, peel, seeds, leaves, bark, wood, roots, or from resinous exudates
- Animal products and their extracts (ambergris from the sperm whale, tonkin musk from the testes of musk deer, castoreum from beaver glands, beeswax absolute from beeswax, and civet from glands of the civet cat)
- Numerous synthetic fragrance chemicals

Because of the difficulties in testing with individual fragrances, a perfume screening mixture for patch testing was developed to increase the ability to detect perfume allergy [5]. The current fragrance mix 8% in petrolatum consists of eight ingredients, each at a concentration of 1%:

- Amyl cinnamal
- Cinnamal
- Cinnamyl alcohol
- Eugenol
- *Evernia prunastri* (oak moss)
- Geraniol
- Hydroxycitronellal
- Isoeugenol

The fragrance mix from Hermal and Chemotechnique contains sorbitan sesquioleate as an emulsifier. This fragrance mix has been shown to be a valuable screening agent for perfume dermatitis: most reactions have been caused by oak moss (Fig. 2), isoeugenol, and cinnamal. The test concentration in the TRUE Test is 430 µg/cm².

In most centers, fragrance mix ranks second only to nickel as the most common contact allergen, with a response rate in dermatological patients of between 6% and 11% (Fig. 3). Fragrance allergy is more common among women than men due to greater exposure, though the differences are small [3, 6–8] and may increase with age [9]. Clinical studies have shown a highly significant association between re-

Fig. 1a, b.
Contact allergy to fragrances in deodorants can be very severe: formation of large blisters (**a**) and erythema-multiforme-like lesions with spreading (**b**). (Courtesy of P.J. Frosch)

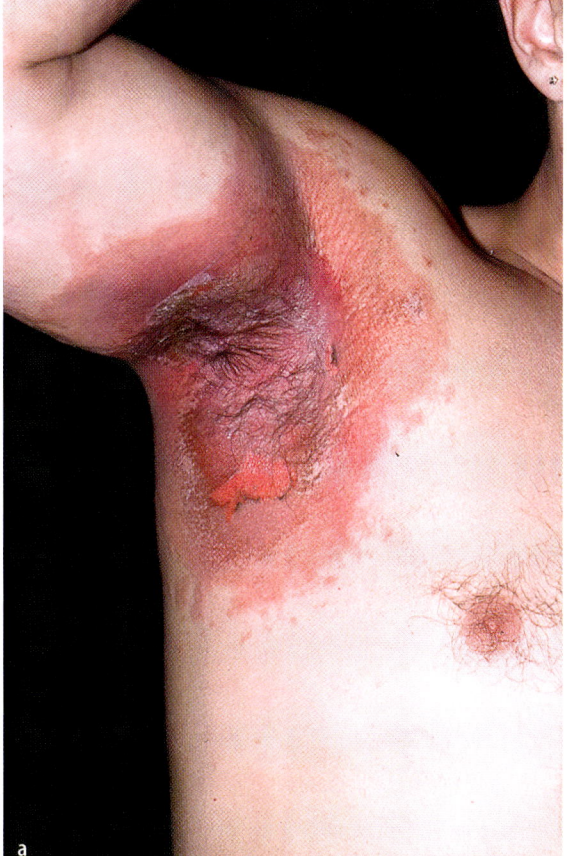

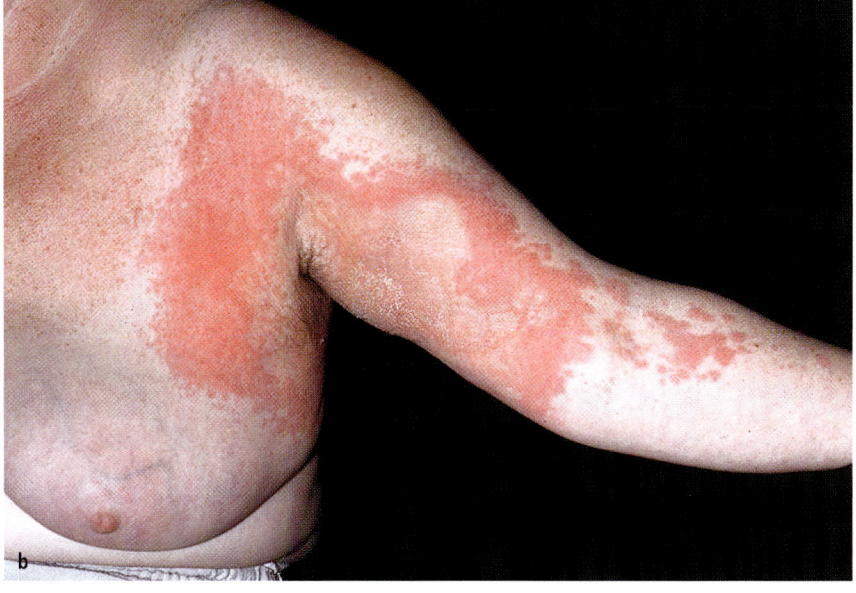

porting a history of visible skin symptoms from using scented products and a positive patch test to the fragrance mix (Fig. 4) [10]. Provocation studies with perfumes and deodorants have also shown that fragrance-mix-positive eczema patients often react to use tests with the products, and subsequent chemical analysis of such products has detected significant amounts of one or more fragrance mix ingredients, confirming the relevance of positive patch tests to fragrance mix in these patients [11, 12].

29

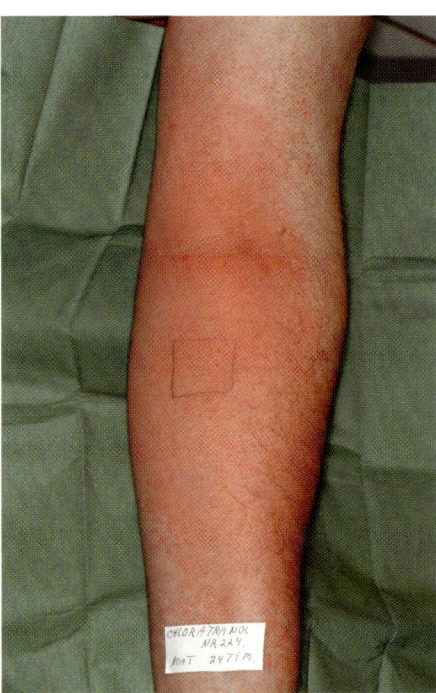

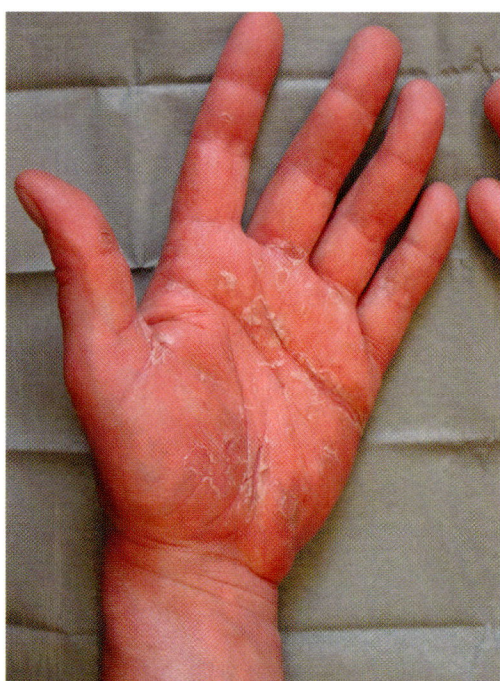

Fig. 2. Strongly positive ROAT to 5 ppm chloratranol solution in ethanol one day after one application of two drops in a male patient with oak moss allergy

Fig. 3. Forty-year-old man with long-lasting hand eczema and strong allergic reactions to fragrance mix and balsam of Peru. Eczema cleared completely after elimination of skin contact with perfumed products

Fig. 4.
Severe long-standing cheilitis in a patient allergic to iso-eugenol present in her lipstick. (Courtesy of P.J. Frosch)

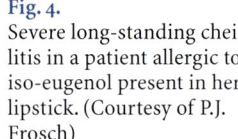

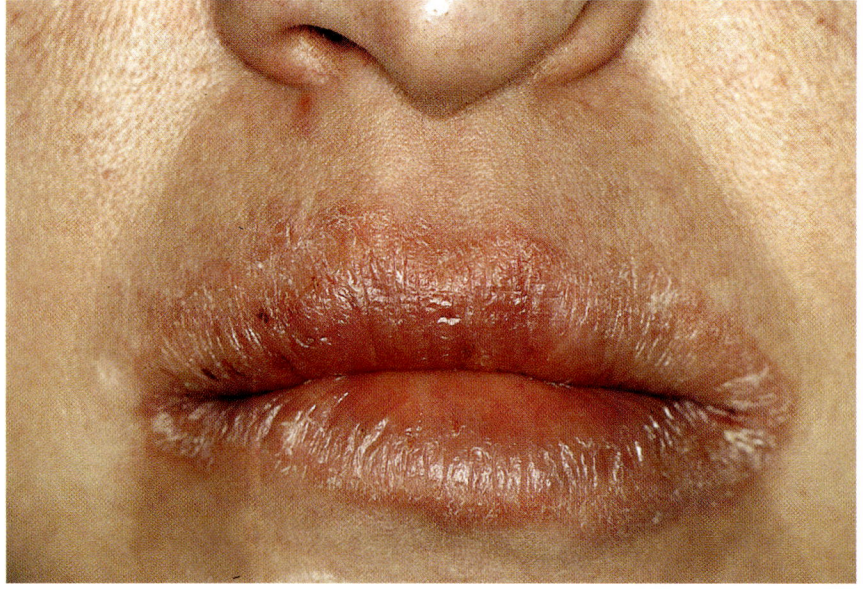

It is estimated that the fragrance mix detects about 75% of all cases of fragrance sensitivity [13, 14]. A second mix has been developed to improve on this [15].

False-positive and false-negative reactions to the mix are common. Marginal reactions may, in some cases, be regarded as irritant, while in other cases, re-

testing with the ingredients of the mix may reveal positive patch tests to one or more of them. To avoid false-negative reactions, ingredient testing is necessary, but evaluation of the patch test results may be difficult because it appears that patch tests in perfume-sensitive patients with fragrance allergens in combination give additive responses compared to patch tests with the allergens separately [16]. Thus, it is important to test patients with their own products.

Evaluation of perfume allergy within Europe is being eased by the mandatory listing on the ingredients label of the fragrance mix substances present in cosmetics and detergents (together with other household products) if present at 10 ppm or more in a finished leave-on cosmetic product, or 100 ppm or more in a rinse-off product.

- Alpha-isomethyl ionone
- Amyl cinnamal*
- Amylcinnamyl alcohol
- Anisyl alcohol
- Benzyl alcohol
- Benzyl benzoate
- Benzyl cinnamate
- Benzyl salicylate
- Butylphenyl methylpropional (lilial)
- Cinnamal*
- Citral
- Citronellol
- Coumarin
- D-Limonene
- Eugenol*
- Hydroxycitronellal*
- Iso-eugenol*
- Farnesol
- Geraniol*
- Hexyl cinnamal
- Hydroxyisohexyl-3-cyclohexene carboxaldehyde (Lyral)
- Linalool
- Methyl heptine carbonate
- 2-(4-*tert*-Butylbenzyl) propionaldehyde
- 3-Methyl-4-(2,6,6-tri-methyl-2-cyclohexen-1-yl)-3-buten-2-one
- Oak moss* [*Evernia prunastri*]

* Present in fragrance mixture

References

1. Bauer K, Garbe D, Surburg H (1988) Flavors and fragrances. In: Ullmann's encyclopedia of industrial chemistry, Chap 3, vol A 11. VCH, Weinheim, Germany, pp 144–246
2. Heydorn S, Menne T, Johansen JD (2003) Fragrance allergy and hand eczema – a review. Contact Dermatitis 48: 59–66
3. de Groot AC, Frosch PJ (1997) Adverse reactions to fragrances: a clinical review. Contact Dermatitis 36:57–86
4. Larsen WG (1994) Perfumes. In: Baran R, Maibach HI (eds) Cosmetic dermatology. Dunitz, London, pp 21–26
5. Larsen WG (1977) Perfume dermatitis. A study of 20 patients. Arch Dermatol 113:623–627
6. Johansen JD, Menné T (1995) The fragrance mix and its constituents: a 14-year material. Contact Dermatitis 32: 18–23
7. Marks JG, Belsito DV, DeLeo VA, Fowler JF, Fransway AF, Maibach HI, Mathias CG, Nethercott JR, Rietschel RL, Sherertz EF, Storrs FJ, Taylor JS (1998) North American Contact Dermatitis Group patch test results for the detection of delayed-type hypersensitivity to topical allergens. J Am Acad Dermatol 38:911–918
8. Katsarou A, Kalogeromitros D, Armenaka M, Koufou V, Davou E, Koumantaki E (1997) Trends in the results of patch testing to standard allergens over the period 1984–1995. Contact Dermatitis 37:245–246
9. Buckley DA, Rycroft RJ, White IR, McFadden JP (2003) The frequency of fragrance allergy in patch-tested patients increases with their age. Br J Dermatol 149:986–989
10. Johansen JD, Andersen TF, Veien N, Avnstorp C, Andersen KE, Menné T (1997) Patch testing with markers of fragrance contact allergy. Do clinical tests correspond to patients' self-reported problems? Acta Derm Venereol (Stockh) 77:149–153
11. Johansen JD, Rastogi SC, Menné T (1996) Contact allergy to popular perfumes; assessed by patch test, use test and chemical analysis. Br J Dermatol 135: 419–422
12. Johansen JD, Rastogi SC, Bruze M, Andersen KE, Frosch P, Dreier B, Lepoittevin JP, White IR, Menné T (1998) Deodorants: a clinical provocation study in fragrance-sensitive patients. Contact Dermatitis 39:161–165
13. Frosch PJ, Pilz B, Andersen KE, Burrows D, Camarasa JG, Dooms-Goossens A, Ducombs G, Fuchs T, Hannuksela M, Lachapelle JM et al. (1995) Patch testing with fragrances: results of a multicenter study of the European Environmental and Contact Dermatitis Research Group with 48 frequently used constituents of perfumes. Contact Dermatitis 33:333–342
14. Larsen W, Nakayama H, Fischer T, Elsner P, Frosch PJ, Burrows D, Jordan W, Shaw S, Wilkinson J, Marks J Jr, Sugawara M, Nethercott M, Nethercott J (1998) A study of a new fragrance mix. Am J Contact Dermat 9:202–206
15. Frosch PJ, Pirker C, Rastogi SC, Andersen KE, Bruze M, Svedman C, Goossens A, White IR, Uter W, Arnau EG, Lepoittevin JP, Menné T, Johansen JD (2005) Patch testing with a new fragrance mix detects additional patients sensitive to perfumes and missed by the current fragrance mix. Contact Dermatitis 52:201–215
16. Johansen JD, Skov L, Vølund AA, Andersen KE, Menné T (1998) Allergens in combination have a synergistic effect on the elicitation response: a study of fragrance-sensitized individuals. Br J Dermatol 139:264–270

29.6 Balsam of Peru

Balsam of Peru (INCI name: *Myroxylon pereirae*) is the natural resinous balsam which exudes from the trunk of the Central American tree *Myroxylon pereirae* after scarification of the bark. It consists of essential oil and resin and is, thus, of the oleoresin type. The composition varies and standardization is based on physical characteristics and the identification of some major chemical constituents. Balsam of Peru contains 30% to 40% resins of unknown composition, while the remaining 60% to 70% consist of well-known chemicals: benzyl benzoate, benzyl cinna-

29

mate, cinnamic acid, benzoic acid, vanillin, farnesol (which is also increasingly being used in deodorants) [1], and nerolidol. In a series of 93 patients with contact allergy to balsam of Peru, reactions were seen, in decreasing order, to the following components: cinnamic alcohol, cinnamic acid, coniferyl alcohol, benzoic acid, cinnamyl cinnamate, eugenol, resorcinol monobenzoate, coniferyl alcohol, and benzyl alcohol [2]. Many perfumes and flavorings contain components either identical to, or cross-reacting with, materials contained in balsam of Peru and other natural resins. Positive patch tests with one or more of these substances may be an indication of perfume allergy. In medicinal preparations, balsam of Peru is still used for its dermatological effects. Some chemicals present in balsam of Peru and similar resinous substances may also have antimicrobial effects and be used as preservatives.

The early epidemiology of perfume allergy is based on Hjorth's [3] classic monograph on balsam of Peru. It gave positive reactions in 4.0% of males and 4.0% of females in a Danish epidemiological study consisting of 2,166 eczema patients [4]. However, the importance of balsam of Peru as a marker for perfume allergy is now questionable, as the incidence of concomitant positive patch tests to balsam of Peru in fragrance-sensitive patients shows wide variation [5, 6]. Contact allergy to this compound is relevant to leg ulcer patients [7]. Immediate reactions to patch tests with balsam of Peru occur. Systemic contact-dermatitis-type reactions, like aggravation of vesicular hand dermatitis following ingestion of related compounds, has been reported in previously sensitized patients [8–11], but the benefits of a flavor-avoidance diet may not be obvious [9]. Because of its sensitizing properties, balsam of Peru is prohibited from use in Europe as a fragrance ingredient. Balsam of Peru 25% pet. is the standard dilution for patch testing, and 800 μg/cm² in the TRUE Test.

References

1. Goossens A, Merckx L (1997) Allergic contact dermatitis from farnesol in a deodorant. Contact Dermatitis 37: 179–180
2. Hausen BM (2001) Contact allergy to balsam of Peru. II. Patch test results in 102 patients with selected balsam of Peru constituents. Am J Contact Dermat 12: 93–102
3. Hjorth N (1961) Eczematous allergy to balsams, allied perfumes and flavouring agents. Munksgaard, Copenhagen, Denmark
4. Christophersen J, Menné T, Tanghøj P, Andersen KE, Brandrup F, Kaaber K, Osmundsen PE, Thestrup-Pedersen K, Veien NK (1989) Clinical patch test data evaluated by multivariate analysis. Contact Dermatitis 21: 291–297
5. Buckley DA, Wakelin SH, Seed PT, Holloway D, Rycroft RJ, White IR, McFadden JP (2000) The frequency of fragrance allergy in a patch-test population over a 17-year period. Br J Dermatol 142: 279–283
6. Johansen JD, Andersen TF, Veien N, Avnstorp C, Andersen KE, Menné T (1997) Patch testing with markers of fragrance contact allergy. Do clinical tests correspond to patients' self-reported problems? Acta Derm Venereol (Stockh) 77: 149–153
7. Machet L, Couhe C, Perrinaud A, Hoarau C, Lorette G, Vaillant L (2004) A high prevalence of sensitization still persists in leg ulcer patients: a retrospective series of 106 patients tested between 2001 and 2002 and a meta-analysis of 1975–2003 data. Br J Dermatol 150: 929–935
8. Veien N (1989) Systemically induced eczema in adults. Acta Derm Venereol Suppl (Stockh) 147: 1–58
9. Niinimaki A (1995) Double-blind placebo-controlled peroral challenges in patients with delayed-type allergy to balsam of Peru. Contact Dermatitis 33: 78–83
10. Salam TN, Fowler JF Jr (2001) Balsam-related systemic contact dermatitis. J Am Acad Dermatol 45: 377–381
11. Pfutzner W, Thomas P, Niedermeier A, Pfeiffer C, Sander C, Przybilla B (2003) Systemic contact dermatitis elicited by oral intake of Balsam of Peru. Acta Derm Venereol (Stockh) 83: 294–295

29.7 Colophony

Colophony (rosin) (INCI name: colophonium) is a widespread, naturally occurring material that is the residue from the distillation of the volatile oil from the oleoresin obtained from trees of the *Pinaceae* family. Its chemical composition is complex and variable, depending on the manufacturing process, geographical area, and storage conditions. There are three kinds of colophony: gum rosin from the tops of living trees, the resin being distilled to yield turpentine oil and the gum resin residue; wood rosin, a distillate from pine tree stumps; and tall oil rosin, a by-product from pine wood pulp (see [1] for a review).

Colophony is composed of about 90% resin acids and 10% neutral substances. The principal allergens in colophony have not yet been determined. Oxidation products of abietic acid and dehydroabietic acid have been identified as allergens, but synthetically prepared derivatives and the neutral fraction also contain allergenic compounds [1]. In a 5-year retrospective study involving 16,210 consecutive eczema patients, 4.5% were colophony-sensitive [2]. In addition to contact eczema, it may also cause type I hypersensitivity [1] and photosensitivity [1, 3].

Concomitant and/or cross-reactions between colophony (rosin), balsam of Peru, oil of turpentine, wood tar, pine resin, spruce resin [4], sesquiterpene lactone mix [5], propolis, and fragrance mix may occur, often in the context of a fragrance allergy [6]. The presence of terpenes [5] in some of these materials, as well as contamination by resin acids in oak moss [7], a component of fragrance mix, only partly explain this phenomenon.

Table 3. Products commonly containing colophony

Adhesives	Paper
Chewing gums	Polishes
Cleansing agents	Printing inks
Cosmetics	Rosin (used by, e.g., violinists, sportspersons)
Cutting fluids	Soldering flux
Dentistry products	Surface coatings
Glues (shoes!)	Ulcer bandages
Insulating tapes	Varnishes
Ostomy appliances	Wood wool

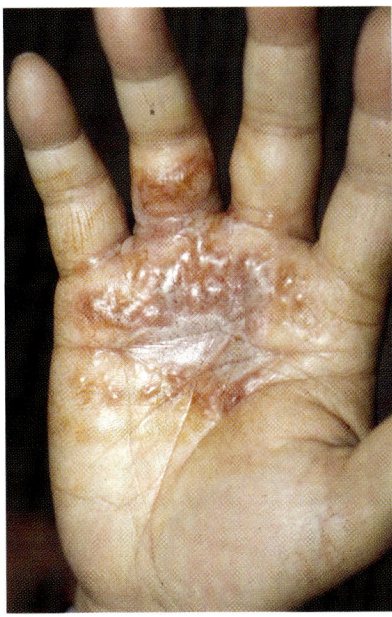

Fig. 5. Severe allergic contact dermatitis from colophonium in a Chinese balsam. (Courtesy of A. Goossens)

Exposure to colophony and its derivatives [1] is likely during both work and leisure hours (Table 3; Fig. 5). In cosmetics, colophony occurs in depilatories, tonics, dressing and hair grooming aids, make-up, mascara, and hair products. In pharmaceutical products, it is used in topical medicaments, including surgical paints [8] and Chinese herbal medicine [9].

Colophony allergy from adhesives has been known for nearly a century, but the use of adhesives based on acrylate polymers has reduced the incidence of contact dermatitis from this source. However, when strong adhesive effects are desired, such as in footwear, colophony or its derivatives may still be used [10–12]. Furthermore, their presence has also been detected in paper, including "no carbon required" (NCR) paper [13], as well as in diapers [14] and sanitary pads [15]. In the modern electronics industry, the use of colophony as a fluxing agent in assembly work produces a significant number of contact allergies appearing as allergic hand [16] and airborne facial [17] dermatitis. Airborne dermatitis may also result from exposure to sawdust – even associated with leukoderma [18] – cutting oils [19], and even jewelry [20].

The occurrence of contact allergy to colophony has been increasing over the past few decades (see [1]). The allergenicity of colophony can be reduced by chemical modification, i.e., by hydrogenation of the nonaromatic double bonds in the resin, which minimizes the content of easily oxidized acids of the abietic type [21]. A mixture of unmodified Chinese and Portuguese gum rosin is used in the standard series at a concentration of 20% pet. [22], and in the TRUE Test, the concentration is 850 µg/cm². Further studies are necessary to improve our understanding of colophony contact allergy and the optimal patch test material [23, 24]. Indeed, if the patient's history indicates heavy exposure to rosin, additional testing with other types of gum rosin and also tall oil rosin may be indicated. If negative responses are still obtained, the possibility of sensitivity to components of modified rosin must be considered [24], since tests with unmodified rosin (in the standard series) are most often negative in patients who react to modified-rosin derivatives, the latter probably being stronger sensitizers [25, 26].

References

1. Downs AMR, Sansom JE (1999) Colophony allergy: a review. Contact Dermatitis 41:305–310
2. Bruynzeel DP, Diepgen TL, Andersen KE, Brandão FM, Bruze M, Frosch PJ, Goosssens A, Lahti A, Mahler V, Maibach HI, Menné T, Wilkinson JD (2005) Monitoring the European Standard series in 10 centres: 1996–2000. Contact Dermatitis (in press)
3. Kuno Y, Kato M (2001) Photosensitivity from colophony in a case of chronic actinic dermatitis associated with contact allergy from colophony. Acta Derm Venereol 81: 442–443
4. Hjorth N (1961) Eczematous allergy to balsams, allied perfumes and flavouring agents. Munksgaard, Copenhagen, Denmark
5. Paulsen E, Andersen KE, Brandão FM, Bruynzeel DP, Ducombs G, Frosch PJ, Goossens A, Lahti A, Menné T, Shaw S, Tosti A, Wahlberg JE, Wilkinson JD, Wrängsjö K (1999) Routine patch testing with the sesquiterpene lactone mix in Europe: a 2-year experience. A multicentre study of the EECDRG. Contact Dermatitis 40:72–76
6. Wöhrl S, Hemmer W, Focke M, Götz M, Jarisch R (2001) The significance of fragrance mix, balsam of Peru, colophony and propolis as screening tools in the detection of fragrance allergy. Br J Dermatol 145:268–273

29

7. Lepoittevin J-P, Meschkat E, Huygens S, Goossens A (2000) Presence of resin acids in "Oakmoss" patch test material: a source of misdiagnosis? J Invest Dermatol 115: 129–130

8. Reichert-Pénétrat S, Barbaud A, Pénétrat E, Granel F, Schmutz JL (2001) Allergic contact dermatitis from surgical paints. Contact Dermatitis 45:116–117

9. Li LF, Wang J (2002) Patch testing in allergic contact dermatitis caused by topical Chinese herbal medicine. Contact Dermatitis 47:166–168

10. Saha M, Srinivas CR, Shenoy SD, Balachandrar C, Acharya S (1993) Footwear dermatitis. Contact Dermatitis 28: 260–264

11. Lyon CC, Tucker SC, Gäfvert E, Karlberg A-T, Beck MH (1999) Contact dermatitis from modified rosin in footwear. Contact Dermatitis 41:102–103

12. Strauss RM, Wilkinson SH (2002) Shoe dermatitis due to colophonium used as leather tanning or finishing agent in Portuguese shoes. Contact Dermatitis 47:59

13. Lange-Ionescu S, Bruze M, Gruvberger B, Zimerson E, Frosch P (2000) Kontaktallergie durch kohlefreies Durchschlagpapier. Dermatosen Beruf Umwelt 48:183–187

14. Karlberg AT, Magnusson K (1996) Rosin components identified in diapers. Contact Dermatitis 34:176–180

15. Kanerva L, Rintala H, Henriks-Eckerman K, Engström K (2001) Colophonium in sanitary pads. Contact Dermatitis 44:59–60

16. Färm G (1996) Contact allergy to colophony and hand eczema. A follow-up study of patients with previously diagnosed contact allergy to colophony. Contact Dermatitis 34:93–100

17. Karlberg AT, Gäfvert E, Meding B, Stenberg B (1996) Airborne contact dermatitis from unexpected exposure to rosin (colophony). Rosin sources revealed with chemical analyses. Contact Dermatitis 35:272–278

18. Kumar A, Freeman S (1999) Leukoderma following occupational allergic contact dermatitis. Contact Dermatitis 41:94–98

19. Corazza M, Borghi A, Virgili A (2004) A medicolegal controversy due to a hidden allergen in cutting oils. Contact Dermatitis 50:254–255

20. Agarwal S, Gawkrodger DJ (2002) Occupational allergic contact dermatitis to silver and colophonium in a jeweler. Am J Contact Dermatitis 13:74

21. Karlberg AT, Boman A, Nilsson JLG (1988) Hydrogenation reduces the allergenicity of colophony. Contact Dermatitis 19:22–29

22. Karlberg A-T, Gäfvert E (1996) Isolated colophony allergens as screening substances for contact allergy. Contact Dermatitis 35:201–207

23. Sadhra S, Foulds IS, Gray CN (1998) Oxidation of resin acids in colophony (rosin) and its implications for patch testing. Contact Dermatitis 39:58–63

24. Gäfvert E, Bordalo O, Karlberg A-T (1996) Patch testing with allergens from modified rosin (colophony) discloses additional cases of contact allergy. Contact Dermatitis 35: 290–298

25. Hausen BM, Mohnert J (1989) Contact allergy due to colophony. (V) Patch test results with different types of colophony and modified-colophony products. Contact Dermatitis 20:295–301

26. Goossens A, Armingaud P, Avenel-Audran M, Begon-Bagdassarian I, Constandt L, Giordano-Labadie F, Girardin P, Le Coz CJ, Milpied-Homsi B, Nootens C, Pecquet C, Tennstedt D, Vanhecke E (2002) An epidemic of allergic contact dermatitis due to epilating products. Contact Dermatitis 47:67–70

29.8 Neomycin

Neomycin is a widely used aminoglycoside antibiotic produced from *Streptomyces fradiae*. The frequency of neomycin sensitivity varies from clinic to clinic, depending to a large extent on local referral and prescription habits [1]. In a series of 40,000 consecutive eczema patients, the patch-test results of which were published in 1997, 1% to 6% had neomycin contact allergy. This is comparable to the results obtained in a recent study by the EECDRG concerning 26,210 consecutive eczema patients tested in 10 different centers [2], in which the frequency was 3%, with individual frequencies varying from 1.6% to 7.7%. Several patch test studies demonstrated that there is an upward trend in the occurrence of neomycin sensitivity over the years, probably due to increased use of topical drugs containing this antibiotic [3, 4]. The patients particularly at risk of neomycin sensitivity appear to be those with chronic and recurrent dermatitis in skin areas where occlusion or bandaging is prone to occur or is used, as in stasis dermatitis, but also those with otitis externa [5, 6] and perianal eczema. Occupational contact dermatitis, as well as systemic reactions, may occur.

The diagnosis of neomycin allergy may be difficult because the dermatitis is not vesicular or bullous, but often appears instead as aggravation or simply chronicity of a pre-existing dermatitis. It is instructive to note that the therapeutic concentration of neomycin is often 0.5%, while the patch test concentration is 20% in petrolatum. Even at this concentration (and in this vehicle) [7], some positives may be missed; the positive neomycin patch test appears late, after 3–4 days in many cases, and there are many inter-individual variations [7]. The neomycin concentration in the TRUE Test is 230 µg/cm².

The cross-sensitization pattern of neomycin is complex. Cross-sensitivity occurs, although not with the same frequency, between neomycin, amikacin, arbekacin, dibekacin, framycetin, gentamycin, isepamicin, kanamycin, paromomycin, ribostamycin, sisomycin, spectinomycin, and tobramycin [8].

References

1. Schnuch A, Geier J, Uter W, Frosch PJ, Lehmacher W, Aberer W, Agathos M, Arnold R, Fuchs T, Laubstein B, Lischka G, Pietrzyk, PM Rakoski J, Richter G, Rueff F (1997) National rates and regional differences in sensitization to allergens of the standard series. Population-adjusted frequencies of sensitization (PAFS) in 40,000 patients from a multicenter study (IVDK). Contact Dermatitis 37:200–209

2. Bruynzeel DP, Diepgen TL, Andersen KE, Brandão FM, Bruze M, Frosch PJ, Goosssens A, Lahti A, Mahler V, Maibach HI, Menné T, Wilkinson JD (2004) Monitoring the Eu-

ropean Standard series in 10 centres: 1996–2000. Contact Dermatitis (in press)

3. Edman B, Möller H (1982) Trends and forecasts for standard allergens in a 12-year patch test material. Contact Dermatitis 8:95–104
4. Gollhausen R, Enders F, Przybilla B, Burg G, Ring J (1988) Trends in allergic contact sensitization. Contact Dermatitis 18:147–154
5. van Ginkel CJ, Bruintjes TD, Huizing EH (1995) Allergy due to topical medications in chronic otitis externa and chronic otitis media. Clin Otolaryngol Allied Sci 20:326–328
6. Hillen U, Geier J, Goos M (2000) Kontaktallergien bei Patienten mit Ekzemen des äußeren Gehörgangs. Hautarzt 51:239–243
7. Bjarnason B, Flosadóttir E (2000) Patch testing with neomycin sulfate. Contact Dermatitis 43:295–302
8. Kimura M, Kawada A (1998) Contact sensitivity induced by neomycin with cross-sensitivity to other aminoglycoside antibiotics. Contact Dermatitis 39:148–150

29.9 Benzocaine (Ethylaminobenzoate)

Benzocaine is a para-aminobenzoic acid (PABA) derivative and is used as a local anesthetic.

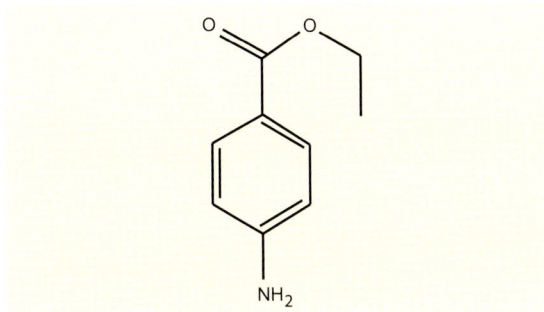

Scheme 1. 4-Aminobenzoic acid ethyl ester

The incidence of contact sensitivity reported varies widely from country to country, probably depending on the level of use of benzocaine in the community [1, 2]. The incidence of positive reactions to topical anesthetics in eczema patients ranges from 0.5% to 2% [2]. In some countries, such as the United States, it is widely used in over-the-counter preparations, whereas in others, such as the United Kingdom, its use is much less common [3].

According to Sidhu et al. [3], and in agreement with previous studies [4, 5], it would be good to include a "caine mix" in the standard series consisting of benzocaine, tetracaine HCl, and dibucaine HCl [each 5% pet.), since benzocaine [5% petrolatum) alone is inadequate. The TRUE test includes a caine mix containing benzocaine, dibucaine hydrochloride, and tetracaine hydrochloride (5:1:1) 630 μg/cm². In order to detect more patients sensitive to topical anesthetics, it is necessary to test with other

"caine" anesthetics [5, 6]. Benzocaine-sensitive individuals can safely use amide derivatives, such as lidocaine (lignocaine).

Benzocaine can cross-react with compounds other than local anesthetics, such as para-phenylenediamine, sunscreens such as para-aminobenzoic acid esters used as sunscreens, sulfonamides, and certain dyes.

References

1. Placucci F, Lorenzi S, La Placa M, Vincenzi C (1996) Sensitization to benzocaine on a condom. Contact Dermatitis 34:293
2. Bruynzeel DP, Diepgen TL, Andersen KE, Brandão FM, Bruze M, Frosch PJ, Goossens A, Lahti A, Mahler V, Maibach HI, Menné T, Wilkinson JD (2004) Monitoring the European Standard series in 10 centres: 1996–2000. Contact Dermatitis (in press)
3. Sidhu SK, Shaw S, Wilkinson J (1999) A 10-year retrospective study on benzocaine allergy in the United Kingdom. Am J Contact Dermat 10:57–61
4. Wilkinson JD, Andersen KE, Lahti A, Rycroft RJG, Shaw S, White I (1990) Preliminary patch testing with 25% and 15% "caine" mixes. The EECDRG. Contact Dermatitis 22:244–245
5. Beck MH, Holden A (1988) Benzocaine – an unsatisfactory indicator of topical local anaesthetic sensitization for the UK. Br J Dermatol 118:91–94
6. van Ketel WG, Bruynzeel DP (1991) A "forgotten" topical anaesthetic sensitizer: butyl aminobenzoate. Contact Dermatitis 25:131–132

29.10 Clioquinol

Synonyms for clioquinol are: chinoform, chloroiodoquine, cliochinolum, iodochlorhydroxyquin, iodochlorhydroxyquinoline, and 5-chloro-7-iodoquinolin-8-ol.

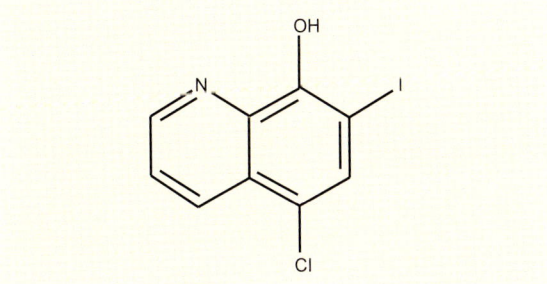

Scheme 2. Clioquinol

Because of manufacturing problems, clioquinol 5% pet. replaced the quinoline mix in the standard series. The mix contained a mixture of clioquinol and chlorquinaldol [1]. These substances have both antibacterial and antifungal activity, and are commonly used in creams and ointments to treat skin conditions in which an anti-infective agent is required. A concentration of 3% in such preparations is usual, and they are often combined with a topical corticosteroid. Clioquinol has been used in orally. Chlorquinaldol is 5,6-dichloro-2-methylquinolin-8-ol. These quinolines are not potent allergens. The acquisition of allergic sensitivity to them does not generally cause a marked worsening of eczema, and, when combined with a topical corticosteroid, the steroid will cause some suppression of the inflammatory response. Although Cronin [2] found that no particular pattern of eczema predisposed to clioquinol sensitivity, it may be more common in relation to stasis dermatitis and otitis externa [3, 4]. Geographical variation in the incidence depends on the types of products locally available and the type of patient being investigated. The prevalence of contact allergy to clioquinol is about 0.7% [5]. The oral administration of either clioquinol or chlorquinaldol has resulted in a generalized eruption in individuals allergic to these compounds [6–8]. A first drug eruption due to clioquinol has been reported [9]. An immediate-type reaction occurred in a woman intolerant of oral quinine when clioquinol was applied topically [10]; a quinoline ring is common to both. It may cause contact urticaria on patch testing [11]. Cross-reactions between clioquinol and chlorquinaldol are not common, and clioquinol is the more important of the two allergens. In patients tested consecutively to both quinoline mix and clioquinol, it was found that clioquinol alone missed 34% of the patients reacting to quinoline mix [1]. However, in three patients believed to have been sensitized previously to clioquinol, a spectrum of reactions was recorded to other halogenated hydroxyquinolines [12]. Irritant reactions to clioquinol-containing products have also been described, particularly when used in sensitive skin areas, such as the perineum [13, 14].

References

1. Agner T, Menné T (1993) Sensitivity to clioquinol and chlorquinaldol in the quinoline mix. Contact Dermatitis 29:163
2. Cronin E (1980) Contact dermatitis. Churchill Livingstone, Edinburgh, UK, p 219
3. Goh CL, Ling R (1998) A retrospective epidemiology study of contact eczema among the elderly attending a tertiary dermatology referral centre in Singapore. Singapore Med J 39:442–446
4. Van Ginkel CJ, Bruintjes TD, Huizing EH (1995) Allergy due to topical medications in chronic otitis externa and chronic otitis media. Clin Otolaryngol 20:326–328
5. Morris SD, Rycroft RJ, Wakelin SH, McFadden JP (2002). Comparative frequency of patch test reactions to topical antibiotics. Br J Dermatol 146:1047–1051
6. Ekelund A, Möller H (1969) Oral provocation in eczematous contact allergy to neomycin and hydroxy-quinolines. Act Derm Verereol (Stockh) 49:422–426
7. Skog E (1975) Systemic eczematous contact-type dermatitis induced by iodochlorhydroxyquin and chloroquine phosphate. Contact Dermatitis 1:187
8. Silvestre JF, Alfonso R, Moragón M, Ramón R, Botella R (1998) Systemic contact dermatitis due to norfloxacin with a positive patch test to quinoline mix. Contact Dermatitis 39:83
9. Janier M, Vignon MD (1995) Recurrent fixed drug eruption due to clioquinol. Br J Dermatol 133:1013–1034
10. Simpson JR (1974) Reversed cross-sensitisation between quinine and iodochlorhydroxyquinoline. Contact Dermatitis Newslett 15:431
11. Katsarou A, Armenaka M, Ale I, Koufou V, Kalogeromitros D (1999) Frequency of immediate reactions to the European standard series. Contact Dermatitis 41:276–279
12. Allenby CF (1965) Skin sensitisation to Remederm and cross-sensitisation to hydroxyquinoline compounds. Br Med J ii:208–209
13. Kero M, Hannuksela M, Sothman A (1979) Primary irritant dermatitis from topical clioquinol. Contact Dermatitis 5:115–117
14. Beck MH, Wilkinson SM (1994) A distinctive irritant contact reaction to Vioform (clioquinol). Contact Dermatitis 31:54–55

29.11 Wool Wax Alcohols (Lanolin)

Lanolin is a natural product from sheep fleece and consists of a complex mixture of esters and polyesters of high-molecular-weight alcohols and fatty acids. The composition varies from time to time and from place to place. Wool wax alcohols (INCI name: lanolin alcohol) are a complex mixture of esters of alcohols and fatty acids derived from hydrolysis of the oily, waxy fraction of sheep fleece. The general incidence of lanolin allergy in consecutively tested eczema patients is around 2% to 3% [1, 2]. Lanolin and wool wax alcohols are weak allergens and experimental sensitization cannot be achieved in humans and animals [3].

The use of lanolin extends from topical preparations to industrial lubricants, polishes, anti-corrosives, printing inks, leather and textile finishes, and paper constituents. The literature on contact allergy to lanolin has been extensively reviewed [4–6].

Lanolin allergy is uncommon on normal skin and with cosmetic usage, but is common when applied to leg ulcers and other diseased skin, such as in the anogenital area [6]. Because of the rarity of lanolin sensitization when applied to normal skin, every positive patch test to wool wax alcohols and lanolin should be verified to determine whether it represents an allergy or nonspecific reactivity (e.g., the excited skin syndrome) [5, 7].

To detect contact allergy cases, wool wax alcohols at a concentration of 30% pet. are tested in the standard series, and the concentration in the TRUE Test is 1,000 µg/cm². Other derivatives have also been tested, among them include hydrogenated lanolin and Amerchol L-101 (mineral oil and lanolin alcohol), the latter having been found to be an additional marker for lanolin sensitivity [6, 8, 9]. However, irritant reactions with these compounds are not excluded [5].

The lanolin allergens are unknown, although they are probably present in the alcoholic fraction. Several modifications of lanolin have been tested to produce one with a less sensitizing capacity [10, 11].

References

1. Schnuch A, Geier J, Uter W, Frosch PJ, Lehmacher W, Aberer W, Agathos M, Arnold R, Fuchs T, Laubstein B, Lischka G, Pietrzyk PM, Rakoski J, Richter G, Rueff F (1997) National rates and regional differences in sensitization to allergens of the standard series. Population-adjusted frequencies of sensitization (PAFS) in 40,000 patients from a multicenter study (IVDK). Contact Dermatitis 37: 200–209
2. Bruynzeel DP, Diepgen TL, Andersen KE, Brandão FM, Bruze M, Frosch PJ, Goosssens A, Lahti A, Mahler V, Maibach HI, Menné T, Wilkinson JD (2005) Monitoring the European Standard series in 10 centres: 1996–2000. Contact Dermatitis (in press)
3. Kligman AM (1983) Lanolin allergy: crisis or comedy. Contact Dermatitis 9: 99–107
4. Breit R, Bandmann HJ (1973) Contact dermatitis XXII. Dermatitis from lanolin. Br J Dermatol 88: 414–416
5. Kligman AM (1998) The myth of lanolin allergy. Contact Dermatitis 39: 103–107
6. Wakelin SH, Smith H, White IR, Rycroft RJG, McFadden JP (2001) A retrospective analysis of contact allergy to lanolin. Br J Dermatol 145: 28–31
7. Gallenkemper G, Rabe E, Bauer R (1998) Contact sensitization in chronic venous insufficiency: modern wound dressings. Contact Dermatitis 38: 274–278
8. Carmichael AJ, Foulds IS, Bransbury DS (1991) Loss of lanolin patch-test positivity. Br J Dermatol 125: 573–576
9. Matthieu L, Dockx P (1997) Discrepancy in patch test results with wool wax alcohols and Amerchol-L101. Contact Dermatitis 36: 150–151
10. Clark EW, Blondeel A, Cronin E, Oleffe JA, Wilkinson DS (1981) Lanolin of reduced sensitizing potential. Contact Dermatitis 7: 80–83
11. Edman B, Moller H (1989) Testing a purified lanolin preparation by a randomized procedure. Contact Dermatitis 20: 287–290

29.12 Paraben Mix

The most widely used preservatives in foods, drugs, and cosmetics are the parabens (alkyl esters of *p*-hydroxybenzoic acid) [1].

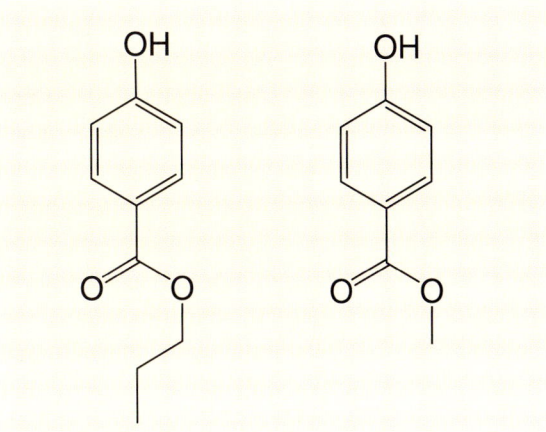

Scheme 3. Propylparaben and methylparaben

This group of preservatives has been used for more than 60 years and includes methyl-, ethyl-, propyl-, and butylparaben (INCI names). They are also marketed under a number of trade names for use in noncosmetic products, i.e., Solbrol, Tegosept, Betacide, Bonomold, Chemoside, Nipagin, and Propagin. The parabens are most often used in combination due to their different solubility and action spectrum. They are less efficient against gram-negative bacteria; therefore, parabens are often used in cosmetic products in combination with other biocides. The vast majority of the cosmetics registered at the FDA contain parabens and the use concentration is usually in the range 0.1% and 0.8%. Cross-reactions between the four paraben esters methyl-, ethyl-, propyl- and butylparaben are common, but exceptions can occur. The paraben mix used to contain these four esters plus benzylparaben. Benzylparaben has been removed because it is no longer allowed for use in cosmetics and drugs as it is suspected to be a carcinogen. Further, butylparaben is now in discredit because of estrogenic effects in animal models; however, the clinical implications of this suspicion has not yet been determined [2].

In diagnostic patch testing, Menné and Hjorth [3] found that approximately 1.0% of more than 8,000 eczema patients tested were sensitized. Similar frequencies are reported in other large-scale patch test studies [4–6]. The frequency of positive reactions has been remarkably constant over a 15-year period [5]. In spite of the extensive use of parabens, it must be regarded as a very safe preservative in topical products and allergic contact dermatitis, as it is relatively rare. In animal experiments, they also seem to be

29

weak allergens; propylparaben was not able to show any sensitization in a guinea pig maximization test [7]. Clinical experience shows that the incidence of paraben sensitization in healthy persons is small, and agrees with the impression that occasional cases of paraben sensitivity occur and are important to the particular patient's welfare [8]. Cosmetics seems to be an uncommon source of sensitization. Clinical experience shows that patients with chronic dermatitis are at risk, particularly patients with stasis dermatitis and leg ulcers [9, 10]. Fisher coined the term "paraben paradox," denoting the fact that many leg ulcer patients with a paraben allergy tolerate paraben-preserved cosmetics on healthy skin [11, 12]. In spite of the low frequency of paraben contact allergy, it is important to keep the allergen in the standard series, since it is difficult to verify the suspicion of the existence of paraben allergy. Often, the sufferers are patients with long lasting dermatitis that do not get better under normal treatment and skin care. If the allergen is not included in the standard battery series, the diagnosis will be missed.

Fisher et al. [8] and Schorr [13] assumed that repeated topical application of low concentrations of parabens in medicaments or cosmetics could cause sensitization, while Hjorth and Trolle-Lassen [14] stated that higher concentrations were necessary for the majority of cases. They reported a 1% incidence of paraben sensitivity, suggesting that this was due to the frequent use in Denmark of topical antifungal agents containing up to 5% paraben (Amycen). Cross-reactions have been described to other para compounds, such as benzocaine, para-phenylenediamine, and sulfonamides, but they are rare [15]. It has been reported that paraben-sensitive patients may experience flares of dermatitis from parabens in food and systemic medicaments [16, 17]. Placebo-controlled oral challenge with methyl-p-hydroxybenzoate in 14 paraben-sensitive patients was negative in 11, doubtful in one, and two had a flare of dermatitis. However, subsequent low-paraben diet had no effect on the dermatitis [18]. Immediate-type reactions (both systemic and contact urticaria) from parabens have been reported, but are very rare and not related to paraben-induced allergic dermatitis [19, 20].

In the European standard series, the parabens are tested as a mix of 4% of methyl-, ethyl-, propyl-, and butylparaben, a total of 16% pet., and in the TRUE Test, the concentration is 1,000 $\mu g/cm^2$ (Table 1). In Menné and Hjorth's study [2], two-thirds of the patients reacting to the mix showed positive reactions to one or more of the individual esters. Multiple patch test reactivity is probably due to cross-sensitization, but concomitant sensitization to individual

esters is a possibility because the esters are often used in combination. Patch testing with products preserved with parabens is often negative in paraben-sensitized patients because the paraben concentration is too low to elicit dermatitis on normal skin, even under occlusive conditions.

The final details of the paraben story remain to be elucidated. Except for high concentration (i.e., >1%) drug use and application to leg ulcers, the parabens are rare contact sensitizers. Combined with the extensive chronic toxicity data available on their systemic effects, these compounds set the standard for relative safety that new preservatives will have difficulty matching. It is too early to say if the estrogenic effect story changes this view. Technical and microbiological considerations sometimes make alternative preservatives necessary. However, the paraben mix is important in the standard series because paraben allergy is difficult to detect from the history or clinical appearance of dermatitis.

References

1. Rastogi SC, Schouten A, de Kruijf N, Weijland JW (1995) Contents of methyl-, ethyl-, propyl-, butyl- and benzylparaben in cosmetic products. Contact Dermatitis 32:28–30
2. Harvey PW, Everett DJ (2004) Significance of the detection of esters of p-hydroxybenzoic acid (parabens) in human breast tumours. J Appl Toxicol 24:1–4
3. Menné T, Hjorth N (1988) Routine patch testing with paraben esters. Contact Dermatitis 19:189–191
4. Schnuch A, Geier J, Uter W, Frosch PJ (1998) Patch testing with preservatives, antimicrobials and industrial biocides. Results from a multicentre study. Br J Dermatol 138:467–476
5. Jacobs MC, White IR, Rycroft RJ, Taub N (1995) Patch testing with preservatives at St John's from 1982 to 1993. Contact Dermatitis 33:247–254
6. Wilkinson JD, Shaw S, Andersen KE, Brandao FM, Bruynzeel DP, Bruze M, Camarasa JM, Diepgen TL, Ducombs G, Frosch PJ, Goossens A, Lachapelle JM, Lahti A, Menne T, Seidenari S, Tosti A, Wahlberg JE (2002) Monitoring levels of preservative sensitivity in Europe. A 10-year overview (1991–2000). Contact Dermatitis 46:207–210
7. Andersen KE, Volund A, Frankild S (1995) The guinea pig maximization test – with a multiple dose design. Acta Derm Venereol (Stockh) 75:463–469
8. Fisher AA, Pascher F, Kanof NB (1971) Allergic contact dermatitis due to ingredients of vehicles. A "vehicle tray" for patch testing. Arch Dermatol 104:286–290
9. Gallenkemper G, Rabe E, Bauer R (1998) Contact sensitization in chronic venous insufficiency: modern wound dressings. Contact Dermatitis 38:274–278
10. Praditsuwan P, Taylor JS, Roenigk HH Jr (1995) Allergy to Unna boots in four patients. J Am Acad Dermatol 33:906–908
11. Fisher AA (1973) The paraben paradox. Cutis 12:830–832
12. Fisher AA (1979) Paraben dermatitis due to a new medicated bandage: the "paraben paradox". Contact Dermatitis 5:273–274

13. Schorr WF (1968) Paraben allergy. A cause of intractable dermatitis. JAMA 204:859–862
14. Hjorth N, Trolle-Lassen C (1963) Skin reactions to ointment bases. Trans St Johns Hosp Dermatol Soc 49:127–140
15. Maucher OM (1974) Beitrag zur Kreuz- oder Kopplingsallergie zur parahydroxybenzoe-säure-ester. Berufsdermatosen 22:183–187
16. Fisher AA (1975) Letter: Paraben-induced dermatitis. Arch Dermatol 111:657–658
17. Carradori S, Peluso AM, Faccioli M (1990) Systemic contact dermatitis due to parabens. Contact Dermatitis 22:238–239
18. Veien NK, Hattel T, Laurberg G (1996) Oral challenge with parabens in paraben-sensitive patients. Contact Dermatitis 34:433
19. Henry JC, Tschen EH, Becker LE (1979) Contact urticaria to parabens. Arch Dermatol 115:1231–1232
20. Nagel JE, Fuscaldo JT, Fireman P (1977) Paraben allergy. JAMA 237:1594–1595

29.13 Formaldehyde

Formaldehyde is a ubiquitous and potent sensitizer, industrially, domestically, and medically. Lowering its usage concentration to 30 ppm could decrease the cases of allergy observed [1]. Formaldehyde exposure is difficult to estimate because the chemical – besides being manufactured, imported, and used as such – is incorporated into a large variety of products and reactants in many chemical processes, including formaldehyde releasers, polymerized plastics, metalworking fluids, medicaments, fabrics, cosmetics, and detergents (Table 4) [2]. Therefore, the detection of the formaldehyde content by chemical analysis, such as e.g., the closed container diffusion method (CCD) as proposed by Karlberg et al., would be interesting

Table 4. Formaldehyde uses and exposure

Clothing, wash and wear, crease-resistant clothing
Medications: wart remedies, anhidrotics
Antiperspirants
Preservative in cosmetics
Photographic paper and solutions
Paper industry
Disinfectants and deodorizers
Cleaning products
Polishes
Paints and coatings
Printing etching materials
Tanning agents
Dry cleaning materials
Chipboard production
Mineral wool production
Glues
Phenolic resins and urea plastics in adhesives
  and footwear
Fish meal industry
Smoke from wood, coal, and tobacco
  (relevance is controversial)

for the prevention of recurrence of allergic contact dermatitis in formaldehyde-allergic patients [3]. Shampoos may contain formaldehyde, but because they are quickly diluted and washed off, only exquisitely formaldehyde-sensitive consumers develop dermatitis on the scalp and face from them. However, hairdressers may get hand dermatitis from similar products due to their more intense exposure.

Formaldehyde dermatitis from textiles is rare today because the manufacturers have improved the fabric finish treatment and have reduced the amount of formaldehyde residues in new clothing. Garments made from 100% acrylic, polyester, linen, silk, nylon, and cotton are generally considered to be formaldehyde free [4, 5]. Formaldehyde sensitivity is not necessarily accompanied by a simultaneous sensitivity to formaldehyde resins and formaldehyde releasers, and vice versa [6–9]. Forty five percent of the subjects tested in St John's were positive to formaldehyde alone, whereas 47% of the subjects reacted simultaneously to quaternium-15 [10]. Indeed, some of the formaldehyde releasers might act as prohaptens. It depends on the exposure conditions and the actual release of formaldehyde. The frequency of formaldehyde-positive patch tests in consecutive eczema patients is around 2–3% [11–13].

Inexplicable positive patch test reactions frequently occur where no clinical relevance is found. A deeper search, however, might often reveal it. Hidden sources of formaldehyde in the home may be a cause of hand eczema in some women with formaldehyde allergy. In certain cases, the positive patch test should be confirmed by a repeated test and by a use test, since false-positive reactions may occur; this may explain why about one-third of allergies reported to formaldehyde and its releasers can be lost on repeated patch testing, although a lack of reproducibility in patch testing might also account for this phenomenon [9, 14, 15]. In a detailed clinical experiment, the eliciting closed patch test threshold concentration was 10,000 ppm formaldehyde in 10 of 20 formaldehyde-sensitive individuals, 9 reacted to 5,000 ppm, 3 reacted to 1,000 ppm, 2 reacted to 500 ppm, and 1 reacted to 250 ppm (Fig. 6). Positive reactions were not observed in nonoccluded patch test with a dilution series from 25 ppm to 10,000 ppm, or in a repeated open application test (ROAT) with a leave-on cosmetic product containing a formaldehyde releaser (an average of 300 ppm formaldehyde) [16]. Thus, the threshold concentration for occluded patch test to formaldehyde in formaldehyde-sensitive patients seems to be around 250 ppm. The threshold level of formaldehyde required to elicit an eczematous reaction in the axilla of formaldehyde-sensitive volunteers was 30 ppm [17].

Fig. 6.
Lowest formaldehyde concentration giving positive reactions in occluded patch testing, compared to the strength of the reactions in diagnostic patch testing (10,000 ppm) among 19 formaldehyde-sensitive eczema patients. (From [16])

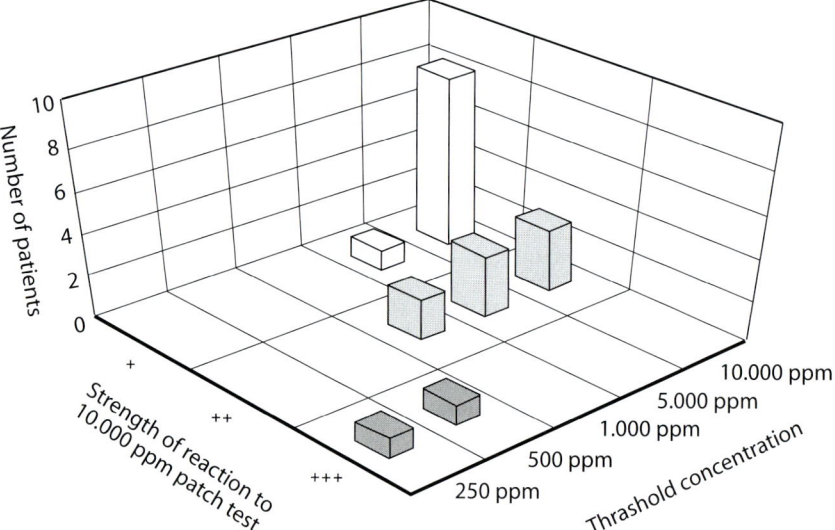

29

A follow-up study of 57 formaldehyde-sensitive eczema patients interviewed and examined 1–5 years after initial diagnosis showed that many of the patients were still exposed to formaldehyde-containing products. However, those who paid attention to their allergy had significantly fewer exacerbations of dermatitis than those who did not, and there was a trend that severe eczema was found more often in patients still exposed to formaldehyde. This study also showed that formaldehyde is widely distributed in the environment and is difficult to avoid because many finished products may contain small amounts of formaldehyde. It may not appear on the label though, as formaldehyde can be present in raw materials that may be released during storage and use [18].

Immediate reactions from formaldehyde may also occur, both of presumably allergic and nonallergic nature [19–21].

Formaldehyde releasers used as preservatives in cosmetics and technical products are often concealed by trade names or synonyms (Table 5) [22]. The epidemiology of formaldehyde sensitization requires re-evaluation. Most early studies utilized irritant patch test concentrations. The current recommended patch test concentration is 1% aq. [9, 23], and the TRUE Test contains 180 µg/cm².

Table 5. Formaldehyde releasers (from [22]

Bakzid P (mixture of cyclic aminoacetals
   and organic amine salts)
Biocide DS 5249 (1,2-benzisothiazolin-3-one
   and a formaldehyde releaser)
Bronopol (2-bromo-2-nitropropane-1.3-diol)
Dantoin MDMH (methylaldimethyoxymethan formal)
DMDM hydantoin (dimethyloldimethyl hydantoin)
Dowicil 200, Quaternium-15
Germall 115 (imidazolidinyl urea)
Germall II (diazolidinyl urea)
Grotan BK [1,3,5-tris(hydroxyethyl)hexahydrotriazine]
Hexamethylentetramine, methenamine [1,3,5,7-tetraaza-
   adamantan –1,3,5,7-tetraazatricyclo(3,3,1,1³·⁷)decan]
KM 103 (substituted triazine)
Paraformaldehyde (polyoxymethylene)
Parmetol K50 (*N*-methylolchloracetamid,
   O-formal of benzyl alcohols)
Polynoxylin (polyoxymethylene urea)
Preventol D 1 [1-(3-chlorallyl)-3,5,7-triaza-1- azonia-
   adamantanchloride benzyl formal]
Preventol D 2 (benzylhemiformal)
Preventol D 3 (chlormethylacylamino methanol)

References

1. Flyvholm MA, Menne T (1992) Allergic contact dermatitis from formaldehyde. A case study focussing on sources of formaldehyde exposure. Contact Dermatitis 27:27–36
2. Feinman SE (1988) Formaldehyde sensitivity and toxicity. CRC, Boca Raton, Fla.
3. Karlberg AT, Skare L, Lindberg I, Nyhammar E (1998) A method for quantification of formaldehyde in the presence of formaldehyde donors in skin-care products. Contact Dermatitis 38:20–28
4. Adams RM, Fisher AA (1986) Contact allergen alternatives: 1986. J Am Acad Dermatol 14:951–969
5. Scheman AJ, Carroll PA, Brown KH, Osburn AH (1998) Formaldehyde-related textile allergy: an update. Contact Dermatitis 38:332–336
6. Ford GP, Beck MH (1986) Reactions to Quaternium-15, Bronopol and Germall 115 in a standard series. Contact Dermatitis 14:271–274
7. de Groot AC, van Joost T, Bos JD, van der Meeren HL, Weyland JW (1988) Patch test reactivity to DMDM hydantoin. Relationship to formaldehyde allergy. Contact Dermatitis 18:197–201

8. Storrs FJ, Bell DE (1983) Allergic contact dermatitis to 2-bromo-2-nitropropane-1,3-diol in a hydrophilic ointment. J Am Acad Dermatol 8:157–170

9. Kranke B, Szolar-Platzer C, Aberer W (1996) Reactions to formaldehyde and formaldehyde releasers in a standard series. Contact Dermatitis 35:192–193

10. Jacobs MC, White IR, Rycroft RJ, Taub N (1995) Patch testing with preservatives at St John's from 1982 to 1993. Contact Dermatitis 33:247–254

11. Christophersen J, Menne T, Tanghoj P, Andersen KE, Brandrup F, Kaaber K, Osmundsen PE, Thestrup-Pedersen K, Veien NK (1989) Clinical patch test data evaluated by multivariate analysis. Danish Contact Dermatitis Group. Contact Dermatitis 21:291–299

12. Schnuch A, Geier J, Uter W, Frosch PJ, Lehmacher W, Aberer W, Agathos M, Arnold R, Fuchs T, Laubstein B, Lischka G, Pietrzyk PM, Rakoski J, Richter G, Rueff F (1997) National rates and regional differences in sensitization to allergens of the standard series. Population-adjusted frequencies of sensitization (PAFS) in 40,000 patients from a multicenter study (IVDK). Contact Dermatitis 37:200–209

13. Wilkinson JD, Shaw S, Andersen KE, Brandao FM, Bruynzeel DP, Bruze M, Camarasa JM, Diepgen TL, Ducombs G, Frosch PJ, Goossens A, Lachappelle JM, Lahti A, Menne T, Seidenari S, Tosti A, Wahlberg JE (2002) Monitoring levels of preservative sensitivity in Europe. A 10-year overview (1991–2000). Contact Dermatitis 46:207–210

14. Uter W, Geier J, Land M, Pfahlberg A, Gefeller O, Schnuch A (2001) Another look at seasonal variation in patch test results. A multifactorial analysis of surveillance data of the IVDK. Information Network of Departments of Dermatology. Contact Dermatitis 44:146–152

15. Kang KM, Corey G, Storrs FJ (1995) Follow-up study of patients allergic to formaldehyde and formaldehyde releasers: retention of information, compliance, course, and persistence of allergy. Am J Contact Dermat 6:209–215

16. Flyvholm MA, Hall BM, Agner T, Tiedemann E, Greenhill P, Vanderveken W, Freeberg FE, Menne T (1997) Threshold for occluded formaldehyde patch test in formaldehyde-sensitive patients. Relationship to repeated open application test with a product containing formaldehyde releaser. Contact Dermatitis 36:26–33

17. Jordan WP Jr, Sherman WT, King SE (1979) Threshold responses in formaldehyde-sensitive subjects. J Am Acad Dermatol 1:44–48

18. Agner T, Flyvholm MA, Menne T (1999) Formaldehyde allergy: a follow-up study. Am J Contact Dermat 10:12–17

19. Maurice F, Rivory JP, Larsson PH, Johansson SG, Bousquet J (1986) Anaphylactic shock caused by formaldehyde in a patient undergoing long-term hemodialysis. J Allergy Clin Immunol 77:594–597

20. Orlandini A, Viotti G, Magno L (1988) Anaphylactoid reaction induced by patch testing with formaldehyde in an asthmatic. Contact Dermatitis 19:383–384

21. Andersen KE, Maibach HI (1984) Multiple application delayed onset contact urticaria: possible relation to certain unusual formalin and textile reactions? Contact Dermatitis 10:227–234

22. Fiedler HP (1983) Formaldehyde and formaldehyde releasers (in German). Derm Beruf Umwelt 31:187–189

23. Trattner A, Johansen JD, Menne T (1998) Formaldehyde concentration in diagnostic patch testing: comparison of 1% with 2%. Contact Dermatitis 38:9–13

29.14 Quaternium-15

Quaternium-15 is a quaternary ammonium salt that conforms to the formula:

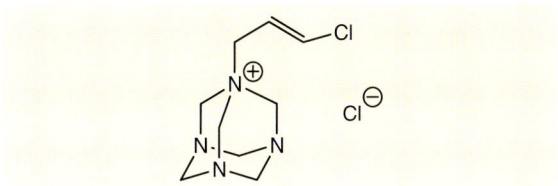

Scheme 4. Quaternium-15

It is a formaldehyde releaser used chiefly as a cosmetic preservative, and it is also an antistatic agent [1]. Formaldehyde releasers are in widespread usage in industry, household products, and cosmetics. They are marketed under a multitude of trade names. Chemically, they are linear or cyclic reversible polymers of formaldehyde, and formaldehyde is formed in different amounts, depending mainly on temperature and pH.

Quaternium-15 has several synonymous names: Dowicil 200, 100, and 75, CoSept 200, Preventol D1, 1-(3-chloroallyl)-3,5,7-triaza-1-azonia – adamantane chloride, chloroallyl methanamine chloride, N-(3-chlorallyl)-hexamine chloride, chlorallyl methenamine chloride. Formaldehyde is released in small amounts and formaldehyde-sensitive patients may react simultaneously to this preservative [2]. However, quaternium-15 sensitivity may also be directed towards the entire molecule. Allergic contact dermatitis from a formaldehyde-releasing agent may, thus, be due to the entire molecule, to formaldehyde, or to both [3–5]. Positive quaternium-15 patch tests are often of clinical relevance [6]. In about 50% of the cases, simultaneous reactivity is seen to formaldehyde [7]. The usual preservative concentration of 0.1% releases about 100 ppm free formaldehyde and this concentration can elicit dermatitis in formaldehyde-sensitive patients [8].

The repeated use of lotions and creams with this preservative may provoke dermatitis by mild irritation from the vehicles and subsequent sensitivity to the preservative. Sensitive patients should request cosmetics without formaldehyde releasers, even though some alternative formaldehyde releasers might be tolerated due to reduced formaldehyde production. Full cosmetic ingredients labeling, as that required today, makes it easy to avoid the use of specific ingredients in sensitized subjects (e.g., [9]). Occupational contact dermatitis due to quaternium-15 is extremely uncommon; two cases of hand dermatitis in hairdressers, one case of nail dystrophy in an

29

engineer, and a case of periorbital and hand dermatitis from an electrode gel in an electroencephalogram technician, and airborne dermatitis from a photocopier toner containing quaternium-15 have been reported [10–13]. The frequency of positive reactions varies from country to country, possibly due to variations in the frequency of use [14–17]. The patch test concentration is 1% pet. and 100 μg/cm² in the TRUE Test.

References

1. Anonymous (1997) International cosmetic ingredients dictionary and handbook, 7th edn. The Cosmetic, Toiletry, and Fragrance Association, Washington, DC
2. Dickel H, Taylor JS, Bickers DR, Merk HF, Bruckner TM (2003) Multiple patch-test reactions: a pilot evaluation of a combination approach to visualize patterns of multiple sensitivity in patch-test databases and a proposal for a multiple sensitivity index. Am J Contact Dermat 14: 148–153
3. Storrs FJ, Bell DE (1983) Allergic contact dermatitis to 2-bromo-2-nitropropane-1,3-diol in a hydrophilic ointment. J Am Acad Dermatol 8: 157–170
4. de Groot AC, van Joost T, Bos JD, van der Meeren HL, Weyland JW (1988) Patch test reactivity to DMDM hydantoin. Relationship to formaldehyde allergy. Contact Dermatitis 18: 197–201
5. Kranke B, Szolar-Platzer C, Aberer W (1996) Reactions to formaldehyde and formaldehyde releasers in a standard series. Contact Dermatitis 35: 192–193
6. Maouad M, Fleischer AB Jr, Sherertz EF, Feldman SR (1999) Significance-prevalence index number: a reinterpretation and enhancement of data from the North American contact dermatitis group. J Am Acad Dermatol 41: 573–576
7. Kang KM, Corey G, Storrs FJ (1995) Follow-up study of patients allergic to formaldehyde and formaldehyde releasers: retention of information, compliance, course, and persistence of allergy. Am J Contact Dermat 6: 209–215
8. Jordan WP Jr, Sherman WT, King SE (1979) Threshold responses in formaldehyde-sensitive subjects. J Am Acad Dermatol 1: 44–48
9. Boffa MJ, Beck MH (1996) Allergic contact dermatitis from quaternium-15 in Oilatum cream. Contact Dermatitis 35: 45–46
10. Tosti A, Piraccini BM, Bardazzi F (1990) Occupational contact dermatitis due to quaternium-15. Contact Dermatitis 23: 41–42
11. Marren P, de Berker D, Dawber RP, Powell S (1991) Occupational contact dermatitis due to quaternium-15 presenting as nail dystrophy. Contact Dermatitis 25: 253–255
12. Finch TM, Prais L, Foulds IS (2001) Occupational allergic contact dermatitis from quaternium-15 in an electroencephalography skin preparation gel. Contact Dermatitis 44: 44–45
13. Zina AM, Fanan E, Bundino S (2000) Allergic contact dermatitis from formaldehyde and quaternium-15 in photocopier toner. Contact Dermatitis 43: 241–242
14. Perrenoud D, Bircher A, Hunziker T, Suter H, Bruckner-Tuderman L, Stager J, Thurlimann W, Schmid P, Suard A, Hunziker N (1994) Frequency of sensitization to 13 common preservatives in Switzerland. Swiss Contact Dermatitis Research Group. Contact Dermatitis 30: 276–279
15. Jacobs MC, White IR, Rycroft RJ, Taub N (1995) Patch testing with preservatives at St John's from 1982 to 1993. Contact Dermatitis 33: 247–254
16. Schnuch A, Geier J, Uter W, Frosch PJ (1998) Patch testing with preservatives, antimicrobials and industrial biocides. Results from a multicentre study. Br J Dermatol 138: 467–476
17. Wilkinson JD, Shaw S, Andersen KE, Brandao FM, Bruynzeel DP, Bruze M, Camarasa JM, Diepgen TL, Ducombs G, Frosch PJ, Goossens A, Lachappelle JM, Lahti A, Menne T, Seidenari S, Tosti A, Wahlberg JE (2002) Monitoring levels of preservative sensitivity in Europe. A 10-year overview (1991–2000). Contact Dermatitis 46: 207–210

29.15 Chloromethyl- and Methylisothiazolinone (MCI/MI)

The isothiazolinones (5-chloro-2-methyl-4-isothiazolin-3-one and 2-methyl-4-isothiazolin-3-one, 3:1 ratio by weight) are the active ingredients in Kathon CG (Rohm and Haas, Philadelphia), a cosmetic preservative. The INCI-adopted names for the active chemicals are methylchloroisothiazolinone and methylisothiazolinone (MCI/MI), and they appear in the preservative in the ratio of 3:1.

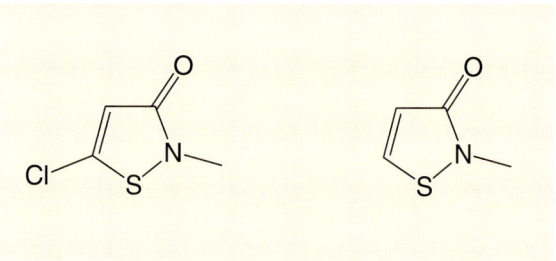

Scheme 5. Methylchloroisothiazolinone and methylisothiazolinone

Isothiazolinones are used extensively as effective biocides to preserve the water content of cosmetics, toiletries, household, and industrial products, such as metalworking fluids, water-based paints (Fig. 7), cooling tower water, latex emulsions, and for slime control in paper mills (Table 6) [1]. Also, other isothiazolinone derivatives, such as e.g., 2-methyl-4,5 trimethylene-4-isothiazolin-3-one (MTI) and 2-octyl-4-isothiazolin-3-one (Skane M8) are used as biocides for paints and latex emulsions [2,3].

Isothiazolinones are marketed under many brand names [4], which make it easy to overlook the presence of these chemicals in the formulations. Approximately 25% of all cosmetic products and toiletries – in particular, rinse-off products – in the Netherlands in the late 1980s contained Kathon CG and synonymous preservatives [1]. A Danish study examined the content of Kathon CG in 156 of the most commonly used cosmetic products in 1990. Kathon CG was

Fig. 7.
Painter with occupational hand eczema and contact allergy to Bronopol and Kathon CG used as preservatives in water-based paints

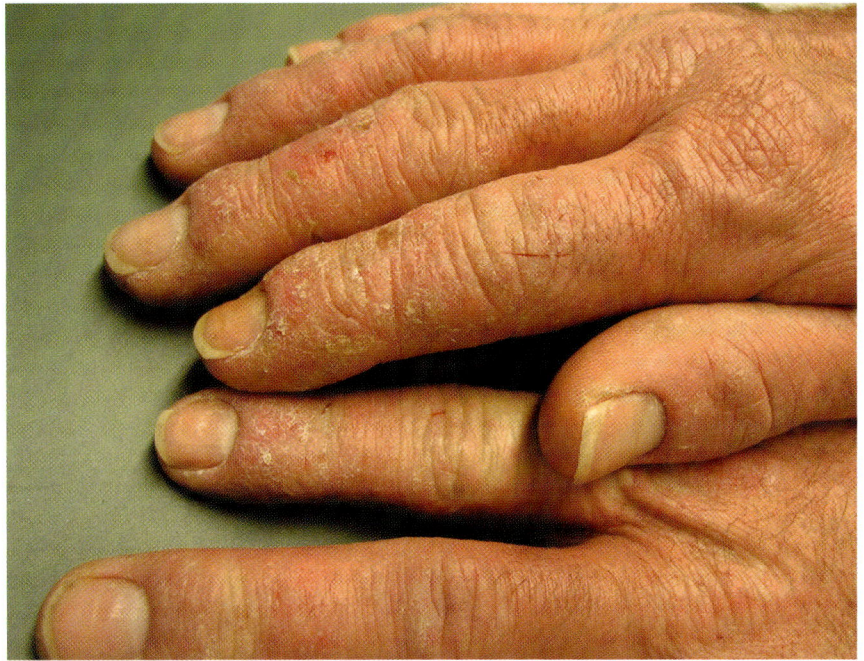

present in 48% of wash-off and 31% of leave-on cosmetic products [5]. A search of the chemical products database (PROBAS) in Denmark, containing information about approximately 30,000 products, showed that MCI/MI was registered in 550 products; 64% of them (paints, shampoos, skin care products, and cleaning agents) contained concentrations above or equal to 10 ppm. The authors also draw the attention to occupational exposure from isothiazolinones, as they may occur in many industrial categories, e.g., preservatives may contain up to 13.9% MCI/MI [6].

Methylchloroisothiazolinone and methylisothiazolinone are strong sensitizers in guinea pig allergy tests [7], and multiple reports have documented a varying and, in some countries in the late 1980s, an increasing incidence of allergic contact dermatitis from these chemicals, probably explained by increased exposure [8, 9]. Over the last 10 years, the incidence of MCI/MI contact allergy has remained stable around 2.0–2.5% of consecutively tested eczema patients in Europe [10]. MCI/MI is an important allergen for the hands and the face, and it may also cause urticaria [11, 12] and airborne contact dermatitis [13]. The airborne MCI/MI dermatitis may appear in the face of sensitized individuals who stay in newly painted rooms, and the diagnosis is easily missed unless specifically considered [14, 15]. In cosmetic products, the permissible level of MCI/MI is 15 ppm, and it appears that this concentration in rinse-off products is rather safe, since most subjects previously sensitized to MCI/MI tolerated the use of a shampoo preserved with MCI/MI for 2 weeks [16]. In leave-on products, a maximum concentration of 7.5 ppm is recommended.

Patch test reactions to MCI/MI may show unusually sharp borders and can still be true allergic reactions. The patch test concentration is 100 ppm aq. This is the best compromise, as higher concentrations (200–300 ppm) may produce irritation and patch test sensitization [1, 17]. On the other hand, 100 ppm may, in some cases, perhaps give false-negative test results on normal back skin in patients with an isothiazolinone-induced aggravation of hand dermatitis. A use test is helpful in doubtful cases of allergy. Due to the activity of isothiazolinones on the skin, it is imperative that exact dosing be used when iso-

Table 6. Biocides containing methylchloroisothiazolinone/ methylisothiazolinone. Some of these products may also contain other ingredients

Kathon CG	Metat GT
Kathon DP	Metatin GT
Kathon 886 MW	Mitco CC 31 L
Kathon LX	Mitco CC 32 L
Kathon WT	Special Mx 323
Acticide	Parmetol DF 35
Algucid CH 50	Parmetol DF 12
Amerstat 250	Parmetol A 23
Euxyl K 100	Parmetol K 50
Fennosan IT 21	Parmetol K 40
GR 856 Izolin	Parmetol DF 18
Grotan TK 2	P 3 Multan D
Grotan K	Piror P 109
Mergal K 7	

thiazolinones are used for patch testing. In the TRUE Test, the concentration is 4 µg/cm². Patch testing with products preserved with MCI/MI is often negative in sensitized patients, while a use test may be positive. With regard to the prevention of chemical burns and allergic contact dermatitis from higher concentrations, addition of sodium bisulfite seems to have the capacity to "deactivate" the MCI/MI mixture [18]. There is no cross-sensitization between MCI/MI and two other isothiazolinones, benzisothiazolinone (Proxel) and octylisothiazolinone (Kathon 893, Skane M8) [19].

References

1. de Groot AC, Weyland JW (1988) Kathon CG: a review. J Am Acad Dermatol 18:350–358
2. Burden AD, O'Driscoll JB, Page FC, Beck MH (1994) Contact hypersensitivity to a new isothiazolinone. Contact Dermatitis 30:179–180
3. Mathias CG, Andersen KE, Hamann K (1983) Allergic contact dermatitis from 2-n-octyl-4-isothiazolin-3-one, a paint mildewcide. Contact Dermatitis 9:507–509
4. Bjorkner B, Bruze M, Dahlquist I, Fregert S, Gruvberger B, Persson K (1986) Contact allergy to the preservative Kathon CG. Contact Dermatitis 14:85–90
5. Rastogi SC (1990) Kathon CG and cosmetic products. Contact Dermatitis 22:155–160
6. Nielsen H (1994) Occupational exposure to isothiazolinones. A study based on a product register. Contact Dermatitis 31:18–21
7. Andersen KE, Volund A, Frankild S (1995) The guinea pig maximization test – with a multiple dose design. Acta Derm Venereol (Stockh) 75:463–469
8. Cronin E, Hannuksela M, Lachapelle JM, Maibach HI, Malten K, Meneghini CL (1988) Frequency of sensitisation to the preservative Kathon CG. Contact Dermatitis 18:274–279
9. Bruze M, Dahlquist I, Fregert S, Gruvberger B, Persson K (1987) Contact allergy to the active ingredients of Kathon CG. Contact Dermatitis 16:183–188
10. Wilkinson JD, Shaw S, Andersen KE, Brandao FM, Bruynzeel DP, Bruze M, Camarasa JM, Diepgen TL, Ducombs G, Frosch PJ, Goossens A, Lachappelle JM, Lahti A, Menne T, Seidenari S, Tosti A, Wahlberg JE (2002) Monitoring levels of preservative sensitivity in Europe. A 10-year overview (1991–2000). Contact Dermatitis 46:207–210
11. de Groot AC (1997) Vesicular dermatitis of the hands secondary to perianal allergic contact dermatitis caused by preservatives in moistened toilet tissues. Contact Dermatitis 36:173–174
12. Gebhardt M, Looks A, Hipler UC (1997) Urticaria caused by type IV sensitization to isothiazolinones. Contact Dermatitis 36:314
13. Schubert H (1997) Airborne contact dermatitis due to methylchloro- and methylisothiazolinone (MCI/MI). Contact Dermatitis 36:274 med
14. Bohn S, Niederer M, Brehm K, Bircher AJ (2000) Airborne contact dermatitis from methylchloroisothiazolinone in wall paint. Abolition of symptoms by chemical allergen inactivation. Contact Dermatitis 42:196–201
15. Finkbeiner H, Kleinhans D (1994) Airborne allergic contact dermatitis caused by preservatives in home-decorating paints. Contact Dermatitis 31:275–276
16. Frosch PJ, Lahti A, Hannuksela M, Andersen KE, Wilkinson JD, Shaw S, Lachapelle JM (1995) Chloromethylisothiazolone/methylisothiazolone (CMI/MI) use test with a shampoo on patch-test-positive subjects. Results of a multicentre double-blind crossover trial. Contact Dermatitis 32:210–217
17. Farm G, Wahlberg JE (1991) Isothiazolinones (MCI/MI): 200 ppm versus 100 ppm in the standard series. Contact Dermatitis 25:104–107
18. Gruvberger B, Bruze M (1998) Can chemical burns and allergic contact dermatitis from higher concentrations of methylchloroisothiazolinone/methylisothiazolinone be prevented? Am J Contact Dermat 9:11–14
19. Geier J, Schnuch A (1996) No cross-sensitization between MCI/MI, benzisothiazolinone and octylisothiazolinone. Contact Dermatitis 34:148–149

29.16 Paraphenylenediamine

Para-phenylenediamine (PPD) is a colorless compound that acts as a primary intermediate in hair dyes. It is oxidized by hydrogen peroxide and then polymerized to a color within the hair by a coupler (such as resorcinol). In Europe, it is permitted in amounts of up to 6% free base in hair dyes before the addition of peroxide. This equates to 3%, but, in practice, is not used at greater than 2%.

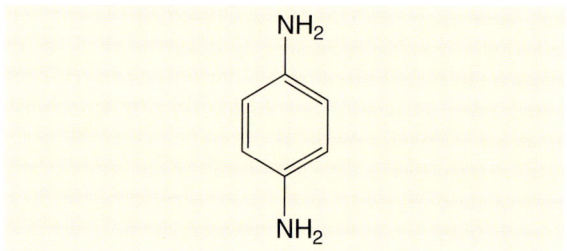

Scheme 6. *para*-Phenylenediamine

Most cases of contact allergy to PPD occur from contact with hair dyes, in either the consumer or the hairdresser [1]. In the United States, it is one of the three substances most useful in the initial patch test screening of hairdressers with dermatitis (besides glyceryl thioglycolate and formaldehyde) [2]. In a study performed in nine European centers, PPD was found to be the second most important allergen in hairdressers (after glyceryl thioglycolate), though marked regional variations were observed [3]. The information network of the Departments of Dermatology in Germany (IVDK) reported that PPD was the fifth most common allergen (4.8%) in 40,000 patients, again with considerable geographical variation in frequency, ranging from 2.8% to 7.1% [4]. The frequency of PPD allergy is high in India [5]. Many cases of PPD allergy are seen in men from the Indian subcontinent who are resident in the United Kingdom, due to the fact that they dye their hair and beard.

PPD is an important occupational allergen in hair-dressers in relation to hand dermatitis. In this group, sensitization may be facilitated by irritation of the hands from wetness, shampoos, and perming lotions. The most important measures to reduce the risk of allergic reactions from hair dyes include, besides improved products, effective removal of excess hair dye formulation from newly dyed hair, the use of protective gloves, and adequate education and information. A multicenter German study of hairdressers with hand dermatitis showed that the prevalence of contact allergy to PPD dropped from 26.6% to 17.2% between 1995 and 2002 [6]. Amongst a series of 40 hairdressers with a known contact allergy to PPD, none reacted to a new generation of hair dyes containing FD&C and D&C colors, which suggests a possible safer alternative [7].

In consumers, allergic contact dermatitis caused by PPD can be severe [8], with edema of the face, scalp, and ears that may be clinically mistaken for angio-edema [9]. Although not legal in Europe, active sensitization to PPD has been increasingly observed from its use as a skin paint in so-called *temporary tattoos* when *black henna* is used [10, 11].

PPD often gives rise to strong patch test reactions in sensitive patients. The reactions may appear after a very short patch test application time. In six of 16 PPD-sensitive patients, 15 min exposure to 1% PPD was sufficient to elicit an eczematous reaction [12]. Patients with PPD allergy may show cross-reactions with benzocaine, procaine, sulfonamides and PABA sunscreens, azo and aniline dyes, anthraquinone, antihistamines, and the rubber antioxidant 4-isopropylaminodiphenylamine [13]. However, Cronin did not find that any of 47 hairdressers positive to PPD reacted to the PPD–rubber mix [14]. Cross-reactions occur to other related hair dyes, such as *p*-toluenediamine, *p*-aminodiphenylamine, 2,4-diaminoanisole, and *o*-aminophenol are seen. Also, cross-reactivity between azo dyes and *para*-amino compounds are common. Seidenari et al. [15] studied 236 consecutively tested dermatitis patients sensitized to at least one of six azo textile dyes. Co-sensitizations to *para*-phenylenediamine were present in most subjects sensitized to *p*-aminoazobenzene (75%) and Disperse Orange 3 (66%), while the following gave lower rates of co-sensitization; Disperse Yellow 3 (36%), Disperse Red 1 (27%), and Disperse Blue 124 (only 16%) [15]. Apart from the hands and face, the neck and axilla were the most frequently involved skin sites in these patients. Cross-sensitizations between azo dyes and *para*-amino compounds can partly be explained on the basis of structural affinities or metabolic conversion in the skin [16]. Further, clinical experiments in selected patients with contact allergy to *para*-group haptens have shown that patch test reactivity to oxidizable aromatic haptens depends on the amount of freshly reduced substance, the rate of oxidation on the skin, and, therefore, the quantity of reactive intermediates, such as quinones [17]. This cross-reactivity pattern may explain the difficulty in finding the relevance of some PPD positives. Immediate-type hypersensitivity to PPD, with urticarial reactions, have been reported [18, 19], including anaphylaxis. PPD base 1% pet. was replaced by PPD dihydrochloride 0.5% pet. in the standard series in 1984. There was a general impression that this led to fewer positives. A multicenter trial showed that the dihydrochloride missed some true positives, and so, it was replaced in 1988 by PPD free base 1% pet. [20]. The TRUE Test contains 90 µg/cm².

References

1. Guerra L, Bardazzi F, Tosti A (1992) Contact dermatitis in hairdressers' clients. Contact Dermatitis 26:108–111
2. Holness DL, Nethercott JR (1990) Epicutaneous testing results in hairdressers. Am J Contact Dermatitis 1:224–234
3. Frosch PJ, Burrows D, Camarasa JG, Dooms-Goossens A, Ducombs G, Lahti A, Menné T, Rycroft RJG, Shaw S, White I, Wilkinson JD (1993) Allergic reactions to a hairdressers' series: results from 9 European centres. Contact Dermatitis 28:180–183
4. Schnuch A, Geier J, Uter W, Frosch PJ, Lehmacher W, Aberer W, Agathos M, Arnold R, Fuchs T, Laubstein B, Lischka G, Pietrzyk PM, Rakoski J, Richter G, Rueff F (1997) National rates and regional differences in sensitization to allergens of the standard series. Population-adjusted frequencies of sensitization (PAFS) in 40,000 patients from a multicenter study (IVDK). Contact Dermatitis 37:200–209
5. Sharma VK, Chakrabarti A (1998) Common contact sensitizers in Chandigarh, India. Contact Dermatitis 38:127–131
6. Uter W, Lessmann H, Geier J, Schnuch A (2003) Contact allergy to ingredients of hair cosmetics in female hairdressers and clients – an 8-year analysis of IVDK data. Contact Dermatitis 49:236–240
7. Fautz R, Fuchs A, van der Walle H, Henny V, Smits L (2002) Hair dye-sensitized hairdressers: the cross-reaction pattern with new generation hair dyes. Contact Dermatitis 46:319–324
8. Sosted H, Rastogi SC, Andersen KE, Johansen JD, Menne T (2004) Hair dye contact allergy: quantitative exposure assessment of selected products and clinical cases. Contact Dermatitis 50:344–348
9. Sosted H, Agner T, Andersen KE, Menne T (2002) 55 cases of allergic reactions to hair dye: a descriptive, consumer complaint-based study. Contact Dermatitis 47:299–303
10. Wakelin SH, Creamer D, Rycroft RJG, White IR, McFadden JP (1998) Contact dermatitis from paraphenylenediamine used as a skin paint. Contact Dermatitis 39:92–93
11. Nawaf AM, Joshi A, Nour-Eldin O (2003) Acute allergic contact dermatitis due to para-phenylenediamine after temporary henna painting. J Dermatol 30:797–800

29

12. McFadden JP, Wakelin SH, Holloway DB, Basketter DA (1998) The effect of patch duration on elicitation of para-phenylenediamine contact allergy. Contact Dermatitis 39 : 79–81
13. Herve-Bazin B, Gradiski D, Duprat P, Marignac B, Fousse-reau J, Cavelier C, Bieber P (1977) Occupational eczema from N-isopropyl-N'-phenyl-paraphenylenediamine (IPPD) and N-dimethyl-1,3-butyl-N'-phenylparapheny-lenediamine (DMPPD) in tyres. Contact Dermatitis 3 : 1–15
14. Cronin E (1980) Contact dermatitis. Churchill Livingstone, Edinburgh, UK, p 137
15. Seidenari S, Mantovani L, Manzini BM, Pignatti M (1997) Cross-sensitizations between azo dyes and para-amino compound. A study of 236 azo-dye-sensitive subjects. Contact Dermatitis 36 : 91–96
16. Goon AT, Gilmour NJ, Basketter DA, White IR, Rycroft RJ, McFadden JP (2003) High frequency of simultaneous sensitivity to Disperse Orange 3 in patients with positive patch tests to para-phenylenediamine. Contact Dermatitis 48 : 248–250
17. Picardo M, Cannistraci C, Cristaudo A, De Luca C, Santuc-ci B (1990) Study on cross-reactivity to the para group. Dermatologica 181 : 104–108
18. Edwards EK Jr, Edwards EK (1984) Contact urticaria and allergic contact dermatitis caused by paraphenylenediamine. Cutis 34 : 87–88
19. Wong GA, King CM (2003) Immediate-type hypersensitivity and allergic contact dermatitis due to para-phenylenediamine in hair dye. Contact Dermatitis 48 : 166
20. Andersen KE, Burrows D, Cronin E, Dooms-Goossens A, Rycroft RJG, White IR (1988) Recommended changes to standard series. Contact Dermatitis 19 : 389–390

29.17 Thiuram Mix

The thiuram mix used in the standard series contains the following four compounds, each at a dilution of 0.25%. The concentration in the TRUE Test is 25 μg/cm^2:

- Tetraethylthiuram disulfide (TETD, disulfiram)
- Tetramethylthiuram disulfide (TMTD)
- Tetramethylthiuram monosulfide (TMTM)
- Dipentamethylenethiuram disulfide (PTD)

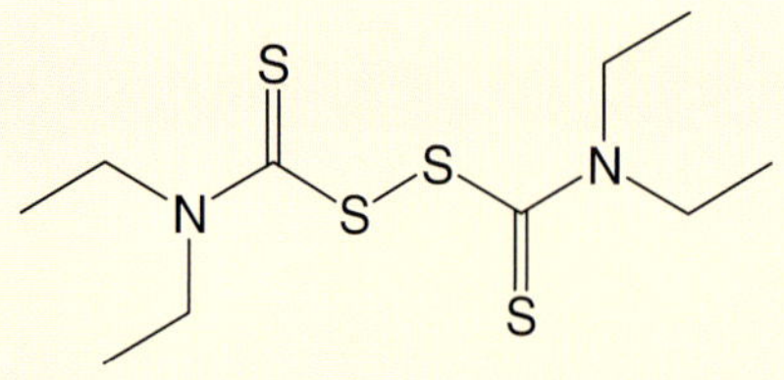

Scheme 7. TETD

These chemicals are accelerating agents used in the vulcanization of rubber. They increase the rate of cross-linking by sulfur between the hydrocarbon chains of the uncured rubber and may also donate some sulfur to the reaction. In the fully cured product, unreacted accelerators remain. Over time, some of these may migrate onto the surface of the finished article, together with other rubber chemicals. By thorough washing with hot water of thin rubber items, such as latex-dipped gloves or condoms, it is possible to leach out most of these thiuram residues. Some hypoallergenic rubber articles are accelerated by thiurams, but have been treated by washing as described.

The use of thiurams is ubiquitous in the rubber industry. The compounds are encountered in rubbers for both industrial and domestic use. Different manufacturers have preferences for the particular thiurams that they use for particular applications. This fact may explain geographical variations in the incidence of sensitivity to components of the mix [1]. Gloves are the most common cause of rubber dermatitis, and the allergen is usually a thiuram [2, 3]. Rubber glove dermatitis is important in the healthcare setting [4], where an increase in thiuram allergy in healthcare workers with hand dermatitis has been reported [5]. Release of thiuram from rubber gloves into synthetic sweat may vary between brands [6]. Thiuram sensitivity is more common in women than in men. Foot dermatitis, particularly in children, may be caused by the rubber in shoes [7]. Construction workers also constitute a risk group regarding the development of rubber allergy due to frequent use of gloves and boots [8].

An allergic contact dermatitis from a thiuram in rubber often has no clear clinical pattern, and, in a glove dermatitis, the classical distribution of the eczematous reaction may not be present. This classical pattern consists of a diffuse eczema over the back of the hands and a band of eczema to the mid-forearm at the level of the cuff of the glove. Rubber sensitivity is often clinically significant for eczema.

In individuals who are sensitive to thiurams, the use of vinyl gloves, shoes with leather or polyurethane soles, and clothing elasticated with Lycra (a polyurethane elastomer) may be required where indicated to reduce personal exposure to the allergens.

Thiurams have found wide use as fungicides, particularly for agricultural purposes, but also for such applications in wallpaper adhesives and paints. They have also been used in animal repellents. TETD has been used in scabicidal soap. TETD, when administered systemically, causes inhibition of the enzyme aldehyde dehydrogenase. On taking an alcoholic drink, there is a build-up of acetaldehyde, which causes skin irritation, erythema, and urticaria. In the form of Antabuse, TETD is used to treat alcohol dependence. Topical exposure to TETM and oral intake of alcohol has caused a similar toxic reaction, as has the taking of Antabuse and topical exposure to alcohol in toiletries [9–12]. TETD has been used to treat vesicular hand eczema in nickel-sensitive individuals [13]. A widespread eczematous reaction may develop after systemic administration of TETD to previously sensitized individuals [14, 15].

The carbamates are no longer included in the standard series of contact allergens [16, 17]. It has been shown that the majority of individuals who gave an allergic reaction to carbamix (diphenylguanidine, zinc dibutyl dithiocarbamate, zinc diethyl dithiocarbamate) also reacted to the thiuram mix. The thiuram mix is, therefore, a good detector of rubber sensitivity to this group of rubber chemicals, to which they are chemically similar – although a concomitant sensitization cannot always be excluded, since rubber gloves usually contain more than one accelerator [17]. However, a more extensive series of rubber components may be useful in selected risk groups of dermatitis patients with significant exposure to rubber in an industrial setting [18].

Both thiuram mix and the carbamates may cause false-positive patch test results [3, 19]. The carbamate mix produced false-positive irritant reactions, which were frequently misinterpreted.

References

1. Cronin E (1980) Contact dermatitis. Churchill Livingstone, Edinburgh, UK, pp 716–745
2. Estlander T, Jolanki R, Kanerva L (1994) Allergic contact dermatitis from rubber and plastic gloves. In: Mellström G, Wahlberg JE, Maibach HI (eds) Protective gloves for occupational use. CRC, Boca Raton, Fla., pp 221–240
3. Geier J, Lessmann H, Uter W, Schnuch A (2003) Occupational rubber glove allergy: results of the Information Network of Departments of Dermatology (IVDK), 1995–2001. Contact Dermatitis 48:39–44
4. Nettis E, Assennato G, Ferrannini A, Tursi A (2002) Type I allergy to natural rubber latex and type IV allergy to rubber chemicals in health care workers with glove-related skin symptoms. Clin Exp Allergy 32:441–447
5. Gibbon KL, McFadden JP, Rycroft RJ, Ross JS, White IR (2001) Changing frequency of thiuram allergy in healthcare workers with hand dermatitis. Br J Dermatol 144:347–350
6. Knudsen BB, Larsen E, Egsgaard H, Menné T (1993) Release of thiurams and carbamates from rubber gloves. Contact Dermatitis 28:63–69
7. Cockayne SE, Shah M, Messenger AG, Gawkrodger DJ (1998) Foot dermatitis in children: causative allergens and follow-up. Contact Dermatitis 38:203–206
8. Conde-Salazar L, del-Rio E, Guimaraens D, Gonzalez Domingo A (1993) Type IV allergy to rubber additives: a 10-year study of 686 cases. J Am Acad Dermatol 29:176–180
9. Frosch PJ, Born CM, Schultz R (1987) Kontaktallergien auf Gumini-, Operations- und Vinylhandschuhe. Hautarzt 38:210–217
10. Gold S (1966) A skinful of alcohol. Lancet 2:1417
11. Stole D, King LE Jr (1980) Disulfiram-alcohol skin reaction to beer-containing shampoo. J Am Med Assoc 244:2045
12. Rebandel P, Rudzki E (1996) Secondary contact sensitivity to TMTD in patients primarily positive to TETD. Contact Dermatitis 35:48
13. Kaaber K, Menné T, Veien N, Hougaard P (1983) Treatment of dermatitis with Antabuse; a double blind study. Contact Dermatitis 9:297–299
14. Gamboa P. Jauregui I, Urrutia I, Antepara I, Peralta C (1993) Disulfiram-induced recall of nickel dermatitis in chronic alcoholism. Contact Dermatitis 28:255
15. van Hecke E, Vermander F (1984) Allergic contact dermatitis by oral disulfiram. Contact Dermatitis 10:254
16. Andersen KE, Burrows D, Cronin E, Dooms-Goossens A, Rycroft RJG, White IR (1988) Recommended changes to the standard series. Contact Dermatitis 19:389–390
17. Logan RA, White JR (1988) Carbamix is redundant in the patch test series. Contact Dermatitis 18:303–304
18. Holness DL, Nethercott JR (1997) Results of patch testing with a special series of rubber allergens. Contact Dermatitis 36:207–211
19. Geier J, Gefeller O (1995) Sensitivity of patch tests with rubber mixes. Results of the Information Network of Departments of Dermatology from 1990 to 1993. Am J Contact Dermatitis 6:143–149

29.18 Mercapto Mix and Mercaptobenzothiazole

The mercapto mix contains the following four compounds, each at a concentration of 0.5% pet.:

- 2-mercaptobenzothiazole (MBT)
- N-cyclohexyl-2-benzothiazole sulfenamide (CBS)
- 2,2'-dibenzothiazyl disulfide (MBTS)
- Morpholinyl mercaptobenzothiazole [2-(morpholinothio) benzothiazole, N-oxydiethylene benzothiazole sulfenamide, MBS, MMBT]

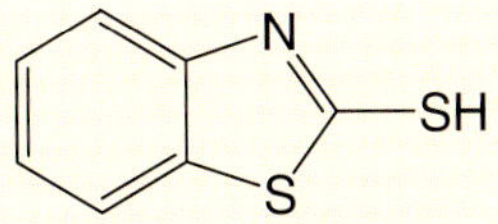

Scheme 8. MBT

Mercaptobenzothiazole is tested alone at a concentration of 2% pet. The TRUE Test includes MBT 75 µg/cm² and MBS, MBTS, and CBS (1:1:1) 75 µg/cm² in two separate patches. These chemicals

29

are present in many rubbers, to which they are added as accelerators before vulcanization takes place (see Sect. 29.17 on Thiuram Mix), and, like thiurams, are ubiquitous in rubber products. The majority of individuals who react to the mix react to MBT if tested to the individual components of the mix, and it is, therefore, not possible to identify the primary allergen. Fregert [1] observed that benzene with a thiazole ring and a thiol group in the 2 position was required for cross-sensitization to occur.

According to Cronin [2], gloves or shoes have probably sensitized women who react to MBT, but, in men, the sensitization is mainly from footwear, in which MBT is one of the most important allergens [3]. Among the numerous other sources of contact with rubbers containing MBT are rubber handles, masks, elastic bands, tubing, elasticated garments, artificial limbs [4], and even cosmetic sponges [5]. MBT may be present in a variety of nonrubber products, including cutting oils, greases, coolants, antifreezes, fungicides, adhesives, and veterinary medicaments [6].

As well as the mercapto mix, MBT is included on the standard series at 2% pet. The mix failed to detect 30% of patients who were MBT-allergic when compared to simultaneous testing with 1% MBT, and 12 of 24 individuals who reacted to 2% MBT did not react to the mix [7].

The mercapto mix used in North America does not contain MBT, which is tested separately at 1% pet., the concentration of the remaining three allergens being 0.33%. On reviewing the sensitivity of patch test material, the German Contact Dermatitis Research Group (DKG) has recommended testing with the components of the mercapto mix when there is a reaction to either the mix or MBT itself [8]. Analysis of the stability of the mercaptobenzothiazole compounds has shown that the so-called cross-sensitivity reported for this group may be the result of chemical interaction resulting in one main hapten in the presence of reducing sulfhydryl compounds [9].

References

1. Fregert S (1969) Cross-sensitivity pattern of 2-mercaptobenzothiazole (MBT). Acta Derm Venereol (Stockh) 49: 45–48
2. Cronin E (1980) Contact dermatitis. Churchill Livingstone, Edinburgh, UK, pp 734–735
3. Mancuso G, Reggiani M, Berdondini RM (1996) Occupational dermatitis in shoemakers. Contact Dermatitis 34: 17–22
4. Condè-Salazar L, Llinas Volpe MG, Guimaraens D, Romero L (1988) Allergic contact dermatitis from a suction socket prosthesis. Contact Dermatitis 19:305–306
5. Maibach HI (1996) Possible cosmetic dermatitis due to mercaptobenzothiazole. Contact Dermatitis 34:72
6. Taylor JS (1986) Rubber. In: Fisher AA (ed) Contact dermatitis, 3rd edn. Lea and Febiger, Philadelphia, Pa., p 623
7. Andersen KE, Burrows D, Cronin E, Dooms-Goossens A, Rycroft RJG, White IR (1988) Recommended changes to standard series. Contact Dermatitis 5:389–390
8. Geier J, Uter W, Schnuch A, Brasch J; German Contact Dermatitis Research Group (DKG); Information Network of Departments of Dermatology (IVDK) (2002) Diagnostic screening for contact allergy to mercaptobenzothiazole derivatives. Am J Contact Dermat 13:66–70
9. Hansson C, Agrup G (1993) Stability of the mercaptobenzothiazole compounds. Contact Dermatitis 28:29–34

29.19 N-Isopropyl-N′-phenyl-p-phenylenediamine (IPPD)

N-Isopropyl-N′-phenyl-p-phenylenediamine (IPPD) 0.1% pet. replaced, in the standard series, the PPD–black-rubber mix, which contained the following three compounds in pet.:

- N-Isopropyl-N′-phenyl-p-phenylenediamine (IPPD), phenylisopropyl-p-phenylenediamine, 4-isopropylamino-diphenylamine: 0.1%
- N-phenyl-N′-cyclohexyl-p-phenylenediamine (CPPD): 0.25%
- N,N′-diphenyl-p-phenylenediamine (DPPD): 0.25%

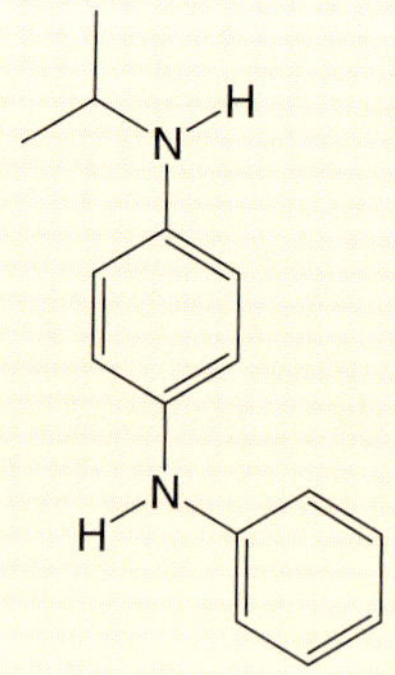

Scheme 9. IPPD

Although IPPD is the most important allergen in the PPD–black-rubber mix, by testing only with IPPD in the standard series, approximately 10% of allergy to these industrial rubber chemicals may escape detection [1]. The TRUE Test includes IPPD, CPPD, and DPPD (2:5:5) 75 µg/cm². With time, vulcanized rubber gradually reacts with atmospheric oxygen and ozone to crack and crumble, a process known as perishing. To reduce this effect, antioxidants and antiozonants may be added before vulcanization, particularly to those rubbers intended for heavy and stressful uses, such as in tires and industrial applications. A number of antiozonant types are available, but those based on derivatives of *p*-phenylenediamine (PPD derivatives, staining antidegradants) are in common use [2]. The chemicals used as antiozonants are not related in use to *p*-phenylenediamine, which is a hair dye. IPPD was established as a contact allergen in heavy-duty rubber goods when Bieber and Foussereau [3] reported nine cases, including four men who had occupational contact with tires.

Manufacturers of rubber chemicals have attempted to produce an antiozonant with the desired technical properties of IPPD, but having a reduced potential for inducing sensitization. A substitute that has been proposed for IPPD is *N*-(1,3-dimethylbutyl)-*N'*-phenyl-*p*-phenylenediamine (DMPPD), which has been claimed to have a lower potential for inducing cutaneous sensitization and, as a result, it has replaced IPPD and some of its derivatives in many applications. However, in practice, it has been noted that individuals who are allergic to IPPD usually react to DMPPD on patch testing [4]. Herve-Bazin et al. [5] evaluated 42 tire handlers who were IPPD-sensitive and found that all 15 who were also tested to DMPPD reacted to it. Guinea-pig maximization performed independently by this group showed DMPPD to be a more potent allergen than IPPD in this animal model. DMPPD was not present in the standard series mix.

In factories where IPPD continues to be used as an antiozonant, no significant excess of allergic reactions to it was found [6]; this may be related to the considerably improved hygiene in rubber factories and automation in recent years. The hand dermatitis induced by hypersensitivity to PPD-derived antiozonants often has a palmar distribution, because this is the usual area of skin contact with rubbers most likely to contain these agents. Clinically, a PPD-derivative hand dermatitis can look endogenous. The prognosis of such a PPD-derivative hand dermatitis can be adversely affected by allowing chronic exposure to the offending allergen and may cause the dermatitis to persist after avoidance of further contact. IPPD has been shown to be an important occupational allergen for construction workers and farmers [7, 8]. Although PPD-derived antiozonants are commonly present in rubbers for heavy-duty applications, they may also be present in other rubbers. Examples of these include squash balls, scuba masks [9], motorcycle handles [10], boots [11, 12], watch straps [13], rubber bracelets [14], eyelash curlers [15], spectacle chains [16], and orthopedic bandages [17]. A purpuric contact dermatitis has been described in some individuals sensitive to IPPD. The dermatitis was summarized by Fisher [18] as being pruritic, petechial, and purpuric. The reaction is usually localized to the area of skin contact, but may also be widespread. Purpuric patch tests to IPPD have been reported. A lichenoid contact dermatitis from IPPD has been observed [19], although the histological features of the reaction were those of a lichenified dermatitis.

References

1. Menné T, White IR, Bruynzeel DP, Goossens A (1992) Patch test reactivity to the PPD-black-rubber-mix (industrial rubber chemicals) and individual ingredients. Contact Dermatitis 26:354
2. Fisher AA (1991) The significance of a positive reaction to the "black rubber mix". Am J Contact Dermatitis 2:141–142
3. Bieber MP, Foussereau J (1968) Role de deux amines aromatiques dans l'allergie au caoutchouc; PBN et 4010 NA, amines anti-oxydantes dans l'industrie du pneu. Bull Soc Franc Dermatol Syphilogr 75:63–67
4. Hansson C (1994) Allergic contact dermatitis from N-(1,3-dimethylbutyl)-N'-phenyl-p-phenylenediamine and from compounds in polymerized 2,2,4- trimethyl-1,2-dihydroquinoline. Contact Dermatitis 30:114–115
5. Herve-Bazin B, Gradiski D, Marignac B, Foussereau J (1977) Occupational eczema from N-isopropyl-N'-phenyl-paraphenylenediamine (IPPD) and N-dimethyl-1,3-butyl-N'-phenylparaphenylenediamine (DMPPD) in tyres. Contact Dermatitis 3:1–15
6. White IR (1988) Dermatitis in rubber manufacturing industries. Dermatol Clin 6:53–59
7. Uter W, Ruhl R, Pfahlberg A, Geier J, Schnuch A, Gefeller O. (2004) Contact allergy in construction workers: results of a multifactorial analysis. Ann Occup Hyg 48:21–27
8. Rademaker M (1998) Occupational contact dermatitis among New Zealand farmers. Australas J Dermatol 39:164–167
9. Tuyp E, Mitchell JC (1983) Scuba diver facial dermatitis. Contact Dermatitis 9:334–335
10. Goh CL (1987) Hand dermatitis from a rubber motorcycle handle. Contact Dermatitis 16:40–41
11. Ho VC, Mitchell JC (1985) Allergic contact dermatitis from rubber boots. Contact Dermatitis 12:110–111
12. Nishioka K, Murata M, Ishikawa T, Kaniwa M (1996) Contact dermatitis due to rubber boots worn by Japanese farmers, with special attention to 6-ethoxy-2,2,4-trimethyl-1,2-dihydroquinoline (ETMDQ) sensitivity. Contact Dermatitis 35:241–245
13. Romaguera C, Aguirre A, Diaz Perez JL, Grimalt F (1986) Watch strap dermatitis. Contact Dermatitis 14:260–261
14. Lodi A, Chiarelli G, Mancini LL, Coassini A, Ambonati M, Crosti C (1996) Allergic contact dermatitis from a rubber bracelet. Contact Dermatitis 34:146
15. McKenna KE, McMillan C (1992) Facial contact dermatitis due to black rubber. Contact Dermatitis 26:270–271
16. Conde-Salazar L, Guimaraens D, Romero LV, Gonzalez MA (1987) Unusual allergic contact dermatitis to aromatic amines. Contact Dermatitis 17:42–44
17. Carlsen L, Andersen KE, Egsgaard H (1987) IPPD contact allergy from an orthopedic bandage. Contact Dermatitis 17:119–121
18. Fisher AA (1984) Purpuric contact dermatitis. Cutis 33:346, 349, 351
19. Ancona A, Monroy F, Fernandes-Diez J (1982) Occupational dermatitis from IPPD in tyres. Contact Dermatitis 8:91–94

29.20 Epoxy Resin

Some 95% of all epoxy resins consist of a glycidyl ether group formed by reaction of bisphenol A with epichlorohydrin.

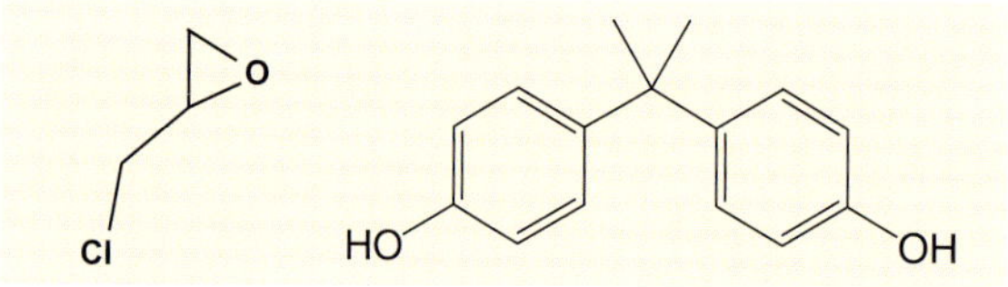

Scheme 10. Bisphenol A, epichlorohydrin polymer

Theoretically, there are many different chemical compositions that can be used to make an epoxy resin. Until recently, these have not been important, but they are rapidly becoming so as epoxy resins with different properties are being used. Epoxy resins are commonly used in everyday life as adhesives. Along with the resin itself in these compounds, there are fillers, pigments, plasticizers, reactive diluents, and solvents, and these compounds are then mixed with a hardening/curing agent that polymerizes the resin.

Epichlorohydrin/bisphenol A epoxy resin can vary in molecular weight from 340 to much larger polymers, the larger polymers having much less sensitizing capacity [1]. Epoxy resin compounds should, therefore, contain little or no low-molecular-weight epoxy resin.

Epoxy resins are used as adhesives (also in shoes!), in paints requiring hardness and durability, for instance in ships, in electrical insulation, as an additive to cement for quick bonding and strength, as well as in fiberglass (e.g., in boats), and for impregnating carbon fiber cloth [2, 3] used in situations of stress and heat, such as airplanes. They are all potential sources of contact allergy (Fig. 8). Epoxy resin has been reported to be the cause of occupational contact dermatitis in the production of skis [4] and in a windmill factory [5]. An unexpected source of epoxy allergy, epoxy compounds present in an immersion oil, caused a worldwide epidemic among laboratory technicians performing microscopy (see [6] for a review).

Epoxy resin systems are important sensitizers and are often responsible for occupational airborne dermatitis. Vitiligo, both to epoxy resin and reactive diluents, has been reported [7, 8].

In the standard series, it is the epoxy resin of the bisphenol A type that is tested (1% pet). The TRUE Test contains 50 µg/cm². In a recent retrospective study in 26,210 consecutively tested patients [9], the frequency was 1.3%. A negative patch test to epoxy resin does not mean that the patient is not allergic to the epoxy product that they have been using for the

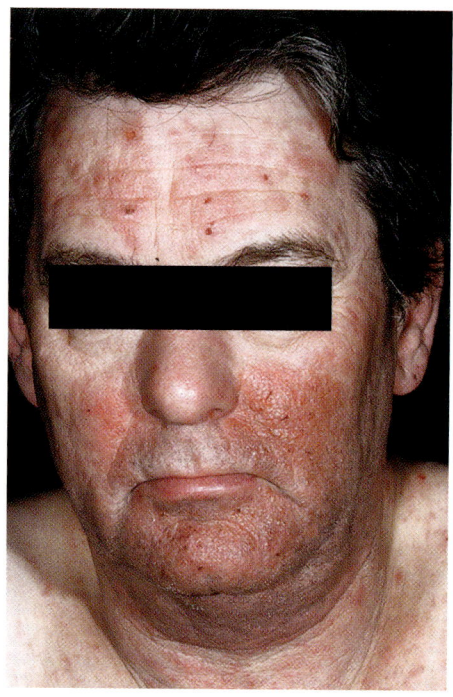

Fig. 8. Airborne contact dermatitis from epoxy resin in a patient who frequently repaired models (airplanes, ships) in his toy shop. He wore glasses due to presbyopia, explaining the sparing of the ocular region (Courtesy of P.J. Frosch)

following reasons: (1) there may be some other epoxy resin in the compound; (2) they may be allergic to some other compound in the resin, for instance, dyes, fillers, plasticizers, etc. (uncommon); or (3) they may be allergic to the hardener. If epoxy allergy is suspected, it is very important to test for other types of epoxy resins, such as bisphenol F-based resins [10, 11], dimethacrylated epoxy resins, which are used extensively in dental composite resins (e.g., [12]), UV-cured inks [13], which have become important allergens, as well as other epoxy systems [14]. Moreover, the specific compounds used by the patients [7] should also be tested, but extreme care must be taken to avoid primary sensitization [6].

Hardeners cannot be contained in the standard series because, although 95% of epoxy resins are one particular chemical, very many different hardeners are used. Both epoxy resins and hardeners can be irritant – also in patch testing – as well as sensitizing, although isolated contact allergy to hardeners without an allergy to epoxy resins is rare. Here too, patch testing with the hardeners to which the patients have been exposed may be advisable in order to detect the allergen [15, 16].

Many patients give a positive patch test to epoxy resin without any obvious contact with uncured epoxy resin. It may be that the source of sensitization is contact with the so-called cured epoxy, which may contain pockets of uncured resin. Fregert and Truls-son [17, 18] have suggested that chemical tests may be of value in demonstrating uncured resin. There are two tests for epoxy resin, one a simple color reaction, which is not specific for uncured resin, the other thin-layer chromatography, which is specific.

References

1. Fregert S, Thorgeirsson A (1977) Patch testing with low molecular oligomers of epoxy resin in humans. Contact Dermatitis 3:301–303
2. Koch P (2002) Occupational allergic contact dermatitis from epoxy resin systems and possibly acetone in a shoe-maker. Contact Dermatitis 46:362–363
3. Burrows D, Campbell H, Fregert S, Trulsson L (1984) Contact dermatitis from epoxy resins, tetraglycidal-4,4'-meth-ylene dianiline and o-diglycidyl phthalate in composite material. Contact Dermatitis 11:80–83
4. Jolanki R, Tarvainen R, Tatar T, Estlander T, Henricks-Eckerman M-L, Mustakallio KK, Kanerva L (1996) Occupational dermatoses from exposure to epoxy resin compounds in a ski factory. Contact Dermatitis 34:390–396
5. Pontén A, Carstensen O, Rasmussen K, Gruvberger B, Isaksson M, Bruze M (2004) Epoxy-based production of wind turbine rotor blades: occupational dermatoses. Contact Dermatitis 50:329–338
6. Kanerva L, Jolanki R, Estlander T (2001) Active sensitization by epoxy in Leica immersion oil. Contact Dermatitis 44:194–196
7. Kumar A, Freeman S (1999) Leukoderma following occupational allergic contact dermatitis. Contact Dermatitis 41:94–98
8. Silvestre JF, Albares MP, Escutia B, Vergara G, Pascual JC, Botella R (2003) Contact vitiligo appearing after allergic contact dermatitis from aromatic reactive diluents in an epoxy resin system. Contact Dermatitis 49:113–114
9. Bruynzeel DP, Diepgen TL, Andersen KE, Brandão FM, Bruze M, Frosch PJ, Goosssens A, Lahti A, Mahler V, Maibach HI, Menné T, Wilkinson JD (2004) Monitoring the European Standard series in 10 centres: 1996–2000. Contact Dermatitis (in press)
10. Géraut C, Seroux D, Dupas D (1989) Allergie cutanée aux nouvelles résines époxydiques. Arch Mal Prof 50:187–188
11. Pontén A, Zimerson E, Bruze M (2004) Contact allergy to the isomers of diglycidyl ether of bisphenol F. Acta Derm Venereol (Stockh) 84:12–17
12. Koch P (2003) Allergic contact dermatitis from BIS-GMA and epoxy resins in dental bonding agents. Contact Dermatitis 49:104–105
13. Kanerva L, Estlander T, Jolanki R, Alanko K (2000) Occupational allergic contact dermatitis from 2,2-bis (4-(2-hy-droxy-3-acryloxypropoxy) phenyl) propane (epoxy diacrylate) in ultraviolet-cured inks. Contact Dermatitis 43:56–59
14. Jolanki R, Estlander T, Kanerva L (2001) 182 patients with occupational allergic epoxy contact dermatitis over 22 years. Contact Dermatitis 44:121–123
15. Kanerva L, Jolanki R, Estlander T (1991) Allergic contact dermatitis from epoxy resin hardeners. Am J Contact Dermatitis 2:89–97
16. Kanerva L, Jolanki R, Estlander T (1998) Occupational epoxy dermatitis with patch test reactions to multiple hardeners including tetraethylenepentamine. Contact Dermatitis 38:299–301
17. Fregert S, Trulsson L (1978) Simple methods for demonstration of epoxy resins in bisphenol A type. Contact Dermatitis 4:69–72
18. Fregert S (1988) Physicochemical methods for detection of contact allergens. Dermatol Clin 6:97–104

29.21 Para-Tertiary-Butylphenol-Formaldehyde Resin

Para-tertiary-butylphenol-formaldehyde resin (PTBP resin) is made by reacting the substituted phenol p-tert-butylphenol with formaldehyde.

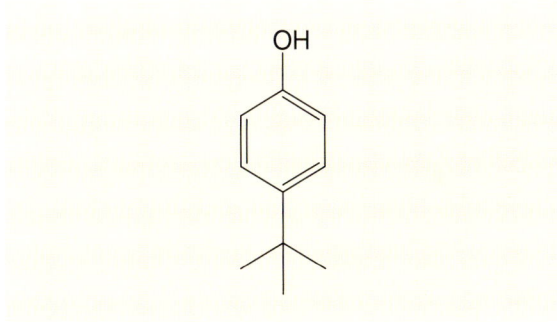

Scheme 11. PTBP

It is a useful adhesive that sticks rapidly, is durable and pliable, and has high strength at raised temperatures. Because of its flexibility, it is used in shoe construction and in leather goods. It is also used in other contact adhesives, such as those used in laminating surfaces and in the rubber industry for bonding rubber to rubber and rubber to metal [1]. These contact adhesives based on PTBP resins are often formulated with neoprene (a synthetic rubber), which provides the initial bonding until the resin cures.

PTBP resins have commonly been reported as causes of both occupational and nonoccupational allergic contact dermatitis. The first occupational cases were described in individuals making or repairing shoes [2], who developed hand eczema, but PTBP resins are also among the most important allergens in those who wear shoes containing this adhesive [2–4].

There are, however, many other occupational sensitizing sources to PTBP resin, such as adhesives for fixing rubber weather-strip car-door seals in place in car assembly plants [5] and finishes for glass wool causing airborne dermatitis [6]. PTBP resin in athletic tape has been reported as an occupational sensitization source in female athletes in Japan [7]. Nonoccupational sources of hypersensitivity to PTBP resin include an adhesive of the pads of a derotation brace and a finishing agent in a raincoat fabric [8], leather watchstraps glued with the adhesive [9], some brands of plastic fingernail adhesive [10], and domestic

29

PTBP resin adhesives [11]. It may also be present on adhesive labels [12, and even in the adhesive dressing used to secure an intravenous canula [13]. More recent reports concern a wetsuit [14], a knee brace [15], a limb prosthesis [16, 17], and electrodes [18].

The frequency of PTBP-resin sensitivity reported by the Information Network of Departments of Dermatology (IDVK) in Germany was 0.9% in 40,000 patients [19] and 1.3% in a recent study by the EECDRG of 26,210 consecutively tested eczema patients [20].

There are many allergens in PTBP resin, including low-, medium-, and high-molecular-weight fractions, for which the pattern of reactivity differs among patients hypersensitive to the resin [21], but PTBP itself is a rare allergen (as is formaldehyde in the resin). Para-tertiary-butylcatechol (PTBC), a potent sensitizer used in paint manufacture and in the rubber and plastics industries [22], was found to be present in some PTBP-F resins and to cross-react with a strong allergenic monomer present in the resin [23]. This explains the statistically significant overrepresentation of simultaneous patch test reactions to PTBP resin and PTBC in contact dermatitis patients [22].

In a polychloroprene/PTBP resin adhesive that caused an allergic contact dermatitis, the allergens were found to be 2-hydroxy-5-tertiary-butyl benzylalcohol and a condensate of 4-*para*-tertiary-butyl-phenol molecules joined by methylene bridges [24]. In a case of contact allergy to a phenolic resin used as a tackifier in a marking pen, the patient reacted to PTBP resin in the standard series and to 2-hydroxy-5-tertiary-butyl benzylalcohol and 2,6-bis(hydroxy-methyl)-4-tert-butylphenol identified in the phenolic resin [25]. Depigmentation of the skin caused by PTBP and other substituted phenols has been reported to occur in workers manufacturing the chemical when exposure has been excessive. Such depigmentation also occurred in those using PTBP resin adhesives in a car factory, where the problem was probably due to the excess PTBP in the adhesive. It has been pointed out that such depigmentation can occur without any accompanying skin irritation [26, 27]. Exceptionally, noneczematous pigmented [28] and lymphomatoid [29] contact dermatitis have also been described.

The patch test concentration of PTBP resin is 1% pet. It has been pointed out, however, that patch testing with PTBP resin is not sufficient to detect allergy to phenol-formaldehyde resins based on phenols other than para-tertiary butyl phenol [30]. The TRUE Test contains 45 µg/cm².

References

1. van der Willingen AH, Stolz E, van Joost T (1987) Sensitization to phenol formaldehyde in rubber glue. Contact Dermatitis 16 : 291–292
2. Foussereau J, Cavelier C, Selig D (1976) Occupational eczema from para-tertiary-butylphenol formaldehyde resins: a review of the sensitizing resins. Contact Dermatitis 2 : 254–258
3. Freeman S (1997) Shoe dermatitis. Contact Dermatitis 36 : 247–251
4. Rani Z, Hussain L, Haroon TS (2003) Common allergens in shoe dermatitis: our experience in Lahore, Pakistan. Int J Dermatol 42 : 605–607
5. Engel HO, Calnan CD (1966) Resin dermatitis in a car factory. Br J Ind Med 23 : 62–66
6. Wollina U (2002) Contact sensitization to para-tertiary butylphenol formaldehyde resin possibly due to glass wool exposure. Exogenous Dermatol 1 : 265
7. Shono M, Ezoe K, Kaniwa M, Ikarashi Y, Kojima S, Nakamura A (1991) Allergic contact dermatitis from para-tertiary-butylphenol-formaldehyde resin (PTBP-FR) in athletic tape and leather adhesive. Contact Dermatitis 24 : 281–288
8. Hayakawa R, Ogino Y, Suzuki M, Kaniwa M (1994) Allergic contact dermatitis from para-tertiary-butylphenol-formaldehyde resin (PTBP-F-R). Contact Dermatitis 30 : 187–188
9. Mobacken H, Hersle K (1976) Allergic contact dermatitis caused by para-tertiary-butylphenol-formaldehyde resin in watch straps. Contact Dermatitis 2 : 59
10. Rycroft RJG, Wilkinson JD, Holmes R, Hay RJ (1980) Contact sensitization to p-tertiary butylphenol (PTBP) resin plastic nail adhesive. Clin Exp Dermatol 5 : 441–445
11. Moran M, Pascual AM (1978) Contact dermatitis to para-tertiary-butylphenol formaldehyde. Contact Dermatitis 4 : 372–373
12. Dahlquist I (1984) Contact allergy to paratertiary butyl-phenol formaldehyde resin in an adhesive label. Contact Dermatitis 10 : 54
13. Burden AD, Lever RS, Morley WN (1994) Contact hypersensitivity induced by p-tert-butylphenol-formaldehyde resin in an adhesive dressing. Contact Dermatitis 31 : 276–277
14. Nagashima C, Tomitaka-Yagami A, Matsunaga K (2003) Contact dermatitis due to para-tertiary-butylphenol-formaldehyde resin in a wetsuit. Contact Dermatitis 49 : 267–268
15. Bredlich RO, Gall H (1998) Generalisiertes allergisches Kontaktekzem durch Kniebandagen. Dermatosen Beruf Umwelt 46 : 125–128
16. Sood A, Taylor J, Billock JN (2003) Contact dermatitis to a limb prosthesis. Am J Contact Dermat 14 : 169–171
17. Romaguera C, Grimalt F, Vilaplana J (1985) Paratertiairy butylphenol formaldehyde resin in prosthesis. Contact Dermatitis 12 : 174
18. Avenel-Audran M, Goosssens A, Zimerson E, Bruze M (2003) Contact dermatitis from electrocardiograph-monitoring electrodes: role of p-tert-butylphenol-formaldehyde resin. Contact Dermatitis 48 : 108–111
19. Schnuch A, Geier J, Uter W, Frosch PJ, Lehmacher W, Aberer W, Agathos M, Arnold R, Fuchs T, Laubstein B, Lischka G, Pietrzyk PM, Rakoski J, Richter G, Rueff F (1997) National rates and regional differences in sensitization to allergens of the standard series. Population-adjusted frequencies of sensitization (PAFS) in 40,000 patients from a

20. Bruynzeel DP, Diepgen TL, Andersen KE, Brandão FM, Bruze M, Frosch PJ, Goosssens A, Lahti A, Mahler V, Maibach HI, Menné T, Wilkinson JD (2005) Monitoring the European Standard series in 10 centres: 1996–2000. Contact Dermatitis 53:146–149

21. Zimerson E, Bruze M (2002) Low-molecular-weight contact allergens in p-tert-butylphenol-formaldehyde resin. Am J Contact Dermat 13:190–197

22. Zimmerson E, Bruze M, Goossens A (1999) Simultaneous p-tert-butylphenol-formaldehyde resin and p-tert-butyl-catechol contact allergies in man and sensitizing capacities of p-tert-butylphenol and p-tert-butylcatechol in guinea pigs. J Occup Environ Med 41:23–28

23. Zimerson E, Bruze M (1999) Demonstration of the contact sensitizer p-tert-butylcatechol in p-tert-butylphenol-formaldehyde resin. Am J Contact Dermat 10:2–6

24. Schubert H, Agatha G (1979) Zur Allergennatur der paratert. Butylphenolformaldehydharze. Dermatosen Beruf Umwelt 27:49–52

25. Hagdrup H, Egsgaard H, Carlsen L, Andersen KE (1994) Contact allergy to 2-hydroxy-5-tert-butyl benzylalcohol and 2,6-bis(hydroxymethyl)-4-tert-butylphenol, components of a phenolic resin used in a marking pen. Contact Dermatitis 31:154–156

26. Malten KE, Rath R, Pastors PMH (1983) p-tert.-Butylphenol formaldehyde and other causes of shoe dermatitis. Dermatosen Beruf Umwelt 31:149–153

27. Bajaj AK, Gupta SC, Chatterjee AK (1990) Contact depigmentation from free para-tertiary-butylphenol in bindi adhesive. Contact Dermatitis 22:99–102

28. Özkaja-Bayazit N, Büjükbabani N (2001) Non-eczematous pigmented interface dermatitis from para-tertiary-butyl-phenol-formaldehyde resin in a watchstrap adhesive. Contact Dermatitis 44:45–46

29. Evans AV, Banerjee P, McFadden JP, Calonje E (2003) Lymphomatoid contact dermatitis to para-tertyl-butylphenol resin. Clin Exp Dermatol 28:272–273

30. Bruze M (1987) Contact dermatitis from phenol-formaldehyde resins. In: Maibach HI (ed) Occupational and industrial dermatology, 2nd edn. Year Book Medical, Chicago, Illinois, pp 430–435

29.22 Primin

Primin or 2-methoxy-6-*n*-pentyl-*p*-benzoquinone is the major allergen in *Primula* dermatitis.

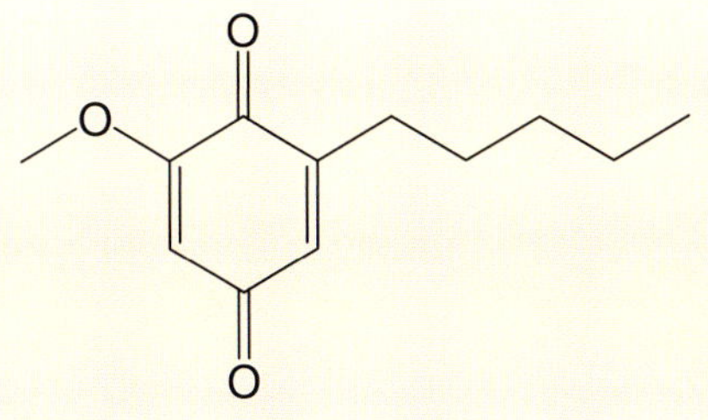

Scheme 12. Primin

Primin is included in the European standard series because it is an important allergen in certain countries, e.g., in Northern Europe. The frequency of positive primin patch tests in European clinics varies from 0.1% to 1.2% of consecutively tested eczema patients. The vast majority of patch test positive patients are women. Florists, nursery workers, and housewives are particularly at risk when exposed to primula plants. Primin sensitization seems to be relatively more common in elderly patients [1], and primin allergy may be difficult to suspect because the patients may not be aware of contact with the plant. It is recommended to show color photos of the plant as a routine procedure in cases where there are positive patch test reactions to primin [2–4].

However, the sensitization rate is so low in some countries, for example, the USA, that it is not incorporated into the local standard series [5].

Primula obconica, which has round leaves covered with fine hairs, is the usual culprit, but other species of *Primula* may cause dermatitis. *Primula auricula*, *P. vulgaris*, and *P. forrestii* have been reported to cause dermatitis [6], and it may be more frequent than previously recorded. On the other hand, primin-free *P. obconica* have been introduced to the European market, and they mimic the allergenic variety in color and appearance [7].

Primin is a powerful sensitizer contained in the fine hairs, and the content varies with the season, hours of sunshine, and the care of the plant [4, 8]; the primin content is highest in warm summer and lowest during winter [9]. Besides primin, also, a potential other allergen is present in primula, i.e., miconidin, which is biogenetically related to primin [9, 10]. Primin may be emitted to the surrounding air from intact plants and plant parts, and may be a source of airborne contact dermatitis [11].

In *Primula* dermatitis, lesions are often arranged in linear streaks and most often appear on exposed skin. The parts most often affected are the eyelids, cheeks, chin, neck, fingers, hands, and arms. Sometimes, severe reactions, such as erythema-multiforme-like lesions [12] and photodermatitis have been observed [13]. Other plants and woods containing quinones may show cross-reactivity with primin [9].

The patch test concentration is 0.01% pet. Testing with synthetic primin is preferable to an extract of the plant for various reasons: standardization, decreased risk of active sensitization, avoidance of irritant or false-positive reactions, and of seasonal variation in the allergenicity of the plant [14, 15]. Testing may invoke flare reactions. However, we should take into account that testing with primin alone might miss allergy to the plant itself [4, 16].

References

1. Piaserico S, Larese F, Recchia GP, Corradin MT, Scardigli F, Gennaro F, Carriere C, Semenzato A, Brandolisio L, Peserico A, Fortina AB; North-East Italy Contact Dermatitis Group (2004) Allergic contact sensitivity in elderly patients. Aging Clin Exp Res 16:221–225

2. Paulsen E (1994) Primula eczema – well-known and overlooked. Ugeskr Laeger 156:1147–1148

3. Britton JE, Wilkinson SM, English JS, Gawkrodger DJ, Ormerod AD, Sansom JE, Shaw S, Statham B (2003) The British standard series of contact dermatitis allergens: validation in clinical practice and value for clinical governance. Br J Dermatol 148:259–264

4. Christensen LP (2000) Primulaceae. In: Avalos J, Maibach HI (eds) Dermatologic botany. CRC, Boca Raton, Fla., pp 201–235

5. Mowad CM (1998) Routine testing for Primula obconica: is it useful in the United States? Am J Contact Dermat 9:231–233

6. Aplin CG, Lovell CR (2001) Contact dermatitis due to hardy Primula species and their cultivars. Contact Dermatitis 44:23–29

7. Christensen LP, Larsen E (2000) Primin-free Primula obconica plants available. Contact Dermatitis 43:45–46

8. Hjorth N (1967) Seasonal variations in contact dermatitis. Acta Derm Venereol (Stockh) 47:409–418

9. Krebs M, Christensen LP (1995) 2-methoxy-6-pentyl-1,4-dihydroxybenzene (miconidin) from Primula obconica: a possible allergen? Contact Dermatitis 33:90–93

10. Hausen BM (1978) On the occurrence of the contact allergen primin and other quinoid compounds in species of the family of primulaceae. Arch Dermatol Res 261:311–321

11. Christensen LP, Larsen E (2000) Direct emission of the allergen primin from intact Primula obconica plants. Contact Dermatitis 42:149–153

12. Virgili A, Corazza M (1991) Unusual primin dermatitis. Contact Dermatitis 24:63–64

13. Ingber A (1991) Primula photodermatitis in Israel. Contact Dermatitis 25:265–266

14. Fregert S, Hjorth N, Schulz KH (1968) Patch testing with synthetic primin in persons sensitive to Primula obconica. Arch Dermatol 98:144–147

15. Tabar AI, Quirce S, Garcia BE, Rodriguez A, Olaguibel JM (1994) Primula dermatitis: versatility in its clinical presentation and the advantages of patch tests with synthetic primin. Contact Dermatitis 30:47–48

16. Dooms-Goossens A, Biesemans G, Vandaele M, Degreef H (1989) Primula dermatitis: more than one allergen? Contact Dermatitis 21:122–124

29.23 Sesquiterpene Lactone Mix (SL Mix)

The SL mix contains the following three sesquiterpene lactones in pet.:

- Alantolactone 0.033%
- Dehydrocostus lactone 0.033%
- Costunolide 0.033%

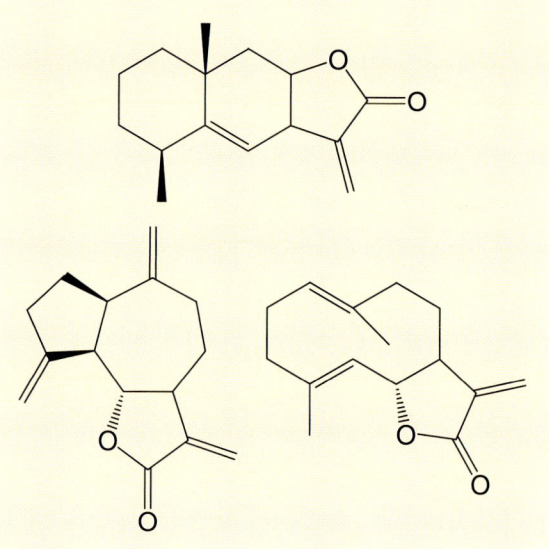

Scheme 13. Alantolactone. dehydrocostus lactone and costunolide

The SL mix was developed by Ducombs et al. [1]. These sesquiterpene lactones are contact allergens present in Compositae plants (syn. Asteraceae), which constitute one of the largest plant families in the world. More than 200 of the ~25,000 known Compositae species have caused allergic contact dermatitis. The Compositae family includes many of the common weeds, milfoil, yarrow (*Achillea millefolium* L.), tansy (*Tanacetum vulgare* L.), mugwort (*Artemisia vulgaris* L.), wild chamomile [*Chamomilla recutita* (L.) Rauschert], and feverfew [*Tanacetum parthenium* (L.) Schultz-Bip.] – and many cultivated garden flowers, such as chrysanthemum (*Chrysanthemum indicum* L.), marguerite, ox-eye daisy (*Leucanthemum vulgare* L.), marigold (*Calendula officinalis* L.), goldenrod (*Solidago virgaurea* L.), African marigolds (*Tagetes*), and sunflowers (*Helianthus annuus* L.). The edible types of Compositae include ordinary lettuce [2,3], endive, and artichoke [4]. Cross-sensitivity between Compositae plants is common [4–6]. The SL mix detected about 65% of Compositae-allergic patients in a Danish investigation comprising of more than 4,000 consecutively tested eczema patients [7]. The remaining cases were diagnosed by testing with the Hausen Compositae mix and other Compositae extracts [8].

The Compositae are the most frequent cause of occupational allergic plant dermatitis in gardeners and greenhouse workers in Denmark, and important sensitizers are chrysanthemums, marguerite, daisies, and lettuce [9]. Besides localized eczema, most often hand eczema, caused by direct contact between the skin and the plants, the Compositae may give rise to a more widespread dermatitis localized to light- and air-exposed skin areas causing suspicion towards an airborne contact dermatitis [10, 11]. However, that it is an airborne allergic contact dermatitis to sesquiterpene lactones remains to be proven [12]. So far, only emission of terpenes from feverfew plants have been documented, and these terpenes have only elicited few positive reactions in Compositae-sensitive patients [13]. Seasonal variation in the severity of the eczema with summer exacerbation is frequently seen [14,15]. A number of patients have had localized eczema, particular hand eczema, for a number of years when it suddenly turns into a widespread dermatitis one summer [11]. The duration of exposure as well as a history of childhood eczema or hay fever, seem to be significant risk factors for the development of Compositae-related symptoms [9]. Compositae sensitivity may also predispose to photosensitivity [16]. Many Compositae-sensitive patients have multiple contact allergies. The high prevalence of other contact allergies in Compositae gardeners may reflect the impact of strongly allergenic sesquiterpene lactones [17]. They may also be responsible for severe systemically induced skin eruptions [18]. The allergens are present in all parts of the plant and also in dead plant material and dust. The SL mix reveals about 60% to 70% of all cases of Compositae contact allergy and it is important to supplement testing with the plants in suspicion and ether extracts of Compositae plants, such as the Hausen Compositae mix [8, 9, 19]. Paulsen et al. [9] found that, among gardeners, the Compositae extract mix detected twice as many of the sensitized as the SL mix. However, the Compositae mix seems to be more irritating and the overall detection rate with the two mixes was still not higher than 76% in the group of gardeners. The detection rate of both mixes was raised to 93% in the series of consecutive eczema patients [7]. It has been claimed that the Compositae mix 6% pet. may cause patch test sensitization [20, 21], and a reduced concentration of extracts in the mix has been proposed. However, this also reduced the sensitivity of the mix [22]. Late-appearing reactivation patch reaction to Compositae allergens is also documented in previously sensitized patients, and this phenomenon should be differentiated from patch test sensitization [7]. The mixes have their limitations and the importance of aimed patch testing in persons with specific exposures is emphasized. The addition of parthenolide, the main allergen in feverfew, to the existing SL mix did not turn out to be of great value, although it was a fairly good screen on its own, detecting 75% of the cases positive to the SL mix [23]. Therefore, the creation of another sesquiterpene lactone mix might be appropriate. Further, it is important to emphasize that the content of allergenic sesquiterpene lactones in plants may vary from season to season and from area to area. A European multicenter patch test study with the SL mix in 11 clinics showed 1% of patients as positive in more than 10,000 consecutively tested patients, three-quarters of which were of current or of old relevance. The prevalence varied between 0.1% and 2.7% in different centers; it was highest in areas with pot flower and cut plant industries. More than one-third were positive to perfume and/or colophony, possibly reflecting cross reactivity [24]. The SL mix is non-sensitizing and non-irritating.

References

1. Ducombs G, Benezra C, Talaga P, Andersen KE, Burrows D, Camarasa JG, Dooms-Goossens A, Frosch PJ, Lachapelle JM, Menne T et al. (1990) Patch testing with the "sesquiterpene lactone mix": a marker for contact allergy to Compositae and other sesquiterpene-lactone-containing plants. A multicentre study of the EECDRG. Contact Dermatitis 22:249–252
2. Hausen BM, Andersen KE, Helander I, Gensch KH (1986) Lettuce allergy: sensitizing potency of allergens. Contact Dermatitis 15:246–249
3. Oliwiecki S, Beck MH, Hausen BM (1991) Compositae dermatitis aggravated by eating lettuce. Contact Dermatitis 24:318–319
4. Paulsen E (1992) Compositae dermatitis: a survey. Contact Dermatitis 26:76–86
5. Paulsen E, Andersen KE, Hausen BM (2001) Sensitization and cross-reaction patterns in Danish Compositae-allergic patients. Contact Dermatitis 45:197–204
6. Nandakishore T, Pasricha JS (1994) Pattern of cross-sensitivity between 4 Compositae plants, Parthenium hysterophorus, Xanthium strumarium, Helianthus annuus and Chrysanthemum coronarium, in Indian patients. Contact Dermatitis 30:162–167
7. Paulsen E, Andersen KE, Hausen BM (2001) An 8-year experience with routine SL mix patch testing supplemented with Compositae mix in Denmark. Contact Dermatitis 45:29–35
8. Hausen BM (1996) A 6-year experience with compositae mix. Am J Contact Dermat 7:94–99
9. Paulsen E, Sogaard J, Andersen KE (1998) Occupational dermatitis in Danish gardeners and greenhouse workers (III). Compositae-related symptoms. Contact Dermatitis 38:140–146
10. Fitzgerald DA, English JS (1992) Compositae dermatitis presenting as hand eczema. Contact Dermatitis 27:256–257
11. Paulsen E, Andersen KE (1993) Compositae dermatitis in a Danish dermatology department in 1 year (II). Clinical features in patients with Compositae contact allergy. Contact Dermatitis 29:195–201
12. Christensen LP, Jakobsen HB, Paulsen E, Hodal L, Andersen KE (1999) Airborne Compositae dermatitis: monoterpenes and no parthenolide are released from flowering Tanacetum parthenium (feverfew) plants. Arch Dermatol Res 291:425–431
13. Paulsen E, Christensen LP, Andersen KE (2002) Do monoterpenes released from feverfew (Tanacetum parthenium)

plants cause airborne Compositae dermatitis? Contact Dermatitis 47:14–18

14. Wrangsjo K, Ros AM, Wahlberg JE (1990) Contact allergy to Compositae plants in patients with summer-exacerbated dermatitis. Contact Dermatitis 22:148–154

15. Paulsen E, Andersen KE, Hausen BM (1993) Compositae dermatitis in a Danish dermatology department in one year (I). Results of routine patch testing with the sesquiterpene lactone mix supplemented with aimed patch testing with extracts and sesquiterpene lactones of Compositae plants. Contact Dermatitis 29:6–10

16. Murphy GH, White IR, Hawk JL (1990) Allergic airborne contact dermatitis to Compositae with photosensitivity – chronic actinic dermatitis in evolution. Photodermatol Photoimmunol Photomed 7:38–39

17. Paulsen E (1998) Occupational dermatitis in Danish gardeners and greenhouse workers (II). Etiological factors. Contact Dermatitis 38:14–19

18. Mateo MP, Velasco M, Miquel FJ, de la Cuadra J (1995) Erythema-multiforme-like eruption following allergic contact dermatitis from sesquiterpene lactones in herbal medicine. Contact Dermatitis 33:449–450

19. Goulden V, Wilkinson SM (1998) Patch testing for Compositae allergy. Br J Dermatol 138:1018–1021

20. Kanerva L, Estlander T, Alanko K, Jolanki R (2001) Patch test sensitization to Compositae mix, sesquiterpene-lactone mix, Compositae extracts, laurel leaf, Chlorophorin, Mansonone A, and dimethoxydalbergione. Am J Contact Dermat 12:18–24

21. Wilkinson SM, Pollock B (1999) Patch test sensitization after use of the Compositae mix. Contact Dermatitis 40:277–278

22. Bong JL, English JS, Wilkinson SM; British Contact Dermatitis Group (2001) Diluted Compositae mix versus sesquiterpene lactone mix as a screening agent for Compositae dermatitis: a multicentre study. Contact Dermatitis 45:26–28

23. Orion E, Paulsen E, Andersen KE, Menne T (1998) Comparison of simultaneous patch testing with parthenolide and sesquiterpene lactone mix. Contact Dermatitis 38:207–208

24. Paulsen E, Andersen KE, Brandao FM, Bruynzeel DP, Ducombs G, Frosch PJ, Goossens A, Lahti A, Menne T, Shaw S, Tosti A, Wahlberg JE, Wilkinson JD, Wrangsjo K (1999) Routine patch testing with the sesquiterpene lactone mix in Europe: a 2-year experience. A multicentre study of the EECDRG. Contact Dermatitis 40:72–76

29.24 Budesonide

The corticoid budesonide is used topically (0.025% in a cream or ointment) in the treatment of various skin disorders, but is more often used by inhalation in the form of a metered aerosol, a dry powder inhaler, or a nebulized solution for the management of asthma, and as a nasal spray for the prophylaxis and treatment of allergic rhinitis [1]. It is also used in rectal preparations to treat inflammatory bowel diseases.

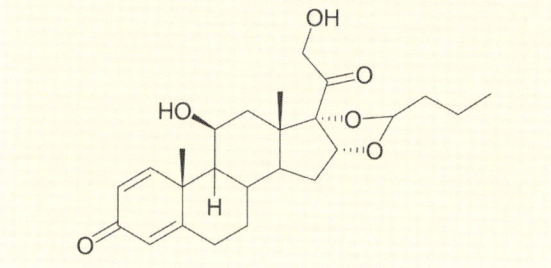

Scheme 14. Budesonide

Beginning in 1986, several publications appeared reporting budesonide-containing aerosols and sprays as the cause of eczematous eruptions, sometimes associated with endonasal complaints, with, in a few cases, indications of both type I and IV allergic mechanisms (for a review, see [2]). Although reactions to inhalation products do occur [3], sometimes, reactivating previous contact dermatitis lesions [4, 5], they seem to be infrequent relative to the large scale of their use [6], and, in most cases, they are secondary to sensitization via skin application of budesonide or a cross-reacting corticosteroid. Indeed, budesonide has been recognized as an important screening agent for the detection of contact allergy of corticosteroids of group B (acetonides) and of group D2 (the labile prodrug esters) [7]. Budesonide allergy has been detected in 1.0% to 1.5% of consecutively tested dermatitis patients [8].

As most contact allergies are missed if corticosteroids are not routinely tested, it has been recommended [9] that budesonide (0.01% pet.) be added to the standard series, although a uniform agreement on the patch test concentration has not been achieved with some authors favoring lower [10, 11] and others favoring higher [12, 13] patch test concentrations. With respect to the vehicle, several studies have shown equivalent patch test results when testing with budesonide in ethanol or petrolatum [13]. With respect to the reliability and adverse effects of the patch test, irritant reactions are not common. Reactions such as blanching, reactive vasodilation, and "edge" effects often occur and are the result of the pharmacological characteristics of the corticosteroid, which also make patch test readings necessary not only on D3 or D4 but also on D7 [9].

References

1. Parfitt K (ed) (1999) Martindale, the complete drug reference, 32nd edn. Pharmaceutical Press, London, pp 1034–1035
2. Dooms-Goossens A (1995) Allergy to inhaled corticosteroids: a review. Am J Contact Dermat 6:1–3
3. Pirker C, Misic A, Frosch PJ (2002) Angioedema and dysphagia caused by contact allergy to inhaled budesonide. Contact Dermatitis 49:77–79
4. Isaksson M, Bruze M (2002) Allergic contact dermatitis in response to budesonide reactivated by inhalation of the allergen. J Am Acad Dermatol 46:880–885
5. Bennett ML, Fountain JM, McCarty MA, Sheretz EF (2001) Contact allergy to corticosteroids in patients using inhaled or intranasal corticosteroids for allergic rhinitis or asthma. Am J Contact Dermatitis 12:193–196
6. Goossens A, Matura M, Degreef H (2000) Reactions to corticosteroids: some new aspects regarding cross-sensitivity. Cutis 65:43–46
7. Isaksson M, Andersen KE, Brandão FM, Bruynzeel DP, Camarasa JG, Diepgen T, Ducombs G, Frosch PJ, Goossens A, Lahti A, Menné T, Rycroft RJG, Seidenari S, Shaw S, Tosti A, Wahlberg J, White IR, Wilkinson JD (2000) Patch testing with corticosteroid mixes in Europe. A multicentre study of the EECDRG. Contact Dermatitis 42:27–35
8. Isaksson M, Brandão FM, Bruze M, Goossens A (2000) Recommendation to include budesonide and tixocortol pivalate in the European standard series. Contact Dermatitis 43:41–42
9. Isaksson M, Andersen KE, Brandão FM, Bruynzeel DP, Camarasa JG, Diepgen T, Ducombs G, Frosch PJ, Goossens A, Lahti A, Menné T, Rycroft RJG, Seidenari S, Shaw S, Tosti A, Wahlberg J, White IR, Wilkinson JD (2000) Patch testing with budesonide in serial dilutions. A multicentre study of the EECDRG. Contact Dermatitis 42:352–354
10. Isaksson M, Bruze M, Björkner B, Hindsén M, Svensson L (1999) The benefit of patch testing with a corticosteroid at a low patch concentration. Am J Contact Dermat 10:31–33
11. Wilkinson SM, Beck MH (2000) Patch testing for corticosteroids using high and low concentrations. Contact Dermatitis 42:350–351
12. Chowdhury MMU, Statham BN, Sansom JE, Foulds IS, English JSC, Podmore P, Bourke J, Orton D, Ormerod AD (2002) Patch testing for corticosteroid allergy with low and high concentrations of tixocortol pivalate and budesonide. Contact Dermatitis 46:311–312
13. Wilkinson SM, Beck MH (1996) Corticosteroid hypersensitivity: what vehicle and concentration? Contact Dermatitis 34:305–308

29.25 Tixocortol Pivalate

The corticoid tixocortol pivalate is used in buccal, nasal, throat, and rectal preparations [1], but not for the treatment of skin diseases.

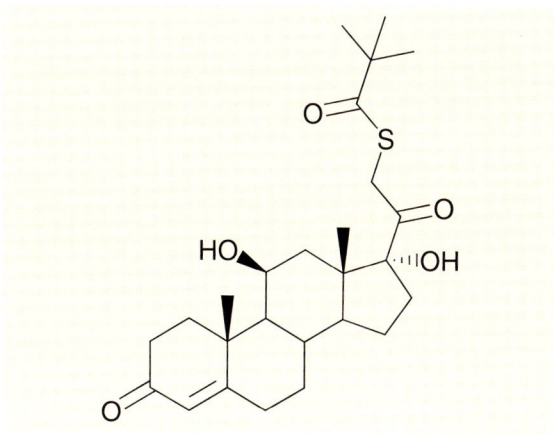

Scheme 15. Tixocortol pivalate

It is, however, a good marker for detecting contact allergy to group A corticosteroids (e.g., hydrocortisone and derivatives) [2–4], which has been confirmed in guinea pig maximization tests [5]. Primary sensitization due to mucosal preparations, however, are clearly not excluded. Tixocortol pivalate allergy has been detected in 0.9% to 4.4% of consecutive dermatitis patients [6–8].

With respect to the vehicle, equivalent patch test results were found for both ethanol and petrolatum [9]. Based on a study performed by the EECDRG [8], testing with 0.1% pet. has been recommended. However, in selected cases in which tixocortol pivalate is strongly suspected and testing with the routine concentration is negative, additional testing with 1.0% pet. should be performed [10], which is the concentration is preferred by some other authors [11, 12]. Tixocortol pivalate does not produce irritant patch test reactions, and, the same as for budesonide, late readings should be performed.

References

1. Parfitt K (ed) (1999) Martindale, the complete drug reference, 32nd edn. Pharmaceutical Press, London, pp 1034–1035
2. Lauerma AI (1991) Screening for corticosteroid contact sensitivity. Comparison of tixocortol pivalate, hydrocortisone-17-butyrate and hydrocortisone. Contact Dermatitis 24:123–130
3. Goossens A, Matura M, Degreef H (2000) Reactions to corticosteroids: some new aspects regarding cross-sensitivity. Cutis 65:43–45
4. Isaksson M, Bruze M, Goossens A, Lepoittevin JP (2000) Patch-testing with serial dilutions of tixocortol pivalate and potential cross-reactive substances. Acta Derm Venereol (Stockh) 80:33–38

29

5. Frankild S, Lepoittevin JP, Kreilgaard B, Andersen KE (2001) Tixocortol pivalate contact allergy in the GPMT: frequency and cross-reactivity. Contact Dermatitis 44: 18–22
6. Burden AD, Beck MH (1992) Contact hypersensitivity to topical corticosteroids. Br J Dermatol 127: 497–500
7. Lutz ME, el-Azhary RA, Gibson LE, Fransway AF (1998) Contact hypersensitivity to tixocortol pivalate. J Am Acad Dermatol 38: 691–695
8. Isaksson M, Andersen KE, Brandão FM, Bruynzeel DP, Camarasa JG, Diepgen T, Ducombs G, Frosch PJ, Goossens A, Lahti A, Menné T, Rycroft RJG, Seidenari S, Shaw S, Tosti A, Wahlberg J, White IR, Wilkinson JD (2000) Patch testing with corticosteroid mixes in Europe. A multicentre study of the EECDRG. Contact Dermatitis 42: 27–35
9. Wilkinson SM, Beck MH (1996) Corticosteroid contact hypersensitivity: what vehicle and concentration? Contact Dermatitis 34: 305–308
10. Isaksson M, Brandão FM, Bruze M, Goossens A (2000) Recommendations to include budesonide and tixocortol pivalate in the European standard series. ESCD and EECDRG. European Society of Contact Dermatitis. Contact Dermatitis 43: 41–42
11. Wilkinson SM, Beck MH (2000) Patch testing for corticosteroid allergy using high and low concentrations. Contact Dermatitis 42: 350–351
12. Chowdhury MMU, Statham BN, Sansom JE, Foulds IS, English JSC, Podmore P, Bourke J, Orton D, Ormerod AD (2002) Patch testing for corticosteroid allergy with low and high concentrations of tixocortol pivalate and budesonide. Contact Dermatitis 46: 311–312

29.26 Ethylenediamine Dihydrochloride

(No longer included in standard series)

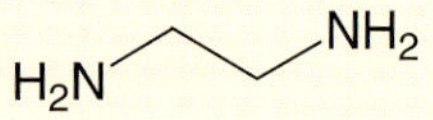

Scheme 16. Ethylenediamine

When patch testing, 1% pet. is the standard test concentration. The TRUE test contains 50 µg/cm². Allergy to this compound is commonest by far in the United States and Belgium where Mycolog cream, a preparation containing neomycin, nystatin, and triamcinolone, is widely used. A similar preparation is used in Britain – Tri-Adcortyl cream. In these preparations it is used as a stabilizer. The corresponding ointment does not contain it as a stabilizer.

Ethylenediamine has other uses, and dermatitis has been described due to its presence in the following sources – floor polish remover [1], epoxy hardener, and coolant oil [2–4]. Its use has also been described in a number of other industries, rubber, dyes, insecticides, and synthetic waxes. Occupational dermatitis has been reported in nurses and a laboratory technician working with theophylline and aminophylline [5, 6].

There is a potential problem with systemic administration in those sensitized, either with drugs that contain ethylenediamine, for instance aminophylline, or with drugs chemically related to it, including various antihistamines, among which are hydroxyzine hydrochloride and its active metabolite ceterizine, piperazine, and cyclizine [7–10]. Cases have been described with generalized erythroderma in patients who have become allergic to piperazine in local applications, who received piperazine phosphate to treat worms [11]. Patients seldom, if ever, become sensitized through systemic administration and problems only arise in those already sensitized who receive the drugs, and it is surprising how few reactions occur considering the number of patients sensitized. Immediate-type reactions have also been reported [12]. Few patients become sensitized through contact in industry, and ethylenediamine is a rare sensitizer outside the local application that contains it.

References

1. English JS, Rycroft RJ (1989) Occupational sensitization to ethylenediamine in a floor polish remover. Contact Dermatitis 20: 220–221
2. Chieregato C, Vincenzi C, Guerra L, Farina P (1994) Occupational allergic contact dermatitis due to ethylenediamine dihydrochloride and cresyl glycidyl ether in epoxy resin systems. Contact Dermatitis 30: 120 med.tss./MAG
3. Crow KD, Peachey RD, Adams JE (1978) Coolant oil dermatitis due to ethylenediamine. Contact Dermatitis 4: 359–361
4. Angelini G, Meneghini CL (1977) Dermatitis in engineers due to synthetic coolants. Contact Dermatitis 3: 219–220
5. Dias M, Fernandes C, Pereira F, Pacheco A (1995) Occupational dermatitis from ethylenediamine. Contact Dermatitis 33: 129–130
6. Dal Monte A, de Benedictis E, Laffi G (1987) Occupational dermatitis from ethylenediamine hydrochloride. Contact Dermatitis 17: 254 med.tss./MAG
7. Stingeni L, Caraffini S, Agostinelli D, Ricci F, Lisi P (1997) Maculopapular and urticarial eruption from cetirizine. Contact Dermatitis 37: 249–250
8. Walker SL, Ferguson JE (2004) Systemic allergic contact dermatitis due to ethylenediamine following administration of oral aminophylline. Br J Dermatol 150: 594
9. Ash S, Scheman AJ (1997) Systemic contact dermatitis to hydroxyzine. Am J Contact Dermat 8: 2–5
10. Guin JD, Fields P, Thomas KL (1999) Baboon syndrome from i.v. aminophylline in a patient allergic to ethylenediamine. Contact Dermatitis 40: 170–171
11. Price ML, Hall Smith SP (1984) Allergy to piperazine in a patient sensitive to ethylenediamine. Contact Dermatitis 10: 120 med.tss./MAG
12. De la Hoz B, Perez C, Tejedor MA, Lazaro M, Salazar F, Cuevas M (1993) Immediate adverse reaction to aminophylline (see comments). Ann Allergy 71: 452–454

Chapter 30

Cosmetics and Skin Care Products* 30

Ian R. White, Anton C. de Groot

* In this chapter, the nomenclature used is according to the International Nomenclature
of Cosmetic Ingredients (INCI), as required for ingredient labeling in Europe.

Contents

30.1 What Are Cosmetics?

In European legislation, a "cosmetic product" is any substance or preparation intended to be placed in contact with the various external parts of the human body (epidermis, hair system, nails, lips, and external genital organs) or with the teeth and the mucous membranes of the oral cavity with a view exclusively or mainly to cleaning them, perfuming them, changing their appearance and/or correcting body odors and/or protecting them or keeping them in good condition (**Cosmetics Directive 76/768/EEC; article 1**).

Included within the definition of a cosmetic are the following:

- Soaps, shampoos, toothpastes, and cleansing and moisturizing creams for regular care
- Color cosmetics, such as eye shadows, lipsticks, and nail varnishes
- Hair colorants and styling agents
- Fragrance products, such as deodorants, aftershaves, and perfumes
- Ultraviolet light (UV light) screening preparations

30.2 Epidemiology of Side-Effects from Cosmetics

30.2.1 The General Population

Everyone uses cosmetics and, given the enormous volume of sales and the range of products available, there is remarkably little information on the incidence of adverse reactions to them. Most individuals who experience an adverse reaction to a cosmetic have a mild reaction and simply change to another product. Only rarely is an adverse reaction reported to a manufacturer, unless discomfort is marked or significant. In Europe, the industry is required to record adverse reactions reported to it and make the

30

register available to the appropriate "competent authority." Individuals are also unlikely to present to a dermatologist for evaluation, unless an adverse reaction is severe, as in the case of contact allergy to a hair dye, or persistent.

Several thousand substances are available to the cosmetic scientist for incorporation into cosmetics. The European Commission publishes an indicative but not exhaustive list of general ingredients and fragrance substances – known as the Inventory [1]. Many of these ingredients have had a long and established use, and are recognized as being safe or having a low toxicological profile. Some substances, however, pose a significant risk of causing adverse reactions, and, for these other substances, little is known about their safety. Regulatory aspects are discussed in Chap. 45.

In the general population, a questionnaire survey of 1,022 individuals in the United Kingdom found 85 people (8.3%) who claimed to have experienced an adverse reaction related to the use of a cosmetic [2]. Of these 85 individuals, 44 were patch tested and in 11 (1.1%), a significant reaction was obtained to a cosmetic ingredient. In Holland, a survey of 982 individuals attending beauticians found 254 (26%) who claimed to have experienced an adverse reaction to a cosmetic [3]. Evaluation of 150 cases of this group by patch testing demonstrated 10 individuals, 1% of the total, with an allergic reaction attributable to a cosmetic ingredient. These and other studies give an idea of the proportion of the population who may have experienced an allergic contact reaction to a cosmetic ingredient at some time. An estimated 1% is allergic to fragrances [4] and 2–3% are allergic to substances that may be present in cosmetics and toiletries [5].

30.2.2 Patients Seen by Dermatologists

Detailed information is available regarding the prevalence of contact allergy to some cosmetic ingredients amongst individuals who have been patch tested as an investigation for their dermatitis (of whatever type). The European standard series of contact allergens includes the following substances which may be used in cosmetics: fragrance mix, balsam of Peru (INCI name: Myroxylon pereirae; not used as such in cosmetics, but included as an indicator of fragrance sensitivity), formaldehyde, quaternium-15, methylchloroisothiazolinone (and) methylisothiazolinone (MCI/MI), parabens, lanolin (wool alcohols), colophonium (colophony), and p-phenylenediamine. Many centers also routinely test with the preservatives methyldibromo glutaronitrile, imidaz-

Table 1. Frequency of reactions (mean from all centers and range) to cosmetic ingredients in the standard series ($n=20,791$) [5]

Substance	Mean (%)	Range (%)
Fragrance mix	7.0	6.4–9.4
Balsam of Peru (*Myroxylon pereirae*)	5.8	4.0–6.7
Colophony (colophonium)	3.4	1.7–4.7
p-Phenylenediamine	2.8	0.3–4.9
Wool wax alcohols (lanolin alcohol)	2.8	1.2–3.9
Formaldehyde	2.2	1.4–5.2
Parabens	1.1	0.5–2.6
Quaternium-15	0.9	0.3–2.2

olidinyl urea, and diazolidinyl urea, and some include iodopropynyl butylcarbamate and others. A European study of the frequency of hypersensitivity to some of these agents in a patch-tested population totaling 20,791 individuals showed the incidence of reactions as listed in Table 1 [5]. Of dermatological patients patch tested for suspected allergic contact dermatitis, about 10% are allergic to cosmetic ingredients [5].

Women are more at risk of acquiring hypersensitivity to cosmetic ingredients than men, due to their greater product use. Variability in the frequency of reactions reported is partially attributable to different patient selection between centers. True temporal and geographical variations in the frequency of hypersensitivity to cosmetic ingredients occur because of differences in ingredient use. These differences involve marketing strategies, local product preference, and preferred ingredient usage by manufacturers. Additionally, changes in legislation, recommendations on ingredient use, and availability are further important factors. Dillarstone [6] has pointed out the phasic nature of the prevalence of contact allergy to preservatives that results from these latter factors.

30.3 Clinical Picture

Sometimes, allergic contact dermatitis from cosmetic products can easily be recognized. Examples include reactions to deodorant, eye shadow, perfume dabbed behind the ears or on the wrist, and lipstick. In more than half of all cases, however, the diagnosis of cosmetic allergy is not clinically suspected [7].

The clinical picture of allergic cosmetic dermatitis depends on the type of products used (and, consequently, the sites of application), exposure, and the patient's sensitivity. Usually, a cosmetic contains only weak allergens or stronger ones present at low dilution, and the dermatitis resulting from cosmetic allergy is mild: erythema, minimal edema, desquamation, and papules. Weeping vesicular dermatitis rarely occurs, although some products, especially the permanent hair dyes, may cause fierce reactions, notably on the face, ears, and scalp. Allergic reactions on the scalp may be seborrhö dermatitis-like with (temporary) hair loss.

Contact allergy to fragrances may resemble an endogenous eczema [8]. Lesions in the skin folds may be mistaken for atopic dermatitis. Dermatitis due to perfumes or toilet water may be "streaky." Allergy to tosylamide/formaldehyde resin in nail polish may affect the fingers [9], but most allergic reactions are located on the eyelids, in and behind the ears, on the neck, and sometimes around the anus or vulva. Eczema of the lips and the perioral region (cheilitis) [10] may be caused by toothpastes [11], notably from the flavors contained therein [12].

The face itself is frequently involved, and often, the dermatitis is limited to the face and/or eyelids. Other predilection sites for cosmetic dermatitis are the neck, arms, and hands. However, all parts of the body may be involved. Most often, the cosmetics have been applied to previously healthy skin (especially the face), nails, or hair. However, allergic cosmetic dermatitis may be caused by products used on previously damaged skin, for example, to treat or prevent dry skin of the arms and legs or irritant or atopic hand dermatitis.

30.4 The Products Causing Cosmetic Allergy

Most allergic reactions are caused by those cosmetics that remain on the skin: "stay-on" or "leave-on" products such as skin care products (moisturizing and cleansing creams, lotions, milks, tonics), hair cosmetics (notably hair dyes), nail cosmetics (nail varnish), deodorants and other perfumes, and facial and eye make-up products [13–15]. "Rinse-off" or "wash-off" products, such as soap, shampoo, bath foam, and shower foam, less commonly elicit or induce contact allergic reactions. This is explained by the dilution of the product (and, consequently, of the [potential] allergen) under normal circumstances of use, and because the product is removed from the skin by rinsing after a short period. An exception to this general rule was allergy to a fraction in some commercial grades of the surfactant cocamidopropyl betaine, which caused reactions to shampoo in consumers and occupational dermatitis in hairdressers, and to shower gels [16–18].

Trends in cosmetic usage, e.g., the expansion of the cosmetic market for men and the targeting of products specifically for children, may influence the situation.

30.5 The Allergens

Although there are numerous publications on contact allergy to the ingredients of cosmetics, the systematic investigation of the allergens in such products has been rare [7, 15]. Fragrances and preservatives (and in recent years, the preservative methyldibromo glutaronitrile [18–20] has emerged as an important cosmetic allergen) are the most common causative ingredients in allergic cosmetic dermatitis. Other important allergens are the hair color p-phenylenediamine (and related permanent dyes), the nail varnish resin tosylamide/formaldehyde resin [21], and uncommonly to UV filters, lanolin and other substances.

30.5.1 Fragrances

Adverse reactions to fragrances in perfumes and in fragranced cosmetic products include allergic contact dermatitis, irritant contact dermatitis, photosensitivity, immediate contact reactions (contact urticaria), and pigmented contact dermatitis [22]. Reviews of the adverse effects of fragrances (and essential oils) are available [14, 23]. The history of fragrances has been well described [24, 25].

Considering the enormous use of fragrances, the frequency of contact allergy to them is relatively small. In absolute numbers, however, fragrance allergy is common. In a group of 90 student nurses, 12 (13%) were shown to be fragrance allergic [26]. In a group of 567 unselected individuals aged 15–69 years, 6 (1.1%) were shown to be allergic to fragrances, as evidenced by a positive patch test reaction to the fragrance mix [4].

In dermatitis patients seen by dermatologists, the prevalence of contact allergy to fragrances is between 6–14% [27]; only nickel allergy occurs more frequently. When tested with 10 popular perfumes, 6.9% of female eczema patients proved to be allergic to them [28] and 3.2–4.2% were allergic to fragrances from perfumes present in various cosmetic products [29].

When patients with suspected allergic cosmetic dermatitis are investigated, fragrances are identified as the most frequent allergens, not only in perfumes, aftershaves and deodorants, but also in other cosmetic products not primarily used for their smell [21, 30]. Occupational contact with fragrances is rarely significant [14].

Contact allergy to fragrances usually causes dermatitis of the hands, face, and/or axillae. Patients appear to become sensitized to fragrances, particularly from the use of deodorant sprays and/or perfumes, and, to a lesser degree, from cleansing agents, deodorant sticks, or hand lotions [31]. Thereafter, eczema may appear or be worsened by contact with other fragranced products: cosmetics, toiletries, household products, industrial contacts, and flavorings in foods and drinks.

Over 100 fragrance chemicals have been identified as allergens [14]. Most reactions have been identified as the substances in the standard perfume mix, and of these, *Evernia prunastri* (oak moss), iso-eugenol, and cinnamal are the main sensitizers. Most recently, hydroxyisohexyl-3-cyclohexene carboxaldehyde (Lyral) has been identified as an important fragrance allergen [32]. An exhaustive review of fragrance allergens is available [33] and was the tool used by the European Commission in evaluating the need for the introduction of fragrance ingredient labeling.

Contact allergy to a particular product or chemical is established by means of patch testing. A perfume may contain as many as 200 or more individual ingredients. This makes the diagnosis of perfume allergy by patch test procedures complicated. The fragrance mix, or perfume mix, was introduced as a screening tool for fragrance sensitivity in the late 1970s [34]. It contains eight commonly used fragrance substances:

- Amyl cinnamal
- Cinnamyl alcohol
- Cinnamal
- *Evernia prunastri* (oak moss)
- Eugenol
- Geraniol
- Hydroxycitronellal
- Iso-eugenol

Between 6% and 14% [27] of patients routinely tested for suspected allergic contact dermatitis react to it. It has been estimated that this mix detects 70–80% of all cases of fragrance sensitivity; this may be an overestimation, as it was positive in only 57% of patients who were allergic to popular commercial fragrances [28]. Testing with the components of the mix is required when a positive reaction to the mix is found.

Although the fragrance mix remains an extremely important tool for the detection of cases of contact allergy to fragrances, it is far from ideal: it misses 20–30% of relevant reactions or more, and may cause both false-positive (i.e., a "positive" patch test reac-

tion in a non-fragrance-allergic individual) and false-negative (i.e., no patch test reaction in an individual who is actually allergic to one or more of the ingredients of the mix) reactions. The routine testing with hydroxyisohexyl-3-cyclohexene carboxaldehyde (Lyral) and/or a second fragrance mix developed by Frosch [35] should improve the rate of detection.

In addition to patch testing, another useful test in cases of doubt (for example, with weakly positive patch test reactions, which are difficult to interpret) is the repeated open application test (ROAT; see below).

The finding of a positive reaction to the fragrance mix should be followed by a search for its relevance, i.e., is fragrance allergy the cause of the patient's current or previous complaints, or does it at least contribute to it? Often, however, correlation with the clinical picture is lacking and many patients can tolerate perfumes and fragranced products without problems [14]. This may sometimes be explained by irritant (false-positive) patch test reactions to the mix. Alternative explanations include the absence of relevant allergens in those products or a concentration too low to elicit clinically visible allergic contact reactions.

Between 50% and 65% of all positive patch test reactions to the mix are relevant. There is a highly significant association between the occurrence of self-reported visible skin symptoms to scented products earlier in life and a positive patch test to the fragrance mix, and most fragrance-sensitive patients are aware that the use of scented products may cause skin problems [36].

For perfume-mix-allergic patients with concomitant positive reactions to perfumes or scented products, interpretation of the reaction as relevant is highly likely. For such patients, the incriminated cosmetics very often contain fragrances present in the mix and, thus, the fragrance mix appears to be a good reflection of actual exposure [37]. Indeed, one or more of the ingredients of the mix are present in nearly all deodorants [38], popular prestige perfumes [28], perfumes used in the formulation of other cosmetic products [29], and natural-ingredient-based cosmetics [39], often at levels high enough to cause allergic reactions [40, 41]. Thus, fragrance allergens are ubiquitous and virtually impossible to avoid if perfumed cosmetics are used.

Determination of relevance has now been made easier by ingredients listing of well recognized fragrance allergens when present at 10 ppm or more in leave-on cosmetic products and at 100 ppm or more in rinse-off products:

- Amyl cinnamal
- Cinnamyl alcohol
- cinnamal
- *Evernia prunastri* (oak moss)
- *Evernia furfuracea* (tree mass)
- Eugenol
- Geraniol
- Hydroxycitronellal
- Iso-eugenol
- Alpha-isomethyl ionone
- Amylcinnamyl alcohol
- Anisyl alcohol
- Benzyl alcohol
- Benzyl benzoate
- Benzyl cinnamate
- Benzyl salicylate
- Citral
- Citronellol
- Coumarin
- d-limonene
- Farnesol
- Hexyl cinnamal
- Hydroxyisohexyl-3-cyclohexene carboxaldehyde (Lyral)
- Butylphenyl methylpropional (lilial)
- Linalool
- Methyl heptine carbonate

30.5.2 Preservatives

Preservatives are added to water-containing cosmetics to inhibit the growth of non-pathogenic and pathogenic micro-organisms, which may cause degradation of the product or be harmful to the consumer. After fragrances, they are the most frequent cause of allergic cosmetic dermatitis. Important review articles on the subject of preservative allergy have been published [42–44].

30.5.2.1 Methylchloroisothiazolinone (and) Methylisothiazolinone

Methylchloroisothiazolinone (and) methylisothiazolinone (MCI/MI) is a preservative system containing, as active ingredients, a mixture of methylchloroisothiazolinone and methylisothiazolinone. The most widely used commercial product contains 1.5% active ingredients; the methylchloroisothiazolinone moiety is the prime allergenic fraction. This highly effective preservative remains an important cosmetic allergen in most European countries. Allergic reactions on the face to cosmetics preserved with MCI/MI can have

unusual clinical presentations that are very similar to seborrheic dermatitis and other dermatoses [45]. In the United States, a prevalence rate of 3% [27] has been observed. The concentration of MCI/MI used is usually between 3 ppm and 15 ppm, which is normally far below the threshold for the detection of allergy with patch tests, indicating that most allergic patients will not react to the cosmetic product upon patch testing. Therefore, MCI/MI is tested separately at 100 ppm in water in the European standard series (but tested at 200 ppm in Sweden). Currently, MCI/MI is primarily used in rinse-off cosmetic products at low concentrations, which infrequently leads to the induction or elicitation of contact allergy [46]. As a consequence, prevalence rates in Europe are static. The subject of contact allergy to isothiazolinones has been reviewed [47, 48]. Methylisothiazolinone itself is now permitted as a cosmetic preservative; it is, however, a much weaker allergen than methylchloroisothiazoline.

30.5.2.2 Methyldibromo Glutaronitrile

Methyldibromo glutaronitrile (synonym: 1,2-dibromo-2,4-dicyanobutane) is a preservative that has been widely used in cosmetics and toiletries. It was thought to be a suitable alternative to the MCI/MI, but, unfortunately, soon proved to be a frequent cause of contact allergy to cosmetics [19] and, in the Netherlands, to moistened toilet tissues [20]. Prevalence rates of sensitization in patients routinely investigated for suspected allergic contact dermatitis were 4% in the Netherlands [20], 2.9% in Italy [49], 2.3% in Germany [50], and 2% [27] to 11.7% in the United States [51]. Between 23% and 75% of positive patch test reactions are considered to be relevant.

Although there is some controversy as to the optimal patch test concentration, 0.5% pet. [52, 53] has been recommended, but 0.3% is also used [54]. False-negative and false-positive reactions may occur [52].

In Europe, methyldibromo glutaronitrile is now only permitted in rinse-off products at a maximum of 0.1%, but even this use may be curtailed.

30.5.2.3 Formaldehyde

Formaldehyde is a frequent sensitizer and ubiquitous allergen, with numerous non-cosmetic sources of contact. Routine testing in patients with suspected allergic contact dermatitis yields prevalence rates of sensitization of 3% [5] to as much as 9% in the United States [27]. Because of this, the cosmetic industry uses small but effective concentrations, with the amount of free formaldehyde not exceeding 0.2% and its use is restricted almost exclusively to rinse-off products. In recent years, it has largely been replaced by other preservatives (such as MCI/MI); the literature on formaldehyde allergy has been reviewed [43, 44].

30.5.2.4 Formaldehyde Donors

Formaldehyde donors are preservatives that, in the presence of water, release formaldehyde. Therefore, cosmetics preserved with such chemicals will contain free formaldehyde, the amount depending on the preservative used, its concentration, and the amount of water present in the product. The antimicrobial effects of formaldehyde donors are said to be intrinsic properties of the parent molecules and are not related to formaldehyde release. Formaldehyde donors used in cosmetics and toiletries include quaternium-15, imidazolidinyl urea, diazolidinyl urea, 2-bromo-2-nitropropane-1,3-diol, and DMDM hydantoin. In anionic shampoos, the amount of formaldehyde released by such donors increases in the order: imidazolidinyl urea < DMDM hydantoin < diazolidinyl urea <quaternium-15 [55]. Contact allergy to formaldehyde donors may be due either to the preservative itself or to formaldehyde sensitivity [43, 44].

30.5.3 Quaternium-15

Patients sensitized to formaldehyde may experience cosmetic dermatitis from using leave-on preparations containing quaternium-15. The threshold for eliciting allergic contact dermatitis in the axillae is approximately 30 ppm formaldehyde. At a concentration of 0.1% (1,000 ppm), quaternium-15 releases about 100 ppm of free formaldehyde. Routine testing with quaternium-15 in the United States yielded a prevalence rate of 9.2% in patients suspected of allergic contact dermatitis [27]. Half of these reactions may have been caused by formaldehyde sensitivity [56]. In Europe, sensitization to quaternium-15 is less frequent [57].

30.5.4 Imidazolidinyl Urea

Imidazolidinyl urea releases only small amounts of formaldehyde, and, consequently, poses little threat to formaldehyde-sensitive subjects. Contact allergy to imidazolidinyl urea occurs occasionally [58]. In 1,175 patients tested with the preservative 2% aq. in Belgium, only eight (0.7%) positive reactions were observed, of which, one was accompanied by a reaction to formaldehyde [58]. In the United States, where imidazolidinyl urea is part of the routine series, 3.1% of patients patch tested reacted to the preservative [27]. Cross-reactions to and from the structurally related diazolidinyl urea may be observed [57].

30.5.5 Diazolidinyl Urea

Diazolidinyl urea is the most active member of the imidazolidinyl urea group, and a number of case reports of cosmetic allergy from diazolidinyl urea have been published [59]. In a Dutch study of 2,142 patients with eczema, patch tested with diazolidinyl urea 2% aq, 12 (0.6%) reacted. In 5 of these 12 cases, the patients were also allergic to formaldehyde and formaldehyde donors [60]. The members of the North American Contact Dermatitis Group tested 3,085 patients with diazolidinyl urea 1% in water, and obtained 3.7% positive reactions [27]. Of 58 individuals with diazolidinyl urea sensitivity seen at the Mayo Clinic, 47 (81%) also reacted to formaldehyde [61]. Cross-reactions to and from imidazolidinyl urea occur [59, 61]. Diazolidinyl urea appears to be a stronger sensitizer than imidazolidinyl urea.

30.5.6 2-Bromo-2-Nitropropane-1,3-Diol (Bronopol)

2-Bromo-2-nitropropane-1,3-diol is not a frequent cause of contact allergy in Europe [17, 62]. In the United States, however, it was found to be such a common cause of cosmetic allergy in one cosmetic cream [63], that the manufacturer decided to replace it. Recently, 2.3% of patients routinely tested in the United States were allergic to it [27]. Because interaction with amines and amides can result in the formation of nitrosamines or nitrosamides, suspected carcinogens, there is restriction in the formulations that may contain this preservative.

30.5.7 DMDM Hydantoin

DMDM hydantoin itself is probably not an allergen, but may cause reactions in formaldehyde-allergic individuals by virtue from the release of formaldehyde. Routine testing with DMDM hydantoin 3% aq. in 501 patients resulted in four positive reactions; all four were also allergic to formaldehyde [64]. Subsequent testing in patients allergic to formaldehyde resulted in positive reactions to DMDM hydantoin at concentrations as low as 0.3% [65]. Also, repeated open application to the skin of a cream containing 0.25% w/w DMDM hydantoin elicited a positive response in some patients. Consequently, patients sensitized to formaldehyde may experience cosmetic dermatitis from using leave-on products preserved with DMDM hydantoin. In the United States, a prevalence rate of 2.3% positive reactions has been observed [27].

30.5.7.1 Parabens

The paraben esters (methyl, ethyl, propyl, butyl) are widely used preservatives in cosmetic products. Parabens have had an unwarranted reputation as sensitizers. However, most cases of paraben sensitivity are caused by topical medicaments applied to leg ulcers or stasis dermatitis. Routine testing in the European standard series yields low prevalence rates of sensitization [66]. At the usual concentration of 0.1–0.3% in cosmetics, parabens rarely cause adverse reactions. Parabens are not included in the North American standard series of contact allergens as the allergen causes problems only rarely [27].

Sensitized individuals may be able to tolerate products containing parabens, a phenomenon which has been called the *paraben paradox* [67]. Tolerance is related to concentration, duration and site of application, and skin status. The subject of paraben sensitivity has been reviewed [44].

30.5.7.2 Iodopropynyl Butylcarbamate

This preservative was popular in many skin care and hair care products, and contact allergy to it from cosmetic use has been reported [68, 69]. The recommended patch test concentration, based on an analysis of concurrent testing with several dilutions, is 0.2%. However, because of concerns about the bioavailability of iodine, there has been considerable reduction in its use in cosmetics.

30.5.7.3 Miscellaneous Preservatives

Preservatives used in cosmetics that have occasionally caused allergy include benzyl alcohol, chloroacetamide, chlorphenisin [70], phenoxyethanol, and triclosan.

30.5.8 Tosylamide/Formaldehyde Resin

Contact allergy to the main allergen in nail varnish, tosylamide/formaldehyde resin, is common [9,

71–75]. Up to 6.6% of women habitually or occasionally using nail cosmetics and presenting with dermatitis are allergic to it [71], and the prevalence in patients routinely tested in the United States was 1.6% [27]. Eighty percent of all reactions are observed as a dermatitis of the face and neck, with many cases manifesting as an eyelid dermatitis. Occasionally, other parts of the body are involved, including the thighs, the genitals, and the trunk; generalized dermatitis is rare. Periungual dermatitis may be far more common (60%) than previously thought [9]. Desquamative gingivitis was the sole manifestation in a compulsive nail-biter [76]. Partner ("connubial") dermatitis has been observed. Other, but rarely reported, allergens in nail lacquers include formaldehyde, nitrocellulose [77], polyester resin, phthalates, and o-toluenesulfonamide [72, 73].

Important sociomedical consequences of nail varnish allergy have been reported [9]. Allergic patients should stop using nail varnishes or use varnishes free from tosylamide/formaldehyde resin. However, some products claiming not to contain the resin may still do so [78]. Also, such nail varnishes may contain other sensitizers, such as methyl acrylate and epoxy resin [79]. Useful review articles on adverse reactions to nail cosmetics [80, 81] and sculptured nails [82] are available.

30.5.9 *p*-Phenylenediamine and Related Hair Dyes

p-Phenylenediamine and related hair dyes are very common and important sensitizers. Safer permanent dyes with a lower risk of contact allergy, but with the same technical qualities, are not available. Many cases of sensitization were reported in the 1930s, and sensitization was considered so great a hazard that the use of *p*-phenylenediamine in hair dyes was prohibited in several countries. Currently, its incorporation in cosmetic products is allowed in the European Union up to a maximum concentration of 6% (as free base), which equates, after mixing with the oxidizing agent, to 3%; in practice, the maximum level to which the consumer is exposed is 2%.

p-Phenylenediamine remains an important cause of cosmetic allergy, with a 6.8% prevalence rate of sensitization in routinely tested patients in the United States [27]. The clinical features of hair dye allergy are discussed in Chap. 29.

These oxidation dyes are also an occupational hazard for hairdressers and beauticians [83]. The chemistry of, and adverse reactions to, oxidation coloring agents have been reviewed [84]. Semi-permanent and temporary dyes rarely cause allergic cos-

Table 2. Examples of hair colors that have caused cosmetic allergy

1-Hydroxy-3-nitro-4-aminobenzene
1-Hydroxyethylamino-3-nitro-4-aminobenzene
2-Nitro-*p*-phenylenediamine
Basic blue 99
Henna
m-Aminophenol
N-(b-Hydroxyethyl)-2-nitro-4-hydroxyaminobenzene
Naphthalenediol
N-Phenyl-*p*-phenylenediamine
p-Aminophenol
p-Phenylenediamine
Pyrocatechol
Resorcinol
Toluene-2,4-diamine
Toluene-2,5-diamine

30

metic dermatitis. Examples of hair colors that have caused cosmetic allergy are listed in Table 2.

30.5.10 Cocamidopropyl Betaine

Cocamidopropyl betaine is an amphoteric surfactant, which is widely present in shampoos and bath products, such as bath and shower gels [16–18]. Residues in some commercial grades, dimethylaminopropylamine [85] and cocamidopropyl dimethylamine ("amidoamine") [86], were responsible for prevalence rates of sensitization to cocamidopropyl betaine in a range from 3.7% to 5% [85, 87, 88]. Due to its presence in shampoos, cocamidopropyl betaine was an important occupational hazard to hairdressers. Consumers became sensitized to shampoos and a variety of other hygiene products, such as liquid shower soaps and facial cleansers [85]. Since the allergenic fractions were removed, the problem has disappeared.

30.5.11 UV Filters

Ultraviolet light filters (UV filters) are used in sunscreens to protect the consumer from harmful UV irradiation from the sun and are also incorporated in some cosmetics, notably facial skin care products, to inhibit UV photo-degradation of the product and protect the skin of the user. The main classes of sunscreens are PABA and its esters (amyl dimethyl, glyceryl, octyl dimethyl), cinnamates, salicylates, anthranilates, benzophenones, and dibenzoylmethanes [89]. The latter have become very popular, since they absorb mainly in the UVA range (315–400 nm).

The most frequent adverse reaction to sunscreen preparations is irritation, which occurs in over 15% of users [90]. UV filters have also been identified as allergens and photoallergens, but such reactions are uncommon. Patients who regularly use sunscreens because they suffer from the photosensitivity dermatitis/actinic reticuloid syndrome may have an increased risk for developing allergic side effects to sunscreens [91]. (Photo)allergic reactions can easily be overlooked, as the resulting dermatitis may be interpreted by the patient or consumer as failure of the product to protect against sunburn or as worsening of the (photo)dermatosis for which the sunscreen was used.

Currently, the most frequent cause of (photo)contact allergy to UV filters is benzophenone-3 (oxybenzone) [92]. Cross-reactions between benzophenones appear to be rare [93]. A number of UV filters are reported to have caused (photo)contact allergy [13, 89, 93–96] and these are discussed further in Chap. 27.

30.5.12 Lanolin and Derivatives

Lanolin and lanolin derivatives are used extensively in cosmetic products as emollients and emulsifiers. However, the majority of individuals have been sensitized by using topical pharmaceutical preparations containing lanolin, especially for treating varicose ulcers and stasis dermatitis (a similar situation to that of parabens) [97].

Additionally, many "positive" patch test reactions are not reproducible [98]. Thus, it appears that the currently used test allergen (30% wool wax alcohols) may cause false-positive, irritant, patch test reactions [98, 99]. Possibly, the same applies to the lanolin derivative Amerchol L-101, which is often used in addition to patch testing [100].

The presence of lanolin or its derivatives in cosmetics may cause cosmetic dermatitis in lanolin-sensitive individuals, but the risk of sensitization from using such products is small [101]. In the general population, contact allergy to lanolin is considered to be rare [98, 99].

30.5.13 Glyceryl Thioglycolate

Glyceryl thioglycolate, a waving agent used in acid permanent waving products, occasionally sensitizes consumers [102], but it is usually an occupational hazard for the hairdresser [83]. Patients allergic to glyceryl thioglycolate infrequently react to ammonium thioglycolate, also a contact allergen, used in "hot" permanent wave procedures.

30.5.14 Propylene Glycol

Propylene glycol is widely used in dermatologic and non-dermatologic topical formulations, including cosmetics, as well as in numerous other products [103–105]. Propylene glycol may cause irritant contact dermatitis, allergic contact dermatitis, non-immunologic immediate contact reactions, and subjective or sensory irritation [103].

Allergic contact dermatitis is uncommon and its clinical significance has been overestimated. In earlier studies, higher concentrations of propylene glycol may have induced many irritant patch test reactions. Currently, a concentration of 1–10% [105] is advised in order to avoid such irritation, but cases of contact allergy are probably missed as a result (false-negative reactions). A diagnosis of allergic contact dermatitis should never be made on the basis of one positive patch test alone. Testing should be repeated after several weeks. In addition, repeat tests with serial dilutions down to 1% propylene glycol helps in discriminating between irritant responses and true allergic ones. Repeated open application tests (ROAT) and/or provocative use tests (PUT) can be conducted to verify the allergic basis of a positive patch test result.

30.5.15 Antioxidants

Antioxidants are added to cosmetics to prevent the deterioration of unsaturated fatty acids and are an occasional cause of cosmetic allergy [7, 15], though the actual prevalence may be underestimated [106]. Antioxidants that have caused cosmetic allergy include: BHA (butylated hydroxyanisole) [106], BHT (butylated hydroxytoluene) [106], t-butylhydroquinone [106, 107], gallates (dodecyl, octyl, propyl) [108], tocopherol (vitamin E), and its esters [109, 110].

30.5.16 Miscellaneous Allergens

Examples of other, infrequent causes of cosmetic allergy include oleamidopropyl dimethylamine [111], ceteayl alcohol [112], maleated soya bean oil [113], dicapryl maleate [114], diisostearyl malate [115], triethanolamine, and methyl glucose dioleate, castor oil [116], ricinoleates [117], polyvinylpyrrolidone (PVP) eicosene copolymer [118], polyvinylpyrrolidone triacontene copolymer [119], polyoxyethylene lauryl ether [120], tetrahydroxypropyl ethylenediamine, 1,3-butylene glycol [121], shellac [122], phthalic anhydride/trimellitic anhydride/glycols copolymer [123], colophonium [124], propolis [125], colors [126], and botanicals [127].

The depigmenting agent kojic acid is a common allergen in Japan [128].

A comprehensive literature survey on cosmetic allergy has been published [13, 129].

30.6 Diagnostic Procedures

The diagnosis of cosmetic allergy should strongly be suspected in any patient presenting with dermatitis of the face, eyelids, lips, and neck [13, 130]. Cosmetic allergic dermatitis may develop on previously healthy skin of the face or on already damaged skin (irritant contact dermatitis, atopic dermatitis, seborrheic dermatitis, allergic contact dermatitis from other sources). Also, dermatitis of the arms and hands may be caused or worsened by skin care products used to treat or prevent dry skin, irritant, or atopic dermatitis. Patchy dermatitis on the neck and around the eyes is suggestive of cosmetic allergy from nail varnish or hardeners. More widespread problems may be caused by ingredients in products intended for general application to the body. Hypersensitivity to other products, such as deodorants, usually causes a reaction localized to the site of application. A thorough history of cosmetic usage should always be obtained.

When the diagnosis of cosmetic allergy is suspected, patch tests should be performed to confirm the diagnosis and identify the sensitizer. Only in this way can the patient be counseled about their future use of cosmetic (and other) products, and the prevention of recurrences of dermatitis from cosmetic or non-cosmetic sources. Patch tests should be performed with the European (or other national) standard series, a "cosmetics series" containing established cosmetic allergens, and the products used by the patient.

The European routine series contains a number of cosmetic allergens and "indicator" allergens: colophonium, *Myroxylon pereirae* (balsam of Peru), fragrance mix, formaldehyde, quaternium-15, methylchloroisothiazolinone (and) methylisothiazolinone, lanolin, and *p*-phenylenediamine.

Although the patient's products should always be tested (for test concentrations, see Table 3 and Chap. 50), patch testing with cosmetics has problems. Both false-negative and false-positive reactions occur frequently. False-negative reactions are due to the low concentration of some allergens and the usually weak sensitivity of the patient. Classic examples of false-negative reactions have occurred with methylchloroisothiazolinone (and) methylisothiazolinone [47, 48] and paraben sensitivity. False-positive reactions may occur with any cosmetic product, but especially with products containing detergents or surfac-

Table 3. Recommended test concentrations for cosmetic products [130]

Cosmetic product	Test concentration and vehicle
Depilatory	Thioglycolate 1% pet.
Foaming bath product	1% water
Foaming cleanser	1% water
Hair bleach	Ammonium persulfate 1% pet.
Hair dyes	2% water
Hair straightener	Individual ingredients
Mascara	Pure (allow to dry)
Nail cuticle remover	Individual ingredients
Nail glue	Individual ingredients
Nail varnish remover	Individual ingredients
Nail varnish	Pure (allow to dry)
Permanent wave solution	Glyceryl thioglycolate 1% pet.
Shampoo	1% water
Shaving lather or cream	1% water
Skin lightener	Hydroquinone 1% pet.
Soap or detergent	1% water
Toothpaste	2% water

Most cosmetics not mentioned in this table can be tested undiluted

30

tants, such as shampoos, soaps, and bath and shower products. As a consequence, these products must be diluted (1% in water) before testing. Even then, mild irritant reactions are observed frequently, and, of course, the (necessary) dilution of these products may result in false-negative results in patients actually allergic to them. Testing such products is, therefore, highly unreliable.

In many cases, testing with the European standard series, suspected products, and a cosmetics screening series will establish the diagnosis of cosmetic allergy and identify one or more contact allergens. The label on the incriminated product will indicate whether or not the product actually contains the allergen(s). If not, the possibility of a false-positive reaction to the product should be suspected. The test should be repeated and/or control tests on non-exposed individuals should be performed. If an allergy is confirmed, an ingredient not included in the European series or the cosmetics screening series may be responsible. In such cases, the manufacturer should be asked for samples of the ingredients, and these can be tested on the patient after proper dilution [131].

In certain cases, an allergy to cosmetics is strongly suspected, but patch testing remains negative. In such patients, ROAT and/or usage tests can be performed. In the ROAT, the product is applied twice daily for a maximum of 14 days to the antecubital fossa. A negative reaction after 2 weeks indicates that sensitivity is highly unlikely. This procedure should be performed with all suspected products, except detergent-containing cosmetics, such as soap, shampoo, and shower products.

During the usage test, the use of all cosmetic products is stopped until the dermatitis has disappeared. The cosmetics are then reintroduced as normally used, one at a time, with an interval of 3 days for each product, until a reaction develops. Photopatch testing should be performed whenever photo-allergic cosmetic dermatitis is suspected. When all tests remain negative, the possibility of seborrheic dermatitis (scalp, eyelids, face, axillae, trunk), atopic dermatitis (all locations), irritant contact dermatitis (also from cosmetic products), and allergic contact dermatitis from other sources should be considered.

30.7 Ingredient Labeling in the European Union

Cosmetic ingredient labeling (introduced voluntarily in the United States in the 1970s) was a constant demand of European dermatologists for years. On 1 January 1997, the 6th Amendment to the Cosmetics Directive (76/768/EEC) in Europe became effective. This directive requires all cosmetic products marketed in the European Union to display their ingredients on the outer package or, in certain cases, in an accompanying leaflet, label, tape, or tag. The primary purpose of ingredient labeling is to allow dermatologists to identify specific ingredients that cause allergic responses in their patients, and to enable such patients to avoid cosmetic products containing the substances to which they are allergic.

The mandatory nomenclature used throughout the European Union for labeling is the International Nomenclature of Cosmetic Ingredients (INCI), based on the American Cosmetic, Toiletry, and Fragrance Association (CTFA) system. Most CTFA terms have been retained unchanged. However, all colorants are listed as color index (CI) numbers, except hair dyes, which have INCI names. Plant ingredients are declared as genus/species names using the Linnaean system. The source of information on ingredients is the European Inventory [1] published by the European Commission. Provided are the INCI names (in alphabetical order), CAS number, EINECS/ELINCS numbers, chemical/IUPAC names, and functions.

Patients allergic to certain ingredients of cosmetics must be supplied with the INCI names of their allergens, otherwise, they may fruitlessly seek for well-known names such as Kathon CG, oxybenzone, balsam of Peru, Amerchol L-101, dibromodicyanobutane, or orange oil. Dermatologists should be familiar with the INCI nomenclature. However, the relevant names are sometimes difficult to find, but a list of substances which can be present in cosmetics and have been described as allergens has been generated and their names [CTFA, Merck Index, names provided by the producers of commercially available allergens (e.g., Chemotechnique, Trolab), "common names," and commonly used trade names] compared with those of the INCI [132].

References

1. The European Commission's Inventory of Ingredients http://pharmacos.eudra.org/F3/cosmetic/cosm_inci_index.htm
2. Consumers' Association (1979) Reactions of the skin to cosmetics and toiletry products. Consumers' Association, London
3. de Groot AC, Beverdam EG, Ayong CT, Coenraads PJ, Nater JP (1988) The role of contact allergy in the spectrum of adverse effects caused by cosmetics and toiletries. Contact Dermatitis 19:195–201
4. Nielsen NH, Menné T (1992) Allergic contact sensitization in an unselected Danish population. Acta Derm Venereol (Stockh) 72:456–460
5. de Groot AC (1990) Labelling cosmetics with their ingredients. Br Med J 300:1636–1638
6. Dillarstone A (1997) Letter to the editor. Contact Dermatitis 37:190
7. Adams RM, Maibach HI (1985) A five-year study of cosmetic reactions. J Am Acad Dermatol 13:1062–1069
8. Meynadier J-M, Raison-Peyron N, Meunier L, Meynadier J (1997) Allergie aux parfums. Rev Fr Allergol 37:641–650
9. Lidén C, Berg M, Färm G, Wrangsjö K (1993) Nail varnish allergy with far-reaching consequences. Br J Dermatol 128:57–62
10. Ophaswongse S, Maibach HI (1995) Allergic contact cheilitis. Contact Dermatitis 33:365–370
11. Sainio EL, Kanerva L (1995) Contact allergens in toothpastes and a review of their hypersensitivity. Contact Dermatitis 33:100–105
12. Skrebova N, Brocks K, Karlsmark T (1998) Allergic contact cheilitis from spearmint oil. Contact Dermatitis 39:35
13. de Groot AC, Weyland JW, Nater JP (1994) Unwanted effects of cosmetics and drugs used in dermatology, 3rd edn. Elsevier, Amsterdam, the Netherlands
14. de Groot AC, Frosch PJ (1997) Adverse reactions to fragrances. A clinical review. Contact Dermatitis 36:57–86
15. de Groot AC, Bruynzeel DP, Bos JD, van der Meeren HLM, van Joost T, Jagtman BA, Weyland JW (1988) The allergens in cosmetics. Arch Dermatol 124:1525–1529
16. de Groot AC (1997) Cocamidopropyl betaine: a "new" important cosmetic allergen. Dermatosen 45:60–63
17. de Groot AC, van der Walle HB, Weyland JW (1995) Contact allergy to cocamidopropyl betaine. Contact Dermatitis 33:419–22
18. de Groot AC (1997) Contact allergens – what's new? Cosmetic dermatitis. Clin Dermatol 15:485–492
19. de Groot AC, van Ginkel CJW, Weyland JW (1996) Methyldibromo glutaronitrile (Euxyl K 400): an important "new" allergen in cosmetics. J Am Acad Dermatol 35:743–747
20. de Groot AC, de Cock PAJJM, Coenraads PJ, van Ginkel CJW, Jagtman BA, van Joost T, van der Kley AMJ, Meinardi MMHM, Smeenk G, van der Valk PGM, van der Walle HB, Weyland JW (1996) Methyldibromo glutaronitrile is an important contact allergen in the Netherlands. Contact Dermatitis 34:118–120
21. Berne B, Boström Å, Grahnén AF, Tammela M (1996) Adverse effects of cosmetics and toiletries reported to the Swedish Medical Product Agency 1989–1994. Contact Dermatitis 34:359–362
22. de Groot AC, Frosch PJ (1998) Fragrances as a cause of contact dermatitis in cosmetics: clinical aspects and epidemiological data. In: Frosch PJ, Johansen JD, White IR (eds) Fragrances. Beneficial and adverse effects. Springer, Berlin Heidelberg New York, pp 66–75
23. Frosch PJ, Johansen JD, White IR (eds) (1998) Fragrances. Beneficial and adverse effects. Springer, Berlin Heidelberg New York
24. Guin JD (1982) History, manufacture, and cutaneous reactions to perfumes. In: Frost P, Horwitz SW (eds) Principles of cosmetics for the dermatologist. Mosby, St. Louis, Calif., pp 111–129
25. Scheinman PL (1996) Allergic contact dermatitis to fragrance: a review. Am J Contact Dermatitis 7:65–76
26. Guin JD, Berry VK (1980) Perfume sensitivity in adult females. A study of contact sensitivity to a perfume mix in two groups of student nurses. J Am Acad Dermatol 3:299–302
27. Marks JG Jr, Belsito DV, DeLeo VA, Fowler JF Jr, Fransway AF, Maibach HI, Mathias CGT, Nethercott JR, Rietschel RL, Sheretz EF, Storrs FJ, Taylor JS (1998) North American Contact Dermatitis Group patch test results for the detection of delayed-type hypersensitivity to topical allergens. J Am Acad Dermatol 38:911–918
28. Johansen JD, Rastogi SC, Menné T (1996) Contact allergy to popular perfumes; assessed by patch test, use test and chemical analysis. Br J Dermatol 135:419–422
29. Johansen JD, Rastogi SC, Andersen KE, Menné T (1997) Content and reactivity to product perfumes in fragrance mix positive and negative eczema patients. A study of perfumes used in toiletries and skin-care products. Contact Dermatitis 36:291–296
30. Dooms-Goossens A, Kerre S, Drieghe J, Bossuyt L, Degreef H (1992) Cosmetic products and their allergens. Eur J Dermatol 2:465–468
31. Johansen JD, Andersen TF, Kjøller M, Veien N, Avnstorp C, Andersen KE, Menné T (1998) Identification of risk products for fragrance contact allergy: a case-referent study based on patients' histories. Am J Contact Dermatitis 9:80–86
32. Frosch PJ, Johansen JD, Menne T, Rastogi SC, Bruze M, Andersen KE, Lepoittevan JP, Gimenez Arnau E, Pirker C, Goossens A, White IR (1999) Lyral is an important sensitizer in patients sensitive to fragrances. Br J Dermatol 141:1076–1083
33. The Scientific Committee on Cosmetic Products and Non-Food Products intended for Consumers (1999) Concerning Fragrance Allergy in Consumers. Available at http://europa.eu.int/comm/health/ph_risk/committees/sccp/documents/out98_en.pdf
34. Nethercott JR, Larsen WG (1997) Contact allergens – what's new? Fragrances. Clin Dermatol 15:499–504
35. Frosch PJ, Pirker C, Rastogi SC, Andersen KE, Bruze M, Svedman C, Goossens A, White IR, Uter W, Arnau EG, Lepoittevin JP, Menné T, Johansen JD (2005) Patch testing with a new fragrance mix detects additional patients sensitive to perfumes and missed by the current fragrance mix. Contact Dermatitis 52:207–215

30

36. Johansen JD, Andersen TF, Veien N, Avnstorp C, Andersen KE, Menné T (1997) Patch testing with markers of fragrance contact allergy. Do clinical tests correspond to patients' self-reported problems? Acta Derm Venereol (Stockh) 77:149–153

37. Johansen JD, Rastogi SC, Menné T (1996) Exposure to selected fragrance materials. A case study of fragrance-mix-positive eczema patients. Contact Dermatitis 34:106–110

38. Rastogi SC, Johansen JD, Frosch PJ, Menné T, Bruze M, Lepoittevin JP, Dreier B, Andersen KE, White IR (1998) Deodorants on the European market: quantitative chemical analysis of 21 fragrances. Contact Dermatitis 38:29–35

39. Rastogi S, Johansen JD, Menné T (1996) Natural ingredients based cosmetics. Content of selected fragrance sensitizers. Contact Dermatitis 34:423–426

40. Johansen JD, Andersen KE, Menné T (1996) Quantitative aspects of iso-eugenol contact allergy assessed by use and patch tests. Contact Dermatitis 34:414–418

41. Johansen JD, Andersen KE, Rastogi SC, Menné T (1996) Threshold responses in cinnamic-aldehyde-sensitive subjects: results and methodological aspects. Contact Dermatitis 34:165–171

42. Fransway AF (1991) The problem of preservation in the 1990 s. I. Statement of the problem, solution(s) of the industry, and the current use of formaldehyde and formaldehyde-releasing biocides. Am J Contact Dermat 2:6–23

43. Fransway AF, Schmitz NA (1991) The problem of preservation in the 1990 s. II. Formaldehyde and formaldehyde-releasing biocides: incidences of cross-reactivity and the significance of the positive response to formaldehyde. Am J Contact Dermat 2:78–88

44. Fransway AF (1991) The problem of preservation in the 1990 s. III. Agents with preservative function independent of formaldehyde release. Am J Contact Dermatitis 2:145–174

45. Morren MA, Dooms-Goossens A, Delabie J, De Wolf-Peeters C, Marien K, Degreef H (1992) Contact allergy to isothiazolinone derivatives: unusual clinical presentations. Dermatology 184:260–264

46. Frosch PJ, Lahti A, Hannuksela M, Andersen KE, Wilkinson JD, Shaw S, Lachapelle JM (1995) Chloromethylisothiazolone/methylisothiazolinone (CMI/MI) use test with a shampoo on patch-test-positive subjects. Results of a multicentre double-blind crossover trial. Contact Dermatitis 32:210–217

47. de Groot AC, Weyland JW (1988) Kathon CG: a review. J Am Acad Dermatol 18:350–358

48. de Groot AC (1990) Methylisothiazolinone/methylchloroisothiazolinone (Kathon CG) allergy: an updated review. Am J Contact Dermat 1:151–156

49. Tosti A, Vincenzi C, Trevisi P, Guerra L (1995) Euxyl K 400: incidence of sensitization, patch test concentration and vehicle. Contact Dermatitis 33:193–195

50. Schnuch A, Geier J (1994) Die häufigsten Kontaktallergene im zweiten Halbjahr 1993. Dermatosen 42:210–211

51. Jackson JM, Fowler JF (1998) Methyldibromoglutaronitrile (Euxyl K400): a new and important sensitizer in the United States? J Am Acad Dermatol 38:934–937

52. de Groot AC, van Ginkel CJW, Weyland JW (1996) How to detect sensitization to Euxyl K 400. Contact Dermatitis 34:373–374

53. Bruze M, Goossens A, Gruvberger B; ESCD; EECDRG (2005) Recommendation to include methyldibromo glutaronitrile in the European standard patch test series. Contact Dermatitis 52:24–28

54. Banerjee P, McFadden JP, Ross JS, Rycroft RJG, White IR (2003) Increased positive patch test reactivity to methyldibromo glutaronitrile. Contact Dermatitis 49:111–113

55. Rosen M, McFarland AG (1984) Free formaldehyde in anionic shampoos. J Soc Cosmet Chem 35:157–169

56. Parker LU, Taylor JS (1991) A 5-year study of contact allergy to quaternium-15. Am J Contact Dermat 2:231–234

57. Jacobs M-C, White IR, Rycroft RJG, Taub N (1995) Patch testing with preservatives at St John's from 1982 to 1993. Contact Dermatitis 33:247–254

58. Dooms-Goossens A, de Boulle K, Dooms M, Degreef H (1986) Imidazolidinyl urea dermatitis. Contact Dermatitis 14:322–324

59. de Groot AC, Bruynzeel DP, Jagtman BA, Weyland JW (1988) Contact allergy to diazolidinyl urea (Germall II). Contact Dermatitis 18:202–205

60. Perret CM, Happle R (1989) Contact sensitivity to diazolidinyl urea (Germall II). In: Frosch PJ, Dooms-Goossens A, Lachapelle J-M, Rycroft RJG, Scheper RJ (eds) Current topics in contact dermatitis. Springer, Berlin Heidelberg New York, pp 92–94

61. Hectorne KJ, Fransway AF (1994) Diazolidinyl urea: incidence of sensitivity, patterns of cross-reactivity and clinical relevance. Contact Dermatitis 30:16–19

62. Frosch PJ, White IR, Rycroft RJG, Lahti A, Burrows D, Camarasa JG, Ducombs G, Wilkinson JD (1990) Contact allergy to Bronopol. Contact Dermatitis 22:24–26

63. Storrs F, Bell DE (1983) Allergic contact dermatitis to 2-bromo-2-nitropane-1,3-diol in a hydrophilic ointment. J Am Acad Dermatol 8:157–164

64. de Groot AC, Bos JD, Jagtman BA, Bruynzeel DP, van Joost T, Weyland JW (1986) Contact allergy to preservatives – II. Contact Dermatitis 15:218–222

65. de Groot AC, van Joost T, Bos JD, van der Meeren HLM, Weyland JW (1988) Patch test reactivity to DMDM hydantoin. Relationship to formaldehyde. Contact Dermatitis 18:197–201

66. Menné T, Hjorth N (1988) Routine patch testing with paraben esters. Contact Dermatitis 19:189–191

67. Fisher AA (1993) The parabens: paradoxical preservatives. Cutis 51:405–406

68. Brasch J, Schnuch A, Geier J, Aberer W, Uter W; German Contact Dermatitis Research Group; Information Network of Departments of Dermatology (2004) Iodopropynylbutyl carbamate 0.2% is suggested for patch testing of patients with eczema possibly related to preservatives. Br J Dermatol 151:608–615

69. Schollnast R, Kranke B, Aberer W (2003) Anal and palmar contact dermatitis caused by iodopropynyl butylcarbamate in moist sanitary wipes. Hautarzt 54:970–110

70. Wakelin SH, White IR (1997) Contact dermatitis from chlorphenisin in a facial cosmetic. Contact Dermatitis 37:138–139

71. Tosti A, Guerra L, Vincenzi C, Piraccini BM, Peluso AM (1993) Contact sensitization caused by toluene sulfonamide-formaldehyde resin in women who use nail cosmetics. Am J Contact Dermat 4:150–153

72. Hausen BM (1994) Nagellack-Allergie. HG Z Hautkr 69:252–262

73. Hausen BM, Milbrodt M, Koenig WA (1995) The allergens of nail polish (I). Allergenic constituents of common nail polish and toluenesulfonamide-formaldehyde resin (TS-F-R). Contact Dermatitis 33:157–164

74. Giorgini S, Brusi C, Francalanci S, Gola M, Sertoli A (1994) Prevention of allergic contact dermatitis from nail varnishes and hardeners. Contact Dermatitis 31:325–326

75. Kardorff B, Fuchs M, Kunze J (1995) Kontaktallergien auf Nagellack. Aktuel Dermatol 21:349–352

76. Staines KS, Felix DH, Forsyth A (1998) Desquamative gingivitis, sole manifestation of tosylamide/formaldehyde resin allergy. Contact Dermatitis 39:90

77. Castelain M, Veyrat S, Laine G, Montastier C (1997) Contact dermatitis from nitrocellulose in a nail varnish. Contact Dermatitis 36:266–267

78. Hausen BM (1995) A simple method of determining TS-F-R in nail polish. Contact Dermatitis 32:188–190

79. Kanerva L, Lauerma A, Jolanki R, Estlander T (1995) Methyl acrylate: a new sensitizer in nail lacquer. Contact Dermatitis 33:203–204

80. Rosenzweig R, Scher RK (1993) Nail cosmetics: adverse reactions. Am J Contact Dermat 4:71–77

81. Barnett JM, Scher RK (1992) Nail cosmetics. Int J Dermatol 31:675–681

82. Kanerva L, Lauerma A, Estlander T, Alanko K, Henriks-Eckerman M-L, Jolanki R (1996) Occupational allergic contact dermatitis caused by photobonded sculptured nails and a review of (meth) acrylates in nail cosmetics. Am J Contact Dermat 7:109–115

83. Conde-Salazar L, Baz M, Guimaraens D, Cannavo A (1995) Contact dermatitis in hairdressers: patch test results in 379 hairdressers. Am J Contact Dermat 6:19–23

84. Marcoux D, Riboulet-Delmas G (1994) Efficacy and safety of hair-coloring agents. Am J Contact Dermat 5:123–129

85. Pigatto PD, Bigardi AS, Cusano F (1995) Contact dermatitis to cocamidopropylbetaine is caused by residual amines: relevance, clinical characteristics, and review of the literature. Am J Contact Dermat 6:13–16

86. Fowler JF, Fowler LM, Hunter JE (1997) Allergy to cocamidopropyl betaine may be due to amidoamine: a patch test and product use test study. Contact Dermatitis 37:276–281

87. Fowler JF Jr (1993) Cocamidopropyl betaine: the significance of positive patch test results in twelve patients. Cutis 52:281–284

88. Angelini G, Foti C, Rigano L, Vena G (1995) 3-Dimethylaminopropylamine: a key substance in contact allergy to cocamidopropylbetaine? Contact Dermatitis 32:96–99

89. Funk JO, Dromgoole SH, Maibach HI (1995) Sunscreen intolerance. Contact sensitization, photocontact sensitization, and irritancy of sunscreen agents. Dermatol Clin 13:473–481

90. Foley P, Nixon R, Marks R, Frowen K, Thompson S (1993) The frequency of reactions to sunscreens: results of a longitudinal population-based study on the regular use of sunscreens in Australia. Br J Dermatol 128:512–518

91. Bilsland D, Ferguson J (1993) Contact allergy to sunscreen chemicals in photosensitivity dermatitis/actinic reticuloid syndrome (PD/AR) and polymorphic light eruption. Contact Dermatitis 29:70–73

92. Darvay A, White IR, Rycroft RJG, Jones AB, Hawk JLM, McFadden JP (2001) Photoallergic contact dermatitis is uncommon. Br J Dermatol 145:597–601

93. Manciet JR, Lepoittevin JP, Jeanmougin M, Dubertret L (1994) Study of the cross-reactivity of seven benzophenones between themselves and with fenofibrate. Nouv Dermatol 13:370–371

94. Pons-Guiraud A, Jeanmougin M (1993) Allergie et photoallergie de contact aux crèmes de photoprotection. Ann Derm Venereol (Stockh) 120:727–731

95. Gonçalo M, Ruas E, Figueiredo A, Gonçalo S (1995) Contact and photocontact sensitivity to sunscreens. Contact Dermatitis 33:278–280

96. Theeuwes M, Degreef H, Dooms-Goossens A (1992) Para-aminobenzoic acid (PABA) and sunscreen allergy. Am J Contact Dermat 3:206–207

97. Wilson CI, Cameron J, Powell SM, Cherry G, Ryan TJ (1997) High incidence of contact dermatitis in leg-ulcer patients – implications for management. Clin Exp Dermatol 16:250–261

98. Nachbar F, Korting HC, Plewig G (1993) Zur Bedeutung des positiven Epicutantests auf Lanolin. Dermatosen 41:227–236

99. Kligman AM (1998) The myth of lanolin allergy. Contact Dermatitis 39:103–107

100. Matthieu L, Dockx P (1997) Discrepancy in patch test results with wool wax alcohols and Amerchol L-101. Contact Dermatitis 36:150–151

101. Wolf R (1996) The lanolin paradox. Dermatology 192:198–202

102. Guerra L, Bardazzi F, Tosti A (1992) Contact dermatitis in hairdressers' clients. Contact Dermatitis 26:108–111

103. Funk JO, Maibach HI (1994) Propylene glycol dermatitis: re-evaluation of an old problem. Contact Dermatitis 31:236–241

104. Aberer W, Fuchs T, Peters KP, Frosch PJ (1993) Propylenglykol: kutane Nebenwirkungen und Testmethodik. Dermatosen 41:25–27

105. Wahlberg JE (1994) Propylene glycol: search for a proper and nonirritant patch test preparation. Am J Contact Dermat 5:156–159

106. White IR, Lovell CR, Cronin E (1984) Antioxidants in cosmetics. Contact Dermatitis 11:265–267

107. Le Coz CJ, Schneider G-A (1998) Contact dermatitis from tertiary-butylhydroquinone in a hair dye, with cross-sensitivity to BHA and BHT. Contact Dermatitis 39:39–40

108. Serra-Baldrich E, Puig LL, Gimenez Arnau A, Camarasa JG (1995) Lipstick allergic contact dermatitis from gallates. Contact Dermatitis 32:359–360

109. Parsad D, Saini R, Verma N (1997) Xanthomatous reaction following contact dermatitis from vitamin E. Contact Dermatitis 37:294

110. Wyss M, Elsner P, Homberger H-P, Greco P, Gloor M, Burg G (1997) Follikuläres Kontaktekzem auf eine Tocopherol-linoleat-haltige Körpermilch. Dermatosen 45:25–28

111. Foti C, Rigano L, Vena GA, Grandolfo M, Liguori G, Angelini G (1995) Contact allergy to oleamidopropyl dimethylamine and related substances. Contact Dermatitis 33:132–133

112. Tosti A, Vincenzi C, Guerra L, Andrisano E (1996) Contact dermatitis from fatty alcohols. Contact Dermatitis 35:287–289

113. le Coz CJ, Lefebvre C (2000) Contact dermatitis from maleated soybean oil: last gasps of an expiring cosmetic allergen. Contact Dermatitis 43:118–119

114. Laube S, Davies MG, Prais L, Foulds IS (2002) Allergic contact dermatitis from medium-chain triglycerides in a moisturizing lotion. Contact Dermatitis 47:171

115. Guin JD (2001) Allergic contact cheilitis from di-isostearyl malate in lipstick. Contact Dermatitis 44:375

116. le Coz CJ, Ball C (2000) Recurrent allergic contact dermatitis and cheilitis due to castor oil. Contact Dermatitis 42:114–115

117. Magerl A, Heiss R, Frosch PJ (2001) Allergic contact dermatitis from zinc ricinoleate in a deodorant and glyceryl ricinoleate in a lipstick. Contact Dermatitis 44:119–121

118. le Coz CJ, Lefebvre C, Ludmann F, Grosshans E (2000) Polyvinylpyrrolidone (PVP)/eicosene copolymer: an emerging cosmetic allergen. Contact Dermatitis 43:61–62

119. Stone N, Varma S, Hughes TM, Stone NM (2002) Allergic contact dermatitis from polyvinylpyrrolidone (PVP)/1-triacontene copolymer in a sunscreen. Contact Dermatitis 47:49

120. Kimura M, Kawada A (2000) Follicular contact dermatitis due to polyoxyethylene laurylether. J Am Acad Dermatol 42:879–880

121. Diegenant C, Constandt L, Goossens A (2000) Allergic contact dermatitis due to 1,3-butylene glycol. Contact Dermatitis 43:234–235

122. Le Coz CJ, Leclere JM, Arnoult E, Raison-Peyron N, Pons-Guiraud A, Vigan M; Members of Revidal-Gerda (2002) Allergic contact dermatitis from shellac in mascara. Contact Dermatitis 46:149–152

123. Moffitt DL, Sansom JE (2002) Allergic contact dermatitis from phthalic anhydride/trimellitic anhydride/glycols copolymer in nail varnish. Contact Dermatitis 46:236

124. Batta K, Bourke JF, Foulds IS (1997) Allergic contact dermatitis from colophony in lipsticks. Contact Dermatitis 36:171–172

125. Hausen BM, Wollenweber E, Senff H, Post B (1987) Propolis allergy (I). Origin, properties, usage and literature review. Contact Dermatitis 17:163–170

126. Guin JD (2003) Patch testing to FD&C and D&C dyes. Contact Dermatitis 49:217–218

127. Kiken DA, Cohen DE (2002) Contact Dermatitis to botanical extracts. Am J Contact Dermat 13:148–152

128. Nakagawa M, Kawai K, Kawai K (1995) Contact allergy to kojic acid in skin care products. Contact Dermatitis 32:9–13

129. de Groot AC (1988) Adverse reactions to cosmetics. Thesis, State University of Groningen, the Netherlands

130. De Groot AC (1998) Fatal attractiveness: the shady side of cosmetics. Clin Dermatol 16:167–179

131. De Groot AC (1994) Patch testing. Test concentrations and vehicles for 3700 allergens, 2nd edn. Elsevier, Amsterdam, The Netherlands

132. de Groot AC, Weijland JW (1997) Conversion of common names of cosmetic allergens to the INCI nomenclature. Contact Dermatitis 37:145–150

30

Chapter 31

Allergens of Special Interest

31

JEANNE DUUS JOHANSEN, JEAN-PIERRE LEPOITTEVIN, DAVID BASKETTER, JOHN MCFADDEN, HEIDI SØSTED

Contents

31.1 Fragrances

JEANNE DUUS JOHANSEN, JEAN-PIERRE LEPOITTEVIN

31.1.1 Introduction

The applications of fragrances are numerous and contact may be difficult to avoid, if one should wish so. Fragrances are used in all kinds of cosmetics and toiletries, in cleansing agents, air fresheners, toys and textiles, and in industrial settings. Many fragrance ingredients are also used as flavors in food and some are naturally occurring in spices. Fragrance products are used in aromatherapy, may be contained in herbal remedies, and, in some regions, natural fragrance products are used as topical medicaments for their antiseptic properties. Fragrances are capable of neutralizing unpleasant odors. They are added to products to produce a pleasant scent, add special character to the product, or as functional ingredients, e.g., providing antibacterial effects.

31.1.2 Fragrance Ingredients

The International Fragrance Association (IFRA) defines fragrance ingredients as any basic ingredient used in the manufacture of fragrance materials for its odorous, odor enhancing, or blending properties [1]. A fragrance ingredient may be a chemically defined substance or a natural product.

Natural fragrance products are obtained by processing material from fragrance-producing plants. The fragrance can be present in almost any part of the plant and is obtained by pressing or steam distillation to give essential oils or by organic solvent extraction to give concretes and absolutes [2]. The content and consistency of the naturals depends on climatic and soil conditions for the plant, as well as many other factors, which makes it very difficult, if not impossible, to fully standardize the contents and quality of the end product.

The volatile fragrance product obtained from plants usually contains numerous ingredients. The characteristic odor of the fragrance product may be due either to a particular ingredient, or, in the case of a complex composition, the blending of a number of ingredients [3]. Oak moss absolute contains at least 250 ingredients and has several odor-determining agents [4], while clove oil contains up to 80% eugenol, which is the determining odor agent [5].

Previously, also animal secretions, such as musk from deer and ambergris from the sperm whale, were used as the basis for the production of natural fragrance ingredients. These are now mostly replaced by blends of fragrance chemicals.

Originally, all perfumes were composed of natural products, but with the scientific and technical developments in the first half of the 19th century, chemists were able to identify the odor-determining major ingredients of natural fragrance materials. Following this development, industrial production of synthetic fragrance materials began. The synthesized ingredients are often nature-identical chemicals, that is, imitations of naturally occurring substances; however, also, the production of entirely new chemicals takes place.

The EU Commission has issued two inventories of fragrance ingredients, both of which are currently in use, one of the chemical substances and one of the natural products, also named botanicals. The lists are based on information from the industry and contain about 2,500 different ingredients [6].

Core Message

■ Two thousand five hundred (2,500) fragrance ingredients are in current use for compounding perfumes. The ingredients are natural extracts of plant products, nature-identical, or entirely synthetic chemicals.

31.1.3 The Fragrance Formula

A fragrance formula consists of a mixture of 10–300 or more different fragrance ingredients, naturals, and/or chemicals. The fragrance formula is incorporated into the end product, e.g., a cosmetic. Some cosmetic products are used primarily for their scent, such as perfumes, eau de cologne, and aftershaves. These products consist mainly of fragrance ingredients diluted with alcohol/water. A perfume usually contain 15–30% fragrance ingredients, a cologne about 3–5%, a deodorant 1%, a cream 0.4%, and undiluted soaps 0.5–2% [7].

The creation of a perfume, the fragrance formula, is regarded as an art. In designing a perfume, components from different odor families and of different volatilities are combined to form an esthetic whole. The most volatile ingredients are called top notes, usually fruity and spicy, which is followed by the heart note, built up by floral accords, forming the most essential part of the perfume; the long-lasting materials are known as the bottom notes. These include woody, moss-like, and sweet vanilla-like ingredients [8]. The basic pattern and principal structure of perfumes has not changed dramatically throughout the history of perfumery. The difference lies in the quality and availability of the raw materials and a different way of compounding [8].

31.1.4 Chemistry

Fragrance ingredients are organic compounds and must be volatile to be perceived. Therefore, in addition to the nature of the functional groups and the molecular structure of a substance, the molecular mass is an important factor. Molecular masses of about 200 occur relatively frequently [5]; further, many of the fragrance ingredients are lipophilic in nature and, thus, have good penetration abilities, even of intact skin [9].

A fragrance formula is a mixture of molecules with very different physico-chemical properties; allergens may be formed in the mixture, e.g., by oxidization [10] or in the skin by metabolism [11]. The mixture of molecules may result in interactions during skin penetration, skin metabolism, and epitope formation [9]. These interactions may lead to a change in sensitization and elicitation potential [12–15], effects, which, as yet, have only been seldom investigated [9].

31.1.5 Fragrance Contact Allergens

Allergenic fragrance ingredients have been identified by predictive assays in humans [16], in guinea pigs [17], and in mice [18]. A number of these studies are produced by the fragrance industry itself. In the past, most of such studies have remained unpublished, in-house data. Recently, the industry has changed this policy and has published data in review form.

Due to the high number of fragrance ingredients in use, structure activity relationship (SAR) analysis has been employed to identify potential allergens, e.g., in deodorants [19]. Testing a series of individual aldehydes in the animal assay, local lymph node assay (LLNA), and combining these results with reactivity and lipophilicity parameters has developed further quantitative SARs (QSARs). Equations derived from these QSARs allow improvement of the predictions made based on chemical structure alone of new aldehydes [18, 20]. However, most clinically relevant knowledge comes from patch testing eczema patients with fragrance ingredients suspected of causing allergic reactions. In this way, the first screening test for fragrance contact allergy was designed [21], an approach followed by others [22–33]. This first true screening test for fragrance allergy, called the fragrance mix (FM I), was composed in the late 1970s by Larsen [21]. It consists of a mixture of eight ingredients: seven chemicals and a natural extract with the addition of an emulsifier (Table 1.1). Among the ingredients of FM I, the natural oak moss absolute has, for some years, been the top ranking, usually followed by isoeugenol, cinnamal, and/or hydroxycitronellal (Fig. 1.1). In recent multinational studies, addi-

Table 1.1. Ingredients of fragrance mix I (FM I)

Fragrance ingredients, INCI name (chemical name)	Concentration in FM I (%)
α-Amyl cinnamal (α-amylcinnamic aldehyde)	1
Cinnamal (cinnamic aldehyde)	1
Eugenol (eugenol)	1
Geraniol (geraniol)	1
Hydroxycitronellal (hydroxycitronellal)	1
Isoeugenol (iso-eugenol)	1
Evernia prunastri (oak moss absolute)	1
Emulsifier Sorbitan sesquioleate	5

Each ingredient is tested at the same concentration in FM I as individually, except sorbitan sesquioleate, which is individually tested at 20% in petrolatum

tional important allergens have been identified [26–30]. Among these are both chemicals, such as hydroxyisohexyl 3-cyclohexene carboxaldehyde (Lyral) [34], farnesol, citral, α-hexylcinnamic aldehyde [26], as well as natural extracts, such as ylang ylang oil, lemongrass oil, narcissus absolute, sandalwood oil, and jasmine absolute [27]. The following sections are comments on selected fragrance chemicals and naturals of special interest.

31.1.5.1 Fragrance Chemicals

Cinnamal (chemical name cinnamic aldehyde) is a strong allergen [16] and has, for many years, been a

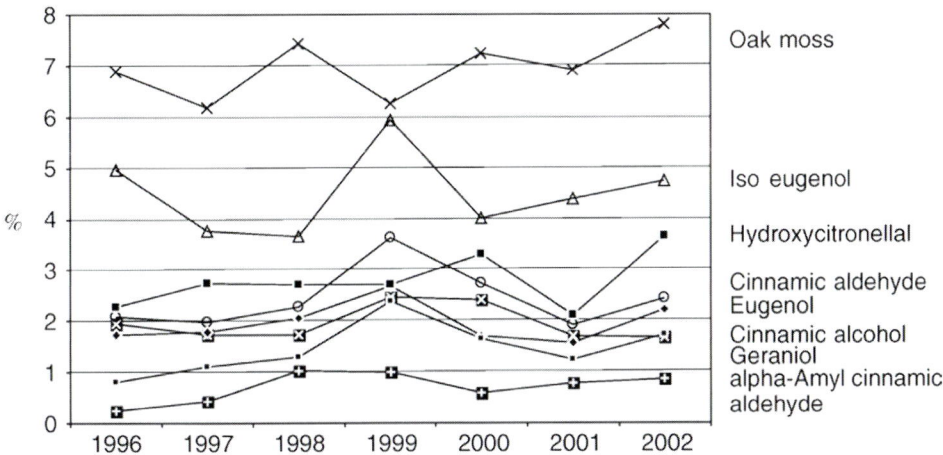

Fig. 1.1. Time trend of reactions to ingredients of fragrance mix (FM I). Data collected by the Information Network of Departments of Dermatology (IVDK), University of Göttingen, Germany. Testing performed in selected patient numbers of between 1,083 and 1,924 yearly, adapted from Schnuch et al. [61]

top ranking fragrance allergen [35], though recently a decline in reactions has been seen [36]. Cinnamal is the main component of cinnamon oil. It is also used as a flavoring and is described as an occupational allergen in bakers on a case basis [37, 38]. In newer investigations, cinnamal was found only rarely in cosmetic products [39–42]; however, the chemically related substance, cinnamic alcohol, seems to be converted in the skin to cinnamal [11, 43]. Cinnamal is restricted to 0.1% in the Cosmetic Directive [44].

Isoeugenol is a strong allergen [16]. It caused contact allergy in 1.7% of 2,261 consecutively tested eczema patients in a European multi-center study [45]. It is found in many cosmetic products and may be present in relatively high concentrations, especially in colognes and similar products [42]. There seems to be no relation between the metabolism of eugenol, which is also a constituent of fragrance mix, and isoeugenol [46, 47]. Isoeugenol is restricted to 0.02% in cosmetic products in the Cosmetic Directive [44]. Recent studies have shown that patients with isoeugenol contact allergy react to esters, but not ether derivatives of isoeugenol [45], providing a basis for allergen substitution.

Hydroxycitronellal is classified as a relatively weak allergen based on its inherent properties [48]; even so, it is one of the top ranking causes of fragrance contact allergy. It is widely used in cosmetic products, both perfumes and deodorants, and often in relatively high concentrations. It is restricted to 1% in cosmetic products [44].

Hydroxyisohexyl 3-cyclohexene carboxaldehyde (Lyral) has been used for many years without restrictions. It is related to hydroxycitronellal and has probably been used as a substitute in many cases as hydroxycitronellal was restricted [49]. The use concentrations have generally been very high; more than 3.0% in perfumes have been reported [49]. A series of systematic investigations under the leadership of Frosch has shown that Lyral is one of the most fre-

quent allergens, giving positive reactions in 1–2.7% of consecutively patch tested patients [25, 26, 29, 34] (Table 1.2).

Farnesol is both used as a fragrance ingredient and as a biocide, e.g., in deodorants [50]. It is has been shown to cause allergy in 1.1% of patients consecutively patch tested by the German Information Network of Departments of Dermatology (IDVK) [51]. Those positive to farnesol were characterized by being young females and having hands and face more often affected than patients negative to farnesol [51]. Probably, many cases of deodorant contact allergy due to farnesol have been missed in the past, as most of the patients reacting to farnesol are negative to the fragrance mix [29, 51].

Citral is a relatively weak allergen, which also has irritant properties. It has a steep dose–response curve [52] and has been shown to be of possible significance in patients with long-term chronic hand eczema, which may be due to its combined allergenic and irritant effects [52, 53]. The irritant properties of citral have been shown to be temperature dependent [54]. In European multi-center studies, 0.7–1.1% of consecutively tested eczema patients gave a positive reaction to citral 2% [26, 29].

Coumarin is the subject of several studies and case investigations [26, 55]. It has been reported to cause reactions in 0.4% of consecutively tested patients [56] and also gave rise to positive reactions in 0.3% of patients in a European multi-center study [26]. However, in the most recent European investigation, it gave no reactions among 1,701 patients [29]. The reason for this is unknown, but may be related to the use of a better quality of coumarin containing fewer sensitizing impurities.

Table 1.2. Ingredients of fragrance mix II (*FM II*) and reactivity

Ingredient (INCI name)	Patch test concentration in FM II (14% in petrolatum) [28]	Patch test concentration at individual ingredient testing in petrolatum	Frequency of reactions to individual ingredients [26] ($N=1,855$)	Frequency of reactions to individual ingredients [29] ($N=1,701$)
Lyral[a]	2.5%	5.0%	50 (2.7%)	28 (1.6%)
Citral	1.0%	2.0%	21 (1.1%)	12 (0.7%)
Farnesol	2.5%	5.0%	10 (0.5%)	6 (0.4%)
Citronellol	0.5%	1.0%	7 (0.4%)	4 (0.2%)
α-Hexyl cinnamal	5.0%	10%	6 (0.3%)	1 (0.06%)
Coumarin	2.5%	5.0%	5 (0.3%)	0

[a] INCI name: hydroxyisohexyl 3-cyclohexene carboxaldehyde

31

31.1.5.2 Oxidation Products

d-Limonene is obtained as a by-product from the citrus juice industry. Peal oil from the skins of citrus fruits contains normally more than 95% D-limonene. It is used as a fragrance ingredient, but also has many other applications. In itself, it is not a sensitizer, but it rapidly oxidizes when in contact with air [10]. Antioxidants such as butylated hydroxytoluene (BHT) are, therefore, often added to commercial products. However, once the antioxidant is consumed, the oxidation starts immediately. The allergens formed are mainly hydroperoxides [57], with strong sensitizing potential. Testing consecutive patients in different clinics with oxidized d-limonene gave positive results in 0.3–6.5% of cases [58].

Recently, similar findings have been obtained for linalool, another terpene [59, 60]. This emphasizes the need for testing with the chemicals that are in the products and not just what was originally added. Patch test material of the oxidized forms of linalool and limonene are not commercially available yet. In terms of prevention, expiry dates taking auto-oxidation into consideration will help solve the problem.

31.1.5.3 Fragrance Naturals

Oak moss absolute is derived from the lichen *Evernia prunastri*. It has been used as a basic ingredient and a fixative in many perfumes. It is a constituent of the fragrance mix and it is a top ranking allergen when the single ingredients are tested [36, 61] (Fig. 1.1). A systematic search of the allergens in the extract has recently been performed. A bio-guided fractionation procedure was used based on the testing of patients sensitized to oak moss absolute with fractions of the natural in question. This was combined with chemical analysis and SAR analysis to ultimately identify the allergens in oak moss absolute [4]. Several allergens were identified, and among these chloroatranol, atranol, and methyl-β-orcinol carboxylate gave the most reactions. These allergens are formed during the processing of the lichen (Fig. 1.2). Chloroatranol and atranol have been further studied and are shown to be strong allergens and potent elicitors, giving reactions at extremely low levels [62]. An explanation of the high rates of sensitization to oak moss absolute was found by assessing exposure. Chloroatranol and/or atranol were found in 87% of 31 investigated products, mostly perfumes [63].

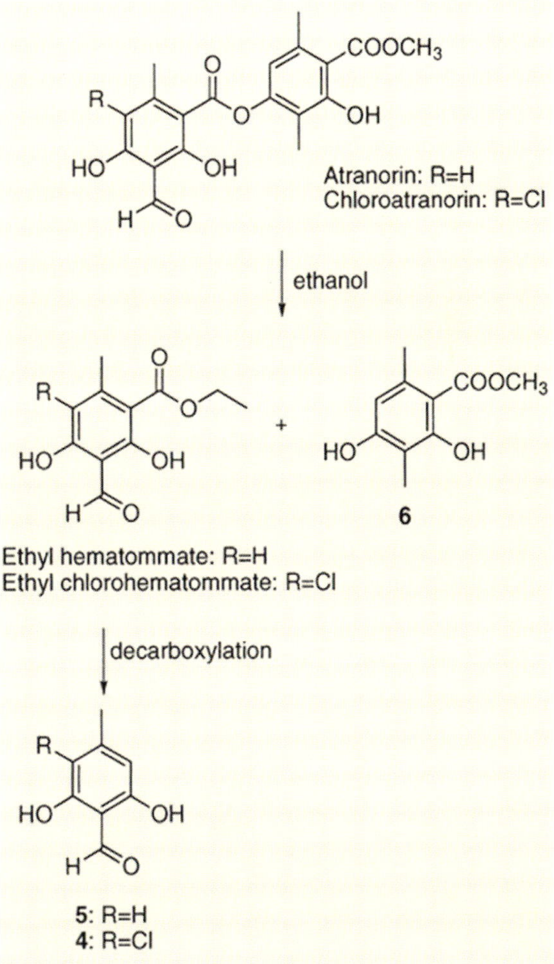

Fig. 1.2. Degradation products of atranorin and chloroatranorin formed during oak moss processing. R=H: atranorin, R=Cl: chloroatranorin. Adopted from Bernard et al. [4].

Based on these investigations, the Scientific Committee on Consumer Products (SCCP) advisory to the EU Commission has expressed an opinion that neither chloroatranol nor atranol should be present in consumer products [64].

Ylang ylang oil is produced by steam distillation of the flowers of *Cananga odorata*. Four grades are produced, which differ in odor, price, and composition. Ylang ylang oil is a major cause of allergic contact dermatitis in Asian countries, where it is frequently followed by hyper-pigmentation [65]. In a European multi-center study including 1,606 patients, ylang ylang oils of grades I and II were tested and gave a positive patch test reaction in 2.6% and 2.5% of patients, respectively, with the highest frequency in London, possibly due to the city's large Asian population; detailed information can be found in a paper by Frosch et al. [27].

Lemongrass oil, narcissus absolute, jasmine absolute, geranium oil bourbon, spearmint oil, sandalwood oil, lavender oil, and others have also been reported as frequent sensitizers [27, 30–32, 65] (Table 1.3).

Myroxylon pereirae (balsam of Peru) is derived from the sap of a tree, *Myroxylon pereirae* (MP) and is composed of 250 constituents, of which 189 are known structurally [66]. MP has been used in topical medicaments, such as wound treatment, for its antibacterial properties [67], but also as a flavor and perfume ingredient. In many countries, the use of MP in topical medicaments has been discontinued due to its sensitizing properties; however, it may still occur in herbal and natural products [68]. The crude form of MP has been banned from use in perfumes by the fragrance industry since 1974 [69]; however, the extent of the use of modified MP in perfumes is unknown. MP has been in the standard series since its first edition and is still causing many reactions [61].

Colophony (rosin) is a resin obtained from different species of coniferous trees. It is a complex mixture of resin acids and natural substances. Its composition varies with the species from which it is obtained and also depends on the recovery processes and storage conditions [70]. Unmodified colophony is known to cause contact allergy. The main allergenic components are oxidized resin acids formed on exposure to air. The allergenicity can be changed by chemical modification, e.g., it can be decreased by hydrogenation, while other kinds of modifications may enhance the allergenicity [70]. Colophony has many applications and has also been used as a fragrance ingredient. The use of unmodified colophony in perfumes was banned in 1992 by the industry [71]; however, it is unknown to what extent modified forms of colophony are used in perfumes.

An extensive review has been published listing fragrance ingredients, chemicals, and natural products identified in the available literature as allergens in clinical studies of groups of patients or single cases [72]; about 100 chemicals and a similar number of natural products are in these lists.

Table 1.3. Patch test reactions to selected natural ingredients [27, 30–31, 33]. (*NT* Not tested)

Ingredient	*N*=1,606 [27][a] *N*=218 [30][b] *N*=178 [31][c]
Ylang ylang oil I	2.6%[a]
Ylang ylang oil II	2.5%[a]
Ylang ylang oil (unspecified)[d]	NT
Lemongrass oil	1.6%[a]
Narcissus abs.[d]	1.3%[a]
Jasmine abs.[d]	1.2%[a], 16.9%[c]
Sandalwood oil[d]	0.9%[a]
Patchouli oil	0.8%[a]
Spearmint oil[d]	0.8%[a], 5.0%[c]
Dwarf pine needle oil	0.7%[a]
Cedarwood oil	0.6%[a]
Peppermint oil	0.6%[a]
Clove bud oil	19.3%[b]
Lavender oil	2.8%[b]
Eucalyptus oil	1.8%[b]
Geranium oil bourbon	8.4%[c]

[a]　Consecutively tested patients
[b, c]　Selected patients with fragrance sensitivity
[d]　Tested as a natural mix in 752 fragrance-sensitive subjects, gave a response in 47% of cases [33]

Core Message

■ The main allergens in the natural extract oak moss absolute have been identified as chloroatranol and atranol, which elicit contact allergy at very low levels. A ban on those ingredients in cosmetics has been proposed.

31.1.6 Epidemiology of Fragrance Contact Allergy

Frequencies of sensitization to perfume ingredients were previously difficult to estimate due to the lack of a reliable test substance to screen for this allergy, but it was regarded as a common condition [73]. MP was shown by Hjorth to be a marker of contact allergy to fragrances in the 1960s [67], and later the fragrance mix (FM I) was developed, which enabled assessment of the problem [21].

Contact allergy to fragrance ingredients as identified with FM I is seen in all geographical regions of the industrialized world [28, 74–77].

Studies of the general population show that about 2% of adolescents and 1–4% of adults have fragrance contact allergy in Denmark [78–80], depending on the age group of investigation. One-third of 12- to 16-year-old children had, at the time of diagnosis, symptoms of their allergy, as did half of the adult population [78, 79]. An estimation based on the sales of patch test materials in Germany and patient data gave similar results. It showed that 1.8–4.2% of the German population is sensitized to fragrance mix, amounting to 1.4–3.4 million people in the German population of 82 million inhabitants [81]. In adults with contact eczema undergoing patch testing contact allergy, FM is one of the most frequent causes of contact allergy, often next to nickel. In the most recent multi-center investigations in Europe, 6.5% of adult eczema patients reacted to the fragrance mix and 10.9% in North America [28, 82], which was a decrease compared to previous findings [26, 82]. The frequency of fragrance allergy in patch-tested patients increases with age [83, 84]; nevertheless, FM I is also among the top-ranking allergens in children with eczema [85, 86], and cases down to 2 years of age have been reported, even though it is rare [83]. In eczema patients, the female : male ratio of FM I allergy is usually 2 : 1 [36, 61, 87], while in the general population, especially in the younger years, a more equal sex distribution is seen [78]. While an increase in FM I allergy was described in the 1990s, at least in some geographical regions [61, 87, 88], the most recent investigations from the German surveillance system (IVDK) shows a statistically significant decrease in the frequency of FM I allergy among eczema patients in recent years from 13.1% in 1999 to 7.8% in 2002 [61]. This is in accordance with a chemical analysis of ten prestige perfumes, showing that fewer FM allergens were present in newly launched perfumes in comparison with perfumes manufactured more than 10 years ago [89]. MP showed a similar trend, but to a lesser extent and surpassed the FM I in frequency in 2002 [61]. This may be a reminder that the use of other allergenic fragrance compounds, structurally similar to ingredients in MP, may have increased [61]. Certainly, high frequencies of contact allergy to natural extracts such as ylang ylang oil and jasmine absolute have been demonstrated [27, 30, 31] and, in addition, a number of chemicals not included in FM I have been shown to be important allergens [26, 30–32]. Thus, the epidemiology of fragrance contact allergy is only partly displayed by the results from

testing with FM I, which should be borne in mind both in assessing the size of the problem on a community level and in the diagnostic workup of the individual patient.

31.1.7 Clinical Aspects

Allergic contact dermatitis may develop as itchy eczematous patches where perfume has been applied, usually behind the ears, on the neck, the upper chest, and sometimes the elbow flexures and wrists [73]. Another typically presenting feature is a bilateral axillary dermatitis caused by perfume in deodorants; if the reaction is severe, it may spread down the arms and to other areas of the body [73] (Fig. 1.3). It is not always that such patients will consult a dermatologist, but a history of such first-time symptoms have been shown to be statistically significantly related to the diagnosis of perfume allergy by FM I in eczema patients [90].

Facial eczema is a classical manifestation of fragrance allergy from the use of different fragranced cosmetic products [33, 91, 92]. In men, aftershave lotion may cause a eczematous eruption of the beard area and adjacent part of the neck [73] (Fig. 1.4) and

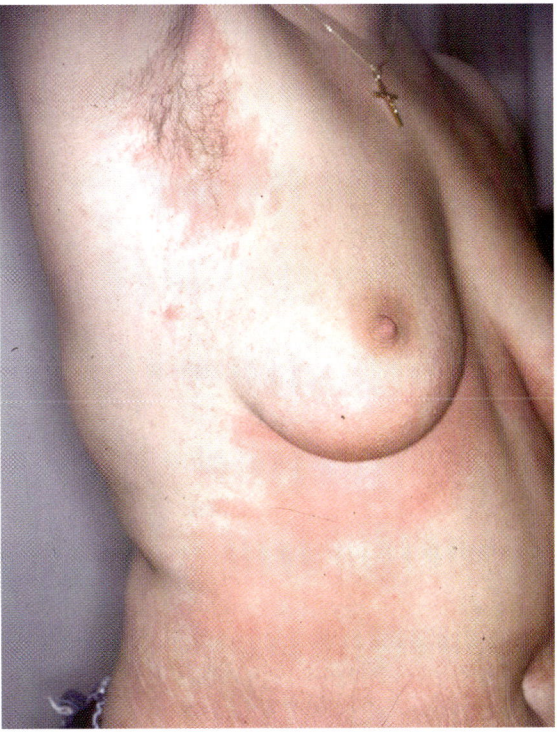

Fig. 1.3. Allergic contact dermatitis from perfume in deodorant (courtesy of N. Veien)

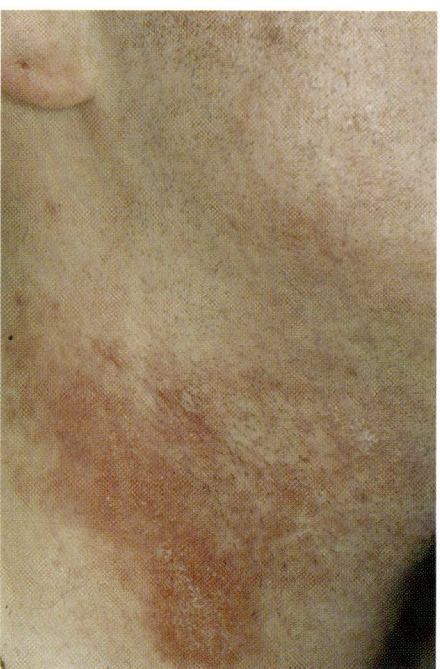

Fig. 1.4. Allergic contact dermatitis from perfume in aftershave (courtesy of N. Veien)

31

men using wet shaving opposed to dry have been shown to have an increased risk of 2.9 of being fragrance allergic [93].

Data from St Johns in London in 1980s showed that perfumes and deodorants were the most frequent sources of sensitization in women and aftershave lotions and deodorants were usually the most responsible in men [73]. More recent investigations have confirmed that this is still the case [42, 94–98].

Primary hand eczema or aggravation of hand eczema can be caused by contact to fragranced products, as seen in occupational settings [99]. Also, a significant relationship between hand eczema and fragrance contact allergy has been found in some studies based on patients investigated for contact allergy [100–102]. However, hand eczema is a multi-factorial disease and the clinical significance of fragrance contact allergy in (severe) chronic hand eczema is controversial. A review on the subject has been published by Heydorn et al. [99].

Pigmented contact dermatitis has been described in Japan as a manifestation of contact allergic reaction to a range of contact allergens, e.g., ylang ylang oil and jasmine absolute [65]. The pigmentation disappears or improves upon avoidance.

Systemic contact dermatitis may occur in selected cases. The phenomenon that patients, sensitized by skin contact, react with a rash to oral intake of fla-vored food has especially been described in conjunction with MP sensitivity [68, 103–105]. In general, the problem is to quantify exposure and determine the relevance to chronic eczema. Systemic contact dermatitis is the subject of a separate chapter in this book, Chap. 16.

Core Message

■ Deodorants and perfumes/aftershaves are frequent sources of perfume allergy.

31.1.8 Exposure to Fragrance Allergens

31.1.8.1 Consumer Products

Exposure may be by direct skin contact, and, the longer time of contact, the higher the risk of sensitization and elicitation, even though the frequency of applications also plays a role. The most significant nonoccupational exposure is from cosmetics products. Chemical analysis of more than 150 different cosmetic products has shown that the fragrance mix ingredients occur widely and, in some products, in high concentrations (Table 1.4). Isoeugenol was found in 24% of products in a concentration of between <0.001% and 0.34% [7]. Also, an important allergen, Lyral, has been shown to be widely distributed in cosmetic products and, in particular, in high concentrations of 3% or more in fine fragrances [34, 49, 106]. Natural-ingredient-based cosmetic perfumes have been shown to contain fragrance allergens to the same degree or more than ordinary products [39], which perhaps is not so surprising, since most fragrance ingredients and, thus, allergens are nature-identical. Children's products may also contain fragrance allergens; however, in an investigation of 25 children's products, the fragrance mix ingredients were either not present or present in fairly low concentrations [41]. The highest levels of fragrance mix allergens were found in perfumes and extreme levels were seen in a toy perfume [41]. Chemical analysis of 59 household products showed that the most commonly detected fragrance allergen was limonene, which was found in 78% of products, followed by linalool in 61%, and citronellol in 47% [107], while the ingredients of the fragrance mix were found less frequently than expected from the analysis of cosmetic products. Some of the investigated household products were also for occupational use. The exposure to naturals extracts, which may have a signifi-

Table 1.4. Exposure assessment of fragrance allergens in cosmetics and household products by chemical analysis and information from the industry. [*ND* Not done. *NQ* not quantified, *NG* not given, *PPM* µg/ml (10,000 ppm=1%)]

Ingredient	Prestige perfumes, $N=10^a$; $N=NG^b$; $N=31^c$; [42]^a; [49]^b; [62]^c		Natural-ingredient-based perfumes $N=22$ [39]		Deodorants $N=73$ [40]		Household products $N=59$ [107]	
	In % of analyzed products	Concentration range (ppm)	In % of analyzed products	Concentration range (ppm)	In % of analyzed products	Concentration range (ppm)	In % of analyzed products	Concentration range (ppm)
α-Amyl cinnamal	30^a	300–6,900	36	1,940–30,390	31	1–617	8	NQ
Cinnamal	0^a		0		17	1–424	3	NQ
Cinnamyl alcohol	60^a	300–7,900	14	890–21,010	39	6–1,169	2	NQ
Eugenol	90^a	400–8,900	36	350–22,890	57	1–2,355	27	32–349
Geraniol	90^a	800–4,800	63	NQ	76	1–1,178	41	53–1,758
Hydroxycitronellal	90^a	2,500–11,900	23	1,350–60,440	50	1–1,023	12	15–140
Isoeugenol	70^a	500–3,400	9	270–1,390	29	1–458	5	NQ
Lyral	46^b	32,000 (mean)	ND		53	1–1,874	10	36–103
Farnesol	ND		ND		ND		25	48–1,088
Citral	ND		ND		ND		78	6–9,443
Limonene	ND		ND		ND		78	6–9,443
Linalool	90^b	47,000 (mean)	ND		97	9–1,927	61	3–439
Chloroatranol^d	87^c	0.004–53	ND		ND		ND	
Atranol^d	77^c	0.012–190	ND		ND		ND	

^{a} Consecutively tested patients
^{b,c} Selected patients with fragrance sensitivity
^{d} Allergens in oak moss absolute

cant allergenic potential, is virtually unknown, as it is only possible to quantify the exposure to identified chemicals. The demonstration of the main allergens in the extract oak moss absolute and their presence in almost all investigated perfumes/aftershaves is an example of a hidden exposure to important allergens in naturals [4, 63].

> **Core Message**
>
> ■ Fragrance allergens are widespread in consumer products.

31.1.8.2 Occupational Exposure

There are a number of occupations where fragrance exposure may occur from cosmetic or domestic products, e.g., in hairdressers, beauticians, aromatherapists, masseurs, and cleaners. Chefs and bakers are exposed to spices and flavors, which may contain fragrance allergens, e.g., cinnamal from cinnamon. Eugenol is used for dental fillings and is a rare cause of contact allergy in dentists [108]. Multivariate anal-

ysis of associations between occupation and contact allergy to the fragrance mix showed that the highest occupational risk of fragrance contact allergy was associated with work as a masseur, physiotherapist, metal furnace operator, potter or glass marker, or geriatric nurse, when using data on 57,779 patients from the German surveillance system (IVDK) [109]. In an English investigation, healthcare worker (medicine, dentistry, nursing, veterinary) was also the occupation with the highest overall prevalence of sensitization to FM I [83]. Metalworkers exposed to metalworking fluids and with occupational skin diseases were found to have an increased risk of sensitization to fragrances in terms of a positive patch test to FM I and MP, when compared to metalworkers with occupational disease, but not exposed to metalworking fluids [110]; this could not be explained by the use of skin care and protecting creams. According to recent information from the lubricants-producing industry, fragrances are no longer usually added to metalworking fluid concentrate. However, it may be that masking fragrances are added during usage [110]. It is recommended that cases of fragrance allergy in metal workers should be thoroughly investigated for a causal relationship [111]. Another association to fragrance allergy was found in workers producing rotor blades for wind turbines with an epoxy-based technology [112]. A significant relationship between contact allergy to epoxy resins and FM I was found, and the same association was found among male eczema patients undergoing patch testing, possibly caused by cross-reactivity [112].

31.1.9 Diagnosis of Fragrance Contact Allergy

The basic investigation of suspected fragrance contact allergy is made by patch testing with the standard patch test series, which currently entail three potential indicators of fragrance contact allergy: FM I, MP, and colophony. FM I has been used as an indicator of fragrance contact allergy since the late 1970s. The ingredients of the mix have remained unchanged since, while the test concentration of the mix was lowered from 16% originally to 8% in 1984, as data suggested that the higher concentration gave irritant reactions [113]. Thus, the individual ingredients were lowered from 2% to 1%, which may give rise to false-negative results when testing the ingredients separately [114]. The emulsifier sorbitan sesquioleate was later added to the individual ingredients, as it was shown to improve the positive rate [115]. FM I is a heterogeneous mix, which means that it contains molecules that differ widely in size and reactivity [9]. In this way, it is a realistic imitation of perfumes. Further, its composition has been shown to be a relevant reflection of exposure [116]. It has been assessed that FM I detects 50–80% of eczema patients with reactions to perfumes in cosmetics [42, 74, 117]. The same applies if individual fragrance allergens are tested [23, 26, 27, 30–32]. However, the developments in the fragrance industry, changing fashion, and regulatory interventions mean that the exposure pattern is constantly changing and fragrance ingredients other than FM I are relevant to test [22, 25–27, 30–32, 74, 102, 118].

An EU-funded research program was aimed at designing an additional screening test for fragrance allergy, fragrance mix II (FM II) [28, 29]. Based on previous investigations [22, 23, 25, 30–32, 49], published information in general and the IFRA guidelines, a selection of candidates for testing was made, chemicals [26] and naturals [27]. Fourteen chemical were tested in 1,855 patients; the six chemicals with the highest reactivity following FM were Lyral (2.7%), citral (1.1%), farnesol (0.5%), citronellol (0.4%), α-hexylcinnamal (0.3%), and coumarin (0.3%) [26]. These six chemicals were further tested as a mixture in three different concentrations, and with the corresponding individual ingredients in 1,701 consecutive patients [28]. Positive reactions to the FM II were

dose-dependent and 2.9% reacted to the FM II in a test concentration of 14%, which was recommended as an additional diagnostic screening tool [28]. About one-third of those reacting to FM II 14% were negative at testing with FM I. In breakdown testing of the single ingredients, 74% gave a response, if doubtful reactions were included [29], and the rank order of the ingredients was as in the first study [26], except that no unequivocal positive reaction to coumarin was observed. Lyral was the dominant single constituent, with positive reactions in 36% of patients reacting to 14% FM II. Assessments made of clinical relevance by different methods showed that FM II detects additional relevant cases of contact allergy to fragrances [28, 29].

It is recommended to supplement the standard patch test series with FM II 14%, when available, and Lyral 5% pet., as a fragrance ingredient of special importance. Lyral is already included in the standard series in Germany [119] and many other clinics. The allergens present in FM I and II also cover the most frequent fragrance allergens detected in patients with hand eczema: citral, hydroxycitronellal, Lyral, and eugenol [53], though oxidized limonene, which gave positive patch tests in 0.9% of chronic hand eczema patients [53], is not commercially available.

The function of MP as an indicator of fragrance contact allergy is more complex and heterogeneous than FM and may vary in different parts of the world due to local habits. MP contains ingredients also present in FM I, such as cinnamates, which comprise more than 35% of the MP constituents and isoeugenol/eugenol [68]. Hausen has hypothesized that the pattern of reactions may indicate sources of exposure, so that contact allergy to MP and isoeugenol/eugenol can be traced back to fragrances, especially if the reaction to FM I is moderate or strong, while reactions to cinnamal/cinnamates can be traced to essential oils and possible sunscreens [68].

A statistically significant relationship between reactions to FM I and MP was seen in a study covering several countries [29]. This may be explained by the contents of mutual allergens, while only a weak association was seen with FM II, the ingredients of which are not in MP, except for farnesol in trace amounts [68].

Some advances in the diagnostics of contact allergy to natural fragrance ingredients have also been attempted [27, 30–32]. Larsen tested a natural mix consisting of jasmine absolute, ylang ylang oil, narcissus absolute, sandalwood oil, and spearmint oil, and found that it identified 84% of perfume-allergic patients [33]. Natural extracts, such as ylang ylang oil, narcissus oil, sandalwood oil, and jasmine absolute, were identified as frequent sensitizers by Frosch [27],

Fig. 1.5a, b.
Patch test reaction to the new fragrance mix (FM II) in dose-dependent intensity (day 3) (**a**). Breakdown testing revealed high sensitivity to Lyral. The repeated open application test (ROAT) with Lyral was strongly positive already on day 4 (**b**) (courtesy of PJ Frosch)

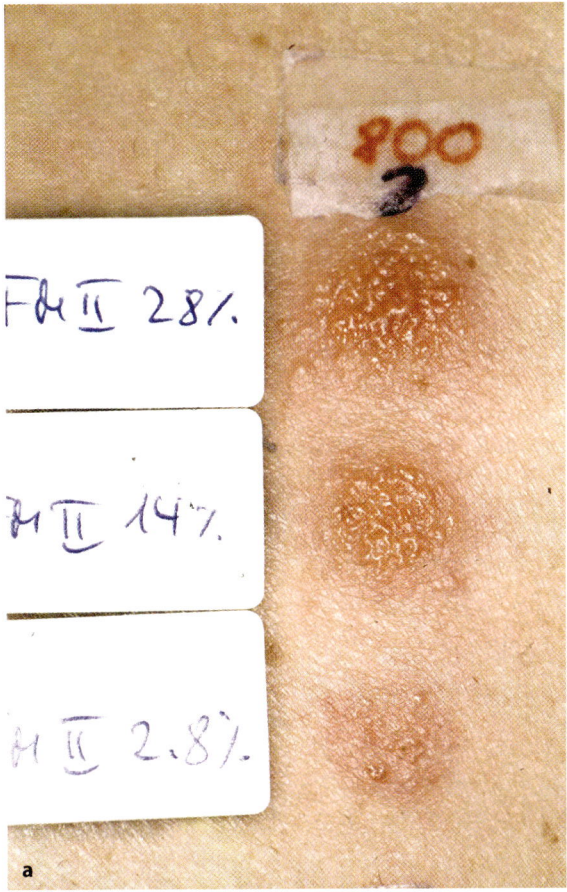

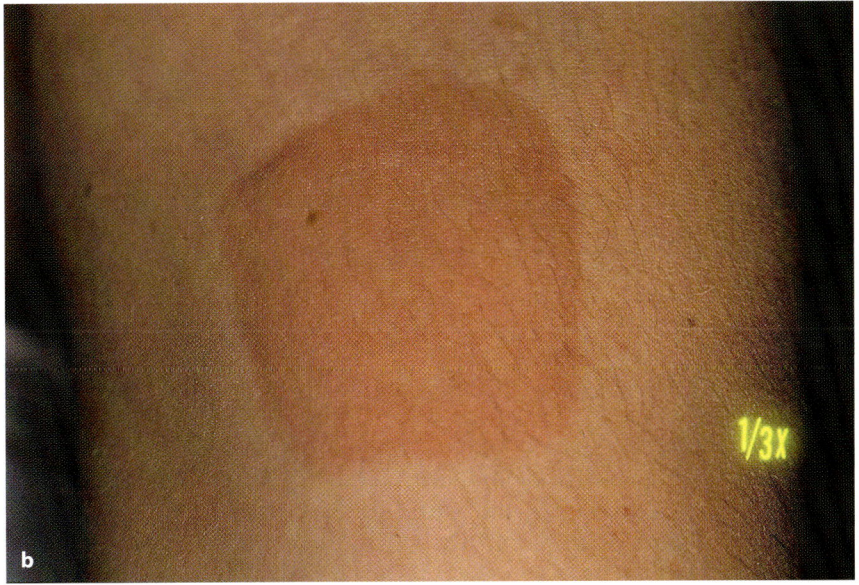

and relevant cases are missed by only testing with FM I. Still, a screening series of naturals awaits development and it is not known to which extent MP and oil of turpentine are good indicators of fragrance allergy to natural extracts in general, as has been suggested previously [61].

The role of colophony in detecting fragrance contact allergy is minor compared to MP, FM I, and FM

31

II. Colophony has many different applications and it is uncertain if it is used in fragrances; however, ingredients of colophony may be present in fragrances or cross-reactivity may occur. No relationship between reactions to FM I or FM II and colophony was found in consecutive eczema patients tested in a European multi-center study [29]. While a significant relationship between colophony and FM I, as well as colophony and MP, was found in 747 patients suspected of fragrance contact allergy [92], it was also shown that the probability of a reaction to an extended fragrances series increased with the number of positive reactions to the fragrance indicators of the standard series [92].

As none of the current diagnostic tools is perfect, it is important to test with the cosmetic products, fine fragrances, essential oils, etc. used by the patient. It should generally be confined to stay-on products, as wash-off products, due to their irritant nature, make the interpretation of patch test reactions difficult. Further investigations of reactions to commercial products can be made based on the ingredient labeling of sensitizing fragrance substances introduced for cosmetics and detergents in the EU region in 2005 [44] (Table 1.5), by obtaining information/ingredients from the manufacturer [120] or by chemical fractionation in special cases [55, 121, 122].

Core Message

■ A new fragrance mix (FM II) has been developed, which will detect additional relevant cases of fragrance contact allergy. A validated screening agent or screening series for contact allergy to natural fragrance extracts is needed.

31.1.10 Clinical Relevance and Patient Advice

Clinical relevance can be assessed based on the patient's history of rashes to perfumes/perfumes products. A significant relationship between such a history and positive patch test to FM I has been shown previously [90, 115]. Currently, a higher proportion of patients giving a positive history is found among those reacting to the newly developed FM II than those reacting to FM I [28]. Other ways of determining relevance is by exposure assessment. In a case study, all patients with a positive patch test to FM I ingredients were shown to be exposed to these aller-

Table 1.5. Fragrance ingredients to be labeled as ingredients if present in cosmetics [44]

INCI name	CAS no.
α-Isomethyl ionone	127–51–5
Amyl cinnamal	122–40–7
Amylcinnamyl alcohol	101–85–9
Anisyl alcohol	105–13–5
Benzyl alcohol	100–51–6
Benzyl benzoate	120–51–4
Benzyl cinnamate	103–41–3
Benzyl salicylate	118–58–1
Butylphenyl methylpropional	80–54–6
Cinnamal	104–55–2
Cinnamyl alcohol	104–54–1
Citral	5392–40–5
Citronellol	106–22–9
Coumarin	91–64–5
Eugenol	97–53–0
Evernia prunastri (oak moss) extract	90028–68–5
Evernia furfuracea (tree moss) extract	90028–67–4
Farnesol	4602–84–0
Geraniol	106–24–1
Hexyl cinnamal	101–86–0
Hydroxycitronellal	107–75–5
Hydroxyisohexyl 3-cyclohexene carboxaldehyde	31906–04–4
Isoeugenol	97–54–1
Limonene	5889–27–5
Linalool	78–70–6
Methyl 2-octynoate	111–12–6

The presence of the substance must be indicated in the list of ingredients when its concentration exceeds 0.001% in leave-on products and 0.01% in rinse-off products according to the Cosmetic Directive [44]. The list was complied from information in [71] regarding fragrance chemicals reported as allergens in cosmetic and toiletries and based on World Health Organization (WHO) criteria for contact allergens [142]. Oak moss/tree moss absolute were included as they were relevant for FM I

Information regarding the presence of other fragrance ingredients in cosmetics may be made available by the fragrance industry on a case basis [120]

gens in cosmetic products causing eczema [116]. Similar findings exist for Lyral [34, 106] and other FM II ingredients [29]. Simulations of exposure by repeated open application tests (ROAT) with commercial products containing FM I allergens have been shown to cause eczema in 60% of exposed patients who patch tested positive to FM I [42, 95]. Dummy products spiked with a single fragrance allergen in realistic concentrations have also been tested. In a series of deodorant exposure studies with cinnamal and hydroxycitronellal, 94–100% of eczema patients sensitized to the ingredient in question reacted, while all controls were negative [96, 97]. ROAT with realistic concentrations of Lyral applied in ethanol caused reactions in 16 of 18 (89%) sensitized patients [106].

Clinical relevance can be determined by one or all of the above-mentioned methods in the individual patient. Another indicator of clinical relevance is the strength of the patch reaction. Patients with strong reactions to the standard patch test FM I are more likely to react to the individual ingredients of the mix, to a low level of allergen [123], and to give a positive ROAT with the allergen in question [124]. Further, they are more likely to have a positive history of adverse reactions to fragranced products [115].

Thus, the advice given to the patient depends on the clinical presentation and the degree of allergy. Some patients have a weak degree of allergy and no chronic eczema problem; they can usually tolerate (some) scented products on the skin. Others are more sensitive and have to abstain from stay-on products, while some cannot use any scented products at all, including wash-off products, such as shampoos. Patients with a chronic or relapsing eczema disease should be advised to use unscented emollients, regardless of whether they are allergic to fragrances or not, due to the risk of becoming sensitized and aggravation of their disease. In this context, it is important for the patient to know that the labeling "fragrance-free" may be misleading [125, 126]. Such products may contain fragrance ingredients, which are often various flower or plant extracts or chemicals acting as preservatives, e.g., geraniol and farnesol.

A change in cosmetic legislation in Europe has been made [44] and also concerns detergents [127]. A series of 26 selected fragrance ingredients, mostly chemicals, known to cause allergic reactions in humans are mandated on the label, if present in more than 10 ppm in stay-on products and 100 ppm in wash-off products. These limits are administrative and decided, as, otherwise, a labeling of all perfumed cosmetics was expected due to the presence of chemical allergens in trace amounts in essential oils. This legislation is expected to be in full force in 2005. It entails all the ingredients of FM I and FM II, and will enable the fragrance-allergic patient, who wishes to use fragranced cosmetics, to make a pre-selection of products based on the ingredient information. Further, it will provide the dermatologists with a tool for improving diagnostics and assessing clinical relevance.

Clinical relevance is not a static phenomenon, especially not in the area of fragrance allergy. It is a question of interaction between individual predisposition (genetics)/susceptibility and environmental exposures. Changes in general exposure to the allergens by interventions, e.g., legislation or just changes of fashion, will affect the clinical consequences of being contact allergic, defined by a positive patch test. These dynamics mean that assessment of the value of a diagnostic test such as FM I or FM II at a given time is only a snapshot. The focus, which has been on the ingredients of FM I and FM II by research programs on an EU-commission-level and by consumer organizations, means that exposure has or will be decreased [89], as actually intended by these initiatives. The consequence is that fewer individuals will become sensitized to the allergens in question, as already indicated for FM I [61], and that fewer of those already sensitized will have clinical problems, which is possibly seen in the most current assessments of clinical relevance [28].

This should not lead to the confusion that the lack of clinical relevance is a sign of false-positive patch tests. It is a consequence of changing exposures and may be different in other geographical regions or may change again with time and exposure.

Core Message

■ Twenty six fragrance ingredients with a sensitization potential are mandated on the label of cosmetics and detergents from 2005 as information to the consumer.

31.1.11 Other Skin Effects

31.1.11.1 Immediate Reactions

Fragrances have been reported to cause contact urticaria of the nonimmunological type. This is a high-dose effect and cinnamal, cinnamic alcohol, and MP are known causes of contact urticaria, but others have been reported also [128–130]. The reactions to MP may be due to its containing cinnamates [68]. A relationship to delayed contact hypersensitivity has been suggested [131], but in a recent study no significant difference was found between a fragrance-allergic group and a control group in the frequency of immediate reactions to fragrance ingredients [130]. This is in keeping with a nonimmunological basis for the reactions seen [130].

31

31.1.11.2 Photoallergy/ Phototoxic Reactions

Musk ambrette produced a considerable number of photocontact allergic reactions in the 1970s [132, 133] and was later banned. Today, photoallergic contact dermatitis is uncommon [134]. Psoralens in naturally occurring fragrance ingredients were previously the cause of phototoxic reactions, giving rise to erythema, followed by hyperpigmentation in its characteristic form, called Berloque dermatitis [135]. There are now limits of the amount of psoralens in fragrance products. Phototoxic reactions still occur but are rare [136].

31.1.11.3 Irritant Contact Dermatitis

Irritant effects of single fragrance ingredients are well known, e.g., citral [52, 54]. Probably, irritant contact dermatitis is frequent, however no investigations exist substantiating this [72]. Many more people complain about rashes to perfumes/perfumed products than are proven allergic by testing [90]. This may be due to irritant effects or insufficient diagnostic apparatus.

31.1.12 Airway Symptoms

Fragrances are intended for skin application in order to give a volatile perception. In addition to skin exposure, the wearing of perfumes exposes the eyes and airways. Many people are bothered by respiratory or eye symptoms caused by the volatile fragrance ingredients and it is estimated that 2–4% of the adult population is affected in their daily life by this exposure [137]. It is known that exposure to fragrances may exacerbate pre-existing asthma [138]; further asthma-like symptoms can be provoked possibly by sensory mechanisms [139, 140]. In an epidemiological investigation, a significant association was found between respiratory issues elicited by fragrances and contact allergy to fragrance ingredients, as well as hand eczema, which were independent risk factors in a multivariate analysis [141]. This indicates a relationship between the airways and the skin caused by fragrance ingredients [141], which opens up a new understanding of these disease entities.

31.1.13 Case Reports

Case Reports

- A 23-year-old woman presented with a long history of axillary dermatitis. Symptoms improved on changing to a different deodorant spray and worsened again with reuse of the former deodorant. Patch testing with the deodorant "as is" showed a ++ reaction, no reaction was seen to FM I 8% or colophony, while a ?+ was seen to *Myroxylon pereirae*. The perfume of the deodorant was tested in the same concentration as in the product and showed a + reaction. Farnesol was present in the deodorant and gave ++ reaction upon testing at 1% in pet. [141].
  Comment: Many cases of perfume allergy due to farnesol in deodorants have probably been overlooked in the past. It is important to test with the relevant products used by the patient and to use this test as guidance for further investigation. Farnesol is a constituent of the new diagnostic test FM II and is entailed by the new ingredient labeling of selected fragrance allergens.

- A 50-year-old woman presented with an erythematous eruption, characterized by papules, vesicles, and crusting over the neck and chest. At patch testing, initially, the only positive reaction observed was with her own eau de toilette, named Women. FM I was negative. Chemical fractionation of the Women perfume concentrate was combined with a sequenced patch testing procedure and with SAR studies. Ingredients supplied by the manufacturer were also included in the study. Benzophenone-2, Lyral, α-hexyl cinnamic aldehyde, and alpha-damascone were found to be responsible for the patient's contact allergy to the eau de toilette, Women [121].
  Comment: It is important to test with relevant products used by the patient. Light absorbers, such as benzophenone-2, are used in perfumes to protect against degradation. These may also be the cause of contact allergy. Some patients are allergic to several fragrance ingredients. Information about the contents of fragrance ingredients can be obtained from the fragrance manufacturer [120] and for selected fragrance allergens on the label of the product.

References

1. International Fragrance Association (IFRA). Code of practice. Definitions. Home page at: http://www.ifraorg. org

2. Müller J (1992) The H&R book of perfume. Understanding fragrance. Origin, history, development. Guide to fragrance ingredients. Glöss, Hamburg, Germany

3. Poucher WA (1993) Poucher's perfumes, cosmetics and soaps. The production, manufacture and application of perfumes, 9th edn, vol 2. Chapman and Hall, London

4. Bernard G, Giménez-Arnau E, Rastogi SC, Heydorn S, Johansen JD, Menné T, Goossens A, Andersen K, Lepoittevin JP (2003) Contact allergy to oak moss: search for sensitizing molecules using combined bioassay-guided chemical fractionation, GC-MS, and structure–activity relationship analysis. Arch Dermatol Res 295:229–235

5. Bauer K, Garbe D, Surburg H (1990) Common fragrance and flavor materials, 2nd edn. VCH Verlagsgesellschaft, Weinheim, Germany

6. SCCNFP (1998) The Scientific Committee on Cosmetic Products and Non-Food Products Intended for Consumers. Opinion concerning fragrance inventory. Adopted by the SCCNFP during the plenary session of 23 September 1998

7. Johansen JD (2002) Contact allergy to fragrances: clinical and experimental investigations of the fragrance mix and its ingredients. Contact Dermatitis 46 (Suppl 3):4–31

8. Harder U (1998) The art of creating a perfume. In: Frosch PJ, Johansen JD, White IR (eds) Fragrances –beneficial and adverse effects. Springer, Berlin Heidelberg New York, pp 3–5

9. Lepoittevin JP, Mutterer V (1998) Molecular aspects of fragrance sensitisation. In: Frosch PJ, Johansen JD, White IR (eds) Fragrances – beneficial and adverse effects. Springer, Berlin Heidelberg New York, pp 49–56

10. Karlberg AT (1998) d-limonene – an old perfume ingredient introduced as a "natural" solvent in industry: is there a risk of sensitization? In: Frosch PJ, Johansen JD, White IR (eds) Fragrances – beneficial and adverse effects. Springer, Berlin Heidelberg New York, pp 106–112

11. Basketter DA (1992) Skin sensitization to cinnamic alcohol: the role of skin metabolism. Acta Derm Venereol (Stockh) 72:264–265

12. Nilsson AM, Jonsson C, Luthman K, Nilsson JL, Karlberg AT (2004) Inhibition of the sensitizing effect of carvone by the addition of non-allergenic compounds. Acta Derm Venereol (Stockh) 84:99–105

13. Karlberg AT, Nilsson AM, Luthman K, Nilsson JL (2001) Structural analogues inhibit the sensitizing capacity of carvone. Acta Derm Venereol (Stockh) 81:398–402

14. Johansen JD, Skov L, Volund A, Andersen K, Menné T (1998) Allergens in combination have a synergistic effect on the elicitation response: a study of fragrance-sensitized individuals. Br J Dermatol 139:264–270

15. Grabbe S, Steinert M, Mahnke K, Schwarz A, Luger TA, Schwarz T (1996) Dissection of antigenic and irritative effects of epicutaneously applied haptens in mice. Evidence that not the antigenic component but nonspecific proinflammatory effects of haptens determine the concentration-dependent elicitation of allergic contact dermatitis. J Clin Invest 98:1158–1164

16. Marzulli FN, Maibach HI (1980) Contact allergy: predictive testing of fragrance ingredients in humans by Draize and maximization methods. J Environ Pathol Toxicol 3:235–245

17. Frankild S (1999) Dose–response studies in guinea pig allergy tests. PhD thesis, Faculty of Health Sciences, University of Southern Denmark, Denmark

18. Patlewicz GY, Wright ZM, Basketter DA, Pease CK, Lepoittevin JP, Arnau EG (2002) Structure–activity relationships for selected fragrance allergens. Contact Dermatitis 47:219–26

19. Rastogi SC, Lepoittevin JP, Johansen JD, Frosch P, Menné T, Bruze M, Dreier B, Andersen KE, White I (1998) Fragrances and other materials in deodorants – search for potentially sensitizing molecules using combined GC-MS and structure activity relationship (SAR) analysis. Contact Dermatitis 39:293–303

20. Patlewicz GY, Basketter DA, Pease CK, Wilson K, Roberts DW, Bernard G, Arnau EG, Lepoittevin JP (2004) Further evaluation of quantitative structure activity relationship models for the prediction of the skin sensitization potency of selected fragrance allergens. Contact Dermatitis 50:91–97

21. Larsen WG (1977) Perfume dermatitis. A study of 20 patients. Arch Dermatol 113:623–626

22. Malten KE, van Ketel WG, Nater JP, Liem DH (1984) Reactions in selected patients to 22 fragrance materials. Contact Dermatitis 11:1–10

23. de Groot AC, Liem DH, Nater JP, van Ketel WG (1985) Patch tests with fragrance materials and preservatives. Contact Dermatitis 12:87–92

24. Wilkinson JD, Andersen KE, Camarasa J, Ducombs G, Frosch PJ, Lahti A, Menné T, Rycroft RJG, White I (1989) Preliminary results on the effectiveness of two forms of fragrance mix as screening agents for fragrance sensitivity. In: Frosch PJ, Dooms-Goossens A, Lachapelle JM, Rycroft RJG, Sheper RJ (eds) Current topics in contact dermatitis. Springer, Berlin Heidelberg New York, pp 127–131

25. Frosch PJ, Pilz B, Andersen KE, Burrows D, Camasara JG, Dooms-Goossens A, Ducombs G, Fuchs T, Hannuksela M, Lachapelle JM, Lahti A, Maibach HI, Menne T, Rycroft RJG, Shaw S, Wahlberg JE, White IR, Wilkinson JD (1995) Patch testing with fragrances: results of a multicenter study of the European Environmental and Contact Dermatitis Research Group with 48 frequently used constituents of perfumes. Contact Dermatitis 33:333–342

26. Frosch PJ, Johansen JD, Menné T, Pirker C, Rastogi SC, Andersen KE, Bruze M, Goossens A, Lepoittevin JP, White IR (2000) Further important sensitizers in patients sensitive to fragrances. I. Reactivity to 14 frequently used chemicals. Contact Dermatitis 47:78–85

27. Frosch PJ, Johansen JD, Menné T, Pirker C, Rastogi SC, Andersen KE, Bruze M, Goossens A, Lepoittevin JP, White IR (2002) Further important sensitizers in patients sensitive to fragrances. II. Reactivity to essential oils. Contact Dermatitis 47:279–287

28. Frosch PJ, Pirker C, Rastogi SC, Andersen KE, Bruze M, Svedman C, Goossens A, White IR, Uter W, Arnau EG, Lepoittevin JP, Menné T, Johansen JD (2005) Patch testing with a new fragrance mix detects additional patients sensitive to perfumes and missed by the current fragrance mix. Contact Dermatitis 52:207–215

29. Frosch PJ, Rastogi SC, Pirker C, Brinkmeier T, Andersen KE, Bruze M, Svedman C, Goossens A, White IR, Uter W, Arnau EG, Lepoittevin JP, Johansen JD, Menné T (2005) Patch testing with a new fragrance mix – reactivity to the single constituents and chemical detection in relevant cosmetic products. Contact Dermatitis 52:216–225

30. Larsen W, Nakayama H, Lindberg M, Fischer T, Elsner P, Burrows D, Jordan W, Shaw S, Wilkinson J, Marks J Jr, Su-

31

gawara M, Nethercott J (1996) Fragrance contact dermatitis: a worldwide multicenter investigation, part I. Am J Contact Dermatitis 7:77–83

31. Larsen W, Nakayama H, Fischer T, Elsner P, Frosch P, Burrows D, Jordan W, Shaw S, Wilkinson J, Marks J Jr, Sugawara M, Nethercott M, Nethercott J (2001) Fragrance contact dermatitis: a worldwide multicenter investigation, part II. Contact Dermatitis 44:344–346

32. Larsen W, Nakayama H, Fischer T, Elsner P, Frosch P, Burrows D, Jordan W, Shaw S, Wilkinson J, Marks J Jr, Sugawara M, Nethercott M, Nethercott J (2002) Fragrance contact dermatitis: a worldwide multicenter investigation, part III. Contact Dermatitis 46:141–144

33. Larsen W, Nakayama H, Fischer T, Elsner P, Frosch P, Burrows D, Jordan W, Shaw S, Wilkinson J, Marks J Jr, Sugawara M, Nethercott M, Nethercott J (1998) A study of new fragrance mixtures. Am J Contact Dermat 9:202–206

34. Frosch PJ, Johansen JD, Menné T, Rastogi SC, Bruze M, Andersen KE, Lepoittevin JP, Arnau EG, Pirker C, Goossens A, White IR (1999) Lyral is an important sensitizer in patients sensitive to fragrances. Br J Dermatol 141:1076–1083

35. Enders F, Przybilla B, Ring J (1989) Patch testing with fragrance mix 16% and 8%, and its individual constituents. Contact Dermatitis 20:237–238

36. Buckley DA, Wakelin SH, Holloway D, Rycroft RJG, White IR, McFadden JP (2000) The frequency of fragrance allergy in a patch test population over a 17-year period. Br J Dermatol 142:279–283

37. Meding B, Wrangsjo K, Brisman J, Jarvholm B (2003) Hand eczema in 45 bakers – a clinical study. Contact Dermatitis 48:7–11

38. Bauer A, Geier J, Elsner P (2002) Type IV allergy in the food processing industry: sensitization profiles in bakers, cooks and butchers. Contact Dermatitis 46:228–235

39. Rastogi SC, Johansen JD, Menné T (1996) Natural ingredient based cosmetics. Content of selected fragrance sensitizers. Contact Dermatitis 34:423–426

40. Rastogi SC, Johansen JD, Frosch PJ, Menné T, Bruze M, Lepoittevin JP, Dreier B, Andersen KE, White IR (1998) Deodorants on the European market: quantitative chemical analysis of 21 fragrances. Contact Dermatitis 38:29–35

41. Rastogi SC, Johansen JD, Menné T, Frosch PJ, Bruze M, Andersen KE, Lepoittevin JP, Wakelin S, White IR (1999) Contents of fragrance allergens in children's cosmetics and cosmetic-toys. Contact Dermatitis 41:84–88

42. Johansen JD, Rastogi SC, Menné T (1996) Contact allergy to popular perfumes; assessed by patch test, use test and chemical analysis. Br J Dermatol 135:419–422

43. Elahi EN, Wright Z, Hinselwood D, Hotchkiss SA, Basketter DA, Pease CK (2004) Protein binding and metabolism influence the relative skin sensitization potential of cinnamic compounds. Chem Res Toxicol 17:301–310

44. European Communities (2004) Council directive 76/768/EEC of 27 July 1976 on the approximation of the laws of the member states relating to cosmetic products. European Communities Official Journal, L262

45. Tananka S, Royds C, Buckley D, Basketter DA, Goossens A, Bruze M, Svedman C, Menné T, Johansen JD, White IR, McFadden JP (2004) Contact allergy to isoeugenol and its derivatives: problems with allergen substitution. Contact Dermatitis 51:288–291

46. Barratt MD, Basketter DA (1992) Possible origin of the skin sensitization potential of isoeugenol and related compounds, (I). Preliminary studies of potential reactions mechanisms. Contact Dermatitis 27:98–104

47. Bertrand F, Basketter DA, Roberts DW, Lepoittevin JP (1997) Skin sensitization to eugenol and isoeugenol in mice: possible metabolic pathways involving ortho-quinone and quinone methide intermediates. Chem Res Toxicol 10:335–343

48. Basketter DA, Wright ZM, Warbrick EV, Dearman RJ, Kimber I, Ryan CA, Gerberick GF, White IR (2001) Human potency predictions for aldehydes using the local lymph node assay. Contact Dermatitis 45:89–94

49. Fenn RS (1989) Aroma chemical usage trends in modern perfumery. Perfumer Flavorist 14:1–10

50. Goossens A, Merckx L (1997) Allergic contact dermatitis from farnesol in a deodorant. Contact Dermatitis 37:179–180

51. Schnuch A, Uter W, Geier J, Lessmann H, Frosch PJ (2004) Contact allergy to farnesol in 2021 consecutively patch tested patients. Results of the IVDK. Contact Dermatitis 50:117–121

52. Heydorn S, Menné T, Andersen KE, Bruze M, Svedman C, White IR, Basketter DA (2003) Citral a fragrance allergen and irritant. Contact Dermatitis 49:32–36

53. Heydorn S, Johansen JD, Andersen KE, Bruze M, Svedman C, White IR, Basketter DA, Menné T (2003) Fragrance allergy in patients with hand eczema – clinical study. Contact Dermatitis 48:317–323

54. Rothenborg HW, Menné T, Sjolin KE (1977) Temperature dependent primary irritant dermatitis from lemon perfume. Contact Dermatitis 3:37–48

55. Mutterer V, Gimenez Arnau E, Lepoittevin JP, Johansen JD, Frosch PJ, Menné T, Andersen KE, Bruze M, Rastogi SC, White IR (1999) Identification of coumarin as the sensitizer in a patient sensitive to her own perfume but negative to the fragrance mix. Contact Dermatitis 40:196–199

56. Kunkeler AC, Weijland JW, Bruynzeel DP (1998) The role of coumarin in patch testing. Contact Dermatitis 39:327–328

57. Matura M, Goossens A, Bordalo O, Garcia-Bravo B, Magnusson K, Wrangsjo K, Karlberg AT (2003) Patch testing with oxidized R-(+)-limonene and its hydroperoxide fraction. Contact Dermatitis 49:15–21

58. Matura M, Goossens A, Bordalo O, Garcia-Bravo B, Magnusson K, Wrangsjo K, Karlberg AT (2002) Oxidized citrus oil (R-limonene): a frequent skin sensitizer in Europe. J Am Acad Dermatol 47:709–714

59. Skold M, Borje A, Matura M, Karlberg AT (2002) Studies on the autoxidation and sensitizing capacity of the fragrance chemical linalool, identifying a linalool hydroperoxide. Contact Dermatitis 46:267–272

60. Skold M, Borje A, Harambasic E, Karlberg AT (2004) Contact allergens formed on air exposure of linalool. Identification and quantification of primary and secondary oxidization products and effects on skin sensitization. Chem Res Toxicol 17:1697–1705

61. Schnuch A, Lessmann, Geier J, Frosch PJ, Uter W: IDVK (2004) Contact allergy to fragrances: frequencies of sensitization from 1996 to 2002. Results of the IVDK. Contact Dermatitis 50:65–76

62. Johansen JD, Andersen KE, Svedman C, Bruze M, Bernard G, Gimenez-Arnau E, Rastogi SC, Lepoittevin JP, Menné T (2003) Chloroatranol, an extremely potent allergen hidden in perfumes: a dose–response elicitation study. Contact Dermatitis 49:180–184

63. Rastogi SC, Bossi R, Johansen JD, Menné T, Bernard G, Giménez-Arnau E, Lepoittevin JP (2004) Content of oak moss allergens atranol and chloroatranol in perfumes and similar products. Contact Dermatitis 50:367–370

64. Scientific Committee on Consumer Products (SCCP) (2004) Opinion on atranol and chloroatranol present in natural extracts (e.g. oak moss and tree moss extract). Adopted by SCCP during the 2nd plenary meeting of 7 Dec 2004

65. Nakayama H (1998) Fragrance hypersensitivity and its control In: Frosch PJ, Johansen JD, White IR (eds) Fragrances – beneficial and adverse effects. Springer, Berlin Heidelberg New York, pp 83–91

66. Hausen BM, Simatupang T, Bruhn G, Evers P, Koenig WA (1995) Identification of new allergens constituents and proof of evidence for coniferyl benzoate in balsam of Peru. Am J Contact Dermat 6:199–208

67. Hjorth N (1961) Eczematous allergy to balsams. Allied perfumes and flavoring agents – with special reference to balsam of Peru. Thesis. University of Copenhagen, Denmark

68. Hausen BM (2001) Contact allergy to balsam of Peru. II. Patch test results in 102 patients with selected balsam of Peru constituents. Am J Contact Dermat 12:93–102

69. International Fragrance Association (IFRA) (1974) Recommendations concerning Peru balsam. Code of Practice. October 1974, last amended December 1991. Home page at http://www.ifraorg.org

70. Karlberg AT (2000) Colophony. In: Kanerva L, Elsner P, Wahlberg J, Maibach H (eds) Handbook of occupational dermatology, vol 64. Springer, Berlin Heidelberg New York, pp 509–516

71. International Fragrance Association (IFRA) Standards. Colophony. Last amended December 1991. Home page at <url>http://www.ifraorg.org</url>

72. de Groot AC, Frosch PJ (1997) Adverse reactions to fragrances. A clinical review. Contact Dermatitis 36:57–87

73. Cronin E (1980) Perfumes. Contact dermatitis. Churchill Livingstone, Edinburgh, pp 158–170

74. Trattner A, David M (2003) Patch testing with fine fragrances: comparison with fragrance mix, balsam of Peru and a fragrance series. Contact Dermatitis 49:287–289

75. Maouad M, Fleischer AB, Sherertz EF, Feldman SR (1999) Significance-prevalence index number: a reinterpretation and enhancement of data from the North American Contact Dermatitis group. J Am Acad Dermatol 41:573–576

76. Li LF, Guo J, Wang J (2004) Environmental contact factors in eczema and the results of patch testing Chinese patients with a modified European standard series of allergens. Contact Dermatitis 51:22–25

77. Greig JE, Carson CF, Stuckey MS, Riley TV (2000) Prevalence of delayed hypersensitivity to the European standard series in a self-selected population. Australas J Dermatol 41:86–89

78. Mortz CG, Lauritsen JM, Bindslev-Jensen C, Andersen KE (2002) Contact allergy and allergic contact dermatitis in adolescents: prevalence measures and associations. The Odense Adolescence Cohort Study on Atopic Diseases and Dermatitis (TOACS). Acta Derm Venereol (Stockh) 82:352–358

79. Nielsen NH, Menné T (1992) Allergic contact sensitization in an unselected Danish population. The Glostrup Allergy Study. Acta Derm Venereol (Stockh) 72:456–460

80. Nielsen NH, Linneberg A, Menné T, Madsen F, Frolund L, Dirksen A, Jorgensen T (2001) Allergic contact sensitization in an adult Danish population: two cross-sectional surveys eight years apart (the Copenhagen Allergy Study). Acta Derm Venereol (Stockh) 81:31–34

81. Schnuch A, Uter W, Geier J, Gefeller O; IDVK study group (2002) Epidemiology of contact allergy: an estimation of morbidity employing the clinical epidemiology and drug-utilization research (CE-DUR) approach. Contact Dermatitis 47:32–39

82. Marks JG, Belsito DV, DeLeo VA, Fowler JF, Fransway AF, Maibach H I, Mathias Toby CG, Pratt MD, Rietschel RL, Sherertz EF, Storrs FJ, Taylor J (2003) North American Contact Dermatitis Group patch-test results, 1998 to 2000. Am J Contact Dermat 14:59-62

83. Buckley DA, Rycroft RJG, White IR, McFadden JP (2003) The frequency of fragrance allergy in patch-tested patients increases with their age. Br J Dermatol 149:986–989

84. Uter W, Schnuch A (2004) Fragrance allergy increases with age. Br J Dermatol 150:1212–1234

85. Mortz C, Andersen KE (1999) Allergic contact dermatitis in children and adolescents. Contact Dermatitis 41:121–30

86. Heine G, Schnuch A, Uter W, Worm M (2004) Frequency of contact allergy in German children and adolescents patch tested between 1995 and 2002: results from the Information Network of Departments of Dermatology and the German Contact Dermatitis Group. Contact Dermatitis 51:111–117

87. Johansen JD, Menné T, Christophersen J, Kaaber K, Veien N (2000) Changes in the sensitization pattern to common allergens in Denmark between 1985–1986 and 1997–1998, with a special view to the effect of preventive strategies. Br J Dermatol 142:490–495

88. Scheinman PL (2002) Prevalence of fragrance allergy. Dermatology 205:98–102

89. Rastogi SC, Menné T, Johansen JD (2003) The composition of fine fragrances is changing. Contact Dermatitis 48:130–132

90. Johansen JD, Andersen TF, Veien N, Avnstorp C, Andersen KE, Menné T (1997) Patch testing with markers of fragrance contact allergy. Do clinical tests correspond to patients' self-reported problems? Acta Derm Venereol (Stockh) 77:149–153

91. Katz AS, Sheretz F (1999) Facial dermatitis: patch test results and final diagnosis. Am J Contact Dermat 10:153–156

92. Wöhrl S, Hemmer W, Focke M, Görtz M, Jarisch R (2001) The significance of fragrance mix, balsam of Peru, colophony and propolis as screening tools in the detection of fragrance allergy. Br J Dermatol 145:268–273

93. Edman B (1994) The influence of shaving method on perfume allergy. Contact Dermatitis 31:291–292

94. Johansen JD, Andersen TF, Kjøller M, Veien N, Avnstorp C, Andersen KE, Menné T (1998) Identification of risk products for fragrance contact allergy: a case-referent study based on patients' histories. Am J Contact Dermat 2:80–87

95. Johansen JD, Rastogi SC, Bruze M, Andersen KE, Frosch PJ, Dreier B, Lepoittevin JP, White IR, Menné T (1998) Deodorants: a clinical provocation study in fragrance-sensitive individuals. Contact Dermatitis 39:161–165

96. Svedman C, Bruze M, Johansen JD, Andersen KE, Goossens A, Frosch PJ, Lepoittevin JP, Rastogi S, White IR, Menne T (2003) Deodorants: an experimental provocation study with hydroxycitronellal. Contact Dermatitis 48:217–223

97. Bruze M, Johansen JD, Andersen KE, Frosch P, Lepoittevin JP, Rastogi S, Wakelin S, White I, Menne T (2003) Deodorants: an experimental provocation study with cinnamic aldehyde. J Am Acad Dermatol 48:194–200

98. von Peter C, Hoting E (1993) Anwendungstest mit parfümierten Kosmetika bei Patienten mit positivem Epikutantest auf Duftstoff-Mischung. Dermatosen 41:237–241

99. Heydorn S, Menné T, Johansen JD (2003) Fragrance allergy and hand eczema – a review. Contact Dermatitis 48: 59–66

100. Buckley DA, Rycroft RJG, White IR, McFadden JP (2000) Contact allergy to individual fragrance mix constituents in relation to primary site of dermatitis. Contact Dermatitis 43:304–305

101. Christophersen J, Menne T, Tanghoj P, Andersen KE, Brandrup F, Kaaber K, Osmundsen PE, Thestrup-Pedersen K, Veien NK (1989) Clinical patch test data evaluated by multivariate analysis. Danish Contact Dermatitis Group. Contact Dermatitis 21:291–299

102. Katsarma G, Gawkrodger DJ (1999) Suspected fragrance contact allergy requires extended patch testing to individual fragrance allergens. Contact Dermatitis 41:193–197

103. Veien NK (1989) Systemically induced eczema in adults. Acta Derm Venereol Suppl (Stockh) 147:1–58

104. Niinimaki A (1995) Double-blind placebo-controlled peroral challenges in patients with delayed-type allergy to balsam of Peru. Contact Dermatitis 33:78–83

105. Veien NK, Hattel T, Laurberg G (1996) Can oral challenge with balsam of Peru predict possible benefit from a low-balsam diet? Am J Contact Dermat 7:84–87

106. Johansen JD, Frosch PJ, Svedman C, Andersen KE, Bruze M, Pirker C, Menné T (2003) Hydroxyisohexyl 3-cyclohexene carboxaldehyde – known as Lyral: quantitative aspects and risk assessment of an important fragrance allergen. Contact Dermatitis 48:310–316

107. Rastogi SC, Heydorn S, Johansen JD, Basketter D (2001) Fragrance chemicals in domestic and occupational products. Contact Dermatitis 45:221–225

108. Wallenhammar LM, Ortengren U, Andreasson H, Barregard L, Bjorkner B, Karlsson S, Wrangsjo K, Meding B (2000) Contact allergy and hand eczema in Swedish dentists. Contact Dermatitis 43:192–199

109. Uter W, Schnuch A, Geier J, Pfahlberg A, Gefeller O; IVDK study group. Information Network of Departments of Dermatology (2001) Association between occupation and contact allergy to the fragrance mix: a multifactorial analysis of national surveillance data. Occup Environ Med 58: 392–398

110. Geier J, Lessmann, Schnuch A, Uter W (2004) Contact sensitization in metalworkers with occupational dermatitis exposed to water-based metalworking fluids: results of the research project "FaSt". Int Arch Occup Environ Health 77:543–551

111. Owen CM, August PJ, Beck MH (2000) Contact allergy to oak moss resin in a soluble oil. Contact Dermatitis 43:112

112. Pontén A, Björk J, Carstensen O, Gruvberger B, Isaksson M, Rasmussen K, Bruze M (2004) Associations between contact allergy to epoxy resin and fragrance mix. Acta Derm Venereol (Stockh) 84:151–175

113. Larsen WG (1987) Detection of allergic dermatitis to fragrances. Acta Derm Venereol (Stockh) 134:83–86

114. de Groot AC, van der Kley AM, Bruynzeel DP, Meinardi MM, Smeenk G, van Joost T, Pavel S (1993) Frequency of false-negative reactions to the fragrance mix. Contact Dermatitis 28:139–140

115. Frosch PJ, Pilz B, Burrows D, Camarasa JG, Lachapelle J-M, Lahti A, Menné T, Wilkinson JD (1995) Testing with fragrance mix. Is the addition of sorbitan sesquioleate to the constituents useful? Contact Dermatitis 32:266–272

116. Johansen JD, Rastogi SC, Menné T (1996) Exposure to selected fragrance materials. A case study of fragrance-mix-positive eczema patients. Contact Dermatitis 34:106–110

117. Johansen JD, Rastogi SC, Andersen KE, Menné T (1997) Content and reactivity to product perfumes in fragrance mix positive and negative eczema patients. A study of perfumes used in toiletries and skin-care products. Contact Dermatitis 36:291–296

118. de Groot AC, Coenraads PJ, Bruynzeel DP, Jagtman BA, van Ginkel CJ, Noz K, van der Valk PG, Pavel S, Vink J, Weyland JW (2000) Routine patch testing with fragrance chemicals in the Netherlands. Contact Dermatitis 42: 184–185

119. Geier J, Brasch J, Schnuch A, Lessmann H, Pirker C, Frosch PJ; For the Information Network of Departments of Dermatology (IVDK) and the German Contact Dermatitis Research Group (DKG) (2002) Lyral has been included in the patch test standard series in Germany. Contact Dermatitis 46:295–297

120. Roberts G (2002) Procedures for supplying fragrance information to dermatologists. Letter to the editor. Am J Contact Dermat 13:206–207

121. Gimenez-Arnau A, Gimenez-Arnau E, Serra-Baldrich E, Lepoittevin JP, Camarasa JG (2002) Principles and methodology for identification of fragrance allergens in consumer products. Contact Dermatitis 47:345–352

122. Arnau EG, Andersen KE, Bruze M, Frosch PJ, Johansen JD, Menné T, Rastogi SC, White IR, Lepoittevin JP (2000) Identification of Lilial as a fragrance sensitizer in a perfume by bioassay-guided chemical fractionation and structure-activity relationships. Contact Dermatitis 43:351–358

123. Johansen JD, Andersen KE, Rastogi SC, Menné T (1996) Threshold responses in cinnamic-aldehyde-sensitive subjects: results and methodological aspects. Contact Dermatitis 34:165–171

124. Johansen JD, Andersen KE, Menné T (1996) Quantitative aspects of isoeugenol contact allergy assessed by use and patch tests. Contact Dermatitis 34:414–418

125. Scheinman PL (2001) Exposing covert fragrance chemicals. Am J Contact Dermat 12:225–228

126. Scheinman PL (1999) The foul side of fragrance-free products: what every clinician should know about managing patients with fragrance allergy. J Am Acad Dermatol 41:1020–1024

127. European Communities (2004) Detergents directive 73/404/EEC of 22 Nov 1973, amended 2004

128. Safford RJ, Basketter DA, Allenby CF, Goodwin BF (1990) Immediate contact reactions to chemicals in the fragrance mix and a study of the quenching action of eugenol. Br J Dermatol 123:595–606

129. Temesvari E, Nemeth I, Balo-Banga MJ, Husz S, Kohanka V, Somos Z, Judak R, Remenyik EVA, Szegedi A, Nebenführer L, Meszaros C, Horvath A (2002) Multicentre study of fragrance allergy in Hungary. Immediate and late type reactions. Contact Dermatitis 46:325–330

130. Tanaka S, Matsumoto Y, Dlova N, Ostlere LS, Goldsmith PC, Rycroft RJG, Basketter DA, White IR, Banerjee P, McFadden JP (2004) Immediate contact reactions to fragrance mix constituents and Myroxylon pereirae resin. Contact Dermatitis 51:20–21

131. Katsarou A, Armenaka M, Ale I, Koufou V, Kalogeromitros D (1999) Frequency of immediate reactions to the European standard series. Contact Dermatitis 41:276–279

132. Kroon S (1979) Musk Ambrette, a new cosmetic sensitizer and photo sensitizer. Contact Dermatitis 5:337–338

133. Cronin E (1984) Photosensitivity to musk ambrette. Contact Dermatitis 11:88–92

134. Darvay A, White IR, Rycroft RJ, Jones AB, Hawk JL, McFadden JP (2001) Photoallergic contact dermatitis is uncommon. Br J Dermatol 145:597–601

135. Cronin E (1980) Phototoxic reactions. Contact dermatitis. Churchill Livingstone, Edinburgh, pp 417–432

31

136. Wang L, Sterling B, Don P (2002) Berloque dermatitis induced by "Florida water". Cutis 70 : 29–30
137. Elberling J, Linneberg A, Dirksen A, Johansen JD, Frolund L, Madsen F, Nielsen NH, Mosbech H (2005) Mucosal symptoms elicited by fragrance products in a population-based sample in relation to bronchial hyper-reactivity. Clin Exp Allergy 35 : 75–81
138. Kumar P, Caradonna-Graham VM, Gupta S, Cai X, RAO PN, Thompson J (1995) Inhalation challenge effects of perfume scent strips in patients with asthma. Ann Allergy Asthma Immunol 75 : 429–433
139. Millqvist E, Lowhagen O (1996) Placebo-controlled challenges with perfume in patients with asthma-like symptoms. Allergy 51 : 434–439
140. Millqvist E, Bende M, Lowhagen O (1998) Sensory hyperreactivity – a possible mechanism underlying cough and asthma-like symptoms. Allergy 53 : 1208–1212
141. Elberling J, Linneberg A, Mosbech H, Dirksen A, Frolund L, Madsen F, Nielsen NH, Johansen JD (2004) A link between skin and airways regarding sensitivity to fragrance products? Br J Dermatol 151 : 1197–1203
142. World Health Organization (1997) Criteria for classification of skin- and airway-sensitizing substances in the work and general environments. Flyvholm M (ed) EUR/ICP/EHPM 050201

31.2　Hair Dyes

David Basketter, Jeanne Duus Johansen,
John McFadden, Heidi Søsted

31.2.1　Introduction

Henna was originally used in ancient Egypt to stain the fingers and toes of the Pharaohs prior to mummification. This goes back 4,000 years, and today, in the 21st century, people still color their body and hair with henna. By the end of the 19th century, the oxidative hair dye process had been invented. Reactions with aromatic amines, such as *para*-phenylenediamine (PPD), toluene-2,5-diamine and *m*-aminophenols, resorcinol, and hydrogen peroxide made it possible to make a permanent coloring of hair [1]. Contact dermatitis to synthetic hair dyes has been known for many years, and in 1939, Bonnevie suggested resorcinol, PPD, and aminophenol as part of a patch test standard series for identifying patients sensitized to PPD by furs, hair dyes, or occupational exposure [2]. Today, PPD still is allowed for the coloring of human hair and the sales of hair dyes containing aromatic amines are very substantial. A recent Danish-population-based study showed that almost 75% of women and 20% of men had dyed their hair at some point in their lives [3]. It seems that cosmetics are used neither more nor less in Denmark compared to the rest of Europe, so these results may also be valid for other countries in Europe. It was also found that the median age for the first hair dyeing was 16 years [3]. This means that hair coloring is not just used for covering gray hair, but is also a fashion among teenagers.

Hair dyes are found in three common classes and allergic contact dermatitis has been observed for all kinds of hair dyes. *Oxidative dyes* produce a permanent dyeing of the hair that cannot be washed out. They consist of two components that are mixed before use. They contain a precursor/primary intermediates; these substances could be, for example, PPD, toluene-2,5-diamine, *p*-aminophenol, or *o*-aminophenol, and a coupler, typically, *m*-phenylenediamine, *m*-aminophenol, resorcinol, or others, all of which have been described as contact sensitizers. Couplers determine the final shade by reaction with the oxidized form of primary intermediates, followed by further oxidative coupling reactions. Oxidants could be hydrogen peroxide, urea peroxide, or sodium percarbonate or perborate. Some oxidative dyes contain alkalinizing agents, such as ammonia, mono-ethanolamine, or aminomethylpropanol. *Semi-permanent hair dyes* are nitrophenylenediamine, nitro-aminophenol, or azo dyes [4], which, because of their low molecular weight, enters the hair straw. *Temporary dyes* contain larger molecules and the dye does not enter the hair follicle, but stays as a layer around each follicle.

A questionnaire study in Denmark showed that 5.3% of the people who have dyed their hair reported an adverse skin reaction compatible with allergic origin, and only about 1 in 6 of these people contacted the health care services [3]. Other studies confirm that only a minority of patients with hair dye reactions are investigated by a dermatologist [5]. Results from patch testing female patients between 1995 and 2002 in whom hair cosmetics have been considered as being causative of their contact dermatitis showed no trend over the period in the number of women sensitized to PPD, but a significant increase from 3.1% to 6.8% in women sensitized to toluene-2,5-diamine [6].

Core Message

- Allergic contact dermatitis has been seen to occur from all kind of hair dyes (permanent oxidative, semi-permanent, and temporary dyes), but is believed to be the most common with permanent dyes.

31

31.2.2 Clinical Picture

31.2.2.1 Allergic Contact Dermatitis

The severity of clinical symptoms from hair dyeing may vary considerably. There may be intense edema of the face, particularly of the eyes, with exudation of the scalp. Erythema and swelling may extend down the neck, on to the upper chest and arms, and can even become generalized. The swelling of the face may be so striking that a mistaken diagnosis of angioneurotic edema is made (see Fig. 2.1) [5, 7]. Less dramatic symptoms are periodic swelling of the eyes related to hair dyeing or acute eczema at the scalp margins, sometimes extending to the neck or face (see Fig. 2.2) [2,7]. Men dyeing their beard may have similar symptoms, also with varying severity [8]. In hairdressers, the most common regions affected are the hands and arms [9]; however, even though patients who apply the dye themselves wear gloves, their hands and arms occasionally may be affected [7]. The onset of symptoms may be from a few hours to the following day(s). The symptoms can be long lasting, even though hair dyeing is avoided. In a study concerning 55 cases of hair dye allergy, 23 had symptoms for more than 3 weeks [5], and hair loss has been reported following severe scalp reactions [5,10]. A number of morphological variants of disease expression occur, including leukoderma, lichenoid, and erythema multiforme-like rash [11–13].

> ### Core Message
>
> ■ Hair dye allergy may cause severe clinical reactions, with edema of the face, eyelids, and scalp. More moderate reactions are seen as erythema, suppuration, and ulceration, typically at the scalp margin, on the ears, and sometimes with evidence of eczema where the dye has run down the neck.

31.2.3 Temporary Tattoos

Temporary black henna tattoos may contain PPD and give rise to the induction of PPD allergy. The level of PPD in tattoo paint has been measured to be 0.43% [14]. Typically, an eczematous reaction occurs in the original tattoo days to weeks after the tattoo has been made, as a sign of primary sensitization. Individuals sensitized to PPD by semi-permanent tattoos cannot tolerate hair dyes and may experience very severe clinical reactions [15].

> ### Core Message
>
> ■ Temporary black henna tattoos may contain PPD and cause primary sensitization.

31.2.4 Diagnosis

A key step in the diagnosis of hair dye allergy involves patch testing with commercially available screening series of hair dye ingredients for routine investigations or by workup of the individual case by obtaining the exact components in the hair dye from the producer [16]. PPD is a part of the standard patch test and screening trays with PPD-related substances are commercially available.

Based on retrospective collected data on PPD allergy, it nevertheless represents a fairly good screen for clinical hair dye dermatitis [17]. However, the existing patch test trays for diagnosing hair dye allergy may have been focused to too great an extent on PPD and PPD-related substances. More than 200 ingredients are in use currently and, by a chemical structure activity analysis based on results from predictive testing in animals, many of these substances are predicted to be strong/moderate sensitizers [18]. In Table 2.1, a list is given of the substances that, based on predicted potency and volume of use, are currently being considered for clinical validation as an additional screening tray for hair dye allergy.

Toluene-2,5-diamine, p-aminophenol, and m-aminophenol are all available as patch test preparations, while the commonly used 4-amino-3-nitrophenol and 3-nitro-p-hydroxyethylamino-phenol, which have been reported positive in PPD-negative patients, are not routinely used for the investigation of hair dye allergy [18]. If the ingredients in a hair dye are not available commercially, they may be requested from the producers. Even though the diagnostic workup of individual cases may be valuable, the complicated procedure for acquiring substances for testing probably means that patients with contact allergy to hair dyes not reacting to PPD or only giving weak allergic reactions to PPD are overlooked [16, 19].

PPD may give very strong patch test reactions, bullous or erosive, at the standard concentration of 1%. This has been observed especially in patients with PPD allergy following skin painting with temporary black henna tattoos. A new method of using PPD at lower concentrations for the investigation of such patients has been proposed, starting with 0.01% PPD; if the result is negative at the first reading, the concentration is stepped up to 0.1%, or even 1% [20].

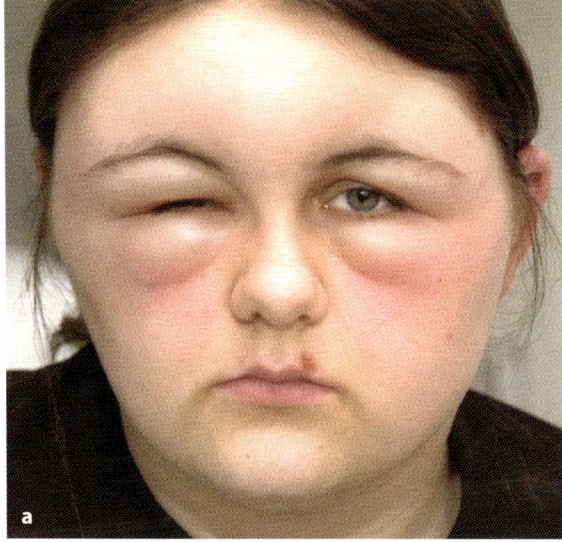

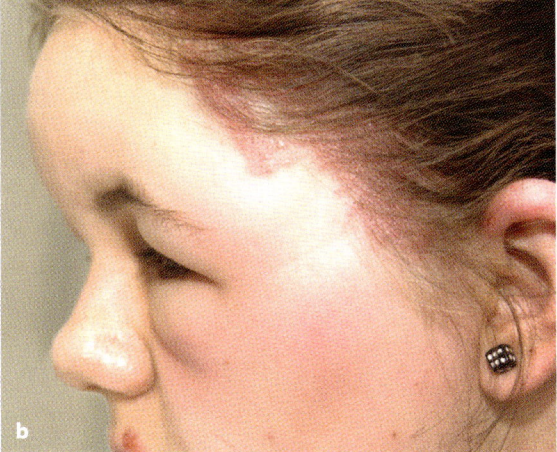

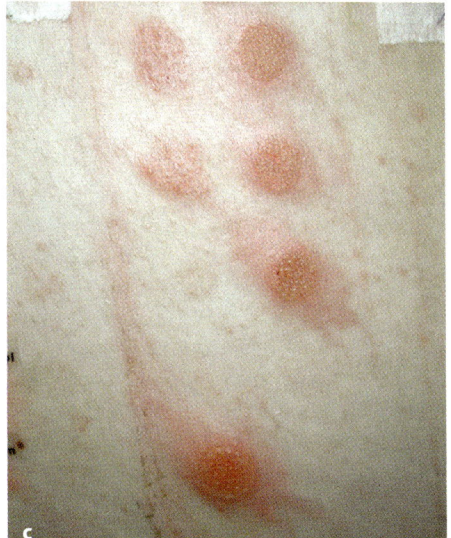

Fig. 2.1a–c. Severe edema of the face 2 days after dyeing the hair at home (a). The patient was referred by the emergency physician as erysipelas because she had slight fever, nausea, and lymphadenopathy. Close inspection revealed eczematous lesions at the hairline and on the scalp (b). Patch testing revealed a high degree of sensitization to p-phenylenediamine, toluene-2.5-diamine, hydroquinone, resorcinol, benzocaine, Disperse Orange 3, and to the used hair dye (2% aqueous) (c) (courtesy of P.J. Frosch).

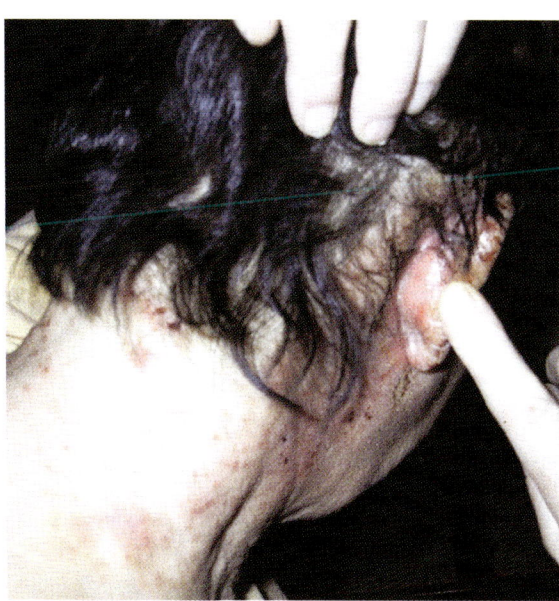

Fig. 2.2. Hair dye dermatitis with eczema at the scalp margins, extending to the neck and suppuration on the ears. The symptoms were caused by a permanent oxidative hair dye on a hairdresser's client

Table 2.1. List of commonly used hair dye ingredients, which are considered for clinical validation as an additional screening tray for hair dye allergy

INCI name	INCI name
1-Hydroxyethyl-4,5-diaminopyrazole sulfate	4-Hydroxypropylamino-3-nitrophenol
1-Naphthol	Acid Violet 43
2,4,5,6-Tetraaminopyrinidine	Disperse Violet 1
2,4-Diaminophenoxyethanol HCl	HC Red no. 3
2,7-Naphthalenediol[c]	HC Blue no. 2
2-Amino-3-hydroxypyridine	m-Aminophenol[abc]
2-Amino-6-chloro-4-nitrophenol	N, N-bis(2-Hydroxyethyl)-p-phenylenediamine
2-Methyl-5-hydroxyethylaminophenol	o-Aminophenol[c]
3-Nitro-p-hydroxyethylaminophenol[c]	p-Aminophenol[abc]
4-Amino-3-nitrophenol[c]	p-Methylaminophenol
4-Amino-2-hydroxytoluene	p-Phenylenediamine[abc]
4-Amino-m-cresol	Picramic acid
4-Chlororesorcinol	Resorcinol[ac]
	Toluene-2,5-diamine[abc]

[a] Available from Chemotechnique Diagnostics, Malmö, Sweden
[b] Available from Trolab Hermal, Reinbek, Germany
[c] Reported as clinical contact allergens [16, 18]

31

Patch testing may be supplemented with the dyed hair of the patient [7] and/or the hair dye itself. In case severe reactions to the hair dye are anticipated from the original clinical presentation, a stepwise procedure can be applied as for PPD [20] by just adjusting the exposure time instead of the concentration, e.g., starting with a 30-min open exposure, followed by normal occluded exposure, if negative at the first reading. It is not known whether the optimal procedure for testing permanent hair dyes is in their oxidized or unoxidized states, or if the site of application, rather than on the back, should be behind the ears [21] or in the neck hairline in order to mimic as much as possible normal exposure.

Core Message

■ Hair dye allergy cannot always be detected by patch testing with PPD alone.

31.2.4.1 Immediate Reactions

By far the most common allergic reactions to hair dyes are contact dermatitis. However, immediate hypersensitivity reactions, including asthma, contact urticaria, and anaphylactic shock, attributed to hair dyes have been reported [17, 22–24], and even with the very rare possibility of a fatal outcome [25].

31.2.5 PPD – The Archetype

As PPD is really the "classic" hair dye allergen, it is reviewed here in greater detail than other dyes. In the EU, the current maximum use level is 6% (=3% when mixed in use), although in practice the typical maximum level is closer to 4%.

31.2.5.1 Chemistry

Paraphenylenediamine (PPD) belongs to the family of aromatic amines (see Fig. 2.3). Whilst many haptens contain chemically reactive groups that react directly with skin protein, PPD is a member of the class of contact allergens referred to as prohaptens, where an apparently unreactive chemical is converted to a more reactive agent [26]. PPD can be metabolized in the skin to different compounds. Mayer [27] proposed that the formation of p-benzoquinone in vivo is a possible explanation for both the allergenicity and cross-reactivity of aromatic amines, including PPD. However, a number of groups have tried to confirm this theory, both in predictive animal models and in clinical studies, without any success [28, 29]. Of particular note is the failure of the key putative hapten, 1,4-benzoquinone, to give positive patch test reactions in more than a small minority of PPD-allergic individuals. An alternative explanation for the allergenic effect associated with PPD was sought via the formation of Bandrowski's base (BB), which is, essentially, a trimmer of PPD that forms readily when PPD is exposed to air. Evidence for this pos-

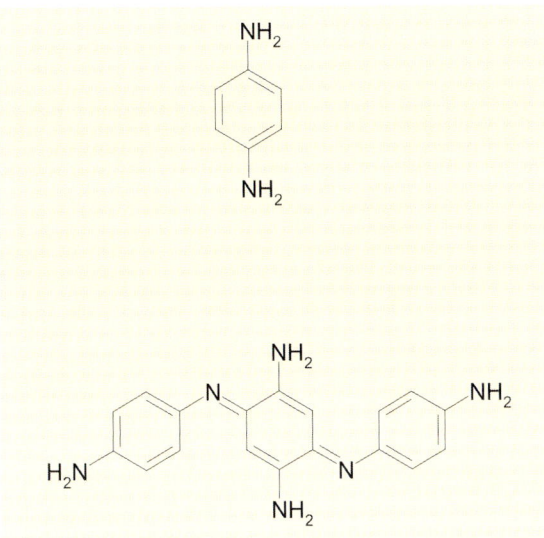

Fig. 2.3. Chemical structures of PPD and the related substance Bandrowski's base (*BB*)

sibility came from in vitro lymphocyte proliferation assays using cells taken from PPD-allergic subjects. Positive in vitro results were obtained with most of the subjects, whereas none of the lymphocyte populations would react to PPD itself [30]. Unfortunately, when PPD-allergic subjects are actually patch tested with BB, the large majority fails to react, and those that do react do so only weakly [31]. In reality, it seems likely that metabolic processes in skin, which, as yet, are not well understood, will play a key role in the induction of PPD allergy [32]. A potential consequence of this is the possibility that it may be feasible to determine genetic markers that will identify individuals likely to develop allergy to PPD [33]. Nevertheless, despite the various pieces of work mentioned above, the true nature of the in vivo hapten(s) associated with PPD remains unknown.

31.2.5.2 Immunology

Although the real in vivo hapten(s) arising from PPD may not be known, a number of other aspects of PPD immunology have been examined. A key factor in the induction of contact allergy is the release of danger signals. Picardo (1996) found that PPD induced oxidative stress in normal human keratinocytes in culture [34]. Exposure to noncytotoxic concentrations of PPD produced lipoperoxidative damage. With the overwhelming free radicals generated, an event cascade with recruitment and activation of the immune system occurs. Other authors also showed activation of multiple dermal enzymes following the applica-

tion of both PPD and PPD in the presence of hydrogen peroxide [35].

Yokozeki et al. looked at the profile of T-cells involved in PPD allergy. Using a mouse model, they showed early (6 h) and late (12–24 h) swellings in adoptive transfer experiments with elicitation challenge [36]. Sieben and colleagues have characterized elements of the antigen presentation pathways used during the elicitation of PPD responses [37].

In predictive allergy tests using humans, PPD has been shown to be strongly positive. Ten percent PPD sensitized all 24 subjects who were exposed to it in a human maximization test [38]. In the human repeated insult patch test, 1% PPD in petrolatum sensitized 54% of the volunteers, 0.1% sensitized 11%, and 0.01% sensitized 7% [39]. Similarly, in predictive animal tests, PPD is also strongly positive, yielding a 100% reaction rate in the guinea pig maximization test [40] and 90% in the Buehler test [41]. Currently, the murine local lymph node assay (LLNA) is the preferred standard for establishment of the relative allergenic potencies of different haptens [42]. Potency is expressed as an EC_3 value, this being the estimated concentration of chemical necessary to cause a threefold increase in proliferation activity. PPD is one of the most potent allergens on this basis, with an EC value of 0.1% [43]. Given the overwhelming evidence that PPD is, indeed, one of the most powerful of contact allergens, it is not surprising that its use at levels of 1–4% in hair dyes is associated with a degree of allergic contact dermatitis.

31.2.5.3 Epidemiology

As with most contact allergens, the true epidemiology of PPD allergy is relatively poorly understood. There is a rather wide variation in the frequency of positive patch test reactions to PPD in patch test clinics around the world, no doubt reflecting in part the varying exposure to PPD which occurs where there is a trend to dye gray hair black, then the use of PPD is likely to be prevalent, as is allergy to it. In London, the frequency of positives remained a little over 3% throughout the 1990s [44]. The North American Contact Dermatitis Group (NACDG) reported a rate of 6.4% in 1998 [45]. In India, an even higher rate of 11.5% was reported [46]. Across Germany, an average rate of 4.6% was reported from an analysis of 9 years of data from 33 clinics [47]. However, of special interest was the attempt made to translate these data into a view of the frequency of contact allergy in the general population. The authors concluded that the prevalence was between 0.7% and 1.6%. This estimate corresponded well with the figure of 1.5%, also from

Germany, where over 1,000 adults from the general population were patch tested [48]. Interestingly, recent data from Thailand indicate that a rather higher percentage of adults there may be sensitized to PPD (2.3%), in line with expectations regarding general use levels of PPD in a very predominantly black-haired population [49]. In this location, the gender ratio was approximately 2:1 female:male, which is similar to the situation in Europe. No doubt, the gender bias in use will vary in different countries: in one location in India, the ratio was 2:1 male:female [46].

31.2.5.4 Cross Reactions

For many years, the concept of "*para* group" cross sensitization has persisted, often despite real evidence. PPD belongs to the group of 1,4-substituted benzenes, along with, e.g., *p*-aminobenzoic acid, benzocaine, procaine, some sulfonamides, sunscreens, anthraquinones, and certain rubber chemicals. The reality is that the majority of 1,4-substituted benzenes most commonly do not cross react; however, there are clear exceptions: individuals sensitized to PPD may react to some other hair dyes, e.g., toluene-2,5-diamine [50], *p*-aminophenol [50], 2-nitro-PPD [50], and to Disperse Orange 3 [51]. PPD is not generally a good screen for azo dyes; however, cross or simultaneous reactions are described to varying degrees [52]. Cross reactions also occur with the black rubber chemical family, including IPPD [53]. As regards to local anesthetics, little evidence is published of cross-sensitization, however this does seem to occur especially in patients highly sensitized to PPD,

e.g., from a temporary tattoo. Such patients may have simultaneous reactions to both local anesthetics and IPPD, without any history of prior exposure to these chemicals (Fig. 2.4). In a recent publication, patch-test-proven reactions to *para*-aminobenzoic acid (PABA), benzocaine, and IPPD in PPD-positive subjects with hair dye allergy were less than 10% [54].

31.2.5.5 Occupational Allergy to PPD

This topic is discussed elsewhere in the relevant sections of this book. However, it is appropriate to mention here that hairdressers are at particular risk of PPD sensitization. Whilst the prevalence of PPD sensitization in hairdressers is not always high [55], it has been reported as a positive patch test from 15% to 45% of those tested, with relevance to ACD being high [6, 56–58].

31.2.6 Substances Other than PPD

Hair dye substances that have caused cosmetic allergic contact dermatitis in humans are listed in Table 2.2.

31.2.6.1 Toluene-2,5-diamine

Many reports on contact allergic reaction to toluene-2,5-diamnine from hair dyes exist either from patients dyeing their own hair or by their occupation as hairdressers. It was the most used hair dye substance

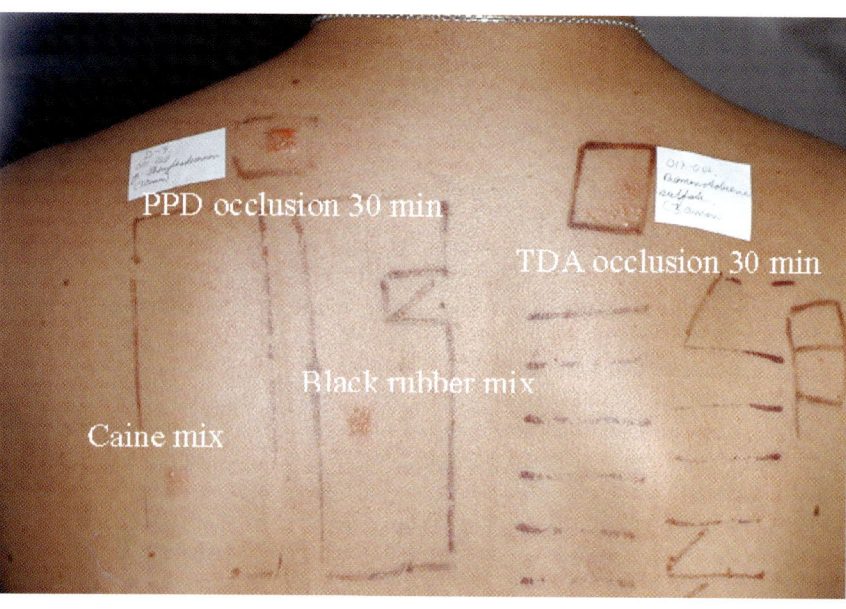

Fig. 2.4.
Strong patch test reaction to PPD, day 3. Exposure time to PPD only 30 min. Cross-reactivity to caine mix (local anesthetics), black rubber mix, and toluene-2,5-diamine (TDA) in a patient sensitized by a temporary black henna tattoo (courtesy of K.E. Andersen)

Table 2.2. INCI names of hair coloring agents that have caused cosmetic allergy in humans

INCI name
2.4-Diaminophenol
2.7-Naphthalenediol
2-Aminomethyl-*p*-aminophenol HCL
2-Chloro-*p*-phenylenediamine
2-Nitro-*p*-phenylenediamine
3-Nitro-*p*-hydroxyethylaminophenol
4-Amino-3-nitrophenol
Basic Blue 99
Basic Red 22
Disperse Brown 1
Disperse Orange 3
Henna
Hydroquinone
Lead acetate
m-Aminophenol
N-Phenyl-*p*-phenylenediamine
o-Aminophenol
p-Aminophenol
p-Phenylenediamine
Resorcinol
Solvent Red 1
Toluene-2,5-diamine

Based on [16, 18, 72]

in 2002. Toluene-2,5-diamine is commercially available as patch test preparation in petrolatum and it often cross-reacts with PPD but seems to give weaker reactions in PPD-positive patients at patch testing than PPD itself [50]. In a QSAR model, toluene-2,5-diamine was predicted to be a strong/moderate sensitizer [18]. Toluene-2,5-diamine is allowed at a concentration of 10% in hair dyes in the EU [59]. Products containing a 0.18% concentration have been reported to cause elicitation [60]. A German study showed that contact allergy to toluene-2,5-diamine is an increasing problem among patch-tested consumers [6].

31.2.6.2 Resorcinol

Resorcinol is known from pharmaceuticals and has been used in hair dyes for more than 100 years. It was the second most used hair dye substance in 2002, but, taking its use into account, it is not a frequent sensitizer when used in hair dyes. However, cases of contact allergy to resorcinol have been reported [61–62].

31.2.6.3 Aminophenol

o-, *p*-, and *m*-aminophenol are frequently used hair dye substances. *m*-Aminophenol is allowed at a concentration of up to 2% in hair dyes within the EU [59] and has elicited allergic contact dermatitis in products containing 0.067% *m*-aminophenol [60]. The number of patients sensitized to *p*-aminophenol, in whom hair cosmetics have been considered as being causative of their contact dermatitis, increased from 3.6% in 1995 to 8.9% in 2002, while no trend was found concerning *m*-aminophenol (0.36–1.04%) [6].

31.2.6.4 Henna

Allergic contact dermatitis to henna from hair dyes is seen, although it is very rare [63, 64]. Allergic contact dermatitis from henna painted on a toe has been described [65]. Immediate-type hypersensitivity with urticaria, rhinitis, and bronchial asthma on exposure to henna has been reported [66, 67].

31.2.6.5 Bleaching Agents

Ammonium persulfate is used to bleach hair and has been identified as the cause of occupational asthma and contact allergy in hairdressers [6, 68]. Consumers have also been found sensitized [6]. A positive patch test to hydrogen peroxide was seen in a housewife who had used a dyeing cream mixed with aqueous solution of 20–40% hydrogen peroxide. Contact dermatitis from handling hairdressers' products that contains hydrogen peroxide is frequently seen [10].

A case report described allergic contact dermatitis to the cream developer trideceth-2-carboxamide MEA from a permanent hair dye product [69].

31.2.6.6 New Generation of Hair Dyes

A new generation of hair dyes (Acid Black 1, Acid Violet 43, Acid Orange 7, and Acid Red 33) seems to have different chemical properties to PPD and toluene-2,5-diamine [18] and a lack of cross-reaction between the two groups is described [50]. All these substances are predicted as potent contact allergens in a QSAR analysis [18].

31.2.7 Pre-testing and Advising Patients

31.2.7.1 Pre-testing

Hair dye allergy may result in very severe reactions. It is, therefore, desirable to predict whether a person has already become sensitized and should not proceed to the full hair dyeing procedure. An open test has been recommended by the hair dye producers to be performed 48 h prior to hair dyeing, both in the case of home coloring and at the hairdressers [21]. The criticism has been that these tests are not validated. One study has been performed in patients with PPD allergy and a history of hair dye dermatitis [21]. The hair dye contained 1.8% PPD, which is not representative of the concentration range of PPD and PPD-like substances found in marketed products [60]. The study showed that patients who had already reacted clinically to a hair dye would be identified by the open test under the given conditions of exposure, so, for diagnostic purposes, in eczema patients, the test may be very useful. However, the pre-test is recommended for use by consumers who have never experienced clinical symptoms, and so, do not know whether they are allergic to hair dyes. Validation of a screening test has to be performed in the target group, as, in this case, consumers dyeing their hair and not yet having had clinical symptoms. A validation should also include an assessment of whether this additional, long-term (48 h) skin exposure to a hair dye containing potent allergens could cause sensitization in healthy consumers, who would otherwise not have become sensitized. The historic experiments by Kligman et al. indicate that this should be a real concern [70].

> **Core Message**
>
> ■ A properly conducted pre-test may provide a potential alert for the highly allergic individual, but the numbers of individuals presenting clinically with allergic eczema to hair dyes suggests that there are clear limitations to its utility/predictivity.

31.2.7.2 Advising Patients

Patients with hair dye allergy are advised to stop dyeing their hair. Some hair dye ingredients are used in both permanent and temporary hair dyes [18] and, therefore, it is not possible to give general advice that one type of hair dye can be tolerated if a reaction has occurred to the other. In addition cross-reactivities may occur. Henna may be used, but it is not always cosmetically acceptable. Some patients weakly sensitized to PPD are known to be able to continue dyeing their hair with PPD with impunity. Chan et al. found that 20 out of 33 patients with PPD allergy had a clinically relevant reaction attributed the use of hair

dyes. Follow-up showed that 3 of the 20 continued dyeing their hair using PPD hair dyes, 2 had recurrent dermatitis and lived with it, 1 had no problems [71], and 2 appeared to be clinically tolerant, as they were using PPD hair dyes at the time of patch testing but did not experience hair dye dermatitis.

A new generation of hair dyes has been developed, Food and Drug and Cosmetic hair dyes (FD and C) [50], but their practical value remains to be fully demonstrated. Forty hairdressers with PPD and PPD-related allergies were patch tested with ingredients and finished formulations of the FD and C dyes. Two had a positive patch test to one or more of the finished formulations. None reacted to the individual ingredients [50]. Time will show whether these hair dyes are a safe alternative to permanent hair dyes based on PPD and PPD-related substances.

Patients sensitized to PPD or PPD-related substances by hair dyeing may have cross or simultaneous sensitivity to textile dyes [52]; however, it rarely causes clinical problems.

31.2.8 Case Reports

Presented below are two case reports whose purpose is to provide a practical illustration of the presentation of hair-dye-related allergic contact dermatitis.

> **Case Reports**
>
> ■ A 50-year-old previously healthy woman had her hair dyed for the first time in her life at a hairdresser. No side-effects occurred. A year later, she dyed her hair with a nonpermanent hair dye at home and made the recommended pre-exposure test without any reaction. The following day, she developed scalp dermatitis with severe itching, spreading to her face, neck, and upper part of the thorax. As a further complication, the patient developed vesicular hand eczema for the first time in her life. Treatment with systemic and topical steroids was given for several months, leading to the gradual clearing of the dermatitis. Patch testing was performed in several sequences with the European Standard Series supplemented with selected cosmetic allergens and a hairdressers' series. At the initial patch testing, there was a +? result to PPD at days 3 and 7. Further, she reacted with a +? to her own hair collected at day 3 after the hair dye dermatitis had erupted.

An open exposure to the product, which had initiated the dermatitis, was negative both before (arm exposure at home) and after (back exposure at dermatological clinic) the allergic reaction to the product. None of the screening chemicals in the hairdressers' series gave a definite positive reaction. Only by patch testing with the individual hair dye ingredients (provided for individual patch testing by the producer) were the patient's reactions explained. The patient gave a positive patch test to 4-amino-3-nitrophenol and 3-nitro-*p*-hydroxyethylaminophenol at readings on days 3–4. These substances are not commercially available and the severe clinical reaction would have remained unexplained if patch testing had only been performed with PPD and PPD-related substances. The two substances are on the list of substances that, based on chemical considerations, have a moderate/strong allergenic potential (Table 2.1) and is considered for validation as a new screening tray [18].

■ A 39-year-old women with no previous skin disease had dyed her hair tips regularly once a year at the hairdressers. Following a dyeing with a permanent hair color of a reasonably fair shade, she developed a facial edema and oozing scalp dermatitis 3 days later. She received medical treatment from emergency service doctors and, later, her general practitioner, who, at first, suspected mumps due to the severe edema of her face. She received treatment with antihistamines only and the symptoms subsided after 1–2 weeks. Testing with the standard series and a hairdressers' series showed positive patch tests to PPD and PPD-related substances (toluene-2,5-diamine, nitro-*para*-toluenediamine) and 4-aminoazobenzene (probably cross-reactivity to textile azo dyes). Chemical analyses of the hair dye showed that it contained 0.27% PPD.

The case shows that the severe angioedema-like symptoms may be mistaken for other diseases and falsely treated as a type I reaction with only anti-histamines. Furthermore, fair colors may also cause severe reactions; in this case, only 0.27% PPD was present in the hair dye, while up to 6% is permitted [59].

References

1. Balzer W, Braun HJ, Chassot L, Clausen T (2001) Diaminopyrazoles: novel primary intermediates for hair dyeing formulations. Söfw J 127:12–16
2. Bonnevie P (1939) Aetiologie und pathogenese der Ekzemkrankheiten. Klinische Studien über die Ursachen der Ekzeme unter besonderer Berücksichtigung des Diagnostischen Wertes der Ekzemproben. Busch, Copenhagen/Barth, Leipzig, Germany
3. Sosted H, Hesse U, Menne T, Andersen KE, Johansen JD (2005) Contact dermatitis to hair dye in an adult Danish population – an interview based study. Br J Dermatol 153:132–135
4. Nohynek GJ, Fautz R, Benech-Kieffer F, Toutain H (2004) Toxicity and human health risk of hair dyes. Food Chem Toxicol 42:517–543
5. Sosted H, Agner T, Andersen KE, Menne T (2002) 55 cases of allergic reactions to hair dye: a descriptive, consumer complaint-based study. Contact Dermatitis 47:299–303
6. Uter W, Lessmann H, Geier J, Schnuch A (2003) Contact allergy to ingredients of hair cosmetics in female hairdressers and clients – an 8-year analysis of IVDK data. Contact Dermatitis 49:236–240
7. Cronin E (1980) Hair preparations. In: Cronin E (ed) Contact dermatitis. Churchill Livingstone, Edinburgh, pp 115–126
8. Hsu TS, Davis MD, el Azhary R, Corbett JF, Gibson LE (2001) Beard dermatitis due to para-phenylenediamine use in Arabic men. J Am Acad Dermatol 44:867–869
9. Frosch PJ, Burrows D, Camarasa JG, Dooms-Goossens A, Ducombs G, Lahti A, Menne T, Rycroft RJ, Shaw S, White IR et al. (1993) Allergic reactions to a hairdressers' series: results from 9 European centres. The European Environmental and Contact Dermatitis Research Group (EECDRG). Contact Dermatitis 28:180–183
10. Aguirre A, Zabala R, Sanz de Galdeano, Landa N, Diaz-Perez JL (1994) Positive patch tests to hydrogen peroxide in 2 cases. Contact Dermatitis 30:113
11. Brancaccio R, Cohen DE (1995) Contact leukoderma secondary to para-phenylenediamine. Contact Dermatitis 32:313
12. Sharma VK, Mandal SK, Sethuraman G, Bakshi NA (1999) Para-phenylenediamine-induced lichenoid eruptions. Contact Dermatitis 41:40–41
13. Tosti A, Bardazzi, F, Valeri F, Toni F (1987) Erythema multiforme with contact dermatitis to hair dyes. Contact Dermatitis 17:321–322
14. Avnstorp C, Rastogi SC, Menné T (2002) Acute fingertip dermatitis from temporary tattoo and quantitative chemical analysis of the product. Contact Dermatitis 47:119–120
15. Marcoux D, Couture-Trudel PM, Riboulet-Delmas G, Sasseville D (2002) Sensitization to para-phenylenediamine from a streetside temporary tattoo. Pediatr Dermatol 19:498–502
16. Sosted H, Menne T (2005) Allergy to 3-nitro-p-hydroxyethylamino-phenol and 4-amino-3-nitrophenol in a hair dye. Contact Dermatitis 52:317–319
17. Koopmans AK, Bruynzeel DP (2003) Is PPD a useful screening agent? Contact Dermatitis 48:89–92
18. Sosted H, Basketter DA, Estrada E, Johansen JD, Patlewicz GY (2004) Ranking of hair dye substances according to predicted sensitization potency: quantitative structure-activity relationships. Contact Dermatitis 51:241–254

19. Blanco R, de la Hoz B, Sanchez-Fernandez C, Sanchez-Cano M (1998) Allergy to 4-amino-3-nitrophenol in a hair dye. Contact Dermatitis 39:136

20. Ho SG, White IR, Rycroft RJ, McFadden JP (2004) A new approach to patch testing patients with para-phenylenediamine allergy secondary to temporary black henna tattoos. Contact Dermatitis 51:213–214

21. Krasteva M, Cristaudo A, Hall B, Orton D, Rudzki E, Santucci B, Toutain H, Wilkinson J (2002) Contact sensitivity to hair dyes can be detected by the consumer open test. Eur J Dermatol 12:322–326

22. Pasche-Koo F, French L, Piletta-Zanin PA, Hauser C (1998) Contact urticaria and shock to hair dye. Allergy 53:904–905

23. Mavroleon G, Begishvili B, Frew AJ (1998) Anaphylaxis to hair dye: a case report. Clin Exp Allergy 28:121–122

24. Fukunaga T, Kawagoe R, Hozumi H, Kanzaki T (1996) Contact anaphylaxis due to para-phenylenediamine. Contact Dermatitis 35:185–186

25. Belton AL, Chira T (1997) Fatal anaphylactic reaction to hair dye. Am J Forensic Med Pathol 18:290–292

26. Landsteiner J, Jacobs JL (1936) Studies on the sensitization of animals with simple chemical compounds. II. J Exp Med 64:625–629

27. Mayer RL (1954) Group-sensitization to compounds of quinone structure and its biochemical basis role of these substances in cancer. Prog Allergy 4:79–172

28. Basketter DA, Liden C (1992) Further investigation into the prohapten concept: reactions to benzene derivatives in man. Contact Dermatitis 27:90–92

29. Lisi P, Hansel K (1998) Is benzoquinone the prohapten in cross-sensitivity among aminobenzene compounds? Contact Dermatitis 39:304–306

30. Krasteva M, Nicolas J-F, Chabeau G, Garrigue JL, Bour H, Thivolet J, Schmitt D (1993) Dissociation of allergenic and immunogenic functions in contact sensitivity to para-phenylenediamine. Int Arch Allergy Immunol 102:200–204

31. McFadden JP, Kullavanijaya P, Duangdeeden I, Fletcher S, Basketter DA (2005) p-Phenylenediamine allergy: the role of Bandrowski's base. J Clin Immunol (in press)

32. Kawakubo Y, Merk HF, Masaoudi TA, Sieben S, Blomeke B (2000) N-acetylation of paraphenylenediamine in human skin and keratinocytes. J Pharmacol Exp Ther 292:150–155

33. Schnuch A, Westphal GA, Muller MM, Schulz TG, Geier J, Brasch J, Merk HF, Kawakubo Y, Richter G, Koch P, Fuchs T, Gutgesell T, Reich K, Gebhardt M, Becker D, Grabbe J, Szliska C, Aberer W, Hallier E (1998) Genotype and phenotype of N-acetyltransferase 2 (NAT2) polymorphism in patients with contact allergy. Contact Dermatitis 38:209–211

34. Picardo M, Zompetta C, Grandinetti M, Ameglio F, Santucci B, Faggioni A, Passi S (1996) Paraphenylenediamine, a contact allergen, induces oxidative stress in normal human keratinocytes in culture. Br J Dermatol 134:681–685

35. Mathur AK, Gupta BN, Singh S, Singh A, Narang S (1992) Dermal toxicity of paraphenylenediamine. Biomed Environ Sci 5:321–324

36. Yokozeki H, Watanabe K, Igawa K, Miyazaki Y, Katayama I, Nishioka K (2001) Gammadelta T cells assist alphabeta T cells in the adoptive transfer of contact hypersensitivity to para-phenylenediamine. Clin Exp Immunol 125:351–359

37. Sieben S, Kawakubo Y, Al Masaoudi T, Merk HF, Blomeke B (2002) Delayed-type hypersensitivity reaction to para-phenylenediamine is mediated by 2 different pathways of antigen recognition by specific alphabeta human T-cell clones. J Allergy Clin Immunol 109:1005–1011

38. Kligman A (1966) The identification of contact allergens by human assay. 3. The maximization test: a procedure for screening and rating contact sensitizers. J Invest Dermatol 47:393–409

39. Marzulli FN, Maibach HI (1974) The use of graded concentrations in studying skin sensitizers: experimental contact sensitization in man. Food Cosmet Toxicol 12:219–227

40. Basketter DA, Scholes EW (1992) Comparison of the local lymph node assay with the guinea-pig maximization test for the detection of a range of contact allergens. Food Chem Toxicol 30:65–69

41. Basketter DA, Gerberick GF (1996) An interlaboratory evaluation of the Buehler test for the identification and classification of skin sensitizers. Contact Dermatitis 35:146–151

42. Kimber I, Basketter DA, Berthold K, Butler M, Garrigue JL, Lea LJ, Newsome C, Roggeband R, Steiling W, Stropp G, Waterman S, Wiemann C (2001) Skin sensitization testing in potency and risk assessment. Toxicol Sci 59:198–208

43. Gerberick GF, Ryan CA, Kern PS, Dearman RJ, Kimber I, Patlewicz GY, Basketter DA (2004) A chemical dataset for the evaluation of alternative approaches to skin-sensitization testing. Contact Dermatitis 50:274–288

44. Armstrong DK, Jones AB, Smith HR, Ross JS, White IR, Rycroft RJ, McFadden JP (1999) Occupational sensitization to p-phenylenediamine: a 17-year review. Contact Dermatitis 41:348–349

45. Marks JG, Belsito DV, DeLeo VA, Fowler JF Jr, Fransway AF, Maibach HI, Mathias CG, Nethercott JR, Rietschel RL, Sherertz EF, Storrs FJ, Taylor JS (1998) North American Contact Dermatitis Group patch test results for the detection of delayed-type hypersensitivity to topical allergens. J Am Acad Dermatol 38:911–918

46. Sharma VK, Chakrabarti A (1998) Contact sensitizers in Chandigarh, India. A study of 200 patients with the European standard series. Contact Dermatitis 38:127–131

47. Schnuch A, Uter W, Geier J, Gefeller O; IVDK study group (2002) Epidemiology of contact allergy: an estimation of morbidity employing the clinical epidemiology and drug-utilization research (CE-DUR) approach. Contact Dermatitis 47:32–39

48. Schafer T, Bohler E, Ruhdorfer S, Weigl L, Wessner D, Filipiak B, Wichmann HE, Ring J (2001) Epidemiology of contact allergy in adults. Allergy 56:1192–1196 (Erratum: Allergy 57:178, 2002)

49. Basketter DA, Duangdeeden I, Gilmour NG, Kullavanijaya P, McFadden J (2004) Prevalence of contact allergy in an adult Thai population. Contact Dermatitis 50:128–129

50. Fautz R, Fuchs A, van der WH, Henny V, Smits L (2002) Hair dye-sensitized hairdressers: the cross-reaction pattern with new generation hair dyes. Contact Dermatitis 46:319–324

51. Goon AT-J, Gilmour NJ, Basketter DA, White IR, Rycroft RJG, McFadden JP (2003) High frequency of simultaneous sensitivity to Disperse Orange 3 in patients with positive patch tests to para-phenylenediamine. Contact Dermatitis 48:248–250

52. Seidenari S, Mantovani L, Manzini BM, Pignatti M (1997) Cross-sensitizations between azo dyes and para-amino compound. A study of 236 azo-dye-sensitive subjects. Contact Dermatitis 36:91–96

53. Herve-Bazin B, Gradiski D, Duprat P, Marignac B, Foussereau J, Cavalier C, Bierber P (1977) Occupational eczema from N-isopropyl-N'-phenylparaphenylenediamine (IPPD) and N-dimethyl-1,3 butyl-N'-phenylparaphenylenediamine (DMPPD) in tyres. Contact Dermatitis 3:1–15

54. Ho SGY, Basketter DA, Jefferies D, Rycroft RJG, White IR, McFadden JP (2005) Analysis of para-phenylenediamine allergic patients in relation to strength of patch test reaction. Br J Dermatol 153:364–367

55. Frosch PJ, Burrows D, Camarasa JG, Dooms-Goossens A, Ducombs G, Lahti A, Menne T, Rycroft RJ, Shaw S, White IR et al. (1993) Allergic reactions to a hairdressers' series: results from 9 European centres. The European Environmental and Contact Dermatitis Research Group (EECDRG). Contact Dermatitis 28:180–183

56. Uter W, Lessmann H, Geier J, Schnuch A (2003) Contact allergy to ingredients of hair cosmetics in female hairdressers and clients – an 8-year analysis of IVDK data. Contact Dermatitis 49:236–240

57. Guerra L, Tosti A, Bardazzi F, Pigatto P, Lisi P, Santucci B, Valsecchi R, Schena D, Angelini G, Sertoli A et al. (1992) Contact dermatitis in hairdressers: the Italian experience. Gruppo Italiano Ricerca Dermatiti da Contatto e Ambientali. Contact Dermatitis 26:101–107

58. Nettis E, Marcandrea M, Colanardi MC, Paradiso MT, Ferrannini A, Tursi A (2003) Results of standard series patch testing in patients with occupational allergic contact dermatitis. Allergy 58:1304–1307

59. European Communities (2004) Council directive 76/768/EEC of 27 July 1976 on the approximation of the laws of the member states relating to cosmetic products, annex III amended. European Communities Official Journal, L262

60. Sosted H, Rastogi SC, Andersen KE, Johansen JD, Menne T (2004) Hair dye contact allergy: quantitative exposure assessment of selected products and clinical cases. Contact Dermatitis 50:344–348

61. Guerra L, Bardazzi F, Tosti A (1992) Contact dermatitis in hairdressers' clients. Contact Dermatitis 26:108–111

62. Vilaplana J, Romaguera C, Grimalt F (1991) Contact dermatitis from resorcinol in a hair dye. Contact Dermatitis 24:151–152

63. Garcia Ortiz JC, Terron M, Bellido J (1997) Contact allergy to henna. Int Arch Allergy Immunol 114:298–299

64. Perez RG, Gonzalez R, Gonzalez M, Soloeta R (2003) Palpebral eczema due to contact allergy to henna used as a hair dye. Contact Dermatitis 48:238

65. Nigam PK, Saxena AK (1988) Allergic contact dermatitis from henna. Contact Dermatitis 18:55–56

66. Bolhaar ST, Mulder M, van Ginkel CJ (2001) IgE-mediated allergy to henna. Allergy 56:248

67. Majoie IM, Bruynzeel DP (1996) Occupational immediate-type hypersensitivity to henna in a hairdresser. Am J Contact Dermat 7:38–40

68. Fisher AA, Dooms-Goossens A (1976) Persulfate hair bleach reactions. Cutaneous and respiratory manifestations. Arch Dermatol 112:1407–1409

69. Bowling JC, Scarisbrick J, Warin AP, Downs AM (2002) Allergic contact dermatitis from trideceth-2-carboxamide monoethanolamine (MEA) in a hair dye. Contact Dermatitis 47:116–117

70. Kligman AM (1966) The identification of contact allergens by human assay. II. Factors influencing the induction and measurement of allergic contact dermatitis. J Invest Dermatol 47:375–392

71. Chan YC, Ng SK, Goh CL (2001) Positive patch-test reactions to para-phenylenediamine, their clinical relevance and the concept of clinical tolerance. Contact Dermatitis 45:217–220

72. Edwards EK Jr, Edwards EK (1982) Allergic contact dermatitis to lead acetate in a hair dye. Cutis 30:629–630

Contents

32.1 Introduction

There exist more than 50 metals and an enormous number of naturally occurring and manmade alloys and metal compounds. A few metals – foremost, ions and compounds of nickel, chromium, and cobalt – belong to the most important contact allergens, causing allergic contact dermatitis in a large proportion of the general population, as well as in large occupational groups.

Metals are present in the Earth's crust, usually as oxides, sulfides, and silicates, and only the precious metals in metallic form. Metallic compounds occur naturally in drinking water and in food, and some are probably essential nutrients for humans. Many metallic metals and metal compounds are toxic to the environment, and some belong to the most important environmental hazards. The industrial use of many metals, their alloys, and their compounds, is extremely important in modern society, as they possess valuable mechanical, electrical, and chemical properties. The most often used metals are iron, chromium, lead, nickel, cobalt, aluminum, and copper. Mining, refining, production, and trading of metals represent enormous economic values. Skin problems related to metals are caused not primarily by metals in the natural environment, but are related to human activity – by metallic metals and metal compounds in consumer products and industrial processes. Some recent reviews and textbooks cover metallurgical, occupational, and toxicological aspects of metals and contact dermatitis [1–9].

Metals are elements with a metallic luster, and they are good conductors of electricity and heat. The metals are divided into different, overlapping groups, depending on their chemical and physical properties and their use. There are 50 metals and a few metalloids, the latter including arsenic. The expression *heavy metals*, which includes most metals, is often used. Toxic and non-essential heavy metals (TNEM) are cadmium, mercury, and lead, which are those often termed heavy metals. The toxicity of metal is, however, quite unrelated to density. Precious metals are gold, silver, rhodium, palladium, platinum, and some other platinum metals.

Metallic items are generally made of alloys, which may be combined, soldered, plated, etc. Common examples of nickel-containing alloys are stainless steels (iron/nickel/chromium), copper-nickel, and nickel-silver (nickel/copper/zinc). Brass (copper/zinc) and red gold (gold/silver/copper) are examples of nickel-free alloys. Alloys are compounds or solid solutions of more than one element in metallic form, but cannot be considered as mixtures of metals. Resistance to corrosion on skin contact varies widely between different alloys, depending on their composition. This is of great importance for the probability of alloys inducing and eliciting allergic contact dermatitis. Metallurgical aspects of nickel and other metals, and their corrosion in contact with sweat have been reviewed [1]. Metal compounds are often referred to by toxicologists as soluble or insoluble. Their solubility in sweat, however, is generally not mentioned.

Why some metals act as potent or clinically important contact allergens and others do not is not fully understood. The question of multiple metal reactivity, cross-reactivity, and multiple sensitizations also remains under discussion. The clinical relevance of some metallic metals and metal compounds as contact allergens is still controversial. Some metal compounds are potent contact allergens in experimental animals, but not all of them present clinically relevant problems.

Several metallic metals and their compounds present important occupational health hazards, and several have been recognized by the International Agency for Research on Cancer (IARC) as human carcinogens [10, 11]. Arsenic and arsenic compounds are unique in the formation of skin cancer, related to oral medical therapy and inhalation exposure. The respiratory system is the most frequent target site of metal-induced cancers in humans, and metal-induced respiratory tumors have occurred only from inhalation exposure. Compounds of arsenic, beryllium, cadmium, chromium, and nickel have been associated with pulmonary carcinomas, and hexavalent chromium compounds and certain nickel compounds have been associated with nasosinal cavity tumors.

Core Message

■ Nickel, chromium, and cobalt, their ions and compounds, belong to the most important skin sensitizers.
Consumer products and occupational skin exposure are the main sources of sensitization and elicitation.
The pure metals, their alloys, platings, and compounds have different abilities to cause allergic contact dermatitis.

References

1. Flint GN (1998) A metallurgical approach to metal contact dermatitis. Contact Dermatitis 39:213–221
2. Rietschel RL, Fowler JF Jr (1995) Contact dermatitis and other reactions to metals. In: Rietschel RL, Fowler JF Jr (eds) Fisher's contact dermatitis, 4th edn. Williams and Wilkins, Baltimore, Md., pp 808–885
3. Burrows D, Adams RM, Flint GN (1999) Metals. In: Adams RM (ed) Occupational skin disease, 3rd edn. Saunders, Philadelphia, Pa., pp 395–433
4. Lidén C (2000) Nickel. In: Kanerva L, Elsner P, Wahlberg JE, Maibach HI (eds) Handbook of occupational dermatology. Springer, Berlin Heidelberg New York, pp 524–533
5. Burrows D (2000) Chromium. In: Kanerva L, Elsner P, Wahlberg JE, Maibach HI (eds) Handbook of occupational dermatology. Springer, Berlin Heidelberg New York, pp 534–540
6. Fischer T (2000) Hard metals. In: Kanerva L, Elsner P, Wahlberg JE, Maibach HI (eds) Handbook of occupational dermatology. Springer, Berlin Heidelberg New York, pp 541–543

32

7. Isaksson M, Bruze M (2000) Gold. In: Kanerva L, Elsner P, Wahlberg JE, Maibach HI (eds) Handbook of occupational dermatology. Springer, Berlin Heidelberg New York, pp 544–550
8. Wahlberg JE (2000) Other metals. In: Kanerva L, Elsner P, Wahlberg JE, Maibach HI (eds) Handbook of occupational dermatology. Springer, Berlin Heidelberg New York, pp 551–555
9. Lidén C, Maibach HI, Wahlberg JE (1995) Skin. In: Goyer RA, Klaassen CD, Waalkes MP (eds) Metal toxicology. Academic, New York, pp 447–464
10. Waalkes MP (1995) Metal carcinogenesis. In: Goyer RA, Klaassen CD, Waalkes MP (eds) Metal toxicology. Academic, New York, pp 47–69
11. Zenz C, Dickerson OB, Horvath EP (1994) Occupational medicine, 3rd edn. Mosby, St Louis, Mo.

32.2 Nickel

Nickel (Ni) was first isolated by the Swedish mineralogist Axel Fredrik Cronstedt in the middle of the 18th century. Since the 19th century, nickel has become widely used in many alloys, particularly in stainless steel [1]. Contact dermatitis from nickel was first recognized in 1889 in the plating industry [2]. Nickel allergy was first verified by patch testing by Schittenhelm and Stockinger in Kiel in 1925 [3]. Nickel has since been established as an important ubiquitous contact allergen.

Most cases of primary nickel sensitization come from exposure to metal items made of nickel alloys designed to be in prolonged and direct skin contact, such as costume jewelry, suspenders, etc. But primary sensitization and elicitation may also take place on the hands as an occupational skin disease. Further to contact allergy, nickel compounds have other toxicological properties, such as carcinogenicity, pulmonary effects, and general toxicity. These various types of toxicological effects are unrelated to contact allergy, as they are caused by different nickel compounds and different exposures [1]. Milestones in our understanding of nickel dermatitis are summarized in Table 2.1.

Core Message

■ Occupational and, later, consumer product nickel contact allergy has been frequent for the last 100 years.

32.2.1 Nickel Use and Exposure

In nature, nickel is present as oxides and sulfides bound in the ore, together with cobalt, copper, and small amounts of platinum, palladium, and gold. Global nickel deposits and reserves are large and are mainly present in Canada, Australia, and Siberia. The main primary and end uses of nickel are shown in Table 2.2 [4]. Nickel is first and foremost used in stainless steel, together with iron and chromium. Stainless steel is one of the backbones in modern society and is widely used in industry, construction, cars, shipbuilding, and private homes. Only a minor part of nickel is used in items designed to be in prolonged skin contact. The nickel sulfides and oxides found in nature are not allergenic. Only the free nickel ion acts as a hapten. The presence of nickel and co-

Table 2.1. Milestones in the history of nickel dermatitis

1889	Description of nickel dermatitis in plating workers
1925	Patch testing with nickel sulfate in plating workers
1935	Large-scale consumer nickel dermatitis
1950s	Suspender dermatitis with secondary spread
1970s	Nickel allergy and hand eczema
	Systemic contact dermatitis
1980s	Epidemiological studies – general population
	Hazard identification – risk assessment
1990s	Strategy for risk management – prevention – legislation
2000	Implementation of EU Nickel Directive

Table 2.2. Distribution and end uses of primary nickel, 1996 [4]

Distribution of primary nickel	%	End uses of primary nickel	%
Stainless steel	65	Consumer products	19
Non-ferrous alloys	13	Building and construction materials	17
Plating	9	Automobile production	11
Alloy steels	8	Process equipment	10
Foundry	3	Chemical industry	8
Other	2	Electronics	8
		General engineering	6
		Other	4
		Railway/transportation equipment	3
		Aerospace materials	3
		Petroleum industry	3
		Electric power generation	2
		Marine equipment	2
		Nickel chemicals	1

balt together in nature explain the frequent occurrence of simultaneous contact allergy. Cobalt is more costly than nickel. The amount of cobalt in nickel is, therefore, decreasing, as also seems the frequency of concomitant nickel and cobalt allergy. Nickel and chromium do not occur together in nature and this combined contact allergy is, consequently, rare and mainly related to certain occupational exposures.

The most important factor for the induction and elicitation of nickel contact allergy is the amount of nickel per skin unit area present in the epidermis as a consequence of nickel exposure. The free nickel ion may be either present in the industrial environment or be leached out of nickel-plated surfaces or nickel alloys easily corroded by the influence of human sweat [5]. The unit for the quantification of exposure to contact allergens is µg/cm². When it comes to nickel exposure from nickel released from metal items designed to be in prolonged skin contact, µg/cm² over time is used as release may vary over time [6].

Bang-Pedersen et al. introduced the idea that the significant risk factor for nickel contact allergy was the amount of nickel released from the alloy in synthetic sweat and not the total concentration of nickel in the alloy [7]. Later studies showed that items such as metal buttons and earrings known to induce and elicit allergic contact dermatitis released large amounts of nickel in synthetic sweat [8, 9]. Menné et al. [6] conceptualized the idea that, by investigating a range of well-defined nickel alloys and coatings, which were known either to induce nickel allergy or to be safe with respect to nickel allergy, in relation to nickel release in synthetic sweat and reactivity in nickel-allergic individuals, operational risk assessments could be obtained. Based on this research, a limit of 0.5 µg/cm² per week of nickel release was suggested as a reasonably safe practical compromise. Alloys releasing less than this amount – typically, stainless steel or white gold – will only rarely elicit a reaction in nickel-sensitive individuals, and alloys releasing more than 0.5 µg/cm² per week, typically nickel-coated items, will provoke a large number of allergic reactions in already sensitized individuals [6, 10–14]. Roughly, the dimethylglyoxime (DMG) test discriminates between these two types of alloy [6], but important exceptions occur, particularly in the borderline area [12].

Nickel is frequently used as an interliner for thin (on the order of µm) gold plating. These are highly porous and do not protect against nickel allergy [5, 10]. If such alloys are used for ear piercing, both gold and nickel may be left in the tissue, probably explaining the high risk of induction of primary sensitization by this procedure [15].

Occupational nickel exposures on the hands are more difficult to quantify. Undoubtedly, industrial exposure, particularly in the plating industry, was previously significant [2, 3, 16], though nickel allergy seems to be a rare problem in nickel refineries. Tolerance developing from inhaled nickel may possibly be an explanation [1]. Quantification of nickel exposure in different industries has been documented [17–19]. Many work tools release large amounts of nickel in synthetic sweat and elicitation of nickel hand eczema is a possibility [20]. The amount of nickel released from coins during normal handling is generally insufficient to elicit a reaction in nickel-sensitized individuals [21, 22]. Nickel exposure today is not only defined as exposures in specific industries, but is more related to the individual job. It is, therefore, important, in the case of a positive patch test to nickel, to trace the source of primary sensitization (typically, costume jewelry, jeans buttons, etc.), evaluate previous and current exposure to metal items in direct skin contact, and, in the case of hand eczema, evaluate personal and occupational exposure using the DMG test and other exposure measurements (see below).

Nickel is frequently found in consumer products, including washing liquids and powders, and other household products, at a concentration of 1–5 ppm as an impurity. Only exceptionally this does give rise to clinical disease in nickel-sensitized individuals [23, 24].

> ### Core Message
>
> ■ The risk of nickel sensitization depends upon nickel release from metal items designed to be in direct and prolonged contact with the skin expressed as µg/cm² over time.

32.2.2 Quantification of Nickel Exposure

The relevant nickel exposure parameter is the free nickel ion in the environment or the nickel skin concentration. Chemical methods have been developed to assess exposure based on atomic absorption and standardized as outlined in Chap. 25. It is particularly important to investigate nickel release from metal surfaces designed to be in direct and prolonged skin contact. The DMG test has been refined and represents a quick and easy spot test. False-positive and false-negative reactions occur (Chap. 25). These

32

methods are not ideal for obtaining an overall impression of exposure in the individual person or worker, as they are exposed to so many different nickel-releasing alloys, as well as to nickel in solutions, e.g., oils [19] and water [18]. To quantify nickel exposure, nickel in nails and in skin may be more relevant parameters. Nickel binds and accumulates in the stratum corneum and the nail plate. A single patch test with nickel sulfate generates a deposit of nickel in the epidermis, with a high concentration in the upper part of the stratum corneum and a declining concentration gradient though the epidermis. Fullerton et al. [25–27] and Hostynek [28] have illustrated that repeated skin tape stripping may be a powerful tool to quantify nickel exposure.

Nickel in nails may be used as a parameter of nickel exposure. Peters et al. [29] found a significant difference in the nail concentrations in differently occupationally exposed groups (Table 2.3). Allenby and Basketter [30] observed that repeated thumb immersion in a 1-ppm nickel solution in sodium lauryl sulfate led to the accumulation of nickel in thumbnails at up to 22.2 ppm. Nielsen et al. [31], in a controlled exposure study, including nickel-allergic patients with hand eczema, showed that repeated skin exposure to 10–100 ppm provoked a flare-up of eczema. The corresponding nickel nail concentrations are shown in Table 2.3, together with other experimental provocation studies and occupational field studies. It appears that moderate nickel exposure, as probably present in many workplaces, gives a nickel nail concentration comparable with those concentrations obtained in experimental exposure studies where a significant flare-up of dermatitis was achieved. Such methods may serve as a more objective evaluation of suspected occupational nickel hand eczema. Similarly, the nickel skin concentration seems to be a useful parameter in experimental exposure studies [32]. Such methods need to be standardized and made generally available for the evaluation of the patients with nickel allergy and hand eczema.

Core Message

■ Nickel exposure can be quantified by nickel skin and nickel nail measurements.

32.2.3 Patch Testing with Nickel

That nickel sulfate, and not the chloride, is used for patch testing is probably accidental. When making the first patch test with nickel sulfate, Schittenhelm and Stockinger [3] simply used the solution from the nickel bath to which the workers were exposed. In the 1930s, Bonnevie with this background included nickel sulfate in the first standard patch test series. Based on this, nickel sulfate 2.5% or nickel sulfate 5% in petrolatum is now used for the standard series in North America and Europe, respectively [33]. The TRUE Test also uses nickel sulfate and tends to elicit stronger reactions. False-positive reactions may occur in atopics, in whom, particularly, follicular irritant reactions are seen [34]. Weak true-positive reactions can also show a follicular pattern. False-negative reactions undoubtedly occur. In such cases, reactions can be obtained with nickel chloride 5% (actually increasing the Ni++ concentration) or by adding penetration enhancers to the patch test, such as DMSO (Chap. 22). None of these approaches are suitable for routine testing, as irritant reactions are common. Patch test sensitization from nickel sulfate 5% in petrolatum has never been documented. This is in agreement with the experiences of Kligman [35] and Vandenberg and Epstein [36], who could only obtain experimental nickel sensitization by repeated exposures to high nickel concentrations in combination with irritants. When a dermatologist-obtained detailed history of nickel exposure is compared with the outcome of patch testing, there is a high degree of

Table 2.3. Nickel in nails reflecting exposure

Type of exposure		Nickel µg/g (mean)	Reference
Occupational	None (controls)	1.19	[29]
Occupational	Moderate	29.20	[29]
Occupational	Heavy	123.00	[29]
Experimental[a]	Immersion of finger in nickel 1 ppm for 23 days, twice a day	7.80	[30]
Experimental	Immersion of finger in 10 ppm nickel once a day for 1 week	5.50	[32]
Experimental	Immersion of finger in 100 ppm nickel once a day for 1 week	12.00	[32]
Experimental	Baseline	1.58	[32]

[a] Four observations

correspondence [18, 37]. If the history is taken via a short questionnaire, both false-positive and false-negative histories of nickel allergy are common. Typically, the nickel-sensitized patients have a history of previous inflammation, related to ear piercing or from exposure to cheap jewelry, and later, repeated instances of eczema related to metal items. False-positive histories typically have only one such incident and typically on hot summer days. The positive nickel patch test is reproducible [38], but its strength varies in the individual patients over time [39].

A locally increased specific hyper-reactivity may persist after nickel dermatitis [40]. This phenomenon is specific both with respect to allergic and irritant contact dermatitis [41]. The association between atopy and nickel allergy is controversial. In general population patch test studies, nickel allergy is equally common among those with and without a positive prick test [42]. Hospital-based materials are more difficult to interpret and both a decreased and increased frequency of positive nickel patch test reactions has been reported in atopic patients (Chap. 9). One explanation may be that active atopic dermatitis tends to down-regulate the type IV response and, thereby, the nickel patch test.

Dose–response studies have been performed with nickel sulfate and nickel chloride using both occluded and non-occluded exposure. The concentration threshold for reactivity to a single exposure has been established to be 1.5 $\mu g/cm^2$ in open testing [43] and 0.5 $\mu g/cm^2$ in closed applications [11, 44, 45]. For the weakest positive reactions, papular/follicular morphology is typical. This is not well described in the literature and both the hair follicle and the sweat duct may be important routes for nickel absorption (Chap. 11).

In vitro testing with haptens is dealt with in Chap. 2. There is comprehensive literature on the diagnosis of nickel allergy by the lymphocyte transformation test. Individuals with a positive history of metal dermatitis, but negative patch test, may have an elevated lymphocyte transformation test. Further, it has been observed that the lymphocyte transformation test to nickel is elevated in non-nickel-sensitive controls, compared to cord blood. The implication of this finding is uncertain, and the consequences for clinical disease are not investigated [46].

Core Message

■ The standard nickel patch test is safe and reproducible.

32.2.4 Clinical Picture

Historically, nickel dermatitis was an occupational hand and forearm eczema seen in workers in the plating industry [2, 3, 16]. The combined effect of irritancy and contact allergy from exposure to high nickel concentrations, combined with low hygiene standards and the unavailability of treatment led to the severe itchy dermatitis seen in these workers. The first cases of consumer nickel dermatitis were seen from nickel released from spectacle frames and wristwatches [47]. Bonnevie [48] was the first to patch test a large group of eczema patients with a standard series containing nickel sulfate. This led to the recognition of suspender dermatitis as a consequence of primary nickel sensitization. In the 1950s and 1960s, Calnan [49] and Marcussen [50] published a large number of nickel dermatitis cases. Separation of nickel dermatitis into the primary and secondary eruption was introduced. The primary eruption meant the place of primary sensitization, typically related to the suspender area or other metal contact sites. The secondary eruptions were symmetrical eruptions with vesicular hand eczema, eczema in the flexural areas, and on the eyelids. It was speculated that this tendency to spread was caused by cutaneous nickel dissemination or a hematogenous spread caused by nickel absorption through the area of suspender dermatitis. Research on systemic contact dermatitis from nickel (see later) in the 1970s and 1980s indicated that the secondary eruptions seen in females with persistent metal object dermatitis (e.g., earrings) are equivalent to systemic contact dermatitis and are caused by systemic nickel exposure from nickel skin absorption. The causes of primary nickel eruptions (sensitization) have changed with fashion, from suspenders to buttons in blue jeans and, more recently, to ear piercing [15, 51–53]. The primary eruption of nickel allergy differs around the world, depending on local fashion and regulation of nickel skin exposure (see later). The severity of nickel dermatitis depends upon whether the condition is recognized and further nickel exposure from metal items, in direct and prolonged skin contact is avoided, and whether occupational nickel hand contact can be minimized.

Core Message

■ Occupational nickel dermatitis presents as chronic hand eczema. Consumer nickel dermatitis is present in skin areas in direct and prolonged contact with costume jewelry, buttons etc., eventually complicated by vesicular hand eczema.

32.2.5 Systemic Contact Dermatitis

Systemic contact dermatitis in general and from medicaments specifically is dealt with in Chaps. 16 and 35, respectively. Systemic contact dermatitis is an eruption, including vesicular hand eczema, flexural eczema, flare-up of earlier eczema sites of contact dermatitis, and the "baboon syndrome" [54, 55], in individuals with a contact allergy if they are exposed systemically (orally, by inhalation or transcutaneously) to the specific hapten. The early reports of nickel dermatitis already described the tendency to a more widespread dermatitis [3]. Christensen and Möller [56] were the first to provoke systemic contact dermatitis experimentally in patients with nickel allergy. A number of later studies have confirmed their observations. There is a clear tendency towards a dose response, with few reacting at a dose below 0.5 mg elemental nickel and the majority reacting at 5.6 mg [57, 58]. Flare-up reactions depend upon the degree of earlier exposure and time period since the last eruption [50]. Experimental provocation doses are higher than the daily nickel intake in food, which ranges between 100–300 μg per day. Under normal circumstances, a number of factors interfere with the amount of nickel absorbed, among them are alcohol intake, atopy [59], medicaments, and the composition of food. Release of nickel from infusion cannulae, dialysis equipment, internal prostheses, and dental braces is a rare cause of systemic nickel contact dermatitis.

Core Message

■ Systemic contact dermatitis should be suspected in chronic cases of nickel dermatitis with vesicular hand eczema and, eventually, a more widespread dermatitis where external nickel exposure is excluded.

32.2.6 Epidemiology

Earlier, it was believed that the number of patients receiving medical treatment reflected the number of individuals with a contact allergy to nickel. Based upon this assumption, Marcussen [60] estimated the frequency of nickel allergy to be one in ten thousand females. In the 1970s, ideas arose that contact allergy to nickel, and also to other haptens, were probably very common and that those cases seen by dermatologists represented only the most severe and complicated cases. Independent studies in Scandinavia and the US [61–63] disclosed a population frequency for nickel allergy of approximately 10% in females and 1–2% in males. Later, more comprehensive studies have confirmed these findings and illustrated a higher frequency, particularly in the youngest age groups [64]. Recently, this picture has changed and nickel allergy seems to decrease in the younger age groups, probably reflecting exposure regulation [65–67]. Most of those in the general population who have a positive patch test to nickel have a healthy skin at the time of examination, but give a history of earlier ear piercing, jewelry dermatitis, and/or hand eczema. In those countries where studies of the general population have been done, the figures are relatively similar worldwide.

Clinical patch test data published over the last 50 - years have invariably put nickel as the most common contact allergen in women worldwide. While most other allergens in the standard series react at a frequency of 2–4%, nickel is at a level of 15–25%. This is not because nickel is a particularly strong allergen. The human maximization test [35] classified nickel as a medium–strong sensitizer. The reason for the high frequency has been the uncontrolled nickel exposure in females from costume jewelry, suspenders, and ear piercing. Explanations for differences in frequencies between patients patch tested at different centers can be large, and may not necessarily reflect real differences either in frequency or in exposure pattern.

Data over time from the same patch test center may be more interesting, as major variables are controlled. Such data from Malmö, Sweden [39], illustrate an increase in the frequency of positive patch test to nickel in females from 7% in 1962 to 29% in 1997, and from 1% to 6% in males during the same time period.

Three Danish patch test centers, using similar patch test technology with unchanged staff and unchanged referral patterns, have compared their patch data from 1986 to 1998, standardized with respect to sex, age, atopy, leg ulcers, and occupation (MOAHL index). The frequency of nickel allergy in children (0–18 years of age) has fallen from 25.8% in 1986 to 9.2% in 1998 [68]. Present or past jewelry dermatitis was identified in most patients with a positive patch test. 33.2% of the nickel-sensitive patients seen in 1998 were judged to have a current non-occupational exposure to nickel, as compared to 73.5% in 1986. A similar trend has been observed in Germany and Aalborg, Denmark [69, 70]. These changes might be a consequence of the regulation of nickel skin exposure (see later).

Core Message

■ Nickel is the most common contact allergen in females, affecting 10% of all women worldwide. Frequencies between 20 and 30% are seen among patch-tested patients.

32.2.7 Hand Eczema and Nickel Allergy

Nickel can induce or aggravate hand eczema by four different pathogenic mechanisms (Table 2.4). Hand eczema is frequently a multifactorial disease and the different types of pathogenesis may operate together. Atopy is not specifically mentioned, but is known to be an aggravating factor for the prognosis of nickel hand eczema [45, 71, 72]. Earlier nickel dermatitis in the same skin region decreases the concentration threshold for reactivity [40]. This mechanism and its combination with irritants might also operate together with the four main etiologies [73].

There is solid historical evidence that high concentrations of nickel sulfate or nickel chloride in the plating industry both induced and elicited hand eczema [2, 3, 16]. Regarding moderate nickel exposure, point two in Table 2.4, the clinical evidence is more limited. Wall and Calnan [17] described seven workers in the electronic industry, in whom allergic nickel eczema was primarily induced on the hands by an exposure concentration of 40 ppm. A controlled hand exposure study in the nickel-sensitive using a 1 ppm concentration did not provoke any aggravation [30]. In a double-blind controlled exposure study over 2 weeks, a statistically significant aggravation was seen from using 10 ppm and 100 ppm nickel in patients with nickel allergy and low-grade hand eczema [31]. This exposure level is probably not uncommon in many industries, as indicated by nickel nail measurements.

Vesicular hand eczema caused by transcutaneous absorption of nickel from jewelry dermatitis, suspender dermatitis, etc., is probably still common today [74, 75]. The vesicular eruption appears on the hands as a systemic contact dermatitis because of transcutaneous absorption of nickel. It has been shown that elimination of metal items causing contact dermatitis may lead to the clearance of hand eczema in a significant number of patients [75].

Finally, nickel hand eczema may be a part of systemic contact dermatitis, with vesicular hand eczema provoked by nickel in food or nickel released from dental braces or metal prostheses (see Chap. 16).

The frequency of occupational nickel hand eczema will vary from one country to the other, depending upon the perception of the disease entity, regional industries, and local laws. Recent reviews include Fischer et al. [76] and Shah et al. [77]. In the period 1984–1991, a total number of 1,486 cases of occupational nickel dermatitis were notified to the Danish authorities in a background population of 5 million [78]. Most cases had been notified by dermatologists based on patch testing, occupational history, and assessment of exposure to nickel at a workplace by using the DMG test. Developments of methods for exposure assessment may improve the quality of the medico-legal process.

A number of epidemiological studies, based both on the general population and selected groups, have shown that subjects with nickel allergy, in general, seem to incur an increased risk of developing hand eczema [62, 79–83]. Other studies have failed to establish such an association [72]. In a study among monozygotic twins, a correlation between nickel allergy and hand eczema was similarly established [84]. Studies investigating the correlation based on patch-tested patients are difficult to interpret [85]. Future studies based on patients classified according to skin exposure assessment will make such data more valid. After the introduction of nickel exposure regulation in Denmark, the statistical association between nickel allergy and hand eczema has weakened [66].

Table 2.4. Mechanisms which can cause and aggravate hand eczema in the nickel-sensitive population

1	Occupational exposure to high (not further defined) concentration of nickel. Where nickel acts both as an allergen and an irritant, e.g., in electroplating
2	Exposure (occupational) to moderate nickel salt concentrations in the region of 10–100 ppm, probably in combination with irritants. Many different jobs in industry
3	Transcutaneous absorption of nickel released from metal items worn in prolonged skin contact, e.g., costume jewelry, suspenders, buttons, etc.
4	Systemic nickel exposure from food or nickel released from, e.g., dental braces

Core Message

■ Nickel allergy can cause hand eczema, either as a consequence of occupational or domestic exposure or as a part of systemic contact dermatitis.

32.2.8 Specific Treatment

Besides general treatment recommendations (Chap. 44), specific treatment modalities partly experimentally exist for nickel dermatitis. Nickel hand eczema as described in the literature is known to have a notoriously bad prognosis, but, undoubtedly, many mild cases exist unnoticed in the population. Contributing to the bad prognosis are secondary bacterial infection, atopy, multiple contact allergies, and frequent nickel exposure, either transcutaneously or systemically. In the evaluation of the patients with nickel hand eczema, all these factors need consideration. If standard evaluation and treatment fails to help patients, a diet with low nickel content may help [86, 87]. The diet is recommended to be evaluated over 1–2 months. Chelating drugs have an effect on nickel dermatitis, both used topically and systemically [88]. Statistically significant effects of systemic diethyldithiocarbamate (Antabuse) have been found in a controlled study [89], but the treatment has not found general acceptances because of possible side-effects, such as flare-up of nickel dermatitis and, in some patients, liver toxicity.

32.2.9 Prevention and Legislation

Based on the evidence that nickel alloys releasing less than 0.5 $\mu g/cm^2$ per week nickel are unlikely to induce primary nickel sensitization and rarely elicit nickel dermatitis in already nickel-sensitized individuals, legislation was passed in Denmark in 1990 [90]. By using the DMG test as a control, metal items designed to be in prolonged skin contact releasing large amounts of nickel are now uncommon in Danish shops. Metal contact dermatitis is now dwindling in Denmark and epidemiological studies indicate that the frequency of nickel allergy has decreased significantly in the youngest age group [68]. European legislation was passed in 1994 modeled on the Danish regulation, but increasing consumer safety still further reduced by regulation of the total amount of nickel permitted in material for ear-piercing (in reality, making them nickel-free), and by setting a 2-year quality demand for eventual coatings (Table 2.5). A group led by Lidén, within the European Committee for Standardization (CEN), has worked out analytical methods for the control of compliance with the requirements of the Directive (Table 2.5). This European regulation developed by collaboration between the industry and dermatologists has come into effect from 2000. Based on the Danish experience and the outcome of other allergen exposure limitations, e.g., the European cosmetics directive and limitation of exposure to hexavalent chromate in cement in Scandinavian countries, a major impact can be expected [67, 69, 70]. Carefully planned follow-up case and epidemiological studies need to be performed to evaluate the effect of this regulation in the future. The frequency on the market of items under part 2 of the Nickel Directive that release nickel was investigated. A baseline study before and a follow-up study 2 years after coming into force of the Nickel Directive showed that there had been significant adaptation to the requirements [91, 92]. It is important to realize that the present regulation concerns well-defined nickel-containing metallic items designed to be in direct and prolonged skin

Table 2.5. The EU Nickel Directive and analytical methods [European Parliament and Council Directive 94/27 EC (Nickel) 1994, European Committee for Standardization (CEN)]

Part	Nickel may not be used	CEN standard for control of limit
1	*To September 2005:* In post assemblies used during epithelization, unless they are homogeneous and the concentration of nickel is less than 0.05%	EN 1810 (nickel content by atomic absorption spectrometry)
1 rev.	*From September 2005:* In all post assemblies which are inserted into pierced ears and other pierced parts (not only during epithelization), unless the nickel release is less than 0.2 $\mu g/cm^2$ per week	EN 1811 (nickel release in artificial sweat)
2	In products intended to come into direct and prolonged contact with the skin, such as earrings, necklaces, wristwatch cases, watch straps, buttons, tighteners, and zips, if nickel release is greater than 0.5 $\mu g/cm^2$ per week	EN 1811 (nickel release in artificial sweat) CR 12471 (screening test by dimethyl-glyoxime)
3	In coated products, unless the coating is sufficient to ensure that the nickel release will not exceed 0.5 $\mu g/cm^2$ per week after two years normal use	EN 12472 (wear and corrosion test)

contact e.g., costume jewelry, buttons, and spectacles. That is to say, occupational exposure from tools and, e.g., coins and other materials, are not included. Whether such items need any kind of regulation may depend upon the future risk assessment.

Core Message

- Regulating nickel release from consumer items designed to be in direct and prolonged skin contact effectively prevents nickel dermatitis.

Suggested Reading

In 1956, Calnan [49] published a large group of patients with nickel dermatitis. He described the primary eruption from metal consumer items and the tendency to secondary eruptions, particularly vesicular hand eczema. Christensen and Möller in 1975 [56] provoked nickel-allergic individuals with an oral nickel dose and observed lesions similar to the secondary eruptions described earlier by Calnan. The studies led to the general understanding that a limited allergic contact dermatitis may lead to a widespread eruption through a systemic exposure based on a transcutaneous absorption. By repeating the oral nickel provocation studies, by Christensen and Möller, we observed skin changes that led to description of the "baboon syndrome" [55] as a part of systemic contact dermatitis.

References

1. Morgan LG, Usher V (1994) Health problems associated with nickel refining and use. Ann Occup Hyg 38:189–198
2. Blaschko A (1889) Die Berufsdermatosen der Arbeiter. Ein Beitrag zur Gewerbehygiene. I. Das Galvanisier-Ekzem. Dtsch Med Wochenschr 15:925–927
3. Schittenhelm A, Stockinger W (1925) Über die Idiosynkrasie gegen Nickel (Nickel-krätze) und ihre Beziehung zur Anaphylaxie. Z Ges Exp Med 45:58–74
4. Nickel Development Institute (1997) Safe use of nickel in the workplace. Nickel Development Institute, Toronto, Canada, pp 1–78
5. Flint GN (1998) A metallurgical approach to metal contact dermatitis. Contact Dermatitis 39:213–221
6. Menné T, Brandrup F, Thestrup-Pedersen K, Veien NK, Andersen JR, Yding F, Valeur G (1987) Patch test reactivity to nickel alloys. Contact Dermatitis 16:255–259
7. Pedersen NB, Fregert S, Brodelius P, Gruvberger B (1974) Release of nickel from silver coins. Acta Derm Venereol (Stockh) 54:231–234
8. Menné T, Solgaard P (1979) Temperature-dependent nickel release from nickel alloys. Contact Dermatitis 5:82–84
9. Fischer T, Fregert S, Gruvberger B, Rystedt I (1984) Nickel release from ear piercing kits and earrings. Contact Dermatitis 10:39–41
10. Lidén C, Menné T, Burrows D (1996) Nickel-containing alloys and platings and their ability to cause dermatitis. Br J Dermatol 134:193–198
11. Emmett EA, Risby TH, Jiang L, Ng SK, Feinman S (1988) Allergic contact dermatitis to nickel: bioavailability from consumer products and provocation threshold. J Am Acad Dermatol 19:314–322
12. Cavelier C, Foussereau J, Massin M (1985) Nickel allergy: analysis of metal clothing objects and patch testing to metal samples. Contact Dermatitis 12:65–75
13. Haudrechy P, Mantout B, Frappaz A, Rousseau D, Chabeau G, Faure M, Claudy A (1997) Nickel release from stainless steels. Contact Dermatitis 37:113–117
14. Hemingway JD, Molokhia MM (1987) The dissolution of metallic nickel in artificial sweat. Contact Dermatitis 16:99–105
15. Suzuki H (1998) Nickel and gold in skin lesions of pierced earlobes with contact dermatitis. A study using scanning electron microscopy and x-ray microanalysis. Arch Dermatol Res 290:523–527
16. Wedroff N (1935) Über Ekzeme bei Vernicklern. Arch Gewerbepathol Gewerbehyg 6:179–196
17. Wall LM, Calnan CD (1980) Occupational nickel dermatitis in the electroforming industry. Contact Dermatitis 6:414–420
18. Clemmensen OJ, Menné T, Kaaber K, Solgaard P (1981) Exposure of nickel and the relevance of nickel sensitivity among hospital cleaners. Contact Dermatitis 7:14–18
19. Wahlberg JE, Lindstedt G, Einarsson O (1977) Chromium, cobalt and nickel in Swedish cement, detergents, mould and cutting oils. Berufsdermatosen 25:220–228
20. Lidén C, Röndell E, Skare L, Nalbanti A (1998) Nickel release from tools on the Swedish market. Contact Dermatitis 39:127–131
21. Fournier P-G, Govers TR (2003) Contamination by nickel, copper and zinc during the handling of Euro coins. Contact Dermatitis 48:181–188
22. Zhai H, Chew AL, Bashir SJ, Reagan KE, Hostynek JJ, Maibach HI (2003) Provocative use test of nickel coins in nickel-sensitized subjects and controls. Br J Dermatol 149:311–317
23. Basketter DA, Briatico-Vangosa G, Kaestner W, Lally C, Bontinck WJ (1993) Nickel, cobalt and chromium in consumer products: a role in allergic contact dermatitis? Contact Dermatitis 28:15–25
24. Basketter DA, Angelini G, Ingber A, Kern PS, Menné T (2003). Nickel, chromium and cobalt in consumer products: revisiting safe levels in the new millennium. Contact Dermatitis 49:1–7
25. Fullerton A, Andersen JR, Hoelgaard A (1988) Permeation of nickel through human skin in vitro – effect of vehicles. Br J Dermatol 118:509–516
26. Fullerton A, Hoelgaard A (1988) Binding of nickel to human epidermis in vitro. Br J Dermatol 119:675–682
27. Fullerton A, Andersen JR, Hoelgaard A, Menné T (1986) Permeation of nickel salts through human skin in vitro. Contact Dermatitis 15:173–177
28. Hostynek JJ (2003) Factors determining percutaneous metal absorption. Food Chem Toxicol 41:327–345
29. Peters K, Gammelgaard B, Menné T (1991) Nickel concentrations in fingernails as a measure of occupational exposure to nickel. Contact Dermatitis 25:237–241
30. Allenby CF, Basketter DA (1994) The effect of repeated open exposure to low levels of nickel on compromised hand skin of nickel-allergic subjects. Contact Dermatitis 30:135–138

31. Nielsen NH, Menné T, Kristiansen J, Christensen JM, Borg L, Poulsen LK (1999) Effects of repeated skin exposures to low nickel concentrations – a model for allergic contact dermatitis to nickel on the hands. Br J Dermatol 141: 676–682

32. Kristiansen J, Christensen JM, Henriksen T, Nielsen NH, Menné T (2000) Determination of nickel in fingernails and forearm skin (stratum corneum). Anal Chim Acta 403: 265–272

33. Cronin E (1975) Patch testing with nickel. Contact Dermatitis 1: 56–57

34. Möller H, Svensson Å (1986) Metal sensitivity: positive history but negative test indicates atopy. Contact Dermatitis 14: 57–60

35. Kligman AM (1966) The identification of contact allergens by human assay. 3. The maximization test: a procedure for screening and rating contact sensitizers. J Invest Dermatol 47: 393–409

36. Vandenberg JJ, Epstein WL (1963) Experimental nickel contact sensitization in man. J Invest Dermatol 41: 413–418

37. Cronin E (1972) Clinical prediction of patch test results. Trans St Johns Hosp Dermatol Soc 58: 153–162

38. Nielsen NH, Linneberg A, Menné T, Madsen F, Frølund L, Dirksen A, Jørgensen T (2001) Persistence of contact allergy among Danish adults: an 8-year follow-up study. Contact Dermatitis 45: 350–353

39. Hindsén M, Bruze M, Christensen OB (1999) Individual variation in nickel patch test reactivity. Am J Contact Dermat 10: 62–67

40. Hindsén M, Bruze M, Christensen OB (1997) The significance of previous allergic contact dermatitis for elicitation of delayed hypersensitivity to nickel. Contact Dermatitis 37: 101–106

41. Hindsén M, Christensen OB (1992) Delayed hypersensitivity reactions following allergic and irritant inflammation. Acta Derm Venereol (Stockh) 72: 220–221

42. Nielsen NH, Menné T (1996) The relationship between IgE-mediated and cell-mediated hypersensitivities in an unselected Danish population: the Glostrup Allergy Study, Denmark. Br J Dermatol 134: 669–672

43. Menné T, Calvin G (1993) Concentration threshold of non-occluded nickel exposure in nickel-sensitive individuals and controls with and without surfactant. Contact Dermatitis 29: 180–184

44. Andersen KE, Lidén C, Hansen J, Vølund A (1993) Dose-response testing with nickel sulphate using the TRUE test in nickel-sensitive individuals. Multiple nickel sulphate patch-test reactions do not cause an 'angry back'. Br J Dermatol 129: 50–56

45. Hindsén M, Bruze M (1998) The significance of previous contact dermatitis for elicitation of contact allergy to nickel. Acta Derm Venereol (Stockh) 78: 367–370

46. Lisby S, Hansen LH, Menné T, Baadsgaard O (1999) Nickel-induced proliferation of both memory and naive T cells in patch test negative individuals. Clin Exp Immunol 171: 217–222

47. McAlester AV Jr, McAlester AW III (1931) Nickel sensitization from white gold spectacle frames. Am J Ophthalmol 14: 925–926

48. Bonnevie P (1939) Ätiologie und Pathogenese der Eczemkrankheiten. Barth, Leipzig

49. Calnan CD (1956) Nickel dermatitis. Br J Dermatol 68: 229–236

50. Marcussen PV (1957) Spread of nickel dermatitis. Dermatologica 115: 596–607

51. Boss A, Menné T (1982) Nickel sensitization from ear piercing. Contact Dermatitis 8: 211–213

52. Larsson-Stymne B, Widström L (1985) Ear piercing – a cause of nickel allergy in schoolgirls? Contact Dermatitis 13: 289–293

53. Brandrup F, Larsen FS (1979) Nickel dermatitis provoked by buttons in blue jeans. Contact Dermatitis 5: 148–150

54. Hindsén M, Bruze M, Christensen OB (2001) Flare-up reactions after oral challenge with nickel in relation to challenge dose and intensity and time of previous patch test reactions. J Am Acad Dermatol 44: 616–623

55. Andersen KE, Hjorth N, Menné T (1984) The baboon syndrome: systemically-induced allergic contact dermatitis. Contact Dermatitis 10: 97–100

56. Christensen OB, Möller H (1975) External and internal exposure to the antigen in the hand eczema of nickel allergy. Contact Dermatitis 1: 136–141

57. Menné T, Veien N, Sjolin KE, Maibach HI (1994) Systemic contact dermatitis. Am J Contact Dermat 5: 1–12

58. Jensen CS, Menné T, Lisby S, Kristiansen J, Veien NK (2003). Experimental systemic contact dermatitis from nickel: a dose-response study. Contact Dermatitis 49: 124–132

59. Hindsén M, Christensen OB, Möller H (1994) Nickel levels in serum and urine in five different groups of eczema patients following oral ingestion of nickel. Acta Derm Venereol (Stockh) 74: 176–178

60. Marcussen PV (1959) Nikkeleksem (Nickel eczema. Survey based on 621 cases. In Danish). Ugeskr Laeger 121: 1349–1353

61. Prystowsky SD, Allen AM, Smith RW, Nonomura JH, Odom RB, Akers WA (1979) Allergic contact hypersensitivity to nickel, neomycin, ethylenediamine, and benzocaine. Relationships between age, sex, history of exposure, and reactivity to standard patch tests and use tests in a general population. Arch Dermatol 115: 959–962

62. Peltonen L (1979) Nickel sensitivity in the general population. Contact Dermatitis 5: 27–32

63. Menné T (1978) The prevalence of nickel allergy among women. An epidemiological study in hospitalized female patients. Derm Beruf Umwelt 26: 123–125

64. Nielsen NH, Menné T (1992) Allergic contact sensitization in an unselected Danish population. The Glostrup Allergy Study, Denmark. Acta Derm Venereol (Stockh) 72: 456–460

65. Nielsen NH, Linneberg A, Menné T, Madsen F, Frølund L, Dirksen A, Jørgensen T (2001) Allergic contact sensitization in an adult Danish population: two cross-sectional surveys eight years apart (the Copenhagen Allergy Study). Acta Derm Venereol (Stockh) 81: 31–34

66. Nielsen NH, Linneberg A, Menné T, Madsen F, Frølund L, Dirksen A, Jørgensen T (2002) The association between contact allergy and hand eczema in 2 cross-sectional surveys 8 years apart. The Copenhagen Allergy Study. Contact Dermatitis 46: 71–77

67. Jensen CS, Lisby S, Baadsgaard O, Vølund A, Menné T (2000) Decrease in nickel sensitization in a Danish schoolgirl population with ears pierced after implementation of a nickel-exposure regulation. Br J Dermatol 46: 636–642

68. Johansen JD, Menné T, Christophersen J, Kaaber K, Veien N (2000) Pattern of sensitization to common contact allergens in Denmark. Changes from 1985–1986 to 1997–1998, with a special view to the effect of preventive strategies. Br J Dermatol 142: 490–495

69. Schnuch A, Uter W (2003) Decrease in nickel allergy in Germany and regulatory interventions. Contact Dermatitis 49: 107–108

70. Veien NK, Hattel T, Laurberg G (2001) Reduced nickel sensitivity in young Danish women following regulation of nickel exposure. Contact Dermatitis 45: 104–106

32

71. Christensen OB (1982) Prognosis in nickel allergy and hand eczema. Contact Dermatitis 8:7–15
72. Diepgen TL, Fartasch M (1994) General aspect of risk factors in hand eczema. In: Menné T, Maibach HI (eds) Hand eczema, 2nd edn. CRC Press, Boca Raton, Florida, pp 141–156
73. Agner T, Johansen JD, Overgaard L, Vølund A, Basketter D, Menné T (2002) Combined effects of irritants and allergens. Synergistic effects of nickel and sodium lauryl sulfate in nickel-sensitized individuals. Contact Dermatitis 47:21–26
74. Ingber A, Klein S, David M (1998) The nickel released from jewelry in Israel and its clinical relevance. Contact Dermatitis 39:195–197
75. Kalimo K, Lammintausta K, Jalava J, Niskanen T (1997) Is it possible to improve the prognosis in nickel contact dermatitis? Contact Dermatitis 37:121–124
76. Fischer T (1989) Occupational nickel dermatitis. In: Maibach HI, Menné T (eds) Nickel and the skin: immunology and toxicology. CRC, Boca Raton, Fla., pp 117–132
77. Shah M, Lewis FM, Gawkrodger DJ (1998) Nickel as an occupational allergen. A survey of 368 nickel-sensitive subjects. Arch Dermatol 134:1231–1236
78. Halkier-Sorensen L (1996) Occupational skin diseases. Contact Dermatitis 35:1–120
79. Menné T, Borgan O, Green A (1982) Nickel allergy and hand dermatitis in a stratified sample of the Danish female population: an epidemiological study including a statistic appendix. Acta Derm Venereol (Stockh) 62:35–41
80. Nilsson E, Bäck O (1986) The importance of anamnestic information of atopy, metal dermatitis and earlier hand eczema for the development of hand dermatitis in women in wet hospital work. Acta Derm Venereol (Stockh) 66:45–50
81. Bryld LE, Hindsberger C, Kyvik KO, Agner T, Menné T (2003) Risk factors influencing the development of hand eczema in a population based twin sample. Br J Dermatol 149:1214–1220
82. Mortz CG, Lauritsen JM, Bindslev-Jensen C, Andersen KE (2002) Nickel sensitization in adolescents and association with ear piercing, use of dental braces and hand eczema. Acta Derm Venereol (Stockh) 82:359–364
83. Meding B, Lidén C, Berglind N (2001) Self-diagnosed dermatitis in adults. Results from a population survey in Stockholm. Contact Dermatitis 45:341–345
84. Menné T, Holm NV (1983) Hand eczema in nickel-sensitive female twins. Genetic predisposition and environmental factors. Contact Dermatitis 9:289–296
85. Wilkinson DS, Wilkinson JD (1989) Nickel allergy and hand eczema. In: Maibach HI, Menné T (eds) Nickel and the skin: immunology and toxicology. CRC, Boca Raton, Fla., pp 133–163
86. Veien NK, Hattel T, Laurberg G (1993) Low nickel diet: an open, prospective trial. J Am Acad Dermatol 29:1002–1007
87. Kaaber K, Veien NK, Tjell JC (1978) Low nickel diet in the treatment of patients with chronic nickel dermatitis. Br J Dermatol 98:197–201
88. Gawkrodger DJ, Healy J, Howe AM (1995) The prevention of nickel contact dermatitis. A review of the use of binding agents and barrier creams. Contact Dermatitis 32:257–265 [published erratum appears in Contact Dermatitis 33:288, 1995]
89. Kaaber K, Menné T, Tjell JC, Veien N (1979) Antabuse treatment of nickel dermatitis. Chelation – a new principle in the treatment of nickel dermatitis. Contact Dermatitis 5:221–228
90. Menné T, Rasmussen K (1990) Regulation of nickel exposure in Denmark. Contact Dermatitis 23:57–58
91. Lidén C, Johnsson S (2001) Nickel on the Swedish market before the Nickel Directive. Contact Dermatitis 44:7–12
92. Lidén C, Norberg K (2005) Nickel on the Swedish market. Follow-up after implementation of the Nickel Directive. Contact Dermatitis 52:29–35

32.3 Chromium

Crocoite – a lead-containing chromium (Cr) ore – was found in Russia by Pallas in 1765. Chromium metal itself was isolated in 1797 in France by Vauqelin [1]. Since the 19th century, chromium has found many industrial uses, including leather tanning, in alloys, and for chrome plating. In 1925, Parkhurst was the first to report chromium contact allergy based on skin testing in a blue print processor [2]. Open testing with a 0.5% aqueous solution of potassium dichromate produced a papulovesicular reaction in 24 h. Thereafter, chromium compounds have been established as important ubiquitous contact allergens.

By far the most common cause of chromium sensitization is contact with hexavalent chromium in wet cement, which means that allergic contact dermatitis from chromate is a significant occupational skin disease in construction workers. Besides contact allergy, chromium compounds have other toxicological properties, such as carcinogenicity, caustic capacity, and general toxicity [3, 4]. A chemical burn from chromic acid can be life-threatening (see Chap. 15). The same type of chromium compounds may induce both contact allergy and cancer, while the other toxicological effects are unrelated to contact allergy. Milestones in our understanding of chromium dermatitis are summarized in Table 3.1.

Table 3.1. Milestones in the history of chromium dermatitis

1900s	"Cement itch" in construction workers
1925	Chromium contact allergy in a blue print processor
1931	Patch testing with potassium dichromate, ammonium chromate, and sodium dichromate
1950	Detection of hexavalent chromium in cement
1970s	Detection of new sources of chromium exposure
	Chemical studies on iron sulfate and cement
1980s	Legislation in Nordic countries – iron sulfate added to cement
1990s	Epidemiological studies – general population and construction workers
2005	EU legislation on hexavalent chromium in cement

Core Message

■ Occupational, and later, consumer product chromium allergy has been frequent for the last 100 years.

32.3.1 Physicochemical Aspects and Sensitizing Potential

Chromium is one of the most widely distributed metals. Chromite ($FeOCr_2O_3$) is the principal ore of chromium. Chromium exists in every oxidation state from 0 to +6, but only the ground states 0, +2, +3, and +6 are common. Many chromium compounds have the capacity to induce sensitization and elicit chromium contact allergy. However, in contrast to other sensitizing metals, metallic chromium (ground state 0) is not sensitizing, due to its capacity to form a poorly soluble layer of oxide on the surface [5]. Therefore, it is probably more accurate to use the term "chromate allergy." The question whether there is one or more chromium haptens is not firmly resolved. Most hexavalent chromium compounds are freely water-soluble and pass through the epidermis more readily than most trivalent chromium compounds, which are insoluble [6, 7]. It is thought that hexavalent chromium penetrates the skin and is then reduced enzymatically to trivalent chromium, which combines with protein as the hapten [8, 9]. It has previously been demonstrated using a standard patch test technique that, if the concentration of trivalent chromium is high enough, and the exposure time sufficiently prolonged, positive tests will also result [10]. More recent data indicate that patch testing with serial dilutions of hexavalent and trivalent chromium may result in positive reactions down to low concentrations [11]. Principally, the capacity to induce and elicit chromium contact allergy depends on the concentration of the chromium compound, oxidation state, and solubility, the latter often being dependent on the pH [12].

Hexavalent chromium exists as chromates and dichromates of potassium, sodium, calcium, and ammonium, which are highly water-soluble, while barium, lead, and zirconium chromates and dichromates are poorly soluble. Zinc dichromate is soluble, while zinc chromate is less soluble.

Trivalent chromium exists as salts of inorganic and organic acids, for example, chlorides, nitrates, sulfates, and oxalates. Most of these salts are water-soluble, but penetrate the skin to a lesser degree than water-soluble hexavalent chromium compounds. In an alkaline environment, poorly soluble chromium hydroxide is precipitated from trivalent chromium salts. On the other hand, basic chromium (III) sulfate used for leather tanning is also water-soluble in an alkaline environment. Chromium (III) oxide and chromium hydroxide are virtually water-insoluble.

Tetravalent chromium compounds, such as chromium dioxide, can be partly transformed to hexavalent and trivalent chromium in the presence of water.

32.3.2 Chromium Use and Exposure

Chromium as a metal is present in various alloys, for example, in stainless steel, together with nickel and iron. Metallic chromium is also present on chrome-plated surfaces.

Chromium compounds are present in the raw materials used for the production of cement. Cement is produced at a high temperature in an alkaline environment and with an excess of oxygen, by which trivalent chromium compounds are partly oxidized to hexavalent chromium. The content of water-soluble hexavalent chromium in cement varies widely in different countries, mainly due to the variation in chromium content of the raw materials used [13, 14], but it is also due to the amount of alkali sulfate in the cement [15]. However, there is no correlation between the total content of chromium compounds in cement and its content of water-soluble hexavalent chromium [12].

Primer paints, usually yellow, red and orange, often contain poorly water-soluble zinc, lead, and barium chromates (VI). Also, freely soluble and, thus, sensitizing alkali chromates (VI) can be present. When iron treated with such anticorrosion paints is tooled, hexavalent chromium can be extracted by the cutting fluids. Chromates in paints for wood do not contain the sensitizing alkali chromates.

Zinc-galvanized sheet metal is often coated (chromated) with trivalent and hexavalent chromium compounds to prevent the metal dulling. When such chromated metal is handled, chromates can leach out and be transferred to volar parts of the hands.

On welding of stainless steel and non-stainless steel, hexavalent chromium can be released and generated, respectively, and distributed to the face via the welding fume.

Hexavalent chromium compounds are used in special tanks for chrome plating, a process consisting of applying a layer of metallic chromium to the surface. To avoid chrome ulcers from skin contact with such caustic chromium compounds, the process is automated, which not only prevents chrome ulcers, but also reduces the risk of chromate sensitization.

Trivalent chromium compounds, such as basic chromium sulfate, are used for leather tanning. White leather and chamois leather are not chrome-tanned. Tannery workers can become sensitized from trivalent chromium [16], but more individuals are sensitized and develop allergic contact dermatitis from trivalent chromium in finished leather products, such as gloves and shoes [17–23]. Apart from trivalent chromium, leather often also contains low amounts of hexavalent chromium, which is formed by oxidation of trivalent chromium during the tannery process [21, 24, 25]. In a recent study on the content of hexavalent chromium in 43 leather products on the Danish market, 35% of the investigated products contained hexavalent chromium above the detection limit of 3 ppm in the range 4 ppm to 15 ppm [26].

Besides the above-mentioned causes of chromate sensitization, there are many other possibilities, including the wood pulp industry, ash either from burnt wood or matches with chromate in the match head, coolants and machine oils, defatting solvents, brine added to yeast residues, the dye industry (due to either a dye, a reducing agent, or a mordant), printing, glues, foundry sand, boiler linings, television work [ammonium dichromate to produce cross-linking of light-sensitive polyvinyl alcohol magnetic tape (chromium dioxide)], solutions used to facilitate tire fitting, and preservatives used in milk testing. More detailed information can be obtained in references [1] and [27].

Clearly, exposure to chromium compounds is most likely to occur occupationally and, above all, in jobs where men traditionally predominate. Examples of occupational exposure to chromium chemicals and work procedures are given in Table 3.2. However, chromate allergy is not uncommon in women, and many times in connection with a foot dermatitis [21] or hand dermatitis [28, 29]. High levels of chromium in detergents and bleaches have been suggested as a possible cause of chromate allergy in women in Spain, France, Belgium, and Israel [28–30], while bleaches had only trace levels of chromate in the USA [31]. When the presence of chromate in detergents and bleaches was investigated chemically in a recent study, chromium above 1 ppm was detected in most of the products and with a top value at 546 ppm for a detergent [28]. The clinical relevance of chromate in household products was investigated in a study including 17 dermatitis patients with contact allergy to hexavalent chromium [32]. The patients were patch tested with serial dilutions of potassium dichromate and repeated open application test (ROAT) was per-

Table 3.2. Occupational exposure to chromium is possible during contact with the following chemicals and work procedures (from [49])

Analytic standards reagents
Anticorrosion agents
Batteries
Catalysts (for hydrogenation, oxidation, polymerization)
Ceramics
Drilling muds
Chromium lignosulfonates (from sodium dichromate using lignosulfate waste)
Electroplating and anodizing agents
Engraving
Explosives
Fire retardant
Magnetic tapes
Metallic chromium
Milk preservatives
Paints and varnishes
Paper
"Chrome cake" (containing sodium sulfate and small amounts of sodium dichromate)
Photography
Roofing
Sutures
Tanning leather
Textile mordants and dyes
Television screens
Wood preservatives

formed with aqueous solutions containing 1% sodium lauryl sulfate (SLS) and potassium dichromate in the concentration range 5–50 ppm. The respective solution was applied to the antecubital fossa twice daily for 1 week. Fifty seven percent of the patients failed to react to 50 ppm while 20% tested positively to 5 ppm.

In certain areas of the USA, Scotland, Mexico, and Japan, large volumes of chromite ore-processing residue (COPR) containing hexavalent chromium have been used to fill low-lying areas [33]. Because of concern about the potential risk of chromate allergy, sensitization, and, particularly, elicitation in already-sensitized individuals, several reports and studies have been conducted to elucidate the problem in the 1990s [33–40]. Based on the results of the patch test study in which the threshold dose (g/cm^2) (MET) for allergic contact dermatitis was measured among those who had previously been sensitized [34], and estimations and assumptions on exposure assessment regarding soil-on-skin adherence and the bio-

32

availability of hexavalent chromium in COPR, it was concluded that direct contact with soil concentrations at least as high as 1,240 ppm should not elicit allergic contact dermatitis in sensitized individuals [35]. In a recent study, the potential for the elicitation of allergic contact dermatitis from skin contact with chromium in standing water in the environment was investigated [33]. Twenty six persons known to be allergic to hexavalent chromium were exposed to 25–29 ppm chromium by immersion of one arm for 30 min per day on three consecutive days in a potassium dichromate bath [33]. Ten of the volunteers developed a few papules or vesicles, mild redness, and pruritus on the chromate-challenged arm. Histopathologically, there was perieccrine and perivascular inflammation with spongiosis, consistent with an allergic mechanism, but in some specimens, epidermal necrosis spoke more in favor of an irritant mechanism. Generally, participants with the lowest MET to hexavalent chromium were more likely to react [33]. Due to the lack of a control group of non-sensitized individuals, it was impossible to tell whether the reactions were allergic or irritant in nature. In spite of the development of inflammatory reactions in 10 out of 26 (38%) volunteers, the authors state: "Based on these data, concentrations of 25–29 mg/l Cr (VI) in water can be considered the no-effect levels for allergic contact dermatitis and irritant contact dermatitis for Cr-sensitized persons for nearly all plausible environmental exposures to standing water" [33]. However, our interpretation is that these inflammatory reactions in the ten volunteers were allergic in nature, as the concentration of aqueous potassium dichromate needed to cause irritant reactions on patch testing is around 1,000 ppm and allergic patch test reactions can be elicited by concentrations lower than 25 ppm [41, 42].

Sometimes, chemical investigations are required to demonstrate present exposure to chromium in a chromate-sensitive person. Most often, atomic absorption spectroscopy is used, but it is important to stress that this method measures the total chromium level, while it is only the chromate level that is of interest from a contact allergic standpoint. Atomic absorption spectroscopy has been used by Nielsen et al. [43] to demonstrate the accumulation of chromium in the fingernails of chromate-sensitive patients with hand dermatitis, after the fingers had been immersed in aqueous chromate solutions for 10 min per day for a period of 2 weeks. In Chap. 25, a method to evaluate hexavalent chromium content is described.

> ## Core Message
>
> ■ Particularly hexavalent chromium compounds are significant for chromium allergy. Cement and leather are important sources of hexavalent chromium.

32.3.3 Patch Testing with Chromate

In 1931, there were three publications on allergic contact dermatitis from chromate and in which hexavalent chromium compounds, ammonium chromate 1% [44], potassium dichromate 0.5% [45], and sodium dichromate 0.1% [46], respectively, were used for patch testing. Also in the 1930s, Bonnevie included potassium dichromate in the first standard patch test series [47]. Today, potassium dichromate 0.5% in petrolatum is still present in the standard series for Europe, while the same salt at 0.25% is recommended in North America [48, 49]. The TRUE Test also uses potassium dichromate. There is a major problem with these standard test preparations, as irritant reactions can be elicited; reactions which morphologically resemble allergic reactions and can, therefore, be interpreted as allergic reactions. Whenever an irritant reaction is a possibility, retesting is recommended, if possible, both epicutaneously and intracutaneously [50, 51]. When lower concentrations of potassium dichromate, 0.375% and 0.25%, are used there will be fewer irritant reactions, but these preparations will also miss some true chromate allergies [52, 53]. Patch testing with trivalent salts such as chromium trichloride and chromium sulfate produces a high percentage of false-negatives [34, 54]. Compared to hexavalent chromium, the patch test activity of trivalent compounds has been reported to be in the order of 1/10 for oxalate, 1/100 for chloride, and 1/1,000 for the acetate [10], which is in contrast with the results of a recent study in which patients hypersensitive to hexavalent chromium were patch tested with dilutions of both hexavalent chromium (potassium dichromate) and trivalent chromium (chromium trichloride hexahydrate) [11]. Both compounds were capable of eliciting dermatitis at low concentrations.

There are several reports of patch test studies performed to determine the threshold concentration of hexavalent chromium to elicit erythema or dermatitis [11, 32, 34, 38, 41, 42, 55, 56]. Expectedly, the results vary with the population studied, patch test technique and vehicles used, and the definition of end point. In the presence of sodium lauryl sulfate (SLS), the threshold was lowered almost ten times [32]. Based on the literature, the threshold for elicitation of allergic contact dermatitis from hexavalent chromium is 1–10 ppm (corresponding to 0.03–0.3 µg/cm² for a Finn Chamber with a diameter of 0.8 cm and application of 15 µl to the patch unit) [41, 42]. With the TRUE Test technique, the concentration threshold for a single exposure has been established at 0.089 g/cm² [34].

Leucocyte migration inhibition and lymphocyte blast transformations tests have been used to examine contact sensitivity to chromium. These tests can supplement patch testing. Equivalent results for trivalent and hexavalent chromium compounds have been reported [57, 58].

> **Core Message**
>
> ■ Patch testing with 0.5% potassium dichromate is needed to not miss chromium allergy, but this concentration can elicit an irritant reaction.

32

32.3.4 Clinical Picture

Allergic contact dermatitis from chromate is eczematous, sometimes widespread and very persistent [59–62]. Although the reasons for the persistence of chrome dermatitis are unknown, a common explanation is the presence of unrecognized chromium in the environment. A pattern resembling nummular eczema may be seen. Frequent and marked dryness and lichenification makes it resemble atopic dermatitis. Cement eczema caused by hexavalent chromium is initially localized to the dorsal aspect of the hands, and often has a nummular pattern. Later, the cement eczema can also involve the volar parts of the hands.

> **Core Message**
>
> ■ Allergic contact dermatitis from chromate may present as a widespread persistent dermatitis, resembling nummular eczema.

32.3.5 Systemic Contact Dermatitis

Chromium, trivalent or hexavalent, is an essential element required for normal carbohydrate and lipid metabolism. Studies on patients under total parenteral nutrition have indicated that a lack of chromium may cause disturbances in glucose metabolism [63]. The chromium intake of healthy subjects consuming normal diets is suboptimal [63]. There is a great difference in chromium intake depending more on the menu than on cooking in stainless steel utensils [64]. Yet, the fact that minute chromium compounds are present in food and water have made some authors speculate that oral ingestion may cause or contribute to the persistence of allergic contact dermatitis from chromium [65]. This has been questioned by others [37], since in vivo data have demonstrated that hexavalent chromium is readily reduced to trivalent chromium in the gastric fluid of the stomach before being systemically absorbed [66, 67]. However, in provocation studies with oral hexavalent chromium [65, 68], this reduction in the gastric fluid does not seem to affect the capacity of oral hexavalent chromium to elicit a systemic contact dermatitis. In patients with nickel or chromium allergy and dyshidrotic hand eczema, elbow eruptions have been reported to be characteristic of systemic allergic contact dermatitis from these metals [68, 69].

32.3.6 Epidemiology

Expectedly, the prevalence of chromium allergy varies widely in different countries due to many factors related not only to the degree and type of exposure, but also to factors related to diagnostic testing. Proctor et al. [37] have summarized the prevalence rates of chromium (VI) contact allergy in more than 30 studies published since 1950. These studies consist mostly of persons who have attended dermatological clinics in Europe and North America. The prevalence rates for specific cohorts range from 19.5% in workers with cement eczema in Switzerland in 1950 [70] to a prevalence rate of 1% for a clinical population tested from 1992 to 1996 in North America [58]. Although the prevalence of chromium allergy in dermatitis patients has been steadily decreasing over the past 25 years, several reports demonstrate that chromium allergy still is significant [16–18, 22, 23, 71–75]. Several investigators have suggested that the decline in chromium allergy is most likely due to improved workplace hygiene, decreased contact with construction materials [76], and the addition of iron sulfate to cement to reduce most of the hexavalent chromium to an insoluble trivalent salt, which has negligible potential for sensitization and elicitation [77–81]. In countries where iron sulfate is not added to cement, chromate allergy may still be common in construction workers. Irvine et al. reported a high prevalence (17%) of chromate allergy among underground workers during the construction of the Channel Tunnel [82]. Sixty five percent of grouters patch tested had chromate allergy. The suggested causes for the decline in chromium allergy refer mainly to men. The frequency has also decreased in women, which has been attributed to the replacement of dichromate-containing bleaches with other detergents [78]. Still, there are countries where this has not been implemented, probably contributing to a high frequency of chromium allergy in housewives [28].

There are some investigations studying the prevalence of chromium allergy in the European general population. In Finland, Peltonen and Fräki [83] have evaluated the prevalence of chromium (VI) sensitivity among 822 human volunteers. An overall prevalence of 1.7% was found. Seidenari et al. conducted a study in which 593 Italian cadets were patch tested with 0.5% potassium dichromate [84]. None tested positively. Lantinga et al. assessed the prevalence of allergic contact dermatitis for the general adult population in one defined area in the Netherlands [85]. Of the 1,992 individuals examined, 141 were identified as having episodes of eczema within the past 3 years. These individuals were patch tested and 9 of the 1,992 cases (0.5%) tested positively to hexavalent chromium. Nielsen and Menné assessed the distribution of allergic contact dermatitis in an unselected population living in western Copenhagen, Denmark [86]. In 567 adults patch tested, a prevalence of 0.5% was noted; 0.7% in men and 0.3% in women. A higher frequency of chromium allergy was noted in a western Australasian community, where 9.1% of 219 adult volunteers were contact allergic [87]. According to a recent review on allergic contact dermatitis in children and adolescents, the prevalence of chromate allergy in these groups has been reported to be between 0.2% and 7.6%, the latter frequencies seeming, according to our experience, highly unlikely [88].

Core Message

■ In construction workers exposed to hexavalent chromium, contact allergy rates exceeding 10% are seen, while the contact allergy rate in the European general population is around 1%.

32.3.7 Prevention and Legislation

Wass and Wahlberg have adopted a simple extraction procedure for the determination of leachable hexavalent chromium that could be used in industrial applications to check the quality of chromated products and to establish a "threshold limit value" for such products [89]. Based on the results of occlusive tests with chromated discs in chromate-sensitive individuals, it was proposed that the mean release of hexavalent chromium from chromated parts should not exceed 0.3 $\mu g/cm^2$. Release above this value was found in approximately one out of four yellow chromated parts collected from a chromating plant and a car assembly plant. Wass and Wahlberg suggested that their method should be added to the tests performed to evaluate the technical quality of the chromate layers to reduce the risk of causing chromate allergy.

Basketter et al. reviewed the literature on published and unpublished industry data on transition metal contamination of consumer products and assessed the hazard in man [78]. Based on information on sensitization potential, including dose–response data, the levels of chromium found in consumer products and in relation to the known epidemiology of allergic contact dermatitis from chromium and in the context of the nature and extent of consumer exposure, Basketter et al. stated that good manufacturing practice in 1993 ensured that the chromium concentration in consumer products was less than 5 ppm. It was recommended that this was accepted as a standard for maximum concentration and that the target should be to achieve a concentration as low as 1 ppm. With these concentrations, it was thought that there will be no induction of chromate sensitization and that it is very unlikely that dermatitis will be elicited in already-sensitized individuals [78]. However, the maximum concentration should be lower than 5 ppm, as a ROAT study showed that 20% of the chromium-allergic patients reacted to an aqueous solution containing 5 ppm potassium dichromate as, well as 1% SLS [32].

In men, Portland cement has been, and still is in many countries, one of the most common causes of occupational skin conditions. In the beginning of the previous century, there were severe outbreaks of "cement itch" during the building of the Underground in London and of "la gâle du ciment" when the Métro in Paris was constructed. Although several investigators in the 1930s and 1940s reported that cement eczema was frequently combined with positive patch test reactions to chromate, it was not until 1950 that Jaeger and Pelloni first demonstrated the presence of hexavalent chromium in cement [70]. The content of hexavalent chromium in cement and concrete varies widely due to the source of the cement and additives used [13, 14]. It was previously demonstrated by Burckhardt that iron sulfate has the capacity to reduce hexavalent chromium to a trivalent form [90], and chemical analysis showed no demonstrable water-soluble chromium in cement to which iron sulfate had been added [91]. It is known that trivalent chromium will precipitate as chromium hydroxide in an alkaline solution. As cement has high alkalinity, this chemical process is most likely the reason that it is impossible to demonstrate water-soluble chromium in cement to which iron sulfate has been added [41]. Chromic hydroxide is also virtually insoluble in human sweat [41]. Because of this, iron sulfate has been added to all cement in connection with the manufacturing process in Scandinavian countries, since 1981 in Denmark and since 1983 in Sweden.

Denmark passed legislation requiring the use of cement with lower levels of hexavalent chromium (<2 ppm) in 1983. Finland followed in 1987 and Sweden in 1989. Cement eczema is steadily decreasing in prevalence, and had been doing so before the introduction of iron sulfate, and a decline is also occurring in countries where iron sulfate has not been added [92, 93]. Therefore, it had been questioned whether the decrease of hexavalent chromium in cement was a major cause of the decline in chromate allergy. However, some recent studies strongly indicate that the decrease of hexavalent chromium in cement is a significant and major factor in explaining the decreasing chromate allergy. In Singapore, a change in the manufacturing process of cement giving a lower content of hexavalent chromium has accompanied a decline in the prevalence of chromate allergy among construction workers [94]. In Denmark and Finland, where the content of hexavalent chromium in cement is below 2 ppm, the results of epidemiological investigations in construction workers concerning irritant and allergic contact dermatitis from cement strongly indicate that the decrease in chromate allergy has, to a large extent, been caused by the addition of iron sulfate [77, 79–81]. Furthermore, during the Channel Tunnel project, 332 out of 1,138 construction workers exposed to cement/concrete to which iron sulfate had not been added were diagnosed as having an occupational dermatitis [82]. Of these, 180 were patch tested and 96 (53%) were allergic to chromate. In similar building projects in Denmark and Sweden, during the construction of the combined tunnel and bridge of the Great Belt in Denmark and of the combined tunnel and bridge over Öresund, the strait between Denmark and Sweden, occupational dermatitis and chromate allergy has not been a problem ([79], B.H. Nielsen, Sundlink Contractors HB, Malmö, Sweden,

1999, personal communication). Recently, it was decided in the EU that cement which human skin may be exposed to must not contain more than 2 ppm hexavalent chromium from 17 January 2005 [95].

Thus, it is highly unlikely that cement with iron sulfate added will sensitize and it is likely that such cement will be of minor significance for elicitation in already-chromate-sensitized persons [41]. However, chromate sensitization from cement may still occur in countries with legislation demanding the addition of iron sulfate, due to reluctance in the addition of iron sulfate to imported cement [79] or due to storage conditions leading to oxidation of trivalent chromium to hexavalent [96].

Core Message

■ Regulating the content of hexavalent chromium in cement effectively prevents chromium dermatitis.

References

1. Burrows D, Adams RM (1990) Metals. In: Adams RM (ed) Occupational skin disease, 2nd edn. Saunders, Philadelphia, Pa., pp 349–386
2. Parkhurst HJ (1925) Dermatosis industrialis in a blue print worker due to chromium compounds. Arch Dermatol 12: 253–256
3. Hayes RB (1997) The carcinogenicity of metals in humans. Cancer Causes Control 8:371–385
4. Costa M (1998) Carcinogenic metals. Sci Prog 81:329–339
5. Flint GN (1998) A metallurgical approach to metal contact dermatitis. Contact Dermatitis 39:213–221
6. Samitz MH, Katz SA (1964) A study of the chemical reaction between chromium and skin. J Invest Dermatol 43: 35–43
7. Gammelgaard B, Fullerton A, Avnstorp C, Menné T (1992) Permeation of chromium salts through human skin in vitro. Contact Dermatitis 27:302–310
8. Burrows D (1984) The dichromate problem. Int J Dermatol 23:215–220
9. Polak L, Turk JL, Frey JR (1973) Studies on contact hypersensitivity to chromium compounds. Prog Allergy 17: 145–226
10. Fregert S, Rorsman H (1966) Allergic reactions to trivalent chromium compounds. Arch Dermatol 93:711–713
11. Hansen MB, Johansen JD, Menné T (2003) Chromium allergy: significance of both Cr (III) and Cr(VI). Contact Dermatitis 49:206–212
12. Fregert S (1981) Chromium valencies and cement dermatitis. Br J Dermatol 21:7–9
13. Fregert S, Gruvberger B (1972) Chemical properties of cement. Berufsdermatosen 20:238–248
14. Turk K, Rietschel RL (1993) Effect of processing cement to concrete on hexavalent chromium levels. Contact Dermatitis 28:209–211

32

15. Fregert S, Gruvberger B (1973) Correlation between alkali sulphate and water-soluble chromate in cement. Acta Derm Venereol (Stockh) 53:225–228
16. Estlander T, Jolanki R, Kanerva L (2000) Occupational allergic contact dermatitis from trivalent chromium in leather tanning. Contact Dermatitis 43:114
17. Freeman S (1997) Shoe dermatitis. Contact Dermatitis 36:247–251
18. Geijer J, Schnuch A, Frosch PJ (2000) Contact allergy to dichromate in women. Derm Beruf Umwelt 48:4–10
19. Oumeish OY, Rushaidat QM (1980) Contact dermatitis to military boots in Jordan. Contact Dermatitis 6:498
20. Rudzki E, Kozlowska A (1980) Causes of chromate dermatitis in Poland. Contact Dermatitis 6:191–196
21. Hansen MB, Rydin S, Menné T, Duus Johansen J (2002) Quantitative aspects of contact allergy to chromium and exposure to chrome-tanned leather. Contact Dermatitis 47:127–134
22. Shackelford KE, Belsito DV (2002) The etiology of allergic-appearing foot dermatitis: a 5-year retrospective study. J Am Acad Dermatol 47:715–721
23. Rani Z, Hussain I, Haroon TS (2003) Common allergens in shoe dermatitis: our experience in Lahore, Pakistan. Int J Dermatol 42:605–607
24. Graf D (2001) Formation of Cr(VI) traces in chrome-tanned leather: causes, prevention and latest findings. J Am Leather Chem Assoc 96:169–179
25. Nygren O, Wahlberg JE (1998) Speciation of chromium in tanned leather gloves and relapse of chromium allergy from tanned leather samples. Analyst 123:935–937
26. Rydin S (2002) Investigation of the content of CrVI and CrIII in leather products on the Danish market. Danish Environmental Protection Agency, Denmark
27. Burrows D (1983) Chromium: metabolism and toxicity. CRC, Boca Raton, Fla.
28. Ingber A, Gammelgaard B, David M (1998) Detergents and bleaches are sources of chromium contact dermatitis in Israel. Contact Dermatitis 38:101–104
29. García-Pérez A, Martín-Pascual A, Sánchez-Misiego A (1973) Chrome content in bleaches and detergents. Its relationship to hand dermatitis in women. Acta Derm Venereol (Stockh) 53:353–358
30. Lachapelle J M, Lauwerys R, Tennstedt D, Andanson J, Benezra C, Chabeau G, Ducombs G, Foussereau J, Lacroix M, Martin P (1980) Eau de Javel and prevention of chromate allergy in France. Contact Dermatitis 6:107–110
31. Hostynek JJ, Maibach HI (1988) Chromium in US household bleach. Contact Dermatitis 18:206–209
32. Basketter D, Horev L, Slodovnik D, Merimes S, Trattner A, Ingber A (2001) Investigation of the threshold for allergic reactivity to chromium. Contact Dermatitis 44:70–74
33. Fowler JF Jr, Kauffman CL, Marks JG Jr, Proctor DM, Fredrick MM, Otani JM, Finley BL, Paustenbach DJ, Nethercott JR (1999) An environmental hazard assessment of low-level dermal exposure to hexavalent chromium in solution among chromium-sensitized volunteers. J Occup Environ Med 41:150–160
34. Nethercott J, Paustenbach D, Adams R, Fowler J, Marks J, Morton C, Taylor J, Horowitz S, Finley B (1994) A study of chromium induced allergic contact dermatitis with 54 volunteers: implications for environmental risk assessment. J Occup Environ Med 51:371–380
35. Horowitz SB, Finley BL (1994) Setting health-protective soil concentrations for dermal contact allergens: a proposed methodology. Regul Toxicol Pharmacol 19:31–47
36. Fagliano J, Savrin J, Udasin I, Gochfeld M (1997) Community exposure and medical screening near chromium waste sites in New Jersey. Regul Toxicol Pharmacol 26:S13–S22
37. Proctor D, Fredrick M, Scott P, Paustenbach D, Finley B (1998) The prevalence of chromium allergy in the United States and its implications for setting soil clean up: a cost-effectiveness case study. Regul Toxicol Pharmacol 28:27–37
38. Stern AH, Bagdon RE, Hazen RE, Marzulli FN (1993) Risk assessment of the allergic dermatitis potential of environmental exposure to hexavalent chromium. J Toxicol Environ Health 40:613–641
39. Bagdon RE, Hazen RE (1991) Skin permeation and cutaneous hypersensitivity as a basis for making risk assessments of chromium as a soil contaminant. Environ Health Perspect 92:111–119
40. Paustenbach DJ, Sheehan PJ, Paull JM, Wisser LM, Finley BL (1992) Review of the allergic contact dermatitis hazard posed by chromium-contaminated soil: identifying a "safe" concentration. J Toxicol Environ Health 37:177–207
41. Bruze M, Fregert S, Gruvberger B (1990) Patch testing with cement containing iron sulfate. Dermatol Clin 8:173–176
42. Eun HC, Marks R (1990) Dose–response relationships on topically applied antigens. Br J Dermatol 122:491–499
43. Nielsen NH, Kristiansen J, Borg L, Christensen JM, Poulsen LK, Menné T (2000) Repeated exposures to cobalt or chromate on the hands of patients with hand eczema and contact allergy to that metal. Contact Dermatitis 43:212–215
44. Smith AR (1931) Chrome poisoning with manifestations of sensitization. J Am Med Assoc 97:95–98
45. Englehardt WE, Mayer RL (1931) Über Chromekzeme im Graphischen Gewerbe. Arch Gewerbepath Hyg 2:140–168
46. Kesten B, Laszlo E (1931) Dermatitis due to sensitization to contact substances: Dermatitis venenata occupational dermatitis. Arch Dermatol 23:221–237
47. Bonnevie P (1939) Ätiologie und Pathogenese der Eczemkrankheiten. Barth, Leipzig
48. Marks JG, Belsito DV, DeLeo VA, Fowler JF Jr, Fransway AF, Maibach HI, Mathias CG, Nethercott JR, Rietschel RL, Sherertz EF, Storrs FJ, Taylor JS (1998) North American Contact Dermatitis Group patch test results for the detection of delayed-type hypersensitivity to topical allergens. J Am Acad Dermatol 38:911–918
49. Andersen KE, Burrows D, White IR (1992) Allergens from the standard series. In: Rycroft RJG, Menné T, Frosch PJ, Benezra C (eds) Textbook of contact dermatitis. Springer, Berlin Heidelberg New York, pp 412–456
50. Möller H (1989) Intradermal testing in doubtful cases of contact allergy to metals. Contact Dermatitis 20:120–123
51. Bruze M, Conde-Salazar L, Goossens A, Kanerva L, White IR (1999) Thoughts on sensitizers in a standard patch test series. The European Society of Contact Dermatitis. Contact Dermatitis 41:241–250
52. Andersen KE, Burrows D, Cronin E, Dooms-Goossens A, Rycroft RJ, White IR (1988) Recommended changes to standard series. Contact Dermatitis 19:389–390
53. Burrows D, Andersen KE, Camarasa JG, Dooms-Goossens A, Ducombs G, Lachapelle JM, Menne T, Rycroft RJ, Wahlberg JE, White IR, et al (1989) Trial of 0.5% versus 0.375% potassium dichromate. European Environmental and Contact Dermatitis Research Group (EECDRG). Contact Dermatitis 21:351
54. Frosch PJ, Aberer W (1988) Chrom-Allergie. Dermatosen 36:168–169
55. Allenby CF, Goodwin BFS (1983) Influence of detergent washing powders on minimal eliciting patch test concentration of nickel and chromium. Contact Dermatitis 9:491–499

56. Skog E, Wahlberg JE (1969) Patch testing with potassium dichromate in different vehicles. Arch Dermatol 99: 697–700

57. Al-Tawil NG, Marcusson JA, Möller E (1983) Lymphocyte stimulation by trivalent and hexavalent chromium compounds in patients with chromium sensitivity. An aid to diagnosis. Acta Derm Venereol (Stockh) 63:296–303

58. Räsänen L, Sainio H, Lehto M, Reunala T (1991) Lymphocyte proliferation test as a diagnostic aid in chromium contact sensitivity. Contact Dermatitis 25:25–29

59. Thormann J, Jespersen NB, Joensen HD (1979) Persistence of contact allergy to chromium. Contact Dermatitis 5: 261–264

60. Fregert S (1975) Occupational dermatitis in a 10-year material. Contact Dermatitis 1:96–107

61. Burrows D (1972) Prognosis in industrial dermatitis. Br J Dermatol 87:145–148

62. Wall LM, Gebauer KA (1991) A follow-up study of occupational skin disease in Western Australia. Contact Dermatitis 24:241–243

63. Anderson RA (1995) Chromium and parenteral nutrition. Nutrition 11:83–86

64. Accominotti M, Bost M, Haudrechy P, Mantout B, Cunat PJ, Comet F, Mouterde C, Plantard F, Chambon P, Vallon JJ (1998) Contribution to chromium and nickel enrichment during cooking of foods in stainless steel utensils. Contact Dermatitis 38:305–310

65. Kaaber K, Veien NK (1977) The significance of chromate ingestion in patients allergic to chromate. Acta Derm Venereol (Stockh) 57:321–323

66. Kerger B, Finley B, Corbett G, Paustenbach D (1996) Absorption and elimination of trivalent and hexavalent chromium in humans following ingestion of a bolus dose in drinking water. J Appl Toxicol 141:145–158

67. Kerger B, Finley B, Corbett G, Dodge D, Paustenbach D (1997) Ingestion of chromium (VI) in drinking water by human volunteers: absorption, distribution, and excretion of single and repeated doses. J Appl Toxicol 50:67–95

68. Kaaber K, Sjolin, Menné T (1983) Elbow eruptions in nickel and chromate dermatitis. Contact Dermatitis 9:213–216

69. Costa M (1998) Carcinogenic metals. Sci Prog 81:329–339

70. Jaeger J, Pelloni E (1950) Tests épicutanés aux bichromates, postifs dans l'eczéma au ciment (Positive skin tests with bichromates in cement eczema). Dermatologica 100: 207–216

71. Uter W, Ruhl R, Pfahlberg A, Geier J, Schnuch A, Gefeller O (2004) Contact allergy in construction workers: results of a multifactorial analysis. Ann Occup Hyg 48:21–27

72. Goon TJA, Goh C-L (2000) Epidemiology of occupational skin disease in Singapore 1989–1998. Contact Dermatitis 43:133–136

73. Kanerva L, Jolanki R, Estlander T, Alanko K, Savela A (2000) Incidence rates of occupational allergic contact dermatitis caused by metals. Am J Contact Dermat 11: 155–160

74. Balasubramaniam P, Gawkrodger P (2003) Chromate: still an important occupational allergen for men in the UK. Contact Dermatitis 49:162–163

75. Bock M, Schmidt A, Bruckner T, Diepgen TL (2003) Occupational skin disease in the construction industry. Br J Dermatol 149:1165–1171

76. Estlander T (1990) Occupational skin disease in Finland. Observations made during 1974–1988 at the Institute of Occupational Health, Helsinki. Acta Derm Venereol Suppl (Stockh) 155:1–85

77. Avnstorp C (1991) Risk factors for cement eczema. Contact Dermatitis 25:81–88

78. Basketter DA, Briatico-Vangosa G, Kaestner W, Lally C, Bontinck WJ (1993) Nickel, cobalt and chromium in consumer products: a role in allergic contact dermatitis? Contact Dermatitis 28:15–25

79. Zachariae COC, Agner T, Menné T (1996) Chromium allergy in consecutive patients in a country where ferrous sulfate has been added to cement since 1981. Contact Dermatitis 35:83–85

80. Roto P, Sainio H, Reunala T, Laippala P (1996) Addition of ferrous sulfate to cement and risk of chromium dermatitis among construction workers. Contact Dermatitis 34: 43–50

81. Johansen J, Menné T, Christophersen J, Kaaber K, Veien N (2000) Changes in the pattern of sensitization to common contact allergens in Denmark between 1985–1986 and 1997–1998, with a special view to the effect of preventive strategies. Br J Dermatol 142:490–495

82. Irvine C, Pugh CE, Hansen E, Rycroft RJG (1994) Cement dermatitis in underground workers during construction of the Channel Tunnel. Occup Med 44:17–23

83. Peltonen L, Fräki J (1983) Prevalence of dichromate sensitivity. Contact Dermatitis 9:190–194

84. Seidenari S, Manzini BM, Danese P, Motolese A (1990) Patch and prick test study of 593 healthy subjects. Contact Dermatitis 23:162–167

85. Lantinga H, Nater JP, Coenraads PJ (1984) Prevalence, incidence and course of eczema on the hands and forearms in a sample of the general population. Contact Dermatitis 10:135–139

86. Nielsen NH, Menné T (1992) Allergic contact sensitization in an unselected Danish population. The Glostrup Allergy Study, Denmark. Acta Derm Venereol (Stockh) 72: 456–460

87. Greig JE, Carson CF, Stuckey MS, Riley TV (2000) Prevalence of delayed hypersensitivity to the European standard series in a self-selected population. Australas J Dermatol 41:86–89

88. Mortz CG, Andersen KE (1999) Allergic contact dermatitis in children and adolescents. Contact Dermatitis 41: 121–130

89. Wass U, Wahlberg JE (1991) Chromated steel and contact allergy. Recommendation concerning a "threshold limit value" for the release of hexavalent chromium. Contact Dermatitis 24:114–118

90. Burckhardt W, Frenk E, de Sépibus D, Paschoud JM, Szadurski J, Schwarz K (1971) Abschwächung der ekzematogenen Wirkung des Zementes durch Ferrosulfat (Decrease of the eczematous effect of dement by ferrous sulphate, in German). Dermatologica 142:271–273

91. Fregert S, Gruvberger B, Sandahl E (1979) Reduction of chromate in cement by iron sulfate. Contact Dermatitis 5: 39–42

92. Färm G (1986) Changing patterns in chromate allergy. Contact Dermatitis 15:298–299

93. von Gailhofer G, Ludvan M (1987) Zur Änderung des Allergenspektrums bei Kontaktekzemen in den Jahren 1975–1984. Berufsdermatosen 35:12–16

94. Goh CL, Gan SL (1996) Change in cement manufacturing process, a cause for decline in chromate allergy? Contact Dermatitis 34:51–54

95. EU directive 2003/53/EG (18 June 2003)

96. Bruze M, Gruvberger B, Hradil E (1990) Chromate sensitization and elicitation with iron sulfate. Acta Derm Venereol (Stockh) 70:160–162

32

32.4 Cobalt

Cobalt (Co) is a silvery metal which belongs, together with nickel and chromium, to the transition elements. Cobalt is a skin and respiratory allergen. Occupational exposure to cobalt occurs mainly through the respiratory tract. Pulmonary effects, particularly in the hard-metal industry, are hard-metal pneumoconiosis and occupational asthma. Inhalation of hard-metal dust induces asthma, in some cases, by a type I immunological mechanism. Cardiomyopathy has been described among heavy consumers of cobalt-contaminated beer. Cobalt is genotoxic. It is controversial whether cobalt can give rise to human cancer. Cobalt is an essential trace element, as it occurs in vitamin B12.

32.4.1 Cobalt Use and Exposure

Since the 1930s, there has been a large increase in cobalt production, which reached 24,500 tonnes in 1995. Cobalt is now mainly a by-product of nickel and copper mining, 50% of world production being based on the copper ores of central Africa. Cobalt has been used for thousands of years [1] (Table 4.1). The oxidation states of cobalt are 0, +1, +2, and +3.

The main uses of cobalt are in the production of superalloys (Ni/Co/Fe; 25%), hard materials, carbides and diamond tooling (15%), colors (12%), magnets (10%), and adhesives, soaps, and driers (10%) [1] (Table 4.2). Hard metal is manufactured by combining tungsten and carbon with cobalt as a binder. The product has 90–95% of the hardness of diamond and is used for the cutting edges of tools and drills. Cobalt is used in different electroplatings to produce hard, wear-resistant, and bright coatings.

Table 4.1. Timetable for cobalt [1]

2600 BC	Cobalt coloring of pottery and glass
1735	Metallic cobalt was isolated by G Brandt
1780	Cobalt was proved as an element
1842	Cobalt electroplating
Up to the 20th century	Coloring from cobalt oxides and silicates was the main use
1901	Use as paint dryer
1933	Alnico magnets
1936	Dental alloy
1953	Extensive use as catalyst
1980	Co–Cr alloys in prosthetics
1991	Growth of catalyst chemical market

Table 4.2. Main uses of cobalt [1]

Metallurgical	Superalloys
	Wear-resistant coatings
	High-speed steels
	Prosthetic alloys
	Low-expansion alloys
	Steels
	Corrosion-resistant alloys
Magnetic alloys	Hard and soft magnets
Chemicals	Catalysts
	Adhesives, cobalt soaps
	Driers, pigments, colors
	Electroplating
	Agriculture and medicine
	Electromagnetic recording
Cemented carbides	Cobalt-bonded diamonds
Electronics	Recording material (mainly Co–Ni)
	Matched-expansion alloys
	Leads
Ceramics and enamels	Colors in glass, enamels, pottery, china

The use of cobalt in objects intended for direct and prolonged contact with the skin may increase, as a substitute for nickel, which is limited by the Nickel Directive.

Based on risk assessment addressing allergic contact dermatitis, it was recommended that consumer products such as household products and personal care items should not contain more than 5 ppm of each of nickel, chromium, or cobalt, and that the ultimate target level should be 1 ppm [2]. Only minor traces of cobalt, 0–5 ppm, were found in such consumer products [2, 3].

Knowledge about skin exposure to cobalt is limited and is often associated with simultaneous exposure to nickel or chromate. Nickel-containing alloys generally contain traces of cobalt. Cement may contain cobalt and nickel as well as chromate [4, 5]. Exposure to cobalt and its compounds alone is said to occur mainly in the hard-metal and ceramics industries. To increase knowledge about cobalt in relation to skin exposure, 20 cobalt-containing alloys were stored in synthetic sweat for 1 week. The content of different metals in the solution was analyzed. The study showed that the release of cobalt varied significantly from different materials, from 0.1 µg/cm² per week through 400 µg/cm² per week (C. Lidén, unpublished).

Atomic absorption spectroscopy was used to study the accumulation of cobalt in fingernails after immersion of a finger in aqueous cobalt solutions for 10 min per day during 2 weeks [6].

> ### Core Message
>
> ■ Cobalt is used in the production of alloys, magnets, dental and surgical implants, and in hard metals. Cobalt compounds are used as catalysts and as drying agents in paints, etc. Cobalt may also be present at a low level in nickel alloys, consumer products, and cement.

32.4.2 Allergic Contact Dermatitis

Contact allergy to cobalt chloride is common and is generally associated with concomitant contact allergy to nickel or chromate. Routine patch testing, including nickel, cobalt, and chromium compounds, was carried out in 1960–1964 on 5,416 patients with suspected contact dermatitis [7]. Ten percent of the patients were positive to one or more of the three metal compounds. Allergy to cobalt was equally common in both sexes – chromium/cobalt was common in men and nickel/cobalt in women. Contact allergy to cobalt chloride was found among 5–8% of patch-tested dermatitis patients, and generally at a higher rate in women than in men [8].

Far too little is known about cobalt allergy, although cobalt is one of the major contact allergens. Until now, we have often had difficulty in explaining to patients induction, elicitation, and possible cross-reactivity. Solitary cobalt allergy is seen mainly among hard-metal workers and in the glass and pottery industries, but it is often difficult to identify the source of isolated positive cobalt patch tests [9–12].

Occupational allergic contact dermatitis caused by metallic cobalt dust in a factory producing tungsten carbide alloys was described in 1945 [13]. Eight hundred and fifty three hard-metal workers were examined and patch tested with metals and other substances from their environment [10, 11]. Five percent of the workers were allergic to cobalt. Individuals with concomitant nickel and cobalt allergy had more severe hand eczema than those with isolated cobalt or nickel sensitivity, or irritant contact dermatitis. The authors concluded that nickel sensitivity and irritant hand eczema had preceded cobalt sensitization.

In a Finnish pottery factory, positive patch test reactions to cobalt and dermatitis on the arms and hands were related to exposure to wet, alkaline clay containing cobalt [12].

Cobalt is an important occupational contact allergen in construction workers. In Northern Bavaria, Germany, during 1990 to 1999, 335 cases of occupational skin disease in the construction industry were recorded [14]. Allergic contact dermatitis was found in 62%, chromate caused half of the cases, followed by epoxy and cobalt. In Germany, during the period 1989 to 1993, contact allergy to cobalt was found in 15% of 205 male dermatitis patients working in the construction industry compared to 5% among 5,706 male patients not working in this industry [15]. Corresponding figures from Germany and Austria during 1992 to 2000 show that contact allergy to cobalt was found in 8.6% of construction workers compared to 4.9% of the remaining dermatitis patients [16]. Cobalt allergy in construction workers was strongly associated with allergy to chromate [15, 16]. When 449 male construction workers in Spain who were dermatitis patients were patch tested, contact allergy to cobalt chloride was found in 20% [17]. Only single cases were allergic to cobalt chloride alone.

Case reports on dermatitis related to occupational exposure to cobalt-containing materials, such as black ink, animal feeds, and cement, have been published, and stomatitis related to cobalt-containing dentures and dermatitis related to orthopedic prostheses have also been reported [18]. A blue pigment used for tattoos (cobaltous aluminate) may cause allergic granulomatous reactions [19]. Chronic photocontact dermatitis has been reported in patients who were sensitive to cobalt [20, 21]. They were exposed to cement products or pig fodder.

Contact allergy to cobalt chloride was found in 1.1% when 567 persons, a sample of the general population in Denmark, were patch tested [22].

The simultaneous reactivity to cobalt chloride and nickel sulfate or chromate is not believed to be due to cross-reactivity, but rather, due to combined exposure. This is based partly on knowledge of use and exposure, and partly on results from animal studies.

Cobalt chloride was used in a human maximization test and it sensitized 10 out of 25 volunteers [23]. It was reported to be a grade 3 allergen (highest grade being 5). Cobalt chloride is a potent sensitizer in the guinea pig. In a guinea pig maximization test, all animals were sensitized and cobalt chloride was reported to be a grade 5 allergen [24]. Animals induced with cobalt chloride did not react to nickel sulfate or chromate – the results speaking in favor of multiple sensitization rather than cross-reactivity [25, 26]. Guinea pigs sensitized to nickel sulfate were found to be more easily sensitized to cobalt chloride [27]. Cross-sensitization experiments in guinea pigs with cobalt chloride and rhodium chloride, however, indicate cross-reactivity [28].

Core Message

■ The contact allergy rate to cobalt in the general population is around 1% and in patch-tested dermatitis patients 5–8%. Cobalt is an important contact allergen in construction workers and hard-metal workers. Allergy to cobalt is often seen together with allergy to nickel or to chromate. Solitary cobalt allergy is rare.

32.4.3 Patch Testing with Cobalt

The diagnostic patch test concentration used in the European standard series is cobalt chloride 1% in petrolatum. However, 0.5% in petrolatum has often been used in the Swedish standard series, due to the fact that 1% may produce porous reactions [29]. The TRUE Test also uses cobalt chloride.

A study was carried out to establish the minimum levels of cobalt chloride required to elicit a positive patch test response. On normal skin, the minimum eliciting concentration was 2,260 ppm. When the skin was pretreated for 24 h with sodium dodecyl sulfate (SDS), the minimum eliciting level was 2.3–226 ppm cobalt chloride [30].

Patch testing was carried out with a metallic cobalt disc containing 100% cobalt, supplementary to the standard series including 1% cobalt chloride in petrolatum [31]. In all, 458 consecutive dermatitis patients were patch tested and 23 were positive to cobalt chloride, of whom, 11 were positive to the cobalt disc. No positive reactions were recorded for the cobalt disc in patients with a negative patch test to cobalt chloride.

Core Message

■ Patch testing with 1% cobalt chloride is recommended. This concentration may, however, elicit non-allergic porous reactions.

32.4.4 Prevention and Legislation

There is no regulatory limitation in the use of cobalt for the prevention of contact dermatitis, such as for nickel and chromium in cement. These regulations may, however, affect exposure and sensitization to cobalt. If the use of cobalt increases, as a substitute for nickel in the items covered by the Nickel Directive, this may result in an increase in allergic contact dermatitis due to cobalt. The risk is obvious, as cobalt is a potent skin sensitizer. It has been speculated that the limitation of chromium in cement may decrease also the risk of cobalt allergy in construction workers, secondary to the reduction of chromate dermatitis [16, 32].

Core Message

■ To avoid an increase in cobalt allergy, it is essential that cobalt is not used instead of nickel in items in contact with the skin.

References

1. Clark B (1996) Cobalt facts. The Cobalt Development Institute (CDI), Wickford, Essex
2. Basketter DA, Briatico-Vangosa G, Kaestner W, Lally C, Bontinck WJ (1993) Nickel, cobalt and chromium in consumer products: a role in allergic contact dermatitis? Contact Dermatitis 28:15–25
3. Basketter DA, Angelini G, Ingber A, Kern PS, Menné T (2003). Nickel, chromium and cobalt in consumer products: revisiting safe levels in the new millennium. Contact Dermatitis 49:1–7
4. Goh CL, Kwok SF, Gan SL (1986) Cobalt and nickel content of Asian cements. Contact Dermatitis 15:169–172
5. Tandon R, Aarts B (1993) Chromium, nickel and cobalt contents of some Australian cements. Contact Dermatitis 28:201–205
6. Nielsen NH, Kristiansen J, Borg L, Christensen JM, Poulsen LK, Menné T (2000) Repeated exposures to cobalt and chromate on the hands of patients with hand eczema and contact allergy to that metal. Contact Dermatitis 43:212–215
7. Fregert S, Rorsman H (1966) Allergy to chromium, nickel and cobalt. Acta Derm Venereol (Stockh) 46:144–148
8. Fowler JF Jr (1990) Allergic contact dermatitis to metals. Am J Contact Dermat 1:212–223
9. Rystedt I (1979) Evaluation and relevance of isolated test reactions to cobalt. Contact Dermatitis 5:233–238
10. Fischer T, Rystedt I (1983) Cobalt allergy in hard metal workers. Contact Dermatitis 9:115–121
11. Rystedt I, Fischer T (1983) Relationship between nickel and cobalt sensitization in hard metal workers. Contact Dermatitis 9:195–200
12. Pirilä V (1953) Sensitivity to cobalt in pottery workers. Acta Derm Venereol (Stockh) 33:193–198

32

13. Schwartz L, Peck SM, Blair KE et al (1945) Allergic dermatitis due to metallic cobalt. J Allergy Clin Immunol 16: 51–53

14. Bock M, Schmidt A, Bruckner T, Diepgen TL (2003) Occupational skin disease in the construction industry. Br J Dermatol 149:1165–1171

15. Geier J, Schnuch A (1995) A comparison of contact allergies among construction and nonconstruction workers attending contact dermatitis clinics in Germany: results of the Information Network of Departments of Dermatology from November 1989 to July 1993. Am J Contact Dermat 6: 86–94

16. Uter W, Rühl R, Pfahlberg A, Geier J, Schnuch A, Gefeller O (2004) Contact allergy in construction workers: Results of a multifactorial analysis. Ann Occup Hyg 48:21–27

17. Condé-Salazar L, Guimaraens D, Villegas C, Romero A, Gonzalez MA (1995) Occupational allergic contact dermatitis in construction workers. Contact Dermatitis 33: 226–230

18. Burrows D, Adams RM, Flint GN (1999) Metals. In: Adams RM (ed) Occupational skin disease, 3rd edn. Saunders, Philadelphia, Pa., pp 395–433

19. Levy J, Sewell M, Goldstein N (1979) A short history of tattooing. J Dermatol Surg Oncol 5:851–856

20. Camarasa JG, Alomar A (1981) Photosensitization to cobalt in a bricklayer. Contact Dermatitis 7:154–155

21. Romaguera C, Lecha M, Grimalt F, Muniesa AM, Mascaro JM (1982) Photocontact dermatitis to cobalt salts. Contact Dermatitis 8:383–388

22. Nielsen NH, Menné T (1992) Allergic contact sensitization in an unselected Danish population. The Glostrup Allergy Study, Denmark. Acta Derm Venereol (Stockh) 72: 456–460

23. Kligman AM (1966) The identification of contact allergens by human assay. 3. The maximization test: a procedure for screening and rating contact sensitizers. J Invest Dermatol 47:393–409

24. Wahlberg JE, Boman A (1978) Sensitization and testing of guinea pigs with cobalt chloride. Contact Dermatitis 4: 128–132

25. Lidén C, Wahlberg JE (1994) Cross-reactivity to metal compounds studied in guinea pigs induced with chromate or cobalt. Acta Derm Venereol (Stockh) 74:341–343

26. Wahlberg JE, Lidén C (2000) Cross-reactivity patterns of cobalt and nickel studied with repeated open applications (ROATs) to the skin of guinea pigs. Am J Contact Dermat 11:42–48

27. Lammintausta K, Pitkänen OP, Kalimo K, Jansen CT (1985) Interrelationship of nickel and cobalt contact sensitization. Contact Dermatitis 13:148–152

28. Lidén C, Wahlberg JE, Maibach HI (1995) Skin. In: Goyer RA, Klaassen CD, Waalkes MP (eds) Metal toxicology. Academic Press, New York, pp 447–464

29. Fischer T, Rystedt I (1985) False-positive, follicular and irritant patch test reactions to metal salts. Contact Dermatitis 12:93–98

30. Allenby CF, Basketter DA (1989) Minimum eliciting patch test concentrations of cobalt. Contact Dermatitis 20: 185–190

31. de Fine Olivarius F, Menné T (1992) Skin reactivity to metallic cobalt in patients with a positive patch test to cobalt chloride. Contact Dermatitis 27:241–243

32. Kanerva L, Jolanki R, Estlander T, Alanko K, Savela A (2000) Incidence rates of occupational allergic contact dermatitis caused by metals. Am J Contact Dermat 11: 155–160

32.5 Aluminum

Aluminum (Al) is widely used and contact with aluminum in its elemental form or it salts is unavoidable.

32.5.1 Allergic Contact Dermatitis

Few case reports of contact allergy to aluminum exist. It is considered a weak contact allergen. Occupational contact dermatitis due to aluminum exposure has been reported in aluminum production [1], in aircraft manufacture [2], and in a machine construction plant [3]. A rather new method for aluminum production, cold sealing, with nickel floride, constitutes a new risk of dermatitis from working with aluminum. The risk is not from the aluminum itself, however, but from nickel sulfate on the surface of cold-sealed aluminum objects [4].

Water-soluble aluminum salts in antiperspirants may cause axillary dermatitis [5], but this is usually irritant. Reactions to aluminum-absorbed vaccines may induce allergic contact dermatitis [6–11]. Reactions to aluminum from the Finn Chambers used for patch testing have rarely been recorded [12]. Systemic aluminum contact dermatitis from toothpaste has been reported [13].

References

1. Johannessen H, Bergan-Skar B (1980) Itching problems among potroom workers in factories using recycled alumina. Contact Dermatitis 6:42–43

2. Hall AF (1944) Occupational contact dermatitis among aircraft workers. J Am Med Assoc 125:179–185

3. Peters T, Hani N, Kirchberg K, Gold H, Hunzelmann N, Scharffetter-Kochanek K (1998) Occupational contact sensitivity to aluminium in a machine construction plant worker. Contact Dermatitis 39:322–323

4. Lidén C (1994) Cold-impregnated aluminium. A new source of nickel exposure. Contact Dermatitis 31:22–24

5. Williams S, Freemont AJ (1984) Aerosol antiperspirants and axillary granulomata. Br Med J (Clin Res Ed) 288: 1651–1652

6. Frost L, Johansen P, Pedersen S, Veien N, Ostergaard PA, Nielsen MH (1985) Persistent subcutaneous nodules in children hyposensitized with aluminium-containing allergen extracts. Allergy 40:368–372

7. Veien NK, Hattel T, Justesen O, Norholm A (1986) Aluminium allergy. Contact Dermatitis 15:295–297

8. Clemmensen O, Knudsen HE (1980) Contact sensitivity to aluminium in a patient hyposensitized with aluminium precipitated grass pollen. Contact Dermatitis 6:305–308

9. Bohler-Sommeregger K, Lindemayr H (1986) Contact sensitivity to aluminium. Contact Dermatitis 15:278–281

10. Fawcett HA, McGibbon D, Cronin E (1985) Persistent vaccination granuloma due to aluminum sensitivity. Br J Dermatol 113(Suppl 29):101–102

11. Nielsen AO, Kaaber K, Veien NK (1992) Aluminum allergy caused by DTP vaccine. Ugeskr Laeger 154:1900–1901
12. Dwyer CM, Kerr RE (1993) Contact allergy to aluminium in 2 brothers. Contact Dermatitis 29:36–38
13. Veien NK, Hattel T, Laurberg G (1993). Systemically aggravated contact dermatitis caused by aluminium in toothpaste. Contact Dermatitis 28:199–200

32.6 Beryllium

Beryllium (Be) is a ubiquitous metal present in soil and as soluble and insoluble salts in waste and salt water. Most beryllium is used as an alloy or in specialty ceramics for electrical and electronic applications, while pure beryllium finds use in the nuclear industry, aircraft, and medical devices, including dental alloys.

Beryllium has been clearly established as a human carcinogen [1]. Beryllium is extremely toxic, resulting in acute and chronic respiratory disease [2]. Chronic beryllium disease is characterized by non-caseating granulomas and interstitial pulmonary infiltrates, where the diagnosis is based on the demonstration of a cell-mediated immune response to beryllium salts, either in vitro with the beryllium lymphocyte proliferation test or in vivo with a patch test to beryllium sulfate [3].

Chemical burns, contact dermatitis, and granulomatous lesions may result from skin exposure to beryllium compounds. Soluble beryllium salts, such as beryllium chloride and beryllium fluoride, are caustic at high concentrations. Cutaneous findings were emphasized in a recent paper on occupational chronic beryllium disease [4].

32.6.1 Allergic Contact Dermatitis

In 1951, Curtis was the first to diagnose beryllium contact allergy in workers at two beryllium plants by patch testing with various beryllium salts [5]. Beryllium present in dental alloys has been reported to cause contact allergic reactions of the oral mucosa [6, 7]. In Spain, three patients tested positively to beryllium chloride 1% in petrolatum [6]. One patient suffered from a stomatitis adjacent to a beryllium-containing prosthesis. When the prosthesis was replaced with one not containing beryllium, the symptoms disappeared. A dental mechanic making beryllium-containing prostheses presented with a hand dermatitis that was diagnosed as an occupational allergic contact dermatitis from beryllium [6]. Haberman et al. reported two patients who developed gingivitis adjacent to a beryllium-containing alloy in their dental prostheses [7]. Patch testing demonstrated positive reactions to beryllium sulfate 1% in petrolatum in the two patients, while none of the 30 controls tested positively to this preparation.

Using the guinea pig maximization test, beryllium sulfate has been demonstrated to be a sensitizer [8].

References

1. Costa M (1998) Carcinogenic metals. Sci Prog 81:329–339
2. Kriebel D, Sprince NL, Eisen EA, Greaves IA (1988) Beryllium exposure and pulmonary function: a cross-sectional study of beryllium workers. Br J Ind Med 45:167–173
3. Bobka CA, Stewart LA, Engelken GJ, Golitz LE, Newman LS (1997) Comparison of in vivo and in vitro measures of beryllium sensitization. J Occup Environ Med 39:540–547
4. Berlin JM, Taylor JS, Sigel JE, Bergfeld WF, Dweik RA (2003) Beryllium dermatitis. J Am Acad Dermatol 49:939–941
5. Curtis CH (1951) Cutaneous hypersensitivity to beryllium: a study of 13 cases. Arch Dermatol Syphilol 64:470–482
6. Vilaplana J, Romaguera C, Grimalt F (1992) Occupational and non-occupational allergic contact dermatitis from beryllium. Contact Dermatitis 26:295–298
7. Haberman AL, Pratt M, Storrs FJ (1993) Contact dermatitis from beryllium in dental alloys. Contact Dermatitis 28:157–162
8. Zissu D, Binet S, Cavelier C (1996) Patch testing with beryllium alloy samples in guinea pigs. Contact Dermatitis 34:196–200

32.7 Cadmium

Cadmium (Cd) is one of the most toxic metals and environmental poisons. Cadmium is used in pigments for plastics, paints, glass and ceramics, in alloys, solders and platings, and in nickel–cadmium batteries. The main industrial exposure is to fumes and dust by inhalation, and environmental exposure is via food and smoking. Acute toxicity causes nausea, vomiting, and pneumonitis and may be fatal, and chronic toxicity affects many organs (kidney, lung, bones, hematopoietic system). The itai-itai disease affected mainly women, probably due to higher gastro-intestinal absorption at low iron stores [1].

32.7.1 Allergic Contact Dermatitis

When cadmium chloride (2% in water) was included in the standard patch test used in 1,502 dermatitis patients, 25 were patch test positive [2]. Further testing with serial dilutions was not interpreted in favor of contact allergy, as only 1 of 6 patients was positive to 1% cadmium chloride. The reactions were regarded as non-relevant and probably irritant in nature. Cadmium chloride 0.5% in petrolatum was, based on testing in 662 dermatitis patients, recommended for patch testing [3]. In total, 791 patients, among them 59 dental technicians, were patch tested with a dental materials series including cadmium chloride (1% in petrolatum) [4]. Of the patients, 9% were patch test positive to cadmium chloride. The reactions were judged non-relevant, as the rates were equal among dental technicians (possibly exposed) and other patients (probably not exposed). Cadmium red (cadmium selenide) has previously been used for the coloration of dentures and it was not evaluated as an allergen [5].

Yellow cadmium sulfide is used as a pigment for yellow and red tattoos, and it may cause phototoxic reactions and sarcoid-like granulomas [6].

The sensitizing potential of cadmium chloride was evaluated in a guinea pig maximization test, and cadmium chloride caused no statistically significant reactivity in induced animals compared to control animals [7].

References

1. Vahter M, Berglund M, Åkesson A, Lidén C (2002) Metals and women's health. Environ Res 88:145–155
2. Wahlberg JE (1977) Routine patch testing with cadmium chloride. Contact Dermatitis 3:293–296
3. Geier J, Vieluf D, Fuchs T (1996) Patch testing with cadmium chloride. Contact Dermatitis 34:73–74
4. Gebhart M, Geier J (1996) Evaluation of patch test results with denture material series. Contact Dermatitis 34:191–195
5. Kaaber S, Cramers M, Jepsen FL (1982) The role of cadmium as a skin sensitizing agent in denture and non-denture wearers. Contact Dermatitis 8:308–313
6. Björnberg A (1963) Reaction to light in yellow tattoos from cadmium sulfide. Arch Dermatol 88:267–271
7. Wahlberg JE, Boman A (1979) Guinea pig maximization test method – cadmium chloride. Contact Dermatitis 5:405

32.8 Copper

Copper (Cu) is an important metal in industry. The primary use of copper, approximately half its production, is in electrical equipment. Copper is widely used in alloys together with tin, zinc, silver, and cadmium. Copper/tin alloys are called bronzes, and may also contain other metals. Copper-containing alloys are used for coins, jewelry, pipes, roofs, etc., and may be used in some dental materials. Copper sulfate and organic copper salts are used in agriculture as fungicides and algicides. Copper is an essential trace element that is crucial in hemoglobin synthesis and in other enzyme functions.

32.8.1 Allergic Contact Dermatitis

Copper has been considered a rare skin sensitizer [1]. This was concluded also in a recent review of publications on copper hypersensitivity [2]. Reports of positive patch test reactions in patients with dermatitis related to the use of copper-containing intrauterine contraceptive devices (IUCD) [3, 4] have been published. Single cases of contact stomatitis [5], oral pain [6], and oral lichen planus [7] have been described. When copper sulfate (2% in petrolatum) was included in the standard patch test used in 1,190 dermatitis patients in Sweden, 1% positive reactions were recorded, but they were considered non-relevant [1]. When copper sulfate (2% in petrolatum) was included in the patch test series in Austria, 3.5% were positive [8]. The authors suggested 5% copper sulfate for patch testing, but stated that positive reactions are usually of low clinical relevance, and that the reproducibility of test reactions was considered modest.

The sensitizing potential of copper sulfate was evaluated in a series of guinea pig maximization tests, and it was classified as a weak sensitizer or a grade I allergen [1]. Local lymph node assay (LLNA) in mice was positive [9].

32.8.2 Irritant Contact Dermatitis

Concentrated solutions of copper sulfate are corrosive and cause primary irritation on skin contact.

References

1. Karlberg A-T, Boman A, Wahlberg JE (1983) Copper – a rare sensitizer. Contact Dermatitis 9:134–139
2. Hostynek JJ, Maibach HI (2003) Copper hypersensitivity: dermatologic aspects – an overview. Rev Environ Health 18:153–183
3. Barranco VP (1972) Eczematous dermatitis caused by internal exposure to copper. Arch Dermatol 106:386–387
4. Romaguera C, Grimalt F (1981) Contact dermatitis from a copper-containing intrauterine contraceptive device. Contact Dermatitis 7:163–164
5. Nordlind K, Lidén S (1992) Patch test reactions to metal salts in patients with oral mucosal lesions associated with amalgam restorations. Contact Dermatitis 27:157–160
6. Santosh V, Ranjith K, Shenoi SD, Sachin V, Balachandran C (1999) Results of patch testing with dental materials. Contact Dermatitis 40:50–51
7. Frykholm KO, Frithiof F, Fernström AI, Moberger G, Blohm SG, Bjorn E (1969) Allergy to copper derived from dental alloys as a possible cause of oral lesions of lichen planus. Acta Derm Venereol (Stockh) 49:268–281
8. Wöhrl S, Hemmer W, Focke M, Götz M, Jarisch R (2001) Copper allergy revisited. J Am Acad Dermatol 45:863–870
9. Basketter DA, Gerberick GF, Kimber I, Loveless SE (1996) The local lymph node assay: a viable alternative to currently accepted skin sensitization tests. Food Chem Toxicol 34:985–997

32.9 Gold

Many persons are or may be exposed to metallic gold (Au) as it is present in jewelry and dental materials. Currently, gold is a controversial sensitizer [1]. The reason for this is understandable. Until recently, gold allergy was considered to be extremely rare, so it was remarkable when a contact allergy rate to gold of around 10% was reported in consecutively patch tested dermatitis patients [2]. Gold, maybe the most beloved and precious metal, has been used and worshipped for thousands of years without any obvious complaints of skin problems, either in those participating in mining and other ways of prospecting, or in those wearing jewelry.

32.9.1 Gold Use and Exposure

Gold is the only metal except copper that is markedly colored. It is abundant in low concentrations over almost all the Earth's crust and in seawater, above all in metallic form and also as gold telluride. Gold is found as grains in the bottom of rivers, above all in California, Australia, Alaska, and Russia, while gold ore in South Africa is harvested from mines with auriferous leaders. Gold is also produced as a by-product from the production of copper, nickel, and lead. The world's yearly production of gold is 1,000 tons, of which, 150 tons are used in the electronics industry [3].

Pure gold is very soft but malleable and ductile. To increase its strength, alloys with other metals, such as silver, copper, nickel, palladium, and zinc, are common. The color of gold is influenced by the alloy addition, where silver gives a greenish yellow, copper a reddish, and nickel a light yellow to whitish gold.

Gold is resistant to corrosion as it does not combine with oxygen or other substances in the atmosphere, not even at elevated temperatures. Gold occurs in oxidation states 0, +I, and +III, the latter being most stable, and the equilibrium between these states can be altered easily [4]. All halogens attack gold, and so do halogen acids mixed with nitric acid or other oxidizers. Aqua regia, a mixture of hydrochloric and nitric acids, as well as cyanide solutions attack gold. To be a hapten, gold has to be ionized. When subjecting gold-containing jewelry alloys to artificial sweat for 1 and 3 weeks, no release of gold was detected [5]. However, this does not mean that metallic gold cannot be of significance for gold sensitization, as the absence of amino acids in the synthetic sweat used [5] could affect the release rate of gold ions [6]. It has been demonstrated that gold can dissolve in water

solutions that contain thiol-substituted amino acids (cysteine, glutathione) and be absorbed through animal skin [4, 6]. Actually, in a use test study with two types of visually indistinguishable earrings made of titanium nitride with and without coating with 24-carat gold in 60 gold-hypersensitive females, more statistically significantly reactions were noted in those using the gold-plated earrings [7]. Furthermore, the blood level of gold is higher in dermatitis patients with dental gold compared to those without dental gold and with a correlation between the gold blood level and the number of dental gold restorations, strongly suggesting that gold is released from dental gold [8]. Studies have also demonstrated the significance of dental gold for sensitization [9–12]. In a double blind study including patch testing as well as clinical and radiological investigation of the oral cavity, a dose–response relationship was found for gold allergy and dental gold; the more dental gold, the higher contact allergy rate [12].

Gold is found in jewelry, either as an alloy, as gold plating, or as rolled gold. In plating, a base metal such as copper is electrolytically covered with nickel and then gold of varying thickness is added. Gold is also present in alloys in dentistry to make crowns, bridges, etc. Gold hydroxide, gold oxide, and various gold salts, such as potassium and sodium gold trichloride, sodium tetrachloroaurate dihydrate, potassium dicyanoaurate, and gold sodium sulfite, find their uses to make ruby glass and to color enamel and porcelain, as well as for other decorative applications in photography, in printed circuit boards, and in electronics manufacture. In the medical profession, both elemental gold and various gold compounds are used for various purposes, above all, to treat rheumatoid arthritis [13].

Core Message

■ Dental gold is significant for gold sensitization.

32.9.2 Patch Testing with Gold and Gold Compounds

Elemental gold has been used for patch testing, but it has only occasionally elicited a positive patch test. Various gold salts/compounds, both monovalent and trivalent, such as potassium dicyanoaurate, gold sodium thiosulfate, gold sodium thiomalate, and gold chloride, have been used for patch testing. Gold (III) chloride has often been used. However, it is important to stress that a test solution of gold chloride is a solution of gold chloride in hydrochloric acid, since it is insoluble in water, and, hence, it is a strong irritant with a risk of false-positive reactions. Nevertheless, gold chloride is a sensitizer, which has been demonstrated by Kligman in a human maximization test in the 1960s [14]. In the late 1980s, Fowler reported that gold sodium thiosulfate at 0.5% in petrolatum was a good screening preparation for tracing contact allergy to gold [15]. At the Jadassohn Congress in London in 1996, gold sodium thiosulfate in petrolatum at 2% was reported to elicit higher numbers of positive patch test reactions without giving more irritant reactions or patch test sensitization [16]. Whenever patch testing with gold sodium thiosulfate, keep in mind that a test reading should also be performed after 1 week [17]. In fact, even readings on days 14–21 may be indicated. Currently, we do not recommend including gold sodium thiosulfate in the standard series [1]. It should be applied for scientific purposes and when allergic contact dermatitis from gold is suspected.

Positive test reactions to gold sodium thiosulfate and gold sodium thiomalate have also been obtained when tested intracutaneously [2, 17, 18], as well as with in vitro tests [18–21].

> ### Core Message
>
> ■ Gold sodium thiosulfate is not recommended for the standard series. It should be applied for scientific purposes and when allergic contact dermatitis from gold is suspected. Positive test reactions to gold sodium thiosulfate may appear late, which is why readings should also be performed after 1 week.

32.9.3 Clinical Picture

In patients hypersensitive to gold sodium thiosulfate, dermatitis has been reported to be over-represented in certain locations, such as the fingers, earlobes, the and eye area [9, 22]. Gold dermatitis has also been reported to resemble seborrheic dermatitis [23]. In patients with gold allergy and pierced ears, persistent papular elements and nodules on the earlobes have developed [24–28]. Recently, a patient with orofacial granulomatosis caused by contact allergy to dental gold and manifesting with erythema and swelling of the upper lips and cheek was presented [29].

The oral clinical manifestations of dental gold in hypersensitive persons have included ulcerations, erosions, and erythematous lesions [18, 30].

32.9.4 Systemic Contact Dermatitis

Experimentally, the drug Myocrisin (gold sodium thiomalate) has been demonstrated to elicit systemic contact dermatitis in gold-sodium-thiosulfate-hypersensitive individuals [31–33]. Besides flare-up reactions of previous positive patch tests to gold compounds and of previous sites of gold dermatitis, the patients have experienced "fever" reactions and, biochemically, a significant rise in inflammatory mediators has been demonstrated [32, 33]. However, there are currently no data indicating that systemic administration of gold, except for gold drug administration and the consumption of a gold-containing liquor [34, 35], has any clinical significance for the elicitation or deterioration of contact dermatitis.

32.9.5 Epidemiology

When gold sodium thiosulfate was introduced in the standard test series in Malmö, Sweden, in the early 1990s, a contact allergy rate of 9% was noted [2]. Thereafter, contact allergy rates to gold sodium thiosulfate in the range 1–23% were reported from various countries, and in most studies with a female predominance. Similar figures have been obtained when patch testing subgroups of the general population [36–38].

There are several case reports, both occupational and non-occupational, on allergic contact dermatitis and allergic contact stomatitis from gold. Elemental gold found in jewelry such as earrings, rings, and necklaces seems to make up the majority of cases. Sporadic cases of occupational contact dermatitis from gold salts have been reported in electroplaters, guilders, and those manufacturing and selling jewelry. Irritant contact dermatitis from gold salts, particularly potassium dicyanoaurate, has been reported. Allergic contact stomatitis and glossitis from gold have been caused by gold-containing alloys in dental appliances, such as crowns, bridges, and dentures. More information on contact allergy rates and allergic as well as irritant manifestations from gold compounds are given in [1, 3, 30, 39].

Core Message

■ Contact allergy to gold sodium thiosulfate in the range 1–23% was seen in dermatitis patients and most often with a female predominance. Similar rates have been noted in groups of the general population. Cases of occupational contact dermatitis from gold salts have been reported.

References

1. Bruze M, Andersen KE (1999) Gold – a controversial sensitizer. European Environmental and Contact Dermatitis Research Group. Contact Dermatitis 40:1–5
2. Björkner B, Bruze M, Möller H (1994) High frequency of contact allergy to gold sodium thiosulfate. An indication of gold allergy? Contact Dermatitis 30:144–151
3. Isaksson M, Bruze M (2000) Gold. In: Kanerva L, Elsner P, Wahlberg JE, Maibach HI (eds) Handbook of occupational dermatology. Springer, Berlin Heidelberg New York
4. Brown DH, Smith WE, Fox P, Sturrock RD (1982) The reactions of gold (o) with amino acids and the significance of these reactions in the biochemistry of gold. Inorg Chim Acta 67:27–30
5. Lidén C, Nordenadler M, Skare L (1998) Metal release from gold-containing jewelry materials: no gold release detected. Contact Dermatitis 39:281–285
6. Flint GN (1998) A metallurgical approach to metal contact dermatitis. Contact Dermatitis 39:213–221
7. Ahnlide I, Björkner B, Bruze M, Möller H (2000) Exposure to metallic gold in patients with contact allergy to gold sodium thiosulfate. Contact Dermatitis 43:344–350
8. Ahnlide I, Ahlgren C, Björkner B, Bruze M, Lundh T, Möller H, Nilner K, Schütz A (2002) Gold concentration in blood in relation to the number of gold restorations and contact allergy to gold. Acta Odontol Scand 60:301–305
9. Bruze M, Edman B, Björkner B, Möller H (1994) Clinical relevance of contact allergy to gold sodium thiosulfate. J Am Acad Dermatol 31:579–583
10. Schaffran RM, Storrs FJ, Schalock P (1999) Prevalence of gold sensitivity in asymptomatic individuals with gold dental restorations. Am J Contact Dermat 10:201–206
11. Vamnes JS, Morken T, Helland S, Gjerdet NR (2000) Dental gold alloys and contact hypersensitivity. Contact Dermatitis 42:128–133
12. Ahlgren C, Ahnlide I, Björkner B, Bruze M, Liedholm R, Möller H, Nilner K (2002) Contact allergy to gold is correlated to dental gold. Acta Derm Venereol (Stockh) 82:41–44
13. Eisler R (2003) Chrysotherapy: a synoptic review. Inflamm Res 52:487–501
14. Kligman AM (1966) The identification of contact allergens by human assay. 3. The maximization test: a procedure for screening and rating contact sensitizers. J Invest Dermatol 47:393–409
15. Fowler JF Jr (1987) Selection of patch test materials for gold allergy. Contact Dermatitis 17:23–25
16. Bruze B, Björkner B, Möller H (1999) Patch testing with gold sodium thiosulfate. Jadassohn Centenary Congress, London, UK (abstract book 14)
17. Bruze M, Hedman H, Björkner B, Möller H (1995) The development and course of test reactions to gold sodium thiosulfate. Contact Dermatitis 33:386–391
18. Räsänen L, Kalimo K, Laine J, Vainio O, Kotiranta J, Pesola I (1996) Contact allergy to gold in dental patients. Br J Dermatol 134:673–677
19. Silvennoinen-Kassinen S, Niinimäki A (1984) Gold sensitivity blast transformation. Contact Dermatitis 11:156–158
20. Räsänen L, Kaipiainen-Seppänen O, Myllykangas-Luosujärvi R, Käsnänen T, Pollari P, Saloranta P, Horsmanheimo M (1999) Hypersensitivity to gold in gold sodium thiomalate-induced dermatosis. Br J Dermatol 141:683–688
21. Vamnes JS, Gjerdet NR, Morken T, Moe G, Matre R (1999) In vitro lymphocyte reactivity to gold compounds in the diagnosis of contact hypersensitivity. Contact Dermatitis 41:156–160
22. Fowler JF Jr, Taylor J, Storrs F, Sherertz E, Rietschel R, Pratt M, Mathias CG, Marks J, Maibach H, Fransway A, DeLeo V, Belsito D (2001) Gold allergy in North America. Am J Contact Dermat 12:3–5
23. McKenna KE, Dolan O, Walsh MY, Burrows D (1995) Contact allergy to gold sodium thiosulfate. Contact Dermatitis 32:143–146
24. Iwatsuki K, Tagami H, Moriguchi T, Yamada M (1982) Lymphadenoid structure induced by gold hypersensitivity. Arch Dermatol 118:608–611
25. Kobayashi Y, Nanko H, Nakamura J, Mizoguchi M (1992) Lymphocytoma cutis induced by gold pierced earrings. J Am Acad Dermatol 27:457–458
26. Fleming C, Burden D, Fallowfield M, Lever R (1997) Lymphomatoid contact reaction to gold earrings. Contact Dermatitis 37:298–299
27. Armstrong DKB, Walsh MY, Dawson JF (1997) Granulomatous contact dermatitis due to gold earrings. Br J Dermatol 136:776–778
28. Park YM, Kang H, Kim HO, Cho BK (1999) Lymphomatoid eosinophilic reaction to gold earrings. Contact Dermatitis 40:216–217
29. Lazarov A, Kidron D, Tulchinsky Z, Minkow B (2003) Contact orofacial granulomatosis caused by delayed hypersensitivity to gold and mercury. J Am Acad Dermatol 49:1117–1120
30. Möller H (2002) Dental gold alloys and contact allergy. Contact Dermatitis 47:63–66
31. Möller H, Björkner B, Bruze M (1996) Clinical reactions to systemic provocation with gold sodium thiomalate in patients with contact allergy to gold. Br J Dermatol 135:423–427
32. Möller H, Ohlsson K, Linder C, Björkner B, Bruze M (1998) Cytokines and acute phase reactants during flare-up of contact allergy to gold. Am J Contact Dermat 9:15–22
33. Möller H, Ohlsson K, Linder C, Björkner B, Bruze M (1999) The flare-up reactions after systemic provocation in contact allergy to nickel and gold. Contact Dermatitis 40:200–204
34. Möller H, Björkner B, Bruze M, Hagstam Å (1996) Flare-up at contact allergy sites in a gold-treated rheumatic patient. Acta Derm Venereol (Stockh) 76:55–58
35. Russell MA, Langley M, Truett AP 3rd, King LE, Boyd AS (1997) Lichenoid dermatitis after consumption of gold-containing liquor. J Am Acad Dermatol 36:841–844

36. Gruvberger B, Bruze M, Almgren G (1998) Occupational dermatoses in a plant producing binders for paints and glues. Contact Dermatitis 38:71–77

37. Fleming C, Lucke T, Forsyth A, Rees S, Lever R, Wray D, Aldridge R, MacKie R (1998) A controlled study of gold contact hypersensitivity. Contact Dermatitis 38:137–139

38. Isaksson M, Zimerson E, Bruze M (1999) Occupational dermatoses in composite production. J Occup Environ Med 41:261–266

39. Fowler JF Jr (2001) Gold. Am J Contact Dermat 12:1–2

32.10 Mercury

Mercury (Hg) exists in three chemical forms; elemental, organic, and inorganic. Currently, the main sources of mercury exposure are: (1) dental amalgam restorations; (2) in various industries, including the manufacture of insecticides, fungicides, paper, paint, jewelry, chlorine, caustic soda, and in dentistry; and (3) mercury-containing vaccines, eye and ear drops, contact lens cleaning and storage solutions, skin-lightening creams, emulsion paints, and fungicides and herbicides used in the home [1–3].

Chronic exposure to either inorganic or organic mercury can permanently damage the brain, kidneys, and the developing fetus. The most sensitive target of low-level exposures to metallic and organic mercury, following short- or long-term exposure, appears to be the nervous system, whereas the most sensitive target of low-level exposure to inorganic mercury appears to be the kidney [3]. Mercury poisoning can result in different clinical conditions with assorted cutaneous findings [4].

32.10.1 Allergic Contact Dermatitis

All three chemical forms of mercury can sensitize. Clinically, mercury allergy can manifest as allergic contact dermatitis, allergic gingivostomatitis, and systemic contact dermatitis [4] with malaise and fever [5]. There is no general consensus regarding which mercury compounds to use for patch testing patients with suspected mercury hypersensitivity. Mercury compounds may be highly irritant to the skin and aqueous solutions of mercury salts may react with aluminum in Finn Chambers to produce irritant compounds [2]. In a report on mercury allergy, both metallic mercury and ammoniated mercury were recommended for patch testing when mercury allergy is suspected [2]. More information on mercury allergy is given in the chapter on skin disease from dental materials (Chaps. 36).

References

1. Langan DC, Fan PL, Hoos AA (1987) The use of mercury in dentistry: a critical review of the recent literature. J Am Dent Assoc 115:867–880

2. Handley J, Todd D, Burrows D (1993) Mercury allergy in a contact dermatitis clinic in Northern Ireland. Contact Dermatitis 29:258–261

3. al-Saleh I, al-Doush I (1997) Mercury content in skin-lightening creams and potential hazards to the health of Saudi women. J Toxicol Environ Health 51:123–130

4. Boyd AS, Seger D, Vannucci S, Langley M, Abraham JL, King LE Jr (2000) Mercury exposure and cutaneous disease. J Am Acad Dermatol 43:81–90

5. Lerch M, Bircher AJ (2004) Systemically induced allergic exanthem from mercury. Contact Dermatitis 50:349–353

32.11 Palladium

Palladium (Pd) belongs to the platinum group of metals. Palladium is an inexpensive precious metal, which is less resistant to corrosion than platinum. The main uses are for electrical components alloyed with copper and silver, and as a catalyst. Smaller amounts are used in jewelry, where it is used as a whitener in white gold. Palladium is increasingly used in cast dental alloys and in dental prostheses.

32.11.1 Allergic Contact Dermatitis

A case of contact dermatitis from palladium was reported in 1969. A chemist working on precious metals analysis developed dermatitis on his hands and face, and he was patch test positive to nickel chloride and palladium chloride [1]. The dermatitis cleared up on avoidance of exposure to these metals. Since the beginning of the 1990s, palladium chloride has been included in the standard series of many patch test clinics. Few reports on work-related dermatitis have been published, but several reports on positive patch test reactions to palladium chloride have been released. The frequency of contact allergy to palladium chloride among dermatitis patients has been reported to be approximately 3–8% [2]. One study reported increasing frequency of contact allergy to palladium chloride over the period 1991 to 2000, with 9.7% in year 2000 [3]. Of nickel-sensitive individuals, 30–40% are also sensitive to palladium chloride [4, 5]. In almost every case of allergy to palladium chloride, simultaneous reactivity to nickel is shown. Patch testing with palladium chloride is generally performed at 1% in petrolatum.

Some authors have related palladium allergy to dental alloys. Few cases of contact stomatitis or oral lichen planus related to palladium and patch test re-

32

activity to palladium chloride have been reported. One case with positive reactions to palladium chloride, palladium metal plate, a platinum compound, and nickel sulfate has been described [6]. The stomatitis disappeared after replacing the palladium and platinum-containing prosthesis.

Patch testing with elemental palladium has been carried out, but the results do not support clinical reports of allergy to elemental palladium. None of the 12 patients who were patch test positive to palladium chloride reacted to pure palladium metal foil [7]. Metal discs made of palladium were tested in 103 nickel-sensitive patients [8]. Only one reaction was recorded in a patient who did not react to palladium chloride.

The clinical relevance of palladium chloride or elemental palladium as sensitizers is not fully understood. Cross-reactivity to palladium chloride in nickel-sensitive persons seems the most likely, but concomitant sensitivity, or contamination of palladium chloride by nickel sulfate have also been discussed [4, 7, 9].

Palladium chloride has been shown to be a potent sensitizer in the guinea pig [10]. Animals induced with palladium chloride also reacted to nickel sulfate [11], and to a higher degree on closed patch testing than when challenge was carried out as ROATs [12]. The results speak in favor of cross-reactivity. Guinea pigs induced with nickel sulfate have shown a variable degree of responsiveness on challenge with palladium chloride [11, 12].

References

1. Munro-Ashman D, Munro DD, Hughes TH (1969) Contact dermatitis from palladium. Trans St Johns Hosp Dermatol Soc 55:196–197
2. Aberer W, Holub H, Strohal R, Slavicek R (1993) Palladium in dental alloys – the dermatologists' responsibility to warn? Contact Dermatitis 28:163–165
3. Larese Filon L, Uderzo D, Bagnato E (2003) Sensitization to palladium chloride: a ten-year evaluation. Am J Contact Dermat 14:78–81
4. Kanerva L, Kerosuo H, Kullaa A, Kerosuo E (1996) Allergic patch test reactions to palladium chloride in schoolchildren. Contact Dermatitis 34:39–42
5. Brasch J, Geier J (1997) Patch test results in schoolchildren. Results from the Information Network of Departments of Dermatology (IVDK) and the German Contact Dermatitis Research Group (DKG). Contact Dermatitis 37:286–293
6. Koch P, Baum H-P (1996) Contact stomatitis due to palladium and platinum in dental alloys. Contact Dermatitis 34:253–257
7. Todd DJ, Burrows D (1992) Patch testing with pure palladium metal in patients with sensitivity to palladium chloride. Contact Dermatitis 26:327–331
8. Uter W, Fuchs T, Häusser M, Ippen H (1995) Patch test results with serial dilutions of nickel sulfate (with and without detergent), palladium chloride, and nickel and palladium metal plates. Contact Dermatitis 32:135–142
9. Kränke B, Aberer W (1996) Multiple sensitivities to metals. Contact Dermatitis 34:225
10. Wahlberg JE, Boman A (1990) Palladium chloride – a potent sensitizer in the guinea pig. Am J Contact Dermat 1:112–113
11. Wahlberg JE, Boman AS (1992) Cross-reactivity to palladium and nickel studied in the guinea pig. Acta Derm Venereol (Stockh) 72:95–97
12. Wahlberg JE, Lidén C (1999) Cross-reactivity patterns of palladium and nickel studied by repeated open applications (ROATs) to the skin of guinea pigs. Contact Dermatitis 41:145–149

32.12 Platinum

Platinum (Pt) salts can induce allergic responses of the immediate hypersensitivity type, including rhinitis and asthma [1]. On the other hand, platinum as a cause of contact allergic sensitization has been questioned. Koch and Baum reported a patient with contact stomatitis due to combined sensitization to palladium and platinum, both metals being present in dental alloys in the patient's mouth [2]. In contrast to the positive patch test to ammonium tetrachloroplatinate 0.25% in petrolatum, the palladium chloride test was strongly positive. Because of this, together with doubtful reactions to platinum metal discs in the patient and controls, as well as the knowledge that the platinum test preparation was contaminated with palladium, the authors concluded that a platinum allergy was strongly suspected but not confirmed. Recently, occupational contact allergy to platinum traced by patch testing with platinum salts was reported in refinery workers [3] and in a chemical process worker [4]. The recommended patch test preparation is ammonium tetrachloroplatinate 0.25% in petrolatum.

References

1. Baker DB, Gann PH, Brooks SM, Gallagher J, Bernstein IL (1990) Cross-sectional study of platinum salts sensitization among precious metals refinery workers. Am J Ind Med 18:653–664
2. Koch P, Baum H-P (1996) Contact stomatitis due to palladium and platinum in dental alloys. Contact Dermatitis 34:253–257
3. Santucci B, Valenzano C, de Rocco M, Cristaudo A (2000) Platinum in the environment: frequency of reactions to platinum-group elements in patients with dermatitis and urticaria. Contact Dermatitis 43:333–338
4. Dastychová E, Semrádová V (2000) A case of contact hpersensitivity to platinum salts. Contact Dermatitis 43:226

32.13 Rhodium

Rhodium (Rh) is one of the platinum-group metals. Little is known about the toxicology of rhodium. It is used in alloys and platings for jewelry and in some dental materials. Rhodium is also used in catalysts, high-temperature furnaces, electrical contacts, high-reflective mirrors and other optical surfaces, and in nozzles for glass-fiber spinning.

32.13.1 Allergic Contact Dermatitis

Elemental rhodium has not been described as a sensitizer. Single reports on contact allergy to rhodium salts, in platers and silversmiths, have been published. A goldsmith was patch test positive to rhodium sulfate 0.05% in water and to cobalt chloride, while 40 controls were negative to rhodium sulfate at a higher concentration [1]. Contact dermatitis, contact urticaria, and asthma among 17 out of 50 workers in a precious metals factory were reported [2]. Patch tests for delayed hypersensitivity and scratch-patch tests for immediate-type hypersensitivity were positive in 7 out of 12 patients.

Rhodium chloride has been shown to be a potent sensitizer in guinea pigs [3, 4]. Challenge was carried out with rhodium chloride, and with cobalt chloride, nickel sulfate and palladium chloride. Animals induced with rhodium chloride also reacted to cobalt chloride, the clinical relevance of which is not known.

References

1. de la Cuadra J, Grau-Massanés M (1991) Occupational contact dermatitis from rhodium and cobalt. Contact Dermatitis 25:182–184
2. Nakayama H, Imai T (1982) Occupational contact urticaria, contact dermatitis and asthma caused by rhodium hypersensitivity. In: Proceedings of the 6th international symposium on contact dermatitis and joint meeting between ICDRG and JCDRG, Tokyo, Japan
3. Lidén C, Karlberg A-T (1992) Rhodium chloride – a potent sensitizer in guinea pigs. In: Proceedings of the 1st congress of the European Society of Contact Dermatitis, Brussels, Belgium, October 1992
4. Lidén C, Maibach HI, Wahlberg JE (1995) Skin. In: Goyer RA, Klaassen CD, Waalkes MP (eds) Metal toxicology. Academic Press, New York, pp 447–464

32.14 Tin

Tin (Sn) is widely used in metal alloys and most humans are exposed intraorally from the tin present in amalgam.

Nielsen and Skov [1] described a worker with an airborne pattern contact dermatitis caused by exposure to dust from a tin containing metal alloy. A positive patch test with $SnCl_2 \cdot 2H_2O$ 1% in petrolatum was present. A dilution series support an allergic reaction. Allergy could not be supported by the attempted lymphocytic transformation test.

Earlier non-relevant cutaneous reactivity has been seen in consecutive patients, tested with metallic, tin, and tin chloride [2]. The recommended patch test concentration is 1% tin chloride in petrolatum, but it is only based on a single case with a relevant positive patch test.

References

1. Nielsen NH, Skov L (1998) Occupational allergic contact dermatitis in a patient with a positive patch test to tin. Contact Dermatitis 39:99–100
2. Menné T, Andersen KE, Kaaber K, Osmundsen PE, Andersen JR, Yding F, Valeur G (1987) Tin: an overlooked contact sensitizer? Contact Dermatitis 16:9–10

Chapter 33

Metalworking Fluids

33

Johannes Geier, Holger Lessmann

Contents

oils in cutting, grinding, and honing. Their complex composition is commonly based on mineral oils or (semi-) synthetic hydrocarbon compounds. Various admixtures, such as emulsifiers, buffers, stabilizers, anti-fog-additives, foam inhibitors, tensides, solubility enhancers, lubricants, corrosion inhibitors, extreme-pressure-additives, and biocides (bactericides and fungicides), are usually added, according to the respective needs [3, 5, 6, 20, 30, 70, 72]. In the comments on the German occupational exposure threshold limit values (MAK-Werte) published in 2000, more than 200 components used in MWF are listed [6]. During the working process, wb MWF are subject to change: the concentration may rise due to the vaporization of water, the emulsion might break, and the pH may shift due to heating at the workpiece or due to bacterial contamination. Biocides other than those contained in the original MWF may be added to prevent microbial growth during the long time of use, and slideway oils or hydraulic oils from the processing machines may be introduced into the MWF by leakage [26, 30, 70, 72].

Core Message

- Two types of metalworking fluids (MWF) can be distinguished: water-based MWF (wb MWF) and neat oils. Their composition is complex. Many components and additives are in use. Wb MWF are subject to change during the working process.

33.1 Metalworking Fluids: Usage and Ingredients

Metalworking fluids (MWF) are used in metal processing for cooling and lubricating purposes, for corrosion inhibition, and for flushing away of metal chips. Two groups of MWF can be distinguished: water-based MWF (wb MWF), usually emulsions, which are prepared at the metalworking company by aqueous dilution of a concentrate delivered by the lubricant producer, and neat oils, which are non-water-miscible oily preparations used as obtained from the manufacturer. Wb MWF are used in the drilling, cutting, turning, and grinding of metal parts, neat

33.2 Occupational Skin Disease due to Metalworking Fluids

Occupational contact dermatitis (OCD) is common in metalworkers exposed to MWF [2, 9, 14, 15, 22, 34, 35, 61, 62]. In an epidemiological study on 286 metalworkers exposed to MWF, de Boer et al. found hand dermatitis in 26% of the employees [14, 15]. Of 201 trainees, 47 (23%) had had hand dermatitis at least once during the study period of 2.5 years in the Swiss Prospective Metal Worker Eczema Study (PRO-METES) [9]. The 3-year-incidence of hand eczema was 15.3% among metalworker apprentices in a German prospective cohort study in the car industry (PACO-study) [22]. Recently, in a Swedish cross-sectional study on 163 MWF-exposed metalworkers with skin complaints, OCD was diagnosed in 14.1% [35]. In these and other studies on OCD in metalworkers [2, 34], irritant contact dermatitis (ICD) was more frequently observed than allergic contact dermatitis (ACD). However, as in any other comparable occupational situation, irritant contact dermatitis promotes, and often precedes, sensitization [39]. Hence, the frequency of ACD in a given study population depends on the average duration of exposure and skin disease. Moreover, a simple dichotomization in ICD and ACD does not reflect reality, since other factors such as atopy are also important, and in most cases, the occupational skin disease is a mixture of constitutional and irritant and/or allergic contact dermatitis [5, 30, 34, 61, 62, 69]. It is likely that contact allergy due to MWF is under-diagnosed because not every possible allergenic substance is being tested in the patients concerned [26, 66].

Clinically, OCD due to MWF usually presents as vesicular or rhagadiform eczema of the web spaces, the lateral aspects of the fingers, and the backs of the hands. Often, the dermatitis spreads to the palms and the wrists up to the forearms. Bacterial superinfections are possible [2, 20, 61, 62]. MWF dermatitis may have an unsatisfactory prognosis. Pryce et al. performed a follow-up study on 121 metalworkers concerned, and found skin symptoms in more than 70% of the patients still present after two years, partly in spite of job discontinuation [61]. Shah et al. made similar findings [68]. However, the authors admit that the outcome depends very much on the individuals concerned, particularly on the patients' understanding of the cause of the disease and on their willingness to change their behavior at the workplace.

Core Message

■ MWF are a frequent cause of occupational contact dermatitis (OCD), with irritant contact dermatitis (ICD) being diagnosed more often than allergic contact dermatitis (ACD). However, in most cases, the occupational skin disease is a mixture of constitutional dermatitis, ICD, and/or ACD. Contact allergy due to MWF may be under-diagnosed.

33.3 Irritant Contact Dermatitis due to Metalworking Fluids

MWF, in particular wb MWF, exhibit irritant effects to the skin. Due to the risk of injury from rotating tools, it is prohibited to wear protective gloves at most MWF workplaces (Fig. 1). Skin irritation by wb MWF is not only caused by wet work, but also by the alkaline pH, usually ranging from 8.5 to 9.6 [72]. Additionally, emulsifiers damage the epidermal barrier and biocides have irritant properties [61, 62]. In many workplaces, there is no continuous exposure to wb MWF, but the skin is contaminated at some repetitive operations, e.g., when changing the workpiece. Mostly, the wb MWF splashes are not removed for other operations, such as control measurements or burr removing. They dry up on the skin within few minutes, and, as a consequence, the wb MWF is concentrated due to vaporization, and irritancy increases [48]. Additionally, it could be shown in the PROMETES study that not only chemical irritation, but also mechanical factors play a role in the damage of the epidermal barrier in metalworkers [9]. Moreover, in metal processing, as in any other comparable occupational setting, a too short recovery time after repetitive minor irritant exposures eventually leads to clinically visible irritant skin damage, following the model described by Malten [9, 52].

Core Message

■ In most MWF workplaces, no gloves are allowed. Irritant effects of wb MWF are due to wet work, alkalinity, emulsifiers, and biocides. In wb MWF splashes that dry up on the skin, concentration of the components increases within minutes, thus, enhancing irritancy.

33.4 Contact Allergy due to Metalworking Fluids

In 1985, Alomar et al. found an increased number of contact allergies to *para*-phenylenediamine (PPD), dichromate, and cobalt in the standard series, and to benzisothiazolinone (BIT), 1,3,5-tris(2-hydroxyethyl)-hexahydrotriazine (Grotan BK), and triethanolamine (TEA) in a MWF test series in their study on 230 MWF-exposed metalworkers with OCD [2]. However, the clinical relevance of the positive reactions to the standard series allergens could not be stated def-

Fig. 1.
Drilling with wb MWF. The worker's hand is permanently wetted with MWF. No gloves are allowed at this workplace because of the risk of injury from rotating tools (courtesy of Dr. H.-G. Englitz)

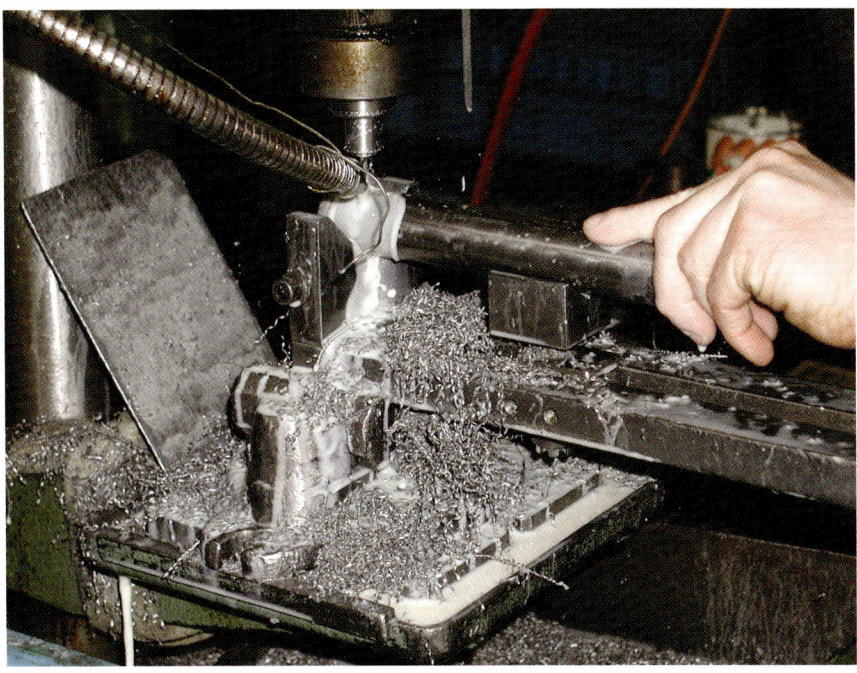

initely in most cases [2]. In a study performed in 1986/1987 on 174 patients with suspected MWF dermatitis, Grattan et al. saw an increase of sensitizations to nickel, colophonium, formaldehyde, the formaldehyde releaser Dowicil 200 (Quaternium 15), and other biocides [34]. In 1989, de Boer et al. published an investigation on 286 metalworkers exposed to MWF, of which, 75 had had hand eczema. A patch test was performed in 40 of these 75 patients, and 8 of them had a contact allergy [15]. Occupational sensitizations in these cases were due to formaldehyde and 5-chloro-2-methylisothiazol-3-one/2-methylisothiazol-3-one (MCI/MI) [15]. Nethercott et al. investigated 27 metalworkers exposed to MWF with hand dermatitis in 1990. Thirteen of these patients had had ACD, and 11 of them were sensitized to MCI/MI, which was used in the MWF [57]. At the beginning of the 1990s, two retrospective studies on contact allergies in metalworkers were published by the Information Network of Departments of Dermatology (IVDK). However, these data analyses were focused neither on patients exposed to MWF nor on those with OCD. In both analyses, a surprisingly high frequency of sensitizations to p-aminoazobenzene (PAAB) was found [73, 74]. Brinkmeier et al. performed an investigation on 408 metalworkers and found positive patch test reactions to Biobans P 1487, CS 1246, and CS 1135 in 13 patients (3.4%). Most of the test reactions were weak positive and could be reproduced on re-testing in only 2 out of 10 patients [11]. In the course of a large German study on contact aller-

gies among patients with OCD (FaSt study), 160 metalworkers were investigated from 1999 to 2001 [32]. Most frequently, sensitizations to monoethanolamine (MEA), colophonium/abietic acid, and fragrance mix were observed. Additionally, cobalt, diethanolamine (DEA), formaldehyde, formaldehyde releasers, and other biocides were important allergens in these patients. Metalworkers exposed to wb MWF with OCD had a significantly increased risk of sensitization to colophonium, formaldehyde, and fragrance mix when compared to metalworkers with OCD who were *not* exposed to wb MWF, or men not working in the metal industry [32]. Recently (2003), a Swedish study on OCD among the employees of a metalworking plant was published by Gruvberger et al. [35]. Of 164 metalworkers with skin complaints, 10 were found to have occupationally induced ACD, and 4 of them were sensitized to BIT, while 3 patients had a contact allergy due to the extreme-pressure-additive ethylhexylzinc dithiophosphate (EHZDTP) [35].

During the last decade, sensitizations to the following MWF components have been reported in case reports of metalworkers with OCD: diglycolamine [28], ethylenediamine [13], also possibly as indicator for a sensitization to other amines [19], MEA [47, 58], alkanolamineborates [12], a condensate of boric acid, MEA, and fatty acids [43], fatty acid polydiethanolamide [45], oleyl alcohol [47], tertiary-butylhydroquinone [54], imazalil [60], iodopropynyl butylcarbamate [51], sodium pyrithione [41, 49], ethylhexylzinc dithiophosphate [42, 45], and oak moss resin [58].

33

33.5 Important Allergens in Metalworking Fluids

33.5.1 Monoethanolamine (MEA), Diethanolamine (DEA), Triethanolamine (TEA), and Diglycolamine

In wb MWF, MEA, DEA, and TEA are used as rust preventive agents with emulsifying properties, while diglycolamine serves as emulsifier. MEA ranked first among the allergens in wb MWF in two recent studies [31, 32]. MEA may be present in the MWF as reaction products of MEA with boric acid or other MWF components, and probably only a certain fraction of MEA is present as such. Cases of contact allergy due to such reaction products have been reported, partly without reaction to MEA [12, 43]. Due to a potential formation of carcinogenic N-nitrosamines, the concentration of DEA is limited to 0.2% in the MWF concentrate in Germany by law since 1993 [4]. Due to this limitation, the use of DEA in wb MWF has declined in the following years. This is probably reflected by the far lower frequency of sensitizations to DEA compared to MEA in the two above-mentioned recent German studies [31, 32]. TEA, which is also frequently used as an emulsifier in creams and cosmetics, was found to be a rare MWF allergen. However, we have no information on the extent of its use in MWF currently on the market. Thus, the very low proportion of patients allergic to TEA may be either due to a lower sensitizing capacity, which could be explained by a lower reactivity due to its chemical structure, or due to a less frequent use in wb MWF. Diglycolamine was first described as an MWF aller-

gen in 2002 [28], and was not included in a MWF test series before 2003 [31]. Hence, experience with this substance is still limited, but it seems to be an important MWF allergen though.

33.5.2 Colophonium/Abietic Acid

A positive patch test reaction to colophonium indicates a sensitization to oxidation products of abietic acid and other resin acids which are contained in colophonium [38]. The concentrate of a wb MWF may contain 4–8% (in some cases, up to 10%) distilled tall oil (DTO). Usually, this concentrate is diluted with water down to 5%. In this case, the concentration of DTO in the final wb MWF (to which the metalworker is exposed) is in the range 0.2–0.4%. According to information from the industry, about 30% of the DTO are resin acids, and of these, about one third is abietic acid. In other words: the content of resin acids in the wb MWF is 0.06–0.12%, the content of abietic acid is 0.02–0.04%. On exposure to air, which occurs during normal use of wb MWF, the resin acids oxidize rather quickly [36, 37, 46]. The fact that resin acids form alkanolamine salts in the wb MWF probably has no influence on the oxidation because different parts of the resin acid molecules are involved in the formation of salts and the oxidation process, respectively [37]. The concentration of resin acids in the wb MWF may seem rather low. However, in most workplaces, the wb MWF dries up on the contaminated skin, and the concentration rises within minutes [48]. If, furthermore, the irritant damage to the epidermal barrier of the exposed skin is taken into account, occupational exposure to wb MWF carries a high risk of sensitization. This is illustrated by epidemiological data. In the above-mentioned FaSt study (1999 to 2001), metalworkers with OCD and exposure to wb MWF had an eightfold increased risk of sensitization to colophonium [odds ratio (OR) 8.0; 95% confidence interval (CI) 1.7–73.5] when compared to metalworkers with OCD who were *not* exposed to wb MWF [32].

33.5.3 Fragrances

In the same study, metalworkers exposed to wb MWF with OCD had an increased risk of sensitization to fragrances in terms of positive patch test reactions to fragrance mix and to *Myroxylon pereirae* (MPR; balsam of Peru) when compared to metalworkers with OCD who were *not* exposed to wb MWF [32]. If the use of barrier creams or emollients was taken into account in an adjusted logistic regression analysis, the risk estimate was somewhat even higher. This strongly indicated that the exposure to wb MWF itself was the relevant risk factor. Until about 1990, fragrances or odor masks, even MPR, were mentioned as common components of wb MWF [15, 40, 62]. According to recent information from the lubricant producing industry, normally, no fragrances are added to the MWF concentrate nowadays. However, it cannot be excluded that odor masks are added by the metalworking companies during the usage of the wb MWF. Corresponding products are being offered on the market. Of course, this does not imply that every fragrance allergy in exposed metalworkers is acquired by wb MWF. In every individual case, a complete history has to be taken carefully, particularly with respect to other allergen sources (aftershave, deodorant etc.). Sometimes, however, this investigation will reveal occupational causation of fragrance allergy induced by wb MWF [58].

33.5.4 Cobalt, Nickel, Dichromate

Six comprehensive studies on cobalt, nickel, and dichromate in MWF have been published so far [16, 17, 50, 55, 59, 79]. In most of these studies, analyses were performed by atomic absorption spectrometry (AAS), and mostly, it was not stated whether the contents of metal particles (abrasion of tools or workpieces) or of metal ions was determined. The valence state of the metal ions was not investigated. The "bioavailability" was not fully elucidated; hence, it cannot be excluded that, in some cases, hardly soluble metal oxides or metal sulfides were described, which are not as important from the allergological point of view. The results of these studies can be summarized as follows: cobalt, nickel, and chromium are not present in fresh, unused MWF (concentration <1 ppm). The presence of cobalt in used MWF mainly depends on the metals or alloys processed. If no cobalt-containing hard metals were processed, the cobalt concentration was usually below 3 ppm. When processing hard metals containing cobalt, the cobalt concentration was up to 300 ppm, in single cases, even up to 550 ppm. The elicitation threshold in patients allergic to cobalt is regarded to be about 100 ppm to 1,000 ppm cobalt ions [65, 78]. In predamaged skin, reactions could even be elicited with 10 ppm cobalt [1]. Hence, if cobalt is present as dissolved ions, concentrations found in MWF which are used in hard metal processing could be sufficient to elicit an allergic reaction, possibly even to induce sensitization. In the above-mentioned studies, concentrations of nickel and chromium in used MWF were usually below 1 ppm. However, there were some

exceptions, with concentrations of nickel up to 130 ppm and of chromium up to 280 ppm, which might be sufficient for elicitation in high-grade sensitized individuals, provided the metals are present in a suitable, ionized form. If chromium is present in the hexavalent state, an induction of contact allergy seems possible with the exceptionally high concentrations mentioned, whereas the induction of nickel allergy seems unlikely this way.

In two studies, an increased frequency of cobalt allergies among metalworkers with OCD exposed to MWF was found [2, 32], and in one study each, an increase of sensitizations to nickel [34] and dichromate [2], respectively, was described. However, the clinical relevance of these findings could not be clearly established. In a multifactorial analysis of data from the IVDK in more than 80,000 patients, Uter et al. could not find an increased risk of sensitization to cobalt, nickel, or dichromate in metalworkers [76]. Hence, in each case of contact allergy to these metals in metalworkers exposed to MWF, it is mandatory to elucidate the source of exposure and to establish clinical relevance of the positive test reaction. Occupational exposure other than MWF (e.g., workpieces, tools, handles) or private exposure (e.g., jeans button, costume jewelry, piercing) has to be considered.

33.5.5 Formaldehyde and Formaldehyde Releasers

Several years ago, it was common to use formaldehyde solution for additional preservation of wb MWF during usage, but this seems to be obsolete today. Nowadays, usually formaldehyde releasers, mainly O-formals (acetals, semiacetals) and N-formals (aminals, semiaminals) are used for the preservation of wb MWF and in system cleansers [26, 71]. The amount of formaldehyde released varies, depending on various factors such as pH, temperature, microbial contamination, etc. [25]. Peak formaldehyde concentrations may arise from additional preservation during the usage. An increased frequency of sensitizations to formaldehyde among metalworkers with OCD exposed to wb MWF has been known from studies in the 1980s [15, 34]. In the FaSt study (1999 to 2001), it could be shown that the risk of formaldehyde allergy was significantly increased in these patients when compared to men not working in the metal industry (OR 4.1; 95% CI 1.5–9.2) [32]. In the above-mentioned multifactorial IVDK data analysis of 80,000 patients, the metalworkers' risk of formaldehyde allergy ranked second after health care workers, who are exposed to it by disinfectants [76]. Sensitizations to formaldehyde releasers may be directed against the whole molecule or the formaldehyde released. There is only a limited correlation between the ability to release formaldehyde and concomitant patch test reactions to formaldehyde and the releaser [25]. Studies on this subject are hampered by the fact that patch test reactions to formaldehyde releasers are often weak and poorly reproducible [11, 25].

33.5.6 Methyldibromo Glutaronitrile (MDBGN) and 2-phenoxyethanol (PE)

Methyldibromo glutaronitrile (MDBGN) has been used some years ago for the preservation of wb MWF. According to information from the lubricant industry, it is currently not in use for this purpose [26]. However, the occurrence of MDBGN as a preservative in creams, cosmetics, and skin care products dramatically increased in the 1990s, and the frequency of corresponding sensitizations rose in parallel [24, 80]. Hence, metalworkers may have acquired sensitization to MDBGN by protective creams or emollients, or by private skin care products as well as by wb MWF formerly. In the standard series, MDBGN is routinely tested in combination with PE at a total concentration of 1% because this mixture has frequently been used as a preservative. However, PE, which, in contrast to MDBGN, is still in use as a preservative in wb MWF, plays no role as a sensitizer. So, in the vast majority of the cases, MDBGN is the relevant allergen in positive test reactions to MDBGN/PE [24, 27]. In the MDBGN/PE combination used, MDBGN has a test concentration of 0.2%. Patch testing with MDBGN 0.3% leads to more positive reactions, of which, according to a study of the German Contact Dermatitis Research Group (DKG), many are probably irritant, i.e., false-positive [27]. Hence, particularly when testing with MDBGN in high concentrations, the clinical relevance of every positive reaction has to be established, taking into account both domestic and occupational exposure, including skin care at work.

33.5.7 5-Chloro-2-methylisothiazol-3-one/ 2-methylisothiazol-3-one (MCI/MI)

Due to its chemical properties, MCI/MI is not used as a preservative in the MWF concentrate, but it may be added to the wb MWF at the workplace as an additional biocide (top up biocide) [26]. Particularly in the beginning of the 1990s, MCI/MI was very frequently found as a preservative in skin care products,

but in the following years, its use declined dramatically due to the "epidemic" of sensitization in these years [56]. Recently, MCI/MI has come back into this field, albeit with lower concentrations, which will probably not induce new sensitizations [18, 63]. Hence, the particular exposure to MCI/MI has to be established in every metalworker sensitized with special regard to additional preservation of the wb MWF during its use. Benzisothiazolinone (BIT) and octylisothiazolinone (OIT), which are also currently used for the preservation of wb MWF, do not cross react with MCI/MI [23].

33.5.8 Other Biocides

As mentioned above, various other biocides, particularly formaldehyde releasers and other isothiazolinones, such as BIT and OIT, are being, or have been, used as preservatives in wb MWF, and cases of sensitization have been observed. Corresponding test substances are part of the respective MWF test series (see below). Iodopropynyl butylcarbamate (IPBC) had been tested at 0.1% pet., which was too low a test concentration. Hence, sensitizations remained undetected [67]. As the result of a corresponding study, the DKG recommends to test IPBC at 0.2% pet. [10]. In every case of a metalworker with OCD, a detailed history including additional preservation of the MWF during its use has to be taken and, in case of a weak or doubtful patch test reaction to biocides, a repeated open application test (ROAT) or provocative use test (PUT) can be recommended.

33.5.9 *p*-Aminoazobenzene (PAAB)

p-Aminoazobenzene (PAAB) is tested as a marker for contact allergy to para di-substituted aromatic amines or azo dyes [77], and was part of the MWF patch test series. Until the beginning of the 1990s, it was common to dye MWF [40, 62] partly with azo dyes. Nowadays, MWF are produced without dye, but occasionally, some metalworking companies add colors to their MWF systems. In contrast, most technical oils, such as hydraulic oils or slideway oils, are colored, but azo dyes should not be used for this purpose [30]. MWF often become contaminated with these technical oils by leakage and, thus, they might be a source of exposure to dyes for the metalworker. However, while concomitant reactions to PAAB and PPD are frequent and probably indicate a contact allergy to para-amino compounds [77], we know from the analysis of data concerning allergic reactions to textile dyes that PAAB is not a reliable marker for contact allergy to azo dyes [8]. An increased risk of active sensitization has been described when PAAB and PPD are patch tested in parallel [7]. In view of these circumstances, PAAB should be deleted from the MWF test series, although it was one of the frequent allergens in a recent IVDK data analysis [31]. In the cases concerned, which may, however, not easily be suspected, the actual dyes in technical oils from the patients' workplace should be tested instead.

33.6 MWF Patch Test Series

Patch test series for diagnostics in metalworkers are commercially available. However, regarding the wide variety of substances and components used in MWF [6], it seems likely that relevant contact allergies may be overlooked because far from all potentially allergenic MWF components are available as standardized patch test preparations. Additionally, the composition of MWF changes with time, due to technological progress. Hence, for a valid allergy diagnostic in this field, it is important to continuously adapt the MWF test series to the current spectrum of occupational exposure. In 2000, the interdisciplinary working party on allergy diagnostics in the metal branch compiled two lists of MWF allergens commercially available as patch test substances [26]. The first list contains substances currently used in MWF, and the second list contains substances that have only been used previously, mostly before 1994 [26]. Based on this information, at the end of 2001, the DKG established two corresponding MWF series. These series are to be tested in patients with suspected ACD and exposure to MWF in addition to the standard series, the ointment base series, and the preservative series. This design was chosen because it usually makes sense also to test the latter two series, as skin care products are another possible allergen source in metalworkers with suspected OCD. To avoid duplicate patch tests, the DKG omitted from the MWF series those potential MWF allergens that are contained in the standard, ointment base, or preservative series. Recently, results with these test series have been evaluated [31]. Based on this data, current and former MWF allergens which should be tested in metalworkers with suspected MWF dermatitis are compiled in Tables 1 and 2.

The allergological diagnostic in MWF dermatitis has improved a great deal during the last years. Principally, there are two possible ways to maintain its diagnostic value. First, frequently used MWF components that are not investigated sufficiently regarding their allergenic potential can be tested systematically in clinical studies. In a study of that kind, diglycola-

mine has been found to be a relevant MWF allergen recently [29]. Second, MWF from the patient's workplace and their components should be tested in every case concerned.

33.7 Patch Testing with MWF from the Patient's Workplace

Patch testing with MWF from the patient's workplace is an important additional diagnostic tool in patients with suspected MWF dermatitis, which has been employed in several studies on occupational dermatitis in metalworkers [2, 15, 34, 35]. However, in these studies, as in published recommendations for patch testing with MWF, test concentrations and vehicles have varied greatly [2, 15, 20, 21, 34, 35, 44]. A recent retrospective study on MWF patch tests in 141 metalworkers showed that MWF can be tested at workplace concentration and neat oils at 50% in olive oil without undue risk of irritant test reactions [33]. With lower concentrations, relevant allergic reactions might be missed.

The interdisciplinary working party on allergy diagnostics in the metal branch has published recommendations on how to patch test MWF from the patient's workplace in 2002 [72]. The essential points of these recommendations, which are as yet published in German only, are: of every MWF used by the patient, two samples should be taken, i.e., one fresh and one used sample. In the case of wb MWF, a sample of the fresh, undiluted MWF concentrate should be obtained. The used samples are to be taken from the inflows of the machines (and not from the so-called sumps) to avoid contamination with metal chips, which might cause irritant patch test reactions. Samples of used wb MWF must be stored in a refrigerator, and be tested within 3–5 days, as otherwise, microbial contamination will change or even destroy the emulsion. Fresh concentrate of the wb MWF should be tested 5% aq., which is an average workplace concentration. Used wb MWF can be patch tested as is, provided that the concentration at the workplace is ≤8%. In the case of higher workplace concentrations, further dilution to an end concentration of 4–8%, as required, is recommended. As a rule of thumb, this can be achieved by a 1:1 aqueous dilution of the wb MWF. Usually, wb MWF are alkaline (pH 8.6–9.5), but experience shows that this is tolerated by patients on patch testing. Neat oils should be tested 50% in olive oil. Used wb MWF samples must be accompanied by information about the concentration and pH at the time of sampling, date of the last change of the MWF, system cleaner used, date of last preservation, name of bactericide and fungicide

Table 1. Current MWF allergens to be tested in metalworkers with suspected MWF dermatitis (modified from [26, 30, 31])

No.	Substance	Occurrence in MWF	Function in MWF	Patch test concentration
	MWF series (current allergens)			
1	Benzylhemiformal	wb MWF	Biocide, formaldehyde releaser	1% pet.
2	4,4-Dimethyl-1,3-oxazolidine/3,4,4-trimethyl-1,3-oxazolidine (Bioban CS 1135)	wb MWF	Biocide, formaldehyde releaser	1% pet.
3	7-Ethylbicyclooxazolidine (Bioban CS 1246)	wb MWF	Biocide, formaldehyde releaser	1% pet.
4	Iodopropynyl butylcarbamate (IPBC)	wb MWF	Biocide	0.2% pet.
5	N,N'-Methylene-bis-5-methyl-oxazolidine	wb MWF	Biocide, formaldehyde releaser	1% pet.
6	1,2-Benzisothiazolin-3-one, sodium salt	wb MWF	Biocide	0.1% pet.
7	Octylisothiazolinone	wb MWF	Biocide	0.025% pet.
8	2-Phenoxyethanol	wb MWF	Biocide	1% pet.
9	Sodium-2-pyridinethiol-1-oxide (sodium omadine)	wb MWF	Biocide	0.1% aq.
10	1,3,5-Tris(2-hydroxyethyl)-hexahydrotriazine (Grotan BK®)	wb MWF	Biocide, formaldehyde releaser	1% pet.
11	Benzotriazole	wb MWF and neat oils	Rust preventive	1% pet.
12	Diethanolamine (DEA)[a]	wb MWF	Rust preventive	2% pet.
13	Monoethanolamine (MEA)	wb MWF	Rust preventive	2% pet.
14	p-tert-Butylphenol	neat oils	Antioxidant	1% pet.
15	Abietic acid	wb MWF	Emulsifier/surfactant	10% pet.
16	Diglycolamine [2-(2-aminoethoxy)ethanol]	wb MWF	Emulsifier	1% pet.
	Standard series			
17	Formaldehyde[b]	wb MWF	Top up biocide	1% aq.
18	5-Chloro-2-methylisothiazol-3-one/2-methylisothiazol-3-one (MCI/MI)	wb MWF	Top up biocide	0.01% aq.
19	Lanolin alcohol	wb MWF	Anti-wear additive	30% pet.
20	Zinc diethyldithiocarbamate (ZDEC)[c]	neat oils	Anti-wear additive	1% pet.
21	Cetearyl alcohol	wb MWF	Stabilizer/anti-wear additive	20% pet.
22	Colophonium[d]	wb MWF	Emulsifier/surfactant	20% pet.
23	Mercaptobenzothiazole	wb MWF	Rust preventive	2% pet.
	Ointment base series			
24	Propylene glycol	wb MWF	Stabilizer	5% pet.
25	Polyethylene glycol (tested as polyethylene glycol ointment base)	–	Stabilizer/anti-wear additive	100%
26	Triethanolamine (TEA)	wb MWF	Rust preventive	2.5% pet.
27	Butylhydroxy toluol (BHT)	Neat oils	Antioxidant	2% pet.
	Preservative series			
28	Triclosan	Neat oils	Biocide	2% pet.

[a] Use in MWF limited by law in Germany since 1993
[b] Released from formaldehyde releasers
[c] Tested as a marker for sodium diethyldithiocarbamate
[d] Allergic reaction indicates contact allergy to oxidation products of resin acids

33

Table 2. Former MWF allergens to be tested in metalworkers with suspected MWF dermatitis (modified from [26, 30, 31])

No.	Substance	Occurrence in MWF	Function in MWF	Patch test concentration
MWF series (former allergens)				
1	Chlorocresol	Neat oils	Biocide	1% pet.
2	Chloroxylenol	wb MWF	Biocide	1% pet.
3	Dipentene (d,l-limonene)	wb MWF	Biocide	2% pet.
4	Hexamethylene tetramine	wb MWF	Biocide	1% pet.
5	2-Hydroxymethyl-2-nitro-1,3-propanediol (Tris Nitro)[a].	wb MWF	Biocide, formaldehyde releaser	1% pet
6	Methyldibromo glutaronitrile (MDBGN)	wb MWF	Biocide	0.3% pet.
7	4-(2-Nitrobutyl) morpholine/4,4´-(2-ethyl-2-nitro-trimethylene) dimorpholine (Bioban P 1487)[a]	wb MWF	Biocide, formaldehyde releaser	1% pet.
8	Morpholinyl mercaptobenzothiazole (MOR)	wb MWF	Rust preventive	0.5% pet.
9	Ethylenediamine dihydrochloride	wb MWF	?	1% pet.
Standard series				
10	Paraben mix	wb MWF	Biocide	16% pet.
11	Methyldibromo glutaronitrile/2-phenoxyethanol (MDBGN/PE)[b]	wb MWF	MDBGN: biocide	1% pet.
12	*Myroxylon pereirae* resin (MPR, balsam of Peru)	wb MWF	Odor mask	25% pet.
13	Fragrance mix[c]	wb MWF	Odor mask	8% pet.
Ointment base series				
14	Coconut diethanolamide[a]	wb MWF	Emulsifier	0.5% pet.
Preservative series				
15	Bronopol (2-bromo-2-nitropropane-1,3-diol)[d]	wb MWF	Biocide, formaldehyde releaser	0.5% pet.
16	Chloroacetamide	wb MWF	Biocide	0.2% pet.

[a] Prohibited in MWF by law in Germany since 1993
[b] In contrast to PE, MDBGN is probably no longer used in MWF
[c] It is unclear which fragrances are used in MWF, if at all
[d] No longer used in MWF, but is used in skin care products

used, name of other additives and date of addition, material processed in the machine, and possible influx of hydraulic oils, slideway oils, or other oils by leakage. For neat oils, only data on the last change of the MWF, additives, material processed in the machine, and possible influx of other oils needs to be documented. Drafts of information sheets and test protocols, as well as instructions for patch testing can be downloaded in the German language at http://www.ivdk.org (section on "downloads") or at http://www.hautstadt.de as part of a training course for patch testing with material brought in by the patient.

The interdisciplinary working party emphasizes that false-negative test reactions to MWF may occur, even under the recommended conditions [72]. Allergenic components in the MWF may be diluted too much, and, thus, may elicit no reaction on patch testing in the intact skin of the upper back, although they may cause ACD on the pre-damaged skin of the hands under workplace conditions. Hence, patch testing with the single components of the MWF should not only be performed in case of a positive patch test reaction to the MWF from the workplace, but also in clinically suspected cases, in whom no test reaction to the individual MWF could be seen [53, 64]. However, to obtain maximum benefit from a breakdown test with single components of the MWF, complete information on the ingredients and additives of the MWF must be at hand. To obtain detailed, allergologically useful information about the ingredients and additives of an MWF is a very time-consuming business. First, the patient and his/her employer have to cooperate in providing information about the workplace exposure, in particular, correct identification of the products and batches used and their manufacturers. In the material safety data sheets of the MWF, far from every component that might be responsible for the individual patient's disease is listed. Usually, only those chemicals are named which are known sensitizers, and are present above a threshold concentration which requires labeling with the risk phrase R 43. If mentioned at all, chemicals may be denoted using synonyms not known to the clinician. Some lubricant producers are very co-operative and readily supply additional information, while others are not. As time is limited in the hospital routine, these difficulties are presumably one reason why additional diagnostics are rarely performed, and why the clinical relevance of positive reactions to standardized MWF allergens often remains unclear in the individual case. The adequate concentration for patch testing of many MWF components does not necessarily correspond to their use concentration in the MWF. Thus, performing a breakdown test with the single MWF components is hampered by uncertainty concerning correct patch test concentrations (on the producer's as well as on the physician's part), and, consequently, uncertainty about interpreting test reactions with these preparations. Additionally, often, the producers cannot deliver chemically defined components, since reaction products may be formed in the production process of the MWF which are not completely characterized. In this connection, reaction products of boric acid and alkanolamines may serve as an example: usually, more than one alkanolamine, such as MEA, diglycolamine etc., is added to the MWF base, which contains boric acid, and the reaction products are not analyzed. Hence, contact allergy to these reaction products – although well known from several case reports [12, 43] – is not easy to diagnose.

Against this background, we propose a center for information and documentation of contact allergies due to occupational exposure (German acronym: IDKB, from "Informations- und Dokumentationsstelle für Kontaktallergien durch Berufsstoffe"), which should work like the "IDOK," which successfully does the same work in the field of cosmetics and skin care products [75], and could provide:

- Support in obtaining information on, and samples of, single constituents of the occupational material (workplace MWF)
- Help in finding adequate patch test preparations
- Central documentation of patch test results and detection of new allergens
- Quality control of patch testing by continuous adaptation of test recommendations

Core Message

- Patch testing with MWF from the patients' workplace is a time consuming, but very useful additional diagnostic step which is not easy to perform correctly. Recommendations for the adequate performance are available in German at http://www.ivdk.org (section on "downloads") or at http://www.hautstadt.de as part of a training course for patch testing with material brought in by the patient.

33.8 Preventive Measures

Working with wb MWF is connected with wet work, and corresponding preventive measures have to be taken. Additionally, some peculiarities should be considered. If the skin is wetted with MWF only intermittently, the MWF should not dry up on the skin, but should be removed in order to avoid a rise in concentration by the vaporization of water and the resulting increase of irritancy. Cleaning clothes used for tools or workpieces should easily be distinguishable from those for wiping off the hands. Skin contact with MWF should be minimized by automation, encapsulation of machines, etc. For the degreasing of workpieces, hooks, sieves, or similar devices should be used for immersing, thus, reducing the alternating skin irritation by MWF and solvent.

Pollution of the MWF by dirt, food, etc. has to be avoided. Workplaces have to be kept clean. The concentration and pH of the MWF have to be controlled weekly in order to recognize and eliminate any increase of concentration or pH in time. Bacterial contamination itself does not affect skin irritancy of the MWF. However, there is an indirect effect because, in case of a too high microbial colonization, additional preservation is necessary due to technical reasons. Every additional preservation has to be documented exactly (date, amount, product used). Most suitable, additional preservation is performed after the last shift on Friday, so the biocide is almost completely dispensed at the beginning of work on Monday morning. In companies without a weekend break, as few metalworkers as possible should be exposed to the maximum biocide concentration, and all workers must be informed about the additional preservation. System cleansers should not be used during operation hours as they contain high concentrations of biocides. The same precautions as with additional preservation have to be taken.

At most MWF workplaces, it is prohibited to wear protective gloves because of the risk of injury from rotating tools. If gloves are allowed, a denseness guaranty should be demanded from the glove manufacturer. A skin protection plan has to be set up. For protection against wb MWF, water-in-oil emulsions are recommended. Creams containing tannins may be helpful under gloves. Usually, mild tensides are sufficient for skin cleaning. Regular skin care after work is as important as skin protection before work.

References

1. Allenby CF, Basketter DA (1989) Minimum eliciting patch test concentrations of cobalt. Contact Dermatitis 20: 185–190
2. Alomar A, Conde-Salazar L, Romaguera C (1985) Occupational dermatoses from cutting oils. Contact Dermatitis 12:129–138
3. Anonymous (1991) DIN 51385 Schmierstoffe; Kühlschmierstoffe; Begriffe. Beuth, Berlin, Germany
4. Anonymous (1993) Technische Regeln für Gefahrstoffe (TRGS) 611, Verwendungsbeschränkungen für wassermischbare bzw. wassergemischte Kühlschmierstoffe, bei deren Einsatz N-Nitrosamine auftreten können. Heymanns, Cologne, Germany
5. Anonymous (1999) Berufsgenossenschaftliche Regeln für Sicherheit und Gesundheit bei der Arbeit, BGR 143. Heymanns, Cologne, Germany
6. Anonymous (2000) Kühlschmierstoffe. In: Greim H (ed) Gesundheitsschädliche Arbeitsstoffe. Toxikologisch-arbeitsmedizinische Begründungen von MAK-Werten. 31. Lieferung. VCH, Weinheim, Germany
7. Arnold WP, van Joost T, van der Valk PGM (1995) Adding p-aminoazobenzene may increase the sensitivity of the European standard series in detecting contact allergy to dyes, but carries the risk of active sensitization. Contact Dermatitis 33:444
8. Bauer A, Geier J, Lessmann H, Elsner P (2004) Kontaktallergien gegen Textilfarbstoffe. Ergebnisse des Informationsverbundes Dermatologischer Kliniken (IVDK). Aktuel Dermatol 30:23–27
9. Berndt U, Hinnen U, Iliev D, Elsener P (2000) Hand eczema in metalworker trainees – an analysis of risk factors. Contact Dermatitis 43:327–332
10. Brasch J, Schnuch A, Geier J, Aberer W, Uter W: German Contact Dermatitis Research Group; Information Network of Departments of Dermatology (2004) Iodopropynylbutyl carbamate (IPBC) 0.2% is suggested for patch testing of patients with eczema possibly related to preservatives. Br J Dermatol 151:608–615
11. Brinkmeier T, Geier J, Lepoittevin JP, Frosch PJ (2002) Patch test reactions to Biobans in metalworkers are often weak and not reproducible. Contact Dermatitis 47:27–31
12. Bruze M, Hradil E, Eriksohn IL, Gruvberger B, Widström L (1995) Occupational allergic contact dermatitis from alkanolamineborates in metalworking fluids. Contact Dermatitis 32:24–27
13. Crow KD, Peachey RDG, Adams JE (1978) Coolant oil dermatitis due to ethylenediamine. Contact Dermatitis 4: 359–361
14. de Boer EM, van Ketel WG, Bruynzeel DP (1989) Dermatoses in metal workers. (I). Irritant contact dermatitis. Contact Dermatitis 20:212–218
15. de Boer EM, van Ketel WG, Bruynzeel DP (1989) Dermatoses in metal workers. (II). Allergic contact dermatitis. Contact Dermatitis 20:280–286
16. Einarsson Ö, Kylin B, Lindstedt G, Wahlberg JE (1975) Chromium, cobalt and nickel in used cutting fluids. Contact Dermatitis 1:182–183
17. Einarsson Ö, Eriksson E, Lindstedt G, Wahlberg JE (1979) Dissolution of cobalt from hard metal alloys by cutting fluids. Contact Dermatitis 5:129–132
18. Fewings J, Menné T (1999) An update of the risk assessment for methylchloroisothiazolinone/methylisothiazolinone (MCI/MI) with focus on rinse-off products. Contact Dermatitis 41:1–13
19. Fisher AA (1998) Ethylenediamine hydrochloride versus amines in cutting oils. Am J Contact Dermat 9:139
20. Foulds IS (2000) Cutting fluids. In: Kanerva L, Elsner P, Wahlberg JE, Maibach HI (eds) Handbook of occupational dermatology, Chap 86. Springer, Berlin Heidelberg New York, pp 691–700
21. Frosch PJ, Pilz B, Peiler D, Dreier B, Rabenhorst S (1997) Die Epikutantestung mit patienteneigenen Produkten. In: Plewig G, Przybilla B (eds) Fortschritte der praktischen Dermatologie und Venerologie 15. Springer, Berlin Heidelberg New York, pp 166–181
22. Funke U, Fartasch M, Diepgen TL (2001) Incidence of work-related hand eczema during apprenticeship: first results of a prospective cohort study in the car industry. Contact Dermatitis 44:166–172
23. Geier J, Schnuch A (1996) No cross sensitization between MCI/MI, benzisothiazolinone and octylisothiazolinone. Contact Dermatitis 34:148–149
24. Geier J, Fuchs T, Schnuch A (1996) Zunahme der Kontaktallergien gegen Methyldibromoglutaronitril in Deutschland. Allergologie 19:399–402
25. Geier J, Lessmann H, Schnuch A, Fuchs T (1997) Kontaktallergien durch formaldehydabspaltende Biozide. Eine Analyse der Daten des IVDK aus den Jahren 1992 bis 1995. Allergologie 20:215–224
26. Geier J, Lessmann H, Schumacher T, Eckert C, Becker D, Boveleth W, Buß M, Eck E, Englitz H-G, Koch P, Müller J, Nöring R, Rocker M, Rothe A, Schmidt A, Uter W, Warfolomeow I, Zoellner G (2000) Vorschlag für die Epikutantestung bei Verdacht auf Kontaktallergie durch Kühlschmierstoffe. 1. Kommerziell erhältliche Testsubstanzen. Derm Beruf Umwelt 48:232–236
27. Geier J, Schnuch A, Brasch J, Gefeller O (2000) Patch testing with methyldibromoglutaronitrile. Am J Contact Dermat 11:207–212
28. Geier J, Lessmann H, Graefe A, Fuchs T (2002) Contact allergy to diglycolamine in a water-based metalworking fluid. Contact Dermatitis 46:121
29. Geier J, Lessmann H, Frosch PJ, Pirker C, Koch P, Aschoff R, Richter G, Becker D, Eckert C, Uter W, Schnuch A, Fuchs T (2003) Patch testing with components of water-based metalworking fluids. Contact Dermatitis 49:85–90
30. Geier J, Lessmann H, Schmidt A, Englitz HG, Schnuch A (2003) Kontaktekzeme durch Kühlschmierstoffe in der Metallindustrie. Aktuel Dermatol 29:185–194
31. Geier J, Lessmann H, Dickel H, John SM, Frosch PJ, Koch P, Becker D, Jappe U, Aberer W, Schnuch A, Uter W (2004) Patch test results with the metalworking fluid series of the German Contact Dermatitis Research Group (DKG). Contact Dermatitis 51:118–130
32. Geier J, Lessmann H, Schnuch A, Uter W (2004) Contact sensitizations in metalworkers with occupational dermatitis exposed to water-based metalworking fluids: results of the research project "FaSt". Int Arch Occup Environ Health 77:543–551

33

33. Geier J, Uter W, Lessmann H, Frosch PJ (2004) Patch testing with metalworking fluids from the patient's workplace. Contact Dermatitis 51:172–179

34. Grattan CEH, English JSC, Foulds IS, Rycroft RJG (1989) Cutting fluid dermatitis. Contact Dermatitis 20:372–376

35. Gruvberger B, Isaksson M, Frick M, Pontén A, Bruze M (2003) Occupational dermatoses in a metalworking plant. Contact Dermatitis 48:80–86

36. Hausen BM, Krohn K, Budianto E (1990) Contact allergy due to colophony. (VII). Sensitizing studies with oxidation products of abietic and related acids. Contact Dermatitis 23:352–358

37. Hausen BM, Börries M, Budianto E, Krohn K (1993) Contact allergy due to colophony. (IX). Sensitization studies with further products isolated after oxidative degradation of resin acids and colophony. Contact Dermatitis 29:234–240

38. Hausen BM, Brinkmann J, Dohn W (1998) Lexikon der Kontaktallergene, 6. Ergänzungs-Lieferung, Kolophonium, K 4. Ecomed, Landsberg, Germany, pp 1–15

39. Hornstein OP (1984) Ekzemkrankheiten. Therapiewoche 34:400–409

40. Ippen H (1979) Allergische Hautschäden bei der Metallbearbeitung. Derm Beruf Umwelt 27:71–74

41. Isaksson M (2002) Delayed diagnosis of occupational contact dermatitis from sodium pyrithione in a metalworking fluid. Contact Dermatitis 47:248–249

42. Isaksson M, Frick M, Gruvberger B, Pontén A, Bruze M (2002) Occupational allergic contact dermatitis from the extreme pressure (EP) additive, zinc, bis ((O,O'-di-2-ethylhexyl) dithiophosphate) in neat oils. Contact Dermatitis 46:248–249

43. Jensen CD, Andersen KE (2003) Allergic contact dermatitis from a condensate of boric acid, monoethanolamine and fatty acids in a metalworking fluid. Contact Dermatitis 49:45–46

44. Jolanki R, Estlander T, Alanko K, Kanerva L (2000) Patch testing with a patient's own materials handled at work. In: Kanerva L, Elsner P, Wahlberg JE, Maibach HI (eds) Handbook of occupational dermatology, Chap 47. Springer, Berlin Heidelberg New York, pp 375–383

45. Kanerva L, Tupasela O, Jolanki R (2001) Occupational allergic contact dermatitis from ethylhexylzinc dithiophosphate and fatty acid polydiethanolamide in cutting fluids. Contact Dermatitis 44:193–194

46. Karlberg A-T (1991) Air oxidation increases the allergenic potential of tall oil rosin. Colophony contact allergens also identified in tall oil resin. Am J Contact Dermat 2:43–49

47. Koch P (1995) Occupational allergic contact dermatitis from oleyl alcohol and monoethanolamine in a metalworking fluid. Contact Dermatitis 33:273

48. Krbek F, Schäfer Th (1991) Untersuchungen an Tropfen und Rückständen von wassermischbaren Kühlschmierstoffen. Arbeitsmed Sozialmed Präventivmed 26:411–416

49. le Coz C-J (2001) Allergic contact dermatitis from sodium pyrithione in metalworking fluid. Contact Dermatitis 45:58–59

50. Lehmann E, Fröhlich N (1993) Kühlschmierstoffe – Zusätzliche Belastungen durch Metallionen? Amtliche Mitteilungen der Bundesanstalt für Arbeitsschutz, Januar 1993, pp 1–7

51. Majoie IML, van Ginkel CJW (2000) The biocide iodopropynyl butylcarbamate (IPBC) as an allergen in cutting oils. Contact Dermatitis 43:238–240

52. Malten KE (1981) Thoughts on irritant contact dermatitis. Contact Dermatitis 7:238–247

53. Malten KE (1987) Old and new, mainly occupational dermatological problems in the production and processing of plastics. In: Maibach HI (ed) Occupational and industrial dermatology, 2nd edn. Yearbook Medical, Chicago, Ill., p 310

54. Meding B (1996) Occupational contact dermatitis from tertiary-butylhydroquinone (TBHQ) in a cutting fluid. Contact Dermatitis 34:224

55. Minkwitz R, Fröhlich N, Lehmann E (1983) Untersuchungen von Schadstoffbelastungen an Arbeitsplätzen bei der Herstellung und Verarbeitung von Metallen – Beryllium, Cobalt und deren Legierungen. Schriftenreihe der Bundesanstalt für Arbeitsschutz, Fb 367, Dortmund, Germany

56. Mowad CM (2000) Methylchloro-isothiazolinone revisited. Am J Contact Dermat 11:114–118

57. Nethercott JR, Rothman N, Holness DL, O'Toole T (1990) Health problems in metal workers exposed to a coolant oil containing Kathon 886 MW. Am J Contact Dermat 1:94–99

58. Owen CM, August PJ, Beck MH (2000) Contact allergy to oak moss resin in a soluble oil. Contact Dermatitis 43:112

59. Pfeiffer W, Breuer D, Blome H, Deninger C et al (1996) BIA-Report 7/96 Kühlschmierstoffe. Herausgegeben vom Hauptverband der gewerblichen Berufsgenossenschaften (HVBG), Sankt Augustin, Germany

60. Piebenga WP, van der Walle HB (2003) Allergic contact dermatitis from 1-[2-(2,4-dichlorophenyl)-2-(2-propenyloxy)ethyl]-1H-imidazole in a water-based metalworking fluid. Contact Dermatitis 48:285–286

61. Pryce DW, Irvine D, English JSC, Rycroft RJG (1989) Soluble oil dermatitis: a follow-up study. Contact Dermatitis 21:28–35

62. Pryce DW, White I, English JSC, Rycroft RJG (1989) Soluble oil dermatitis: a review. J Soc Occup Med 39:93–98

63. Robinson MK, Gerberick GF, Ryan CA, McNamee P, White IR, Basketter DA (2000) The importance of exposure estimation in the assessment of skin sensitization risk. Contact Dermatitis 42:251–259

64. Rycroft RJG (1987) Cutting fluids, oil, and lubricants. In: Maibach HI (ed) Occupational and industrial dermatology, 2nd edn. Yearbook Medical, Chicago, Ill., p 289

65. Rystedt I (1979) Evaluation and relevance of isolated test reactions to cobalt. Contact Dermatitis 5:233–238

66. Scheinman PL (1996) Multiple sensitizations in a machinist using a new cooling fluid. Am J Contact Dermat 7:61

67. Schnuch A, Geier J, Brasch J, Uter W (2002) The preservative iodopropynyl butylcarbamate: frequency of allergic reactions and diagnostic considerations. Results from the IVDK. Contact Dermatitis 46:153–156

68. Shah M, Lewis FM, Gawkrodger DJ (1996) Prognosis of occupational hand dermatitis in metalworkers. Contact Dermatitis 34:27–30

69. Skudlik C, Schwanitz H-J (2003) Berufsbedingte Handekzeme – Ätiologie und Prävention. Allergo J 12:513–520

70. Sonnenschein G (1998) Kühlschmierstoffe. In: Konietzko J, Dupuis H (eds) Handbuch der Arbeitsmedizin, 20. Ergänzungslieferung 5/98, Kap IV-2.47.1. Ecomed, Landsberg, Germany, pp 1–15

71. Thamm H (1997) Formaldehyd und Formaldehydabspalter in Kühlschmierstoffen: aktueller Stand. Allergologie 20:232–238

72. Tiedemann K-H, Zoellner G, Adam M, Becker D, Boveleth W, Eck E, Eckert C, Englitz H-G, Geier J, Koch P, Lessmann H, Müller J, Nöring R, Rocker M, Rothe A, Schmidt A, Schumacher T, Uter W, Warfolomeow I, Wirtz C (2002) Empfehlungen für die Epikutantestung bei Verdacht auf

Kontaktallergie durch Kühlschmierstoffe. 2. Hinweise zur Arbeitsstofftestung. Derm Beruf Umwelt 50:180–189

73. Uter W, Schaller S, Bahmer FA, Brasch J et al (1993) Contact allergy in metal workers – a one-year analysis based on data collected by the "Information Network of Dermatological Clinics" (IVDK) in Germany. Derm Beruf Umwelt 41:220–227

74. Uter W, Geier J, Ippen H (1996) Nachrichten aus dem IVDK: Aktuelle Sensibilisierungshäufigkeiten bei der DKG-Testreihe "Metallverarbeitung". Derm Beruf Umwelt 44:34–36

75. Uter W, Geier J, Lessmann H, Schnuch A (1999) Unverträglichkeitsreaktionen gegen Körperpflege- und Haushaltsprodukte: was ist zu tun? Die Informations- und Dokumentationsstelle für Kontaktallergien (IDOK) des Informationsverbundes Dermatologischer Kliniken (IVDK). Deutsche Dermatologe 47:211–214

76. Uter W, Gefeller O, Geier J, Lessmann H, Pfahlberg A, Schnuch A (2002) Untersuchungen zur Abhängigkeit der Sensibilisierung gegen wichtige Allergene von arbeitsbedingten sowie individuellen Faktoren. Schriftenreihe der Bundesanstalt für Arbeitsschutz und Arbeitsmedizin, Forschung, Fb 949. Wissenschaftsverlag NW, Bremerhaven, Germany

77. Uter W, Lessmann H, Geier J, Becker D, Fuchs Th, Richter G; IDVK Study Group; German Contact Dermatitis Research Group (DKG) (2002) The spectrum of allergic (cross-)sensitivity in clinical patch testing with "para amino" compounds. Allergy 7:319–322

78. Wahlberg JE (1973) Thresholds of sensitivity in metal contact allergy. 1. Isolated and simultaneous allergy to chromium, cobalt, mercury and-or nickel. Berufsdermatosen 21:22–33

79. Wahlberg JE, Lindstedt G, Einarsson Ö (1977) Chromium, cobalt and nickel in Swedish cement, detergents, mould and cutting oils. Berufsdermatosen 25:220–228

80. Wilkinson JD, Shaw S, Andersen KE, Brandao FM, Bruynzeel DP, Bruze M, Camarasa JM, Diepgen TL, Ducombs G, Frosch PJ, Goossens A, Lachappelle JM, Lahti A, Menne T, Seidenari S, Tosti A, Wahlberg JE (2002) Monitoring levels of preservative sensitivity in Europe. A 10-year overview (1991–2000). Contact Dermatitis 46:207–210

Chapter 34

Plastic Materials

34

BERT BJÖRKNER, ANN PONTÉN, ERIK ZIMERSON, MALIN FRICK

Contents

Introduction

One of the most important branches of the chemical industry is the polymer industry, which uses a wider variety of chemicals than any other sector. Plastic materials are more frequently used in daily living than ever before. Plastics come from oil and 5% of the total oil production in the world is used by the polymer industry. The number of commercially important plastics today is more than 50. Application areas for plastics are many and varied: the construction industry, packaging, electronics, recreation, medical, etc.; 30% of base plastics are used for packaging and 20% are used in the construction industry.

There are several ways of classifying polymeric materials. Chemically, they are very large molecules (polymers) formed by the linking up of small molecules (monomers) into large chain-like units. If only one type of monomer is involved in forming the polymer, it is called a homopolymer. If two or more different types are involved, it is called a copolymer.

The words "plastic" and "resin" are often used synonymously. However, strictly speaking, plastics are synthetic macromolecular end products, while the term "resin" is used to denote all low-, medium-, and high-molecular-weight intermediate synthetic substances from which plastics are made. Natural rubbers and cellulose do not fit into these definitions because their starting material is of natural origin and not synthetic.

If the monomers that form the final polymer simply link up into long chains by joining bonds, and nothing is eliminated in the process, the polymerization is called an addition reaction. If two or more different monomers react with each other, thereby eliminating a simple molecule such as water, the polymerization is called a condensation reaction.

Traditionally and practically, plastics can be divided into three major categories: thermoplastic, thermosetting, and elastomers. The thermoplastic resins are characterized by softening when exposed to heat, and when soft, they can be made to flow and assume the desired shape. When cooled, they become hard again. Thermoplastic resins are made up of long molecular chains unconnected with each other. When heated, the molecular chains become moveable and the plastic material melts, starts to float, and becomes liquid. The thermoplastic resins, therefore, have different characteristics at different temperatures.

Thermosetting resins have chemical bonds between the long molecular chains. When heated for the first time, they, therefore, undergo further chemical reactions in which cross-links develop between polymer chains, holding them rigid in the desired position. They do not soften on re-heating into the original polymer. Examples of thermoplastic resins are polyethylene, polystyrene, polyvinyl chloride, and saturated polyesters. Examples of thermosetting resins are phenol formaldehyde resins, epoxy resins, polyurethanes, unsaturated polyesters, and acrylates. Synthetic rubbers are examples of elastomers.

The final plastic products, when completely cured or hardened, are generally considered to be inert and non-hazardous to the skin. Skin problems from plastics are almost exclusively related to ingredients such as monomers, hardeners, and other additives, or degradation products of low molecular weight.

34.1　Acrylic Resins

BERT BJÖRKNER

Acrylic resins are thermoplastics formed by derivatives of acrylic acid (CH_2=CH-COOH). The acrylic group is a vinyl group (CH_2=CH-). The monomers in acrylic resins are acrylic acid and methacrylic acid and their esters, cyanoacrylic acid and its esters, acrylamides, and acrylonitrile. Numerous different acrylic monomers, therefore, exist and, as a result, a multitude of different polymers and resins are produced.

The polymerization of acrylic monomers is an addition reaction obtained either at room temperature or by heating. Adding initiators, accelerators, and catalysts usually speeds up the process. Polymerization or curing can also be achieved by ultraviolet (UV) light, visible light, or electron beams (EB), for which initiators are not necessary.

34.1.1　Monoacrylates and Monomethacrylates

Mono(meth)acrylates (monoacrylates and monomethacrylates) are used in the production of a wide variety of polymers.

Polymethyl methacrylate is the most important plastic in the acrylics group, with the following repeating unit: $[CH_2\text{-}CH(CH_3)COOCH_3]_n$. This plastic has excellent transparency and is, therefore, used in products such as roof windows, housewares, watch glasses, bags, lamp housings, and windscreens. A two-component system is used in the manufacture of dentures, hearing aids, noise protectors, and bone cement in orthopedic surgery. The first component is a prepolymer powder of polymethyl methacrylate with benzoyl peroxide as an initiator. The second compo-

Fig. 1.1.
Polymethyl methacrylate
and methyl methacrylate
mixed with sand are some-
times used as flooring. Protective gloves are recom-
mended

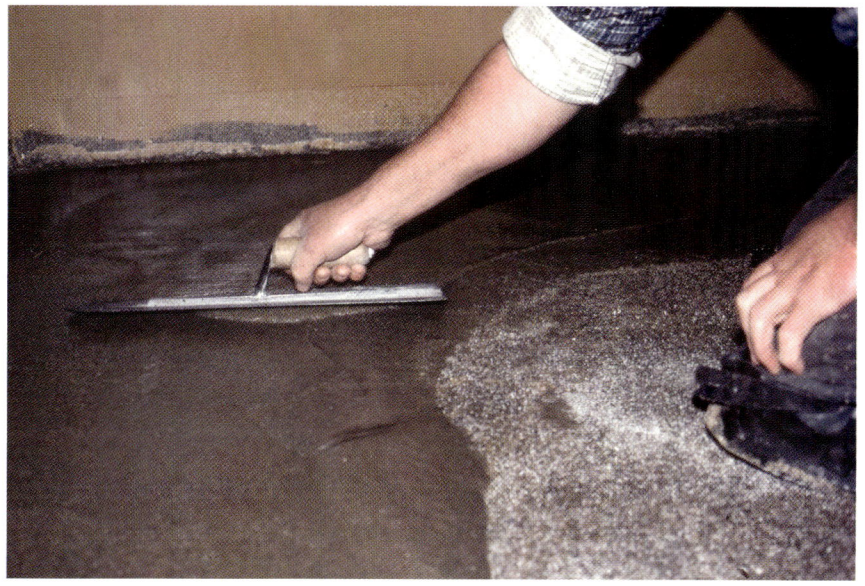

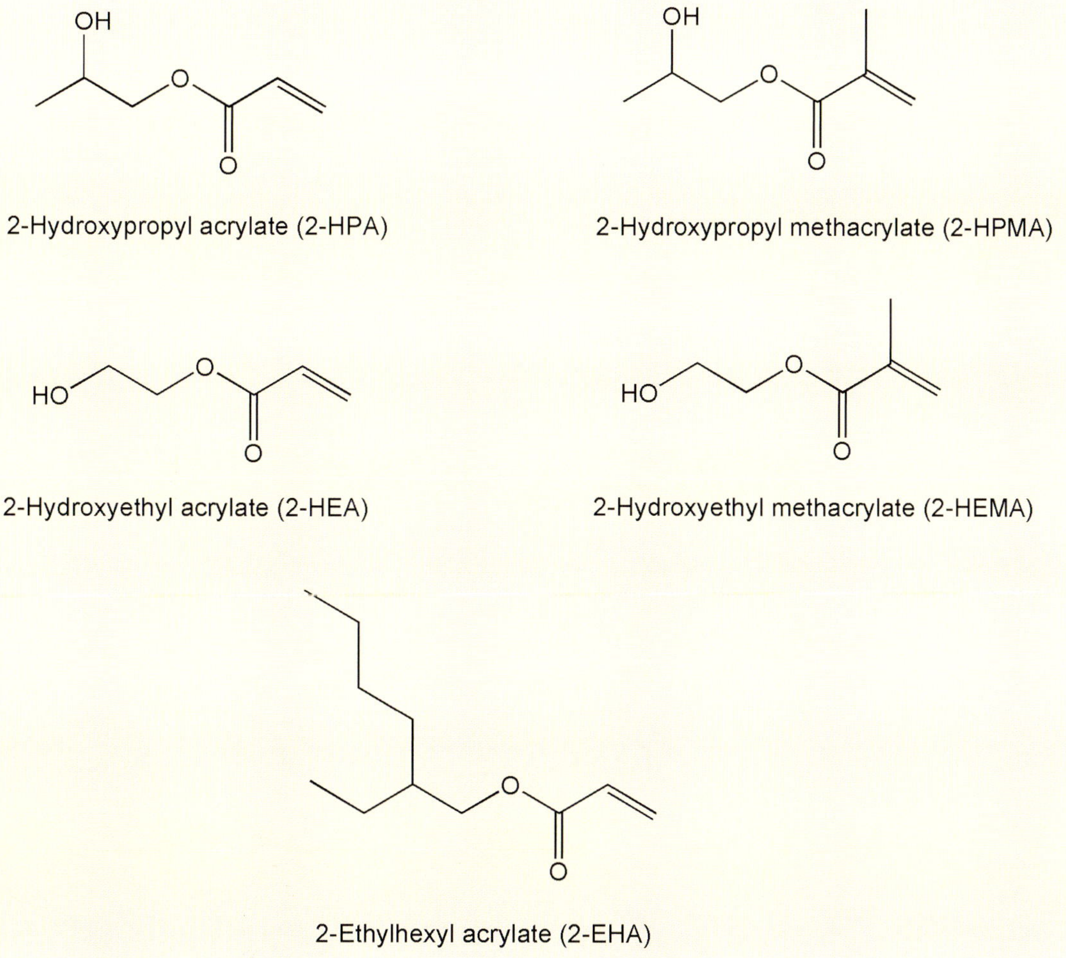

2-Hydroxypropyl acrylate (2-HPA)

2-Hydroxypropyl methacrylate (2-HPMA)

2-Hydroxyethyl acrylate (2-HEA)

2-Hydroxyethyl methacrylate (2-HEMA)

2-Ethylhexyl acrylate (2-EHA)

Fig. 1.2. Chemical formulae of some monofunctional acrylate compounds in UV-curable acrylate-based paints and lacquers nent is a monomeric liquid of methyl methacrylate containing an accelerator, e.g., N, N′-dimethyl-p-toluidine. A two-component methyl methacrylate system mixed with sand is used in flooring (Fig. 1.1).

Other polymers of the mono(meth)acrylate type are mostly used in industry. Leather finishes, adhesives, paints, printing inks and coatings are example of practical applications. Butyl acrylate is sometimes used in spectacle frames. 2-Ethylhexyl acrylate is often used in the manufacturer of pressure-sensitive adhesives, but a wide range of other acrylates are also used in this field.

The acrylic monomers preferred in the preparation of UV-curable inks and coatings or in the photoprepolymer printing plate procedure are 2-hydroxyethyl acrylate (2-HEA), 2-hydroxypropyl acrylate (2-HPA), 2-hydroxypropyl methacrylate (2-HPMA), 2-hydroxyethyl methacrylate (2-HEMA), and 2-ethylhexyl acrylate (2-EHA) (Fig. 1.2). 2-HPMA is also used in light-sensitive compositions for fissure sealants/adhesives or bonding preparations in dentistry and in printing plates. Various mono(meth)acrylates can be used in water-based acrylic latex paints. Plastic dispersions of acrylic polymers are used as binders or thickeners in paints, as well as cosmetic creams. Their monomer content is usually less than 0.3%.

34.1.2 Multifunctional Acrylates

Acrylates with at least two reactive acrylic groups are called multifunctional acrylates. These are, e.g., di(-meth)acrylate esters of dialcohols or tri- and tetra-acrylate esters of polyalcohols. Multifunctional acry-

Table 1.1. Acrylates used in acrylic nail preparations

Methyl methacrylate
Ethyl methacrylate
Ethyl acrylate
2-Hydroxyethyl acrylate
Butyl methacrylate
Isobutyl methacrylate
Methacrylic acid
Tetrahydrofurfuryl methacrylate
Ethylene glycol dimethacrylate
Diethylene glycol dimethacrylate
Triethylene glycol dimethacrylate
Trimethylol propane trimethacrylate
Urethane methacrylate
Tripropylene glycol acrylate

lates are used in formulations for UV-curable inks and coatings, where they act as cross-linking agents and reactive diluents, and become a part of the final coating on UV exposure (Fig. 1.3). The multifunctional acrylates are also important in photopolymers, flexographic printing plates, and photoresists (an etch-resist for printed circuit boards). The multifunctional acrylate esters are useful in acrylic adhesives and anaerobic sealants, as well as in artificial nail preparations. Some of the more commonly used multifunctional acrylates for artificial nail preparations are ethylene glycol dimethacrylate (EGDMA), diethylene glycol dimethacrylate (DEGDMA), and trimethylol propane trimethacrylate (TMPTMA). The various acrylates used in acrylic nail preparations are listed in Table 1.1 [1–5].

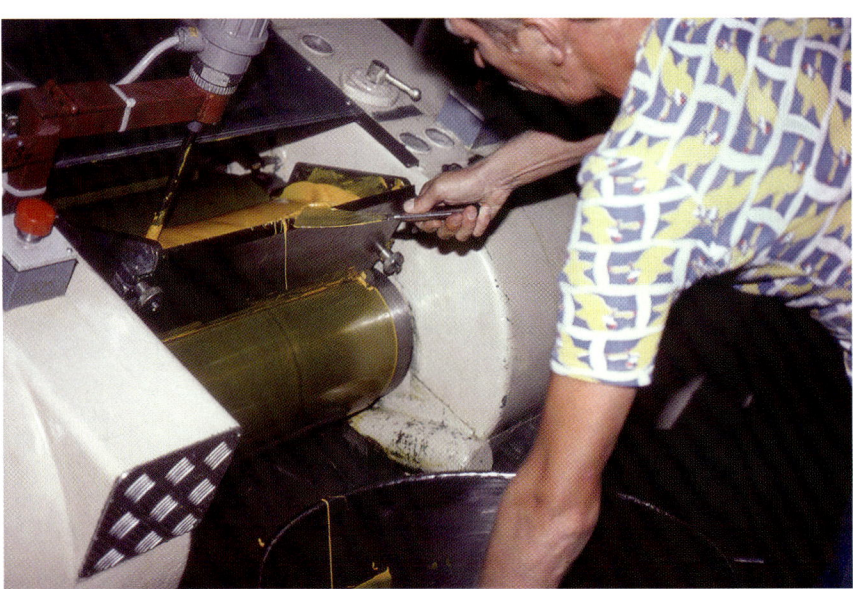

Fig. 1.3.
UV-curable acrylic inks mixed with color pigments. Protective gloves are highly recommended

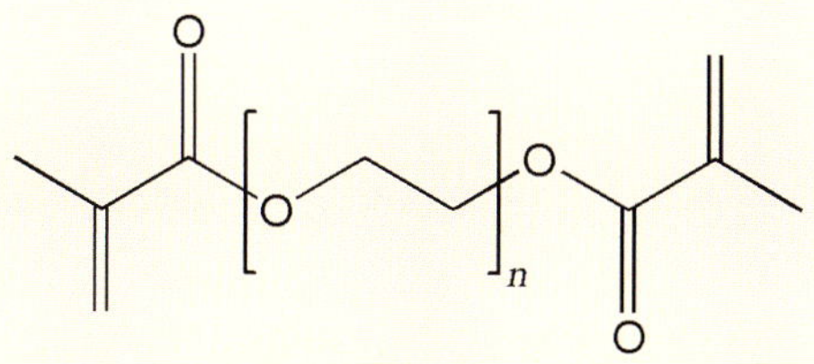

Fig. 1.4.
Chemical formulae of *n*-ethylene glycol di(meth)acrylates

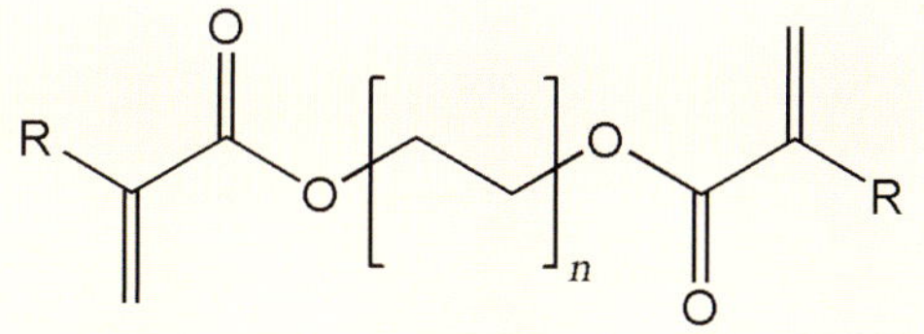

n=1: Ethylene glycol dimethacrylate (EGDMA)
n=2: Diethylene glycol dimethacrylate (DEGDMA)
n=3: Triethylene glycol dimethacrylate (TREGDMA)

Fig. 1.5.
Chemical formulae of 1,6-hexanediol diacrylate and 1,4-butandiol dimethacrylate

R=H, *n*=3:   1,6-Hexanediol diacrylate (HDDA)
R=CH₃, *n*=2: 1,4-Butanediol dimethacrylate (BUDMA)

Most of the dental composite resin materials and denture base polymers are "diluted" with the less viscous, difunctional acrylates. These are the methacrylic monomers, of which EGDMA, DEGDMA, triethylene glycol dimethacrylate (TREGDMA) (Fig. 1.4), and 1,4-butanediol dimethacrylate (BUDMA) (Fig. 1.5) are the most widely used (Table 1.2). Acrylates used in dentistry are an expanding field. Some are also new to dermatology, but others are well-known sensitizers [6–8]. 1,6-Hexanediol diacrylate (HDDA) is used as a dental acrylate, but is a known sensitizer in the printing ink and coating fields (Fig. 1.5).

The simplest UV-curable ink or coating formulations may consist of only three components. In practice, however, a typical industrial formulation contains a much greater number of ingredients. The three essential components are: a UV-reactive prepolymer that provides the bulk of the desired properties, a diluent system composed of multifunctional acrylate esters (and at times, monofunctional acrylic esters), and a photoinitiator system. The most commonly used multifunctional acrylate in a UV-curable ink or coating formulation is an acrylic acid ester of either pentaerythritol (PETA), trimethylolpropane (TMPTA), or hexanediol (HDDA) (Figs. 1.5 and 1.6).

During the past 15–20 years, the use of UV-curable acrylates in inks and coatings has increased tremendously. In the can-coating industry, UV printing inks

Table 1.2. Acrylic compounds used in dental materials

Methyl methacrylate
Triethyleneglycol dimethacrylate
Urethane dimethacrylate
Ethyleneglycol dimethacrylate
BIS-GMA
BIS-MA
BIS-EMA
BIS-PMA
2-(Dimethylamino)ethyl methacrylate
Butyl methacrylate
2-Hydroxyethyl methacrylate
1,6-Hexanediol diacrylate
1,10-Decanediol dimethacrylate
1,4-Butanediol dimethacrylate
1,12-Dodecanediol dimethacrylate
Trimethylolpropane trimethacrylate
Phenylsalicylate glycidyl methacrylate
Tetrahydrofurfuryl methacrylate
Benzaldehyde glycol methacrylate
N-Tolylglycine-glycidylmethacrylate
1,3-Butyleneglycol diacrylate
3,6-Dioxaoctamethylene dimethacrylate
Biphenyl dimethacrylate
Glycerol phosphate dimethacrylate

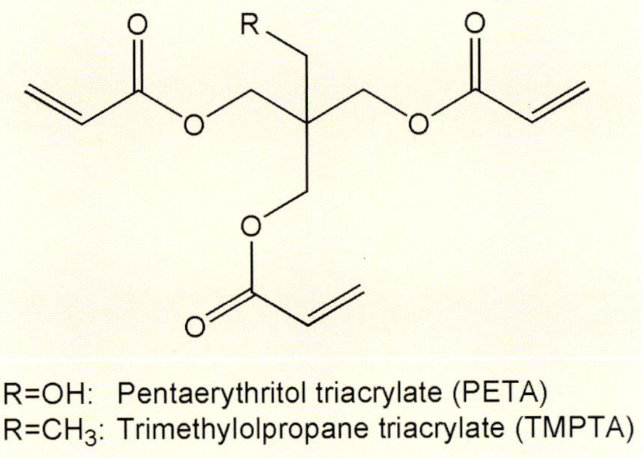

R=OH: Pentaerythritol triacrylate (PETA)
R=CH₃: Trimethylolpropane triacrylate (TMPTA)

Fig. 1.6. Chemical formulae of two common UV-curable multifunctional acrylates

34

are used on beverage and beer cans, as well as on crown caps and aerosol containers. UV-curable acrylate coatings are used as wood finishes, matt varnishes, parquet varnishes and sealers, and as varnishes and coatings in the manufacture of furniture.

TMPTA and PETA can both be used in the production of polyfunctional aziridine, added to paint primer and floor top-coatings as a self-curing crosslinker or hardener [9–11].

In the absence of oxygen and in the presence of metals, anaerobic acrylic sealants, e.g., Loctite, Treebond, and Sta-Lok, polymerize rapidly. Dimethacrylates are their principal components [7, 12–18]. Diethylene glycol dimethacrylate oligomer is most commonly used for screw-thread-locking, whereas urethane dimethacrylate is used for retaining and locking flat metal surfaces.

34.1.3 Prepolymers

Acrylate resins, based on the conventional thermoplastic resins, into which two or more reactive acrylate or methacrylate groups have been introduced, are called prepolymers. The most commonly used prepolymers are acrylated epoxy resins, acrylated polyurethanes, acrylated polyesters, and acrylated polyethers.

Core Message

■ UV-curable acrylic compounds contain three basic components: a reactive base prepolymer, a diluent system of multifunctional acrylic esters, and a photoinitiator system.

34.1.4 Epoxy Acrylates

Epoxy acrylate is another name for beta-hydroxyester acrylate, since it is usually obtained by reacting epoxy resins or glycidyl derivatives with acrylic acid (Fig. 1.7). Both aromatic or aliphatic epoxy acrylates are available, as well as acrylated epoxydized oils. Epoxy acrylates have found a wide range of useful applications in UV- or EB-curing.

The addition-reaction product between bisphenol A and glycidyl methacrylate or an epoxy resin and methacrylic acid is BIS-GMA; 2,2-bis[4-(2-hydroxy-3-methacryloxypropoxy)phenyl]propane (Fig. 1.7). BIS-GMA can, therefore, be classified as a dimethacrylated epoxy, although it does not contain a reactive epoxy group. BIS-GMA is the most commonly used prepolymer in dental composite restorative materials.

Several similar compounds have also appeared as substitutes for BIS-GMA or in addition to BIS-GMA in dental resins (Table 1.2). Such dimethacrylates based on bisphenol A with various chain lengths are BIS-MA; 2,2-bis[4-(methacryloxy)phenyl]-propane and BIS-EMA; 2,2-bis[4-(2-methacryloxyethoxy)phenyl]-propane and BIS-PMA; 2,2-bis[4-(3-methacryloxypropoxy)phenyl]-propane (Fig. 1.7).

The industrial applications of BIS-GMA resins and other similar derivatives are extensive. Acrylates based on bisphenol A or epoxy resin can be polymerized not only by exposure to EB, UV-light, or even visible light, but can also be chemically activated by the use of various peroxides.

34.1.5 Urethane Acrylates

There are many types of acrylated urethanes on the market. While some are based on aromatic isocyanates, others are of the aliphatic type. Acrylated urethanes are used not only in prepolymers in UV-curable inks or coatings, for instance vinyl floorings, but also as resins with dental applications. The acrylated urethanes used in dentistry are of the methacrylated type.

34.1.6 Polyester Acrylates

There are various types of polyester acrylates on the market and they are mostly used in UV-curable lacquers and printing inks for wood and paper coatings.

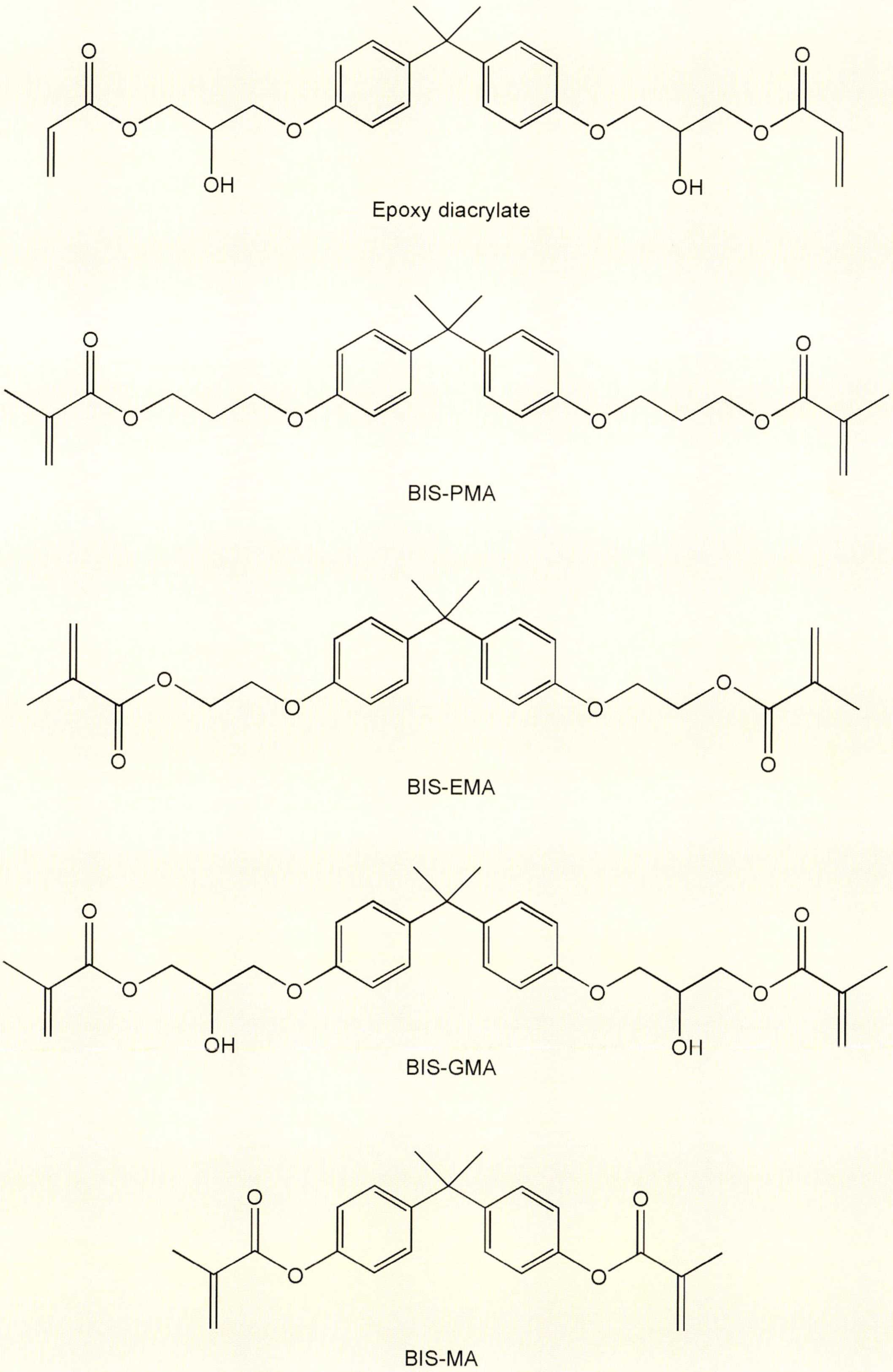

Epoxy diacrylate

BIS-PMA

BIS-EMA

BIS-GMA

BIS-MA

Fig. 1.7. Chemical formulae of di(meth)acrylates based on bisphenol A and epoxy resin

34.1.7 The Effects of Acrylate Esters on the Skin

Evaluation of the irritant potential of various acrylic monomers has shown that the diacrylates are strong irritants, monoacrylates weak to moderate irritants, and monomethacrylates and dimethacrylates non-irritant or weak irritants to guinea-pig skin [19–27]. Multifunctional acrylates as well as acrylated prepolymers seem to be more irritating than the corresponding methacrylates. These effects have been seen when patch testing both humans and guinea pigs [27]. Bullous irritant skin reactions in workers exposed to tetramethylene glycol diacrylate have been reported [28]. A peculiar delayed irritation from butanediol diacrylate and hexanediol diacrylate has been observed by Malten et al. [29]. Tetraethylene glycol diacrylate can cause delayed irritant reactions as well as allergic contact dermatitis [30]. The irritant effect of various acrylate compounds has been reviewed by Kanerva et al. [31, 32].

The sensitizing potential of many mono(meth)acrylates, multifunctional (meth)acrylates, and acrylated resins in guinea pigs has been thoroughly studied by numerous authors [19–27]. Tests have shown that monoacrylates are strong sensitizers while mono(meth)acrylates have weak to moderate sensitizing potential [19, 21, 23, 27]. Thus, the introduction of a methyl group reduces the sensitizing potential of monoacrylates. Of the multifunctional acrylates, the di- and triacrylic compounds should be regarded as potent sensitizers [22, 24, 27]. The methacrylated multifunctional acrylic compounds are weak sensitizers [24, 27].

Among the various di(meth)acrylates based on bisphenol A or epoxy resin, allergenicity seems to diminish if the acrylates have three or more methylene groups in the molecular chain [22–27]. It is more difficult to predict the sensitizing capacity of the various prepolymers. Epoxy acrylates are strong sensitizers and their sensitizing capacity is due to the entire molecule, thereby, excluding the epoxide group as the sole sensitizing part of these compounds [27]. Free epoxy resin may be present in epoxy acrylates, which may sensitize separately or simultaneously [24, 33].

The whole molecular structure of polyester acrylate probably acts as an allergen as well. However, the reactive acrylate and methacrylate terminal groups seem to be of great importance for antigen formation and sensitization [25]. The carboxyethyl side group seems to be of importance for antigenicity [34].

The aliphatic urethane acrylates are more potent sensitizers than the aromatic ones, while the aliphatic urethane methacrylate commonly used in dental resins is a weak sensitizer [26, 35].

There are many reports of contact allergy to mono(meth)acrylates in humans. Contact dermatitis due to 2-HPMA in printers exposed to printing plates, as well as to UV-curing inks, has been reported [36, 37] (Fig. 1.8). Contact allergy to 2-HEMA, one of the ingredients in a photo prepolymer mixture, has been described [38]. 2-HEMA is a water-soluble form of methacrylate resin and is, therefore, commonly used as a dentine-bonding compound. The bonding systems used contain a primer and an adhesive. Primer, followed by the adhesive, first coats the dentine. This is polymerized with a visible-light curing unit and then a dental composite resin is ap-

34

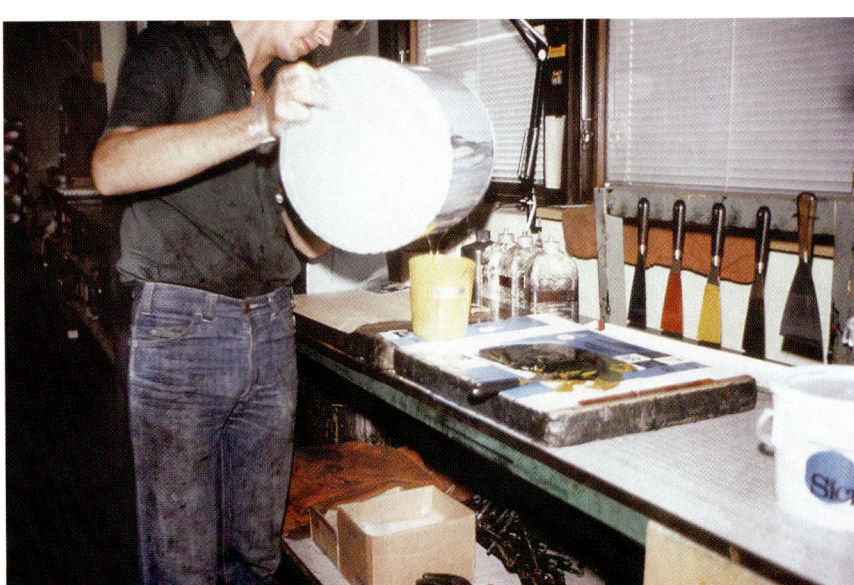

Fig. 1.8.
A printer with contaminated clothes mixing UV-curable acrylics

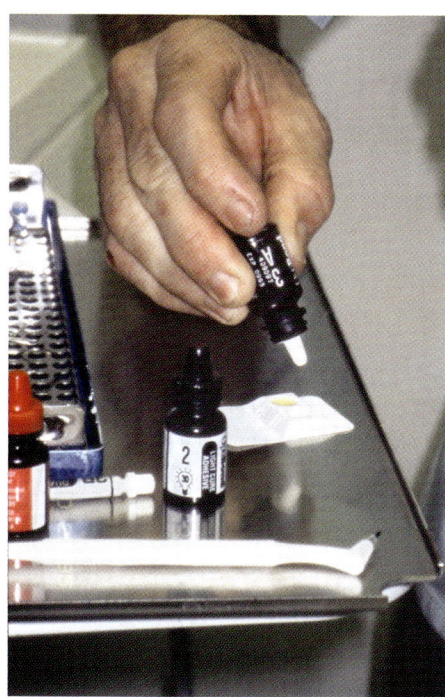

Fig. 1.9. Uncured acrylates that remain on the outside of a bottle used for dental bonding systems can cause fingertip dermatitis

plied to the tooth and cured chemically or with light. 2-HEMA is a common allergen in dental personnel (Fig. 1.9). Fingertip dermatitis is common in dentists and dental nurses allergic to dentine-bonding acrylates [6, 39–42] (Figs. 1.10 and 1.11)

Contact dermatitis from 2-EHA in an acrylic-based adhesive tape has been reported [43]. Orthope-

dic surgeons, surgical technicians, nurses, and dental technicians are exposed to methyl methacrylate monomer when preparing bone cement and dentures. Contact allergy to methyl methacrylate monomer is rare in patients undergoing hip surgery [44].

In recent decades, many reports of contact allergy caused by various multifunctional acrylic compounds have been published [6–8, 27, 45–47]. At risk of developing contact allergy to multifunctional tri- and diacrylates are those working with UV-curable inks or coatings, while contact allergy to dimethacrylates is more commonly seen in dentistry, in those working with anaerobic acrylic sealants and in those exposed to acrylic nails [6, 7, 27, 39–42, 47–55]. In spite of that risk, epoxy acrylates are strong sensitizers in animal studies [27], allergic contact dermatitis caused by epoxy (di)methacrylates seems to be rare in workers exposed to ultraviolet-cured inks [56, 57] There are some reports of allergic contact dermatitis from dimethacrylates based on bisphenol A or epoxy resin in dental composite materials. At risk of developing contact dermatitis are dentists and dental technicians, as well as dental patients [6, 7, 39–42, 53–55]. Methacrylates have also caused asthma and rhinoconjunctivitis in dental personnel [50–52]. Patients allergic to BIS-GMA may also react to epoxy resin MW 340 [24, 54, 58]. It is uncertain whether any residual epoxy resin monomer is left unreacted or whether it is formed in the synthesis of the BIS-GMA monomer [24, 33].

Methyl methacrylate and 2-HEMA can cause paresthesia of the fingertips for months after discontinuation of contact with the monomer [59–61]. An ef-

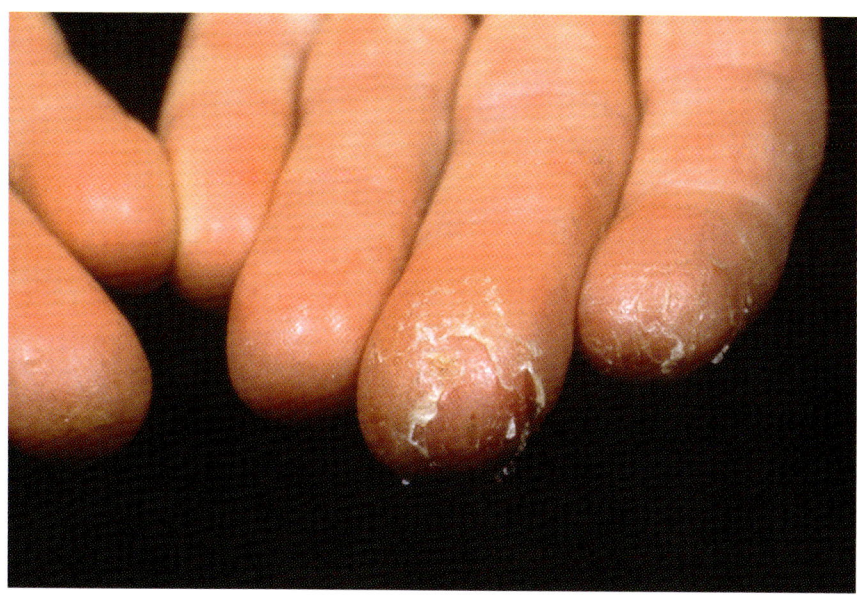

Fig. 1.10.
Severe fingertip dermatitis in a dentist with contact allergy to acrylates used in dentistry

Fig. 1.11.
When grinding prosthesis, uncured acrylates can cause dermatitis in sensitized dental personal

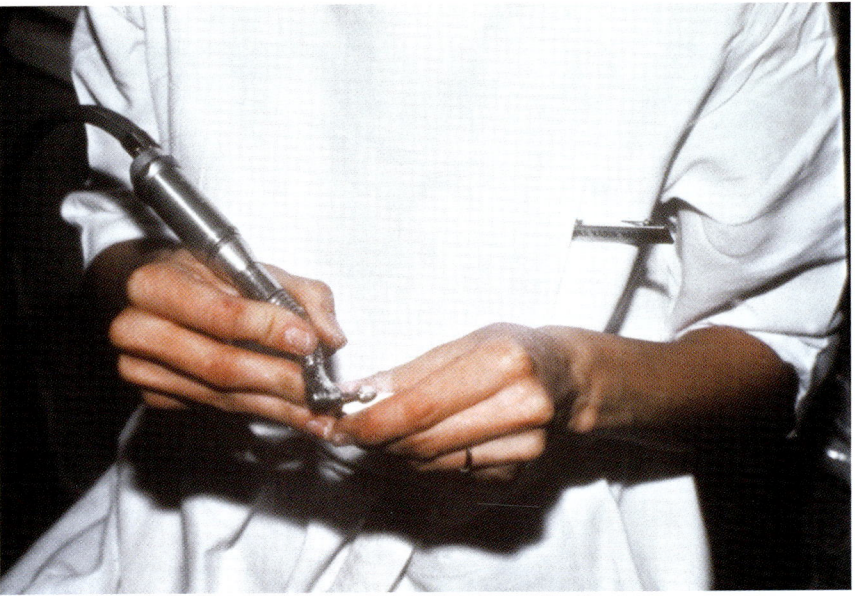

34

fect on the peripheral nervous system has also been described for acrylamide [62] and cyanoacrylates (see later).

> ### Core Message
>
> ■ Free epoxy resin may be present in epoxy acrylates, which may sensitize separately or simultaneously.

34.1.8 Acrylonitrile

Acrylonitrile ($H_2C=CH-CN$) is used as a copolymer in approximately 25% of all synthetic fibers. It is further used for synthetic rubbers and for the production of acrylonitrile-butadiene-styrene and styrene-acrylonitrile plastics. These ter- and copolymers are used in the automobile industry and in the production of housewares, electrical appliances, suitcases, food packaging, and disposable dishes. Acrylonitrile can also be a constituent in fabrics and paints.

34.1.9 Skin Problems from Acrylonitrile

There are a few reports of contact allergy to the acrylonitrile monomer [63–67]. In the guinea pig maximization test, however, acrylonitrile has shown strong allergenic potential [67].

34.1.10 Acrylamide and Derivatives

Acrylamide ($H_2C=CH-CO-NH_2$) is an odorless, white, crystalline solid used as a monomer or as a raw material in the production of polyacrylamides and other compounds. Most of the acrylamide monomer is produced and used as an aqueous solution. The reactive acrylamide monomer is used in the production of other compounds, mostly polymers of acrylamide, and as a grouting agent in the construction or rehabilitation of dams, buildings, sewers, tunnels, and other structures. Acrylamide grouts are used predominantly as barriers against ground-water seepage into sewers. About 95% of the acrylamide produced is consumed in the production of other compounds, including polyacrylamide products that are widely used as flocculents in potable water and waste-water treatment, mineral ore processing and sugar refining, water-flow control agents in oil-well operations, and adhesives in paper making and construction. The remaining 5% is used as a monomer. Acrylamide and its derivatives are also used in the production of photopolymer printing plates. Because acrylamide is produced by catalytic or sulfuric acid hydration of acrylonitrile, acrylamide production workers may also be exposed to acrylonitrile.

34.1.11 Health Effects from Acrylamide and Derivatives

Polyacrylamide products are generally considered non-hazardous. The monomer can be irritating and cause contact allergy. Skin problems are seen among printers exposed to photopolymerizing printing plates. Acrylamide and their acrylamide compounds N, N'-methylene-bis-acrylamide, N-methylol acrylamide and N-[2-(diethylamino) ethyl] acrylamide have been described as allergens [68–76]. N-Methylol acrylamide sensitization has also been observed in workers making PVA-acrylic copolymers for paints. Acrylamide, N-hydroxymethyl acrylamide and N, N'-methylene-bis-acrylamide are moderate sensitizers when tested in guinea pigs [20].

The acrylamide monomer may be neurotoxic, carcinogenic, genotoxic, and hazardous to reproduction. Recent studies confirm that acrylamide exposure causes cancer and has reproductive effects in animals, but epidemiological studies have not demonstrated these effects in humans. The neurotoxic effects from acrylamide exposure include peripheral nerve damage and central nervous system effects [62, 71–73].

Allergic contact dermatitis from piperazine diacrylamide, used as a reagent and as a cross-linker for acrylamide gels in electrophoreses and column chromatography has been described by Wang et al. [77].

Core Message

- The acrylamide monomer may be neurotoxic, carcinogenic, genotoxic, and hazardous to reproduction.

34.1.12 Cyanoacrylates

Cyanoacrylates ($H_2C=C(CN)$-COOR) are also called "super glues." The structure of the side chain (R) defines the different alkyl 2-cyanoacrylates and is dependent on the alcohol that has been used. For instance, methanol gives methyl 2-cyanoacrylate, ethanol gives ethyl 2-cyanoacrylate, etc.

Methyl 2-cyanoacrylate is mainly used in instant glue for household use. Ethyl 2-cyanoacrylate is the most commonly used in industry and the most of the different adhesive products on the market are manufactured by Loctite. n-Butyl 2-cyanoacrylate and isobutyl 2-cyanoacrylate are commonly used in medical adhesives.

Glues based on cyanoacrylates are widely used as contact adhesives for metal, glass, rubber, plastics, and textiles, as well for biological materials, including binding tissues and sealing wounds in surgery.

The bonding action of cyanoacrylates is generally believed to be the result of an anionic polymerization that is highly exothermic and rapidly occurring, within seconds or minutes, even at room temperature. Catalysts are not required for this reaction to occur, since weak bases, such as water and alcohols or nucleophilic groups on proteins, e.g., amine or hydroxyl groups, already present on the adherent surfaces initiate the polymerization.

Vaporized cyanoacrylates are known to irritate the eyes and respiratory tract. Irritation and discomfort of the face and eyes may occur in workers due to associated low humidity [78, 79].

Contact sensitization to cyanoacrylates is considered extremely rare, due to the immediate bonding of the cyanoacrylate to the surface keratin [78]. The adhesive was, therefore, believed to have never come into contact with immunocompetent cells deeper in the epidermis. For instance, Parker and Turk [21] were unable to sensitize guinea pigs with methyl or butyl 2-cyanoacrylate. However, in the last decade, some case reports have been published which strongly indicate that cyanoacrylates are able to induce contact allergy [80–92].

Patch testing with cyanoacrylate glue might give false-negative reactions when dissolved in acetone using the Finn chamber (aluminum) technique. Patch testing with petrolatum as the vehicle in a plastic chamber is recommended [87].

Cyanoacrylates, besides causing skin sensitization and irritation, have also been shown to cause occupational asthma and to be mutagenic. Furthermore, cyanoacrylates are suspected to be carcinogenic and to induce peripheral neuropathy and onychodystrophy [89–92] (Fig. 1.12).

34.1.13 Care in the Handling of Acrylic Resins

Gloves are recommended to protect the hands against the various acrylic compounds. Methyl methacrylate, as well as other acrylic monomers, such as butylacrylate and acrylamide, easily penetrates natural rubber latex gloves, and vinyl gloves are even worse in this respect [20, 93–99]. Polyethylene gloves give the best protection against methyl methacrylate diffusion [20]. Nitrile gloves give better protection than neoprene gloves against UV-curable acrylate resins [94]. New multilayer glove material of the folio type, with ethylene-vinyl-alcohol copolymer laminated with polyethylene on both sides, has especially good chemical resistance [100]. The protective effect of gloves against acrylates in dentine-bonding systems was tested on acrylate-sensitized patients and

Fig. 1.12.
Onychodystrophy in a patient allergic to nail polish based on cyanoacrylate

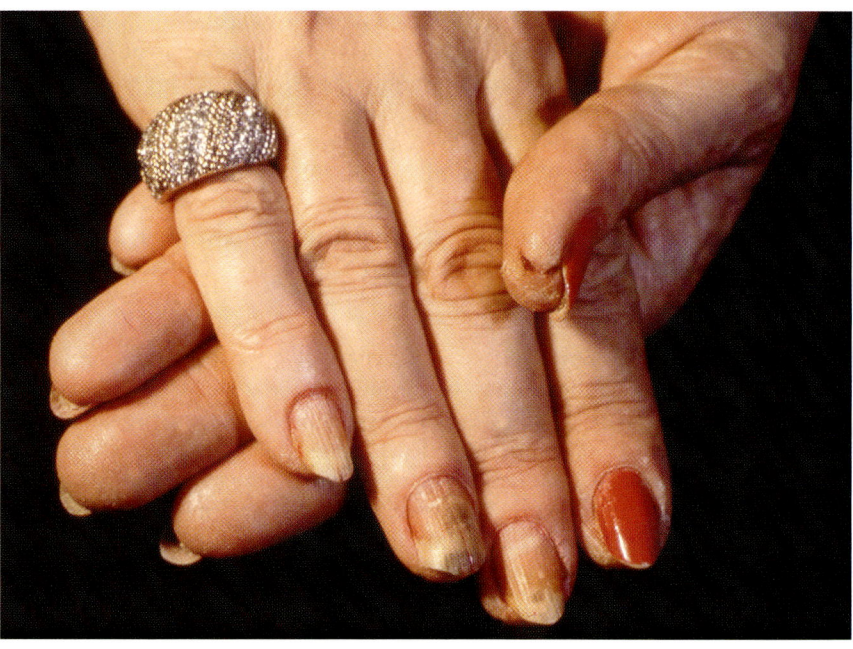

showed clear differences in the protective efficacy between types of gloves [96, 97]. Because acrylics used in dentine-bonding systems are strong sensitizers and quickly penetrate most gloves, dentists and dental personnel should use no-touch techniques [6, 100].

As most of the acrylic compounds used in UV-curable acrylic resins should be regard as irritants and relatively potent sensitizers, care should, thus, be taken accordingly to minimize their contact with the skin.

Measures that seem effective in preventing the occurrence of dermatitis include the use of impermeable protective gloves and protective clothing. Face shields and goggles are recommended whenever there is a risk of splattering. The contaminated skin should be washed with soap and water and contaminated clothing should be removed promptly. It is essential to separate clean from contaminated clothing. Thorough education of employees regarding skin hazards is also recommended.

> **Core Message**
>
> ■ Because acrylics used in dentine-bonding systems are strong sensitizers and quickly penetrate most gloves, dentists and dental personnel should use no-touch techniques.

34.1.14 Patch Testing with Acrylic Compounds

In general, a patch test concentration of 2% in petrolatum is recommended for methacrylated monomers and 0.1% in petrolatum for acrylated monomers, to avoid patch test sensitization [101]. A marked decrease in the number of positive test responses has been noticed when acetone and alcohol has been used as the test vehicle for various acrylic compounds instead of petrolatum [87] The petrolatum vehicle probably prevents the acrylic monomers from polymerizing. A rapid polymerization of acrylic monomers was also seen when an aluminum test chamber was used instead of a plastic test chamber. Aluminum oxide probably enhances the polymerization process [87]. When acrylic compounds are patch tested, it is, thus, recommended to use petrolatum as the test vehicle in a plastic test chamber.

Cross-reactions of multifunctional methacrylates and acrylates has been investigated by Kanerva [102] and Rustemeyer et al. [103].

> **Core Message**
>
> ■ When acrylic compounds are patch tested, it is recommended to use petrolatum as the test vehicle in a plastic test chamber.

34

34.2 Epoxy Resin Systems

Ann Pontén

Epoxy resins and curing agents are the two mandatory components in epoxy resin systems. Additionally, epoxy resin systems may contain several types of modifiers and additives. The term "epoxy resin" is often used to indicate the resins in both the thermoplastic (uncured) and thermoset (cured) states [104].

> ## Core Message
>
> ■ Epoxy resin systems contain epoxy resins and hardeners and may contain modifiers and additives.

34.2.1 Epoxy Resins

Epoxy (or ethoxylin) resins contain at least two epoxy groups, also called oxirane or epoxide groups, in their molecules. The epoxy group is formed when two carbon and one oxygen atoms bind chemically. The commercially most important epoxy resins are produced by polycondensation of compounds with at least two hydroxy groups and epichlorohydrin [104,105]. About 75–90% of epoxy resins are based on diglycidyl ether of the bisphenol A (DGEBA), formed by combining epichlorohydrin and bisphenol A [synonyms: 4,4'-(1-methylethylidene)bisphenol; 4,4'-isopropylidenediphenol; 2,2-*bis*(4-hydroxyphenyl)-propane] [104, 105]. DGEBA resins were first synthesized in the late 1930s. When the proportion of epichlorohydrin and bisphenol A is varied during the manufacturing process, different amounts of low- and high-molecular-weight (MW) resins are formed. The general chemical structure of DGEBA resin is

shown in Fig. 1.13. The repeating part of the resin molecule has MW 284. When $n=0$ (Fig. 1.13), an epoxy resin containing only the monomer DGEBA with MW 340 is obtained. Low-MW epoxy resins are semi-isolid or liquid and have an average MW of less than 900, and a large amount of the monomer DGEBA. Resins with an average MW of more than 900 are solids, but may contain more than 15% DGEBA [106, 107]. Commercial epoxy resins are, thus, mixtures of oligomers of different MWs, 340 ($n=0$), 624 ($n=1$), 908 ($n=2$), 1,192 ($n=3$), etc. Components such as colorants, fillers, tar, UV-light absorbers, flame retardants, solvents, reinforcement agents, and plasticizers can also be added to the raw materials. Epoxy resins may also be blended with formaldehyde resins based on phenol, urea, and melamine.

The total world production of epoxy resins is approximately 1,000,000 tons a year. Epoxy resin systems are used in the casting of models and in electron microscopy, as a glue for metal, rubber, plastics, and ceramics, electric insulation, floor covering, corrosion protection of metals, mending of cracks and fissures both in concrete and emeralds, for laminates, composites, and adhesives. About 40–50% is used in coatings. High-molecular solid epoxy resins in various solvents and solventless low-molecular liquid epoxy resins are used for painting, while solid resins in powder paints are used for electrostatic hard-coating of metal.

When great strength is required, fibers made from carbon, glass, nylon, etc. impregnated with epoxy resin systems are increasingly used as composite materials. Difficulties are encountered, however, with adherence to carbon fibers with DGEBA resins. Epoxy resins based on other epoxy compounds than DGEBA have, thus, been developed. Examples are tetraglycidyl-4,4'-methylenedianiline (TGMDA), triglycidyl *p*-aminophenol (TGPAP), and *o*-diglycidyl phthalate. Applications in which pre-impregnated glass fibers ("prepreg") can be used are the aircraft industry, the manufacture of electronic circuit

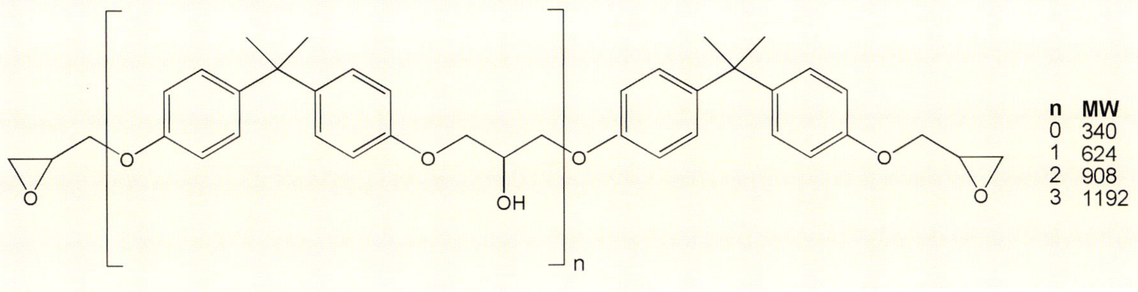

n	MW
0	340
1	624
2	908
3	1192

Fig. 1.13. Diglycidylether of bisphenol A (DGEBA) epoxy resin

boards, and wind turbine rotor blades [108–111]. When needed, diglycidyl ether of tetrabromo-bisphenol A (4Br-DGEBA) is often used as a flame retardant.

Instead of bisphenol A, bisphenol F or phenolic novolak resins can be used for the manufacture of epoxy resins. The monomers of these resins are the three isomers of diglycidyl ether of bisphenol F (DGEBF). The DGEBF resins can be mixed with DGEBA resins and have improved chemical and physical resistance [110]. Other polyhydroxy compounds can also be used, e.g., resorcinol, glycerol, ethylene glycol, pentaerythritol, and trimethylolpropane. Aliphatic epoxy resins are constituents of paints. Cycloaliphatic epoxy resin can occur in neat oils and jet aviation hydraulic fluid [112, 113].

Triglycidyl isocyanate (TGIC) and terephthalic acid diglycidylester are epoxy compounds that may be present in polyester powder paints (see Sect. 34.6) [114–116].

Epoxy acrylates can be obtained by reacting epoxy resin with acrylic acid and, generally, do not contain reactive epoxy groups. They are commonly used as prepolymers in UV-curable printing inks and coatings. Both aromatic and aliphatic epoxy acrylates are available, as well as acrylated epoxidized oils (see Sect. 34.1.4).

34.2.2 Hardeners

Hardeners (curing agents) react with the epoxy groups of the resin and are incorporated in the molecular network. Catalytic curing agents are added in small quantities and act as a catalytic agent for reacting the epoxy groups with one another, as accelerators and co-curing agents, or as activators [117]. The thermoplastic epoxy resins can be cross-linked through the use of a variety of hardeners to form thermoset plastics with insoluble three-dimensional structures. When epoxy resins are used in two-component products, the hardeners are added to the resins immediately preceding the application, and the subsequent cross-linking occurs at either ambient or elevated temperatures. One-component products contain latent curing agents which are inactive at normal storage temperatures, but which initiate cross-linking when heated. Examples of one-component epoxy products include powder paints and special adhesives.

There are many curing agents on the market. In Table 2.1, the commonly used hardeners are listed. The hardeners used in cold-curing are mostly polyamines, polyamides, or isocyanates, and those used

Table 2.1. Commonly used hardeners and catalysts (compiled using [117, 118])

Aliphatic amines and derivatives
Ethylenediamine (EDA)
Diethylenetriamine (DETA)
Triethylenetetramine (TETA)
Tetraethylenepentamine (TEPA)
Dipropylenetriamine (DPTA)
Diethylaminopropylamine (DEAPA)
3-Dimethylaminopropylamine (DMAPA)
Trimethylhexamethylenediamine (TMDA)
Cycloaliphatic polyamines
Isophoronediamine (IPDA)
N-Aminoethylpiperazine
3,3′-Dimethyl-4,4′-diaminodicyclohexylmethane
Menthanediamine
4,4′-Diaminodicyclohexyl methane
Aromatic amines
N, N-Dimethylbenzylamine
4,4′-Diaminodiphenylmethane (DDM)=4,4′-Methylene dianiline (MDA)
m-Phenylenediamine (MPDA)
4,4′-Diaminodiphenylsulphone (DDS)=bis (4-amino phenylsulphone); (Dapsone)
3,3′-Diaminodiphenyl sulfone
2,4,6-Tris-(dimethylaminomethyl)phenol
m-Xylylenediamine
Polyaminoamides
Condensation products of ethyleneamines and carboxylic acids
Adducts
Based on the reaction between aliphatic or aromatic amines and epoxy resin, epoxy-reactive diluents, ethylene oxide, etc.
Acid anhydrides
Phthalic anhydride (PA)
Maleic anhydride (MA)
Hexahydrophthalic anhydride (HHPA)
Methyl nadic anhydride
Tetrahydrophthalic anhydride (THPA)
Methyltetrahydrophthalic anhydride (MTHPA)
Methylhexahydrophthalic anhydride (MHHPA)
Trimellitic anhydride (TMA)
Miscellaneous
Cyanoguanidine (DICY)
Di- and polyisocyanates
Polymercaptans
Polyphenols
Phenolic novolaks
Cresol novolaks
Urea formaldehyde resins
Melamine formaldehyde resins
1,3,5-Triglycidyl isocyanurate[a]
Terephthalic acid diglycidylester[a]
Trimellitic acid triglycidylester[a]

[a] Epoxy compounds in polyester resin systems

for thermal curing are carboxylic acids and anhydrides or aldehyde condensation products, e.g., phenol-formaldehyde resins, melamine-formaldehyde resins, and urea-formaldehyde resins. Aliphatic and cycloaliphatic amines are low-viscosity liquids that react readily with epoxy resins at ambient temperatures; less reactive aromatic amines require an elevated curing temperature [104]. Examples of hardeners for composite epoxy resins are methyl nadic anhydride, *N,N*-dimethylbenzylamine, 4,4′-diaminodiphenyl sulfone (DDS), and dicyandiamide (DICY) [117]. Accelerators, e.g., tertiary amines, can be added to speed up the polymerization of epoxy resins. An example is 2,4,6-tris-(dimethylaminomethyl)phenol [117, 118]. Hexavalent chromate may be present in accelerators of the epoxy resin system [118].

34.2.3 Epoxy-Reactive Diluents

Reactive diluents are used to modify epoxy resins, principally by reducing their viscosity. They contain one or more epoxide groups that react with the hardener at approximately the same rate as the resin. Most of the reactive diluents on the market are used in the cold-curing process. They are blended in with commercial epoxy resin at a concentration of 10–30% [119–121]. The epoxy-reactive diluents are generally glycidyl ethers, but sometimes, are glycidyl esters of aliphatic or aromatic structure. Aliphatic reactive diluents include compounds as 1,4-butanediol diglycidyl ether, *n*-butyl glycidyl ether (BGE), allyl glycidyl ether, or other alkyl glycidyl ethers with longer carbon chains (C_8–C_{14}), e.g., epoxide 7 and epoxide 8. Examples of aromatic reactive diluents are phenyl glycidyl ether (PGE) and cresyl glycidyl ether (CGE) [119, 121].

34.2.4 Skin Hazards
from Epoxy Resin Systems

Epoxy resin systems have been found to be one of the most frequent causes of occupational allergic contact dermatitis [121–124]. Most recorded cases were sensitized to DGEBA resins. In a study performed in an epoxy-based construction industry, it was found that 16.4% of the workers had acquired occupational contact allergy to ERS after one year of employment [125]. An epidemic of occupational contact allergy was caused by DGEBA resin in an immersion oil for microscopy [126].

Core Message

■ Epoxy resin systems are important occupational contact allergens.

Alkaline hardeners were first considered to be responsible for most of the cases of dermatitis observed during the handling of the DGEBA-based resin systems in the 1950s, but later, the resin was identified as the main cause [127, 128]. Gaul [129, 130] suspected that bisphenol A was the sensitizer of the resin, whereas Calnan [131] believed that the epoxy group of epichlorohydrin was more likely to be responsible for contact allergy. In 1977, Fregert and Thorgeirsson [132, 133] finally confirmed that the main sensitizer was the DGEBA monomer with a MW of 340. In the guinea pig maximization test, the oligomer with a MW of 624 was also a sensitizer, but was considerably weaker than the MW 340 oligomer. The sensitizing capacity of epoxy resin decreases as the average MW increases [132–134]. In many cases, allergic epoxy dermatitis develops after accidental contact with epoxy resin, and frequent causative agents for epoxy dermatitis are paints and the raw material for paint [124, 135]. However, it is not unusual to find a positive patch test reaction to DGEBA resin where the cause of the sensitization is unknown. Dermatitis caused by epoxy resin systems is localized mostly to the hands and forearms, but sometimes the face is also involved. If the face and eyelids are involved, the dermatitis may be caused by airborne exposure to hardeners or reactive diluents. These compounds are very volatile compared to epoxy resin [136].

High MW epoxy resin in solvents for painting or epoxy resin powder for electrostatic coating of metals are thought to rarely cause sensitization because of the low content of MW 340 oligomer. However, chemical analyses have shown that a solid epoxy resin, which was not declared as a sensitizer, contained 18% DGEBA [107].

Even if the epoxy resin system is believed to be cured, up to 25% of monomers can remain non-hardened, particularly when cured at room temperature [109]. When DGEBA resins are cured by polyamine hardeners at room temperature, the amounts of unreacted DGEBA or polyamine decrease rapidly within 1 or 2 days, but, thereafter, the decrease is slow. Nevertheless, after 1-week's cure, 0.02–12% of free DGEBA and 0.01–1% of free diethylenetriamine (DETA) were found when six different epoxy resin products were experimentally cured by DETA [121]. Allergic contact dermatitis may, thus, be elicited in previously sensitized individuals. Traces of nonhardened epoxy resin have been found in twist-off caps, film cassettes, furniture, metal pieces, signboards, textile labels, stoma pouches, polyvinylchloride plastic, nasal cannulas, hemodialysis sets, cardiac pacemakers, fiberglass, brass door knobs, and tool handles, among other products [137]. Recent reports involve bowl polish and a bus pass [138, 139]. Epoxy-by-proxy dermatitis is also a possibility [140].

Fregert and Trulsson have described methods used for detecting the presence of epoxy resins of the bisphenol A type [137, 141] (see Sect. 25.1). The thin-layer chromatography method described for DGEBA has 150–200 times lower sensitivity for DGEBF [107].

Non-DGEBA epoxy resins are also potential causes of allergic contact dermatitis. The monomers of epoxy resins of the DGEBF type are strong sensitizers and cross-react to a high degree with DGEBA in animal studies [142], and many patients simultaneously react to both DGEBA and DGEBF resins [143, 144]. A statistically significant association between contact allergy to DGEBA resin and fragrance mix has been found [145].

The composite epoxy resins based on o-diglycidyl phthalate, tetraglycidyl-4,4′-methylenedianiline (TGMDA), triglycidyl p-aminophenol (TGPAP), and 4Br-DGEBA are sensitizers in humans [108, 110]. Testing with DGEBA resin may not reveal contact allergy to the composite epoxy resin [108, 110, 134, 146]. In workers handling fiberglass or carbon fibers, irritant dermatitis can be induced by fiber fragments [111, 147].

Reactive diluents contain epoxy groups and are strong sensitizers that may or may not cross-react with epoxy resins [148, 149]. Several cases with contact allergy to reactive diluents have been described [150, 151]. Reactive diluents may cause airborne allergic contact dermatitis and also depigmentation [150, 152].

Occupational contact allergies can occur to epoxy compounds in products other than epoxy resin systems, such as cycloaliphatic epoxy resin in neat oil and jet aviation hydraulic fluid and 2,3-epoxypropyl trimethyl ammonium chloride (EPTMAC) used in a starch modification factory [112, 113, 153].

Polyamine hardeners can be both sensitizers and irritants (Table 2.1) [32, 118, 154]. In patients with allergic contact dermatitis, isolated contact allergy to the hardeners of the epoxy resin systems is unusual, but may occur [118]. In an industrial investigation among workers exposed to epoxy resins systems, 30% of the workers had contact allergy exclusively to at least one hardener [125]. The most potent sensitizers among the hardeners are the aliphatic polyamines (Table 2.1) [109, 148, 155]. Cycloaliphatic poly-

amines are also strong sensitizers [118, 148, 154, 156–158], and reports on contact allergies to 2,4,6-tris-(dimethylaminomethyl)phenol and m-xylenediamine have been published [118, 159]. Hardeners of the polyaminoamide type are nonsensitizers, but may contain aliphatic amines. Amine-epoxy adducts can contain free amines, but no free DGEBA [106, 121]. Contact allergy to methylhexahydrophthalic anhydride present in epoxy resin systems has been described [160].

Reports of contact allergy to bisphenol A are controversial. In a few studies, a high incidence of bisphenol A allergy was found among those sensitized to epoxy resin [130, 161]. Other investigators have not confirmed these results [162–164]. Bisphenol A has, however, been identified as a contact allergen in vinyl gloves [165, 166].

A rather high risk of sensitization to epichlorohydrin has been reported for workers in plants manufacturing epoxy resin [163, 164, 167].

Contact urticaria can be caused by DGEBA resin, the hardeners methylhexahydrophthalic anhydride and methyltetrahydrophthalic anhydride, as well as by aliphatic polyamine hardeners [124, 168–170].

Photosensitivity has been reported in relation to the heating of DGEBA resin [171] and the use of epoxy powder paints [172]. The photosensitivity has been suspected to be due to bisphenol A contained in the resin [171]. Persistent light reactivity has been found in mice photosensitized by bisphenol A [173].

34.2.5 Patch Testing with Epoxy Resin Systems

Approximately 60–80% of the cases with contact allergy to epoxy resin systems are sensitized to DGEBA resin [125, 174]. A patch test with the low-molecular-weight epoxy resin containing a high amount of oligomer MW 340 is, thus, adequate in the majority of cases. It is recommended to patch test with the epoxy resin 1% in petrolatum and this allergen is included in most standard series. Even if DGEBA resin is non-irritating, other types of epoxy resins can be irritants. For the latter, a patch test concentration of 0.25–1% is recommended [110, 134, 143]. There are too many hardeners and reactive diluents on the market to be used in routine testing. However, if contact allergy to hardeners or reactive diluents is suspected, it is necessary to obtain information and samples from the manufacturer and to test the components of the epoxy resin system separately. The recommended test concentration for hardeners and reactive diluents is 0.1–1% in petrolatum, acetone, or ethanol [118, 121].

■ Epoxy resin in the standard patch test series does not detect all contact allergies to epoxy resin systems

34.2.6 Preventive Measures when Handling Epoxy Resin Systems

Workers handling epoxy resin systems should be informed of the risk of skin sensitization. The simultaneous use of irritant chemicals, e.g., organic solvents and amine hardeners, increases the risk of sensitization. The highly alkaline amine hardeners can be replaced by polyaminoamides or amine-epoxy adducts; this reduces the irritability of the epoxy resin system. Management personnel as well as the workers who come into contact with epoxy resin systems should be advised to refrain from skin contact. Approximately 95% of exposed workers report wearing the gloves as recommended; still, the frequency of occupational contact allergy is high [125]. The use of proper personal protective measures, especially careful hand protection and regular cleaning and maintenance of all contaminated equipment, should be imperative (Fig. 2.1). Epoxy resins are able to penetrate plastic and rubber gloves. Only heavy-duty vinyl gloves provide sufficient protection [175]. Multilayered glove material of folio type (4H gloves) has been shown to give even better protection against epoxy resins and the auxiliary compounds used with them [176]. Barrier creams have been reported to protect against epoxy resins from minutes to some hours [100, 177, 178]. To reduce the allergenic properties of DGEBA resins, the use of the MW 340 oligomer at the lowest possible concentration and the use of high MW reactive diluents is recommended. However, all epoxy resins should be regarded as potential sensitizers, and, preferably, they should be marked with labels specifying the concentrations of epoxy compounds with low MW. In some countries, education prior to being allowed to work with epoxy resin systems is mandatory.

Suggested Reading

Fregert S, Thorgeirsson A (1977) Patch testing with low molecular oligomers of epoxy resins in humans. Contact Dermatitis 3 : 301–303

When patients with contact allergy to epoxy resin in the standard patch test series were patch tested with the isolated oligomers of an epoxy resin based on bisphenol A, all patients with contact reacted to the monomer diglycidyl ether of bisphenol A (DGEBA) with molecular weight (MW) 340. No patient reacted to oligomers with higher MW. The results were in accordance with results from a guinea-pig maximization test published in the same year by the same authors. Thus, it was shown that, in the quantitatively most important epoxy resin on the market, the monomer DGEBA was the main allergen. These results still hold true.

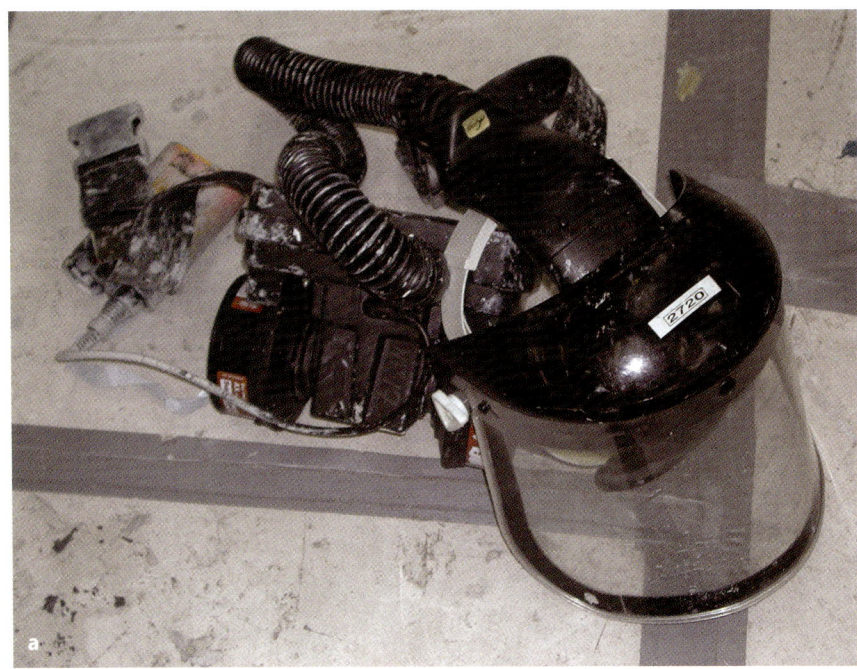

Fig. 2.1a–c.
Contamination in the epoxy industry

Fig. 2.1b, c.

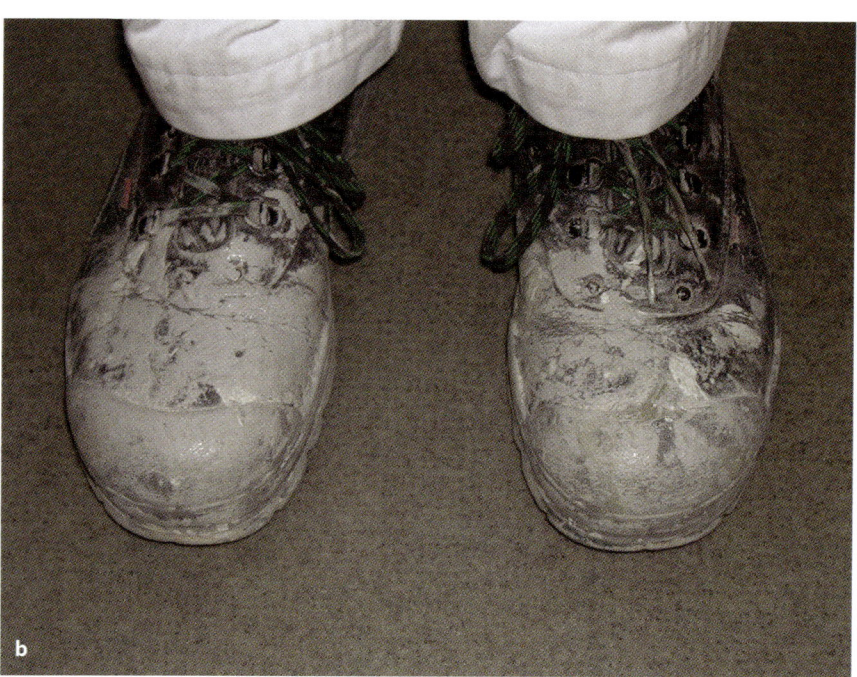

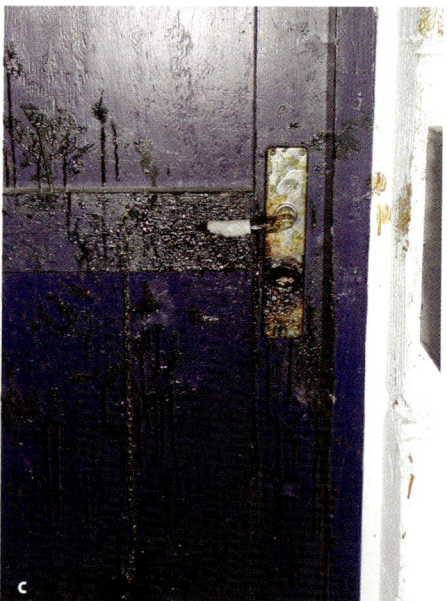

34.3 Phenol-Formaldehyde Resins

Erik Zimerson

Phenol-formaldehyde resins (phenolic resins) are polycondensation products of phenols and aldehydes, in particular, phenol and formaldehyde. They are divided into resols and novolaks. When phenol reacts with an excess of formaldehyde under alkaline conditions, a resol resin is produced. As formaldehyde is in excess in the process, various methylolphenol compounds are formed, such as monomers, dimers, and molecules of higher molecular weight. The base-catalyzed polycondensation of the products is stopped deliberately before complete curing. During processing, the polycondensation can be restarted by heating to achieve curing of the resin. This means that the resols are self-cross-linking and can be considered as prepolymers. [179, 180].

Novolak resins are formed when formaldehyde reacts with an excess of phenols under acidic conditions. Mainly, dimers such as dihydroxydiphenylmethanes (bisphenol F isomers) are formed, but also are trimers and molecules of higher molecular weight. However, the formed molecules in this case have no or few methylol groups. The novolaks can only be cured by the addition of curing agents, such as formaldehyde, paraformaldehyde, or hexamethylenetetramine, in addition to heating. The cured polymer for both novolaks and resols is called resite or C-stage resin [179, 180].

Commercially available phenol-formaldehyde resins are most commonly based on phenol itself, but other phenols such as cresols, xylenols, resorcinol (1,3-dihydroxybenzene), bisphenol A (4,4'-isopropylidenediphenol), p-tert-butylphenol, 4-isooctylphenol, and 4-nonylphenol can be used. Besides formaldehyde, other aldehydes, e.g., acetaldehyde, glyoxal, and furfural (2-furancarboxaldehyde) can also be used [179, 180]. Phenolic resins are available as solids (fragments, flakes, pastilles, or granules), or as solutions and liquids [180].

Phenol-formaldehyde and p-tert-butylphenol-formaldehyde resins still have many industrial applications, although other plastics nowadays have replaced the use of these resins in many applications. Glues and glue films based on phenol-formaldehyde resins are used in the plywood industry. Because of their moisture resistance, the glues and laminates are used in the building industry, and in boat and aircraft construction. The resins are also good insulators against electricity; they are thus used in electronic and electric appliances. In addition, they can be used for the production of decorative laminates and coatings, and to coat rigid constructions, e.g., pipelines and reaction vessels, because of their high chemical resistance. They are also used as binders for glass and mineral fibers in the production of heat-, noise-, and fire-insulating materials, as well as in foundry molding sand and abrasives, such as sandpaper, abrasive cloth, and flexible sanding discs. Novolak resins can be used in the production of grinding wheels, brake linings, and clutch facings. They are also used as raw materials for polyfunctional epoxy resins [179–181].

p-tert-Butylphenol-formaldehyde resins are used in adhesives based on neoprene and other rubbers. These adhesives can be used in shoes, leather products, automobile interior upholstery, furniture, adhesive tapes and labels, and in the gluing of certain floor coverings [179, 180]. p-tert-Butylphenol-formaldehyde resins are also used as adhesives for leather, artificial fingernails, and labels.

The third largest group is phenolic resins modified by natural resins. Rosin-modified phenolic resins are used as binders for book offset-printing inks [179].

34.3.1 Skin Hazards from Phenol-Formaldehyde Resins

The adverse effects in workers handling phenol-formaldehyde resins are mostly skin problems. Contact dermatitis is common and is usually caused by the development of contact allergy. Most of the reported cases of contact dermatitis are due to sensitization to p-tert-butylphenol-formaldehyde resins. Reviews on p-tert-butylphenol-formaldehyde resin-induced occupational eczema have been published [179, 182–184]. In general, population allergy frequencies of 0.5–2.1% are reported from different European countries [185–187].

Many of the substances found in p-tert-butylphenol-formaldehyde resin are allergens. However, patch testing with dilution series of components from the resin in sensitized patients and sensitization studies in animals have shown that the methylol-substituted dimers, 4-tert-butyl-2-(5-tert-butyl-2-hydroxy-3-hydroxymethyl-benzyloxymethyl)-6-hydroxymethyl-phenol (Fig. 3.1a), and 4-tert-butyl-2-(5-tert-butyl-2-hydroxy-3-benzyloxymethyl)-6-hydroxymethyl-phenol (Fig. 3.1b) are major sensitizers in this type of resin [188, 189]. Among the monomers 2,6-dimethylol-p-tert-butylphenol (Fig. 3.1c) and 5-tert-butyl-2-hydroxy-3-hydroxymethyl-benzaldehyde (Fig. 3.1d) are considered to be the most important allergens [190–193]. The strong sensitizer p-tert-butylcatechol (Fig. 3.1e) has been shown to be present in p-tert-butylphenol-formaldehyde resin and to be of relevance considering allergic reactions to this resin. p-tert-Butylcatechol is also an antioxidant used as a stabilizer for a number of other monomers used in the production of plastics. The raw materials for the production of p-tert-butylphenol-formaldehyde resin are formaldehyde and p-tert-butylphenol (Fig. 3.1f, PTBP). Few patients allergic to p-tert-butylphenol-formaldehyde resin are reported to react positively to the raw materials, indicating that these substances are not important allergens in the resin [191, 194]. However, guinea pigs sensitized to p-tert-butylcatechol showed cross-reactions when tested with p-tert-butylphenol [195].

The allergens in resins based on phenol and formaldehyde have also been investigated, and several substances among the monomers and the dimers have been shown to be allergens. Methylol-substitut-

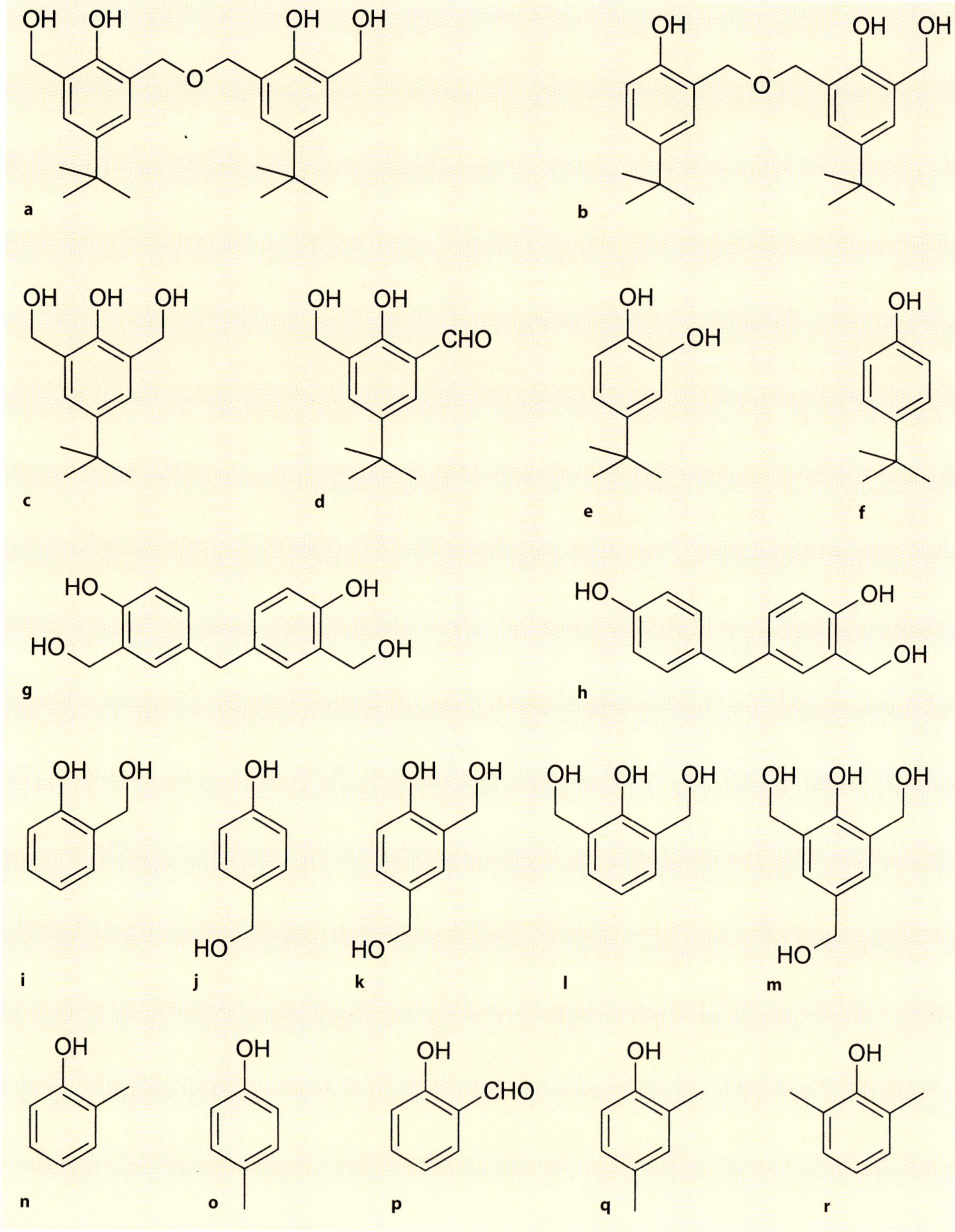

Fig. 3.1a–r. Chemical structures of allergens in p-*tert*-butyl-phenol-formaldehyde resin (**a–f**), phenol-formaldehyde resin (**g–n**) and substances which are cross-reactors in patients allergic to phenol-formaldehyde resin (**o–r**). **a** 4-*tert*-Butyl-2-(5-*tert*-butyl-2-hydroxy-3-hydroxymethyl-benzyloxymethyl)-6-hydroxymethyl-phenol; **b** 4-*tert*-butyl-2-(5-*tert*-butyl-2-hydroxy-3-benzyloxymethyl)-6-hydroxymethyl-phenol; **c** 2,6-dimethylol-*p*-*tert*-butylphenol; **d** 5-*tert*-butyl-2-hydroxy-3-hy-droxymethyl-benzaldehyde; **e** *p*-*tert*-butylcatechol; **f** *p*-*tert*-butylphenol; **g** 4,4′-dihydroxy-3,3′-dihydroxymethyl-diphenylmethane; **h** 4,4′-dihydroxy-3-hydroxymethyl-diphenylmethane; **i** 2-methylolphenol; **j** 4-methylolphenol; **k** 2,4-dimethylolphenol; **l** 2,6-dimethylolphenol; **m** 2,4,6-trimethylolphenol; **n** *o*-cresol; **o** *p*-cresol; **p** salicylaldehyde; **q** 2,4-dimethylphenol; **r** 2,6-dimethylphenol

ed dimers were found to be major allergens in these resins, such as 4,4′-dihydroxy-3,3′-dihydroxymethyl-diphenylmethane (Fig. 3.1g) and 4,4′-dihydroxy-3-hydroxymethyl-diphenylmethane (Fig. 3.1h). Examples of allergens among the monomers are 2-methylolphenol (Fig. 3.1i), 4-methylolphenol (Fig. 3.1j), 2,4-dimethylolphenol (Fig. 3.1k), 2,6-dimethylolphenol (Fig. 3.1l), 2,4,6-trimethylolphenol (Fig. 3.1m), and o-cresol (Fig. 3.1n). The monomers were, however, weaker allergens than the dimers. [179, 196–203]. A patch test study in patients with contact allergy to phenol-formaldehyde resin indicates that p-cresol (Fig. 3.1o), salicylaldehyde (Fig. 3.1p), 2,4-dimethylphenol (Fig. 3.1q), and 2,6-dimethylphenol (Fig. 3.1r) are cross-reacting substances, possibly after metabolic conversion into the corresponding methylolphenols in the skin. The observed cross-reactions can indicate a connection between allergy to phenol-formaldehyde resin and tar as the methylphenols (Fig. 3.1n, o, q, and r) can be found in tar [204]. Formaldehyde is not the main sensitizer in phenol-formaldehyde resins [194]. Simultaneous reactions to phenol-formaldehyde resins, colophony/hydroxy-abietyl alcohol, and balsam of Peru/fragrance mix may occur [205].

Phenol-formaldehyde resins may also irritate the skin and cause chemical burns and depigmentation. Phenols and aldehydes are primary skin irritants and concentrated phenol may even cause corrosive chemical burns. Besides being a potent sensitizer, formaldehyde is also a skin irritant.

Irritant contact dermatitis has been reported in the manufacture of an electric insulation material (Bakelite), which is phenol-formaldehyde resin made of incompletely condensed resin powder in molds [206]. Irritant contact dermatitis was also common among workers in the manufacture of decorative laminates made of paper sheets impregnated with phenol-formaldehyde resins [194, 207].

Immediate contact reactions to p-tert-butylphenol-formaldehyde resin have also been reported [208, 209].

34.3.2 Patch Testing with Phenol-Formaldehyde Resins

In addition to p-tert-butylphenol-formaldehyde resin, it is also necessary to patch test with the actual resin to which the worker is exposed, as there is no single reliable test substance to detect allergy to the wide variety of phenolic resin types. Bruze found 2.5 times more patients with contact allergy to phenol-formaldehyde resins when routinely patch testing with a resin based on phenol and formaldehyde

(P-F-R-2) in addition to p-tert-butylphenol-formaldehyde resin [210].

When detecting contact allergy to p-tert-butylphenol-formaldehyde resin in patients for whom no clinically relevant contact with the resin can be found, the possibility of p-tert-butylcatechol as the eliciting factor should be considered and patch testing with this substance should be performed when indicated. However, due to observed active sensitization when using a patch test concentration of 1% p-tert-butylcatechol in pet., Estlander et al. recommend a lower concentration of 0.25% pet. [211].

34.4 Polyurethane Resins

MALIN FRICK

Polyurethanes (PUR) are plastics formed by addition reaction between isocyanates with di- or polyfunctionality and polyhydroxy compounds (polyols). When one or both components are polyfunctional, the PUR polymer cross-links and thermosetting end products are produced. However, if both components are only difunctional, the PUR polymer can have a linear arrangement that does not cross-link, resulting in a thermoplastic product. The polyols used are mainly polyesters or polyethers, but isocyanates can also react with other molecules if they carry active hydroxyl groups, such as, for example, water and amines. Isocyanates are low-molecular-weight aromatic, aliphatic, or cycloaliphatic compounds which are characterized by a highly reactive -N=C=O group. Some diisocyanates used in the production of polyurethane products are shown in Fig. 4.1. Aromatic diisocyanates dominate the market, but since they undergo oxidative discoloration upon exposure to light and moisture, aliphatic isocyanates are used in applications that are exposed to a lot of light [212]. The most commonly used aromatic diisocyanate is diphenylmethane diisocyanate (MDI), followed by toluene diisocyanate (TDI). They are frequently used in the production of rigid and flexible foam, but are also used in coatings, adhesives, binders, and elastomers. Technical qualities of MDI used in industry contain a complex mixture of 25–80% monomeric 4,4′-MDI and oligomers containing 3–6 rings, as well as other minor monomeric isomers, such as 2,4′-MDI and 2,2′-MDI (Fig. 4.1). The exact composition varies with the manufacturer [213]. These mixtures are usually referred to as polymeric MDI (PMDI), but the synonyms crude MDI and polymethylene polyphenyl isocyanate (PAPI or PMPPI) are also used. Phenyl isocyanate can be a contaminant in PMDI. TDI is industrially available as mixtures of the isomers 2,4-

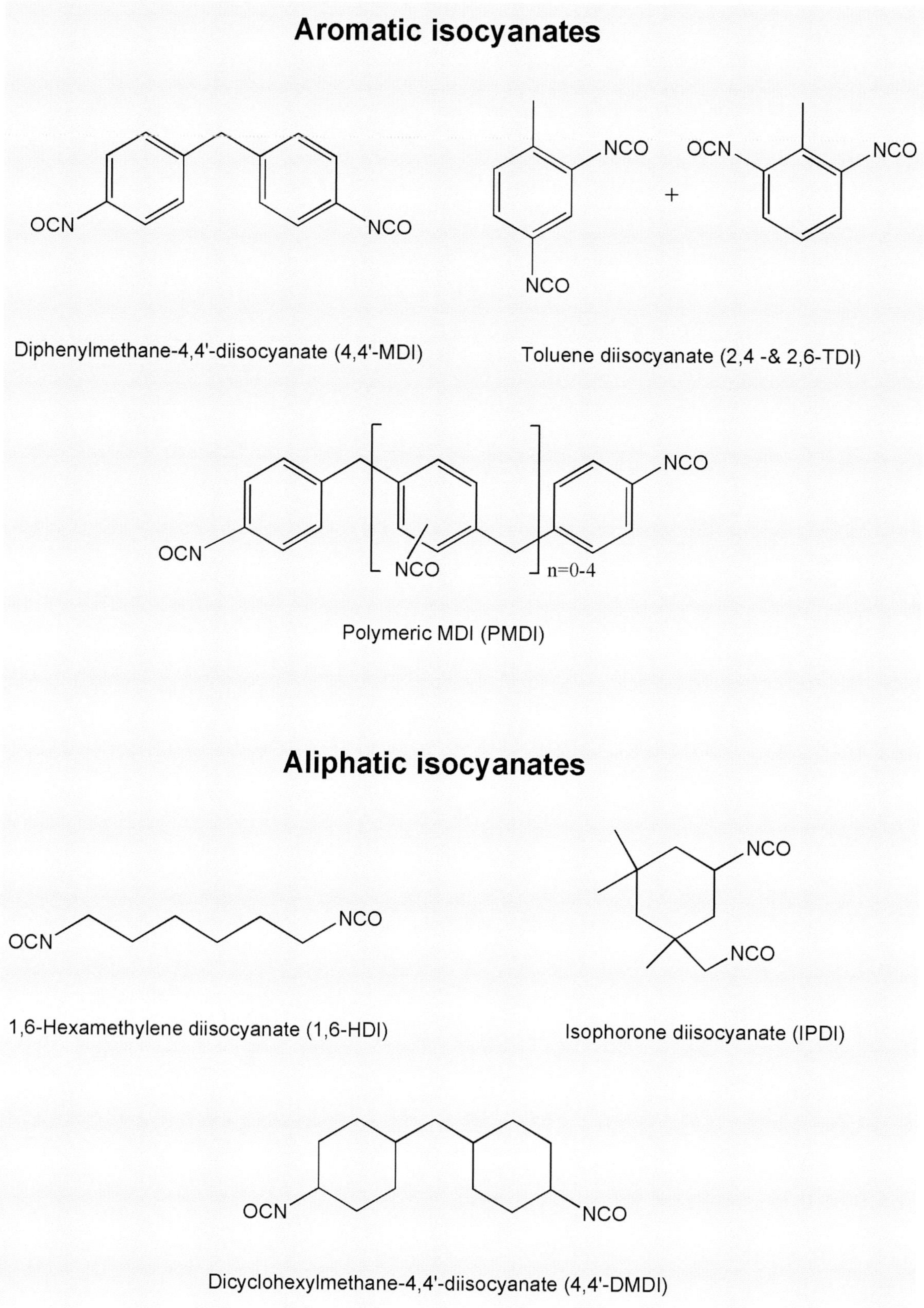

Aromatic isocyanates

Diphenylmethane-4,4'-diisocyanate (4,4'-MDI)   Toluene diisocyanate (2,4 -& 2,6-TDI)

Polymeric MDI (PMDI)

34

Aliphatic isocyanates

1,6-Hexamethylene diisocyanate (1,6-HDI)   Isophorone diisocyanate (IPDI)

Dicyclohexylmethane-4,4'-diisocyanate (4,4'-DMDI)

Fig. 4.1. Chemical formulae of various isocyanates used in the production of polyurethane plastics

TDI and 2,6-TDI in the ratio 80:20 or 65:35 (2,4:2,6), or as pure 2,4-TDI. Due to their light and weather resistance, the aliphatic diisocyanates 1,6-hexamethylene diisocyanate (HDI) and isophorone diisocyanate (IPDI) is commonly used in lacquers, coatings, and paints. Industrially, they are often used as modified higher molecular weight polyisocyanates (biuret or isocyanurate derivatives) to decrease their volatility [214]. Examples of other diisocyanates used in special products include trimethyl hexamethylene diisocyanate (TMDI), which is a mixture of the two isomers 2,2,4-TMDI and 2,4,4-TMDI, naphthalene diisocyanate (NDI), triphenylmethane triisocyanate (TPMTI), and dicyclohexylmethane diisocyanate (DMDI) [68, 79, 215]. When producing diisocyanates monomers, the corresponding diamines are typically used as starting materials [214].

Many auxiliary substances are also used in the manufacture of PUR products. The hardening process can be modified by heat or with a catalyst, usually tertiary amines and/or organometallics (primarily tin compounds) [216]. Other additives, e.g., fire retardants, fillers, coloring agents, and cross-linking agents, can be added to modify the polyurethane reaction, as well as the properties of the final product. In the production of foamed plastics, blowing agents, e.g., pentane, carbon dioxide, or water, is also added [217].

In many applications, diisocyanates are used in a prepolymerized form. The prepolymers are produced by mixing small amounts of di- or polyfunctional alcohols with an excess of isocyanate. This is done for reasons such as to add cross-linking, to modify the chemical reactivity of the isocyanate groups, or to decrease the volatility of the isocyanate, etc. [214]. In heat-setting applications, the isocyanate groups can also be blocked, i.e., temporarily inactivated. When heated, the blocking groups escape, thereby, releasing the isocyanate groups and enabling them to react [217]. When used as activators or hardeners, diisocyanates are often dissolved in aliphatic or aromatic hydrocarbon solvents, or a mixture of different organic solvents, e.g., aliphatic hydrocarbon solvents, petroleum, and butyl acetate. Adhesives, varnishes, and paints may also contain solvents. Polyurethanes occur in many forms, such as coatings, paints, lacquers, adhesives (one- or two-component glue), binding agents, castings, elastomers, foams, fibers, and synthetic rubbers. Flexible polyurethane foams are used for mattresses, cushions, dashboards, and packages [215].

Core Message

■ Polyurethanes (PUR) are formed by reacting a di- or polyfunctional isocyanate with a polyol in the presence of suitable catalysts and additives.

34.4.1 Skin Problems from Polyurethane Resins

The main occupational hazard associated with PUR is the presence of isocyanates, which can cause asthma and rhinitis, hypersensitive pneumonitis or alveolitis, conjunctivitis, and chronic obstructive lung diseases [218–220]. Isocyanates are considered toxic and poisonous chemicals [219].

Exposure to isocyanates may result in both allergic and irritant contact dermatitis, as well as urticaria [79, 221–225], and the typical localization are the hands and face. Diisocyanates are strong contact sensitizers, in accordance with the results of animal studies [226, 227]. Animal experiments have also shown that polyisocyanate prepolymers are capable of causing skin sensitization in guinea pigs [228]. However, in spite of this, reports on allergic contact dermatitis are few in number, considering the extensive use of these chemicals in manufacturing processes and other applications. The rigorous rules that the workers have to follow when working with polyurethanes to minimize the hazardous effect of isocyanates on the respiratory tract have probably also decreased the amount of all forms of skin conditions.

Isocyanates are described as mild to strong irritants and irritant contact dermatitis seems to have been more common than allergic contact dermatitis [32]. Amine accelerators, e.g., diaminodiphenylmethane (MDA), triethylenediamine, and triethylamine, can also cause skin irritation. Contact allergy to MDI, TDI, IPDI, HDI, TMDI, and DMDI have been reported [79, 215, 221, 222, 229–241]. Most recorded cases were sensitized to MDI or DMDI.

DMDI has been reported as a very potent sensitizer [229, 235, 242–245]. In a company manufacturing medical equipment, 13 out of 100 workers were sensitized to DMDI, which was used in a glue [235]. At a factory making car badges, two out of seven workers showed positive patch-test reactions to DMDI. It was also believed that irritant contact dermatitis from DMDI was the cause of three of the workers' skin problems [229].

MDI-positive patients may also react to MDA [215, 221, 234, 239, 246, 247]. In 1967, Fregert [246] was the first to report these simultaneous reactions. He attributed this to cross-reactivity. In 1976, Rothe [221] suggested that MDA might be the actual allergen and that it is formed from hydrolysis of MDI when MDI comes into contact with the skin. Several reports describe workers exposed to MDI with positive patch-test reactions to MDA, but negative reactions to MDI [215, 234, 239, 248–250], and it has been proposed that MDA might be an important marker for MDI hypersensitivity [215, 234, 239]. MDA may also represent cross-allergy to *para*-phenylenediamine [221, 251]. Heavy exposure to diisocyanates may result in a rapid sensitization within a week to some months after exposure [215, 234, 235].

Completely hardened polyurethane products usually do not cause skin problems. Unreacted isocyanate monomer may, however, remain in excess inside polyurethane foams, even after curing. This can create a health hazard due to isocyanate exposure when polyurethane dust is produced during machining or cutting [41, 241, 242]. If polyurethanes are heated to above 250°C, they decompose into isocyanates and nitrogen oxides and may, again, cause dermatitis.

34.4.2　Patch Testing with Polyurethane Resins

Commercially available patch-test preparations of TDI and MDI only contain one isomer of the respective monomers. Therefore, patients are generally tested with the isomers 4,4′-MDI, and 2,4-TDI. Patch-test preparations of DMDI are not commercially available, but is normally tested as the 4,4′-DMDI isomer. Therefore, most reports refer to contact allergy to these specific isomers. However, when previously described, the general abbreviations MDI, TDI, and DMDI have been used.

Isocyanates are highly reactive and their stability in patch-test preparations have been discussed. In 1992, Estlander et al. [215] suggested that preparations of TDI and 4,4-MDI could be used for over a year, since preparations that were 5.5 and 15.5 months old had elicited positive reactions in two patients. No chemical analyses were done. In 2004, Frick et al. [213] performed chemical analysis on commercially available patch-test preparations of 4,4′-MDI that were obtained from 12 dermatology departments and two major suppliers of patch test allergens. Seven of the preparations were analyzed before the expiry date, yet, only one came close to the stated concentration. In most cases, the concentration was only a few

percent or less than the concentration stated on the label. It was concluded that there is a high risk of false-negative reactions when using these preparations and, therefore, additional patch testing with the patients' own fresh work material was recommended. The same recommendation was given by Gossens et al. [239] when reporting 13 patients with positive patch-test reactions to isocyanate-based products and where only one of these patients reacted to any commercially available patch-test preparation of diisocyanates.

Patch testing workers exposed to polyurethane chemicals should include relatively fresh preparations of the most common diisocyanates MDI, TDI, HDI, and IPDI, as well as MDA and the actual chemicals to which the workers have been exposed. It has been proposed that positive reactions to isocyanates appear late and, therefore, it is advisable that isocyanate patch tests are also read on day 7 and that patients should be advised to make contact with the clinic if any reactions appear after day 7 [234].

One case of a possible active patch-test sensitization with TDI 1% in pet. has been reported [252].

Core Message

■ When patch testing workers exposed to polyurethane chemicals, it is advisable to test with their own work material in addition to the commercially available patch-test preparations of diisocyanates. A second reading on day 7 is advisable since positive reactions may appear late. Positive reactions to MDA should be taken into account, as it may be an important marker for MDI sensitivity.

Suggested Reading

Fregert S (1967) Allergic contact dermatitis to diphenyl-4,4′-diisocyanate. Contact Dermatitis Newsletter 2:17
This is a case report describing three men who developed dermatitis of the hands and face when they handled a mixture of diphenylmethane-4,4′-diisocyanate (4,4′-MDI), castor oil, and coaltar during two weeks. Only one of the workers was patch tested. He showed positive reactions to 4,4′-MDI 1% in acetone, coaltar, phenol-formaldehyde resin, and diaminodiphenylmethane (MDA). The simultaneous reactions between 4,4′-MDI and MDA were attributed to cross-reactivity. This is the first report to note the simultaneous reactions between 4,4′-MDI and MDA. Since then, several reports describing these concurrent reactions have occurred.

34.5 Other Plastics

Bert Björkner

34.5.1 Amino Plastics

Amino plastics is the common name for plastics formed by the reaction between an aldehyde and a compound with one or more amino groups. The most common aldehyde is formaldehyde, but sometimes, hexamethylenetetramine, which is a formaldehyde releaser, can be used. Amino plastics always contain an excess of formaldehyde. The most common amino-containing compounds are urea (carbamide), $H_2N-CO-NH_2$, and melamine, 2,4,6-triamino-1,3,5-triazine. The reaction with formaldehyde produces thermosetting urea-formaldehyde and melamine-formaldehyde resins by a polycondensation type reaction. The amino resins are cured by heat, commonly with an inorganic acid as catalyst. Although both resins are quite similar in appearance, the melamine-formaldehyde resins have superior water resistance to cured urea-formaldehyde resins. Both amino plastics are relatively unaffected by common organic solvents, oils, and greases, and are widely used as laminating and bonding materials in the wood and furniture industry. They are used as wood glues and surface coatings. They are also utilized to improve the wet strength of paper and the crease-resistance of textiles. Powders from urea-formaldehyde resins can be molded and used as containers of cosmetics products, electric fittings, and bottle caps. Urea-formaldehyde foams have found applications as insulation in refrigerators and within the walls of houses. Other typical uses of urea-formaldehyde resins are clock cases, lavatory seats, and buttons. Melamine-formaldehyde resin powders filled with cellulose are used for tableware. High-quality decorative laminates are made of melamine-formaldehyde resins. Amino plastics are often used in conjunction with fillers and reinforcements, such as glass mat and cloth, silica, cotton fabrics, and certain synthetic fibers.

34.5.1.1 Skin Problems from Amino Plastics

Usually, the finished product does not cause primary sensitization, but occasionally, the uncured substance does. Textile dermatitis caused by urea- and melamine-formaldehyde resins is rare. Contact allergy to amino resins is often combined with formaldehyde allergy [253, 254].

Urea and melamine do not cause contact allergy. Sensitization to amino plastics has developed from urea-formaldehyde resin used in fiberboard [255] as a textile finish [254, 256], and from melamine-formaldehyde resin in orthopedic casts [257], gypsum molds [254], or in the coating of plastic tubes intended for cosmetics.

The irritancy of amino plastic is mainly due to formaldehyde, which can be released from plastics. Nowadays, resins used in textiles release lower levels of free formaldehyde than previously [254]. Occupational irritant contact dermatitis from fiberboard containing urea-formaldehyde resin has been reported [258]. Dust from urea-formaldehyde insulating foam has caused airborne irritancy [259].

34.5.2 Polyester Resins

Polyester resins are polycondensation thermosetting compounds in two different forms: saturated and unsaturated.

The saturated polyesters, also termed unmodified alkyd resins, are produced from dicarboxylic acids, usually phthalic acid or maleic acid, mainly used in their anhydride forms, and polyalcohols, usually glycerol, pentaerythritol, or trimethylolpropane.

The saturated polyesters synthesized in this way are macromolecules, commonly used as plasticizers for other plastic materials. Alkyd resins are formed by modification with oils containing fatty acids, which bind to free hydroxyl groups on the polyfunctional alcohol. In this form, the resin is often used in modern water-based paints and surface coatings.

Unsaturated polyesters are produced through esterification of organic acids or their anhydrides, e.g., maleic anhydride, phthalic anhydride, or fumaric acid, and diols, e.g., diethylene glycol or 1,2-propylene glycol. Cross-linking between parts of the linear macromolecule cures the unsaturated polyester. Unsaturated monomers, e.g., styrene, are used as solvents and for copolymerization with unsaturated groups along the polyester chain. Vinyl toluene and methyl methacrylate may be also used for cross-linking. An initiator or catalyst is required to start the cross-linking process. The catalyst is usually a peroxide, such as benzoyl peroxide or methyl ethyl ketone peroxide. Accelerators, e.g., cobalt naphthenate, or tertiary amines, such as dimethyl aniline, diethyl aniline, and dimethyl-*p*-toluidine, are necessary for the curing of plastics at room temperature. In styrene, there are usually inhibitors, e.g., *p-tert*-butylcatechol or hydroquinone. The peroxide-cured unsaturated polyesters have been used commercially for many years, but unsaturated polyesters cured by UV-light have equivalent properties. The UV-curable polyester system is used in the furniture industry as topcoats and for orthopedic casts. Casts cured by UV-light usually consist of unsaturated polyester with vinyl toluene as the cross-linking agent and a benzoin-ether molecule as the photo-initiator. The resin is impregnated into woven glass fiber. Reactive (meth)acrylate groups can be attached to the molecular backbone of the unsaturated polyesters through functional groups, such as hydroxyl and anhydride, forming acrylated polyesters used in UV-curable inks or coatings for wood and paper.

Unsaturated polyesters have been used extensively in the reinforced plastics industry in the manufacture of products for transportation, construction, and marine applications. They are also used for coatings, finishes, lacquers, cements, and glues.

34.5.2.1 Skin Problems from Polyester Resins

Contact dermatitis from saturated polyesters appears to be very rare. Allergic contact dermatitis has, however, been caused by a trifunctional epoxy compound, triglycidyl isocyanurate (TGIC), used as cross-linker in heat-cured polyester paints [114, 115, 260–262] and to terephthalic acid diglycidylester in powder coating [116] (Fig. 5.2) Phthalic anhydrides have been reported to cause irritation [263], immediate IgE-mediated hypersensitivity, asthma, allergic rhinitis, and urticaria [160, 168, 264, 265]. Alkyd resins are not sensitizing, but phthalic anhydrides used in the manufacture of alkyd resins can cause irritation. Unsaturated polyester resin is a rare sensitizer. Those at risk are workers employed in the manufacturing industry, with a few exceptions [32, 266–271]. According to Malten, unsaturated polyester no longer appears to have sensitizing capacity, presumably because the formation of sensitizing, free maleic acid esters is prevented by the avoidance of monoalcoholic impurities [230]. Should the diols contain monoalcohols like ethanol and butanol, then ethyl maleate and dibutyl maleate can be formed, which are strong contact sensitizers. Diethyl maleate was reported to be a sensitizer in four men working with unsaturated polyester resins [266]. Allergic contact dermatitis from unsaturated polyester resins has more frequently been reported to be due to the auxiliary ingredients, such as catalysts [266, 272] and cross-linking agents [272–280]. Unsaturated polyester dust from reinforced plastic products [281, 282] or unsaturated polyester in automobile repair putty [271, 283] have also caused allergic contact dermatitis.

The main irritants in unsaturated polyester resin systems are styrene and organic peroxides. Unsaturated polyester resin may contain 30–60 wt% styrene. Styrene is classified as a mild skin irritant [32, 284]. Repeated skin contact with liquid styrene, however, causes drying of the skin and may also cause irritant contact dermatitis [272, 285–287]. In addition, workers in the reinforced plastics industry are exposed to numerous other skin irritants, such as glass fiber, organic solvents, and other additives.

Peroxides are used at 3–10 wt% to catalyze the hardening process of unsaturated polyester resins. These reactive organic peroxides are weak sensitizers but strong irritants [288], and have also been reported to cause stinging on uncovered skin areas during spray lamination [284].

34.5.3 Polyvinyl Resins

The chemical structure of a vinyl compound is $CH_2=CH-R$, where $CH_2=CH-$ is the vinyl group and the R is the symbol for different chemical groups used to synthesize various polyvinyl resins. Some examples of vinyl compounds are vinyl chloride (R: Cl-), vinyl acetate (R: CH_3COOH-), vinyl acetal (R: CH_3 $(CH_2)_n-O-$, $n=0,1,2…$), vinyl alcohol (R: OH-), and vinylidene chloride (R: $CH_2=CCl_2$). The polyvinyl resins are polymerized through a polyaddition reaction and belong to the group of thermoplastics. Vinyl chloride ($CH_2=CH-Cl$) is a gaseous monomer, polymerized by suspension, emulsion, solution, and bulk processes. The repeating unit of polyvinyl chloride (PVC) is $-CH_2-CHCl-$.

There are various additives in PVC plastics, such as antioxidants, light stabilizers, initiators, plasticizers, flame-retardants, and pigments. As initiators, potassium persulfate, benzoyl peroxide, lauryl peroxide, percarbonate, and some azo compounds can be used. The presence of chlorine in the hydrocarbon backbone gives rigidity and toughness to the polymer, but PVC liberates hydrogen chloride when exposed to high temperatures. To prevent this, stabilizers are added to the polymer. There are several kinds of stabilizers on the market. The most important contain lead, tin, calcium and zinc, and barium and zinc. Plasticizers, mainly phthalates, are added to almost all PVC to impart flexibility to the finished products and to improve processing of the melt. Hard PVC contains approximately 10% and soft PVC up to 60–70% plasticizers. The plasticizers are mostly in the form of phthalic acid esters, most commonly diethylhexyl phthalate (DEHP), often termed dioctyl phthalate (DOP). However, more than one plasticizer is usually used when properties other than flexibility are also required in the end product. Sometimes, uncured epoxy resin is added as a plasticizer and stabilizer to PVC. Soft or plasticized PVC is very popular in applications such as artificial skin, wallpapers, laminated table cloths, carpets, toys, garden hoses, wire coatings for electric cables, shower curtains, adhesive plasters, foils, bandages, casts, and protective gloves.

PVC is one of the most inexpensive thermoplastics and is the most used plastic after polyethylene. The toughness and rigidity of hard PVC give rise to applications in sewage systems, agricultural products, drinking water pipes, furniture, window frames, dishes, and packages of various shapes.

34.5.3.1 Skin Problems from Polyvinyl Resins

Workers processing PVC plastics can develop contact dermatitis [289, 290]. The vinyl chloride polymer (PVC) does not sensitize, and its additives only seldom cause skin issues. In the final PVC product, there are always molecules of the monomer as well as a number of additives that may cause allergic contact dermatitis [289, 291–295], irritant contact dermatitis [290, 296], and contact urticaria [297, 298]. Allergic contact reactions to epoxy resin in PVC plastic film and to phenylthiourea and phenylisothiocyanate in PVC adhesive tape have been reported [293, 299]. Diphenylthiourea is a heat stabilizer in PVC and is partly decomposed to phenyl isothiocyanate.

The irritancy of polyvinyl resins is due to the plasticizers and stabilizers, dibutyl thiomalate, dibutyl sebacate, or dioctyl phthalate [32, 296]. PVC powder may irritate in a particular environment: an outbreak of acneiform eruptions that occurred in a PVC manufacturing factory has been reported [300]. The cause was probably the combination of heat, high humidity, and irritation from the PVC powder. Toxic polyvinyl chloride disease, from the manufacturing of PVC, consisting of Raynaud's phenomenon, lytic disease of bone, and scleroderma, has been reported.

> ### Core Message
>
> ■ In the final PVC product, there are always molecules of the monomer, as well as a number of additives which may cause allergic contact dermatitis.

34.5.4 Polystyrene

Polystyrene (PS) is a hard and transparent plastic. It is manufactured by polyaddition polymerization of styrene, $CH_2=CH-C_6H_5$, using peroxide as an initiator. Polystyrene resin is one of the thermoplastics. As a foam, polystyrene plastic is an important packaging and insulation material. Modified polystyrene plastics with a co- or ter-polymer structure, e.g., styrene-butadiene (SB), styrene-acrylonitrile (SAN), acrylonitrile-butadiene-styrene (ABS), are used in household utensils, toys, electrical appliances, handles, bags, and pipes. Polystyrene products are also widely used in food packaging and disposable tableware. Polystyrene products can usually be identified by their metallic sound when dropped on a hard surface.

To increase the light stability of styrene-based plastics, stabilizers such as benzophenones, benzotriazoles, and organic nickel compounds are usually added.

34.5.4.1 Skin Problems from Polystyrene Resins

Contact allergy to styrene is extremely rare. One patient, sensitive to styrene, cross-reacted on patch testing to 2-, 3-, and 4-vinyltoluene (2-, 3-, and 4-methylstyrene) and to the metabolites styrene epoxide and 4-vinylphenol (4-hydroxy-styrene). It is assumed that styrene is a pro-hapten metabolized in the skin by arylhydrocarbon hydroxylase to styrene epoxide, which acts as a true hapten. Styrene occurs both in nature and as a synthetic product and vinyltoluenes (methylstyrenes) occur as synthetic products in plastics [274]. Cases of immediate allergy to styrene have also been reported [272, 274, 285, 286].

Though styrene is generally classified as a mild irritant [32, 284], it has, on occasions, been reported to cause chemical burns [272, 287].

34.5.5 Polyolefins

Polyolefins belong to a group of thermoplastics polymerized through polyaddition reaction of olefins (unsaturated hydrocarbons). The most important polyolefins are ethylene (ethene), $CH_2=CH_2$, which gives polyethylene, and propylene (propene) $CH_2=CHCH_3$, which gives polypropylene, when polymerized.

Polyethylene is the largest-volume plastic among those that have been known for more than half a century. The repeating unit of polyethylene is $-CH_2-CH_2-$. Polymerization is produced at high or low pressures, aided by catalysts and initiators. According to their density, polyethylenes are grouped into three main categories: low-density polyethylenes, linear low-density polyethylenes, and high-density polyethylenes.

All of these types are lighter than water and belong to the most inexpensive group of plastics. Films and sheets for packaging uses are the most widespread forms of polyethylene plastics. Because low-density polyethylene is soft, flexible, transparent, and nontoxic due to the absence of plasticizers, it is used for food packaging. In addition, shopping bags and sacks are the most popular applications of low-density polyethylenes. Linear low-density polyethylene is the main plastic in the film manufacturing industry, due to its greater mechanical strength. Because low-density polyethylene has outstanding chemical and frost resistance, its main applications are for hoses, sleeves of electric cables and wires, and many kinds of household utensils, such as jars, containers, deep-freeze boxes, and cases. High-density polyethylenes are used mainly for bottles and containers, but also for shopping bags and pipes.

Polypropylene has the repeating unit $-CH_2-CH(CH_3)-$ and is similar to high-density polyethylene, but slightly harder and tougher. In addition to filament applications, such as home furnishings, non-woven products, and carpets, polypropylene is generally used for pipes and films.

34.5.5.1 Skin Problems from Polyolefins

Irritant and allergic contact dermatitis from polyethylene and polypropylene are rare. Contact urticaria due to polyethylene gloves has been reported [301]. Incompletely cured resins may cause contact dermatitis, which is most likely to be caused by additives such as catalysts and initiators. When sawing and grinding polyolefins, the frictional heat may cause depolymerization and release chemicals, e.g., aldehydes, ketones, and acids, which might cause airborne contact dermatitis. Itching caused by the irritancy of heat-decomposed polyethylene plastics has been reported [302].

Core Message

- Irritant and allergic contact dermatitis from polyethylene and polypropylene are rare.

34.5.6 Polyamides

The polyamides are thermoplastics manufactured by condensation polymerization of adipic acid, $HOOC-(CH_2)_4-COOH$, and hexamethylenediamine, $H_2N-(CH_2)_6-NH_2$. The resulting polymer has a linear structure with repeating unit $-OC-(CH_2)_4CONH-(CH_2)_6-NH-$. Other polyamides can be polymerized from caprolactam and water.

The polyamides are made into fibers known as nylons. The transparency of polyamide films makes them very useful for packaging purposes. Hospital wares made of polyamide plastics have good stability at sterilization temperatures, and combined films of laminates are used, for example, in vacuum packaging of meat.

34.5.6.1 Skin Problems from Polyamides

Irritant and allergic contact dermatitis from polyamides are rare. Contact dermatitis caused by polyamide trousers pockets has been described [303]. Contact dermatitis in nylon production is usually caused by various additives [304–307]. Contact urticaria due to nylon has been reported [308].

34.5.7 Polycarbonates

The $-O-CO-O-$ group characterizes a polycarbonate plastic. It can be made from phosgene ($COCl_2$) and bisphenol A ($4,4'$-dihydroxydiphenyl-2,2-propane) and has the structure $-O-(C_6H_4)-C(CH_3)_2-(C_6H_4)-O-CO-$. Bisphenols other than bisphenol A can also be used. Polycarbonate plastic is a very transparent, tough, and inert material that is extremely resistant to sunlight and weather. It is used, among other things, in safety helmets, bullet-proof windows, shields, doors, bottles, and lamp globes. However, the plastic is relatively expensive and, therefore, has limited applications.

34.5.7.1 Skin Problems from Polycarbonates

Irritant and allergic contact dermatitis from polycarbonates are rare.

34.5.8 Rare Plastic Materials

Plastics of less dermatological importance are coumarone-indene polymers, cellulose polymers, and cyclohexanone resins. It is not fully known if the monomers, additives, or impurities are the cause of dermatitis in reported cases [309, 310].

34.6 Plasticizers and other Additives in Synthetic Polymers

BERT BJÖRKNER

Additives are used to modify the properties of the plastic material. The major classes of additives to plastics are plasticizers, fillers and reinforcements, biocides, flame retardants, heat stabilizers, antioxidants, UV-light absorbers, blowing agents, initiators, lubricants and flow-control agents, antistatic agents, curing agents, colorants, solvents, and optical brighteners.

There are nearly 2,500 individual chemicals or mixtures that are utilized in the above major classes of additives. In the plastics industry, the word "compound" is used for a chemical product of plastic resin mixed with additives. Compounds are delivered to the plastic industry as powders or pellets. Masterbatch is a concentrated mixture of additives in the plastics.

34.6.1 Plasticizers

Plasticizers constitute a broad range of chemically and thermally stable products of a variety of chemical classes that are added to improve the flexibility, softness, and processing of plastics. Their principal use is in thermoplastic resins and 80–85% of the world's production of plasticizers is used in PVC manufacturing. Approximately 450 plasticizers are commercially available. Many are esters of carboxylic acids (e.g., phthalic, isophthalic, adipic, benzoic, abietic, trimellitic, oleic, sebacic acids) or phosphoric acid. Other plasticizers are chlorinated paraffins, epoxidized vegetable oils, and adipate polymers.

Although there are about 100 phthalates that have been employed as plasticizers, around 14–15 phthalates account for over 90% of commercial phthalate production. The most commonly used phthalate is diethylhexyl phthalate (DEHP), which is often called dioctyl phthalate (DOP). Other plasticizers used are butyl benzyl phthalate (BBP), diisononyl phthalate (DINP), diisodecyl phthalate (DIDP), methyl-, ethyl-, butyl phthalate, dialkyl (C_6C_{11}) phthalate, and diethylhexyl adipate. Adipates and other aliphatic diesters are used in low-temperature applications, while trimellitates are used for high-temperature applications. Methyl-, ethyl-, and butyl phthalates are more often used as solvents than plasticizers in the plastics industry.

34.6.2 Flame Retardants

Flame retardants are required for high-performance thermoplastic resins because of their use in electrical and high-temperature applications. Numerous chemicals are used as flame retardants. Chlorine- and bromine-containing aliphatic, cycloaliphatic, and aromatic compounds are the most widely used. Others are antimony trioxide, aluminum hydrate, and chloroparaffins. A more fire-resistant epoxy resin can be produced by brominating bisphenol A in epoxy resins to tetrabromobisphenol A.

34.6.3 Heat Stabilizers

Plastics, particularly chlorine-containing polymers, are susceptible to thermal decomposition when exposed to high temperatures or prolonged heating. There are several kinds of stabilizers on the market. The most important contain lead, tin, calcium and zinc, or barium and zinc. Epoxidized oils and esters are also used. Diphenylthiourea is used as a heat stabilizer in PVC.

34.6.4 Antioxidants

Oxidative degradation of polymers during the manufacturing process or during their useful lifetime is a major industrial concern. Examples of antioxidants are alkylated phenols and polyphenols (e.g., butylated hydroxytoluenes (BHT) and 4-tertiary-butylcatechol), epoxidized soyabean oil, propylphenol phosphite, thiobisphenol, organic phosphates, bisphenol A, benzophenone, hydroquinones, and triazoles.

34.6.5 Ultraviolet Light Absorbers

Radiation from the sun or fluorescent light rapidly degrades most plastics. The most widely used UV absorbers belong to six distinct chemical classes:

- Benzophenones
- Benzotriazoles
- Salicylates
- Acrylates
- Organo-nickel derivatives
- Hindered amines
- Metal complexes with dialkyldithiocarbamate

The most widely used UV absorbers are 2-hydroxy-benzophenones, 2-hydroxy-phenyl-benzotriazoles, and 2-cyanodiphenyl-acrylate.

34.6.6 Initiators

A chain reaction polymerization process produces most commercial synthetic polymers. Some of the many initiators used are various peroxides (e.g., benzoyl peroxide, di-tertiary-butyl peroxide, cyclohexanone peroxide, and methyl ethyl ketone peroxide). There are more than 65 commercially available organic peroxides in over 100 formulations.

34.6.7 Curing Agents

The usefulness of a number of plastics, such as unsaturated polyester, epoxy, and phenolic resins, is limited, unless their linear polymer chains are cross-linked or cured. The various curing agents and compounds used as initiators (accelerators or catalysts) are discussed under the various plastics.

34.6.8 Biocides

Biostabilizers will prevent the growth of micro-organisms on the surface and in the pores of plastics. Plastic materials easily attacked by micro-organisms are PVC, polyurethane, silicon products, and fiber products based on polypropene and polyamide. Micro-organisms usually cause discoloration, but can also cause cracks in plastic materials. Biocides are usually added to plastic products used in environments of high temperature and humidity, e.g., saunas, showers, pools, and boats. The most widely used biocides are methyl and octyl isothiazolinones and oxybisphenoxarsine (OBPA).

34.6.9 Colorants (Dyes and Pigments)

Pigments are inert and, unlike dyes, insoluble in the medium in which they are incorporated. Both inorganic and organic pigments are used in plastics. Most colorants are inorganic pigments, with titanium dioxide being the most commonly used and iron oxides the second most common.

34.6.10 Metals and Metal Salts

Many metals, metal salts, and metallic compounds are used as additives in plastics. They act as stabilizers, pigments, fillers, flame retardants, and antistatics. The most commonly used metals are aluminum, titanium, lead, zinc, antimony, tin, chromium, and molybdenum. Nickel, copper, and zirconium compounds are used to a lesser degree.

34.6.11 Skin Problems from Additives

Allergic and irritant contact dermatitis from various additives were briefly mentioned in connection with the various plastics. In spite of phthalates being the most widely used additives in plastics, there are only a few reports in the literature of skin problems caused by them. Allergic contact dermatitis from dibutyl phthalate has been reported when used in a plastic watchstrap, an antiperspirant spray, and a corticosteroid cream [311–314]. Contact dermatitis from diethyl phthalate has been reported from spectacle frames and a hearing aid of cellulose ester plastics [315, 316]. Two cases of contact allergy to dimethyl phthalate in computer "mice" have been reported [317].

An outbreak of dermatitis occurring in an aircraft factory was caused by o-diglycidyl phthalate, among other chemicals [108]. Burrows and Rycroft have reported contact allergy to tricresyl ethyl phthalate in a plastic nail adhesive [318], and Hills and Ive observed allergic contact dermatitis from di-isodecylphthalate in an PVC identity band [294].

Phthalates can also appear in deodorant formulations, perfumes, emollients, and insect repellents [319]. A case of contact urticaria syndrome due to di(2-ethylhexyl)phthalate (DOP) in work clothes has been described [298]. Triphenylphosphate allergy from spectacle frames has been reported [320, 321].

In 1976, the International Contact Dermatitis Research Group (ICDRG) examined the incidence of sensitization to the flame retardant tris(2,3-dibromopropyl)phosphate and found two positives among 1,103 patients. One of these two cases has been reported in detail by Andersen [322].

Contact allergy to ultraviolet light absorbers like 2-hydroxybenzophenone, resorcinol monobenzoate, 2-(2-hydroxy-5-methylphenyl)benzotriazole (Tinuvin P), and bis-(2,2,6,6)-tetramethyl-4-piperidyl-sebacate has been encountered [323, 324].

Organic pigments, mostly of the azo type, are potentially sensitizing additives in plastics [325, 326]. Allergic contact dermatitis from perinone-type plastic dyes, C.I. Solvent Orange 60, and C.I. Solvent Red

179 used in spectacle frames has been described [327, 328]. C.I. Solvent Orange 60 has also been found to cause contact allergy in workers exposed to polyamide plastics (E. Zimerson, personal communication).

Cobalt, nickel and mercury used in plastic shoes, personal computer (PC) mice, and in polyester resins have been reported [329–331].

Other additives of dermatological importance are hydroquinone, *p-tert*-butyl-catechol, cobalt naphthenate, benzoyl peroxide, dimethylaniline, methyl-4-toluene sulfonate, *p*-tolyl-diethanolamine, and dimethyl-, diethyl-, and diphenylthiourea. These agents may cause both allergic and irritant contact dermatitis [32].

Core Message

■ In spite of phthalates being the most widely used additives in plastics, there are only a few reports in the literature of skin problems caused by them.

References

1. Freeman S, Lee MS, Gudmundsen K (1995) Adverse contact reactions to sculptured acrylic nails: 4 case reports and a literature review. Contact Dermatitis 33:381–385
2. Koppula S, Feldman J, Storrs F (1995) Screening allergens for acrylate dermatitis associated with artificial nails. Am J Contact Dermat 6:78–85
3. Kanerva L, Lauerma A, Estlander T, Alanko K, Henriks-Eckerman ML, Jolanki R (1996) Occupational allergic contact dermatitis caused by photobonded sculptured nails and a review of (meth) acrylates in nail cosmetics. Am J Contact Dermat 7:109–115
4. Hemmer W, Focke M, Wantke F, Gotz M, Jarisch R (1996) Allergic contact dermatitis to artificial fingernails prepared from UV light-cured acrylates. J Am Acad Dermatol 35:377–380
5. Fischer A (1990) Adverse nail reactions and paresthesia from "photobonded acrylate 'sculptured' nails". Cutis 45: 293 294
6. Kanerva L, Estlander T, Jolanki R, Tarvainen K (1994) Dermatitis from acrylates in dental personnel. In: Menne T, Maibach HI (eds) Hand eczema. CRC, Boca Raton, Fla., pp 231–273
7. Kanerva L, Estlander T, Jolanki R (1989) Occupational allergic contact dermatitis from acrylates: observations concerning anaerobic acrylic sealants and dental composite resins. In: Frosch PJ, Dooms-Goossens A, Lachapelle JM, Rycroft RJG, Scheper RJ (eds) Current topics in contact dermatitis. Springer, Berlin Heidelberg New York, pp 352–359
8. Geukens S, Goossens A (2001) Occupational contact allergy to (meth)acrylates. Contact Dermatitis 44:153–159
9. Dahlquist I, Fregert S, Trulson L (1983) Contact allergy to trimethylolpropane triacrylate (TMPTA) in an aziridine plastic hardener. Contact Dermatitis 9:122–124
10. Cofield BG, Storrs FJ, Strawn CB (1985) Contact allergy to aziridine paint hardener. Arch Dermatol 121:373–376
11. Kanerva L, Estlander T, Jolanki R, Tarvainen K (1995) Occupational allergic contact dermatitis and contact urticaria caused by polyfunctional aziridine hardener. Contact Dermatitis 33:304–309
12. Dempsey KJ (1982) Hypersensitivity to Sta-Lok and Loctite anaerobic sealants. J Am Acad Dermatol 7: 779–784
13. Ranchoff RE, Taylor JS (1985) Contact dermatitis to anaerobic sealants. J Am Acad Dermatol 13:1015–1020
14. Conde-Salazar L, Guimaraens D, Romero LV (1988) Occupational allergic contact dermatitis from anaerobic acrylic sealants. Contact Dermatitis 18:129–132
15. Kanerva L, Jolanki R, Leino T, Estlander T (1995) Occupational allergic contact dermatitis from 2-hydroxyethyl methacrylate and ethylene glycol dimethacrylate in a modified acrylic structural adhesive. Contact Dermatitis 33:84–89
16. Corazza M, Bacilieri S, Virgili A (2000) Anaerobic sealants: still a problem today. Eur J Dermatol 10:468–469
17. Kanerva L, Estlander T, Jolanki R (2001) Optician's occupational allergic contact dermatitis, paresthesia and paronychia caused by anaerobic acrylic sealants. Contact Dermatitis 44:117–119
18. Brooke RC, Beck MH (2002) A new source of allergic contact dermatitis from UV-cured (meth)acrylate adhesive. Contact Dermatitis 47:179–180
19. van der Walle HB (1982) Sensitizing potential of acrylic monomers in guinea pigs. Katholieke Universiteit te Nijmegen, Holland, Kripps Repro, Meppel, The Netherlands
20. Waegemaekers T (1985) Some toxicological aspects of acrylic monomers, notably with reference to the skin. Katholieke Universiteit te Nijmegen, The Netherlands
21. Parker D, Turk JL (1983) Contact sensitivity to acrylate compounds in guinea pigs. Contact Dermatitis 9:55–60
22. Björkner B (1981) Sensitization capacity of acrylated prepolymers in ultraviolet curing inks tested in the guinea pig. Acta Derm Venereol (Stockh) 61:7–10
23. Cavelier C, Jelen G, Herve-Bazin B, Foussereau J (1981) Irritation et allergie aux acrylates et methacrylates. Premiere partie: monoacrylates et monomethacrylates simples. Ann Dermatol Venereol (Stockh) 108:549–556
24. Björkner B, Niklasson B, Persson K (1984) The sensitizing potential of di-(meth)acrylates based on bisphenol A or epoxy resin in the guinea pig. Contact Dermatitis 10: 286–304
25. Björkner B (1982) Sensitization capacity of polyester methacrylate in ultraviolet curing inks tested in the guinea pig. Acta Derm Venereol (Stockh) 62:153–154
26. Bjorkner B (1984) Sensitizing potential of urethane (meth)acrylates in the guinea pig. Contact Dermatitis 11: 115–119
27. Björkner B (1984) Sensitizing capacity of ultraviolet curable acrylic compounds. Thesis, University of Lund, Lund, Sweden
28. Beurey J, Mougeolle JM, Weber M (1976) Accidents cutanes des resines acryliques dans l'imprimerie. Ann Dermatol Syphiligr (Paris) 103:423–430
29. Malten KE, den Arend JA, Wiggers RE (1979) Delayed irritation: hexanediol diacrylate and butanediol diacrylate. Contact Dermatitis 5:178–184

34

30. Nethercott JR, Gupta S, Rosen C, Enders LJ, Pilger CW (1984) Tetraethylene glycol diacrylate. A cause of delayed cutaneous irritant reaction and allergic contact dermatitis. J Occup Med 26:513–516

31. Finnish Advisory Board of Chemicals (1992) Acrylate compounds: uses and evaluation of health effects. Government Printing Office, Helsinki, Finland

32. Kanerva L, Björkner B, Estlander T (1996) Plastic materials: occupational exposure, skin irritancy and its prevention. In: van der Valk PGM, Maibach HI (eds) The irritant contact dermatitis syndrome. CRC, Boca Baton, Fla., pp 127–155

33. Niinimaki A, Rosberg J, Saari S (1983) Traces of epoxy resin in acrylic dental filling materials. Contact Dermatitis 9:532

34. Roberts DW (1987) Structure–activity relationships for skin sensitisation potential of diacrylates and dimethacrylates. Contact Dermatitis 17:281–289

35. Nethercott JR, Jakubovic HR, Pilger C, Smith JW (1983) Allergic contact dermatitis due to urethane acrylate in ultraviolet cured inks. Br J Ind Med 40:241–250

36. Pedersen NB, Senning A, Nielsen AO (1983) Different sensitising acrylic monomers in Napp printing plate. Contact Dermatitis 9:459–464

37. Björkner B (1984) Contact allergy to 2-hydroxypropyl methacrylate (2-HPMA) in an ultraviolet curable ink. Acta Derm Venereol (Stockh) 64:264–267

38. Malten KE, Bende WJ (1979) 2-Hydroxy- ethyl-methacrylate and di- and tetraethylene glycol dimethacrylate: contact sensitizers in a photoprepolymer printing plate procedure. Contact Dermatitis 5:214–220

39. Kanerva L, Estlander T, Jolanki R (1994) Occupational skin allergy in dental profession. In: Taylor S (ed) Dermatologic clinics. Saunders, Philadelphia, Pa., pp 517–532

40. Kanerva L, Henriks-Eckerman M, Estlander T (1994) Occupational allergic contact dermatitis and composition of acrylates in dental bonding systems. J Eur Acad Derm Venereol 3:157–168

41. Kanerva L, Jolanki R, Estlander T (1997) 10 years of patch testing with the (meth)acrylate series. Contact Dermatitis 37:255–258

42. Kanerva L, Estlander T, Jolanki R (1995) Dental problems. In: Guin JD (ed) Practical contact dermatitis. McGraw-Hill, New York, p 137

43. Whittington CV (1981) Dermatitis from UV acrylate in adhesive. Contact Dermatitis 7:203–204

44. Fregert S (1983) Occupational hazards of acrylate bone cement in orthopaedic surgery. Acta Orthop Scand 54:787–789

45. Estlander T, Jolanki R, Kanerva L (1998) Occupational allergic contact dermatitis from UV-cured lacquer containing dipropylene glycol diacrylate. Contact Dermatitis 39:36

46. Moffitt DL, Sansom JE (2001) Occupational allergic contact dermatitis from tetrahydrofurfuryl acrylate in a medical-device adhesive. Contact Dermatitis 45:54

47. Goon AT, Rycroft RJ, McFadden JP (2002) Allergic contact dermatitis from trimethylolpropane triacrylate and pentaerythritol triacrylate. Contact Dermatitis 47:249

48. Henriks-Eckerman ML, Alanko K, Jolanki R, Kerosuo H, Kanerva L (2001) Exposure to airborne methacrylates and natural rubber latex allergens in dental clinics. J Environ Monit 3:302–305

49. Kanerva L, Rantanen T, Aalto-Korte K, Estlander T, Hannuksela M, Harvima RJ, IIasan T, Horsmanheimo M, Jolanki R, Kalimo K, Lahti A, Lammintausta K, Lauerma A, Niinimaki A, Turjanmaa K, Vuorela AM (2001) A multi-

center study of patch test reactions with dental screening series. Am J Contact Dermat 12:83–87

50. Piirila P, Hodgson U, Estlander T, Keskinen H, Saalo A, Voutilainen R, Kanerva L (2002) Occupational respiratory hypersensitivity in dental personnel. Int Arch Occup Environ Health 75:209–216

51. Lindstrom M, Alanko K, Keskinen H, Kanerva L (2002) Dentist's occupational asthma, rhinoconjunctivitis, and allergic contact dermatitis from methacrylates. Allergy 57:543–545

52. Kanerva L, Estlander T, Jolanki R, Pekkarinen E (1992) Occupational pharyngitis associated with allergic patch test reactions from acrylics. Allergy 47:571–573

53. Wrangsjö K, Swartling C, Meding B (2001) Occupational dermatitis in dental personnel: contact dermatitis with special reference to (meth)acrylates in 174 patients. Contact Dermatitis 45:158–163

54. Kanerva L, Alanko K, Estlander T (1999) Allergic contact gingivostomatitis from a temporary crown made of methacrylates and epoxy diacrylates. Allergy 54:1316–1321

55. Koch P (2003) Allergic contact stomatitis from BIS-GMA and epoxy resins in dental bonding agents. Contact Dermatitis 49:104–105

56. Carmichael AJ, Gibson JJ, Walls AW (1997) Allergic contact dermatitis to bisphenol-A-glycidyldimethacrylate (BIS-GMA) dental resin associated with sensitivity to epoxy resin. Br Dent J 183:297–298

57. Jolanki R, Kanerva L, Estlander T (1995) Occupational allergic contact dermatitis caused by epoxy diacrylate in ultraviolet-light-cured paint, and bisphenol A in dental composite resin. Contact Dermatitis 33:94–99

58. Kanerva L, Estlander T, Jolanki R (1989) Allergic contact dermatitis from dental composite resins due to aromatic epoxy acrylates and aliphatic acrylates. Contact Dermatitis 20:201–211

59. Bohling HG, Borchard U, Drouin H (1977) Monomeric methylmethacrylate (MMA) acts on the desheathed myelinated nerve and on the node of Ranvier. Arch Toxicol 38:307–314

60. Kanerva L, Verkkala E (1986) Electron microscopy and immunohistochemistry of toxic and allergic effects of methylmethacrylate on the skin. Arch Toxicol Suppl 9:456–459

61. Mathias CG, Caldwell TM, Maibach HI (1979) Contact dermatitis and gastrointestinal symptoms from hydroxyethylmethacrylate. Br J Dermatol 100:447–449

62. Edwards PM (1975) Neurotoxicity of acrylamide and its analogues and effects of these analogues and other agents on acrylamide neuropathy. Br J Ind Med 32:31–38

63. Balda BR (1971) Allergic contact dermatitis due to acrylonitrile. Contact Dermatitis Newslett 9:219

64. Balda BR (1975) Akrylnitril als Kontaktallergen. Hautarzt 26:599–601

65. Romaguera C, Grimalt F, Vilaplana J (1985) Methyl methacrylate prosthesis dermatitis. Contact Dermatitis 12:172

66. Chu CY, Sun CC (2001) Allergic contact dermatitis from acrylonitrile. Am J Contact Dermat 12:113–114

67. Bakker JG, Jongen SM, van Neer FC, Neis JM (1991) Occupational contact dermatitis due to acrylonitrile. Contact Dermatitis 24:50–53

68. Malten KE (1987) Printing plate manufacturing processes. In: Maibach HI (ed) Occupational and industrial dermatology, 2nd edn. Year Book Medical, Chicago, Ill., pp 351–366

69. Malten KE, van der Meer-Roosen CH, Seutter E (1978) Nyloprint-sensitive patients react to N,N′-methylene bis acrylamide. Contact Dermatitis 4:214–222

70. Pedersen NB, Chevallier MA, Senning A (1982) Secondary acrylamides in Nyloprint printing plate as a source of contact dermatitis. Contact Dermatitis 8:256–262

71. Dooms-Goossens A, Garmyn M, Degreef H (1991) Contact allergy to acrylamide. Contact Dermatitis 24:71–72

72. Lambert J, Matthieu L, Dockx P (1988) Contact dermatitis from acrylamide. Contact Dermatitis 19:65

73. Pye RJ, Peachey RD (1976) Contact dermatitis due to Nyloprint. Contact Dermatitis 2:144–146

74. Beyer DJ, Belsito DV (2000) Allergic contact dermatitis from acrylamide in a chemical mixer. Contact Dermatitis 42:181–182

75. Aalto-Korte K, Jolanki R, Suuronen K, Estlander T (2002) Biochemist's occupational allergic contact dermatitis from iodoacetamide and acrylamide. Contact Dermatitis 47:361–362

76. Garnier R, Levy-Amon L, Malingrey L (2003) Occupational contact dermatitis from N-(2-(diethylamino)-ethyl) acrylamide. Contact Dermatitis 48:343–344

77. Wang MT, Wenger K, Maibach HI (1997) Piperazine diacrylamide allergic contact dermatitis. Contact Dermatitis 37:300

78. Calnan CD (1979) Cyanoacrylate dermatitis. Contact Dermatitis 5:165–167

79. Malten KE (1982) Old and new, mainly occupational dermatological problems in the production and processing of plastics. In: Maibach HI, Gellin GA (eds) Occupational and industrial dermatology. Year Book Medical, Chicago, Ill., pp 237–238

80. Jacobs MC, Rycroft RJ (1995) Allergic contact dermatitis from cyanoacrylate? Contact Dermatitis 33:71

81. Fitzgerald DA, Bhaggoe R, English JS (1995) Contact sensitivity to cyanoacrylate nail-adhesive with dermatitis at remote sites. Contact Dermatitis 32:175–176

82. Tomb RR, Lepoittevin JP, Durepaire F, Grosshans E (1993) Ectopic contact dermatitis from ethyl cyanoacrylate instant adhesives. Contact Dermatitis 28:206–208

83. Belsito DV (1987) Contact dermatitis to ethyl-cyanoacrylate-containing glue. Contact Dermatitis 17:234–236

84. Pigatto PD, Giacchetti A, Altomare GF (1986) Unusual sensitization to cyanoacrylate ester. Contact Dermatitis 14:193

85. Fisher AA (1985) Reactions to cyanoacrylate adhesives: "instant glue". Cutis 35:18

86. Bruze M, Björkner B, Lepoittevin JP (1995) Occupational allergic contact dermatitis from ethyl cyanoacrylate. Contact Dermatitis 32:156–159

87. Björkner B, Niklasson B (1984) Influence of the vehicle on elicitation of contact allergic reactions to acrylic compounds in the guinea pig. Contact Dermatitis 11:268–278

88. Conde-Salazar L, Rojo S, Guimaraens D (1998) Occupational allergic contact dermatitis from cyanoacrylate. Am J Contact Dermat 9:188–189

89. Guin JD, Baas K, Nelson-Adesokan P (1998) Contact sensitization to cyanoacrylate adhesive as a cause of severe onychodystrophy. Int J Dermatol 37:31–36

90. Kanerva L, Estlander T (2000) Allergic onycholysis and paronychia caused by cyanoacrylate nail glue, but not by photobonded methacrylate nails. Eur J Dermatol 10:223–225

91. Foti C, Cassano N, Conserva A, Vena GA (2003) Irritant paronychia with onychodystrophy caused by cyanoacrylate nail glue. Contact Dermatitis 48:274–275

92. Guin JD, Wilson P (1999) Onycholysis from nail lacquer: a complication of nail enhancement? Am J Contact Dermat 10:34–36

93. Pegum JS, Medhurst FA (1971) Contact dermatitis from penetration of rubber gloves by acrylic monomer. Br Med J 2:141–143

94. Rietschel RL, Huggins R, Levy N, Pruitt PM (1984) In vivo and in vitro testing of gloves for protection against UV-curable acrylate resin systems. Contact Dermatitis 11:279–282

95. Munksgaard EC (1992) Permeability of protective gloves to (di)methacrylates in resinous dental materials. Scand J Dent Res 100:189–192

96. Andersson T, Bruze M, Björkner B (1999) In vivo testing of the protection of gloves against acrylates in dentin-bonding systems on patients with known contact allergy to acrylates. Contact Dermatitis 41:254–259

97. Andersson T, Bruze M, Gruvberger B, Björkner B (2000) In vivo testing of the protection provided by non-latex gloves against a 2-hydroxyethyl methacrylate-containing acetone-based dentin-bonding product. Acta Derm Venereol (Stockh) 80:435–437

98. Andreasson H, Boman A, Johnsson S, Karlsson S, Barregard L (2003) On permeability of methyl methacrylate, 2-hydroxyethyl methacrylate and triethyleneglycol dimethacrylate through protective gloves in dentistry. Eur J Oral Sci 111:529–535

99. Nakamura M, Oshima H, Hashimoto Y (2003) Monomer permeability of disposable dental gloves. J Prosthet Dent 90:81–85

100. Estlander T, Jolanki R (1988) How to protect the hands. In: Taylor JS (ed) Occupational dermatoses. Saunders, Philadelphia, Pa., pp 105–114 (Dermatological clinics, vol 6)

101. Kanerva L, Estlander T, Jolanki R (1988) Sensitization to patch test acrylates. Contact Dermatitis 18:10–15

102. Kanerva L (2001) Cross-reactions of multifunctional methacrylates and acrylates. Acta Odontol Scand 59:320–329

103. Rustemeyer T, de Groot J, von Blomberg BM, Frosch PJ, Scheper RJ (1998) Cross-reactivity patterns of contact-sensitizing methacrylates. Toxicol Appl Pharmacol 148:83–90

104. Muskopf JW, McCollister SB (1987) Epoxy resins. In: Gerhartz W, Yamamoto YS, Kaudy L, Rounsaville JF, Schulx G (eds) Ullmann's encyclopedia of industrial chemistry, 5th completely revised edn, vol A9. VCH Verlagsgesellschaft, Weinheim, Germany, pp 547–569

105. Ellis B (1993) The synthesis and manufacture of epoxy resins. In: Ellis B (ed) Chemistry and technology of epoxy resins, 1st edn. Blackie Academic and Professional, Glasgow, pp 16–36

106. Henriks-Eckerman M-L, Laijoki T (1986) Glycidyl ethers in epoxy resin products (in Finnish with English summary). Työterveyslaitoksen Tutkimuksia 4:41–46 (summary p 70)

107. Pontén A, Zimerson E, Sörensen Ö, Bruze M (2004) Chemical analysis of monomers in epoxy resins based on bisphenols F and A. Contact Dermatitis 50:289–297

108. Burrows D, Fregert S, Campbell H, Trulsson L (1984) Contact dermatitis from the epoxy resins tetraglycidyl-4,4′-methylene dianiline and o-diglycidyl phthalate in composite material. Contact Dermatitis 11:80–82

109. Fregert S (1981) Manual of contact dermatitis, 2nd edn. Munksgaard, Copenhagen, Denmark

110. Kanerva L, Jolanki R, Estlander T, Henriks-Eckerman M, Tuomi M, Tarvainen K (2000) Airborne occupational allergic contact dermatitis from triglycidyl-p-aminophenol and tetraglycidyl-4,4′-methylene dianiline in preimpregnated epoxy products in the aircraft industry. Dermatology 201:29–33

111. Bruze M, Edenholm M, Engström K, Svensson G (1996) Occupational dermatoses in a Swedish aircraft plant. Contact Dermatitis 34:336–340

112. Jensen CD, Andersen KE (2003) Two cases of occupational allergic contact dermatitis from a cycloaliphatic epoxy resin in a neat oil: case report. Environ Health 2:3

113. Maibach HI, Mathias CT (2001) Allergic contact dermatitis from cycloaliphatic epoxide in jet aviation hydraulic fluid. Contact Dermatitis 45:56

114. Mathias CG (1988) Allergic contact dermatitis from triglycidyl isocyanurate in polyester paint pigments. Contact Dermatitis 19:67–68

115. Allmaras S (2003) Worker exposure to 1,3,5-triglycidyl isocyanurate (TGIC) in powder paint coating operations. Appl Occup Environ Hyg 18:151–153

116. Geier J, Oestmann E, Lessmann H, Fuchs T (2001) Contact allergy to terephthalic acid diglycidylester in a powder coating. Contact Dermatitis 44:43–44

117. Ashcroft WR (1993) Curing agents for epoxy resins. In: Ellis B, (ed) Chemistry and technology of epoxy resins, 1st edn. Blackie Academic and Professional, Glasgow, pp 37–71

118. Kanerva L, Estlander T, Jolanki R (1996) Occupational allergic contact dermatitis caused by 2,4,6-tris-(dimethylaminomethyl)phenol, and review of sensitizing epoxy resin hardeners. Int J Dermatol 35:852–856

119. Shaw SJ (1993) Additives and modifiers for epoxy resins. In: Ellis B (ed) Chemistry and technology of epoxy resins, 1st edn. Blackie Academic and Professional, Glasgow, pp 117–143

120. Thorgeirsson A, Fregert S, Magnusson B (1975) Allergenicity of epoxy-reactive diluents in the guinea pig. Berufsdermatosen 23:178–183

121. Jolanki R (1991) Occupational skin diseases from epoxy compounds. Epoxy resin compounds, epoxy acrylates and 2,3-epoxypropyl trimethyl ammonium chloride. Acta Derm Venereol Suppl (Stockh) 159:1–80

122. Uter W, Ruhl R, Pfahlberg A, Geier J, Schnuch A, Gefeller O (2004) Contact allergy in construction workers: results of a multifactorial analysis. Ann Occup Hyg 48:21–27

123. Dickel H, Kuss O, Schmidt A, Diepgen TL (2002) Occupational relevance of positive standard patch-test results in employed persons with an initial report of an occupational skin disease. Int Arch Occup Environ Health 75:423–434

124. Jolanki R, Estlander T, Kanerva L (1987) Occupational contact dermatitis and contact urticaria caused by epoxy resins. Acta Derm Venereol Suppl (Stockh) 134:90–94

125. Pontén A, Carstensen O, Rasmussen K, Gruvberger B, Isaksson M, Bruze M (2004) Epoxy-based production of wind turbine rotor blades: occupational dermatoses. Contact Dermatitis 50:329–338

126. Le Coz CJ, Coninx D, van Rengen A, El Aboubi S, Ducombs G, Benz MH, Boursier S, Avenel-Audran M, Verret JL, Erikstam U, Bruze M, Goossens A (1999) An epidemic of occupational contact dermatitis from an immersion oil for microscopy in laboratory personnel. Contact Dermatitis 40:77–83

127. Birmingham DJ (1959) Clinical observations on the cutaneous effects associated with curing epoxy resins. AMA Arch Ind Health 19:365–367

128. Bourne LB, Milner FJ, Alberman KB (1959) Health problems of epoxy resins and amine-curing agents. Br J Ind Med 16:81–97

129. Gaul LE (1957) Sensitizing structure in epoxy resin. J Invest Dermatol 29:311–313

130. Gaul LE (1960) Sensitivity to bisphenol A. Arch Dermatol 82:1003

131. Calnan CD (1975) Epoxy resin dermatitis. J Soc Occup Med 25:123–126

132. Thorgeirsson A, Fregert S (1977) Allergenicity of epoxy resins in the guinea pig. Acta Derm Venereol (Stockh) 57:253–256

133. Fregert S, Thorgeirsson A (1977) Patch testing with low molecular oligomers of epoxy resins in humans. Contact Dermatitis 3:301–303

134. Jolanki R, Sysilampi ML, Kanerva L, Estlander T (1989) Contact allergy to cycloaliphatic epoxy resins. In: Frosch PJ, Dooms-Goossens A, Lachapelle JM, Rycroft RJG, Scheper RJ (eds) Current topics in contact dermatitis. Springer, Berlin Heidelberg New York, pp 360–367

135. Kanerva L, Tarvainen K, Pinola A, Leino T, Granlund H, Estlander T, Jolanki R, Forstrom L (1994) A single accidental exposure may result in a chemical burn, primary sensitization and allergic contact dermatitis. Contact Dermatitis 31:229–235

136. Dahlquist I, Fregert S (1979) Allergic contact dermatitis from volatile epoxy hardeners and reactive diluents. Contact Dermatitis 5:406–407

137. Fregert S (1988) Physicochemical methods for detection of contact allergens. In: Taylor JS (ed) Occupational dermatoses, dermatological clinics, vol 6. Saunders, Philadelphia, Pa., pp 97–104

138. Lyon CC, O'Driscoll J, Erikstam U, Bruze M, Beck MH (1998) Bowlers' grip. Contact Dermatitis 38:223

139. Sasseville D, Hakim M, Muhn C (2002) Bus pass dermatitis. Am J Contact Dermat 13:146–147

140. Lyon CC, Beck MH (2000) Epoxy-by-proxy dermatitis. Contact Dermatitis 42:306

141. Fregert S, Trulsson L (1978) Simple methods for demonstration of epoxy resins of bisphenol A type. Contact Dermatitis 4:69–72

142. Pontén A, Zimerson E, Sorensen O, Bruze M (2002) Sensitizing capacity and cross-reaction pattern of the isomers of diglycidyl ether of bisphenol F in the guinea pig. Contact Dermatitis 47:293–298

143. Pontén A, Bruze M (2001) Contact allergy to epoxy resin based on diglycidyl ether of bisphenol F. Contact Dermatitis 44:98–99

144. Lee HN, Pokorny CD, Law S, Pratt M, Sasseville D, Storrs FJ (2002) Cross-reactivity among epoxy acrylates and bisphenol F epoxy resins in patients with bisphenol A epoxy resin sensitivity. Am J Contact Dermat 13:108–115

145. Pontén A, Bjork J, Carstensen O, Gruvberger B, Isaksson M, Rasmussen K, Bruze M (2004) Associations between contact allergy to epoxy resin and fragrance mix. Acta Derm Venereol (Stockh) 84:151–152

146. Lembo G, Balato N, Cusano F, Baldo A, Ayala F (1989) Contact dermatitis to epoxy resins in composite material. In: Frosch PJ, Dooms-Goossens A, Lachapelle JM, Rycroft RJG, Scheper RJ (eds) Current topics in contact dermatitis. Springer, Berlin Heidelberg New York, pp 377–380

147. Eedy DJ (1996) Carbon-fibre-induced airborne irritant contact dermatitis. Contact Dermatitis 35:362–363

148. Thorgeirsson A (1978) Sensitization capacity of epoxy resin hardeners in the guinea pig. Acta Derm Venereol (Stockh) 58:323–326

149. Pontén A, Zimerson E, Sörensen Ö, Bruze M (2005) Contact allergy to phenyl glycidyl ether in relation to the main contact allergens in common epoxy resins studied in humans and in the guinea pig (in press)

150. Angelini G, Rigano L, Foti C, Grandolfo M, Vena GA, Bonamonte D, Soleo L, Scorpiniti AA (1996) Occupational

34

sensitization to epoxy resin and reactive diluents in marble workers. Contact Dermatitis 35:11–16

151. Jolanki R, Tarvainen K, Tatar T, Estlander T, Henriks-Eckerman ML, Mustakallio KK, Kanerva L (1996) Occupational dermatoses from exposure to epoxy resin compounds in a ski factory. Contact Dermatitis 34:390–396

152. Silvestre JF, Albares MP, Escutia B, Vergara G, Pascual JC, Botella R (2003) Contact vitiligo appearing after allergic contact dermatitis from aromatic reactive diluents in an epoxy resin system. Contact Dermatitis 49:113–114

153. Estlander T, Jolanki R, Kanerva L (1997) Occupational allergic contact dermatitis from 2,3-epoxypropyl trimethyl ammonium chloride (EPTMAC) and Kathon LX in a starch modification factory. Contact Dermatitis 36:191–194

154. Jolanki R, Kanerva L, Estlander T, Tarvainen K, Keskinen H, Henriks-Eckerman ML (1990) Occupational dermatoses from epoxy resin compounds. Contact Dermatitis 23:172–183

155. Mathias CG (1987) Allergic contact dermatitis from a nonbisphenol A epoxy in a graphite fiber reinforced epoxy laminate. J Occup Med 29:754–755

156. Lachapelle JM, Tennstedt D, Dumont-Fruytier M (1978) Occupational allergic contact dermatitis to isophorone diamine (IPD) used as an epoxy resin hardener. Contact Dermatitis 4:109–112

157. Dahlquist I, Fregert S (1979) Contact allergy to the epoxy hardener isophoronediamine (IPD). Contact Dermatitis 5:120–121

158. Jolanki R, Estlander T, Kanerva L (1987) Contact allergy to an epoxy reactive diluent: 1,4-butanediol diglycidyl ether. Contact Dermatitis 16:87–92

159. Sommer S, Wilkinson SM (2001) Occupational contact dermatitis due to the epoxy hardener m-xylylenediamine. Contact Dermatitis 44:374

160. Kanerva L, Hyry H, Jolanki R, Hytonen M, Estlander T (1997) Delayed and immediate allergy caused by methylhexahydrophthalic anhydride. Contact Dermatitis 36:34–38

161. Krajewska D, Rudzki E (1976) Sensitivity to epoxy resins and triethylenetetramine. Contact Dermatitis 2:135–138

162. Fregert S, Rorsman H (1962) Hypersensitivity to epoxy resins with reference to the role played by bisphenol A. J Invest Dermatol 39:471–472

163. Prens EP, de Jong G, van Joost T (1986) Sensitization to epichlorohydrin and epoxy system components. Contact Dermatitis 15:85–90

164. van Joost T, Roesyanto ID, Satyawan I (1990) Occupational sensitization to epichlorohydrin (ECH) and bisphenol-A during the manufacture of epoxy resin. Contact Dermatitis 22:125–126

165. Matthieu L, Godoi AF, Lambert J, van Grieken R (2003) Occupational allergic contact dermatitis from bisphenol A in vinyl gloves. Contact Dermatitis 49:281–283

166. Aalto-Korte K, Alanko K, Henriks-Eckerman ML, Estlander T, Jolanki R (2003) Allergic contact dermatitis from bisphenol A in PVC gloves. Contact Dermatitis 49:202–205

167. van Joost T (1988) Occupational sensitization to epichlorohydrin and epoxy resin. Contact Dermatitis 19:278–280

168. Tarvainen K, Jolanki R, Estlander T, Tupasela O, Pfaffli P, Kanerva L (1995) Immunologic contact urticaria due to airborne methylhexahydrophthalic and methyltetrahydrophthalic anhydrides. Contact Dermatitis 32:204–209

169. Kanerva L, Jolanki R, Tupasela O, Halmepuro L, Keskinen H, Estlander T, Sysilampi ML (1991) Immediate and delayed allergy from epoxy resins based on diglycidyl ether of bisphenol A. Scand J Work Environ Health 17:208–215

170. Kanerva L, Pelttari M, Jolanki R, Alanko K, Estlander T, Suhonen R (2002) Occupational contact urticaria from diglycidyl ether of bisphenol A epoxy resin. Allergy 57:1205–1207

171. Allen H, Kaidbey K (1979) Persistent photosensitivity following occupational exposure to epoxy resin. Arch Dermatol 115:1307–1310

172. Göransson K, Andersson R, Andersson G, Marklund S et al. (1984) An outbreak of occupational photodermatosis of the face in a factory in northern Sweden. In: Berglund B, Lindvall T, Sundell J (eds) Indoor air, vol 3. Swedish Council for Building Research, Stockholm, Sweden, pp 367–375

173. Maguire HC Jr (1988) Experimental photoallergic contact dermatitis to bisphenol A. Acta Derm Venereol (Stockh) 68:408–412

174. Jolanki R, Estlander T, Kanerva L (2001) 182 patients with occupational allergic epoxy contact dermatitis over 22 years. Contact Dermatitis 44:121–123

175. Pegum JS (1979) Penetration of protective gloves by epoxy resin. Contact Dermatitis 5:281–283

176. Roed-Petersen J (1989) A new glove material protective against epoxy and acrylate monomer. In: Frosch PJ, Dooms-Goossens A, Lachapelle JM, Rycroft RJG, Scheper RJ (eds) Current topics in contact dermatitis. Springer, Berlin Heidelberg New York, pp 603–606

177. Blanken R, Nater JP, Veenhoff E (1987) Protection against epoxy resins with glove materials. Contact Dermatitis 16:46–47

178. Blanken R, Nater JP, Veenhoff E (1987) Protective effect of barrier creams and spray coatings against epoxy resins. Contact Dermatitis 16:79–83

179. Bruze M (1985) Contact sensitizers in resins based on phenol and formaldehyde. Acta Derm Venereol Suppl (Stockh) 119:1–83

180. Elvers B, Hawkins S, Schulz G (1991) Ullmann's encyclopedia of industrial chemistry, 5th completely revised edn, vol A19. VCH Verlagsgesellschaft, Weinheim, Germany, p 371

181. Estlander T, Tarvainen K, Jolanki R, Kanerva L (1993) Occupational sensitization to a resin binder used in rock wool. In: Books of abstracts, 3rd congress of the European Academy of Dermatology and Venereology, 26–30 September, Copenhagen, Denmark, p 283

182. Foussereau J, Cavelier C, Selig D (1976) Occupational eczema from para-tertiary-butylphenol formaldehyde resins: a review of the sensitizing resins. Contact Dermatitis 2:254–258

183. Schubert H, Agatha G (1979) Zur Allergennatur der paratert. Butylphenolformaldehydharze (The allergenic nature of p-tert-butylphenolformaldehyde resin, in German). Derm Beruf Umwelt 27:49–52

184. White IR (1990) Adhesives. In: Adams RM (ed) Occupational skin disease. Saunders, Philadelphia, Pennsylvania, pp 395–407

185. Barros MA, Baptista A, Correia TM, Azevedo F (1991) Patch testing in children: a study of 562 schoolchildren. Contact Dermatitis 25:156–159

186. Nielsen NH, Menne T (1992) Allergic contact sensitization in an unselected Danish population. The Glostrup Allergy Study, Denmark. Acta Derm Venereol (Stockh) 72:456–460

187. Dotterud LK, Falk ES (1995) Contact allergy in relation to hand eczema and atopic diseases in north Norwegian schoolchildren. Acta Paediatr 84:402–406

188. Zimerson E, Bruze M (2000) Sensitizing capacity of 5,5'-di-*tert*-butyl-2,2'-dihydorxy-(hydroxymethyl)-dibenzyl ethers in the guinea pig. Contact Dermatitis 43:72–78

189. Zimerson E, Bruze M (2000) Contact allergy to 5,5'-di-*tert*-butyl-2,2'-dihydroxy-(hydroxymethyl)-dibenzyl ethers, sensitizers, in p-*tert*-butylphenol-formaldehyde resin. Contact Dermatitis 43:20–26

190. Zimerson E, Bruze M (2002) Low-molecular-weight contact allergens in p-*tert*-butylphenol-formaldehyde resin. Am J Contact Dermat 13:190–197

191. Zimerson E, Bruze M (2002) Contact allergy to the monomers in p-*tert*-butylphenol-formaldehyde resin. Contact Dermatitis 47:147–153

192. Zimerson E, Bruze M (2002) Sensitizing capacity of two monomeric aldehyde components in p-*tert*-butylphenol-formaldehyde resin. Acta Derm Venereol (Stockh) 82:418–422

193. Zimerson E, Bruze M (1998) Contact allergy to the monomers of p-*tert*-butylphenol-formaldehyde resin in the guinea pig. Contact Dermatitis 39:222–226

194. Bruze M, Fregert S, Zimerson E (1985) Contact allergy to phenol-formaldehyde resins. Contact Dermatitis 12:81–86

195. Zimerson E, Bruze M, Goossens A (1999) Simultaneous p-*tert*-butylphenol-formaldehyde resin and p-*tert*-butylcatechol contact allergies in man and sensitizing capacities of p-*tert*-butylphenol and p-*tert*-butylcatechol in guinea pigs. J Occup Environ Med 41:23–28

196. Bruze M, Zimerson E (2002) Contact allergy to o-cresol – a sensitizer in phenol-formaldehyde resin. Am J Contact Dermat 13:198–200

197. Bruze M, Zimerson E (1985) Contact allergy to 3-methylol phenol, 2,4-dimethylol phenol and 2,6-dimethylol phenol. Acta Derm Venereol 65:548–551

198. Bruze M (1986) Sensitizing capacity of 4,4(1)-dihydroxy-(hydroxymethyl)-diphenyl methanes in the guinea pig. Acta Derm Venereol (Stockh) 66:110–116

199. Bruze M, Fregert S, Persson L, Zimerson E (1987) Contact allergy to 2,4'-dihydroxy-(hydroxymethyl)-diphenyl methanes. Sensitizers in a phenol-formaldehyde resin. Derm Beruf Umwelt 35:52–55

200. Bruze M, Fregert S, Persson L, Zimerson E (1986) Contact allergy to 4,4'-dihydroxy-(hydroxymethyl)-diphenyl methanes: sensitizers in a phenol-formaldehyde resin. J Invest Dermatol 87:617–623

201. Bruze M (1986) Sensitizing capacity of dihydroxydiphenyl methane (bisphenol F) in the guinea pig. Contact Dermatitis 14:228–232

202. Bruze M (1986) Sensitizing capacity of 2-methylol phenol, 4-methylol phenol and 2,4,6-trimethylol phenol in the guinea pig. Contact Dermatitis 14:32–38

203. Bruze M, Zimerson E (1985) Contact allergy to dihydroxydiphenyl methanes (bisphenol F). Derm Beruf Umwelt 33:216–220

204. Bruze M, Zimerson E (1997) Cross-reaction patterns in patients with contact allergy to simple methylol phenols. Contact Dermatitis 37:82–86

205. Bruze M (1986) Simultaneous reactions to phenol-formaldehyde resins colophony/hydroabietyl alcohol and balsam of Peru/perfume mixture. Contact Dermatitis 14:119–120

206. Fregert S (1980) Irritant dermatitis from phenol-formaldehyde resin powder. Contact Dermatitis 6:493

207. Bruze M, Almgren G (1988) Occupational dermatoses in workers exposed to resins based on phenol and formaldehyde. Contact Dermatitis 19:272–277

208. Kalimo K, Saarni H, Kytta J (1980) Immediate and delayed type reactions to formaldehyde resin in glass wool. Contact Dermatitis 6:496

209. Katsarou A, Armenaka M, Ale I, Koufou V, Kalogeromitros D (1999) Frequency of immediate reactions to the European standard series. Contact Dermatitis 41:276–279

210. Bruze M (1988) Patch testing with a mixture of 2 phenol-formaldehyde resins. Contact Dermatitis 19:116–119

211. Estlander T, Kostiainen M, Jolanki R, Kanerva L (1998) Active sensitization and occupational allergic contact dermatitis caused by para-tertiary-butylcatechol. Contact Dermatitis 38:96–100

212. Ulrich H (2001) Diisocyanates. In: Ulrich H (ed) Chemistry and technology of isocyanates, 1st edn. Wiley, Chichester, pp 315–467

213. Frick M, Zimerson E, Karlsson D, Marand A, Skarping G, Isaksson M, Bruze M (2004) Poor correlation between stated and found concentrations of diphenylmethane-4,4'-diisocyanate (4,4'-MDI) in petrolatum patch-test preparations. Contact Dermatitis 51:73–78

214. Thorpe D (2002) Isocyanates. In: Lee S (ed) The Huntsman polyurethanes book, 1st edn. Wiley, Chichester, pp 63–88

215. Estlander T, Keskinen H, Jolanki R, Kanerva L (1992) Occupational dermatitis from exposure to polyurethane chemicals. Contact Dermatitis 27:161–165

216. Zimmerman R (2002) Catalysts. In: Lee S (ed) The Huntsman polyurethanes book, 1st edn. Wiley, Chichester, pp 137–150

217. Anonymous (1996) Thermosetting plastics. Statue Book of the Swedish National Board of Occupational Safety and Health. AFS 1996:4

218. Zeiss CR, Kanellakes TM, Bellone JD, Levitz D, Pruzansky JJ, Patterson R (1980) Immunoglobulin E-mediated asthma and hypersensitivity pneumonitis with precipitating anti-hapten antibodies due to diphenylmethane diisocyanate (MDI) exposure. J Allergy Clin Immunol 65:347–352

219. Mowe G (1980) Health risks from isocyanates. Contact Dermatitis 6:44–45

220. Baur X (1991) Isocyanates. Clin Exp Allergy 21(Suppl 1):241–246

221. Rothe A (1976) Zur Frage arbeitsbedingter Hautschadigungen durch Polyurethanchemikalien (Occupational dermatoses due to polyurethane drugs, in German). Berufsdermatosen 24:7–24

222. Kanerva L, Lähteenmäki MT, Estlander T, Jolanki R, Keskinen H (1989) Allergic contact dermatitis from isocyanates. In: Frosch PJ, Dooms-Goossens A, Lachapelle JM, Rycroft RJG, Scheper RJ (eds) Current topics in contact dermatitis. Springer, Berlin Heidelberg New York, pp 366–379

223. Kanerva L, Estlander T, Jolanki R, Lahteenmaki MT, Keskinen H (1991) Occupational urticaria from welding polyurethane. J Am Acad Dermatol 24:825–826

224. Larsen TH, Gregersen P, Jemec GB (2001) Skin irritation and exposure to diisocyanates in orthopedic nurses working with soft casts. Am J Contact Dermat 12:211–214

225. Valks R, Conde-Salazar L, Barrantes OL (2003) Occupational allergic contact urticaria and asthma from diphenylmethane-4,4'-diisocyanatae. Contact Dermatitis 49:166–167

226. Tanaka K, Takeoka A, Nishimura F, Hanada S (1987) Contact sensitivity induced in mice by methylene bisphenyl diisocyanate. Contact Dermatitis 17:199–204

34

227. Thorne PS, Hillebrand JA, Lewis GR, Karol MH (1987) Contact sensitivity by diisocyanates: potencies and cross-reactivities. Toxicol Appl Pharmacol 87:155–165

228. Zissu D, Binet S, Limasset JC (1998) Cutaneous sensitization to some polyisocyanate prepolymers in guinea pigs. Contact Dermatitis 39:248–251

229. White IR, Stewart JR, Rycroft RJ (1983) Allergic contact dermatitis from an organic di-isocyanate. Contact Dermatitis 9:300–303

230. Malten KE (1984) Dermatological problems with synthetic resins and plastics in glues. Part I. Derm Beruf Umwelt 32:81–86

231. Malten KE (1984) Dermatological problems with synthetic resins and plastics in glues. Part II. Derm Beruf Umwelt 32:118–125

232. Rothe A (1992) Contact dermatitis from diisocyanates. Contact Dermatitis 26:285–286

233. Schroder C, Uter W, Schwanitz HJ (1999) Occupational allergic contact dermatitis, partly airborne, due to isocyanates and epoxy resin. Contact Dermatitis 41:117–118

234. Frick M, Isaksson M, Björkner B, Hindsen M, Pontén A, Bruze M (2003) Occupational allergic contact dermatitis in a company manufacturing boards coated with isocyanate lacquer. Contact Dermatitis 48:255–260

235. Frick M, Björkner B, Hamnerius N, Zimerson E (2003) Allergic contact dermatitis from dicyclohexylmethane-4,4′-diisocyanate. Contact Dermatitis 48:305–309

236. Thompson T, Belsito DV (1997) Allergic contact dermatitis from a diisocyanate in wool processing. Contact Dermatitis 37:239

237. Belsito DV (2003) Common shoe allergens undetected by commercial patch-testing kits: dithiodimorpholine and isocyanates. Am J Contact Dermat 14:95–96

238. Morgan CJ, Haworth AE (2003) Allergic contact dermatitis from 1,6-hexamethylene diisocyanate in a domestic setting. Contact Dermatitis 48:224

239. Goossens A, Detienne T, Bruze M (2002) Occupational allergic contact dermatitis caused by isocyanates. Contact Dermatitis 47:304–308

240. Mancuso G, Reggiani M, Berdondini RM (1996) Occupational dermatitis in shoemakers. Contact Dermatitis 34:17–22

241. Wilkinson SM, Cartwright PH, Armitage J, English JS (1991) Allergic contact dermatitis from 1,6-diisocyanatohexane in an anti-pill finish. Contact Dermatitis 25:94–96

242. Emmett EA (1976) Allergic contact dermatitis in polyurethane plastic moulders. J Occup Med 18:802–804

243. Malten KE (1977) 4,4′ diisocyanato dicyclohexyl methane (Hylene W): a strong contact sensitizer. Contact Dermatitis 3:344–346

244. King CM (1980) Contact sensitivity to hylene W. Contact Dermatitis 6:353–354

245. Israeli R, Smirnov V, Sculsky M (1981) Intoxication due to dicyclohexyl-methane-4-4′ diisocyanate exposure (author's translation). Int Arch Occup Environ Health 48:179–184

246. Fregert S (1967) Allergic contact reaction to diphenyl-4,4′-diisocyanate. Contact Dermatitis Newslett 2:17

247. Lidén C (1980) Allergic contact dermatitis from 4,4′-diisocyanatol-diphenyl methane (MDI) in a molder. Contact Dermatitis 6:301–302

248. Alomar A (1986) Contact dermatitis from a fashion watch. Contact Dermatitis 15:44–45

249. Tait CP, Delaney TA (1999) Reactions causing reactions: allergic contact dermatitis to an isocyanate metabolite but not to the parent compound. Australas J Dermatol 40:116–117

250. Bruynzeel DP, van der Wegen-Keijser MH (1993) Contact dermatitis in a cast technician. Contact Dermatitis 28:193–194

251. Van Joost T, Heule F, de Boer J (1987) Sensitization to methylenedianiline and para-structures. Contact Dermatitis 16:246–248

252. Le Coz CJ, El Aboubi S, Ball C (1999) Active sensitization to toluene di-isocyanate. Contact Dermatitis 41:104–105

253. Fregert S (1981) Formaldehyde dermatitis from a gypsum-melamine resin mixture. Contact Dermatitis 7:56

254. Belsito DV (1993) Textile dermatitis. Am J Contact Dermatitis 4:249

255. Bell HK, King CM (2002) Allergic contact dermatitis from urea-formaldehyde resin in medium-density fibreboard (MDF). Contact Dermatitis 46:247

256. Metzler-Brenckle L, Rietschel RL (2002) Patch testing for permanent-press allergic contact dermatitis. Contact Dermatitis 46:33–37

257. Ross JS, Rycroft RJ, Cronin E (1992) Melamine-formaldehyde contact dermatitis in orthopaedic practice. Contact Dermatitis 26:203–204

258. Vale PT, Rycroft RJ (1988) Occupational irritant contact dermatitis from fibreboard containing urea-formaldehyde resin. Contact Dermatitis 19:62

259. Dooms-Goossens AE, Debusschere KM, Gevers DM, Dupre KM, Degreef HJ, Loncke JP, Snauwaert JE (1986) Contact dermatitis caused by airborne agents. A review and case reports. J Am Acad Dermatol 15:1–10

260. Dooms-Goossens A, Bedert R, Vandaele M, Degreef H (1989) Airborne contact dermatitis due to triglycidylisocyanurate. Contact Dermatitis 21:202–203

261. McFadden JP, Rycroft RJ (1993) Occupational contact dermatitis from triglycidyl isocyanurate in a powder paint sprayer. Contact Dermatitis 28:251

262. Munro CS, Lawrence CM (1992) Occupational contact dermatitis from triglycidyl isocyanurate in a powder paint factory. Contact Dermatitis 26:59

263. Tarvainen K (1996) Occupational dermatoses from plastic composites based on polyester resins, epoxy resins and vinyl ester resins. People Work 11:1–66

264. Venables KM (1989) Low molecular weight chemicals, hypersensitivity, and direct toxicity: the acid anhydrides. Br J Ind Med 46:222–232

265. Jolanki R, Kanerva L, Estlander T (1997) Skin allergy caused by organic acid anhydrides. In: Amin S, Lahti A, Maibach HI (eds) Contact urticaria syndrome. CRC, Boca Raton, Fla., pp 217–224

266. Malten KE (1964) Occupational dermatoses in the processing of plastics. Trans St John's Hosp Dermatol Soc 59:78–113

267. Wehle U (1966) Occupational eczema caused by polyester. Allerg Asthma (Leipz) 12:184–186

268. Lidén C, Löfström A, Storgards-Hatam K (1984) Contact allergy to unsaturated polyester in a boatbuilder. Contact Dermatitis 11:262–264

269. Dooms-Goossens A, de Jonge G (1985) Contact allergy to unsaturated polyester in a boat builder. Letter to the editor. Contact Dermatitis 12:238

270. MacFarlane AW, Curley RK, King CM (1986) Contact sensitivity to unsaturated polyester resin in a limb prosthesis. Contact Dermatitis 15:301–303

271. Tarvainen K, Jolanki R, Estlander T (1993) Occupational contact allergy to unsaturated polyester resin cements. Contact Dermatitis 28:220–224

272. Bourne LB, Milner FJ (1963) Polyester resin hazards. Br J Ind Med 20:100–109

34

273. Meneghini CL, Rantuccio F, Riboldi A (1963) Klinisch-allergologische Beobachtungen bei beruflichen ekzematösen Kontakt-Dermatosen. Derm Beruf Umwelt 11:181–244

274. Sjöborg S, Fregert S, Trulsson L (1984) Contact allergy to styrene and related chemicals. Contact Dermatitis 10:94–96

275. Minamoto K, Nagano M, Yonemitsu K, Futatsuka M (2002) Allergic contact dermatitis from unsaturated polyester resin consisting of maleic anhydride, phthalic anhydride, ethylene glycol and dicyclopentadiene. Contact Dermatitis 46:62–63

276. Minamoto K, Nagano M, Inaoka T, Futatsuka M (2002) Allergic contact dermatitis due to methyl ethyl ketone peroxide, cobalt naphthenate and acrylates in the manufacture of fibreglass-reinforced plastics. Contact Dermatitis 46:58–59

277. Guin JD (2001) Sensitivity to adipic acid used in polyester synthesis. Contact Dermatitis 44:256–257

278. Pfaffli P, Jolanki R, Estlander T, Tarvainen K, Kanerva L (2002) Identification of sensitizing diethyleneglycol maleate in a two-component polyester cement. Contact Dermatitis 46:170–173

279. Bhushan M, Craven NM, Beck MH (1998) Contact allergy to methyl ethyl ketone peroxide and cobalt in the manufacture of fibreglass-reinforced plastics. Contact Dermatitis 39:203

280. Kanerva L, Tarvainen K, Estlander T (2000) Polyester resins. In: Kanerva L, Elsner P, Wahlberg JE, Maibach HI (eds) Handbook of occupational dermatology. Springer, Berlin Heidelberg New York, pp 602–606

281. Tarvainen K, Jolanki R, Forsman-Gronholm L, Estlander T, Pfaffli P, Juntunen J, Kanerva L (1993) Exposure, skin protection and occupational skin diseases in the glass-fibre-reinforced plastics industry. Contact Dermatitis 29:119–127

282. Tarvainen K, Kanerva L, Jolanki R (1995) Occupational dermatoses from the manufacture of plastic composite products. Am J Contact Dermatitis 6:95–104

283. Kanerva L, Estlander T, Alanko K, Pfaffli P, Jolanki R (1999) Occupational allergic contact dermatitis from unsaturated polyester resin in a car repair putty. Int J Dermatol 38:447–452

284. Schmunes E (1990) Solvents and plasticizers. In: Adams RM, (ed) Occupational skin diseases, 2nd edn. Saunders, Philadelphia, Pa., pp 439–461

285. Conde-Salazar L, Gonzalez MA, Guimaraens D, Romero L (1989) Occupational allergic contact dermatitis from styrene. Contact Dermatitis 21:112

286. Moscato G, Biscaldi G, Cottica D, Pugliese F, Candura S, Candura F (1987) Occupational asthma due to styrene: two case reports. J Occup Med 29:957–960

287. Bruze M, Fregert S, Gruvberger B (2000) Chemical skin burns. In: Menne T, Maibach HI (eds) Hand eczema. CRC, Boca Raton, Fla., pp 117–127

288. Haustein UF, Tegetmeyer L, Ziegler V (1985) Allergic and irritant potential of benzoyl peroxide. Contact Dermatitis 13:252–257

289. Vidovic R, Kansky A (1985) Contact dermatitis in workers processing polyvinyl chloride plastics. Derm Beruf Umwelt 33:104–105

290. Schulsinger C, Mollgaard K (1980) Polyvinyl chloride dermatitis not caused by phthalates. Contact Dermatitis 6:477–480

291. Tung RC, Taylor JS (1998) Contact dermatitis from polyvinyl chloride identification bands. Am J Contact Dermat 9:234–236

292. Fregert S, Rorsman H (1963) Hypersensitivity to epoxy resins used as plasticizers and stabilizers in polyvinyl chloride (PVC) resins. Acta Derm Venereol 43:10–13

293. Fregert S, Trulson L, Zimerson E (1982) Contact allergic reactions to diphenylthiourea and phenylisothiocyanate in PVC adhesive tape. Contact Dermatitis 8:38–42

294. Hills RJ, Ive FA (1993) Allergic contact dermatitis from di-isodecyl phthalate in a polyvinyl chloride identity band. Contact Dermatitis 29:94–95

295. Huh WK, Masuji Y, Tada J, Arata J, Kaniwa M (2001) Allergic contact dermatitis from a pyridine derivative in polyvinyl chloride leather. Am J Contact Dermat 12:35–37

296. Di Lernia V, Cameli N, Patrizi A (1989) Irritant contact dermatitis in a child caused by the plastic tube of an infusion system. Contact Dermatitis 21:339–340

297. Osmundsen PE (1980) Contact urticaria from nickel and plastic additives (butylhydroxytoluene, oleylamide). Contact Dermatitis 6:452–454

298. Sugiura K, Sugiura M, Hayakawa R, Shamoto M, Sasaki K (2002) A case of contact urticaria syndrome due to di(2-ethylhexyl) phthalate (DOP) in work clothes. Contact Dermatitis 46:13–16

299. Fregert S, Meding B, Trulsson L (1984) Demonstration of epoxy resin in stoma pouch plastic. Contact Dermatitis 10:106

300. Goh CL, Ho SF (1988) An outbreak of acneiform eruption in a polyvinyl chloride manufacturing factory. Derm Beruf Umwelt 36:53–57

301. Sugiura K, Sugiura M, Shiraki R, Hayakawa R, Shamoto M, Sasaki K, Itoh A (2002) Contact urticaria due to polyethylene gloves. Contact Dermatitis 46:262–266

302. Thestrup-Pedersen K, Madsen JB, Rasmussen K (1989) Cumulative skin irritancy from heat-decomposed polyethylene plastic. In: Frosch PJ, Dooms-Goossens A, Lachapelle JM, Rycroft RJG, Scheper RJ (eds) Current topics in contact dermatitis. Springer, Berlin Heidelberg New York, pp 412–416

303. Grimalt F, Romaguera C (1981) Contact dermatitis caused by polyamide trouser pockets. Derm Beruf Umwelt 29:35–39

304. Tanaka M, Kobayashi S, Miyakawa S (1993) Contact dermatitis from nylon 6 in Japan. Contact Dermatitis 28:250

305. Valsecchi R, Leghissa P, Piazzolla S, Cainelli T, Seghizzi P (1993) Occupational dermatitis from isothiazolinones in the nylon production. Dermatology 187:109–111

306. Savage J (1978) Chloracetamide in nylon spin finish. Contact Dermatitis 4:179

307. Batta K, McVittie S, Foulds IS (1999) Occupational allergic contact dermatitis from N,N-methylene-bis-5-methyl-oxazolidine in a nylon spin finish. Contact Dermatitis 41:165

308. Dooms-Goossens A, Duron C, Loncke J, Degreef H (1986) Contact urticaria due to nylon. Contact Dermatitis 14:63

309. Bruze M, Boman A, Bergqvist-Karlsson A, Björkner B, Wahlberg JE, Voog E (1988) Contact allergy to a cyclohexanone resin in humans and guinea pigs. Contact Dermatitis 18:46–49

310. Heine A, Laubstein B (1990) Contact dermatitis from cyclohexanone-formaldehyde resin (L2 resin) in a hair lacquer spray. Contact Dermatitis 22:108

311. Husain SL (1975) Dibutyl phthalate sensitivity. Contact Dermatitis 1:395

312. Calnan CD (1975) Dibutyl phthalate. Contact Dermatitis 1:388

313. Sneddon IB (1972) Dermatitis from dibutyl phthalate in an aerosol antiperspirant and deodorant. Contact Dermatitis Newslett 12:308

314. Wilkinson SM, Beck MH (1992) Allergic contact dermatitis from dibutyl phthalate, propyl gallate and hydrocortisone in Timodine. Contact Dermatitis 27:197

315. Smith EL, Calnan CD (1966) Studies in contact dermatitis. XVII. Spectacle frames. Trans St Johns Hosp Dermatol Soc 52:10–34

316. Oliwiecki S, Beck MH, Chalmers RJ (1991) Contact dermatitis from spectacle frames and hearing aid containing diethyl phthalate. Contact Dermatitis 25:264–265

317. Capon F, Cambie MP, Clinard F, Bernardeau K, Kalis B (1996) Occupational contact dermatitis caused by computer mice. Contact Dermatitis 35:57–58

318. Burrows D, Rycroft RJ (1981) Contact dermatitis from PTBP resin and tricresyl ethyl phthalate in a plastic nail adhesive. Contact Dermatitis 7:336–337

319. Hamanaka S, Hamanaka Y, Otsuka F (1992) Phthalic acid dermatitis caused by an organostannic compound, tributyl tin phthalate. Dermatology 184:210–212

320. Carlsen L, Andersen KE, Egsgaard H (1986) Triphenyl phosphate allergy from spectacle frames. Contact Dermatitis 15:274–277

321. Camarasa JG, Serra-Baldrich E (1992) Allergic contact dermatitis from triphenyl phosphate. Contact Dermatitis 26:264–265

322. Andersen KE (1977) Sensitivity to a flame retardant, Tris(2,3-dibromopropyl)phosphate (Firemaster LVT 23 P). Contact Dermatitis 3:297–300

323. Niklasson B, Björkner B (1989) Contact allergy to the UV-absorber Tinuvin P in plastics. Contact Dermatitis 21:330–334

324. Ikarashi Y, Tsuchiya T, Nakamura A (1994) Contact sensitivity to Tinuvin P in mice. Contact Dermatitis 30:226–230

325. Kanerva L, Jolanki R, Estlander T (1985) Organic pigment as a cause of plastic glove dermatitis. Contact Dermatitis 13:41–43

326. Jolanki R, Kanerva L, Estlander T (1987) Organic pigments in plastics can cause allergic contact dermatitis. Acta Derm Venereol Suppl (Stockh) 134:95–97

327. Shono M, Kaniwa MA (1999) Allergic contact dermatitis from a perinone-type dye C.I. Solvent Orange 60 in spectacle frames. Contact Dermatitis 41:181–184

328. Tsunoda T, Kaniwa MA, Shono M (2001) Allergic contact dermatitis from a perinone-type dye C.I. Solvent Red 179 in spectacle frames. Contact Dermatitis 45:166–167

329. Koch P, Nickolaus G (1996) Allergic contact dermatitis and mercury exanthem due to mercury chloride in plastic boots. Contact Dermatitis 34:405–409

330. Kanerva L, Kanervo K, Jolanki R, Estlander T (2001) Cobalt – a possible sensitizer in personal computer (PC) mouse and polyester resins. Contact Dermatitis 45:126–127

331. Goossens A, Bedert R, Zimerson E (2001) Allergic contact dermatitis caused by nickel and cobalt in green plastic shoes. Contact Dermatitis 45:172

Chapter 35

Topical Drugs

35

FRANCISCO M. BRANDÃO, AN GOOSSENS, ANTONELLA TOSTI

Contents

35.1 Incidence and Prevalence

Cutaneous adverse drug reactions are usually an iatrogenic disease induced in patients. More rarely, they are an occupational disease, either in health care personnel or in pharmaceutical industry employees.

The incidence of topical reactions to drugs varies from one area to another, and from one country to another, depending on local prescribing and self-medication habits. Prescribing habits are changing, and some medicaments that were common allergens 20–30 years ago, such as sulfonamides, penicillin, and antihistamines, have now been replaced by other allergenic drugs, such as nonsteroidal anti-inflammatory drugs (NSAID), and corticosteroids.

The real incidence of adverse reactions to topical medicaments is not known, and most of the data about prevalence are quite old. Bandmann et al. [1] found that 14% of 4,000 patients tested in several European countries were allergic to medicaments. Blondeel et al. [2] found a much higher incidence – 54.6%. Still, in Belgium [3], 17% of 2,025 patients were allergic to the ingredients of pharmaceutical products, while in Italy, in the 1980s [4], about 20.5% of 8,230 patients were allergic to topical drugs. In Sweden, 40% of all recorded allergic reactions were due to medicaments [5], which was equivalent to an annual incidence of 43/100,000. More recently, in Singapore [6], 22.5% of patients tested at a contact dermatitis clinic had medicament sensitivity. A more recent survey in Italy (1984–1993) disclosed a prevalence of 13.2% in patients with nonoccupational allergic contact dermatitis [7], while in Portugal, over a 6-year period (1998–2003), 18.0% of all patch-tested patients were sensitized to medicaments (Table 1). Such a high figure may be due to the existence and use of several topical medications still containing mercury compounds, neomycin, and other common sensitiz-

Table 1. Incidence of medicament contact allergy in Portugal, 1998–2003 (data from the Portuguese Contact Dermatitis Group)

Year	Total patients patch tested	Patch tests positive to medicaments	%
1998	4,154	740	17.8
1999	3,990	755	18.9
2000	3,625	675	18.6
2001	3,361	635	18.9
2002	2,681	490	18.3
2003	2,849	426	14.9
Total	20,660	3,721	18.0

ers. However, there is a trend of these figures to decrease in future.

These differences are due not only to geographic differences, but also to the type of patient selection – leg ulcer patients, anogenital dermatitis, for example – and to the specific interests of some investigators. A prevalence of allergic reactions to medicaments of about 15%, excluding leg ulcers or other high-risk patients, seems a realistic figure to be expected in a contact dermatitis clinic. However, this figure does not include other clinical entities, such as irritant contact dermatitis or contact urticaria, among others.

Core Message

■ A prevalence of up to 15% of allergic contact dermatitis to topical medicaments is, probably, a realistic figure in most contact clinics.

35.2 Factors Predisposing to Medicament Contact Dermatitis

Many factors may contribute, in various ways, to cutaneous drug sensitization. The environment, on the whole, must be considered to be the more important contributing factor, although there is some individual predisposition, which mainly depends on genetic factors. The intrinsic sensitizing potential of each drug is by far the most important factor (see Chap. 3), although sometimes impurities, contaminants, and degradation of products may be the allergenic material [4]. Moreover, compound allergy [8] and quenching phenomena [9] may interfere with this intrinsic capacity. However, many of the more potent allergens, such as sulfonamides and penicillin, have now been almost banished from our prescribing habits and from the market; on the other hand, some weak sensitizers, such as neomycin, are so widely used that several new cases are seen every year.

The use of medicaments in high concentrations or in vehicles that increase skin penetration favors their irritant and sensitizing capacities. The same applies when medications are used in folds, under occlusive dressings or in transdermal devices, both of which lead to a much greater skin absorption and, thus, increase the probability of developing contact allergy.

Damage to the skin barrier is another very important factor favoring sensitization. Leg ulcer and stasis dermatitis patients are known to have a very high incidence of medicament allergy [3, 4]. In addition, patients with otitis externa, eye problems, perianal and vulval dermatoses, and chronic hand and foot dermatitis are known to frequently develop secondary medicament allergy.

In other chronic dermatological conditions, however, such as atopic dermatitis and psoriasis, this possibly increased contact allergy seems to be an open question. In atopic patients, the defective T-cell population and the difficulty in sensitizing patients to dinitrochlorobenzene (DNCB) would suggest that these patients would not develop allergic contact dermatitis as often as nonatopic individuals [10]. This seems to be confirmed in some reports [11, 12], although others consider that atopic patients become sensitized to topical medicaments at least as often as nonatopic patients [13–15].

It has also been suggested that psoriatic patients are not easily sensitized [16, 17], and that sensitization could be associated with certain localizations (palmoplantar and flexural [18]), although this could not be confirmed by other authors [19, 20]. Sensitization was found to be equal in other patients, especially to antipsoriatic medicaments [21–24], although seemingly less to corticosteroids [19, 25].

Core Message

■ The use of medicaments under occlusion or in folds increases its absorption and allergenic potential. It is not unanimous if atopic and psoriatic patients really do sensitize more or less to topical medicaments.

35.3 Clinical Patterns of Contact Reactions

Allergic contact dermatitis is by far the more common and more important clinical entity caused by topical drugs. However, other pathological clinical entities, through direct cutaneous aggression, by immunoallergic mechanisms, or by local or systemic pharmacological effects, may be caused by medicaments (Table 2) [26–29].

35.3.1 Irritant Contact Dermatitis

There are several medicaments that can irritate the skin [26, 30] (Table 3). Most are well-known mildly irritant drugs, and their irritancy is usually expected,

35

Table 2. Clinical patterns of eruptions caused by topical medicaments [26–29]

Allergic contact dermatitis
Irritant contact dermatitis
Photoallergic contact dermatitis
Phototoxic contact dermatitis
Contact urticaria
Photocontact urticaria
Dermographism
Airborne allergic contact dermatitis
Airborne irritant contact dermatitis
Airborne photoallergic contact dermatitis
Airborne phototoxic contact dermatitis
Erythema-multiforme-like eruptions
Lichenoid contact dermatitis
Purpuric contact dermatitis
Skin necrosis
Dyschromia
Pustular contact dermatitis
Lymphomatoid contact dermatitis
Acne/folliculitis/rosacea
Granulomatous eruption
Interactions with cutaneous microbial flora
Pharmacological local effects
Systemic side-effects

Table 3. Topical drugs that can induce irritant contact dermatitis (adapted from [26, 30])

Oxidizing agents	Hydrogen peroxide, benzoyl peroxide, cantharidin, sodium hypochlorite, potassium permanganate, bromine, iodine, povidone-iodine
Denaturing agents	Formaldehyde, mercuric chloride
Keratolytic drugs	Salicylic acid, sulfur compounds, resorcinol, pyrogallol
Organic solvents	Alcohols, propylene glycol, ethyl ether, chloroform, acetone
Antineoplastic drugs	Carmustine, mechlorethamine, 5-fluorouracil
Other compounds	Quaternary ammonium compounds, tar, dithranol, thimerosal, gentian violet, brilliant green, hexachlorophene, mercurial compounds, chlorhexidine, capsaicin, nonsteroidal anti-inflammatory drugs, tretinoin, calcipotriol, urea, lactic acid and other α-hydroxy acids, dimethylsulfoxide, phenol, monobenzone, podophyllotoxin, selenium sulfide, methyl nicotinate

and sometimes desired, as part of their therapeutic action – tretinoin, benzoyl peroxide, 5-fluorouracil, dithranol, sulfur compounds, and others. The first contact usually does not produce any visual alteration or abnormal subjective sensation. However, after repeated contact, the skin becomes dry, erythematous, and scaly, with pruritus or burning sensation, usually confined to the application area [26]. If applied for a longer time, in higher concentrations, or in occluded areas, they may cause acute irritant contact dermatitis with edema, erythema, vesicles, or bullae that may be difficult to differentiate from allergic contact dermatitis.

Airborne irritant contact dermatitis predominates in exposed areas, but, as opposed to photosensitive dermatitis, it does not spare areas such as the upper eyelids, retroauricular folds, or submental area.

The subjective irritant sensation of "stinging" may be immediate or delayed, and may be caused by several drugs (see Chap. 15).

35.3.2 Contact Urticaria

Since the first reports [31], the contact urticaria syndrome (CUS) has been frequently studied. It includes the localized cutaneous forms (immunological and nonimmunological), as well as a broad spectrum of noncutaneous involvement (generalized urticaria, asthma, and anaphylaxis). The list of medicaments causing immunological contact urticaria (ICU) or nonimmunological contact urticaria (NICU) is very long (Table 4) [32–37] (see also Chap. 5). Chlorpromazine has been reported as causing photocontact urticaria [38].

35.3.3 Other Important Clinical Patterns

Topical medicaments may cause other noneczematous contact reactions (see Chap. 21). Erythema-multiforme-like eruptions or urticarial papular and plaque eruption may be caused by several drugs [26–28, 39–41] (Table 5). This eruption is usually preceded by an eczematous allergic reaction, which becomes urticarial, disseminates after a few days, and persists longer than the initial reaction.

Skin necrosis induced by medicaments is a rare event. Gentian violet and brilliant green may cause necrosis, especially when applied in the genital area [42]. Quaternary ammonium compounds in high concentration [43], dichlorhexidine, 5-fluorouracil, phenol, and povidone iodine have also been incriminated as causing skin necrosis [26, 44].

Purpuric reactions may be due to proflavine [45] and benzoyl peroxide [46]. Aminoglycoside antibiotics can cause lichenoid reactions [47], as can mercury in dental amalgams; its removal sometimes improves the oral lesions [48, 49]. Mercury salts may also cause either hyper- or hypopigmentation [50].

Table 4. Topical drugs that can induce immunological contact urticaria (ICU) and nonimmunological contact urticaria (NICU) [32–37]

NICU	ICU
Alcohols	Alcohols
Benzoic acid/sodium benzoate	Antibiotics
Benzocaine	Ampicillin
Camphor	Bacitracin
Capsaicin	Cephalosporins
DMSO	Chloramphenicol
Formaldehyde	Clioquinol
Nicotinic acid esters	Gentamicin
Sorbic acid/sorbates	Mezlocillin
Tar extracts	Neomycin
Tincture of benzoin	Penicillin
	Rifamycin
	Streptomycin
	Virginiamycin
	Aescin
	Benzocaine
	Lidocaine
	Carboxymethyl cellulose
	Benzophenone
	Phenothiazines
	Promethazine
	Chlorpromazine
	Levomeprazine
	Nonsteroidal anti-inflammatory drugs
	Aminophenazone
	Diclofenac
	Etofenamate
	Ketoprofen
	Loxoprofen
	Propoxyphen butazone
	Salicylic acid
	Mechlorethamine
	Ketoconazole
	Clobetasol propionate
	Polyethylene glycol
	Polysorbate 60
	Parabens
	Cetyl alcohol
	Nicotine
	Pentamidine
	Pilocarpine
	Polyvinyl pyrrolidone

Table 5. Topical drugs inducing erythema-multiforme-like eruptions [26–28, 39–41]

Ethylenediamine	Phenylbutazone
Pyrrolnitrin	Econazole
Sulfonamides	IDU
Promethazine	Furazolidone
Mephenesin	Nifuroxime
Mafenide	Scopolamine hydrobromide
Proflavine	Mechlorethamine
Clioquinol	Povidone iodine
Chloramphenicol	DNCB
Neomycin	Diphenylcyclopropenone
Lincomycin	Ketoprofen
Vitamin E	Bufexamac
Tea tree oil	

35

The effects of the application of topical corticosteroids, mainly potent fluorinated steroids, over long periods are well known. Women with a seborrheic diathesis, using steroids on the face, may develop acneiform or rosaceiform eruptions, perioral dermatitis, or hypertrichosis, leading to so-called topical drug addiction [51]. On the face, as well as in other areas, they induce cutaneous atrophy, telangiectasia, purpura, ecchymoses (which evolve into pseudostellariae scars), susceptibility to minor trauma, striae distensae, and vellus hair growth [26, 52]. When applied on skin infections, mainly tinea, but also other fungal, viral, or parasitic diseases, they can mask and aggravate the pre-existing disease, leading, for example, to "tinea incognito" or converting common scabies into the "Norwegian" type.

Long-term application of potent corticosteroids to the whole skin promotes skin absorption of large amounts of the drug, which may induce Cushing's syndrome [53].

The percutaneous absorption of other drugs can rarely provoke toxic systemic effects. The degree of absorption depends on the physicochemical properties of the substance, the use of occlusive dressings, the vehicle in which the substance is incorporated, the drug concentration, the site of application, age, temperature, and the integrity of the skin barrier [26]. Boric acid, carmustine, clindamycin, gentamicin, hexachlorphene, lindane, malathion, mercurial compounds, phenol, salicylic acid, and selenium sulfide [26] represent some of the drugs that have been noted to cause systemic toxicity.

Core Message

- Beyond allergic contact dermatitis, topical drugs may induce several other clinical patterns, like irritant dermatitis, contact urticaria, erythema multiforme, skin necrosis, purpuric and lichenoid reactions, hyper and hypopigmentation, and others.

35.3.4 Allergic Contact Dermatitis

Most contact reactions to medicaments are of the allergic type, whether by direct contact, or an airborne or photoallergic mechanism. They usually arise as a complication of a pre-existing, possibly eczematous, dermatosis.

The clinical picture is usually an acute dermatitis – erythema, edema, papules, and vesicles, sometimes with exudation and scaling, and always accompanied by intense pruritus. When a previous dermatosis is being treated, aggravation of the picture may suggest superimposed sensitization. However, particularly if the sensitization is due to a corticosteroid or to an ingredient of a corticosteroid cream, this acute picture is usually mild or absent due to the anti-inflammatory properties of the steroid. In these circumstances, if the dermatosis does not improve, despite correct treatment, a secondary contact allergy should be suspected.

In patients with stasis dermatitis and/or leg ulcers, or other chronic eczemas, it is not rare to see dissemination of the eczema (hematogenous route – systemic contact dermatitis) to the other leg at first, then to the entire integument, leading sometimes to erythroderma; this is mainly seen in older patients with long-standing eczemas. Sometimes, there is scant local symptomatology, and the first acute symptoms are seen at a distance, usually by ectopic dissemination (on the face, for example). In our experience, elderly patients with eyelid dermatitis should arouse the suspicion of allergy to topical drugs applied on the lower limbs, i.e., NSAID and venotropic drugs.

Airborne [54] and photoallergic contact dermatitis have a similar clinical expression – acute or subacute dermatitis on exposed areas. They differ from toxic dermatitis because they have a more polymorphic clinical picture, not precisely limited to exposed areas. However, as stated with the irritant type, there are some locations spared in photodermatitis, which may be affected in the airborne type, such as the upper eyelids, under the chin, behind the ears, the back of the neck, or even the scalp.

35.4 Allergens

Topical medicaments include active principles and ingredients of the vehicles, many of which are found in cosmetics. Most substances in a medicament may, at some point, induce cutaneous sensitization.

35.4.1 Local Anesthetics

The esters of p-aminobenzoic acid (PABA), benzocaine, procaine (Novocaine), and amethocaine (tetracaine) are allergenic topical anesthetics [55, 56]. They were often used to treat pruritus ani, hemorrhoids [57, 58], or pruritus vulvae [59], but occupational cases have been reported [60]. Nowadays, they have largely been replaced by anesthetics of other groups. They may cross-react with other components of the para-group, especially with p-phenylenediamine.

Dibucaine (cinchocaine), a quinoline derivative, is currently more frequently used in such medicaments. It can also cause allergic contact dermatitis [55, 61–64] and systemic contact dermatitis [65].

The amide derivative group, lidocaine (lignocaine, xylocaine), bupivacaine (Marcaine), mepivacaine (Carbocaine), and prilocaine (Citanest), are less potent sensitizers. However, as they are now more often used than p-aminobenzoic esters, there have been several cases of sensitization reported. Since the first descriptions [66, 67], many other cases of allergy to lidocaine have been reported [68, 69], mainly from Australia [68], where there are several over-the-counter products containing lidocaine. It cross-reacts with mepivacaine and less often with bupivacaine and prilocaine [68]. Contact sensitization to prilocaine is rare [70], and it has been primarily induced by EMLA cream [71, 72]; in none of these cases was there cross-reaction with lidocaine.

Several other, mainly local, anesthetics, including butacaine, proxymetacaine (proparacaine) [73], oxybuprocaine (in ophthalmic preparations) [74], propipocaine, pramocaine (pramoxine), amylocaine, cyclomethycaine, propanidid (intravenous anesthetic), diclonine hydrochloride [26, 55], and butylaminobenzoate [75] have been reported as sensitizers.

Core Message

■ Benzocaine and other p-aminobenzoic derivatives may cross-react with components of the para-group, but are less used nowadays. Dibucaine and lidocaine and derivatives, which are more often used, are less potent sensitizers, but several cases of allergic contact dermatitis have been reported.

35.4.2 Antibiotics and Antimicrobials

Antibiotics and other antimicrobials and antiseptics that are used on the skin may cause contact allergy. Their sensitizing capacity is quite variable, depending not only on their intrinsic potential, but also on percutaneous penetration, site of application, and frequency of prescription and use.

Aminoglycoside antibiotics, especially neomycin, form the most important group of topical antibiotics. Neomycin, which is included in the standard series, has a wide range of use and is rarely used systemically. It is often combined with topical corticosteroids, not only for use on the skin, but also in many eye and ear preparations (Fig. 1). This association may mask the neomycin sensitization, due to the corticosteroid anti-inflammatory activity. In most statistics, neomycin appears as the leading allergenic medicament [1, 3, 4, 76–79]. Gentamicin is less often used and seems to be less allergenic than neomycin [77, 78, 80], with which it may cross-react [76, 81]. Other less frequently used aminoglycosides are mainly found in ophthalmic and ear preparations, or sensitize through occupational medical or veterinary contact – streptomycin, tobramycin, kanamycin, paromomycin, ribostamycin, amikacin, sisomicin, framycetin (neomycin B, soframycin). With the exception of streptomycin, aminoglycosides often cross-react [76, 78, 81–83].

Tylosin tartrate, virginiamycin, and spiramycin are mainly of veterinary use. Veterinary surgeons and farmers are those usually affected [84, 85]. Virginiamycin can cross-react with pristinamycin.

Bacitracin causes contact urticaria [86] and contact allergy, especially in leg ulcers/stasis dermatitis patients [87–91]. The concomitance of reactions to both neomycin and polymyxin B [88, 91] is not due to cross-reaction, but to their frequent association in topical medicaments [92]. Contact allergy to chloramphenicol is uncommon and is usually due to the use of eye preparations [77, 93]. As with other antimicrobials, allergy to sodium fusidate seems to occur especially in leg ulcer patients [79, 90, 94]. Tetracyclines [95], clindamycin [96] (which may cross-react with lincomycin), and mupirocin [97] are generally rare sensitizers. Erythromycin base is a weak sensitizer [98], but its salts (sulfate, stearate, and ethylsuccinate) may more readily induce contact allergy [99].

In the past, penicillin became a frequent sensitizer in some countries [1], but nowadays, it is hardly used topically. Semi-synthetic penicillins and derivatives – ampicillin, amoxycillin, pivampicillin, cloxacillin, and cephalosporins (first, second, or third generation) – can cause either allergic contact dermatitis [100–104] or contact urticaria [105, 106] in health care personnel, pharmaceutical industry workers, veterinary surgeons, or farmers.

Having been one of the major sensitizers some decades ago [1, 4], topical sulfonamides are now very little used in skin products. They are still present in ophthalmic preparations (sulfathiazole and sulfacetamide) and vaginal creams (sulfathiazole), but reports of sensitization are scarce. Sulfanilamide-containing powders and creams may, however, be a problem in leg ulcer patients [89], and mafenide (4-homosulphanilamide) can still be a common allergen in some countries [107]. Silver sulfadiazine, marketed in some countries for use on burns, seems to be almost nonallergenic and does not cross-react with other sulfonamides [108].

Nitrofurazone is a local antiseptic used in ointment or lubricated dressings for wounds and burns. It is a well known sensitizer that can induce very severe reactions in some patients [76, 109]. Clioquinol (Vioform) and chlorquinaldol (Sterosan) are usually combined with corticosteroids in topical preparations. They are weak sensitizers and may cross-react, clioquinol being the more important of the two allergens [79, 110].

One of the most extensively used local antiseptics in the present day is povidone iodine. Besides skin irritation and necrosis, there have been a few reports of contact allergy [89, 111] and contact urticaria [36]. Thimerosal (thiomersal) contains two sensitizing

35

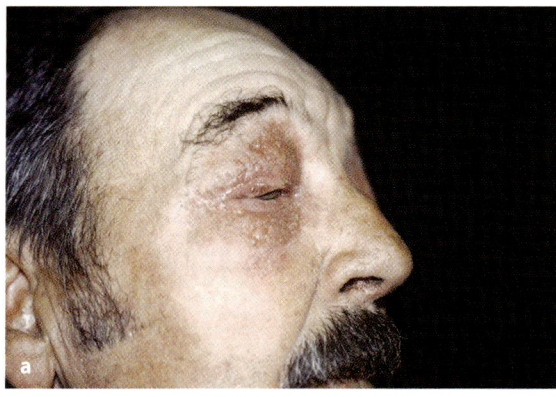
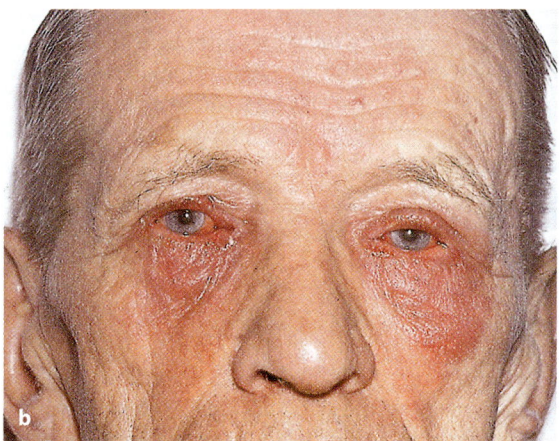

Fig. 1a, b. Allergic contact dermatitis from neomycin in eyedrops (**a**) and associated with severe conjunctivitis (**b**) (courtesy of P.J. Frosch)

moieties, mercury and thiosalicylic acid [112]. It is used in merthiolate tincture, and as a preservative in vaccines, toxoids, contact lens solutions, and other eye preparations. The relevance of a positive patch test to thimerosal is usually very difficult to establish. Most cases seem to be due either to vaccines or to ophthalmic products [113–115]. Patients sensitized to the thiosalicylic moiety of thimerosal are at risk of developing photosensitization to piroxicam [112, 116]. Other mercury compounds include merbromin and phenylmercury salts. Merbromin (mercurochrome) had wide use in Portugal, Spain, and certain other countries, but its use has now almost been abandoned; it may cause anaphylaxis [117]. Quaternary ammonium compounds are widely used antiseptics and disinfectants, and can cause irritation and necrosis, as well as contact sensitization [118].

Triphenylmethane dyes include gentian violet (pyoctanin), brilliant green, malachite green, methyl green, rosaniline, chrysoidine, and eosin. They are rare sensitizers [119, 120].

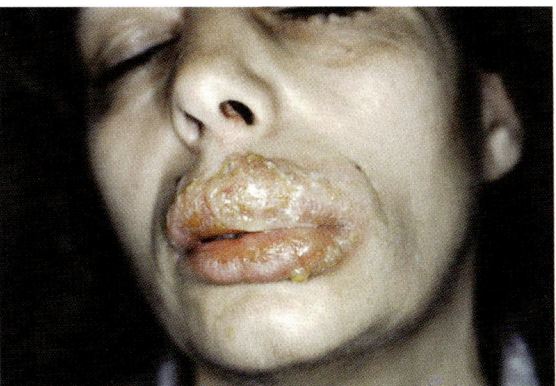

Fig. 2. Acute allergic contact dermatitis from tromantadine HCl

Core Message

■ Neomycin is still a frequent allergen and may cross-react with most aminoglycosides, with the exception of streptomycin. Penicillin and sulfonamides are, currently, rare sensitizers. Bacitracin can cause immediate and delayed reactions and, often, reacts simultaneously with neomycin and polymyxin B.

35.4.3 Antivirals

Tromantadine hydrochloride and acyclovir are the two most widely prescribed antiviral drugs. Tromantadine is a potent sensitizer, with several cases of contact allergy reported [121–123]. It usually causes a very severe acute exudative eczema around the lips, characteristically in patients who have already used tromantadine several times for treatment of recurrent herpes simplex (Fig. 2). Acyclovir, although much more extensively used, is a weak sensitizer [124, 125]. Some of the cases of contact dermatitis from Zovirax cream are probably due to compound allergy [126]. Patients with allergic contact dermatitis to acyclovir may develop systemic contact dermatitis to valaciclovir, ganciclovir, and famciclovir [127–129], the only valid alternatives being foscarnet and cidofovir [129]. Idoxuridine (IDU) [123, 130] and triflu-

ridine [131] are mainly used in ophthalmologic preparations.

Core Message

■ Acyclovir is a weak allergen. Patients sensitized to this antiviral may develop systemic contact dermatitis if administered valaciclovir, ganciclovir, or famciclovir.

35.4.4 Antimycotics

Most antimycotics can cause contact allergy, among them are hydroxyquinoline, undecylenic acid [132] and its derivatives, pyrrolnitrin, nystatin [133], tolnaftate [134], naftifine [135], and amorolfine [136, 137], as well as several imidazole derivatives, for which contact and cross-allergic reactions have been missed because of problems with the correct choice of vehicle for patch testing [138]. An extensive study on the sensitizing capacity (in guinea pigs) of imidazoles [139, 140], triazoles – mostly used in agriculture [140] – and azoles [141] was performed by Hausen et al. and they could demonstrate that imidazoles, the most commonly used antimycotics, have only very weak sensitization properties compared to, for example, naftifine [139]. The most frequently reported imidazoles having caused allergic contact dermatitis [see 138–140 for a review] are the substances most commonly used, i.e., miconazole, econazole, isoconazole – which may provoke pustular contact dermatitis [142] – and tioconazole [143] (probably due to its use at a 28% concentration in a nail solution) (Fig. 3). Croconazole, which is only marketed in the Far East,

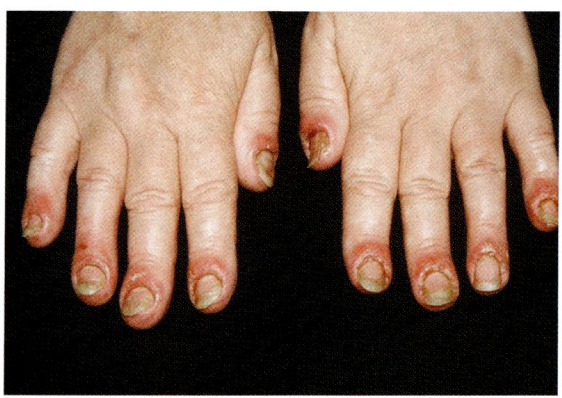

Fig. 3. Paronychia due to allergic contact dermatitis from tioconazole nail solution (courtesy of O. Bordalo)

seems to be a strong allergen, both clinically and experimentally [see 140 for a review]. Clotrimazole, considered to be an unusual allergen [144], but reported as an occupational allergen in a nurse [145], sulconazole, ketoconazole, oxiconazole, bifonazole – which showed a moderate sensitizing capacity [140] – enilconazole, and fenticonazole [138,146] have been less frequently reported as causes of contact allergy.

Cross-sensitivity has been reported mainly within the group of the phenylmethylimidazoles, for example, between miconazole, econazole, and isoconazole, as well as sulconazole, and also between isoconazole and tioconazole [138,147], but not ketoconazole. They do not seem to cross-react with the phenylmethylimidazoles, i.e., clotrimazole, bifonazole, and croconazole, for which cross-reactions between them may [148], but not necessarily [149], occur. The more recent reports concern neticonazole [150–152] (with possible cross-reactivity with econazole and sulconazole [150]), lanoconazole [152–156] – all from Japan – and sertaconazole (cross-reactivity to miconazole and econazole) [157].

Drug eruptions after systemic administration have been described, such as immediate reactions to ketoconazole [158,159], systemic reactions to nystatin – also in lozenges [160] – and a generalized exanthematous pustulosis (confirmed by a positive patch test result) to terbinafine [161].

Core Message

■ The imidazoles are not strong sensitizers, but as they are very extensively used, several cases have been described. Cross-reaction between them has been reported mainly within the group of

phenylethylimidazoles (miconazole, econazole, isoconazole, sulconazole, and tioconazole). Systemic contact dermatitis may occur with antimycotics.

35.4.5 Corticosteroids

Contact allergy to corticosteroids is now a well established phenomenon, and cases from all over the world have been reported in the literature. The incidence of the reactions observed, however, varies and depends on several factors, such as the nature and amount of corticosteroids used in each country, prescription habits, the awareness among the medical profession of the importance of corticosteroid sensitivity, the selection of the patients and their referral to test centers, the routine testing of screening agents for corticosteroid sensitivity, as well as of all the corticosteroids used by the patient, and the test and reading methods used (see [162, 163] for a review, [164,165]).

Patients with contact allergy to corticosteroids generally present with a chronic dermatitis that is not exacerbated by, but fails to respond to, corticosteroid therapy. Indeed, the allergenic and simultaneous anti-inflammatory effects of topical corticosteroids cause a nonspecific self-supporting eczematous condition, which is rarely recognized as a potentially iatrogenic sensitivity [162–164].

Although infrequent relative to the large scale of their use, allergic reactions may also arise to the corticosteroids administered by inhalation in the treatment of rhinitis or bronchial asthma [162–164]. Generalized reactions may, of course, also occur after systemic administration (oral, intravenous, intra-articular). The lesions may manifest themselves mainly as eczema, exanthema, purpura, urticaria, and so on [163, 166, 167], with type IV or delayed hypersensitivity [168] being much more common than type I or immediate hypersensitivity [169, 170].

In general, corticosteroid-sensitive patients react upon patch testing to several corticosteroids. This may, in part, be because most of them have used large numbers of corticosteroids and would, thus, be vulnerable to concomitant sensitization. However, irrefutable proof for the existence of cross-reactions is provided by reactions to substances to which the patient has never been exposed. Studies in this regard can have practical consequences for the identification of screening agents and for advice regarding the topical and systemic corticosteroids that the corticosteroid-sensitive patient can safely use. Our earlier

Table 6. The new classification of corticosteroids based on cross-reaction patterns

	Characteristics of the group	Typical members	Possible cross-reactions with corticosteroids outside the group
Group A	No methyl substitution on C16, no side chain on C17, possibly short side chain on C21	Cloprednol, fludrocortisone acetate, hydrocortisone, methylprednisolone, prednisolone, tixocortol pivalate	D2 group labile steroids: hydrocortisone aceponate, hydrocortisone-17-butyrate, methylprednisolone aceponate, prednicarbate
Group B	Cis diol or ketal function on C16 and C17, possibly a side chain on C21	Budesonide (R-isomer), amcinonide, desonide, fluocinolone acetonide, triamcinolone acetonide	–
Group C	Methyl substitution on C16, no side chain on C17, possibly a side chain on C21	Betamethasone dexamethasone, flumethasone pivalate, halomethasone	–
Group D1	Methyl substitution on C16 (so far halogenation on the basic structure), side-chain ester on C17, and often also on C21	Betamethasone, dipropionate, betamethasone-17-valerate, clobetasol propionate, fluticasone propionate, momethasone furoate	–
Group D2	No methyl substitution on C16 (up to now no halogenation of the four-ring structure), side-chain ester on C17, possibly a side chain on C21	Hydrocortisone aceponate, hydrocortisone buteprate, hydrocortisone-17-butyrate, methylprednisolone aceponate, prednicarbate	Budesonide S-isomer, Group A corticosteroids

studies led us to suggest four groups of cross-reacting molecules [171], which, in the light of new findings [172], were subclassified as regards to the ester-type corticosteroids (Table 6).

Indeed, when testing Group D molecules, contact-allergic reactions are frequently observed with substances such as hydrocortisone-17-butyrate, -aceponate, and -buteprate, as well as methylprednisolone aceponate and prednicarbate, rather than with molecules as betamethasone and its esters, such as valerate and dipropionate, diflucortolone valerate, diflorasone diacetate, clobetasol propionate, clobetasone butyrate, and also the newer mometasone furoate and fluticasone propionate (now classified as Group D1). The former esters can be classified as the more sensitizing D2 corticosteroid molecules. They are "pro-drug" corticosteroids that, because of their high lipophilicity, easily penetrate the skin, where they break down into the corresponding structures with the hydroxyl group at the C21 and/or C17 positions. As regards the influence of the skin metabolization of corticosteroids, patch test results have shown [172] that, for instance, positive reactions to "labile" molecules such as prednicarbate and methylprednisolone aceponate correlate significantly with reactions obtained with Group A corticosteroids ($P<0.01$), to

which the metabolized prednisolone [173] and methylprednisolone [174] belong. This mechanism might also account for cross-reactions that have been observed between hydrocortisone and hydrocortisone-17-butyrate (our own data and [175]), the latter being able to be converted to hydrocortisone-21-butyrate, which is rapidly hydrolyzed to form hydrocortisone [176]. However, individual skin metabolization characteristics certainly influence the cross-sensitivity patterns observed [172, 177].

Thus, not only the molecular configuration, but also other factors, such as the presence of certain substituents, the role of which is still being discussed and more than one site of immune recognition might be involved [177], the solubility in the vehicle used, the patch-test conditions [178], and the skin penetration [177] seem to be critical for the allergenic and the cross-reaction potential of individual corticosteroids.

As most contact allergies are missed if corticosteroids are not routinely tested, it has been recommended [179] to add tixocortol pivalate (0.1% pet.) (screening agent for Group A) [180, 181] and budesonide (0.01% pet.) (screening agent for acetonides and the labile esters [182]) to the standard series, although a uniform agreement on the patch-test concentration has not been achieved, with some authors favoring lower [183, 184] and others higher [185, 186] patch-test concentrations.

Should a corticosteroid sensitivity be detected, more extensive corticosteroid series should be tested, if possible, to determine cross-reactivity patterns, so that appropriate advice for the future can be given both for local and for systemic corticosteroid therapy [187].

> **Core Message**
>
> ■ Allergic contact dermatitis to corticosteroids is more common than previously judged, and should be suspected whenever a chronic dermatitis is exacerbated by or does not respond to local corticosteroid therapy. Four groups of cross-reacting molecules have been proposed. It has been recommended that budesonide and tixocortol pivalate should be added to the standard series as screening agents for corticosteroid allergy.

35.4.6 Antihistamines

Topical antihistamines are mainly used for their antipruritic properties. However, their sensitizing capacity greatly exceeds their beneficial effects. Beyond that, oral antihistamines or chemically related substances may induce systemic contact dermatitis in patients topically sensitized. Thus, they are now becoming less frequently used [188]. Diphenhydramine (which belongs to the ethanolamine group) can cause allergic [189] and photoallergic contact dermatitis [190], chorpheniramine is a sensitizer, either in topical application [62] or in eye drops [191], and promethazine and chlorpromazine (which are phenothiazines) are well known sensitizers and photosensitizers. Promethazine cream still exists in some European countries, including Portugal, and several cases of allergy and photoallergy are seen every year. Chlorpromazine, which is now much less employed, previously sensitized mainly health care personnel handling this medicament and pharmaceutical industry workers [192].

More recently, doxepin, a tricyclic antidepressive drug with antihistamine activity, has been widely used for pruritus relief. Some cases of allergic and systemic contact dermatitis have been reported [193–197].

35.4.7 Nonsteroidal Anti-Inflammatory Drugs

Topical nonsteroidal anti-inflammatory drugs (NSAIDs) have been introduced to the market in the past few decades for the treatment of soft tissue trauma, inflammatory and musculoskeletal disorders, and some inflammatory skin diseases as an alternative to topical corticosteroids. They have the advantage of being simple to apply, of having low systemic absorption, and of avoiding the well known systemic side-effects [198, 199]. However, they do cause frequent local side effects, which led to the withdrawal of some of these substances from the market – benoxaprofen, suprofen, and, in some countries, phenylbutazone and oxyphenbutazone [198].

They belong to eight different groups [198]: salicylates, pyrazolone derivatives, p-aminophenol derivatives, indometacin and sulindac, arylacanoic acid, tolmetins, arylpropionic acid derivatives, and oxicans. Cutaneous side effects include skin irritation, phototoxicity, contact urticaria, erythema-multiforme-like eruptions, and, mainly, allergic and photoallergic contact dermatitis. Since many of these compounds may also be used systemically, the possibility of the development of systemic contact dermatitis, in patients topically sensitized, must always be borne in mind [200–202].

With the exception of pyrazolones and bufexamac, which are used in northern European countries, most of the reports in the literature were coming from the Mediterranean area. This could partially be explained by the former extensive use of these drugs in these countries and also by the higher UV radiance in southern Europe, contributing to the development of photosensitization [203]. However, they are currently used in many other countries.

Arylpropionic acid derivatives, mainly ketoprofen, are responsible for the great majority of cases of allergy and photoallergy reported to date (Fig. 4 a, b). Since the first reports [204, 205] to the present day [206–209], several dozen cases have been published. Cross-reactivity of ketoprofen with other drugs of the same group is controversial. Although cross-reactivities have been reported for ibuproxam [210], flubiprofen [211, 212], and suprofen [201, 213], they were not found by Le Coz et al. [207], who regarded them as concomitant reactions. These authors suggested that benzophenone is the sensitizing moiety of ketoprofen, which could explain the almost constant cross-reaction with tiaprofenic acid [202, 214] and with unsubstituted benzophenone, and the frequent cross-reaction with fenofibrate [202, 215] and other monosubstituted benzophenones, such as oxybenzone [202, 203, 216, 217].

profen [201], piketoprofen [220, 221], and tiaprofenic acid [207]. Dexketoprofen is a new arylpropionic acid derivative NSAID that induces photoallergic contact dermatitis and cross-reacts with ketoprofen [222, 223].

From the other groups, some emphasis should be given to etofenamate, which can cause contact dermatitis [224, 225], contact urticaria [226], and photocontact allergy [227, 228], and to bufexamac. This is widely used in some northern countries as an alternative to topical corticosteroids. Bufexamac seems to have a high sensitizing capacity [229–231] (Fig. 5), and may cause erythema-multiforme-like eruptions [39]. Although it has been suggested that it should be added to the standard series in some countries [231], because of the high rate of sensitization and the serious clinical pictures of bufexamac allergy, the use of this drug should be critically reassessed [232]. Diclofenac, which is now being used for the treatment of actinic keratoses, and aceclofenac have also been reported as sensitizers [233, 234].

Benzydamine hydrochloride is mainly a photoallergen [235]. Piroxicam is usually a systemic photosensitizer in patients allergic to the thiosalicylic acid moiety of thimerosal [116, 236], but it also can sensitize and photosensitize topically [218].

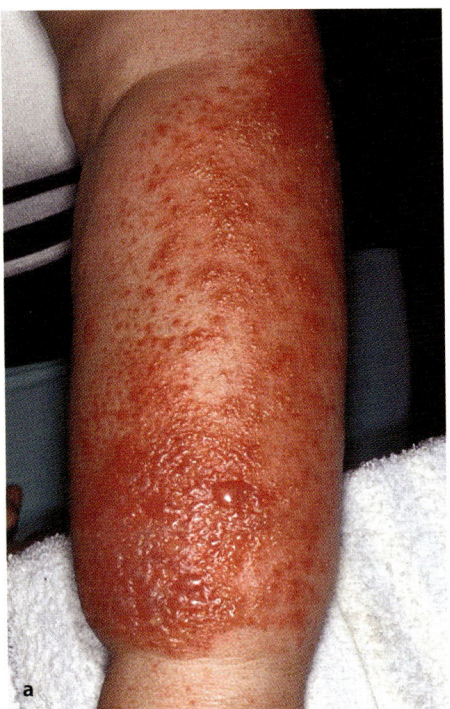

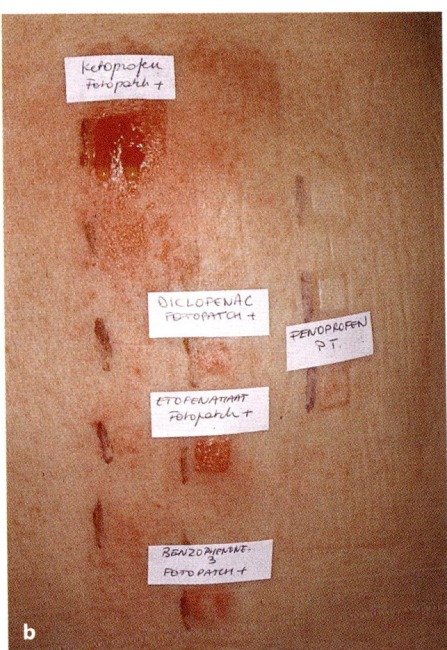

Fig. 4a, b. Photoallergic contact dermatitis from ketoprofen (a). Positive photopatch test to ketoprofen and related materials (b) (courtesy of A. Dooms-Goossens)

Ibuproxam is another arylpropionic acid derivative which sensitizes mainly by contact [214, 218]. Isolated reports of allergy or photoallergy to other NSAIDs of this group include ibuprofen [219], su-

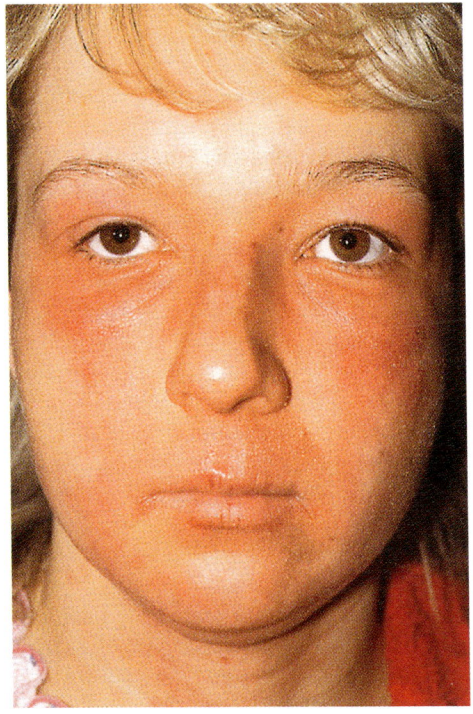

Fig. 5. Allergic contact dermatitis from bufexamac in a patient with atopic dermatitis (courtesy of PJ Frosch)

Indomethacin [237] and the pyrazolone derivatives are now less often used, but can cause allergic contact dermatitis [200, 238] and erythema-multiforme-like reactions [40]. Thiocolchicoside, not exactly an NSAID, is a muscle relaxant that was reported as a contact allergen [239] and photoallergen [240].

Core Message

■ Nonsteroidal anti-inflammatory drugs (NSAIDs) are very widely used and are frequent sensitizers. Ketoprofen induces allergic and photoallergic contact dermatitis and cross-reacts with arylpropionic acid derivatives, tiaprofenic acid, as well as with benzophenone, oxybenzone, and fenofibrate. Bufexamac is strongly allergenic and its use should, probably, be discontinued.

35.4.8 Ingredients of the Vehicles

Active products are incorporated in vehicles, which may contain several different substances, with different purposes – preservatives, emollients, emulsifiers, humectants, antioxidants, perfumes – which may also induce contact allergy.

Sensitization to white and yellow petrolatum is rare [241–243], but white petrolatum, which is purer than yellow petrolatum, seems to be less allergenic [4]. Lanolin is a natural product from sheep fleece and consists of a complex mixture of sterols (wool wax alcohols), fatty alcohols, and fatty acids, whose composition varies from time to time and from place to place [244]. It is an important sensitizer in patients with long-standing eczemas, especially in leg ulcer patients, in whom it is usually one of the main allergens. However, it seems to be a very weak allergen when used on noneczematous skin or in cosmetics [244–247]. The allergen fraction resides mainly in the wool wax alcohols. Therefore, 30% wool wax alcohols in petrolatum is the recommended concentration for patch testing. Acetylated lanolin [248, 249], dewaxed lanolin, hydrogenated lanolin [250], and a purified anhydrous lanolin [251] have been claimed to cause less sensitization, although they may reduce the effectiveness of lanolin as an excipient [252].

Propylene glycol (PPG) is a viscous hygroscopic liquid. It may cause irritant and allergic contact dermatitis, as well as NICU and subjective or sensory irritation [253, 254]. PPG patch test reactions are often difficult to evaluate and reports of contact allergy in the literature must, therefore, be interpreted with caution. Cases of allergy to PPG in corticosteroid creams, EEC electrodes and gel, and other creams have been reported [255–258]. Polyethylene glycols (PEG) are the condensation products of glycols with ethylene oxide, with variable molecular weight (200–6,000 Da), depending on the condensation degree. Their sensitizing capacity is higher for lower molecular weights [259]. Emulsifiers and emollients, like long-chain aliphatic fatty alcohols – lauryl, myristyl, oleyl, cetyl, and stearyl alcohols – may sensitize, especially in leg ulcer patients [260]. Oleyl alcohol seems to be the stronger sensitizer [261]. Contact sensitivity to other emulsifiers, like sorbitan sesquioleate (Arlacel 83), sorbitan stearate and oleate (Span 60 and 80), and polysorbates (Tween 40 and 80) has also been reported [262, 263].

Parabens are the most widely used preservatives, either in cosmetics or in topical medicaments. There are four esters (methyl, ethyl, propyl, and butyl), which are used in combination, mainly methyl and propyl esters, in concentrations up to 0.1–0.3%. Some decades ago, they were used in much higher concentrations (up to 5%), but in the currently used concentrations, the benefits largely exceed the risks of sensitization, which remains at about 0.5–1% of all patch-tested patients [264–266]. The paraben paradox is well known [267] – patients sensitized topically through medicaments can tolerate cosmetics preserved with parabens.

Sorbic acid, which induces NICU and contact allergy [268], chlorocresol [269], and nonoxynols [270] are other preservatives reported as causes of contact allergy.

Formaldehyde and formaldehyde releasers, isothiazolinones, and methyldibromoglutaronitrile, as well as a few other preservatives are mainly used in cosmetics (see Chap. 30).

Core Message

■ Lanolin is an important allergen in patients with stasis dermatitis and leg ulcers, but it rarely induces allergy when used in noneczematous skin or in cosmetics. Similarly, parabens may be safely used in cosmetics, but can induce sensitization in patients with long-standing eczemas.

35.4.9 Other Allergens

Several other topical drugs, either in therapeutic or occupational use, may sensitize. Psoriatic patients may become topically sensitized, which can aggravate and possibly be, in some cases, a trigger factor for their skin disease [21]. Although extensively used, corticosteroids rarely seem to sensitize these patients [19, 25], but two cases have been reported by Heule et al. [21]. More often, tars [21, 25], dithranol [25, 271, 272], calcipotriol [273–276], and tacalcitol [277] are the main offenders. From the recently introduced topical immunomodulators, a case of allergic contact dermatitis to tacrolimus has been reported [278], but no known cases from pimecrolimus.

Antineoplastic drugs may induce contact urticaria (cisplatin [279] and mechlorethamine [280]) and allergic contact dermatitis {5-fluorouracil [281], (Fig. 6), mitomycin C [282], mechlorethamine [283], and azathioprine [284]}.

Other possible allergenic topical drugs include proflavine [77], minoxidil [285] (which can also photosensitize [286] and cause pigmentation [287]), metronidazole [288], retinoic acid [289], zinc pyrithione [290], salicylic acid [291], acaricides like crotamiton [292], benzyl benzoate and mesulfen [293], resorcinol [294], ethanol [295], and benzoyl peroxide, mainly when used for leg ulcer treatment [296].

Topical traditional Chinese medicaments are largely sold as over-the-counter products, not only in the Far East, but also in Asian communities in some European countries and in the USA. The components usually include terpenes, salicylates, and essential oil extracts [297]. They may irritate [298] and sensitize [297, 299, 300] (Fig. 7). Colophony, fragrance, and myrrh seem to be rather frequent allergens in these preparations [300–303]. Four patients who reacted to five Chinese medicaments were also allergic to fragrance mix, and three to *Myroxylon pereirae* (balsam of Peru), which strongly suggests cross-sensitization with the plant extracts contained in these medicaments [297]. In a study conducted in Taiwan, 30 patients were tested with 27 traditional Chinese crude drugs and other selected material. Fifteen out of the 30 patients reacted to at least one of 23 crude drugs; seven were positive to Myroxylon Pereirae resin and six to colophony, which was a much higher incidence than in the patients without contact dermatitis to Chinese medicaments [304].

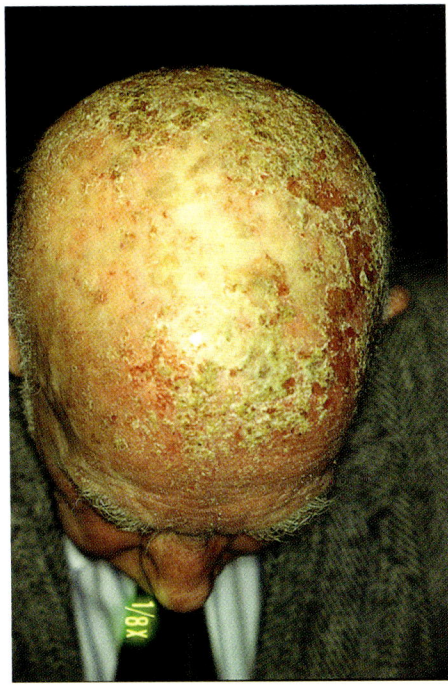

Fig. 6. Severe infected allergic contact dermatitis from fluorouracil ointment used for the treatment of actinic keratoses (courtesy of PJ Frosch)

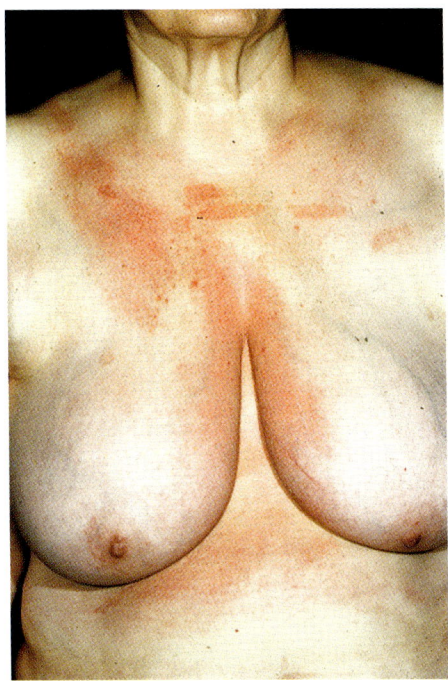

Fig. 7. Allergic contact dermatitis from tea-tree oil used by the patient to treat seborrheic keratosis (courtesy of PJ Frosch)

> **Core Message**
>
> ■ Traditional Chinese medicaments can induce sensitization. They contain several different chemical products, with colophony, fragrances, and myrrh being the main sensitizers.

> **Core Message**
>
> ■ The occlusion these systems provoke predisposes to inducing hypersensitivity. Several different drugs have been reported to cause allergy – scopolamine, clonidine, nitroglycerin, estradiol, norethisterone, nicotine, and testosterone.

35.4.10 Transdermal Therapeutic Systems

These therapeutic devices were introduced to the market more than two decades ago, and an increasing number of drugs are being used this way. They have made possible effective rate-controlled transcutaneous administration of the drugs. In addition, gastro-intestinal absorption and first-pass hepatic metabolism is avoided and an improved compliance, with decreased administration cycle, is obtained. However, they also have some disadvantages. The effect of occlusion for 1–7 days may induce miliaria and irritant contact dermatitis, and these conditions predispose to inducing hypersensitivity to one or more components [305, 306].

There are now reports of allergy to six different transdermal therapeutic systems. Contact allergy may be due to a component of the adhesive layer – ethanol, hydroxypropyl cellulose, polyisobutylene, methacrylates – or, more commonly, to the drug itself – scopolamine [307], clonidine [308, 309], nitroglycerin [310, 311] (Fig. 8), estradiol [312–315], and norethisterone [314], nicotine [316], and testosterone [317, 318].

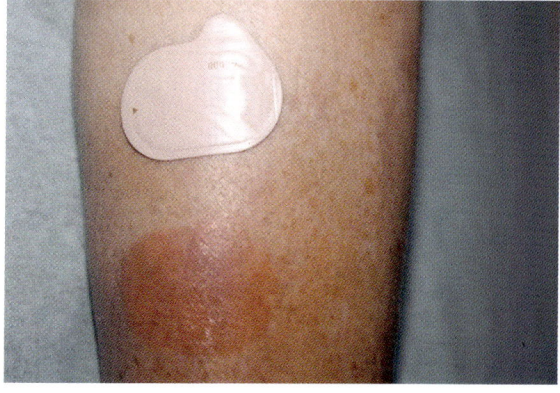

Fig. 8. Allergic contact dermatitis to a transdermal device containing nitroglycerin (courtesy of O Bordalo)

35.5 Sites at Risk

Several skin sites, for one reason or another, may be at special risk of developing contact sensitization. They are usually sites where skin conditions are prone to be chronic and, for that reason, many topical medicaments are applied over the course of time. Besides that, particular anatomical and pathological conditions, or special application methods, can increase skin penetration, which also increases the sensitizing capacity of pharmaceutical products. In this short review, we will consider three special sites and pathological conditions – ophthalmic preparations, anogenital dermatoses and stasis dermatitis, and leg ulcers.

35.5.1 Ophthalmic Preparations

Such medicaments are quite a common cause of contact sensitization [93, 319–321]. Patients with glaucoma who are chronically treated with several ophthalmic drugs are likely to become sensitized [322]. Symptoms may be limited to the eye (allergic contact conjunctivitis) or may involve the periocular skin and the eyelids. Allergic contact conjunctivitis often goes undiagnosed, since it usually occurs in patients who are already affected by ocular inflammation due to other causes, and its clinical features are not specific. Clinical examination reveals pronounced vasodilatation and chemosis of the conjunctiva. Watery discharge and papillary response can be present. Possible complications include punctate keratitis and corneal opacities.

Patch tests should be carried out with the eye preparations used by the patient and their individual ingredients (Table 7). Patch testing only the preparations may give false-negative results, especially when the responsible allergen is a preservative. The diagnosis of allergic contact conjunctivitis may be confirmed by a provocative test with the responsible eye preparation.

Table 7. Substances reported to have caused contact allergy in ophthalmics (modified from [93, 319–321, 323])

Preservatives	Antiviral drugs
Benzalkonium chloride	Idoxiuridine
Benzethonium chloride	Trifluridine
Chlorhexidine gluconate	β-interferon
Cetalkonium chloride	
Phenylmercuric nitrate	Antihistaminics
Sorbic acid	Chlorpheniramine
Thimerosal	Sodium cromoglycate
	Amlexanox
Beta-blockers	N-Acyl-aspartyl glutamic acid (NAAGA-DCI)
Befunolol	Ketotifen
Betaxolol	
Carteolol	Anesthetics
Levobunolol	Benzocaine
Metipranol	Procaine
Metoprolol	Oxybuprocaine
1-Pentbutol	Proxymetacaine
Timolol	Proparacaine
	Tetracaine
Mydriatics	
Atropine	Enzymatic cleaners
Cyclopentolate	Papain
Dipivalyl-epinephrine	Tegobetaine L7
Homatropine	
Phenylephrine	Others
Scopolamine	Apraclonidine
Tropicamide	Boric acid
	Brominidine
Antibiotics	D-Penicillamine
Bacitracin	Diclofenac
Chloramphenicol	Dorzolamide
Gentamicin	Echothiopate iodine
Kanamycin	e-Aminocaproic acid
Neomycin	Pilocarpine
Polymyxin B	Prednisolone
Oxytetracycline	Resorcinol
Penicillin	Rubidium iodide
Sulfathiazole	Tolazoline
Cefradine	
Tobramycin	

Both preservatives and active ingredients may produce contact sensitization. Preservatives are certainly the most important sensitizers in eye drops, and since each preservative is contained in a large number of ophthalmic preparations, not only does allergic conjunctivitis due to these compounds frequently go undetected, but it can actually be prolonged by the very eye drops that are prescribed to relieve the patient's ocular discomfort. Thimerosal sensitization is probably the main allergological problem in eye drop users, as it is also in contact lens wearers [115]. Preservative-free monodose eye drops are now available for the most important ophthalmic ingredients.

Active ingredients of the ophthalmic products that may cause sensitization include beta-adrenergic blocking agents, mydriatics, antibiotics, antiviral drugs, antihistamines, anti-inflammatory drugs, corticosteroids, and anesthetics [93, 319–321, 323].

35.5.2 Vulval and Perianal Dermatoses

Patients with chronic vulval dermatoses, mainly pruritus vulvae, lichen sclerosus, and lichen simplex chronicus, frequently apply several topical preparations that may contribute to maintain, prolong, and aggravate the local symptomatology. Vulval skin is hyper-reactive to local irritants [324], which, in conjunction with the local conditions – occlusion and high temperature – and an increased permeability of vulvovaginal mucosa compared to that of keratinized skin [325], are factors that predispose to inducing sensitization. Contact allergy incidence in these patients is high (29–58%) [59, 326–328] and is higher in patients with simultaneous anogenital dermatoses [64, 329].

Fragrances and topical medicaments are the main relevant allergens. Among topical drugs, antibiotics, particularly neomycin, local anesthetics, corticosteroids [330], antiseptics, and preservatives should be highlighted.

Patients with pruritus ani and hemorrhoids are submitted to the same local and general conditions, as well as to the application of multiple topical drugs. Therefore, allergic contact eczema is frequently seen in these patients [64, 329]. Local anesthetics are, by far, the more common allergens [57, 58, 64, 331–333], but several other topical drugs or components of medicaments have been reported as contact allergens in this area – clobetasone butyrate [334], nifuratel [335], sodium metabisulfite [336], glyceryl trinitrate [337], enoxolone [338], trimebutine [339], and bufexamac [232]. This induced a generalized eruption, "baboon-syndrome"-like, similar to the one induced by 5-aminosalicylic acid enemas [340].

Core Message

■ A hyperreactive skin mucosa, in conjunction with local conditions like occlusion and high temperature, and an increased permeability are factors that predispose to sensitization in these patients. Local anesthetics are the more common allergens, but antibiotics, corticosteroids, antiseptics, and preservatives should not be forgotten.

35.5.3 Stasis Dermatitis and Leg Ulcer Patients

Stasis dermatitis and leg ulcer patients have a well known increased risk of becoming sensitized. The long course of these pathological conditions, the damage to the skin barrier, and the use of occlusive bandages promoting skin penetration are all factors that favor polysensitization. There is usually a very high incidence of medicament contact allergy in these patients, varying in different series from 58% to 86% [3, 4, 89, 90, 94, 341–345].

The more important allergen groups are the following:

■ Lanolin: despite all the polemics around its sensitizing capacity [94, 244–246], lanolin remains a constant finding as one of the main sensitizers in these patients
■ Antibiotics and other chemotherapeutic agents: neomycin, bacitracin, polymyxin B, chloramphenicol, nitrofurazone, clioquinol, sodium fusidate
■ Corticosteroids [346] (Fig. 9)
■ Preservatives and antiseptics: parabens, benzalkonium chloride, cetrimide, povidone iodine, benzoyl peroxide
■ Emollients and emulsifiers: cetearyl alcohol (Lanette O), Lanette N, and Lanette E, sorbitan sesquioleate and others [260, 347, 348]

In the last two decades, new wound dressings, such as hydrocolloids, hydrogels, alginates, and polyurethane foams, have been used with increasing frequency. They are generally well tolerated, but can occasionally cause irritant contact dermatitis. Some recent publications report allergic contact dermatitis from components of these dressings, mainly from hydrocolloids. Pentalin (pentaerythritol ester of hydrogenated rosin), a tackifying agent that usually cross-reacts with colophony, and Vistanex (polyisobutylene), another tackifier, are the main allergens reported [349–353]. PPG proved to be the sensitizer in

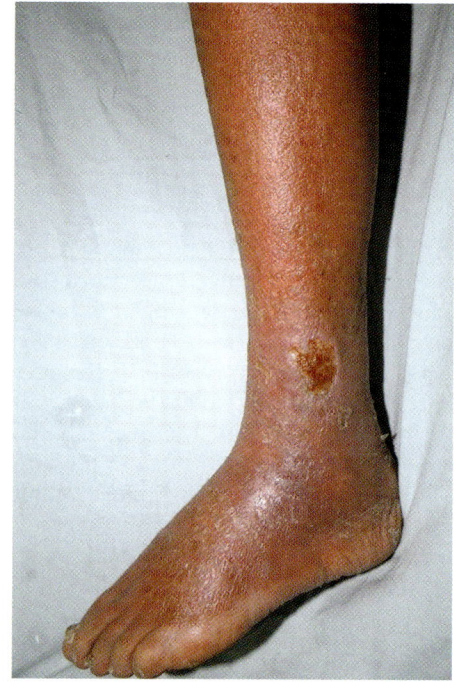

Fig. 9. Allergic contact dermatitis from methylprednisolone aceponate in a patient with leg ulcer (courtesy of O Bordalo)

35

three patients allergic to hydrogels [344]. Carboxymethyl cellulose in a hydrocolloid dressing induced a generalized urticarial rash [35].

Core Message

◼ A high percentage of stasis dermatitis and leg ulcer patients are contact allergic to several topical drugs – lanolin, topical antibiotics, corticosteroids, and emulsifiers are the main allergens. Some components of recent wound dressings may rarely sensitize.

35.6 Systemic Contact Dermatitis

This very important matter is dealt with in much more detail elsewhere in this textbook (Chap. 16). It is an inflammatory skin disease that may develop from the systemic administration of a substance in patients topically sensitized to it or to a chemically related substance [354]. The route of administration may be oral, rectal, vaginal, parenteral, intra-articular, by inhalation, or through percutaneous penetration.

Drugs are, by far, the most frequent causes of systemic contact dermatitis, and because of the possibility of severe generalized reactions, one should always bear this clinical entity in mind. The more important drugs and chemically related substances that may cause systemic contact dermatitis are listed in Table 8.

Systemic contact dermatitis may assume several different clinical cutaneous manifestations, which, in some severe cases, may be accompanied by general symptomatology, like fever, malaise, headache, nausea, vomiting, diarrhea, or even syncope [26, 354, 355]:

◼ Flare-up of previous eczema or patch-test reaction sites.
◼ Vesicular hand eczema, with or without erythema, localized to the palms, volar aspects, and sides of the fingers.
◼ Generalized maculopapular rash – this is the commonest eruption, which may become more severe and lead to erythroderma [356] (Fig. 10).
◼ Erythema multiforme, purpura, vasculitis.
◼ Generalized acute exanthematic pustulosis [161].
◼ Urticaria and anaphylaxis.
◼ The "baboon syndrome" [357]: this well recognized syndrome has a characteristic distribution pattern, with diffuse pink or dark violet erythema of the buttocks and inner thighs, like an inverted triangle or V-shaped; sometimes, the axilla are also involved. Several drugs may cause the baboon syndrome, particularly ampicillin, erythromycin, other antibiotics, and mercury.

Mercury may induce other exanthematic reactions, such as mercury exanthema – a diffuse symmetrical erythema predominantly of major flexures [358, 359] – and even acute generalized exanthematic pustulosis. These eruptions, which are currently much less common than some years ago, were usually due to

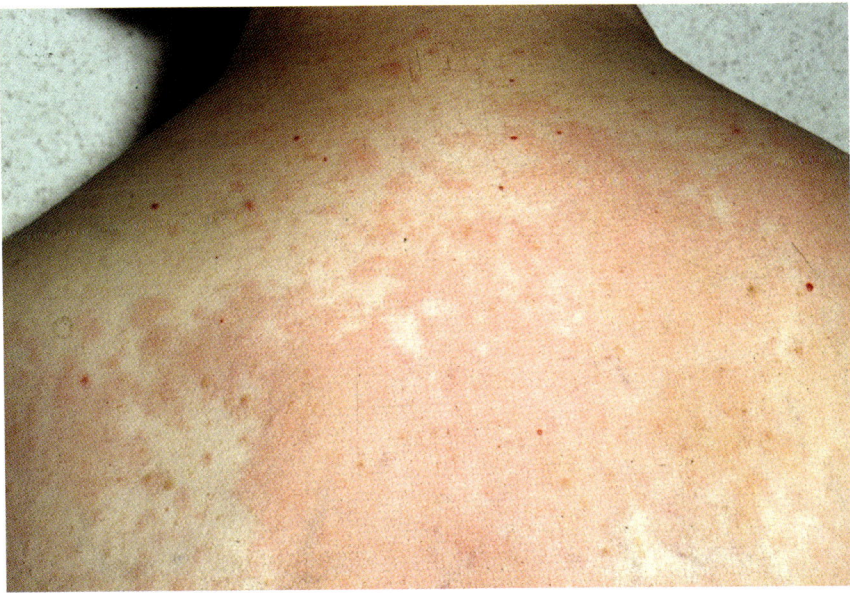

Fig. 10.
Systemic reaction to an injection of methylprednisolone in a patient previously sensitized by a topical preparation containing the same corticosteroid (courtesy of A. Dooms-Goossens)

Table 8. Drugs and chemically related substances that may cause systemic contact dermatitis [26, 354–359]

Topical drugs	Substances (groups) that can induce systemic contact dermatitis
Acyclovir	Acyclovir
Antimycotic imidazoles	Antimycotic imidazoles, metronidazole
Benzocaine	Para-amino compounds
Captopril	Captopril
Chloramphenicol	Chloramphenicol
Cinchocaine	Cinchocaine
Clonidine	Clonidine
Corticosteroids	Corticosteroids
Diphenhydramine	Diphenhydramine
Doxepin	Doxepin
Ephedrine	Pseudoephedrine
Estradiol	Estradiol
Ethyl alcohol	Alcohol-containing medicaments and beverages
Ethylenediamine	Ethylenediamine antihistamines (hydroxyzine), aminophylline
Famciclovir	Acyclovir
5-Fluorouracil	5-Fluorouracil
Gentamycin	Neomycin and other aminoglycoside antibiotics
Halogenated hydroxyquinolines	Vioform, chlorquinaldol
Iodine	Iodides, iodinated organic compounds
Mercury compounds	Mercury compounds (organic and inorganic)
Methyl salicylate	Acetyl salicylic acid
Mitomycin C	Mitomycin C
Neomycin	Aminoglycoside antibiotics, except streptomycin
Nitroglycerin	Nitroglycerin
Nonsteroidal anti-inflammatory drugs	Nonsteroidal anti-inflammatory drugs
Norfloxacin	Clioquinol
Nystatin	Nystatin
Parabens	Parabens
Penicillin/semi-synthetic penicillins	Penicillin/semi-synthetic penicillins
Phenothiazines	Phenothiazines (antihistamines and other)
Propylene glycol	Propylene glycol (in foods)
Pseudoephedrine	Ephedrine, phenylephrine
Sorbic acid	Sorbic acid, sorbates
Sulfonamides	Sulfonamides, sulfonylureas, para-amino compounds
Terbinafine	Terbinafine
Thimerosal	Thimerosal, piroxicam
Valaciclovir	Acyclovir
Vitamin B6	Vitamin B6
Vitamins B1/C	Vitamins B1/C

35

the inhalation of mercury vapors resulting from broken thermometers and, less often, following dental treatments.

> ### Core Message
>
> ■ Several topical medicaments can induce systemic contact dermatitis in sensitized patients, if administered by other routes. Multiple different clinical patterns may be seen, with the "baboon syndrome" being a well recognized manifestation that can be provoked by several medicaments.

35.7 Diagnosis and Prognosis

Correct diagnosis of the many cutaneous drug reactions is not always an easy task. Nonallergic reactions are, in most cases, diagnosed on a presumptive basis, according to the clinical history and course, with reference to the available literature. The evaluation of immediate reactions (ICU/NICU) should follow the test procedures suggested by Amin et al. [33]. Other allergic noneczematous patterns, like erythema multiforme, purpura, or lymphomatoid reactions, may be diagnosed by patch tests, although patch test reactions are usually eczematous, not reproducing the clinical features.

In cases of suspected allergic contact dermatitis, besides the history and the whole clinical picture, patch tests are of utmost importance. The patient must be tested with all and every medicament that he has applied, as well as all the active principles and other suspected substances. This may prove rather difficult in many instances because patients may often use many different medicaments and, in cases of ectopic dermatitis, the offending drugs may be disregarded.

Several difficulties arise in testing these patients:

- Some allergenic drugs are also irritants or, at least, marginal irritants – propylene glycol, dithranol, calcipotriol, 5-fluorouracil, some counterirritants, and others. Patch test interpretation may be quite difficult and false-positive reactions may be misinterpreted.
- Most commercial medicaments have a complex composition. False-negative reactions may be expected from the whole medicament, if the allergenic substance is used at a low concentration in the final product.
- The possibility of testing all the components of a commercial product depends largely on the manufacturer's goodwill. This may make the identification of individual allergens impossible.
- Contact allergy to some medicaments may be due to compound allergy [8, 126]. Here, again, the identification of the allergenic substance may prove a hard task.
- Correct concentrations and vehicles for patch testing have not yet been determined for many drugs, which can lead to false-positive/negative reactions. In the case of a positive reaction to an uncommon allergen, the use of serial dilutions and patch tests in controls is mandatory.
- In polysensitized patients, the occurrence of an excited skin syndrome must not be overlooked.

Patients with medicament contact allergy usually have a good prognosis. However, in some circumstances, there is a high propensity for relapse – in patients with long-standing eczemas, this is a rather common phenomenon due to possible cross-reactions with other drugs, the difficulty in completely avoiding some allergens, like lanolin, or the possibility of systemic contact dermatitis.

35.8 Appendix: Allergens in Medicaments (*pet.* petrolatum, *aq.* aqueous, *eth.* ethanol, *o.o.* olive oil)

1. Anesthetics
   a. Amethocaine (tetracaine) – 1% pet.
   b. Amylocaine – 5% pet.
   c. Benzamine lactate – 1% pet.
   d. Benzocaine – 5% pet.
   e. Bupivacaine – 1% pet.
   f. Butacaine – 5% pet.
   g. Butethamine – 5% pet.
   h. Butyl aminobenzoate – 5% pet.
   i. Cyclomethycaine – 1% pet.
   j. Dibucaine (cinchocaine) – 5% pet.
   k. Diperocaine – 1% pet.
   l. Lidocaine – 5% pet.
   m. Mepivacaine – 1% pet.
   n. Orthocaine – 1% pet.
   o. Oxybuprocaine – 1% pet.
   p. Polidocanol – 3% pet.
   q. Pramocaine – 1% pet.
   r. Prilocaine – 5% pet.
   s. Procaine – 1% pet.
   t. Propanidid – 5% pet.
   u. Proparacaine (proxymetacaine) – 2% pet.
   v. Propipocaine – 1% pet.

2. Antibiotics
   a. Ampicillin – 5% pet.
   b. Amikacin – 20% pet.
   c. Azidamfenicol – 2% pet.
   d. Bacitracin – 20% pet.
   e. Cephalosporins – 5%–20% aq. or pet.
   f. Chloramphenicol – 5% pet.
   g. Clindamycin – 1% aq.
   h. Erythromycin base – 1% pet.
   i. Erythromycin salts – 1% aq.
   j. Framycetin – 20% pet.
   k. Gentamicin – 20% pet.
   l. Kanamycin – 10% pet.
   m. Lincomycin – 1% aq.
   n. Mafenide – 10% pet.
   o. Mupirocin – 10% pet.
   p. Neomycin – 20% pet.
   q. Paromomycin – 10% pet.
   r. Penicillin (benzyl) – 10.000 U/g pet.
   s. Polymyxin B – 3% pet.
   t. Pristinamycin – 5% pet.
   u. Ribostamycin – 20% pet.
   v. Rifamycin – 2.5% pet.
   w. Sisomicin – 20% pet.
   x. Sodium fusidate – 2% pet.

y. Spiramycin – 10% pet.
z. Streptomycin – 2.5% pet.
aa. Sulfonamides – 5% pet.
ab. Tetracyclines – 3% pet.
ac. Thiamphenicol – 5% pet.
ad. Tobramycin – 20% pet.
ae. Tylosin tartrate – 5% pet.
af. Virginiamycin – 5% pet.

3. Antivirals
   a. Acyclovir – 5% pet.
   b. Famciclovir – 10% aq.
   c. Ganciclovir – 20% aq.
   d. Idoxuridine – 1% pet.
   e. Trifluridine – 5% pet.
   f. Tromantadine – 1% pet.
   g. Valaciclovir – 10% aq.

4. Antiseptics/antibacterials
   a. Ammoniated mercury – 1% pet.
   b. Chlorquinaldol – 5% pet.
   c. Clioquinol – 5% pet.
   d. Cycloheximide – 1% pet.
   e. Ethacridine – 2% pet.
   f. Merbromin – 2% aq. or pet.
   g. Mercuric chloride – 0.1% pet.
   h. Nitrofurazone – 1% pet.
   i. Phenylmercuric salts – 0.05% pet. (acetate, borate, nitrate)
   j. Povidone iodine – 10% aq.
   k. Proflavine HCl – 1% pet.
   l. Triphenylmethane dyes – 2% aq.
   m. Thimerosal – 0.1% pet.
5. Antimycotics
   a. Amorolfine – 1% pet.
   b. Chlorphenesin – 1% pet.
   c. Dibenzthione – 3% pet.
   d. Haloprogin – 1% pet.
   e. Imidazoles
      – bifonazole – 1% eth.
      – clotrimazole – 1% eth.
      – croconazole – 1% eth.
      – econazole – 1% eth.
      – enilconazole – 1% eth.
      – fenticonazole – 1% eth.
      – isoconazole – 1% eth.
      – ketoconazole – 1% eth.
      – lanoconazole – 1% eth.
      – miconazole – 1% eth.
      – neticonazole – 1% eth.
      – oxiconazole – 1% eth.
      – sertaconazole – 1% eth.
      – sulconazole – 1% eth.
      – tioconazole – 1% eth.

f. Naftifine – 5% eth.
g. Nystatin – 2% pet.
h. Pecilocin – 1% pet.
i. Pyrrolnitrin – 1% pet.
j. Tolnaftate – 1% pet.
k. Undecylenic acid – 2% pet.

6. Antihistamines
   a. Amlexanox – 1% pet.
   b. Antazoline – 1% pet.
   c. Chlorpheniramine – 5% pet.
   d. Chlorpromazine – 0.1% pet.
   e. Diphenhydramine – 1% pet.
   f. Doxepin – 5% pet.
   g. Ketotifen – 0.7% aq.
   h. Promethazine – 1% pet.
   i. Pyrilamine – 2% pet.
   j. Sodium cromoglycate – 2% aq.
   k. Tripelennamine – 1% pet.

7. Antineoplastic drugs
   a. Azathioprine – 1% pet
   b. Chlorambucil – 2% pet.
   c. Fluorouracil – 1% pet.
   d. Mechlorethamine – 0.02% aq
   e. Mitomycin C – 0.1% pet.

8. Antiparasitics
   a. Benzyl benzoate – 5% pet.
   b. Crotamiton – 3% pet.
   c. Mesulfen – 5% pet.
   d. Metronidazole – 1% pet.

9. NSAIDs
   a. Aceclofenac – 1% pet.
   b. Benzydamine – 5% pet.
   c. Bufexamac – 5% pet.
   d. Carprofen – 5% pet.
   e. Cinnoxicam – 1% pet.
   f. Dexketoprofen – 1% pet.
   g. Diclofenac – 1% pet.
   h. Etofenamate – 2% pet.
   i. Fenoprofen – 5% pet.
   j. Feprazone – 5% pet.
   k. Flufenamic acid – 1% pet.
   l. Flurbiprofen – 5% pet.
   m. Ibuprofen – 5% pet.
   n. Ibuproxam – 2.5% pet.
   o. Indomethacin – 5% pet.
   p. Ketoprofen – 2.5% pet.
   q. Mefenamic acid – 1% pet.
   r. Mofebutazone – 1% pet.
   s. Naproxen – 5% pet.
   t. Oxyphenbutazone – 1% pet.

u. Phenylbutazone – 1% pet.
v. Piketoprofen – 2.5% pet.
w. Piroxicam – 1% pet.
x. Sulindac – 1% pet.
y. Suprofen – 0.1% pet.
z. Tenoxicam – 1% pet.
aa. Tiaprofenic acid – 1% pet.
ab. Thiocolchicoside – 1% pet.

10. Antipsoriatic drugs
    a. Calcipotriol – 2 µg/ml eth.
    b. Dithranol – 0.02% pet.
    c. Tacalcitol – 2 µg/ml eth.
    d. Tars (coal tar) – 5% pet.

11. Corticosteroids
    a. Alclometasone dipropionate – 1% eth.
    b. Amcinonide – 0.1% eth.
    c. Betamethasone dipropionate – 1% eth
    d. Betamethasone-17-valerate – 1% eth.
    e. Budesonide – 0.1% pet.
    f. Clobetasol propionate – 1% eth.
    g. Clobetasone butyrate – 1% eth.
    h. Cloprednol – 1% eth.
    i. Desonide – 1% eth.
    j. Desoxymethasone – 1% eth.
    k. Dexamethasone acetate – 1% eth.
    l. Dexamethasone phosphate – 1% eth.
    m. Diflorasone diacetate – 1% eth.
    n. Diflucortolone pivalate – 1% eth.
    o. Fludrocortisone acetate – 1% eth.
    p. Flumethasone acetate – 1% eth.
    q. Fluocinolone acetonide – 1% eth.
    r. Fluocinonide – 1% eth.
    s. Fluocortolone – 1% eth.
    t. Fluticasone propionate – 1% eth.
    u. Halcinonide – 1% eth.
    v. Halomethasone – 1% eth.
    w. Hydrocortisone – 1% eth.
    x. Hydrocortisone aceponate – 1% eth.
    y. Hydrocortisone acetate – 1% eth.
    z. Hydrocortisone buteprate – 1% eth.
    aa. Hydrocortisone-17-butyrate – 1% eth.
    ab. Methylprednisolone aceponate – 1% eth.
    ac. Methylprednisolone acetate. – 1% eth.
    ad. Mometasone furoate – 1% eth.
    ae. Prednicarbate – 1% eth.
    af. Prednisolone – 1% eth.
    ag. Tixocortol pivalate – 1% pet.
    ah. Triamcinolone acetonide – 1% eth.
12. β-Blockers
    a. Befulenol – 1% aq.
    b. Betaxolol – 1% aq.
    c. Carteolol – 1% aq

d. Levobunolol – 1% aq.
e. Metipranolol – 2% aq.
f. Metopronolol – 3% aq.
g. 1-Pentbutolol – 2% aq.
h. Timolol – 0.5% aq.

13. Mydriatics
    a. Atropine – 1% pet.
    b. Cyclopentolate – 0.5% aq.
    c. Dipivalyl-epinephrine – 1% aq.
    d. Homatropine – 1% aq.
    e. Phenylephrine –10% aq.
    f. Scopolamine – 0.25% aq.
    g. Tropicamide – 1% pet.

14. Preservatives/antioxidants
    a. Benzyl alcohol – 1% pet.
    b. Bithionol – 1% pet.
    c. Butylated hydroxyanisol – 2% pet.
    d. Butylated hydroxytoluene – 2% pet.
    e. Chloroacetamide – 0.2% pet.
    f. Chlorhexidine gluconate – 0.5% aq.
    g. Chlorocresol – 1% pet.
    h. Chloroxylenol – 1% pet.
    i. Dichlorophene – 1% pet.
    j. Ethyl alcohol – 10% aq.
    k. Nonoxynols – 5% aq.
    l. Nordihydroguaiaretic acid – 2% pet.
    m. Quaternary ammonium compounds – 0.1% aq.
    n. Propyl gallate – 1% pet.
    o. Sorbic acid – 2% pet.
    p. Alpha-tocopherol – 10% pet.
    q. Triclocarban – 1% pet.
    r. Triclosan – 1% pet.
    s. Zinc pyrithione – 1% pet.

15. Vehicle ingredients
    a. Amerchol L-101 – 50% pet.
    b. Carbowaxes – as is
    c. Castor oil – as is
    d. Cetyl alcohol – 5% pet.
    e. Cetearyl alcohol – 20% pet.
    f. Ethyl sebacate – 2% eth.
    g. Ethylenediamine – 1% pet.
    h. Eucerin – as is
    i. Lanette E – 20% pet.
    j. Lanette N – 20% pet.
    k. Lanolin – as is
    l. Myristyl alcohol – 5% pet.
    m. Oleyl alcohol – 30% pet.
    n. Petrolatum – as is
    o. Polyethylene glycols – pure
    p. Polysorbate [20, 40, 80] – 5% pet.

q. Propylene glycol – 5% aq.
r. Sesame oil – as is
s. Sodium lauryl sulfate – 0.1% aq.
t. Sorbitan laureate – 5% aq.
u. Sorbitan oleate – 5% aq.
v. Sorbitan palmitate – 5% aq.
w. Sorbitan sesquioleate – 20% pet.
x. Stearyl alcohol – 30% pet.
y. Triethanolamine – 2.5% pet.
z. Wool wax alcohols – 30% pet.

16. Miscellaneous
a. Allantoin – 0.5% aq.
b. e-Aminocaproic acid – 1% aq.
c. Benzoyl peroxide – 1% pet
d. Boric acid – 10% pet.
e. Clonidine – 1% pet.
f. Cocamidopropyl betaine – 1% aq.
g. Dexpanthenol – 50% aq.
h. Echothiopate iodine – 1% aq.
i. Ephedrine – 1% pet.
j. Epinephrine – 1% aq.
k. Estradiol – 2% eth.
l. Ichthammol – 10% pet.
m. Methyl salicylate – 2% pet.
n. Minoxidil – 5%: 20% PPG/aq.
o. Monobenzylether hydroquinone – 1% pet.
p. Nicotine – 10% pet.
q. Nitroglycerin – 1% pet.
r. Norethisterone acetate – 1% eth.
s. Papain – 1% pet.
t. D-Penicillamine – 1% aq.
u. Pilocarpine – 1% pet.
v. Resorcinol – 1% pet.
w. Retinoic acid – 0.005% pet.
x. Rubidium iodide – 1% pet.
y. Salicylic acid – 1% pet.
z. Scopolamine hydrobromide – 0.25% aq.
aa. Tacrolimus – 2.5% eth.
ab. Testosterone propionate – 1% eth.
ac. Thioxolone – 0.5% eth.
ad. Tolazoline – 10% aq.
ae. Triethanolamine polypeptide oleate condensate – 25% o.o.

References

1. Bandmann HJ, Calnan CD, Cronin E, Fregert S, Hjorth N, Magnusson B, Maibach HI, Malten E, Meneghini CL, Pirila V, Wilkinson DS (1972) Dermatitis from applied medicaments. Arch Dermatol 106:335–337
2. Blondeel A, Oleffe J, Achten G (1978) Contact allergy in 330 patients. Contact Dermatitis 4:270–276
3. Dooms-Goossens A (1982) Allergic contact dermatitis to ingredients used in topically applied pharmaceutical products and cosmetics. Katholieke Universitat Leuven, Leuven, Belgium
4. Angelini G, Vena GA, Meneghini CL (1985) Allergic contact dermatitis to some medicaments. Contact Dermatitis 12:263–269
5. Edman B, Moller H (1986) Medicament contact allergy. Derm Beruf Umwelt 34:139–143
6. Goh CL (1989) Contact sensitivity to topical medicaments. Int J Dermatol 28:25–28
7. Sertoli A, Francalanci S, Acciai MC, Gola M (1999) Epidemiological survey of contact dermatitis in Italy (1984–1993) by GIRDCA (Gruppo Italiano Ricerca Dermatiti da Contatto e Ambientali). Am J Contact Dermat 10:18–30
8. Smeenk G, Kerckoffs HP, Schreurs PH (1987) Contact allergy to a reaction product in Hirudoid cream: an example of compound allergy. Br J Dermatol 116:223–231
9. Fisher AA, Dooms-Goossens A (1976) The effect of perfume "ageing" on the allergenicity of individual perfume ingredients. Contact Dermatitis 2:155–159
10. Beltrani VS (1996) Clinical manifestations of atopic dermatitis. In: Leung DYM (ed) Atopic dermatitis: from pathogenesis to treatment. Springer, Berlin Heidelberg New York, p 24
11. Jones HE, Lewis CW, McMarlin SL (1973) Allergic contact dermatitis in atopic patients. Arch Dermatol 107:217–222
12. Angelini G, Meneghini CL (1977) Contact and bacterial allergy in children with atopic dermatitis. Contact Dermatitis 3:163–167
13. Lammintausta K, Kalimo K, Fagerlund VL (1992) Patch test reactions in atopic patients. Contact Dermatitis 26:234–240
14. Klas PA, Corey G, Storrs FJ, Chan SC, Hanifin JM (1996) Allergic and irritant patch test reactions in atopic disease. Contact Dermatitis 34:121–124
15. Giordano-Labadie F, Rance F, Pellegrin F, Bazex J, Dutau G, Schwarze HP (1999) Frequency of contact allergy in children with atopic dermatitis: results of a prospective study of 137 cases. Contact Dermatitis 40:192–195
16. Fedler R, Stromer K (1993) Nickel sensitivity in atopic, psoriatics and healthy subjects. Contact Dermatitis 29:65–69
17. Henseler T, Christophers E (1995) Disease concomitance in psoriasis. J Am Acad Dermatol 32:982–986
18. Fransson J, Storgards A, Hammer H (1985) Palmoplantar lesions in psoriatic patients and their relation to inverse psoriasis, tinea infection and contact allergy. Acta Derm Venereol (Stockh) 65:218–223
19. Fleming CJ, Burden AD (1997) Contact allergy in psoriasis. Contact Dermatitis 36:274–276
20. Stinco G, Frattasio A, De Francesco V, Bragadin G, Patrone P (1999) Frequency of delayed-type hypersensitivity to contact allergens in psoriatic patients. Contact Dermatitis 40:323–324

35

21. Heule F, Tahapary GJM, Bello CR, van Joost T (1998) Delayed-type hypersensitivity to contact allergens in psoriasis. A clinical evaluation. Contact Dermatitis 38: 78–82

22. Barile M, Cozzani E, Anonide A, Usiglio D, Burroni A, Guarrera M (1996) Is contact allergy rare in psoriatics? Contact Dermatitis 35: 111–114

23. Pigatto P (2000) Atopy and contact sensitization in psoriasis. Acta Derm Venereol Suppl 211: 19–20

24. Malhotra V, Kaur I, Saraswat A, Kumar B (2002) Frequency of patch-test positivity in patients with psoriasis: a prospective controlled study. Acta Derm Venereol (Stockh) 82: 432–435

25. Burden AD, Muston H, Beck MH (1994) Intolerance and contact allergy to tar and dithranol in psoriasis. Contact Dermatitis 31: 185–186

26. de Groot AC, Weyland JW, Nater JP (1994) Unwanted effects of cosmetics and drugs used in dermatology, 3rd edn. Elsevier, Amsterdam, The Netherlands

27. Goh CL (1999) Noneczematous contact reactions. In: Rycroft RJG, Menné T, Frosch PJ, Lepoittevin J-P (eds) Textbook of contact dermatitis, 3rd edn. Springer, Berlin Heidelberg New York, pp 413–431

28. Rietschel RL, Fowler JF (1995) Noneczematous contact dermatitis. In: Rietschel RL, Fowler JF (eds) Fisher's contact dermatitis. Williams and Wilkins, Baltimore, Md., pp 92–113

29. Watsky KL, McGovern T (2003) Intolerance to topical products may be due to dermographism. Am J Contact Dermat 14: 35–36

30. Frosch PJ (1999) Clinical aspects of irritant contact dermatitis. In: Rycroft RJG, Menné T, Frosch PJ, Lepoittevin J-P (eds) Textbook of contact dermatitis, 3rd edn. Springer, Berlin Heidelberg New York, pp 311–354

31. Maibach HI, Johnson HL (1975) Contact urticaria syndrome: contact urticaria to diethyltoluamide (immediate-type hypersensitivity). Arch Dermatol 111: 726–730

32. von Krogh G, Maibach HI (1981) The contact urticaria syndrome–an update review. J Am Acad Dermatol 5: 328–342

33. Amin S, Tanglertsampan C, Maibach HI (1997) Contact urticaria syndrome: 1997. Am J Contact Dermat 8: 15–19

34. Escribano MM, Muñoz-Bellido FJ, Velazquez E, Delgado J, Serrano P, Guardia J, Condé J (1997) Contact urticaria to aescin. Contact Dermatitis 37: 233

35. Johnson M, Fiskerstrand EJ (1999) Contact urticaria syndrome due to carboxymethylcellulose in a hydrocolloid dressing. Contact Dermatitis 41: 344–345

36. Adachi A, Fukunaga A, Hayashi K, Kunisada M, Horikawa T (2003) Anaphylaxis to polyvinylpyrrolidone after vaginal application of povidone-iodine. Contact Dermatitis 48: 133–136

37. Suzuki T, Kawada A, Hashimoto Y, Isogai R, Aragane Y, Tezuka T (2003) Contact urticaria due to ketoprofen. Contact Dermatitis 48: 284–285

38. Lovell CR, Cronin E, Rhodes EL (1986) Photocontact urticaria from chlorpromazine. Contact Dermatitis 14: 290–291

39. Koch P, Bahmer FA (1994) Erythema-multiforme-like, urticarial papular and plaque eruptions from bufexamac: report of 4 cases. Contact Dermatitis 31: 97–101

40. Kerre S, Busschotts A, Dooms-Goossens A (1995) Erythema-multiforme-like contact dermatitis due to phenylbutazone. Contact Dermatitis 33: 213–214

41. Khanna M, Qasem K, Sasseville D (2000) Allergic contact dermatitis to tea tree oil with erythema multiforme-like id reaction. Am J Contact Dermat 11: 238–242

42. Bjornberg A, Mobacken H (1976) Necrotic skin reactions caused by 1 per cent gentian violet and brilliant green. Acta Derm Venereol (Stockh) 52: 55–60

43. Armijo Moreno M, Gutierrez Salméron MT, Camacho Martinez F, Naranjo Sintes R, Armijo Lozano R, Garcia Mellado V, De Dulanto F (1976) Necrose de pene por dequalinium (Necrosis of the penis caused by dequalinim, in Spanish). Act Dermosifiliogr 67: 547–552

44. Corazza M, Bulciolu G, Spisani L, Virgili A (1997) Chemical burns following irritant contact with povidone-iodine. Contact Dermatitis 36: 115–116

45. Goh CL (1987) Erythema multiforme-like and purpuric eruption due to contact allergy to proflavine. Contact Dermatitis 17: 53–54

46. van Joost T, van Ulsen J, Vuzevski VD, Naafs B, Tank B (1990) Purpuric contact dermatitis to benzoyl peroxide. J Am Acad Dermatol 22: 359–361

47. Lembo G, Balato N, Patruno C, Pini D, Ayala F (1987) Lichenoid contact dermatitis due to aminoglycoside antibiotics. Contact Dermatitis 17: 122–123

48. Laine J, Kalimo K, Happonen RP (1997) Contact allergy to dental restorative materials in patients with oral lichenoid lesions. Contact Dermatitis 36: 141–146

49. Dunsche A, Kastel I, Terheyden H, Springer IN, Christophers E, Brasch J (2003) Oral lichenoid reactions associated with amalgam: improvement after amalgam removal. Br J Dermatol 148: 70–76

50. Garcia-Bravo B, Martinez-Falero AA (1998) Reacciones por mercuriales. Mapfre Med 9(Suppl 1): 16–20

51. Burry JN (1973) Topical drug addiction: adverse effects of fluorinated corticosteroid creams and ointments. Med J Aust 1: 393–396

52. Robertson DS, Maibach HI (1982) Topical corticosteroids. Int J Dermatol 21: 59–67

53. Staughton RC, August P (1975) Cushing's syndrome and pituitary-adrenal suppression due to clobetasol propionate. Br Med J 2: 419–421

54. Dooms-Goossens A, Deleu H (1991) Airborne contact dermatitis: an update. Contact Dermatitis 25: 211–217

55. Cronin E (1980) Contact dermatitis. Churchill Livingstone, Edinburgh, pp 193–202

56. Rietschel RL, Fowler JF (1995) Local anesthetics. In: Fisher's contact dermatitis, 4th edn. Williams and Wilkins, Baltimore, Md., pp 236–248

57. van Ketel WG (1983) Contact allergy to different antihaemorrhidal anaesthetics. Contact Dermatitis 9: 512–513

58. Lodi A, Ambonati M, Coassini A, Kouhdari Z, Palvarini M, Crosti C (1999) Contact allergy to 'caines' caused by antihemorrhoidal ointments. Contact Dermatitis 41: 221–222

59. Lewis FM, Harrington CD, Gawkrodger DJ (1994) Contact sensitivity in pruritus vulvae: a common and manageable problem. Contact Dermatitis 31: 264–265

60. Dawe RS, Watt D, O'Neill S, Forsyth A (2002) A laser-clinic nurse with allergic contact dermatitis from tetracaine. Contact Dermatitis 46: 306

61. Nakada T, Iijima M (2000) Allergic contact dermatitis from dibucaine hydrochloride. Contact Dermatitis 42: 283

62. Hayashi K, Kawachi S, Saida T (2001) Allergic contact dermatitis due to both chlorpheniramine maleate and dibucaine hydrochloride in an over-the-counter medicament. Contact Dermatitis 44: 38–39

63. Fernandez-Redondo V, Léon A, Santiago T, Toribio J (2001) Allergic contact dermatitis from local anaesthetic on peristomal skin. Contact Dermatitis 45: 238

64. Bauer A, Geier J, Elsner P (2000) Allergic contact dermatitis in patients with anogenital complaints. J Reprod Med 45: 649–654

65. Marques C, Faria E, Machado A, Gonçalo M, Gonçalo S (1995) Allergic contact dermatitis and systemic contact dermatitis from cinchocaine. Contact Dermatitis 33:443

66. Turner TW (1977) Contact dermatitis to lignocaine. Contact Dermatitis 3:210–211

67. Fregert S, Tegner E, Thelin I (1979) Contact allergy to lidocaine. Contact Dermatitis 5:185–188

68. Weightman W, Turner T (1998) Allergic contact dermatitis from lignocaine: report of 29 cases and review of the literature. Contact Dermatitis 39:265–266

69. Mackley CL, Marks JG, Anderson BE (2003) Delayed-type hypersensitivity to lidocaine. Arch Dermatol 139:343–346

70. Suhonen R, Kanerva L (1997) Contact allergy and cross-reactions caused by prilocaine. Am J Contact Dermat 8:231–235

71. van den Hove J, Decroix J, Tennstedt D, Lachapelle JM (1994) Allergic contact dermatitis from prilocaine, one of the local anaesthetics in EMLA cream. Contact Dermatitis 30:239

72. le Coz CJ, Cribier BJ, Heid E (1996) Patch testing in suspected allergic contact dermatitis due to EMLA cream in haemodialyzed patients. Contact Dermatitis 35:316–317

73. Dannaker CJ, Maibach HI, Austin E (2001) Allergic contact dermatitis to proparacaine with subsequent cross-sensitization to tetracaine from ophthalmic preparations. Am J Contact Dermat 12:177–179

74. Blaschke V, Fuchs T (2001) Periorbital allergic contact dermatitis from oxybuprocaine. Contact Dermatitis 44:198

75. van Ketel WG, Bruynzeel DP (1991) A 'forgotten' topical anaesthetic sensitizer: butyl aminobenzoate. Contact Dermatitis 25:131–132

76. Bajaj AK, Gupta SC (1986) Contact hypersensitivity to topical antibacterial agents. Int J Dermatol 25:103–105

77. Goh CL (1989) Contact sensitivity to topical antimicrobials. I. Epidemiology in Singapore. Contact Dermatitis 21:46–48

78. Bajaj AK, Gupta SC, Chatterjee AK (1992) Contact sensitivity to topical aminoglycosides in India. Contact Dermatitis 27:204–205

79. Morris SD, Rycroft RJ, White IR, Wakelin SH, McFadden JP (2002) Comparative frequency of patch test reactions to topical antibiotics. Br J Dermatol 146:1047–1051

80. van Ketel WG, Bruynzeel DP (1989) Sensitization to gentamicin alone. Contact Dermatitis 20:303–304

81. Rudzki E, Zakrzewski Z, Rebandel P, Grzywa Z, Hudymowicz W (1988) Cross reactions between aminoglycoside antibiotics. Contact Dermatitis 18:314–316

82. Rudzki E, Rebandel P (1996) Cross-reactions with 4 aminoglycoside antibiotics at various concentrations. Contact Dermatitis 35:62

83. Kimura M, Kawada A (1998) Contact sensitivity induced by neomycin with cross-sensitivity to other aminoglycoside antibiotics. Contact Dermatitis 39:148–150

84. Hjorth N, Weissmann K (1973) Occupational dermatitis among veterinary surgeons caused by spiramycin, tylosin and penethamate. Acta Derm Venereol (Stockh) 5:229–232

85. Veien NK, Hattel T, Justesen O, Norholm A (1980) Occupational contact dermatitis due to spiramycin and/or tylosin among farmers. Contact Dermatitis 6:410–413

86. Farley M, Pak H, Carregal V, Engler R, James W (1995) Anaphylaxis to topically applied bacitracin. Am J Contact Dermat 6:28–31

87. Katz BE, Fisher AA (1987) Bacitracin: a unique topical antibiotic sensitizer. J Am Acad Dermatol 17:1016–1024

88. Kleinhans D (1989) Bacitracin and polymyxin B: important contact allergens in patients with leg ulcers. In: Frosch PJ, Dooms-Goossens A, Lachapelle JM (eds) Current topics in contact dermatitis. Springer, Berlin Heidelberg New York, pp 258–260

89. Faria A (1992) Dermite de contacto em doentes com úlcera de perna (contact dermatitis in patients with leg ulcers, in Portuguese). Trab Soc Port Dermatol Venereol L [Suppl]:481–489

90. Zaki I, Shall L, Dalziel KL (1994) Bacitracin: a significant sensitizer in leg ulcer patients? Contact Dermatitis 31:92–94

91. Sood A, Taylor JS (2003) Bacitracin: allergen of the year. Am J Contact Dermat 14:3–4

92. Grandinetti PJ, Fowler JF Jr (1990) Simultaneous contact allergy to neomycin, bacitracin, and polymyxin. J Am Acad Dermatol 23:646–647

93. Tabar I, Garcia BE, Rodriguez E, Quirce S, Olaguibel JM (1990) Etiologic agents in allergic contact dermatitis by eyedrops. Contact Dermatitis 23:50–51

94. Tavadia S, Bianchi J, Dawe RS, McEvoy M, Wiggins E, Hamill E, Urcelay M, Strong AM, Douglas WS (2003) Allergic contact dermatitis in venous leg ulcer patients. Contact Dermatitis 48:261–265

95. Rudzki E, Rebandel P (1997) Sensitivity to oxytetracycline. Contact Dermatitis 37:136

96. Coskey RJ (1978) Contact dermatitis due to clindamycin. Arch Dermatol 114:446

97. Zappi EG, Brancaccio RR (1997) Allergic contact dermatitis from mupirocin ointment. J Am Acad Dermatol 36:266

98. Fisher AA (1976) The safety of topical erythromycin. Contact Dermatitis 2:43–44

99. Martins C, Freitas JD, Gonçalo M, Gonçalo S (1995) Allergic contact dermatitis from erythromycin. Contact Dermatitis 33:360

100. Conde-Salazar L, Guimaraens D, Romero LV, Gonzalez MA (1986) Occupational dermatitis from cephalosporins. Contact Dermatitis 14:70–71

101. Moller NE, Nielsen B, von Wurden K (1986) Contact dermatitis to semisynthetic penicillins in factory workers. Contact Dermatitis 14:307–311

102. Gamboa P, Jauregui I, Urrutia I (1995) Occupational sensitization to aminopenicillins with oral tolerance to penicillin. Contact Dermatitis 32:48–49

103. Foti C, Bonamonte D, Trenti R, Vena GA, Angelini G (1997) Occupational contact allergy to cephalosporins. Contact Dermatitis 36:104–105

104. Häusermann P, Bircher AJ (2002) Immediate and delayed hypersensitivity to ceftriaxone, and anaphylaxis due to intradermal testing with other beta-lactam antibiotics, in a previously amoxicillin-sensitized patient. Contact Dermatitis 47:311–312

105. Miyahara H, Koga T, Imayama S, Hori Y (1993) Occupational contact urticaria syndrome from cefotiam hydrochloride. Contact Dermatitis 29:210–211

106. Conde-Salazar L, Guimaraens D, Gonzalez MA, Mancebo E (2001) Occupational allergic contact urticaria from amoxicillin. Contact Dermatitis 45:109

107. Breit R, Seiffert P (1989) Mafenide – still an allergen of importance? In: Frosch PJ, Dooms-Goossens A, Lachapelle JM (eds) Current topics in contact dermatitis. Springer, Berlin Heidelberg New York, pp 222–224

108. Degreef H, Dooms-Goossens A (1985) Patch testing with silver sulfadiazine cream. Contact Dermatitis 12:33–37

109. Rietschel RL, Fowler JF (1995) Reactions to topical antimicrobials. In: Rietschel RL, Fowler JF (eds) Fisher's contact dermatitis. Williams and Wilkins, Baltimore, pp 205– 225

35

110. Agner T, Menné T (1993) Sensitivity to clioquinol and chlorquinaldol in the quinoline mix. Contact Dermatitis 29:163
111. Marks JG (1982) Allergic contact dermatitis to povidone iodine. J Am Acad Dermatol 6:473–475
112. Gonçalo M, Figueiredo A, Gonçalo S (1996) Hypersensitivity to thimerosal: the sensitizing moiety. Contact Dermatitis 34:201–203
113. Moller H (1980) Why thimerosal allergy? Int J Dermatol 19:29
114. Forstrom L, Hannuksela M, Kousa M, Lehmuskallio E (1980) Merthiolate hypersensitivity and vaccination. Contact Dermatitis 6:241–245
115. Tosti A, Tosti G (1988) Thimerosal: a hidden allergen in ophthalmology. Contact Dermatitis 18:268–272
116. de Castro JLC, Freitas JP, Brandao FM, Themido R (1991) Sensitivity to thimerosal and photosensitivity to piroxicam. Contact Dermatitis 24:187–192
117. Camarasa JMG (1976) Contact dermatitis from mercurochrome. Contact Dermatitis 2:120–121
118. Afzelius H, Thulin H (1979) Allergic reactions to benzalkonium chloride. Contact Dermatitis 5:60
119. Koch P, Bahmer FA, Hausen BM (1995) Allergic contact dermatitis from purified eosin. Contact Dermatitis 32:92–95
120. Schoppelrey HP, Mily H, Agathos M, Breit R (1997) Allergic contact dermatitis from pyoctanin. Contact Dermatitis 36:221–224
121. Fanta D, Mischer P (1976) Contact dermatitis from tromantadine hydrochloride. Contact Dermatitis 2:282–284
122. Brandão FM, Pecegueiro M (1982) Contact dermatitis from tromantadine hydrochloride. Contact Dermatitis 8:140–141
123. Angelini G, Vena GA, Meneghini CL (1986) Contact allergy to antiviral agents. Contact Dermatitis 15:114–115
124. Camarasa JMG, Serra-Baldrich E (1988) Allergic contact dermatitis from acyclovir. Contact Dermatitis 19:235–236
125. Tennstedt D, Lachapelle JM (1992) Patch testing and oral challenge with acyclovir in allergic contact dermatitis to Zovirax cream: a spectrum of reactions. In: Lachapelle JM (ed) Abstract book, 1st Congress of the European Society of Contact Dermatitis, Brussels, Belgium, 8–10 October 1992
126. Koch P (1995) No evidence of contact sensitization to acyclovir in acute dermatitis of the lips following application of Zovirax cream. Contact Dermatitis 33:255–257
127. Bayrou O, Gaouar H, Leynadier F (2000) Famciclovir as a possible alternative treatment in some cases of allergy to acyclovir. Contact Dermatitis 42:42
128. Lammintausta K, Mäkelä L, Kalimo K (2001) Rapid systemic valaciclovir reaction subsequent to acyclovir contact allergy. Contact Dermatitis 45:181
129. Vernassiere C, Barbaud A, Trechot PH, Weber-Muller F, Schmutz JL (2003) Systemic acyclovir reaction subsequent to acyclovir contact allergy: which systemic antiviral drug should then be used? Contact Dermatitis 49:155–157
130. van Ketel WG (1977) Allergy to idoxuridine eyedrops. Contact Dermatitis 3:106–107
131. Millan-Parrilla F, de la Cuadra J (1990) Allergic contact dermatitis from trifluoridine in eye drops. Contact Dermatitis 22:289
132. Anguita JL, Escutia B, Mari JI, de la Cuadra J, Aliaga A (2002) Allergic contact dermatitis from undecylenic acid in a common antifungal nail solution. Contact Dermatitis 46:109
133. Cooper SM, Shaw S (1999) Contact allergy to nystatin: an unusual allergen. Contact Dermatitis 41:120
134. Gonzalez Perez R, Aguirre A, Oleaga JM, Eizaguirre X, Diaz Perez JL (1995) Allergic contact dermatitis from tolnaftate. Contact Dermatitis 32:173
135. Willa-Craps C, Wyss M, Elsner P (1995) Allergic contact dermatitis from naftifine. Contact Dermatitis 32:369–370
136. Kramer K, Paul E (1996) Contact dermatitis from amorolfine-containing cream and nail lacquer. Contact Dermatitis 34:145
137. Fidalgo A, Lobo L (2004) Allergic contact dermatitis due to amorolfine nail lacquer. Am J Contact Dermat 15:54
138. Dooms-Goossens A, Matura M, Drieghe J, Degreef H (1995) Contact allergy to imidazoles used as antimycotic agents. Contact Dermatitis 33:73–77
139. Hausen BM, Heesch B, Kiel U (1990) Studies on the sensitizing capacity of imidazole derivatives, part I. Am J Contact Dermat 1:25–33
140. Hausen BM, Angel M (1992) Studies on the sensitizing capacity of imidazole and triazole derivatives, part II. Am J Contact Dermat 3:95–101
141. Hausen BM, Lücke R, Rothe E, Erdogan A, Rinder H (2000) Sensitizing capacity of azole derivatives, part III. Investigations with antihelmintics, antimycotics, fungicides, antithyroid compounds, and proton pump inhibitors. Am J Contact Dermat 11:80–88
142. Lazarov A, Ingber A (1997) Pustular allergic contact dermatitis to isoconazole nitrate. Am J Contact Dermat 8:229–230
143. Heikkila H, Stubb S, Reitamo S (1996) A study of 72 patients with contact allergy to tioconazole. Br J Dermatol 134:678–680
144. Cooper SM, Shaw S (1999) Contact allergy to clotrimazole: an unusual allergen. Contact Dermatitis 41:168
145. Nöhle M, Straube MD, Czliska C, Schwanitz HJ (1997) Beruflich erworbene sensibilisierung gegen clotrimazole. Derm Beruf Umwelt 45:232–234
146. Guidetti HS, Vicenzi C, Guerra L, Tosti A (1995) Contact dermatitis due to imidazole antimycotics. Contact Dermatitis 33:282
147. Faria A, Gonçalo S, Gonçalo M, Freitas C, Baptista AP (1996) Allergic contact dermatitis from tioconazole. Contact Dermatitis 35:250–252
148. Erdmann S, Hertl M, Merk HF (1999) Contact dermatitis from clotrimazole with positive patch-test reactions also to croconazole and itraconazole. Contact Dermatitis 40:47–48
149. Steinmann A, Mayer G, Breit R, Agathos M (1996) Allergic contact dermatitis from croconazole without cross sensitivity to clotrimazole and bifonazole. Contact Dermatitis 35:255–256
150. Kawada A, Hiruma M, Fujioka A, Tajima S, Ishibashi A, Kawada I (1997) Contact dermatitis from neticonazole. Contact Dermatitis 36:106–107
151. Shono M (1997) Allergic contact dermatitis from neticonazole hydrochloride. Contact Dermatitis 37:136–137
152. Umebayashi Y, Ito S (2001) Allergic contact dermatitis due to lanoconazole and neticonazole. Contact Dermatitis 44:48–49
153. Tanaka N, Kawada A, Hiruma M, Tajima S, Ishibashi A (1996) Contact dermatitis from lanoconazole. Contact Dermatitis 35:256–257
154. Nakano R, Miyoshi H, Kanzaki T (1996) Allergic contact dermatitis from lanoconazole. Contact Dermatitis 35:63
155. Umebayashi Y (1999) Three cases of contact dermatitis due to lanoconazole. Environ Dermatol (Jpn) 6:122

156. Soga F, Katoh N, Kishimoto S (2004) Contact dermatitis due to lanoconazole, cetyl alcohol and diethyl sebacate in lanoconazole cream. Contact Dermatitis 50:49–50

157. Goday JJ, Yanguas I, Aguirre A, Ilardia R, Soloeta S (1995) Allergic contact dermatitis from sertaconazole with cross sensitivity to miconazole and econazole. Contact Dermatitis 32:370–371

158. van Ketel WG (1983) An allergic eruption probably caused by ketoconazole. Contact Dermatitis 9:113

159. van Dijke CPH, Veerman FR, Haverkamp HC (1983) Anaphylactic reactions to ketoconazole. Br Med J 287:1673

160. Cooper SM, Reed J, Shaw S (1999) Systemic reaction to nystatin. Contact Dermatitis 41:345–346

161. Kempinaire A, de Raeve L, Merckx M, de Coninck A, Bauwens M, Roseeuw D (1997) Terbinafine-induced acute generalized exanthematous pustulosis confirmed by a positive patch test result. J Am Acad Dermatol 37:653–655

162. Matura M, Goossens A (2000) Contact allergy to corticosteroids. Allergy 55:698–704

163. Scheuer E, Warshaw E (2003) Allergy to corticosteroids: update and review of epidemiology, clinical characteristics and structural cross-reactivity. Am J Contact Dermat 14:179–187

164. Corazza M, Mantovani C, Maranini C, Bacilieri S, Virgili A (2000) Contact sensitization to corticosteroids: increased risk in long term dermatoses. Eur J Dermatol 10:533–535

165. Keegel T, Saunders H, Milne R, Sajjachareonpong P, Fletcher A, Nixon R (2004) Topical corticosteroid allergy in an urban Australian centre. Contact Dermatitis 50:6–14

166. Uter W (1990) Allergische reaktionen auf glukokorticoide (Allergic reaction to glucocorticoids, in German). Derm Beruf Umwelt 38:75–90

167. Lauerma AI, Reitamo S (1994) Allergic reactions to topical and systemic corticosteroids. Eur J Dermatol 5:354–358

168. Whitmore SE (1995) Delayed systemic allergic reactions to corticosteroids. Contact Dermatitis 32:193–198

169. Butani L (2002) Corticosteroid-induced hypersensitivity reaction. Ann Allergy Asthma Immunol 89:439–445

170. Karsh J, Yang W (2003) An anaphylactic reaction to intra-articular triamcinolone: a case report and review of the literature. Ann Allergy Asthma Immunol 90:254–258

171. Coopman S, Degreef H, Dooms-Goossens A (1989) Identification of cross-reaction patterns in allergic contact dermatitis from topical corticosteroids. Br J Dermatol 121:27–34

172. Goossens A, Matura M, Degreef H (2000) Reactions to corticosteroids: some new aspects regarding cross-sensitivity. Cutis 65:43–45

173. Barth J, Lehr KH, Derendorf H, Möllmann HW, Höhler T, Hochhaus G (1993) Studies on the pharmacokinetics and metabolism of prednicarbate after cutaneous and oral administration. Skin Pharmacol 6:179–186

174. Töpert M, Olivar A, Optiz D (1990) New developments in corticosteroid research. J Dermatol Treat 1(Suppl 3):S5–S9

175. Wilkinson SM, Hollis S, Beck MH (1995) Reaktionen auf andere Kortikosteroide bei Patienten mit allergischer Kontaktdermatitis infolge Hydrocortison. Z Haut Geschlechtskr 70:368–372

176. Täuber U (1994) Dermatocorticosteroids: structure, activity, pharmacokinetics. Eur J Dermatol 4:419–429

177. Wilkinson SM (2000) Corticosteroid cross-reactions: an alternative view. Contact Dermatitis 42:59–63

178. Isaksson M, Bruze M (2003) Corticosteroid cross-reactivity. Contact Dermatitis 49:53–54

179. Isaksson M, Brandao FM, Bruze M, Goossens A (2000) Recommendation to include budesonide and tixocortol pivalate in the European standard series. Contact Dermatitis 43:41–42

180. Wilkinson SM, English JSC (1991) Hydrocortisone sensitivity: a prospective study of the value of tixocortol pivalate and hydrocortisone acetate as patch test markers. Contact Dermatitis 25:132–133

181. Lauerma AI, Tarvainen K, Forström L, Reitamo S (1993) Contact hypersensitivity to hydrocortisone-free alcohol in patients with allergic patch test reactions to tixocortol pivalate. Contact Dermatitis 28:10–14

182. Lepoittevin J-P, Drieghe J, Dooms-Goossens A (1995) Studies in patients with corticosteroid contact allergy. Understanding cross-reactivity among different steroids. Arch Dermatol 131:31–37

183. Isaksson M, Bruze M, Björkner B, Hindsén M, Svensson L (1999) The benefit of patch testing with a corticosteroid at a low concentration. Am J Contact Dermat 10:31–33

184. Isaksson M, Andersen KE, Brandao FM, Bruynzeel DP, Bruze M, Diepgen T, Ducombs G, Frosch PJ, Goossens A, Lahti A, Menné T, Seidenari S, Tosti A, Wahlberg J, Wilkinson JD (2000) Patch testing with budesonide in serial dilutions. A multicentre study of the EECDRG. Contact Dermatitis 42:352–354

185. Wilkinson SM, Beck MH (2000) Patch testing for corticosteroids using high and low concentrations. Contact Dermatitis 42:350–351

186. Chowdhury MMU, Statham BN, Sansom JE, Foulds IS, English JSC, Podmore P, Bourke J, Orton D, Ormerod AD (2002) Patch testing for corticosteroid allergy with low and high concentrations of tixocortol pivalate and budesonide. Contact Dermatitis 46:311–312

187. Bircher AJ, Levy F, Langauer S, Lepoittevin J-P (1995) Contact allergy to topical corticosteroids and systemic contact dermatitis from prednisolone with tolerance of triamcinolone. Acta Derm Venereol (Stockh) 75:490–493

188. Goossens A, Linsen G (1998) Contact allergy to antihistamines is not common. Contact Dermatitis 39:38

189. Heine A (1996) Diphenhydramine: a forgotten allergen? Contact Dermatitis 35:311–312

190. Yamada S, Tanaka K, Kawahara Y, Inada M, Ohata Y (1998) Photoallergic contact dermatitis due to diphenhydramine hydrochloride. Contact Dermatitis 38:282

191. Parente G, Pazzaglia M, Vincenzi C, Tosti A (1999) Contact dermatitis from pheniramine maleate in eye drops. Contact Dermatitis 40:338

192. Calnan CD, Frain-Nell W, Cuthbert JW (1962) Occupational dermatitis from chlorpromazine. Trans St John Derm Soc 48:49

193. Greenberg JH (1995) Allergic contact dermatitis from topical doxepin. Contact Dermatitis 33:281

194. Taylor JS, PradiTsuwan P, Handel D, Kuffner G (1996) Allergic contact dermatitis from doxepin cream. One-year patch test clinic experience. Arch Dermatol 132:515–518

195. Bilbao I, Aguirre A, Vicente JM, Raton JA, Zabala R, Diaz Perez JL (1996) Allergic contact dermatitis due to 5% doxepin cream. Contact Dermatitis 35:254–255

196. Buckley DA (2000) Contact allergy to doxepin. Contact Dermatitis 43:231–232

197. Horn HM, Tidman MJ, Aldridge RD (2001) Allergic contact dermatitis due to doxepin cream in a patient with dystrophic epidermolysis bullosa. Contact Dermatitis 45:115

35

198. Ophaswongse S, Maibach HI (1993) Topical nonsteroidal antiinflammatory drugs: allergic and photoallergic contact dermatitis and phototoxicity. Contact Dermatitis 29: 57–64

199. Achten B, Bourlond A, Haven E, Lapière CM, Piérard G, Reynaers H (1973) Étude du bufexamac crème et du bufexamac onguent dans le traitement de diverses dermatoses (Bufexamac cream and ointment for the treatment of various dermatoses, in French). Dermatologica 146:1–7

200. Pigatto PD, Riboldi A, Morelli M, Altomare GF, Polenghi MM (1985) Allergic contact dermatitis from oxyphenbutazone. Contact Dermatitis 12:236–237

201. Kurumaji Y, Ohshiro Y, Miyamoto C, Keong CH, Katoh T, Nishioka K (1991) Allergic photocontact dermatitis due to suprofen. Contact Dermatitis 25:218–223

202. Bagheri H, Lhiaubet V, Montrastuc JL, Chouini-Lalanne N (2000) Photosensitivity to ketoprofen: mechanisms and pharmacoepidemiological data. Drug Saf 22:339–349

203. Horn HM, Humphreys F, Aldridge RD (1998) Contact dermatitis and prolonged photosensitivity induced by ketoprofen and associated with sensitivity to benzophenone-3. Contact Dermatitis 38:353–354

204. Valsecchi R, Falghieri G, Cainelli T (1983) Contact dermatitis from ketoprofen. Contact Dermatitis 9:163–164

205. Alomar A (1985) Ketoprofen photodermatitis. Contact Dermatitis 12:112–113

206. Adamski H, Benkalfate L, Delaval Y, Ollivier I, le Jean S, Toubel G, le Hir-Garreau I, Chevrant-Breton J (1998) Photodermatitis from non-steroidal anti-inflammatory drugs. Contact Dermatitis 38:171–174

207. le Coz CJ, Bottlaender A, Scrivener JN, Santinelli F, Cribier B, Heid E, Grosshans E (1998) Photocontact dermatitis from ketoprofen and tiaprofenic acid: cross-reactivity study in 12 consecutive patients. Contact Dermatitis 38: 245–252

208. Durieu C, Marguery MC, Giordany-Labadie F, Journe F, Loche F, Bazex J (2001) Allergies de contact photoaggravées et photoallergies de contact au ketoprofène: 19 cas. Ann Dermatol Venereol 128:1020–1024

209. Matthieu L, Meuleman L, van Hecke E, Blondeel A, Dezfoulian B, Constandt L, Goossens A (2004) Contact and photocontact allergy to ketoprofen. The Belgian experience. Contact Dermatitis 50:238–241

210. Cusano F, Capozzi M (1992) Photocontact dermatitis from ketoprofen and cross-reactivity to ibuproxam. Contact Dermatitis 27:50–51

211. Mozzanica N, Pigatto PD (1990) Contact and photocontact allergy to ketoprofen: clinical and experimental study. Contact Dermatitis 23:336–340

212. Kawada A, Aragane Y, Maeda A, Yudate T, Tezuka T (2000) Contact dermatitis due to flurbiprofen. Contact Dermatitis 42:167–168

213. Sugiyiama M, Nakada T, Hosaka H, Sueki H, Iijima M (2001) Photocontact dermatitis to ketoprofen. Am J Contact Dermat 12:180–181

214. Pigatto PD, Bigardi A, Legori A, Valsecchi R, Picardo M (1996) Cross-reactions in patch testing and photopatch testing with ketoprofen, thiaprophenic acid, and cinnamic aldehyde. Am J Contact Dermat 7:220–223

215. Serrano G, Fortea JM, Latasa JM, Millan F, Janes C, Bosca F, Miranda MA (1992) Photosensitivity induced by fibric acid derivatives and its relation to photocontact dermatitis to ketoprofen. J Am Acad Dermatol 27: 204–208

216. Jeanmougin M, Petit A, Manciet JR, Sigal M, Dubertret L (1996) Eczema photoallergique de contact au ketoprofène. Ann Dermatol Venereol 123:251–255

217. Kawada A, Aragane Y, Asai M, Tezuka T (2001) Simultaneous photocontact sensitivity to ketoprofen and oxybenzone. Contact Dermatitis 44:370

218. Pigatto PD, Mozzanica N, Bigardi AS, Legori A, Valsecchi R, Cusano F, Tosti A, Guarrera M, Balato N, Sertoli A (1993) Topical NSAID allergic contact dermatitis. Italian experience. Contact Dermatitis 29:39–41

219. Valsecchi R, Cainelli T (1985) Contact dermatitis from ibuprofen. Contact Dermatitis 12:286–287

220. Navarro LA, Jorro G, Morales LC, Pelaez A (1995) Allergic contact dermatitis due to piketoprofen. Contact Dermatitis 32:181

221. Goday JJ, Oleaga M, Gonzalez M, del Pozo JDP, Fonseca E (2000) Photoallergic contact dermatitis from piketoprofen. Contact Dermatitis 43:115

222. Valenzuela N, Puig L, Barnadas MA, Alomar A (2002) Photocontact dermatitis due to dexketoprofen. Contact Dermatitis 47:237

223. Cuerda E, Goday JJ, del Pozo JDP, Garcia J, Peña C, Fonseca E (2003) Photocontact dermatitis due to dexketoprofen. Contact Dermatitis 48:283–284

224. Vanhee J, Gevers D, Dooms-Goossens A (1981) Contact dermatitis from an antirheumatic gel containing etofenamate. Contact Dermatitis 7:50–51

225. Hergueta JP, Ortiz FJ, Iglesias L (1994) Allergic contact dermatitis from etofenamate: report of 9 cases. Contact Dermatitis 31:60–62

226. Piñol J, Carapeto FJ (1984) Contact urticaria to etofenamate. Contact Dermatitis 11:132–133

227. Montoro J, Rodriguez-Serna M, Liñara JJ, Ferre MA, Sanchez-Motilla JM (1997) Photoallergic contact dermatitis due to flufenamic acid and etofenamate. Contact Dermatitis 37:139–140

228. Sanchez-Perez J, Sanchez TS, Garcia-Diez A (2001) Combined contact and photocontact allergic dermatitis to etofenamate in flogoprofen gel. Am J Contact Dermat 12: 215–216

229. Smeenk G (1973) Contact allergy to bufexamac. Dermatologica 147:334–337

230. Frosch PJ, Raulin C (1987) Kontaktallergie auf bufexamac (Contact allergy to bufexamac, in German). Hautarzt 38: 331–334

231. Kranke B, Szolar-Platzer C, Komericki P, Derhaschnig J, Aberer W (1997) Epidemiological significance of bufexamac as a frequent and relevant contact sensitizer. Contact Dermatitis 36:212–215

232. Proske S, Uter W, Schnuch A, Hartschuh W (2003) Severe allergic contact dermatitis with generalized spread due to bufexamac presenting as the "baboon" syndrome (in German). Dtsch Med Wochenschr 128:545–547

233. Kerr OA, Kavanagh G, Horn H (2002) Allergic contact dermatitis from topical diclofenac in Solaraze gel. Contact Dermatitis 47:175

234. Goday JJ, Garcia GM, Martinez W, del Pozo J, Fonseca E (2001) Photoallergic contact dermatitis from aceclofenac. Contact Dermatitis 45:170

235. Fernandez de Corres L (1980) Photodermatitis from benzydamine. Contact Dermatitis 6:285

236. Figueiredo A, Ribeiro CF, Gonçalo S, Caldeira MM, Poiares-Baptista AP, Teixeira F (1987) Piroxicam-induced photosensitivity. Contact Dermatitis 17:73–79

237. Beller V, Kaufmann R (1987) Contact dermatitis to indomethacin. Contact Dermatitis 17:121

238. Walchner M, Rueff F, Przybilla B (1997) Delayed-type hypersensitivity to mofebutazone underlying a severe drug reaction. Contact Dermatitis 36:54–55

35

239. Foti C, Cassano N, Mazzarella F, Bonamonte D, Vena GA (1997) Contact allergy to thiocolchicoside. Contact Dermatitis 37:134

240. Foti C, Vena GA, Angelini G (1992) Photocontact allergy due to thiocolchicoside. Contact Dermatitis 27:201–202

241. Grimalt F, Romaguera C (1978) Sensitivity to petrolatum. Contact Dermatitis 4:377

242. Dooms-Goossens A, Degreef H (1980) Sensitization to yellow petrolatum used as a vehicle for patch testing. Contact Dermatitis 6:146–147

243. Conti A, Manzini BM, Schiavi ME, Motolese A (1995) Sensitization to white petrolatum used as vehicle for patch testing. Contact Dermatitis 33:201–202

244. Andersen KE, Maibach HI (1983) Drugs used topically. In: de Weck AL, Bundgaard H (eds) Allergic reactions to drugs. Springer, Berlin Heidelberg New York, pp 313–372

245. Kligman AM (1983) Lanolin allergy: crisis or comedy? Contact Dermatitis 9:99–107

246. Kligman AM (1998) The myth of lanolin allergy. Contact Dermatitis 39:103–107

247. Wakelin SH, Smith H, White IR, Rycroft RJG, McFadden JP (2001) A retrospective analysis of contact allergy to lanolin. Br J Dermatol 145:28–31

248. Clark EW, Blondeel A, Cronin E, Oleffe JA, Wilkinson DS (1981) Lanolin of reduced sensitizing potential. Contact Dermatitis 7:80–83

249. Schlossman ML, McCarthy JP (1979) Lanolin and derivatives chemistry: relationship to allergic contact dermatitis. Contact Dermatitis 5:65–72

250. Oleffe JA, Blondeel A, Boschmans S (1978) Patch testing with lanolin. Contact Dermatitis 4:233–247

251. Edman B, Moller H (1989) Testing a purified lanolin preparation by a randomized procedure. Contact Dermatitis 20:287–290

252. Rietschel RL, Fowler JF (1995) Dermatitis to preservatives and other additives in cosmetics and medications. In: Rietschel RL, Fowler JF (eds) Fisher's contact dermatitis. Williams and Wilkins, Baltimore, Md, pp 257–329

253. Hannuksela M, Pirila V, Salo OP (1975) Skin reactions to propylene glycol. Contact Dermatitis 1:112–116

254. Funk JO, Maibach HI (1994) Propylene glycol dermatitis: re-evaluation of an old problem. Contact Dermatitis 31:236–241

255. Fowler JF (1993) Contact allergy to propylene glycol in topical corticosteroids. Am J Contact Dermat 4:37

256. Uter W, Schwanitz HJ (1996) Contact dermatitis from propylene glycol in ECG electrode gel. Contact Dermatitis 34:230–231

257. Connolly M, Buckley DA (2004) Contact dermatitis from propylene glycol in ECG electrodes, complicated by medicament allergy. Contact Dermatitis 50:42

258. Farrar CW, Bell HK, King CM (2003) Allergic contact dermatitis from propylene glycol in Efudix cream. Contact Dermatitis 48:345

259. Bajaj AK, Gupta SC, Chatterjee AK, Singh KG (1990) Contact sensitivity to polyethylene glycols. Contact Dermatitis 22:291–292

260. Pasche-Koo F, Piletta PA, Hunziker N, Hauser C (1994) High sensitization rate to emulsifiers in patients with chronic leg ulcers. Contact Dermatitis 31:226–228

261. Tosti A, Vicenzi C, Guerra L, Andrisano E (1996) Contact dermatitis from fatty alcohols. Contact Dermatitis 35:287–289

262. Hannuksela M, Kousa M, Pirilä V (1976) Contact sensitivity to emulsifiers. Contact Dermatitis 2:201–204

263. Tosti A, Guerra L, Morelli R, Bardazzi F (1990) Prevalence and source of sensitization to emulsifiers: a clinical study. Contact Dermatitis 23:68–72

264. Menné T, Hjorth N (1988) Routine patch testing with paraben esters. Contact Dermatitis 19:189–191

265. Goossens A, Claes L, Drieghe J (1998) Antimicrobials: preservatives, antiseptics and disinfectants. Contact Dermatitis 39:133–134

266. Wilkinson JD, Shaw S, Andersen KA, Brandao FM, Bruynzeel DP, Bruze M, Camarasa JMG, Diepgen T, Ducombs G, Frosch PJ, Goossens A, Lachapelle J-M, Lahti A, Menné T, Seidenari S, Tosti A, Wahlberg JE (2002) Monitoring levels of preservative sensitivity in Europe. A 10-year overview (1991–2000). Contact Dermatitis 46:207–210

267. Fisher AA (1973) The paraben paradox. Cutis 12:830–832

268. Ramsing DW, Menné T (1993) Contact sensitivity to sorbic acid. Contact Dermatitis 28:124–125

269. Oleffe JA, Blondeel A, de Connick A (1979) Allergy to chlorocresol and propylene glycol in a steroid cream. Contact Dermatitis 5:53–54

270. Dooms-Goossens A, Deveylder H, de Alam AG, Lachapelle JM, Tennstedt D, Degreef H (1989) Contact sensitivity to nonoxynols as a cause of intolerance to antiseptic preparations. J Am Acad Dermatol 21:723–727

271. de Groot AC, Nater JP (1981) Contact allergy to dithranol. Contact Dermatitis 7:5–8

272. Chadha V, Shenoi SD (1999) Allergic contact dermatitis from dithranol. Contact Dermatitis 41:166

273. Zollner TM, Ochsendorf FR, Hensel O, Thaci D, Diehl S, Kalveram CM, Boehncke W-H, Wolter M, Kaufmann R (1997) Delayed-type reactivity to calcipotriol without cross-sensitization to tacalcitol. Contact Dermatitis 37:251

274. Frosch PJ, Rustemeyer T (1999) Contact allergy to calcipotriol does exist. Report of an unequivocal case and review of the literature. Contact Dermatitis 40:66–71

275. Krayenbühl BH, Elsner P (1999) Allergic and irritant contact dermatitis from calcipotriol. Am J Contact Dermat 10:78–80

276. Park YK, Lee JH, Chung WJ (2002) Allergic contact dermatitis from calcipotriol. Acta Derm Venereol (Stockh) 82:71–72

277. Kimura K, Katayama I, Nishioka K (1995) Allergic contact dermatitis from tacalcitol. Contact Dermatitis 33:441–442

278. Shaw DW, Eichenfield LF, Shainhouse T, Maibach HI (2004) Allergic contact dermatitis from tacrolimus. J Am Acad Dermatol 50:962–965

279. Schena D, Barba A, Costa G (1996) Occupational contact urticaria to cisplatin. Contact Dermatitis 34:220–221

280. Daughters D, Zackheim H, Maibach HI (1973) Urticaria and anaphylactoid reactions after topical applications of mechlorethamine. Arch Dermatol 107:429–430

281. Anderson LL, Welch ML, Grabski WJ (1997) Allergic contact dermatitis and reactivation phenomenon from iontophoresis of 5-fluorouracil. J Am Acad Dermatol 36:478–479

282. Valsecchi R, Imberti G, Cainelli T (1991) Mitomycin C contact dermatitis. Contact Dermatitis 24:70–71

283. Vonderheid EC, van Scott EJ, Johnson WC, Grekin DA, Asbell SO (1977) Topical chemotherapy and immunotherapy of mycosis fungoides: intermediate-term results. Arch Dermatol 113:454–462

284. Burden A, Beck MH (1992) Contact hypersensitivity to azathioprine. Contact Dermatitis 27:329–330

285. Suzuki K, Suzuki M, Akamatsu H, Matsungaga K (2002) Allergic contact dermatitis from minoxidil: study of the cross-reaction to minoxidil. Am J Contact Dermat 13: 45–46

286. Tosti A, Bardazzi F, de Padova MP, Caponeni GM, Melino M, Veronesi S (1985) Contact dermatitis to minoxidil. Contact Dermatitis 13: 275–276

287. Trattner A, David M (2002) Pigmented contact dermatitis from topical minoxidil 5%. Contact Dermatitis 46: 246

288. Vicenzi C, Lucente P, Ricci C, Tosti A (1997) Facial contact dermatitis to metronidazole. Contact Dermatitis 36: 116–117

289. Balato N, Patruno C, Lembo G, Cuccurullo FM, Ayala F (1995) Allergic contact dermatitis from retinoic acid. Contact Dermatitis 332: 51

290. Pereira F, Fernandes C, Dias M, Lacerda MH (1995) Allergic contact dermatitis from zinc pyrithione. Contact Dermatitis 33: 131

291. Goh CL, Ng SK (1986) Contact sensitivity to salicylic acid. Contact Dermatitis 14: 114

292. Baptista A, Barros MA (1992) Contact dermatitis to crotamiton. Contact Dermatitis 27: 59

293. Meneghini CL, Vena GA, Angelini G (1982) Contact dermatitis to scabicides. Contact Dermatitis 8: 285–286

294. Fisher AA (1982) Resorcinol – a rare sensitizer. Cutis 29: 331

295. Okazawa H, Aihara M, Nagatani T, Nakajima H (1998) Allergic contact dermatitis due to ethyl alcohol. Contact Dermatitis 38: 233

296. Agathos M, Bandmann HJ (1984) Benzoyl peroxide contact allergy in leg ulcer patients. Contact Dermatitis 11: 316–317

297. Leow YH, Ng SK, Wong WK, Goh CL (1995) Contact allergic potential of topical traditional Chinese medicaments in Singapore. Am J Contact Dermat 6: 4–8

298. Lee TY, Lam TH (1988) Irritant contact dermatitis due to a Chinese herbal medicine Lu-Shen-Wan. Contact Dermatitis 18: 213–218

299. Lee TY, Lam TH (1991) Contact dermatitis due to Chinese orthopaedic tincture, Zheng Gu Shui. Contact Dermatitis 24: 64–65

300. Barbaud A, Mougeolle JM, Tang JQ, Protois JC (1991) Contact allergy to colophony in Chinese Musk and Tiger-Bone Plaster. Contact Dermatitis 25: 324–326

301. Koh D, Lee BL, Ong HY, Ong CN (1997) Colophony in topical traditional Chinese medicaments. Contact Dermatitis 37: 243

302. Lee TY, Lam TH (1993) Myrrh is the putative allergen in bonesetter's herbs dermatitis. Contact Dermatitis 29: 279

303. Li L-F, Wang J (2002) Patch testing in allergic contact dermatitis caused by topical Chinese herbal medicine. Contact Dermatitis 47: 166–168

304. Chen HH, Sun CC, Tseng MP, Hsu CJ (2003) A patch test study of 27 crude drugs commonly used in Chinese topical medicaments. Contact Dermatitis 49: 8–14

305. Holdiness MR (1989) A review of contact dermatitis associated with transdermal therapeutic systems. Contact Dermatitis 20: 3–9

306. Hogan DJ, Maibach HI (1990) Adverse dermatologic reactions to transdermal drug delivery systems. J Am Acad Dermatol 22: 811–814

307. Gordon DR, Shupak A, Doweck I, Spitzer O (1989) Allergic contact dermatitis by transdermal hyoscine. Br Med J 298: 1220–1221

308. Corazza M, Mantovani L, Virgili A, Strumia R (1995) Allergic contact dermatitis from a clonidine transdermal delivery system. Contact Dermatitis 32: 246

309. Prisant LM (2002) Transdermal clonidine skin reactions. J Clin Hypertens (Greenwich) 4: 136–138

310. Torres V, Lopes JC, Leite L (1992) Allergic contact dermatitis from nitroglycerin and estradiol transdermal therapeutic systems. Contact Dermatitis 26: 53–54

311. Perez-Calderon R, Gonzalo-Garijo MA, Rodriguez-Nevado I (2002) Generalized allergic contact dermatitis from nitroglycerin in a transdermal therapeutic system. Contact Dermatitis 46: 203

312. Boehncke W-H, Gall H (1996) Type IV hypersensitivity to topical estradiol in a patient tolerant to it orally. Contact Dermatitis 35: 187–188

313. Gonçalo M, Oliveira HS, Monteiro C, Clerins I, Figueiredo A (1999) Allergic and systemic contact dermatitis from estradiol. Contact Dermatitis 40: 58–59

314. Koch P (2001) Allergic contact dermatitis from estradiol and norethisterone acetate in a transdermal hormonal patch. Contact Dermatitis 44: 112–113

315. Corazza M, Mantovani L, Montanari A, Virgili A (2002) Allergic contact dermatitis from transdermal estradiol and systemic contact dermatitis from oral estradiol. A case report. J Reprod Med 47: 507–509

316. Farm G (1993) Contact allergy to nicotine from a nicotine patch. Contact Dermatitis 29: 214–215

317. Buckley DA, Wilkinson SM, Higgins EM (1998) Contact allergy to a testosterone patch. Contact Dermatitis 39: 91–92

318. Shouls J, Shum KW, Gadour M, Gawkrodger DJ (2001) Contact allergy to testosterone in an androgen patch: control of symptoms by pre-application of topical corticosteroid. Contact Dermatitis 45: 124–125

319. Herbst RA, Maibach HI (1991) Contact dermatitis caused by allergy to ophthalmic drugs and contact lens solutions. Contact Dermatitis 25: 305–312

320. Herbst RA, Maibach HI (1992) Contact dermatitis caused by allergy to ophthalmics: an update. Contact Dermatitis 27: 335–336

321. Herbst RA, Maibach HI (1997) Allergic contact dermatitis from ophthalmics: update 1997. Contact Dermatitis 37: 252–253

322. Manni G, Centofanti M, Sacchetti M, Oddone F, Bonini S, Parravano M, Bucci MG (2004) Demographic and clinical factors associated with the development of brimonidine tartrate 0.2%-induced ocular allergy. J Glaucoma 13: 163–167

323. Friedlaender MH (1995) A review of the causes and treatment of bacterial and allergic conjunctivitis. Clin Ther 17: 800–810

324. Britz MB, Maibach HI (1979) Human cutaneous vulvar reactivity to irritants. Contact Dermatitis 5: 375–377

325. Farage MA, Bjerke DL, Mahony C, Blackburn KL, Gerberick GF (2003) Quantitative risk assessment for the induction of allergy contact dermatitis: uncertainty factors for mucosal exposure. Contact Dermatitis 49: 140–147

326. Marren P, Wojnarowska F, Powell SM (1982) Allergic contact dermatitis and vulvar dermatoses. Br J Dermatol 126: 52–56

327. Virgili A, Corazza M, Bacilieri S, Califano A (1997) Contact sensitivity in vulvar lichen simplex chronicus. Contact Dermatitis 37: 296–297

328. Lewis FM, Shah M, Gawkrodger DJ (1997) Contact sensitivity in pruritus vulvae: patch test results and clinical outcome. Am J Contact Dermat 8: 137–140

329. Goldsmith PC, Rycroft RJG, White IR, Ridley CM, Neill SM, McFadden JP (1997) Contact sensitivity in women with anogenital dermatoses. Contact Dermatitis 36: 174–175

35

330. Chow ET (2001) Multiple corticosteroid allergies. Australas J Dermatol 42:62–63

331. Black RJ, Dawson TAJ, Strang WC (1990) Contact sensitivity to lignocaine and prilocaine. Contact Dermatitis 23:117–118

332. Urrutia I, Jauregui I, Gamboa P, Gonzalez G, Antepara I (1998) Photocontact dermatitis from cinchocaine (dibucaine). Contact Dermatitis 39:139–140

333. Lee AY (1998) Allergic contact dermatitis from dibucaine in Proctosedyl ointment without cross-reaction. Contact Dermatitis 39:261

334. Corbett JR (1985) Allergic contact dermatitis to Trimovate. Contact Dermatitis 13:281

335. Valsecchi R, Imberti GL, Cainelli T (1990) Nifuratel contact dermatitis. Contact Dermatitis 23:187

336. Sanchez-Perez J, Abajo P, Córdoba S, Garcia-Diez A (2000) Allergic contact dermatitis from sodium metabisulfite in an antihemorrhoidal cream. Contact Dermatitis 42:176–177

337. McKenna KE (2000) Allergic contact dermatitis from glyceryl trinitrate ointment. Contact Dermatitis 42:246

338. Tanaka S, Otsuki T, Matsumoto Y, Hayakawa R, Sugiura M (2001) Allergic contact dermatitis from enoxolone. Contact Dermatitis 44:192

339. Reyes JJ, Fariña MC (2001) Allergic contact dermatitis due to trimebutine. Contact Dermatitis 45:164

340. Gallo R, Parodi A (2002) Baboon syndrome from 5-aminosalicylic acid. Contact Dermatitis 46:110

341. Pecegueiro M Brandão FM (1983) Alergia de contacto em doentes com úlcera de perna (contact allergy in patients with leg ulcers, in Portuguese). Trab Soc Port Dermatol Venereol XLI:37–46

342. Schupp DL, Winkelmann RK (1988) The role of patch testing in stasis dermatitis. Cutis 42:528–530

343. Wilson CL, Cameron J, Powell SM, Cherry G, Ryan TJ (1991) High incidence of contact dermatitis in leg-ulcer patients – implications for management. Clin Exp Dermatol 16:250–253

344. Gallenkemper G, Rabe E, Bauer R (1998) Contact sensitization in chronic venous insufficiency: modern wound dressings. Contact Dermatitis 38:274–278

345. Machet L, Couhe C, Perrinaud A, Hoarau C, Lorette G, Vaillant L (2004) A high prevalence of sensitization still persists in leg ulcer patients: a retrospective series of 106 patients tested between 2001 and 2002 and a meta-analysis of 1975–2003 data. Br J Dermatol 150:929–935

346. Wilkinson SM (1994) Hypersensitivity to topical corticosteroids. Clin Exp Dermatol 19:1–11

347. Keilig W (1983) Kontaktallergie auf cetylstearyl alkohol (Lanette O) als therapeutisches problem bei stauungsdermatitis und ulcus cruris (Contact allergy to cetylstearylalcohol (Lanette O) as a therapeutic problem in stasis dermatitis and leg ulcer, in German). Derm Beruf Umwelt 31:50–54

348. Mallon E, Powell SM (1994) Sorbitan sesquioleate: a potential allergen in leg ulcer patients. Contact Dermatitis 30:180–181

349. Mallon E, Powell SM (1994) Allergic contact dermatitis from Granuflex hydrocolloid dressing. Contact Dermatitis 30:110–111

350. Schliz M, Rauterberg A, Weiss J (1996) Allergic contact dermatitis from hydrocolloid dressings. Contact Dermatitis 34:146–147

351. Molin L, Stymne S, Stark HU, Eriksson IL (1996) Allergic contact dermatitis induced by tackifying agents in hydrocolloid dressings. J Eur Acad Dermatol Venereol 7(Suppl 2):S142–S143

352. Sasseville D, Tennstedt D, Lachapelle JM (1997) Allergic contact dermatitis from hydrocolloid dressings. Am J Contact Dermat 8:236–238

353. Downs AMR, Sharp LA, Sansom JE (1999) Pentaerythritol-esterified gum rosin as a sensitizer in Granuflex hydrocolloid dressing. Contact Dermatitis 41:162–163

354. Menné T, Veien N, Sjolin K-E, Maibach HI (1994) Systemic contact dermatitis. Am J Contact Dermat 5:1–12

355. Rietschel RL, Fowler JF (1995) Systemic contact-type dermatitis. In: Rietschel RL, Fowler JF (eds) Fisher's contact dermatitis. Williams and Wilkins, Baltimore, Md., pp 114–129

356. Guin JD, Phillips D (1989) Erythroderma from systemic contact dermatitis: a complication of systemic gentamicin in a patient with contact allergy to neomycin. Cutis 43:564–567

357. Andersen KE, Hjorth N, Menné T (1984) The baboon syndrome: systemically-induced allergic contact dermatitis. Contact Dermatitis 10:97–100

358. Nakayama H, Niki F, Shono M, Hada S (1983) Mercury exanthema. Contact Dermatitis 9:411–417

359. Bártolo E, Brandão FM (1988) Mercury exanthema. Contact Dermatitis 18:172

Chapter 36

Dental Materials

36

TUULA ESTLANDER, KRISTIINA ALANKO, RIITTA JOLANKI

Contents

36.1 Introduction

Dental care personnel and dental laboratory workers are exposed daily to several allergens or irritants that cause delayed- or immediate-type allergic or irritant contact dermatitis. In addition, the hands of workers are repeatedly exposed at short intervals to water and cleansing agents. Even the use of plastic or rubber protective gloves is not without problems. Water- and air-tight gloves may hydrate and irritate the skin. In the worst case, allergy to glove materials may develop. Gloves permeable to chemicals used at work may even promote the development of allergy to these chemicals.

The same dental care products may also elicit allergic or irritant reactions in dental patients. They usually cause delayed-type allergic contact stomatitis (ACS) reactions, but immediate reactions are also possible. Patch testing is essential in distinguishing delayed allergic reactions from irritant ones. A biopsy may sometimes be necessary to exclude other oral diseases.

36.2 Dental Care Personnel and Dental Laboratory Workers

Nowadays, it is known worldwide that dentists, dental nurses, and other dental workers are at considerable risk of developing occupational contact dermatitis from the materials used in their work, whereas their patients only rarely develop contact stomatitis from dental materials [1–17]. Other occupational diseases may also develop, for instance bronchial asthma, rhinitis, conjunctivitis, pharyngitis, and laryngitis [18–23].

During the past decades, the frequency of occupational contact dermatitis has increased steadily in dental care personnel and was considered to be about 40% in the first part of the 1990s [11]. In the 1990s, three times as many occupational diseases of dentists and dental nurses compared to earlier were reported to the Finnish Register of Occupational Diseases

(FROD). In the same period, plastic materials had taken the place of amalgam in dental restoration, and the use of protective gloves [usually natural rubber latex (NRL) gloves] had become common practice because of the increased risk of HIV (human immunodeficiency virus) and hepatitis virus infections. In particular, allergic contact dermatitis (ACD) caused by methacrylates and NRL gloves, as well as contact urticaria due to NRL gloves had increased [14–15].

According to the information obtained from the FROD in 1990–2000, and from the study on dental nurses, two-thirds of all occupational diseases of dental care personnel were cases of contact dermatitis, with ACD being the most common of them. Typically, the number of cases of ACD is more than two-thirds, and the cases of irritant contact dermatitis is less than one-third of all the cases of contact dermatitis. Dental care workers belong to the eight most risky occupations concerning occupational allergic contact dermatitis. The risk of developing ACD is six times more common in dental care work compared to the average risk in all occupations [14–15].

Similar results concerning the sensitization of dental care personnel have been obtained in other studies as well [6–7, 17]. The frequency of type-IV sensitivity in dentists, dental hygienists, dental assistants, or dental students attending annual health screenings in 1997, 1998, 2000, 2002, and 2003 arranged by the American Dental Association (ADA) Annual Sessions, held in various major American cities, was determined by patch testing. One hundred and seventy eight (178) dentists and 51 non-dentists participated, and 49% of the patch-tested participants displayed positive reactions to at least one allergen. The most prominent allergens derived from dental materials were rubber chemicals and methacrylates [17].

In 1990–2000, a total of 151 cases of dermatosis among dentists and cases among 302 dental nurses were reported to the FROD. The number of cases of contact dermatitis was 349, of which more than two-thirds (255 cases) were cases of allergic contact dermatitis (type-IV allergy). Ninety-four (94) were cases of contact urticaria or protein contact dermatitis (type-I allergy) [14].

Dental laboratory workers have a similar risk of developing hand eczema as other dental personnel [24–26]. At the beginning of the 1980s, a Finnish questionnaire study of dental technicians [24] revealed the frequency of their hand dermatitis, both present and previous, to be about 30%. These technicians were mainly men (80%). In a Danish cross-sectional questionnaire study among dental technicians [27], the 1-year prevalence of skin problems of the hands was 43%, which was eight times as high as among the general population. More than half (60%) of the study participants were women. Another study with the same group showed that there was a rapid increase in the skin problems of dental technician trainees [28].

In a Swedish retrospective cohort study [26] of former dental technician students (n=2,139), a postal questionnaire inquired about the factors for the occurrence of hand eczema, including age of onset, occupational exposure, and use of protective gloves. In dental technicians, the incidence of hand eczema was 7.1 cases/1,000 person years among men and 10.8 among women during the time that they were exposed to acrylates. Based on the results, the risk of hand eczema was stated to be more than doubled in dental technicians.

36.3 Allergic Contact Dermatitis

36.3.1 Clinical Picture

The hands, and especially the fingers of dentists, dental nurses, orthodontists, and dental technicians, are most exposed to hazardous chemicals, which are often both allergens and irritants. Allergic contact dermatitis (ACD) caused by chemicals is typically located on the fingertips, which may become very dry, hyperkeratotic, chapped, smarting or itching, and reddish (pulpitis). There may also be vesicles or scaling. Stinging or burning sensations are also quite common, especially in cases caused by acrylics. ACD caused by methacrylates can be followed by mild paresthesia. The symptoms of paresthesia may last for weeks, even for half a year after the dermatitis has disappeared. These symptoms can also appear without previous development of contact allergy [29]. Also, the nail folds may become inflamed and red, swollen, and chapped [30]. Dermatitis may also appear in other locations, including the face, eyelids, and other exposed skin areas by airborne contact or by contaminated hands or gloves [5, 11].

ACD caused by rubber or plastic gloves appears typically on the skin areas covered by the gloves. Separate, itching eczematous areas may occur on the backs of the hands or on the wrists, or there may be reddish, swollen, and scaling dermatitis throughout the glove-covered areas. The dermatitis is usually the worst in skin areas that are in close contact with the gloves. Sometimes edema of the face and eyelids may be associated [31].

After contact with the causative agent has stopped, the dermatitis will disappear in different ways, de-

36

pending on its location. Even very mild pulpitis may take 2 or 3 weeks to cure, whereas dermatitis on the backs of the hands may disappear in a week. The skin usually remains symptomless if it is not in contact with the causative allergen, but one contact a week with the allergen makes dermatitis recur and may induce chronic dermatitis.

36.3.2 Causative Agents

36.3.2.1 Acrylics and Other Plastic Chemicals

Methacrylates and Acrylates

The methacrylates and acrylates contained in uncured dental plastic materials are the most common causes of ACD in dental personnel, including dentists, orthodontists, and dental nurses, and in dental laboratory workers, such as dental technicians and dental laboratory assistants [1–5, 7, 11, 14–15, 17, 25–26].

Up until the 1980s, knowledge of the irritant and sensitizing effects of dental materials was scarce. However, hypersensitivity to methylmethacrylate (MMA) in the manufacture of prostheses was reported as early as in 1941 [32, 33]. In 1954, Fisher and Woodside [34] described two dentists and two dental mechanics (technicians) who were occupationally sensitized to methylmethacrylate and who also had positive patch test reactions. The number of reports on dental personnel occupationally sensitized to acrylics was still small in the 1970s. Knowledge about the sensitizing capacity of acrylics was lacking and MMA was widely used as a standard allergen in revealing sensitization to dental acrylics. Better possibilities for investigating and understanding allergies associated with dental materials were not discovered until the beginning of the 1980s. New information was obtained about the sensitizing capacity of methacrylate and acrylate compounds in two theses using guinea pig maximization tests [35, 36]. At the same time, Tony Axell, together with Bert Björkner, Sigfrid Fregert, and Bo Niklasson in co-operation with the Scandinavian Institute of Dental Materials (NIOM), began to develop a patch test series suitable for examining stomatitis patients as well as dental care personnel [37]. The series contained 21 patch test substances, which were selected based on reported cases of contact allergy to dental materials, and the most frequently used components with documented or suspected potential contact allergens in dental practice. Most of these substances are still included in commercially available dental screening series, e.g., Chemotechnique Diagnostics, Malmö, Swe-

den and Trolab, Hermal, Reinbeck, Germany. In the 1990s, several clinical studies showed that MMA is a rather poor screening allergen for acrylics, and confirmed previous guinea pig sensitization studies on acrylics indicating that especially low-molecular-weight (LMW) methacrylates, such as 2-hydroxyethylmethacrylate (2-HEMA), triethylene glycol dimethacrylate (TREGDMA), and ethyleneglycol dimethacrylate (EGDMA) in the dental materials are stronger contact sensitizers than MMA, and also need to be used for patch testing [1–2, 4, 38–44] (see also Table 1).

Dental Composite Resins

The plastic products used in dental restoration can be dental composite resins (DCR), glass ionomers, glass-ionomer cements with plastic reinforcement, and compomers (glass ionomer added to DCR). DCR based on bisphenol A and methacrylates, e.g., 2,2-bis[4-(2-Hydroxy-3-methacryloxypropoxy)phenyl]-propane (Bisphenol A glycidyl methacrylate or bis-GMA), have been used since 1962 [46]. bis-GMA is the most extensively used hardening binder of DCR, which can also be replaced by urethane dimethacrylate (UEDMA), which has similar properties. bis-GMA and epoxy diacrylate sensitized four out of eight dental patients having occupational ACD in the 1980s [38]. Thereafter, new cases have not been reported from dental practice. High-molecular-weight (HMW) bis-GMA and UEDMA are probably not as common a sensitizer as LMW methacrylates. Allergy to UEDMA may be even less common than allergy to epoxy dimethacrylate [5].

Because HMW methacrylates have high viscosity, LMW methacrylates, including TREGDMA and EGDMA, are added to dilute these HMW monomers. The most commonly used dimethacrylate is TREGDMA. When water solubility is necessary, 2-HEMA is added, e.g., in glass ionomers and compomers. DCR may also contain chemically reactive prepolymers as allergens, usually methacrylated epoxies and urethanes, methacrylates, and dimethacrylates.

Concomitant positive patch test reactions to sensitizing methacrylates are common [2, 4, 25], which can be ascribed to multiple sensitization or cross-reactions based on animal tests [2, 47, 48]. Patch test results of sensitized workers with large (meth)acrylate series of Chemotechnique Diagnostics indicate that inter-patient cross-reactions to acrylics vary. During their work, career dental personnel are exposed to various DCR products, which may differ in composition from one batch to another [4–5].

DCR also contain inorganic fillers, e.g., fine particles of glass or quartz, pigments, nonreactive inert

Table 1. Allergic (meth)acrylate reactions in a 10-year study (October 1994 – September 2004) at the Finnish Institute of Occupational Health. At least one allergic patch test reaction was shown by 53 patients. The results have been compared to the sensitizing capacity of (meth)acrylates, based on animal studies, according to Björkner [45]. Source of (met)acrylates: *C* Chemotechnique Diagnostics AB, Malmö, Sweden; *T* Trolab, Hermal, Reinbeck, Germany; *O* manufactured by the Finnish Institute of Occupational Health (FIOH). Sensitizing capacity: *NG* not given; *I* weak; *II* mild; *III* moderate; *IV* strong; *V* extreme

(Meth)acrylate series	Abbreviation	Source	Patch test concentration (%, w/w)	Allergic/ tested	Allergic (%)	Rank order	Sensitizing capacity
Ethyl acrylate	EA	C	0.1	13/404	3.2	7	NG
Butyl acrylate	BA	C	0.1	4/403	1.0	20	NG
2-Ethylhexyl acrylate	2-EHA	C	0.1	0/403	0	–	V
Methyl methacrylate	MMA	C/T	2	7+4/258+305	2.0	10	NG
Ethyl methacrylate	EMA	C	2	14/402	3.5	6	NG
n-Butyl methacrylate	BMA	C	2	3/402	0.7	24	NG
2-Hydroxyethyl methacrylate	2-HEMA	C/T	2/1	12+18/93+304	7.6	2	I
2-Hydroxypropyl methacrylate	2-HPMA	C	2	33/403	18.2	1	I
Ethyleneglycol dimethacrylate	EGDMA	C/T	2	11+16/91+302	6.9	3	I
Triethyleneglycol dimethacrylate	TREGDMA	C/T	2	3+7/92+306	2.5	8	I
1,4-Butanediol dimethacrylate	BUDMA	C	2	7/397	1.8	12	I
Urethane dimethacrylate	UDMA	C	2	3/397	0.8	22	II
2,2-bis[4-(2-Methacryloxyethoxy)-phenyl]propane	bis-EMA	C	1	3/403	0.7	24	IV
2,2-bis[4-(Methacryloxy)phenyl]propane	bis-MA	C	2	0/332	0	–	V
2,2-bis[4-(2-Hydroxy-3-methacryloxypropoxy) phenyl]propane	bis-GMA	C/T	2	1+2/90+303	0.8	22	I
1,4-Butanediol diacrylate	BUDA	C	0.1	8/402	2.0	10	III-V
1,6-Hexanediol diacrylate	HDDA	C	0.1	5/396	1.3	16	III-V
Diethyleneglycol diacrylate	DEGDA	C	0.1	16/403	4.0	4	II
Dipropyleneglycol diacrylate	DPGDA	O	0.1	2/174	1.1	18	NG
Tripropyleneglycol diacrylate	TPGDA	C	0.1	6/403	1.5	14	IV
Triethyleneglycol diacrylate	TREGDA	C	0.1	3/77	3.9	5	I
Trimethylolpropane triacrylate	TMPTA	C	0.1	5/403	1.2	17	IV
Pentaerythritol triacrylate	PETA	C	0.1	7/403	0.5	13	V
Oligotriacrylate 480	OTA 480	C	0.1	2/403	0.5	28	III
Epoxy diacrylate {2,2-bis[4-(2-hydroxy-3-acryloxypropyl)phenyl]propane}	bis-GA	C	0.5	3/401	0.7	24	III-V
Urethane diacrylate (aliphatic)	al-UDA	C	0.1	1/403	0.2	31	V
Urethane diacrylate (aromatic)	ar-UDA	C	0.05	4/403	1.0	20	II
N,N-Methylenebisacrylamide	MBAA	C	1	1/403	0.2	31	NG
Tetrahydrofurfuryl methacrylate	THFMA	C	2	10/396	2.5	8	NG
N,N-Dimethylaminoethyl methacrylate	DMAEMA	O	0.2	0/66	0	–	NG
Glycidyl methacrylate	GMA	O	0.1	5/324	1.5	14	NG
Ethoxylated bisphenol-A dimethacrylate	EBADMA	O	0.2	2/175	1.1	18	NG
Ethoxyethyl acrylate	EEA	O	0.1	1/324	0.3	29	NG
2-Phenoxyethyl acrylate	PEA	O	0.1	2/338	0.6	27	NG
Isobornyl acrylate	IBA	O	0.1	0/338	0	–	NG
Ethyl cyanoacrylate	ECA	O	10	1/341	0.3	29	NG

36

polymers, and polymeric waxes that necessarily are not allergens [38]. When these additional substances are missing, the product is called a resin [4–5, 14].

Polymerization of the DCR mixture may take place by using chemicals or visible light. Double curing materials are cured using both chemicals and light. DCR may, therefore, contain various additives, such as photoinitiators (e.g., camphoroquinone), other initiators [e.g., (di)benzoylperoxide], activators (e.g., tertiary aromatic amines), and inhibitors (e.g., hydroquinone or methylhydroquinone), which may also sensitize [5, 11, 14].

Light-cured glass ionomers contain similar sensitizing methacrylates as DCR, and may cause allergy. A dental nurse had daily handled light-cured hybrid glass ionomers and developed occupational fingertip dermatitis, typical of ACD caused by acrylate compounds. On patch testing, she reacted to several acrylics, including 2-HEMA. Her hybrid glass ionomer primer and liquid also provoked an allergic patch test reaction [49].

Dentin bonding systems are needed to ensure firm adhesion of the DCR to the tooth. The first dentin-resin bonding agent was N-phenyl glycine glycidyl methacrylate, developed by Bowen in 1962 [46]. Since then, a large number of new dentin bonding compounds have been developed [51]. In 1978, a bonding system with a hydrophobic resin (methacryloxyethyl phenyl phosphate), phenyl P, mixed with a water-soluble form of methacrylate resin, i.e., 2-HEMA, was marketed in Japan. In 1983, the 3M Company introduced a bonding system using a phosphate ester of bis-GMA, and in 1988 saw a new system based on maleic acid and 2-HEMA. Eleven patients were sensitized to acrylics in dentin bonding systems. Four dental nurses and five dentists developed ACD, one dentist had pharyngitis, but no skin symptoms, and one dental nurse was probably sensitized from patch testing with her own undiluted acrylate products [51]. Concentrations of methacrylates identified in dental restorative materials are given in Table 2. However, the composition may change and new products are continuously being developed.

Before the restorative material (e.g., DCR) is applied into the teeth, the cavity is treated with an acidic etching agent and a bonding system, e.g., with a primer followed by an adhesive. The curing takes place with visible light. 2-HEMA is commonly used in both primers and adhesives. Nowadays more often one-component bonding systems are used [4, 5].

Prostheses

The composition of the basement sheets of dental prostheses has been almost the same for decades.

Table 2. Concentrations of methacrylates identified in dental restorative materials [142]. For the abbreviations of (meth)acrylates, see Table 1

Identified methacrylate	Concentration (%, w/w)	
	Range	Median
Bonding materials (seven products)		
2-HEMA	0.3–28	17
bis-GMA	21–40	27
EGDMA	0.05–0.4	<0.3
TREGDMA	4–46	
UDMA	2–29	
Diethyleneglycol dimethacrylate	0.05–5	
Trimethylolpropane trimethacrylate	3–7	
EMA	1	
Glycerine dimethacrylate	4–8	
Methacrylic acid	Not quantified	
2-HPMA	0.3	
1-Chloromethyl-2-hydroxy-ethyl methacrylate	Not quantified	
Composite resins (8 products)		
bis-GMA	6–21	10
TREGDMA	3–7	6
EGDMA	0.05–5	
UDMA	8–15	11
bis-EMA	6–8	
Decamethylene dimethacrylate	0.05–1	
2-HEMA	7	
DMAEMA	2	
bis-MA	5	
Diethyleneglycol dimethacrylate	Not quantified	
Methacrylic acid	Not quantified	
Glass ionomers (2 products)		
2-HEMA	0.2–23	
EGDMA	0.1–0.2	
Methacrylic acid	Not quantified	
TMPTMA	9	
2-HPMA	0.3	

They are prepared from a mixture of polymethyl methacrylate (PMMA) powder and liquid MMA, and the mass is molded manually or mechanically. The components of the powder and liquid of an acrylic denture base material are shown in Table 3. The powder may also contain copolymers with different acrylates, e.g., polybutyl acrylate, or methacrylates, e.g., polyethyl methacrylate and polyisobutyl methacrylate or polystyrene, initiators [(di)benzoylperoxide, barbiturates], colors, pigments (salts of cadmium, calcium, and zinc), butyl hydroxytoluene (BHT), and various filling agents, such as silicone dioxide [4, 5, 11, 25, 52].

Table 3. Components of the powder and liquid of an acrylic denture base material [5]

Powder	Liquid
Polymethyl methacrylate or polymer	Methyl methacrylate or monomer
Organic peroxide initiator	Hydroquinone inhibitor
Titanium dioxide for control translucency	Dimethacrylate or cross-linking agent[a]
Inorganic pigments for color	Organic amine accelerator[b]
Dyed synthetic fibers for appearance	

[a] A cross-linking agent is present if the manufacturer indicates that the material is a cross-linked acrylic
[b] The amine is present only if the material is labeled as a product to be processed at room temperature. Some manufacturers list them as cold-curing or self-curing materials

When PMMA powders melted at lower temperatures than usual are used, they can contain, in addition, copolymers of MMA, e.g., ethylmethacrylate (EMA). The powders may also contain small amounts of monomer impurities, e.g., MMA and ethylacrylate (EA). N-Butyl methacrylate, isobutyl methacrylate, and other methacrylates can be used to replace liquid MMA. After molding, the acrylate mixture polymerizes. The reaction is based on the use of heat, chemicals, light (UV or visible), or microwaves. (di)Benzoylperoxide is used in mixtures that polymerize at room temperature (cold-cured or self-cured) or at higher temperatures (heat-cured) to initiate the hardening process [4, 5, 11, 25].

If the manufacturer indicates that the material is a cross-linked acrylic, then 1,4-butanediol dimethacrylate (BUDMA), EGDMA, or ethylene glycol methacrylate can be used., e.g., the monomer liquid in heat-polymerizable products contains 1,4-butanediol dimethacrylate or EGDMA as cross-linkers. Monomer liquids may also contain 2-HEMA and other dimethacrylates. Cold-curable liquids may contain allergenic activators such as N, N-dimethyl-p-toluidine, 4-tolyldiethanolamine, and diethanol-p-toluidine. Liquids may also contain stabilizers (polymerization inhibitors), such as (methyl)hydroquinone, p-methoxyphenol or butylated cresols (BHT). Other components include ethyl alcohol and plasticizers, such as phthalates (dibutyl phthalate). In addition, benzophenones or benzotriazoles, phenyl salicylate, methyl salicylate, resorcinol monobenzoate, or stilbene can be added as UV-absorbers [3–5, 24, 25, 52–55].

Also, complex light-curable (UV or visible) acrylics similar in composition to DCR are used by dental technicians, and this may mean an increased risk of sensitization to these materials. According to some safety data sheets, these products may contain urethaneacrylates, e.g., polyester urethaneacrylate, dimethacrylates, e.g., diurethane dimethacrylate, 1,6-hexanedioldimethacrylate, methacrylates, e.g., MMA, dimethylaminoethyl methacrylate, acrylates, e.g., 3-dimethyaminoneopentylacrylate, and accelerators,

photoinitiators, e.g., camphoroquinone, and other compounds, including fillers, pigments, and BHT [4, 5].

Crown and bridge materials can contain, in addition to MMA, e.g., tetrafurfuryl methacrylate, EGDMA, TREGDMA, I, 4-BUDMA and UEDMA [5, 25, 53].

Fasting cements for prostheses usually contain similar acrylate compounds as DCR.

Dental technicians and other dental laboratory workers also use daily many other materials, such as glues, plasters, waxes, dental alloys, polishing pastes, and enamel. Molding plasters can contain melamine-formaldehyde resin, which has sensitized dental technicians [25].

Cyanoacrylate glues are used almost daily in dental laboratories. They are usually used to repair cracks in plaster and stone (hard) plaster models, but can also be used to glue together broken acrylic prostheses. Cyanoacrylate glues seldom sensitize. Cases have been reported from glueing artificial nails [56–58] and attaching false hair with the glues [59]. The allergens in these cases were ethyl cyanoacrylate and MMA. Cyanoacrylate glues may also irritate the skin and induce chemical burns as a result of accidental exposure [57]. Nail dystrophy has been described after the use of artificial nails [58]. Asthma caused by cyanoacrylate exposure is also well known [60].

In a German study, out of 55 patch tested dental technicians, 16% reacted to MMA, 33% to 2-HEMA, and 27% to EGDMA. Positive reactions to other methacrylates, e.g., to EMA (11%) and TREGDMA (4%), and to acrylates, e.g., EA (6%) and pentaerythritol triacrylate (PETA) (4%), were less common. The study also demonstrated high cross-reactivity between 2-HEMA and EGDMA and moderate cross-reactivity between MMA and 2-HEMA. Only two positive reactions to TREGDMA were observed and one to BUDMA, suggesting that these are less sensitizing compounds than MMA, 2-HEMA, and EGDMA [25]. MMA, 2-HEMA, and EGDMA were also the most common reactors in a previous German study of dental technicians [55].

Additives in Dental Acrylics

Additives used in dental restoration and prosthetic materials are seldom the cause of ACD.

(di)Benzoyl peroxide is an essential part of these materials. An appreciable amount of benzoylperoxide can be present in dentures [61]. However, only solitary cases of sensitization have been reported. Two cases of ACD from manufacturing dental prostheses were reported by Calnan [62]. Kanerva et al. 1994 [63] described a dentist who was sensitized to mercury and benzoyl peroxide. Benzoyl peroxide has also caused sensitization in other exposures, including acrylic bone cement, an arm prosthesis, acne treatment preparations, baking additives, and the treatment of leg ulcers [64–66]. It has also caused airborne ACD [67]. On patch testing, benzoyl peroxide is an irritant that easily causes false-positive reactions. The frequency of 11% positive reactions of the participants in an American patch test study of dental personnel suggests several irritant reactions [17].

Also N,N-dimethyl-p-toluidine and 4-tolyl diethanolamine are very rare sensitizers in dental personnel. A dentist with occupational ACD had positive patch tests reactions to 4-tolyl diethanolamine, as well as to coconut diethanolamide and N-ethyl-4-toluene sulfonamide [68].

Methylhydroquinone and hydroquinone are used to prevent unintended polymerization, but sensitization in dental personnel has not been reported. Other stabilizers, p-methoxy phenol and BHT, are also very rare sensitizers [5, 24].

Plasticizers are added to improve the flexibility, softness, and pliability of plastics. Dibutyl phthalate has been added as a plasticizer at various times to denture base resins by the manufacturer or by the dental technician. In general, allergy to dibutylphthalate is very rare [5].

Camphoroquinone is used as an initiator for visible-light-cured DCR materials and primers. It has been considered as a nonsensitizer, but one case of active sensitization from patch testing has been reported [69].

Various UV-absorbers are incorporated in DCR products, other plastics, textiles, and sunscreens. They include, e.g., 2-hydroxy-4-methoxy-benzophenone (Eusolex 4360), 2-(2-hydroxy-5-methylphenyl)benzotriazole (Tinuvin P), phenyl salicylate, methyl salicylate, resorcinol monobenzoate, and stilbene. Sporadic cases of sensitization have been reported, but not in dental personnel [4, 5, 53].

Epoxy Resin and Bisphenol A

Sensitizing diglycidylether-of-bisphenol-A epoxy resin (DGEBA-ER) is, nowadays, used as a component of a root canal sealant. Some of the dental workers sensitized to DCR also reacted to DGEBA-ER on patch testing [45]. DCR may contain DGEBA-ER as an impurity. Possibly, DGEBA-ER and bis-GMA cross-react in some individuals, although there is also evidence that they do not cross-react [5, 45, 70].

Bisphenol A is a raw material in the production of epoxy and acrylic resins. A dental nurse was sensitized to bisphenol A, possibly as an impurity in the DCR products that she had handled at work [71].

Bisphenol A can also be used as an additive in the manufacture of PVC plastics. A dentist and an oral hygienist were sensitized from the use of PVC gloves of the same trademark. However, it cannot be ruled out that the DCR which they had handled during their restorative work may have contributed to their sensitization. After these cases, the disposable PVC gloves on the Finnish markets were analyzed, but bisphenol A could no longer be found [72].

36.3.2.2 Rubber Chemicals

Protective gloves are the most common source of occupational allergic contact dermatitis from rubber chemicals [31]. They are among the most common causes of ACD in dental care personnel, in addition to methacrylate and acrylate compounds [6, 14, 15, 17]. They have to be taken into account also in dental laboratory work, even though gloves are not used as consistently as in dental restoration work [24–26, 53]. There may also be other causes of rubber sensitization among dentists, e.g., dams and polishing discs made of rubber [38].

Rubber gloves are usually manufactured using various automated processes. The primary ingredient is rubber polymer, which is blended with 15–20 additives, including vulcanizing agents, accelerators, antioxidants, pigments, fillers, and oils. Rubber polymer can be a natural product made from milky liquid (natural latex) of the rubber tree, or it can be manufactured synthetically. Whether a rubber glove is called natural (NRL) or synthetic depends on the origin of the polymer used in its manufacture [31].

Sensitizing chemicals are contained in gloves made of both natural and synthetic rubbers. However, natural rubber gloves are commonly used gloves, and are, therefore, probably the main cause. The three most important allergenic causative chemicals include thiuram, dithiocarbamate, and benzothiazole accelerators [31]. In an American patch test study of dental personnel, 10% reacted to thiurams and 12% to carbamates [17].

In 1990–2000, a total of 61 (18%) out of 255 cases of allergic contact dermatitis in dental personnel reported to the FROD were caused by rubber chemicals [14, 15].

36.3.2.3 Antimicrobials

Antimicrobials are also an important group of sensitizers among dental care and dental laboratory workers [5, 14, 15, 17]. They can be components of disinfectants and cleansing agents, e.g., glutaraldehyde, formaldehyde and formaldehyde-releasing agents, glyoxal, chloramine-T, and persulfates. They can also be used as components of tooth bleaching agents (persulfates), and they may be present in medicines used to cure gingivitis, disinfectant liquids of implants, and mouth and hand washes (chlorhexidine). All antimicrobials used in hand cleansing agents and hand creams can also be causes of contact allergy in dental work (e.g., isothiazolinones, methyldibromo glutaronitrile, and formaldehyde liberators).

Glutaraldehyde is widely used as an antimicrobial agent in the cold sterilization of dental equipment and in hospitals, e.g., for disinfecting metal parts of beds and in hospital laboratories. It may be present in dental acrylic adhesives and bonding agents at concentrations of 0.7–5%. It is also an irritant, and has previously been considered to be a weak sensitizer [73]. However, more recent reports suggest it to be a stronger sensitizer [74–76]. Glutaraldehyde, in addition to other antimicrobials, has induced sensitization in dental nurses [38, 76, 77]. Glutaraldehyde and formaldehyde do not cross-react, but concomitant sensitization is common [3, 64]. In an American patch test study, glutaraldehyde and formaldehyde each produced 3.5% positive reactions with no evidence of cross-reactivity [17].

Formaldehyde is a commonly used chemical and a frequent sensitizer in many countries [78]. Paraformaldehyde, previously commonly used to treat root canals, has been an important source of formaldehyde allergy in dentistry [15, 38]. Formaldehyde as such is possibly no longer a component in disinfecting and cold-sterilizing liquids in dental practice. Various formaldehyde-releasing agents are probably the source of formaldehyde in some cleansing agents and soaps. According to Flyvholm's investigation in Danish markets [79], bromonitropropanediol, bromonitrodioxane, and trihydroxyethylhexahydro s-triazine were the most common formaldehyde releasers in cleansing agents, and bromonitrodioxane, imidazolidinyl urea, and bromonitropropanediol in

soaps and other skin care products. Patients allergic to formaldehyde will benefit from information on exposure to formaldehyde releasers. In addition, some formaldehyde releasers can act as allergens themselves [14, 15, 79].

Minimal amounts of formaldehyde which possibly leach from acrylics are not important in the development of allergy to the chemical.

Glyoxal (ethanediol) is a dialdehyde, which can be a component in many disinfectants used to disinfect equipment and rooms in hospitals and in dental practices. Elsner et al. [80] reported on seven health care workers sensitized to the chemical. Two of these seven also reacted to formaldehyde and three of six to glutaraldehyde. One report describes a dental nurse who had developed occupational ACD from glyoxal, glutaraldehyde, and neomycin sulfate [77].

TEGO, the commercial name of certain disinfectants sold in many countries under various trade names, has been the cause of several cases of ACD [38, 81, 82]. The active ingredient of TEGO is dodecyl-di-(aminoethyl)glycine (DDAG), but is not present in all TEGO products. It has been widely used in Europe as an antiseptic for instruments in hospitals and in dental practices [38]. From the 1970s to the 1990s, it was the most common antimicrobial agent causing ACD in Finnish dental personnel [15, 38, 83]. Since 1991, TEGO products have not been available in Finland.

Chlorhexidine, 1,6-di-(4-chlorophenyldiguanido)-hexane was introduced in the 1950s. It is a guanidin disinfectant. Chlorhexidine diacetate, digluconate, or hydrochloride can be used as an antimicrobial, e.g., in topical antiseptics, for disinfectants, e.g., in ointments, mouth, and hand washes. It is also used to cure gingivitis. Despite its widespread use, delayed allergic reactions, as well as photoallergic reactions can be considered rare. Immediate reactions due to exposure to the chemical are more important [5, 84].

Quaternary ammonium compounds classified in cationic detergents are, nowadays, increasingly used as disinfectants for various dental instruments and equipment. They are irritants that can also cause delayed irritation reactions. A delayed irritant reaction may be difficult to distinguish from true allergic reactions on patch testing.

Benzalkonium chloride is the most extensively used quaternary ammonium compound in medical use. It has been classified as weak allergens in animal experiments [85]. It has been concluded that, in the average population, benzalkonium chloride is not a relevant allergen, whereas in medical professionals and in ophthalmological patients, it is possibly a relevant one, but only some cases of allergy to the compound have been reported. A dental nurse having contact allergy to benzalkonium chloride from a sterilizing solution has been reported. [5, 76, 84].

Placucci et al. [86] reported hand dermatitis in a dental nurse from *N*-benzyl-*N*, *N*-dihydroxyethyl-*N*-cocosalkyl-ammonium chloride, present in disinfectant wipes used in dentistry.

ACD from polyvinylpyrrolidone-iodine (*povidone-iodine*, Betadine) has rarely been reported. It is used at a concentration of 4% as a skin cleanser. Those sensitized to povidone-iodine are usually not allergic to iodine [87, 88]. The chemical is possibly a weak sensitizer. Occupational ACD is rare [89–91], but has been reported in a dentist and in an operating room nurse [92].

Products containing *potassium persulfate* are used to disinfect surfaces, but not instruments in dental practice. It is also used in toothpastes and other bleaching agents of teeth. The chemical may irritate the skin and cause delayed and immediate allergic reactions, as well as asthma [5, 93–95].

36.3.2.4 Metals

Metallic *mercury* has been used, e.g., in dental amalgams, thermometers, pharmaceuticals, antifouling agents, and agricultural chemicals. Mercury unites with many metals to form an amalgam. Amalgams prepared from zinc, tin, and mercury have been used as dental cements, and amalgams of mercury with gold, silver, or copper have been used as fillings for teeth [3]. The composition of amalgams used in different countries varies and there has also been variation over time [96]. Occupational amalgam allergy is relatively rare, but has been reported in dentists and dental nurses [2, 5, 97, 98].

Gold in dentistry is used in the form of alloys with silver, copper, palladium, platinum, and zinc to make, e.g., crowns and bridges. Previously, contact allergy to metallic gold and gold salts was considered to be low, but during the past 10 years, a high frequency of positive reactions among dermatitis patients patch tested with gold sodium thiosulfate have been reported [99–107]. Patch testing with the salt may cause a long-lasting patch test reaction [108]. Hypersensitivity to gold may be seen, together with contact allergy to other metals, including mercury, nickel, and palladium [109–111].

Several sporadic cases of ACD from both metallic gold and gold salts have been reported. Occupational gold allergy has been reported in the electronics and gold-plating industry [111]. A dental nurse working in a special dental laboratory polished gold crowns and bridges in periods of 2 weeks, and was exposed to fine metal dust. She developed itching dermatitis on her hands and face when polishing the pieces, and the dermatitis faded soon after she had stopped the work. On patch testing, she showed a positive reaction to gold sodium thiosulfate, probably from exposure to the dust containing gold (unpublished).

Orthodontists are increasingly applying braces to children and adults. Since at least 10% of women are allergic to *nickel*, a nickel-allergic orthodontist may get hand dermatitis when bending the metal parts of braces. Dental technicians may use instruments releasing nickel, and they can also be exposed to materials containing nickel, resulting in sensitization and ACD to nickel, or their pre-existing nickel allergy may worsen [3, 5, 11, 14].

Palladium is a metal found most commonly in ore combined with platinum, gold, and copper. It is used in varying amounts (4–82%) in cast dental restorations. It has also been used instead of amalgam in dental fillings to avoid the possible toxicity of mercury. Dermatitis from palladium was previously considered rare, but nowadays, about one-third of the patients allergic to nickel sulfate also show positive patch test reactions to palladium, possibly as a sign of cross-reactivity. There are no convincing reports on occupational dermatitis caused by palladium [3, 5, 112, 113].

Cobalt–chromium alloys, which form the framework of partly metal dentures, and base metal alloys contain about 60% cobalt. Dental technicians may have a risk of developing sensitivity to *cobalt*, e.g., when exposed to the polishing dust of these alloys. However, none of the 55 dental technicians in a German study reacted to cobalt [25]. It is often not clear whether *chromium* or other metals or metal salts have caused the allergic reactions elicited by dental metals [5, 25].

Aluminum is used as pure metal or as an alloy, e.g., in dental materials. Aluminum salts can be used in dental ceramics. Allergy is very rare, and has not been reported from dental aluminum [5, 113].

Dental amalgam may also contain *copper*, but allergic reactions to copper are rarely reported. Many of the patients who are patch test positive to copper are concomitantly positive to nickel sulfate, and the question of cross-reactivity has, therefore, been raised. On the other hand, the copper patch test substance may contain nickel, and the positive reaction may represent allergy to nickel. However, copper allergy has been reported [5, 113–115]. Metallic platinum is also used in dentistry, but it rarely causes ACD [113].

Dental amalgam also contains *silver* and *tin*. Metallic silver has not been reported to cause ACD.

There is no convincing evidence of sensitization caused by tin [113].

Titanium frameworks with removable partial dentures have been recommended for use in patients allergic to other metals. Titanium is also used in dental implants. Some reports indicate that the metal can act as an allergen. Its use in these applications is still recommended [5, 113].

36.3.2.5 Colophony, Eugenol, and Balsam of Peru

Colophony or rosin is a resin obtained from different species of coniferous trees. There are three types of rosin, depending on the method of recovery. Colophony is a complex mixture of resin acids (about 90%) and neutral substances. The major acids are abietic acid and dehydroabietic acid. As a result of exposure to air, oxidized components are present in colophony. The oxidized components are important sensitizers. The major allergen is the primary oxidation product, 15-hydroperoxyabietic acid. Patients with positive patch test reactions to colophony often also react to balsam of Peru and fragrance mix [116]. Colophony is present in dental materials, e.g., in periodontal dressings, impression materials, cavity varnishes (cements), and temporary filling materials. Zinc-oxide-eugenol (ZOE) cements may also contain colophony. Even more than 30% colophony may be present in Duraphat, a fluoride varnish. Occupational dermatitis caused by colophony has been reported in dental nurses [117, 118] and in a dental technician [119].

In dentistry, essential oils are chiefly used as pharmaceutical aids and mild antiseptics. Eugenol is an important chemical constituent of clove oil. It is also present in many other products, including cinnamon oil, perfumes, soaps, bay rum, pimento oil (allspice), flower oils, food spices, and flavoring agents [64]. It is one of the eight components in the fragrance mixture of the standard patch series used to detect fragrance allergy. In dentistry, eugenol is mixed with zinc oxide to form ZOE cement. It can also be used in toothache drops, antiseptics, and mouth washes. ZOE has beneficial physical and therapeutic effects, making it suitable for use as a provisional restorative material, base material, and root canal filling material. Eugenol can also be combined with colophony and used as an intermediate two-component restorative material with polymethylmethacrylate powder, e.g., in IRM liquid. The two components of IRM are mixed before use. Also, eugenol-free IRM liquid is available. When eugenol is used in dental preparations, including impression pastes, surgical packing, and cements and provisional restorative fillings, it may also be the cause of occupational ACD in dental personnel [120, 121].

Other sensitizing oils can also be constituents of dental products, e.g., cinnamon, peppermint, anise, and spearmint oil. Balsam of Peru can be present in liquids mixed in surgical and impression pastes. Also, other balsams, e.g., Canada balsam, can be used [14, 122].

36.3.2.6 Impression Compounds and Resin Carriers

Silicon-based materials, alginate, and beeswax are commonly used as impression compounds. Silicon-based materials have probably not caused sensitization in dental personnel. Two cases of contact allergy have been reported, caused by a catalyst in a silicon-based material [123]. Alginates have not caused any definite cases of sensitization [124]. Beeswax is a sensitizer, and occupational dermatitis has been reported [125]. Dental modeling waxes may contain at least 17% beeswax [5].

Resin carriers are used to isolate cavities under restorations, e.g., N-ethyl-4-toluene-sulphonamide. A dentist with multiple sensitivities to materials that she had used in her dental practice also displayed a positive reaction to the chemical [68]. In a Swedish multicenter study, 9 of 1,657 patch-tested patients with oral symptoms reacted to N-ethyl-4-toluene-sulphonamide [5].

36.3.2.7 Local Anesthetics

Local anesthetics can be divided into two groups, amides and esters, based on their structure. Allergies to local anesthetics were common earlier, when the ester group of anesthetics, e.g., benzocaine was used, but allergy from amides is rare. Up to 1991, only 18 cases had been reported since the 1940s, when amide anesthetics were more extensively used [126]. Cross-reactions may occur between structurally related ester anesthetics, but not between structurally unrelated groups. Cross-reactions between amide anesthetics are not well known.

Dentists' sensitization to local anesthetics was rather common earlier [64]; nowadays, sensitization to these products is probably unusual. Benzocaine, tetracaine, and procaine used to be the sensitizers in these cases [64]. Lidocaine (xylocaine, lignocaine) is an amide anesthetic and does not cross-react with benzocaine or tetracaine. It is safe to both dentists and their patients because allergic reactions are rare

[127]. Mepivacaine and prilocaine have caused a few solitary cases of sensitization [127, 128].

36.4 Contact Urticaria, Protein Contact Dermatitis, and Other Immediate Reactions

Contact urticaria (CU) may be an immunological (allergic) or a nonimmunological reaction. IgE-mediated (type-I) allergic reactions are usually caused by proteins, but certain LMW chemicals may also elicit similar immediate hypersensitivity reactions caused by both allergic and unknown mechanisms [5].

36.4.1 Clinical Picture

Contact urticaria reaction as a result of type-I allergy develops in minutes, usually in less than half an hour, after the skin of the hands, especially the back of the hands and fingers and wrists and forearms, has come into contact with the causative allergen. Sometimes, the eyelids can be the worst affected, probably by airborne contact or by the hands. Typically, there is redness and whealing on the skin of the contact areas, which may also be swollen and itching or smarting. A contact urticaria reaction also disappears quickly, usually in the course of a few hours, leaving the affected skin completely symptomless. Sometimes, a local contact urticaria reaction may elicit generalized urticaria. Other symptoms of type-I allergy are also common, including itching and running of the eyes or nose, conjunctivitis, rhinitis, coughing, dyspnea, or asthma. In the worst case, a life-threatening anaphylactic reaction may develop.

Type-I allergy may also lead to so-called protein contact dermatitis. When the skin is repeatedly in contact with proteinaceous causative agents, whealing may no longer be seen on the skin. The appearance of dermatitis resembles that of eczema and cannot be distinguished from allergic or irritant contact eczema caused by chemicals.

36.4.2 Causative Agents

36.4.2.1 Protective Gloves

Proteins in *natural rubber latex* (NRL) are the most important cause of contact urticaria in general, especially in dental personnel [129], and NRL gloves are the most important source. Tarlo et al. [130] reported that 10% of dental students and staff had NRL sensi-

tivity. Safadi et al. [131] reported that 12% of oral health care workers had positive skin prick tests to latex protein. Heese et al. [132] reported positive prick tests to NRL in 8.7% of 296 dental students. Lindberg and Silverdahl [13], in a study of 527 dental professionals (192 dentists, 269 nurses, 64 hygienists, 2 in administrative work), tested 389 participants with CAP-RAST (Pharmacia Upjohn Diagnostics, Uppsala, Sweden) to estimate the prevalence of NRL allergy: 7.2% were found positive in the test. There was a significant difference among the three professions: 10.2% positive dentists (13 of 128 tested), 6.0% positive nurses (13 of 216 tested), and 4.4% positive hygienists (2 of 45 tested). In Finland, dentists and dental nurses have been estimated to have the greatest risk of all occupations investigated of getting immediate allergy to latex proteins. Based on the cases reported to the FROD in 1991–1996, the incidence rate of NRL allergy in dental nurses was 11.8 cases/10,000 workers and in dentists 6.0 cases/10,000 workers. Dental nurses had 50 times as much contact urticaria and protein contact dermatitis caused by NRL proteins as all the occupations on average [129]. Also, occupational asthma caused by NRL is possible. In a study based on the cases reported to the FROD in 1990–1998, 62 cases of occupational respiratory hypersensitivity were observed in dental personnel. NRL caused ten cases of occupational rhinitis and two cases of asthma [23].

The *cornstarch powder* in NRL gloves has very seldom been reported as a cause of contact urticaria [133, 134]. On rare occasions, *chemicals* have been reported to cause contact urticaria from rubber products. A case of contact urticaria caused by latex-free nitrile gloves has been reported [5].

36.4.2.2 Low-Molecular-Weight Chemicals

Haptens may also cause IgE-mediated reactions. The hapten binds to protein or another macromolecule, and the resulting hapten–carrier conjugate acts as an allergen [135].

Chloramine-T (sodium-*N*-chlorine-*p*-toluene sulfonamide), used in dental work as a disinfectant of instruments, boxes, and surfaces, can cause occupational contact urticaria, as can persulfates used for the same purposes. In addition, they can be the cause of occupational rhinitis and asthma. At the Finnish Institute of Occupational Health (FIOH) in 1990–1998, three cases of asthma and one case of rhinitis in dental personnel were diagnosed as being caused by chloramine-T [23].

Chlorhexidine can be present in agents used to cure gingivitis and as a constituent of hand washes.

As an acetate or gluconate salt, it is used for topical application, on skin or mucous membranes, wounds, burns, surgical instruments, and surfaces. It can cause contact urticaria and asthma [136]. It can also be the cause of photosensitivity and fixed drug eruptions [136].

Colophony and eugenol have also caused immediate-type hypersensitivity reactions. In a Finnish study of dental personnel [23], one case of occupational rhinitis caused by Nobetec containing colophony was diagnosed. Contact urticaria from eugenol has been considered to be a nonimmunological reaction, but recently, it has been reported to cause type-I sensitivity and contact urticaria in a dental patient [137].

Acrylics may cause immediate hypersensitivity as well. Contact urticaria, conjunctivitis, rhinitis, pharyngitis, and asthma from cyanoacrylates, MMA, acrylic acid, and nonspecified acrylics have been reported [18–22], but the mechanism of the reactions is not known. According to the FROD, a total of 64 cases of occupational respiratory diseases were diagnosed in dental personnel in Finland; two cases were diagnosed in 1975–1989 and 62 in 1990–1998. There were 28 cases of occupational asthma (18 caused by methacrylates), 28 occupational rhinitis (6 caused by methacrylates), 7 allergic alveolitis, and 1 organic toxic syndrome. This study shows the increasing frequency of respiratory hypersensitivity in dental personnel [23].

36.5 Irritant Contact Dermatitis

Dental workers are exposed to many skin irritants. The most common irritants include cleaning agents (detergents) and disinfectants used for hands, as well as for surfaces and instruments, wet work, hydrating effect of protective gloves, and dental acrylics.

Occupational irritant contact dermatitis is, in general, more common than allergic contact dermatitis. However, according to information obtained from the FROD concerning occupational dermatoses of dentists and dental nurses in 1990–2000, only 19% of the reported 86 cases were due to irritation [14]. Detergents were reported as the main causes of irritant contact dermatitis in half of the cases (51%), wet work in 19%, and methacrylates in 10% of the cases. In a study on Finnish dental nurses, frequent hand washing was considered to be the main cause of irritant dermatitis. Half of the nurses reporting work-related hand dermatitis said that using protective gloves aggravated their hand dermatitis [15].

Corresponding results were obtained in a study of 55 patch tested dental technicians; 13 (24%) had irritant contact dermatitis and 2 had allergic/irritant contact dermatitis [25]. The causative agents were metals and plastics (acrylics), plasters, and ceramics. The most important agents causing irritant contact dermatitis to dental technicians have been wet work, work with plaster, grinding, and physical irritation, as caused by polishing metal and plastic materials. Hand washing up to 100 times a day was considered to contribute as well [24, 25]. Mürer et al. [27] studied Danish dental technicians and found acrylates to be the most important cause of their hand problems. Of the 69 having hand dermatitis at the time of the questionnaire study, 64 reported using MMA or cyanoacrylate glue daily or almost daily. Three reported allergy to MMA. A study on dental technician trainees [28] showed that, shortly after beginning their education, the trainees had the same high proportion of skin problems as the dental technicians at work.

36.6 Photo-Related Reactions

Phototoxic or photoallergic reactions may represent a new problem in dentistry as a result of extensive powerful light sources in the curing of dental resins. Many substances, including sulfonamides present in some cavity liners, phenothiazines, griseofulvin, and tetracyclines, used in dentistry may have phototoxic properties. Photoallergic compounds in dentistry include eugenol, chlorhexidine, derivatives of 4-aminobenzoic acid (PABA), sulfonamides, and phenothiazines. A generalized erythematous eruption of the face and submental area in a dental hygienist was caused by trimethoprim medication and exposure to a photocuring unit [5, 138].

36.7 Investigations

In investigations, the determination of exposure to chemicals, explanation of the work techniques used, as well as skin tests (patch and prick test) are the most important tasks, supplemented by clinical examination of the skin (localization and type of eruption), and follow-up of the course of dermatitis during working days and weekends, as well as during holiday periods and sick leave. Sometimes, the determination IgE-specific antibodies in the serum of the patient will be added to examinations.

Safety data sheets (SDSs) may be helpful in detecting exposing chemicals, but it should be remembered that not all components are given in the sheets [139–142]. In a recent study [142], acetone-soluble methacrylates in commercial dental restorative ma-

36

Table 4. Dental screening series of Chemotechnique Diagnostics (Malmö, Sweden) (*C*), Hermal (Trolab, Reinbeck/Hamburg, Germany) (*T*), and the Finnish Contact Dermatitis Group (*F*). For the abbreviations of (meth)acrylates, see Table 1. Chemotechnique Diagnostics has three dental screening series: a broad series (*B*), and specific series for patients (*P*), and for staff (*S*) (*NI* not included)

Test substance	Concentration in petrolatum or in water (aq.) (%)		
	C	T	F
(Meth)acrylates			
MMA	2 (B, P, S)	2	2
TREGDMA	2 (B, P, S)	2	2
UDMA	2 (B)	NI	2
EGDMA	2 (B, P, S)	2	2
bis-GMA	2 (B, P, S)	2	2
bis-EMA	2 (P)	NI	NI
BUDMA	2 (B, P, S)	NI	2
bis-MA	2 (B)	NI	NI
2-HEMA	2 (B, P, S)	1	2
DMAEMA	0.2 (B, P)	NI	0.2
HDDA	0.1 (B, P)	NI	NI
THFMA	2 (B, P, S)	NI	2
Diurethane dimethacrylate	NI	2	NI
Epoxy resin compounds			
Bisphenol A	NI	1	1
Epoxy resin	0.1 (P)	NI	NI
Acrylate activators, inhibitors, UV filters			
N,N-Dimethyl-4-toluidine	5 (B)	2	NI
2-Hydroxy-4-methoxy-benzophenone	10 (B)	NI	NI
N-Ethyl-4-toluenesulphonamide	0.1 (B, P)	NI	0.1
4-Tolyldiethanolamide	2 (B)	NI	2
Methylhydroquinone	1 (B)	NI	1
Hydroquinone	NI	1	1
Camphoroquinone	1 (B)	NI	NI
2(2-Hydroxy-5-methylphenyl)benzotriazol	1 (B, P)	NI	NI
Benzoyl peroxide	NI	1	NI
Metals			
Potassium dichromate	0.5 (B, P)	NI	0.5
Cobalt chloride	1 (B, P)	NI	1
Gold sodium thiosulfate	2 (B, P)	0.25	NI
Potassium dicyanoaurate	NI	0.002 aq.	NI
Nickel sulfate	5 (B, P)	NI	5
Copper sulfate	2 (B)	NI	NI
Palladium chloride	2 (B, P)	1	1
Aluminum chloride hexahydrate	2 (B)	NI	NI
Tin	50 (B)	NI	NI
Mercury	0.5 (B, P, S)	NI	0.5
Ammoniated mercury	NI	1	NI
Mercuric chloride	NI	NI	0.1
Mercury ammonium chloride	NI	NI	1
Amalgam	NI	5	NI
Amalgam alloying metals	NI	20	NI
Ammonium tetrachloroplatinate	NI	0.25	NI
Fragrances, colophony			
Eugenol	2 (B, P, S)	1	2
Colophony	20 (B, P)	NI	20
Balsam of Peru	25 (P)	NI	NI
Menthol	NI	1	NI
Peppermint oil	NI	2	NI
R-(L)-Carvone	5 (P)	NI	NI
Antimicrobials			
Formaldehyde	1 aq. (B)	NI	1 aq.
Glutaraldehyde	0.2 (S)	NI	0.2
Chlorohexidine digluconate	NI	NI	0.5 aq.
Ammonium persulfate	NI	NI	2.5
Anesthetics			
Caine mix III (benzocaine, dibucaine, tetracaine)	NI	NI	10
Rubber chemicals			
Thiuram Mix	NI	NI	1

terials – seven bonding materials, eight DCRs, and two glass ionomers – were identified by gas chromatography with mass-selective detection, and were quantified with liquid chromatography with ultraviolet detection. Information about methacrylates was given in the SDSs for only about half of the products that, according to the analysis, contained methacrylates. This result and corresponding previous results indicate that SDSs need to be improved.

If available, a special data base for dental materials, e.g., the German Info-Dent, would give more detailed information about the products. All the information in Info-Dent about the ingredients of the product was obtained from the manufacturer, mostly in confidence [11].

The clinical diagnosis of occupational ACD is confirmed by patch testing. The dental screening series of Chemotechnique Diagnostics, Trolab, and the Finnish Contact Dermatitis Group are shown in Table 4. These series contain the most common sensitizers in dental materials. If dental acrylics allergy is suspected, but methacrylate compounds in a dental screening series have, nevertheless, displayed negative results, an extensive methacrylate series (one example in Table 1) may give more information about the causative agent. Patch testing with a rubber chemical series (Chemotechnique or Trolab) may also be decisive in some cases [31].

Skin prick tests with or without determination of IgE-specific antibodies in the patient's serum are necessary when type-I allergy is suspected.

Some cases of active sensitization caused by commercial (meth)acrylate patch test substances and the patient's own acrylic products have been reported [143–147]. Previously, three patients at the FIOH were sensitized when higher patch test concentrations of certain acrylate patch test substances were used.

Despite excellent screening series, patch testing with suspected materials, such as dental acrylics and rubber and plastic glove materials, may be necessary. This is because minor components or impurities, and not the main components, may be the cause of sensitization, and also it may reveal new allergenic components. An analysis of the suspected product may also be necessary to detect special impurities possibly left in the manufacturing processes of separate acrylate compounds, e.g., epoxy resin or bisphenol A in the production of epoxy acrylates.

Patch testing with suspected acrylic products is a difficult task because too low a concentration may cause a false-negative patch test result, and too high a concentration may sensitize. It has been suggested that DCRs should be tested at 1–2% petrolatum [148]. In possible further tests with the products, the concentration should not exceed that of any acrylics.

Patch tests or use tests with undiluted acrylic products should never be performed, as even a single exposure with undiluted allergen may sensitize [146, 147]. Reports include a patient who had been sensitized from patch testing with undiluted dentin bonding acrylics, and another patient with contact leucoderma from undiluted DCR [5, 147]. In patch testing materials other than those containing acrylics, the recommendations of Jolanki et al. [148] should be followed.

36.8 Hand Protection

In the prevention of occupational contact dermatitis in dental care and laboratory work, it is of essential importance to ensure the cleanliness of the work environment, and to use technical aids that lessen the handling of reactive chemicals and encourage the use of nontouch techniques. Highly sensitizing DCRs containing various methacrylates and other products in dental restoration and monomer liquids containing MMA and other acrylate compounds should never be handled with the bare hands. However, it is difficult to select disposable gloves to protect against chemicals. Many chemicals permeate thick industrial gloves, and thin gloves made basically from the same material are permeated even more rapidly. Thin gloves also break more easily under chemical or mechanical stress and, similar to thick gloves, they may also have holes or defects. Many acrylics quickly penetrate all disposable gloves [149–155].

Permeation studies of NRL and PVC disposable examination gloves showed that these gloves do not give sufficient protection against methacrylates, such as 2-HEMA contained in primers used in dental restoration. Solvents in materials, e.g., acetone or ethyl alcohol, markedly worsen the protection given by the glove [153]. Acetone should be omitted from the dentin bonding materials, as it can penetrate even thick industrial gloves in less than 5 min. It would, therefore, be better to use ethyl alcohol instead, if possible [149–151, 153, 155, 156].

At least double gloving with PVC or NRL gloves should be used for a 15-min task. For tasks lasting 15 min to 30 min, good quality nitrile rubber gloves should be used, preferably as a double layer with other gloves. A simple PE (polyethene) glove under another glove may improve the protection considerably when performing longer tasks. Double-gloving becomes easier if the inner gloves are of a larger size. Against MMA in liquids used in the manufacture of basement sheets of prostheses or bridges, there are hardly any protective glove alternatives available, except laminated gloves, e.g., PE/EVAL(ethylene vinyl alcohol)/PE at present [155]. Gloves contaminated with uncured acrylic materials should be removed immediately, and the hands washed with water and cleansing agents.

Common protective glove materials usually give sufficient protection against cleansing agents and X-ray developers. Recent studies of the permeation of common hospital chemicals through surgical single-layered and double-layered NRL gloves and single-layered chloroprene (neoprene) gloves showed that potassium hydroxide (45%), sodium hypochlorite (13%), or hydrogen peroxide (30%) did not permeate the gloves. Furthermore, none of glutaraldehyde, chlorhexidine digluconate, or povidone-iodine in the commercial disinfectant solutions studied permeated the gloves [157].

Based on permeation studies, disposable gloves made of NRL or PVC, for example, provide sufficient protection against occasional splashes of disinfectants. Alcohols and formaldehyde permeate these gloves rapidly, and contaminated gloves must be replaced quickly and the hands must be washed. However, in continuous contact, even diluted glutaraldehyde and concentrated hydrogen peroxide permeate thin examination gloves. Chlorhexidine digluconate or povidone are not likely to permeate intact gloves [155].

To prevent NRL allergy, PVC gloves, synthetic rubber gloves, or NRL gloves with a low protein content are recommended. PE gloves under NRL gloves increase the protection and prevent sensitization to glove proteins and chemicals [15, 31, 158].

36.9 Patients

36.9.1 Oral Mucosa

The oral mucosa, like the skin, is exposed to irritants and sensitizers. The allergic reactions can be immediate, type-I reactions, e.g., from contact with NRL, or delayed, type-IV reactions, e.g., from contact with dental metals or acrylics. The term mucosal contact dermatitis has been used for delayed reactions. There is a lesser tendency to sensitization through the mucous membrane than through the skin. A chronic irritant reaction may develop due to repeated or constant exposure to irritant or toxic agents at low concentrations over long periods. Chronic irritant reactions can be seen in areas of the oral mucosa that are in close contact with amalgam or other fillings, possibly from mechanical causes. The clinical appearance of these lesions may be difficult to distinguish from those caused by contact allergy. The diagnosis is based on the exclusion of contact allergy with negative patch tests [5].

The mucosa is considered to be more resistant to irritants than the skin. The reactions to contactants are lessened by saliva, buffers, and possibly yeasts, which can modify the appearance of stomatitis. Regions with inflammation with or without ulcerations beneath removable partial dentures have caused problems for prosthodontists. Potential factors include microbial infection, obstructive sialadenitis, and allergic or irritant reactions to metal frameworks [159].

Contact allergy has been described as a factor in oral lichenoid reactions and recurrent oral ulceration. Some investigators have suggested that allergic factors are involved in patients with the burning mouth syndrome [160], while others have not [161]. Allergic factors are probably of minor importance in most cases of burning mouth syndrome, but may have contributed to the symptoms of some patients [5].

36.9.2 Allergic Contact Stomatitis and Cheilitis

36.9.2.1 Clinical Picture and Symptoms

The subjective symptoms of patients with allergic contact stomatitis (ACS) are often more prominent than the clinical signs. The complaints include burning and stinging sensations, numbness, soreness, and loss of taste. The clinical appearance varies from barely visible changes to mild or severe erythema and edema. Lingual papillae may disappear and the mucosa may look smooth, waxy and glazy, and show edema. If vesicles appear, they rupture quickly and form erosions [162].

In allergic reactions to base materials of dentures, there is a clear border between the reddish inflamed mucosa covered by the denture and the adjacent uninvolved area. The clinical appearance due to an ill-fitting plate may be similar, and patch testing is, therefore, necessary. Similarly, ACS or allergic contact cheilitis from dental metals or acrylics often shows a distinct border just around the treated tooth, but lichenoid reactions without allergy are also possible. ACS may also mimic oral changes caused by vitamin deficiency and some systemic diseases. ACS is often accompanied by cheilitis [163]. The clinical appearance includes dryness, scaling, fissuring, and angular cheilitis. It can also be caused by contactants applied to the lips. Lips rarely show edema or vesiculation. Allergic contact cheilitis does not have a boundary of normal skin immediately adjacent to the vermilion border, in contrast to perioral dermatitis, which is an endogenous skin disease. Exogenous perioral dermatitis, on the other hand, can develop from allergy to dental products [5, 164].

36.9.2.2 Causative Agents

Acrylics and Other Plastic Chemicals

Dental patients are exposed to uncured acrylic monomers for only short periods. Therefore, they are at much less risk of developing allergy than the dentists or dental nurses. Accordingly, sensitization of patients from dental acrylics other than prosthetic devices is rare [164, 165].

In the manufacture of removable dental prostheses, polymerization may remain incomplete and leave, e.g., MMA monomer in the denture, possibly causing sensitization. The heat-cured method of dentures induces more complete polymerization than the cheaper cold-cured methods, which may leave more residual monomer in the acrylate-based denture. In a German study, 0.3–4.4% residual MMA monomer was identified in all of the dental plastics investigated [54, 166].

Fisher showed that the sensitizing agent of acrylic prostheses was MMA monomer, but thought that heat-cured dentures were not allergenic [34]. Later, Crissey [167] reported allergic denture sore mouth or stomatitis from heat-cured prostheses. Kaaber [168] has reported 18 cases of MMA-induced prosthesis stomatitis. Aphthous ulcerations have been reported from TREGDMA [169]. Edema and burning sensations in both lips have been reported from a prosthesis, which, according to the manufacturer, contained in its powder component polymethylmethacrylate, benzoyl peroxide, cadmium, and ferric salts, and in the liquid MMA, EGDMA, and hydroquinone. On patch testing, the patient reacted to MMA, 2-HEMA, 2-HPMA, and EGDMA. When she started to use a dental prosthesis made of nickel and chromium, the edema of the lips resolved [170]. Edema and ulceration of the lips from 2-HEMA and TREGDMA was reported by Agner and Menné [171], and vesiculation of the lips and perioral skin from TREGDMA and bis-GMA was reported by Niinimäki et al. [172]. Also, more generalized reactions from the use of prostheses have been described, i.e., chronic urticaria without mucosal or perioral symptoms [173], and stomatitis and edema of the tongue, lips, eyelids, and hands [174]. Dental prostheses with 5–11 times higher content of residual monomer than in heat-cured dentures are also in general use. Allergic denture stomatitis may be encountered more often than previously believed [5]. Several other case reports have been published [96, 169, 175–179].

A female patient displaying a positive patch test to MMA first developed contact stomatitis from one prosthesis, but became symptomless when she used a prosthesis made of Vulcanite rubber. After more teeth were removed, a new complete upper and lower prosthesis was needed. The new prosthesis gradually began to cause worsening stomatitis with burning, itching, and erythema of the oral mucous membrane. The patient also had itching on her lips and on a small skin area around the mouth. The oral symptoms were accompanied by generalized itching and occasional whealing on her lower elbows. On patch testing, she reacted to MMA, EGDMA, 1,4-butanediol diacrylate, and 2-HEMA. In addition, her prostheses also gave positive reactions. The patient's prosthesis was coated with LPH Lack, and UV-light curing was performed for 7 h. She was able to use her prosthesis for half a year without any symptoms of stomatitis, and after relaquering for at least 8 months more [54].

Another female patient developed gingivitis, stomatitis, and perioral dermatitis after insertion of a temporary crown made of restorative two-component material. The base paste and catalyst of the crown contained three methacrylates, i.e., a proacrylate, which is a modification of bis-GMA; a triacrylate, which is saturated aliphatic tricyclic methacrylate; and urethane methacrylate. On patch testing, she reacted to bis-GMA, and other epoxy diacrylates and methacrylates, as well as to the base paste and catalyst of the crown. Allergic reactions were probably elicited by bis-GMA, a cross-reacting methacrylate or other methacrylates in the temporary crown [165].

Only two cases of extra-oral manifestations of delayed allergy ascribed to bis-GMA have been reported. One patient, who developed a measles-like rash, itching, open blisters, and mild respiratory distress but not stomatitis, was reported at the end of the 1970s. After the allergen was removed, complete recovery occurred in 6 months [180]. A recent report described a 12-year-old boy with itchy, relapsing dermatitis on his limbs, trunk, and face. A few days after remodeling of the connections of his orthodontic device, a new, more severe vesicular eruption appeared. He had worn this appliance for over 1 year without any changes in the oral mucosa. On patch testing, he reacted to bis-GMA and *p-tert*-butyl-phenolformaldehyde resin. He also reacted to the bonding paste, which contained bis-GMA. After removal of the orthodontic prosthesis, the dermatitis disappeared within 2 months [181].

Mucosal symptoms caused by *additives* in dental plastics are even rarer than those caused by dental acrylics. Kaaber et al. [182] reported one positive patch test reaction to *N, N*-dimethyl-4 toluidine among 53 denture wearers. Tosti et al. [183] and Verschueren and Bryunzeel [184] reported on patients who had denture sore mouth syndrome from the same chemical. (di)Benzoylperoxide has also been described as a cause of stomatitis [64]. Hydroquinone has been reported on rare occasions to cause gingivostomatitis [185].

Bisphenol A has been reported to cause burning mouth syndrome in a patient. The denture used was of unknown composition, but the patient showed a positive patch reaction to bisphenol A and epoxy resin. It was hypothesized that the epoxy resin used for repairing the denture caused the sensitization [186].

A patient possibly sensitized to epoxy resin at the age of 15 developed painful swelling of oral mucosa for half a day following root canal treatment with product AH 26 (Dentsply De Trey, Germany), which, according to the manufacturer, contains DGEBA-epoxy resin, but not bis-GMA. Two years later, she had developed chronic stomatitis, beginning a few hours after insertion of provisional dental bondings, which were subsequently removed. Patch testing in two sessions showed positive reactions to bis-GMA, and epoxy resin, bisphenol F epoxy resin, and a weak reaction to diphenylmethane-4,4´-diisocyanate. Dental restorations free of plastic materials and new amalgam fillings were inserted, and these were tolerated without any side-effects [187]. Allergic contact dermatitis caused by bis-GMA and associated with sensitivity to epoxy resin has been reported in dental patients by Carmichael et al. [188].

Metals

Mercury amalgam allergy has aroused a great deal of controversy. Previously, it was considered to be a rare sensitizer, but later several studies have shown it to be much more common [189–193]. Many patients with allergic ACS or oral lichen planus (OLP) have become symptomless after the removal of their amalgam restoration [189–193]. The role of dental amalgam in the etiology of OLP or oral lichenoid lesions (OLLs) remains controversial. Some authors have reported that two-thirds of the patients with OLP or OLL have allergy to mercury, whereas other studies show much lower figures [194, 195]. Martin et al. [196] suggest that the corrosion of amalgams and the presence of a galvanic effect from dissimilar metals in continuous contact (bimetallism) are associated with an increased risk of OLL. Amalgam may induce OLL without an allergic mechanism too. OLL may be one disease or a number of similar immunologic or other responses to various stimuli, such as mercury from corroding amalgam fillings [197].

In a study by Athavale et al. [198], 55 patients with OLL were referred for patch testing due to suspected allergy to dental metals (ammoniated and metallic mercury, salts of gold, platinum, palladium, zinc, and copper). Of these 55 patients, 25 (45%) had a relevant positive reaction. Allergy to mercury, and to a lesser extent to gold, was potentially relevant to OLL. Compared with other studies [109], the proportion of patients who were patch test positive to mercury was lower, but more patients reacted to gold. On follow-up, eight of the nine who had their dental metals removed improved after 1 year. The possibility also remained that the replacement of the amalgam removed a physical agent that was causing OLL by an irritant mechanism. The authors concluded that type-IV allergy to mercury in dental amalgam, or to a lesser extent to gold in dental restorations seems to be relevant to the causation of OLL in some patients, but would not be the only mechanism for inducing the condition [198].

In a previous study [199] of 84 patients with typical OLL lesions adjacent to amalgam fillings, encouraging results were obtained. The patch tested metals or metal salts included metallic mercury, ammoniated mercury, mercuric chloride, in some cases phenyl mercuric nitrate, and amalgam discs. Of 84 patients, 33 (39%) had positive patch test findings. Of the 33 patch tested patients, 30 underwent replacement of their amalgam fillings, and 28 (87%) patients experienced improvement of their symptoms and signs within 3 months. The authors concluded that, in some cases, mercury allergy is a factor in the pathogenesis of OLL. It has also been suggested that the removal of dental amalgam is an important therapeutic procedure, even if OLLs are not adjacent to the dental amalgam fillings [200].

Gold salts can be strong sensitizers, but allergy to metallic gold has been considered to be rare. In a study by Ahlgren et al. [201], 102 patients referred for patch testing due to suspected contact dermatitis showed that there was a positive relationship between contact allergy to gold and the presence and amount of dental gold alloys. Metallic gold in dental crowns and restorations has been reported to cause stomatitis and gingivitis [108, 202]. Patch tests for allergy to gold should include gold sodium thiosulfate, GSTS [203], but not gold trichloride [204]. Instead, gold leaf, metallic gold, or gold scrapings may give false-negative results [64]. Metals other than gold may also be the cause of gold jewelry dermatitis or stomatitis, because gold alloys contain variable amounts of other metals as well, including nickel, copper, zinc, silver, or palladium. In a Finnish study [105], 12.4% of patients were positive to GSTS; 25%

had symptoms from jewelry or dental restorations. As in the above-mentioned study, dental gold was concluded to be able to cause OLL [198] and possibly to contribute to burning mouth syndrome in some patients. However, mechanisms other than allergy are often involved in OLL and burning mouth syndrome. Despite this fact, it may not be wise to use golden dental restorations for patients with allergic patch test reactions to GSTS, or to remove restorations from symptomless GSTS allergic patients [5].

In general, *nickel*-sensitive persons have been found to tolerate orthodontic treatment with nickel-containing devices without symptoms. However, stomatitis and systemically induced contact dermatitis from metal wire in orthodontic devices have been reported [191, 205]. Stainless steel tools have very seldom been reported to cause allergic contact dermatitis, although intraoral stainless steel appliances may, in even rarer cases, induce systemic contact dermatitis without stomatitis [206, 207]. On the other hand, nickel allergy may be local and appear only as mucosal inflammation.

Palladium is being used increasingly in industry, jewelry making, and dentistry, and is becoming more common after the EU directive restricted the use of nickel in all products that are in direct contact with the skin. In a study [208] of 4,446 patients patch tested during 1991–2000, 2.3% of the men and 6.7% of the women showed a positive reaction to palladium. Simultaneous sensitization to nickel was common, and the number of those sensitized only to palladium was small. Patch test reactions to palladium chloride may reflect cross-reactivity to nickel sulfate [112, 209]. Patients allergic to palladium chloride tolerate skin contact and, apparently, also mucosal contact with metallic palladium [210]. It is, therefore, uncertain whether metallic palladium in the mouth could be dissolved into its salts and induce stomatitis in patients with dental devices containing palladium. Relatively few cases of relevant palladium-induced allergy have been reported [209, 211]. Koch and Baum [212] reported a patient with ACS due to combined allergy to palladium and platinum from a dental alloy. In addition, contact stomatitis, urticarial, and lichenoid reactions have also been reported [213, 214].

Cobalt and *chromium* allergy seldom originate from dental devices. Fisher reported on a patient whose chrome-cobalt pins used to fasten porcelain teeth to acrylic dentures induced extensive stomatitis and cheilitis [64]. A patient allergic to cobalt in a metal denture developed hand dermatitis [215]. A few cases of systemic contact dermatitis from dental products containing chromium have been reported [205, 216, 217].

Although allergy to *copper* can be considered rare [114, 115], sensitization to copper may have contributed to OLL at least in some cases [64, 218–222]. Koch and Baum [212] reported on a patient who had ACS due to concomitant sensitization to palladium and *platinum*. Some reports suggest that *titanium* may act as an allergen [223, 224]. *Indium* and *iridium* can be used in dental amalgams, as well as in white gold, onto which porcelain is fused in making dental crowns and bridges. Marcusson et al. [225] reported several patients with suspected sensitivity to dental materials, and who, on patch testing, reacted to indium and iridium. Indium isotopes used medically have been reported to cause anaphylactoid reactions.

Vilaplana et al. [96] reported allergic patch test reactions to various *rare metals*, such as rhodium, beryllium, copper, and zinc, in addition to allergic reactions to nickel and mercury. A report on two patients indicates that beryllium may cause ACS and gingivitis [226]. It has also been suggested that beryllium should not be used in dental alloys [227]. Müller-Quernheim et al. [228] reported on a dental technician who was thought to have developed berylliosis from occupational exposure to beryllium.

Manganese will, in future, be increasingly used in the manufacture of dental prostheses [229]. Although manganese has been suggested to have limited potential to cause sensitization [230], sensitization to manganese should, nevertheless, be remembered as a cause of stomatitis in patients wearing dental prostheses. Recently [231], a patient with ACS probably from sensitization to manganese has been reported. The prosthesis was made of chromium-cobalt alloy, which contained 64.8% cobalt, 28.5% chromium, 5.3% molybdenum, 0.5% silica, 0.5% manganese, and 0.4% carbon. On extensive patch testing, the patient reacted only to manganese chloride at 5% in pet. and 15 controls were negative to manganese. She was fitted with a manganese-free denture and remained symptomless thereafter.

Other Compounds

Impression compounds are rare agents that cause oral mucosal symptoms. Two cases of contact allergy have been caused by a catalyst in a silicon-based material [123]. Beyer and Belsito [232] reported allergic gingival hyperplasia from silicon tetrachloride used as curing cement in a porcelain crown. Alginates have not caused any definite cases of sensitization [124].

Propolis, made by bees to build, protect, and repair hives, is used in cosmetic and medicinal preparations because of its antiseptic, anti-inflammatory, and anesthetic properties. Its therapeutic qualities have been well documented for intraoral treatment [233]. A patient treating her recurrent oral ulcerations with an alcoholic solution of propolis 25% as a mouthwash twice daily has been reported. Two days after starting the treatment, she developed labial edema, oral pain and swelling, dysphonia, and mild dyspnea. On patch testing, propolis as well as 25% mouthwash produced a positive reaction. A few cases of cheilitis and other intraoral conditions have been reported. As a result of its possibly increased use in oral preparations, propolis should be taken into consideration as a possible cause of intraoral allergic symptoms [234].

When *eugenol* is used in dental preparations, including impression pastes, surgical packing, and cements, it may cause contact urticaria, gingivitis, and stomatitis [120, 121, 235, 236]. Three cases of eugenol allergy have been reported; in one of the patients, a eugenol impression paste produced allergic cheilitis and ACS [120].

Colophony or rosin may also be included in various dental materials (see Sect. 36.3.2, Causative Agents). A patient with contact stomatitis from colophony has been reported [117], as well as a case of systemically induced contact dermatitis caused by dental rosin [236].

Rubber chemicals in dentists' rubber gloves coming into contact with the skin of rubber-chemical-allergic patients during operations or restorative treatment may induce relatively long-lasting swollen dermatitis on the contact areas on the face.

Allergenic compounds in *toothpastes* may also cause cheilitis [237, 238].

36.9.3 Immediate Reactions

36.9.3.1 Proteins in Natural Rubber Latex

NRL gloves are, generally, the most common cause of type-I allergy and contact urticaria on the skin, especially in health care workers and dental personnel [129]. Because immediate allergy to NRL is quite common in the general population, dental patients are also a special risk group when one remembers that mucosal contact usually gives a stronger reaction than skin contact. Dental patients should always be asked about their possible NRL allergy. No other NRL rubber materials, e.g., dams, should be used if latex allergy is present.

36.9.3.2 Gutta-Percha

Boxer et al. [239] reported on an NRL-allergic dental hygienist who underwent root canal surgery. During the operation, gutta-percha points were inserted into a maxillary molar. Despite of the avoidance of NRL gloves, the patient reported immediate discomfort, lip and gum swelling, a throbbing sensation around the tooth, and diffuse urticaria. Persistent oral discomfort and urticaria followed. The gutta-percha was removed 4 weeks later, and the patient experienced immediate relief of her oral discomfort. Urticarial lesions disappeared in a few hours. The authors were not able to demonstrate an allergic prick test or IgE antibodies to gutta-percha. NRL and gutta-percha represent examples of isomerism. Both are HMW polymers and are structured from the same basic units [240]. They are derived from trees of the same botanical family, and may, thus, have potential for cross-reactivity [239].

36.9.3.3 Fibrin Tissue

A patient who developed urticaria and shortness of breath 1 h after dental examination and tooth extraction has been reported [241]. The patient's extraction socket had been filled with a commercial fibrin tissue to stop bleeding. The cause was believed to be the bovine protein of the fibrin tissue. Another similar case has also been reported [242].

36.9.3.4 Metals

Nickel and cobalt are not common causes of contact urticaria. In rare cases, nickel has caused both delayed and immediate allergy with contact urticaria, rhinitis, asthma, and contact dermatitis [243]. A case of chronic urticaria has been reported from a nickel-containing dental prosthesis [5]. Platinum is a strong type-I allergen [244, 245]. Iridium, another metal of the platinum group, has been reported to induce respiratory allergy and contact urticaria [246]. Also, other metals of the platinum group, such as ruthenium, rhodium, and palladium, have caused immediate allergy [247, 248]. Mercury salts [249] and sodium fluoride [250] present in 31% of the toothpastes sold in Finland [237] have caused contact urticaria.

36.9.3.5 Formaldehyde

Formaldehyde is a rather rare cause of immediate allergy [251], but has caused anaphylaxis after the application of formaldehyde-containing tooth fillings [252]. The patient also had specific serum IgE antibodies to formaldehyde, but prick and patch tests were negative. At least 15 patients [253] have been reported to have developed urticaria or anaphylaxis from formaldehyde released from root-canal disinfectants, and most of these cases were due to paraformaldehyde-containing root canal fillings. Of the 15 reported cases, 11 displayed anaphylaxis to formaldehyde, suggesting that type-I allergy caused by formaldehyde in tooth fillings tends to provoke life-threatening symptoms. Specific IgE to formaldehyde in the patients' sera was clearly elevated in all six cases tested, and three other patients showed positive formaldehyde prick tests. A characteristic feature of the type-I allergic response was that at least 7 of the 15 reported patients presented with allergic symptoms 2–12 h after dental treatment with paraformaldehyde. This is probably because formaldehyde is gradually released from water-soluble paraformaldehyde, and gradually penetrates the dentin, and is, thus, increasingly being present in the circulating blood, finally in amounts able to trigger symptoms. Of 13 tested patients, 7 also showed positive reactions to formaldehyde, indicating they had combined type-I and type-IV allergy to formaldehyde. The authors also suggest that direct mucous membrane contact or direct infusion into the blood plays an important role in the development of type-I allergy [253]. Paraformaldehyde-containing root canal medications have not been used in Finland, for example, for about 15 years.

36.9.3.6 Chlorhexidine

The potential risk of anaphylactic reactions from the application of chlorhexidine has been well known since the 1980s [254, 255]. In 1986, Ohtoshi et al. [256] demonstrated IgE antibodies in the sera of eight patients with anaphylaxis caused by chlorhexidine. Today, there are numerous reports of anaphylaxis due to the chemical (reviewed by Krautheim et al. [136]). Chlorhexidine has caused severe anaphylactic reactions in two dental patients [257, 258]. Both were healthy and unaware of their sensitivity. The first patient developed anaphylaxis when chlorhexidine liquid was sprayed into the cavity after the extraction of a wisdom tooth, the other one suffered from pericoronitis and developed anaphylaxis when Hibitane Dental Gel 1% (chlorhexidine) was applied to the gingival pocket. Krautheim et al. [136] analyzed the reported previous anaphylactic reactions caused by chlorhexidine and suggested that patients with previous sensitization to chlorhexidine and with relatively mild contact dermatitis are at risk of severe immediate-type reactions during their following contacts with the chemical. Chlorhexidine may cause anaphylaxis through the mucosal route at a much lower concentration than elsewhere, generally as low

as 0.05%. The Japanese Ministry of Health recommended avoiding the use of chlorhexidine on mucous membranes in 1984.

36.9.4 Investigations

The investigations have focused on the same work tasks as in the cases of suspected occupational dermatoses of dental care and dental laboratory personnel. In addition to patch and prick tests, as well as determinations of specific IgE antibodies in the sera, the examination and follow-up of the mucous membranes of the mouth is important. In some cases, biopsies are necessary to exclude other diseases of the mucous membranes.

References

1. Estlander T (1990) Occupational skin disease in Finland. Observations made during 1974–1988 at the Institute of Occupational Health, Helsinki (thesis). Acta Derm Venereol Suppl (Stockh) 155:1–263
2. Kanerva L, Estlander T, Jolanki R (1994) Occupational skin allergy in dental profession. Dermatol Clin 12: 517–532
3. Kanerva L, Estlander T, Jolanki R (1995) Dental problems. In: Guin JD (ed) Practical contact dermatitis: a handbook for the practitioner. McGraw-Hill, New York, pp 397–432
4. Kanerva L, Estlander T, Jolanki R, Alanko K (2000) Dermatitis from acrylate compounds in dental personnel. In: Menné T, Maibach HI (eds) Hand eczema, 2nd edn. CRC Press, Boca Raton, Fla., pp 251–274
5. Kanerva L (2001) Skin disease from dental Materials. In: Rycroft RJG, Menné T, Frosch PJ, Lepoittevin J-P (eds) Textbook of contact dermatitis. Springer, Berlin Heidelberg New York, pp 841–881
6. Wrangsjö K, Österman K, van Hage-Hamsten M (1994) Glove-related skin symptoms among operating theatre and dental care unit personnel (II). Clinical examinations, tests and laboratory findings indicating latex allergy. Contact Dermatitis 30:139–143
7. Wrangsjö K, Swartling C, Meding B (2001) Occupational dermatitis in dental personnel: contact dermatitis with special reference to (meth)acrylates in 174 patients. Contact Dermatitis 45:158–161
8. Munksgaard EC, Hansen EK, Engen T, Holm U (1996) Self reported occupational dermatological reactions among Danish dentists. Eur J Oral Sci 104:396–402
9. Hill JV, Grimwood RE, Hermesch CB, Marks JG Jr (1998) Prevalence of occupationally related hand dermatitis in dental workers. J Am Dent Assoc 129:212–217
10. Lönnroth EC, Shahnavaz H (1998) Adverse health reactions in skin, eyes, and respiratory tract among dental personnel in Sweden. Swed Dent J 22:33–45
11. Rustemeyer T, Frosch PJ (2000) Occupational contact dermatitis in dental personnel. In: Kanerva L, Elsner P, Wahlberg JE, Maibach HI (eds) Handbook of occupational dermatology. Springer, Berlin Heidelberg New York, pp 899–905

36

12. Wallenhammar LM, Örtengren U, Andreasson H, Barregard L, Bjorkner B, Karlsson S, Wrangsjo K, Meding B (2000) Contact allergy and hand eczema in Swedish dentists. Contact Dermatitis 43:192–199

13. Lindberg M, Silverdahl M (2000) The use of protective gloves and the prevalence of hand eczema, skin complaints and allergy to natural rubber latex among dental personnel in the county of Uppsala, Sweden. Contact Dermatitis 43:4–8

14. Alanko K, Estlander T, Jolanki R (2003) Allergologia hammashoidossa (Allergology in dental care, in Finnish). In: Autti H, LeBell Y, Meurman JH, Murtomaa H (eds) Therapia odontologica. Academica, Helsinki, pp 288–296

15. Alanko K, Susitaival P, Jolanki R, Kanerva L (2004) Occupational skin disease among dental nurses. Contact Dermatitis 50:77–82

16. Rao R, Shenoi SD (2004) Dermatological problems in dental health personnel. Contact Dermatitis 50:252

17. Hogan D, Hamman C, Rodgers P, Siew C (2004) Occupationally based type IV hypersensitivity in dental professionals. Contact Dermatitis 50:141

18. Kanerva L, Estlander T, Jolanki R, Pekkarinen E (1992) Occupational pharyngitis associated with allergic patch test reactions from acrylics. Allergy 47:571–573

19. Estlander T, Kanerva L, Kari O, Jolanki R, Mölsa K (1996) Occupational conjunctivitis associated with type IV allergy to methacrylates. Allergy 51:56–59

20. Sala E, Hytönen M, Tupasela O, Estlander T (1996) Occupational laryngitis with immediate or immediate type specific chemical hypersensitivity. Clin Otolaryngol Allied Sci 21:1404–1411

21. Savonius B, Keskinen H, Tuppurainen M, Kanerva L (1993) Occupational respiratory disease caused by acrylics. Clin Exp Allergy 23:416–424

22. Piirilä P, Kanerva L, Keskinen H, Estlander T, Hytönen M, Tuppurainen M, Nordman H (1998) Occupational respiratory hypersensitivity caused by preparations containing acrylates in dental personnel. Clin Exp Allergy 28:1404–1411

23. Piirilä P, Hodgson U, Estlander T, Keskinen H, Saalo A, Voutilainen R, Kanerva L (2002) Occupational respiratory hypersensitivity in dental personnel. Int Arch Occup Environ Health 75:209–216

24. Estlander T, Rajaniemi R, Jolanki R (1984) Hand dermatitis in dental technicians. Contact Dermatitis 10:201–205

25. Rustemeyer T, Frosch PJ (1996) Occupational skin disease in dental laboratory workers. (I) Clinical picture and causative factors. Contact Dermatitis 34:123–133

26. Meding B, Hosseiny S, Wrangsjö K, Andersson E, Hagberg S, Wass U, Toren K, Brisman J (2004) Hand eczema, skin exposure and glove use in dental technicians. Contact Dermatitis 50:203

27. Mürer AJL, Poulsen OM, Roed-Petersen J, Tüchsen F (1995) Skin problems among Danish dental technicians. A cross-sectional study. Contact Dermatitis 33:42–47

28. Mürer AJL, Poulsen OM, Tüchsen F, Roed-Petersen J (1995) Rapid increase in skin problems among dental technician trainees working with acrylates. Contact Dermatitis 33:106–111

29. Kanerva L, Mikola H, Henriks-Eckerman M-L, Jolanki R, Estlander T (1998) Fingertip paresthesia and occupational allergic contact dermatitis caused by acrylics in a dental nurse. Contact Dermatitis 38:114–116

30. Kanerva L, Henriks-Eckerman M-L, Estlander T, Jolanki R (1997) Dentist's occupational allergic paronychia and contact dermatitis caused by acrylics. Eur J Dermatol 7:177–180

31. Estlander T, Jolanki R (2005) Allergic contact dermatitis from rubber and plastic gloves In: Boman A, Estlander T, Wahlberg JE, Maibach HI (eds) Protective gloves for occupational use, 2nd edn. CRC Press, Boca Raton, Fla., pp 27–144

32. Stevenson WJ (1941) Methyl-methacrylate dermatitis. Contact Point 18:171–173

33. Moody WL (1941) Severe reaction from acrylic liquid. Dent Digest 47:305

34. Fisher AA (1954) Allergic sensitization of skin and oral mucosa to acrylic denture materials. J Am Med Assoc 156:238–242

35. van der Walle HB (1982) Sensitizing potential of acrylic monomers in guinea pigs. Thesis, Katholieke Universiteit Nijmegen, Krips Repro, Meppel, The Netherlands, pp 1–112

36. Björkner B (1984) Sensitizing capacity of ultraviolet curable acrylic compounds. Thesis, Lund, Sweden, pp 1–78

37. Axell T, Björkner B, Fregert S, Niklasson B (1983) Standard patch test series for screening contact allergy dental materials. Contact Dermatitis 9:82

38. Kanerva L, Estlander T, Jolanki R (1989) Allergic contact dermatitis from dental composite resins due to aromatic epoxy acrylates and aliphatic acrylates. Contact Dermatitis 20:201–211

39. Kanerva L, Turjanmaa K, Estlander T, Jolanki R (1991) Occupational allergic contact dermatitis from 2-hydroxyethyl methacrylate (2-HEMA) in a new dentin adhesive. Am J Contact Dermat 2:24–30

40. Kanerva L, Henriks-Eckerman M-L, Estlander T, Jolanki R, Tarvainen K (1994) Occupational allergic contact dermatitis and composition of acrylates in denting bonding systems. J Eur Acad Derm Venereol 3:157–169

41. Guerra L, Vincenzi C, Peluso AM, Tosti A (1993) Prevalence and sources of occupational contact sensitization to acrylates in Italy. Contact Dermatitis 28:101–103

42. Tosti A, Guerra L, Vincenzi C, Peluso AM (1993) Occupational health hazards from synthetic plastics. Toxicol Ind Health 9:493–502

43. Cleenewerk MB (1997) Current features of allergic occupational dermatoses. Rev Fr Allergol Immunol Clin 37:617–633

44. Kanerva L Jolanki R, Estlander T (1997) 10 years of patch testing with the (meth)acrylate series. Contact Dermatitis 37:255–258

45. Björkner B (1989) Kontaktallergi för ultraviolett härdande akrylatprodukter I färger och lacker (in Swedish). Arbete och Hälsa 20:1–39

46. Bowen RL (1962) Dental filling material comprising vinyl silane treated fused silica and a binder consisting of the reaction product of bisphenol A and glycidyl acrylate. US Patent 3,066,112

47. Rustemeyer T, de Groot A, von Blomberg BME, Frosch PJ, Scheper RJ (1998) Cross-reactivity patterns of contact sensitizing methacrylates. Toxicol Appl Pharmacol 148:83–90

48. van der Walle HB, Bensink T (1982) Cross reaction pattern of 26 acrylic monomers in guinea pig skin. Contact Dermatitis 8:376–382

49. Kanerva L, Estlander T, Jolanki R (1997) Occupational allergic contact dermatitis of dental nurse caused by acrylic tri-cure glass ionomer. Contact Dermatitis 37:49–50

50. ADEPT report (1990) Pertinent information on cosmetic, adhesive, and restorative dentistry. ADEPT Institute, Santa Rosa, Calif., 1:33–44

36

51. Kanerva L, Henriks-Eckerman M-L, Estlander T, Jolanki R, Tarvainen K (1994) Occupational allergic contact dermatitis and composition of acrylates in dentin bonding systems. J Eur Acad Derm Verereol 3:157–168

52. Finnish Advisory Board of Chemicals (1992) Acrylate compounds: uses and evaluation of health effects. Government Printing Centre, Helsinki, Finland, pp 1–60

53. Kanerva L, Estlander T, Jolanki R, Tarvainen K (1993) Occupational contact dermatitis caused by exposure to acrylates during work with dental prostheses. Contact Dermatitis 28:268–275

54. Kanerva l, Tarvainen K, Jolanki R, Estlander T (1995) Successful coating of an allergenic acrylate-based dental prosthesis. Am J Contact Dermat 6:24–27

55. Schnuch A, Geier J (1994) Kontaktallergene bei Dental-berufen. Dermatosen 42:253–255

56. Belsito DV (1987) Contact dermatitis to ethyl-cyanoacrylate-containing glue. Contact Dermatitis 17:234–236

57. White IR (1990) Adhesives. In: Adams RM (ed) Occupational skin disease, 2nd edn. Saunders, Philadelphia, Pa., pp 395–407

58. Guin JD, Baas K, Nelson-Adesokan P (1998) Contact sensitization to cyanoacrylate adhesive as a cause of severe onychodystrophy. Int J Dermatol 37:31–36

59. Tomb RR, Lepoittevin J-P, Durepaire F, Grosshans E (1993) Ectopic contact dermatitis from ethyl cyanoacrylate instant adhesives. Contact Dermatitis 28:206–208

60. Lozewicz S, Davison AG, Hopkirk A, Burge PS, Boldy DA, Riordan JF, McGivern DV, Platts BW, Davies D, Newman Taylor JA (1985) Occupational asthma due to methyl methacrylate and cyanoacrylates. Thorax 40:836–839

61. Smith DC (1959) The acrylic denture base – the peroxide concentration in dental polymers. Br Dent J 107:62–67

62. Calnan CD, Stevenson CJ (1963) Studies in contact dermatitis XV: dental materials. Trans St John's Hosp Dermatol Soc 49:9–26

63. Kanerva L, Tarvainen K, Estlander T, Jolanki R (1994) Occupational allergic contact dermatitis caused by mercury and benzoyl peroxide. Eur J Dermatol 4:359–361

64. Fisher AA (1986) Contact dermatitis, 3rd edn. Lea and Febiger, Philadelphia, Pa.

65. Jager M, Balda BR (1979) Loosening of hip prosthesis at contact allergy to benzoyl peroxide. Arch Orthop Trauma Surg 94:175–8

66. Vincenzi G, Cameli N, Vassipoulou A, Tosti A (1991) Allergic contact dermatitis due to benzoyl peroxide in arm prosthesis. Contact Dermatitis 24:66–67

67. Quirce S, Olaguibel JM, Garcia BE, Tabar AI (1993) Occupational airborne contact dermatitis due to benzoylperoxide. Contact Dermatitis 29:165

68. Kanerva L, Jolanki R, Estlander T (1993) Dentist's occupational allergic contact dermatitis caused by coconut diethanolamide, N-ethyl-4-toluene sulfonamide and 4-tolyldiethanolamine. Acta Derm Venereol (Stockh) 73:126–129

69. Malanin K (1993) Active sensitization to camphoroquinone and double active sensitization to acrylics with long-lasting patch test reactions. Contact Dermatitis 29:284–285

70. Jolanki R (1991) Occupational skin diseases from epoxy compounds. Epoxy resin compounds, epoxy acrylates and 2,3-epoxypropyl trimethyl ammonium chloride (thesis). Acta Derm Venereol Suppl (Stockh) 169:1–80

71. Jolanki R, Kanerva L, Estlander T (1995) Occupational allergic contact dermatitis caused by epoxy diacrylate in ultraviolet-light-cured paint, and bisphenol A in dental composite resin. Contact Dermatitis 33:94–99

72. Aalto-Korte K, Alanko K, Henriks-Eckerman M-L, Estlander T, Jolanki R (2003) Allergic contact dermatitis from bisphenol A in PVC gloves. Contact Dermatitis 49:202–205

73. Cronin E (1980) Contact dermatitis. Churchill Livingstone, Edinburgh, pp 1–915

74. Bardazzi F, Melino M, Alagna G, Veronesi S (1986) Glutaraldehyde dermatitis in nurses. Contact Dermatitis 14:319–320

75. Nethercott JR, Holness DL, Page E (1988) Occupational contact dermatitis due to glutaraldehyde in health care workers. Contact Dermatitis 18:193–196

76. Cusano F, Luciano S (1993) Contact allergy to benzalkonium chloride and glutaraldehyde in a dental nurse. Contact Dermatitis 28:127–127

77. Kanerva L Miettinen P, Alanko K, Estlander T, Tupasela O, Jolanki R (2000) occupational allergic contact dermatitis from glyoxal, glutaraldehyde and neomycin sulfate in a dental nurse. Contact Dermatitis 42:116–117

78. Flyvholm M-A (1997) Formaldehyde exposure at the workplace and in the environment. Allergologie 5:225–231

79. Flyvholm M-A (2000) Formaldehyde and formaldehyde releasers. In: Kanerva L, Elsner P, Wahlberg JE, Maibach HI (eds) Handbook of occupational dermatology. Springer, Berlin Heidelberg New York, pp 474–478

80. Elsner P, Pevny I, Burg G (1990) Occupational contact dermatitis due to glyoxal in health care workers. Am J Contact Dermat 1:250–253

81. Suhonen R (1980) Contact allergy to dodecyl-di-(aminoethyl)glycine (Desimex I). Contact dermatitis 6:290–291

82. Foussereau J, Samsoen M, Hecht MT (1983) Occupational dermatitis to Ampholyt G in hospital personnel. Contact Dermatitis 9:233–234

83. Estlander T, Kanerva L, Jolanki R (1989) Occupational skin sensitization to the antimicrobials ortho-benzyl para-chlorophenol and Ampholyte 103G. In: Frosch P, Dooms-Goossens A, Lachapelle J-M, Rycroft RJG, Scheper RJ (eds) Current topics in contact dermatitis. Springer, Berlin Heidelberg New York, pp 88–91

84. Timmer C (2000) Antimicrobials and disinfectants. In: Kanerva L, Elsner P, Wahlberg JE, Maibach HI (eds) Handbook of occupational dermatology. Springer, Berlin Heidelberg New York, pp 462–473

85. Snuch A (1997) Benzalkonium chloride. Dermatosen 45:179–180

86. Placucci F, Benini A, Guerra L, Tosti A (1996) Occupational allergic contact dermatitis from disinfectant wipes used in dentistry. Contact Dermatitis 35:306–306

87. Lachapelle J-M (1984) Occupational allergic contact dermatitis to povidone-iodine. Contact Dermatitis 11:189–190

88. Ancona A, de la Torre RS, Macotela E (1985) Allergic contact dermatitis from povidone-iodine. Contact Dermatitis 13:66–68

89. Kudo H, Takahashi K, Suzuki Y, Tanaka T, Miyachi Y, Imamura S (1988) Contact dermatitis from a compound mixture of sugar and povidone-iodine. Contact Dermatitis 18:155–157

90. van Ketel WG, van der Berg WH (1990) Sensitization to povidone-iodine. Dermatol Clin 8:107–109

91. Tosti A, Vincenzi C, Bardazzi F, Mariani R (1990) Allergic contact dermatitis to povidone-iodine. Contact Dermatitis 23:197–198

92. Kanerva L Estlander T (1999) Occupational allergic contact dermatitis caused by povidone-iodine (Betadine). Environ Dermatol 6:101–104

93. White IR, Catchpole HE, Rycroft RJG (1982) Rashes amongst persulphate workers. Contact Dermatitis 8: 168–172

94. van Joost T, Roesyanto ID (1991) Sensitization to persulphates in occupational and non-occupational hand dermatitis. Contact Dermatitis 24:376–378

95. Kanerva L, Alanko K, Jolanki R, Aalto-Korte K, Estlander T (1999) Occupational allergic contact dermatitis from potassium persulfate. Contact Dermatitis 40:116–117

96. Vilaplana J, Romaguera C, Cornellana F (1994) Contact dermatitis and adverse oral mucous membrane reactions related to use of dental prostheses. Contact Dermatitis 30:80–84

97. Ancona A, Ramos M, Suarez R, Macotela E (1982) Mercury sensitivity in a dentist. Contact Dermatitis 8: 218

98. Kanerva L, Komulainen M, Estlander T, Jolanki R (1993) Occupational allergic contact dermatitis from mercury. Contact Dermatitis 28:26–28

99. Björkner B, Bruze M, Möller H (1994) High frequency of contact allergy to gold sodium thiosulfate. An indication of gold allergy? Contact Dermatitis 30:144–151

100. Bruze M, Edman B, Björkner B, Möller H (1994) Clinical relevance of contact allergy to gold sodium thiosulfate. J Am Acad Dermatol 31:579–583

101. Möller H, Larsson Å, Björkner B, Bruze M (1994) The histological and immunohistochemical pattern of positive patch test reactions to gold sodium thiosulfate. Acta Derm Venereol (Stockh) 74:417–423

102. Bruze M, Hedman H, Björkner B, Möller H (1995) The development and course of test reactions to gold sodium thiosulfate. Contact Dermatitis 33:386–391

103. McKenna KE, Dolan O, Walsh MY, Burrows D (1995) Contact allergy to gold sodium thiosulfate. Contact Dermatitis 32:143–146

104. Sabroe RA, Sharp LA, Peachey RDG (1996) Contact allergy to gold sodium thiosulfate. Contact Dermatitis 34: 345–348

105. Räsänen LR, Kalimo K, Laine J, Vainio O, Kotiranta J, Pesola I (1996) Contact allergy to gold in dental patients. Br J Dermatol 134:673–677

106. Fleming C, Forsyth A, MacKie R (1997) Prevalence of gold contact hypersensitivity in the west of Scotland. Contact Dermatitis 36:302–304

107. Leow Y-H, Ng S-K, Goh C-L (1998) A preliminary study of gold sensitization in Singapore. Contact Dermatitis 38: 69–70

108. Aro T, Kanerva L, Häyrinen-Immonen R, Silvennoinen-Kassinen S, Konttinen YT, Jolanki R, Estlander T (1993) Long-lasting allergic patch test reaction caused by gold. Contact Dermatitis 28:276–281

109. Koch P, Bahmer FA (1995) Oral lichenoid lesions, mercury hypersensitivity and combined hypersensitivity to mercury and other metals: histologically-proven reproduction of the reaction by patch testing with metal salts. Contact Dermatitis 33:323–328

110. Heise H, Beyer H, Rauschenbach D (1997) Ergebnisse der Epikutantestung auf Goldsalze versus Amalgam. Z Dermatol 183:68–73

111. Isaksson M, Bruze M (2000) Gold. In: Kanerva L, Elsner P, Wahlberg JE, Maibach HI (eds) Handbook of occupational dermatology. Springer, Berlin Heidelberg New York, pp 544–550

112. Liden C (2000) Nickel. In: Kanerva L, Elsner P, Wahlberg JE, Maibach HI (eds) Handbook of occupational dermatology. Springer, Berlin Heidelberg New York, pp 524–533

113. Wahlberg JE (2000) Other metals. In: Kanerva L, Elsner P, Wahlberg JE, Maibach HI (eds) Handbook of occupational dermatology. Springer, Berlin Heidelberg New York, pp 551–555

114. Förström L, Kiistala U, Tarvainen K (1977) Hypersensitivity to copper verified by test with 0.1% CuSO4. Contact Dermatitis 3:280–281

115. Karlberg A, Boman A, Wahlberg JE (1983) Copper – a rare sensitizer. Contact Dermatitis 9:134–139

116. Karlberg A-T (2004) Colophony. In: Kanerva L, Elsner P, Wahlberg JE, Maibach HI (eds) Condensed handbook of occupational dermatology. Springer, Berlin Heidelberg New York, pp 312–330

117. Isaksson M, Bruze M, Björkner B, Niklasson B (1993) Contact allergy to Duraphat. Scand Dent Res 101:49–61

118. Kanerva L, Estlander T (1999) Occupational allergic contact dermatitis from colophony in 2 dental nurses. Contact Dermatitis 41:342–343

119. Cockayne SE, Murphy R, Gawkrodger DJ (2001) Occupational contact dermatitis from colophonium in dental technician. Contact Dermatitis 44:42–43

120. Göransson K, Karltorp N, Ask H, Smedberg O (1967) Några fall av eugenolöverkänsligheter (Some cases of eugenol hypersensitivity; in Swedish with English summary). Svensk Tandläk Tidskr 60:545–549

121. Kanerva L, Estlander T, Jolanki R (1998) Dental nurse's occupational allergic contact dermatitis from eugenol used as a restorative dental material with polymethylmethacrylate. Contact Dermatitis 38:339–340

122. Yli-Urpo et al (2003) Hammashoidon materiaalit (Dental materials, in Finnish). In: Autti H, LeBell Y, Meurman JH, Murtomaa H (eds) Therapia odontologica. Academica, Helsinki, Finland, pp 1019–1037

123. Ölveti E, Hegedus C (1994) Contact allergy reactions to Silodent impression material (in Hungarian). Fogorv Sz 87:115–119

124. Rice CD, Barker BF, Kestenbaum T, Dykstra MA, Lumpkin D (1992) Intraoral vesicles occurring after alginate impressions. Oral Surg Oral Med Oral Pathol 74:698–704

125. Camarasa G (1975) Occupational dermatitis from beeswax. Contact Dermatitis 1:124

126. Klein CE, Gall H (1991) Type IV allergy to amide-type local anesthetics. Contact Dermatitis 25:45–48

127. Curley RK, Macfarlane AW, King CM (1986) Contact sensitivity to amide anesthetics lidocaine, prilocaine, and mepivacaine. Arch Dermatol 122:924–926

128. Suhonen R, Kanerva L (1997) Contact allergy and cross-reactions to prilocaine. Am J Contact Dermat 8:231–235

129. Jolanki R, Estlander T, Alanko K, Savela A, Kanerva L (1999) Incidence rates of occupational contact urticaria caused by natural rubber latex. Contact Dermatitis 40: 329–331

130. Tarlo SM, Sussman GL, Holness DL (1997) Latex sensitivity in dental students and staff: a cross-sectional study. J Allergy Clin Immunol 99:396–401

131. Safadi GS, Safadi TJ, Terezhalmy GT, Taylor JS, Battisto JR, Melton Al Jr (1996) Latex hypersensitivity: its prevalence among dental professionals. J Am Dent Assoc 127:83–88

132. Heese A, Peters KP, Koch HU, Hornstein OP (1995) Häufigkeit und Zunahme von Typ I-Allergien gegen Gummihandschuhe bei Zahnmedizinstudenten (Incidence and increase in type I allergies to rubber gloves in dental medicine students, in German). Hautarzt 46:15–21

133. Hamann C (1993) Hold the talc, pass the cornstarch. J Am Dent Assoc 124:14–16

134. Seggev JS, Mawhinney TP, Yunginger JW, Braun SR (1990) Anaphylaxis due to cornstarch surgical glove powder. Ann Allergy 65:152–155

135. Kanerva L (1997) Contact urticaria from dental products. In: Amin S, Lahti A, Maibach HI (eds) Contact urticaria syndrome. CRC Press/LLC, Boca Raton, Fla., pp 119–128

136. Krautheim AB, Jermann THM, Bircher AJ (2004) Chlorhexidine anaphylaxis: case report and review of the literature. Contact Dermatitis 50:113–116

137. Bhalla M, Thami GP (2003) Acute urticaria due to dental eugenol. Allergy 58:158

138. Hudson LD (1987) Phototoxic reactions triggered by a new dental instrument. J Am Acad Dermatol 17:508–509

139. Foussereau J (1991) Guide de dermato-allergologie professionnelle. Masson, Paris, France

140. Kanerva L, Henriks-Eckerman M-L, Jolanki R, Estlander T (1997) Plastics/acrylics: material safety data sheets need to be improved. Clin Dermatol 15:533–546

141. Henriks-Eckerman M-L, Kanerva L (1997) Product analysis of acrylic resins compared to information given in material safety sheets. Contact Dermatitis 36:164–165

142. Henriks-Eckerman M-L, Suuronen K, Jolanki R, Alanko K (2004) Methacrylates in dental restorative materials. Contact Dermatitis 50:233–237

143. Kanerva L, Estlander T, Jolanki R (1988) Sensitization to patch test acrylates. Contact Dermatitis 18:10–15

144. Kanerva L, Estlander T, Jolanki R (1992) Double active sensitization caused by acrylics. Am J Contact Dermat 3:23–26

145. Kanerva L, Estlander T, Jolanki R (1992) Active sensitization caused by 2-hydroxyethyl methacrylate, 2-hydroxypropyl methacrylate, ethyleneglycol dimethacrylate and N,N-dimethylaminoethyl dimethacrylate. J Eur Acad Derm Venereol I:165–169

146. Kanerva L, Lauerma A (1998) Iatrogenic acrylate allergy complicating amalgam allergy. Contact Dermatitis 38:58–59

147. Kanerva L, Turjanmaa K, Estlander T, Jolanki R (1991) Occupational allergic contact dermatitis from iatrogenic sensitization by a new acrylate dentin adhesive. Eur J Dermatol 1:25–28

148. Jolanki R, Estlander T, Alanko K, Kanerva L (2004) Patch testing with patient's own work materials. In: Kanerva L, Elsner P, Wahlberg JE, Maibach HI (eds) Condensed handbook of occupational dermatology. Springer, Berlin Heidelberg New York, pp 195–205

149. Pegum JS, Medhurst FA (1971) Contact dermatitis from penetration of rubber gloves by acrylic monomer. Br Med J 2:141–143

150. Waegemaekers THJM, Seutter E, den Arend JACJ, Malten KE (1983) Permeability of surgeons' gloves to methyl methacrylate. Acta Orthop Scand 54:790–795

151. Darre E, Vedel P, Jensen JS (1987) Skin protection against methylmethacrylate. Acta Orthop Scand 58:236–238

152. Munksgaard EC (1992) Permeability of protective gloves to (di)methacrylates in resinous dental materials. Scand J Dent Res 100:189–192

153. Munksgaard EC (2000) Permeability of protective gloves by 2-HEMA and TEGDMA in the presence of solvents. Acta Odontol Scand 58:57–62

154. Mäkelä EA, Väänänen V, Alanko K, Jolanki R, Estlander T, Kanerva L (1999) Resistance of disposable gloves to permeation by 2-hydroxyethyl methacrylate and triethyleneglycol dimethacrylate. Occup Hyg 5:121–129

155. Mäkelä EA, Jolanki R (2005) Chemical permeation through disposable gloves. In: Boman A, Estlander T, Wahlberg JE, Maibach HI (eds) protective gloves for occupational used, 2nd edn. CRC Press, Boca Raton, Fla., pp 299–314

156. Mäkelä EA, Vainiotalo S, Peltonen K (2003) Permeation of 70% isopropyl alcohol through surgical gloves: comparison of standard methods ASTM F 739 and EN 374. Ann Occup Hyg 47:305–312

157. Mäkelä EA, Vainiotalo S, Peltonen K (2003) The permeability of surgical gloves to seven chemicals commonly used in hospitals. Ann Occup Hyg 47:313–323

158. Estlander T, Jolanki R, Kanerva L (2000) Protective gloves. In: Menné T, Maibach HI (eds) Hand eczema, 2nd edn. CRC Press, Boca Raton, Fla., pp 309–322

159. Taylor DT, Morton TH (1991) Ulcerative lesion of the palate associated with removable partial denture castings. J Prosthet Dent 66:213–221

160. Shah M, Lewis FM, Gawkrodger DJ (1996) Contact allergy in patients with oral symptoms: a study of 47 patients. Am J Contact Dermat 7:146–151

161. Helton J, Storrs F (1994) The burning mouth syndrome: lack of role for contact urticaria and contact dermatitis. J Am Acad Dermatol 31:201–205

162. Rietschell RL, Fowler JF Jr (1995) Fisher's contact dermatitis, 4th edn. Williams and Watkins, Baltimore, Md.

163. Ophaswongse S, Maibach HI (1995) Allergic contact cheilitis. Contact Dermatitis 33:365–370

164. Kanerva L, Alanko K (1998) Stomatitis and perioral dermatitis caused by epoxy diacrylates in dental composite resins. J Am Acad Derm 38:116–120

165. Kanerva L, Alanko K, Estlander T (1999) Allergic contact gingivostomatitis from a temporary crown made of methacrylates and epoxy diacrylates. Allergy 54:1316–1321

166. Marx H, Fukui M, Stender E (1983) Zur Frage der Restmonomer-Untersuchung von Prosthesenkunststoffen. Dtsch Zahnärtzl Z 38:550–553

167. Crissey JT (1965) Stomatitis, dermatitis, and denture materials. Arch Dermatol 92:45–48

168. Kaaber S (1990) Allergy to dental materials with special reference to the use of amalgam and polymethylmethacrylate. Int Dent J 40:359–365

169. Guerra L, Vincenzi C, Peluso AM, Tosti A (1993) Role of contact sensitizers in the burning mouth syndrome. Am J Contact Dermat 4:154–157

170. Ruiz-Genao DP, Moreno de Vega MJ, Sánchez Pérez J, Garcia-Diez A (2003) Labial edema due to an acrylic dental prosthesis. Contact Dermatitis 48:273–274

171. Agner T, Menné T (1994) Sensitization to acrylates in a dental patient. Contact Dermatitis 30:249–250

172. Niinimäki A, Rosberg J, Saari S (1983) Allergic stomatitis from acrylic compounds. Contact Dermatitis 9:148

173. Lunder T, Rogi-Butina M (2000) Chronic urticaria from acrylic dental prosthesis. Contact Dermatitis 43:232–233

174. Bauer A, Wollina U (1998) Denture-induced local and systemic reactions to acrylate. Allergy 53:722–723

175. Kanzaki T, Kabasawa Y, Jinno T, Isayama K (1989) Contact stomatitis due to methyl methacrylate monomer. Contact Dermatitis 20:146–148

176. Ölveti E (1991) Contact dermatitis from an acrylic-metal dental prosthesis. Contact Dermatitis 24:57

177. Corazza M, Virgili A, Martina S (1992) Allergic contact stomatitis from methyl methacrylate in a dental prosthesis, with persistent patch test reaction. Contact Dermatitis 26:210–211

178. Fowler JF Jr (1992) Burning mouth caused by dentures. Am J Contact Dermat 3:3–4

179. Kobayashi T, Sakuraoka K, Hasegawa Y, Konohana A, Kurihara S (1996) Contact dermatitis to an acrylic dental prosthesis. Contact Dermatitis 35:370–371

180. Nathanson D, Lockhart P (1979) Delayed extraoral hypersensitivity to dental composite material. Oral Surg Oral Med Oral Pathol 47:329–333

181. Menni S, Lodi A, Coassini D, Boccardi P, Rossini P, Crosti C (2003) Unusual widespread vesicular eruption related dental composite resin sensitization. Contact Dermatitis 48:174

182. Kaaber S, Thulin H, Nielsen E (1979) Skin sensitivity to denture base materials in the burning mouth syndrome. Contact Dermatitis 5:90–96

183. Tosti A, Bardazzi F, Piancastelli E, Brasile GP (1990) Contact stomatitis due to N, N-dimethyl-paratoluidine. Contact Dermatitis 22:113

184. Verschueren GLA, Bryunzeel DP (1991) Allergy to N, N-dimethyl-p-toluidine in dental materials. Contact Dermatitis 24:149

185. Torres V, Mano-Azul AC, Correia T, Soares AP (1993) Allergic cheilitis and stomatitis from hydroquinone in an acrylic dental prosthesis. Contact Dermatitis 29:102–103

186. van Joost TH, van Ulsen J, van Loon LAJ (1988) Contact allergy to denture materials in the burning mouth syndrome. Contact Dermatitis 18:97

187. Koch P (2003) Allergic contact stomatitis from BIS-GMA and epoxy resins in dental bonding agents. Contact Dermatitis 49:104–105

188. Carmichael AJ, Gibson JJ, Walls AWG (1997) Allergic contact dermatitis to bisphenol-A-glycidyldimethacrylate (BIS-GMA) dental resin associated with sensitivity to epoxy resin. Br Dent J 183:297–298

189. Pang PK, Freeman S (1996) Oral lichenoid lesions caused by allergy to mercury in amalgam fillings. Contact Dermatitis 33:423–427

190. Smart ER, Macleod RI, Lawrence CM (1995) Resolution of lichen planus following removal of amalgam restorations in patients proven allergy to mercury salts: a pilot study. Br Dent J 178:108–112

191. Alanko K, Kanerva L, Jolanki R, Kannas L, Estlander T (1996). Oral mucosal diseases investigated by patch testing with a dental screening series. Contact Dermatitis 34:263–267

192. Laine J, Kalimo K, Forssell H, Happonen R-P (1992) Resolution of oral lichenoid lesions after replacement of amalgam restorations in patients allergic to mercury compounds. Br J Dermatol 126:10–15

193. Laine J, Kalimo K, Happonen R-P (1997) Contact allergy to dental restorative materials in patients with oral lichenoid lesions. Contact Dermatitis 36:141–146

194. Koch P, Bahmer F (1999) Oral lesions and symptoms related to metals used in dental restorations: clinical, allergological, and histologic study. Am J Acad Dermatol 41:422–430

195. Scalf LA, Fowler JF Jr, Morgan KW, Looney SW (2001) Dental metal allergy in patients with oral, cutaneous and genital lichenoid lesions. Am J Contact Dermat 12:146–150

196. Martin MD, Broughton S, Drangsholt M (2003) Oral lichen planus and dental materials: a case-control study. Contact Dermatitis 48:331–336

197. Östman PO, Anneroth G, Skoglund A (1994) Oral lichen planus lesions in contact with amalgam fillings: a clinical, histologic, and immunohistochemical study. Scand J Dent Res 102:172–179

198. Athavale PN, Shum KW, Yeoman CM, Gawkrodger DJ (2003) Oral lichenoid lesions and contact allergy to dental mercury and gold. Contact Dermatitis 49:264–265

199. Wong L, Freeman S (2003) Oral lichenoid lesions (OLP) and mercury in amalgam fillings. Contact Dermatitis 48:74–79

200. Pigatto P, Passoni E, Crippa R, Tanzi C, Zerboni R, Brambilla L, Guzzi G, Muratori S (2004) Oral lichenoid reactions and amalgams: no topographical relationship. Contact Dermatitis 50:176

201. Ahlgren C, Ahnlide C, Björkner B, Bruze M, Liedholm R, Möller H, Nilner C (2002) Contact allergy to gold is correlated to dental gold. Acta Derm Venereol (Stockh) 82:41–44

202. Laeijendecker R, van Joost T (1994) Oral manifestations of gold allergy. J Am Acad Dermatol 30:205–209

203. Fowler JF Jr (1987) Selection of patch test materials for gold allergy. Contact Dermatitis 17:23–25

204. Möller H, Ahnlide I, Gruvberger B, Bruze M (2004) Gold trichloride as a marker of contact allergy to gold. Contact Dermatitis 50:176

205. Veien NK, Borchorst E, Hattel T, Laurberg G (1994) Stomatitis or systemically-induced contact dermatitis from metal wire in orthodontic materials. Contact Dermatitis 30:210–213

206. Kerosuo H, Kanerva L (1997) Systemic contact dermatitis caused by nickel in a stainless steel orthodontic appliance. Contact Dermatitis 36:112–113

207. Lyzak WA, Flaitz CM, McGuckin RS, Eichmiller F, Brown RS (1994) Diagnosis and treatment of an oral base-metal contact lesion following negative dermatologic patch test. Ann Allergy 73:161–165

208. Larese Filon F, Uderzo D, Bagnato E (2003). Sensitization to palladium chloride: a 10-year evaluation. Am J Contact Dermat 14:78–81

209. Kanerva L, Kerosuo H, Kullaa A, Kerosuo E (1996) Allergic patch test reactions to palladium chloride in schoolchildren. Contact Dermatitis 34:39–42

210. de Fine Olivarius F, Menné T (1992) Contact dermatitis from metallic palladium in patients reacting to palladium chloride. Contact Dermatitis 27:71–73

211. Vincenzi C, Tosti A, Guerra L, Kokelj F, Nobile C, Rivara G, Zangrando E (1995) Contact dermatitis to palladium: a study of 2,300 patients. Am J Contact Dermat 6:110–112

212. Koch P, Baum HP (1996) Contact stomatitis due to palladium and platinum in dental alloys. Contact Dermatitis 34:253–257

213. Camarasa JG, Serra-Baldrich E, Lluch M, Malet A, Garcia Calderon G (1989) Recent unexplained patch test reactions to palladium. Contact Dermatitis 20:388–389

214. Nakayama H, Nogi N, Kasahara N, Matsuo S (1990) Allergen control. An indispensable treatment for allergic contact dermatitis. Dermatol Clin 8:197–204

215. Glendenning WE (1971) Allergy to cobalt in metal denture as cause of hand dermatitis. Contact Dermatitis Newslett 10:255–226

216. Hubler WR Jr, Hubler WR Sr (1983) Dermatitis from chromium dental plate. Contact Dermatitis 9:377–398

217. Guimaraens D, Gonzalez MA, Conde-Salazar L (1994) Systemic contact dermatitis from dental crowns. Contact Dermatitis 30:124–125

218. Frykholm K, Frithiof L, Fernström B, Moberger G, Blohm G, Björn E (1969) Allergy to copper derived from dental alloys as a possible cause of oral lesions of lichen planus. Acta Derm Venereol (Stockh) 49:268–281

219. Santosh V, Ranjith K, Shenoi S, Sachin V, Balachandran C (1999) Results of patch testing with dental materials. Contact Dermatitis 40:50–51

36

220. Wöhrl S, Hemmer W, Focke M, Götz M, Jarish R (2001) Copper allergy revisited. J Am Acad Dermatol 45: 863–870

221. Gerhardsson L, Björkner B, Karlsteen M, Schutz A (2002) Copper allergy from dental copper amalgam? Sci Total Environ 290: 41–46

222. Vergara G, Silvestre JF, Botella R, Albares MP, Pascual JC (2004) Oral lichen planus and sensitization to copper sulfate. Contact Dermatitis 50: 374

223. Dunlap CL, Vincent SK, Barber BF (1989) Allergic reaction to orthodontic wire: report of case. J Am Dent Assoc 118: 449–450

224. Schweitzer A (1997) Erstfeststellung einer Titan-Allergie. Dermatosen 45: 190

225. Marcusson JA, Cederbrant K, Heilborn J (1998) Indium and iridium allergy in patients exposed to dental alloys. Contact Dermatitis 38: 297–298

226. Haberman AL, Pratt M, Storrs FJ (1993) Contact dermatitis from beryllium in dental alloys. Contact Dermatitis 28: 157–162

227. Klotzer WT (1991) Metalle und Legierungen – Korrosion, Toxikologie, sensibiliserande Wirkung (Teil) (Metals and alloys – corrosion, toxicology, sensitivity reactions 1, in German). ZWR 100: 300–304

228. Müller-Quernheim J, Zissel G, Schopf R, Vollmer E, Schlaak M (1996) Differential diagnosis of berylliosis/sarcoidosis in a dental technician (in German). Dtsch Med Wochenschr 121: 1462–1466

229. Vilaplana J, Romaguera C (1998) New developments in jewellery and dental materials. Contact Dermatitis 39: 55–57

230. Motolese A, Truzzi M, Giannini A, Seidenari S (1993) Contact dermatitis and contact sensitization among enamellers and decorators in the ceramic industry. Contact Dermatitis 28: 59–62

231. Pardo J, Rodriguez-Serna M, De La Cuadra J, Fortea JM (2004) Allergic contact stomatitis due to manganese in a dental prosthesis. Contact Dermatitis 50: 41

232. Beyer DJ, Belsito DV (1997) Delayed hypersensitivity to silicon causing gingival hyperplasia. Contact Dermatitis 27: 234

233. Magro-Filho O, de Carvalho AC (1994) Topical effect of propolis in the repair of sulcoplasties by the modified Kazanjian technique. Cytological and clinical evaluation. J Nihon Univ Sch Dent 36: 102–111

234. Garrido Fernández S, Lasa Luaces E, Echechipia Madoz S, Arroabarren Alémán E, Anda Apiñániz M, Tabar Purroy AI (2004) Allergic contact stomatitis due to therapeutic propolis. Contact Dermatitis 50: 321

235. Hensten-Pettersen A, Östavil D, Wennberg A (1985) Allergic potential of root canal sealers. Endod Dent Traumatol 1: 61–65

236. Bruze M (1994) Systemically induced contact dermatitis from dental rosin. Scand J Dent Res 101: 376–378

237. Sainio EL, Kanerva L (1995) Contact allergens in toothpastes and a review of their hypersensitivity. Contact Dermatitis 33: 100–105

238. Veien NK, Hattel T, Laurberg G (1993) Systemically aggravated contact dermatitis by aluminium in toothpaste. Contact Dermatitis 28: 199–200

239. Boxer MB, Grammer LC, Orfan N (1994) Gutta-percha allergy in a health care worker with latex allergy. J Allergy Clin Immunol 93: 943–944

240. Fisher AA (1994) The safety of gutta-percha from root canal use in rubber sensitive individuals. Am J Contact Dermat 5: 188

241. Ockenfels HM, Seemann U, Goos M (1995) Allergy to fibrin tissue in dental medicine. Contact Dermatitis 32: 363–364

242. Wüthrich B, Bianchi-Kusch E, Johansson SG (1996) Allergic urticaria and angioedema caused by a hemostatic sponge of bovine fibrin used in tooth extraction. Allergy 51: 49–51

243. Estlander T, Kanerva L, Tupasela O, Keskinen H, Jolanki R (1993) Immediate and delayed allergy to nickel with contact urticaria, rhinitis, asthma and contact dermatitis. Clin Exp Allergy 23: 306–310

244. Baker DB, Gann PH, Brooks SM, Gallagher J, Bernstein IL (1990) Cross-sectional study of platinum salts sensitization among precious metals refinery workers. Am J Ind Med 18: 653–664

245. Schena D, Barba A, Costa G (1996) Occupational contact urticaria to cisplatin. Contact Dermatitis 34: 220–221

246. Bergman A, Svedberg U, Nilsson E (1995) Contact urticaria and anaphylactic reactions caused by occupational exposure to iridium salt. Contact Dermatitis 32: 14–17

247. Murdoch RD, Pepys J, Hughes EG (1986) IgE antibody responses to platinum group metals: a large scale refinery survey. Br J Ind Med 43: 37–43

248. Murdoch RD, Pepys J (1987) Platinum group metal sensitivity: reactivity to platinum group metal salts in platinum halide salt-sensitive workers. Ann Allergy 59: 464–469

249. Torresani C, Caprari E, Manara GC (1993) Contact urticaria syndrome due to phenylmercuric acetate. Contact Dermatitis 29: 282–283

250. Camarasa JG, Serra-Baldrich E, Lluch M, Malet A (1993) Contact urticaria from sodium fluoride. Contact Dermatitis 28: 294

251. Dykewicz MS, Patterson RP, Cugell DW, Harris KE, Wu AF (1991) Serum IgE and IgG to formaldehyde-human serum albumin: lack of relation to gaseous formaldehyde exposure and symptoms. J Allergy Clin Immunol 87: 48–57

252. Wantke F, Hemmer W, Haglmuller T, Gotz M, Jarisch R (1995) Anaphylaxis after dental treatment with formaldehyde-containing tooth-filling material. Allergy 50: 274–276

253. Kunisada M, Adachi A, Asano H, Horikawa T (2002) Anaphylaxis due to formaldehyde released from root-canal disinfectant. Contact Dermatitis 47: 215–218

254. Nomura M, Okano M, Okada N et al (1983) Four cases with anaphylaxis induced by chlorhexidine. Skin Res 25: 306

255. Nishioka K, Doi T, Katayama I (1984) Histamin release in contact urticaria. Contact Dermatitis 11: 191

256. Ohtoshi T, Yamauchi N, Takodoro K, Miyachi S, Suzuki S, Miyamoto T (1986) IgE antibody-mediated shock reaction caused by topical application of chlorhexidine. Clin Allergy 16: 155–161

257. Petersen JK (1994) Et tilfaelde af akut anafylaktisk shock efter mundskylning med klorheksidinoplosning (in Danish). Tandlaegebladet 98: 335–338

258. Petersen JK, Heiden M (1995) Nyt tilfaelde af anafylaktisk shock over for klorheksidin (in Danish). Tandlaegebladet 99: 733

Chapter 37

Clothing

37

Christophe J. Le Coz

Contents

37.1 Introduction

Clothes help to regulate skin temperature and moisture, and protect from environmental injuries. They should be safe, with no toxicity, carcinogenicity, or allergenicity. Reports of clothing dermatitis are frequently individual, with the exception of rare epidemics [1, 2] occurring from furs dyed by PPD and derivatives in the 1920s [3], from dyed nylon stockings in the 1940s [3, 4], or from black "velvet" clothing and blouses in the 1980s [5, 6]. Epidemiological studies regarding this topic are most often not controlled, and habitually report a frequency of positive patch tests to textile additives, mainly dyes or finishes [7–16]. Thus, the prevalence of sensitization to substances potentially implicated in textile dermatitis is difficult to establish [17], being around 1–5% of tested patients, although the interest and the clinical relevance of such tests are frequently questionable. For example, a recent study in 1,012 patients tested indicated that 31 patients (3%) reacted to at least one clothing dye, but that only 10 reactions were relevant [16]. It is difficult to determine its exact incidence for these reasons, but many data suggest that clothing dermatitis is not exceptional [4, 7, 14, 17].

Changes in fashion, styling, new leisure activities, and technological progress explain the variations of clinical patterns and allergens in clothing dermatitis. For instance, sock suspenders, hats, or corsets are out of fashion in most countries. Conversely, many people wear sports clothing daily and most clothing is treated against shrinkage, creasing, or the development of odors. Concerning allergens, ester gum (abietic acid and alcohol) used as an adhesive was responsible for epidemics of dermatitis in the 1940s [18], allergy to formaldehyde in garments is rarer than previously, since more recent textile finish resins release little or no formaldehyde, as new dye stuffs are regularly synthesized before coming onto the market. It is arduous to detect the newer allergens and the disappearance of the older, since the chemicals used in textiles are not declared, contrary to the case with cosmetics. The manufacturing and legislation modifications in developed countries permit a dramatic reduction of formaldehyde release [19] and the interdiction of textile dyes that are carcinogenic or which can release carcinogenic aromatic amines [20]. Some industrial labels, such as the Oeko-Tex Standard 100, wish to promote "safe textiles" as well [21]. However, such resolutions run the risk of being counterbalanced by the level of imported clothing from the Far East or underdeveloped countries which contain various textile additives.

The diagnosis of clothing dermatitis requires cautious examination both of the patient and of the suspected article. A poor history, lack of clinical information, or no examination of the clothing often lead to a missed diagnosis [3,10]. We have principally considered dermatitis due to clothing itself, and excluded damage from accessories such as jewels or belts, or those provoked by gloves and shoes.

37.2 Clinical Examination

Contact dermatitis from clothing has, generally, the clinical features of a typical eczema [3,10,22], though dry rather than vesicular. The lesions can progress and be severe, generalized or even erythrodermic, as long as contact with the allergen is not avoided. Follicular or nummular eczema is possible with finish resins [14, 22]. Pigmented contact dermatitis arises mainly in patients with phototype IV or V, and has been described from Naphthol AS as well [1]. In some instances, the lesions can be monomorphic and infiltrated [7]. They may simulate an atopic dermatitis in popliteal areas [3], demonstrate a persistent erythematous or urticarial-type dermatitis, or even present solely as diffuse itching [10]. Purpuric clothing dermatitis, described during the Second World War, was due to textile finishes in British soldiers' uniforms. This rare instance occurred with rubber compounds such as isopropyl-phenyl *p*-phenylenediamine (IPPD), with the azo dyes Disperse Blue 85 [23], Disperse Blue 106/124 [24], or Disperse Yellow 27 [25]. It is not clear if purpuric reactions are of allergic and/or toxic mechanisms. Cocarde lesions are rarely described [10].

The dermatitis generally occurs on the sites of intimate contact with the garment [3,13–15], and the lesions are sometimes symmetrical (Figs. 1 and 2). Friction or perspiration sites are preferentially involved, particularly in hypersensitivity from textile finish resins [3, 4, 22, 26], and a clinical pattern of textile dermatitis is generally described: neck, major skin folds, inner thighs. The areas protected by underclothing or the lining of the skirt of the clothing are often free of symptoms [27, 28]. The face can be involved from handling of the dyes. Some peculiar localizations, in accordance with the form of the garment, are reported in Table 1.

Core Message

■ Allergy from textiles frequently offers a typical pattern, mainly located in body areas in contact with the garment. Sweating and friction promote dermatitis.

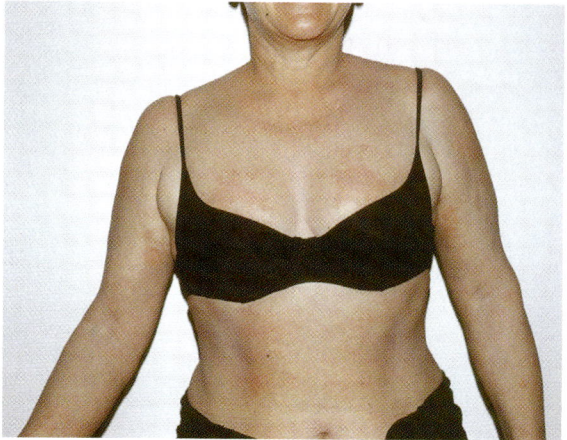

Fig. 1. Allergic contact dermatitis from clothing dye in a black dress containing Disperse Blue 106/124

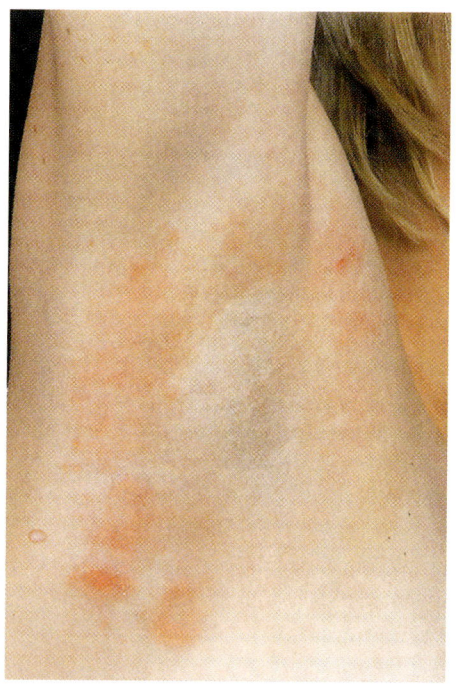

Fig. 2. Allergic contact dermatitis from clothing resin around axillary borders

Dermatitis from *socks* will be distributed on the feet and lower legs [3]. Hypersensitivity to *stockings* or *tights* (panty hose) will start on the lower legs, dorsum of feet, and toes, and then spread to the popliteal fossae [3]. In the case of dermatitis from *blouses* and *dresses*, the back is typically involved.

In addition, dress dermatitis affects the neck, elbows and axilla, predominates around the axillary borders [4], and can involve the forearms and wrists [3].

37

Table 1. Localization of dermatitis according to garment type

Type of garment	Localization of lesions
Socks	Feet, legs
Stockings	Lower legs, feet, toes, popliteal fossae
Blouses	Back, chest, axillary borders
Dresses	Back, neck, elbows, axillary borders, forearms, wrists
Jackets	Dorsum of hands, wrists, and forearms
Trousers	Thighs, lower legs, dorsum of hands

Allergy from *jackets* involves the backs of the hands or wrists [4]. Dermatitis from *trousers* occurs on the thighs and lower legs, and in the popliteal fossae. The dorsum of the hands is affected in patients who often put them in their pockets [3, 4].

Examination of the garment is indispensable. The labeling indicates the fiber composition (if ratio >5%) and can guide to specific dyes or textile finishes. The practitioner should examine the different parts of the fabric and take some of them, of different colors or textures, for patch testing or for further chemical analysis.

37.3 The Inducers of Dermatitis

Irritant dermatitis is more frequent than allergic, either of delayed or of immediate type. In addition, obtaining the final diagnosis by the way of the exact composition of a garment is often a challenge, which necessitates tenacity and cooperation between the practitioner, the patient, and the manufacturer.

37.3.1 Textile Fibers

The exact fiber composition of a garment is generally designated on the label, as long as the fibers are present at a ≥5% amount. Textile fibers are numerous and industrial developments are extensive. Natural fibers are cellulose (cotton, linen) or protein based (wool, silk). Synthetic fibers mainly consist of cellulose derivatives (rayon, acetate, and triacetate), polyamides such as nylon (Perlon, Antron, Quiana), polyesters (Dacron, Tergal, Terylene), acrylics (Acrylan, Acribel, Dralon, Courtelle), elastomers (Lycra, Vyrene) or new fibers derived from nylon such as aramids (Kevlar, Nomex). Fibers are frequently blended, sometimes even with metal. Cosmetics such as deodorants, perfumes, and even moisturizing agents can be added during manufacture: their concentra-

tion generally fades away with wearing or after a few washing.

Textile fibers themselves, rubber excepted, are usually not implicated in allergic contact dermatitis [3, 29]. Observations of allergy from *wool* are often ancient and questionable [29, 30]. *Silk* can seldom provoke immediate or delayed hypersensitivity. Allergens are controversial and could be the fibers, sericin in raw silk, or silkworm protein [31]. Allergic contact dermatitis from *nylon* itself is exceptional [29], but can be due to the monomer of nylon 6, epsilon-aminocaproic acid [32]. *Spandex*, a polyurethane-urea elastomer used in brassieres and girdles, formerly contained mercaptobenzothiazole [29]. *Neoprene rubber* is a synthetic rubber based on polychloroprene polymerized with sulfur and 2,3-dichloro-1,3-butadiene. It is used to make wet suits, swimming gear, slimming suits, and clothing for fire fighters and contains, especially, thiourea derivatives such as ethylene-thiourea, and diethyl-, dibutyl-, and diphenyl-thiourea, which have been described as allergens [33–35].

Textile fibers are mainly responsible for irritant contact dermatitis and patients suffering from atopic dermatitis or dry skin often complain of intolerance to garments. The irritant potential of wool and that of synthetic fibers is significantly higher in such patients, while cotton garments are best tolerated [36]. This is due to the structure of wool and many synthetic fibers that have a thorny surface. Irritation can be diffuse or much localized, occurring, for example, at the site of cutaneous contact with clothing tags, frequently made of synthetic coarse fibers. This has been described as "label dermatitis" [37].

Nylon, because of a poor sweat absorption, can promote miliaria-like eruptions [30]. Other synthetic fibers, such as rayon, polyester, and acrylics can be irritant, and provoke pruritus and maceration [30, 36].

Core Message

■ With the exception of rubber derivatives, textile fibers induce mostly irritant dermatitis.

37.3.2 Textile Resins and Formaldehyde

Textile finish resins (TFR), also named durable-press resins or permanent press clothing finishes, are especially and widely used for cotton, cotton/polyester, or wrinkle-resistant linen. TFR can facilitate bleaching and dying, and ameliorate nylon and make it electrically antistatic. They give textiles body, and improve their quality, touch, and appearance. Fabrics are crease-resistant, waterproof, non-shrinkable, mothproof, and noniron [3, 22, 38]. It is hard, if ever possible, to know the exact composition of TFR used today by the manufacturers [personal communications]. Two major types of TFR have been developed for the textile industry: the older are formaldehyde-based resins (urea-formaldehyde resins and melamine-formaldehyde resins), as the more recent TFR are cyclized urea derivatives, which are preponderant in Europe. Most TFR release more or less high amounts of formaldehyde, due to the necessity of formaldehyde to synthesize the resin, to a subsequent degradation of the resin during the storage, during wearing because of sweat, during an acid washing [3], or by the use of chlorine during laundry [18]. Industrial washing, although expensive, decreases the presence of unreacted formaldehyde and resins at the surface of the garment. Glyoxal, another aldehyde, is sometimes used as a substitute of formaldehyde in systems which subsequently release no formaldehyde.

Urea formaldehyde (methylolurea) resins derive from the polymerization of urea and formaldehyde with a curing agent. The intermediate products are monomethylolurea CAS [1000–82–4], dimethylolurea (also named carbamol or oxymethurea) CAS [140–95–4], and methyleneurea CAS [13547–17–6]. The second stage consists in the condensation of the methylolureas to low molecular polymers by methylene and methylene-ether linkages that secondarily polymerize within the interstices of the textile fibers [3, 26]. These resins release large amounts of free formaldehyde, particularly under moist and heat conditions, but are no more used for clothing in most countries for clothing.

Melamine formaldehyde resins result from the condensation of formaldehyde and melamine CAS [108–78–1], which is obtained by the dehydratation of urea. Trimethylolmelamine CAS [1017–56–7] and hexamethylolmelamine CAS [531–18–0] are the main compounds, resulting from the condensation of melamine with three and six formaldehyde molecules, respectively. They polymerize into resins in the interstices of the fibers. Some unpolymerized methylol residues (R-CH$_2$-OH) contained in such resins can

37

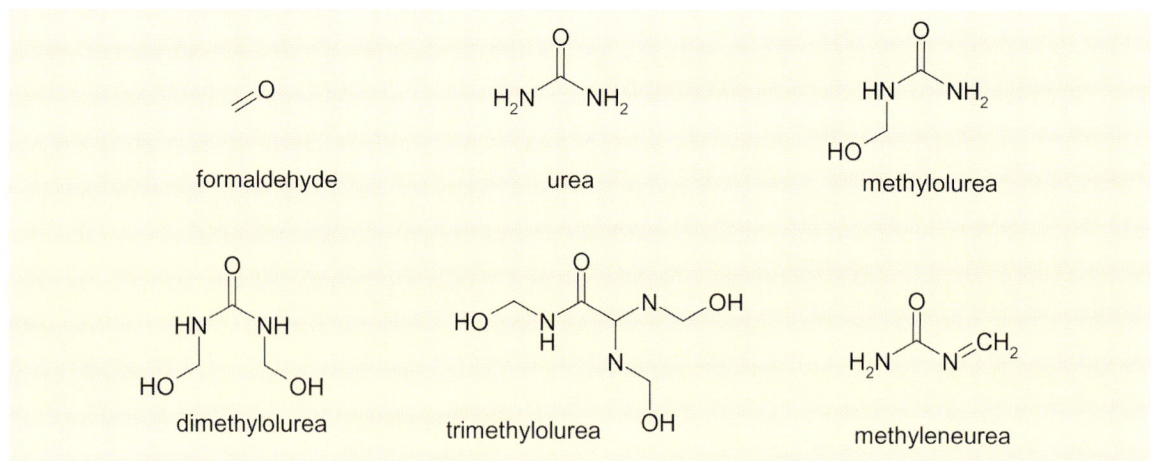

Fig. 3. Structures of formaldehyde, urea, (mono)methylolurea, dimethylolurea, trimethylolurea, and methyleneurea

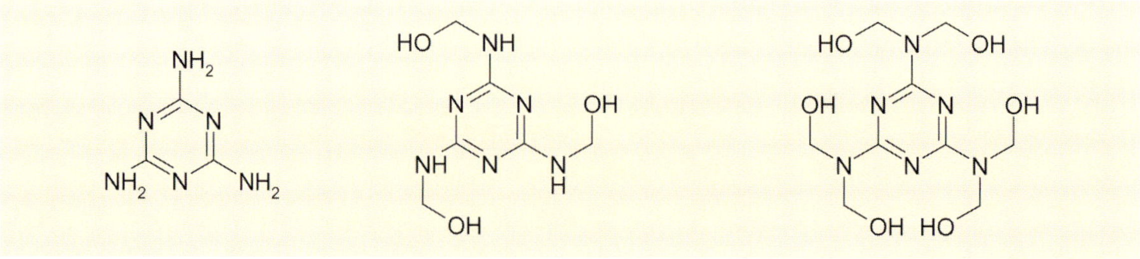

Fig. 4. Structures of melamine, trimethylolmelamine, and hexamethylolmelamine

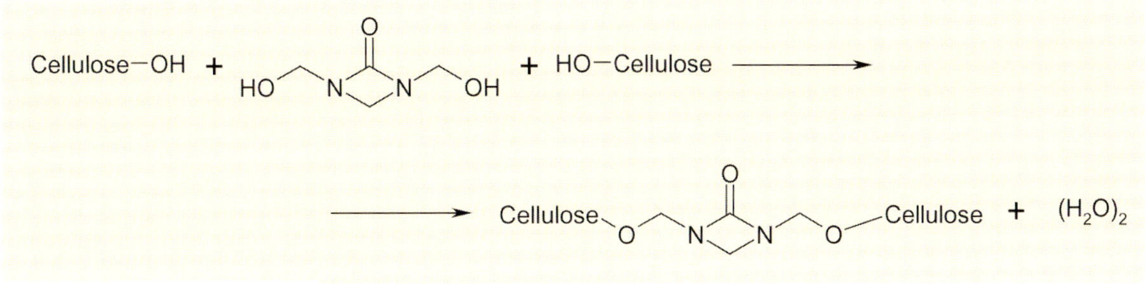

Fig. 5. Simplified schema of the ether reaction between cyclized urea and cellulosic fibers

subsequently be degraded into free formaldehyde (CH$_2$=O). These TFR release large amounts of formaldehyde [26], but are out of fashion in Europe for clothing.

Cyclized urea derivatives, the now current TFR, are reticulating agents based on N-alkoxymethylated cyclized urea. With magnesium chloride to initiate the reaction, their N-methylol (N-CH$_2$-OH) groups cross-link with the hydroxyl (OH) groups of the cellulosic textile fibers to form stable ether bonds.

These numerous molecules mainly consist of substituted ethylene ureas, such as dimethylol ethylene urea (DMEU) CAS [136–84–5], dimethyl-dihydroxy ethylene urea (DMeDHEU) CAS [3923–79–3], and di-methylol-dihydroxy ethylene urea (DMDHEU, CAS [1854–26–8]), and of substituted propylene ureas such as dimethylol propylene urea (DMPU) CAS [3270–74–4], dimethylol-dihydroxy propylene urea (DMDHPU), dimethylol-5-hydroxy propylene urea, and dimethylol-4-methoxy-5,5-dimethyl propylene urea. Other molecules are dimethylol-hexahydrotriazine and urons (uron-formaldehyde), such as dimethoxymethyl uron CAS [7388–44–5]. All of them are marketed with tenths for their names (e.g., >30 for DMDHEU).

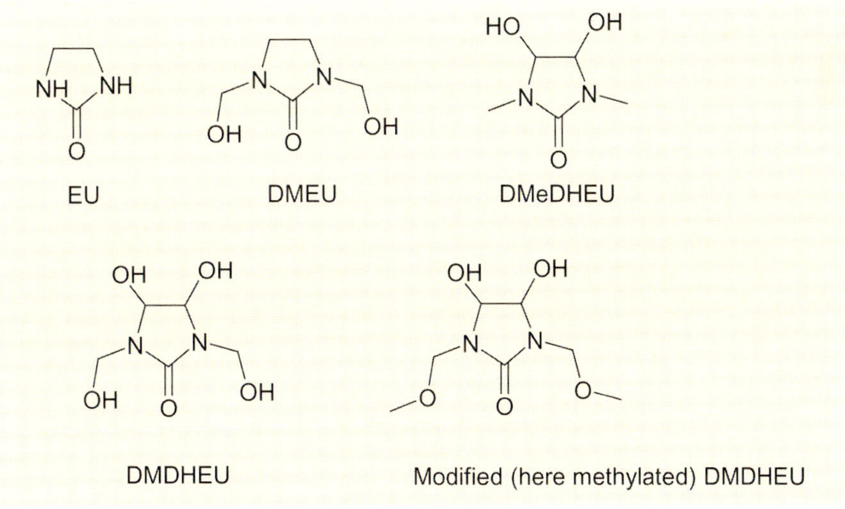

Fig. 6.
Structures of ethylene urea (*EU*), dimethylol ethylene urea (*DMEU*), dimethyl-dihydroxy ethylene urea (*DMeDHEU*), dimethylol-dihydroxy ethylene urea (*DMDHEU*), and modified DMDHEU (here, methylated dimethylol-dihydroxy ethylene urea)

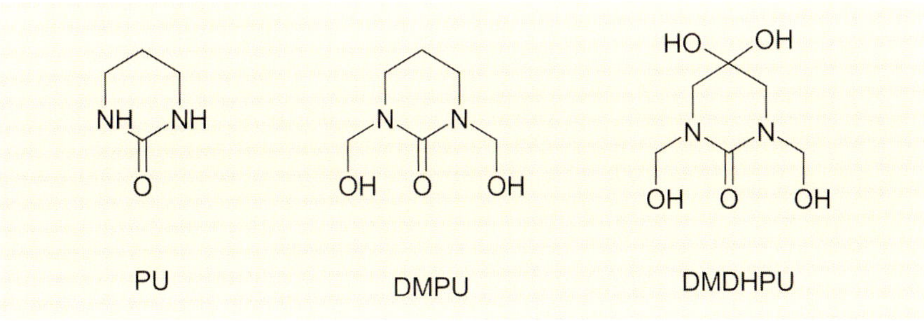

Fig. 7.
Structures of propylene urea (PU), dimethylol propylene urea (DMPU), and dimethylol-dihydroxy propylene urea (DMDHPU)

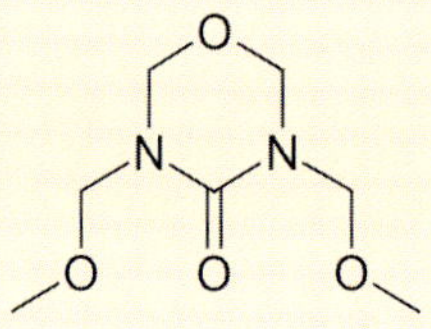

Fig. 8. Dimethoxymethyl uron

DMDHEU and its derivatives are now the main TFR used in Europe. During polymerization, free formaldehyde is released. Inadequate curing also leads to the liberation of formaldehyde at high temperature. A number of approaches have been developed to limit the amount of formaldehyde released, such as after washing of cured fabrics, the addition of formaldehyde scavengers such as carbohydrazide to the bath, the use of urea in the pad-bath, or application through a spray, the modification of DMDHEU. Such substitutions of the molecule are expected to decrease the release of formaldehyde and DMDHEU can be modified to etherized, glycolated, or methylated DMDHEU, so as to give dimethoxymethyl dihydroxyethylene urea, known, e.g., as modified DMDHEU. Commercially, it is the modified DMDHEU (glycolated or methylated) that is most often used today. The product is pre-buffered to prevent premature curing and is also pre-blended with a catalyst, with magnesium-based catalysts being the most popular in use today. Such resins release various amounts of free formaldehyde: a moderate rate (100 to 1,000 ppm) for DMPU, DMEU, and urons, a low rate (<100 ppm) for DMDHEU and DMMDHEU, and a very low rate (<30 ppm) for blended or substituted DMDHEU [26, 30, 38].

Alternatives to DMDHEU are also being researched but *other durable-press resins are of less importance in industry and in allergic contact dermatitis.*

Carbamate derivatives are particularly used in the USA for mixed cotton-polyester. For example, (di)methylolcarbamates are usually used in white shirts [30]. They release moderate amounts of formaldehyde [26, 30, 38].

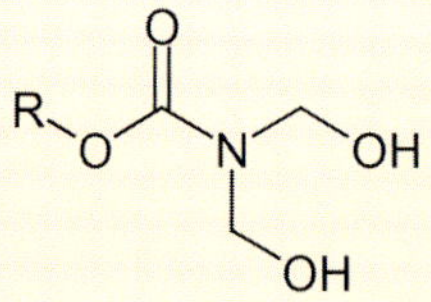

Polycarboxylic acid systems such as butane 1,2,3,4-tetracarboxylic acid (BTCA), citric acid, or modified polycarboxylic acids have been more recently developed. However, BTCA is expensive to use and citric acid causes yellowing. Although they could be "safe" TFR, they are not of interest in allergologic routine [26, 30, 38]. Another approach has been to use polymers of maleic acid to form ester cross-links, and yet another to fix a quaternary group through an epoxidation reaction to the cellulose chain to form cross-links. Research on all these alternatives continues.

The incidence of TFR-related contact dermatitis seems lower than 0.5% of patch tested patients [39], and higher in women than in men [22, 26], probably because of the greater frequency of wearing treated garments in women [18]. Patients positive to TFR are generally allergic to formaldehyde released by TFR [3, 22, 26]. Such people can be sensitive to formaldehyde released by preservatives used in cosmetics and have an associated facial dermatitis [26], which is a source of error in diagnosis. Previous studies have demonstrated the presence of free formaldehyde (1–3,500 ppm) in synthetic and natural fibers, particularly in 100% rayon, or in cotton-blended fabrics [3, 40]. The threshold rate for allergic contact dermatitis is 500 ppm or 750 ppm free formaldehyde in the garment [26, 40]. During recent years, a 10- to 30-fold decrease in free formaldehyde has been noted in fabrics [18, 26]. First regulation was observed in Japan and in Finland. European norms EN ISO 14184 parts 1 and 2 [19] are based on three principles: no detectable formaldehyde in garments for infants (in fact, <20 ppm is the threshold of detection associated to Japanese regulation Law 112), level <75 ppm for garments with direct skin contact, level <300 ppm for clothing that are not in contact with skin. This decrease to 10–100 ppm is due to the use of DMDHEU and derivatives, or to non-formaldehyde-based resins. So, the former estimation that 8.6% of patients sensitized to formaldehyde were sensitive to textiles [39] is currently overestimated. In some instances, patients seem to be allergic to the resin itself, without formaldehyde sensitivity [8, 14, 18, 26, 41].

Fig. 9. Dimethylol carbamates. *R* alkyl, hydroxyalkyl, or alkoxyalkyl chain

Core Message

■ Textile resins are used to enhance the touch and quality of clothing (nonshrinkable and noniron). Some of them (urea-formaldehyde and melamine formaldehyde) significantly release formaldehyde. Current cyclized-urea resins derived from DMDHEU release fewer or no formaldehyde.

37

37.3.3 Textile Dyes

Sensitization to textile dyes in clothing necessitates a transfer of the dye from the garment to the skin. However, "bleeding" of textile dyes, which induces skin discoloration, is a non-allergic phenomenon unnecessary for sensitization [4]. Sensitization occurs from the dye itself, from intermediate products during the dying process or after-treatments, or from metabolites arising in the skin. Attributing an allergy to a textile dye is a hard process and, even if a textile dye is found to be positive on patch testing, the precise identification of the sensitizer in the garment is extremely difficult. There are thousands of textile dyes, marketed under different names (up to 30 for some of them), and the Color Index (CI) does not contain all the information on them. A final textile color often results from a subtle mixture of several dyes. Because of this, a priori unexpected dyes can be employed as yellow, red, orange, or red dyes, for black or blue garments, respectively. For example, Serisol Black L 1944, used to dye black "velvet" clothes, contained five disperse dyes, namely, Blue 124 and 106, Red 1, Yellow 3, and Blue 1 [5]. Moreover, a commercial dye often comprises of one or two major components, and even impurities [42]. If Disperse Yellow 3 is generally pure, Disperse Red 153 or Disperse Blue 35 contain two major fractions, and Disperse Red 1 comprises one major compound and at least two other minor substances [27, 42]. Disperse Blue 124 also contains several dyes and traces of Disperse Blue 106, as ascertained by comparative thin-layer chromatography (TLC) (personal observation). These impurities can also be responsible for sensitization [3, 43]. The manufacturing processes are complex and additional procedures, such as bleaching, can also lead to allergenic products [2]. Skin metabolism may be responsible for the transformation of dyes. For example, Disperse Orange 3 is degraded to p-phenylenediamine (PPD) and nitroaniline in the skin [3, 44] (Fig. 10).

According to their chemical structures and to the Color Index system, dyes can be classified into 12 groups: nitro dyes, triphenylmethane derivatives, xanthenes, acridine derivatives, quinoline derivatives, azines, anthraquinones, indigoid dyes, phthalocyanines dyes, oxidation bases, insoluble azo dye precursors, and azo dyes (classes XII to XVII) [45]. In practice, textile dyes are classified into different application classes: disperse, acid, basic, direct, vat, fiber-reactive, sulfur, premetallic, solvent dyes, and naphthols [11, 30, 45]. The principal allergenic textile dyes are reported in Table 2.

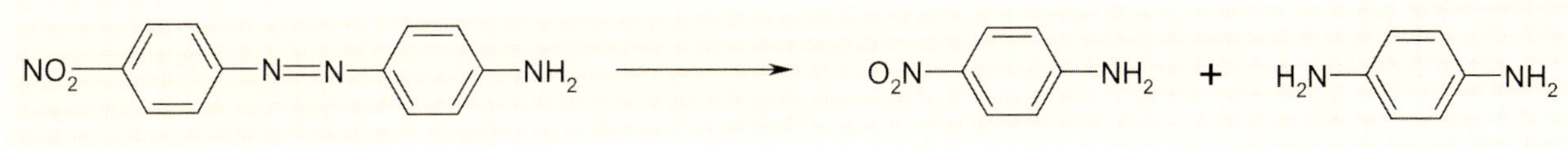

Fig. 10. Degradation of Disperse Orange 3 into nitroaniline and PPD

Table 2. Main textile dyes reported as allergens. [*C* Chemotechnique (Malmö, Sweden), *T* Trolab (Hermal, Reinbeck, Germany), *F* FIRMA (Florence, Italy)]

Names of the dyes	CI no.	CAS no.	Application class	Chemical class	Test concentration	Suppliers
Acid Black 48	65005	1328–24–1	Acid	Anthraquinone	1% pet.	F
Acid Red 118	26410	12217–35–5	Acid	Azoic	5% pet.	C
Acid Red 359	–	–	Premetallic	Azoic (chrome)	5% pet.	C
Acid Violet 17	42650	4129–84–4	Acid	Triphenylmethane	1% pet.	
Acid Yellow 36	13065	587–98–4	Acid	Azoic	1% pet.	T
Acid Yellow 61	18968	12217–38–8	Acid	Azoic	5% pet.	C
Basic Black 1	50431	–	Basic	Azine		
Basic Brown 1 (Bismarck Brown R)	21000	1052–38–6	Basic	(Di)azoic	0.5% pet.	F, T
Basic Red 46	–	12221–69–1	Basic	Azoic	1% pet.	C
Direct Black 38[a]	30235	1937–37–7	Direct	(Tri)azoic	1% pet.	
Direct Orange 34	40215	12222–37–6	Direct	Azo (stilbene)	5% pet.	C
Direct Orange 39	40215	1325–54–8	Direct	Azoic		
Direct Yellow 169	–	–	Direct	Azoic		

Table 2. Continued

Names of the dyes	CI no.	CAS no.	Application class	Chemical class	Test concentration	Suppliers
Disperse Black 1	11365	60–11–7	Disperse	Azoic	1% pet.	F
Disperse Black 2	11255	6232–57–1	Disperse	Azoic	1% pet.	
Disperse Blue 1[a,b]	64500	2475–45–8	Disperse	Anthraquinone	1% pet.	
Disperse Blue 3[c]	61505	2475–46–9	Disperse	Anthraquinone	1% pet.	C, F, T
Disperse Blue 7[c]	62500	3179–90–6	Disperse	Anthraquinone	1% pet.	
Disperse Blue 26[c]	63305	3860–63–7	Disperse	Anthraquinone	1% pet.	
Disperse Blue 35[c]	–	12222–75–2	Disperse	Anthraquinone	1% pet.	C
Disperse Blue 85	11370	3177–13–7	Disperse	Azoic	1% pet.	C
Disperse Blue 102[c]	–	12222–97–8	Disperse	Azoic	1% pet.	
Disperse Blue 106[c] (formerly 357)	111935	12223–01–7; 104573–53–7	Disperse	Azoic (cf. Db 124)	1% pet.	C, T[d]
Disperse Blue 124[c]	–	15141–18–1; 61951–51–7	Disperse	Azoic (cf. Db 106)	1% pet.	C, F, T[d]
Disperse Blue 153	–	–	Disperse	Anthraquinone	1% pet.	C
Disperse Brown 1[c]	11152	23355–64–8	Disperse	Azoic	1% pet.	C
Disperse Orange 1[c]	11080	2581–69–3	Disperse	Azoic	1% pet.	C
Disperse Orange 3[c]	11005	730–40–5	Disperse	Azoic	1% pet.	C, F, T
Disperse Orange 13	26080	6253–10–7	Disperse	Azoic	1% pet.	
Disperse Orange 76[c] (formerly 37)	11132	51811–42–8	Disperse	Azoic	1% pet.	
Disperse Red 1[c]	11110	2872–52–8	Disperse	Azoic	1% pet.	C, F, T
Disperse Red 11[c]	62015	2872–48–2	Disperse	Anthraquinone	1% pet.	T
Disperse Red 17[c]	11210	3179–89–3	Disperse	Azoic	1% pet.	C, F, T
Disperse Red 153	–	78564–87–1	Disperse	Azoic	1% pet.	
Disperse Yellow 1[c]	10345	119–15–3	Disperse	Nitro	1% pet.	
Disperse Yellow 3[a,c]	11855	2832–40–8	Disperse	Azoic	1% pet.	C, F, T
Disperse Yellow 9[c]	10375	6373–73–5	Disperse	Nitro	1% pet.	C, F, T
Disperse Yellow 27	–	73299–30–6	Disperse	Azoic	1% pet	
Disperse Yellow 39[c]	–	12236–29–2	Disperse	Methine	1% pet.	
Disperse Yellow 49[c]	–	54824–37–2	Disperse	Methine	1% pet.	
Disperse Yellow 54	47020	7576–65–0, 12223–85–7	Disperse	Quinoline	1% pet.	
Disperse Yellow 64	47023	10319–14–9, 12223–86–8	Disperse	Quinoline	1% pet.	
Naphthol AS	37505	92–77–3	Coupling agent	Naphthol	1% pet.	T
p-Aminophenol	76550	123–30–8		Related to some azo dyes	1% pet.	F, T
p-Aminoazobenzene (Solvent Yellow 1)	11000	60–09–3		Related to some azo dyes	0.25% pet.; 1% pet.	F, T
p-Phenylenediamine	76060	106–50–3		Related to some azo dyes	1% pet.	C, F, T
Reactive Black 5[b]	20505	17095–24–8	Reactive	Azoic	1% pet.	C
Reactive Blue 21[b]	18097	12236–86–1, 73049–92–0	Reactive	Phthalocyanine	1% pet (copper).	C
Reactive Blue 238[b]	–	149315–83–3	Reactive	(Di)azoic	1% pet.	C
Reactive Orange 107[b]	–	90597–79–8	Reactive	Azoic	1% pet.	C
Reactive Red 123[b]	–	61969–31–1	Reactive	Azoic	1% pet.	C
Reactive Red 228[b]	–	–	Reactive	Azoic	1% pet.	C
Reactive Red 238[b]	–	–	Reactive	Azoic	1% pet.	C
Reactive Violet 5[b]	18097	12226–38–9	Reactive	Azoic	1% pet.	C
Vat Green 1	59825	128–58–5	Vat dye	Anthraquinone	1% pet.	

[a] Also considered as a carcinogenic
[b] Not considered as allergenic for consumers, only if occupational exposure
[c] Dye banned due to being allergenic by the label Oeko-Tex
[d] Disperse Blue mix 106–124

37

37.3.3.1 Disperse Dyes

Disperse dyes are partially soluble in water [46] and are used to color synthetic fibers such as polyester, acrylic, and acetate, and sometimes nylon, particularly in stockings. They are not employed for natural fibers. *These molecules are the main sensitizers.* Women seem to be more prone than men to becoming sensitized [9, 47], but these data are not constant [46].

Core Message

■ Disperse dyes (azo or anthraquinone type) are the most often employed dyes, and the most frequent inducers of textile allergy, due to synthetic fibers.

Anthraquinone Dyes

These dyes consist of substituted anthraquinones [3, 45]. They are plastosoluble and are used to stain synthetic fibers, such as polyester, acetate, or nylon [46].

Disperse Blue 1, also used in coloring fabrics and plastics or for semi permanent hair colorations such as anthraquinone dyes Disperse Blue 3 and 7, Disperse Red 11 and 15, Disperse Violet 1, 4 and 15 [48], induced urinary bladder carcinomas and sarcomas in rats. It is reasonably anticipated to be a human carcinogen [49], such as Disperse Orange 11 (CI 60700).

Among these disperse anthraquinone dyes, *Disperse Red 11*, *Disperse Blue 3*, and *Disperse Blue 35* have been reported as causes of contact dermatitis from dresses, trousers, or nylon stockings [13, 15, 45, 50, 51]. Disperse Blue 35 is also a phototoxic compound [45, 52]. *Disperse Blue 3* has a structure close to that of Disperse Blue 7, and was positive in several patients tested with a dye series [15, 45, 47]. With Disperse Orange 76 (an azo dye), Disperse Red 11 was thought to be one of the most common causes of dye

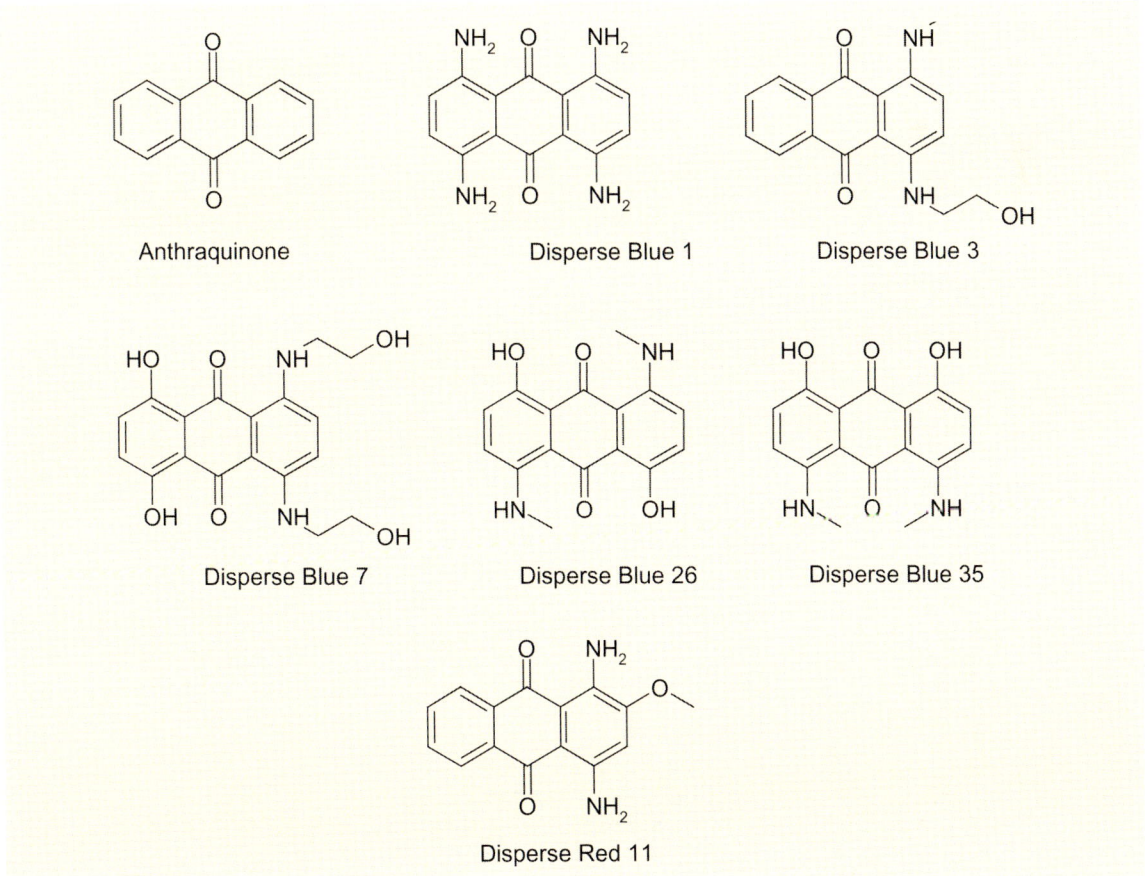

Fig. 11. Anthraquinone disperse dyes: Blue 1, Blue 3, Blue 7, Blue 26, Blue 35 (major compound), and Red 11

allergy in men [47]. Disperse Blue 26, one of the most used dyes in the world, is forbidden in garments with label Oeko-Tex because of its allergenicity [21].

Azo Dyes

Azo dyes are characterized by an R1-N=N-R2 chemical structure. They represent the majority of commercial colorants, enabling a broad spectrum of shades and fastness properties. They are suitable for coloring various substrates, including both synthetic and natural fibers. These molecules are trapped within the fibers in which they are formed during the dying process. Azo dyes, disperse type, are used in synthetic fibers. They are the molecules most often implicated in textile dye dermatitis, mainly in nylon stocking, socks, trousers, dresses, and underwear. Disperse Yellow 3, Disperse Orange 3, and Disperse Red 1 were the principal sensitizers in a retrospective study in 1940–1984 [53]. Today, Disperse Blue 124 and/or 106, Disperse Orange 3, Red 1 or Yellow 3 are frequently encountered [7, 10, 15]. A recent classification divided them into four chemical sub-groups [27].

The monoazoic compound *Disperse Blue 124* is the most frequently positive dye on patch testing with textile series [9, 10, 15, 16, 54], particularly in women [9, 47]. It is probably the main cause of textile contact dermatitis today [5, 55–57]. It is closely related to another azo dye, *Disperse Blue 106*, marketed since 1985, and formerly known as Disperse Blue 357. Both are frequently used together, and Disperse Blue 124 contains traces of Disperse Blue 106, as ascertained by comparative TLC (Fig. 12). The latter seems to have the stronger sensitizing potential [5, 6, 13, 55] and can provoke infiltrated lesions [7, 56]. Concomitant positive reactions to both Disperse Blue 106 and 124 are constant [5, 7].

The delay necessary for the diagnosis may be long [56].

Disperse Blue 102 was detected in suspect fabric of four patients with allergic contact dermatitis. It was always associated to Disperse Yellow 3 in the fabric. The four patients were all sensitized to Disperse Blue 106/124 [58].

Disperse Orange 3 was cited in reports of stocking dermatitis [3, 47] and remains a frequent allergen [12, 15]. Patients are sensitized to PPD at an average of 2/3, and primary sensitization to Disperse Orange 3 seems to be acquired from hair dyes [9, 15]. *para*-Aminoazobenzene (PAAB, Solvent Yellow 1) and *para*-dimethylaminoazobenzene (PDMAAB) are positive in about two/three patients sensitized to Disperse Orange 3 [15].

Disperse Red 1 was implicated in dermatitis from stockings [47], and is frequently observed on patch testing [10, 16], especially in subjects under 12 years of age [15].

Disperse Red 17 gave positive patch test reactions in patients sensitized to other azo dyes [10, 15, 27], and was cited as a stocking dye [3, 22].

Disperse Brown 1 is less frequently positive, as is Disperse Brown 2 [27].

Disperse Orange 76, also formerly named *Disperse Orange 37*, is often positive, and was thought to be one of the main causes of dye allergy in men, together with Disperse Blue 3 (an anthraquinone dye) [3, 15, 47].

Reactions to *Disperse Yellow 3* are frequent [3, 7, 9, 10, 16]. The first cases reported concerned nylon stocking dermatitis, and this azo dye is still currently used to dye such garments [3, 4, 22] (personal observation). This dye is regarded as a carcinogen.

Disperse Red 153 is based on two structurally close compounds [27].

Disperse Black 1 and 2 are rarely positive [13, 15].

Core Message

■ Among disperse azo dyes, Disperse Blue 106/124 are currently the main sensitizers, which are found in synthetic fibers such as cellulose, acetate or polyamide.

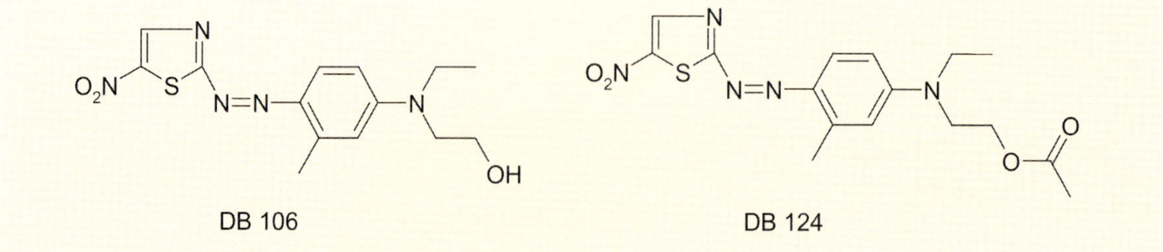

Fig. 12. Azo disperse dyes Disperse Blue 106 and Disperse Blue 124

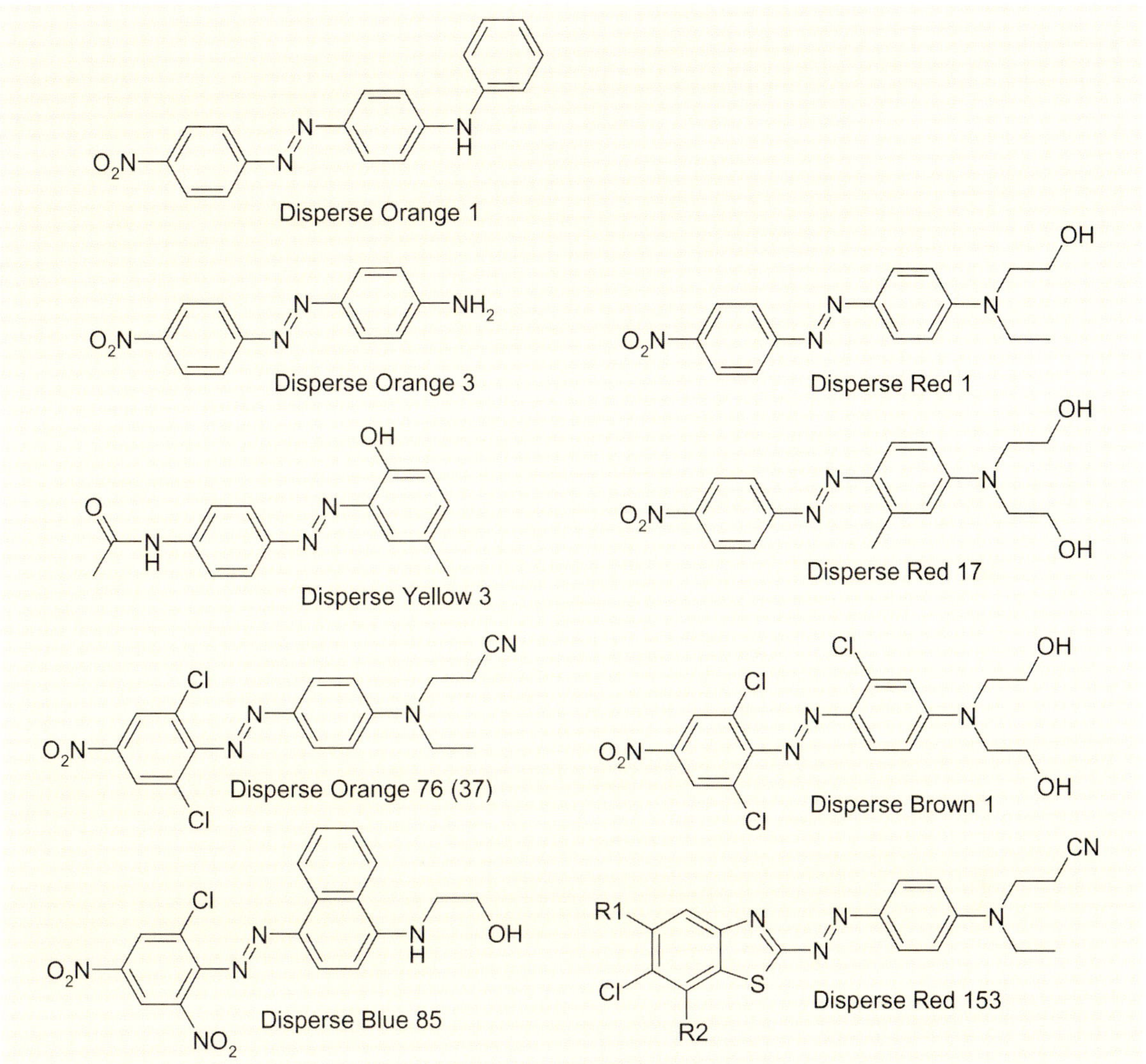

Fig. 13. Azo disperse dyes Orange 1, Orange 3, Red 1, Yellow 3, Red 17, Orange 76 (37), Brown 1, Blue 85, and Red 153 (R1=Cl or H and R2=H or Cl, respectively)

Methine, Nitro, and Quinoline Dyes

Disperse Yellow 39, a methine dye, was implicated in trouser dermatitis [4, 45]. Disperse Yellow 54 and its brominated derivative Disperse Yellow 64 (quinoline), Disperse Yellow 1, and Disperse Yellow 9 (nitro) were cited in some reports [4, 45, 47].

37.3.3.2 Acid Dyes

These are used to color silk, wool, and other animal protein fibers, or nylon (polyamide) when high wet-fastness is needed [30, 46]. Such dyes include mono-azoic, diazoic, triphenylmethane, and anthraquinone compounds. Acid Yellow 23, Acid Black 48, Acid Black 63 [3], and Acid Violet 17 (triphenylmethane derived) were reported in the literature, mainly before 1985 [4, 45]. Acid Yellow 61, Acid Red 359, and Acid Red 118, each tested 5% pet., and removed at 3 days (sic), were positive in five, two, and one out of 1,814 consecutive patients, respectively. Relevance was considered possible in four patients [11]. Acid Red 26 (CI 16150) is regarded as a carcinogen and is forbidden in the EU.

Core Message

■ Acid dyes used for protein or nylon fibers are rare allergens.

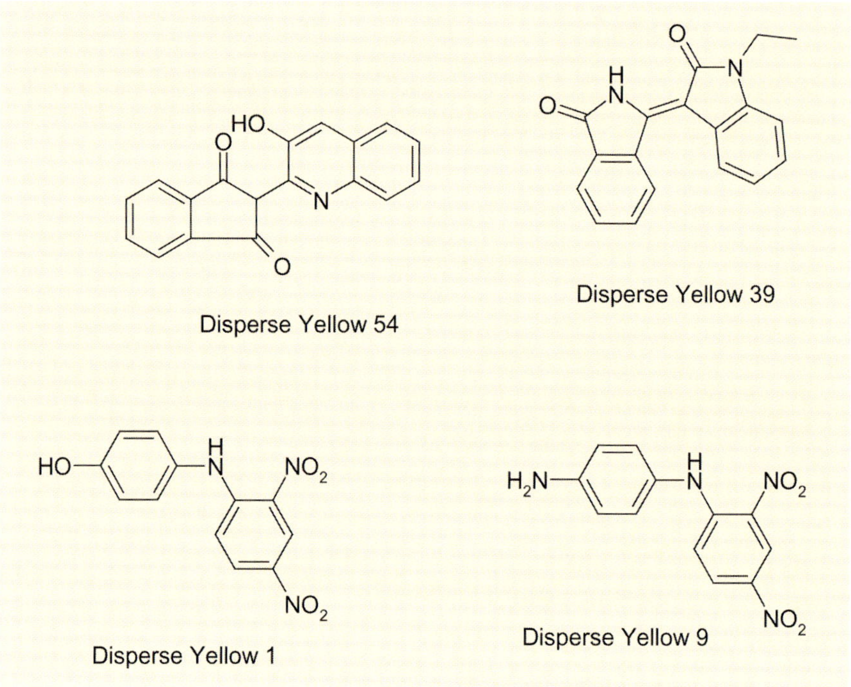

Fig. 14.
Disperse Yellow 54 (quinoleine), Disperse Yellow 39
(quinoleine), Disperse Yellow
1, and Disperse Yellow 9
(nitro)

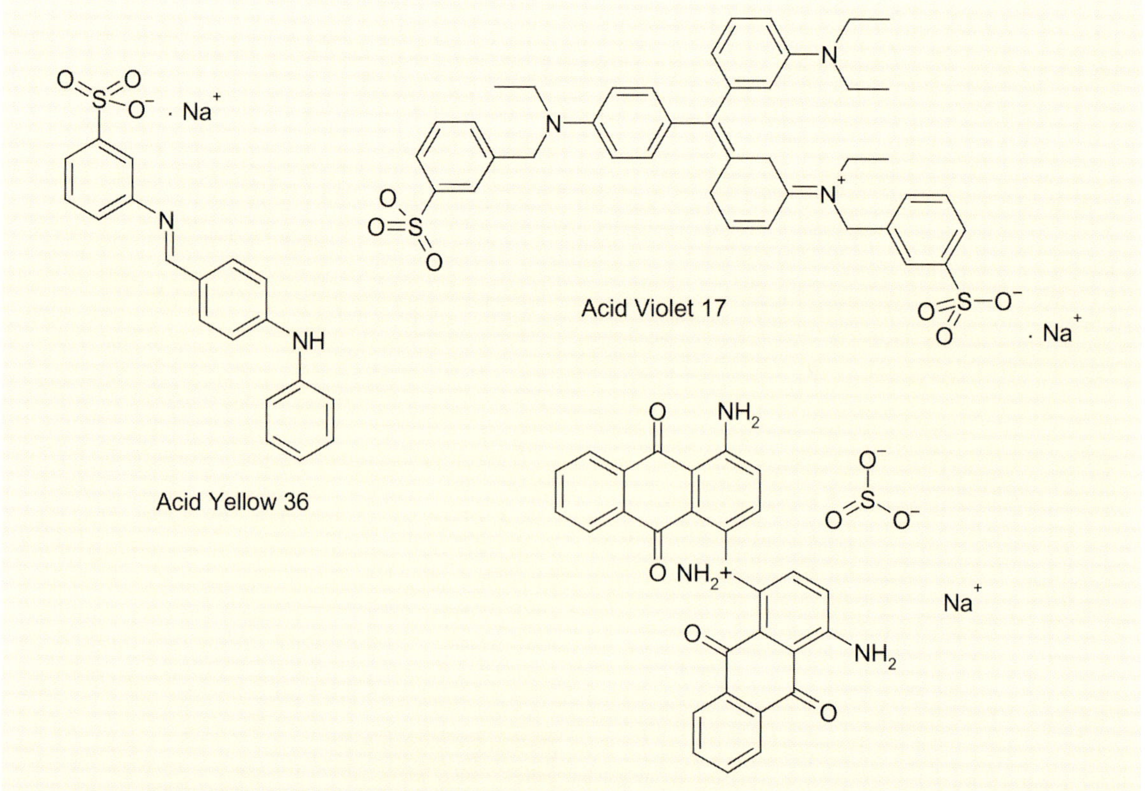

Disperse Yellow 54

Disperse Yellow 39

Disperse Yellow 1

Disperse Yellow 9

37

Acid Yellow 36

Acid Violet 17

Acid Black 48

Fig. 15. Acid yellow 36 (monoazoic), Acid Violet 17 (triphenylmethane), and Acid Black 38 (anthraquinone)

37.3.3.3 Basic Dyes

These are mainly used to dye wool and silk, acrylic, modacrylic, nylon, polyester, and blends of these fibers with cotton. They can be applied to cotton with a mordant [46]. Basic dyes comprise monoazoic, diazoic, and azine compounds. Basic Red 46, a monoazoic dye, was implicated in occupational [59] and in a clothing dermatitis sweater [60]. It seems to be an important cause of foot dermatitis, being a frequent allergen in acrylic socks [61]. Basic Brown 1, Basic Black 1 (CI), Brilliant Green (CI42040), Turquoise Reactive, and Neutrichrome Red have also been reported as allergens [3, 13, 46].

Basic Red 9 (Magenta, CI 42500) and Basic Violet 14 (CI 42510) are regarded as carcinogens.

Core Message

■ Among basic dyes, Basic Red 46 seems to be an important allergen in acrylic socks.

37.3.3.4 Direct Dyes

These dyes are directly applied on fibers, most often, cotton, wool, flax, or leather, in a neutral or alkaline bath. They have low wet-fastness, and frequently need after-treatments [46]. Direct Black 38, a triazoic compound dye used for cotton, wool, and silk [44], has been implicated in patients wearing black clothes, with concomitant immediate-type reactions in some cases [62].

The azo dye Direct Orange 34 (CI 40230) was positive during systematic testing in 8/1,814 patients [11].

Direct Black 38 (CI 30235), Direct Blue 6 (CI 22610), and Direct Red 28 (CI 22120) are regarded as carcinogens.

37.3.3.5 Vat Dyes

Such water-insoluble dyes are applied in a reduced soluble form, and then re-oxidized to the original insoluble form once absorbed into the fiber. They have high wet-fastness and are used to dye cotton, flax, wool, and rayon fibers. They mostly comprise of Vat Blue 6, formerly responsible for cosmetic dermatitis [45], and Vat Green 1. Vat Blue 1 (indigoid dye) is used to dye Levi Strauss 501 "shrink to fit" blue jeans [30].

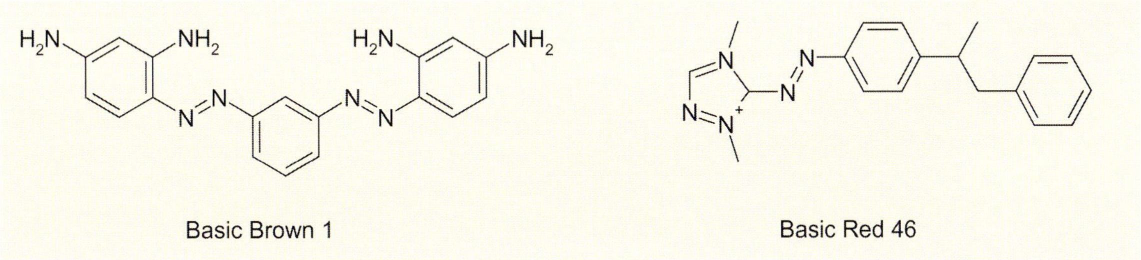

Fig. 16. Basic Brown 1 and Basic Red 46

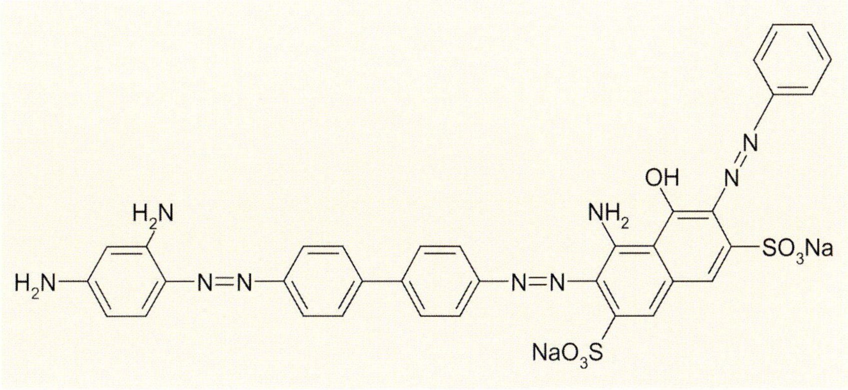

Fig. 17. Direct Black 38

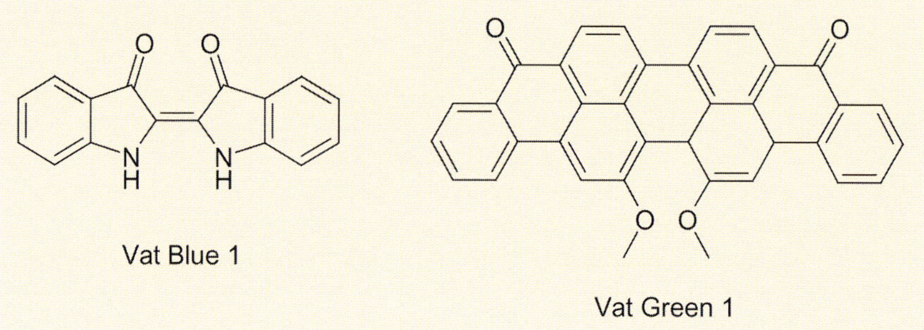

Fig. 18.
Vat Blue 1 (synthetic indigo) and Vat Green 1

Vat Blue 1

Vat Green 1

Vat Green 1, an anthraquinone derivative, has only been reported as a cause of clothing contact dermatitis from navy-blue uniforms in nurses [63].

Core Message

■ Vat dyes are exceptional allergens.

37.3.3.6 Fiber-Reactive Dyes

Reactive dyes consist of a two-part, direct coloring agent. The first moiety is a chromophore with an azo, anthraquinone, or phthalocyanine derivative structure. This moiety is connected to a second reactive group, which is able to form covalent bonds with the amine or sulfhydryl groups of proteins in the textile fibers. Such dyes are used for coloring cellulosic fibers (cotton, silk), wool, or polyamides, and are widely used for the production of clothes, with most sources of sensitization being occupational. In a study of 1,813 consecutive patients tested with an additional textile series of 12 reactive dyes, 18 (0.99%) were found to be sensitized to reactive dyes [8]. However, only five patients had a history of intolerance to garments, and two of four patch tests performed with pieces of garment were positive. In practice, reactive dyes in clothing should not be sensitizers. If they can be extracted from fibers, they are in a hydrolyzed, non-sensitizing form [44]. With the exception of occupational exposure, we think reactive dyes should not be tested in patients, although the risk of active sensitization [64] is, theoretically, of little consequence.

Core Message

■ Reactive dyes cause dermatitis only under their native form, i.e., in occupational circumstances, but not in consumers.

Reactive Black 5

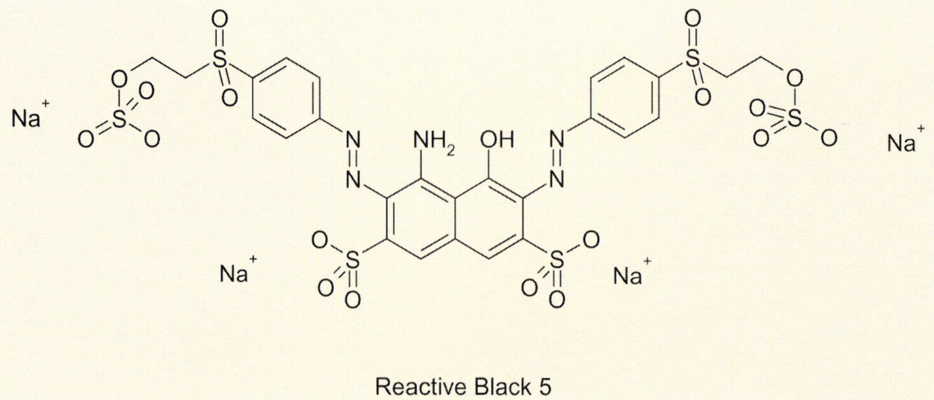

Fig. 19. Structure of Reactive Black 5

37.3.3.7 Sulfur, Solvent, and Non-Disperse Azoic Dyes

Sulfur dyes are used for cotton in work clothes [30]. Solvent dyes are mono- or diazoic compounds used to dye oils, greases, varnishes, solvents, and cosmetics [44]. Solvent Yellow 1 (PAAB), a monoazoic compound, was positive in patients sensitized to stockings [4].

37.3.4 Dye-Fixing and Dye-Coupling Agents

Naphthols are coupling agents, which are used for staining and dyeing. *Beta-naphthol* (2-naphthol, Azoic Coupling Component 1, CAS [135-19-3]) is no longer used in textile industry.

Naphthol AS (3-hydroxy-2-naphthoic acid anilide, Azoic Coupling Component 2), a coupling agent used for cotton dyeing, has replaced beta-naphthol because of a stronger affinity for cellulose. Naphthol AS first caused pigmented contact dermatitis in workers at a textile factory in Mexico in the 1970s, where it was widely used. It was reported as an agent of – sometimes – pigmented contact dermatitis in several patients [1, 46]. We observed a similar case due to a colored foulard imported from India. Patch tests were bullous (+++) to a piece of textile and strongly positive to Naphthol AS 1% pet. The presence of this agent in the foulard was ascertained by a comparative TLC [65].

Several other naphthols are used for textile dyeing, such as Naphthol ASD (3-hydroxy-2-naphthoic acid o-toluidine), Naphthol AS-E [2-naphtalenecarboxamide, 3-(acetyloxy)-N-(4-chloro-phenyl)-, Azoic Coupling Component 10], but they have not been reported as contact allergens.

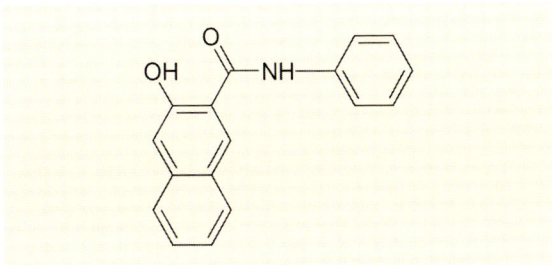

Fig. 20. Naphthol AS

Core Message

■ Naphthol AS is a classical cause of allergic contact dermatitis due to colored cotton clothing.

37.3.5 Rubber

Latex, extracted from *Hevea brasiliensis*, is rarely (and doubtfully) a type IV sensitizer. The main allergens in rubber are vulcanization inhibitors and accelerators, dyes, and antioxidants. Sources are various, such as gloves, boots, or garter belts. They mainly include mercaptobenzothiazole and the components of the mercapto mix (dibenzothiazyl disulfide, N-cyclohexylbenzothiazyl sulfenamide, morpholinylmercaptobenzothiazole (MMBT)), thiurams (tetramethylthiuram monosulfide and disulfide, tetraethylthiuram disulfide, and dipentamethylenethiuram disulfide (PTD)), cyclohexylthiophthalimide, and N,N'-isopropyl-phenyl-paraphenylene diamine (IPPD). This last agent, usually present in grey or black rubber, was formerly implicated in purpuric dermatitis from rubber in the elastic of undergarments [3, 30]. Carbamates (diethyl-, dibutyl-, and dibenzyldithiocarbamates) can be degraded into carbamyl compounds by chlorine used as a bleaching agent and provoke allergic contact dermatitis [3, 30, 66]. The presumed allergen is N,N-dibenzyl carbamyl chloride: patch tests are negative with the standard rubber allergens, but they are positive to the bleached clothing [67].

Neoprene rubber, used to make wet suits, swimming gear, and clothing for fire fighters, contains thiourea derivatives. Diethyl-, dimethyl-, dibutyl-, diphenyl-, and ethylbutyl-thiourea can be responsible for allergic contact dermatitis [33, 34].

37.3.5.1 Other Components of Garments

Trivalent *chromium salts* used to tan leather are sometimes utilized as a mordant in wool dyeing. They caused allergic contact dermatitis from military textiles [4, 30, 63].

Colophony may be present in some garments, particularly in paper-based clothing, such as surgical gowns [68].

Para-tertiary-butylphenol-formaldehyde resin (PTBPFR), the allergen of many neoprene glues, caused contact dermatitis from the adhesive of the pad of a derotation brace in a recently operated patient. The dermatitis relapsed after he wore a raincoat fabric which contained PTBPFR used as a finishing agent [69].

37.3.5.2 Cleaners, Softeners, and Other Auxiliaries

Waterproofing agents and *mothproofing agents* are not sensitizers [18, 30].

Biocides are used for several purposes. Antifungal (antimildew) properties of tributyltin oxide (a strong irritant), mercurial compounds, phenols such as pentachlorophenol, carbamates, or mercaptobenzothiazoles can be contained in outdoor materials, but are no longer allowed in garments, as previously described [19, 47]. Newer molecules and processes have been developed. Triclosan is largely used for its antifungal and antibacterial properties, particularly to prevent odor forming in undergarments such as socks or underpants. It can be applied on the textile or incorporated in a specific thread used during weaving. Only one observation concerned clothing allergy [30].

The *ultraviolet light absorber* 2-(2-hydroxy-5-methylphenyl) benzotriazole (Tinuvin P), used as a photoprotector in plastics and textile fibers, provoked an allergic contact dermatitis from a spandex tape sewn into underwear [70] and from a plastic watch strap [71].

Flame retardants used to treat cotton, rayon, and polyester, in order to retard the different phases of combustion like the presently withdrawn tris (2,3-dibromopropyl) phosphate CAS [126–72–7] or diammonium dihydrogen phosphate, are rare allergens [18, 72]. They are now replaced by fibers that have inherent fireproof properties, for example blends of Kevlar and Nomex.

Cleaners remaining on the fabric, such as 1,1,1-trichloroethane [3], are able to cause irritant contact dermatitis. Contact urticaria was reported from the marking nut *Semecarpus anacardium*, used by the launderer to identify the clothing in his shop [73].

Washing detergents are generally not reported as allergens, excepted rare cases of hypersensitivity to whitening agents. Enzymes are frequently added to enhance the efficacy at lower temperatures, can induce dermatitis by direct contact, but are not harmful for the consumers [74]. Surfactants, especially anionic, can induce irritant dermatitis if they persist on textile after laundry. High doses of detergent, insufficient rinsing, and use of cold tap water for washing and rinsing clothes are promoting factors for dermatitis [75]. The interest of patch testing with detergents [76] is very questionable, since they are firstly irritant, even at low concentrations.

Softeners are frequently suspected by patients and even practitioners. Such products diminish the fiber's coefficient of friction and enhance the pleasant and silky touch of garments. Numerous molecules are used in industry or in consumer goods, consisting of fatty acids, polyethylenes, polymers based on silicon, urethane, or acrylic. Many of them contain preservatives, such as formaldehyde and glutaraldehyde, or fragrances. According to the very low amount of residues on clothing, they seem to be safe [14, 19, 77] and we usually recommend the use of softeners, slightly or not perfumed, in our patients with dermatitis.

Cosmetics can be included in garments, generally, underwear. Allergens include preservatives and perfumes.

Accidental contamination is possible, and clothing may contain various articles or be contaminated by many chemical agents, mainly of occupational origin. They include metalworking fluids, resins and paints, pesticides, insecticides and repellents, plants and plant extracts, metallic particles, and fiberglass [3, 18, 78, 79]. A topical drug applied by the patient can also persist for a long time in a glove, a bandage, a shoe, a slipper, or a garment, and induce a further relapse of allergic contact dermatitis: cases have been observed with ketoprofen or salicylamide ([80], personal observations).

> ### Core Message
>
> ■ Washing detergents and textile softeners are not allergenic.

37.4 Patch Testing

Standard screening patch test series are inadequate for the reliable detection of textile sensitivity [7, 12, 14, 46, 47].

The most essential are the *clothing patch tests*, which remain the gold standard for the diagnosis of clothing allergic contact dermatitis. They are performed with pieces cut from suspected garments (1 × 1 cm to 3 × 3 cm), according to the pattern of eczema. This material may be moistened with a drop of water. In some cases, an extract from clothing (in water, ethanol, or acetone) can be more sensitive than the clothing itself [3, 14]. For "velvet" fabrics, however, testing with pieces may induce active sensitization because of the high level of dyes [5]. Coarse fabrics may irritate the skin and cause a mild erythema or a slight edema at the two-day reading, but it generally faded by four days [47]. Negativity of patch tests with the fabric is frequent, particularly in cases of textile resin sensitivity [3, 14, 30, 47], and does not invalidate the diagnosis of clothing dermatitis [18, 81]. Leaving the fabric patch test on for more than two days or winding a piece of garment around the arm may be helpful. However, negative patch test with the suspected garment makes its responsibility questionable for an allergic phenomenon: other garments or an irritant dermatitis (on atopic skin or, e.g., pilar keratosis) have to be suspected. In such cases, a challenge test (stop and wear again) seems to be more practical to confirm or contradict allergy [10, 47, personal observations].

Core Message

■ The gold standard is patch testing with patient's clothing. Tests are sometimes irritant, inducing slight erythema and edema fading at the second reading.

However, many studies on clothing dermatitis, and even reports which focus on one allergen, do not af-

firm the responsibility of allergens, since they are generally not identified in garments [61, 81]. In a recent study on 20 patients with proved clothing allergic dermatitis, on 32 garments suspected by the patient, 22 actually contained an allergenic dye, and 9 contained a dye that the patient had reacted to [58].

Formaldehyde (1% aq.) is of importance since it can be a marker of sensitivity to textile finishes which release high or medium amounts of free formaldehyde. The cost–benefit ratio of the use of more complete textile finish series seems to be very poor [39]. Urea-formaldehyde resin (dimethylol urea) 10% pet. [39] and the mixture ethylene urea + melamine formaldehyde resin 5% pet. [26, 41] have been good screening agents. Such data are currently doubtful, since formaldehyde resins, ethylene urea, and melamine formaldehyde are no more used for clothing in our countries. DMDHEU [82] or modified DMDHEU could be better screening agents at present. However, all textile resins available for patch testing (Table 3) are under a free, non-fixed form. They can be degraded and release formaldehyde (personal observation, Fig. 21). In fact, most tests positive to TFR are associated and due to sensitization to formaldehyde. So, positive reactions to TFR in patients sensitive to formaldehyde have to be carefully interpreted.

Table 3. Textile finish resin allergens available. (*CU* Cyclized urea derivatives, *MF* melamine formaldehyde resin, *UF* urea formaldehyde resin.) Allergens are available from Chemotechnique (Malmö, Sweden), FIRMA (Florence, Italy), and Trolab (Hermal, Reinbeck, Germany)

Allergen	CAS no.	Concentration	Type	Formaldehyde release	Suppliers
Formaldehyde (methylal)	50–00–0	1% aq.			C, F, T
Urea formaldehyde (dimethylol urea, carbamol, oxymethurea) (UF) (Kaurit S)	140–95–4	10% pet.	UF	High	C, F
Melamine formaldehyde (MF) (Kaurit M70)		7% pet.	MF	High	C
Dimethyl dihydroxy ethylene urea (DMeDHEU) (Fixapret NF)		4.5% aq.	CU	Low	C
Dimethylol dihydroxy ethylene urea (DMDHEU) (Fixapret CPN)	1854–26–8	4.5% aq., 10% pet.	CU	Low	C, F
Dimethylol dihydroxy ethylene urea, modified (modified DMDHEU) (Fixapret ECO)		5% aq.	CU	Low	C
Dimethylol propylene urea (DMPU)	3270–74–4	10% pet.	CU	Medium	F
Ethylene urea *and* melamine formaldehyde		5% pet.[a]	CU + MF	Medium and high	C

[a] Emulsified with sorbitan sesquioleate 5%

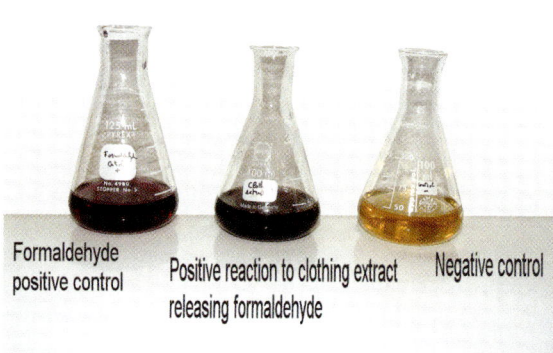

Formaldehyde positive control

Positive reaction to clothing extract releasing formaldehyde

Negative control

Fig. 21. Positive reaction with chromotropic acid method, showing liberation of formaldehyde by textile resins (formaldehyde solution on the *left* as a positive control, negative control on the *right*)

Core Message

■ DMDHEU and modified DMDHEU should be good screeners for sensitivity to textile finish resins (TFR). Patch test reactions to TFR are frequently associated to formaldehyde sensitivity, and it is sometimes difficult to establish the relevance of routinely performed tests.

PPD is an unreliable screening agent for hypersensitivity to textile dyes [5, 7, 13] and should, theoretically, be a detector of some azo dyes only, such as Disperse Orange 3, Disperse Red 1, and Red 17. Patients positive to PPD are frequently sensitized to Disperse Orange 3 [3, 9], but the converse is not so [7]. PPD is hardly ever positive in patients sensitized to the frequently positive Disperse Blue 106 or Disperse Blue 124 [5, 6, 13, 27, 28, 54], to p-aminophenol [7, 28], or to Disperse Yellow 3 [3, 7, 28]. Positive reactions to both diaminodiphenylmethane and Disperse Orange 3 are observed because of their close chemical structures and, probably, a similar metabolite [55]. Cross-reactions are possible among other azo dyes, such as Disperse Orange 3 and Disperse Red 1 [10, 55]. Reactivity is constant to both Disperse Blue 124 and Disperse Blue 106 [5]. Therefore, some authors suggest routine patch testing with a specific textile series containing disperse dyes [8, 10, 46]. Disperse Blue 106 seems to have a good sensitivity [7]. Supplementation of the standard series with four disperse dyes (Disperse Blue 124, Disperse Red 1, Disperse Yellow 3, Disperse

Orange 3) has been useful for some authors [10], but systematic addition of a more complete 16 textile dyes series [12] is of questionable value, although they are scientifically interesting in patients with dye sensitivity [7]. A disperse dye mix has been recommended, but further studies are needed to determine the ideal substances and concentrations [13, 16, 83–85]. This mixture was positive in 26 out of 31 patients positive with individual dyes [16].

Core Message

■ Standards series are unable to detect textile dyes allergy. Systematic addition of textile dye(s) such as Disperse Blue 106 can be recommended.

The practitioner has to be vigilant to the purity of allergens. We could observe in a period of 2002–2004, that several batches of Disperse Orange 3 provided by Chemotechnique, although prepared with both a disperse and orange dye, contained no Disperse Orange 3. The mistake was discovered because successive patients sensitive to PPD and tested with textile series reacted to Disperse Red 1 and Disperse Red 17, but not to the orange dye, as generally observed. Comparative thin-layer chromatographies, nuclear magnetic resonance, and high-performance liquid chromatography detected Disperse Orange 31 that had been wrongly substituted for Disperse Orange 3 [86]. This situation also explained that a relatively low percentage of patients positive to PPD were positive to Disperse Orange 3, although a co-reaction is explained to be very frequent because of skin transformation of Disperse Orange 3 into PPD [86, 87].

Caution is also needed regarding patch testing with dyes series for several reasons. A positive patch test, as a result of sensitivity to a dye, is not always relevant, and can be the result either of a primary sensitization, or of a co- or cross-reaction. For example, a positive reaction to Disperse Orange 3, expected in at least 2/3 of people sensitized to PPD is almost constant in our experience. Therefore, even if a textile dye is found to be positive, this is no guarantee of its presence in the garment. Purity of some dyes in commercial patch test series is doubtful, and only some dyes seem to be pure [44] (Fig. 22). This can lead to false-positive reactions when an impurity is the cause of a positive reaction. In some cases of multiple reactions [13, 54, 55], an "angry back" or excited skin syndrome should also be taken into consideration. Such a situation or non-allergic papular reactions could account for strong differences observed

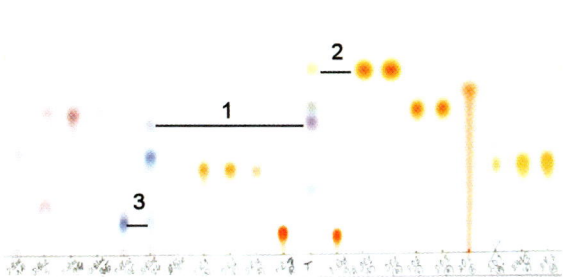

Fig. 22. Thin-layer chromatography performed with acetone extract of a black textile (*T*) and with several disperse dyes. Shown are the different dyed fractions of *T*, corresponding to a component of Disperse Blue 124 (*1*) and to Disperse Orange 1 (*2*). Also noted are the components of "pure" dyes, particularly, Disperse Blue 124, which contains Disperse Blue 106 (*3*)

between frequencies of positive reactions to such close allergens in some observations (12.5% and 20% to Disperse Blue 106 and Disperse Blue 124, respectively, in one study) [88, 89].

Regarding allergens other than textile resins and dyes, rubber compounds are mainly included in the standard series. Thiourea derivatives such as diethyl-, dimethyl-, dibutyl-, diphenyl-, and ethylbutyl-thiourea can also be tested [33, 34].

> **Core Message**
>
> ■ Patch tests with textile dye series have to be cautiously interpreted, according to clinical presentation, particularly + (weakly positive, sometimes irritant) and diffuse (+++ and/or angry-back) reactions.

37.5 Chemical Analyses

37.5.1 Identification of Formaldehyde

In industry and toxicological studies, the most widely used methods for the detection of formaldehyde are based on spectrophotometry, but other methods, such as colorimetry, fluorimetry, high-performance liquid chromatography, polarography, gas chromatography, infrared detection, and gas detector tubes, are also used. The most sensitive of these methods is flow injection, which has a detection limit of 9 ppt

(0.011 µg/m3). Another commonly used method is high-performance liquid chromatography, which offers a detection limit of 0.0017 ppm (0.002 mg/m³). For the practitioner, identification of formaldehyde in garments can be useful for patients suspected of clothing dermatitis and being sensitized to formaldehyde, since it may prevent relapses of their dermatitis. Several methods are available [3, 22, 30].

37.5.1.1 Chromotropic Acid Method

The reaction is exothermic and necessitates caution. Put 2 g of the garment into 100 ml water for 24 h. Filter the solution. Put 1 ml in an Erlenmeyer flask. Add 5 ml distilled water and 1 ml of chromotropic acid (powder stored in the dark and in a fridge) 5% fresh solution plus 5 ml concentrated sulfuric acid. A violet discoloration, due to formation of 3,4,5,6-dibenzoxanthylium, is specific and indicates the presence of formaldehyde at >0.005% (50 ppm) concentration. Other aldehydes or ketones can give a yellowish, orange, reddish, or brownish, but not violet coloration.

37.5.1.2 Schiff's Reagent Method

Cut a small strip of material (8 cm²). Immerse it in about 5 ml of 0.1 N hydrochloric acid (HCl). Heat in water bath for 10 min and remove fabric. Add 5 drops of Schiff's aldehyde reagent (stored in fridge). A violet color indicates the presence of an aldehyde.

37.5.1.3 Acetylacetone Method

Cut a small trip of material (0.5 g) and put it into a glass jar. Add 2.5 ml of Nash reagent (15 g of ammonium acetate, 0.3 ml of glacial acetic acid, 0.2 ml of acetylacetone, and distilled water to 1 l), stick and heat (for low concentrations of formaldehyde) at 60°C for 10 min. Formaldehyde reacting with two molecules of acetylacetone and with one molecule of ammonia will form a yellow compound, 3,5-diacetyl-1,4-dihydrolutidine. Its concentration can be more exactly determined spectrophotometrically at 412 nm. Positive (10, 5, and 2.5 µg/ml formaldehyde solutions) and negative (distilled water) controls are needed. This method, sensitive down to 4 ppm, is contraindicated with dyed clothing [90–92].

Core Message

■ Identification of formaldehyde in textiles is possible for practitioners by chromotropic acid, Schiff's, or acetylacetone methods.

37.5.2 Identification of Dyes

Thin-layer chromatography (TLC) can be carried out with the dye extracted from the textile. It necessitates comparison with one or several dyes, whose chemical composition is known, in order to compare them [3, 5, 42].

In some cases, TLC permits patch testing with different fractions of the dye mixture used in the garment. Pieces of textiles are cut into shreds and extracted with an eluent-like chloroform. TLC is done with the solution put on TLC plates, using chloroform and methanol as eluents. A combination of TLC, magnetic resonance spectroscopy, and infrared spectrometry is sometimes useful to identify some dyes [3].

We recently developed a method, which we named EpiCAT [43], consisting of an epicutaneously chromatogram applied test. The procedure is as follows:

■ Cut a piece of garment (e.g., 1 g) and put it in a weigh filter
■ Add acetone in order to have a 5% solution (here, add 19 g acetone)
■ Leave it until apparition of a colored solution (30 min to 7 days)
■ Perform a TLC with a spot of colored solution on a TLC aluminum sheet with silica gel (Merck, Darmstadt, Germany), and then put in a blend of 60% ethyl acetate and 40% hexane as eluents
■ Vary the eluent proportions in order to well separate the dye spots if necessary
■ Realize the procedure with a band of dye solution in order to obtain bands of separated dyes
■ Put the round-shaped TLC plate on the patient's upper back covered with an adhesive tape for 48 h
■ Read at D2 and D3 or D4; linear positive reaction(s) will occur in front of the allergenic dye (Fig. 23)
■ Realize comparative TLC or further analysis to identify the offending dye

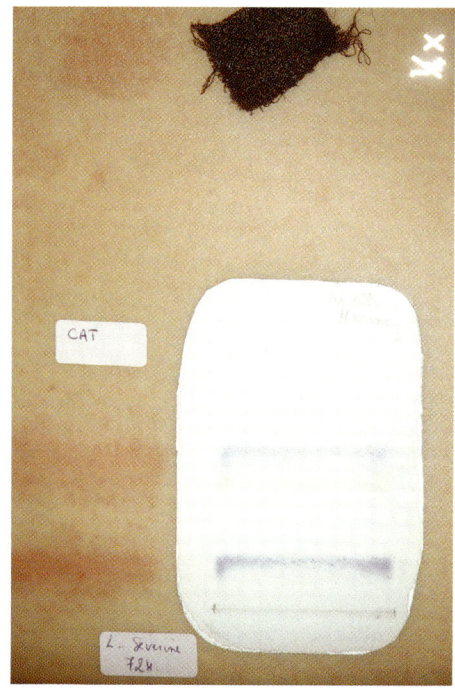

Fig. 23. Patch testing with a piece of garment, and EpiCAT (performed with TLC). Linear allergic reactions occur regarding two components of Disperse Blue 124 present in the textile

Core Message

■ Extraction of dyes from clothing is useful to ascertain the diagnosis of allergy and to identify the offending dye(s) in textiles. Patch tests can be directly realized with the TLC (EpiCAT).

37.6 Patient Advice

Patients sensitized to textile resins (a rare situation, in fact) have to replace their garments with untreated fabrics, and avoid "dry-drip," "crease resistant," "durable-press," "permanent-press," "easy care," "easy to iron," "no iron," "wash and go," or "wash and wear" textiles, particularly rayon, 100% cotton, or blends of those fibers. Most blended textiles are treated and, consequently, have to be avoided, such as permanent press or wrinkle-resistant garments. Wool, linen, denim, nylon, or silk are unlikely to be treated and should be preferred. New textiles can be submitted for chemical analysis in hypersensitive patients (see above). Washing all new textiles at least twice before using is useful because formaldehyde transfer is possible from treated to untreated fabrics [18]. However, free formaldehyde will be washed out in water, but the resin will persist in the garment [22]. Wearing a protective undergarment is sometimes useful [18].

Core Message

■ Patients with textile dermatitis and who are sensitized to finish resins or formaldehyde should avoid "no-iron" clothing.

Concerning textile dye hypersensitivity, it is generally of little importance to the patient to know whether he/she is allergic to one or several textile dyes. Because of cross-reactions, it is frequent to observe that the patients are sensitized to dyes which are not present in a garment, even after TLC [13, 47]. However, cross-reactions occur among the same, but not between different, chemical classes. Strongly colored synthetic textiles should be avoided. Lightly colored garments can be permitted, such as pure (100%) natural fibers (cotton, linen, silk, wool), and even some dark colored [7].

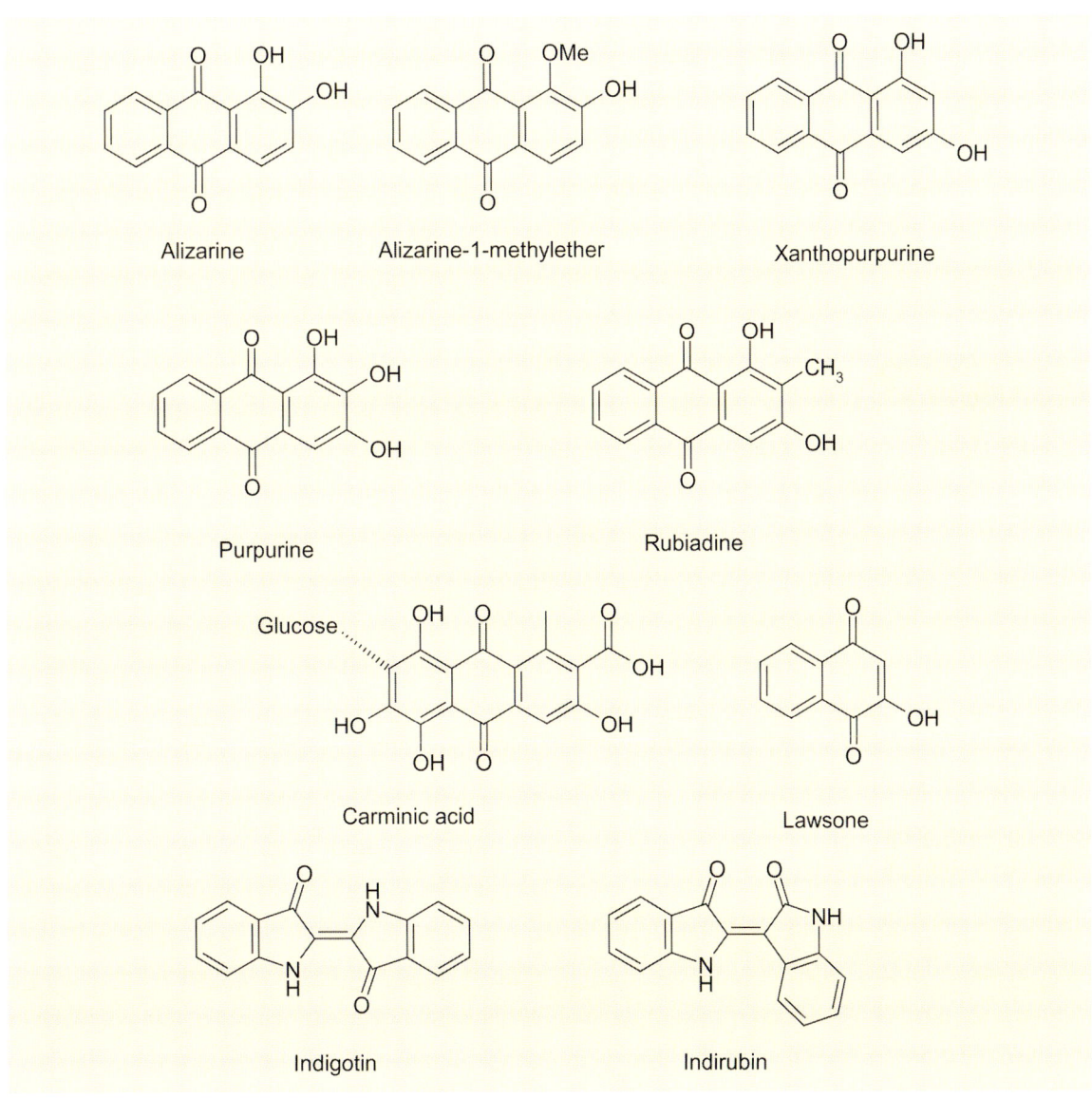

Fig. 24. Natural dyes alizarin, alizarine-1-methylether, xanthopurpurine, purpurine, rubiadine (Rubiaceae), carminic acid (cochineal), lawsone (henna), indigotin, and indirubin (indigo)

Core Message

■ Patients sensitized to textile dyes have to avoid synthetic fibers (if sensitized to disperse dyes), strongly colored or dark synthetic garments (if sensitized only to disperse dyes Blue 106 and 124), or cotton-colored dyes (if positive to Naphthol AS).

Natural clothing dyes of vegetable origin, such as henna – containing lawsone – or indigo – containing indirubine and indigotin (natural indigo or Vat Blue 1) – or of animal source, such as cochineal – containing the anthraquinone compounds carminic and kermesic acids that give the carmine color – can be used to color wool, cotton, and silk fabrics. Among frequent natural dyes, we can cite alizarin and its derivative alizarin-1-methylether, purpurine, xanthopurpurine, and rubiadine contained in the Rubiaceae family, to which belongs madder (*Rubia tinctorum* L.) [93]. Natural dyes are generally not mentioned as a cause of clothing dermatitis, although lawsone and carminic acid can be allergenic [45, 94].

Core Message

■ Clothing treated with natural dyes are well tolerated by patients sensitized to synthetic dyes.

37

We generally propose to our patients sensitive to disperse dyes to perform a spot test with a cotton bud impregnated with acetone. If rubbing on the garment, and particularly on synthetic lining, does not produce any color transfer, it is unlikely that the garment will be allergenic. This was observed and confirmed in our disperse dye(s) allergic patients.

Core Message

■ When negative, a spot-test performed with acetone is, generally, a good indicator of non-allergenicity of dyes in a textile.

References

1. Roed-Petersen J, Batsberg W, Larsen E (1990) Contact dermatitis from Naphthol AS. Contact Dermatitis 22:161–163
2. Kojima S, Momma J, Kaniwa MA, Ikarashi Y, Sato M, Nakaji Y, Kurokawa Y, Nakamura A (1990) Phosgene (chlorophenyl)hydrazones, strong sensitizers found in yellow sweaters bleached with sodium hypochlorite, defined as causative allergens for contact dermatitis by an experimental screening method in animals. Contact Dermatitis 23:129–141
3. Foussereau J (1987) Les eczémas allergiques: cosmétologiques, thérapeutiques et vestimentaires. Masson, Paris, France
4. Hatch KL, Maibach HI (1985) Textile dye dermatitis. A review. J Am Acad Dermatol 12:1079–1092
5. Hausen B M (1993) Contact allergy to Disperse Blue 106 and Blue 124 in black "velvet" clothes. Contact Dermatitis 28:169–173
6. Menezes Brandao F, Altermatt C, Pecegueiro M, Bordalo O, Foussereau J (1985) Contact dermatitis to Disperse Blue 106. Contact Dermatitis 13:80–84
7. Dooms-Goossens A (1992) Textile dye dermatitis. Contact Dermatitis 27:321–323
8. Manzini BM, Motolese A, Conti A, Ferdani G, Seidenari S (1996) Sensitization to reactive textile dyes in patients with contact dermatitis. Contact Dermatitis 34:172–175
9. Balato N, Lembo G, Patruno C, Ayala F (1990) Prevalence of textile dye contact sensitization. Contact Dermatitis 23:111–122
10. Seidenari S, Manzini BM, Danese P (1991) Contact sensitization to textile dyes: description of 100 subjects. Contact Dermatitis 24:253–258
11. Seidenari S, Manzini BM, Schiavi ME, Motolese A (1995) Prevalence of contact allergy to non-disperse azo dyes for natural fibers: a study in 1814 consecutive patients. Contact Dermatitis 33:118–122
12. Borrego L, Ortiz-Frutos J (1996) Textile dye dermatitis: Spanish experience. J Am Acad Dermatol 34:715–716
13. Lisboa C, Barros MA, Azenha A (1994) Contact dermatitis from textile dyes. Contact Dermatitis 31:9–10
14. Sherertz EF (1992) Clothing dermatitis: practical aspects for the clinician. Am J Contact Dermat 3:55–64
15. Seidenari S, Mantovani L, Manzini BM, Pignatti M (1997). Cross-sensitizations between azo dyes and para-amino compound. A study of 236 azo-dye-sensitive subjects. Contact Dermatitis 36:91–96
16. Lodi A, Ambonati M, Coassini A, Chiarelli G, Mancini LL, Crosti C (1998) Textile dye contact dermatitis in an allergic population. Contact Dermatitis 39:314–315
17. Hatch KL, Maibach HI (2000) Textile dye allergic contact dermatitis prevalence. Contact Dermatitis 42:187–195
18. Hatch KL, Maibach HI (1986) Textile chemical finish dermatitis. Contact Dermatitis 14:1–13
19. Le Coz C (1999) Dermites de contact aux apprêts et ennoblisseurs textiles. Progrès en dermato-allergologie, Lyon 1999. John Libbey Eurotext, Paris, France
20. Official Journal of the European Communities (2002) No L 243/15. Directive 2002/61/EC of the European Parliament and of the Council of 19 July 2002 amending for the 19th time Council Directive 76/769/EEC relating to restrictions on the marketing and use of certain dangerous substances and preparations (azocolourants)
21. http://www.oeko-tex.com
22. Cronin E (1963) Formalin textile dermatitis. Br J Dermatol 267–273

23. van der Veen JPW, Neering H, de Haan P, Bruynzeel DP (1988) Pigmented purpuric clothing dermatitis due to Disperse Blue 85. Contact Dermatitis 19:222–223

24. Komericki P, Aberer W, Arbab E, Kovacevic Z, Kränke B (2001) Pigmented purpuric contact dermatitis from Disperse Blue 106 and 124 dyes. J Am Acad Dermatol 45: 456–458

25. Foti C, Elia G, Filotico R, Angelini G (1998) Purpuric clothing dermatitis due to Disperse Yellow 27. Contact Dermatitis 39:273

26. Fowler JF Jr, Skinner SM, Belsito DV (1992) Allergic contact dermatitis from formaldehyde resins in permanent press clothing: an underdiagnosed cause of generalized dermatitis. J Am Acad Dermatol 27:962–968

27. Nakagawa M, Kawai K, Kawai K (1996) Multiple azo disperse dye sensitization mainly due to group sensitizations to azo dyes. Contact Dermatitis 34:6–11

28. Mathelier-Fusade P, Aïssaoui M, Chabane MH, Mounedji N, Leynadier F (1996) Chronic generalized eczema caused by multiple dye sensitization. Am J Contact Dermat 7: 224–225

29. Hatch KL, Maibach HI (1985) Textile fiber dermatitis. Contact Dermatitis 12:1–11

30. Rietschel RL, Fowler JF (1994) Fisher's contact dermatitis, 4th edn, Chap. 19. Williams and Wilkins, Baltimore, Md., pp 358–392

31. Inoue A, Ishido I, Shoji A, Yamada H (1997) Textile dermatitis from silk. Contact Dermatitis 37:185

32. Tanaka M, Kobayashi S, Miyakawa S-I (1993) Contact dermatitis from nylon 6 in Japan. Contact Dermatitis 28: 250

33. Kerre S, Devos L, Verhoeve L, Bruze M, Gruvberger B, Dooms-Goossens A (1996) Contact allergy to diethylthiourea in a wet suit. Contact Dermatitis 35:176–178

34. Reynaers A, Goossens A (1998) La diéthylthiourée: allergène de contact dans divers objets en néoprène. Lettre GERDA 15:60–61

35. Alcántara M, Martínez-Escribano J, Frías J, García-Sellés FJ (2000) Allergic contact dermatitis due to diphenylthiourea in a neoprene slimming suit. Contact Dermatitis 43: 224–225

36. Diepgen TL, Stäbler A, Hornstein OP (1990) Textilunverträglichkeit beim atopischen Ekzem. Eine kontrollierte klinische Studie (Textile intolerance in atopic eczema. A controlled clinical study, in German). Z Hautkr 65: 907–910

37. Veien NK, Hattel T, Laurberg G (1991) Can "label dermatitis" become "creeping neurotic excoriations"? Contact Dermatitis 27:272–273

38. Hatch KL, Maibach HI (1995) Textile dermatitis: an update (I). Resins, additives and fibers. Contact Dermatitis 32: 319–326

39. Andersen KE, Hamann K (1982) Cost benefit of patch testing with textile finish resins. Contact Dermatitis 8:64–67

40. Schorr WF, Keran E, Plotka E (1974) Formaldehyde allergy. The quantitative analysis of American clothing for free formaldehyde and its relevance in clinical practice. Arch Dermatol 110:73–76

41. Marks JG, Belsito DV, DeLeo VA, Fowler JF Jr, Fransway AF, Maibach HI, Mathias CG, Nethercott JR, Rietschel RL, Sherentz EF, Storrs FJ, Taylor JS (1998) North American Contact Dermatitis Group patch test results for the detection of delayed-type hypersensitivity to topical allergens. J Am Acad Dermatol 38:911–918

42. Foussereau J, Dallara J M (1986) Purity of standardized textile dye allergens: a thin layer chromatography study. Contact Dermatitis 14:303–306

43. Le Coz CJ, Lefebvre C, Haberkorn L (2002) Epicutaneous chromatogram applied test (EpiCAT): an original test method for allergic contact dermatitis (ACD) from clothing dyes. Contact Dermatitis 46 [Suppl 4]:34

44. Cavelier C, Foussereau J, Tomb R (1988) Allergie de contact et colorants (2e partie). Cahiers Notes Doc INRS 133: 615–647

45. Cavelier C, Foussereau J, Tomb R (1988) Allergie de contact et colorants (1e partie). Cahiers Notes Doc INRS 132: 421–443

46. Hatch KL, Maibach HI (1995) Textile dye dermatitis. J Am Acad Dermatol 32:631–639

47. Cronin E (1980) Contact dermatitis. Churchill Livingstone, Edinburgh, pp 36–92

48. Wenninger JA, Canterbery RC, McEwen GN Jr (eds) (2000) International cosmetic ingredient dictionary and handbook, 8th edn. The Cosmetic, Toiletry, and Fragrance Association, Washington, DC

49. US Department of Health and Human Services (2002) Public Health Service, National Toxicology Program, Report on Carcinogens, 10th edn, Dec 2002

50. Cronin E (1968) Studies in contact dermatitis. 18. Dyes in clothing. Trans St John's Hosp Derm Soc 54:156–164

51. Cronin E (1968) Studies in contact dermatitis. XIX. Nylon stocking dyes. Trans St John's Hosp Derm Soc 54:165–169

52. Dabestani R, Reszka KJ, Davis DG, Sik RH, Chignell CF (1991) Spectroscopic studies of cutaneous photosensitizing agents – XVI. Disperse blue 35. Photochem Photobiol 54:37–42

53. Hausen BM, Sawall EM (1989) Sensitization experiments with textile dyes in guinea pigs. Contact Dermatitis 20:27–31

54. Dejobert Y, Martin P, Thomas P, Bergoend H (1995) Multiple azo dye sensitization revealed by the wearing of a black "velvet" body. Contact Dermatitis 33:276–277

55. Massone L, Anonide A, Isola V, Borghi S (1991) 2 cases of multiple azo dye sensitization. Contact Dermatitis 24: 60–63

56. Pecquet C, Assier-Bonnet H, Artigou C, Verne-Fourment L, Saïag P (1999) Atypical presentation of textile dye sensitization. Contact Dermatitis 40:51

57. Guin JD, Dwyer G, Sterba K (1999) Clothing dye dermatitis masquerading as (coexisting) mimosa allergy. Contact Dermatitis 40:45

58. Hatch K, Motschi H, Maibach HI (2003) Disperse dyes in fabrics of patients patch-test-positive to disperse dyes. Am J Contact Dermat 14:205–212

59. Chave TA, Nicolaou N, Johnston GA (2003) Hand dermatitis in a student caused by Basic Red 46. Contact Dermatitis 49:161–162

60. Foussereau J (1986) Contact dermatitis to Basic Red 46. Contact Dermatitis 15:106

61. Opie J, Lee A, Frowen K, Fewings J, Nixon R (2003) Foot dermatitis caused by the textile dye Basic Red 46 in acrylic blend socks. Contact Dermatitis 49:297–303

62. Noferi A, Ferrante E, Testa A (1966) Dermatosi allergiche da nero diretto colorante azoico solubile. Folia Allerg 13: 478–480

63. Wilson HTH, Cronin E (1971) Dermatitis from dyed uniforms. Br J Dermatol 85:67–69

64. Sommer S, Wilkinson SM (2000) A series of 3 patients sensitized to reactive dyes during patch testing. Contact Dermatitis 43:227–228

65. Le Coz CJ, Lepoittevin JP (2001) Clothing dermatitis from Naphthol AS. Contact Dermatitis 44:366–367

66. Jordan WP Jr, Bourlas M (1975) Allergic contact dermatitis to underwear elastic. Chemically transformed by laundry bleach. Arch Dermatol 111:593–595

67. Blancas-Espinosa R, Ancona-Alayón A, Arévalo-López A (2000) Allergic contact dermatitis to socks presenting as bleached rubber syndrome. Am J Contact Dermat 11: 97–98

68. Bergh M, Menné T, Karlberg AT (1994) Colophony in paper-based surgical clothing. Contact Dermatitis 31: 332–333

69. Hayakawa R, Ogino Y, Suzuki M, Kaniwa M (1994). Allergic contact dermatitis from para-tertiary-butylphenol-for-maldehyde resin (PTBP-F-R). Contact Dermatitis 30: 187–188

70. Arisu K, Hayakawa R, Ogino Y, Matsunaga K, Kaniwa M-A (1992) Tinuvin P in a spandex tape as a cause of clothing dermatitis. Contact Dermatitis 26:311–316

71. Niklasson B, Björkner B (1989) Contact allergy to the UV-absorber Tinuvin P in plastics. Contact Dermatitis 21: 330–334

72. Moreau A, Dompmartin A, Castel B, Remond B, Michel M, Leroy D (1994) Contact dermatitis from a textile flame retardant. Contact Dermatitis 31:86–88

73. Shankar DS (1992) contact urticaria induced by Semecarpus anacardium. Contact Dermatitis 26:200

74. Andersen PH, Bindslev-Jensen C, Mosbech H, Zachariae H, Andersen KE (1998) Skin symptoms in patients with atopic dermatitis using enzyme-containing detergents. A placebo-controlled study. Acta Derm Venereol (Stockh) 78:60–62

75. Kiriyama T, Sugiura H, Uehara M (2003) Residual washing detergent in cotton clothes: a factor of winter deterioration of dry skin in atopic dermatitis. J Dermatol 30: 708–712

76. Belsito DV, Fransway AF, Fowler JF Jr , Sherertz EF, Maibach HI, Mark JG Jr, Mathias CG, Rietschel RL, Storrs FJ, Nethercott JR (2002) Allergic contact dermatitis to detergents: a multicenter study to assess prevalence. J Am Acad Dermatol 46:200–206

77. Kofoed ML (1984) Contact dermatitis to formaldehyde in fabric softeners. Contact Dermatitis 11:254

78. Hafner J, Ruegger M, Kralicek P, Elsner P (1995) Airborne irritant contact dermatitis from metal dust adhering to semisynthetic working suits. Contact Dermatitis 32: 285–288

79. Le Coz CJ, Lepoittevin JP (2001) Occupational erythema-multiforme-like dermatitis from sensitization to costus resinoid, followed by flare-up and systemic contact dermatitis from beta-cyclocostunolide in a chemistry student. Contact Dermatitis 44:310–311

80. Hindsén M, Isaksson M, Persson L, Zimersson E, Bruze M (2004) Photoallergic contact dermatitis from ketoprofen induced by drug-contaminated personal objects. J Am Acad Dermatol 50:215–219

81. Khanna M, Sasseville D (2001) Occupational contact dermatitis to textile dyes in airline personnel. Am J Contact Dermat 12:208–210

82. Metzler-Brenckle L, Rietschel RL (2002) Patch testing for permanent-press allergic contact dermatitis. Contact Dermatitis 46:33–37

83. Francalanci S, Angelini G, Balato N, Berardesca E, Cusano F, Gaddoni G, Lisi P, Lodi A, Schena D, Sertoli A (1995) Effectiveness of disperse dyes mix in detection of contact allergy to textile dyes: an Italian multicentre study. Contact Dermatitis 33:351

84. Sousa-Basto A, Azenha A (1994) Textile dye mixes: useful screening tests for textile dye allergy. Contact Dermatitis 30:89–190

85. Sertoli A, Francalanci S, Giorgini S (1994) Sensitization to textile disperse dyes: validity of reduced-concentration patch tests and a new mix. Contact Dermatitis 31:47–48

86. Le Coz CJ, Jelen G, Goossens A, Vigan M, Ducombs G, Bircher A et al (2004) Disperse (yes), Orange (yes), 3 (no): what do we test in textile dye dermatitis? Contact Dermatitis 50:126–127

87. Goon AT, Gilmour NJ, Basketter DA, White IR, Rycroft RJ, McFadden JP (2003) High frequency of simultaneous sensitivity to Disperse Orange 3 in patients with positive patch tests to para-phenylenediamine. Contact Dermatitis 48:248–250

88. Lazarov A, Trattner A, David M, Ingber A (2001) Textile dermatitis in Israel: a retrospective study. Am J Contact Dermat 11:26–29

89. Uter W Geier J, Lessmann H, Hausen BM; IDVK and the German Contact Dermatitis Research Group; Information Network of Departments of Dermatology (2001) Contact allergy to Disperse Blue 106 and Disperse Blue 124 in German and Austrian patients, 1995 to 1999. Contact Dermatitis 44:173–177

90. Fregert S, Dahlquist I, Gruvberger B (1984) A simple method for the detection of formaldehyde. Contact Dermatitis 10:132–134

91. Gryllaki-Berger M, Mugny C, Perrenoud D, Pannatier A, Frenk E (1992) A comparative study of formaldehyde detection using chromotropic acid, acetylacetone and HPLC in cosmetics and household cleaning products. Contact Dermatitis 26:149–154

92. Le Coz CJ (2002) Allergie de contact au formaldéhyde (Contact allergy to formaldehyde, in French). Ann Dermatol Venereol 129:68–69

93. Cardon D (2003) Le monde des teintures naturelles. Belin, Paris, France

94. Lepoittevin JP, Le Coz C (2000) Dictionary of occupational allergens. In: Kanerva L, Elsner P, Wahlberg JE, Maibach HI (eds) Handbook of occupational dermatology. Springer, Berlin Heidelberg New York, pp 1125–1191

37

Chapter 38

Shoes

38

James S. Taylor, Emel Erkek, Patricia Podmore

Contents

38.1 Introduction

Allergic contact dermatitis (ACD) of the feet caused by shoe allergens is fairly common [1, 2] and should be considered in all patients with chronic foot eczema. Shoe allergy may be acute, subacute, intermittent or chronic and may appear superimposed on endogenous eczema [3–8]. Thus, the patient may have more than one diagnosis, e.g., both atopic and contact dermatitis and more than one allergen, e.g., shoe component plus a topical medicament.

38.2 Epidemiology

Data on the prevalence of shoe allergy come from patch test clinics and range from 1.5% to 11% [3, 4, 7, 9–14]. The highest prevalence rates have been recorded in warm climates [2, 12, 14]. The disorder may affect both sexes and all age groups, including children [3, 6, 7, 12, 15]. In a study of ACD affecting children, feet were the most common sites of involvement and footwear rated the most frequent cause after imitation jewelry [16].

38.3 Risk Factors

Major risk factors for shoe dermatitis include heat, friction, occlusion, hyperhidrosis and atopy [1, 2, 8]. A hot, humid environment within the shoes provides ideal soil for the development of ACD to shoe ingredients [17, 18]. The allergens leach by sweating in heavy, occlusive footwear and traverse the socks to contact skin [19]. Atopics have a susceptibility for the development of shoe allergy [12], and a history of hay fever, asthma or atopic eczema is common in affected patients [7]. In Freeman's study [3], 43% of patients afflicted with shoe dermatitis were atopic and most had hyperhidrosis.

Sports participation is another risk factor for ACD to shoe ingredients [20, 21] and increases the probability of skin exposure to allergens, particularly to rubber [7, 22] and chromium [23].

ACD to footwear is also commonly observed in military personnel [19, 24]. Army boots are not fully lined with cloth [19], explaining the high frequency of ACD.

> **Core Message**
>
> - Patients with intermittent or chronic foot dermatitis should be considered as having allergic contact dermatitis to shoes until proven otherwise.

38.4 Clinical Presentation and Clues Pointing to Allergens

The onset of shoe dermatitis is often sudden, with a history of reaction to a new pair of shoes. Clinical signs such as erythema, papules, vesicles or blisters, oozing, scaling and crusting at site of contact are presumptive of shoe allergy [8, 25]. There may be lichenification and hyperpigmentation in chronic cases [19]. Pruritus and pain may be devastating [8, 12, 25]. Although any part of the foot may be involved in shoe dermatitis [6], typical localization is on the dorsa of feet and toes [7, 12, 19, 24, 25]. Its large surface area and thin stratum corneum, along with intimate and prolonged contact with the shoe upper [12], makes the dorsum of the foot vulnerable to shoe allergy. The lesions are accentuated around the metatarsophalangeal joints and/or over the central dorsal aspect of the foot and/or over the plantar aspect of the foot [7]. Calves and shins may be affected in military personnel with ACD to boots [19]. Bilateral symmetrical dermatitis is the norm although it may be patchy and unilateral [7, 11, 18]. The instep, interdigital spaces, flexural creases of the toes and thicker-skinned heel area are usually spared in shoe dermatitis [7, 8, 13, 19, 24]. There may be associated hyperhidrosis [3, 12, 19].

In a study by Freeman [3], sites affected in 55 cases of shoe dermatitis, a number of which were associated with endogenous eczema, were: dorsal feet (33%), soles weight-bearing (29%), dorsal toes (18%), sides of feet (16%), all surfaces (15%), sides of heels from adhesive heel stiffener (11%), plantar toes (99%), and ankles (2%).

Shoe allergy is typical of many other instances of ACD in that the pattern of presentation suggests the diagnosis but the causative allergen is elusive. The initial pattern of presentation may hold the clue for the causative allergen and allow aimed patch testing with specific groups of chemicals. Dorsal foot dermatitis (Fig. 1) points to an allergen in the shoe upper or tongue of shoe, a portion or portions of which should also be patch tested. Epidemics of shoe dermatitis attributed to chromates and vegetable tannins used in leather have been characterized by dorsal foot involvement [18]. With plantar dermatitis (Fig. 2) sparing the instep and toe creases, shoe allergy should be suspected to the allergens present in the insole or shoe lining or the adhesive that holds these two layers in place. The anterior portion of the sole may be involved exclusively [11]. Confirmation should be sought by testing the patient to portions of the shoes that are in contact with the area of dermatitis. Instep involvement may suggest athletic shoe dermatitis or endogenous eczema. Eczema across the dorsal toes and around the heels suggests allergy to the heel and toe stiffeners or counters, parts of shoes which contain a wide variety of chemicals. Interdigital dermatitis is more likely to be a microbial infection [26].

38

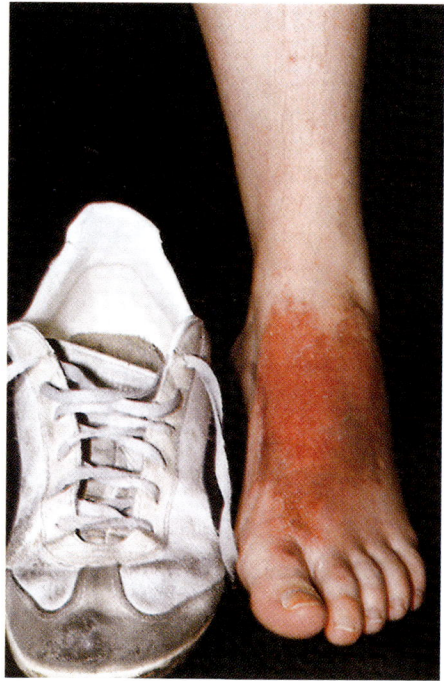

Fig. 1. Dorsal foot allergic contact dermatitis. (Courtesy of P.J. Frosch)

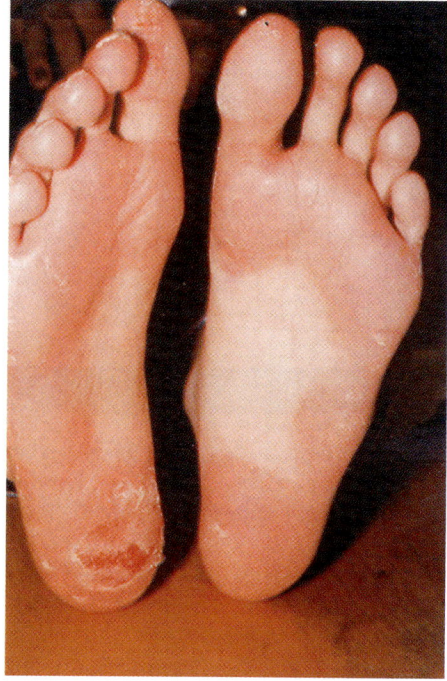

Fig. 2. Plantar foot allergic contact dermatitis

In chronic or severe cases, the presenting pattern may be obscured, making diagnosis more difficult. Shoe allergens can migrate to other parts of the shoe or even to the stockings, disguising the presenting pattern [27, 28]. ACD to medicaments [7, 29] and to socks [11, 30–32] may also confound the clinical presentation. ACD can subsequently spread beyond the initial site of contact by inadvertent exposure or by autosensitization and the dermatitis may be widely and bizarrely distributed [7, 19]. Lear and English [33] reported five patients with mercaptobenzothiazole (MBT) shoe allergy, who had concomitant hand eczema. The hand dermatitis cleared upon resolution of foot eruption. Li and Wang [34] showed that more than one-half of patients with hand and foot dermatitis revealed positive results on patch testing and the main allergens responsible were rubber mix (a mixture of MBT, thiuram and black rubber mixes), paraphenylenediamine (PPDA) and colophony. These findings indicate the importance of considering shoe allergy in cases of foot dermatitis associated with concomitant hand dermatitis [35].

Shoe allergy can mimic other dermatoses of the feet. ACD to MBT is reported to simulate palmoplantar psoriasis or pustular psoriasis [7]. Purpuric eruptions from black rubber boots [36] have been reported. Leukoderma has been seen in Latin America and more commonly in India [37–39]. An Indian report identified monobenzyl ether of hydroquinone in bathroom clogs and rain shoes as the cause of dorsal foot depigmentation [39].

Core Message

■ Shoe allergy may mimic other chronic dermatoses and may be accompanied by hyperhidrosis.

38.5 Shoe Construction and Component Chemicals

Having detailed information on shoe construction and all component chemicals is a helpful and ideal approach in diagnosing shoe allergy. However, this information is often hard to obtain from the manufacturers and identification of all the constituents of a shoe may practically be impossible [1, 7, 40]. Shoes are manufactured all over the world from a vast range of potentially sensitizing chemicals [12, 18, 40]. As many as 3700 allergens have been identified, many of which have clinical relevance to shoe allergy [7].

38.5.1 Shoe Uppers

Shoe uppers can be made from traditional materials such as leather or, in the case of athletic shoes, synthetic materials including polyurethane or neoprene foam. Leather traditionally is chrome tanned, potentially exposing the wearer to the allergen potassium dichromate. However, according to Corey (written communication from Dr Nicholas J Corey, Leather Research Laboratory, University of Cincinnati, Ohio, 27 August, 2004), in almost the entire developed world, chromium tanning is performed exclusively using trivalent chromium, normally in the form of basic chromium sulfate. Corey thus believes that the wearer should not be exposed to potassium dichromate and that reports of traces of Cr VI in leather can be attributed to false-positive test methodology [41, 42]. However chrome allergy in leather has recently been reported from Israel and Pakistan as relevant to foot dermatitis [2, 12]. With the current high-fashion demand of varied finishes, chrome tanning is a multistep process. Leather is tanned and retanned. In approximately 85% of cases, primary tanning is with chrome, but retanning may be with other methods which include vegetable tanning, synthetic tanning, and rarely alum tanning [41]. There is an increasing market from chrome-free leather in the automotive industry. Such chrome-free leather is produced using proprietary formulations that combine modified glutaraldehyde with vegetable tanning agents, primarily Tara powder (written communication from Dr Nicholas J Corey, 27 August, 2004). After tanning, the leather is shaved to a uniform thickness and may be used in athletic shoe uppers, exposing wearers to chrome.

Vegetable tanning is a slow process taking 3 weeks, compared to a few days for chrome tanning. The vegetable tannins are all plant or fruit extracts, with quebracho, wattle, myrobolans, and chestnut extracts being the major ones in use today. These are wood extracts that are approximately 60% tannins. Vegetable tanning is used less commonly but yields highly resilient, hydrophilic leather that is ideal for soles, linings and insoles, but is also harder, less malleable and more difficult to work with than either chrome or synthetic-tanned leathers. It is indicated for chromate-allergic patients. Other uses include automotive leather and clothing belts.

Alum tanning is rarely used nowadays, and the use of free formaldehyde was abandoned in the 1990s. However, formaldehyde is still introduced into leather via the breakdown of synthetic polymerics that are commonly used as retanning agents (written communication from Dr Nicholas J Corey, 27 August, 2004). Concentrations of free formaldehyde typically permitted by leather product manufacturers range from 0.5 to 300 ppm [43]. Alum tanning and glutaraldehyde tanning, which yielded a soft waterproof leather, are now rarely used for shoes. Glutaraldehyde is in widespread use, but its main purpose is to impart perspiration resistance to hat band leather and sports wear such as golf gloves (written communication from Dr Nicholas J Corey, 27 August, 2004). Synthetic tanning is usually used as a final tannage or as an adjunct to primary tanning agents, and utilizes chemicals such as naphthalene, sulfonic acid and phenolic resins, dimethylol urea, dicyandiamide, and melamine-formaldehyde resin. Oxazolidines and tetrakishydroxymethyl phosphonium salts are newer tanning agents that are likely to be used increasingly on lighter leathers such as woolskins and ovine garment leathers (written communication Tony Passman, Director, New Zealand Leather and Shoe Research Association, 26 August, 2004).

Tanning is followed by the application of modern petroleum-based synthetics, including acrylics, that yield waterproof yet breathable, air-permeable leathers. These synthetics have largely replaced a fat liquoring (oiling) process which restored the natural oils leached out by the tanning process, utilizing cod liver oil, synthetic moellon oil (a synthetic fish oil), and sulfonated neatsfoot oil (written communication Dr Nicholas J Corey, 27 August, 2004).

Dyeing is the next process and there are many specific dyestuffs in use. Formerly a rare source of sensitization, dyes are now being manufactured less expensively in third world countries. By-products of the multistep dye production process may persist as impurities and possible allergens. Chrome-tanned leather is best dyed with acid dyes and vegetable-tanned leather with basic dyes. Acid dyes account for approximately 70% of the dyes used to color leather. The other dyestuffs used are: (1) premetalized dyes, which give much improved color uniformity and color fastness, but are more expensive, (2) direct dyes, as used to dye cotton (written communication from Dr Nicholas J Corey, 27 August, 2004), and (3) cationic dyes which are use to increase intensity of acid dyes (written communication Tony Passman, Director New Zealand Leather and Shoe Research Association, 26 August, 2004). Following an initiative by the German government in 1994, the European Union has recently implemented legislation that bans the use of dyes that can break down to release any of 22 specified aromatic amines that are now know to be carcinogenic [44].

Leather finishing is next and is designed to give an attractive but tough outer coat to the leather. The main polymers used are acrylic resins, polyurethanes and nitrocellulose (NC). Diisobutyl ketone is one of several solvents used as a carrier, evaporating after application of the NC. Plasticizers are an essential part of all NC resins and a phthalate ester is added as a plasticizer to prevent cracking of the NC resin. Finishes based on natural protein such as milk casein protein, egg albumin and vegetable wax solids are occasionally used to give a depth of appearance. Other components of finishes may include a spray stain of metal complex pigments to improve the color and a water-repellent coat of alkenyl succinic acid complex, fluorinated acid chromium complex, stearatochromic chloride complex and silicones.

All of these steps may involve chemicals that can cause sensitization and footwear dermatitis. In both the fat liquoring (oiling) and finishing process, biocides, a number of which are also contact allergens, are important additives. Table 1 lists selected biocides which have been used in shoe manufacture. Most are still in use in rubber compounds but only three are allowed for use in leather in the USA. Although trichlorophenol is classified as "reasonably anticipated to be a human carcinogen" by the US National Toxicology Program, it remains one of the most popular fungicides in Australia and other oceanic countries [45]. The use of pentachlorophenol has been almost entirely eradicated following a ban on its use and

Table 1. Biocides which may be used in shoe manufacture[a]

Shoe part	Biocide
Leather upper:	Diiodomethyl-*p*-tolylsulfone (Amical)[b]
	2-(Thiocyanomethylthio) benzothiazole (TCMTM) (Busan)[b]
	Trichlorophenol in Australia and oceanic countries
Heel and toe counter:	*o*-Phenyl phenol (OPP) (Vita-San and Preventol WB)[b]
	1,2-Benzisothiazolin-3-one 10% in an aqueous solution of propylene glycol (Proxel X L2)
Water-based adhesives:	*N*-Trichloro-methyl-thiophthalimide (Fungitrol 11)
	Copper-8-quinolinolate[c]
Lasting board:	Sodium-*o*-phenylphenate (Dowicide A)
	Copper-8-quinolinolate[c]

[a] See text for more detailed discussion
[b] The only fungicides permitted for use with leather in the USA (written communication from Dr Nicholas J Corey, 27 August, 2004)
[c] Mainly used in military footwear (written communication from Barbara Strickland, 26 August, 2004)

presence in leather implemented by Germany in December 1989. This ban was subsequently adopted by all other EU countries, leading to the worldwide withdrawal of PCP as a leather fungicide (written communication from Dr Nicholas J Corey, 27 August, 2004). The use of copper has been discontinued by most adhesive manufacturers, with the notable exception of military footwear, where copper is still on the accepted list as a biocide (written communication Barbara Strickland, Worthen Industries, Nashua, NH, 26 August, 2004).

In recent years, leather uppers have been largely replaced by foam uppers, particularly in athletic footwear. These foams tend to be either polyurethane or neoprene. Polyurethane is a relatively inert substance and includes a wide variety of chemicals in its manufacture, the majority of which are totally polymerized or are absent at the time of wearing. However, it is possible that some catalysts may persist as possible allergens. Common catalysts in use at present in the polyurethane chemical industry are the tertiary or quaternary amines. Ultra-violet light stabilizers, hindered phenols, hindered amines and benzotriazoles are present to a level of 0.5–1% of the final product.

Rubber is a broad term referring to many different polymers, only one of which is natural rubber (Table 2). Natural rubber is derived from the sap of the tree *Hevea brasiliensis* and is composed of *cis* 1,4-polyisoprene monomers. Neoprene is synthetic rubber commonly used as a foam material in shoes. It consists of chloroprene monomers with phenolic resins and thioureas, carbamates and other accelerators and additives which may be contact allergens (also see Sect. 38.5.4, "Adhesives"). Table 3 lists some less familiar rubber chemicals which may be used in shoe manufacture.

Table 2. Rubber polymers. Some formulations may contain a mixture of natural and synthetic rubbers

Polymer	Monomers
Natural rubber	Isoprene
Synthetic rubber	
Styrene-butadiene rubber	Styrene, butadiene
Polybutadiene	Butadiene
Synthetic polyisoprene	Synthetic isoprene
Neoprene	Chloroprene
Thermoplastic elastomers	Styrene, isoprene, butadiene
High-styrene resins	Styrene, butadiene Isoprene, chloroprene

Table 3. Some less familiar rubber chemicals

Chemical category	Chemical
Vulcanizers	Diorthotolyl guanidine
	Dicumyl peroxide
Accelerators	Ethylene thiourea
Antioxidants	Octylated diphenylamines
	2,2,4-Trimethyl-1,2-dihydro-quinoline
	Butylated hydroxytoluene
	Diphenylamines
Pigment	Titanium dioxide
Resins	Coumarone indene resins
	Terpene phenolic resins
	p-tert-Butylphenol-formaldehyde resin
Blowing agents	Azodicarbonamide
	4,4-Oxybis (benzenesulphonyl-hydrazide)

38.5.2 Shoe Soles

Most of the substances used in shoe uppers can also be used in shoe soles, i.e., either chrome- or vegetable-tanned leather or alternatively neoprene or polyurethane as solid foam. The polyurethanes tend to be highly cross-linked, closely packed foams. Other types of rubber may be used in sole manufacture. Natural rubber and synthetic polybutadiene are the popular rubbers for soles and heels. Neoprenes are widely used for oil-resistant work soles, utilizing dibenzothiazyl disulfide as the accelerator. Evaflex soles combine ethyl vinyl acetate (EVA) with rubber polymers.

38.5.3 Shoe Insoles

Shoe insoles, once again, can be made of leather (chrome- or vegetable-tanned) or of polyurethane or neoprene foam. Another material in use, in cheaper shoes particularly, is a fiberboard material. This is a composite material usually made of paper fibers or occasionally wood or even leather fibers, which are solidified in a glue matrix. This biocide-preserved (see Table 1) matrix emulsion consists of various rubber resins, such as neoprene, styrene-butadiene or acrylics. This mixture is set in sheets, and the insoles are cut out of these sheets. Fiberboard can also be used as a lasting board or foundation in cheaper shoes, which in other shoes may be made of thick vegetable-tanned leather. Fiberboard, therefore, exposes patients to a wide range of allergens causing plantar foot dermatitis, including leather chemicals, rubber chemicals, adhesives and biocides.

38.5.4 Adhesives

Adhesives are used throughout the shoe, often in intimate contact with the foot, as when used to glue the shoe insole or shoe lining in place. As a result, they are a major cause of shoe allergy. The main adhesives in use are urethane, neoprene, hot melt and natural rubber; others may include vegetable pastes and nitrocellulose [46].

Hot-melt adhesives are unlikely causes of shoe allergy. They are inert, high molecular weight polymers of EVA, polyamides or polyesters in rod, pellet, or block form. After melting, they are applied hot to the surface, usually in sole and heel attachments.

"Latex" in common parlance often refers to natural rubber latex. However, in the adhesives industry the term is broader, referring to water-based lattices such as natural or synthetic rubber latex. Urethane adhesives are polyurethanes in solution, modified to give the composition tack or adhesion. In special situations, other additives are required: to increase bond strength, isocyanates are added; to apply neoprene, epoxy resins are required; and to apply EVA polymers, tackifiers such as acrylic or phenol-formaldehyde resins are used.

Urethanes, useful as a substitute for rubber allergy, make up 80% of footwear adhesives; whereas solvent-borne or latex neoprenes account for about 15% and solvent-borne or latex rubbers, EVA, pastes (declining use) and hot melts (increased use) account for about 5%. Polyurethanes have taken over from neoprenes as the preferred method of sole attaching because they are faster setting, have higher heat resistance, are clear, do not yellow with age and wear longer. If very high heat or chemical resistance is required then a second adhesive component can be added. In general most higher end shoes selling for more than US$30 per pair will have a polyurethane adhesive. Neoprene is more likely used with custom-made boots or temporary sole-attaching prior to stitching or for less rigorous bonding such as linings to uppers and sock linings(shoe inserts) to insoles. The only definitive way of knowing which adhesive is used is to contact the manufacturer or to pull apart the shoe and perform chemical analysis. Table 4 lists a typical polyurethane adhesive formulation (written communication Barbara Strickland, 26 August, 2004).

Table 4. Typical polyurethane adhesive formulation[a]

Thermoplastic polyurethane resin
Fillers: sodium/calcium/aluminum silicate
Siloxane
Propylene glycol based UV stabilizers
(Rosins and tackifying resins are not normally used; these properties are usually inherent in the selected polyurethane resin)

[a] Formulation provided by Barbara Strickland, Product Development Manager, Worthen Industries, UPACO Adhesives Division, Nashua, NH, 26 August, 2004)

Table 5. Neoprene formulation

Chlorinated rubber (neoprene)
Phenolic resin (*p-tert*-butylphenol-formaldehyde resin or terpene phenolic resin)
Magnesium oxide
Zinc oxide
Ethylene thiourea
Dioctyl-4-phenylenediamine
Fillers: sodium/calcium silicate
Tetramethylthiuram disulfide
Diorthotolyl guanidine
Sodium dibutyldithiocarbamate

Table 6. Natural rubber latex adhesive formulation

Polyoxyethylene	Phenol
Rosin esters	Formaldehyde
Polymerized wood resin	Parachlorometacresol (Collatone)
Triethanolamine	Fatty acid
Diallyl phenyl sulfone	Caustic potash

Table 5 outlines a typical neoprene formulation. Strong neoprene adhesives contain isocyanates, which cause *p*-tert-butylphenol-formaldehyde (PTBP-F) resin to undergo premature cure. Therefore, these strong adhesives either use terpene phenolic resins as tackifiers or consist of two components that are mixed immediately prior to use. Rubber latex adhesives tend to be made of natural rubber, as synthetic rubber is expensive (Table 6). Since they are water-based, they are biocide-preserved and tackifying resins such as colophony are added.

38.5.5 Heel and Toe Counters

If a shoe is to retain its shape, it is necessary to stiffen it at the toe and heel; this leads to the addition of heel and toes stiffeners or counters (Table 7). There are five main types and all serve to strengthen the toes and heels of shoes. The simplest and least problematic type is found in athletic shoes – a layer of hot melt adhesive. However, the other types are more elaborate, consisting of a web polyester or cotton material impregnated with a variety of resins to give stiffness and support. Counters may, therefore, contain a number of potential allergens; natural rubber latex, EVA, hot-melt adhesive, phenol-formaldehyde resin, melamine-formaldehyde resin, urea-formaldehyde resin, pine oil and various biocides [26, 47].

> ## Core Message
>
> ■ Knowledge of shoe construction and composition is helpful when contacting shoe manufacturers and suppliers. This is especially true when obtaining information on shoe chemicals, especially those in shoe components reacting positively on patch testing, and also when ordering special shoes for allergic patients.

Table 7. Heel and toe counters

Type of counter	Composition
Pressed counters	Fiberboard coated with urea- or phenol-formaldehyde resin
	Glue
	Natural rubber latex 95% ethyl vinyl acetate polymer
	Hot melt 5%
Thermoplastic counters	Polyvinylchloride impregnated with rubber resins
	Surlyn (ethylene methacrylic acid)
Solid styrene	Styrene plasticized with methyl ketone
Thermal counters	Woven fabric coated with rubber or melamine-formaldehyde resins
	Glue
	Ethyl vinyl acetate hot melts
Three-part counters	1. Woven fabrics impregnated with urea-formaldehyde resin and natural rubber latex
	2. Ammonium chloride or sodium acetate
	3. Pine oil, sodium-N-methyl-N-oleoyl laurate, dioctyl sodium sulfosuccinate

38.6 Allergens in Shoes

After this detailed look at shoe structure and composition, an extensive list of potential allergens can be compiled (Table 8). The allergens in shoes are gradually changing as a consequence of modifications in footwear manufacture technologies and constant flux in material selection and style design. Leather and shoe dyes were the most common allergens in shoe dermatitis during 1930s and 1940s [7, 22]. Since 1950s and 1960s, rubber allergens and adhesive components have been the leading offenders [6, 7, 22, 32]. The gradual shift from leather to rubber as the most frequent allergen probably reflects improved fixation of chrome in leather and a dramatic change in footwear style with much greater use of rubber components [7, 18, 22].

Currently, the most common causes of shoe allergy are constituents of rubber, adhesives, leather, dyes, biocides, and trim [12, 19]. Allergens include rubber chemicals: thiurams, benzothiazoles, carbamates, and para-phenylenediamine derivatives in rubber or adhesives; chromates in leather; PTBP-F resin in neoprene adhesives; colophony in adhesives; formaldehyde in leather tanning; nickel in decoration and trim; lanolin in some polishes; and para-phenylenediamine in some dyes [11, 13, 26]. Potassium dichromate is the most common sensitizer in leather [19, 24]. Mercaptobenzothiazole (MBT), used as an accelerator, is the leading culprit for rubber [7, 14, 18, 19, 24].

The allergens in 55 patients with shoe dermatitis as reported by Freeman [3] were: rubber chemicals (44%); potassium dichromate (24%); p-tertiary-butylphenol-formaldehyde resin (20%); rosin (colophony) (9%); PPDA (4%); and unknown – patients were positive to shoe pieces (15%). Chemicals in mercapto mix followed by thiuram mix were the most common rubber allergens present mostly in shoe lining adhesives. Other sources of rubber allergy were rubber insoles and elastic in shoe uppers. In the series of Shackelford and Belsito [7], the most common shoe allergens were rubber components, leather, and adhesives. Bacitracin, dithiodimorpholine (a rubber accelerator), potassium dichromate, quaternium-15, neomycin, mercaptobenzothiazole/mercapto mix, p-tertiary-butylphenol-formaldehyde resin, and thiuram mix were the top allergens that produced positive and clinically relevant reactions to shoe components or topical medications. In a study of 119 patients with shoe dermatitis, Rani et al. [12] identified 87 patients (73%) who reacted positively to various allergens; glues (34%), leather (27%), nickel (18%), rubber (8%) and dyes (8%) were noted as the leading causes of shoe allergy. Finally Trattner et al. [2] noted

Table 8. Potential shoe chemical allergens beyond the standard tray

Chemical	Concentration
Tosylamide formaldehyde resin	10% pet.
4,4′-Diaminodiphenylmethane	0.5% pet.
2,2,4-Trimethyl-1,2-dihydroquinoline	1% pet.
1H-Benzotriazole	1% pet.
4,4′-Dithiomorpholine	1% pet.
Coumarone indene resin	20% pet.
Terpene phenolic resin	20% pet.
Tetramethyl butanediamine	1% pet.
N-Octyl-4-isothiazolin-3-one 8% in propylene glycol 92% (Kathon LP)	0.1% pet.
Bismuth neodecanoate	1% pet.
N,N-Diethyl thiourea	1% pet.
Ethylbutyl thiourea	1% pet.
N,N-Dibutyl thiourea	1% pet.
3-Methyl thiazolidine-2-thion (Vulcacit CRU)	1% pet.
Ethylene thiourea	1% pet.
Disperse Orange 3	1% pet.
Disperse Yellow 3	1% pet.
Copper 8-quinolinolate	1% pet.
Diorthotolyl guanidine	1% pet.
Dioctyl phthalate	5% pet.
N-Dodecyl mercaptan	0.1% pet.
Glutaraldehyde	1% aq.
Urea-formaldehyde resin	10% pet.
Dicyandiamide	0.1% aq.
Toluene sulfonhydrazide	0.5% alc.
Dimethylaminoethyl ether (Niax₁)	1% pet.
Azodicarbonamide (Azobisformamide)	0.5% pet.
Styrenated phenol [50]	1% pet.
Cyclohexylthiophtalimide [7, 58]	1% pet.
para-Aminoazobenzene [1, 7, 59].	0.25% pet.
Cinnamic aldehyde [60]	1% pet.
Cinnamic alcohol [60]	5% pet.
Propolis [65]	10% pet.
Ethylcyanoacrylate [62]	5% pet.
Epichlorohydrin [66]	0.1% pet.
Monobenzylether of hydroquinone [29]	1% pet.
Nigrosin [7]	1% pet.
Phenylmercuric acetate [7]	0.01% aq.
Triethylenetetramine [7]	0.5% pet.
Diethylenetriamine [7]	1% pet.
Isophorone diamine [7]	0.1% pet.
Isophorone diisocyanate [7]	1% pet.
Toluene diisocyanate [7]	2% pet.
Diphenylmethane-4, 4-diisocyanate [7]	2% pet.
Triglycidil isocyanurate [7]	0.5% pet.
1,6-Hexamethylenediisocyanate [7]	0.1% pet.
Hexamethylenetetramine [7]	2% pet.
N-Phenyl-2-naphtylamine [7]	1% pet.
Ethoxyquin [7]	0.5% pet.
Kathon CG [7]	100 parts per million aq.

38

positive patch test reactions in 58 of 140 patients (41%) suspected of having shoe dermatitis and the most frequent allergens were documented as potassium dichromate (27%), nickel sulfate (12%), Kathon CG (11%), and PTBP-F (9%).

The most common shoe allergens in diabetic patients were documented as hydroquinone monobenzylether, thiuram mix, potassium dichromate, 4-tert-butylphenol formaldehyde resin, 4-phenylenediamine base, nickel sulfate, colophony, formaldehyde, diphenylthiourea, 2-mercaptobenzothiazole, diethylthiourea, diphenylguanidine, dibutylthiourea, epoxy resin, dodecylmercaptan, Cl+Me-isothiazolinone, 4-aminoazobenzene and 2-n-octyl-4-isothiazolin-3-one [48].

Shoe dermatitis encountered in sporting activities has been attributed to several allergens, including rubber, leather, cobalt, nickel, and PPDA [15, 20]. Among military personnel wearing boots, chromium salts within leather and nickel sulfate have been reported as the most frequent allergens [19].

38.7 Hidden Sources of Shoe Allergens

Despite our knowledge of shoe components, it may be difficult to cure patients completely, perhaps because they continue to encounter their allergens in unexpected places. MBT and thiurams are rubber chemicals, which may not necessarily be limited to soles and heels [49]. Neoprene adhesives have been shown to contain thiuram, and it is not possible to exclude MBT entirely in either synthetic or natural latex [19]. Heel and toe counters, fiberboard lasting boards and leather finish coats all contain rubber resins, which may include MBT or thiurams [40, 50].

Styrenated phenol has been identified as an allergen in athletic shoes in addition to thioureas [51–53].

Diaminodiphenylmethane is a polyurethane precursor and potential allergen in polyurethane upper foam [54]. Polyurethane foam looks more shiny than neoprene foam.

Dodecylmercaptan is a polymerization inhibitor present in polyurethane resins and may be a rare sensitizer [12, 48].

PTBP-F resin is the main tackifier used in neoprene adhesives and is found mainly in shoe-lining and shoe-insole glues. It is also encountered in heel and toe counters [3, 12]. Not all cases of PTBP-F resin sensitivity are detected by testing with the standard series. PTBP itself should be tested, as well as the actual PTBP-F resin used in the shoes [55–57]. Colophony, like PTBP-F resin, is a tackifier occasionally found in heel and toe stiffeners, as well as in rubber latex or neoprene adhesives used to glue shoe insoles and linings in place [3, 13, 40, 58]. It may also be used as a leather tanning or finishing agent in some imported shoes [13]. Patients sensitive to colophony and PTBP-F resin should be advised to wear either unlined shoes or leather-lined shoes with the lining stitched, not glued, in place and shoes with no heel or toe supports.

2-*n*-Octyl-4-isothiazolin-3-one is a biocide used during leather finishing [12]. It is a potential sensitizer [12, 48].

Cyclohexylthiophthalimide is the most widely used vulcanization retarder in the rubber industry. ACD to this substance may develop following exposure to rubber shoes [59].

Allergies to dyes are rarely encountered, with the exception of re-dyed leather or fabric shoes [1, 32]. The most commonly used dyes are azo-aniline group dyes, e.g., para-phenylenediamine and para-aminoazobenzene which are strong sensitizers [1, 60]. PPDA is mainly used as a dye for leather in shoes, while the use of para-aminoazobenzene is extended to the textile and clothing industry [60].

Nickel in shoe trim, eyelets or buckles can be an unexpected cause of dorsal foot dermatitis [12]. Cobalt allergy is often associated with chromium allergy due to leather shoes [12, 17]. Both nickel and cobalt compounds may be used as dyes or pigments within the shoes. Goossens et al. [17] reported a nurse who developed ACD to nickel and cobalt in green plastic shoes.

A vesicular dermatitis of the soles due to ACD to cinnamon powder used as an odor-neutralizing agent in insoles has been reported [61].

According to Storrs [11], Guin described patients who developed positive patch tests to scrapings of scales taken from their foot eruption, suggesting an antigen reservoir in the stratum corneum.

Cotton socks saturated with moisture have been reported to retain some of the allergens, even after thorough washing or boiling [7, 18]. Rietschel [27] proposed that shoe allergens may concentrate in stockings, which may prolong chronic foot eczema. He described two MBT-allergic patients who had positive patch tests to pieces of white socks soaked in 0.1% to 1.0% solutions of MBT.

Reports of occupational dermatitis in shoe production or shoe repair may also point to other shoe allergens [62–69]. These include 1,2-benzisothiazolin-3-one (BIT) [64], ethyl cyanoacrylate [63], propolis [66], epichlorohydrin (a volatile component of epoxy resin) [67] in shoe adhesives; PTBP-F resin [69]; and phthalates in PVC shoes [65]. A study of an Italian shoe factory provides a long list of chemicals in recent use; major occupational allergens were PTBP-F resin and MBT [62]. Other hidden sources of shoe allergens are discussed in Sect. 38.9, "Chemical Analysis" below.

Other potential foot reactions from shoes include contact urticaria and other immediate contact reactions from natural rubber latex and dermatitis as a result of the bleached rubber syndrome [70].

38.8 Patch Testing for Shoe Allergy

The diagnosis of ACD of feet is challenging since the constituents of the shoes are unlabeled [22]. A detailed and compatible history along with characteristic clinical findings may be helpful in diagnosis [7, 25]. Hobbies as well as patient's occupation should be extensively evaluated [25]. Extensive patch testing on healthy skin during disease-free intervals is required for the identification of the offending allergen [3, 7, 25]. Testing for shoe allergy is performed with: (1) chemicals from the standard series; (2) other shoe chemicals present in an expanded shoe series; and (3) pieces of shoes worn by the patient.

Many cases of shoe allergy can be diagnosed by patch testing with the standard series or by the TRUE Test panel [7, 11]. Allergens that are not covered by standard screening series may be identified by additional patch testing with a series of other shoe constituents [2, 6, 11, 22, 26, 41, 71, 72]. Podmore [26] assembled a series of chemicals by breaking down all of the constituents of shoes and identifying all possible culprits. This task is complicated by the fact that today's shoes are manufactured all over the world [40], often in countries from which information on manufacturing components is not readily available. When different components of shoes are derived from different countries, their country of origin may not be recorded [71]. Table 8 lists additional shoe chemicals [26]. These and other lists [6, 11] include resins, rubber accelerators, dyes, plasticizers, tanning agents, antioxidants, and UV stabilizers. In addition to those in Table 8, other authors have included: *p*-aminoazobenzene, a dye; the following biocides: thimerosal, chloroacetamide and phenyl mercuric nitrate; hydroquinone in rubber; vegetable tannins; glutaraldehyde, a rare sensitizer as a leather tannin; other dyes; polyurethane chemicals (Desmodur, Desmocoll 400, Desmodur R and RF and dodecyl mercaptan); and urethane adhesives, and other adhesive components (1,2-benzisothiazolin-3-one, BIT) [1, 8, 11, 54, 73, 74]. Selected shoe chemicals are available from standard patch test suppliers. Testing with additional shoe chemicals may be helpful in confirming an allergen present in patch-test-positive shoe pieces. Alternatively, they may be useful for detecting some patients with false-negative reactions to shoe pieces who are allergic to rubber, adhesives or chrome [75].

In contrast, a sub-group of patients who are suspected of having ACD to shoes may be patch-test-negative to the standard series and to an expanded shoe screening tray, but positive to shoe pieces [1, 3]. In Freeman's study [3], 14.5% of patients reacted positive to shoe pieces, yet had negative patch test results to individual shoe ingredients. This paradox may be attributed to the absence of relevant allergen(s) from the standard and shoe series [1]. Thus careful testing with properly selected pieces of material from the shoe itself is an important adjunct in the diagnosis of shoe allergy [1, 3, 11, 19, 26, 47, 71, 72, 75, 76]. Every effort should be made to obtain a positive patch test response to obtain evidence of delayed type hypersensitivity to relevant portions of the footwear [7, 25]. One should attempt to obtain pieces of the suspect shoe from an area in contact with the affected skin. The pieces should be wafer-thin to avoid false-positive, irritant pressure effects. Since the standard Finn chamber holds portions no larger than 5 mm², many prefer to patch test either with the larger Finn chamber or without a chamber utilizing occlusive tape. With the latter technique, 1 cm² or larger shoe pieces should be used [11, 26]. It may be helpful to leave the shoe pieces in place for 4 or 5 days rather than the usual 2 days [11]. To help replicate the conditions of shoe wearing, Jordan [77] suggests soaking the shoe pieces in water for 15 min before testing, soaking each piece in a separate container. The use of a repetitive open application test as well as testing of volunteers as controls might clarify false-positive reactions to shoe pieces. It must be emphasized that topical medications may be absorbed by the shoes [18], in which case shoe pieces may be false positive from the medication, rather than the shoe itself.

Patch testing with ultrasonic bath extracts of shoe pieces might identify contact allergy which would otherwise go unrecognized. Bruze et al. [78] cited four examples of clinically relevant exposure to rubber bands, gloves, black rubber packing, and paper in which only patch testing with such extracts yielded positive results; tests had been negative to the objects themselves, as well as to the putative chemical allergens.

38

Core Message

■ Patch testing for shoe allergy should ideally include the standard screening tray, a shoe chemical series, pieces from shoes worn by the patient as well as topical medications, foot powders, and shoe inserts used by the patient.

38.9 Chemical Analysis

Detailed chemical analysis of shoe extracts by various types of chromatography and mass spectroscopy and subsequent patch testing of the fractions has identified undetected allergens in several studies. These include dibenzothiazyl disulfide (a dimer of MBT), styrenated phenol, and 6-ethoxy-2,2,4-trimethyl-1,2-dihydroquinoline (ETMDQ). Using this method, unknown shoe allergens were isolated, identified and added to a shoe test series of potential allergens [51, 79, 80].

Mercury chloride, an unexpected allergen, was identified by atomic absorption spectrometry and polarography in new polyvinylchloride boots. The boots were worn by a 5-year-old child, with a history of skin intolerance to Mercurochrome (merbromin), who developed allergic contact dermatitis and a mercury exanthem after wearing the boots [81].

A related study found that the amounts of thioureas and MBT leached from rubber articles were greater than the patch test elicitation threshold for these chemicals. Such studies may be helpful to manufacturers in designing products that do not release allergens in sufficient amounts to cause reactions in consumers [82].

38.10 Differential Diagnosis

Allergy to various textile dyes has been reported to constitute up to 10% of foot ACD. The risk correlates with the ease of leaching of the dye from the fabric [83]. Shoe dermatitis may be imitated by sock or stocking allergy from disperse [11, 31] and non-disperse azo dyes [30, 32]. Although PPDA is traditionally used as an indicator of textile dye dermatitis, it may be negative in azo-dye sensitive patients and is not accepted as a reliable marker [32].

Nylon stocking allergy may spare the toe webs while involving the rest of the feet and legs.

ACD of foot may be an iatrogenic complication of topical medications being used for a preexisting non-allergic foot dermatosis [7, 12]. Topical antibiotics such as neomycin, bacitracin and gentamicin; topical steroids; benzocaine, parabens, lanolin and balsam of Peru (*Myroxylon pereirae*) in topically applied foot medications and *p*-chlorometaxylenol in foot powder may lead to a primary allergic foot dermatitis [7, 29]. It must be noted that the TRUE Test does not include bacitracin or screening agents for topical corticosteroids [7].

Juvenile plantar dermatosis is a condition with distinctive, symmetrical glazed, cracked skin of weight-bearing areas, sparing the web spaces. It presents with erythema and pain, rarely itching, and is found in children usually between ages 3 and 14 years, and rarely in infants and adults. The dermatitis is thought to result from excessive sweating and overdrying of the feet due to modern occlusive footwear in children with atopic background. Patch tests and fungal scrapings are consistently negative in this disorder [8, 84].

Other differential diagnoses include irritant contact dermatitis; atopic eczema, especially involving the ankle and dorsal first toe; tinea pedis; psoriasis, lichen planus, dyshidrotic eczema and id reactions [7, 18].

> ## Core Message
>
> - Differential diagnosis of shoe allergy includes disperse dye allergy in stockings, topical medications used for foot dermatitis, juvenile plantar dermatosis, other eczematous skin disease, and tinea pedis.

38.11 Prognosis and Outcome

Shoe allergy may become chronic and recalcitrant to therapy, disabling with painful fissuring, and may be complicated by secondary infection – cellulitis and lymphangitis [3, 24]. Despite these possibilities, the outcome is generally good. In Freeman's study [3] involving adults, 87.5% of patients afflicted with shoe dermatitis had improved or resolved completely. In a prospective study on children, 72% of patients with foot dermatitis showed improvement or resolution of symptoms at the end of 6 months. However, atopy was a poor prognostic factor [6].

38.12 Allergen Substitution

The only effective treatment that resolves the dermatitis is avoidance of the shoes likely to contain the allergen [7, 8]. Patients with ACD to shoe components are usually advised to use hypoallergenic substitute shoes [1]. Recommendations should be relied on information regarding shoe manufacture in individual countries.

Dermatitis confined to the soles may be treated by replacing the insoles with composition, cork or felt which is glued in with a non-rubber cement. Commercially available insole inserts may be very useful, but one needs to know their composition (e.g., urethane, neoprene, latex, etc.) including additives (fragrance, deodorizers, etc.). Shoe substitution for contact dermatitis of other foot areas may include all-leather shoes such as moccasins with no insole and

no attached outer sole, injection-molded plastic shoes, or wooden shoes for rubber allergy. Vinyl shoes may be an acceptable alternative in patients with allergy to rubber or leather [8, 85].

For patients with chromium allergy and clinically relevant shoe dermatitis, wearing good quality, new, leather shoes and discarding them after a few months (thus preventing the allergens from leaching out), and wearing extra pairs of large cotton socks in shoes (thus preventing contact with the allergens) may help in clearance of foot dermatitis [1, 3]. Although there is skepticism about this, hypoallergenic shoe leather can also be recommended for such patients. The presence of relevant leather-related allergens (e.g., other tanning agents alternative to chromium) and dyes has been documented in hypoallergenic shoe leather, which may cause contact allergies [1]. Alternative in such cases is the use of all-plastic or all-fabric (canvas) shoes. If leather insoles are chrome-tanned, they should be removed. Wooden clogs with vegetable-tanned leather may also be helpful for chrome allergy [1, 11], and, if there is concomitant adhesive allergy, the vegetable-tanned leather uppers can be stapled rather than glued in place.

Pedorthists or orthotists who are knowledgeable about shoe composition may also be helpful in suggesting temporary shoe substitutes such as those made of Plastazote. Some manufacturers will make custom shoes, but these are often expensive [3], and it is important to know as much about the composition of the shoe as possible, especially dyes and adhesives [11, 85] (Table 9). Patch testing with pieces of the substitute shoe in advance of a special order may also be useful. No guarantees should be made about the success of substitute shoes, especially in the case of hybrid eczema in which the patient has both exogenous and endogenous dermatitis. Patch testing with pieces from a number of the patient's shoes may identify patch-test-negative shoes which the patient can continue to wear, discarding those which are patch-test-positive [4]. Concomitant topical therapy is very important; absorbent powders may control hyperhidrosis and topical steroids may help to clear the dermatitis [8].

For army boot dermatitis, the manufacturers should aim at changing the design of boots in order to reduce the allergen load [19].

38.13 Conclusion

Shoe contact dermatitis still remains a difficult condition to manage. It is important to search for patients' known allergens in unexpected places in their shoes and to give patients appropriately detailed advice on avoidance. With proper evaluation, the prognosis of shoe dermatitis remains very good.

Table 9. Sites of common allergens in shoes[a]

Allergen	Location	Avoid
Mercaptobenzothiazole Tetramethylthiuram disulfide	1. Rubber 2. Neoprene adhesives 3. Adhesives + leather treatment biocides 4. Leather finish coats	1. Rubber foam uppers + insoles 2. Solid rubber shoe soles +d heels 3. Sock lining adhesives 4. Fiberboard insoles 5. Highly finished leathers
Dibenzothiazyl disulphide (MBT mix)	1. Solid or adhesive neoprene 2. Rubber	1. Sock lining adhesive 2. Rubber soles or heels 3. Rubber insole sponge
Thiourea	Solid or foam neoprene	EVA-neoprene- nylon combination insole
Diaminodiphenylmethane	Polyurethane	1. Shiny upper foam 2. Combination shoe soles
Colophony	Tackifying resins	1. Natural rubber latex cement (sock lining adhesive) 2. Heel and toe counters
Paratertiary butylphenol formaldehyde resin	Tackifying resins	1. Neoprene adhesives (sock lining adhesive) 2. Heel and toe counters
Nickel	Metal trim	Dimethylglyoxime positive eyelets
Formaldehyde	1. Leather tanning 2. Biocides in natural rubber latex adhesives	Lutidine positive leather or soft perspiration proof leather
Chromate	Leather tanning	1. Leather 2. Athletic shoe uppers

[a] Modified from Patricia Podmore MD, Londonderry, Northern Ireland and Frances J Storrs, MD, Portland, OR

Most patients are successful in finding alternative footwear through a number of different strategies [3, 6]. Even then some cases remain insoluble and must be managed empirically with hypoallergenic footwear, such as plastic shoes or wooden shoes with vegetable-tanned uppers sewn or stapled rather than glued in place.

Case Report

■ **Case Report 1.** A 48-year old consultant developed foot dermatitis with erythematous scaly patches and plaques on her dorsal feet and soles with linear patches corresponding to sites of shoe contact. The eruption began 14 months earlier while she was on vacation and had persisted chronically since then. She was initially treated by her family physician with topical antifungals and topical and systemic corticosteroids with some improvement. A dermatologist diagnosed shoe dermatitis and suggested referral to a center for patch testing. She has a history of allergic rhinitis but no personal or family history of eczema.

■ **Patch testing:** The patient was patch tested with the standard tray and pieces of her shoes and had positive reactions to: thiuram mix (1+), *p*-tertbutylphenol formaldehyde resin (2+), mixed di-alkylthioureas (2+), ethyl acrylate (1+) and methyl methacrylate (1+); additionally she had 1+ to 2+ reactions to pieces of insole and inner foam and other materials from five different pairs of her everyday shoes. She was patch test negative only to pieces of *Think* shoes.

■ **Diagnosis:** Allergic contact dermatitis to neoprene, neoprene adhesives and rubber. The reactions to the shoe components were relevant to the three main allergen groups; she had previously reacted to leather watch bands, foam rubber, foam rubber ear phones as well as her shoes.

■ **Treatment and course:** She was given information on alternative special order shoes without the allergens. Follow-up information 4 months later revealed that she had remained clear by wearing the patch-test-negative *Think* shoes; she also sent her patch test results to several other shoe manufacturers that she identified from the internet and successfully wears these alternative shoes.

■ **Comment:** Prior to patch testing the patient thought that she was allergic to chrome tanned leather. Trial and error changes in shoes along with topical and systemic therapy did not clear her dermatitis. Patch testing allowed her to identify the specific chemicals and shoes to which she was allergic and remain clear of the eruption.

Suggested Reading

1. Calnan CD, Sarkany L (1959) Studies in contact dermatitis: IX. Shoe dermatitis. Tran St John Hosp Derm Soc 43:8–26
   This classic article reviews the shoe dermatitis literature to 1959 and reports the demographics, clinical findings and patch test results from 102 cases of shoe dermatitis seen at the St Johns Hospital for Skin Diseases in London. Shoe allergy occurred in all age groups, was three times more common in women and primarily affected the dorsal feet and toes and anterior soles. Rubber allergy occurred in one-third of cases and leather allergy in two-thirds, with specific allergens often unknown; chromate allergy was uncommon. In addition to patch testing with a small shoe chemical series, the necessity of patch testing with pieces of every shoe warn by the patient is emphasized. Many leather-sensitive patients were able to remain clear of dermatitis by wearing the patch-test-negative shoes.
   This report emphasizes the need to patch test with shoe pieces in order to adequately diagnose and manage shoe allergy and still holds true today and is also emphasized in other "classic" articles on shoe contact allergy [3,75].
2. Freeman S (1997) Shoe dermatitis. Contact Dermatitis 36:247–251
   Follow-up study of 55 cases of shoe allergy published 36 years after the Calnan article [76] emphasizes the chronic disabling nature of shoe allergy, the frequent delay before patch testing is performed, the value of testing standard tray allergens in identifying cases and the absolute necessity of testing with shoe pieces. Follow-up showed that 87.5% of cases improved or resolved completely and most patients were able to find alternative shoes.
   This follow-up study shows that shoe allergy has a good prognosis with careful history and patch testing with the standard screening tray and shoe pieces as well as success in obtaining shoe substitutes.
3. Jung JH, McLaughlin JL, Stannard J, Guin JD (1988) Isolation, via activity-directed fractionation, of mercaptobenzothiazole and dibenzothiazyl disulfide as 2 allergens responsible for tennis shoe dermatitis. Contact Dermatitis 19:254–259
   This article emphasizes the fact that the causative allergen is frequently not known in shoe allergy cases. Reliance cannot always be placed on results of the standard screening tray because such testing may be negative. Even when positive the relevance of the positive screening tests is often unknown since the allergen is almost never extracted from the patient's shoes. Testing with shoe pieces is often positive but the specific allergen is usually never identified. Industrial-grade chemicals may contain contaminants and new allergens may be created via oxidation or other chemical reactions. A case of dermatitis to a tennis shoe insole was studied further by isolating and identifying the causative allergens by step-by-step patch test monitoring of the active fractions obtained by chromatographic separation.
   This is one of the first articles to identify and clarify the allergens in a case of shoe allergy by chemical analysis of the incriminated shoe piece. Since the chemical composition of many shoes is essentially unknown, studies of this type may be the only way to identify shoe allergens in the future.

References

1. van Coevorden AM, Coenraads PJ, Pas HH, van der Valk PG (2002) Contact allergens in shoe leather among patients with foot eczema. Contact Dermatitis 46:145–148
2. Trattner A, Farchi Y, David M (2003) Shoe contact dermatitis in Israel. Am J Contact Dermat 14:12–14
3. Freeman S (1997) Shoe dermatitis. Contact Dermatitis 36:247–251
4. Roul S, Ducombs G, Leaute-Labrege C (1996) Footwear contact dermatitis in children. Contact Dermatitis 34:334–336
5. Cronin E (1966) Shoe dermatitis. Br J Dermatol 78:617–625
6. Cockayne SE, Shok M, Messinger AG (1998) Foot dermatitis in children: causative allergens and followup. Contact Dermatitis 38:203–206
7. Shackelford KE, Belsito DV (2002) The etiology of allergic-appearing foot dermatitis: A 5-year retrospective study. J Am Acad Dermatol 47:715–721
8. Guenst BJ (1999) Common pediatric foot dermatoses. J Pediatr Health Care 13:68–71
9. Lynde CW, Warshawski L, Mitchell JC (1982) Patch test results with a shoe wear screening tray in 119 patients (1977–1980). Contact Dermatitis 8:423–425
10. Saha M, Srinivas CR, Shenoy SD (1993) Footwear dermatitis. Contact Dermatitis 28:260–264
11. Storrs FJ (1986). Dermatitis from clothing and shoes. In: Fisher AA (ed) Contact dermatitis. Lea and Febiger, Philadelphia, Pa., pp 283–337
12. Rani Z, Hussain I, Haroon TS (2003) Common allergens in shoe dermatitis: our experience in Lahore, Pakistan. Int J Dermatol 42:605–607
13. Strauss RM, Wilkinson SM (2002) Shoe dermatitis due to colophonium used as leather tanning or finishing agent in Portuguese shoes. Contact Dermatitis 47:59
14. Chen HH, Sun CC, Tseng MP (2004) Type IV hypersensitivity from rubber chemicals: a 15-year experience in Taiwan. Dermatology 208:319–325
15. Belsito DV (2004) Patch testing with a standard allergen ("screening") tray: rewards and risks. Derm Ther 17:231–239
16. Romaguera C, Vilaplana J (1998) Contact dermatitis in children: 6 years experience (1992–1997). Contact Dermatitis 39:277–280
17. Goossens A, Bedert R, Zimerson E (2001) Allergic contact dermatitis caused by nickel and cobalt in green plastic shoes. Contact Dermatitis 45:172
18. Shoe contact dermatitis (2001) In: Rietschel RL, Fowler JF Jr (eds) Fisher's contact dermatitis. Lippincott Williams and Wilkins, Philadelphia, Pa., pp 305–319
19. Oumeish OY, Parish LC (2002) Marching in the army: common cutaneous disorders of the feet. Clin Dermatol 20:445–451
20. Brooks C, Kujawska A, Patel D (2003) Cutaneous allergic reactions induced by sporting activities. Sports Med 33:699–708
21. Metelitsa A, Barankin B, Lin AN (2004) Diagnosis of sports-related dermatoses. Int J Dermatol 43:113–119
22. Belsito DV (2003) Common shoe allergens undetected by commercial patch-testing kits: dithiodimorpholine and isocyanates. Am J Contact Dermat 14:95–96
23. Hansen MB, Johansen JD, Menne T (2003) Chromium allergy: significance of both Cr(III) and Cr(VI). Contact Dermatitis 49:206–612
24. Wolf R, Orion E, Matz H (2002) Contact dermatitis in military personnel. Clin Dermatol 20:439–444
25. Fishman TD (2000) Wound assessment and evaluation. Dermatol Nurs 12:194–195
26. Podmore P (1995) Shoes. In: Rycroft RJG et al (eds) Textbook of contact dermatitis. Springer, Berlin Heidelberg New York, pp 516–526
27. Rietschel RL (1984) Role of socks in shoe dermatitis. Arch Dermatol 120:398
28. Maibach H (1984) Panty hose dermatitis resembling and complicating tinea pedis. Contact Dermatitis 1:329

29. Saha M, Srinivas CR, Shenoy SD (1993) Sensitivity to topical medicaments among suspected cases of footwear dermatitis. Contact Dermatitis 28:44–45
30. Saha M, Srinivas CR (1993) Footwear dermatitis possibly due to para-phenylenediamine in socks. Contact Dermatitis 28:295
31. Giusti F, Massone F, Bertoni L, Pellacani G, Seidenari S (2000) Contact sensitization to disperse dyes in children. Pediatr Dermatol 20:393–297
32. Wilkinson SM, Thomson KF (2000) Foot dermatitis due to non-disperse azo dyes. Contact Dermatitis 42:162–163
33. Lear JT, English JS (1996) Hand involvement in allergic contact dermatitis from mercaptobenzothiazole in shoes. Contact Dermatitis 34:432
34. Li LF, Wang J (2002) Contact hypersensitivity in hand dermatitis. Contact Dermatitis 47:206–209
35. Warshaw EM (2004) Therapeutic options for chronic hand dermatitis. Derm Ther 17:240–250
36. Calnan CD, Peachey RDG (1972) Allergic contact purpura. Clin Allergy 1:287
37. Zaitz ID, Proenca NG, Broste D (1987) Achromatizing contact dermatitis caused by rubber sandals (Portuguese). Medicina Cutanea Ibero-Latino-Americana 15:1–7
38. Pandhi KK, Kumar AS (1985) Contact leukoderma due to "Bindi" and footwear. Dermatologica 170:260–262
39. Bajaj AK, Supta SC, Challerjee AK (1996) Footwear depigmentation. Contact Dermatitis 35:117–118
40. Koch P (2001) Occupational contact dermatitis. Recognition and management. Am J Clin Dermatol 2:353–265
41. Rutland FH (1991) Environmental compatibility of chromium-containing tannery and other leather product wastes at land disposal sites. J Am Leather Chemists Assoc 86:364–375
42. Long AJ, Corey NJ, Wood CB (2000) Potential chemical mechanisms causing false positive results in hexavalent chromium determinations. J Soc Leather Technol Chemists 84:74–78
43. Corey NJ (2002) An update on environmental constraints. J Am Leather Chemists Assoc 97:496–505
44. Directive 2002/61/EC of the European Parliament and of the Council of 19 July 2002. Official Journal of the European Communities 11/9/2002 L243:15–18
45. Adminis U, Huynh C, Money CA (2002) The need for improved fungicides for wet-blue. J Soc Leather Technol Chemists 86:118–121
46. Harvey AJ (1983) Footwear materials and process technology. LASRA (New Zealand Leather and Shoe Research Association), Palmerston North, New Zealand, pp 257
47. Podmore P (1995) Shoes. In: Guin JD (ed) Practical contact dermatitis. McGraw-Hill, New York, pp 325–332
48. Aye M, Masson EA (2002) Dermatological care of the diabetic foot. Am J Clin Dermatol 3:463–74
49. Lammintausta K, Kalimi K (1995) Sensitivity to rubber. Study with rubber mixes and individual rubber chemicals. Dermatosen 33:204–208
50. Fogh A, Pock-Steen B (1992) Contact sensitivity to thiuram in wooden shoes. Contact Dermatitis 27:348
51. Kaniwa MA, Jsoma K, Nakomura O et al (1994) Identification of causative chemicals of allergic contact dermatitis using a combination of patch testing in patients and chemical analysis. Application to cases from rubber footwear. Contact Dermatitis 30:26–34
52. Roberts JL, Hanifin JM (1979) Athletic shoe dermatitis, contact allergy to ethylbutylthiourea. J Am Med Assoc 241:275–276
53. Roberts JL, Hanifin JM (1980) Contact allergy and cross-reactivity to substituted thiourea compounds. Contact Dermatitis 6:138–139
54. Cronin E (1980) Contact dermatitis. Churchill Livingstone, Edinburgh, p 738
55. Malten K, Seutter E (1985) Allergic degradation products of paratertiary butyl phenol for formaldehyde plastic. Contact Dermatitis 12:222–224
56. Malten KE, Roth R, Pastors PH (1983) Paratertiary butyl phenol formaldehyde and other causes of shoe dermatitis. Derm Beruf Umwelt 31:149–153
57. Malten KE (1967) Contact sensitizations caused by paratertiary butyl phenol and certain phenol formaldehyde-containing glues. Dermatologica 135:541–549
58. Lyon CC, Tucker SC, Gafvert E, Karlberg AT, Beck MH (1999) Contact dermatitis from modified rosin in footwear. Contact Dermatitis 41:102–103
59. Huygens S, Barbaud A, Goossens A (2001) Frequency and relevance of positive patch tests to cyclohexylthiophthalimide, a new rubber allergen. Eur J Dermatol 11:443–445
60. Devos SA, Van Der Valk PG (2001) The risk of active sensitization to PPD. Contact Dermatitis 44:273–275
61. Hartmann K, Hunzelmann N (2004) Allergic contact dermatitis from cinnamon as an odour-neutralizing agent in shoe insoles. Contact Dermatitis 50:253–254
62. Mancuso G, Reggiani M, Berdonidini RM (1996) Occupational contact dermatitis in shoemakers. Contact Dermatitis 34:17–22
63. Bruze M, Bjoskner B, Lepoittevin JP (1995) Occupational allergic contact dermatitis from ethyl cyanoacrylate. Contact Dermatitis 32:156–159
64. Ayadi M, Martin P (1999) Pulpitis of the fingers from a shoe glue containing 1,2-benzisothiazolin-3-one (BIT). Contact Dermatitis 40:115–116
65. Vidovic R, Kansky A (1985) Contact dermatitis in workers processing polyvinyl chloride. Derm Beruf Umwelt 33:104–105
66. Henschel R, Agathos M, Breit R (2002) Occupational contact dermatitis from propolis. Contact Dermatitis 47:52
67. Machado S, Silva E, Sanches M, Massa A (2003) Occupational airborne contact dermatitis. Am J Contact Dermat 14:31–32
68. Adams RM (1990) Shoe repairers. In: Adams RM (ed) Occupational skin disease. WB Saunders, Philadelphia, Pa., pp 662–663
69. White IR (1990) PTBP resins. In: Adams RM (ed) Occupational skin disease. WB Saunders, Philadelphia, Pa., pp 402–403
70. Taylor JS (1986) Rubber. In: Fisher AA (ed) Contact dermatitis. Lea and Febiger, Philadelphia, Pa., pp 603–643
71. Dooms-Goossens A et al (1987) Shoe dermatitis. Boll Dermatol Allergol Profess 2:120–126
72. Grimalt F, Romaguera C (1975) New resin allergens in shoe contact dermatitis. Contact Dermatitis 1:169–174
73. Jelen G, Cavelier C, Protois JP (1989) A new allergen responsible for shoe allergy: chloracetamide. Contact Dermatitis 21:110–111
74. Lynch PJ (1969) Indian sandal strap dermatitis. J Am Med Assoc 209:1906
75. Epstein E (1969) Shoe contact dermatitis. J Am Med Assoc 209:1487–1492
76. Calnan CD, Sarkany L (1959) Studies in contact dermatitis: IX. Shoe dermatitis. Tran St John Hosp Derm Soc 43:8–26
77. Jordan WP (1972) Clothing and shoe dermatitis. Postgrad Med 52:143
78. Bruze M et al (1992) Patch testing with ultrasonic bath extracts. Am J Contact Dermatitis 3:133–137
79. Jung JH, McLaughlin JL, Stannard J, Guin JD (1988) Isolation, via activity-directed fractionation, of mercaptobenzothiazole and dibenzothiazyl disulfide as 2 allergens responsible for tennis shoe dermatitis. Contact Dermatitis 19:254–259
80. Nishioka K et al (1996) Contact dermatitis due to rubber boots worn by Japanese farmers, with special attention to 6-ethoxy-2,2,4-trimethyl-1,2-dihydroquinoline (ETMDQ) sensitivity. Contact Dermatitis 35:241–245
81. Koch P, Nickolaus G (1996) Allergic contact dermatitis and mercury exanthem due to mercury chloride in plastic boots. Contact Dermatitis 34:405–409
82. Emmett EA, Risby TH, Taylor JS (1994) Skin elicitation threshold of ethylbutylthiourea and mercaptobenzothiazole with relative leaching from sensitizing products (published erratum appears in Contact Dermatitis 1994, 31:208). Contact Dermatitis 30:85–90
83. Opie J, Lee A, Frowen K, Fewings J, Nixon R (2003) Foot dermatitis caused by the textile dye Basic Red 46 in acrylic blend socks. Contact Dermatitis 49:297–303
84. Steck WD (1983) Juvenile plantar dermatosis: the "wet and dry foot syndrome". Cleve Clin Q 50:145–149
85. Downs AM, Sansom JE (1999) Severe contact allergy to footwear responding to handmade shoes. Contact Dermatitis 40:218

38

Chapter 39

Occupational Contact Dermatitis **39**

Richard J.G. Rycroft, Peter J. Frosch

Contents

39.1 Introduction

In different ways, occupational contact dermatitis impacts heavily on the working lives of dermatologists, as well as on those of their patients. The clinician should keep in mind the leading role that work plays in people's lives. Patients with occupational contact dermatitis naturally want their dermatitis to be cleared, without their livelihood being lost at the same time [1]. The reduction in the quality of life may be considerable, particularly in severe chronic cases. This is now an area of active research [2–5].

39.2 Definition and Links

A broad definition of occupational contact dermatitis is contact dermatitis due wholly or partly to the patient's occupation. Occupation must be a major factor in stricter definitions, and is essential to causation in a still stricter sense, i.e., an occupational contact dermatitis is a contact dermatitis that would not have occurred if the patient had not been doing the work of that occupation [1]. These medical definitions may deviate considerably from legal definitions, which are the basis for workers' compensation claims (Chap. 46).

Occupational contact dermatitis constitutes over 90% of the wider spectrum of occupational dermatoses [6], with the remainder including contact urticaria, oil folliculitis (oil acne), chloracne, leukoderma, scleroderma-like disease, ulceration (Fig. 1), bacterial, viral, and mycotic infections, as well as epidermal neoplasia [7, 8]. Some substances that cause occupational contact dermatitis also cause other occupational disorders, including: asthma, for example, colophonium [9]; eye irritation, for example, formaldehyde; anosmia, for example, hexavalent chromium; paresthesia, for example, methyl methacrylate; and psychiatric disturbance, for example, organotins.

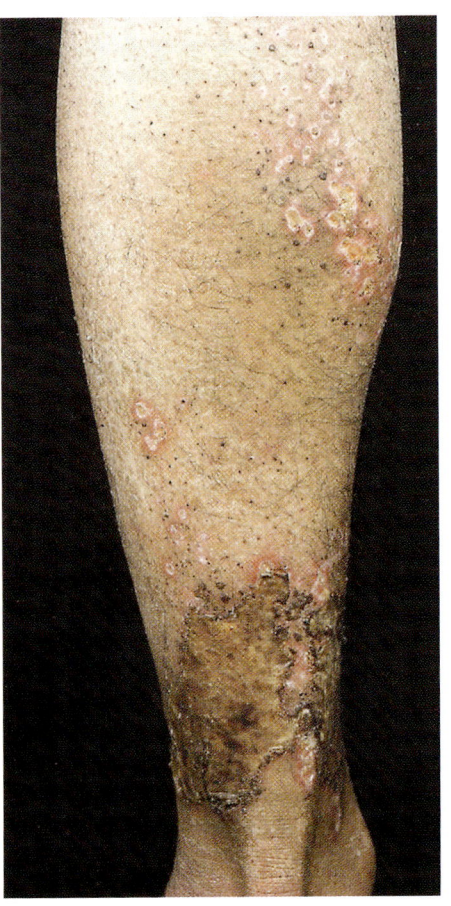

Fig. 1. Cement ulceration (cement burns) from acute occlusion of wet cement (courtesy of St. John's Institute of Dermatology)

39.3　History

The history of modern occupational contact dermatitis began in 1915, with the publication of Prosser White's *The Dermatergoses or Occupational Affections of the Skin* (England), with further impetus being provided in 1939 by Poul Bonnevie's *Aetiologie und Pathogenese der Ekzemkrankheiten* (Denmark) and Louis Schwartz, Louis Tulipan, and Samuel M. Peck's *Occupational Diseases of the Skin* (USA).

Charles Calnan recorded [10] how it was Professor Hageman at the University of Lund in Southern Sweden who gave Sigfrid Fregert the opportunity to make Europe the focus of occupational contact dermatitis over the past 35 years [11], the late Niels Hjorth [12], Helmut Ippen [13], and Veikko Pirilä [14] all striving, among others, to maintain this impetus. Robert Adams [7] in the USA, and Jean Foussereau [15] and Eberhard Zschunke [16] in Europe are the authors of major contemporary texts. Recently, an atlas was also published [17].

39.4　Epidemiology

Coenraads et al. (Chap. 10) and other authors elsewhere in this textbook suggest an incidence of occupational skin disease of 0.5–1.9 cases per 1,000 full-time workers per year. The highest incidence rates are seen in hairdressers (97/10,000 per year), followed by bakers (33/10,000), and florists (24/10,000) [2, 18, 19]. These authors also consider that prevalence studies suggest that age and sex are not risk factors in themselves, but that they are associated instead with different exposures. Evidence remains that black skin tends to be more resistant to contact dermatitis than white [20].

39.5　Etiology

Irritant contact dermatitis remains generally more common occupationally than allergic contact dermatitis, though the more patients who are patch tested, the greater the proportion of allergic contact dermatitis tends to become [11, 21] (Fig. 2). As irritation facilitates the induction of contact allergy [22], many cases of occupational contact dermatitis are likely to be of mixed irritant and allergic etiology (Fig. 3).

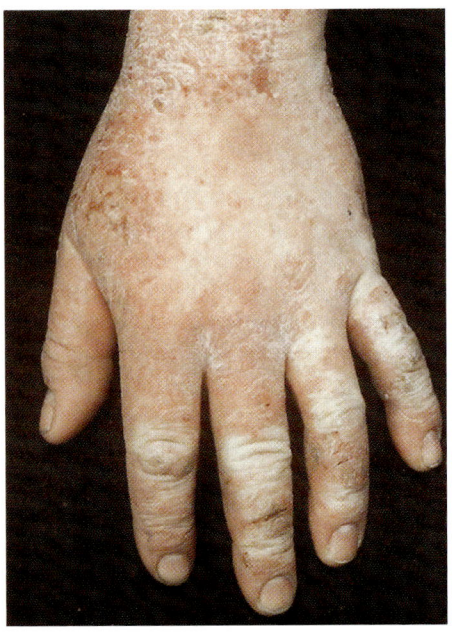

Fig. 2. Allergic contact dermatitis from chromate in cement (courtesy of St. John's Institute of Dermatology)

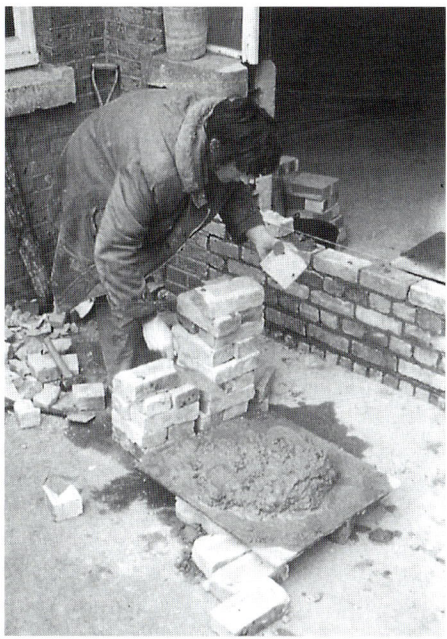

Fig. 3. A bricklayer's apprentice encountering the irritant and allergic risks from cement

The principal occupational contact irritants are:

- Water
- Soaps and detergents
- Alkalis
- Acids
- Metalworking fluids
- Organic solvents
- Other petroleum products
- Oxidizing agents
- Reducing agents
- Animal products
- Physical factors

The wide individual variation in susceptibility to chronic irritant contact dermatitis is gradually becoming better understood. Past or present atopic eczema at least doubles the risk of irritant contact dermatitis of the hands in occupations such as those listed above [23, 24]. A nonatopic genetic marker, involving a tumor necrosis factor (TNF) α polymorphism, has recently been identified as being linked to irritant susceptibility [25] (see also Chaps. 4 and 9).

39.5.1 Irritants

Irritancy in general is covered in Chaps. 4 and 15. The common high-risk occupations for irritant contact dermatitis are:

- Baker
- Butcher
- Caterer
- Cleaner
- Construction worker
- Dental technician
- Florist
- Food producer
- Hairdresser
- Healthcare worker
- Homemaker
- Horticulturist
- Masseur/masseuse
- Metalworker
- Motor mechanic
- Nurse
- Painter
- Printer
- Tiler

39.5.2 Allergens

Common high-risk occupations for allergic contact dermatitis are:

- Adhesives/sealants/resins/plastics worker
- Agriculturalist
- Cement caster
- Construction worker
- Dental technician
- Florist
- Glass worker
- Graphics worker
- Hairdresser and barber
- Horticulturist
- Leather tanner
- Painter
- Pharmaceutical/chemical worker
- Rubber worker
- Textile worker
- Tiler and terrazzo-maker
- Woodworker

The principal occupational contact allergens are:

- Biocides (including isothiazolinones)
- Chromate (cobalt)
- Dyes

- Epoxy resin systems
- Essences and fragrances
- Formaldehyde
- Formaldehyde resins
- (Meth)acrylates
- Nickel (primarily usually nonoccupational)
- Plants and woods
- Rubber-processing chemicals

See also Fig. 4. Atopics do not appear to incur a generally increased risk of allergic contact dermatitis

along with their increased risk of irritant contact dermatitis (see also Chap. 9).

39.6 Clinical Features

The hands are, clearly, by far the most likely primary site of occupational contact dermatitis. Airborne (or exposure-pattern) contact dermatitis is also commonly occupational [26]. Rarer presentations, such as fingernail dystrophies unaccompanied by fingertip dermatitis, are more easily missed [27] (Fig. 5).

Fig. 4.
Allergic contact dermatitis from epoxy resin in a spray paint (courtesy of St. John's Institute of Dermatology)

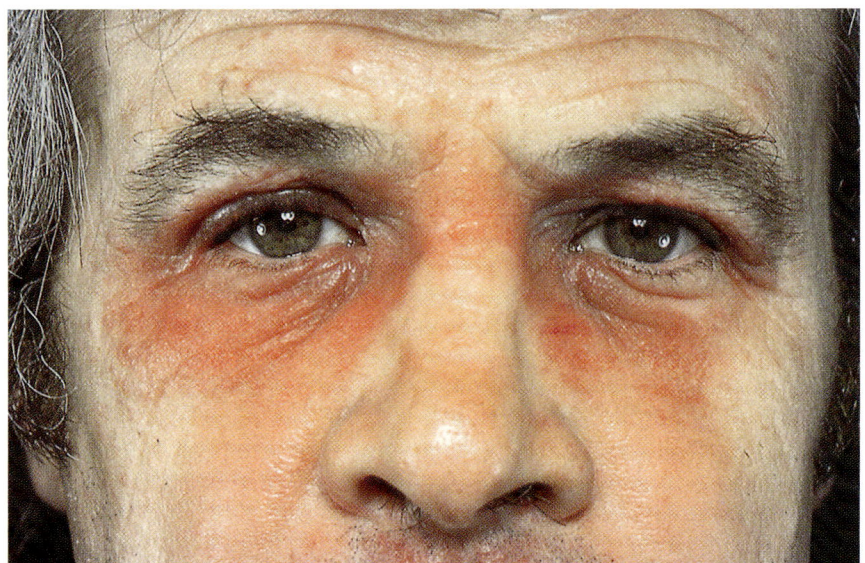

39

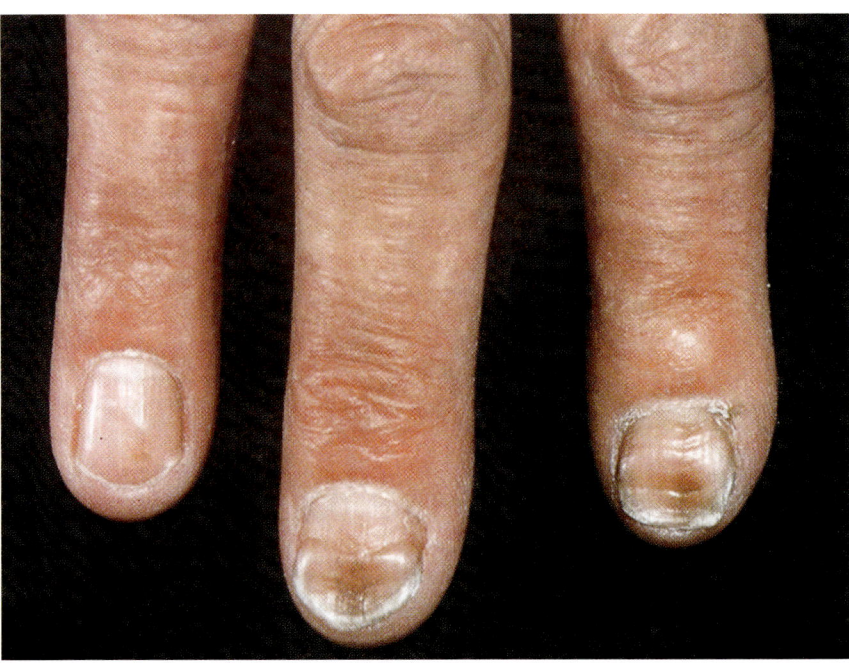

Fig. 5.
Koilonychia from dipping a (gloved) hand into organic solvent (carbitol) (courtesy of St. John's Institute of Dermatology)

39.7 Prognosis

The prognosis of occupational contact dermatitis severe enough to be referred to a specialist dermatologist is one of persistence in more than half of all cases, though with improvement in more than half of these [11, 28, 29]. This applies to irritant as well as to allergic contact dermatitis. Appropriate occupational changes improve the prognosis for most patients, but around 10% of such severe patients develop persistent post-occupational dermatitis [28].

However, many cases less severe than those referred to specialist dermatologists have a much better prognosis. And even in severe cases, dermatitis may become more manageable after thorough investigation and adequate treatment [30]. Improved patient education, via a specially trained nurse, has been shown to improve prognosis [31]. Reasons for the persistence of contact dermatitis, particularly occupational hand dermatitis, are discussed by Hogan et al. [32], who admit that this often remains unexplained.

39.8 Diagnosis

39.8.1 Clinical

Taking the history of a case is a clinical skill requiring adaptation to the individual patient, but every history is based on certain essential facts.

- Time of onset. This is frequently initially set aside by the patient and replaced by the time of onset of the eventual exacerbation that led them to seek medical advice, which may be many months later [11].
- Primary site. The hands or exposed skin favor occupational causation, rather than covered areas of the trunk or feet.
- Secondary spread. Distant spread to the feet or face is more common in allergic than in irritant occupational contact dermatitis [33].
- Occupation. The following are required: the type, the length of time in it, and the precise tasks involved.

There are some particularly useful additional facts to establish:

- Work relatedness. Occupational contact dermatitis initially shows greater and more consistent improvement away from work than nonoccupational dermatitis, though with chronicity such work relatedness may become less clear. Allergic occupational contact dermatitis tends to worsen more rapidly than irritant dermatitis on return to work.
- Prevention. The effects of gloves, other personal protective equipment, or skin care products may help to confirm occupational causation or point to a secondary contact factor.
- Other cases. Involvement of fellow workers (and in what proportion) increases the probability of occupational contact dermatitis (-with larger proportions favoring irritant rather than allergic).

39.8.2 Patch Tests

A standard series is rarely sufficient in occupational cases, and its supplementation with additional series (Table 1) and patients' own samples is frequently required. De Groot's systematic handbook is recommended for readily accessible guidance on appropriate patch test dilutions of individual chemicals [34]. While there is no substitute for practical training and experience in patch testing patients' own samples, certain guidelines are given later in the section on individual occupations (see also Chaps. 49 and 50).

Although not sufficient, the standard series still detects many case of occupational skin diseases, as a

Table 1. Commercially available additional series useful in suspected occupational cases

Series	Supplier[a,b]
Bakery	C
Dental	C,H
Epoxy	C,H
Hairdressing	C,H
Industrial biocides	H
Isocyanates	C
Metal compounds	H
(Meth)acrylate	C
Adhesives, dental, and other	C
Printing	C
Metalworking/oil and cooling fluid	C,H
Photographic chemicals	C,H
Plant	C, H
Rubber additives	C, H
Plastics and glues	C,H
Shoe	C
Textile colors and finishes	C,H

[a] C Chemotechnique Diagnostics, PO Box 80, Edvard Ols väg 2, S-230 42 Tygelsjö, Malmö, Sweden (and national distributors)
[b] H Hermal, D-21465 Reinbek, Germany (and national distributors)

recent evaluation on 4,112 patients reported to health authorities in Northern Bavaria (Germany) shows [35]. Nickel sulfate was the most common sensitizer (29.5%) but had an occupational relevance in only 11% of the cases sensitized. The most occupationally relevant sensitizers were thiuram mix (71%), epoxy resin (67%), PPD free base (59%), PPD black rubber mix/IPPD (53%), potassium dichromate (48%), formaldehyde (38%), chloromethylisothiazolinone/ methylisothiazolinone (37%), and mercapto mix/ mercaptobenzothiazole (35%). Occupational groups at risk of acquiring delayed-type sensitizations were, in particular, electroplaters, tile setters/terrazzo workers, construction and cement workers, solderers, wood processors, and leather industry and fur processors.

39.8.3 Other Tests

Tests for immediate hypersensitivity are described in Chap. 26. Simple chemical tests for the identification of special allergens are described in Chap. 25.

More advanced chemical methods of analysis, such as high-performance liquid chromatography and gas chromatography–mass spectrometry, have contributed greatly to our knowledge of the allergenic fractions of occupational sensitizers, including phenol-formaldehyde resin [36], colophonium [37], D-limonene [38], and the tulip [39]. Dermal exposure assessment techniques [40] to measure the degree of skin contamination have been made more accurate by the further development of video imaging of fluorescent tracers [41]. Recently, a new method for assessing dermal exposure to permanent hair dyes has been described [42].

39.8.4 Workplace Visits

When Fregert et al. were pioneering the practice of occupational dermatology in Southern Sweden, they "soon found that the opportunity of visiting working-places and factories was a requisite for adequate solving of problems of occupational dermatology" [43].

The information useful to be acquired from workplace visits is detailed in Table 2, and the benefits to be gained are listed in Table 3. Similar principles apply to telephoning, faxing, e-mailing, or writing to medical, nursing, employer, or employee representatives. But the answer obtained to a question posed in this way depends greatly on who is asked, whereas trained direct observation is more likely to be accurate (Fig. 6).

Table 2. Information useful to be acquired from workplace visits

Information	Details
Organizational	Name, address (including postal code), telephone and fax numbers, and e-mail address of workplace
	Name and status of all medical, nursing, employer, and employee representatives questioned
Demographic	Numbers employed overall and in the patient's work area
	Current expansion, contraction, and turnover
	Shift pattern and pay scheme
Technical	Broad concept of process as a whole
	Detailed understanding of work carried out by patient and in patient's work area, including all potential irritants and allergens observed and their degree and extent of skin contact
	Names, addresses, telephone and fax numbers, and e-mail addresses of suppliers of materials requiring further identification
Preventive	Broad impression of working conditions (space, lighting, ventilation)
	More detailed review of protective installations, personal protective equipment, skin care products, and education
	Assessment of actual uptake and effectiveness of above
Miscellaneous	Industrial relations, psychological, sociological, and economic factors
	Comparison with sister factory
Clinical	Skin complaints in employees other than the patient
	Their clinical assessment and subdivision into occupational and non-occupational (often provisional)
Epidemiological	Frequency of skin complaints as a proportion of the total number exposed
	Estimate of frequency of occupational dermatoses
Etiological	Opinions of others, with attribution as to source and estimate of reliability
	Own opinion, with grounds for it (may be inconclusive)
Operational	Summary of findings
	Recommendations for future investigation, management, and review
	Follow-up

39

Table 3. Benefits of visiting workplace

Benefits	Reference
Detection of relevance of previously unexplained positive standard patch test reactions	
Detection of missed allergen	[140]
Substantiation of diagnosis of irritant contact dermatitis	
Diagnosis of slight or unfamiliar occupational dermatoses	[120, 140, 141]
Substantiation that various non-occupational dermatoses have been grouped together as a pseudo-occupational dermatosis and why	[142]
Recognition of phenomenon of visible dermatoses, whether occupational or not, causing anxiety and subconsciously imitative symptoms in fellow employees	[141]
Initiation of research on new occupational dermatoses	
Incidental effects, such as improved dermatologist–occupational physician and dermatologist–patient relationships	
Progressive increase in dermatologist's overall knowledge of patients' working contactants	

39.8.5 Epidemiological Surveys

An epidemiological survey of dermatoses within a work area may be needed when the clinical assessment of individual patients fails to delineate an occupational dermatosis clearly enough. Such surveys should always be planned with epidemiological and statistical advice from the very beginning, since this may affect the fundamental design of the study. Coenraads et al. have identified the crucial concepts to be understood in Chap. 10.

Core Message

■ Occupational contact dermatitis is the most frequent cause of occupational skin diseases. It has a major socioeconomic impact. Affected persons often experience severe impairment in the quality of life. The ratio of irritant to allergic contact dermatitis varies considerably among occupations, and depends also on the experience and diagnostic thoroughness of the examining dermatologist.

39.9 Treatment

The treatment of occupational contact dermatitis is founded on accurate diagnosis and subsequent partial or complete separation of the patient from the cause. Besides the treatment principles outlined for contact dermatitis generally in Chap. 44, there are some that are specific for occupational cases.

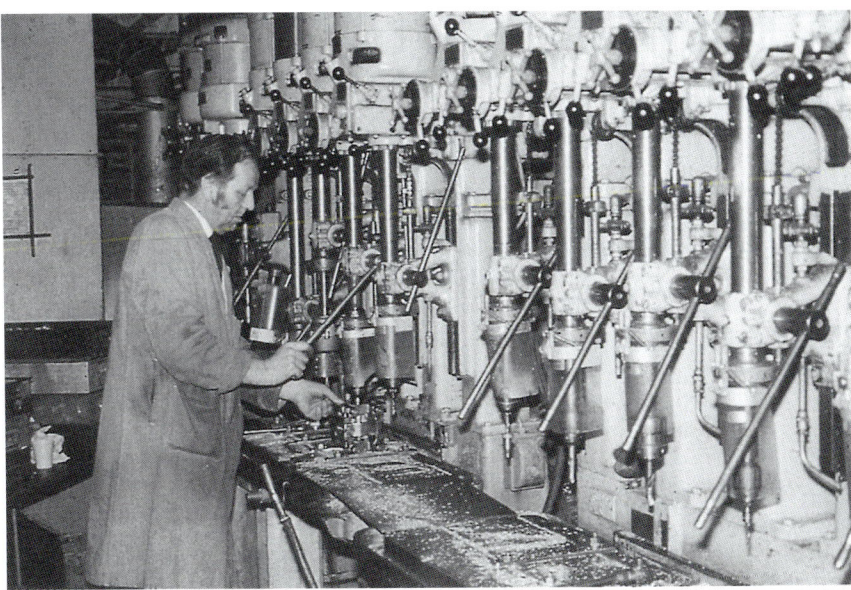

Fig. 6.
Direct observation of machine operators may be needed to explain their dermatitis

39.9.1 Acute

Initial absence from work should be restricted to that required for adequate, rather than necessarily complete, recovery if the resulting disability is to be minimized [1]. In large companies, a temporary transfer to alternative duties allows an early but safe return to work.

39.9.2 Chronic

With certain exceptions, as indicated below, the primary aim of managing the chronic case of occupational contact dermatitis is to return the patient to his or her original job. If this cannot be achieved, the emphasis should then shift to appropriate retraining and redeployment, rather than to lump-sum compensation payment and medical retirement [44].

The first exception to attempting to return patients to their original job is in cases of isolated uncomplicated allergic contact dermatitis from substances such as epoxy resin, biocides, other specific chemicals, or plant allergens. A rapid and permanent change of occupation in such cases usually results in complete clearance, and no change of occupation in almost certain chronicity.

The second such exception is in certain types of wet work, where there is evidence of an increased susceptibility to irritation in those with sensitive skins (see Sect. 39.5.1, Irritants). The prognosis for such individuals tends to be bad, even after a change of occupation, but it is made so much worse by continuation in the same job – for example, catering, hairdressing, and metalworking – that the only realistic option is early redeployment.

In all chronic cases of hand dermatitis, the acquisition of secondary contact allergies to ingredients of skin care products or medicaments must be kept in mind (fragrances, preservatives, rubber allergens, corticosteroids; [45] and Chap. 19).

In hairdressers and other high-risk occupations, the value of teaching programs regarding the avoidance of irritants and allergens as well as the regular use of adequate skin protection and application of skin care products has been well documented (Chap. 44, Sect. 44.3). Chronicity can, thus, often be avoided or minimized in order to keep the worker at his/her job. This is particularly important for employees who seem to be too old or intellectually unsuitable for a retraining procedure.

39.10 Prevention

Because of the poor prognosis associated with well-established occupational contact dermatitis (see Sect. 39.7, Prognosis), its prevention is of great importance (see also Chap. 44).

39.10.1 Pre-Employment Examination

Guidelines have been published on the pre-employment screening of prospective employees with skin disease [46]. Past or present skin atopy at least doubles the risk of irritant contact dermatitis of the hands in occupations such as those listed earlier [23]. Staphylococcal colonization of chronic occupational contact dermatitis may pose threats of cross-infection in health care and of food poisoning in catering [46]. "Rusters" (Fig. 7) should not work with ferrous metals, unless their hyperhidrosis can be successfully treated [47].

39.10.2 Skin Tests

Pre-employment patch testing with potential sensitizers should not be performed. Tests of irritant susceptibility are not yet robust enough for routine use.

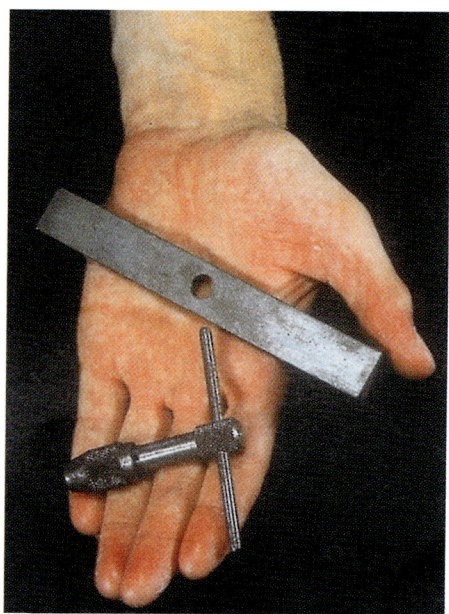

Fig. 7. The hyperhidrotic hand of a "ruster" and the ferrous metal handled by him (courtesy of St. John's Institute of Dermatology)

39

39.10.3 Occupational Hygiene

Substitution of irritants and allergens will always head the hierarchy of exposure controls [48]. Even "automated" processes continue to provide opportunities for skin contact [49], particularly for maintenance fitters (service engineers). Wearing gloves may be considered unsafe in the operation of rapidly rotating machinery.

39.10.4 Personal Hygiene

39.10.4.1 Personal Protective Equipment

Although extensive data are now available on the penetration of protective gloves and clothing by contactants [50], the prevention of contamination of the inside of gloves when putting them on and taking them off is often of even more importance. Detailed guidance as to the suitability of glove material is given in Chap. 44, Sect. 44.2. The actual protection provided depends not only on avoiding inadvertent contamination, but also on factors such as manufacturing quality, glove thickness, chemical concentration, duration of contact, and environmental temperature and humidity.

39.10.4.2 Barrier Creams

"Barrier" creams, in general, are realistically regarded as assisting in the prevention of contact dermatitis by their beneficial effects on the stratum corneum as moisturizers [51, 52], more than as barriers in their own right [53]. Skin care products with specific activities such as the chelation of nickel [54] or the inactivation of methylchloroisothiazolinone + methylisothiazolinone [55] may have a future role. Barrier creams may give weak irritant reactions on patch testing. True sensitization is rare. A critical update according to the criteria of evidence-based medicine has recently been published [56] (see also Chaps. 15 and 44).

39.10.5 Dermatitic Potential

Methods for assessing the irritant and allergic potential are reviewed in Chap. 12.

39.11 Medical Report

The demands on the dermatologist in the preparation of medical reports for compensation purposes vary from country to country. The items listed in Table 4 cover many of the areas requiring consideration for inclusion. It is helpful if medical terms not of common currency are explained as they occur.

> **Core Message**
>
> ■ The main goal in treatment and prevention is avoiding chronicity of the contact dermatitis. After a working diagnosis has been established, this goal can only be achieved by intensive cooperation with the patient and the employer. All contact irritants (chemical, thermal, mechanical) and contact allergens (workplace, skin care products, protective garments, etc.) must be evaluated as the cause or as contributory factors. Together with the employer and safety engineer, these factors must be scrutinized and, if possible, reduced or eliminated.

The worker's motivation and knowledge about his/her disease must be increased in training schools.

39.12 The Major Occupational Problem Areas

39.12.1 Agriculture

The wide variety of contactants in farming raises a large number of possible causes of occupational dermatitis. Irritant contact dermatitis (ICD) can be caused by milking equipment, cleansers, tractor and machinery fuels, chemical fertilizers, animal feed preservatives [57, 58], and pesticides. Allergic contact dermatitis (ACD) arises from: rubber chemicals, including N-isopropyl-N'-phenyl-p-phenylenediamine (IPPD), as well as thiurams, in milking equipment, lambing rings [59], boots and gloves; plants, including members of the Compositae family, more commonly than pesticides; antibiotics in animal feeds and veterinary use [60]; animal feed additives, such as cobalt, vitamin K_3, ethoxyquin, olaquindox [61], dinitolmide, and phenothiazines; and chromate in cement. Contact urticaria (CU)/protein contact dermatitis (PCD) may be caused by animal hair and dander [62, 63].

Table 4. Items to consider including in a medical report

Item	Notes
Qualifications	Sufficient detail to demonstrate expertise
Instructions	Sufficient detail to indicate purpose of report
Sources of information other than the patient	Previous medical records, previous medical reports, workplace inspections
Personal history	Atopy, other allergies, other dermatoses
Family history	Atopy, other allergies, other dermatoses
Occupational history	Job titles, employers, types of contact, dates
Present occupation	Job title, employer's name and full address, dates
Time in contact with suspected causal factors	May be shorter (or longer) time than time in present occupation
Description of the working process	Sufficient detail to give accurate assessment of degree and extent of skin contact, as well as range of skin contactants
Broader working background	Skin care products, personal protective equipment
	Other cases of dermatitis?
Time and site of initial skin complaint	Previous injury at initial site? To whom reported? What treatment given?
Progress, with approximate dates	Gradual/sudden exacerbations/improvements; influence of weekends, holidays, sickness absence; early on, later on
Degree of incapacity during course	Dates of absence from work; level of earnings before and after dermatosis
Changes in occupation since onset	Job titles, dates, details of changes in contactants
Treatment and its effectiveness	Patient may need to obtain details from attending physician
Clinical findings	Present state. Have lesions been suppressed by treatment?
Special investigations	Patch tests, prick tests, open tests, repeated open application tests (positive and negative results, times of readings, concentrations, vehicles, application method, site). Who performed and read such tests? Hematological/bacteriological/myco-logical test results
Intercurrent diseases	Mycotic infections, light eruptions, fever
Diagnosis/diagnoses	
Common knowledge of risk	Could the employer reasonably have been expected to have foreseen any risk to the skin?
Conclusions in terms understandable to non-medical readers	Probable connection between occupation and dermatosis: balanced against predisposing and contributory factors. Possibility of continuing in occupation: prospect of rehabilitation if required
	Probable medical prognosis (likelihood of relapse)
	Probable socioeconomic prognosis (capacity for work)

39

39.12.2 Arts and Crafts

Wet clay, plaster, and organic solvents are potential irritants. This remains one of the few areas of work where turpentine is a potential allergen [64]. Nickel, cobalt, and chromium can all be relevant allergens in pigments, together with colophonium and epoxy resin in the standard series. (Meth)Acrylates, formaldehyde resins, and polyurethane (diisocyanate) resins may all be used in modeling and repairs, requiring additional series to be tested. Azo and phthalocyanine dyes may be used in the creation of pigments [65].

39.12.3 Automotive and Aerospace Assembly and Maintenance

As in many other occupations, the difficulty the dermatologist has here is to identify the rarer cases of contact sensitization against a background of irritancy provided by mechanical wear and tear, light oils, degreasing solvents, and synthetic mineral fibers [66]. Chromate is particularly important because of its use as an anticorrosive [67]. As well as standard (DGEBA) epoxy resin, the aerospace industry uses nonstandard epoxies, such as triglycidyl-*p*-aminophenol (TGPAP) and tetraglycidyl-4,4′-methylenediamine (TGMDA), which cannot be relied upon to cross-react. (Meth)acrylates are widely used as sealants and threadlockers. Unsaturated polyester (UP) resin systems, widely used on automobiles, rarely cause contact dermatitis, and a commercial plastics and glues series is a reasonably good screen for sensitization to their additives (see also Chap. 34).

39.12.4 Baking and Patisserie

CU/PCD must be looked for as well as ICD and ACD. Automation has reduced exposure to dough in many larger bakers, but irritation from the degree of such contact still commonly occurs in smaller and specialist establishments. Cleaning the equipment and surfaces is another common source of irritancy. Spices and essences (cinnamon, cardamom) are important type-I as well as type-IV sensitizers, while flour [68] and flour improvers, such as α-amylase [69], can cause CU/PCD. Skin atopy is probably a significant risk factor in such work [70], where irritancy still seems to predominate over sensitization [71, 72].

39.12.5 Catering and Food Production

Cronin's [73] review remains an extremely good starting point when approaching this large group of workers: "Chefs and kitchen staff handle raw, moist food for many hours each day. The work is wet, they use detergents and cleansers, they rarely wear gloves, and the insult to their hands is considerable." Against this background of commonly occurring chronic ICD, both type-I (CU/PCD) and type-IV (ACD) sensitization require thorough investigation.

Garlic and onion (Alliaceae) are the most important foods to patch test with, their juices diluted to 50% in petrolatum, reducing the irritancy that they otherwise can cause. Diallyl disulfide is a useful additional test for garlic dermatitis, though it is not the only allergen in garlic [74]. Hardwood knife handles can sensitize and should be patch tested as fine scrapings. Compositae mix positives in food handlers with hand dermatitis have been interpreted as indicating lettuce allergy [75], which is, therefore, also important to patch test with as well as to prick test

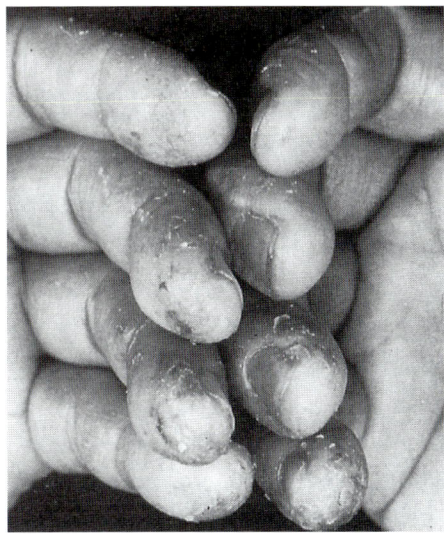

Fig. 8. Irritant catering workers' dermatitis, with heavy staphylococcal colonization (courtesy of St. John's Institute of Dermatology)

with as a known type-I sensitizer (the leaf, as is, is not irritant). Other particularly important foods to prick test with are fish and shellfish [76], cucumber, tomato, and potato [73]. Staphylococcal colonization of food handlers' hand dermatitis carries the public health risk of food poisoning [46] (Fig. 8).

39.12.6 Chemical and Pharmaceutical Production

Irritants and sensitizers are specific to each process and the dermatologist is often left with preparing cautious serial dilutions of unfamiliar chemicals. For example, they may often apply 0.1% and 0.01% initially, adding in 1% at the day-2 reading if 0.1% and 0.01% are negative. Halogenated chemical intermediates tend to be potent allergens. Many transient rashes, even if recurrent, turn out to be negative on both patch testing and prick testing, and are probably due to irritancy enhanced by local factors such as sweating and occlusion. Airborne ACD and erythema-multiforme-like eruptions in chemistry students from an aniline dye [77] and costus resinoid [78] have recently been observed.

39.12.7 Cleaning

Type-I and type-IV allergies to rubber gloves are the only major rivals to chronic ICD in this huge, mainly female, workforce [79]. The standard series can probably be relied on to detect most other contact allergens, such as biocides and fragrances, in cleaning products. D-Limonene, as a component of environmentally friendly cleaning agents, is a currently important exception to this [80]. The relevance of nickel is controversial [81, 82].

39.12.8 Construction, Tunneling, and Mining

The role of chromate in wet cement as the main cause of dermatitis in the construction industry has now disappeared in countries where cement has ferrous sulfate added to it [83], though not necessarily in others [84]. Chronic ICD can also occur from wet cement. Pneumatic drills can release irritant mineral oil and, under extreme winter conditions, ethylene glycol [85]. Machinery fuels and hydraulic oils are further sources of irritancy. The standard series can be relied on to detect the common sensitizations other than chromate, which are rubber processing chemicals (gloves *and* boots) and epoxy resin (flooring and civil engineering) [86].

39.12.9 Electrics and Electronics

This is one of the industries where itchy skin may be caused by low-humidity environments contrived to protect the product [87]. Automation diminishes many of the risks, but ICD can still arise from organic solvents and synthetic mineral fibers, chemical burns from hydrofluoric acid, and ACD from colophonium (rosin) in soldering flux (may be airborne) and epoxy resin and hardeners. Fiber optics manufacture involves UV-curing (meth)acrylates that the standard series would not detect (see Table 1).

39.12.10 Floristry and Horticulture

This group of workers is used to their hands showing wear-and-tear from tasks such as stripping off leaves and wiring stems, and they are familiar with many irritant plants, so that, when they do present to dermatologists, their dermatitis is frequently allergic [11]. Plant material and extracts [88], though bearing risks of false-negative and false-positive reactions and active sensitization, are frequently helpful. Compositae dermatitis can be screened for with the sesquiterpene lactone mix (Hermal) and, while some prefer the Compositae mix (Hermal), the latter has been reported to bear a substantial risk of active sensitization [89]. The standard series may provide fur-

ther indications of sensitization with reactions to balsam of Peru (*Myroxylon pereirae* resin), fragrance mix, and colophonium, as well as primin (if included). The most common additional plant sensitizers currently are probably tulips [74] and alstroemerias [90].

39.12.11 Hairdressing and Beauty

This is another group of workers whose familiarity with low-grade chronic ICD, mainly from shampooing, makes allergy likely if they come to patch testing. Glyceryl thioglycolate (GTG) in acid perming solutions is currently the most common cause of ACD in European hairdressers [91] (Fig. 9), and should, therefore, be present in all hairdressers' series (Table 1), which are essential to patch testing hairdressers. However, major manufacturers of hair care products have stopped the production of GTG because of the high prevalence of sensitization in hairdressers, but which is less frequent in clients. We may, therefore, see a decline in sensitization figures in the near future. *para*-Phenylenediamine (PPD) in the standard series remains the other allergen of major importance [92]. Some hairdressers and beauticians acquire sensitization to PPD not in the professional way by dyeing hair, but privately by a so-called temporary black henna tattoo, which contains a large amount of PPD (see Chaps. 14 and 29). The standard series will also detect relevant allergies to preservatives, such as formaldehyde, formaldehyde releasers and methylchloroisothiazolinone/ methylisothiazolinone (MCI/MI), fragrances and rubber chemicals, with type-I allergy to natural rubber latex also requiring consideration [93]. Sensitization to methyldibromo glutaronitrile in shampoos and leave-on

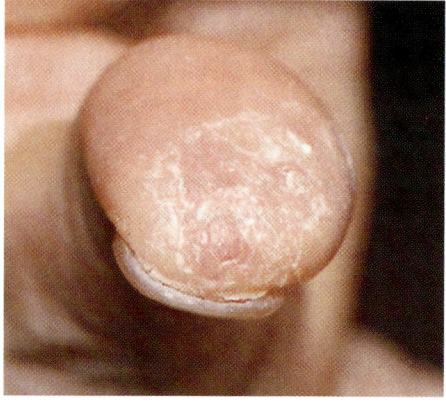

Fig. 9. Allergic contact dermatitis on pulps of hairdresser's hands from glyceryl thioglycolate (courtesy of PJ Frosch)

39

products has become an increasing problem and has led to legislative action (see Chap. 29 and [94, 95]). Previously, cocamidopropyl betaine [96] in shampoos was relevant in some hairdressers, but, due to different manufacturing processes, the major allergen 3-dimethylaminopropylamine (DMAPA) in this surfactant is eliminated or greatly reduced in quantity [97]. The significance of nickel as an occupational allergen is controversial [98] – most hairdressers acquire this sensitization by wearing costume jewelry; nickel-containing objects and tools in hairdressing have virtually vanished [35]. Aromatherapy is increasing the exposure of beauticians to fragrance allergens [99, 100], for whom colophonium can also be relevant from its presence in depilatory wax [101].

processing chemicals remaining important. This group of workers also has a higher risk of sensitization to fragrances and methyldibromo glutaronitrile in liquid soaps, hand creams, and various other materials [103–105]. Relevant allergens not detected by the standard series include, most importantly, glutaraldehyde (endoscopic and dental cold sterilant, X-ray developing systems) and (meth)acrylates (orthopedic and dental reconstruction) [106–108]. Glutaraldehyde, as well as chlorhexidine-containing and povidone-iodine-containing skin cleansers, often cause ICD rather than ACD [109]. Individual drugs – some of which, such as propacetamol [110], can cause airborne ACD – may also need to be tested for, as indicated by the history.

39.12.12 Health Care

CU/PCD from type-I allergy to natural rubber latex (NRL) is more common in this group of workers than in any other [102] (Fig. 10), with ACD from rubber-

39.12.13 Laboratory

Hand washing and cleaning equipment commonly causes chronic ICD. This is another occupational group at risk of type-I NRL allergy and in whom ACD

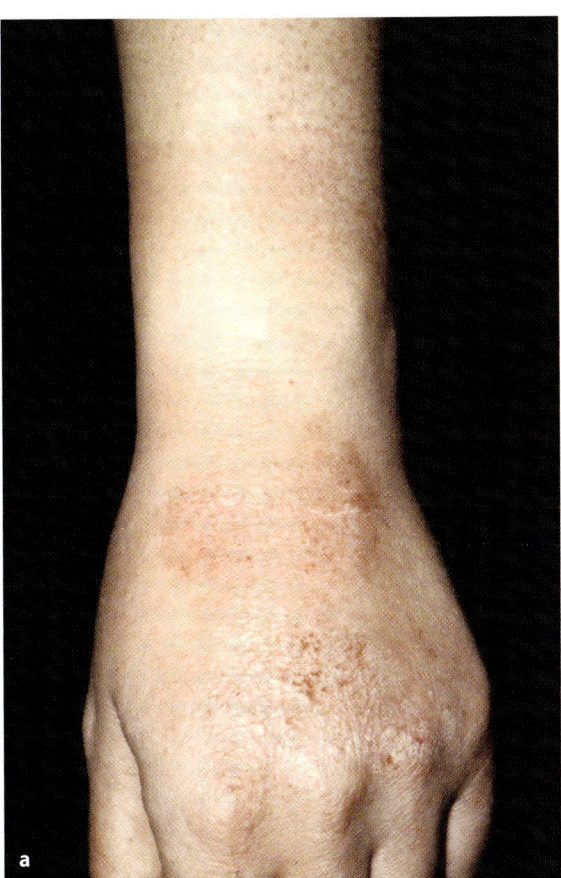 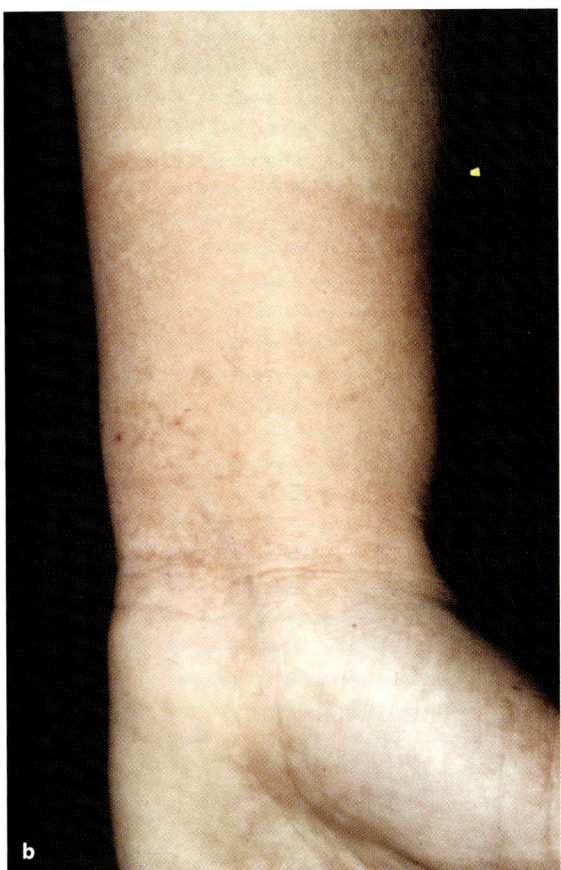

Fig. 10a, b. Occupational allergic contact dermatitis from gloves in a female surgeon (a). She was patch test positive to thiuram mix and the glove's manufacturer confirmed the presence of a thiuram derivative. Note that the dermatitis is the most severe on the back of the hands and least so on the palms (b)

from rubber-processing chemicals also occurs [111]. The standard series will usefully pick up allergens such as epoxy resin, which, recently, caused an epidemic of ACD from its addition to a microscopy immersion oil [112]. Innumerable other allergens are used in laboratories [113], and many may require individual patch and/or prick testing.

39.12.14 Metalworking

It is the metalworking fluids (MWFs) (Fig. 11), rather than the metals, that are a major problem for these workers, with ICD being more common than ACD, though sensitization occurs particularly from water-based MWFs [114, 115] (Fig. 12). Oil-based MWFs (neat oils) can be patch tested at from 1% (low viscosity) to 25% (high viscosity), while the concentrates of water-based MWFs (soluble oils) require ideally a 10%, 5%, 2.5% serial dilution. Recently, a German working party on allergy diagnostics in the metals branch has published guidelines for testing with fresh and used samples of the patients' MWFs [116]. Fresh concentrate of the water-based MWF should be tested at 5% aq., which is an average workplace concentration. Used water-based MWF can be patch tested as is, provided that the concentration at the work-

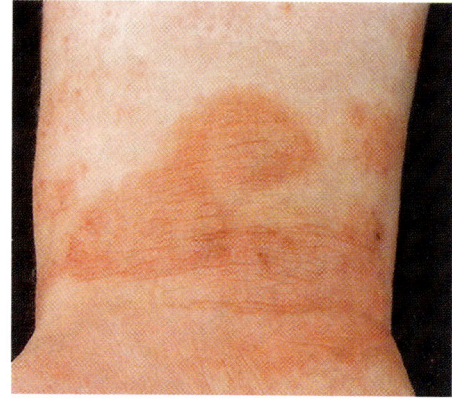

Fig. 12. Patches of soluble oil dermatitis on the flexor aspect of the wrist (courtesy of St. John's Institute of Dermatology)

place is ≤8%. In the case of higher workplace concentrations, further dilution to an end concentration of 4–8% is recommended. As a rule of thumb, this can be achieved by a 1:1 aqueous dilution of the water-based MWF. Neat oils should be tested 50% in olive oils according to this report [116]. It is often the biocides that are the sensitizers in water-based MWFs, and additional series (Table 1) are helpful in identifying these. Alkanolamine borate corrosion inhibitors may sensitize and are difficult to patch test with, a buffered dilution series being recommended [117]. The standard series will identify colophonium-positive individuals who may have been sensitized by chemically related tall-oil-based emulsifiers in water-based MWFs. Mercaptobenzothiazole and ethylenediamine [118] may also be present in water-based MWFs. Fragrances are often added to MWF in order to mask the odor. This explains the higher prevalence of sensitization to the fragrance mix in metal workers ([115] and Chap. 33). Unless they occur in electroplaters, reactions to nickel, cobalt, and chromate require careful assessment as to their relevance, and can be incidental. Degreasing solvents are another common cause of ICD and are usually best left untested.

39.12.15 Office

Office workers are another group who may experience itchy skins from low-humidity environments. Carbonless copy paper and visual display terminals have now largely been exonerated as dermatological hazards. Carbonless paper may contain colophonium and, thus, cause very circumscribed lesions on the hands that have come into contact with the paper [119]. Multiple factors, not all of them medical, may

39

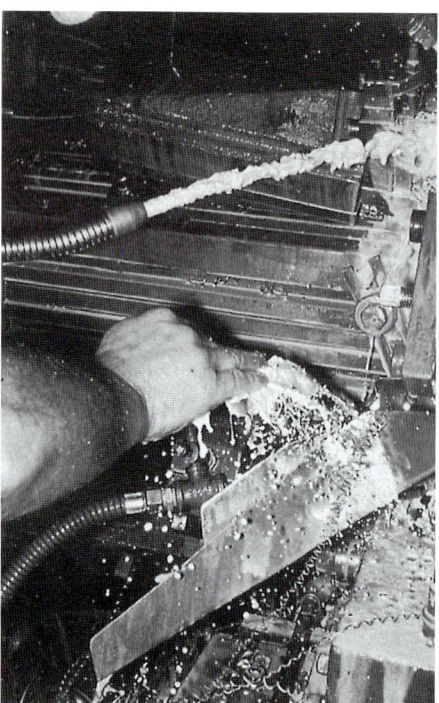

Fig. 11. A machine tool operator deflecting soluble oil to check the machine setting

conspire to produce outbreaks of symptoms misinterpreted as insect bites in such workers [120]. Individual instances of ACD from standard allergens such as nickel and rubber chemicals [121] occur in the office environment. ACD as well as ICD from computer mice and/or the mouse pad have been reported [122–124]. Skin lesions may also consist of blanchable erythematous patches with telangiectases on the ulnar aspect of the palms or eczematous lesions with fissures on the fingertips ("mouse fingers") [125–127]. Although reactions to plastic materials are rare in comparison to the extensive contacts in virtually every occupation, occupational contact dermatitis from headphones containing diethylhexyl phthalate has recently been described [128].

39.12.16 Petroleum Recovery

Drillers are at considerable risk of ICD from drilling "muds," acids, detergents, and organic solvents. ACD has also been reported from polyamines in the emulsifiers of oil-based muds [129]. Further details about this industry are to be found in Rycroft [130].

39.12.17 Photographic

Even with increasing automation, contact sensitization still occurs from both black-and-white and color processing [131]. Additional series (Table 1) are extremely useful and are usually adequate for patch testing. A recent update [132] included formaldehyde and methylchloroisothiazolinone/methylisothiazolinone in the standard series as allergens relevant to color processing.

39.12.18 Printing

The organic solvents used for cleaning down machinery remain a major cause of chronic ICD. Allergens in conventional printing technology are largely covered by the standard series, including formaldehyde, methylchloroisothiazolinone/methylisothiazolinone, chromate, and cobalt [133, 134], whereas UV-curing printing systems [135] require the addition of a (meth)acrylate series (Table 1). Frequent hand washing may sometimes cause ACD from preservatives (e.g., methyldibromo glutaronitrile), as well as, more commonly, ICD [136].

39.12.19 Veterinary, Slaughtering, and Butchery

This somewhat anomalous grouping of occupations is prompted by their overlapping sources of ICD and CU/PCD, with ICD arising from animal fluids and entrails [137] and disinfectants, and CU/PCD from animal tissues/meats, obstetric fluids, animal hair, and dander [62], as well as NRL in rubber gloves. ACD [138] is caused mainly by rubber gloves, and by veterinary medicaments [139] and sterilants.

References

1. Calnan CD, Rycroft RJG (1981) Rehabilitation in occupational skin disease. Trans Coll Med S Afr 25(Suppl Rehabil):136–142
2. Diepgen TL (2003) Occupational skin-disease data in Europe. Int Arch Occup Environ Health 76:331–338
3. Dickel H, Kuss O, John SM, Blome O, Hagemann KH, Schwanitz HJ (2004) Early secondary prevention of occupational skin disease in Germany: the dermatologist's procedure in perspective. Int Arch Occup Environ Health 77:142–149
4. Adisesh A, Meyer JD, Cherry NM (2002) Prognosis and work absence due to occupational contact dermatitis. Contact Dermatitis 46:273–279
5. Hutchings CV, Shum KW, Gawkrodger DJ (2001) Occupational contact dermatitis has an appreciable impact on quality of life. Contact Dermatitis 45:17–20
6. Mathias CGT (1988) Occupational dermatoses. J Am Acad Dermatol 19:1107–1114
7. Adams RM (1990) Occupational skin disease, 2nd edn. Saunders, Philadelphia, Pa.
8. Gawkrodger DJ (2004) Occupational skin cancers. Occup Med (Lond) 54:458–463
9. Brauel P, Brauel R, Stresemann E (1995) Aerogenes Kontaktekzem und Bronchialasthma durch Kolophonium-Sensibilisierung. Arbeitsmed Sozialmed Umweltmed 30:549–551
10. Calnan CD (1977) Prosser White Oration 1977. Dermatology and industry. Clin Exp Dermatol 3:1–16
11. Fregert S (1975) Occupational dermatitis in a 10-year material. Contact Dermatitis 1:97–107
12. Obituary (1991) N. Hjorth, 1919–1990. Contact Dermatitis 24:161–163
13. Obituary (1998) H. Ippen, 1914–1993. Contact Dermatitis 39:159–160
14. Obituary (1999) V. Pirilä, 1915–1998. Contact Dermatitis 40:231
15. Foussereau J (1991) Guide de dermato-allergologie professionnelle. Masson, Paris, France
16. Zschunke E (1985) Grundriss der Arbeitsdermatologie. VEB Verlag Volk und Gesundheit, Berlin, Germany
17. English JSC (1998) A colour handbook of occupational dermatology. Manson, London
18. Dickel H, Schmidt A, Kretz J, Diepgen TL (2002) Importance of irritant contact dermatitis in occupational skin disease. Am J Clin Dermatol 3:283–289
19. Dickel H, Kuss O, Blesius CR, Schmidt A, Diepgen TL (2001) Occupational skin diseases in Northern Bavaria between 1990 and 1999: a population-based study. Br J Dermatol 145:453–462

20. Robinson MK (1999) Population differences in skin structure and physiology and the susceptibility to irritant and allergic contact dermatitis: implications for skin safety testing and risk assessment. Contact Dermatitis 41: 65–79
21. Dickel H, John SM (2003) Ratio of irritant contact dermatitis to allergic contact dermatitis in occupational skin disease. J Am Acad Dermatol 49:360–361, author reply 361–362
22. McFadden JP, Basketter DA (2000) Contact allergy, irritancy and 'danger'. Contact Dermatitis 42:123–127
23. Coenraads PJ, Diepgen TL (1998) Risk for hand eczema in employees with past or present atopic dermatitis. Int Arch Occup Environ Health 71:7–13
24. Dickel H, Bruckner TM, Schmidt A, Diepgen TL (2003) Impact of atopic skin diathesis on occupational skin disease incidence in a working population. J Invest Dermatol 121:37–40
25. Allen MH, Wakelin SH, Holloway D, Lisby S, Baadsgaard O, Barker JNWN, McFadden JP (2000) Association of TNFα gene polymorphism at position –308 with susceptibility to irritant contact dermatitis. Immunogenetics 51: 201–205
26. Dooms-Goossens A, Deleu H (1991) Airborne contact dermatitis: an update. Contact Dermatitis 25: 211–217
27. Rycroft RJG, Baran R (1994) Occupational abnormalities and contact dermatitis. In: Baran R, Dawber RPR (eds) Diseases of the nails and their management, 2nd edn. Blackwell Science, Oxford, pp 263–284
28. Wall LM, Gebauer KA (1991) A follow-up study of occupational skin disease in Western Australia. Contact Dermatitis 24:241–243
29. Rosen RH, Freeman S (1993) Prognosis of occupational contact dermatitis in New South Wales, Australia. Contact Dermatitis 29:88–93
30. Jungbauer FH, van der Vleuten P, Groothoff JW, Coenraads PJ (2004) Irritant hand dermatitis: severity of disease, occupational exposure to skin irritants and preventive measures 5 years after initial diagnosis. Contact Dermatitis 50:245–251
31. Kalimo K, Kautiainen H, Niskanen T, Niemi L (1999) 'Eczema school' to improve compliance in an occupational dermatology clinic. Contact Dermatitis 41:315–319
32. Hogan DJ, Dannaker CJ, Maibach HI (1990) Contact dermatitis: prognosis, risk factors, and rehabilitation. Semin Dermatol 9:233–246
33. Meneghini CL, Angelini G (1984) Primary and secondary sites of occupational contact dermatitis. Derm Beruf Umwelt 32:205–207
34. De Groot AC (1994) Patch testing. Test concentrations and vehicles for 3700 chemicals, 2nd edn. Elsevier, Amsterdam, The Netherlands
35. Dickel H, Kuss O, Schmidt A, Diepgen TL (2002) Occupational relevance of positive standard patch-test results in employed persons with an initial report of occupational skin disease. Int Arch Occup Environ Health 75: 423–424
36. Bruze M, Zimerson E (1997) Cross-reaction patterns in patients with contact allergy to simple methylol phenols. Contact Dermatitis 37:82–86
37. Karlberg A-T (1991) Air oxidation increases the allergenic potential of tall-oil rosin. Colophony contact allergens also identified in tall-oil rosin. Am J Contact Dermat 2: 43–49
38. Karlberg A-T, Magnusson K, Nilsson U (1992) Air oxidation of d-limonene (the citrus solvent) creates potent allergens. Contact Dermatitis 26:332–340
39. Christensen LP, Kristiansen K (1999) Isolation and quantification of tuliposides and tulipalins in tulips (Tulipa) by high-performance liquid chromatography. Contact Dermatitis 40:300–309
40. Fenske RA (1993) Dermal exposure assessment techniques. Ann Occup Hyg 37:687–706
41. Fenske RA, Birnbaum SG (1997) Second generation video imaging technique for assessing dermal exposure (VITAE System). Am Ind Hyg Assoc J 58:636–645
42. Lind ML, Boman A Surakka J, Sollenberg J, Meding B (2004) A method for assessing occupational dermal exposure to permanent hair dyes. Ann Occup Hyg 48: 533–539
43. Fregert S (1963) The organization of occupational dermatology in Lund. Acta Derm Venereol (Stockh) 43:203–205
44. Lobel E (1995) Post-contact chronic eczema: pension or rehabilitation. Aust J Dermatol 36:59–62
45. Geier J, Lessmann H, Uter W, Schnuch A; Information Network of Departments of Dermatology (IDVK) (2003) Occupational rubber glove allergy: results of the Information Network of Departments of Dermatology (IVDK), 1995–2001. Contact Dermatitis 48:39–44
46. Davies NF, Rycroft RJG (2000) Dermatology. In: Cox RAF, Edwards FC, Palmer K (eds) Fitness for work, 3rd edn. Oxford University Press, Oxford, pp 453–462
47. Zschunke E (1978) Metal corrosion (rust) as a result of hyperhidrosis. Dermatol Monatsschr 164:727–728
48. Calnan CD (1970) Studies in contact dermatitis. XXIII. Allergen replacement. Trans St John's Hosp Dermatol Soc 56:131–138
49. Fregert S (1980) Possibilities of skin contact in automatic processes. Contact Dermatitis 6:23
50. Forsberg K, Keith LH (1999) Chemical protective clothing performance index, 2nd edn. Wiley, New York
51. Zhai H, Maibach HI (1998) Moisturizers in preventing irritant contact dermatitis: an overview. Contact Dermatitis 38:241–244
52. Held E, Agner T (1999) Comparison between 2 test models in evaluating the effect of a moisturizer on irritated human skin. Contact Dermatitis 40:261–268
53. Schlüter-Wigger W, Elsner P (1996) Efficacy of 4 commercially available protective creams in the repetitive irritation test (RIT). Contact Dermatitis 34:278–283
54. Healy J, Johnson S, Little MC, MacNeil S (1998) An in vitro study of the use of chelating agents in clearing nickel-contaminated human skin: an alternative approach to preventing nickel allergic contact dermatitis. Contact Dermatitis 39:171–181
55. Gruvberger B, Bruze M (1998) Can glutathione-containing emollients inactivate methyl-chloroisothiazolinone/methylisothiazolinone? Contact Dermatitis 38:261–265
56. Kütting B, Drexler H (2003) Effectiveness of skin protection creams as a preventive measure in occupational dermatitis: a critical update according to criteria of evidence-based medicine. Int Arch Occup Environ Health 76:253–259
57. Henschel R, Agathos M, Breit R (1999) Acute irritant contact dermatitis from propionic acid used in animal feed preservation. Contact Dermatitis 40:328
58. Spiewak R (2001) Pesticides as a cause of occupational skin diseases in farmers. Ann Agric Environ Med 8:1–5
59. Bransbury A, Burge S (1998) Rubber allergy in a shepherdess. Contact Dermatitis 39:45
60. Gauchia R, Rodriguez-Serna M, Silvestre JF, Linana JJ, Aliaga A (1996) Allergic contact dermatitis from streptomycin in a cattle breeder. Contact Dermatitis 35: 374–375

39

61. Schauder S, Schröder W, Geier J (1996) Olaquindox-induced airborne photoallergic contact dermatitis followed by transient or persistent light reactions in 15 pig breeders. Contact Dermatitis 35:344–354

62. Kanerva L, Susitaival P (1996) Cow dander: the most common cause of occupational contact urticaria in Finland. Contact Dermatitis 35:309–310

63. Mahler V, Diepgen TL, Hesse A, Peters K-P (1998) Protein contact dermatitis due to cow dander. Contact Dermatitis 38:47–48

64. Vente C, Fuchs T (1997) Contact dermatitis due to oil of turpentine in a porcelain painter. Contact Dermatitis 37:187

65. Raccagni AA, Baldari U, Righini MG (1996) Airborne dermatitis in a painter. Contact Dermatitis 35:119–120

66. Eedy D (1996) Carbon-fibre-induced airborne irritant contact dermatitis. Contact Dermatitis 35:362–363

67. Hjerpe L (1986) Chromate dermatitis in an engine assembly department. Contact Dermatitis 14:66–67

68. Kanerva L (1998) Occupational fingertip protein contact dermatitis from grain flours and natural rubber latex. Contact Dermatitis 38:295–296

69. Kanerva L, Vanhanen M, Tupasela O (1997) Occupational allergic contact urticaria from fungal but not bacterial alpha-amylase. Contact Dermatitis 36:306–307

70. Bauer A, Bartsch R, Stadeler M, Schneider W, Grieshaber R, Wollina U, Gebhardt M (1998) Development of occupational skin diseases during vocational training in baker and confectioner apprentices: a follow-up study. Contact Dermatitis 39:307–311

71. Nethercott JR, Holness DL (1989) Occupational dermatitis in food handlers and bakers. J Am Acad Dermatol 21:485–490

72. Bauer A, Kelterer D, Stadeler M, Schneider W, Kleesz P (2001) The prevention of occupational hand dermatitis in bakers, confectioners and employees in the catering trades. Preliminary results of a skin prevention program. Contact Dermatitis 44:85–88

73. Cronin E (1989) Dermatitis in food handlers. Adv Dermatol 4:113–123

74. Bruynzeel DP (1997) Bulb dermatitis. Dermatological problems in the flower bulb industries. Contact Dermatitis 37:70–77

75. Shum KW, English JSC (1998) Allergic contact dermatitis in food handlers, with patch tests positive to Compositae mix but negative to sesquiterpene lactone mix. Contact Dermatitis 39:207–208

76. Hjorth N, Roed-Petersen J (1976) Occupational protein contact dermatitis in food handlers. Contact Dermatitis 2:28–42

77. Verlinden V, Goossens A (2003) Airborne occupational allergic contact dermatitis from N,N-bis[2-bromo-ethyl]aniline and N,N-bis [2-[(methylsulfonyl)-oxy]ethyl]aniline in a chemistry student. Contact Dermatitis 49:169

78. Le Coz CJ, Lepoittevin JP (2001) Occupational erythema-multiforme-like dermatitis from sensitization to costus resinoid, followed by flare-up and systemic contact dermatitis from beta-cyclocostunolide in a chemistry student. Contact Dermatitis 44:310–311

79. Nielsen J (1996) The occurrence and course of skin symptoms on the hands among female cleaners. Contact Dermatitis 34:284–291

80. Karlberg A-T, Dooms-Goossens A (1997) Contact allergy to oxidized d-limonene among dermatitis patients. Contact Dermatitis 36:201–206

81. Allenby CF, Basketter DA (1994) The effect of repeated open exposure to low levels of nickel on compromised hand skin of nickel-allergic subjects. Contact Dermatitis 30:135–138

82. Nilsson EJ, Knutsson A (1995) Atopic dermatitis, nickel sensitivity and xerosis as risk factors for hand eczema in women. Contact Dermatitis 31:401–406

83. Zachariae COC, Agner T, Menné T (1996) Chromium allergy in consecutive patients in a country where ferrous sulfate has been added to cement since 1981. Contact Dermatitis 35:83–85

84. Olsavszky R, Rycroft RJG, White IR, McFadden JP (1998) Contact sensitivity to chromate: comparison at a London contact dermatitis clinic over a 10-year period. Contact Dermatitis 38:329–331

85. Skogstad M, Levy F (1994) Occupational irritant contact dermatitis and fungal infection in construction workers. Contact Dermatitis 31:28–30

86. Condé-Salazar L, Guimaraens D, Villegas C, Romero MA, Gonzalez MA (1995) Occupational allergic contact dermatitis in construction workers. Contact Dermatitis 33:226–330

87. Koh D, Foulds IS, Aw TC (1990) Dermatological hazards in the electronics industry. Contact Dermatitis 22:1–7

88. Lovell CR (1993) Plants and the skin. Blackwell Scientific, Oxford, pp 97–105

89. Wilkinson SM, Pollock B (1999) Patch test sensitization after use of the Compositae mix. Contact Dermatitis 40:277–291

90. Scales JW, Sherertz EF (1997) Occupational dermatitis transferred with job duties. Am J Contact Dermatitis 8:179–180

91. Leino T, Estlander T, Kanerva L (1998) Occupational allergic dermatoses in hairdressers. Contact Dermatitis 38:166–167

92. Armstrong DKB, Jones AB, Smith HR, Ross JS, White IR, Rycroft RJG, McFadden JP (1999) Occupational sensitization to p-phenylenediamine: a 17-year review. Contact Dermatitis 41:348–349

93. Kanerva L, Leino T (1999) Prevalence of natural rubber latex allergy in hairdressers. Contact Dermatitis 41:168–169

94. Wilkinson JD, Shaw S, Andersen KE, Brandao FM, Bruynzeel DP, Bruze M, Camarasa JM, Diepgen TL, Ducombs G, Frosch PJ, Goossens A, Lachapelle JM, Lahti A, Menne T, Seidenari S, Tosti A, Wahlberg JE (2002) Monitoring levels of preservative sensitivity in Europe. A 10-year overview (1991–2000). Contact Dermatitis 46:207–210

95. Armstrong DKB, Smith HR, Rycroft RJG (1999) Contact allergy to methyldibromo glutaronitrile presenting as severe scalp seborrhoeic eczema. Contact Dermatitis 40:335

96. Armstrong DKB, Smith HR, Ross JS, White IR (1999) Sensitization to cocamidopropylbetaine: an 8-year review. Contact Dermatitis 40:335–336

97. Foti C, Bonamonte D, Mascolo G, Corcelli A, Lobasso S, Rigano L, Angelini G (2003) The role of 3-dimethylaminopropylamine and amidoamine in contact allergy to cocamidopropylbetaine. Contact Dermatitis 48:194–198

98. Shah M, Lewis FM, Gawkrodger DJ (1996) Occupational dermatitis in hairdressers. Contact Dermatitis 35:364–365

99. Cockayne SE, Gawkrodger DJ (1997) Occupational contact dermatitis in an aromatherapist. Contact Dermatitis 37:306–307

100. Keane FM, Smith HR, White IR, Rycroft RJ (2000) Occupational allergic contact dermatitis in two aromatherapists. Contact Dermatitis 43:49–51

101. O'Reilly FM, Murphy GM (1996) Occupational contact dermatitis in a beautician. Contact Dermatitis 35:47–48

102. Wakelin SH, White IR (1999) Natural rubber latex allergy. Clin Exp Dermatol 24:245–248
103. Uter W, Schnuch A, Geier J, Pfahlberg A, Gefeller O; IDVK study group; Information Network of Departments of Dermatology (2001) Association between occupation and contact allergy to the fragrance mix: a multifactorial analysis of national surveillance data. Occup Environ Med 58:392–398
104. Diba VC, Chowdhury MM, Adisesh A, Statham BN (2003) Occupational allergic contact dermatitis in hospital workers caused by methyldibromo glutaronitrile in a work soap. Contact Dermatitis 48:118–119
105. Sanchez-Perez J, Garcia-Diez A (1999) Occupational allergic contact dermatitis from eugenol, oil of cinnamon and oil of cloves in a physiotherapist. Contact Dermatitis 41:346–347
106. Kanerva L, Mikola H, Henriks-Eckerman M-L, Jolanki R, Estlander T (1998) Fingertip paresthesia and occupational allergic contact dermatitis caused by acrylics in a dental nurse. Contact Dermatitis 38:114–116
107. Alanko K, Susitaival P, Jolanki R, Kanerva L (2004) Occupational skin diseases among dental nurses. Contact Dermatitis 50:77–82
108. Wrangsjö K, Swartling C, Meding B (2001) Occupational dermatitis in dental personnel: contact dermatitis with special reference to (meth)acrylates in 174 patients. Contact Dermatitis 45:158–163
109. Stingeni L, Lapomarda V, Lisi P (1995) Occupational hand dermatitis in hospital environments. Contact Dermatitis 33:172–176
110. Berl V, Barbaud A, Lepoittevin J-P (1998) Mechanism of allergic contact dermatitis from propacetamol: sensitization to activated N,N-diethylglycine. Contact Dermatitis 38:185–188
111. de Groot H, de Jong NW, Duijster E, van Wijk RG, Vermeulen A, van Toorenenbergen AW, Geursen L, van Joost T (1998) Prevalence of natural rubber latex allergy (type I and type IV) in laboratory workers in The Netherlands. Contact Dermatitis 38:159–163
112. Le Coz C-J, Coninx D, Van Rengen A, El Aboubi S, Ducombs G, Benz M-H, Boursier S, Avenel-Audran M, Verret J-L, Erikstam U, Bruze M, Goossens A (1999) An epidemic of occupational contact dermatitis from an immersion oil for microscopy in laboratory personnel. Contact Dermatitis 40:77–83
113. Jolanki R, Estlander T, Kanerva L (1999) Occupational dermatoses among laboratory assistants. Contact Dermatitis 40:166–168
114. Pryce DW, White J, English JSC, Rycroft RJG (1989) Soluble oil dermatitis: a review. J Soc Occup Med 39:93–98
115. Geier J, Lessmann H, Schnuch A, Uter W (2004) Contact sensitization in metalworkers with occupational dermatitis exposed to water-based metalworking fluids: results of the research project "FaSt". Int Arch Occup Environ Health 77:543–551
116. Geier J, Uter W, Lessmann H, Frosch PJ (2004) Patch testing with metalworking fluids from the patient's workplace. Contact Dermatitis 51:172–179
117. Bruze M, Hradil E, Eriksohn I-L, Gruvberger B, Widström L (1995) Occupational allergic contact dermatitis from alkanolamineborates in metalworking fluids. Contact Dermatitis 32:24–27
118. Sasseville D, al-Khenaizan S (1997) Occupational contact dermatitis from ethylenediamine in a wire-drawing lubricant. Contact Dermatitis 36:228–229
119. Lange-Ionescu S, Bruze M, Gruvberger B, Zimmerson E, Frosch PJ (2000) Kontaktallergie durch kohlefreies Durchschlagpapier. Dermatosen 48:183–187
120. Lewis RD, Feir D, Roegner K, Nayan A, Vordtriede S (1999) Investigation of bites and itching in a word processing department. Am Ind Hyg Assoc J 60:310–316
121. Corazza M, Maranini C, Venturini D, Virgili A (1999) Contact allergy to mercaptobenzothiazole in a bank clerk from a wet sponge. Contact Dermatitis 41:105–106
122. Kanerva L, Estlander T, Jolanki R (2000) Occupational contact dermatitis caused by a personal-computer mouse. Contact Dermatitis 43:362–363
123. Garcia-Morales I, Garcia Bravo B, Camacho Martinez F (2003) Occupational dermatitis caused by a personal-computer mouse mat. Contact Dermatitis 49:172
124. Capon F, Cambie MP, Clinard F, Bernardeau K, Kalis B (1996) Occupational contact dermatitis caused by computer mice. Contact Dermatitis 35:57–58
125. Lewis AT, Hsu S, Phillips RM, Lee JA (2000) Computer palms. J Am Acad Dermatol 42:1073–1075
126. Vermeer MH, Bruynzeel DP (2001) Mouse fingers, a new computer-related skin disorder. J Am Acad Dermatol 45:477
127. Romaguera C, Vilaplana J (2000) Occupational contact dermatitis from ylang-ylang oil. Contact Dermatitis 43:251
128. Walker SL, Smith HR, Rycroft RJ, Broome C (2000) Occupational contact dermatitis from headphones containing diethylhexyl phthalate. Contact Dermatitis 42:164
129. Ormerod AD, Wakeel RA, Mann TAN, Main RA, Aldridge RD (1989) Polyamine sensitization in offshore workers handling drilling muds. Contact Dermatitis 21:326–329
130. Rycroft RJG (1999) Petroleum and petroleum derivatives. In: Adams RM (ed) Occupational skin disease, 3rd edn. Saunders, Philadelphia, Pennsylvania, pp 553–566
131. Marconi PMB, Campagna G, Fabri G, Schiavino D (1999) Allergic contact dermatitis from colour developers used in automated photographic processing. Contact Dermatitis 40:109–117
132. Scheman AJ, Katta R (1997) Photographic allergens: an update. Contact Dermatitis 37:130
133. Kanerva L, Jolanki R, Estlander T (1996) Offset printer's occupational allergic contact dermatitis caused by cobalt-2-ethylhexoate. Contact Dermatitis 34:67–68
134. Livesley EJ, Rushton L, English JS, Williams HC (2002) The prevalence of occupational dermatitis in the UK printing industry. Occup Environ Med 59:487–492
135. Goossens A, Coninx D, Rommens K, Verhamme B (1998) Occupational dermatitis in a silk-screen maker. Contact Dermatitis 39:40–42
136. Aalto-Korte K, Jolanki R, Estlander T, Alanko K, Kanerva L (1996) Occupational allergic contact dermatitis caused by Euxyl K 400. Contact Dermatitis 35:193–194
137. Hjorth N (1978) Gut eczema in slaughterhouse workers. Contact Dermatitis 4:49–52
138. Hjorth N, Roed-Petersen J (1980) Allergic contact dermatitis in veterinary surgeons. Contact Dermatitis 6:27–29
139. Dwyer CM, Ormerod AD (1997) Allergic contact dermatitis from thiuram in a veterinary medication. Contact Dermatitis 37:132
140. Rycroft RJG (1988) Looking at work dermatologically. Dermatol Clin 6:1–5
141. Veien N, Hattel T, Laurberg G (1997) Low-humidity dermatosis from car heaters. Contact Dermatitis 37:138
142. Rycroft RJG (1980) Occupational dermatoses in perspective. Lancet 2:24–26
143. Maguire A (1978) Psychic possession among industrial workers. Lancet 1:376–378

39

Chapter 40

Health Personnel

Ana M. Giménez-Arnau

Contents

40.1 Introduction

Health personnel carry out a wide spectrum of jobs. All of them are susceptible to various forms of contact dermatitis. A hospital is like a large factory; many substances found in a hospital can be harmful to the skin. This group of workers belong to the fifth highest occupational risk category [1]. Mahler et al [2]. reported an average annual incidence of occupational skin diseases of 7.3 per 10,000 health workers, with the highest incidence among younger people. The biological and physical causes of these will not be considered in this chapter. Radiation and viral, fungal, bacterial or animal factors may all cause occupational dermatoses in health personnel, but rarely of the contact dermatitis type. Protective measures and general prevention must be organized for the health services, just as in big enterprises [3].

> ### Core Message
>
> ■ Health workers have high occupational risk, mainly in younger people.

40.1.1 Range of Occupations

Health personnel can be divided into three main groups. The first of these includes physicians, surgeons, medical specialists, radiologists, laboratory specialists, and dental personnel. The second group includes nurses, clinical assistants, laboratory and radiology technicians, biologists, pharmacists, physiotherapists, and dialysis workers. The third group includes office personnel, technical service workers, kitchen and laundry workers, cleaners and disinfection area and sterilization area workers. Veterinarians deserve special attention because of their wide spectrum of work.

40.1.2 Type of Cutaneous Disease

Health care workers mainly suffer from irritant and/or allergic contact dermatitis and contact urticaria. The prevalence of such diseases (assessed using patch and prick tests) in health care workers ($n=55$) was found to be: 61% with irritant contact dermatitis, 31% with allergic contact dermatitis, and 27% with contact urticaria to latex [4]. Eleven percent of them showed both allergic contact dermatitis related to thiuram and contact urticaria to latex [4]. Ninety five percent of these cases were deemed to be work-related [4]. Nettis et al [5] found irritant and allergic contact dermatitis to be work-related in 44.4% and 16.5% of diagnoses respectively. Mahler et al [2] observed rates of 54% for irritant and 51% for contact dermatitis.

> **Core Message**
>
> ■ Health workers mainly suffer from irritant and/or allergic contact dermatitis and contact urticaria.

40.1.3 Irritant Contact Dermatitis

Health care personnel are exposed to a variety of cutaneous irritants. The most common type of contact dermatitis in health workers is irritant contact dermatitis. The frequent use of disinfectant solutions, detergents and soaps for hand washing can induce stratum corneum lipid disturbances and consequently a skin barrier defect [6]. Transepidermal water loss (TEWL) is increased with brush washing compared to simple hand washing [7]. Cumulative irritant contact dermatitis favour sensitization to a wide range of common substances.

40.1.4 Atopy as a Risk Factor

Atopy is a risk factor. Personal or family background of atopy favors the development of hand dermatitis and contact urticaria [8]. Hand dermatitis occurred in 65% of those with atopic symptoms and in 75% of those who had unusually dry skin and atopic relatives. Among the remaining workers, only 33% had suffered from eczema elsewhere on the skin or on the hands [9,10].

40.1.5 Wet Work

Hospital wet work also increases the risk of hand eczema. Previous irritant contact dermatitis produced by wet working predisposes to allergic reactions, mostly to nickel, fragrances or rubber chemicals. Of persons with allergic contact dermatitis, 55% had previously suffered irritant hand dermatitis, compared to 44% of those without positive patch test reactions. Of those with sensitivity to fragrance, 70% had suffered from hand dermatitis [11].

> **Core Message**
>
> ■ Atopy and wet work increases the risk of hand eczema in health workers.

40.1.6 Hand Dermatitis

As many as 75% of the occupational skin diseases in hospital cleaners were hand irritant contact dermatitis, 21% were allergic contact dermatitis and 4% were candidosis of the finger webs. The causes of irritant contact dermatitis were detergents, alkaline soaps, acids, sodium perborate and hypochlorite and hypobromite compounds [12–14]. Among these causes, the frequency of type IV thiuram allergy hand dermatitis has increased significantly (odds ratio 2.55, 95% confidence interval 1.25–5.20, $P=0.01$) since 1983 [15]. Euxyl K-400 is a preservative that is recognized as being a sensitizer, but it is only occasionally involved in occupational cases. Its presence in a liquid detergent named Prilan caused allergic contact dermatitis on the fingers of a female hospital cleaner [16]. Local and general prophylactic measures must be extended in order to reduce occupational hand dermatitis among hospital workers, including surgeons, nurses, cleaning personnel, kitchen workers, and clinical assistants, among many others.

40.2 Nurses, Clinical Assistants, and Cleaners

Nurses, clinical assistants and cleaners commonly have their hands exposed to irritants, and so often suffer irritant contact dermatitis of the hands and forearms. This is significantly more frequent in women under 30 years of age, mostly workers in training grades and surgical fields. In the majority of cases (90%) the lesions are irritant, and mainly related to disinfectants. Nevertheless, the importance of natural rubber latex allergy, both delayed and immediate, is well established for nurses [17]. In some special cases, individual allergic contact reactions appear with drugs. Some pharmaceutical products have special relevance for them. (Table 1) As a result of this, the risk of sensitization is high.

Table 1. Special allergens for nurses [1]

	Test
Cetrimide	0.25% pet.
Chlorhexidine digluconate	0.5% aq.
Chlorpromazine	0.1% pet.
Chloroxylenol	1% pet.
Glutaraldehyde	1% aq. or pet.
Penicillin	10,000 IU/g pet.[a]
Povidone-iodine	10% pet.

[a] See section "Medicaments" in text

Core Message

■ Irritant contact dermatitis, delayed and immediate latex allergy, and contact reactions with drugs are common among nurses. The risk of sensitization is very high.

40.2.1 Medicaments

Occupation-related reactions to medications mainly occur in two exposed groups. The first group comprises employees of pharmaceutical and chemical companies that are involved in their manufacture. The second group includes professionals who use the drugs in a therapeutic setting. Of 14,689 patients (1978–2001) suspected of contact allergy, 33 were healthcare workers that exhibited occupational allergic contact dermatitis from drugs [18]. The most common sensitizers are antibiotics such as penicillins, cephalosporins, and aminoglycosides.

Streptomycin is a particularly important contact sensitizer, because of the severity of the reaction to it. Minimal contact is needed to elicit the disease and the symptoms persist long after avoiding contact with the antibiotic (test 1% pet.) [19]. *Aminoglycosides* are a closely related group of bactericidal antibiotics derived from bacteria of genus *Streptomyces*. Cross-reactions between aminoglycosides have been described in the literature. Aminoglycosides are commonly constructed from a disaccharide containing glucosamine and deoxystreptamine linked by a glycoside bond. Two nurses with positive patch tests to amikacin and gentamicin has been reported [18].

Penicillin sensitizes through contact during injections. Contact allergy to penicillin and its derivatives (ampicillin, amoxycillin, cloxacillin, oxacillin, flu-cloxacillin) may be associated with immediate reactions of the anaphylactic type. Therefore, general measures for preventing anaphylactic shock must also be observed in people with penicillin contact dermatitis. Testing with penicillin must be done with extreme care. In vivo tests for allergy to penicillin have not been developed yet. Because of the risk of severe acute generalized reaction, testing with penicillin must only be done in hospitals. An open test with penicillin should be made prior to any other. A closed patch test should be carried out only when an open test is negative, and should be removed immediately if any generalized response is observed. Faced with an obvious and severe history of contact allergy to penicillin, the closed patch test should not be done, even if the open test is negative. There is no agreement on penicillin patch test concentration. Penicillin at 10,000 IU/g pet. is used at St John's Institute of Dermatology, London. Patch testing can also detect generalized immediate allergies to penicillin, without contact dermatitis from this antibiotic [20, 21].

Cephalosporins are also contact allergens. A fairly significant number of cases have been reported in the last few years. The majority of those have occurred in nurses, although they also occur in laboratory analysts and in patients. Usually patients reactive to cephalosporins do not react to penicillin, suggesting that the β-lactam ring does not cause the sensitization. The tetrazolic ring or amino-thiazol-alkoxy-iminicol group presumably constitutes the allergenic portion of the molecule. It is therefore common to obtain positive reactions in these patients to ceftizoxime, cefotaxime, cefodizime, ceftazidime, cephazolin, cefuroxime, and ceftriaxome. Cephalosporins can be tested at 10% to 20% in pet., or from 1% to 10% in aqueous solution [22–25].

The antipneumocystis drug *pentamidine isethionate* has been described as a cause of immunologic contact urticaria in nurses [26].

Meropenem is a β-lactam. *Carbapenem* is an antibiotic used parenterally for pneumonias, especially in cystic fibrosis. Cutaneous adverse events include pruritus, urticaria, Stevens–Johnson syndrome and toxic epidermal necrolysis. Occupational allergic contact dermatitis has been observed in a nurse who reconstituted medications from powdered form into solution. The allergen could leak onto the nurse's hands, either when the solution was drawn up the syringe or during its injection. Face dermatitis was probably due to involuntary contact with the hands or airborne contact [27].

Propacetamol hydrochloride is a water soluble *N,N*-diethylglycidyl ester of paracetamol. After intravenous administration, it is hydrolyzed into paracetamol and *N,N*-diethylglycine by nonspecific plasma esterases. Occupational allergic contact dermatitis was first described by Barbaud et al [28]. Since then, mainly palm and finger hand contact dermatitis and rare back or face dermatitis have been reported [29, 30]. Gielen et al consider this prodrug as an important cause of contact allergy (16.4%) [18]. The *N,N*-diethylglycidyl ester function of the propacetamol molecule is the most reactive part. Allergic contact dermatitis from propacetamol is not related to sensitization to paracetamol but to *N,N*-diethylglycine [31].

Chlorpromazine causes allergic contact dermatitis in nurses who inject or give out the drug in tablet form to patients, thus handling it with their fingers. This is a particularly common occurrence when pulverizing the tablets. This drug can sensitize by itself or in combination with photoallergic mechanisms (test 0.1% pet. or photopatch test if unexpectedly negative result appears) [32, 33].

Diacetylmorphine (heroin), morphine, and codeine are known for their histamine-releasing effects, causing (nonimmunological) contact urticaria. Anaphylactoid reactions, especially severe asthma, have been documented from inhaling heroin. Occupational contact dermatitis consists of redness and swelling, accompanied by severe itching on the eyelids, with subsequent spread to the face and neck. The nurses affected opened capsules containing a mixture of caffeine and diacetylmorphine (heroin) powder and handed it over to the patients [34].

Meclofenoxate is an analeptic of the central nervous system that may also sensitize nurses who inject it into patients [35].

Cyanamide (carbodiimide) is still used in some countries such as Spain for the treatment of alcoholism. Nurses can be sensitized from contact with tablets containing this drug when handling them in psychiatric wards. In many other countries tetraethylthiuram disulfide (Antabuse) represents a similar risk to nurses [36–38].

Potassium chloride has been reported as causing contact dermatitis in a nurse handling it in solution [39].

Ranitidine hydrochloride is an H2-receptor antagonist commonly used for the treatment of peptic ulcers. It is structurally related to cimetidine and famotidine. Chemical structure differences among these H2-receptor antagonists are too great for cross-reaction to occur. Two chemical groups could act as haptens: the terminal unsubstituted amino group and the furan group [40, 41]. Gielen et al reported seven cases of occupational allergic contact dermatitis by ranitidine in healthcare workers [18].

Occupational allergic contact dermatitis from handling other medicaments also has been reported for nurses. Ethylenediamine sensitized a nurse who prepared and administered systemic *aminophylline* in a department of pneumology. Aminophylline is a 2 :1 mixture of theophylline and ethylenediamine, which is used to make theophylline soluble [42].

Mesna (sodium 2-mercaptoethane sulfonate) is a mucolytic, administered by oral or intravenous routes, for example, as a uroprotective in combination with cyclophosphamide. Besides other skin reactions, it can produce allergic contact dermatitis in nurses from handling [43].

Many neoplastic drugs have been reported as being responsible for irritant and allergic contact dermatitis, or contact urticaria (mitomycin, nitroureas, methotrexate, and nitrogen mustard). Occupational contact urticaria in a nurse from cisplatin prepared in infusion solution has been described. Cisplatin is used to treat solid tumors including ovarian cancer and testicular teratoma. Ammonium tetrachloroplatinate 0.25% aq. and ammonium hexachloroplatinate 0.1% aq. were positive [44].

Vitamin B_6 was responsible for contact dermatitis on the hands, face and neck of a paramedical worker who injected vitamins B_1, B_6, and B_{12} into his patient [45]. Allergic contact dermatitis induced by pyrithioxine (pyritinol hydrochloride), the active ingredient in Encephabol, has been described [18]. It is the dihydrochloride monohydrate of pyritinol, a compound of pyridoxine (vitamin B_6). The free sulfydryl (SH) group in thiol drugs may be an inducer of skin lesions.

Nurses widely use formaldehyde as a disinfectant. It is a strong irritant in high concentrations, and a sensitizer, even in weak solutions. The nails are also affected, losing their color and hardness, and paronychia may be produced on the fingers. Its high sensitization power can result in disseminated skin reactions from only local skin contact or inhalation in very sensitive persons (test 1% aq.) [46].

Among others, individual cases of occupational contact dermatitis induced by drugs such as meglumine diatrizoate (used in Angiografin, Urografin and contrast media), papain (immediate and delayed allergic reactions), dipyridamole, tylosin, boldo (diuretic herbal medicine), cascara (anthraquinone stimulant laxative) or methylprednisolone have been reported in nurses, pharmacists or veterinarians.

40.2.2 Glutaraldehyde

1,5-Pentanedial (glutaraldehyde) is a pharmacological agent used for the treatment of hyperhidrosis, as an antifungal agent, and for the treatment of warts and some bullous diseases such as Weber–Cockayne syndrome, porphyria cutanea tarda, and epidermolysis bullosa acquisita. It has also been recommended for herpes zoster, herpes simplex and *Pseudomonas* infections.

Glutaraldehyde is an aliphatic dialdehyde, soluble in water, alcohol and many other solvents. It is employed at 2% as a cold sterilizer for many instruments in hospitals (in bronchoscopy, cytoscopy, anesthetics, renal dialysis, and so on). Unbuffered solutions of glutaraldehyde are stable and have little antimicrobial potential. When sodium bicarbonate is added, an alkaline pH of 8 results and a strong antimicrobial effect is obtained. Its antiviral, fungicidal and bactericidal activity is enhanced, but it remains stable for only 10–15 days. Activated glutaraldehyde retains the allergenic contact capacity of 1,5-pentanedial [47, 48].

Glutaraldehyde causes brown discoloration, irritant and allergic contact dermatitis, mainly in nurses, clinical assistants and cleaning workers in hospitals due to various sources of exposure [49, 50] (Table 2). Cases of hand eczema produced by this biocide are increasing. Clinical symptoms often show some chronicity, perhaps because glutaraldehyde is also employed as a leather tanning agent, in wallpaper, in photographic film and in other industries. Although glutaraldehyde and formaldehyde do not seem to cross-react [51, 52], some patients show positive allergic reactions to both substances [53, 54] (test 1% aq. or pet., but beware false-positive reactions [55]).

Waters et al [56] investigated work practices and glutaraldehyde exposure in relation to cutaneous symptoms and lung function. Disinfection activities were timed and counted, personal exposures established, and control measures documented. Skin problems were defined as "an itchy rash that was coming and going for six months." Bodily location was categorized as local (hand and forearm) or remote (distant from hand and forearm) symptoms.

Exposure values were above the exposure limit (0.10 ppm). Skin symptoms were 3.6 times more likely to be reported by exposed workers. Hand and forearm cutaneous symptoms were significantly associated with glutaraldehyde exposure. Significant cross-shift reductions in lung function parameters were observed.

Although the National Institute of Occupational Safety and Health in the USA has published guidelines for the safe handling of glutaraldehyde, the number of incidences of allergic reaction to it appears to be rising. In Australia, the occupational exposure standard, expressed as a permissible exposure limit ceiling value, was reduced from 0.20 to 0.10 ppm. In the USA it is 0.05 ppm [56]. Natural rubber latex glove material is more permeable to glutaraldehyde than styrene-ethylene-butadiene-styrene thermoplastic elastomer material [57]. Exposure controls for glutaraldehyde are required to improve skin care. Exposure monitoring methods also need to be reviewed.

Core Message

- Cases of hand eczema produced by glutaraldehyde are increasing. Clinical symptoms often show some chronicity, perhaps because glutaraldehyde is also employed in other industries. Although glutaraldehyde and formaldehyde do not seem to cross-react, some patients show positive allergic reactions to both substances.

40.2.3 Ampholytes, Surfactants, Soaps

Ampholytes are used as disinfectants in many different places, but have been widely used by hospital personnel. Desimex, Ampholyt G and Tego 103 G are dodecyldiaminoethylglycine hydrochloride. Ampholyt G does not contain benzyl alcohol or formaldehyde. Tego 103 G contains the active ingredients 9-lauryl-3,6,9-triazanonanoic acid and 7-dilauryl-1,4,7-triazaheptane, benzyl alcohol, and a small quantity of formaldehyde. Cases of allergic contact dermatitis have been described. Because of the chemical nature of these substances, some patients may also be reactive to ethylenediamine, but this special cross-reaction is rare [58, 59].

Dodecyl-dimethyl-ammonium chloride and bis-(aminopropyl)-laurylamine are detergents, disinfectants, and amphoteric tensioactives used to clean op-

Table 2. Sources of glutaraldehyde exposure in healthcare workers [50]

Instrument sterilization
Embalming
Tissue fixation
Radiographic development
Preparation of allergen and collagen extracts for injection
Medical treatment of
Epidermolysis bullosa
Herpes simplex
Hyperhidrosis
Onychomycosis
Warts

erating rooms and other areas. They are bactericidal, virucidal and active against HIV₁. They are used at concentrations of 0.25%. Both may cause allergic contact dermatitis in hospital workers. Patch tests must be from 0.01% aq. to 0.1% and 1% aq. [60]. The use of protective gloves and systematic prevention of contact is recommended. Dinitrochlorobenzene, nitrogen mustards and squaric acid diethylester are examples of such substances.

Gigasept AF, a detergent-disinfectant for surgical instruments, is capable of inducing burning eyes and coughing fits after direct exposure to its vapor. Despite protective measures (gloves and masks), skin lesions and other symptoms can persist. The allergens were dimethyldidecylammonium chloride 0.1%, N,N-bis(3-aminopropyl)dodecylamine 1.0% and N,N-bis(3-aminopropyl)dodecylamine [61].

Antiseptics that commonly cause contact dermatitis in nurses, clinical assistants and cleaners are widely used in different hospital wards. The majority of exposures occur in dental and surgical personnel. Chloramine-T (sodium p-toluenesulfonchloramine) has been found to be a sensitizer for nurses [62]. Chloramine-T is used as sterilizer, disinfectant, antiseptic and chemical reagent (test 0.05% aq.). Allergic contact dermatitis from undecylenamide diethanolamide in a liquid soap has been described in a hospital worker [63].

Methyldibromo glutaronitrile (1,2-dibromo-2,4-dicyanobutane) is used as preservative in soaps and many other products. It is found mainly in the preservative Euxyl K400 combined with phenoxyethanol. Occupational allergic contact dermatitis from this agent is increasing in frequency. Patch test of 0.1%, 0.3% and 0.5% in pet. was positive in two nurses sensitized to methyldibromo glutaronitrile at work [64]. The British Contact Dermatitis Society have recommended adding methyldibromo glutaronitrile to standard series in all UK patch testing centers.

> ### Core Message
>
> - Occupational allergic contact dermatitis from methyldibromo glutaronitrile is increasing in frequency.

40.2.4 Diisocyanates

Diisocyanates are a group of substances widely used as hardeners in paints, surface coatings and foams.

In hospitals, diisocyanates also are found as a constituent of soft casts. They are a cause of occupational asthma and have been described as causing cutaneous problems, both as irritants and as sensitizers.

When using soft casts, the extremity is covered by a layer gauze. The cast is dipped into water and applied while wearing rubber gloves and sometimes a barrier cream. Because of the potential for asthma, the ventilation is often switched on during the casting. When dipping the cast, the forearms above the level of the gloves often get into contact with the water. Having applied the cast, the extremity of the patient is rubbed in light circular motions, so that the cast fits perfectly. The dipping water is reused several times, accumulating diisocyanates from each use.

The sensitizing potential of diisocyanates has previously only been described sporadically. Few studies in animals or in exposed populations support diisocyanates as sensitizers. Larsen et al [65] conducted a study among the nursing staff of an orthopedic outpatient, clinic patch testing five types of diisocyanates. Just one nurse presented a doubtful reaction towards diaminophenylmethane and isophorene diisocyanate. Nine had no reactions to the five diisocyanates used in the patch test. Their observations suggest that diisocyanates are primarily irritants rather than sensitizers in the professional setting studied. No relationship between exposure time and severity of symptoms was observed.

40.2.5 Thiomersal/Mercury

Thiomersal was originally found to induce an allergy when a nurse was vaccinated against viral hepatitis. As a result of further contact with this preservative during the vaccination of schoolchildren, she showed allergic contact dermatitis on the hands. The vaccines from Biomed that she had been exposed to contained 0.01% thiomersal [66]. Two cases (an ophthalmologist and a nurse) of occupational dermatitis due to mercury vapor from a broken sphygmomanometer has been described. Patients suffered from itchy erythema with high fever followed by generalized exanthem. The air concentration of mercury vapor was higher than permissible levels (0.05 mg/m³ at a concentration of 9.9 mg/m³) [67].

40.3 Surgeons

Chemical components of rubber gloves commonly cause allergic contact dermatitis of the hands and forearms in surgeons. Although many different substances can sensitize, the most frequent are those

40

tested in the thiuram mix of the standard series. Less frequent are mercaptobenzothiazole and others tested in the mercapto mix. Release of thiurams and carbamates from rubber gloves varies between brands. Glove powder could enhance contact dermatitis and urticaria. Knowledge about cutaneous reactions from gloves has increased enormously in recent years. The main reason is the broad knowledge of type I allergy to natural rubber latex and recognition of the relatively large number of patients and health care personnel who suffer from this hypersensitivity.

Orthopedic surgeons use acrylic bone cement for fixation of prostheses to the bone of the hip joint. Bone cement contains methyl methacrylate monomer and polymethyl methacrylate. The monomer is a strong lipid solvent. The hand dermatitis caused by allergy to methacrylate is usually a dry, pruriginous, fissured, chronic eczema of the fingertips, sometimes with paresthesia and tingling or burning sensations. Gloves usually do not protect the hands from acrylic bone cement. Indeed, even if two pairs of rubber gloves are worn, the sensitized surgeon may still suffer from contact with the acrylic cement because enough acrylic penetrates both pairs if the surgeon makes contact for a sufficient duration [68–70]. Colophony has also been identified as a causative agent of allergic contact dermatitis in an orthopedic surgeon who suspected paper-based surgical clothing to be the cause [71].

40.3.1 Antiseptics

Antiseptics are present in surgical scrubbing agents in the preoperating room. Some surgeons contract chronic, dry, pruritic, irritant contact dermatitis of the dorsum of the hand from such agents. It is not infrequent for superimposed allergic contact dermatitis to appear, because these substances also have allergic capacity. The most commonly employed are: hexachlorophene G 11 (test 1% pet.), dichlorophene G 4 (test 1% aq.), tribromosalicylanilide (TCSA) (test 1% pet.), dibromosalicylanilide (test 1% pet.), triclosan (Irgasan DP 300) (test 2% pet.), Fentichlor (test 1% pet.), chlorhexidine (test both acetate and gluconate 0.5% aq.) [72], p-cresol (test 1% aq.), Dowicides (phenolic substances) (test 1% pet.), imidazolidinyl urea (test 2% pet.), sodium hypochlorite (test 0.5% aq.), sodium hyposulfite (test 1% aq.), and benzydamine hydrochloride (test 5% aq. or pet.) [73].

Some quaternary ammonium compounds are of special interest. The most common and widely used is benzalkonium chloride (alkylbenzyldimethylammonium chloride), a cationic detergent used as a preoperative skin disinfectant, and also for surgical instruments. Its presence in cosmetics, soaps, medicaments and its capacity to sensitize are well known. Some people allergic to benzalkonium chloride may need to avoid other quaternary ammonium compounds because of cross-reaction [74–77]. Patch testing with 0.1% aq. can also provoke irritant reactions. True allergic responses may be obtained by testing with 0.01% aq., but a dilution series plus ROAT is recommended.

Core Message

■ Chemical components of rubber gloves commonly cause allergic contact dermatitis of the hands and forearms in surgeons. Antiseptics present in surgical scrubbing agents in the preoperating room induce irritant contact dermatitis of the dorsum of the hand.

40.4 Laboratory Personnel

In pharmaceutical laboratories, mainly in product synthesis areas, contact dermatitis may arise in the pharmacologists who synthesize such products. Very often the sensitizers are not the final compounds. Sensitizations have been published as individual case reports, and substances mentioned include vitamin K_3 sodium bisulfite [78, 79], codeine [80], cephalosporins, cytosine arabinoside [81], 3,4-dicarbethoxyhexane-2,5-dione [82], 2-aminophenyldisulfide [83], ethyl-2-bromo-p-methoxyphenylacetate [84], ethyl-chlorooximidoacetate [85], pyridine in Karl Fischer reagent [86, 87], simvastatin [88] and n-acetyl-cysteine [88].

Hypersensitivity to azathioprine is well known, but not that to an intermediate product (5-chloro-1-methyl-4-nitroimidazole) which has been shown to be present in the end product of azathioprine tablets in a sufficient amount to induce allergic contact dermatitis in a man working on its synthesis (test at 0.1% pet.) [89]. Vitamin A acetate has also been reported to be a sensitizer in the industrial production of vitamins (test at 1% pet.) [90]. DDC (dicyclohexyl carbodiimide), diisopropyl carbodiimide and dimethylaminopropylethyl carbodiimide are compounds widely used in peptide chemistry as coupling reagents. Sensitization occurred in two laboratory workers. Because they are highly toxic substances, patch tests must be done from 0.1% acet. or lower concentration [91].

Contact dermatitis caused by alcohols is of special interest. Amyl, butyl, ethyl, methyl, and isopropyl alcohols can all cause allergic contact dermatitis, though rarely. Contact allergy to alcohols may cause a generalized allergic reaction when alcohol is ingested. Nevertheless, contact reactions to alcohol do not necessarily signify that a systemic reaction will develop after drinking alcoholic liquor [92–94]. Alcohol can be an allergen for nurses, physicians and laboratory technicians. It can produce irritant contact dermatitis and nonimmunological contact urticaria. Its effects can be produced by external or internal exposure. Contaminants are common in alcohol. Pure ethanol should be used for patch testing. Because of its volatility, interpreting the results can be difficult. In occlusive patch testing, immediate fading of the reaction suggests irritancy. If the reaction remains clearly visible after 4 days, it may be allergic. Repeated testing with lower dilutions may confirm this. Alcohols can be tested undiluted, although many different concentrations have been used, the lowest being 1% [95].

Laboratories use many other different substances capable of producing dermatitis in their personnel. As the working environments are so diverse, aimed patch testing needs to be performed, guided by a careful history. The substances that have been described as causing allergic contact dermatitis in laboratory technicians are, for example, propylene oxide in preparing tissue specimens in a histopathological laboratory (test in ethanol at 0.1–11%) [96].

DL-Limonene (dipentene) has been used as a nontoxic substitute for xylene as a wax solvent and a cleaning agent for use by laboratory technicians. Hydroperoxides in autoxidized D-limonene have also been identified as potent contact sensitizers in laboratory workers, and they may be present in new solvents such as Parasolve [97].

Pyridine-related molecules [98], and a new isothiazolinone [99] also produce allergic contact dermatitis in such workers.

New immersion oils were recently introduced in order to address ecological concerns. Allergic contact dermatitis to oils is a well recognized phenomenon (Fig. 1). It was initially described in 1997 by Sommer et al [100] and in 1998 by LeCoz and Goossens [101]. Many cases have been reported since then [102–112]. Technicians and physicians working in cytogenetic, bacteriology, and hematology laboratories were the workers affected. Contact dermatitis or airborne allergy mainly involves the forearms and hands, as well as the face and neck. Irritant reactions must also be considered. The product responsible was usually Leica immersion oil (Leica Microsystems, Wetzler, Germany). According to the material safety data sheet,

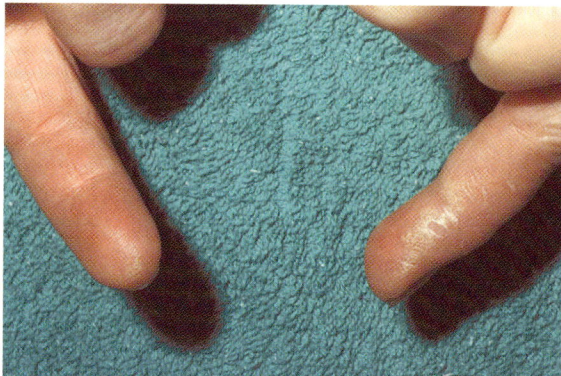

Fig. 1. Chronic allergic contact dermatitis with dyshidrotic features in a laboratory technician, due to epoxy resin in immersion oil (Leica) (courtesy of A. Goossens)

the oil content is: modified cyclohexyl epoxy resin (45%), modified bisphenolic epoxy resins (35%), 1,4-butanediol diglycidylether (10%) and phthalates (4%). A breakdown performed with the oil's ingredients confirmed sensitization to liquid modified epoxy resin components contained at >80% concentration. Diglycidyl ether of bisphenol A (DGBEA) (Mol. Wt. 340 Da), a low molecular weight monomer, was probably the main sensitizer [100]. Positive reactions have also been described to cycloaliphatic epoxy resin and to the diluents phenyl glycidyl ether and cresyl glycidyl ether. Epoxy resin is a strong contact allergen that can induce sensitization after a single exposure in about 50% of those exposed. Their incorporation into microscopic immersion oil was, unfortunately, not needed and could have been avoided [113].

Core Message

■ New ecological immersion oils induce allergic contact dermatitis. Diglycidyl ether of bisphenol A was probably the main sensitizer. Epoxy resin is a strong contact allergen. Their incorporation into microscopic immersion oil was an unnecessary and avoidable oversight.

40.5 Other Therapists

Some substances have been reported to be responsible for occupational contact dermatitis in other personnel involved in special therapeutic procedures.

A physiotherapist suffered allergic contact dermatitis from benzydamine hydrochloride and lavender fragrance, contained in Difflam gel, a topical nonsteroidal anti-inflammatory agent [114].

Isothiazolinone derivatives contained in Parmetol caused allergic contact dermatitis in a radiology technician. Parmetol is used in radiographic developing solutions [115].

Metaproterenol produced airborne contact dermatitis in a respiratory therapist who routinely administered Alupent (metaproterenol sulfate), Mucomyst (acetylcysteine) and Bronkosol (isoetharine) in aerosolized forms [116].

Benzoyl peroxide included in a hardener substance, Lucidol hardening gel, has been demonstrated to induce recurrent eczema of the face, neck and arms for 2 years in an orthopedic technician [117].

40.6 Veterinarians

Veterinarians are exposed to many organic, biological and chemical substances that may produce allergic contact dermatitis. Occupational dermatoses have been reported in 48–77% of veterinarians. Sensitized veterinarians can suffer asthma, rhinitis and contact dermatitis from dander, hair, bristles, or saliva from cows, horses, cats or dogs [118, 119]. Specific IgE and prick/scratch tests are diagnostic. Clinically, allergic contact urticaria, allergic contact dermatitis, or both reactions can be observed [120]. Bovine amniotic fluid (BAF) caused a severe and extensive eruption in a 30-year-old nonatopic veterinarian. Patch test and prick test proved negative, though a weak reaction to the patch was visible by the fourth day. Only an intradermal test was positive to BAF pure and at 1/10. In other similar patients, RAST has been useful for confirming the allergic nature of the relatively common protein contact dermatitis [121].

40.6.1 Antibiotics

Certain antibiotics are used more often in veterinary than in human medicine. Spiramycin, tylosin and benzyl penicillin diethylaminoethylester (penethamate) are the most important. Spiramycin and tylosin [18] are used to treat enteritis in pigs, mastitis in cows, and respiratory infections in household pets [122]. Penethamate hydriodide is used for local or intralesional treatment of mastitis in cows. It cross-reacts with penicillin [123].

40.6.2 Feed Additives and Other Medicaments

Hormones, vitamins, minerals, antibiotics, growth stimulants, preservatives, metals, antioxidants and certain other substances are present in animal feeds (Table 3). Health personnel who handle these additives may experience allergic contact dermatitis. For example, vitamin A and vitamin D_3 contain 5% ethoxyquin as an antioxidant preservative. Ethoxyquin (6-ethyl-1,2-dihydro-2,2,4-trimethylquinoline) is a contact sensitizer. Quindoxin, a growth-promoting factor, is a common sensitizer and it also induces photodermatitis [124, 125, 128]. Quindoxin is an anti-

Table 3. Animal feed additives [135, 136]

	Function	Test
Amprolium	Growth promoter	10% aq.
Arsanilic acid	Growth promoter	10% pet.
Bacitracin zinc	Growth promoter	20% pet.
Chlortetracycline hydrochloride	Growth promoter	5% pet.
Sulfacetamide	Growth promoter (prevents enteral infections)	5% pet.
Tylosin tartrate	Growth promoter (prevents Gram-negative infections)	5% pet.
Diethylstilboestrol	Fattening cattle	1% pet.
Ethoxyquin	Antioxidant preservative	1% pet.
Ethylenediamine	Antiseptic	1% pet.
Medroxyprogesterone acetate	Abortions	1% pet.
Neomycin sulfate	Prevention of dysentery	20% pet.
Nitrofurazone	Prevention of *Salmonella* infection	1% pet.
Penicillin	Prevention of mastitis	10,000 IU/g[a]
Thiabendazole	Worm control	1% pet.
Piperazine	Worm control	1% pet.
Phenothiazines	Worm control	1% pet.

[a] See Sect. 40.2.1, "Medicaments"

biotic of the quinoxaline family, a growth promoter. It has been reported to induce contact and photocontact dermatitis. Its derivatives olaquindox and carbadox have been used as feed additives for growth promotion in pigs, rabbits and other animals. It is extremely difficult for breeders to avoid exposure to dust containing relatively highly concentrations of olaquindox. A very low dose of olaquindox produces contact dermatitis, mainly by phototoxic or photoallergic mechanisms. In some cases persistent light reactors are developed. Olaquindox has an absorption spectrum between 256 nm and 373 nm.

The patients suffer eczema of the hands, wrists, forearms, face and neck with severe itching and light intolerance. In some cases farmers have a history of other photoallergies, for example to chlorpromazine, sunscreens, cosmetics and others. Halquinol, a chlorinated derivative of 8-hydroxyquinoline, is added to animal feeds to prevent *Escherichia coli* and *Salmonella* infections. Halquinol causes irritant, allergic and photoallergic dermatitis, and sometimes allergic contact urticaria and airborne dermatitis [126].

Dinitolmide, which is used to control coccidiosis in chicken factories [127], and nitrofurazone, used for the treatment of salmonellosis in pigs and as a growth promoting factor for cattle and swine, can also cause allergic contact dermatitis in veterinarians [128]. Chlorpromazine and other phenothiazine derivatives are used by veterinarians and farmers for the sedation of animals. The occurrence of contact dermatitis and photodermatitis in a farmer due to chlorpromazine used for the sedation of pigs suggests that this type of medicament should be included in a patch test series for veterinarians (Table 4) [129]. Occupational contact allergy to lincomycin and spectinomycin in chicken vaccinators has been documented [137].

40.7 Laboratory Animal Handlers

Allergic disease is a serious occupational health concern for individuals who have contact with laboratory animals. Urticaria is the most common skin manifestation, although contact dermatitis may also occur [130]. The overall prevalence of allergic disease among laboratory animal handlers is about 23% and respiratory allergy is much more common than skin allergy. There are few data on the incidence or prevalence of skin conditions. A study performed in Sweden by Agrup and Sjöstedt [131] revealed a prevalence of 14% of contact urticaria to rats, but this appears to be an unusually high rate. Another study of pharmaceutical industry and university laboratory workers found no increase in urticaria [132]. Evidence from the study of Aoyama et al indicates that skin allergy tends to be accompanied by respiratory allergy symptoms [137].

40.8 Dental Workers

Dentistry is a high-risk occupation for irritant and allergic hand eczema and also contact urticaria induced by latex allergy. Irritant contact dermatitis is most common. In 1947, Stevenson [138] and Moody [139] reported, for the first time, on an occupationally acquired allergic contact dermatitis in a dental technician. Many reports on allergies of dental personnel to (meth)acrylates have been published [140–142].

A recent Swedish study showed a prevalence of contact allergy to acrylates of below 1% among dentists, and in most cases this did not have serious medical, social or occupational consequences [143]. On patch testing, 50% of dentists studied presented at least one positive reaction. The most frequent allergens were nickel sulfate, fragrance mix, gold sodium thiosulfate and thiuram mix. Similar results were obtained from a Korean study of dental technicians [144]. Metals including potassium dichromate, nickel sulfate, mercury ammonium chloride, cobalt chloride and palladium chloride showed high positive rates. A lower patch-positive reaction to acrylics was observed.

A different picture of the influence of sensitization to dental composite resins upon working ability is given in Finnish study, in which 6/7 dental personnel

Table 4. Contact allergens reported in veterinarians [133, 134]

Penicillin	10,000 IU (g pet.[a])
Formaldehyde	1% aq.
Streptomycin	1% pet.
Mercaptobenzothiazole	2% pet.
Dihydrostreptomycin	0.1% pet.
Merthiolate	0.1% pet.
Erythromycin base	1% pet.
Piperazine	1% aq.
Oxytetracycline	3% pet.
Tuberculin	10% aq.
Penethamate	1% pet.
Bovine tuberculin	10% aq.
Spiramycin (Rovamycin)	10% pet.
Ethoxyquin	1% pet.
Tylosin (tartrate)	5% pet.
Quindoxin	0.1% pet.
Procaine HCl	1% pet.
Chlorpromazine	0.1% pet.
Benzocaine	5% pet.

[a] See Sect. 40.2.1, "Medicaments"

40

could not continue in clinical dentistry. Contact allergy to (meth)acrylate was seen in around 20% of the tested patients in another Swedish study, with allergy to three predominance test substances: 2-hydroxyethyl metacrylate, ethyleneglycol dimethacrylate and methyl methacrylate. A third of the patients allergic to (meth)acrylates had been on sick leave due to dermatitis [145].

Among acrylates, the unpolymerized products are the most allergenic, whereas the end-products obtained after polymerization have little or no allergenic capacity. The usual clinical appearance is a scaly, fissured dermatitis of finger pulps, sometimes accompanied by sensations like burning, tingling or numbness, which can last for several weeks after the dermatitis subsides [146]. The dominant hand is mainly affected. An uncommon clinical picture involves the left palm and fingers [147, 148]. Very late reactions are rare and can be considered as true sensitization or active sensitization [149].

Occupational contact dermatitis in a dental technician from the colophonium at dental baseplates [150] and in a dental nurse from the glutaraldehyde and glyoxal from cold sterilization of instruments [151] has been described.

Work-related face dermatitis has been reported in Swedish dentist; 4.5% from composite and bonding materials, compared to 3.1% from other materials (nickel sulfate) [152]. Finnish dental nurses considered their masks to be the main cause (5.4%) [153]. The face mask was also the most common cause of face dermatitis in Norwegian dental hygienists [154].

The importance of skin protection by gloves, no-touch product packaging and careful work techniques not questioned. But its usefulness is questionable [155]. The type of protective glove that should be recommended for dentistry is not clear. Medical gloves for single use are not impermeable to various acrylate monomers. A combination of a thin copolymer glove under a medical glove for single use offers good protection [156].

Core Message

■ Dentistry is a high-risk occupation for irritant contact hand eczema dermatitis. Among acrylates, it is the unpolymerized products that are the most allergenic. The importance of skin protection by gloves, no-touch product packaging and careful work techniques is not questioned. But its usefulness is questionable.

40.9 Conclusion

Healthcare workers are exposed to many agents capable of inducing irritant or allergic contact dermatitis and also contact urticaria. Skin complaints should be assessed with both prick and patch testing. It is necessary to identify the agents responsible in order to learn how to avoid them. Nevertheless, we need to develop effective prophylactic and preventive measures.

■ **Acknowledgements.** I dedicate this review chapter to Professor Jose G. Camarasa. He taught us to understand and to love immunodermatology.

References

1. Stingeni L, Lapomarda V, Lisi P (1995) Occupational hand dermatitis in hospital environments. Contact Dermatitis 33:172–176
2. Mahler V, Bruckner T, Schmidt A, Diepgen TL (2004) Occupational contact dermatitis in health care workers (ESCD Meeting, Copenhagen). Contact Dermatitis 50:158–159
3. Camarasa JG, Conde Salazar L (1988) Occupational dermatoses in sanitary workers. In: Orfanos CE, Stadler R, Gollnick H (eds) Dermatology in five continents. Proceedings of the XVIIth World Congress of Dermatology, Berlin, 24–29 May 1987. Springer, Berlin Heidelberg New York, pp 1045–1048
4. Holness DL, Mace SR (2001) Results of evaluating health care workers with Prick and Patch testing. Am J Contact Dermat 12:88–92
5. Nettis E, Colanardi MC, Soccio AL, Ferrannini A, Tursi A (2002) Occupational irritant and allergic contact dermatitis among healthcare workers. Contact Dermatitis 46:101–107
6. Kikuchi-Numagami K, Saishu T, Fukaya M, Kanazawa E, Tagami H (1999) Irritancy of scrubbing up for surgery with or without a brush. Acta Derm Venereol (Stockh) 79:230–232 d)
7. Hachem JP, de Paepe K, Sterckx G, Kaufman L, Rogiers V, Roseeuw D (2002) Evaluation of biophysical and clinical parameters of skin barrier function among hospital workers. Contact Dermatitis 46:220–223
8. Valsecchi R, Leghissa P, Cortinovis R, Cologni L, Pomesano A (2000) Contact urticaria from latex in healthcare workers. Dermatology 201:127–131
9. Lammintausta K, Kalimo K (1981) Atopy and hand dermatitis in hospital wet work. Contact Dermatitis 7:301–308
10. Nilson E, Mikaelsson B, Andersson S (1985) Atopy, occupation and domestic work as risk factors for hand eczema in hospital workers. Contact Dermatitis 13:216–223
11. Lammintausta K, Kalimo K, Havu VK (1982) Occurrence of contact allergy and hand eczemas in hospital wet work. Contact Dermatitis 8:84–90
12. Hansen KS (1983) Occupational dermatoses in hospital cleaning women. Contact Dermatitis 9:343–351
13. Singgih SIR, Lantinga H, Nater JP, Woest, Kruyt-Gaspersz JA (1986) Occupational hand dermatoses in hospital cleaning personnel. Contact Dermatitis 14:14–19

14. Gawkrodger DJ, Lloyd MH, Hunter JAA (1986) Occupational skin disease in hospital cleaning and kitchen workers. Contact Dermatitis 15:132–135

15. Gibbon KL, McFadden JPM, Rycroft RJG, Ross JS, Chinn S, White IR (2001) Changing frequency of thiuram allergy in healthcare workers with hand dermatitis. Br J Dermatol 144:347–350

16. Aalto-Korte K, Jolanki R, Estlander T, Alanko K, Kanerva L (1996) Occupational allergic contact dermatitis caused by Euxyl K 400. Contact Dermatitis 35:193–194

17. Strauss RM, Gawkrodger DJ (2001) Occupational contact dermatitis in nurses with hand eczema. Contact Dermatitis 44:293–296

18. Gielen K, Goossens A (2001) Occupational allergic contact dermatitis from drugs in healthcare workers. Contact Dermatitis 45:273–279

19. Sidi E, Longueville R, Hincky M (1958) Occupational eczema in therapists. Thomas, Springfield, Ill., p 196

20. Blanton WB, Blanton FM (1953) Unusual penicillin hypersensitiveness. J Allergy 24:405–406

21. Pecegueiro M (1990) Occupational contact dermatitis from penicillin. Contact Dermatitis 23:190–1991

22. Miyahara H, Koga T, Imayama S, Hori Y (1993) Occupational contact urticaria syndrome from cefotiam hydrochloride. Contact Dermatitis 29:210–211

23. Foti C, Vena GA, Cucurachi R, Angelini G (1994) Occupational contact allergy from cephalosporins. Contact Dermatitis 31:129–130

24. Foti C, Bonamante D, Trenti R, Vena GA, Angelini G (1997) Occupational contact allergy to cephalosporins. Contact Dermatitis 36:104–119

25. Filipe P, Almeida RS, Rodrigo FG (1996) Occupational allergic contact dermatitis from cephalosporins. Contact Dermatitis 34:226

26. Belsito DV (1993) Contact urticaria from pentamidine isothionate. Contact Dermatitis 29:158–159

27. Yesudian PD, King CM (2001) Occupational allergic contact dermatitis from meropenem. Contact Dermatitis 45:53

28. Barbaud A, Tréchot P, Bertrand O, Schmutz J-L (1995) Occupational allergy to propacetamol. Lancet 346:902

29. Lehners-Weber C, de la Brassine M (1996) Allergie au prodafalgan. Lettre GERDA 13:4–5

30. Szczurko C, Dompmartin A, Michel M, Castel B, Leroy D (1996) Occupational contact dermatitis from propacetamol. Contact Dermatitis 35:299–301

31. Berl V, Barbaud A, Lepoittevin J-P (1998) Mechanissm of allergic contact dermatitis from propacetamol: sensitisation to activated N,N-diethylglycine. Contact Dermatitis 38:185–188

32. Calnan CD, Frain-Bell W, Cuthbert JW (1962) Occupational dermatitis from chlorpromazine. Trans St Johns Hosp Dermatol Soc 48:49

33. Camarasa JG (1976) Contact dermatitis to phenothiazines Nemactil and Decentan. Contact Dermatitis 2:123

34. Coenraads PJ, Hogen Esch AJ, Prevoo RLMA (2001) Occupational contact dermatitis from diacetylmorphine (heroin). Contact Dermatitis 45:114

35. Foussereau J, Lautz JP (1972) Allergy to maclofenoxate in nurses. Contact Dermatitis Newslett 6:231

36. Conde Salazar L, Guimaraens D, Romero L, Harto A (1981) Allergic contact dermatitis to cyanamide (carbodiimide). Contact Dermatitis 7:329–330

37. Goday JJ, Yanguas I, Soloeta R (1994) Allergic contact dermatitis from cyanamide: report of three cases. Contact Dermatitis 31:331–332

38. Mathelier-Fusade P, Leynadier F (1994) Occupational allergic contact reaction to disulfiram. Contact Dermatitis 31:121–122

39. Zabala R, Aguirre A, Eizaguirre X, Diaz Perez JL (1993) Contact dermatitis from potassium chloride. Contact Dermatitis 29:218–219

40. Camarasa JG, Alomar A (1980) Contact dermatitis to H2-antagonist. Contact dermatitis to an H2-antagonist. Contact Dermatitis 6:152–153

41. Goh CL, Ng SK (1984) Allergic contact dermatitis to ranitidine. Contact Dermatitis 11:252

42. Corazza M, Mantorani L, Trimurti S, Virgili A (1994) Occupational contact sensitization to ethylenediamine in a nurse. Contact Dermatitis 31:328–329

43. Benyoussef K, Bottlaender A, Pfister HR, Caussade P, Heid E, Grosshans E (1996) Allergic contact dermatitis from mesna. Contact Dermatitis 34:228–229

44. Bajaj AK, Rastogi S, Misra A, Misra K, Bajaj S (2001) Occupational and systemic contact dermatitis with photosensitivity due to vitamin B6. Contact Dermatitis 44:184

45. Schena D, Barba A, Costa G (1996) Occupational contact urticaria due to cisplatin. Contact Dermatitis 34:320–321

46. Torresani C, Periti I, Beski L (1996) Contact urticaria syndrome from formaldehyde with multiple physical urticarias. Contact Dermatitis 35:174–175

47. Sanderson KV, Cronin E (1968) Glutaraldehyde and contact dermatitis. Contact Dermatitis Newslett 4:79

48. Lyon TC (1971) Allergic contact dermatitis due to Cidex. Oral Surg 32:895

49. Schnuch A, Geier J, Uter W, Frosch PJ (1998) Patch testing with preservatives, antimicrobials and industrial biocides. Results from a multicentric study. Br J Dermatol 138:467–476

50. Shaffer MP, Belsito DV (2000) Allergic contact dermatitis from glutaraldehyde in health-care workers. Contact Dermatitis 43:150–156

51. Neering H, van Ketel WG (1974) Glutaraldehyde and formaldehyde allergy. Contact Dermatitis Newslett 16:518

52. Maibach HI (1975) Glutaraldehyde: cross-reaction to formaldehyde. Contact Dermatitis 1:326

53. Nethercott JR, Holness DL, Page E (1988) Occupational contact dermatitis due to glutaraldehyde in health care workers. Contact Dermatitis 18:193–197

54. Hansen KS (1983) Glutaraldehyde occupational dermatitis. Contact Dermatitis 9:81–82

55. Hansen EM, Menné T (1990) Glutaraldehyde: patch test, vehicle and concentration. Contact Dermatitis 23:369–370

56. Waters A, Beach J, Abramson M (2003) Symptoms and lung function in health care personnel exposed to glutaraldehyde. Am J Ind Med 43:196–203

57. Lehman PA, Franz TJ, Guin JD (1994) Penetration of glutaraldehyde through glove material: Tactylon versus natural rubber latex. Contact Dermatitis 30:176–177

58. Foussereau J, Samsoen M, Hecht MT (1983) Occupational dermatitis to Ampholyt G in hospital personnel. Contact Dermatitis 9:233–234

59. Suhonen R (1980) Contact allergy to dodecyldi(aminoethyl)glycine (Desimex i). Contact Dermatitis 6:290–291

60. Dejobert Y, Martin P, Piette F, Thomas P, Bergoend H (1997) Contact dermatitis from didecyldimethylammonium chloride and bis(aminopropyl)-laurylamine in a detergent-disinfectant used in hospital. Contact Dermatitis 37:95–96

61. Dibo M, Brasch J (2001) Occupational allergic contact dermatitis from N,N-bis(3-aminopropyl)dodecylamine

and dimethyldidecylammonium chloride in 2 hospital staff. Contact Dermatitis 45:40

62. Lombardi P, Gola M, Acciai MC, Sertoli A (1984) Unusual occupational allergic contact dermatitis in a nurse. Contact Dermatitis 20:302

63. Cristersson S, Wrangsjö K (1991) Contact allergy to undecylenamide diethanolamide in a liquid soap. Contact Dermatitis 27:191–192

64. Diba VC, Chowdhury MMU, Adisesh A, Statham BN (2003) Occupational allergic contact dermatitis in hospital workers caused by methyldibromoglutaronitrile in a work soap. Contact Dermatitis 48:118–119

65. Larsen TH, Gregersen P, Jemec GBE (2001) Skin irritation and exposure to diisocyanates in orthopedic nurses working with soft casts. Am J Contact Dermat 12:211–214

66. Kiec-Swierczynska M, Krecisz B, Swierczynska-Machura D (2003) Occupational allergic contact dermatitis due to thiomerosal. Contact Dermatitis 48:337–338

67. Suzuki K, Matsunaga K, Umemura Y, Ueda H, Sasaki K (2000) Two cases of occupational dermatitis due to mercury vapor from a broken sphygmomanometer. Contact Dermatitis 43:175–177

68. Pegum J, Medhurst FA (1971) Contact dermatitis from penetration of rubber gloves by acrylic monomer. Br Med J 2:141

69. Fries JB, Fisher AA, Salvati EA (1975) Contact dermatitis in surgeons from methylmethacrylate bone cement. J Bone Joint Surg (Am) 57:547

70. Fisher AA (1979) Paresthesia of the fingers accompanying dermatitis due to methylmethacrylate bone cement. Contact Dermatitis 5:56

71. Bergh M, Menné T, Karlberg AT (1994) Colophony in paper-based surgical clothing. Contact Dermatitis 31:332–333

72. Knudsen BB, Avnstorp C (1991) Chlorhexidine gluconate and acetate in patch testing. Contact Dermatitis 24:45–49

73. Foti C, Vena GA, Angelini G (1992) Occupational contact allergy to benzydamine hydrochloride. Contact Dermatitis 27:328–329

74. Afzelius H, Thulin H (1979) Allergic reactions to benzalkonium chloride. Contact Dermatitis 5:60

75. Fisher AA, Stillman MA (1972) Allergic contact sensitivity to benzalkonium chloride. Arch Dermatol 106:169–171

76. Wahlberg JE (1962) Two cases of hypersensitivity to quaternary ammonium compounds. Acta Derm Venereol (Stockh) 42:230

77. Holness DL, Tarlo SM, Sussman G, Nethercott JR (1995) Exposure characteristics and cutaneous problems in operating room staff. Contact Dermatitis 32:352–358

78. Romaguera C, Grimalt F, Conde Salazar L (1980) Occupational dermatitis from vitamin K_3 sodium bisulfite. Contact Dermatitis 6:355

79. Camarasa JG, Barnadas M (1982) Occupational dermatosis by vitamin K_3 sodium bisulfite. Contact Dermatitis 8:268

80. Romaguera C, Grimalt F (1983) Occupational dermatitis from codeine. Contact Dermatitis 9:170

81. Conde Salazar L, Guimaraens D, Romero L (1984) Occupational dermatitis from cytosin arabinoside synthesis. Contact Dermatitis 1:44

82. Niklasson B, Björkner B (1990) Contact allergy to 3,4-dicarbethoxyhexane-2,5-dione. Contact Dermatitis 23:46–47

83. Tob RR, Lepoittevin J-P, Caussade P (1991) Contact allergy to 2-aminophenyl disulfide. Contact Dermatitis 25:196–197

84. Kanzaki T, Sakakibara N (1992) Occupational allergic contact dermatitis from ethyl-2-bromo-*p*-methoxyphenylacetate. Contact Dermatitis 26:204–205

85. Haussen BM (1992) Occupational allergic contact dermatitis from ethylchlorooximidoacetate. Contact Dermatitis 27:277–278

86. Knegt-Junk C, Geursen-Reitsma L, van Joost T (1993) Allergic contact dermatitis from pyridine in Karl Fischer reagent. Contact Dermatitis 28:252

87. Sasseville D, Balbul A, Kwong P, Kui Yu (1996) Contact sensitization to pyridine derivatives. Contact Dermatitis 35:100–101

88. Serra Baldrich E, Alomar A (2004) Occupational allergic contact dermatitis from drugs in pharmaceutical workers. Contact Dermatitis 50:59

89. Jolanki R, Alanko K, Pfaffli P, Estlander T, Kanerva L (1997) Occupational allergic contact dermatitis from 5-chloro-1-methyl-4-nitroimidazole. Contact Dermatitis 36:53–54

90. Heidenheim M, Jemec GBE (1995) Occupational allergic contact dermatitis from vitamin A acetate. Contact Dermatitis 33:439–440

91. Poesen N, De Moor A, Busschots A, Dooms Goossens A (1995) Contact allergy to dicyclohexyl carbodiimide and diisopropylcarbodiimide. Contact Dermatitis 32:368–369

92. Fregert S, Kokanson R, Rosman H et al (1963) Dermatitis from alcohols. J Allergy 34:404

93. Martin Scott I (1960) Contact dermatitis from alcohol. Br J Dermatol 72:372

94. Van Ketel WG, Tan Lim KN (1979) Contact dermatitis from ethanol. Contact Dermatitis 1:7

95. Ophaswongse S, Maibach HI (1994) Alcohol dermatitis: allergic contact dermatitis and contact urticaria syndrome, a review. Contact Dermatitis 30:1–6

96. Steinkraus V, Hansen BM (1994) Contact allergy to propylene oxide. Contact Dermatitis 31:120

97. Wakelin SH, McFadden JP, Leonard JN, Rycroft RJG (1998) Allergic contact dermatitis from D-limonene in a laboratory technician. Contact Dermatitis 38:164–165

98. Le Coz CJ, Caussade P, Bottlaender A (1998) Occupational contact dermatitis from methyl-ter-pyridine in a chemistry laboratory technician. Contact Dermatitis 38:214–215

99. Burden AD, O'Driscoll JB, Page FC, Beck MH (1994) Contact hypersensitivity to a new isothiazolinone. Contact Dermatitis 30:179–180

100. Sommer S, Wilkinson SM, Wilson CL (1998) Airborne contact dermatitis caused by microcopy immersion fluid containing epoxy resin. Contact Dermatitis 39:141–142

101. Le Coz C, Goossens A (1998) Contact dermatitis from an immersion oil for microscopy. N Engl J Med 339:406–407

102. Downs AM, Sansom JE (1998) Airborne occupational contact dermatitis from epoxy resin in an immersion oil used for microscopy. Contact Dermatitis 39:267

103. Le Coz CJ, Coninx D, van Rengen A, El Aboubi S, Ducombs G, Benz MH, Boursier S, Avenel-Audran M, Verret JL, Erikstam U, Bruze M, Goosens A (1999) An epidemic of occupational contact dermatitis from an immersion oil for microscopy in laboratory personnel. Contact Dermatitis 40:77–83

104. Lee YC, Gordon DL, Gordon LA (1999) Epoxy resin allergy from microscopy immersion oil. Aust J Dermatol 40:228–229

105. Geraut C, Tripodi D (1999) "Airborne" contact dermatitis due to Leica immersion oil. Int J Dermatol 38:676–679

106. Hasan T (1999) Immersioöljystä epoksihartsiallergia (Epoxy resin allergy from immersion oil; in Finnish). Duodecim 115:1101–1102

107. Crepy MN, Bazire A, Bayeaux-Dunglas MC, Cohen-Jonathan AM, Ratheau MC, Ameille J (2000) Immersion oils for microscopy: a new source of occupational eczema. Ann Derm Venereol (Stockh) 127:210–211
108. Sasseville D, Moreau L, Brassard J, Leclerc G (2000) Allergic contact dermatitis to epoxy resin in microscopy immersion oil: cases from Canada. Am J Contact Dermat 11:99–103
109. Ahmed I, Ilchyshyn A (2000) Immersion oil allergy with no reaction to epoxy resin in standard series. Contact Dermatitis 43: 125–126
110. Andersen KE, Clemmensen OJ (2000) Immersion oil contact allergy, an unsuspected source of epoxy allergy. Am J Contact Dermat 11:133
111. Kanerva L, Jolanki R, Estlander T (2001) Active sensitisation by epoxy in Leica immersion oil. Contact Dermatitis 44:194
112. El-Azhary RA, Yiannias JA (2002) Allergic contact dermatitis to epoxy resin in immersion oil for light microscopy. J Am Acad Dermatol 47:954–955
113. Hughes R, Taylor JS (2002) Surveillance of allergic contact dermatitis: epoxy resin and microscopic immersion oil. J Am Acad Dermatol 47:965–966
114. Rademaker M (1994) Allergic contact dermatitis from lavender fragrance in Difflam gel. Contact Dermatitis 31: 58–59
115. Pazzaglia M, Vincenzi C, Gasparri F, Tosti A (1996) Occupational hypersensitivity to isothiazolinone derivatives in a radiology technician. Contact Dermatitis 34:143
116. Fung MA, Geisse JK, Maibach HI (1996) Airborne contact dermatitis from metaproterenol in a respiratory therapist. Contact Dermatitis 35:317–318
117. Forschner K, Zuberbier T, Worm M (2002) Benzoyl peroxide as a cause of airborne contact dermatitis in an orthopaedic technician. Contact Dermatitis 47:241
118. Camarasa JG (1986) Contact eczema from cow saliva. Contact Dermatitis 2:117
119. Prahl P, Roed-Petersen J (1979) Type I allergy from cows in veterinary surgeons. Contact Dermatitis 5:33–36
120. Roger A, Guspi R, Garcia Patos V, Barriga A, Rubira N, Nogueiras C, Castells A, Cadahia A (1995) Occupational protein contact dermatitis in a veterinary surgeon. Contact Dermatitis 32:248–249
121. Hjorth N, Weissmann K (1972) Occupational dermatitis among veterinary surgeons caused by spiramycin and tylosin. Contact Dermatitis Newslett 12:320
122. Hjorth N (1967) Occupational dermatitis among veterinary surgeons caused by penethamate. Berufsdermatosen 15:163
123. Melhorn HC, Beetz D (1971) Das Antioxydant Aethoxyquin als berufliches Ebenzatogen bei einem Futtermitteldosierer. Berufsdermatosen 19:84
124. Burrows D (1975) Contact dermatitis in animal feed mill workers. Br J Dermatol 92:167
125. Caplan RM (1973) Contact dermatitis from animal feed additives (letter to editor). Arch Dermatol 107:918
126. Bleumink E, Nater JP (1973) Allergic contact dermatitis to dinitolmide (letter to editor). Arch Dermatol 108: 423–424
127. Nelder KM (1972) Contact dermatitis from animal feed additives. Arch Dermatol 106:722–723
128. Shander S, Schröder W, Geier J (1996) Olaquindox-induced airborne photoallergic contact dermatitis followed by transient or persistent light reactors in 15 pig breeders. Contact Dermatitis 35:344–354
129. Hjorth N (1975) Battery for testing veterinary surgeons. Contact Dermatitis 1:122
130. Rudzki E, Rebandel P, Grzywa Z, Pomorski Z, Jakiminska B, Zawisza E (1982) Occupational dermatitis in veterinarians. Contact Dermatitis 8:72
131. Malten KE (1978) Therapeutics for pets as neglected causes of contact dermatitis in housewives. Contact Dermatitis 4:296–299
132. Fisher AA (1973) Allergic contact dermatitis in animal feed handlers. Cutis 16:20
133. Vilaplana J, Romaguera C, Grimalt F (1991) Contact dermatitis from lincomycin and spectinomycin in chicken vaccinators. Contact Dermatitis 24:225–22
134. Seward JP (2001) Medical surveillance of allergy in laboratory animal handlers. ILAR J 42:47–54
135. Agrup G, Sjöstedt L (1985) Contact urticaria in laboratory technicians working with animals. Acta Derm Venereol (Stockh) 65:111–115
136. Davies GE, McArdle LA (1981) Allergy to laboratory animals: A survey by questionnaire. Int Arch Allergy Appl Immunol 64:302–307
137. Aoyama K, Ueda A, Manda F, Matsushita T, Ueda T (1992) Allergy to laboratory animals: an epidemiological study. Br J Ind Med 49:41–47
138. Stevenson WJ (1941) Methyl methacrylate dermatitis. Contact Point 18:171
139. Moody WL (1941) Severe reaction from acrylic liquid. Dent Digest 47:305–307
140. Kanerva L, Estlander T, Jolanki R (1994) Occupational skin allergy in the dental profession. Dermatol Clin 12: 517–532
141. Hensten-Pettersen A, Jacobsen N (1991) Perceived side effects of biomaterials in prosthetic dentistry. J Prosthet Dent 65:138–144
142. Kanerva L, Estlander T, Jolanki R (1989) Allergic contact dermatitis from dental composite resins due to aromatic epoxy acrylates and aliphatic acrylates. Contact Dermatitis 20:201–211
143. Wallenhammar L.M-, Örtengren U, Andreasson H, Barregård L, Björkner B, Karlsson S, Wrangsjö K, Meding B (2000) Contact allergy and hand eczema in Swedish dentists. Contact Dermatitis 43:192–199
144. Lee JY, Yoo JM, Cho BK, Kim HO (2001) Contact dermatitis in Korean dental technicians. Contact Dermatitis 45: 13–16
145. Wrangsjö K, Swartling C, Meding B (2001) Occupational dermatitis in dental personnel: contact dermatitis with special reference to (meth)acrylates in 174 patients. Contact Dermatitis 45:158–163
146. Geukens S, Goossens A (2001) Occupational contact allergy to (meth)acrylates. Contact Dermatitis 44:153–159
147. Pegum J, Medhurst FA (1971) Contact dermatitis from penetration of rubber gloves by acrylic monomer. Br Med J 2:141–143
148. Brandao FM (2001) Palmar contact dermatitis due to (meth)acrylates. Contact Dermatitis 44:186
149. Fowler JF (1999) Late patch test reaction to acrylates in a dental worker. Am J Contact Dermat 10:224–225
150. Cockayne SE, Murphy R, Gawkrodger DJ (2001) Occupational contact dermatitis from colophonium in a dental technician. Contact Dermatitis 44:42
151. Kanerva L, Miettinen P, Alanko K, Estlander T, Jolanki R (2000) Occupational allergic contact dermatitis from glyoxal, glutaraldehyde and neomycin sulfate in dental nurse. Contact Dermatitis 42:116
152. Örtengren U, Andreasson H, Karlsson S, Meding B, Barregård L (1999) Prevalence of self-reported hand eczema and skin symptoms associated to dental materials among Swedish dentists. Eur J Oral Sci 106:496–505

40

153. Kanerva L, Alanko K, Jolanki R, Kanervo K, Susitaival P, Estlander T (2001) The dental face mask–the most common cause of work-related face dermatitis in dental nurses. Contact Dermatitis 44:261–662

154. Jacobsen N, Hensten-Pettersen A (1995) Occupational health problems among dental hygienists. Community Dent Oral Epidemiol 23:177–181

155. Boyle DK, Forsyth A, Bagg J, Stroubou K, Griffiths CEM, Burke FJT (2002) An investigation of the effect of prolonged glove wearing on the hand skin health of dental healthcare workers. J Dent 30:233–241

156. Boman A, Röndell E, Sandborgh-Englund G, Wiatr-Admczak E, Liden C (1999) Contamination and protection during dental work. 12th International Contact Dermatitis Symposium, 15–18 Oct 1999, San Francisco, Calif., USA

Chapter 41

Plants and Plant Products

41

Christophe J. Le Coz, Georges Ducombs

Contents

41.1 Introduction

Contact dermatitis from plants or plant products, *phytodermatitis*, is frequently observed in clinical practice. It is likely that the most frequent reactions of this type, which occur due to occasional and irritant contacts such as those encountered during leisure activities, are not seen by dermatologists. Practitioners usually see more severe dermatitis cases, with irritant or allergic mechanisms, of immediate or delayed type, and sometimes photoworsened or even photoinduced dermatitis.

The exact incidence of dermatitis from plants and plant products is not known, but this problem is not rare. Many patients likely self-medicate following self-diagnosis or diagnosis by a pharmacist, or attend their family doctor who prescribes palliative treatment without necessarily ascertaining the cause of the skin reaction. In other instances, cases do reach the dermatologist. For example, among 1752 patients considered to have occupational dermatitis, Fregert found that 8% of women and 6% of men were reacting to plant-derived products [1]. We can therefore estimate that, among patients attending dermatologic clinics for dermatitis, an average of 5–10% suffer from dermatitis caused by plants or plant products. It is, however, evident that geographical variations in flora considerably influence the epidemiology of plant dermatitis.

In Europe, many phytodermatitis cases are occupationally acquired. Florists, gardeners, horticulturists, foresters, woodworkers, farmers, cookers and people in contact with food preparation are at risk, as described by Paulsen [2–4]. Hobby gardeners, housewives and those who handle or come into contact with plant materials non-occupationally are also at risk. Indeed, any persons enjoying leisure pursuits in the garden or countryside (children playing, campers, walkers and so on) are likely to come into contact with plant material with the potential to cause contact dermatitis.

For plants and plant products, reactions of mixed aetiology are frequent, like allergic reactions superimposed on irritant reactions due to Asteraceae, or mechanical plus chemical irritations evoked by stinging nettles. It is frequently hard to distinguish between allergic and irritant mechanisms in clinical examination and during patch test procedure, and the reader will have to bear this in mind constantly. We will limit this chapter to plant contact, and will not consider the effect of systemic administration of plants of plant extracts.

It is clearly impossible to provide an exhaustive catalog of cutaneous side-effects of plants in this chapter (which owes much to the previous edition by Georges Ducombs and Richard J. Schmitt), and the reader will sometimes be invited to examine the question in more detail using other sources. Some books are prominent in botanical dermatology, like those written by Mitchell and Rook [5], Lovell [6], Sell [7], or Benezra, Ducombs, Sell and Foussereau [8]. Others focus on, are devoted to, or are restricted to geographical areas [9]. Many (but not all) important medical articles and reviews are indexed in international databases like the United States National Library of Medicine (see http://www.nlm.nih.gov/). We also warmly recommend the website BoDD (Bo-

tanical Dermatology Database, owner Richard J. Schmitt, see http://bodd.cf.ac.uk/index.html) for its interesting content [10].

41.2 Clinical Pictures

41.2.1 Immediate-Type Reactions

The types of reaction reviewed in this section belong to the class of immediate responses that have immunological or nonimmunological mechanisms.

41.2.1.1 Contact Urticaria

Contact urticaria appears within minutes following contact with the plant. It has been described for various species [11, 12].

Nonimmunological Contact Urticaria

Probably the best known urticant plants are the nettles belonging to family Urticaceae, like *Urtica dioica* L., *U. urens* L., and *U. pilulifera* L. The stinging hairs are disposed on the ventral faces of the leaves, permitting skin penetration of histamine, acetylcholine and 5-hydroxytryptamine after only a very slight touch. Nettles are used for rheumatic disorders in folk medicine [7,13].

Among other nonprotein substances, plant-derived pharmacological elicitors of urticaria are numerous, and include *Myroxylon pereirae* (balsam of Peru) and the cinnamic acid derivatives contained therein (Fig. 1), thapsigargin from *Thapsia garganica* L. (family Apiaceae) [11, 14, 15], and capsaicin from different species of capsicum, such as paprika and cayenne (*Capsicum* spp., family Solanaceae). The mechanism by which nonimmunologic urticant agents elicit their effect (at least for those agents listed above) appears to involve the release of histamine from mast cells.

Core Message

■ Contact urticaria from nonprotein chemicals is most often due to a non-immunological mechanism.

Immunological (IgE-mediated) Contact Urticaria

Fruits and vegetables may induce allergic contact urticaria, mainly in people with previous dermatitis,

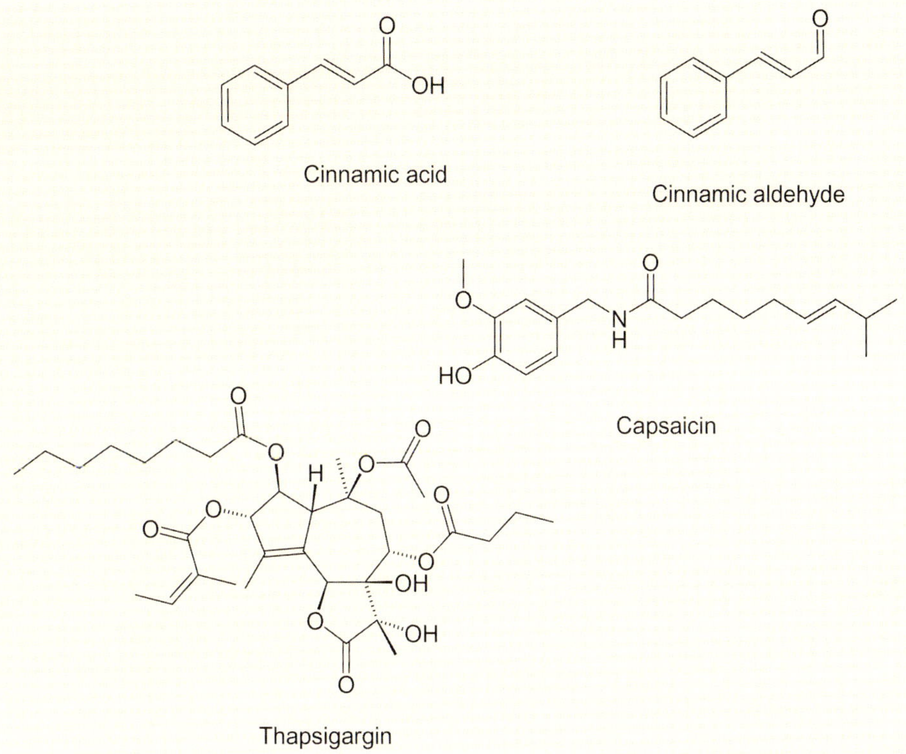

Fig. 1. Cinnamic acid, CAS 621–82–9, cinnamic aldehyde, CAS 104–55–2, thapsigargin, CAS 67526–95–8 and capsaicin CAS 404–86–4

like atopic dermatitis (see Sect. 41.2.1.2, Protein Contact Dermatitis). For example, sensitization from birch pollen (*Betula alba* L., family Betulaceae) may be complicated by immediate symptoms occurring after ingestion (mouth swelling) or skin contact (contact urticaria) due to apples, hazelnuts, almonds, plums, apricot, peach, cherries, or celery and carrot. This is due to strong homologies with the birch pollen allergens Bet v 1 and/or Bet v 2.

A case report of occupational contact urticaria and type I sensitization attributable to a gerbera (probably *Gerbera jamesonii* Bolus, family Asteraceae) has been reported. Conjunctivitis and respiratory symptoms are possible [16].

Airborne contact urticaria can be associated with rhinitis, conjunctivitis or asthma. This has been largely reported as an occupational problem in health workers with hypersensitivity to latex proteins from rubber gloves made with natural latex (usually derived from *Hevea brasiliensis* Muell.Arg., family Euphorbiaceae). Airborne transmission of the latex allergens is enhanced by their adsorption onto the cornstarch (derived from *Zea mays* L., family Gramineae) used as glove powder [17]. Airborne contact urticaria reported in a warehouseman resulted from

exposure to dust derived from cinchona bark (*Cinchona* spp., family Rubiaceae) [18].

Allergic urticaria may spread from the initial site of contact, become generalized or be associated with systemic symptoms of anaphylaxis.

Core Message

- Immunologic-type contact urticaria is due to specific IgE synthesis, mainly to proteins, and can be severe, with generalized or systemic symptoms.

41.2.1.2 Protein Contact Dermatitis

Protein contact dermatitis is mostly seen in persons (with atopy in 50% of cases) who handle foods, meat or vegetables, and has been described with frequent foods like onion, lettuce, potato, carrot or more rarely with asparagus (personal observation). It generally consists of a chronic dermatitis, mainly located on hands and forearms, with acute urticaria appearing within minutes of contact with food proteins, which rapidly disappears. It is followed by worsening of the dermatitis within hours or days [19–23]. Protein contact dermatitis can be of irritant (nonspecific) or allergic (IgE-mediated) type. In such cases, atopy with immediate-type sensitizations to pollens is frequent.

> ## Core Message
>
> ■ Protein contact dermatitis due to plant or plant products consists of contact urticaria followed by worsening of a previous dermatitis, mainly occurring in food handlers.

41.2.2 Irritant Contact Dermatitis

41.2.2.1 Mechanical Irritation

A number of plants can provoke "macrotraumatic" injury by mechanical means due to their armament of prickles, spines or thorns. Others, because of the knife-like morphologies of their leaf edges, may lacerate the skin. Although typically a trivial and self-limiting event, such mechanical damage may lead to the development of sores, secondary infections such as pyodermitis or tetanus, and granulomatous lesions that may develop insidiously some time after the initial trauma, after it has been forgotten. In arid regions of the Americas for example, cacti (family Cactaceae) are responsible for injuries that may become granulomatous, after dermal embedding of plant material [24, 25] (Fig. 2).

Certain plants are injurious because their bristles or barbs (named *trichomes* or *glochids*, respectively) can cause "microtrauma." These structures can penetrate the outer layer of the skin and cause papular dermatitis, prurigo and even symptoms of urticaria. In 1956, Shanon and Sagher [26] described "Sabra dermatitis," due to occupational contact with the prickly pear, also named the Indian or Barbary fig (*Opuntia ficus-indica* Miller, family Cactaceae) (Fig. 3). Dermatitis is caused by penetration of glochids from the spine cushions of the plants and their fruits through the skin, and it simulates chronic eczema or scabies.

Microtrauma (and chemical irritant action) from calcium oxalate needle crystals (named *raphides*) also causes a characteristic dermatitis resembling that from glass fiber [27]. Irritant contact dermatitis occurs almost systematically in people who handle

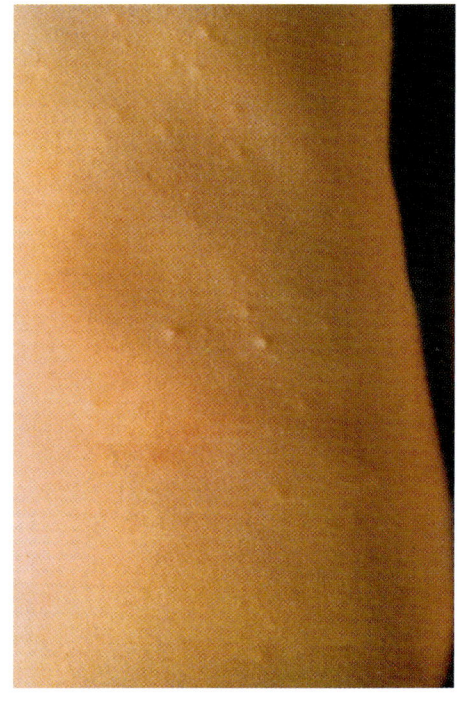

Fig. 2. Granulomatous lesions on a child's arm from cactus (courtesy of F. Vakilzadeh)

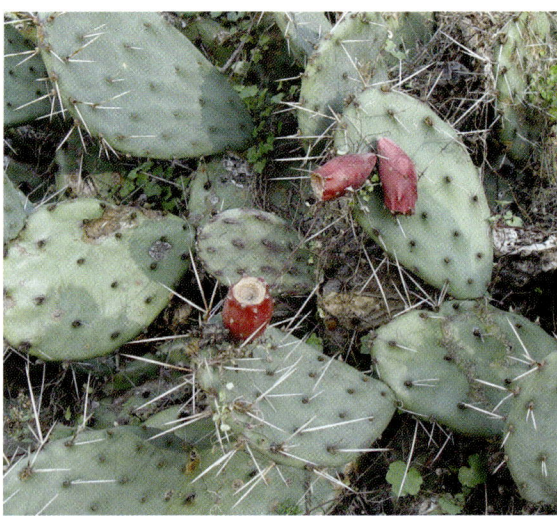

Fig. 3. Indian or Barbary fig (*Opuntia ficus-indica* Miller, family Cactaceae)

plants that contain crystals such as blue agave (*Agave tequilana* Weber) [28]. Penetration of the skin by such raphides may be accompanied by intracutaneous injection of plant sap. This can result in an irritant or allergic skin reaction to one or more of the sap constituents. Thus, preparation of the tubers of various aroids (plants of Araceae family) for food use

41

(for example the malanga or cocoyam, *Xanthosoma sagittifolium* L.) carries with it the risk of dermatitis from the calcium oxalate needle crystals and the saponins it contains [29]. Similarly, calcium oxalate raphides in dumbcanes (*Dieffenbachia* spp., family Araceae), which are commonly grown as decorative house plants, are responsible for an edematous urticaria-like dermatitis, and/or an edematous and bullous stomatitis in people who have handled damaged plant material or accidentally chewed the leaves. The reaction in the mouth renders the victim speechless (hence the common name of the plant, dumbcanes) and may even be life-threatening if the airway becomes obstructed. The severity of the reaction has been ascribed to the presence of a protease named dumbcain in the plant sap, which contributes to the irritant reaction [30].

Core Message

- Trauma due to plants may be due several mechanisms. Prickles, spines or thorns provoke macrotraumas, and leaves may act like knifes. Microtrauma may be due to dermo-epidermic penetration of trichomes (bristles), glochids (barbs), or raphides (calcium oxalate needle crystals).

41.2.2.2 Chemical Irritation

Many plants contain irritant substances (Table 1) which vary from weakly irritant compounds, requiring repeated exposure or a damaged skin barrier to exert their effects, to some of the most irritant compounds known to Man, which can elicit inflammation in microgram quantities, like these contained in Euphorbiaceae. Such potent skin irritants are also mucous membrane irritants, and can cause violent purgation after ingestion, and intense ocular irritation that may lead to blindness when there is contact with the eyes. The mechanical role of calcium oxalate needles has been described above: they moreover enhance the action of toxic chemicals such as the proteloytic enzyme bromelain (of pineapple), or the toxic glucosides contained herein, the so-called saponins.

Acute irritant dermatitis can arise after some minutes or hours. Chronic dermatitis develops after repeated contact with the irritant agent or on the background of previous contact with weakened skin. The clinical presentation of irritant contact dermatitis is various, but lesions are generally monomorphous in a patient (as with burns) and are limited to sites of contact, such as the hands, forearms, mucous membranes, perioral regions, buttocks, and so on. They consist of simple dryness of the skin, cracking and hyperkeratosis, inflammatory reactions with edema, erythema, papules, and vesicles. Pain rather than itching is also a feature. Strong irritant plants like spurges (*Euphorbia* spp., family Euphorbiaceae) may induce blisters, ulceration, or necrosis by the way of their acrid milky juice. Ranunculaceae, such as *Ranunculus bulbosus* L. or *R. repens* L., are sometimes used in traditional medicine, have been reported to be strong irritants, inducing bullous or even necrotizing dermatitis by the way of ranunculin [7, 13, 31].

Core Message

- Chemical irritation from plants (such as Euphorbiaceae) may induce severe chemical burns.

41.2.3 Allergic Contact Dermatitis

Allergic contact dermatitis (ACD) from plants can present in many forms, depending upon both the allergen and the method of exposure. Typical forms are represented by acute ACD, fingertips or periungueal chronic ACD, airborne ACD, contact urticaria, and erythema multiforme-like eruptions.

41.2.3.1 Acute ACD: Acute Eczema

The normal presentation is that of a typical ACD, involving exposed parts such as the hands, forearms, eyelids, and sometimes the genitals if the allergen is conveyed by the hands or clothing. Lesions onset at the site of contact are frequently diffuse, spreading on unexposed areas. The initial maculopapular or vesicular eruption may provoke blisters or develop into a full-blown erythroderma as, for example, with *Frullania* (Jubulaceae family) dermatitis.

41.2.3.2 Chronic ACD and the Example of "Tulip Fingers"

A number of examples of usually occupationally acquired finger dermatitis have been described, with some typical features. This takes the form of fingertip dermatitis, painful rather than pruritic, fissured

Table 1. Main plants responsible for chemical irritant contact dermatitis

Family	Botanical name	English name	French name	German name	Offending chemicals
Agavaceae	*Agave americana* Linné.	Agave	Agave d'Amérique	Amerikanische Agave	Calcium oxalate Sapogenins
Amaryllidaceae	*Narcissus pseudo-narcissus*	Daffodil	Jonquille	Gelbe Narzisse	Calcium oxalate
	Narcissus poeticus L.	Poet's narcissus	Narcisse des poètes	Dichternarzisse	Calcium oxalate
Araceae	*Dieffenbachia picta* Schott	Dumb cane	Dieffenbachia	Dieffenbachie	Calcium oxalate
	Philodendron spp.	Philodendron	Philodendron	Baumlieb	
Bromeliaceae	*Ananas cosmosus*	Pineapple	Ananas	Ananas	Calcium oxalate Bromel(a)in
Brassicaceae	*Armoracia rusticana*	Horse radish	Raifort	Meerrettich	Isothiocyanates
	Brassica oleracea var. *italica*	Broccoli	Brocoli	Brokkoli	
	Brassica nigra L.	True mustard	Moutarde noire	Schwarzer Senf	
	Raphanus sativus L. var. *sativus*	Small radish	Radis	Radieschen	
	Sinapis alba L.	White mustard	Moutarde blanche	Weisser Senf	
Euphorbiaceae	*Euphorbia* spp.	Spurge	Euphorbe	Wolfsmilch	Latex:
	Euphorbia pulcherrima Willdenow	Poinsettia	Poinsettia	Weinachtsstern	esters of phorbol
	Codiaeum variegatum	Croton	Croton	Wunderstrauch	esters of ingenol
	Hippomane mancinella	Manchineel tree	Mancellinier	Manzanillbaum	
	Ricinus communis L.	Castor bean	Ricin	Rizinus, Wunderbaum	
Liliaceae	*Hyacinthus orientalis* L.	Hyacinth	Jacinthe	Gartenhyazinthe	Calcium oxalate
Polygonaceae	*Rheum rhaponticum* L.	Rhubarb	Rhubarbe	Rhabarber	Calcium oxalate
Ranunculaceae	*Anemone pavonina* Lam.	Anemone	Anémone	Anemone	Protoanemonin
	Ranunculus acer L.	Meadow butter-cup	Bouton d'or	Butterblume	
	Aquilegia vulgaris L.	Columbine	Ancolie des jardins	Gemeine Akelei	
	Caltha palustris L.	Yellow marsh marigold	Souci d'eau	Sumpfdotterblume	
Solanaceae	*Capsicum frutescens* L.	Chillies	Piment de Cayenne, langue d'oiseau	Cayennepfeffer	Capsaici
	Capsicum annuum L.	Sweet pepper, capsicum	Poivron, piment doux and piment fort	Tachepfeffer, Paprika	

41

and hyperkeratotic, of which the best-known example is "tulip fingers," seen in tulip pickers (*Tulipa* spp. and cultivars, family Liliaceae). Lesions frequently spread on periungueal sites, inducing onychosis. Similar reactions may arise in persons handling daffodil and narcissus bulbs (*Narcissus* spp. and cultivars, family Amaryllidaceae), Alstroemeria flowers (*Alstroemeria* spp. and cultivars, family Alstroemeri-

aceae) (Fig. 4a, b), garlic (*Allium sativum* L., family Alliaceae), and so on. The most frequently involved fingers are those that are in direct and prolonged contact with the bulb. For garlic dermatitis in cooks, the nondominant hand is generally involved, since it is the one used to maintain the bulb. Although nominally an immunological delayed-type reaction, tulip fingers and related eruptions such as "daffodil itch"

Fig. 4a, b.
a *Alstroemeria* spp. family
Alstroemeriaceae. **b** Allergic
contact dermatitis in a nursery gardener from Alstroemeria (courtesy of P.J.
Frosch)

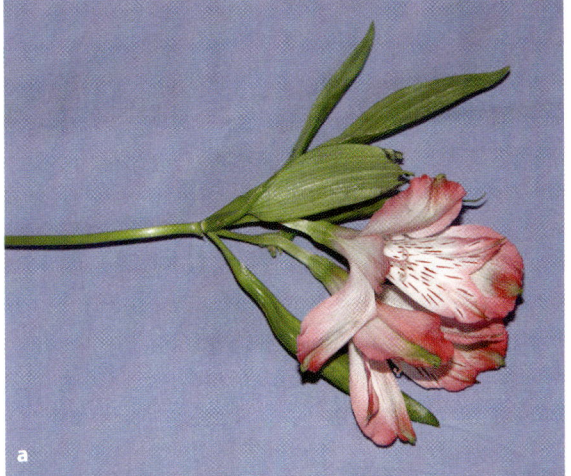

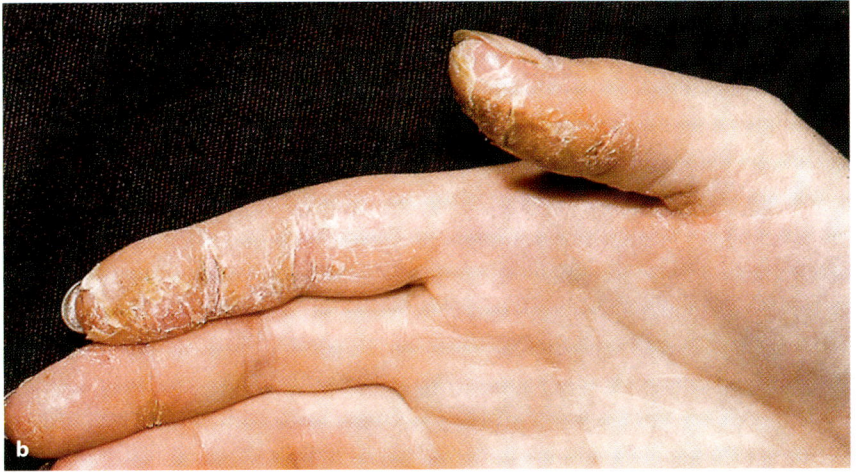

or "lily rash" in daffodil bulb or flower handlers [32] may arise in part from mechanical and/or chemical irritation.

41.2.3.3 Erythema Multiforme-like and Atypical Dermatitis

Bonnevie first described an erythema multiforme-like rash that developed after contact with leaves of *Primula obconica* Hance (family Primulaceae) [33]. The clinical picture resembles that of a drug erup-tion, with confluent pseudo-cockades arising on the contact area. Histopathological features are those of allergic contact dermatitis with severe edema and keratinocyte necrosis. Several authors have reported similar features following contact with poison ivy [34] or tropical woods such as Rio rosewood (*Dalber-gia nig*ra Allemão; pao ferro, *Machaerium scleroxy-lon* Tul., family Leguminosae) [35–38] (Fig. 5). Fur-ther nonoccupational cases have been reported in

the literature. An occupationally acquired airborne erythema multiforme-like eruption was due to py-rethrum (*Tanacetum* spp., family Compositae) used as a pesticide [39].

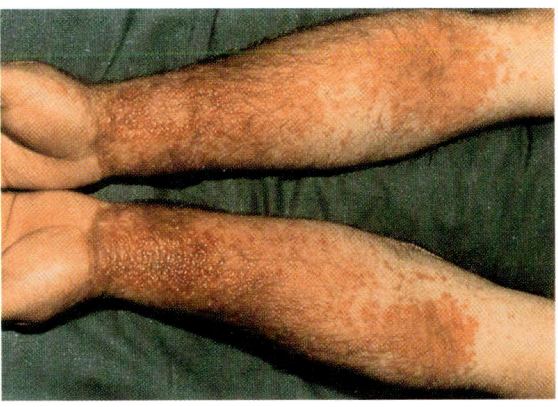

Fig. 5. Erythema-multiforme-like reaction in a carpenter caused by wood dust (pao ferro) (courtesy of P.J. Frosch)

Erythema multiforme-like dermatitis can be the expression of an active sensitization for several days following initial contact [40].

Intense blistering can evoke pemphigoid, as was observed in the wife of a woodworker who had been helping her husband work with bois d'Olon, a kind of satinwood (*Fagara heitzii* Aubrév. and Pellegrin, family Rutaceae) [41].

41.2.3.4 Airborne Contact Dermatitis

Hjorth et al [42] described an airborne ACD of plant origin, due to air-conveyed oleoresins of Compositae, mimicking and often misdiagnosed as a photodermatitis. However, some features may differentiate it from photodermatitis, since airborne contact dermatitis involves the upper eyelids, the triangle of skin behind the earlobe, the backs of facial folds without respect for the triangle under the chin (Fig. 6). Although pollens were usually incriminated as the causative agents of airborne phytodermatitis, it is likely that finely pulverized materials derived from dead plants are the more likely etiological agents in the case of ragweeds (*Ambrosia* spp.) and related members of the Compositae family. Vaporized allergens may be responsible for airborne contact derma-titis in florists exposed to chrysanthemums (*Dendranthema* cultivars, family Compositae) [43] or to *Alstroemeria* L. [44]. It was also noted that simply walking in a forest may bring on an attack of eczema in patients who are sensitized to liverworts of the genus Frullania (*Frullania dilatata Dum.*, family Jubulaceae for example), suggesting that either particles of liverwort or vaporized allergens are the causative agents [45]. Other reports describe airborne contact dermatitis from lichen particles [46, 47] or pine dust (unidentified species of the family Pinaceae) [48]. The last cases exhibited positive patch test reactions to colophony.

In North America and elsewhere it is recognized that the smoke from burning poison ivy (*Toxicodendron* spp.) and related plants in the Anacardiaceae family may sensitize if the allergenic oleoresin is vaporized rather than pyrolyzed [49]. Airborne contact dermatitis to feverfew or congress grass (*Parthenium hysterophorus* L., Asteraceae family) is a major dermatological problem, particularly in northern India. The classical form involves exposed areas, but seborrheic-like dermatitis, widespread dermatitis, photosensitive lichenoid reactions and prurigo nodularis-like eruptions have been reported [9, 50]. Patients suffer seasonal relapses but sensitivity is lifelong, and sometimes complicated by the development of photosensitivity [50, 51].

41.2.4 Photodermatitis (Phytophotodermatitis)

41.2.4.1 Phytophototoxicity

Oppenheim first described dermatitis bullosa striata pratensis, or "meadow dermatitis," in 1926 [52, 53]. The condition only develops under particular circumstances. The individual, having been out in the sun for some time with areas of bare skin and having been sunbathing on damp grassy vegetation, notices the appearance, over several hours, of a pruritic erythematous and bullous rash in a distribution pattern mimicking the shape of the grass or the veins of leaves (Fig. 7). Damp vegetation may be replaced by atmospheric humidity or perspiration. The linear, figurate, and vesiculobullous nature of the lesions on sun-exposed skin leads one to suspect the phototoxic nature of the dermatitis. Dermatitis generally peaks around 72 h, and healing is accompanied by postinflammatory hyperpigmentation. Currently, Oppenheim dermatitis occurs frequently after gardening, and the so-called strimmer rash appears to be a variant of this condition, having a diffuse rather than striated or figurate presentation; a "strimmer"

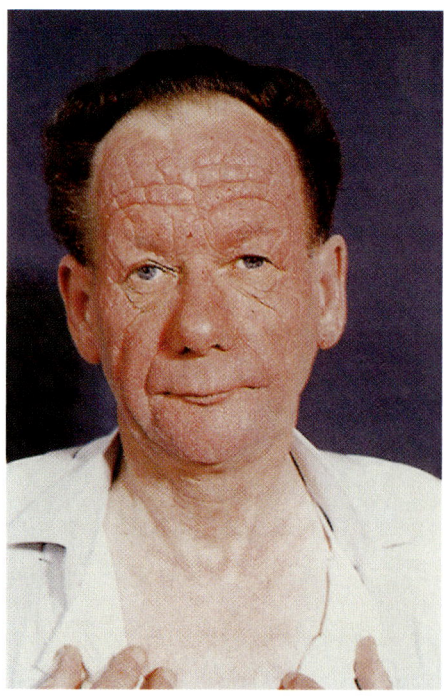

Fig. 6. Airborne contact dermatitis from Compositae in a farmer. Note the marked infiltration on the forehead and the sharp upper border from wearing a hat (courtesy of N. Hjorth)

41

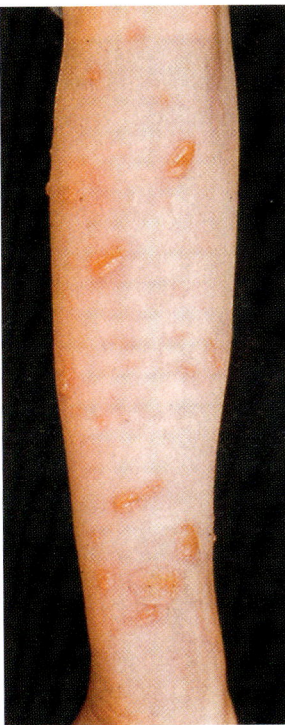

Fig. 7. Phototoxic dermatitis from furocoumarin-containing plants (courtesy of P.J. Frosch)

(string trimmer) is an ingenious hand-held device for cutting vegetation with a mechanically whirled string (nylon filament) [54, 55]. Oppenheim dermatitis can easily be reproduced in individuals exposed to the same conditions [56], rapidly suggesting a nonallergic mechanism. Some peculiar situations have been reported, such as the epidemic of Oppenheim dermatitis in 58 soldiers on an exercise in open country [57], or the phytophototoxicity with extensive linear and blistering skin lesions on the back of an 8-year-old girl that was mistaken for signs of whipping by her father [58].

Meadow dermatitis and associated conditions are commonly ascribed to contact with members of the Asteraceae/Umbelliferae plant family that grow in grassy meadows. In Europe in late summer these plants are in fact a common cause of bullous dermatitis, which may present in a wide variety of circumstances. Such dermatitis is caused by furocoumarins (also known as furanocoumarins or psoralens) (Fig. 8), which are present in the implicated plants and cause exaggeration of the burning potential of sunlight or artificial ultraviolet light, generally UVA. Numerous plants contain psoralens, although they have a limited distribution in the plant kingdom, the most important sources being the families Apiaceae/Umbelliferae, Fabaceae/Leguminosae, Moraceae, and Rutaceae [5, 8, 59].

Coumarin derivatives such as isopimpinellin and limettin also possess photosensitizing properties, and large amounts have been isolated from citrus peels [60].

Another category of photosensitizers are the furoquinolines, among them dictamnine, which is isolated from the roots of Rutaceae such as *Dictamnus albus* L., *Skimmia repens* Nakai, *Aegle marmelos* Correa, *Zanthoxylum alatum* Roxb., and *Ruta graveolens* L. [61–63] (Fig. 9). Important examples of phototoxic plants are reported in Table 2.

Phototoxic contact dermatitis may present as the so-called berloque dermatitis, induced by perfumes or perfumed cosmetics containing high amounts of psoralens, in particular oil of bergamot. Berloque dermatitis normally begins in the neck or décolleté, with erythema at the site where perfume runs down the skin and is irradiated by the sun. Again, this is normally followed by postinflammatory hyperpigmentation, which may last months or years. This dermatitis is currently rare due to the avoidance of fragrances containing psoralens, but it can be observed with artisan or traditional fragrances [64].

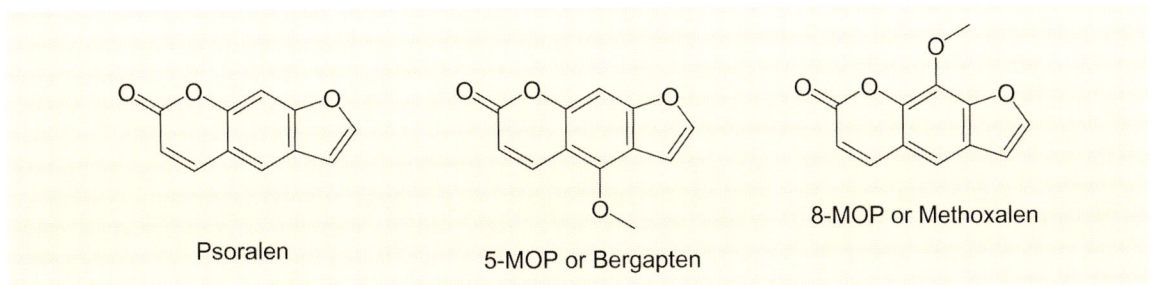

Psoralen   5-MOP or Bergapten   8-MOP or Methoxalen

Fig. 8. Structures of psoralens. Psoralen (ficusin) CAS 66–97–7, 5-methoxypsoralen (bergapten) CAS 484–20–8, and 8-methoxypsoralen (xanthotoxin or methoxalen) CAS 298–81–7

Table 2. Main phototoxic plants

Family	Botanical name	English name	French name	German name
Apiaceae or Umbelliferae	*Ammi majus* L.	Bullwort, Bishop's weed	Ammi élevé	Grosse Knorpelmöhre
	Angelica archangelica L.	Garden angelica	Angélique	Engelwurz, Garten Angelik
	Angelica sylvestris L.	Wild angelica	Angélique des bois	Wilde Engelwurz
	Anthriscus sylvestris Hoffmann	Cow parsley	Chérophylle sauvage, cerfeuil sauvage	Wiesen-Kerbel
	Apium graveolens L.	Wild celery	Céleri sauvage, ache puante	Echte Sellerie, Epf
	Apium graveolens var. *dulce* Persoon	Celery	Céleri à côtes	Stielsellerie
	Daucus carrota L. ssp *sativus* Hayek	Common garden carrot	Carotte	Karotte, Möhre
	Foeniculum vulgare Miller	Fennel	Fenouil	Gemeiner Fenchel
	Heracleum lanatum Michaux.	Cow parsnip, masterwort	Grande berce laineuse	Herkulesstaude, Bärenklau
	Heracleum mantegaz-zianum Somm and Lev.	Giant hogweed, parsnip tree	Berce du Caucase	Kaukasicher Bärenklau
	Heracleum sphondylium L.	Hogweed	Grance berce	Wiesen-Bärenklau
	Heracleum stevenii Manden	Palm of Tromsø	–	–
	Pastinaca sativa L.	Parsnip, madnep queenweed	Panais, pastenade	Pastinak, Hammelmöhre
	Petroselinum crispum	Parsley	Persil	Petersilie
Fabaceae or Leguminosae	*Psoralea corylifolia* L.	Babchi, bakuci	Psoralier	Harzklee
	Myroxylon peirerae Klotzsch.	Balsam tree	Baume du Pérou	Balsam Baum
Moraceae	*Ficus carica* L.	Fig tree	Figuier	Feigenbaum
Rutaceae	*Citrus aurantifolia* Swingle	Lime	Citron vert	Limone
	Citrus aurantium L.	Bitter orange	Bigaradier, orange amère	Bittere Orange, Pomeranze,
	Citrus bergamia Risso and Poit.	Bergamot orange	Bergamote	Bergamottzitronen, Bergamotte
	Citrus limetta Riss.	Sweet lemon	Citron doux	Süsse Zitrone
	Citrus limon (L.) Burm.	Lemon	Citron	Zitrone
	Citrus paradisi Macfad.	Grapefruit	Pamplemousse	Pumpelmuss
	Citrus sinensis Osbeck	Sweet orange	Orange douce	Apfelzine
	Cneoridium dumosum	Bushrue, berryrue	–	–
	Dictamnus albus L.	Gasplant, fraxinella, burning bush	Fraxinelle, buisson ardent	Weisser Diptam
	Pelea anisata H. Mann	Mokihana fruits	Mokihana	Mokihana
	Ruta chalepensis L.	Fringed rue	Rue à feuilles étroites, rue d'Alep	Aleppo-Raute
	Ruta graveolens L.	Rue, Herb of grace	Rue fétide, rue des jardins	Weinraute, Garten-Raute

41

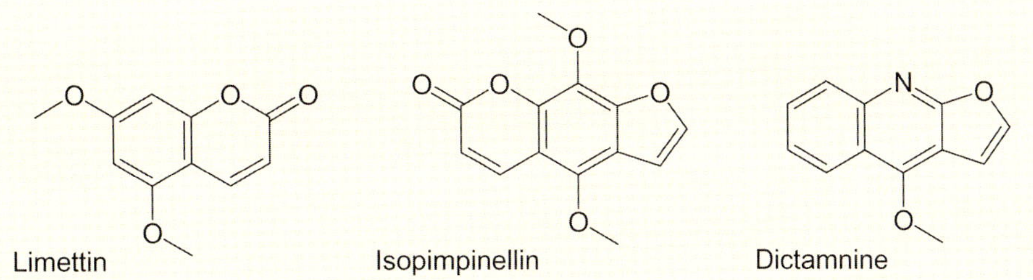

Fig. 9. Structures of limettin CAS 487–06–9, isopimpinellin CAS 482–27–9, and dictamnine, CAS 482–27–9

41.2.4.2 Phytophotoallergic Contact Dermatitis

Plant or plant-product-induced photoallergic dermatitis occurs only very rarely. Perhaps the only well-authenticated cases are a reaction to *Parthenium hysterophorus* L. (family Asteraceae) [65] and a photoallergy to psoralens [66]. However, experimentally induced photoallergies to psoralens and to other coumarins known to occur naturally have been described [67]. It is difficult to differentiate between a photoworsened allergic contact dermatitis and a true photoallergy. Photoworsening of an allergic contact dermatitis is the more likely diagnosis than true photoallergy when plant material is implicated as the cause of a photosensitivity reaction of the skin [46, 47] in lichen pickers with a history of photosensitivity.

A rather different relationship between contact allergy and photosensitivity is seen in chronic actinic dermatitis (persistent light reaction, photosensitive eczema, or actinic reticuloid). In such patients, generally men over 50 years, dermatitis occurs in photoexposed areas during the sunny season, which then worsens with a chronic course, including itching, lichenified, and extensive lesions or even erythroderma. Patients have a marked broad spectrum photosensitivity to UVB, UVA or even visible radiations. It is frequent to observe contact sensitivity (but not photoallergic reactions) to oleoresins from members of the plant family Asteraceae and sesquiterpene lactones contained herein, or photosensitivity to photoallergens such as musk ambrette or sunscreens, but the disease expresses itself even in the absence of exposure to the plant material. It appears that an initial contact sensitization progresses to a generalized photosensitivity state with a relationship between plants of the family Compositae, the sesquiterpene lactones they contain, and chronic actinic dermatitis [68–71].

41.3 Inducers of Dermatitis

It is not possible to consider the whole panorama of plants liable to elicit contact dermatitis here, but the plants most often incriminated are described below. Occupational contacts [12, 72] are usually the most frequent inducers of plant contact dermatitis.

41.3.1 Alliaceae (Onion Family)

Members of the family Alliaceae are widely grown and used for culinary purposes. In addition, garlic (*Allium sativum* L.) has both a contemporary and a folkloric history of use as a medicinal agent. Whilst the lachrymatory properties of onions (*Allium cepa* L.) are widely appreciated, they are rarely discussed in the medical literature. Most commonly reported is occupational dermatitis from garlic and to a lesser extent from onion; this includes both immediate and delayed reactions [19, 73–78]. A typical presentation is a circumscribed irritable hyperkeratotic eczema on the fingers of one or both hands; sometimes the thumb, index and middle fingers of the nondominant (usually left) hand which may be used to grasp the garlic bulb whilst the knife is held in the right hand [79]. Less distinct patterns of eczema are likely more frequent than the presentation described above, but remarkable situations can occur, such as haemorrhagic and blistering contact dermatitis [80], cheiropompholyx associated with the ingestion of garlic extract [81], dermatitis of the elbow flexures, lower back and periorbital regions with cheilitis [82], or airborne dermatitis due to garlic powder, which was also reported as a cause of immediate-type reactions such as conjunctivitis, rhinitis and asthma [83].

Garlic and other *Allium* species have often been reported to have both irritant and allergenic properties, due to phytochemicals not present in undamaged plant material, but released as a response to damage. They are derived from a variety of sulfur-containing amino acids present in the intact plants. A

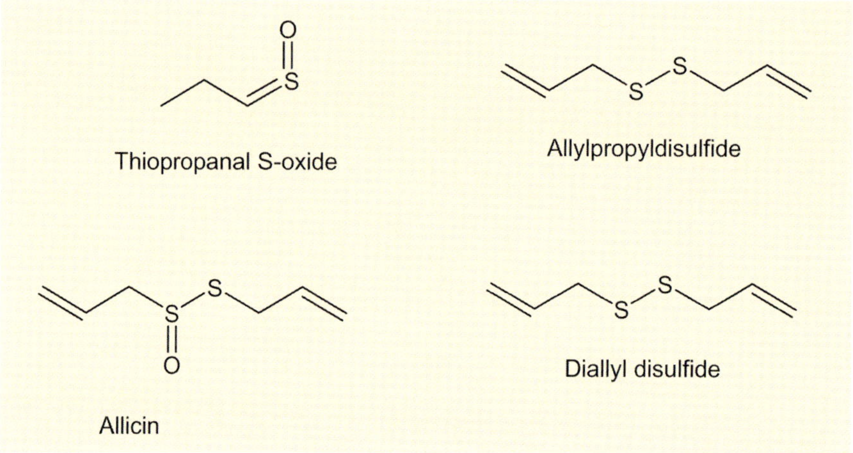

Fig. 10.
Structures of thipropanal
S-oxide CAS 32157–29–2,
allicin CAS 539–86–6, diallyl
disulfide CAS 2179–57–9, and
allypropyl disulfide CAS
2179–59–1

Thiopropanal S-oxide

Allylpropyldisulfide

Allicin

Diallyl disulfide

minor structural difference between the principal precursor compounds, namely S-(1-propenyl)-L-cysteine sulfoxide and S-(2-propenyl)-L-cysteine sulfoxide or alliin for garlic, results in an enzymatic transformation by the thermolabile alliinase: the lachrymatory thiopropanal-S-oxide from onion, but allicin and diallyldisulfide from garlic, as illustrated in Fig. 10 [84]. Diallyldisulfide, allylpropyldisulfide, and allicin have been identified as the principal low molecular weight allergens of garlic [85]. Commercial diallyldisulfide seems to be a suitable preparation for the investigation of garlic dermatitis, although 1% pet. may carry a lower risk of irritancy or can be negative. Irritant reactions with plants are expected with fresh garlic concentrations higher than 10% but concentrations up to 50% for garlic and onion in arachnid oil were considered to be safe [78]. It is likely that each different extraction procedure affects the manner in which the irritants/allergens are released, making it virtually impossible to produce a standard extract. So, patch tests with plant extracts or plant material used as is must be interpreted with some caution [86]. Delayed-type cross-reactions between garlic and onion, although occasionally described, are unlikely.

41.3.2 Alstroemeriaceae (Alstroemer Family) and Liliaceae (Lily Family)

These two families are considered together because members of the genera *Alstroemeria* L. (Peruvian lily, Inca lily) and *Bomarea* Mirb. (family Alstroemeriaceae), and the genus *Tulipa* L. (family Liliaceae) produce the same allergen, tulipalin A (Fig. 11). The substance is released when the plant material (flowers, stems and leaves) is damaged [87–90]. Tulipalin A, otherwise known as α-methylene-γ-butyrolactone, is

obtained from a glucoside precursor known as tuliposide A. This one can be present as 1-tuliposide A [91] or more frequently identified as 6-tuliposide A [92–94].

Tulips contain a second glucoside, 6-tuliposide B [89], which is classically considered to be a nonsensitizer and has antibiotic properties, protecting the plant against bacteria [95]. Patients sensitive to tulips reportedly do not react to either tuliposide B or tulipalin B. However, it was demonstrated that tulipalin B (β-hydroxy-α-methylene-γ-butyrolactone) is a sensitizer in guinea pigs, and that cross-reactivity between tulipalins A and B does occur [96]. Other tuliposides have been detected in *Alstroemeria* species, for example tuliposide D [94]. There is evidence that the tuliposides themselves can elicit allergic contact dermatitis [88, 92], but this may be the outcome of some spontaneous degradation to tulipalin A on the skin [97].

Garden tulips are available both as "species tulips" and as cultivars of hybrid origin. Dermatitis among bulb handlers and florists is a frequent but unpleasant occupational hazard. Bulb collectors, sorters and packers develop a characteristic dermatitis called "tulip fingers," a painful dry fissured hyperkeratotic eczema, at first underneath the true margin of the nails, spreading to the periungueal regions, fingers and hands [98]. Sometimes the dermatitis spreads to the face, forearms, and genital region. It seems certain that both irritant and allergic contact dermatitis occurs. "Tulip fingers" is common in the Netherlands and other parts of Europe. The allergen is found mainly in the epidermis of the bulb, but dermatitis may also occur in those who handle the cut flowers [99].

Alstroemeria hybrids have been popular in the cut-flower trade since the 1980s due to their long lasting and colored flowers (Fig. 4a, b). Horticulturists

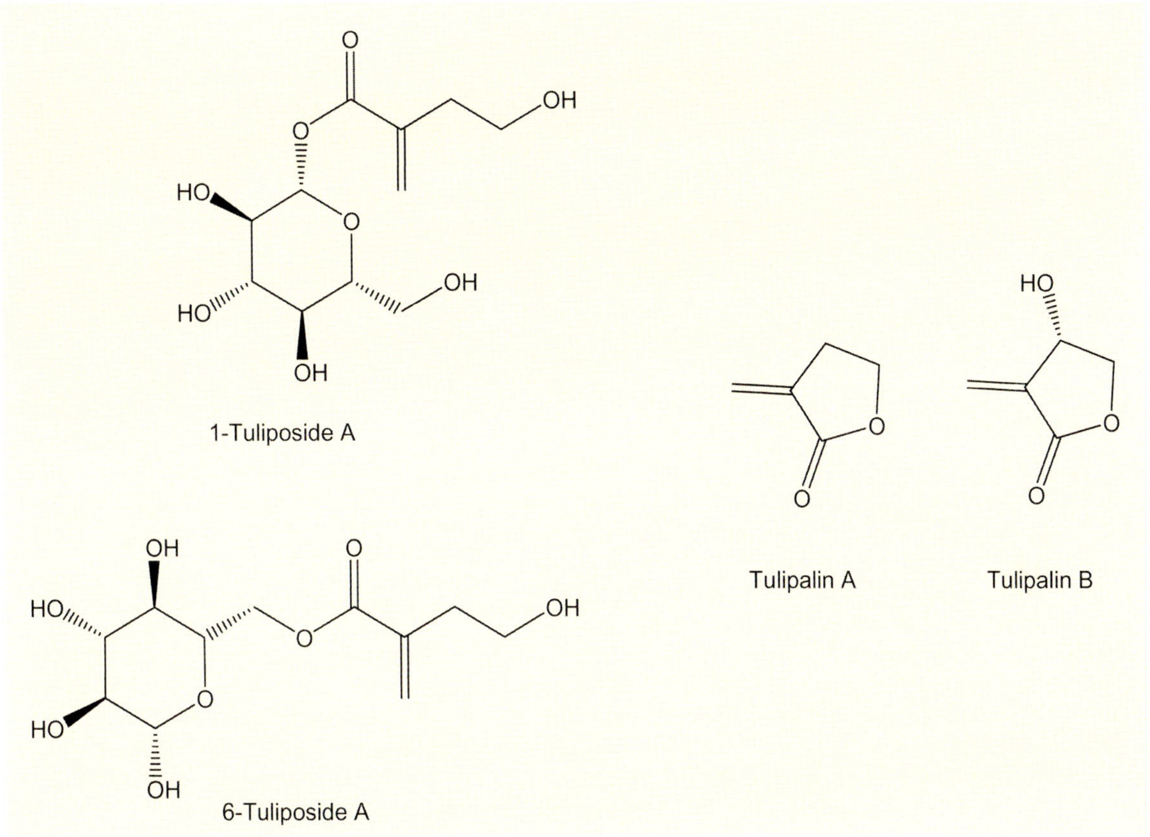

1-Tuliposide A

Tulipalin A

Tulipalin B

6-Tuliposide A

Fig. 11. Structures of 1- and 6-tuliposides A (glycosidic precursors of tulipalin A) CAS 19870-30-5 and CAS 19870-31-6 respectively, tulipalin A (α-methylene-γ-butyrolactone) CAS 547-65-9 and tulipalin B (β-hydroxy-α-methylene-γ-butyrolactone) CAS 38965-80-9

and florists are at high risk of both irritant and allergic contact dermatitis, and the rate of sensitization for tulipalin A can exceed 50% in workers of *Alstroemeria* cultivation [100]. Handling of cut flowers provokes a dermatitis affecting mainly the fingertips, which is similar to "tulip fingers" [101–103]. Depigmentation may follow the resolution of *Alstroemeria* dermatitis or a positive patch test to plant [104]. Contact urticaria and rhinoconjunctivitis, with positive prick tests, were described for *Alstroemeria* [105].

In the preparation of plant material for patch testing, it should be remembered that the various cultivars of *Alstroemeria* and *Tulipa* do not necessarily contain similar levels of tuliposide A or associated contact allergens. For example, the cultivar Rose Copeland is a notorious sensitizer [106], whereas *Tulipa fosteriana* Hoog cv Red Emperor has been found to contain very much less tuliposide than other cultivars [98]. Nonsystematic concomitant patch test reactions between tulips and *Alstroemeria* [101, 104] may be due to differences in amount of allergens. Different ways of performing patch testing have been recommended, since the so-called short ether extracts of *Alstroemeria* are too rich in tulipalin A and carry the risk of active sensitization [91]: a filtered 96% ethanol extract of the reference bulb of *Tulipa* cv Apeldoorn or an 80% acetone extract of the bulbs diluted with 70% ethanol immediately prior to use [98], a tuliposide-rich methanolic extract incorporated into petrolatum [91], a 50-µl application of 6-tuliposide A at 0.01% or an α-methylene-γ-butyrolactone at 0.001% in ethanol [92]. Currently, the 0.01% concentration in petrolatum seems to be effective and safe for detecting sensitive people [91, 107].

Core Message

■ Tulipalin A (α-methylene-γ-butyrolactone) is the main contact allergen in *Alstroemeria* and *Tulipa* species. It frequently induces a fingertip allergy known as "tulip fingers," mostly in people who have occupational contact with flowers and bulbs.

Common hyacinth (*Hyacinthus orientalis* L.) have been described above as inducers of irritant contact dermatitis, due to calcium oxalate present in their bulbs. It is noteworthy that bulbs evoke pruritus in almost all workers who manipulate them, but dermatitis is less frequent [108]. We observed an unusual exposure in two schoolteachers who decided to describe the structure of bulbs and explained in detail the way to cultivate hyacinth bulbs to their pupils (personal observations). Hyacinths likely contain as-yet unidentified allergens [106].

41.3.3 Amaryllidaceae (Daffodil Family)

The Amaryllidaceae family comprises some 1100 species of plant in 85 genera, many of which are cultivated for their showy flowers. Amongst these, daffodils (*Narcissus* spp. and cultivars) are the most common, this term indicating several species such as trumpet narcissi (*Narcissus pseudo-narcissus* L.), narcissi (other species, e.g., *N. poeticus*) and jonquils (*Narcissus jonquilla* L.), which constitute a significant dermatological hazard because of their irritant and allergenic properties. An important bulb and cut flower industry exists in the Netherlands and the Isles of Scilly in the United Kingdom, and with it the occupational disease known as "daffodil itch" or "lily rash" [98, 106], sometimes clinically close to "tulip fingers."

The rash has long been ascribed in part to the calcium oxalate needle crystals present in both the dry outer scales of the bulbs and in the sap exuding from cut flower stems [98]. Observation in the field related the method of picking and then gathering the flowers to the development of the daffodil pickers' rash, at the points of contact of plant sap with the skin like the finger webs, the dorsum of the hand and the anterior aspect of the wrist [109]. Dermatitis may involve the

neck, face, and the genitals [8]. It is likely that the "lily rash" is mainly caused by an irritant mechanism [108], but that an allergic reaction is possible [110]. Among many irritant alkaloids, two allergenic ones were identified from *N. pseudonarcissus* L., namely masonin and homolycorine (Fig. 12) [32]. Patch tests may be performed with leaves, stems and flowers, or with ethanol, acetone or water [8].

41.3.3.1 Anacardiaceae, Ginkgoaceae, and Proteaceae

These plant families are considered together because they contain similar contact allergens and hence cause similar dermatitis. Nevertheless, the clinical picture may vary depending upon the precise mode of contact.

Anacardiaceae (Cashew Family)

The Anacardiaceae family includes 60 genera comprising some 600 species of trees and shrubs, distributed throughout the tropics, and also found in warm temperate regions of Europe, eastern Asia, and the Americas. They are considered to cause more dermatitis than all other plant families combined [5]. Some tropical species are of economic importance, such as *Mangifera indica* L., which provides mango fruits, *Anacardium occidentale* L., which yields cashew nuts, cashew nut shell oil, which is used in the manufacture of brake linings, *Semecarpus anacardium* L.f., which is known as the Indian marking nut tree that provides black juice used as an indelible ink when labeling clothing, the Japanese lacquer tree *Toxicodendron vernicifluum* F. Barkley, or several other species used for dying or tanning. The main dermatologically important plants are reported in Table 3.

41

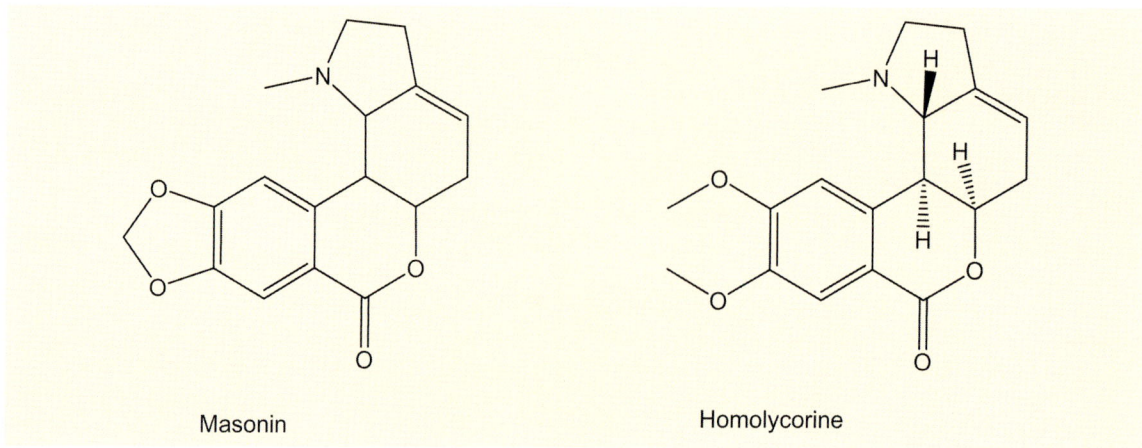

Masonin Homolycorine

Fig. 12. Structures of masonin CAS 568–40–1 and homolycorine, CAS 477–20–3

Table 3. Dermatologically important Anacardiaceae plants

Botanical name	Synonyms	English name	French name	German name
Anacardium occidentale L.		Cashew nut tree	Anacardier, noix de cajou, pomme cajou	Kaschu, Elefantenlaus Baum, westindischer Nierenbaum
Comocladia dodonaea Urban	*Comocladia ilicifolia* Sw., *Ilex dodonaea* L.	Christmas bush, poison ash	Bois de houx	
Gluta laccifera Ding Hou	*Melanorrhoea laccifera* Pierre	Camboge lacquer	Arbre à laque du Cambodge	
Gluta renghas L.		East coast rengas, ape-nut		
Gluta usitata Ding Hou	*Melanorrhoea usitata* Wallich.	Burmese lacquer tree, theetsee	Arbre à laque de Birmanie	
Holigarna ferruginea March.				
Lithraea caustica Hook. and Arn.	*Lithraea venenosa* Miers.	Litre, aroeira		
Mangifera indica L.		Mango tree	Manguier	Mangobaum
Metopium toxiferum Krug and Urban	*Rhus metopium* L.	Poisonwood, coral sumac, Florida poison tree, Honduras walnut		
Semecarpus anacardium L.	*Anacardium orientale* Auct.	Indian marking nut tree, bhilawa tree	Anacarde d'Orient	Tintenbaum
Smodingium argutum E. Mey.		African poison ivy, um-tovane, tovana, rainbow leaf	Smodingie, lierre toxique d'Afrique	Afrikanischer Giftefeu
Toxicodendron diversilobum Greene	*Rhus diversiloba* Torr. & Gray. *R. toxicodendron* L. ssp. *diversiloba* Engl.	Western poison oak, Pacific poison oak	Sumac irrégulièrement lobé, sumac de l'ouest	Sumach, verschieden-lappiger Sumach
Toxicodendron radicans L. ssp. *barkleyi* Gillis	*Rhus villosum* Sessé & Moçiño	Western poison oak		
Toxicodendron radicans L. ssp. *divaricatum* Gillis	*T. divaricatum* Greene, *Rhus divaricata* Greene	Western poison oak		
Toxicodendron radicans L. ssp. *eximium* Gillis	*T. eximium* Greene, *Rhus eximia* Stanley	Western poison oak		
Toxicodendron radicans L. ssp. *hispidum* Gillis	*Rhus toxicodendron* L. var. *hispida* Engl., *R. intermedia* Hayata	Taiwan tsuta-urushi		
Toxicodendron radicans L. ssp. *negundo* Gillis	*T. negundo* Greene, *T. arborigunum* Greene	Taiwan tsuta-urushi	Herbe à puce grimpante	
Toxicodendron radicans L. ssp. *orientale* Gillis	*T. orientale* Greene, *Rhus orientalis* Schneider	Tsuta-urushi		
Toxicodendron radicans L. ssp. *pubens* Gillis	*R. toxicodendron* L. var. *pubens* Engelm.	Tsuta-urushi		
Toxicodendron radicans L. ssp. *radicans* Gillis	*T. radicans* Kuntze, *Rhus radicans* L., *Rhus toxicodendron* L.	Poison ivy, three-leaved ivy, eastern poison ivy, poison vine, black vine, markweed	Sumac radicant, lierre toxique, herbe à puce de l'est	Sumach, Kletter-Gift-sumach, Rankender Sumach, Giftefeu
T. radicans L. ssp. *verrucosum* Gillis	*T. verrucosum* Greene, *Rhus verrucosa* Scheele	Poison ivy, three-leaved ivy, poison vine, black vine, markweed		

Table 3. Continued

Botanical name	Synonyms	English name	French name	German name
Toxicodendron rydbergii Greene poison ivy	*T. radicans* Kuntze var. *rydbergii* Erskine, *Rhus rydbergii* Small, *R. toxicodendron* L. var. *rydbergii* Garnett	Rydberg's poison ivy, western poison ivy	Herbe à puce de Rydberg	
Toxicodendron striatum Kuntze	*Rhus striata* Ruiz and Pavón, *R. juglandifolia* Willd.	Manzanillo, hinchador		
Toxicodendron succedaneum Kuntze	*Rhus succedanea* L.	Japanese wax tree		
Toxicodendron toxicarium Gillis	*T. quercifolium* Greene, *T. toxicodendron* L. Britten, *Rhus quercifolia* Steudel, *R. toxicodendron* L. var. *quercifolium* Michx., *R. toxicarium* Salisb.	Eastern poison oak, oak leaf ivy	Sumac véneneux à feuilles de chêne	Echter Gifstsumac
Toxicodendron vernicifluum F. Barkley	*Rhus verniciflua* Stokes, *R. vernicifera* DC.	Japanese lacquer tree, varnish tree	Sumac à laque, vernis vrai	Lacksumach
Toxicodendron vernix Kuntze	*Rhus vernix* L., *R. venenata* DC.	Poison sumac, poison dogwood, swamp sumac, poison elder	Sumac à vernis, bois chandelle	Giftsumach

Although these and many other species in the family Anacardiaceae are dermatologically hazardous [111–120], perhaps the most important genus is *Toxicodendron*. This genus includes the poison ivy complex (*Toxicodendron radicans* Kuntze and subspecies such as *T. radicans* Kuntze *var. rydbergii* Erskine), the poison oak complex with *Toxicodendron diversilobum* Greene (in western North America) and *Toxicodendron toxicarium* Gillis (in eastern North America), and the poison sumac (*Toxicodendron striatum* Kuntze, *T. vernix* Kuntze) of North America and elsewhere [121–125]. Over half of the population of the United States is sensitive to poison ivy and its relatives [126] while, because the plants are not a part of the natural flora, poison ivy dermatitis is generally unknown in Europe [127]. Clinical aspects vary with exposure. Dermatitis initially appears on the fingers, forearms, arms, legs, and sometimes genitalia [8, 126]. Lesions consist of papules, vesicles, and/or blisters. Erythema multiforme-like eruption is sometimes observed. Systemic contact dermatitis may occur after accidental, medicinal or alimentary ingestion of plant materials. It may present as eczema, as a generalized maculopapular eruption or as erythroderma occurring generally within 48 h following administration. When generalized rash occurs, leukocytosis and neutrophilia are frequent, and liver dysfunction is possible [128, 129]. The same features with eczematous eruption of flex-

ural regions, mouth, and anal itching may occur after ingestion of cashew nuts in people previously sensitized to poison ivy [130]. The "black spot poison ivy dermatitis" is a rarer condition, consisting of black enamel spots, due to colored and dried plant sap, secondarily surrounding patch dermatitis, mainly of allergic origin [131].

Early literature refers to poison ivy and its relatives as species of *Rhus*. On the basis of morphological grounds and phytochemical distinction, it appears that *Toxicodendron* is more suited, and that the genus *Rhus* must be distinguished from the genus *Toxicodendron* [10, 132], although other authors argue for using the term *Rhus* [7]. There is consequently a frequent nomenclatural confusion in the dermatological literature, especially with the numerous synonyms. Individual subspecies of *Toxicodendron* rarely appear in the dermatological literature, largely because case reports of poison ivy dermatitis hardly warrant publication, partly because of the difficulty in precisely identifying the subspecies of the plants. The distributions of the various *Toxicodendron* species and subspecies have been described for the United States [132–134]. The "black spot test" consists of carefully crushing sap from the leaves of the plant onto white paper: the test is positive with *Toxicodendron*, the stain darkening on exposure to the air [135]. The same phenomenon occurs with wood sap (Fig. 13). Poison ivy, poison oak, and poison sumac

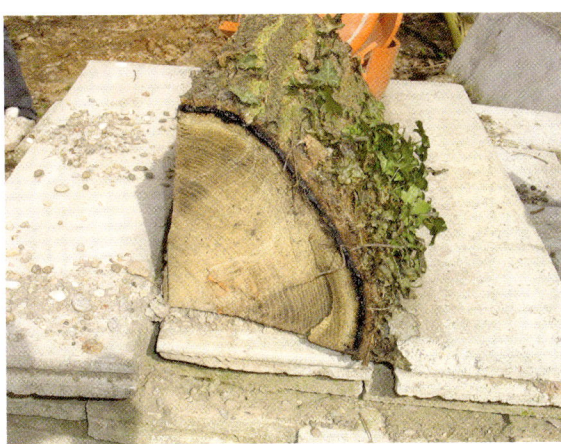

Fig. 13. Stain darkening of sap of *Toxicodendron* species is the basis of the "black spot test", here demonstrated with sap of here demonstrated with sap of a recently cut down Japanese lacquer tree (*Toxicodendron vernicifluum* F. Barkley)

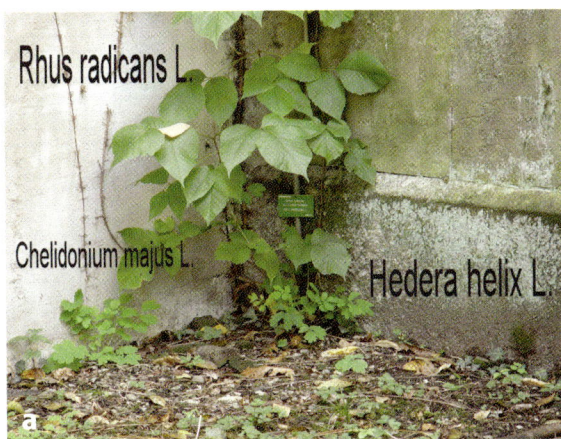

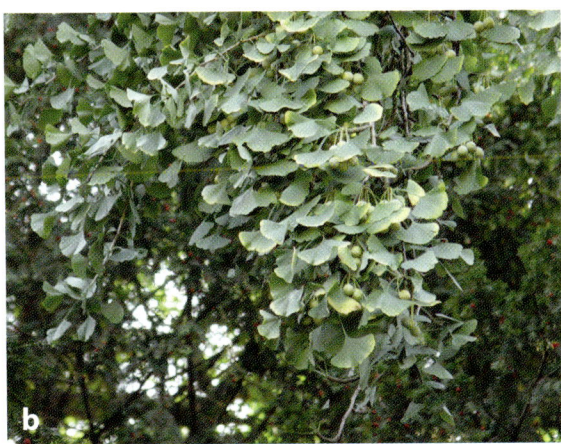

Fig. 14a, b. a *Toxicodendron radicans* growing in the botanical garden of Strasbourg, France. **b** Female Ginkgo tree (*Ginkgo biloba* L.) bearing ovules (Jardin botanique, Strasbourg, France)

are native to North America but can be exported. The dermatitis can present after an individual has been in contact with the plant whilst visiting an endemic area. As the plant has the potential to grow in Europe too (Fig. 14a), it is possible for an individual to be sensitized and subsequently to develop the rash without leaving their country [136], particularly in the case of workers at botanical gardens (personal observations).

Cross-reactivity between Anacardiaceae has been reported for a long time. Similarities between urushiols from poison ivy and cashew nut shell oil are well known. In South America, species of *Lithraea*, and especially *L. caustica* Hook. and Arn. [10], are a frequent cause of a poison ivy-like dermatitis. In 17 *Lithraea*-sensitized subjects, reactions to poison oak urushiol were constant, and reactions to extracts prepared from *Lithraea molleoides* Engl. and *Lithraea brasiliensis* Marchand occurred in 13/17. The responses to poison oak urushiol were stronger and occurred at lower concentrations than those to *Lithraea* extracts [137]. Similar studies of cross-reactivity between *Lithraea* and other members of the Anacardiaceae were reported [138, 139]. Concomitant reactions have been observed, but without systematic cross-reactivity, as in a patient sensitized to poison ivy or poison oak (*Toxicodendron* spp.) whilst in the United States and who subsequently showed apparent cross-reactions to *Rhus copallina* L., *R. semialata* Murray (syn. *R. javanica* L.), and *R. trichocarpa* Miq. [127].

Ginkgoaceae (Maidenhair Family)

Ginkgo biloba L., the ginkgo tree, is the solitary representative of the family Ginkgoaceae and is regarded as one of the world's oldest surviving tree species. Contact dermatitis from the ginkgo tree is not due to its leaves but to its malodorous fruits [140], in fact to the ovules exclusively borne by female trees (Fig. 14b). Contact occurs through inadvertent contamination of the skin with the fruit pulp [141], collecting and using the nut within the fruit in an Asian cooking style [141, 142], or in children through playing marbles with the fallen fruits. The lesions consist of erythematous papules and vesicles, with severe swelling in severe cases. They usually affect the face, the forearms and the thighs, and sometimes the genitalia [142, 143]. Stomatitis, cheilitis, and proctitis following ingestion of ginkgo fruit were described [144].

Cross-reactions between ginkgo fruit pulp, poison ivy, or ginkgo and cashew nut have been discussed [145]. They were, however, not supported by a recent study of the ginkgolic acids found in *Ginkgo* fruits and urushiol from *Toxicodendron* [146]. Patch testing can be performed with fruit pulp in 1% acetone [144].

Proteaceae

The Proteaceae family comprises 1050 species in 62 genera found in tropical areas. In Australia, members of the family Proteaceae are the cause of a poison ivy-like dermatitis. The best known are probably the so-called silky oak or silver oak (*Grevillea robusta* Cunn.) and related *Grevillea* species and cultivars. Contact with the wild and cultivated tree [147–149], as well as with objects made from the wood [150], have been recorded as being allergenic. "Grevillea poisoning" was described as a severe contact dermatitis on exposed areas in people cutting trees or maintaining electric power lines in the Los Angeles area [151]. Allergic dermatitis following contact with

flowers of Kahili or Bank's Grevillea (*Grevillea banksii* R. Br.) was described in Hawaii [152].

Allergens

The allergenic agents in all these members of the Anacardiaceae, Ginkgoaceae and Proteaceae are derivatives of catechol, phenol, resorcinol or salicylic acid with a side chain (-R) (Fig. 15). This side chain is mostly a C_{15} (sometimes a C_{17}) alkyl (saturated) or alkenyl (one, two or three double bonds C=C) chain [4, 8]. The alk(en)yl catechols are also known as *urushiol*, a generic name that in fact refers to the blend of several close molecules (urushiols) naturally contained in the plant. An urushiol with a C_{15} side chain is named pentadecylcatechol (a term sometimes employed in medical literature for poison ivy urushiol), and an urushiol with a C_{17} side chain is a heptadecyl-

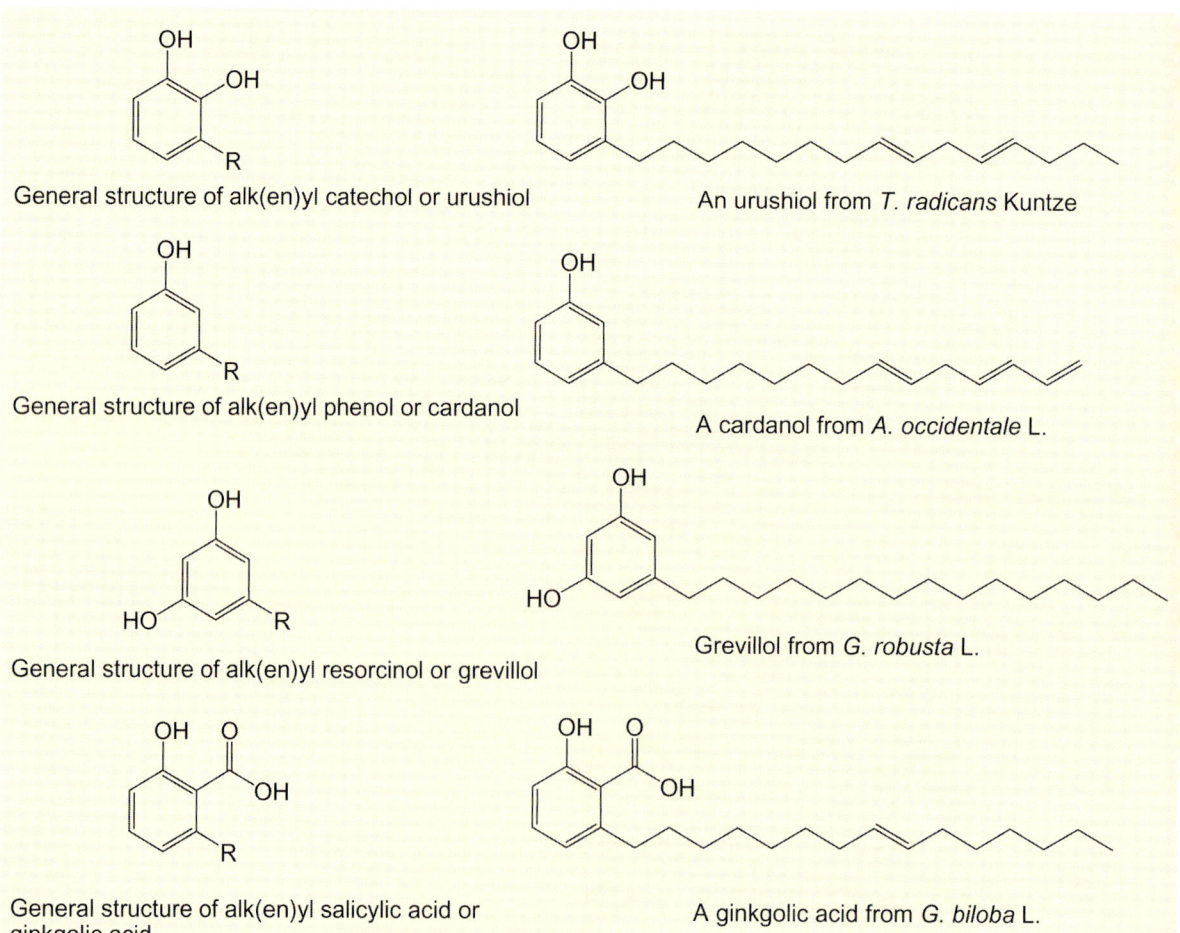

General structure of alk(en)yl catechol or urushiol

An urushiol from *T. radicans* Kuntze

General structure of alk(en)yl phenol or cardanol

A cardanol from *A. occidentale* L.

General structure of alk(en)yl resorcinol or grevillol

Grevillol from *G. robusta* L.

General structure of alk(en)yl salicylic acid or ginkgolic acid

A ginkgolic acid from *G. biloba* L.

Fig. 15. Structures of urushiol and related allergens from Anacardiaceae (*T. radicans* Kuntze, *A. occidentale* L.), Proteaceae (*G. robusta* L.), and Ginkgoaceae (*G. biloba* L.) families

41

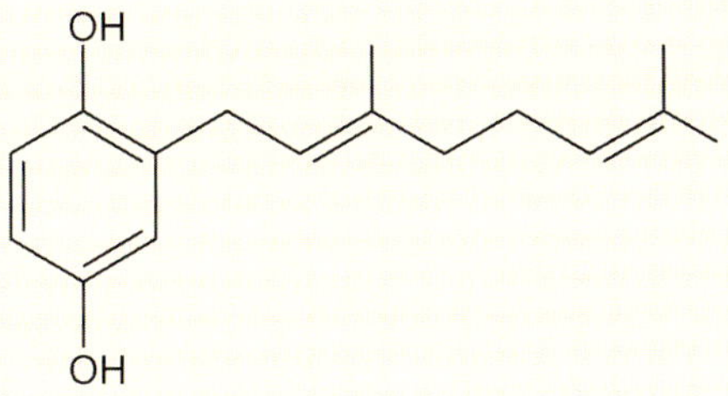

Fig. 16. Structure of geranylhydroquinone CAS 10457–66–6, from *Phacelia crenulata* Torrey

catechol (mostly encountered in poison oak uru- shiol). Phenol, resorcinol, and salicylic acid com- pounds substituted with an alk(en)yl chain have tra- ditionally been called *cardanol, grevillol* and *gink- golic acid*, respectively. Because the allergenic natural plant material is a mixture of closely related com- pounds, and because of the close similarity between individual compounds from a variety of botanical sources, there is the possibility of cross-sensitization between different species throughout the world [153].

The risk of cross-sensitization extends to families other than those described in this section. The genus *Philodendron* (family Araceae) yields sensitizing al- kyl resorcinols [154]. The genera *Phacelia* and *Wi- gandia* belonging to the Hydrophyllaceae family yield alkenyl hydroquinones. Prenylated quinones and prenylated phenols were identified in *W. caraca- sana* Kunth [155], and geranylhydroquinone in *P. cre- nulata* Torrey (Fig. 16); this molecule does not cross- react with poison oak or ivy [156].

Core Message

- Plants of the family Anacardiaceae are frequent cause of contact dermatitis. The skin reaction occurs following sensiti zation to various alkyl or alkenyl catechols (urushiol), phenols, resorcinols or salicylic acid derivatives. These compounds are also primary irritants.

41.3.4 Compositae (Asteraceae) and Liverworts

The two families are considered together because they contain sesquiterpene lactones as allergens.

41.3.4.1 Asteraceae/Compositae (Daisy Family)

The family Asteraceae/Compositae comprises some 13,000 to 20,000 species in over 900 genera. Repre- sentatives are found throughout the world, and ex- amples may be found living in almost every situa- tion, the majority being herbaceous plants. The fam- ily provides a number of food plants, for example let- tuce, endive, chicory, dandelion, salsify, scorzonera, and artichoke. Many more are grown for their deco- rative flowers, such as chrysanthemums, dahlias, and heleniums. Others are widespread and common weeds [157]. Additionally, some species such as arni- ca, chamomile or feverfew are used medicinally, by skin application or systemic administration. It is therefore difficult to avoid contact with these plants. Plants of dermatological interest are indicated in Table 4.

Allergic contact dermatitis from Asteraceae has several clinical presentations (Fig. 6). Accidentally exposed subjects can develop an acute and single epi- sode of dermatitis. Chronic exposure, of occupation- al origin for example, can induce acute dermatitis that can often relapse, or a primary chronic and sec- ondarily lichenified dermatitis. When the lesions are localized to the elbow or knee flexures, they can sim- ulate atopic dermatitis. The eczema, which may be lo- calized initially on the face, hands, and genitals, can become generalized as an erythroderma and can even be, in rare instances, fatal [158].

Exposure to the sesquiterpene lactones by the way of airborne plant material produces an airborne con- tact dermatitis (sometimes mistaken for a photoder- matitis). In the United States, this is known as "rag- weed dermatitis" because it is largely caused by rag- weeds, which are species of *Ambrosia* [159, 160] or "weed dermatitis" in regions where other composite weeds predominate [161], such as *Ambrosia, Artemi- sia, Helenium*, and *Iva* [162–171] species. For example, cases of severe airborne ACD from triangle-leaf bur- sage (*Ambrosia deltoidea*) were reported in the USA, with positive reactions to ether extracts of the plant [172].

In Australia, the same condition is described as "bush dermatitis" due to species such as *Arctotheca, Cassinia, Conyza, Cynara*, and *Dittrichia* [167, 173–176]. In India, another variant has been called "parthenium dermatitis" [9, 177, 178] after the offend- ing plant (*Parthenium hysterophorus* L.).

The environmental conditions favoring ragweed dermatitis and its variants in hot and arid climates are not normally encountered in the temperate re- gions of Europe. Nevertheless, there are also Europe-

Table 4. Dermatologically important Apiaceae/Umbelliferae plants Asteraceae/Compositae

Correct name	Synonyms	English name	French name	German name
Achillea millefolium L.	*Achillea lanulosa* Nuttall	Yarrow, nosebleed, milfoil, thousand leaf	Achilée mille-feuille, herbe à la coupure	Gemeine Schafgarbe
Ambrosia acanthicarpa Hook.	*Franseria acanthicarpa* Cov.	Bur-ragweed, sandbur	Franserie lampourde	Falsche Ambrosie
Ambrosia artemisiifolia L.	*Ambrosia elatior* L.	Short ragweed, common ragweed	Ambroisie à feuille d'armoise, ambroisie élevée	Beifussblättrige Ambrosie, hohes Taubenkraut, Wermutblättrige Ambrosie
Ambrosia psilostachya DeCambolle		Western ragweed, perennial ragweed, common ragweed	Herbe à poux vivace	Ausdauernde Ambrosie
Ambrosia trifida L.	*Ambrosia aptera* DC.	Giant ragweed, tall ragweed		Dreispaltige Ambrosie
Anthemis arvensis L. ssp. arvensis		Field chamomile, corn chamomile (scentless)	Fausse camomille, camomille sauvage, anthémis des champs	Acker Hundskamille
Anthemis cotula L.	*Maruta cotula* DC.	Stinking chamomile, corn chamomile (scented)	Anthémis cotule, anthémis fétide	Stinkende Hundskamille
Arctotheca calendula Levyns	*Arctotis calendulacea* L., *Cryptostemma calendulacea* R. Br.	Capeweed	Artothèque souci	Dune Calendula
Arnica montana L.		Arnica, mountain tobacco, wolf's bane	Arnica, tabac des Vosges, quinquina des pauvres	Berg-Wohlverleih, Arnika
Artemisia ludoviciana Nutt.	*Artemisia ludoviciana* Nutt., *Artemisia purshiana*	Dark-leafed mugwort, prairie sage	Armoise argentée	Edelraute
Artemisia vulgaris L.		Common mugwort	Armoise vulgaire, herbe aux cent goûts	Gewöhnlicher Beifuss, Fliegenkraut
Cassinia aculeata R. Br.		Common cassinia, dogwood, cauliflower bush		
Chamaemelum nobile All.	*Anthemis nobilis* L.	Roman chamomile, dog fennel	Camomille romaine	Römische Kamille
Cichorium endivia L. spp. *endivia* L.		Common endive	Endive, chicorée des jardins	Winter Endivie
Cichorium intybus L.		Chicory, wild chicory	Chicorée sauvage, barbe de capucin	Wilde Zichorie, gemeine Wegwarte, Sonnenwedel
Conyza bonariensis Cronq.	*Erigeron bonariensis* L. *Conyza ambigua* DC., *Conyza crispa* Rupr.	Fleabane	Érigéron crépu	Südamerikanisches Berufskraut
Cynara cardunculus L.	*Cynara cardunculus* L. ssp. *cardunculus*; *Cynara cardunculus* L. ssp. *flavescens*	Cardoon	Cardon, carde	Kardone, Gemüse-Artischocke
Cynara scolymus L.	*Cynara cardunculus* L. ssp. *scolymus*; *Cynara cardunculus* L. ssp. *flavescens*	Globe artichoke	Artichaut	Artischoke, Alcachofra
Dahlia variabilis Desf.	*Dahlia* x *hortensis*	Dahlia	Dahlia	Dahlia
Dendranthema	*Chrysanthemum* x *hortorum* W. Miller, *Chrysanthemum morifolium* Ramat.	Autumn flowering chrysanthemum	Chrysanthème de Chine, chrysanthème d'automne	Chrysanthemen, Allerseelen-Aster

41

Table 4. Continued

Correct name	Synonyms	English name	French name	German name
Dittrichia graveolens Greuter	*Inula graveolens* Desf, *Erigeron graveolens* L.	Stinkwort	Inule fétide	Duftender Alant
Gaillardia pulchella Foug.	*Gaillardia picta* Sweet Foug.	Showy gaillardia	Gaillarde pulchella	Kurzlebige Kokardenblume
Helenium autumnale L.		Sneezeweed, swamp sunflower, false sunflower	Hélénie automnale	Sonnenbrot
Helenium amarum H. Rock	*Helenium tenuifolium* Nutt., *Gaillardia amara* Raf.	Sneezeweed, bitterweed	–	–
Helianthus annuus L.		Sunflower	Tournesol, soleil	Einjährige Sonnenblume
Inula helenium L.		Elecampane, horseheal, scabwort	Aunée officinale, grande aunée, inule aulnée	Echter Alant, Muxiang
Iva angustifolia Nutt.		Narrow-leaf marshelder		
Iva xanthifolia Nutt.		Marshelder		
Lactuca sativa L.		Lettuce	Laitue	Lattich
Leucanthemum vulgare Lam.	*Tanacetum leucanthemum* Schultz-Bip, *Chrysanthemum leucanthemum* L.	Marguerite, ox-eye daisy	Marguerite	Gemeine Wucherblume, Wissen-Margerite
Matricaria chamomilla L. var *recutita* Grieson	*Matricaria chamomilla* L., *Matricaria recutita* L., *Chamomilla recutita* Rauschert	German chamomile, wild chamomile	Matricaire, camomille allemande	Echte Kamille, deutsche Kamille
Parthenium argentatum A. Gray		Guayule	Guayule	Guayule
Parthenium hysterophorus L.		Congress grass, Santa Maria, whitetop	Absinthe bâtard	Parthenium hysterophorus
Petasites albus Gaertner		White butterbur	Pétasite blanc	Weisse Pestwurz
Saussurea lappa C.B. Clarke	*Saussurea costus* Lipsch.	Costus	Costus	Costus
Silybum marianum Gaertn.		Blessed milk-thistle, holy thistle	Chardon de Marie	Mariendistel
Tagetes minuta L.	*Tagetes glandulifera* Schrank	Small-flowered marigold, stinking roger	Tagète des décombres	Tagetes
Tanacetum cinerariifolium Schultz-Bip.	*Chrysanthemum cinerariifolium* Vis., *Pyrethrum cinerariifolium* Trevir.	Pyrethrum, Dalmatian pyrethrum	Pyrèthre	Dalmatinische Insektenblume
Tanacetum parthenium Schultz-Bip.	*Chrysanthemum parthenium* Bernh., *Matricaria parthenium* L.	Feverfew	Grande camomille	Mutterkraut, Falsche Kamille
Tanacetum vulgare L.	*Chrysanthemum tanacetum* Karsch., *C. vulgare* Bernh.	Tansy, bitter buttons	Tanaisie, tanacée, herbe aux vers	Gemeiner Rainfarn, Wurmkraut
Taraxacum officinale Weber	*Leontodon taraxacum* L., *Taraxacum densleonis* Desf., *T. taraxacum* Karst	Dandelion, blowball	Pissenlit, laitue de chien, dent de lion	Gebräulicher Löwenzahn, Kuhlblume
Xanthium spinosum L.		Spiny cocklebur	Lampourde épineuse, petite bardane	Dornige Spitzklette
Xanthium strumarium L.		Noogoora burr	Lampourde ordinaire, herbe aux écrouelles	Gemeine Spitzklette, Kropfspitzklette
X. italicum Moretti	*X. californicum* Greene, *Xanthium strumarium* L. ssp *italicum* D. Löve	Californian burr	Lampourde d'Italie	Italienische Spitzklette

an variants of ragweed dermatitis which have been described in rather specialized circumstances, with feverfew (*Tanacetum parthenium* Schultz-Bip.) [179, 180], chicory (*Cichorium intybus* L.) and lettuce (*Lactuca sativa* L.) [181–183], liverworts of the genus *Frullania* [45], and the chrysanthemums of florists [43]. Contact dermatitis from ragweed particularly affects male subjects and spares women and children [158] but Compositae-induced dermatitis generally appears to be rare in childhood [184].

Many cases have been described with sensitization to Asteraceae [8, 5] like with yarrow (*Achillea millefolium* L.) [162], chamomile (*Anthemis* spp L.) [166], arnica (*Arnica montana* L.) [168], small-flowered marigold (*Tagetes minuta* L.) [185], pyrethrum (*Tanacetum cinerariifolium* Schultz-Bip) [186], dandelion (*Taraxacum officinale* Wiggers) [187], elecampane (*Inula helenium* L.) [188, 189], sunflower (*Helianthus annuus* L.) [190], guayule (*Parthenium argentatum* Gray) [191], or Noogoora Burr (*Xanthium strumarium* L.) [192]. Cultivated plants, such as dahlia or chrysanthemum cultivars, are an important source of occupational contact allergy [193–197]. Botanical and vernacular names of dermatologically important Asteraceae are reported in Table 4.

Phototoxicity may theoretically occur following contact with α-terthienyl, a natural phototoxic thiophene compound of many Asteraceae species [198], but no authentic clinical cases appear to have been described in the literature.

Contact urticaria has been described with this family [12, 199].

> ### Core Message
>
> ■ The large Asteraceae/Compositae family is a frequent inducer of allergic contact dermatitis, due to the sesquiterpene lactones contained in the plants.

41.3.4.2 Liverworts (Jubulaceae)

Liverworts, together with mosses and hornworts, comprise a group of small, nonvascular plants known as bryophytes [200]. Typically they grow as epiphytes in damp locations, although they can withstand periods of desiccation. Of the liverworts, only a few species of *Frullania* have been described as causes of allergic contact dermatitis. These are found on trees in several regions of the world, notably in British Columbia in Canada, the Pacific North-West of the

United States (Oregon), and in the Bordeaux and Strasbourg regions of France. They are a cause of occupational contact dermatitis in forest workers and woodcutters [201, 202], and domestic allergy in people who use lobe-leaved trees as firewood. *Frullania dilatata* Dum., *F. tamarisci* Dum. and *F. tamarisci* Dum. ssp. *nisquallensis* Hatt. are the most aggressive species. Instances of cross-sensitivity reactions between *Frullania* species and members of the Compositae family are accounted for by the occurrence of structurally similar sesquiterpene lactones in the plants concerned, such as costunolide [8, 203]. More specifically, *Frullania dilatata* Dum. and *tamarisci* Dum. are sources of (+)- and (–)-frullanolide, respectively [204, 205]. There is a risk of active sensitization by patch testing [201], sometimes occult, as revealed by a new patch test session (personal observations).

> ### Core Message
>
> ■ The liverwort *Frullania* spp. induces contact allergy in foresters and people who are in contact with raw woods (firewood).

41.3.4.3 Sesquiterpene Lactone Allergens

The main allergens of Asteraceae are sesquiterpene lactones, and different ones may occur in a single species. They are characterized by the presence of a γ-butyrolactone ring bearing an exocyclic α-methylene group (Fig. 17). Hundreds of molecules have been (and continue to be) identified to date [206]. They are also present in related plant families such as Magnoliaceae, Winteraceae, Jubulaceae and Lauraceae [207].

The range of structures encountered among sesquiterpene lactones known to be allergenic is very wide, and each individual species contains a more or less complex mixture of these compounds. So, cross-sensitivity between various species in the Asteraceae is common but neither complete nor predictable [169, 196, 208]. This unpredictability may be exemplified by the fact that individual cultivars of the autumn-flowering chrysanthemums (*Dendranthema* cultivars) do not necessarily cross-react [43, 195, 209], whilst cross-reactions between members of the Compositae and liverworts of the genus *Frullania* (family Jubulaceae), laurel (*Laurus nobilis* L., family Lauraceae) and various members of the family Mag-

41

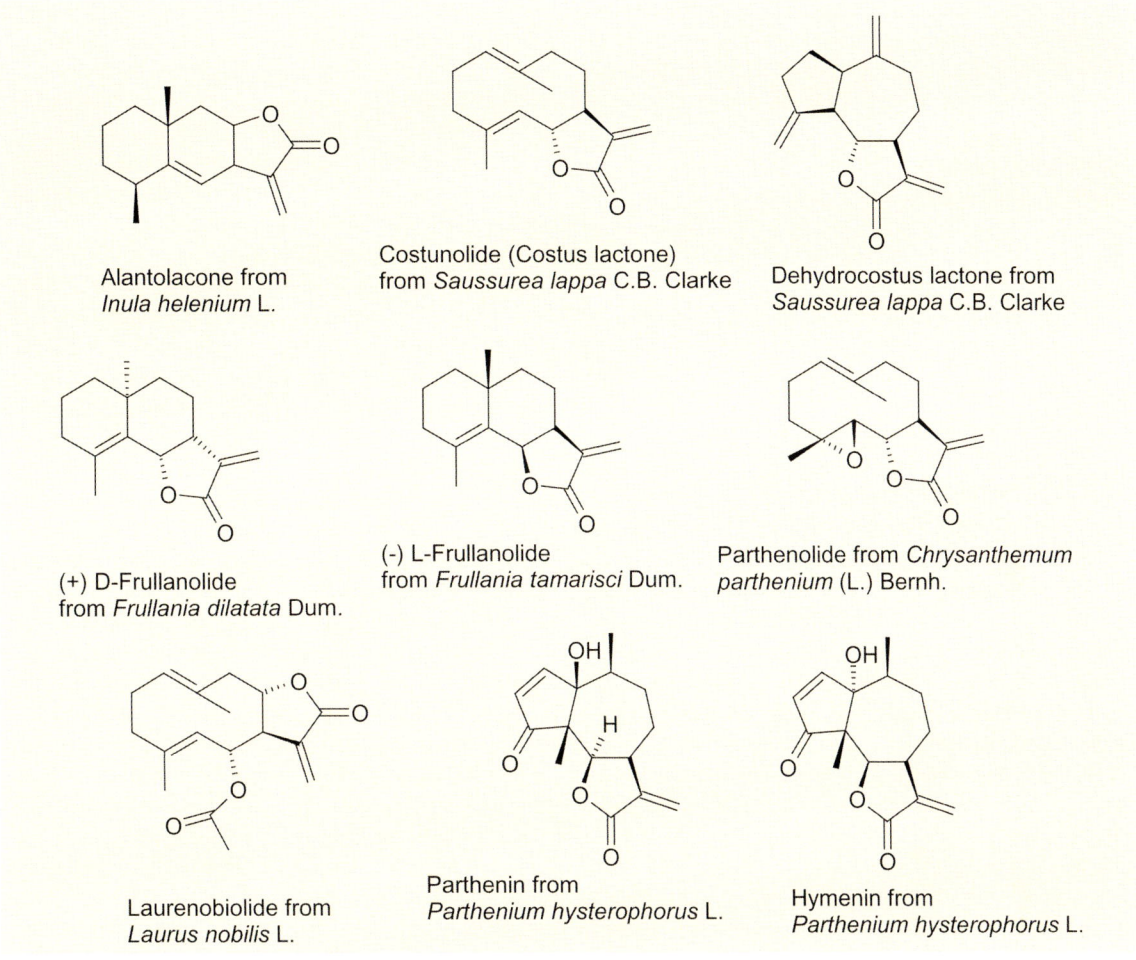

Fig. 17. Structures of some allergenic sesquiterpene lactones. Alantolactone CAS 546–43–0, costunolide CAS 553–21–9, dehydrocostus lactone CAS 477–43–0, D-frullanolide CAS 40776–40–7, L-frullanolide CAS 27579–97–1, parthenin CAS 508–59–8 and its diastereoisomer hymenin, parthenolide CAS 20554–84–1, and laurenobiolide

noliaceae, such as *Michelia lanuginosa* have been reported [5, 45, 210–214]. Data have been reviewed in the literature [215]. Cross-reactivity between sesquiterpene lactones largely depends on their stereochemistry. Parthenin and hymenin are examples of diastereoisomers found in the same plant (*Parthenium hysterophorus* L.) but not produced in the same region, since parthenin is found in India, but hymenin is found in South America. There is no cross-reactivity between the disatereoisomers parthenin and hymenin [216].

A vast number of species in the Compositae family have been described either as causes of contact dermatitis or as elicitors of positive patch test reactions. Many more may be regarded as potential contact allergens on the basis of their reported content of sesquiterpene lactones bearing an α-methylene-γ-butyrolactone ring.

In order to facilitate the diagnosis of sesquiterpene lactone-induced allergic contact dermatitis, a mixture of three representative lactones from various structural classes (alantolactone, costunolide, and dehydrocostus lactone) has been made available for testing. This mixture, called *Sesquiterpene lactone mix*, has been widely tested but detects only about 30% of cases of sensitization [217–220]; this poor sensitivity is partially explained by phytogeographic variations [221]. *Compositae mix* is an alternative preparation comprising a mixture of plant extracts (arnica, yarrow, tansy, German chamomile, and feverfew), which seems to detect a higher proportion of cases [218]. Other blends have been proposed, such as a blend of *Achillea millefolium* L., *Chamaemelum nobile* All. (syn. *Anthemis nobilis* L.), *Helianthus annuus* L., *Tagetes minuta* L., and *Tanacetum vulgare* L. [222], or a mixture of short ether extracts of arnica,

German chamomile, feverfew, tansy, and yarrow [223]. Dandelion and feverfew extracts, together or individually [224, 225], also appear to be more useful than sesquiterpene lactone mix alone.

> ### Core Message
>
> ■ Sesquiterpene lactones are potent contact allergens in Asteraceae/Compositae and liverworts. The numerous molecules generally do not cross-react.

41.3.5 Cruciferae (Cabbage or Mustard Family, Brassicaceae)

The Brassicaceae family contains about 3200 species in 375 genera, covering a large number of food plants such as cabbages (*Brassica oleracea* L.) with several varieties, for example, curly kale (*B. oleracea* var. *fimbriata* Miller), cauliflower (*B. oleracea* var. *botrytis* L.), Brussels sprouts (*B. oleracea* var. *gemmifera* DC.), kohl rabi (*B. oleracea* var. *gongyloides* L.), broccoli (*B. oleracea* var. *botrytis* ssvar. *Cymosa* Lam), turnips (Brassica *campestris* L. *var rapifera* Metz), radishes, rutabagas, mustard, and cress.

Together with the smaller Cleomaceae (which comprises the increasingly popular garden flower cleome or Spider flower, *Cleome spinosa* Jacq., syn. *C.*

pungens) and Capparaceae (Capparidaceae) families, Cruciferae characteristically contain glucosidic compounds (glucosinolates) which, in many species, release mustard oils (isothiocyanates, Fig. 18) when the plant material is damaged. These mustard oils impart pungency to the Cruciferae that contributes to the value of many in food or as irritants in traditional counterirritant remedies and rubefacient ointments. The most commonly used compound is the oil from black mustard seed (*Brassica nigra* Koch), which principally contains allyl isothiocyanate. This isothiocyanate is produced from its glucosinolate precursor sinigrin [226] by the action of an enzyme named myrosinase, activated when the plant material is damaged.

Notwithstanding the irritant properties of mustard oils and pharmaceutical preparations made from them, Coulter [227] observed no irritant reactions following rough handling of Cruciferae. Clinically, these plants are more commonly found to be responsible for allergic contact dermatitis in food handlers [7]. Radishes induced finger dermatitis in a waitress who chopped them (*Raphanus sativus* L.) [228]. Cabbages (*Raphanus sativus* var. *capitata* Alef.) provoked occupational contact dermatitis [229], and cabbage juice produced positive patch test reactions in 5/53 patients with hand dermatitis suspected to have been caused by vegetables [75].

To avoid irritant reactions, patch test concentrations with isothiocyanates should be prepared in the range 0.1–0.05% pet. [5, 230]. Positive patch test reactions to all four of these isothiocyanates have been

41

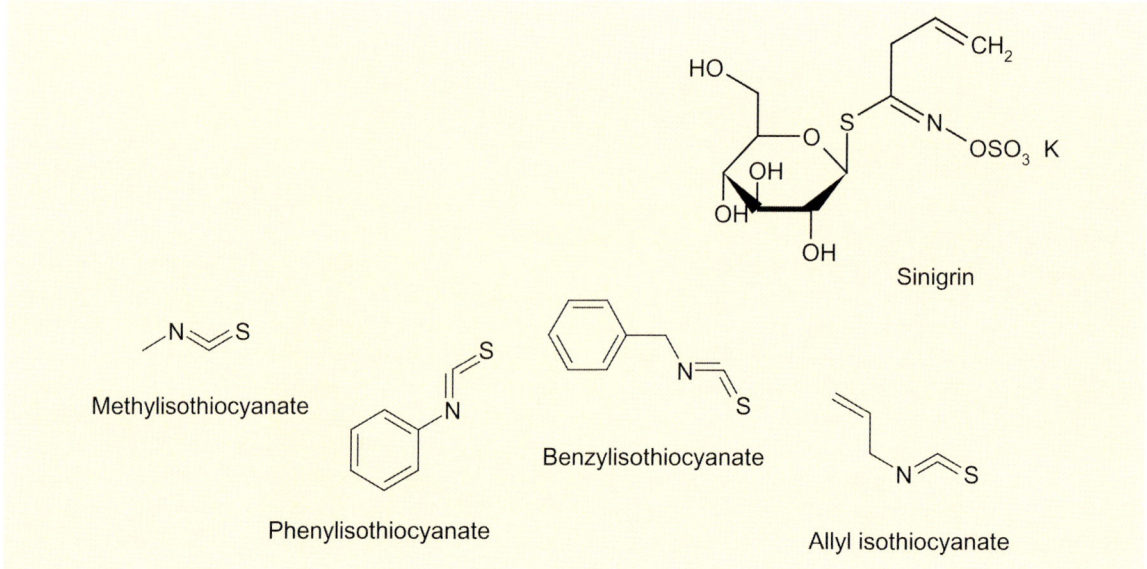

Fig. 18. Structures of methyl isothiocyanate CAS 556–61–6, phenyl isothiocyanate CAS 103–72–0, benzyl isothiocyanate CAS 622–78–6 and ally isothiocyanate CAS 57–06–7, and its precursor sinigrin CAS 3952–98–5

reported in various circumstances, but cross-reactions, if they exist, are not systematic [228, 231]. Methyl isothiocyanate [232] should be tested if plants belonging to the Capparaceae family are suspected as being the cause of dermatitis.

Core Message

■ Brassicaceae are irritant and allergenic, due to the isothiocyanates they release when the plant is damaged.

41.3.6 Euphorbiaceae (Spurge Family)

The Euphorbiaceae family comprises some 5000 species in about 300 genera which, with the exception of the polar regions, are found throughout the world. The largest and most widely distributed genus is *Euphorbia*. In Europe, euphorbias are small weeds known as spurges; tropical species are shrubs or trees, often resembling cacti in arid parts of Africa. They contain a latex which, in many species, is a skin irritant. The irritant compounds are diterpene esters belonging to three general classes: the tiglianes, ingenanes, and daphnanes. These irritant diterpenes are also found in other genera of the Euphorbiaceae and, interestingly, in the unrelated family Thymelaeaceae (daphne family). Reviews deal with the distributions of these compounds within the two families, their irritant properties and their tumor-promoting and other biologically hazardous properties [233–235].

Irritant contact dermatitis from Euphorbiaceae and Thymelaeaceae is rarely seen by European practitioners, but it is likely that accidental skin contact occurs quite frequently. As the irritant reaction resolves spontaneously within 1–2 days, it is unlikely to be seen in a dermatology clinic. Thus, whilst there is extensive anecdotal literature supported by numerous scientific studies of the irritant compounds, clinical studies and case reports are rare: 60 cases of irritant contact dermatitis from the infamous manchineel tree (*Hippomane mancinella* L.) of tropical America [236], irritant contact dermatitis from the African milk bush (*Synadenium grantii* Hook.f.) in a gardener [237], an irritant patch test reaction to the petty spurge (*Euphorbia peplus* L.), a garden weed presented by the patient as a house plant [238], perioral dermatitis from a pencil tree (*Euphorbia tirucalli* L.) [239]. Several authors described the irritant properties of the friendship cactus (*Euphorbia hermentiana* Lemaire) following the use of this plant by

a bank as an inducement to open a savings account [240], examined the irritant properties of a number of tigliane, ingenane and daphnane polyol esters in humans [241], or described a case of an 8-year-old girl who developed irritation and swelling of the face and eyelids as a result of a fight in which a boy beat her with snow-on-the-mountain (*Euphorbia marginata* Pursh) [242]. We have observed irritant dermatitis in a botanist who had botanized and made contact with euphorbia (Fig. 19).

It is frequently difficult to ascertain whether Euphorbiaceae are responsible for irritant or allergic contact dermatitis. Allergy rather than irritation is documented for two common ornamental Euphorbiaceae, namely croton (*Codiaeum variegatum* Blume var. *pictum* Muell. Arg.), and poinsettia (*Euphorbia pulcherrima* Willd.), although the allergens have not yet been characterized [243–247]. Out of 305 cases of contact dermatitis presented at the dermatology clinic on the Hawaiian island of Kauai, 61 were attributable to contact with plants. Among the most frequently blamed, Mango (*Mangifera indica* L., family Anacardiaceae) caused allergic contact dermatitis, and mokihana (*Pelea anisata* H. Mann, family Rutaceae) induced irritant photodermatitis, but the mechanism of the reactions to the euphorbias, allergic or irritant, was not stated [248]. It should be remembered that the irritant properties of these plants are sometimes utilized in popular remedies, for treating warts and basal cell carcinomas [249]. The potential for using euphorbias to produce dermatitis artefacta should also be recognized.

Among the irritants isolated from Euphorbiaceae (Fig. 20), 12-Deoxyphorbol-13-phenylacetate is an example of a tigliane polyol ester, found in the common sun spurge (*Euphorbia helioscopia* L.) [250]. Resiniferatoxin, a daphnane polyol ester that is one of the most irritant compounds known to Man, is found in official spurge (*Euphorbia resinifera* Berg) [251,

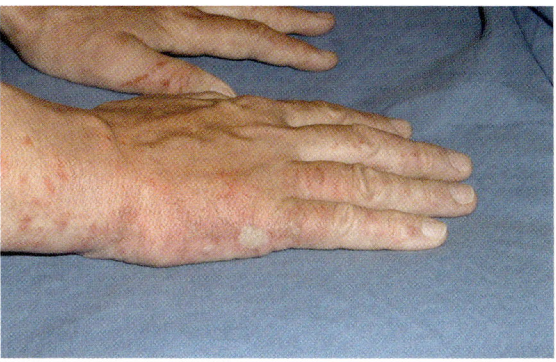

Fig. 19. Bullous irritant hand dermatitis due to *Euphorbia* spp.

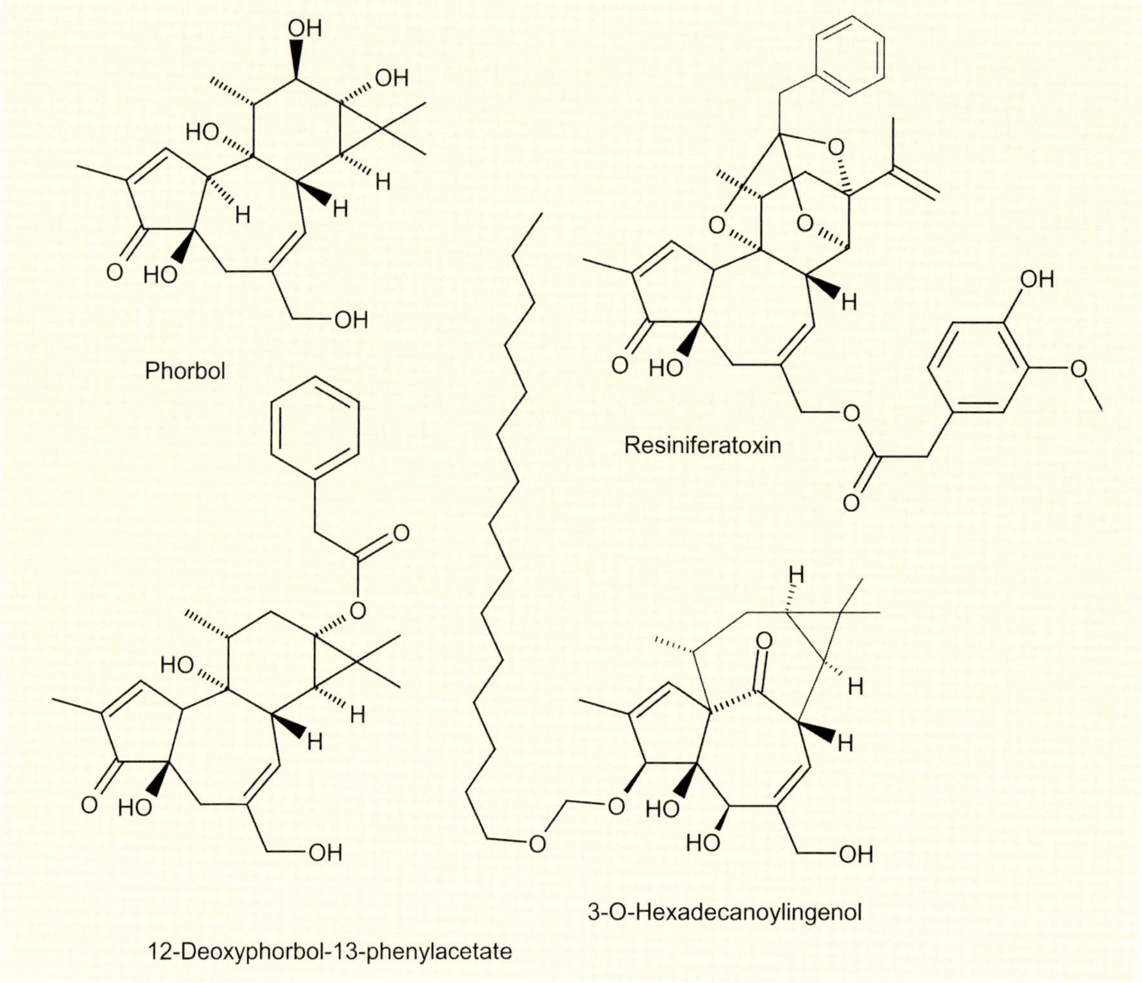

Fig. 20. Structures of the irritant phorbol CAS 17673–25–5 and representative irritants from the Euphorbiaceae and Thymelaeaceae: resiniferatoxin CAS 57444–62–9, 12-deoxyphorbol-13-phenylacetate, and 3-*O*-hexadecanoylingenol

252]. The ingenane polyol ester 3-*O*-hexadecanoyl ingenol is found in the caper spurge (*Euphorbia lathyris* L.) [170]. Readers interested in a comprehensive survey of the occurrence of such compounds in the Euphorbiaceae and Thymelaeaceae are referred to works by Evans [253] and Schmidt [10, 254, 255].

Core Message

■ Euphorbiaceae are very strong irritant and sometimes allergenic plants.

41.3.7 Lichens

Lichens are not really plants, and consist of a symbiotic association of a fungus (mycosymbiont, Kingdom Fungi) and an alga (phytosymbiont, Kingdom Protoctista), the first one providing morphology and sexual reproduction via spores, the second one producing organic materials by the way of photosynthesis [256]. Lichens grow on walls, roofs, trees, and rocks.

Several species are sensitizing, and those most often found to be the causes of allergic contact dermatitis are species of *Cladonia*, *Evernia*, and *Parmelia*, although reactions have been described with other species such as *Hypogymnia*, *Platismatia*, *Physconia*, *Usnea*, and *Alectoria* (*Bryoria*) [201]. Frequent sensitizing compounds from lichens are described in

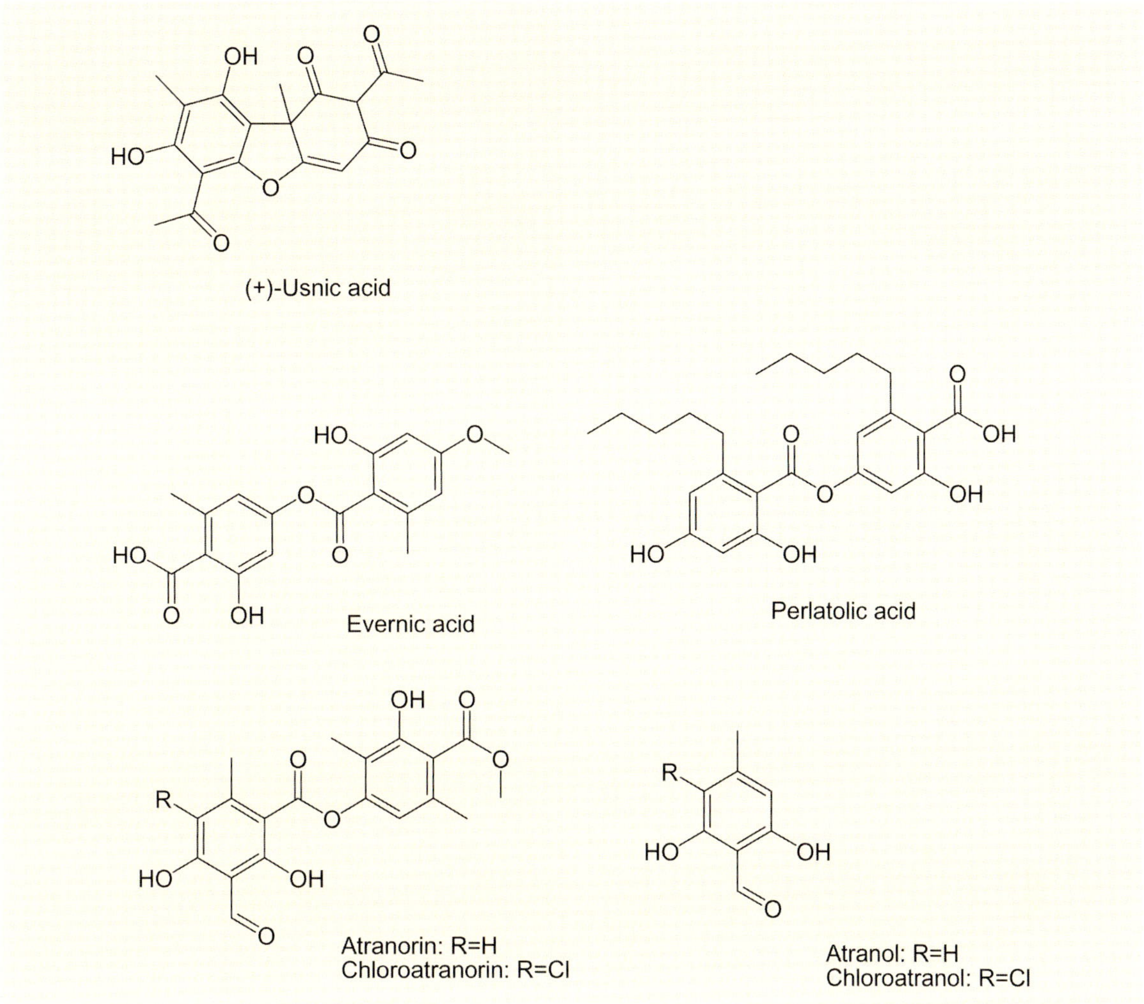

Fig. 21. Structure of some sensitizing lichen compounds. (+)-Usnic acid CAS 125–46–2, evernic acid, CAS 537–09–7, perlatolic acid, atranorin CAS 479–20–9, chloroatranorin, atranol CAS 526–37–4 and chloroatranol CAS 57074–21–2

Fig. 21. Dermatitis usually affects forestry workers and lichen pickers, and appears on the hands, forearms, face and other exposed areas [257, 258]. Allergy to lichens may also be observed following exposure to perfumes containing oak moss (which is not a moss!), which is extracted from *Evernia prunastri* (L.) Ach. and related species [259, 260]. *E. prunastri* contains atranorin and chloroatranorin, depsides that lead to the formation of atranol and chloroatranol during preparation of oak moss absolute. With methyl-β-orcinol carboxylate, they are potent allergens identified in oak moss absolute [261–263].

A history of abnormal photosensitivity is associated with lichen sensitivity, and has been discussed below. Irradiation of patch tests to lichens and their extracts may elicit enhanced responses [264–267]. An airborne contact dermatitis simulating photoderma-

titis has also been suggested to contribute to the clinical features seen in patients with lichen allergy [46]. Immediate-type allergies with asthma and urticaria were described following inhalation of, or direct contact with, algae from lichens [268].

Lichens can be tested "as is," but irritant reactions may occur. Oak moss is present in the fragrance mix of the European standard series, as a mixture of mainly *Evernia prunastri* Ach. (oak moss stricto sensu) and *Pseudevernia furfuracea* Zopf. (syn. *Parmelia furfuracea* Ach., tree moss). As tree moss, growing on both lobe-leaved trees and conifers, is frequently automatically picked with bark, it may contain derivatives of colophony. Such resinic acids are responsible for some positive reactions to fragrance mix in colophony-sensitive patients [269]. Lichen-derived compounds such as atranorin, usnic acid and evernic acid can be tested at 0.1% or 1% pet. Whether cross-sensitization occurs between structurally related lichen compounds is not clear. Because of the common occurrence of some of the lichen compounds in a number of species, concomitant sensitization is possible [257, 258].

> ### Core Message
>
> ■ Lichens are responsible for some cases of contact allergy from plants or from plant extracts in perfumes.

41.3.8 Primulaceae (Primrose Family)

This family of cosmopolitan distribution comprises 1000 species in 20 genera (among them *Cyclamen* spp), but only *Primula* (*Primula obconica* Hance) presents a common dermatological hazard. *P. obconica* is popularly grown in Europe as a house and greenhouse plant for its showy and long-lasting flowers, and the first report of contact allergy in 1888 by White has since been followed by many other reports [5, 270, 271]. Dermatitis (Fig. 22) generally affects the eyelids, face, neck, fingers, hands, and forearms, but *P. obconica* can also cause conjunctivitis and erythema-multiforme-like eruption [272]. The most important allergen of *Primula* is a quinone named primin [273], formed by oxidation of its biosynthetic precursor miconidin (which is also allergenic [274]) in minute glandular hairs (trichomes) present at the surface of the plant (Fig. 23). Dermatitis may be due to direct contact with plants, dust particles or to primin released directly from intact *P. obconica* plants [275]. This explains flares of dermatitis in highly sensitized patients after entering a room containing *P. obconica*. The presence of other allergens has been suggested [271, 276], for example the quinhydrone formed from primin and miconidin [183], the flavone primetin present in *Primula mistassinica* Michaux, and skin oxidized into a quinone derivative [277]. These could explain allergic contact dermatitis with positive allergic patch test reactions to fragments of the plant but negative to primin ([278], personal observation, Fig. 24). Other species of *Primula* are reported to be allergenic, such as *P. auricula* and *P. denticulata* [279, 280]. For a number of years, *P. obconica* was the most common cause of plant-induced contact dermatitis in Europe, but has become less of a problem in recent years, as its reputation has stimulated a widespread avoidance response. It is noteworthy that

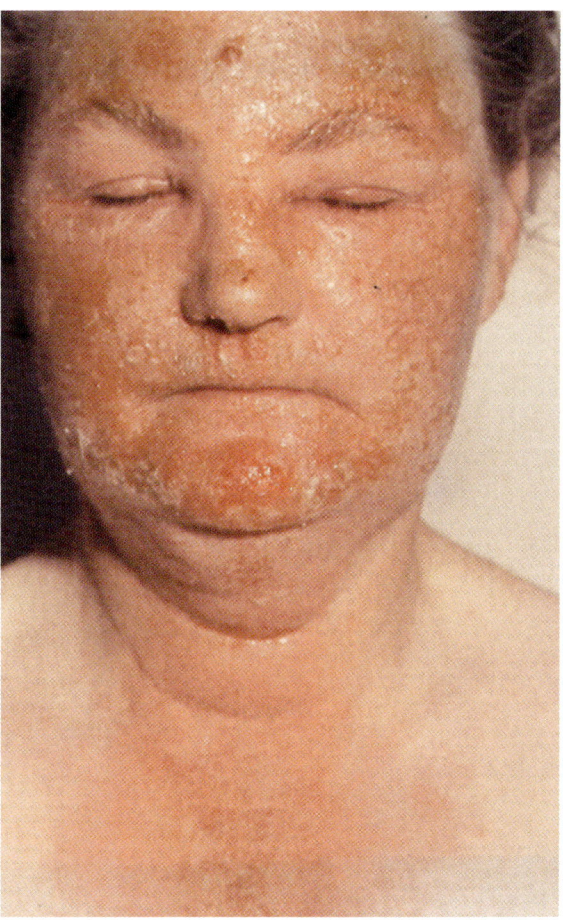

Fig. 22. Unusually severe exudative edematous primula dermatitis on the face (courtesy of N. Hjorth)

primin-free *Primula* have recently been developed, among them the "Touch Me" cultivar [281].

Because the content of primin in the leaves varies with the season, method of cultivation and cultivar identity [282, 283], the outcome of using fresh plant material as such for patch testing varies from the occurrence of false negatives during the winter months [284] to active sensitization between the months of April to August, when primin levels are at their highest [283, 285]. It was previously recommended that an ether extract of the leaves harvested in spring (60 g fresh weight dipped in 100 ml ether before concentrating to 50 ml at room temperature) should be used [286]. Patch testing with commercially available synthetic primin carries a real risk of active sensitization if concentrations greater than the usual (0.01%) are used.

41

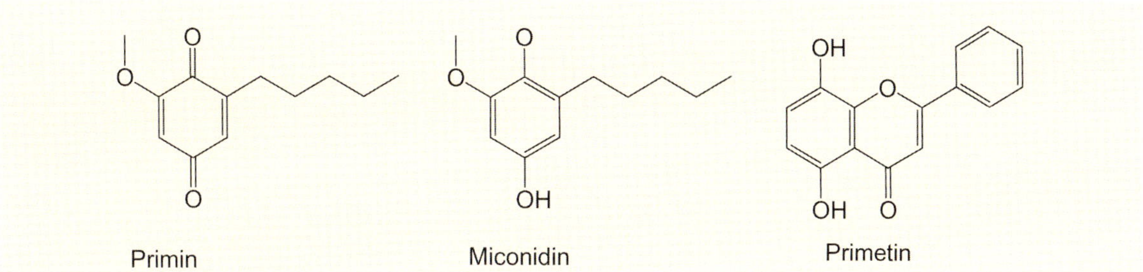

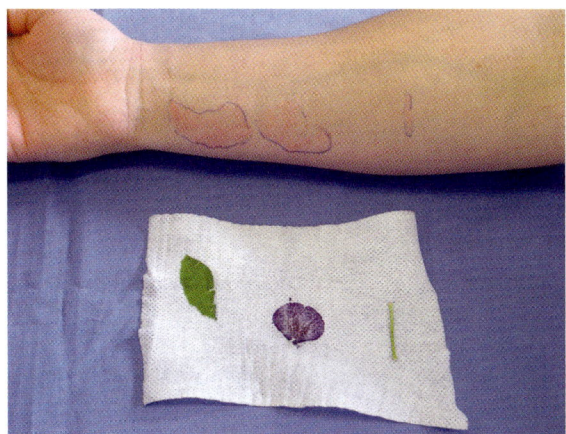

Fig. 23. Chemical structures of primin CAS 15121–94–5, miconidin CAS 34272–58–7 and primetin CAS 548–58–3

Fig. 24. Positive patch test reactions to *Primula obconica* Hance, performed in a horticulturist negative to primin

---

Core Message

■ Primulaceae are a source of contact sensitization, mainly in florists who handle *Primula obconica* Hance.

41.3.9 Ranunculaceae (Buttercup Family)

The family contains 1900 species in 50 genera. Mostly herbaceous with rhizomes, Ranunculaceae chiefly grow in northern temperate regions. Many members of the family are very caustic, and can cause skin or mucous membrane irritation [10, 29, 31]. This has led to the use of poultices of the plants as counterirritants in traditional medicine for the treatment of rheumatic joints, and severe adverse cutaneous reactions, with skin necrosis, may occur [287–291].

Systemic symptoms may occur after accidental ingestion of fresh plants by humans or animals, with systemic, digestive, renal, cardiorespiratory, neurologic and possibly life-threatening symptoms.

Protoanemonin is the irritant agent in Ranunculaceae. It is released from its precursor ranunculin by an enzymatic cleavage when the plant material is damaged [292–295]. Protoanemonin rapidly loses its irritant properties by dimerization into anemonin (Fig. 25). Dried plants are therefore inoffensive.

The following genera are representative members of the Ranunculaceae that have to be regarded as possible causes of irritant contact dermatitis:

■ *Anemone* spp. with wood anemone (*Anemone nemorosa* L.)
■ *Actaea* spp. with baneberry or herb Christopher (*Actaea spicata* L.), and white baneberry (*Actaea alba* Miller)
■ *Caltha* spp. with marsh marigold or kingcup (*Caltha palustris* L.)
■ *Clematis spp.* with Traveller's Joy, called "Old Man's Beard" because of long and feathery achenes or "herbe aux gueux" because middle age mendicants scrubbed their face with sap to provoke dermatitis and pity (*Clematis vitalba* L.)
■ *Pulsatilla* spp. such as prairie crocus (*Pulsatilla patens* Miller, syn. *Anemone patens* L.), Pasque flower (*Pulsatilla vulgaris* Mill., syn. *Anemone pulsatilla* L.)
■ *Ranunculus* such as common meadow buttercup (*Ranunculus acris* L., syn. *Ranunculus acer* Auct.), corn buttercup (*Ranunculus arvensis* L.), bulbous buttercup (*Ranunculus bulbosus* L.) or creeping buttercup (*Ranunculus repens* L.)
■ *Helleborus* spp. with Christmas rose (*Helleborus niger* L.).

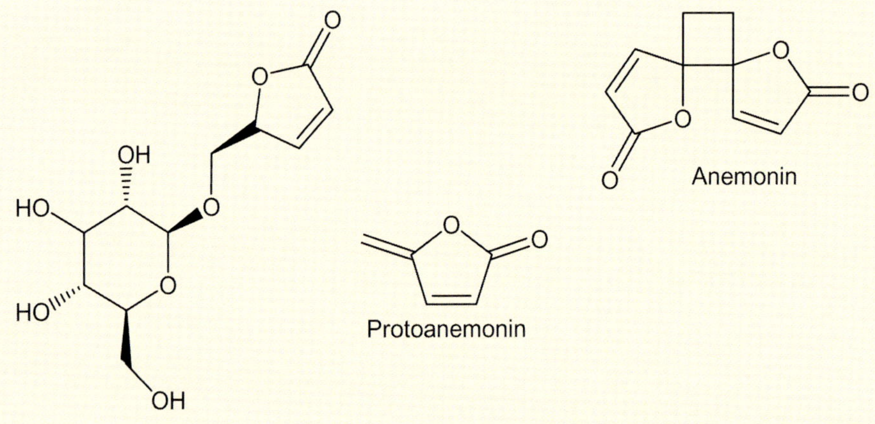

Fig. 25. Structure of ranunculin CAS 644–69–9, precursor of the strong irritant protoanemonin CAS 108–28–1, loses irritancy after dimerization into anemonin CAS 508–44–1

Core Message

- Ranunculaceae are very strong irritants, containing protoanemonin. They can induce severe skin damage, as systemic intoxication after ingestion.

41.3.10 Umbelliferae/Apiaceae (Carrot Family), Rutaceae (Rue Family) and Moraceae (Mulberry Family)

Members of these families have been considered together because of their capacity to induce photodermatitis, of phototoxic origin. The phototoxicity is due to furocoumarins contained in them. The synonym psoralen is derived from the Latin name of the Indian plant babchi or bakuchi (*Psoralea corylifolia* L., Leguminosae family), a plant that was used for treatment of vitiligo [296]. The most classical feature is Oppenheim dermatitis and its variants, discussed below. Children using the stems of hogweeds (*Heracleum mantegazzianum* Somm. and Lev. and *H. sphondylium* L.) as toy telescopes or peashooters in late summer typically develop bullous and erythematous lesions around the eyes and mouth [297, 298]. Other exposed areas of skin may be affected if contact with the sap occurs during horseplay amongst these plants, which are weeds of uncultivated land along roads, railways, and streams [55]. Because several members of these families are important sources of food, phototoxic reactions may occasionally be observed following occupational or household contact and sun exposure, on areas such as hands, the upper limbs and around the mouth.

The Apiaceae/Umbelliferae family contains 2850 species in 275 genera with a cosmopolitan distribution, chiefly in north temperate regions. Some are food plants such as celery (*Apium graveolens* L. var. *dulce* Pers.) [299–301], parsnip (*Pastinaca sativa* L.syn. *Peucedanum sativum* Benth. and Hook.) [302, 303], carrot (*Daucus carota* L.) [8], angelica (*Angelica archangelica* L.) [8, 304], chervil (*Anthriscus cerefolium* Hoffm.), or parsley (*Petroselinum crispum* A.W. Hill, syns. *Apium crispum* Miller, *Petroselinum sativum* Hoffm.) [305]. Others are medicinal, wild or cultivated plants such as Bishop's weed (*Ammi majus* L.) [306], Palm of Tromsø (*Heracleum stevenii* Manden syn. *Heracleum laciniatum* Hornem.) [307], giant hogweed (*Heracleum mantegazzianum* Somm. and Lev) [55, 297], and hogweed (*Heracleum sphondylium* L.) [308]. Several dermatologically significant plants are reported in Table 2.

Allergic contact dermatitis from Apiceae/Umbelliferae is possible, and has been described for carrot, celery and parsley. Falcarinol, also contained in members of Araliaceae (see later section), is probably the delayed-type allergen present [309, 310].

The Rutaceae family comprises citrus fruits. Many of them have induced phototoxicity, such as lime [59, 60, 311], bergamot [312, 313], and orange [314, 315]. Furanocoumarins are isolated mainly from citrus rind.

41

Pulp also contains photosensitizers, but to a lesser degree, with an average ratio of 1:20 to 1:100 [60]. Garden rue (*Ruta graveolens* L.) grows in gardens and may elicit phototoxic reactions after being picked [316, 317], as may other rue species such as *Ruta chalepensis* L. (syn. *Ruta bracteosa* DC.) [318]. Perfumes with psoralens from bergamot oil (*Citrus bergamia* Risso and Poit.) can induce phototoxicity presenting as "berloque dermatitis." Gas plant (*Dictamnus albus* L., syn. *Dictamnus fraxinella* Pers.) [59, 62, 302, 319], mokihana (*Pelea anisata* H. Mann) [320, 321], blister bush (*Phebalium anceps* DC), and Western Australian blister bush (*Phebalium argenteum* Smith) also contain psoralens [322], which largely account for the (sometimes very severe) bullous dermatitis [60].

The Moraceae family contains edible fig (*Ficus carica* L.) [323–326], breadfruit (*Artocarpus altilis*), other *Ficus* spp (naturally growing or as indoor plants in temperate countries), and the tropical wood iroko or African teak (*Chlorophora excelsa* Benth. and Hook. f.), which contains chlorophorin.

Although allergic reactions to psoralens do not seem to have been described, photoallergic reactions can occur [66, 67]. However, a number of psoralen-containing plants may also sensitize as a result of other compounds that they contain. For example, citrus oils are generally weakly allergenic but they are also irritant and some are phototoxic [327]. Similarly, carrots (*Daucus carota* L., family Umbelliferae) have sensitized workers in the canning industry [328–330], but there is no convincing evidence that they may elicit phototoxic reactions, although weak phototoxicity has been observed experimentally [331]. Thus, if an allergic reaction is suspected, it is important to realize that irritancy and photoaggravation may occur during patch testing.

> ## Core Message
>
> ■ The Apiaceae/Umbelliferae family is
>   mainly responsible for phototoxic contact
>   dermatitis (Oppenheim dermatitis
>   and variants) like Rutaceae (citrus family)
>   and Moraceae (fig family) because of
>   the furocoumarins contained in them.

41.3.11 Woods

Although woods are not derived from a botanically homogeneous source, we will consider them together

for practical reasons. Most dermatoses from contact with woods are occupational and are observed in carpenters, joiners, cabinet-makers and in associated tradespersons [5, 8, 12, 72, 332], as forest workers are generally affected by liverwort and lichens growing on trees. Less commonly, dermatitis is due to finished wood products, such as violin chin-rests [333], necklaces [334], bracelets [335], and knife handles [336].

Woodworkers are highly exposed to sawdust, and contact initially occurs on exposed areas (hands and forearms, face and neck, Fig. 26). Standard clothing is not good protection. Airborne sawdust, however, may drift inside loosely fitting protective clothing, and adhere to sweaty areas of skin like the axillae, waistband, groin and ankles. Such areas can be prone to irritant and/or allergic contact dermatitis.

The additional hazards of asthma and sinus ethmoidal adenocarcinoma from inhaling the sawdust of certain woods, and the higher risks of Hodgkin's disease associated with woodworking as well as of systemic symptoms if the wood contains pharmacologically active constituents have been reviewed [337, 338]. Reviews on wood-induced dermatitis are recommended for detailed information [8, 72, 337–342], like the website (http://biodiversity.bio.uno.edu/delta/wood) [343] to which readers can refer for further information.

The most highly sensitizing woods are of tropical origin, as they commonly contain quinones as sensi-

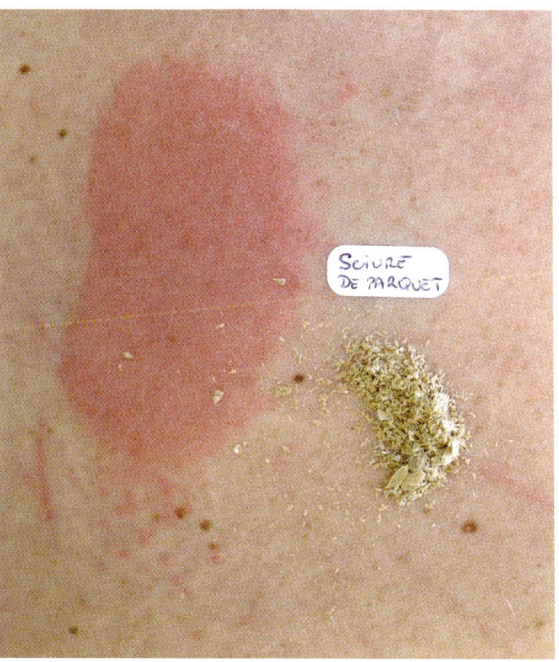

Fig. 26. Positive patch test reaction to woodfloor (wood dust diluted in petrolatum) in a "do it yourself" carpenter

tizers. Because of the wide occurrence of quinones, reactivity to several woods may be expected. For example, 2,6-dimethoxy-1,4-benzoquinone is found in many woods, such as African or American mahogany (*Khaya* spp., Meliaceae family), Bubinga (*Guibourtia spp.*, family Caesalpinaceae), Capomo (*Brosimum alicastrum* Schwartz, family Moraceae), *Bowdichia* spp. (*Bowdichia nitida* Benth.) and *Diplotropis* spp. (*Diplotropis purpurea*), Doussié (*Afzelia* spp.), Afrormosia or Kokrodua *(Pericopsis elata* van Meeuwen), Makoré (*Tieghemella africana* Pierre, *T. heckelii* Pierre ex A. Chev.), Sipo (*Entandrophragma* spp., family Meliaceae) and Wengé (*Millettia* spp. *laurentii* De Wild, *Milettia stuhlmanii* Taub. family Papilionaceae) [342].

In studies with guinea pigs, cross-reactivity between primin, deoxylapachol, various dalbergiones, mansonones and other quinones have been observed [337], but cross-sensitivity between primin and various wood quinones does not seem to occur in humans [344]. In addition to quinonoid allergens, a number of other types of low molecular weight allergens have been identified from woods, reflecting the variety of botanical sources from which exploitable woods are obtained. Structures of some of the best known wood allergens are given in the following figures.

Woods provide some rather significant problems with their identification. Most are transported under a trivial rather than botanical name, and it is not unusual for these trivial names to be misapplied either

inadvertently or deliberately. For example, the single milowood (*Thespesia populnea* Sol. ex Corrêa) is also named Álamo, álamo blanco, algodón de monte, beach maho, bosch-katoen, catalpa, clamor, clemón, cork-tree, cremón, emajagüilla, frescura, grós hahaut, haiti-haiti, jaqueca, John-Bull-tree, macoi, mahault de Londres, maho, mahot bord-de-mer, majagua de Florida, majagüilla, otaheita, palo de jaqueca, palu santu, portiatree, santa maría, seaside mahoe, Spanish cork, and tuliptree. It is imperative, for serious diagnosis and exploration, that a solid sample of a wood believed to be the cause of contact dermatitis (or any other pathological lesion) is sent to a wood anatomist for identification [337]. Its origin and any available trade names should also be made known to the wood anatomist.

41.3.11.1 American and Australian Woods

A variety of American and Australian woods deserve a mention in this context [10, 72, 342–346].

Australian blackwood (*Acacia melanoxylon* R. Br., Mimosaceae family), is a very important wood in Australia, inducing occupational contact dermatitis due to 2,6-dimethoxy-1,4-benzoquinone, acamelin, and melacacidin.

The Australian silky oak (*Grevillea robusta* A. Cunn., Proteaceae family) has been discussed above.

Brazilian rosewood or palissander (*Dalbergia nigra* All., Papillionaceae family) such as East India

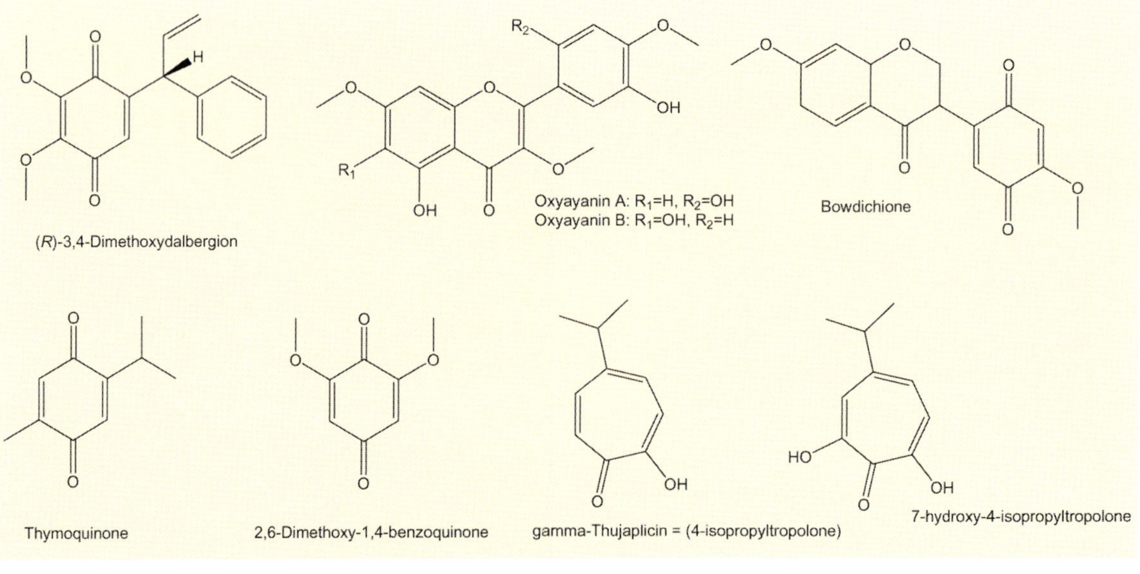

Fig. 27. Allergens from American and Australian woods: (*R*)-3,4-dimethoxydalbergion CAS 3755–64–4, oxyayanin A CAS and oxyayanin B CAS, bowdichione, thymoquinone CAS 490–91–5, 2,6-dimethoxy-1,4-benzoquinone CAS 530–55–2, γ-thujaplicin CAS 672–76–4, and 7-hydroxy-4-isopropyltropolone

rosewood (*Dalbergia latifolia* Roxb.), cocolobo (*Dalbergia retusa* Hemsl., *Dalbergia granadilla*, and *Dalbergia hypoleuca*) or grenadil (*Dalbergia melanoxylon* Guill. and Perr.) are used for high-class furniture such as wooden jewels and musical instruments. Dalbergiones such as (R)-3,4-dimethoxydalbergione, (R)- and (S)-4-methoxydalbergione, (S)-4-methoxydalbergione, (S)-4,4′-dimethoxydalbergione and (S)-4′-hydroxy-4-methoxydalbergione are the sensitizers (Fig. 27).

Grapia is a Brazilian wood (*Apuleia leiocarpa* Macbr., Caesalpinioideae family) that can induce contact dermatitis and mucous membrane symptoms. Main allergens are likely ayanin, oxyayanin-A and oxyayanin-B, the latter also being an allergen in movingui (*Distemonanthus benthamianus* Baill., family Caesalpinioideae).

Incense cedar (*Calocedrus decurrens* Florin, Cupressaceae family) used for pencils, chests or toys is a cause of contact dermatitis due to the allergen thymoquinone.

Pao ferro, "Santos-palissander" or caviuna vermelha (*Machaerium scleroxylon* Tul., Papilionaceae family) is frequently used as a substitute of rosewood. The sensitizers are dalbergiones, including (R)-3,4-dimethoxydalbergione, which is very potent allergen.

Polynesian rosewood or milowood (*Thespesia populnea* Sol., Malvaceae family) is a wood used for small articles and wood jewels. It contains mansonones such as mansonone X.

Sucupira (*Bowdichia nitida* Spruce, Fabaceae family) is a Brazil wood, used for flooring, responsible for allergic contact dermatitis in joiners and flooring workers. Among the allergens present, 2,6-dimethoxy-p-benzoquinone and Bowdichione are the best known.

Western cedar (*Thuja plicata* Donn., family Cupressaceae) is used as a hardwood in construction work or on boats. Its main contact allergen is thymoquinone. It also contains γ-thujaplicin and 7-hydroxy-4-isopropyl-tropolone.

41.3.11.2 Asian Woods

Several Asian woods are reported to be sources of allergens [10, 72, 343, 346].

Teak (*Tectona grandis* L., Verbenaceae family) is largely used for various indoor and outdoor applications (such as in doors and windows) due to its high durability. The sensitizers are naphthoquinones named deoxylapachol and lapachol, which have similar reactivities [72, 346] (Fig. 28).

East-Indian rosewood is similar to Brazilian rosewood in terms of use and allergens.

Macassar (*Diospyros celebica* Bakh., family Ebenaceae) is related to coromandel and ebony.

41.3.11.3 African Woods

The following African woods are the most relevant to this discussion [10, 72, 343, 347].

African ebony (*Diospyros crassifolia* Hiern., family Ebenaceae), coromandel (*Diospyros melanoxylon* Roxb.) are wood species with black heartwood used for precious works.

African mahogany (*Khaya grandiflora* DC.), Khaya mahogany (*Kahya ivorensis* A. Chev.), Krala (*Khaya anthotheca* C. DC.) and Senegal mahogany (*Khaya senegalensis* A. Juss., Meliaceae family) are sensitizers by the way of allergens such as anthothecol (Fig. 29).

African red padauk wood (*Pterocarpus soyauxii* Taub., Papillonaceae family), is a hardwood tree used to manufacture veneer, furniture and musical instruments.

Ayan (*Distemonanthus benthamianus* Baillon, Caesalpinaceae family) is used for flooring or windows. Its allergens are oxyayanin A and B.

Iroko, African teak or kambala (*Chlorophora excelsa* Benth and Hook. f., Moraceae family) has good strength and durability and is used for indoor and

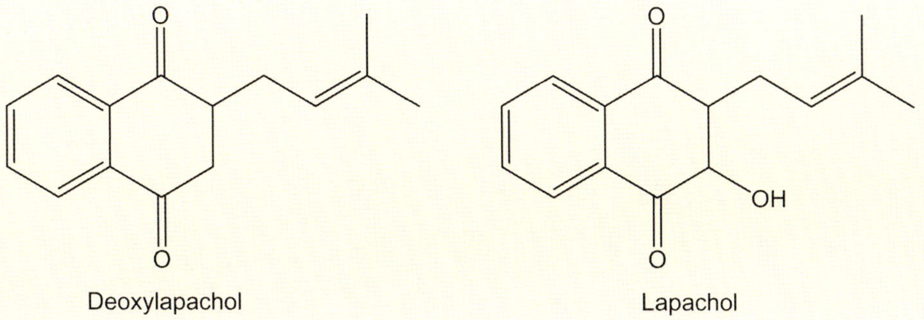

Deoxylapachol   Lapachol

Fig. 28. Structure of deoxylapachol CAS 3568–90–9, and lapachol CAS 84–79–7

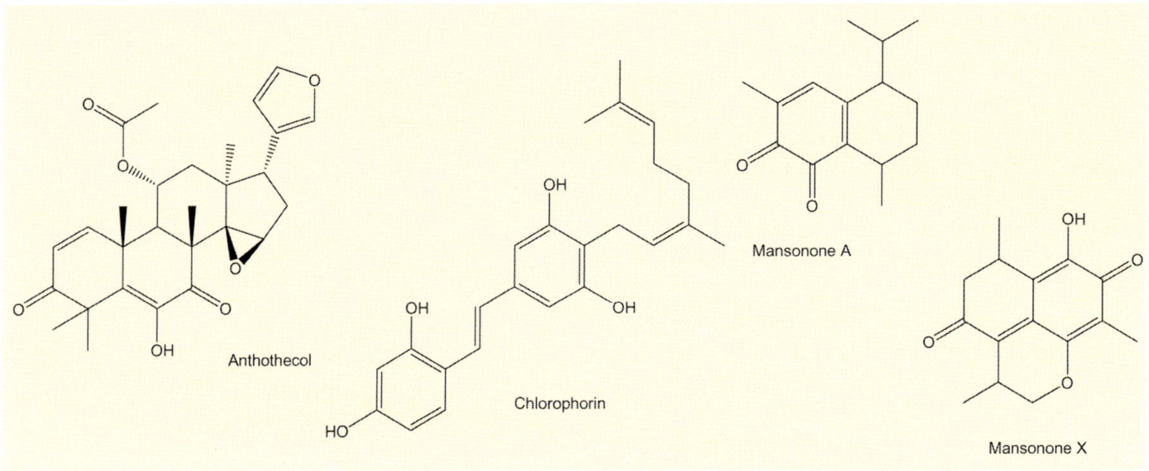

Fig. 29. Structures of some allergens in African woods: anthothecol CAS 10410–83–0, chlorophorin CAS 537–41–7, mansonone A CAS 7715–94–8, and mansonone X

outdoor constructional work. Chlorophorin is its main allergen.

Mansonia or bete (*Mansonia altissima* A. Chev, Sterculiaceae family) is used as a substitute for walnut. It has several sensitizers called sesquiterpenoid mansonones, with the *ortho*-quinone mansonone A being the main allergen.

41.3.11.4 European Woods

Woods derived from trees growing in temperate regions in Europe are also sensitizers [72, 346, 348, 349]. Dermatitis has been reported in association with alder (*Alnus* sp., Betulaceae family), ash (*Fraxinus* sp., Oleaceae family), beech (*Fagus* sp., Fagaceae family), birch (*Betula* sp. Betulaceae family) and poplar (*Populus* sp., Salicaceae family) woods.

The most extensively grown and exploited trees in temperate regions are the pines (*Pinus* spp.), spruces

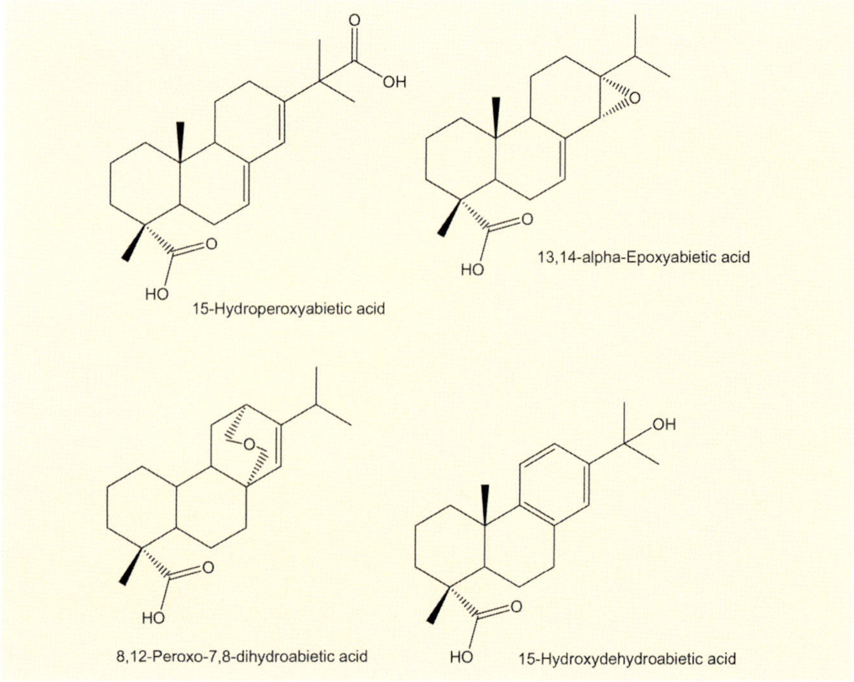

41

Fig. 30. Examples of oxidation products of colophony, responsible for sensitization

(*Picea* spp.), firs (*Abies* spp.), and related conifers (family Pinaceae). These are rarely implicated as causes of allergic contact dermatitis. It is worth noting that patients with dermatitis from pine or spruce have positive reactions to colophony. Pines are sources of turpentine oil and of colophony, both of which are well-known sensitizers. In both of these wood-derived products, the actual sensitizers are the hydroperoxidic autoxidation products that are formed in contact with the air, rather than the major constituents from which they are derived.

The major resinic acids in colophony are abietic and dehydroabietic acids. Abietic acid was formerly claimed to be the cause of colophony (rosin) dermatitis. However, it appears to be neither a sensitizer nor an elicitor of colophony dermatitis if rigorously purified, whereas numerous oxidation products such as 15-hydroperoxyabietic acid or products from secondary oxidation are the allergens responsible (Fig. 30) [350–352].

In turpentine oil, hydroperoxides of 3-carene, and not Δ3-carene itself, are sensitizers [353, 354].

Core Message

■ Woods induce contact dermatitis, mainly in woodworkers. Irritation is frequent, and contact allergy can be severe due to potent allergens like quinones.

41.3.12 Mushrooms

Several cases of occupational allergic contact dermatitis have been described from mushrooms, which mainly induce immediate-type symptoms. The best known manifestation is likely shiitake dermatitis, due to contact or ingestion of raw or half-cooked black mushrooms (*Lentinula edodes* Pegler) [355]. Other mushrooms have been reported as being allergenic, such as yellow boletus (*Boletus luteus* L., syn. *Suillus luteus* Gray), cep or Polish mushroom (*Boletus* edulis Bull.Fr), meadow mushroom (*Agaricus campestris* L.), cultivated mushroom (white type: *Agaricus hortensis* Imai; brown type: *Agaricus bisporus* Pilát), orange agaric (*Lactarius deliciosus* Gray), pine yellow clavaria or fairy clubs (*Clavaria flava* Fr., syn. *Ramaria flava* Quélet), oyster (*Pleurotus ostreatus* Kummer, and yamabushitake or monkey's head mushroom (*Hericicum erinaceum* Pers.) [356–359].

41.3.13 Ferns

Ferns and related plants [360] have rarely been implicated in plant dermatitis. Leatherleaf or Baker fern (*Arachnoides adiantiformis* Tindale, Aspidiaceae or Dryopteridaceae family) provoked allergic contact dermatitis in a flower shop worker [361].

41.3.14 Miscellaneous Plants

Many plants have been described as inducing dermatitis. Case reports are sometime scarce or even unique. Many are reported in dermato-botanical books, but it is interesting to cite some recent reports of dermatitis due to plants belonging to families not mentioned above.

41.3.14.1 Araliaceae (Ginseng, Aralia, Ivy Family)

Common ivy (*Hedera helix* L.) is a very common plant in Europe that may induce contact irritation and more rarely sensitization. It contains three powerful irritants and weak sensitizers, namely didehydrofalcarinol and falcarinol (Fig. 31) that have mod-

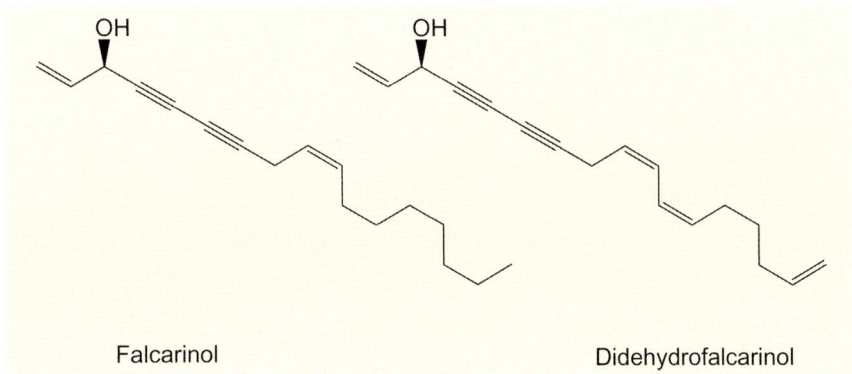

Fig. 31.
Falcarinol, CAS 21852–80–2, and didehydrofalcarinol, CAS 110927–49–6

Falcarinol　　　　　Didehydrofalcarinol

erate sensitizing potentials [310, 362, 363]. These allergens or related molecules are also present in other members of this family, such as ginseng (*Panax ginseng* C. Meyer), *Schefflera arboricola* Hayata [310] or kakuremino (*Dendropanax trifidus* Makino) [364]. Falcarinone, an oxidation product of falcarinol, is commonly found in the Apiaceae/Umbelliferae family [310], and falcarinol is likely a delayed-type allergen of Apiaceae/Umbelliferae, as in carrot, celery, and parsley [309, 310].

41.3.14.2 Papaveraceae (Poppy Family)

Greater celandine, sometimes named "wart plant" (*Chelidonium majus* L., Papaveraceae family), is well known in traditional topical treatments of warts, epithelial tumors, and hyperkeratotic lesions [365]. Its orange-colored juice has irritant properties and has been reported to be a probable allergenic [366]. Systemic (liver) toxicity is possible after ingestion [367].

41.3.14.3 Guttiferae (St John's Wort or Mangosteen Family)

This family comprises herbs, lianes, shrubs, and trees that have a colored resinous juice. They are used for timbers, drugs, dyes, gums, pigments, and resins.

St John's wort (*Hypericum perforatum* L.) has been used for centuries for wounds, burns or dermatitis [365]. It has recently been used systemically for depression. It contains hyperforin, which has antibacterial or claimed antidepressant properties, and the phototoxic substance hypericin (Fig. 32), which is re-

sponsible for cutaneous side-effects such as contact dermatitis and photosensitivity [368–371].

Tamanu oil (Calophyllum inophyllum), extracted from the fruits or seeds of *Calophyllum tacamahaca* L. and used as a cosmetic or traditional medicine ingredient, has been reported to be a cause of allergic contact dermatitis, with photoworsening of patch tests [372].

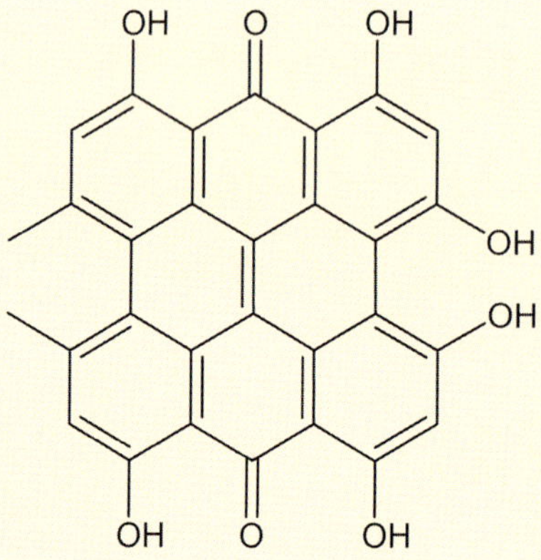

41.3.14.4 Hydrangeaceae

Dermatitis due to *Hydrangea macrophylla* Thunb (Hydrangeaceae family) appears as a chronic, fissuring and scaling dermatitis of hand and finger. Irritant dermatitis is possible, but allergy is not rare and is due to hydrangenol (Fig. 33). Occupational exposure is mainly found in nursery workers, florists or gardeners. Patch tests with leaves and stems are strongly positive, as hydrangenol 0.1% pet., which gives strongly positive reactions [373].

41.3.14.5 Iridaceae (Iris Family)

Contact dermatitis to iris (safflower) (*Iris germanica* var *florentina* Dykes) was reported, with positive reactions to petals [374], but not to leaves in one observation [375].

41.3.14.6 Solanaceae (Nightshade Family)

The family contains more than 2000 species in 90 genera, providing numerous food plants such as tomatoes (*Lycopersicon lycopersicum*), potatoes (*Solanum tuberosum* L.), paprika and pepper (*Capsicum*), and tobacco (*Nicotiana tabacum*).

Occupational hand contact dermatitis is frequent in pickers or harvesters [376], mainly irritant, but sometimes allergic. Leaves of eggplants or brinjal (*Solanum melongena* L.) were tested positive when

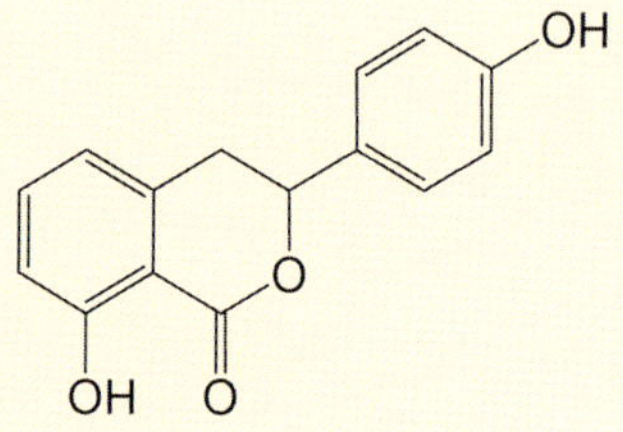

Fig. 32. Hypericin, CAS 548–04–9, extracted from *Hypericum perforatum* L.

Fig. 33. Hydrangenol, CAS 480–87–7 the allergen of hydrangea

41

chopped in petrolatum [377]. Fruits (aubergine) and pollens may induce immediate symptoms.

41.4 Diagnosis of Plant Dermatitis

Finding the source of a plant-induced contact dermatitis is often difficult. A provisional diagnosis may be made by asking patients about their occupation, hobbies and recent excursions during which plant contact may have occurred. It is often necessary to enlist the help of a botanist to identify plants brought in by patients. If the results of an investigation of a plant-induced dermatitis are to be published, it is essential to identify the plant precisely. Whilst photographs of plants are helpful, they are usually less helpful than accurate drawings showing features that enable similar species to be distinguished one from another. There is no substitute for a botanist who is familiar with the taxonomic literature on the plant concerned, but just as there are specialities in the medical profession, no one botanist is an expert on all plants.

41.4.1 Raw Plants

41.4.1.1 Plant Identification

The practitioner has to consider not only the plant species itself, but also its generic and familial identity. The genetic information that groups plants into species, genera and families actually determines to a large extent the nature of the plant's secondary metabolites. Thus, sesquiterpene lactones are a common feature of members of the family Compositae, whilst mono- and dihydroxyalk(en)ylbenzenes are commonly found in members of the family Anacardiaceae. Once a plant has been implicated and identified, reference to the literature should reveal whether or not it has been recorded as an allergenic plant.

41.4.1.2 Prick Tests

Pricks can be performed through the crude material as is, or by the "prick by prick" method (prick into the plant, and then into the skin). Plant materials can be crushed and diluted with saline (for example, 1:9 parts) in order to obtain a solution that can be easily pricked (Fig. 34, rose).

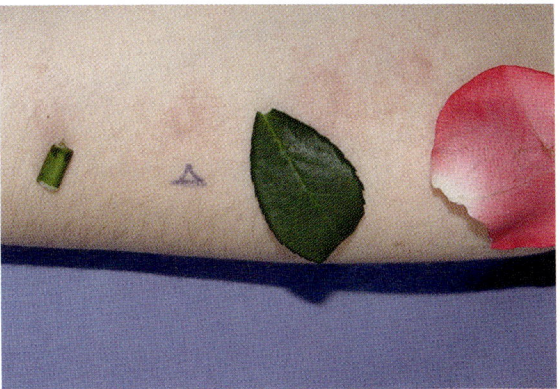

Fig. 34. Positive prick tests to rose (petal, stem, leave and thorn) in a florist with immediate symptoms following contact with roses

41.4.1.3 Patch Tests

It is often possible to carry out tests with plant material "as is," and a diagnosis of plant dermatitis can usually be established with a few grams of fresh plant material. The practitioner has to patch test several plant pieces such as roots, stems, leaves, and reproductive organs (flowers and/or fruits). It is sometimes useful to patch test crushed leaves or slices of stem [378].

It is important to use, whenever possible, the actual plant material that is believed to be responsible for the current dermatitis. This is because distinct chemical races may exist in outwardly identical plants, where one specimen contains the allergen whilst the second does not. As noted above, cultivars of plants such as tulips and chrysanthemums exhibit varying propensities to induce and elicit allergic contact dermatitis. If an inappropriate sample of plant material is tested, the risk of a missed diagnosis clearly exists.

Woods should not be tested as is, because of the risk of irritation and active sensitization. Wood dust can be tested diluted in white petrolatum, 10–20% (weight/weight). Extracts obtained with solvents such as acetone or ethanol can be used. Controls are useful when they are negative because of the high incidence of irritancy [38, 339, 345], but they raise ethical considerations. When purified isolates from woods are available for patch testing, these may be prepared according to the recommendations of Hausen [340]. Here too, the risk of active sensitization is real ([345]; A. Goossens, personal communication).

Care should be taken with plants known to contain either irritant compounds (such as *Euphorbia* spp.) or highly allergenic compounds (such as *Pri-*

mula), where the past experiences of other dermatologists (reported in the literature, at congresses or via networks) should be heeded.

Irritant reactions are frequent with plant materials and have to be considered when doubtful or weakly positive (edema and erythema) reactions are observed.

Core Message

■ Patch tests with plant or wood materials have to be performed cautiously, heeding recommendations, and interpreted carefully because of the irritant and sensitizing risk.

41.4.2 Plant Extracts

Plant allergens, which are generally low molecular weight secondary plant metabolites, are likely to be soluble in acetone, ethanol or ether. Thus, a filtered acetone or ethanol extract of dried plant material, or a short ether extract of fresh material usually produces a solution suitable for patch testing. Producing water extracts of fresh plant material is not recommended, although this is often carried out and can produce active substances. Water extracts seem to degrade rapidly and lose their sensitizing power within a month [170], due to chemical degradation and/or to microbial contamination. For example, acetone extracts of *Parthenium hysterophorus* have been demonstrated to be more sensitive than water extracts, with very good sensitivity to 1% acetone extract [50].

Extracts in organic solvents are generally more stable, but they should not be regarded as having an indefinite shelf life. Moreover, with time, evaporation of the solvent may increase the concentration and the sensitizing effect of the allergen(s). Incorporating an evaporated extract into petrolatum represents a standard means of retaining material for patch testing, but it is questionable whether this extra manipulation of the extract confers any benefit over the application of a known volume of the extract onto a standard occlusive patch chamber.

41.4.3 Allergen Identification

Identification of the phytochemical(s) responsible requires either a supply of the purified sensitizers known to be present in the plant, or a somewhat laborious extraction, isolation, purification, and characterization procedure using, ideally, several kilograms of fresh plant material.

41.4.4 Commercial Allergens

Relatively few plant constituents are available commercially for patch testing. Table 5 indicates the main plant allergens available from Chemotechnique, Firma, and Hermal. Some of them are natural extracts that contain the major allergen as well as other impurities. Volatile oil constituents, which are found in the aromatic oils of plants, are unstable to air oxidation and are generally virtually impossible to purify (except through derivatization and resynthesis) if liquid at room temperature. It should be remembered that the air oxidation products themselves may be the sensitizers. Synthetic or purified extracts contain one or a mixture of molecules.

There is an ongoing search to identify mixtures of compounds that can be used to reliably detect particular common types of plant- or plant product-induced dermatitis. Thus, various authors have recommended mixtures to detect colophony allergy, sesquiterpene lactone allergy, lichen allergy, and so on. It is likely that none of these mixtures will ever be regarded as an absolutely certain means of detecting the group allergy in question. For example, allergy to Asteraceae is difficult to screen, as discussed above. The Compositae mix gives more frequent patch test reactions than sesquiterpene lactone mix [379, 380], but its sensitivity, ascertained by relevance of positive reactions, seems lower than that of SLM [379].

41.4.5 Photopatch Testing

Airborne contact dermatitis from plants can closely simulate photocontact dermatitis, but plant-induced photoallergy is actually very rare. However, patients with photosensitivity have frequent positive reactions to plants or plant extracts. Photoworsening of patch test reactions may be indicative of an underlying acquired photosensitivity, a state that may or may not be causally associated with contact with the plant material being investigated.

Photopatch tests have to be performed in duplicate, one series being a dark (non irradiated) control removed after 48 h as in usual patch tests. The series that will be irradiated is removed after 24 or 48 h, and irradiated by a UVA source, generally with a dose of 5 J/cm^2. When a total spectrum irradiation is possible, which allows us to test both UVA and UVB sen-

41

Table 5. Commercially available plant allergens (*C* Chemotechnique Diagnostics, Malmö, Sweden, *F* Firma, Italy, *T* Trolab Hermal, Reinbeck, Germany)

Allergens	Concentration (%)	Sources of exposure	Providers
Achillea millefolium extract	1	Yarrow	C, T
Alantolactone	0.1		C, F
α-methylene-γ-butyrolactone**	0.01 (C), 0.005 (F)	*Tulipa, Alstroemeria, Bomarea, Disocorea Hispida, Erythronium, Gagea, Fritillaria*	C, F
Arnica montana extract	0.5	Mountain tobacco	C, T
Chamomilla romana (Anthemis nobilis) extract	1 (C), 2.5 (T)	Roman chamomile	C, T
Chrysanthemum cinerariifolium extract	1	Pyrethrum	C
Compositae mix (emulsified with sorbitan sesquioleate)	6 (T), 5 (F)		T, F
Costunolide			
Diallyl disulfide	1 (C), 2 (F)	Garlic	C, F
Lichen acid mix (atranorin, usnic acid, evernic acid)	0.3		C
Parthenolide	0.1	*Tanacetum parthenium* (feverfew), *Parthenium hysterophorus* L. (congress grass)	C
Primin	0.01	*Primula obconica*, Primulaceae	C, F, T
Propolis	10	Beekeepers, medications	C
Sesquiterpene lactone mix (Alantolactone, costunolide, dehydrocostus lactone, each 0.033%)	0.1	Asteraceae/Compositae, Jubulaceae (*Frullania*)	C
Tanacetum parthenium extract	1	Feverfew	T
Tanacetum vulgare extract	1	Tansy	T, C
Taraxacum officinale extract	2.5	Dandelion	C
Usnic acid	0.1 (T), 1 (F)	Lichens	T, F

** Only 0.01% can be considered safe [91])

sitivity, a third series has to be applied. Two series are removed after 24 h and then the first one is irradiated with UVA, and the second one with a sunlight system, delivering 75% of the minimal erythematous dose (MED).

41.4.6 Results and Relevance

Contact urticaria appears within minutes of patch testing and disappears rapidly. Patient interrogatory, literature data, and if necessary results from open tests, prick tests or a search for a specific IgE will lead to the diagnosis of immunologic or nonimmunologic contact urticaria.

Contact dermatitis is much more difficult to explore. The realization of patch tests, their readings and the validity of patch test results are often hard to determine. The relevance of positive test reactions can be difficult to establish because the patient may have handled several plants over a period of time and become sensitized to some or all. The phenomenon of cross-sensitization adds a further dimension to the problem of relevance.

False-positive reactions may be due to an irritant reaction, and it is useful to refer to guidelines before testing plants. Testing with numerous plants or extracts can cause an angry back or excited skin syndrome. Each plant part or plant extract must then be tested again separately. Sometimes, positive reactions arise from contamination of the plant material with pesticides or other agricultural/horticultural chemicals [381], or from fungal contamination. Another cause of positive reactions is the use of an extract at a concentration that is too high, whereby a subclinical sensitivity may be unmasked.

Active sensitization to the material should not be overlooked, but patch test reactions are generally delayed, occurring after 7–10 days. They are theoretically (and practically) possible with many plant materials, such as plant extracts.

False-negative reactions may arise if an inappropriate sample of plant material is tested (such as patch testing with a leaf when the allergen is contained in the stem), or if the extract contains an insufficient concentration of the allergen, perhaps as a result of using a stored extract or of seasonal variations of allergen content.

41.4.7 Multiple Plant Reactions and Cross-sensitivity

In most cases, reactions to several plants in the same patient are not due to cross-sensitization. First, cosensitization is frequent, particularly in people who are frequently in contact with plants. Many plants contain the same hapten, and so a patient sensitized to a particular compound in one plant will react to another plant containing the same compound. Moreover, he or she will react to plants that present a different compound, but one that will be still metabolized into the same allergen. Such situations are false cross-reactions.

In rarer cases, true cross-sensitization arises, when the immune surveillance process misidentifies a second compound due to its structural similarity to the primary sensitizer. Difficult and long procedures, for example chemical studies of spatial molecular structures, correlated to clinical reactivity patterns, and clinical experimentation such as cross-retests permit us to assume a true cross-reactivity between different molecules.

Clearly, false cross-reactions and cross-reactions are almost impossible to detect with certainty in humans because the primary sensitizer cannot easily be determined. Thus, reactions may occur to plants not previously encountered by the patient, as well as to isolates that are not actually present in the sensitizing plant.

41.5 Prevention and Treatment

41.5.1 Removal of the Allergens and Irritants

As soon as the plant responsible for contact dermatitis has been identified, steps should be taken to avoid further contact. In cases of occupational phytodermatitis, work practices and occupational hygiene measures should first be reviewed because of the employer's legal responsibility to provide a safe working environment. However, the patient may have to consider a change of workplace (for example, in the case of *Primula* dermatitis), and sometimes leave his or her occupation (as in the case of foresters allergic to *Frullania*).

41.5.2 Barrier Creams

Barrier creams, used as recommended, can be helpful in the prevention of irritant dermatitis. The practitioner must carefully read their composition in relation to some allergens such as lanolin, methyldibromoglutaronitrile and other allergens.

Their use in primary and secondary prevention of allergic contact dermatitis is discussed [382].

41.5.3 Gloves

It has been demonstrated that wearing gloves is a useful approach.

However, tuliposide A (present in *Alstroemeria* and Liliaceae) readily penetrates through vinyl gloves [103]. Nitrile gloves may prevent contact with tuliposide A [103]. A recent study shows that vinyl, polyethylene and latex gloves are likely permeable to plant allergens such as α-methylene-γ-butyrolactone, primin and diallyldisulfide. Nitrile gloves could protect from primin [383].

41.5.4 Acute Dermatitis

Acute dermatitis has to be rapidly treated with potent topical corticosteroids, such as betamethasone esters. They have to be applied once (or twice) a day, in adequate quantities (for example, an average of 20 g/day of topical 0.05% betamethasone dipropionate cream for each upper limb), every day until total healing. Pulverization, or compresses with saline (around 10 g NaCl per liter of fresh or warm water), are frequently useful. Systemic corticosteroids are used by some authors for severe cases. A high daily dose for a short period, until healing (1 mg/kg per day prednisone) is better than a lower regimen that requires a longer duration.

41.5.5 Chronic Dermatitis

Treatment is symptomatic too. We use topical corticosteroids in the same manner as described below, sometimes with emollients, until healing.

41

Other solutions such as UV therapy are helpful for diffuse dermatitis. Photochemotherapy with UVA and 8-MOP, or even systemic immunosuppressive chemicals such as azathioprine or ciclosporin can be discussed for severe and intractable phytophotodermatitis with or without persistent light reactions [384].

Preventive measures (wearing gloves, removal of allergens or irritants) are always indispensable.

41.5.6 Hyposensitization

Hyposensitization measures have been attempted with limited success when avoidance of contact is impractical, such as with poison ivy in certain outdoor occupations. After a note by R. Dakin in 1829, the first attempts in this direction were attributed to Schamberg in 1919 [385]. Other authors have then carried out oral or parenteral hyposensitization with varied results and sometimes severe side-effects, with reports of fatal renal complications [386–388]. Oral desensitization with daily intake of leaf extract in water has been reported as being beneficial on skin lesion and patch test results [389]. A similar approach was attempted in 24 Indian patients positive to *P. hysterophorus*, with increasing amounts of plant extracts. Of 20 who completed the study, six suffered worsened dermatitis and stopped treatment. In the remaining 14 patients, a progressive fall in the mean clinical severity score was noted, but no significant change in the titer of test reactivity. Long-term results are unspecified, with 3/7 patients free of symptoms after 1 year [51]. Currently, there is no scientific basis behind this practice, and the risk of toxic side effects should be considered [388, 390]. Induction of tolerance in naive subjects appears to be a more successful strategy than desensitization of those already sensitized [391].

So-called hardening is also a procedure that has been discussed, and it has been described as an external topical hyposensitization. It consists of repeated patch test application, until the reactivity progressively fades [388].

41.6 Example of Botanical Nomenclature

The plant *kingdom*, which comprises around 350,000 species, is divided into five *divisions*: phycophytes (seaweeds or algae), bryophytes (mosses, liverworts/hepatics and hornworts), mycophytes (fungi or mycetes), pteridophytes (ferns and related) and spermatophytes (seed plants) [7, 8]. Spermatophytes are divided into two *groups*:

- Gymnosperms: conifers, cycads, ginkgos, ephedras, chlamydosperms
- Angiosperms (Magnoliophyta) group: plants with flowers, which are divided into two *classes*:
  - Dicotyledon (Magnoliopsidae) class, subdivided into nine *subclasses*
  - Monocotyledon (Liliopsidae) class, subdivided into three subclasses

Subclasses are subdivided into *orders*
Orders are divided into *families*
Each family is made up of *genera* (singular: *genus*)
Each genre is divided into *species*

Ideally, to identify a plant, we need information on its roots, stems (aerian or underground), leaves (insertion, venation, arrangement, simple or compound organization, margins) and its reproductive organs (flowers, fruits).

Following the considerable work of the Swedish naturalist Dr. Carl von Linné (1707–1778), each species is characterized by two names written in Latin: the first name is the genus, the second the species. These are often related to the name of the author who first described the species, and are frequently abbreviated.

The purple foxglove (*Digitalis purpurea* L.) belongs to the plant kingdom, the Spermatophyta division, the Angiospermae subdivision, the Dicotyledonae class, the Gamopetalae subclass, the Tubiflorales order, the Scrophulariaceae family, the Rhinanthoideae family, the genus *Digitalis*, and the species *purpurea*, as described by Linné [8]. The white dead nettle (*Lamium album* L.) belongs to the Lamiaceae family, the *Lamium* genus, and the *album* species [7].

References

1. Fregert S (1975) Occupational dermatitis in a 10-year material. Contact Dermatitis 1:96–107
2. Paulsen E, Sogaard J, Andersen KE (1997) Occupational dermatitis in Danish gardeners and greenhouse workers. I. Prevalence and possible risk factors. Contact Dermatitis 37:263–270
3. Paulsen E (1998) Occupational dermatitis in Danish gardeners and greenhouse workers. II. Etiological factors. Contact Dermatitis 38:14–29
4. Evans FJ, Schmidt RJ (1980) Plants and plant products that induce contact dermatitis. Planta Med 38:289–316
5. Mitchell J, Rook A (1979) Botanical dermatology. Plants and plant products injurious to the skin. Greengrass, Vancouver
6. Lovell CR (1993) Plants and the skin. Blackwell Scientific, Oxford

41

7. Sell Y, Benezra C, Guérin B (2002) Plantes et réactions cutanées. John Libbey Eurotext, Paris

8. Benezra C, Ducombs G, Sell Y, Foussereau J (1985) Plant contact dermatitis. Decker, Toronto

9. Behl PN, Captain RM (1979) Skin-irritant and sensitizing plants found in India. Chand, Ram Nagar, New Delhi

10. Schmidt RJ (2005) The botanical dermatology database: homepage. (See http://bodd.cf.ac.uk/index.html)

11. Bourrain JL (2001) Les agents étiologiques des urticaires de contact. Ann Derm Venereol (Stockh) 128:1363–1366

12. Guin JD (2000) Occupational contact dermatitis to plants. In: Kanerva L, Elsner P, Wahlberg JE, Maibach HI (eds) Handbook of occupational dermatology. Springer, Berlin Heidelberg New York, pp 730–766

13. Couplan F, Styner E (1004) Guide des plantes sauvages comestibles et toxiques. Delachaux et Niestlé, Lausanne

14. Norup E, Smitt UW, Brøgger Christensen S (1986) The potencies of thapsigargin and analogues as activators of rat peritoneal mast cells. Planta Med 52:251–255

15. Brøgger Christensen S, Norup E, Rasmussen U (1984) Chemistry and structure-activity relationship of the histamine secretagogue thapsigargin and related compounds. In: Krogsgaard-Larsen P, Brøgger Christensen S, Kofod H (eds) Natural products and drug development. Munksgaard, Copenhagen, pp 405–418 (Alfred Benzon Symposium 20)

16. Estlander T, Kanerva L, Tupasela O, Jolanki R (1988) Occupational contact urticaria and type I sensitization caused by gerbera. Contact Dermatitis 38:118–120

17. Le Coz CJ (2001) Fiche d'éviction. Hypersensibilité au latex ou caoutchouc naturel. Ann Dermatol Venereol 128:577–578

18. Dooms-Goossens A, Deveylder H, Duron C, Dooms M, Degreef H (1986) Airborne contact urticaria due to cinchona. Contact Dermatitis 15:258

19. Hjorth N, Roed-Petersen J (1976) Occupational protein contact dermatitis in food handlers. Contact Dermatitis 2:28–42

20. Hannuksela M, Lahti A (1977) Immediate reactions to fruits and vegetables. Contact Dermatitis 3:79–84

21. Kaupinnen K, Kousa M, Reunala T (1980) Aromatic plants – a cause of severe attacks of angio-edema and urticaria. Contact Dermatitis 6:251–254

22. Veien NK, Hattel T, Justesen O, Norholm A (1983) Causes of eczema in the food industry. Derm Beruf Umwelt 31:84–86

23. Janssens V, Morren M, Dooms-Goossens A, Degreef H (1995) Protein contact dermatitis: myth or reality? Br J Dermatol 132:1–6

24. Karpman RR, Spark RP, Fried M (1980) Cactus thorn injuries to the extremities: their management and etiology. Ariz Med 37:849–851

25. Spoerke DG, Spoerke SE (1991) Granuloma formation induced by spines of the cactus, *Opuntia acanthocarpa*. Vet Hum Toxicol 33:342–344

26. Shanon J, Sagher F (1956) Sabra dermatitis. An occupational dermatitis due to prickly pear handling simulating scabies. AMA Arch Dermatol 74:269–275

27. Snyder DS, Hatfield GM, Lampe KF (1979) Examination of the itch response from the raphides of the fishtail palm *Caryota mitis* Lour. Toxicol Appl Pharmacol 48:287–292

28. Salinas ML, Ogura T, Soffchi L (2001) Irritant contact dermatitis caused by needle-like calcium oxalate crystals, raphides, in *Agave tequilana* among workers in tequila distilleries and agave plantations. Contact Dermatitis 44:94–96

29. Morton JF (1972) Cocoyams (*Xanthosoma caracu, X. atrovirens* and *X. nigrum*), ancient root- and leaf-vegetables, gaining in economic importance. Proc Fl State Hort Soc 85:85–94

30. Walter WG, Khanna PN (1972) Chemistry of the aroids. I. *Dieffenbachia seguine, amoena,* and *pitta.* Econ Bot 26:364–372

31. Metin A, Çalka O, Behçet L, Yildirim E (2001) Phytodermatitis from *Ranunculus damascenus.* Contact Dermatitis 44:183

32. Gude M, Hausen BM, Heitsch H, König WA (1988) An investigation of the irritant and allergenic properties of daffodils (*Narcissus pseudonarcissus* L., Amaryllidaceae. A review of daffodil dermatitis. Contact Dermatitis 19:1–10

33. Bonnevie P (1939) Aetiologie und Pathogenese der Ekzemkrankheiten. Nyt Nordisk Forlag, Copenhagen

34. Schwartz RS, Downham TF (1981) Erythema multiforme associated with *Rhus* contact dermatitis. Cutis 27:85–86

35. Holst R, Kirby J, Magnusson B (1976) Sensitization to tropical woods giving erythema multiforme-like eruptions. Contact Dermatitis 2:295–296

36. Martin P, Bergoend H, Piette F (1980) Erythema multiforme-like eruption from Brasilian rosewood. 5th International Symposium on Contact Dermatitis, 28–30 March 1980, Barcelona, Spain

37. Irvine C, Reynolds A, Finlay AY (1988) Erythema multiforme-like reaction to "rosewood". Contact Dermatitis 19:224–225

38. Athavale PN, Shum KW, Gasson P, Gawkrodger DJ (2003) Occupational hand dermatitis in a wood turner due to rosewood (*Dalbergia latifolia.* Contact Dermatitis 48:345–346

39. García-Bravo B, Rodriguez-Pichardo A, Fernandez de Pierola S, Camacho F (1995) Airborne erythema-multiforme-like eruption due to pyrethrum. Contact Dermatitis 33:433

40. Le Coz CJ, Lepoittevin JP (2001) Occupational erythema-multiforme-like dermatitis from sensitization to costus resinoid, followed by flare-up and systemic contact dermatitis from β-cyclocostunolide in a chemistry student. Contact Dermatitis 44:310–311

41. Ducombs G, Félix B, Allery JP (1996) Erythème polymorphe-like dû au bois d'Olon. A propos d'un nouveau cas. Lettre GERDA 13:70–71

42. Hjorth N, Roed-Petersen J, Thomsen K (1976) Airborne contact dermatitis from Compositae oleoresins simulating photodermatitis. Br J Dermatol 95:613–620

43. Schmidt RJ (1986) Compositae. Clin Dermatol 4:46–61

44. Christensen LP (1999) Direct release of the allergen tulipalin A from *Alstroemeria* cut flowers: a possible source of airborne contact dermatitis? Contact Dermatitis 41:320–324

45. Foussereau J, Muller JC, Benezra C (1975) Contact allergy to *Frullania* and *Laurus Nobilis*: cross-sensitization and chemical structure of the allergens. Contact Dermatitis 1:223–230

46. Thune PO, Solberg YJ (1980) Photosensitivity and allergy to aromatic lichen acids, Compositae oleoresins and other plant substances. Contact Dermatitis 6:64–71

47. Thune PO, Solberg YJ (1980) Photosensitivity and allergy to aromatic lichen acids, Compositae oleoresins and other plant substances. Contact Dermatitis 6:81–87

48. Watsky KL (1997) Airborne allergic contact dermatitis from pine dust. Am J Contact Dermat 8:118–120

49. Fisher AA (1965) The poison "Rhus" plants. Cutis 1:230–236

50. Sharma VK, Sethuraman G, Tejasvi T (2004) Comparison of patch test contact sensitivity to acetone and aqueous extracts of *Parthenium hysterophorus* in patients with airborne contact dermatitis. Contact Dermatitis 50:230–232

51. Handa S, Sahoo B, Sharma VK (2001) Oral hyposensitization in patients with contact dermatitis from *Parthenium hysterophorus*. Contact Dermatitis 44:279–282

52. Oppenheim M (1932) Dermatite bulleuse striée, consécutive aux bains de soleil dans les prés. (Dermatitis bullosa striata pratensis.) Ann Derm Venereol (Stockh) 3:1–7

53. Kissmeyer A (1933) Dermatite bulleuse striée des prés. Bull Soc Fr Dermatol Syphiligr 40:1486–1489

54. Freeman K, Hubbard HC, Warin AP (1984) Strimmer rash. Contact Dermatitis 10:117–118

55. Ippen H (1984) Photodermatitis bullosa generalisata. Derm Beruf Umwelt 32:134–137

56. Tunget CL, Turchen SG, Manoguerra AS, Clark RF, Pudoff DE (1994) Sunlight and the plant: a toxic combination: severe phytophotodermatitis from *Cneoridium dumosum*. Cutis 54:400–402

57. Qadripur SA, Gründer K (1975) Kasuistischer Beitrag über Gruppenerkrankung mit Photodermatitis bullosa striata pratensis (Oppenheim). Hautarzt 26:495–497

58. Campbell AN, Cooper CE, Dahl MGC (1982) "Non-accidental injury" and wild parsnips. Br Med J 284:708

59. Pathak MA, Daniels F, Fitzpatrick TB (1962) The presently known distribution of furocoumarins (psoralens) in plants. J Invest Dermatol 39:225–239

60. Wagner AM, Wu JJ, Hansen RC, Nigg HN, Beiere RC (2002) Bullous phytophotodermatitis associated with high natural concentrations of furanocoumarins in limes. Am J Contact Dermat 13:10–14

61. Schemp P CM, Schöpf E, Simon JC (1999) Dermatitis bullosa striata pratensis durch *Ruta graveolens* L. (Gartenraute). Hautarzt 50:432–434

62. Schempp CM, Sonntag M, Schöpf E, Simon JC (1996) Dermatitis bullosa striata pratensis durch *Dictamnus albus* L. (Brennender Busch). Hautartz 47:708–710

63. El Sayed K, Al-Said MS, El-Feraly FS, Ross SA (2000) New quinoline alkaloids from *Ruta chalepensis*. J Nat Prod 63:995–997

64. Wang L, Sterling B, Don P (2002) Berloque dermatitis induced by "Florida Water". Cutis 70:29–30

65. Bhutani LK, Rao DS (1978) Photocontact dermatitis caused by *Parthenium hysterophorus*. Dermatologica 157:206–209

66. Ljunggren B (1977) Psoralen photoallergy caused by plant contact. Contact Dermatitis 3:85–90

67. Kaidbey KH, Kligman AM (1981) Photosensitization by coumarin derivatives. Arch Dermatol 117:258–263

68. Frain-Bell W, Johnson BE (1979) Contact allergic sensitivity to plants and the photosensitivity dermatitis and actinic reticuloid syndrome. Br J Dermatol 101:503–512

69. Lim HW, Cohen D, Soter NA (1998) Chronic actinic dermatitis: results of patch tests with Compositae, fragrances, and pesticides. J Am Acad Dermatol 38:108–111

70. Du P Menagé H, Ross JS, Norris PG, Breathnach SM, Hawk JLM, White IR (1995) Contact and photocontact sensitization in chronic actinic dermatitis: sesquiterpene lactone mix is an important allergen. Br J Dermatol 132:543–547

71. Du P Menagé H, Hawk JLM, White IR (1998) Sesquiterpene lactone mix contact sensitivity and its relationship to chronic actinic dermatitis: a follow-up study. Contact Dermatitis 39:119–122

72. Hausen BM (2000) Woods. In: Kanerva L, Elsner P, Wahlberg JE, Maibach HI (eds) Handbook of occupational dermatology. Springer, Berlin Heidelberg New York, pp 771–780

73. Bleumink E, Doeglas HMG, Klokke AH, Nater JP (1972) Allergic contact dermatitis to garlic. Br J Dermatol 87:6–9

74. Bleumink E, Nater JP (1973) Contact dermatitis to garlic: cross reactivity between garlic, onion, and tulip. Arch Dermatol Forsch 247:117–124

75. Sinha SM, Pasricha JS, Sharma RC, Kandhari KC (1977) Vegetables responsible for contact dermatitis of the hands. Arch Dermatol 113:776–779

76. Van KeteL WG, de Haan P (1978) Occupational eczema from garlic and onion. Contact Dermatitis 4:53–54

77. Campolmi P, Lombardi P, Lotti T, Sertoli A (1982) Immediate and delayed sensitization to garlic. Contact Dermatitis 8:352–353

78. Cronin E (1987) Dermatitis of the hands in caterers. Contact Dermatitis 17:265–269

79. Burks JW Jr (1954) Classic aspects of onion and garlic dermatitis in housewives. Ann Allergy 12:592–596

80. Eming SA, Piontek JO, Hunzelmann, Rasokat H (1999) Severe toxic contact dermatitis caused by garlic. Br J Dermatol 141:391–392

81. Burden AD, Wilkinson SM, Beck MH, Chalmers RJ (1994) Garlic-induced systemic contact dermatitis. Contact Dermatitis 30:299–300

82. Pereira F, Hatia M, Cardoso J (2002) Systemic contact dermatitis from diallyl disulfide. Contact Dermatitis 46:124

83. Bassioukas K, Orton D, Cerio R (2004) Occupational airborne allergic contact dermatitis from garlic with concurrent Type I allergy. Contact Dermatitis 50:39–41

84. Freeman GG, Whenham RJ (1976) Nature and origin of volatile flavour components of onion and related species. Int Flavours Fd Addit 7:222–227, 229

85. Papageorgiou C, Corbet JP, Menezes-Brandao F, Pecegueiro M, Benezra C (1983) Allergic contact dermatitis to Garlic (*Allium sativum* L.). Identification of the allergens: the role of mono-di-, and trisulfides present in garlic. A comparative study in man and animal (guinea-pig). Arch Dermatol Res 275:229–234

86. Mitchell JC (1980) Contact sensitivity to garlic (*Allium*). Contact Dermatitis 6:356–357

87. Brongersma-Oosterhoff UW (1967) Structure determination of the allergenic agent isolated from tulip bulbs. Recl Trav Chim Pays-Bas Belg 86:705–708

88. Verspyck Mijnssen GAW (1969) Pathogenesis and causative agent of "tulip finger". Br J Dermatol 81:737–745

89. Slob A (1973) Tulip allergens in *Alstroemeria* and some other Liliiflorae. Phytochemistry 12:811–815

90. Slob A, Jekel B, de Jong B, Schlatmann E (1975) On the occurrence of tulliposides in the Liliiflorae. Phytochemistry 14:1997–2005

91. Hausen BM, Prater E, Schubert H (1983) The sensitizing capacity of *Alstroemeria* cultivars in man and guinea pig. Remarks on the occurrence, quantity and irritant and sensitizing potency of their constituents tuliposide A and tulipalin A (α-methylene-γ-butyrolactone. Contact Dermatitis 9:46–54

92. Santucci B, Picardo M, Iavarone C, Trogolo C (1985) Contact dermatitis to *Alstroemeria*. Contact Dermatitis 12:215–219

93. Christensen LP, Kristiansen K (1995) A simple HPLC method for the isolation and quantification of the allergens tuliposide A and tulipalin A in *Alstroemeria*. Contact Dermatitis 32:199–203

94. Christensen LP, Kristiansen K (1995) Isolation and quantification of a new tuliposide (tuliposide D) by HPLC in *Alstroemeria*. Contact Dermatitis 33:188–192

95. Shoji M, Kazuaki A (2003) Antimicrobial activities of anthers in tulips. Plant Biology 2003, 25–30 July 2003, Honolulu, Hawaii, USA

96. Barbier P, Benezra C (1986) Allergenic α-methylene-γ-butyrolactones. Study of the capacity of β-acetoxy- and β-hydroxy-α-methylene-γ-butyrolactones to induce allergic contact dermatitis in guinea pigs. J Med Chem 29: 868–871

97. Beijersbergen JCM (1972) A method for determination of tulipalin A and B concentrations in crude extracts of tulip tissues. Recl Trav Chim Pays-Bas Belg 91:1193–1200

98. Hjorth N, Wilkinson DS (1968) Contact dermatitis. IV. Tulip fingers, hyacinth itch and lily rash. Br J Dermatol 80:696–698

99. Guin JD, Franks H (2001) Fingertip dermatitis in a retail florist. Cutis 67:328–330

100. Van der Mei IA, de Boer EM, Bruynzeel DP (1998) Contact dermatitis in *Alstroemeria* workers. Occup Med (Lond) 48:397–404

101. Rycroft RJG, Calnan CD (1981) Alstroemeria dermatitis. Contact Dermatitis 7:284

102. Rook A (1981) Dermatitis from *Alstroemeria*: altered clinical pattern and probable increasing incidence. Contact Dermatitis 7:355–356

103. Marks JG (1988) Allergic contact dermatitis to *Alstroemeria*. Arch Dermatol 124:914–916

104. Björkner BE (1982) Contact allergy and depigmentation from alstroemeria. Contact Dermatitis 8:178–184

105. Chan RY, Oppenheimer JJ (2002) Occupational allergy caused by Peruvian lily (*Alstroemeria*). Ann Allergy Asthma Immunol 88:638–639

106. Van der Werff PJ (1959) Occupational diseases among workers in the bulb industries. Acta Allergol 14:338–355

107. Bruze M, Björkner B, Hellstrom AC (1996) Occupational dermatoses in nursery workers. Am J Contact Dermat 7: 100–103

108. Bruynzeel DP (1997) Bulb dermatitis. Dermatological problem in the flower bulb industries. Contact Dermatitis 37:70–77

109. Julian CG, Bower PW (1997) The nature and distribution of daffodil picker's rash. Contact Dermatitis 37:259–262

110. Klaschka F, Grimm WW, Beiersdorff HU (1964) Tulpen-Kontaktekzem als Berufsdermatosen. Hautarzt 15:317–321

111. Pardo-Castello V (1923) Dermatitis venenata: a study of the tropical plants producing dermatitis. Arch Dermatol Syphilol 7:81

112. Bertrand G, Brooks G (1934) Recherches sur le latex de l'arbre à laque du Cambodge (*Melanorrhoea laccifera* Pierre). Bull Soc Chim Fr 5:109–114

113. Ridley HN (1911) Rengas-poisoning. Malay Med J 9:7

114. Watt G (1906) Burmese lacquer ware and Burmese varnish. Kew Bull 5:137–147

115. Srinivas CR, Kulkarni SB, Menon SK, Krupashankar DS, Iyengar MA, Singh KK, Sequeira RP, Holla KR (1987) Allergenic agent in contact dermatitis from *Holigarna ferruginea*. Contact Dermatitis 17:219–222

116. Sprague TA (1921) Plant dermatitis. J Bot 59:308–310

117. Kirby-Smith JL (1938) Mango dermatitis. Am J Trop Med 18:373–384

118. Jackson WPU (1946) Plant dermatitis in the Bahamas. BMJ 2:298

119. King DE, Wolfish PS, Heng MCY (1983) The much-maligned dhobie. J Am Acad Dermatol 8:258

120. Findlay GH, Whiting DA, Eggers SH, Ellis RP (1974) *Smodingium* (African "poison ivy") dermatitis. History, comparative plant chemistry and anatomy, clinical and histological features. Br J Dermatol 90:535–541

121. Corbett M, Billets S (1975) Characterization of poison oak urushiol. J Pharm Sci 64:1715–1718

122. Gross M, Baer H, Fales HM (1975) Urushiols of poisonous Anacardiaceae. Phytochemistry 14:2263–2266

123. De Hurtado I (1965) Contact dermatitis caused by the "manzanillo" (*Rhus striata*) tree. Int Arch Allergy Appl Immunol 28:321–327

124. Nakamura T (1985) Contact dermatitis to *Rhus succedanea*. Contact Dermatitis 12:279

125. Powell SM, Barrett DK (1986) An outbreak of contact dermatitis from *Rhus verniciflua* (*Toxicodendron vernicifluum*). Contact Dermatitis 14:288–289

126. Kligman AM (1958) Poison ivy (*Rhus*) dermatitis. An experimental study. AMA Arch Dermatol 77:149

127. Ippen H (1983) Kontaktallergie gegen Anacardiaceae. Übersicht und Kasuistik zur "Poison Ivy"-Allergie in Mitteleuropa. Derm Beruf Umwelt 31:140–148

128. Oh SH, Haw CR, Lee MH (2003) Clinical and immunologic features of systemic contact dermatitis from ingestion of *Rhus* (*Toxicodendron*. Contact Dermatitis 48: 251–254

129. Cardinali C, Francalanci S, Giomi B, Caproni M, Sertoli A, Fabbri P (2004) Contact dermatitis from *Rhus toxicodendron* in a homeopathic remedy. J Am Acad Dermatol 50: 150–151

130. Marks JG Jr, DeMelfi T, McCarthy MA, Witte EJ, Castagnoli N, Epstein WL, Aber RC (1984) Dermatitis from cashew nuts. J Am Acad Dermatol 10:627–631

131. Kurlan JG, Lucky AW (2001) Black spot poison ivy: a report of 5 cases and a review of the literature. J Am Acad Dermatol 45:246–249

132. Gillis WT (1971) The systematics and ecology of poison ivy and the poison-oaks (*Toxicodendron,* Anacardiaceae). Rhodora 73:72–159, 161–237, 370–443, 465–540

133. Guin JD, Gillis WT, Beaman JH (1981) Recognizing the Toxicodendrons (poison ivy, poison oak, and poison sumac. J Am Acad Dermatol 4:99–114

134. Guin JD, Beaman JH (1986) Toxicodendrons of the United States. Clin Dermatol 4:137–148

135. Guin JD (1980) The black spot test for recognizing poison ivy and related species. J Am Acad Dermatol 2:332–333

136. Walker S William J, Lear J, Beck M (2004) Toxicodendron dermatitis in the United Kingdom. Contact Dermatitis 50:163

137. Ale SI, Ferreira F, Gonzalez G, Epstein W (1997) Allergic contact dermatitis caused by *Lithraea molleoides* and *Lithraea brasiliensis*: identification and characterization of the responsible allergens. Am J Contact Dermat 8: 144–149

138. Lima AO (1953) Über das antigene Verhalten der Ölharze einiger Gattungen der Familie Anacardiaceae. Int Archs Allergy Appl Immun 4:169–174

139. De Hurtado I (1968) Studies on the biological activity of *Rhus striata* ("manzanillo"). 2. Skin response to patch tests in humans. Int Arch Allergy Appl Immunol 33:209

140. Mitchell JC, Maibach HI, Guin J (1981) Leaves of *Ginkgo biloba* not allergenic for Toxicodendron sensitive subjects. Contact Dermatitis 7:47–48

141. Nakamura T (1985) Ginkgo tree dermatitis. Contact Dermatitis 12:281–282

142. Tomb RR, Foussereau J, Sell Y (1988) Mini-epidemic of contact dermatitis from ginkgo tree fruit (*Ginkgo biloba* L.). Contact Dermatitis 19:281–283

143. Bolus M, Raleigh NC (1939) Dermatitis venenata due to ginkgo berries. Arch Dermatol Syphilol 39:530

144. Becker LE, Skipworth GB (1975) Ginkgo-tree dermatitis, stomatitis, and proctitis. J Am Med Assoc 231:1162–1163

41

145. Sowers WF, Weary PE, Collins OD, Cawley EP (1965) Ginkgo-tree dermatitis. Arch Dermatol 91 : 452–456
146. Lepoittevin JP, Benezra C, Asakawa Y (1989) Allergic contact dermatitis to *Ginkgo biloba* L.: relationship with urushiol. Arch Dermatol Res 281 : 227–230
147. Occolowitz JL, Wright AS (1962) 5-(10-Pentadecenyl)resorcinol from *Grevillea pyramidalis*. Aust J Chem 15 : 858–861
148. Ridley DD, Ritchie E, Taylor WC (1968) Chemical studies of the Proteaceae. II. Some further constituents of *Grevillea robusta* A. Cunn.; experiments on the synthesis of 5-*n*-tridecylresorcinol (grevillol) and related substances. Aust J Chem 21 : 2979–2988
149. Menz J, Rossi ER, Taylor WC, Wall L (1986) Contact dermatitis from *Grevillea* "Robyn Gordon". Contact Dermatitis 15 : 126–131
150. Hoffman TE, Hausen BM, Adams RM (1985) Allergic contact dermatitis to "silver oak" wooden arm bracelets. J Am Acad Dermatol 13 : 778–779
151. May SB (1960) Dermatitis due to *G. robusta* (Australian silk oak. Report of a case. Arch Dermatol 82 : 1006
152. Arnold HL (1942) Dermatitis to the blossom of *Grevillea banksii*. Arch Dermatol 45 : 1037–1051
153. Benezra C, Ducombs G (1987) Molecular aspects of allergic contact dermatitis to plants. Derm Beruf Umwelt 35 : 4–11
154. Knight TE (1991) Philodendron-induced dermatitis: report of cases and review of the literature. Cutis 48 : 375–378
155. Reynolds GW, Gafner F, Rodriguez E (1989) Contact allergens of an urban shrub *Wigandia caracasana*. Contact Dermatitis 21 : 65–68
156. Reynolds G, Rodriguez E (1979) Geranylhydroquinone: a contact allergen from trichomes of *Phacelia crenulata*. Phytochemistry 18 : 1567–1568
157. Aeschimann D, Lauber K, Moser DM, Theurillat JP (2004) Flora alpina. Belin, Paris
158. Arlette J, Mitchell JC (1981) Compositae dermatitis. Current aspects. Contact Dermatitis 7 : 129–136
159. Mitchell JC, Roy AK, Dupuis G, Towers GHN (1971) Allergic contact dermatitis from ragweeds (*Ambrosia* species). The role of sesquiterpene lactones. Arch Dermatol 104 : 73–76
160. Brunsting LA, Anderson CR (1934) Ragweed dermatitis. A report based on eighteen cases. J Am Med Assoc 103 : 1285–1290
161. Shelmire B (1939) Contact dermatitis from weeds: patch testing with their oleoresins. J Am Med Assoc 113 : 1085–1090
162. Mitchell JC (1975) Biochemical basis of geographic ecology, part 2. Int J Dermatol 14 : 301–321
163. Brunsting LA, Williams DH (1936) Ragweed (contact) dermatitis. Observations in forty-eight cases and report of unsuccessful attempts at desensitization by injection of specific oils. J Am Med Assoc 106 : 1533–1535
164. O'Quinn SE, Isbell KH (1969) Influence of oral prednisone on eczematous patch test reactions. Arch Dermatol 99 : 380–389
165. Möslein P (1963) Pflanzen als Kontakt-Allergene. Berufsdermatosen 11 : 24–28
166. Hausen BM, Busker E, Carle R (1984) Über das Sensibilisierungsvermögen von Compositearten VII. Experimentelle Untersuchungen mit Auszügen und Inhaltsstoffen von *Chamomilla recutita* (L.) Rauschert und *Anthemis cotula* L. Planta Med 50 : 229–234
167. Burry JN (1979) Dermatitis from fleabane: compositae dermatitis in South Australia. Contact Dermatitis 5 : 51
168. Hausen BM (1980) Arnikaallergie. Hautarzt 31 : 10–17
169. Mitchell JC, Geissman TA, Dupuis G, Towers GH (1971) Allergic contact dermatitis caused by *Artemisia* and *Chrysanthemum* species. The role of sesquiterpene lactones. J Invest Dermatol 56 : 98–101
170. Shelmire B (1939) Contact dermatitis from weeds; patch testing with their oleoresins. J Am Med Assoc 113 : 1085–1090
171. Mackoff S, Dahl AO (1951) A botanical consideration of the weed oleoresin problem. Minn Med 34 : 1169–1173
172. Schumacher MJ, Silvis NG (2003) Airborne contact dermatitis from *Ambrosia deltoidea* (triangle-leaf bursage). Contact Dermatitis 48 : 212–216
173. Burry JN, Kuchel R, Reid JG, Kirk J (1973) Australian bush dermatitis: compositae dermatitis in South Australia. Med J Aust 1 : 110–116
174. Burry JN, Reid JG, Kirk J (1975) Australian bush dermatitis. Contact Dermatitis 1 : 263–264
175. Maiden JH (1909) On some plants which cause inflammation or irritation of the skin, part II. Agric Gaz NSW 20 : 1073–1082
176. Burry JN, Kloot PM (1982) The spread of composite (Compositae) weeds in Australia. Contact Dermatitis 8 : 410–413
177. Towers GHN, Mitchell JC, Rodriguez E, Bennett FD, Subbarrao PV (1977) Biology and chemistry of *Parthenium hysterophorus* L., a problem weed in India. J Sci Ind Res 36 : 672–684
178. Towers GH, Mitchell JC (1983) The current status of the weed *Parthenium hysterophorus* L. as a cause of contact dermatitis. Contact Dermatitis 9 : 465–469
179. Hausen BM (1981) Berufsbedingte Kontaktallergie auf Mutterkraut (*Tanacetum parthenium* (L.) Schulz-Bip.; Asteraceae). Derm Beruf Umwelt 29 : 18–21
180. Mensing H, Kimmig W, Hausen BM (1985) Airborne contact dermatitis. Hautarzt 36 : 398–402
181. Malten KE (1983) Chicory dermatitis from September to April. Contact Dermatitis 9 : 232
182. Vail JT, Mitchell JC (1973) Occupational dermatitis from *Cichorium intybus*, *C. endivia*, and *Lactuca sativa* var. *longifolia*. Contact Dermatitis Newslett 14 : 413
183. Friis B, Hjorth N, Vail JT Jr, Mitchell JC (1975) Occupational contact dermatitis from *Cichorium* (chicory, endive) and *Lactuca* (lettuce). Contact Dermatitis 1 : 311–313
184. Wakelin SH, Marren P, Young E, Shaw S (1997) Compositae sensitivity and chronic hand dermatitis in a seven-year-old boy. Br J Dermatol 137 : 289–291
185. Verhagen AR, Nyaga JM (1974) Contact dermatitis from *Tagetes minuta*. A new sensitizing plant of the Compositae family. Arch Dermatol 110 : 441–444
186. Mitchell JC, Dupuis G, Towers GHN (1972) Allergic contact dermatitis from pyrethrum (*Chrysanthemum* spp.). The roles of pyrethrosin, a sesquiterpene lactone, and of pyrethrin II. Br J Dermatol 86 : 568–573
187. Hausen BM (1982) Taraxinsäure-1'-*O*-β-D-glucopyranosid, das Kontaktallergen des Löwenzahns (*Taraxacum officinale* Wiggers). Derm Beruf Umwelt 30 : 51–53
188. Gougerot H, Burnier, Boulle (1933) Purpura réticulé et eczéma généralisé à la suite d'application de feuille d'aunée («Inula Helenium»); sensibilisation. Bull Soc Fr Dermatol Syphiligr 40 : 1702–1704
189. P'iankova ZP, Nugmanova ML (1975) Dermatit ot deviasila (dermatitis due to elecampane). Vestn Dermatol Venereol 12 : 53–54
190. Hausen BM, Spring O (1989) Sunflower allergy. On the constituents of the trichomes of *Helianthus annuus* L. (Compositae). Contact Dermatitis 20 : 326–334

191. Rodriguez E, Reynolds GW, Thompson JA (1981) Potent contact allergen in the rubber plant guayule (*Parthenium argentatum*). Science 211:1444–1445

192. Maiden JH (1918) Plants which produce inflammation or irritation of the skin. Agric Gaz NSW 29:344–345

193. Vryman LH (1933) Dahlienwurzelrinden-Dermatitis. Arch Dermatol Syphilol 168:233

194. Calnan CD (1978) Sensitivity to dahlia flowers. Contact Dermatitis 4:168

195. Olivier J, Renkin A (1954) Eczéma par sensibilité à une seule variété de chrysanthèmes. Arch Belg Dermatol Syphiligr 10:296–297

196. Rook A (1961) Plant dermatitis. The significance of variety-specific sensitization. Br J Dermatol 73:283–287

197. Hausen BM, Schulz KH (1976) Chrysanthemum allergy. III. Identification of the allergens. Arch Dermatol Res 255:111–121

198. Towers GHN, Arnason T, Wat CK, Graham EA, Lam J, Mitchell JL (1979) Phototoxic polyacetylenes and their thiophene derivatives. (Effects on human skin.) Contact Dermatitis 5:140–144

199. Quirce S, Tabar AI, Olaguibel JM, Cuevas M (1996) Occupational contact urticaria syndrome caused by globe artichoke (*Cynara scolymus*. J Allergy Clin Immunol 97:710–711

200. Douin I (1986) Nouvelle flore des mousses et des hépatiques pour la détermination facile des espèces. Belin, Paris

201. Schmidt RJ (1996) Allergic contact dermatitis to liverworts, lichens, and mosses. Semin Dermatol 15:95–102

202. Mitchell JC (1986) *Frullania* (liverwort) phytodermatitis (woodcutter's eczema). Clin Dermatol 4:62–64

203. Mitchell JC, Fritig B, Singh B, Towers GH (1970) Allergic contact dermatitis from *Frullania* and Compositae. The role of sesquiterpene lactones. J Invest Dermatol 54:233–239

204. Knoche H, Ourisson G, Perold GW, Foussereau J, Maleville J (1969) Allergenic component of a liverwort: a sesquiterpene lactone. Science 166:239–240

205. Ducombs G, Lepoittevin JP, Berl V, Andersen KE, Brandao FM, Bruynzeel DP, Bruze M, Camarasa JG, Frosch PJ, Goossens A, Lachapelle JM, Lahti A, Le Coz CJ, Maibach HI, Menné T, Seidenari S, Shaw S, Tosti A, Wilkinson JD; European Environmental and Contact Dermatitis Research Group multicentre study (2003) Routine patch testing with frullanolide mix: an European Environmental and Contact Dermatitis Research Group multicentre study. Contact Dermatitis 48:158–161

206. Hindsen M, Christensen LP, Paulsen E (2004) Contact allergy to the sesquiterpene lactone calocephalin. Contact Dermatitis 50:162

207. Mitchell JC, Dupuis G (1971) Allergic contact dermatitis from sesquiterpenoids of the Compositae family of plants. Br J Dermatol 84:139–150

208. Hausen BM (1979) The sensitizing capacity of Compositae plants. III. Test results and cross-reactions in Compositae-sensitive patients. Dermatologica 159:1–11

209. Schmidt RJ (1985) When is a chrysanthemum dermatitis not a *chrysanthemum* dermatitis? The case for describing florists' chrysanthemums as *Dendranthema* cultivars. Contact Dermatitis 13:115–119

210. Asakawa Y, Benezra C, Foussereau J, Muller JC, Ourisson G (1974) Cross-sensitization between *Frullania* and *Laurus nobilis*. Arch Dermatol 110:957

211. Fernandez de Corres L, Corrales Torres JL (1978) Dermatitis from *Frullania*, Compositae and other plants. Contact Dermatitis 4:175–176

212. Hausen BM, Osmundsen PE (1983) Contact allergy to parthenolide in *Tanacetum parthenium (L.)* Schulz-Bip. (feverfew, Asteraceae) and cross-reactions to related sesquiterpene lactone containing Compositae species. Acta Derm Venereol (Stockh) 63:308–314

213. Marzulli FN, Maibach HI (1980) Further studies of effects of vehicles and elicitation concentrations in contact dermatitis testing. Contact Dermatitis 6:131–133

214. Cheminat A, Stampf JL, Benezra C, Farral MJ, Frechet JM (1981) Allergic contact dermatitis to costus: removal of haptens with polymers. Acta Derm Venereol (Stockh) 61:525–529

215. Warshaw EM, Zug KA (1996) Sesquiterpene lactone allergy. Am J Contact Dermat 7:1–23

216. Rao PV, Mangala A, Towers GH, Rodriguez E (1978) Immunological activity of parthenin and its diasteriomer in persons sensitized by *Parthenium hysterophorus* L. Contact Dermatitis 4:199–203

217. Ducombs G, Benezra C, Talaga P, Andersen KE, Burrows D, Camarasa JG, Dooms-Goossens A, Frosch PJ, Lachapelle JM, Menné T, et al. (1990) Patch testing with the "sesquiterpene lactone mix": a marker for contact allergy to Compositae and other sesquiterpene-lactone-containing plants. Contact Dermatitis 22:249–252

218. Paulsen E, Andersen KE, Hausen BM (1993) Compositae dermatitis in a Danish dermatology department in one year. I. Results of routine patch testing with the sesquiterpene lactone mix supplemented with aimed patch testing with extracts and sesquiterpene lactones of Compositae plants. Contact Dermatitis 29:6–10

219. Green C, Ferguson J (1994) Sesquiterpene lactone mix is not an adequate screen for Compositae allergy. Contact Dermatitis 31:151–153

220. Shum KW, English JSC (1998) Allergic contact dermatitis in food handlers, with patch tests positive to Compositae mix but negative to sesquiterpene lactone mix. Contact Dermatitis 39:207–208

221. Lepoittevin JP, Tomb R (1995) Sesquiterpene lactone mix is not an adequate screen for Compositae allergy. Contact Dermatitis 32:254

222. Stingeni L, Lisi P (1996) Airborne allergie contact dermatitis from Compositae. Ann Ital Dermatol Clin Sperim 50:170–173

223. Hausen BM (1996) A 6-year experience with Compositae mix. Am J Contact Dermat 7:94–99

224. Schmidt RJ, Kingston T (1985) Chrysanthemum dermatitis in South Wales; diagnosis by patch testing with feverfew *(Tanacetum parthenium)* extract. Contact Dermatitis 13:120–121

225. Goulden V, Wilkinson SM (1998) Patch testing for Compositae allergy. Br J Dermatol 138:1018–1021

226. Ettlinger MG, Lundeen AJ (1956) The structures of sinigrin and sinalbin; an enzymatic rearrangement. J Ann Chem Soc 78:4172–4173

227. Coulter S (1904) The poisonous plants of Indiana. Proc Indiana Acad Sci 119:51–63

228. Mitchell JC, Jordan WP (1974) Allergic contact dermatitis from the radish, *Raphanus sativus*. Br J Dermatol 91:183–189

229. Leoni A, Gogo R (1964) Dermatite professionale da contatto con cavolo capuccio. Minerva Med (Roma) 39:326–327

230. Gaul LE (1964) Contact dermatitis from synthetic oil of mustard. Arch Dermatol 90:158–159

231. Fregert S, Dahlquist I, Trulsson L (1983) Sensitization capacity of diphenylthiourea and phenylisothiocvanate. Contact Dermatitis 9:87–88

41

232. Richter G (1980) Allergic contact dermatitis from methyl isothiocyanate in soil disinfectants. Contact Dermatitis 6:183–186

233. Schmidt RJ (1986) Biosynthetic and chemosystematic aspects of the Euphorbiaceae and Thymelaeaceae. In: Evans FJ (ed) Naturally occurring phorbol esters. CRC, Boca Raton, Fla., pp 87–106

234. Webster GL (1986) Irritant plants in the spurge family (Euphorbiaceae). Clin Dermatol 1:36–45

235. Evans FJ (1986) Environmental hazards of diterpene esters from plants. In: Evans FJ (ed) Naturally occurring phorbol esters. CRC, Boca Raton, FL, pp 1–31

236. Satulsky EM, Wirts CA (1943) Dermatitis venenata caused by the manzanillo tree. Further observations and report of 60 cases. Arch Dermatol Syphilol 47:797

237. Rook A (1965) An unrecorded irritant plant, *Synadenium grantii*. Br J Dermatol 77:284

238. Calnan CD (1975) Petty spurge (*Luphorbia peplus* L.). Contact Dermatitis 1:128

239. Strobel M, N'Diaye B, Padonou F, Marchand JP (1978) Les dermites de contact d'origine végétale. A propos de 10 cas observés à Dakar. Bull Soc Méd Air Noire Lang Fr 23:124–127

240. Worobec SM, Hickey TA, Kinghorn AD, Soejarto D, West D (1981) Irritant contact dermatitis from an ornamental, *Euphorbia hermentiana*. Contact Dermatitis 7:19–22

241. Hickey TA, Worobec SM, West DP, Kinghorn AD (1981) Irritant contact dermatitis in humans from phorbol and related esters. Toxicon 19:841–850

242. Pinedo JM, Saavedra V, Gonzalez-de-Canales F, Llamas P (1985) Irritant dermatitis due to *Euphorbia marginata*. Contact Dermatitis 13:44

243. D'Arcy WG (1974) Severe contact dermatitis from poinsettia. Arch Dermatol 109:909–910

244. Hausen BM, Schulz KH (1977) Occupational contact dermatitis due to croton (*Codiaeum variegatum* (L.) A. Juss var. *pictum* (Lodd.) Muell. Arg.). Sensitization by plants of the Euphorbiaceae. Contact Dermatitis 3:289–292

245. Schmidt H, Ølholm-Larsen P (1977) Allergic contact dermatitis from croton (*Codiaeum*). Contact Dermatitis 3:100

246. Cleenewerck MB, Martin P (1989) Occupational contact dermatitis due to *Codiaeum variegatum* L., *Chrysanthemum indicum* L., *Chrysanthemum x hortorum* and *Frullania dilatata* L. In: Frosch PJ, Dooms-Goossens A, Lachapelle JM et al (eds) Current topics in contact dermatitis. Springer, Berlin Heidelberg New York, pp 149–157

247. Santucci B, Picardo M, Cristaudo A (1985) Contact dermatitis from *Euphorbia pulcherrima*. Contact Dermatitis 12:285–286

248. Elpern DJ (1984) The dermatology of Kauai, Hawaii, 1981–1982. Int J Dermatol 24:647–652

249. Weedon D, Chick J (1976) Home treatment of basal cell carcinoma. Med J Aust 1:928

250. Schmidt RJ, Evans FJ (1980) Skin irritants of the sun spurge (*Euphorbia helioscopia* L.). Contact Dermatitis 6:204–210

251. Adolf W, Sorg B, Hergenhahn M, Hecker E (1982) Structure-activity relations of polyfunctional diterpenes of the daphnane type. I. Revised structure for resiniferatoxin and structure-activity relations of resiniferonol and some of its esters. J Nat Prod 45:347–354

252. Schmidt RJ, Evans FJ (1979) Investigations into the skin-irritant properties of resiniferonol ortho esters. Inflammation 3:273–280

253. Evans FJ (1986) Phorbol: its esters and derivatives. In: Evans FJ (ed) Naturally occurring phorbol esters. CRC, Boca Raton, Fla., pp 171–215

254. Schmidt RJ (1986) The daphnane polyol esters. In: Evans FJ (ed) Naturally occurring phorbol esters. CRC, Boca Raton, Fla., pp 217–243

255. Schmidt RJ (1986) The ingenane polyol esters. In: Evans FJ (ed) Naturally occurring phorbol esters. CRC, Boca Raton, Fla., pp 245–269

256. Tiévant P (2001) Guide des lichens. 350 espèces de lichens d'Europe. Delachaux et Niestlé, Lausanne

257. Mitchell JC (1965) Allergy to lichens. Arch Dermatol 92:142–146

258. Mitchell JC, Shibata S (1969) Immunologic activity of some substances derived from lichenized fungi. J Invest Dermatol 52:517–520

259. Dahlquist I, Fregert S (1980) Contact allergy to atranorin in lichens and perfumes. Contact Dermatitis 6:111–119

260. Thune P, Solberg Y, Mc Fadden N, Staerfelt F, Standberg M (1982) Perfume allergy due to oak moss and other lichens. Contact Dermatitis 8:396–400

261. Bernard G, Gimenez-Arnau E, Rastogi SC, Heydorn S, Johansen JD, Menné T, Goossens A, Andersen K, Lepoittevin JP (2003) Contact allergy to oak moss: search for sensitizing molecules using combined bioassay-guided chemical fractionation, GC-MS, and structure-activity relationship analysis. Arch Dermatol Res 295:229–235

262. Bossi R, Rastogi SC, Bernard G, Gimenez-Arnau E, Johansen JD, Lepoittevin JP, Menné T (2004) A liquid chromatography-mass spectrometric method for the determination of oak moss allergens atranol and chloroatranol in perfumes. J Sep Sci 27:537–540

263. Johansen JD, Andersen KE, Svedman C, Bruze M, Bernard G, Gimenez-Arnau E, Rastogi SC, Lepoittevin JP, Menné T (2003) Chloroatranol, an extremely potent allergen hidden in perfumes: a dose-response elicitation study. Contact Dermatitis 49:180–184

264. Thune P (1977) Allergy to lichens with photosensitivity. Contact Dermatitis 3:213–214

265. Tan KS, Mitchell JC (1968) Patch and photopatch tests in contact dermatitis and photodermatitis. A preliminary report of investigation of 150 patients, with special reference to "cedar-poisoning". Can Med Assoc J 98:252–255

266. Thune P (1977) Contact allergy due to lichens in patients with a history of photosensitivity. Contact Dermatitis 3:267–272

267. Salo H, Hannuksela M, Hausen B (1981) Lichen pickers' dermatitis (*Cladonia alpestris* (L.) Rab.). Contact Dermatitis 7:9–13

268. Champion RH (1971) Atopic sensitivity to algae and lichens. Br J Dermatol 85:551–557

269. Lepoittevin JP, Meschkat E, Huygens S, Goossens A (2000) Presence of resin acids in "Oak moss" patch test material: a source of misdiagnosis? J Invest Dermatol 115:129–130

270. Hausen BM (1979) Primelallergie. Hintergründe und Aspekte. Mat Med Nordmark 31:57–76

271. Hjorth N (1979) Primula dermatitis. In: Mitchell J, Rook A (eds) Botanical dermatology. Greengrass, Vancouver, pp 554–564

272. Virgili A, Corazza M (1991) Unusual primin dermatitis. Contact Dermatitis 24:63–64

273. Schildknecht H (1957) Struktur des Primelgiftstoffes. Z Naturforsch 22B:36–41

274. Krebs M, Christensen LP (1995) 2-Methoxy-6-pentyl-1,4-dihydroxybenzene (miconidin) from *Primula obconica*: a possible allergen? Contact Dermatitis 33:90–93

275. Christensen LP, Larsen E (2000) Direct emission of the allergen primin from intact *Primula obconica* plants. Contact Dermatitis 42:149–153

276. Cairns R (1964) Plant dermatoses: some chemical aspects and results of patch testing with extracts of *Primula obconica*. Trans St John's Hosp Dermatol Soc 50: 137–143

277. Hausen BM, Schmalle HW, Marshall D, Thomson RH (1983) 5,8-Dihydroxyflavone (primetin) the contact sensitizer of *Primula mistassinica* Michaux. Arch Dermatol Res 275:365–370

278. Dooms-Goossens A, Biesemans G, Vandaele M, Degreff H (1989) Primula dermatitis: more than one allergen? Contact Dermatitis 21:122–124

279. Aplin C, Tan R, Lovell C (2000) Allergic contact dermatitis from *Primula auricula* and *Primula denticulata*. Contact Dermatitis 42:48

280. Aplin CG, Lovell CR (2001) Hardy primula species and allergic contact dermatitis. Contact Dermatitis 42 [Suppl 2]:11

281. Christensen LP, Larsen E (2000) Primin-free *Primula obconica* plants available. Contact Dermatitis 43:45–46

282. Hjorth N (1966) Primula dermatitis: sources of error in patch testing and patch test sensitization. Trans St John's Hosp Dermatol Soc 52:207–219

283. Hjorth N (1967) Seasonal variations in contact dermatitis. Acta Derm Venereol (Stockh) 47:409–418

284. Fregert S, Hjorth N, Schulz KH (1968) Patch testing with synthetic primin in persons sensitive to *Primula obconica*. Arch Dermatol 98:144–147

285. Fernández de Corres L, Leanizbarrutia I, Muñoz D (1987) Contact dermatitis from *Primula obconica* Hance. Contact Dermatitis 16:195–197

286. Agrup G, Fregert S, Hjorth N, Övrum P (1968) Routine patch tests with ether extract of *P. obconica*. Br J Dermatol 80:497–502

287. Frenzl F (1937) Artificial dermatitis caused by *Anemone nemorosa*. Casop Lék Cesk 76:1831–1835

288. Spengler F (1946) Die therapeutische Verwendung der *Anemone nemorosa* des Buschwindröschens. Pharmazie 1:222–223

289. Rodziewicz J, Wlodarczyk S (1961) Zmiany skórne wywolane dzialaniem jaskru. Przegl Dermatol 48:429–434

290. Aaron TH, Muttitt ELC (1964) Vesicant dermatitis due to prairie crocus (*Anemone patens* L.). Arch Dermatol 90: 168–171

291. Rudzki E, Dajek Z (1975) Dermatitis caused by buttercups (*Ranunculus*). Contact Dermatitis 1:322

292. Kipping FB (1935) The lactone of γ-hydroxyvinylacrylic acid, protoanemonin. J Chem Soc 1145–1147

293. Hill R, van Heyingen R (1951) Ranunculin: the precursor of the vesicant substance of the buttercup. Biochem J 49: 332–335

294. Moriarty RM, Romain CR, Karle IL, Karle J (1965) The structure of anemonin. J Am Chem Soc 87:3251–3252

295. Boll PM (1968) Naturally occurring lactones and lactames. 1. The absolute configuration of ranunculin, lichesterinic acid, and some lactones related to lichesterinic acid. Acta Chem Scand Ser B 22:3245–3250

296. Innocenti G, Dall'Acqua F, Guiotto A, Caporale G (1977) Investigation on skin-photosensitizing activity of various kinds of Psoralea. Planta Med 31:151–155

297. Camm E, Buck HWL, Mitchell JC (1976) Phytophotodermatitis from *Heracleum mantegazzianum*. Contact Dermatitis 2:68–72

298. Dreyer JC, Hunter JAA (1970) Giant hogweed dermatitis. Scott Med J 15:315–319

299. Birmingham DJ, Key MM, Tubich GE, Prone VB (1961) Phototoxic bullae among celery harvesters. Arch Dermatol 83:73–87

300. Seligman PJ, Mathias CGT, O'Malley MA, Beier RC, Fehrs LJ, Serrill WS, Halperin WE (1987) Phytophotodermatitis from celery among grocery store workers. Arch Dermatol 123:1478–1482

301. Austad J, Kavli G (1983) Phototoxic dermatitis caused by celery infected by *Sclerotinia sclerotiorum*. Contact Dermatitis 9:448–451

302. Sommer RG, Jillson OF (1967) Phytophotodermatitis (solar dermatitis from plants. Gas plant and the wild parsnip. N Engl J Med 276:1484–1486

303. Picardo M, Cristaudo A, Luca C de et al (1986) Contact dermatitis to *Pastinaca sativa*. Contact Dermatitis 15: 98–99

304. Coste F, Marceron L, Boyer J (1943) Dermite à l'angélique. Bull Soc Fr Dermatol Syphiligr 50:316–317

305. Arvy MP, Gallouin F (2003) Épices, aromates et condiments. Belin, Paris

306. Sidi E, Bourgeois-Gavardin J (1955) Accidents provoqués par les applications locales d' "Ammi majus". In: Tolérance et intolérance aux produits cosmétiques. Masson, Paris, pp 337–338

307. Kavli G, Midelfart K, Raa J et al (1983) Phototoxicity from furocoumarins (psoralens) of Heracleum laciniatum in a patient with vitiligo. Action spectrum studies on bergapten, pimpinellin, angelicin and sphondin. Contact Dermatitis 9:364–366

308. Weimarck G, Nilsson E (1980) Phototoxicity in *Heracleum sphondylium*. Planta Med 38:97–100

309. Machado S, Silva E, Massa A (2002) Occupational allergic contact dermatitis from falcarinol. Contact Dermatitis 47:109–110

310. Hausen BM, Bröhan J, König WA, Faasch H, Hahn H, Bruhn G (1987) Allergic and irritant contact dermatitis from falcarinol and didehydrofalcarinol in common ivy (*Hedera helix* L.). Contact Dermatitis 17:1–9

311. Sams WM (1941) Photodynamic action of lime oil (*Citrus aurantifolia*). Arch Dermatol Syphilol 44:571–587

312. Opdyke DLJ (1973) Fragrance raw materials monographs. Bergamot oil expressed. Fd Cosm Toxicol 11:1031–1033

313. Girard J, Unkovic J, Delahayes J, Lafille C (1979) Étude expérimentale de la phototoxicité de l'essence de bergamote; corrélation entre l'homme et le cobaye. Dermatologica 158:229–243

314. Volden G, Krokan H, Kavli G, Midelfart K (1983) Phototoxic and contact toxic reactions of the exocarp of sweet oranges: a common cause of cheilitis? Contact Dermatitis 9:201–204

315. Fisher JF, Trama LA (1979) High-performance liquid chromatographic determination of some coumarins and psoralens found in citrus peel oils. J Agric Fd Chem 27: 1334–1337

316. Gawkrodger DJ, Savin JA (1983) Phytophotodermatitis due to common rue (*Ruta graveolens*). Contact Dermatitis 9:224

317. Zobel AM, Brown SA (1990) Dermatitis-inducing furanocoumarins on leaf surfaces of eight species of rutaceous and umbelliferous plants. J Chem Ecol 16:693–700

318. Brener S, Friedman J (1985) Phytophotodermatitis induced by *Ruta chalepensis* L. Contact Dermatitis 12: 230–232

319. Möller H (1978) Phototoxicity of *Dictamnus alba*. Contact Dermatitis 4:264–269

320. Elpern DJ, Mitchell JC (1984) Phytophotodermatitis from mokihana fruits (*Pelea anisata* H. Mann, fam. Rutaceae) in Hawaiian lei. Contact Dermatitis 10:224–226

321. Yoke M, Turjman M, Flynn T, Balza F, Mitchell JC, Towers GH (1985) Identification of psoralen, 8-methoxypsoralen,

41

isopimpinellin, and 5,7-dimethoxycoumarin in *Pelea anisata* H. Mann. Contact Dermatitis 12:196–199

322. Jarvis WM (1968) The photosensitizing furanocoumarins of *Phebalium argenteum* (blister bush). Aust J Chem 21: 537–538

323. Zaynoun ST, Aftimos BG, Abi Ali L, Tenekjian KK, Khalidi U, Kurban AK (1984) *Ficus carica*; isolation and quantification of the photoactive components. Contact Dermatitis 11:21–25

324. Ippen H (1982) Phototoxische Reaktion auf Feigen. Hautarzt 33:337–339

325. Kitchevatz M (1934) Etiologie et pathogénèse de la dermite des figues. Bull Soc Fr Dermatol Syphiligr 41:1751–1759

326. Houloussi-Behdjet D (1933) Dermatite des figues et des figuiers. Bull Soc Fr Dermatol Syphiligr 40:787–796

327. Schwartz L (1938) Cutaneous hazards in the citrus fruit industry. Arch Dermatol Syphilol 37:641–649

328. Vickers HR (1941) The carrot as a cause of dermatitis. Br J Dermatol Syph 53:52–57

329. Peck SM, Spolyar LW, Mason HS (1944) Dermatitis from carrots. Arch Dermatol Syphilol 49:266

330. Klauder JV, Kimmich JM (1956) Sensitization dermatitis due to carrots. Report of cross-sensitization phenomenon and remarks on phytophotodermatitis. Arch Dermatol 74:149–158

331. Van Dijk E, Berrens L (1964) Plants as an etiological factor in phytophotodermatitis. Dermatologica 129:321–328

332. Rackett SC, Zug KA (1997) Contact dermatitis to multiple exotic woods. Am J Contact Dermat 8:114–117

333. Haustein UF (1982) Violin chin rest eczema due to East-Indian rosewood (*Dalbergia latifolia* Roxb.). Contact Dermatitis 8:77–78

334. Hausen BM (1997) Contact dermatitis from a wooden necklace. Am J Contact Dermat 8:185–187

335. Dias M, Vale T (1992) Contact dermatitis from a *Dalbergia nigra* bracelet. Contact Dermatitis 26:61

336. Cronin E, Calnan CD (1975) Rosewood knife handle. Contact Dermatitis 1:121

337. Hausen BM (1981) Woods injurious to human health. A manual. De Gruyter, Berlin

338. Willis JH (1982) Nasal carcinoma in woodworkers: a review. J Occup Med 24:526–530

339. Woods B, Calnan CD (1976) Toxic woods. Br J Dermatol 95:1–97

340. Hausen BM (1986) Contact allergy to woods. Clin Dermatol 4:65–76

341. Hausen BM, Adams RM (1990) Woods. In: Adams RM (ed) Occupational skin disease. Saunders, Philadelphia, PA, pp 524–536

342. Foussereau J (1981) Bois exotiques (TA 23). Fiche d'allergologie, Dermatologie professionnell. INRS, Paris, pp 1–5

343. Richter HG, Dallwitz MJ (2005) Commercial timbers: descriptions, illustrations, identification, and information retrieval (homepage). (See http://biodiversity.bio.uno.edu/delta/wood)

344. Fernández de Corres L, Leanizbarrutia I, Muñoz D (1988) Cross-reactivity between some naturally occurring quinones. Contact Dermatitis 18:186–187

345. Dejobert Y, Martin P, Bergoend H (1995) Airborne contact dermatitis from *Apuleia leiocarpa* wood. Contact Dermatitis 32:242–243

346. Estlander T, Jolanki R, Alanko K, Kanerva L (2001) Occupational allergic contact dermatitis caused by wood dusts. Contact Dermatitis 44:213–217

347. Kiec-Swierczynska M, Krecisz B, Swierczynska-Machura D, Palczynski C (2004) Occupational allergic contact dermatits caused by padauk wood (*Pterocarpus soyauxii* Taub.). Contact Dermatitis 50:384–385

348. Weber LF (1953) Dermatitis venenata due to native woods. AMA Arch Dermatol Syphil 67:388–394

349. Majamaa H, Viljanen P (2004) Occupational facial allergic contact dermatitis caused by Finnish pine and spruce wood dusts. Contact Dermatitis 51:157–158

350. Karlberg AT (1988) Contact allergy to colophony. Chemical identification of allergens, sensitization experiments and clinical experiences. Acta Derm Venereol (Stockh) 139:1–43

351. Karlberg AT, Bohlinder K, Boman A et al (1988) Identification of 15-hydroperoxyabietic acid as a contact allergen in Portuguese colophony. J Pharm Pharmacol 40:42–47

352. Karlberg AT (2000) Colophony. In: Kanerva L, Elsner P, Wahlberg JE, Maibach HI (eds) Handbook of occupational dermatology. Springer, Berlin Heidelberg New York, pp 509–516

353. Hellerström S, Thyresson N, Widmark G (1957) Chemical aspects of turpentine eczema. Dermatologica 115: 277–286

354. Pirilä V, Kilpiö O, Olkkonen A et al (1969) On the chemical nature of the eczematogens in oil of turpentine. V. Pattern of sensitivity to different terpenes. Dermatologica 139: 183–194

355. Lippert U, Martin V, Schwertfeger C, Junghans D, Ellinghaus B, Fuchs T (2003) Shiitake dermatitis. Br J Dermatol 148:178–179

356. Korstanje MJ, van de Staak WJBM (1990) A case of hand eczema due to mushrooms. Contact Dermatitis 22: 115–116

357. Kanerva L, Estlander T, Jolanki R (1998) Airborne occupational allergic contact dermatitis from champignon mushroom. Am J Contact Dermat 9:190–192

358. Maes MFJ, Van Baar HMJ, Van Ginkel CJW (1999) Occupational allergic contact dermatitis from the mushroom White Pom Pom (*Hericium eriaceum*). Contact Dermatitis 40:289–290

359. Simeoni S, Puccetti A, Peterlana D, Tinazzi E, Lunardi C (2004) Occupational allergic contact dermatitis from champignon and Polish mushroom. Contact Dermatitis 51:156–157

360. Prelli R (2001) Les fougères et plantes alliées de France et d'Europe ocidentale. Belin, Paris

361. Hausen BM, Schulz KH (1978) Occupational allergic contact dermatitis due to leatherleaf fern *Arachnoides adiantiformis* (Forst) Tindale. Br J Dermatol 98:325–329

362. Özdemir C, Schneider LA, Hinrichs R, Staib G, Weber L, Weiss JM, Scharffetter-Kochanek K (2003) Allergische Kontaktdermatitis auf Efeu (*Hedera helix* L.). Hautarzt 54:966–969

363. Garcia M, Fernandez E, Navarro A, del Pozo MD, Fernandez de Corres L (1995) Allergic contact dermatitis from *Hedera helix* L. Contact Dermatitis 33:133–134

364. Oka K, Saito F (1999) Allergic contact dermatitis from *Dendropanax trifidus*. Contact Dermatitis 41:350–351

365. Leclerc H (1927) Précis de phytothérapie. Essai de thérapeutique par les plantes françaises. Masson et Cie, Paris

366. Etxenagusia MA, Anda M, González-Mahave I, Fernández E, Fernández de Corrès L (2000) Contact dermatitis from *Chelidonium majus* (greater celandine). Contact Dermatitis 43:47

367. Stickel F, Poschl G, Seitz HK, Waldherr R, Hahn EG, Schuppan D (2003) Acute hepatitis induced by greater celandine (*Chelidonium majus*). Scand J Gastroenterol 38:565–568

368. Holme SA, Roberts DL (2000) Erythroderma associated with St John's wort. Br J Dermatol 143:1127–1128

369. Kubin A, Wierrani F, Burner U, Alth G, Grunberger W (2005) Hypericin – the facts about a controversial agent. Curr Pharm Des 11:233–253

370. Lane-Brown MM (2000) Photosensitivity associated with herbal preparations of St John's wort (*Hypericum perforatum*). Med J Aust 172:302

371. Schempp CM, Müller KA, Winghofer B, Schöpf E, Simon JC (2002) Johanniskraut (*Hypericum perforatum* L.) – eine Pflanze mit Relevanz für die Dermatologie. Hautarzt 53:316–321

372. Le Coz CJ (2004) Allergic contact dermatitis from tamanu oil (*Calophyllum inophyllum, Calophyllum tacamahaca*). Contact Dermatitis 51:216–217

373. Avenel-Audran M, Hausen BM, Le Sellin J, Ledieu G, Verret JL (2000) Allergic contact dermatitis from hydrangea – is it so rare? Contact Dermatitis 43:189–191

374. Van der Willigen AH, van Joost T, Stolz E, van der Hoek JCS (1987) Contact dermatitis to safflower. Contact Dermatitis 17:184–186

375. Dejobert Y, Arzur L, Thellart AS, Martin P, Torck M, Frimat P, Piette F, Thomas P (2004) Contact dermatitis to Iris in a florist. Contact Dermatitis 50:163–164

376. Le Coz CJ (2000) Cigarette and cigar makers and tobacco workers. In: Kanerva L, Elsner P, Wahlberg JE, Maibach HI (eds) Handbook of occupational dermatology. Springer, Berlin Heidelberg New York, pp 887–889

377. Kabashima K, Miyachi Y (2004) Contact dermatitis due to eggplant. Contact Dermatitis 50:101–102

378. Schena D, Magnanini M, Rosina P, Chieregato C (1998) Allergic contact dermatitis due to *Hygrophila salicifolia*. Contact Dermatitis 39:132

379. Assier-Bonnet H (2000) Compositae mix versus sesquiterpene lactone mix for patch testing: a French experience. Contact Dermatitis 42 [Suppl 2]:40

380. Bong J, English JS, Wilkinson SM (2001) Diluted Compositae mix versus sesquiterpene lactone mix as a screening agent for Compositae dermatitis: a multicentre study. Contact Dermatitis 42 [Suppl 2]:49

381. Bruynzeel DP, Tafelkruijer J, Wilks MF (1995) Contact dermatitis due to a new fungicide used in the tulip bulb industry. Contact Dermatitis 33:8–11

382. Grevelink SA, Olsen EA (1991) Efficacy of barrier creams in suppression of experimentally induced Rhus dermatitis. Am J Contact Dermat 2:69.

383. Gonçalo M, Mascarenhas R, Vieira R, Figueiredo A (2004) Permeability of gloves to plant allergens. Contact Dermatitis 50:200–201

384. Wrangsjö K, Ros AM (1996) Compositae allergy. Semin Dermatol 15:87–94

385. Schamberg J (1919) Desensitization of persons against poison ivy. JAMA 73:12–13

386. Kligman AM (1958) Cashew nut shell oil for hyposensitization against Rhus dermatitis. AMA Arch Dermatol 78:359–363

387. Kligman AM (1958) Hyposensitization against Rhus dermatitis. AMA Arch Dermatol 78:359–363

388. Guin JD (1991) The case of Dr Shelmire's child's nurse: a historical look at the confusion surrounding hyposensitization to Toxicodendrons. Am J Contact Dermat 2:194–197

389. Hashimoto Y, Kawada A, Aragane Y, Tezuka T (2003) Occupational contact dermatitis from chrysanthemum in a mortician. Contact Dermatitis 49:106–107

390. Watson ES (1986) *Toxicodendron* hyposensitization programs. Clin Dermatol 4:160–170

391. Resnick SD (1986) Poison-ivy and poison-oak dermatitis. Clin Dermatol 4:208–212

41

Chapter 42

Pesticides

42

Carola Lidén

Contents

42.1 Introduction

Most pesticides are chemicals used in agriculture to control of pests, weeds or plant diseases. Some pesticides are used as vector control agents in public health programs. Pesticides are also used in horticulture, forestry and livestock production. Herbicides, insecticides and fungicides are the major groups (Table 1). Most pesticides used are synthetic products, but some are of biological origin, such as plant extracts or microorganisms. Many pesticides are potentially very hazardous to human health (Table 2) and to other organisms in the environment, and they may cause damage to the ecosystem. Human exposure to pesticides is generally unintentional – dermal, oral or respiratory. Dermal exposure is often the major route through which acute and severe toxic effects are initiated, mainly by the skin's absorption of cholinesterase-inhibiting insecticides (organophosphorus compounds). Contact dermatitis and other adverse skin effects are also important (Table 3). Intentional ingestion during a suicide attempt is often fatal. Acute and chronic health effects of exposure to pesticides constitute a large public health problem in developing countries [57].

Core Message

- Dermal exposure to pesticides may cause systemic toxic effects, dermatitis or other adverse skin effects.

Table 1. Main categories of pesticides

Herbicides and desiccants
Insecticides, acaricides, molluscicides and nematicides
Fungicides
Plant grow regulators
Repellents
Rodenticides
Wood preservatives
Slimicides
Products used against microorganisms in chemical toilets, etc.
Anti-fouling products
Other products
Biological pesticides

Table 2. Health effects of pesticides (based on [57])

Bone-marrow effects
Cancer
Developmental effects
Enzyme induction
Eye lesions
Immunological effects
Neurotoxicity
Reproductive dysfunction
Respiratory effects
Skin lesions (see Table 3)
Systemic poisoning

Table 3. Skin effects of pesticides (based mainly on [1, 8, 18, 28])

Absorption through the skin
Accumulation in skin
Chemical burns
Chloracne
Contact dermatitis: allergic and irritant
Hyper- and hypopigmentation
Nail dystrophy
Photosensitivity
Porphyria cutanea tarda
Sclerodermatous changes
Squamous cell carcinoma

42.2 Use of Pesticides and Limitations of Use

Today, about 750 active ingredients are used as pesticides in 50,000 commercial formulations on the world market, and 25% of the world consumption of pesticides occurs in developing countries [56, 57].

Historically, the use of inorganic chemicals, sulfur and arsenic to control insects dates back to classical Greece and Rome. Paris green, an impure copper arsenite, was introduced in 1867 for crop protection. Iron sulfate was found to be useful for weed control. The first organomercury seed dressing was introduced in 1913 in Germany. DDT was developed in 1940. Since then, a wide range of chemical compounds have been introduced as pesticides.

The use of pesticides is, in large parts of the world, surrounded by regulations concerning the substances allowed, methods, indications and periods of application, education and protective equipment for workers. An increasing number of pesticides have, during the last decades, been banned or severely restricted for use in large parts of Europe and in Northern America, mainly due to their unwanted effects on the environment, and in some cases due to their effects on human health. Examples are DDT and other organochlorine insecticides, many mercury compounds, some phenoxy acid herbicides, and the herbicide paraquat. Many of those pesticides are, however, widely exported to and used in developing countries [9, 10, 52, 57].

DDT and the phenoxy acid herbicide 2,4,5-T are banned in all European Union countries. The producers of paraquat are promoting its use all over the world, stating that it is safe to use according to label instructions. The major markets for paraquat are in Asia, Central and South America, which use ~75% of the paraquat produced. Less than 10% of it is used in Europe [10]. Particularly in developing countries, but also elsewhere, conditions are substandard, resulting in substantial skin exposure. Paraquat is banned in 13 countries. Malaysia was the first developing country to decide (in 2002) to ban paraquat. It has been forbidden in Sweden since 1983. The European Commission decided in 2003 to include paraquat in Annex I of Directive 91/414/EEC, and member countries may allow its use. Sweden has applied to the Court of Justice of the European Communities to annul the decision to authorize paraquat, as it would result in an unacceptably low level of protection (P. Bergkvist, Swedish Chemicals Inspectorate, personal communication).

Core Message

■ The use of pesticides in Europe and Northern America is surrounded by regulations for the protection of the environment and human health, while the use of pesticides causes severe problems in developing countries.

42.3 Terminology, Classification, and Formulations

Pesticides are usually categorized according to what they are used against or to protect (Table 1). The active ingredients are often mentioned by their common names or by trivial names, according to the International Organization for Standardization (ISO), which is the terminology used in this chapter as well. Many synonyms occur, and many pesticides are better known by trade names of pesticide products. The WHO classification by degree of acute hazard to humans is widely used: class Ia is extremely hazardous; Ib is highly hazardous; II is moderately hazardous; and III is slightly hazardous.

Pesticides are formulated in different ways – such as solid or liquid concentrates, solutions or emulsions in water or organic solvents, aerosols, granules, powders, or mixed with sand, dusts, and fumigants. It is essential to recall that pesticide products, besides their active ingredients, also contain non-active ingredients and possibly contaminants. Many of the nonactive ingredients and contaminants are toxic substances, and some are known skin irritants or allergens (organic solvents, formaldehyde, isocyanates). The formulants can also act as facilitators for transport into the skin and may therefore worsen a

42

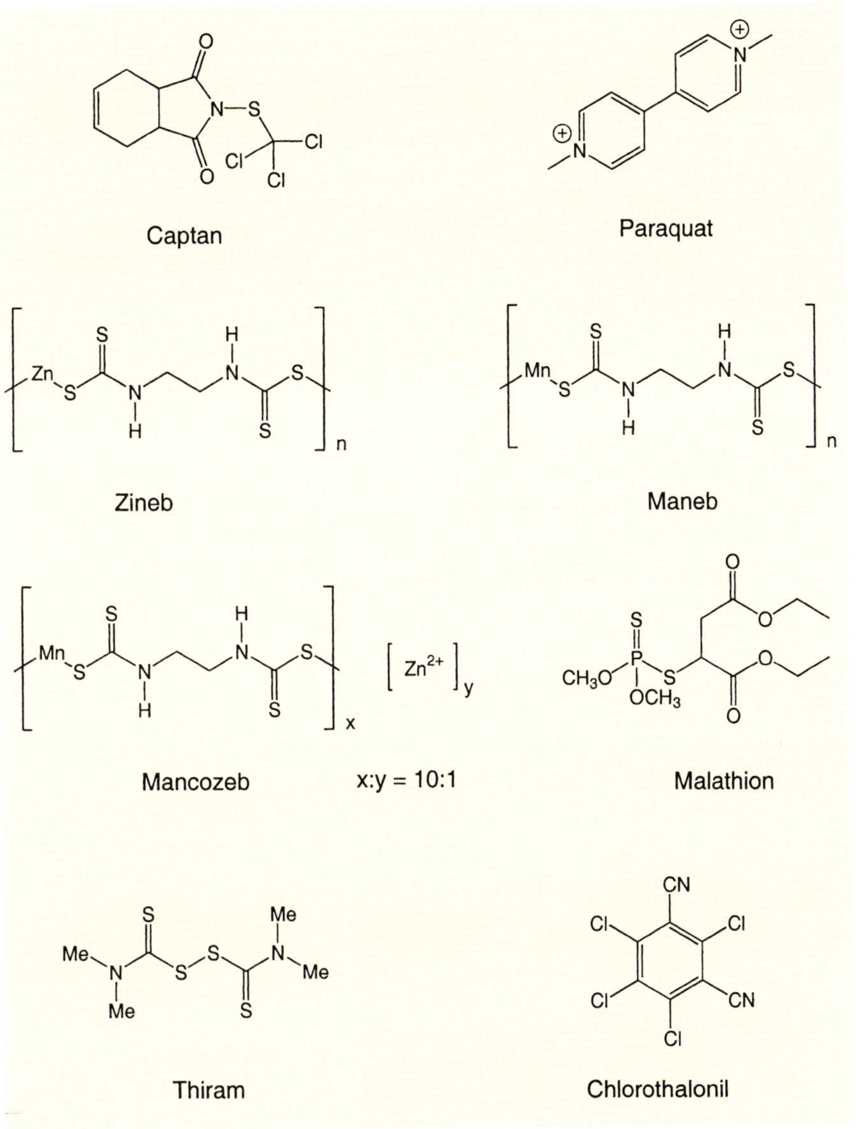

Fig. 1.
Chemical structures of some pesticides

Captan

Paraquat

Zineb

Maneb

Mancozeb   x:y = 10:1   Malathion

Thiram   Chlorothalonil

lesion. The chemical structures of some pesticides are shown in Fig. 1.

42.4 Skin Exposure and Absorption Through Skin

There is a broad variation in the degree of skin exposure to pesticides at work. Sprayers, mixers, loaders, packers, and mechanics perform work with high risk of direct skin contact with pesticides. Sprayers are also exposed to aerosols, during and after application. Workers may be exposed to pesticide residues on treated flowers, crops, bulbs, and wood. Some pesticides are quickly degraded while others are more or less persistent.

A number of methods of exposure assessment have been used for different pesticides [21] (see also Chap. 25, Allergens Exposure Assessment). Cholinesterase activity in erythrocytes or in plasma should be determined in workers using organophosphorus compounds. Paraquat and some other pesticides or their metabolites can be measured in urine. Skin exposure can be studied by hand-wash techniques, by fluorescent tracer technique, and by analysis of pesticide levels in patches on the skin. The hands are generally the part of the body with the highest exposure, but the arms and face and other unprotected or soaked parts are exposed, and with knapsack sprayers, the back and lower legs are too [4].

Percutaneous absorption of pesticides varies considerably from compound to compound, as shown by experimental studies on normal skin of human volunteers, and by in vitro studies [2, 39, 54, 55]. The regional variation in pesticide absorption through the skin is large and highest from scrotal skin, head and neck. Occlusion, skin damage, concentration, contact time, area, humidity and temperature are factors that are important for absorption.

> ### Core Message
>
> ■ Percutaneous absorption of pesticides varies between compounds. Occlusion, skin damage, concentration, contact time and surface area are important factors for absorption. The fluorescent tracer technique and other methods may be used in exposure assessment.

42.4.1 Prevention of Skin Exposure

The most appropriate equipment for protection against exposure to hazardous pesticides depends on the type of work and the properties of the pesticide product. For the most heavily exposed groups, such as applicators, mixers, and producers, the use of coverall, apron, raincoat, gloves, hat, boots, mask and goggles or face shields is often indicated (Fig. 2). For protection it is important that the equipment is used properly, that it is clean and that it is in good shape. The gloves that generally give the best protection are nitrile/butyl rubber gloves or laminate gloves (4H or Barrier). Barrier creams have not been shown to provide effective protection.

In many parts of the world, adequate conditions are not provided for protecting pesticide workers. The reasons for insufficient protection are often a lack of resources and low level of awareness of risks due to skin exposure. It is also uncomfortable to use fully protective equipment in a hot and humid climate. In the poorest developing countries, where many of the most dangerous pesticides are used, workers may have no protection at all. Knapsack sprayers may carry out mixing and spraying dressed in just a T-shirt and shorts (Fig. 3). Spraying by airplane is frequent and people on the ground may be unprotected. This is particularly true for the "flaggers" who are workers in the field guiding the pilot during spraying. Adequate washing conditions for skin, clothes and equipment are often not present.

Skin exposure to pesticides is heavily dependent on how the work is carried out, and on awareness of the risk caused by contamination of the skin. The use of a fluorescent tracer mixed with the pesticide has been introduced for visualization, by UV light, of skin contamination [3, 4, 11]. The method has been very useful for explaining risky techniques and occurrences to workers. Guidelines for personal protection and for field surveys have been published by authorities and organizations such as WHO, US EPA (the U.S. Environmental Protection Agency) and Crop Life International (former GIFAP and GCPF).

> ### Core Message
>
> ■ Adequate protective equipment and working conditions, and awareness of risks and safe handling, are essential for the prevention of severe health effects due to skin exposure to pesticides.

42.5 Skin Effects of Some Pesticides

The true prevalence and incidence of skin disease due to pesticide exposure is not known. It is likely that many of the pesticides cause more dermatitis

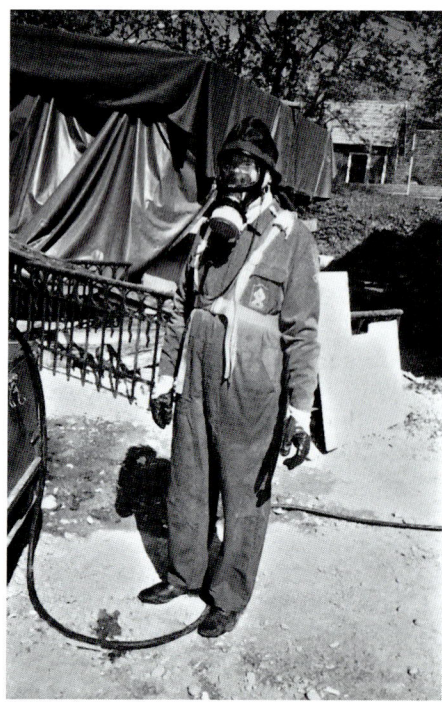

Fig. 2. Well-protected pesticide worker (Photo by Birgitta Kolmodin-Hedmen)

42

Fig. 3.
Unprotected pesticide
worker (Photo by
Carola Lidén)

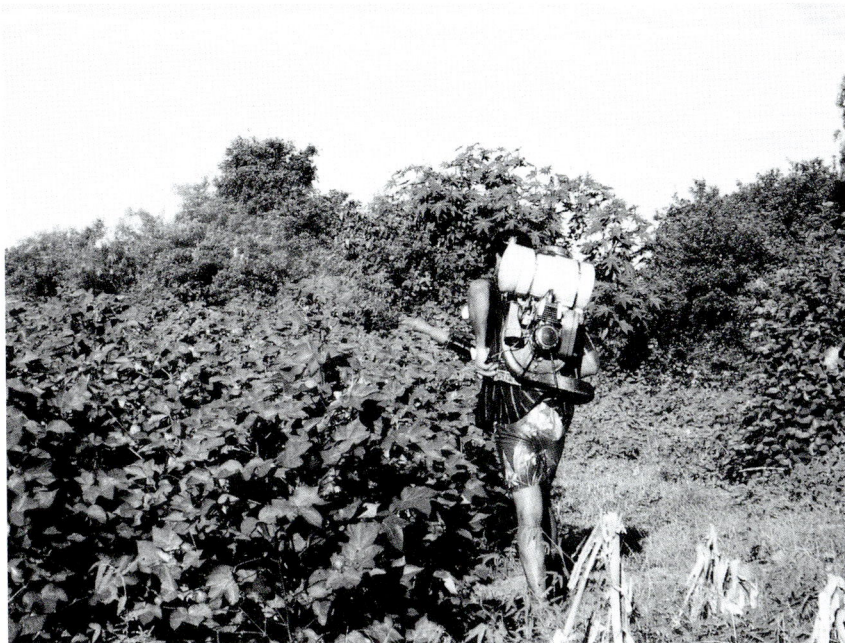

than is reported [8]. Farmers generally do not have easy access to dermatologists; many agricultural workers are temporarily employed and do not seek medical care; and in most developing countries, where skin exposure is expected to be the highest, dermatologists are rare and patch testing is often not done.

Irritant contact dermatitis due to pesticide exposure is believed to be more frequent than allergic contact dermatitis. The most frequently reported cases of allergic contact dermatitis have been related to fungicides and insecticides. The most important fatal effects of skin exposure to pesticides are acute toxic reactions due to skin absorption of organophosphorus compounds. Pesticides are also known to cause other skin effects (Table 3).

The following examples may illustrate how the situation varies globally. In California, adverse health effects due to pesticide exposure have attracted much attention. The agricultural sector has had the highest rate of occupational skin disease of any industry, and epidemics of contact dermatitis have been reported. One third of the illnesses and injuries due to pesticides have been reported to involve the skin [28]. In Japan, contact dermatitis was reported in 27% of 815 patients diagnosed with and treated for pesticide poisoning. The principal pesticides reported to be responsible for the dermatitis cases were fungicides and insecticides, and spraying operations were reported in 78% of cases. Results from patch testing were not given [35]. In Denmark, clinical examina-

tion and patch testing was carried out on 253 gardeners and greenhouse workers with occupational skin symptoms identified by a questionnaire. Contact allergies to the fungicides captan (ten cases) and maneb (three cases) were recorded. The relatively low prevalence of contact allergy to fungicides was thought to reflect the effect of protective measures [41].

Detailed reviews on occupational skin disease related to pesticides, covering large numbers of case reports, as well as more conclusive studies, have been published [1, 8, 18, 28, 47]. The results from the predictive testing of 23 pesticides in guinea-pigs are presented in a review [51]. Some of the most relevant information on the skin effects of commonly used pesticides is summarized below.

Core Message

■ Irritant and allergic contact dermatitis and other skin effects are caused by pesticide exposure. Fungicides and insecticides are the most frequently reported causes of allergic contact dermatitis. Skin absorption of organophosphorus compounds and paraquat cause severe toxic effects.

42.5.1 Herbicides and Desiccants

Glyphosate (Roundup and other trade names) is the largest selling non-selective herbicide applied in agriculture, public areas and for home use. It has been associated with skin disease [40]. Human experimental assays, however, showed no evidence for induction of photo-irritation, allergic or photo-allergic contact dermatitis, and it was a mild irritant [27].

Paraquat (Gramaxone and other trade names) is a nonselective contact herbicide and desiccant. It is one of the most widely used pesticides for weed control. Paraquat is highly toxic when ingested, causing multiple organ failure, and there is no antidote. Irritant contact dermatitis, occupational keratoses, nail lesions with discoloration, deformity and onycholysis, necrotic ulcers and also fatalities have been reported after skin exposure [28]. Fifteen fatal cases of occupational exposure to paraquat in Costa Rica were described, and five were explained by dermal exposure [53]. Considerable amounts may be absorbed through damaged skin and under occlusion, while absorption through intact skin is limited [14].

2,4-D and 2,4,5-T are phenoxy acid herbicides [17, 21]. They are selective against broad-leaved plants and used as defoliants, and are produced in enormous quantities. They may contain TCDD (dioxin), which is often formed during production. This is the explanation for several outbreaks of chloracne and porphyria cutanea tarda among workers in pesticide production, and for the disaster in Seveso, Italy, in 1976. Severe contact dermatitis from a mixture of 2,4-D and 2,4,5-T has been reported. 2,4-D and 2,4,5-T were components of "Agent Orange", used by the United States army to defoliate jungle areas in South Vietnam. "Agent Orange" was contaminated by dioxins and dibenzofurans related to 2,4,5-T.

42.5.2 Insecticides

Many insecticides are very toxic on skin contact, resulting in systemic toxicity; some are skin irritants and some are identified as clinically relevant contact allergens. A substantial number of case reports have been published on different types of skin reaction to several insecticides. Reference is given to reviews [1, 8, 18, 28]. Some illustrative examples are given below.

Pyrethrins are botanical pesticides, and plant extracts. The pyrethrins are obtained from *Chrysanthemum cinerariaefolium* and they are moderately potent allergens. Pyrethroids are synthetic compounds with a longer duration of activity against insects than that of pyrethrum, and less toxicity to mammals than

organophosphorus compounds. Paresthesias following skin exposure has been described, but allergic contact dermatitis due to pyrethroids has not been reported [24, 28].

Malathion, parathion, naled and dichlorvos are examples of organophosphorus pesticides [28]. Parathion is extremely toxic to man and animals, and its use in Europe and Northern America is heavily restricted. Malathion, which is degraded rapidly in the body, is less dangerous. Malathion is a moderate sensitizer according to predictive testing in man and guinea pig ([37], review by [51]). Dichlorvos has been reported to cause irritant contact dermatitis in impregnated flea collars. Allergic contact dermatitis caused by naled, which has a toxicity level between that of malathion and parathion, has been reported in a few cases. Sclerodermatous changes without internal involvement have occurred in workers handling malathion, parathion, DDT and some other pesticides [19].

DDT and lindane are chlorinated hydrocarbons. The use of DDT is banned in the European Union. Allergic contact dermatitis has not been convincingly reported. Lindane is widely used and is a skin irritant, but allergic contact dermatitis is rare [28].

42.5.3 Fungicides

Benomyl, captan, chlorothalonil, difolatan, fluazinam, mancozeb, maneb, zineb, and thiram are some of the fungicides that are most frequently, or convincingly, reported to cause allergic contact dermatitis (reviewed in [1, 8, 18, 28]). Several other fungicides are reported to have caused allergic contact dermatitis in single cases. Some illustrative examples of contact allergy to fungicides are given below.

Benomyl is used for fruits, nuts, vegetables, crops and ornamentals. Several cases of allergic contact dermatitis from exposure to benomyl have been reported. Picking plants containing residues was found to be an important source of sensitization [12, 50].

Mancozeb, maneb, zineb, thiram, and other thiurams are members of the dithiocarbamate group. Cross-reactivity may be present in persons sensitive to these pesticides or chemically related rubber chemicals.

Chlorothalonil (Bravo, Daconil and other trade names) is a broad-spectrum fungicide used on vegetables, fruits, flowers, trees and bananas. Chlorothalonil is also used as a wood preservative and as a fungicide in paints. Allergic contact dermatitis in workers exposed to chlorothalonil in floriculture, banana fields, wood preservation and paints has been described [5, 20, 23, 36, 42, 44, 46]. Chlorothalonil has also been described as a possible cause of skin pigmentation (ashy dermatitis) in 39 banana field workers, of whom 34 were patch test positive [43].

Fluazinam caused outbreaks of contact dermatitis on the arms and face at a tulip processing company and among farmers shortly after it had been introduced. Exposed workers were patch test positive and control persons patch test negative [7, 49].

Predictive testing in animals by the guinea-pig maximization test has shown that benomyl, captan, chlorothalonil, mancozeb, maneb, and zineb are extremely potent sensitizers (reviewed in [51]). The high sensitizing potential of chlorothalonil was further confirmed by testing in mice, using the local lymph node assay, and in the guinea pig, using the cumulative contact enhancement test [5].

42.5.4 Repellents

N,N-Diethyl-*m*-toluamide (DEET) is considered to be the most effective insect repellent against mosquitoes. It has been reported to cause antecubital erythema, progressing to bullae and permanent scarring in American soldiers. It has also been reported to exacerbate seborrhea and acne, and to produce allergic contact dermatitis and contact urticaria [28].

42.5.5 Rodenticides

Warfarin is and antu has been frequently used rodenticides, substances used to kill rats and mice. Only single cases of occupational contact dermatitis due to exposure to Warfarin and antu have been reported [28].

42.5.6 Wood Preservatives, Slimicides, and Anti-fouling Products

Besides its use as a fungicide in agriculture, chlorothalonil is also used as a wood preservative. There are a number of publications concerning allergic contact dermatitis (see Sect. 42.5.3, "Fungicides").

Glutaraldehyde is used as a slimicide and is added to wood pulp slurry in the production of paper. Glutaraldehyde is a known contact allergen and is described in other chapters.

5-Chloro-2-methylisothiazol-3-one/2-methyliso-thiazol-3-one (MCI/MI) is used together with arsenic, chromium, and copper compounds in wood preservation. MCI/MI is also used as a slimicide in the production of paper, added to the wood pulp slurry, and at printing. Contact allergy to MCI/MI (Kathon CG and other trade names), is covered in other chapters.

Tributyltin oxide (TBTO) is used as a wood preservative and in anti-fouling paints. TBTO is a skin irritant and has caused chemical burns, but it is not a skin sensitizer [13, 22].

42.6 Patch Testing

It may be difficult to acquire adequate information concerning possible exposure to pesticide products. It is often even more difficult to obtain detailed information concerning the composition of the actual products, and to achieve access to the active ingredients for patch testing. It is also important to recall that pesticide products, in addition to the active ingredient and possible contaminants, contain other ingredients which may be toxic, irritants or allergens, and that they are often dissolved or mixed in organic solvents or water.

At present, no commercial pesticide patch test series is available. Some patch test clinics have their own pesticides series, composed to correspond to the use of pesticides in their geographical region. As the use of pesticides changes over time and in different areas of application, it is not possible to give definite recommendations.

Patch testing should ideally be carried out with the active ingredients and with other ingredients of the pesticides that the patient is exposed to. It may, however, be extremely difficult to obtain the ingredients. A practical approach is then to patch test with appropriate dilutions of the pesticide product. For many pesticide products, but not all, testing with 1% and 0.3%, and possibly 0.1% of the product in water or petrolatum is possible (D. Bruynzeel, personal communication). It must be stressed, however, that the active ingredient or possibly other ingredients may need further dilution. Positive reactions should be validated by testing on control persons.

Before patch testing, previous experience of testing with the pesticide product or ingredients should be checked in recent reports and reviews. Some of the most well-documented pesticide patch test preparations are listed in Table 4.

Safety is important when testing such potentially hazardous compounds. The recommended amounts applied at patch testing, however, are so small that they are regarded as safe, with no risk of systemic toxicity.

Table 4. Recommended patch test concentrations for some pesticides (based mainly on [1, 8, 18, 28]). (Vehicles: *acet.* Acetone, *aq.* water, *pet.* petrolatum; types of pesticides: *acaricides* Molluscicides and nematicides, *alg* algicides, *fung* fungicides, *herb* herbicides and desiccants, *insect* insecticides, *other* other products, *rod* rodenticides, *slim* slimicides, *wood* wood preservatives)

Active ingredient (CAS number)	Type	Patch test concentration
2,4-DNCB (97–00–7)	Alg	0.01–0.1% aq. or acet.
2-Methyl-4-isothiazolin-3-one (MI) (2682–20–4)	Slim, wood	MI/MCI: 0.01–0.02% aq.
5-Chloro-2-methyl-4-isothiazolin-3-one (MCI) (26172–55–4)	Slim, wood	MI/MCI: 0.01–0.02% aq.
Antu (86–88–4)	Rod	1% pet.
Benomyl (17804–35–2)	Fung	0.1–1% pet.
Captan (133–06–2)	Fung	0.5% aq. or pet.
Chlorothalonil (1897–45–6)	Fung, wood	0.001–0.01% acet.
Dazomet (533–74–4)	Fung, herb, insect	0.1% pet.
DDT (50–29–3)	Insect	1% pet. or acet.
Difolatan (2425–06–1)	Fung	0.1% pet.
Fluazinam (79622–59–6)	Fung	0.5% pet.
Folpet (133–07–3)	Fung	0.1% pet.
Glutaraldehyde (111–30–8)	Slim	0.2–0.3% pet.
Glyphosate (34494–03–6; 38641–94–0; 81591–81–3)	Herb	1–10% aq.
Lindane (58–89–9)	Insect	1% pet.
Malathion (121–75–5)	Insect	0.5% pet.
Maneb (12427–38–2)	Fung	0.5–1% pet.
Paraquat (1910–42–5)	Herb	0.1% pet.
Pentachloronitrobenzene (82–68–8)	Fung	1% pet.
Pyrethrum (several CAS-numbers)	Insect	1% pet.
Thiram (137–26–8)	Fung	1% pet.
Warfarin (81–81–2; 129–06–6)	Rod	0.5% pet.
Zineb (12122–67–7)	Fung	1% pet.
Ziram (137–30–4)	Fung	1% pet.

Core Message

■ Patch testing may be performed with appropriate concentrations of the pesticide product or the active ingredient and other ingredients. Consult the literature for safe handling.

References

1. Adams RM (1995) Occupational dermatitis. In: Rietchel RL, Fowler JF Jr (eds) Fisher's contact dermatitis, 4th edn. Williams and Wilkins, Baltimore, MD, Ch 25, pp 566–572
2. Andersen KE (1999) Systemic toxicity from percutaneous absorption. In: Adams RM (ed) Occupational skin disease, 3rd edn. Saunders, Philadelphia, Pa., pp 69–85
3. Aragón A, Blanco L, López L, Lidén C, Nise G, Wesseling C (2004) Reliability of a visual scoring system with fluorescent tracers to assess dermal pesticide exposure. Ann Occup Hyg 48 : 601–606
4. Blanco LE, Aragón A, Lundberg I, Lidén C, Wesseling C, Nise G (2005) Determinants of dermal exposure among Nicaraguan subsistence farmers during pesticide applications with backpack sprayers. Ann Occup Hyg 49 : 17–24
5. Boman A, Montelius J, Rissanen R-L, Lidén C (2000) Sensitizing potential of chlorothalonil in the guinea pig and the mouse. Contact Dermatitis 43 : 273–279
6. Bruynzeel DP, van Ketel WG (1986) Contact dermatitis due to chlorothalonil in floriculture. Contact Dermatitis 14 : 67–68
7. Bruynzeel DP, Tafelkruijer J, Wilks MF (1995) Contact dermatitis due to a new fungicide used in the tulip bulb industry. Contact Dermatitis 33 : 8–11
8. Cronin E (ed) (1980) Pesticides. In: Contact dermatitis, chap 8. Churchill Livingstone, Edinburgh, pp 391–413
9. Dich J, Hoar Zahm S, Hanberg A, Adami H-O (1997) Pesticides and cancer. Cancer Causes Control 8 : 420–443
10. Dinham B (2003) The perils of paraquat. Sales targeted at developing countries. Pesticide News 60 : 4–7
11. Fenske RA (1993) Dermal exposure assessment techniques. Ann Occup Hyg 37 : 687–706
12. Fregert S (1973) Allergic contact dermatitis from two pesticides. Contact Dermatitis Newslett 13 : 367
13. Gammeltoft M (1978) Tributyltinoxide is not allergenic. Contact Dermatitis 4 : 238
14. Garnier R (1995) Paraquat poisoning by inhalation or skin absorption. In: Bismuth C, Hall AH (eds) Paraquat poisoning – mechanisms, prevention and treatment. Dekker, New York, pp 211–234
15. Grandjean P (1990) Organophosphorus compounds. In: Skin penetration: hazardous chemicals at work. Taylor and Francis, Washington DC, Ch 12, pp 157–170
16. Guo YL, Wang BJ, Lee CC, Wang JD (1996) Prevalence of dermatoses and skin sensitization associated with use of pesticides in fruit farmers of southern Taiwan. Occup Environ Med 53 : 427–431
17. Hayes WJ (1982) Pesticides studies in man. Williams and Wilkins, Baltimore, Md.
18. Hogan DJ, Grafton LH (1999) Pesticides and other agricultural chemicals. In: Adams RM (ed) Occupational skin disease, 3rd edn. Saunders, Philadelphia, Pa., pp 597–622

42

19. Jablonska S (ed) (1975) Scleroderma and pseudoscleroderma. Polish Medical, Warsaw, p 603
20. Johnsson M, Buhagen M, Leira HL, Solvang S (1983) Fungicide-induced contact dermatitis. Contact Dermatitis 9:285–288
21. Legaspi JA, Zenz C (1994) Occupational health aspects of pesticides. Clinical and hygienic principles. In: Zenz C, Dickerson OB, Horvath EP (eds) Occupational medicine, 3rd edn. Mosby, St Louis, Mo., Chap 47, pp 617–653
22. Lewis PG, Emmet EA (1987) Irritant dermatitis from tributyl tin oxide and contact allergy from chlorocresol. Contact Dermatitis 17:129–132
23. Lidén C (1990) Facial dermatitis caused by chlorothalonil in a paint. Contact Dermatitis 22:206–211
24. Lisi P (1992) Sensitization risk of pyrethroid insecticides. Contact Dermatitis 26:349–350
25. Lisi P, Caraffini S, Assalve D (1986) A test series for pesticide dermatitis. Contact Dermatitis 15:266–269
26. Lisi P, Caraffini S, Assalve D (1987) Irritation and sensitization potential of pesticides. Contact Dermatitis 17:212–218
27. Maibach HI (1986) Irritation, sensitization, photoirritation and photosensitisation assays with a glyphosphate herbicide. Contact Dermatitis 15:152–155
28. Manuskiatti W, Abrams K, Hogan DJ, Maibach HI (2000) Pesticide-related dermatoses in agricultural workers. In: Kanerva L, Elsner P, Wahlberg JE, Maibach HI (eds) Handbook of occupational dermatology. Springer, Berlin Heidelberg New York, Chap 92, pp 781–802
29. Mark KA, Brancaccio RR, Soter NA, Cohen DE (1999) Allergic contact and photoallergic contact dermatitis to plant and pesticide allergens. Arch Dermatol 135:67–70
30. Marzulli F, Maguire HC (1982) Usefulness and limitations of various guinea-pig test methods in detecting human skin sensitizers. Validation of guinea-pig tests for skin hypersensitivity. Fd Chem Toxicol 20:67–74
31. Mathias CGT (1997) Allergic contact dermatitis from a lawn care fungicide containing Dyrene. Am J Contact Dermat 8:47–48
32. Mathias CGT (1989) Epidemiology of occupational skin disease in agriculture. In: Dosman JA, Cockroft DW (eds) Principles of health and safety in agriculture. CRC, Boca Raton, Fla., pp 285–287
33. Matsushita T, Aoyama K (1981) Cross-reactions between some pesticides and the fungicide benomyl in contact allergy. Ind Hlth 19:77–83
34. Matsushita T, Arimatsu Y, Nomura S (1976) Experimental study on contact dermatitis caused by dithiocarbamates Maneb, Mancozeb, Zineb and their related compounds. Int Arch Occup Environ Health 37:169–178
35. Matsushita T, Nomura S, Wakatsuki T (1980) Epidemiology of contact dermatitis from pesticides in Japan. Contact Dermatitis 6:255–259
36. Matsushita S, Kanekura T, Saruwatari K, Kanzaki T (1996) Photoallergic contact dermatitis due to Daconil. Contact Dermatitis 35:115–116
37. Milby TH, Epstein WL (1964) Allergic contact sensitivity to malathion. Arch Environ Health 9:434–437
38. Nakamura M, Arima Y, Nobuhara S, Miyachi Y (1999) Airborne photocontact dermatitis due to the pesticides maneb and fenitrothion. Contact Dermatitis 40:222–223
39. Nielsen JB, Nielsen F, Sørensen JA (2004) In vitro percutaneous penetration of five pesticides – effects of molecular weight and solubility characteristics. Ann Occup Hyg 48:697–705
40. O'Malley MAO, Mathias CGT, Coye MJ (1989) Epidemiology of pesticide-related skin disease in California agriculture. In: Dosman JA, Cockroft DW (eds) Principles of health and safety in agriculture. CRC, Boca Raton, Fla., pp 301–304
41. Paulsen E (1998) Occupational dermatitis in Danish gardeners and greenhouse workers. Contact Dermatitis 38:14–19
42. Penagos HG (2002) Contact dermatitis caused by pesticides among banana plantation workers in Panama. Int J Occup Environ Health 8:14–18
43. Penagos H, Jimenez V, Fallas V, O'Malley M, Maibach HI (1996) Chlorothalonil, a possible cause of erythema dyschromicum perstans (ashy dermatitis). Contact Dermatitis 35:214–218
44. Penagos H, Ruepert C, Partanen T, Wesseling C (2005) Pesticide patch test series for the assessment of allergic contact dermatitis among banana plantation workers in Panama. Dermatitis 15:137–145
45. Schuman SH, Dobson RL (1985) An outbreak of contact dermatitis in farm workers. J Am Acad Dermatol 12:220–223
46. Spindeldreier A, Deichmann B (1980) Kontaktdermatitis auf ein Holzschutzmittel mit einer neuer Fungizider Wirksubstans. Dermatosen 28:88–90
47. Susitaival P (2000) Occupational skin diseases in farmers and farm workers. In: Kanerva L, Elsner P, Wahlberg JE, Maibach HI (eds) Handbook of occupational dermatology. Springer, Berlin Heidelberg New York, Chap 130, pp 924–931
48. Tomlin C (ed) (1994) The pesticide manual, 10th edn. British Crop Protection Council / Royal Society of Chemistry, London
49. Van Ginkel CJW, Sabapathy NN (1995) Allergic contact dermatitis from the newly introduced fungicide fluazinam. Contact Dermatitis 32:160–162
50. Van Joost T, Naafs B, van Ketel WG (1983) Sensitization to benomyl and related pesticides. Contact Dermatitis 9:153–154
51. Wahlberg JE, Boman A (1985) Guinea pig maximization test. In: Andersen KE, Maibach HI (eds) Contact allergy predictive tests in guinea pigs. Karger, Basel, pp 59–106 (Current Problems in Dermatology, vol 14)
52. Wesseling C (1997) Health effects from pesticide use in Costa Rica – an epidemiologic approach. Karolinska Institutet, Stockholm, Sweden (Thesis)
53. Wesseling C, Hogstedt C, Picado A, Johansson L (1997) Unintentional fatal paraquat poisonings among agricultural workers in Costa Rica: report of 15 cases. Am J Ind Med 32:433–441
54. Wester RC, Maibach HI (1985) In vivo percutaneous absorption and decontamination of pesticides in humans. J Toxicol Environ Health 16:25–37
55. Wester RC, Maibach HI (1996) Percutaneous absorption: short-term exposure, lag time, multiple exposures, model variations, and absorption from clothing. In: Marzulli FN, Maibach HI (eds) Dermatotoxicology, 5th edn. Taylor and Francis, Washington, DC, Chap 4, pp 35–48
56. Wilkinson CF (1990) Introduction and overview. In: Baker SR, Wilkinson CF (eds) The effects of pesticides on human health. Princeton Scientific Publishing, Princeton, NJ, pp 5–33 (Advances in Modern Environmental Toxicology, vol XVIII)
57. World Health Organization and United Nations Environmental Programme (WHO/UNEP) (1990) Public health impact of pesticides used in agriculture. WHO, Geneva

Chapter 43

Contact Allergy in Children

43

A. Goossens, M. Morren

Contents

43.1 Introduction

Contact allergy has not been studied as extensively in children as in adults. Although there are many similarities between these two patient populations, the results obtained in adults cannot always be applied to children. A child is not simply a small version of an adult.

43.2 Prevalence and Incidence

Allergic contact dermatitis in children has always been considered rare, and their eczematous conditions have mostly been attributed to endogenous factors such as atopic or seborrheic dermatitis, sometimes in association with irritancy induced by soap, clothing, and so on [1–3]. One of the reasons for this would be their reduced exposure to environmental allergens (professional, cosmetic, pharmaceutical) [3, 4]. Some authors also cite a lower reactivity and sensitization capacity for children's skin [5, 6].

Until fairly recently, allergic contact dermatitis was not usually suspected in children, so little patch testing was performed [7]. Since the 1980s, however, this diagnosis has been considered more frequently [8]. Photoallergic contact dermatitis does seem to be rare [1, 7], although it may too be under-diagnosed.

43.2.1 Prevalence of Contact Allergy in an Unselected Population

Data on the prevalence of contact allergy in healthy children are scarce: in a population of 314 healthy children younger than 18 years old, Weston and co-workers [9] found positive patch test results in 20%; Barros and coworkers [10] reported a 13% prevalence in 562 children aged between 5 and 14; while Dotte-rud and Falk [11] observed that 23% of 424 healthy children from 7 to 12 years old had a contact allergy. More recently, Bruckner and coworkers [12] found that 24.5% of 85 children between 6 months and 5 - years of age, attending well-child visits and tested with a TRUE Test panel, presented one (16 infants) or two (4 infants) positive tests. Nickel and thimerosal were the most frequent allergens identified. However, Johnke and coworkers [13] warn for false-positive tests, especially with nickel sulfate in such young children: they found many (111/543 infants) weak transient reactions with the highest (200 $\mu g/cm^2$) nickel concentration tested, of which only 8.6% could be reproduced. Hence, single positive nickel patch tests in small children should be assessed with caution! In a Danish study on adolescents between 12 and 16 years old, a prevalence of 15.2% was found, the

relevance of which was estimated to be 50%, for the present or the past (7.2%). Girls reacted more frequently [14].

43.2.2 Prevalence of Contact Allergy in a Selected Population

Several studies have been performed in children suspected of contact allergy or suffering from atopic or juvenile plantar dermatitis, orofacial granulomatosis, dyshidrosis, psoriasis, photosensitivity, urticaria, or other dermatoses. The studies ([15–37], see Table 1) differ in the numbers and ages of the patients involved, the clinical symptoms, as well as the relevancy and the prevalence of the positive reactions observed. In a study by Pambor and co-workers in 1991 [38], only 3.6% of the children tested showed clinically relevant positive patch tests, whereas Pevny and co-workers observed relevancy rates of up to 71% [16], with the majority around 40%.

Table 1. Incidence of allergic contact dermatitis in selected populations

Author, Reference	Number	Age	Categories	%	Relevancy (%)	Most frequent allergens (% of children with positive test)
Veien et al [15]	168	<14 years	Suspicion of ACD	46	80	Nickel > dichromate > rubber
Pevny et al [16]	147	3–16 years	Suspicion of ACD	71	93	Nickel > cobalt > para-dyes > dichromate
Romaguera et al [17]	1023	<14 years	ACD and others (45% atopics)	31	69.5	Nickel/cobalt > pharmaceutical ingredients > cosmetics > shoes > clothes > professional
Rademaker and Forsyth [18]	129	<12 years	Atopic eczema, eczema, atypical JPD, contact dermatitis, orofacial granulomatosis, other	48	92	Metals > perfume > rubber
Kuiters et al [19]	67	<16 years	Dermatitis	28	84	Nickel > balsam of Peru > fragrance mix > colophony > carba mix
Balato et al [20]	585	<14 years	Eczema	14	?	Nickel > cobalt > ethylenediamine > dichromate > mercury ammonium chloride > mercaptobenzothiazole > neomycin > mercapto mix
Pambor et al [21]	366	2–14 years	Atopic dermatitis (n=214)	25	5	Nickel > chloramphenicol > parabens > turpentine
			Other dermatosis (n=142)	18	7	
Ayala et al [22]	323	<14 years	Atopic dermatitis Contact dermatitis Dyshidrotic eczema Foot, diaper or perioral eczema (palmar/plantar psoriasis)	35.2	61.7	Metals > pharmaceutical ingredients > preservatives > fragrance > shoes
Gonçalo et al [23]	329	<14 years	ACD	51.7	65.3	Nickel, thimerosal, cobalt, mercury ammonium chloride, fragrance mix, dichromate

43

Table 1. Continued

Author, Reference	Number	Age	Categories	%	Relevancy (%)	Most frequent allergens (% of children with positive test)
Sevilla et al [24]	272	2–14 years	ACD	37.1	54.4	Nickel, rubber, mercury chloride, cobalt, thimerosal, benzoyl peroxide, fragrance mix
Motolese et al [25]	53	<3 years	Dermatitis	50	62.5	Thimerosal, nickel, ammoniated mercury
Stables et al. [26]	92	3–14 years	Atopic dermatitis Localized dermatitis JPD Orofacial granulomatosis Reactions to vaccines Atypical psoriasis	32.6	87	Nickel, fragrance mix, balsam of Peru, thimerosal, neomycin, cobalt, lanolin, dichromate, mercapto mix
Rudzki et al [27]	626	3–16 years	?	42.7	?	Nickel, dichromate, cobalt, mercury chloride, fragrance mix, *para*-phenylenediamine, neomycin, balsam of Peru
Wilkowska et al [28]	100	5–15 years	Atopic dermatitis Eczema Nonallergic dermatoses	49	?	Dichromate, cobalt, neomycin
Katsarou et al [29]	232	<16 years	ACD ?	43.5	?	Nickel, cobalt, fragrance mix, dichromate, *para*-phenylenediamine, *para*-tertiary-butyl-phenol-formaldehyde resin, mercapto mix, mercury ammonium chloride, balsam of Peru
Wantke et al [30]	234 72 162	<15 years 0–7 years 7–14 years	ACD	44.65[a] 40.51[a]	?	Ethylmercuric chloride, thimerosal and nickel (girls)
Brasch et al [31]	416	6–15 years	ACD	41	?	Nickel, thimerosal, benzoyl peroxide, fragrance mix, cobalt, amalgam, mercury ammonium chloride, phenyl-mercury acetate, Amerchol L-101, cobalt chloride, dichromate, colophony
Shah et al [32]	83	6–16 years	Atopic dermatitis Hand/feet dermatitis (Peri)oral dermatitis Reactions to local anesthetics Dermatoses with unusual localizations Perianal dermatitis Urticaria Photoreactions	49	?	Nickel, fragrance mix, cobalt, neomycin, *para*-phenylene-diamine, colophony, *para*-tertiary-butylphenol-formaldehyde resin
Manzini et al [33]	670	6 months to 12 years	Dermatitis	42	?	Thimerosal, nickel, methyl(chloro)isothiazolinone, fragrance mix, neomycin, wool alcohols, ammoniated mercury
Romaguera et al [34]	141	<15 years	ACD	50	80	Nickel, cobalt, mercurials, fragrance, rubber
Giordani-Labadie et al [35]	137	<16 years	Atopic dermatitis	43	?	Metals (mainly nickel), fragrance, balsam of Peru, lanolin, neomycin
Roul et al [36]	337	<16 years	ACD	66	?	Nickel, fragrance, rubber
Duarte et al [37]	102	10–19 years	ACD	56	100	Nickel, tosylamide/formaldehyde resin

[a]Boys and girls respectively

Other factors that render comparison of those studies difficult [26] include the different test populations involved (for example the presence or not of atopy, differences in origin and habits), the variability of the test conditions (materials, allergens, concentrations, vehicles, reading times), and the interpretation of the test results (allergic or irritant).

The question arises as to whether contact allergy in children has become more frequent in recent years. According to Björksten [39], its prevalence in 18-year-old Swedish males increased from 0.9% in 1978 to 1.5% in 1993.

> **Core Message**
>
> ■ Contact allergy in children is more frequent than previously suspected, the prevalence in an unselected population being about 20%.

43.2.3 Prevalence in Relation to Genetic Factors

According to Walton and coworkers [40], occupational and environmental factors are essential but the hereditary background can also be important, as could be demonstrated, for example, by the higher prevalence of HLA-B35 and BW22 antigens and their correlation with an increased risk of nickel sensitization in a female population. The importance of genetic factors has also been studied in children [41–43]: these authors conclude that there is a specific genetic selection at the level of the peripheral T-lymphocyte system.

43.2.4 Prevalence Related to Sex

While some authors [9, 10, 26] detected similar prevalence in both boys and girls, others [11, 30] reported a higher prevalence in girls. This is especially the case for nickel [15, 40, 44] and after the age of 12 [18, 27, 29]. Hormonal factors may be a contributory factor here [23, 31]. Kwangsukstith and Maibach [45] have formulated several arguments for the existence of sex-related differences in the prevalence of allergic contact dermatitis: varying test results obtained depending upon the menstrual cycle; increased sensitization liability in females, in general, and enhanced reactivity to dinitrochlorobenzene (DNCB) in females taking contraceptives; allergic contact dermatitis due to transdermal clonidine being more frequently observed in women than in men; and finally, a greater susceptibility of feminine skin to irritation and hence to sensitization.

43.2.5 Prevalence Related to Age

Unlike some authors [10, 26, 36, 44], most report an increasing prevalence of allergic contact dermatitis with age, and attribute it to the increasing exposure to environmental allergens [8, 20, 24, 27, 28, 46]. This also applies to the development of multiple sensitivities [23]. A reduced sensitization potential in younger children has also been suggested [5, 6]. This has been experimentally demonstrated by Uhr and coworkers [47], who showed that sensitization to dinitrofluorobenzene does occur among premature infants but less frequently than among infants carried to term, and in both of these groups less frequently than in children aged 2–12 months. Epstein [48] obtained sensitization to pentadecylcatechol in 44% of children below 1 year of age, in about 58% between 1 and 3 years old, and in 87% of children between 4 and 8 years old. In contrast to this, Moltolese and coworkers [25] found a contact allergy in 32/53 infants (3 months to 2 years) with dermatitis. At least 20 out of the 32 were considered relevant.

Fisher reported several cases of allergic contact dermatitis in neonates and infants [49–52]: epoxy resin in a vinyl identification band in a 1-week-old neonate, three cases of ethylenediamine contact allergy (induced by Mycolog) in children aged 6 weeks to 1 year, one case of nickel allergy due to earrings in a 4-week-old girl, neomycin as a cause of an allergic contact dermatitis on the penis of a 5-week-old boy who was circumcised, balsam of Peru in an ointment to treat diaper rash in an 8-week-old girl (who had received this treatment for only 1 week), and finally nickel in underwear causing a row of contact dermatitis lesions on the back of a 7-month-old boy. Seidenari [53] also described three remarkable contact allergy cases (two of them connubial) in babies: nickel present in the bars of a crib caused dyshidrosis of the hands and feet in a 12-month-old atopic boy; nickel in his mother's jewelry (she wore rings on all her fingers) exacerbated the atopic eczema of a 6-month-old boy; and *para*-phenylenediamine in her mother's dyed hair caused hand dermatitis in a 12-month-old girl. Aihara and Ikezawa [54] have reported a neonate who was allergic to a mydriatic agent used for fundoscopy (the responsible allergen was not detected).

Moreover, several cases of contact allergy in infants have been reported due to the rubber anti-leaking system in their diapers [55–57].

43

Recently, we diagnosed a contact allergy to the electrodes used to monitor an infant for sudden death. An allergy to *para*-tertiary-butylphenol-formaldehyde (PTBPF) resin was found, but we were not able to confirm the presence of this allergen in the electrode.

43.2.6 Prevalence Related to Origin

The exposure of children to certain contact allergens varies throughout the world [8]. For example, in contrast to Europe, poison ivy (and other members of the Rhus family) is particularly apt at inducing sensitization in certain parts of North and South America [1, 8]. In Scandinavian countries, plant dermatitis in children is rare except for reactions to *Heracleum* spp. [3]. Exposure and subsequent sensitivity to neomycin also seems to vary geographically; for example, there is a high prevalence in Portugal [10], Italy [22], and certain areas in the USA such as Denver [9], as opposed to Philadelphia [58]. In contrast to Scandinavian countries [3], shoe dermatitis seems to be particularly common in the USA [59], mainly due to rubber [58]. In developing countries occupational allergy is more common in older children than in Western countries [37].

Regional variations in the type of clothing and living conditions clearly influence the allergen spectrum [15].

43.2.7 Prevalence in Relation to the Sensitization Source

Objects or materials common to the child's environment may give rise to some unusual allergen sources. Diapers [55–57], and, for example, with regard to allergic cheilitis and perioral dermatitis, sucked-on objects are not at all rare causes (also due to rubber allergens), particularly in the younger age group [60]. This also applies to mercurials [31, 59] present in vaccines and topical pharmaceuticals used to treat abrasions and infections of the skin. However, nickel [22, 31], cosmetic ingredients [8], and occupational allergens [5, 16, 37] are causes of allergy more in older children. The prevalence of the allergens found mainly depends on the exposure, which itself varies with the age of the population [30].

43.3 The Clinical Picture

The clinical characteristics of allergic contact dermatitis are, in general, the same in children as in adults.

Table 2. Correlation between the localization of the lesions and the nature of the allergens

Face:	Ingredients of topical pharmaceutical products (e.g., benzoyl peroxide), cosmetics [e.g., methyl(chloro)isothiazolinone], and perfume components; plants
Periorbital area:	Ophthalmic preparations; nickel, cobalt
Perioral area:	Stuck-on objects (rubber additives); nickel, cobalt, and palladium; flavoring agents (cinnamic aldehyde)
Ears:	Nickel and cobalt, eardrops
Neck:	Nickel
Trunk:	Clothing dyes, rubber additives, nickel (periumbilically), PTBP-resin (electrode), PPD and essential oils in temporary tattoos
Arms:	Cosmetics (e.g., sunscreens), aluminum (vaccines), plants, PPD and essential oils (temporary tattoos)
Wrists:	Nickel and cobalt, dichromate (leather watch-strap)
Hands and fingers:	Preservatives (cosmetics, play gels, Plasticine), nickel and cobalt, plants, rubber and resin components
Buttocks and thighs:	Aluminum (vaccines), plastic (toilet seat)
Diaper area:	Topical pharmaceutical (e.g., ethylenediamine, neomycin) and cosmetic products, rubber (or glue) in anti-leaking system from diapers
Legs:	Plants, orthopedic appliances (resins, such as PTBPF and epoxy)
Feet:	Shoe allergens (rubber additives, glues) (PTBP), dichromate, plants, topical pharmaceutical products

It is of the utmost importance to take a detailed history, in order to specify the environment of the child and of those taking care of it, and to examine thoroughly the topography of the lesions. The localization is often an indication of the allergen or allergens involved [8]. Based on data published in the literature, we compiled a list of allergens in relation to specific body sites (see Table 2).

Sometimes the clinical picture is unusual:

- A hypertrophic verrucous cheilitis due to the topical application of thimerosal used to treat fissures [61]
- A bullous dermatitis induced by a neomycin-containing finger bandage; patch tests were positive to neomycin, colophony, and thiuram mix [16]

- A "baboon syndrome" [62, 63] from mercury, due to the intake of erythromycin to treat an infection of the throat [64]
- An EEM-like eruption on the thighs spreading to the trunk after an initial contact eczematous reaction induced by a plant extract containing St John's wort [65], to a temporary henna tattoo [66], to disperse dyes in a 2 year old boy [67], to tea tree oil [68] as well as to mephenesin (own observation)
- A lichenoid contact dermatitis on the feet, hands, and buttocks lasting 6 years, due to topical aminoglycosides in which lichenoid positive patch tests were also obtained [69] (a papular pattern of allergic contact dermatitis does not seem to be rare, such as occurs with nickel [70]); this lichenoid pattern of reaction is also frequently seen in reactions to *p*-phenylene-diamine (PPD) in temporary tattoos [71]. Healing may be with depigmentation [72]
- Itching nodules and granulomas that may persist for months or even years at the injection site of vaccines due to a delayed reaction to aluminum in vaccines [73]
- A generalized nummular dermatitis in both a boy and a girl induced by application of an ethylenediamine-containing preparation to the groins and the feet, respectively [74]; a positive reaction to thimerosal was found in five atopic children (7–28 months old) with nummular eczema on the trunk, limbs and face [75]
- A generalized eczema occurred twice in an 18-month-old boy caused by sensitivity to phenoxyethanol used as a preservative in a DTP vaccine [76]; the third booster vaccine containing thimerosal as the preservative did not produce a reaction
- A systemic contact dermatitis in a 14-year-old boy caused by an orthodontic appliance that contained nickel [77]

43.4 Allergic Contact Dermatitis and Atopy

The association between atopy and contact allergy in children is a controversial subject [78]. The conclusions drawn differ largely according to the allergens investigated and whether the prevalence of contact allergy in atopic children or the prevalence of atopy in children suffering from allergic contact dermatitis children is being investigated [79].

Several authors were unable to detect differences between atopic and nonatopic subjects in this regard [22, 80, 81], but others have. Some authors were able to find a higher prevalence in atopic than in nonatopic children [11, 28, 82] and this was sometimes attributed to the greater permeability of irritated skin [11]. Others report the opposite [26, 29, 31, 47].

Nickel reactions are more often seen in atopics [70, 81, 83], and then mainly in girls [84], which reflects the greater importance of sex and ear piercing than atopy as such. The latter authors (in agreement with, for example, Pambor and coworkers [80]), stress the irritant properties of metals and particularly nickel on atopic skin, and, indeed, papulopustular patch test reactions are a frequent finding [79]. Dotterud and Falk [84] doubt that metal sensitivity is associated with atopy. First, there is the reduced cellular immunity of atopics: positive reactions are found more often in atopic children with moderate dermatitis than in those with severe atopic eczema [85, 86]; second, there is the greater permeability of diseased skin, particularly on the hands, which facilitates the penetration of allergens [85, 87].

Besides nickel, Oranje and co-workers [88] also found cobalt and balsam of Peru (*Myroxylon pereirae*) to be important allergens in an atopic child population; furthermore, they observed few reactions on patch testing with food.

Contact allergy to ingredients of topical medications are also common in atopic dermatitis patients [35, 78].

As with nonatopics, the prevalence of contact allergy was found to increase with age [86, 87].

Core Message

- Certain contactants are characteristic of children (Table 2), and may be responsible for unusual clinical presentations.

Core Message

- Positive reactions in atopics must be interpreted carefully, as atopic skin is readily irritated; this is especially the case for metals.

43.5 Patch Testing in Children

Patch testing is indicated not only when contact allergy is suspected, but also in cases of persistent eczema [20] on specific localizations, such as on the hands and the feet and around the mouth [32] and also in the umbilical region, particularly in atopics [79]. The latter group should certainly be tested when multiple exacerbations occur, even when they are treated, or when the dermatitis is asymmetrical [32].

Most authors agree that patch testing in children is safe [9, 18, 61, 89], the only problems being mainly technical due to the small patch test surface [18], hypermobility (which may result in loss of patch test materials), particularly in younger children [32], and the reluctance of some parents to allow patch testing [4, 32]. Mallory [90] gives the following instructions when testing children:

- Test in different sessions if the test area is very small
- Should the patches come off, ask the parents to report it and instruct them not to reapply them
- It may be necessary to use a stronger adhesive than usual, though this could be irritating [9]
- The application has to be performed as quickly as possible while the child is distracted
- Make a diagram of the tested allergens (this applies for adults, too)
- Inform the parents about the test procedure and the measures that may be taken to optimize the patch test conditions

The patch test concentrations have been discussed in detail in the literature. Some authors have recommended lower concentrations [3, 80, 91, 92], particularly with regard to specific allergens such as nickel and formaldehyde [6, 83], mercurials [61], potassium dichromate, MBT, and thiuram mix [52]. Irritancy problems have been reported with patch testing, especially in the younger age group [6, 9, 11, 21], while others use the same test concentrations as in adults [5, 15, 16, 26, 53, 81, 93]. Wahlberg and Goossens [94] critically reviewed studies on the prevalence of contact allergy, and found that very high prevalences are found in "healthy" children as compared with those found in adults. They suspect that a lot of those reactions might be irritant and therefore conclude that all patch test concentrations used in adults are not necessarily suitable for use in children, as was already suggested for metals by Roul and coworkers [36]. In dubious cases one might have to retest with a lower test concentration [79]. Moreover, as with patch testing in general, false-positive as well as false-negative reactions may occur [1, 49]. It is therefore important that the relevance of the tests are further investigated, if necessary, with a serial dilution test, repeated open application test (ROAT) or a usage test [95]. For marginal irritants such as dichromate, fragrance mix, formaldehyde, mercury compounds and carba mix in particular [94], repeated patch testing with standardized tests (such as TRUE Test) should be performed in order to demonstrate reproducibility and, if necessary, the concentration should be adapted. Johnke and coworkers [13] have already demonstrated that in infants 200 µg/cm² nickel sulfate produces many transient reactions (111/543), whereas reproducible tests were obtained only in 8.6% of the cases. They therefore favor a lower patch concentration for nickel in children.

Core Message

- Patch testing in children is safe, but false-positive reactions are possible. Particularly for children under the age of five, patch testing should only be performed if there is high suspicion by history and clinical picture.

43.6 The Most Frequent Allergens in Children

43.6.1 Metals

43.6.1.1 Nickel

Nickel is the most common allergen both in children and adults in Europe, as it is in many other parts of the world. In the general population, about 10% of females react to it, the prevalence being influenced by the increasing popularity of ear and other piercings [84]. Indeed, ear piercing along with atopy – the latter even in children between 4 and 17 months old [70, 96] – have been regarded as major risk factors for the development of nickel sensitization, especially in girls [84, 97]. Boys may also be affected though [98]. Rademaker and Forsyth [18] could not determine significant differences between boys and girls below the age of 12. Subumbilical and periumbilical, mostly papular reactions are also common and are frequently accompanied by an id-like spread [96, 99, 100].

Veien [101] attributes the high prevalence of nickel allergy in young females to the common habit of wearing cheap jewelry, to reduced suppressor activity correlated with their higher estrogen levels, and to higher skin permeability to nickel. Permeability could be increased by decreased iron levels associated with menarche, as iron is a competitive inhibitor in the skin and on the surface of Langerhans cells.

Nickel sensitization sources in children are numerous: jewelry, even when worn by the mother [53] and particularly earrings [49, 51] (stainless steel, even though silver- or gold-plated is not always "safe" in this regard [102]), metal buttons and snaps in underwear, identification bracelets, safety pins, zippers, jeans and belt buckles [90, 96, 99, 100], metal accessories on shoes, coins, metal toys, magnets, medallions, keys, door handles, and so on [51, 83]. Even bed rails have caused nickel contact allergy [53, 103]. Due to restrictions on the concentration of nickel allowed in jewelry, advised by the authorities in Europe in the beginning of the 1990s, a decline in the prevalence of nickel allergy has been registered in Denmark [104] and Germany [105]. In the USA, Byer et al [100] could only detect nickel in 10% of 74 pairs of jeans buckles, whereas the dimethylglyoxime test was positive in 25 of the 47 belts, indicating that this nickel source is more important for sensitization induction.

Orthodontic appliances may occasionally be at the origin of a nickel allergy, causing cheilitis, perioral eczema [77, 106, 107] and also stomatitis, sometimes associated with systemically induced dermatitis on the eyelids, fingers, ears, periorbital area [107], or more generalized reactions [77], even a severe deterioration of atopic dermatitis [108]. Van Hoogstraten et al [98] were able to show that wearing a dental apparatus before nickel skin contact has occurred may actually induce tolerance to this metal.

A low nickel diet might be useful in resistant nickel allergy cases [15].

43.6.1.2 Cobalt

Cobalt allergies are often found in association with nickel allergies in both adults and children [31]. Not only metallic objects but also certain plastic materials may release cobalt or cobalt salts and induce contact sensitivity. For example, Grimm [109] described the case of an 11-year-old boy who had suffered for 4-years from eczematous lesions at the site of his spectacle frames, on his wrist, and around his mouth. The dermatitis was attributed to cobalt present in the metallic part of his wristwatch, in the polyester resin-type plastics of the spectacle frames, and the ball-point pen which he habitually chewed on.

43.6.1.3 Potassium Dichromate

Leather seems to be the most important cause of chromium allergy; the examples published concern shoes (see below), a body splint [110], and a prayer strap in a 13-year-old Jewish boy [61]. Concomitant reactions to nickel have been observed [31].

43.6.1.4 Mercury

Contact allergy to mercurials is very common in children, particularly in countries where they are still widely used as antiseptics (for example mercurochrome), such as Spain [97, 111] and Italy [112]. Other sensitization sources for mercurials are other topically applied medicaments, such as eye-drops, depigmenting creams [111], pediculosis preparations [113], vaccines [114], as well as broken thermometers [63], amalgam fillings, contact lens solutions, and pesticides. Levy and coworkers [59] warn against the use of mercurials in medications because of their potential systemic toxicity, which may cause kidney damage, particularly when large skin surfaces are treated.

43.6.1.5 Aluminum

For aluminum, vaccines and occasionally also hyposensitization therapy in pollen allergy are reported as being the most important sensitization sources [73, 115–118]. Clinically, the reactions often present as long-lasting, pruritic, excoriated, subcutaneous nodules, occasionally accompanied by hypertrichosis [73, 119]. In many cases, the contact eczema is revealed by positive reactions to Finn chambers used in patch testing or to deodorants [115], eardrops [118], or even toothpaste [116] containing aluminum salts. Flare-ups of previous injection sites may be explained by the persistence of this metal in the skin [115]. The aluminum sensitivity is probably lost with time as this sensitivity is extremely rare in adults [120].

43.6.1.6 Palladium

This metal, shown to be an allergen in animals, is mainly present in orthodontic appliances and jewelry [121]. As with adults, most palladium-allergic children also react to nickel [31, 122], for which cross-sensitization seems to be the most plausible explanation.

43.6.1.7 Iron

There seems to be only one case report of iron contact allergy, which was caused by an orthopedic prosthesis in a 7-year-old boy [123], so this metal seems to be an extremely rare allergen.

43.6.1.8 Copper

According to a Viennese report, copper, present in dental amalgam, caused problems in children [44].

43.6.2 Pharmaceutical Products

Many topical pharmaceutical ingredients have been described as allergens in children and should certainly not be overlooked [124]. They include antibiotics, mainly neomycin [16, 49], which is often used in the treatment of otitis [58]. Leyden and Kligman [58], in contrast to Weston and coworkers [9], suggest that neomycin allergy is less frequently seen in children than in adults. Cross-reactivity with other aminoglycosides does occur [69]; antivirals such as tromantadine (own observations) and Zovirax, of which the responsible allergen could not be identified [125]; antihistamines such as dexchlorpheniramine maleate [126]; nonsteroidal anti-inflammatory agents such as fepradinol [127]; local anesthetics, particularly benzocaine [16], which often cross-reacts with other ester-type anesthetics [90] and also with permanent hair dyes and textile dyes, which may later cause problems due to their chemical relationship [49]. Even corticosteroid preparations may cause contact allergy in children [128], and not infrequently in atopics [129]. Tixocortol pivalate and budesonide may be used as markers in the standard series, but all topical preparations used by the child should be tested as well. Contact allergy to the new class of topical immunomodulatory drugs, especially for tacrolimus, has been reported recently. A provocation test was positive after 1 week for lesions in the face but only after 7 weeks when applied to the antecubital region. Patch tests were only positive after 5 days with tacrolimus 5% and 2.5% in ethanol, but not with Protopic ointment as is, nor with lower concentrations of tacrolimus. The authors suggest that the low percutaneous absorption through intact extrafacial skin is the reason for this delay in positive results and the need for high concentrations [130].

Other agents which have been reported include quinine present in a balsam used in the treatment of respiratory infections (the adult formulation was used and not the one for children which did not contain quinine [131]). Plant extracts may also be responsible for allergic reactions [65].

Certain topical medicaments are specifically used in older children, namely those used to treat acne such as benzoyl peroxide [1, 16].

An allergic dermatitis from the parenteral administration of vitamin K has been reported by Pigatto and coworkers [132].

Not only active principles but also other ingredients may be responsible for allergic reactions in children: emulsifiers and vehicle components, such as wool wax alcohols and derivatives, propyleneglycol and cetostearyl alcohol, as well as a specific ingredient of eardrops – triethanolamine oleyl polypeptide – are typical examples of this [133]. Sometimes, rarer allergens are involved such as laureth-4 [134], ethyl sebacate [128] and Tween 80 [135].

Ethylenediamine, used in Mycolog cream, has been widely used to treat various skin conditions, including diaper dermatitis [50, 74], and may cross-react with some antihistamines and aminophylline to induce severe systemic reactions [50]. This chemical is also used in ophthalmic solutions, insecticides, fungicides, epoxy hardeners, and rubber stabilizers [90].

Preservatives are not at all rare causes of allergic reactions in children [136]. Goulden and Goodfield [137] reported the case of a 12-year-old boy who even reacted to a methylprednisolone injection due to his sensitivity to the preservative myristyl picolinium chloride.

Thimerosal has attracted much attention in the literature, since it is frequently observed as an allergen in young children [138–140], and its inclusion in the standard series has been discussed [141, 142]. It is used as an antiseptic, disinfectant, and preservative agent for contact lens solutions, eyedrops, and vaccines, the last being regarded as the main sensitization source through contamination of the tip of the needle [138, 139, 143, 144]. According to Möller [141] and Aberer [144, 145], the many positive patch test reactions found are in most cases not relevant to the patient's skin condition.

A positive reaction to thimerosal should be taken into account with hyposensitization solutions, eyedrops, eye cosmetics, or contact-lens solutions [144], but does not seem to preclude future vaccinations, provided that they are administered intramuscularly. Furthermore, as this molecule contains two allergenic parts – mercury and thiosalicylic acid – one must consider cross-reactions with other mercurials and with the photoproduct of piroxicam, which is chemically related to the thiosalicylic acid part [114, 138, 146]. Efforts are now being made to omit thimerosal from commonly used vaccines [68].

Phenoxyethanol contact allergy has also been described in relation to a DTP vaccine [76].

Last but not least, adhesive tape can also be a cause of allergy due to colophony and thiuram derivatives [16]. Children may also be exposed to colophony in preparations to treat verrucae [120].

43.6.3 Cosmetics

The market for cosmetic products specially formulated for children is expanding and habits common for adults such as going to "beauty farms" are being adapted for this young age group. Consequently, one can expect cosmetics to become more important causes of contact allergy and they may become the most frequent cause of contact allergy in children [147]. At least one cosmetic or cosmetic ingredient gave a positive reaction in 30% of the children investigated.

Almost every ingredient may be responsible for cosmetic dermatitis. Conti [136] reviewed preservatives and found that 44% of the children reacting to chemicals such as formaldehyde and its releasers, parabens, methyl(chloro)isothiazolinone, Euxyl K400 (methyldibromoglutaronitrile and phenoxyethanol), and the antioxidant butylhydroxyanisole (BHA), were atopic (Fig. 1).

The use of cosmetic products in babies and small children, and particularly those containing balsam of Peru (*Myroxylon pereirae*), has been described as being the cause of a subsequent perfume allergy. Fisher [49, 50] has reported two such cases: one of a 4-month-old baby and another of an 11-year-old girl, both of whom became sensitized by the application of a balsam ointment in the diaper area. One later developed contact eczema from the mother's perfume and the other from a deodorant.

Fisher [60] further stated that children often become allergic to cosmetics used by the mother (or the

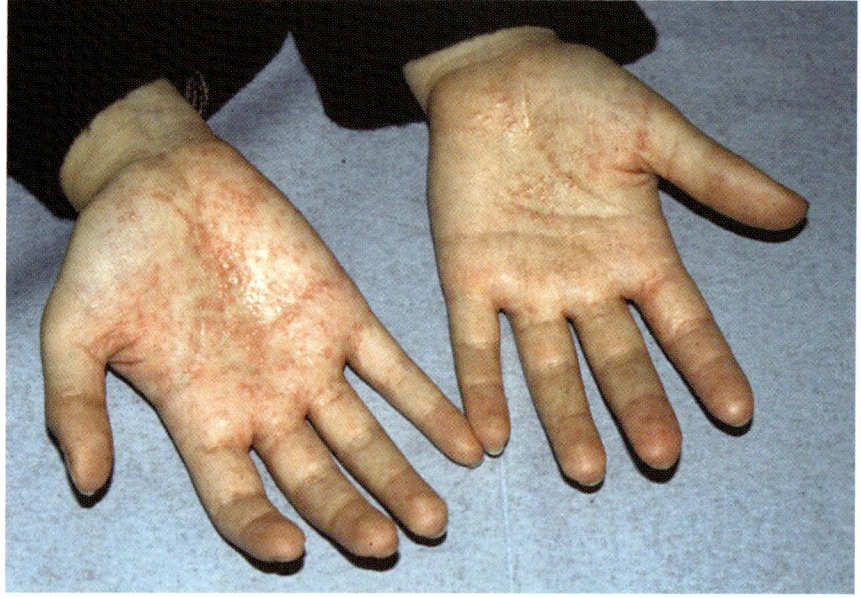

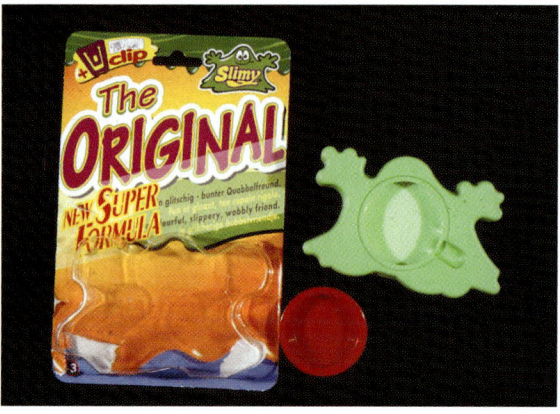

43

Fig. 1.
Allergic contact dermatitis from a play gel containing parabens

person taking care of them). In a 7-year-old girl with allergy to cinnamic aldehyde (cinnamal), cheilitis and perioral dermatitis were caused by the mother's lipstick that was left after she kissed her. The localizations often involved seem to be the forehead and the cheeks, with perfume, lipstick, hairspray, or nail lacquer as the responsible agents. A PPD allergy induced by the mother's dyed hair was observed in a 12-month-old girl [53].

However, children often use cosmetic products themselves, even though this may not always be revealed immediately! An example of "ectopic" dermatitis, localized unilaterally on the face and neck, due to surreptitious use of the mother's nail lacquer illustrates this [61].

Although guidelines for the maximum concentration of preservatives and fragrances in cosmetics have been provided [68], it has been demonstrated that cosmetic toys may contain much higher concentrations of fragrance [148]. No extra safety requirements for those products intended for children are required [120].

Contact allergy to the sunscreen agents 4-methylbenzylidene camphor, isopropyl dibenzoylmethane, and 2-ethylhexyl methoxycinnamate has been described in an 18-month-old boy [149]. Shah and coworkers [32] reported two sunscreen agents as being the cause of photoallergic contact dermatitis. But ingredients other than the sunscreen may also be responsible, such as triethanolamine used as an emulsifier [150], or recently, polymers added to make formulations more water resistant, such as polyvinylpyrrolidone-1-triacontene copolymer [151].

43.6.4 Tattoos

The practice of temporary henna tattooing has gained popularity in Western youngsters, especially when on holiday. Whereas contact allergy to henna itself seems to be rare, in tourist areas additives are added to make the process proceed more rapidly and to obtain a darker pigment. PPD, coffee, oil of eucalyptus, mustard, clove, lemon juice, turpentine, tea and even fresh urine from camels or yaks are examples of such components [66, 71, 72, 152]. It has been demonstrated that the concentration of PPD in some of these tattoos is higher than that allowed for hair dyes [153], even although the use of diaminobenzene derivatives is forbidden in skin dyes [68].

Contact allergies to PPD, and less frequently to essential oils in temporary tattoos are increasingly reported in children [66, 71, 72, 152]. These allergies may have consequences for their future, as certain professions become risky (for instance hairdressing)

in the case of PPD allergy, and potential problems with dark tanned clothing or hair dyes may follow. Eczematous reactions are mostly seen at the site of the tattoo and they may be long-lasting. EEM-like [66] or lichenoid reactions [71] are also described. Moreover, some patients may develop depigmentation [71, 72] following the acute reaction, and this may persist for a period of several months up to over a year.

43.6.5 Toys

Preservatives in play gels have been described as causes of acute eczema on the hands; in the two cases, parabens were found to be the responsible allergens [154, 155]. Tosti [156], too, has described two girls who were sensitized by the preservatives methyl(chloro)isothiazolinone and 2-chloro-N-methylchloroacetamide in Plasticine.

Pevny and coworkers [16] observed a 14-year-old boy with hand eczema from a model kit, glue, and firearm accessories: positive patch tests were found with the plastic materials he had come into contact with and with benzoyl peroxide, p-tert-butyl catechol, and p-tert-butyl phenol (present in the glues), as well as to potassium dichromate in the gun oil.

Facial allergy due to contact with a cuddly toy [90] and from balloons (see below) has been described. An allergy to rubber from his basketball was also the cause of persistent hand eczema in a 9-year old boy [157].

Music playing may also provoke eczema: PPD used to stain the bow used to play the cello provoked eczematous lesions of the first three fingers of the right hand in an 11-year-old girl [158]. Colophony used as rosin for the bow or in the gripping powder used by gymnasts is also a possible allergen [120].

43.6.6 Rubber Items

Additives in the rubber of balloons may occasionally cause a facial dermatitis [2, 159], but they may also be responsible for dermatitis in elastic underwear, particularly when bleached [160, 161], in a ball causing persistent hand eczema [157], in rubber sponges used to apply cosmetics [161], and in gloves [159] (although a preservative in the glove, cetyl pyridinium chloride, may be an exceptional allergen as well [162]). As with balloons, for example, type I allergic reactions may also occur, sometimes associated with a type IV reaction, as was the case in a 6-year-old boy who had undergone multiple surgical operations and who reacted to both gloves and a rubber dam used in dentistry [163]. Moreover, contact urticaria syndrome induced by natural rubber latex proteins is a frequent finding in such children, those suffering from spina bifida being particularly susceptible in this regard.

A particular type of diaper dermatitis reminiscent of a cowboy's gunbelt holsters (hence the term "-Lucky Luke") was reported by Roul et al [55, 56] (Fig. 2). The reaction was provoked by the rubber parts used for the new anti-leaking system in these diapers. The rubber parts were positive in all children and in some MBT, cyclohexyl thiophthalimide [57], and PTBP resin were probably present in the glue.

Rubber additives are also the main allergens responsible for shoe dermatitis (see below).

Thiurams, mercapto chemicals and less commonly carbamates are the responsible allergens in rubber allergy in children; thiourea derivatives in neoprene may also be the cause in for example goggles [172], trainers [120] and diving suits (own case). Polyurethane is usually tolerated and IPPD used in industrial rubbers is unlikely to be the cause [120].

43.6.7 Shoes and Clothes

Shoe dermatitis generally affects the back of the feet (Fig. 3). Mercaptobenzothiazole and thiuram derivatives, which are present not only in rubber shoes but

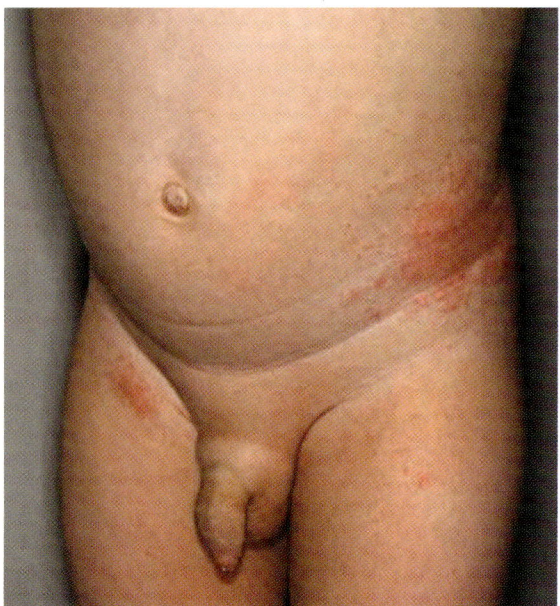

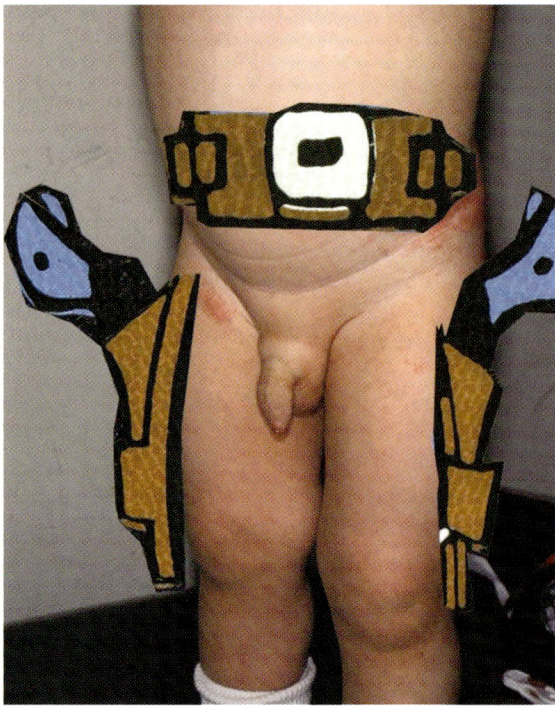

Fig. 2. "Lucky Luke" dermatitis from rubber derivatives in diapers

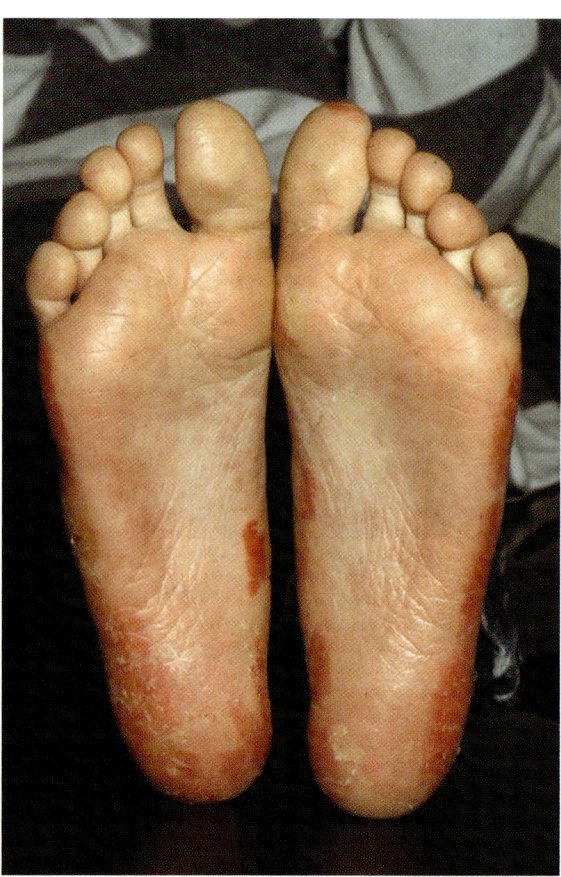

Fig. 3. Shoe dermatitis due to thiuram derivatives in an atopic child, complicated by a corticosteroid (triamcinolone-acetonide) contact allergy

43

also in certain glues [15, 124, 164], are important shoe allergens. Other potential culprits are PPD, which is also a possible dye allergen in socks [165], PPD derivatives such as diaminodiphenylmethane [164], and chromates [140, 166]. Trevistan and Kokelj [140] also consider dodecylmercaptane and thimerosal, used as a preservative in leather or leather cream, to be relevant shoe allergens. Topical medication was the most frequent cause of foot dermatitis in a retrospective study by Shackelford and Belsito [167], the allergens of which persist in shoe material for a long time. On the other hand, shoe allergens may persist in cotton socks even when they are washed.

When only the soles of the feet are affected, especially the first toe and forefoot, particularly in atopics, juvenile plantar dermatosis is more likely.

In Italy, 51 (4.6%) out of 1098 children tested positive to one or more disperse dyes used in synthetic clothes and especially to disperse yellow 3 and disperse orange 3. As only 17% of these children also were positive to PPD in the standard series, the authors suggest adding disperse dyes to the standard series [168].

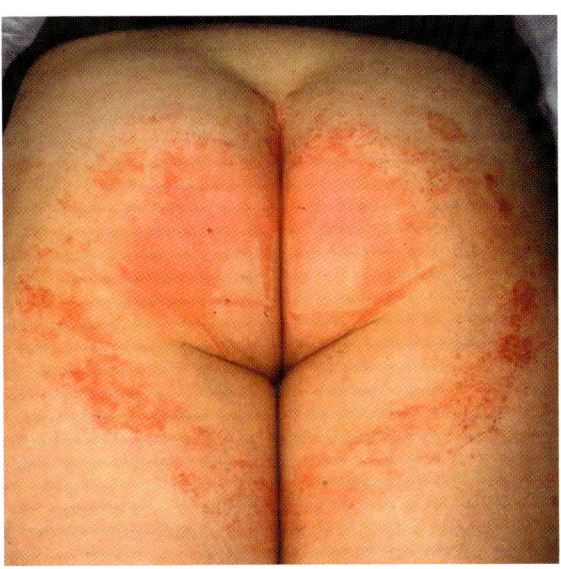

Fig. 4. Allergic contact dermatitis from plastic toilet seat (presence of *para*-tertiary-butylphenol-formaldehyde (*PTBPF*) resin to which the child reacted upon patch testing, however, not confirmed)

43.6.8 Plastic Materials and Resins

Plastic toys as well as glues have been described as typical allergen sources for children [16] (see above). *para*-Tertiary-butylphenol-formaldehyde (PTBPF) resin is the most frequently used phenol-formaldehyde (PF) resin and is mainly used in neoprene-type adhesives and all-purpose glues.

Vincenzi and coworkers [169] reported the case of an adolescent with a linear vesicular dermatitis on the left leg caused by a glue in a knee-guard. There were positive patch tests to PTBPF and PF resins. Shono and coworkers [170] observed four adolescents who reacted to these resins in an adhesive tape used for ankle support. One of them also reacted to sports shoes. It was also reported to be the cause of contact dermatitis to a limb prosthesis in a 5 year old boy [171], and is possibly used as a glue for electrodes to monitor sudden death in infants (personal observation). Phenol-formaldehyde resin and benzoyl peroxide were reported as the cause of contact allergy to swimming goggles in a 12-year old girl; dibutylthiourea in black neoprene rubber may also be the cause [172].

Epoxy resin was the cause of a dermatitis due to the glue used to fix kneepads in trousers [90] as well as an allergy to an identification band [51].

Not just the resins themselves, but also preservatives, such as benzalkonium chloride in plaster of Paris, may cause contact allergy [173].

43.6.9 Plants

Children often come into contact with plants while playing and do not know about their potential irritant, phototoxic (such as in giant hogweed) or allergenic effects. In a review on plant dermatitis in Australia [174], children as well as gardeners were considered at risk.

43.6.9.1 Poison Ivy, Poison Oak, Poison Sumac

Plants belonging to the Rhus family are the ones most often involved in allergic contact dermatitis among children living in northern California. Exposure can be direct or indirect (such as transfer of the allergen via pets), the latter being more difficult to diagnose [1]. Mallory [90] reports the possible presence of black spots on the skin caused by the oleoresin in poison ivy as a clue to its diagnosis.

43.6.9.2 *Toxicodendron succedaneum* (Rhus Tree)

Ten cases of phytophotodermatitis from *Toxicodendron succedaneum* in children under the age of 15 were reported in New Zealand. Generally, the face was involved [175].

43.6.9.3 *Urtica urens*

A combined contact urticarial and contact eczematous reaction on the hands and arms has been described by Edwards [176].

43.6.9.4 Asteraceae or Compositae

Wakelin and coworkers [177] reported the case of an atopic boy with exacerbations of his chronic eczema on the palmar side of his right, dominant hand. Patch tests revealed positivity to sesquiterpene lactones and to chrysanthemums, daisies, and dandelions, some of which he fed his rabbits.

Commens and coworkers [178] discussed the problem of Bindii (*Soliva pterosperma*) dermatitis, which is most often located on the palms, soles, knees and elbows, and tends to occur in Australian children (mainly boys who play sports) in the spring and early summer. The persistence for several months of erythematous papules, and sometimes also squamous and pustular lesions, has been ascribed to a residue of the allergenic seed in the skin. The differential diagnoses include dermatitis herpetiformis.

43.6.9.5 Lichens

Wood and Rademaker [179] reported a facial dermatitis in an 8-year old atopic girl, which occurred whenever she climbed trees. Patch testing was positive to lichens and usnic acid, thus indicating *Parmelia* spp. as the sensitization source.

43.6.9.6 Gingko Fruit

Squashing the fruit of *Gingko biloba* or using it as marbles has been reported as a cause of allergic contact dermatitis in children in France [180].

43.6.9.7 *Dioscorea batatas* Decaisne

Kubo and coworkers [181] described the case of a 9-year-old girl who had accidentally touched her cheek with the rasped root of this plant, which resulted in the development of both an irritant and an allergic contact dermatitis.

43.6.9.8 Protein Contact Dermatitis

Oat-containing moisturizers are used for maintenance therapy in atopic dermatitis. Although allergic reactions to these products are rare, a protein contact dermatitis to avena extract has been reported by Pazzaglia and co-workers [182].

43.6.9.9 Various Plant Materials

Fisher [60] has reported the occurrence of allergic reactions due to the presence of various plant components or extracts in topically applied products. Moreover, as the use of herbal preparations is dramatically increasing, contact allergy to "natural" ingredients such as tea tree oil, especially when photoaged (sun degraded), *Calendula officinalis*, and so on, is becoming more frequent [68].

43.6.10 Occupational Allergens

Among adolescents, certain occupational activities are likely to induce sensitization [23], particularly in hairdressers and construction workers [17, 29] and to a lesser extent in metal workers [17].

Pre-employment patch testing is not recommended, although some authors advocate it, particularly with regard to metal allergy [183].

However, children like to help adults and this may also produce problems, as in the case reported by Corazza and coworkers [184], who reacted to methylchloroisothiazolinone in a beeswax used to polish old wooden furniture.

Core Message

■ Metals, ingredients of pharmaceutical products or cosmetics, rubber additives (in shoes, toys, diapers, sports equipment, and so on), plastics, resins (including those used in glues, orthopedic devices), and plants are allergens in children. In adolescents, sensitization via temporary tattoos or occupational allergens are also possible.

43

43.7 Proposal for a Shortened Standard Series for Children

In view of the lack of chemical exposure of children compared to that of adults and the smaller patch test area, especially with younger children, Vigan [185] and Brasch and Geier [31] proposed testing with an abbreviated standard patch test series of 16 allergens. This was based on the results of four studies [17, 18, 23, 140]. Roul and coworkers [36] also suggest reducing the number of tests: in children up to 6 years old a series of 17 allergens, and in older children a restricted European standard series of 29 allergens. These tests have to be completed with allergens depending on the symptoms and localization of the dermatitis.

A multicenter retrospective study performed by the *Réseau de Vigilance en Dermato-Allergologie* (Revidal) created by the *Groupe d'Etudes et de Recherche en Dermato-Allergologie* (GERDA, France) examined the patch test results of 959 children below the age of 15 tested at 11 different centers from 1995 to 1997. The purpose of this study was mainly to determine the usefulness of standard allergens in children.

The following ten allergens were tested in all centers: potassium dichromate, neomycin, thiuram mix, formaldehyde, colophony, balsam of Peru, paraben mix, woolwax alcohols, fragrance mix, and nickel sulfate. Other standard allergens were often tested too: PPD, cobalt chloride, benzocaine, chinoform, IPPD, mercapto mix, mercaptobenzothiazole, PTBP-FR, epoxy resin, methyl(chloro)isothiazolinone, quaternium-15, sesquiterpene lactone mix, and even primin.

The results [186] were as follows:

- Primine: no reactions
- Benzocaine, chinoform, IPPD, epoxy resin, quaternium-15, sesquiterpene lactone mix: <1%
- All other allergens: >1% of the patients tested.

This argues for the inclusion of PPD, cobalt chloride, mercapto mix, mercaptobenzothiazole, PTBP resin, and methyl(chloro)isothiazolinone in the standard series, because reactions to them occurred in more than 1% of patients tested.

IPPD and sesquiterpene lactone mix can be excluded, which reduces the series to 16 standard allergens (Table 3). In cases where corticosteroids have been used, testing with corticosteroid allergy markers, tixocortol pivalate 0.1% pet. and budesonide

Table 3. Suggested abbreviated standard patch test series for children

1.	Potassium dichromate	0.5% pet.
2.	Neomycin	20% pet.
3.	Thiuram mix	1% pet.
4.	PPD-free base	1% pet.
5.	Cobalt chloride	1% pet.
6.	Formaldehyde	1% aq.
7.	Colophony (colophonium)	20% pet.
8.	Balsam of Peru (*Myroxylon pereirae*)	25% pet.
9.	Woolwax alcohols (lanolin alcohol)	30% pet.
10.	Mercapto mix	2% pet.
11.	Paraben mix	16% pet.
12.	PTBP-FR	1% pet.
13.	Fragrance mix	8% pet.
14.	Nickel sulfate	5% pet.
15.	Chloromethyl- and methyl-isothiazolinone	0.01% aq.
16.	Mercaptobenzothiazole	2% pet.

0.1% pet. (besides the corticosteroids used by the patient) is indicated. Of course, according to the specific history and chemical environment of the patient, other substances should also be tested.

Core Message

- In children, an abbreviated standard series, supplemented with allergens suggested by the history, should be tested.

43.8 Conclusions

Contact allergy in children is more frequent than previously recognized. In an unselected population, for instance one consisting of schoolchildren, the prevalence is about 20%, while in a selected population (children suspected of contact allergy or suffering from atopic or other types of dermatitis) the prevalence is found to be variable, for example related to geographical origin, with a mean of 40%.

Immunological differences between children (especially neonates) and adults do exist, but their impact on the clinical development of contact allergy is still unknown. Although allergic contact dermatitis has occasionally been observed in neonates, it is generally agreed that susceptibility to contact sensitization and certainly also exposure to environmental allergens increase with the child's age.

Whether allergic contact dermatitis is more or less frequently associated with atopy is still a matter of discussion. On the one hand, there is the reduced Th1 response in acute atopic eczema, so atopics are less likely to develop contact allergy; on the other hand, the damaged skin barrier facilitates allergen penetration. The possibility of allergic contact dermatitis in atopic children must be considered, particularly if the distribution of the lesions is asymmetrical, when the dermatitis is located umbilically (nickel!), and when the dermatitis persists when being treated.

As with adults, the history and localization of the dermatitis are crucial for the diagnosis of allergic contact dermatitis, though certain contactants and/or habits that are characteristic of the child or the adolescent may be responsible for unusual clinical presentations.

Patch testing in children is safe; most authors think that irritant reactions are not frequently observed (except in atopics, particularly with metals) and that the same patch test concentrations as used in adults can be applied. However, the possibility of false-positive and false-negative reactions has to be considered and, if there is doubt, lower patch test concentrations should be tested later on.

Due to reduced test surface area, diminished environmental exposure to certain allergens and particularly hypermobility of young children, testing with an abbreviated standard series is recommended.

The most important allergens observed in this population are metals such as nickel (sometimes associated with cobalt), particularly in girls, which is attributed to the popularity of cheap jewelry. The extent to which hormonal factors play a role is still a matter of discussion. Mercury and its derivatives are still used as antiseptic agents in some countries, but the allergic reactions observed to them, even in young children, are often not clinically relevant. This is particularly true for thimerosal, for which vaccines have been regarded as the main sensitization source. However, such an allergy does not seem to preclude future vaccinations, provided the tip of the needle is not contaminated and the injection is administered intramuscularly.

Other allergens identified in children mainly concern ingredients of pharmaceutical products and cosmetics (sometimes via another member of the household), rubber derivatives, which are often responsible for shoe or diaper dermatitis, resins, and plants. Certain occupational allergens (such as those associated with hairdressing, construction, metalworking) are found in adolescents.

Suggested Reading

Brasch J, Geier J (1997) Patch test results in schoolchildren. Contact Dermatitis 37:286–293

In a retrospective study in 22 German centers of the German Contact Dermatitis Research Group, the results from patch tests in children 6–15 years of age were analyzed. The allergens were related to sex and age. Nickel sulfate was the most important allergen (positive in 15.9% of all children), especially in older girls. Mercury components were the second most important group (thimerosal positive in 11.3% of all children tested), and especially important in the younger age group (6–13 years); this was followed by fragrance allergens (fragrance mix positive in 8.2% of all children tested). For screening purposes a shortened standard series comprising nickel, cobalt, dichromate, thimerosal, fragrance-allergens, wool wax alcohols, amerchol and methylchloro- and methylisothiazolinone, all of which produced positive tests in at least 1% of the tested children, was suggested.

Wahlberg JE, Goossens A (2001) Use of patch test concentrations for adults in children and their influence on test reactivity. Occup Environ Dermatol 49:97–101

A comparison between positive patch test results obtained in healthy children with non-eczematous dermatoses and those obtained in adults gave much higher percentages in children than in adults, which indicates that contact allergy was over-diagnosed in children. The authors favored the use of reduced test concentrations in children for allergens, such as potassium dichromate, nickel sulfate, formaldehyde, and possibly also for rubber chemicals. A "wish list" for improving patch testing in children includes: more studies in healthy children, comparison with in vitro tests, defined dosage and dilution series studies, as well as repeated patch testing in order to demonstrate reproducibility. For individual children, serial dilution tests, repeated testing, use tests (though difficult in children), but above all a clinical follow-up are useful if doubt exists about the patch test results.

References

1. Epstein E (1971) Contact dermatitis in children. Pediatr Clin North Am 18:839–852
2. Cronin E (1980) Contact dermatitis. Churchill Livingstone, Edinburgh, pp 20–21
3. Hjorth N (1981) Contact dermatitis in children. Acta Derm Venerol (Stockh) 95:36–39
4. Tennstedt D, Lachapelle JM (1987) Eczéma de contact allergique chez l´enfant. Bull Actual Thérap 32:3223–3228
5. Pevny I, Brennenstuhl M, Razinskas G (1984) Patch testing in children (1). Contact Dermatitis 11:201–206
6. Marcussen PV (1963) Primary irritant patch-test reactions in children. Arch Dermatol 87:378–382
7. Mortz CG, Andersen KE (1999) Allergic contact dermatitis in children and adolescents. Contact Dermatitis 41:121–130
8. Weston WL, Weston JA (1984) Allergic contact dermatitis in children. Am J Dis Child 138:932–936
9. Weston WL, Weston JA, Kinoshita J, Kloepfer S, Carreon L, Toth S, Bullard D, Harper K, Martinez S (1986) Prevalence of positive epicutaneous tests among infants, children, and adolescents. Pediatrics 78:1070–1074

10. Barros MA, Baptista A, Correia TM, Azevedo F (1991) Patch testing in children: a study of 562 schoolchildren. Contact Dermatitis 25:156–159

11. Dotterud LK, Falk ES (1995) Contact allergy in relation to hand eczema and atopic diseases in north Norwegian schoolchildren. Acta Paediat 84:402–406

12. Bruckner AL, Weston WL, Morelli JG (2000) Does sensitization to contact allergens begin in infancy? Pediatrics 105:3–9

13. Johnke H, Norberg LA, Vach W, Bindslev-Jensen C, Host A, Andersen KE (2004) Patch test reactivity to nickel sulphate and fragrance mix in unselected children. Contact Dermatitis 50:131

14. Mortz CG, Lauritsen JM, Bindslev-Jensen C, Andersen KE (2001) Prevalence of atopic dermatitis, asthma, allergic rhinitis, and hand and contact dermatitis in adolescents. The Odense Adolescence Cohort Study on Atopic Diseases and Dermatitis. Br J Dermatol 144:523–532

15. Veien NK, Hattel T, Justesen O, Norholm A (1982) Contact dermatitis in children. Contact Dermatitis 8:373–375

16. Pevny I, Brennenstuhl M, Razinskas G (1984) Patch testing in children (2). Contact Dermatitis 11:302–310

17. Romaguera C, Alomar A, Camarasa JMG, Garcia Bravo B, Garcia Perez A, Grimalt F, Guerra P, Lopez Gorretcher B, Martin Pascual A, Miranda A, Moran M, Pena ML (1985) Contact dermatitis in children. Contact Dermatitis 12:283–284

18. Rademaker M, Forsyth A (1989) Contact dermatitis in children. Contact Dermatitis 20:104–107

19. Kuiters GR, Smitt JH, Cohen EB, Bos JD (1989) Allergic contact dermatitis in children and young adults. Arch Dermatol 125:1531–1533

20. Balato N, Lembo G, Patruno CC, Ayala F (1989) Patch testing in children. Contact Dermatitis 20:305–307

21. Pambor M, Krüger G, Winkler S (1992) Results of patch testing in children. Contact Dermatitis 27:326–328

22. Ayala F, Balato N, Lembo G, Patruno C, Tosti A, Schena D, Pigatto P, Angelini G, Lisi P, Rafanelli A (1992) A multicentre study of contact sensitization in children. Contact Dermatitis 26:307–310

23. Gonçalo S, Gonçalo M, Azenha A, Barros MA, Sousa Bastos A, Brandao FM, Faria A, Marques MSJ, Pecegueiro M, Rodrigues JB, Salgueiro E, Torres V (1992) Allergic contact dermatitis in children. Contact Dermatitis 26:112–115

24. Sevila A, Romaguera C, Vilaplana J, Botella R (1994) Contact dermatitis in children. Contact Dermatitis 30:292–294

25. Motolese A, Manzini BM, Donini M (1995) Patch testing in infants. Am J Contact Dermat 6:153–156

26. Stables GI, Forsyth A, Lever RS (1996) Patch testing in children. Contact Dermatitis 34:341–344

27. Rudzki E, Rebandel P (1996) Contact dermatitis in children. Contact Dermatitis 34:66–67

28. Wilkowska A, Grubska-Suchanek E, Karwacka I, Szarmach H (1996) Contact allergy in children. Cutis 58:176–180

29. Katsarou A, Koufou V, Armenaka M, Kalogeromitros D, Papanayotou G, Vareltzidis (1996) Patch tests in children: a review of 14 years experience. Contact Dermatitis 34:70–71

30. Wantke F, Hemmer W, Jarisch R, Götz M (1996) Patch test reactions in children, adults and the elderly. Contact Dermatitis 34:316–319

31. Brasch J, Geier J (1997) Patch test results in schoolchildren. Contact Dermatitis 37:286–293

32. Shah M, Lewis FM, Gawkrodger DJ (1997) Patch testing in children and adolescents: five years' experience and follow-up. J Am Acad Dermatol 37:964–968

33. Manzini BM, Ferdani G, Simonetti V, Donini M, Seidenari S. (1998) Contact sensitization in children. Pediatr Dermatol 15:12–17

34. Romaguera C, Vilaplana J (1998) Contact dermatitis in children: 6 years experience (1992–1997). Contact Dermatitis 39:277–280

35. Giordano-Labadie F, Rancé F, Pellegrin F, Bazex J, Dutau G, Schwarze HP (1999) Prevalence of contact allergy in children with atopic dermatitis: results of a prospective study of 137 cases. Contact Dermatitis 40:192–195

36. Roul S, Ducombs G, Taïeb A (1999) Usefulness of the European standard series for patch testing in children. A 3-year single-centre study of 337 patients. Contact Dermatitis 40:232–235

37. Duarte I, Lazzarini R, Kobata CM (2003) Contact dermatitis in adolescents. Am J Contact Dermat 14:200–204

38. Pambor M, Krüger G, Winkler S (1991) Results of patch testing in children. Contact Dermatitis 27:326–328

39. Björkstén B (1997) The environment and sensitisation to allergens in early childhood. Pediatr Allergy Immunol 8 [Suppl 10]:32–39

40. Walton S, Nayagam AT, Keczkes K (1986) Age and sex prevalence of allergic contact dermatitis. Contact Dermatitis 15:136–139

41. Walker FB, Smith PD, Maibach HI (1967) Genetic factors in human allergic contact dermatitis. Int Arch Allergy 32:453–462

42. Hawes GE, Struyk L, van den Elsen PJ (1993) Differential usage of T-cell receptor V gene segments in CD4+ and CD8+ subsets of T lymphocytes in monozygotic twins. J Immunol 150:2033–2045

43. Thestrup-Pedersen K (1997) Contact allergy in monozygous twins. Contact Dermatitis 36:52–53

44. Wöhrl S, Hemmer W, Focke M, Götz M, Jarisch R (2003) Patch testing in children, adults and the elderly: influence of age and sex on sensitization patterns. Pediatr Dermatol 20:119–123

45. Kwangsukstith C, Maibach HI (1995) Effect of age and sex on the induction and elicitation of allergic contact dermatitis. Contact Dermatitis 33:289–298

46. Meneghini CL (1995) Contact dermatitis in children. In: Rycroft RJG, Menné T, Frosch PJ (eds) Textbook of Contact Dermatitis. Springer, Berlin Heidelberg New York, pp 403–412

47. Uhr JW, Dancis J, Neumann CG (1960) Delayed-type hypersensitivity in premature neonatal humans. Nature 187:1130–1131

48. Epstein WL (1961) Contact-type delayed hypersensitivity in infants and children: induction of Rhus sensitivity. Pediatrics 27:51–53

49. Fisher AA (1985) Allergic contact dermatitis in early infancy. Cutis 35:315–316

50. Fisher AA (1990) Perfume dermatitis in children sensitized to balsam of Peru in topical agents. Cutis 45:21–23

51. Fisher AA (1994) Allergic contact dermatitis in early infancy. Cutis 54:300–302

52. Fisher AA (1994) Patch testing in children including early infancy. Cutis 54:387–388

53. Seidenari S, Manzini BM, Motolese A (1992) Contact sensitization in infants: report of 3 cases. Contact Dermatitis 27:319–320

54. Aihara M, Ikezawa Z (1988) Neonatal allergic contact dermatitis. Contact Dermatitis 18:105

55. Roul S, Ducombs G, Léauté-Labrèze, Taïeb A (1998) "Lucky Luke" contact dermatitis due to rubber components of diapers. Contact Dermatitis 38:363–364

56. Roul S, Léauté-Labrèze C, Ducombs G, Taïeb A (1998) Eczéma de contact aux changes complets type «Lucky-luke»: un marquer de dermatite atopique? Ann Dermatol Venereol (Stockh) 125[Suppl 3]:3S74

57. Belhadjali H, Giordano-Labadie F, Rancé F, Bazex J (2001) "Lucky Luke" contact dermatitis from diapers: a new allergen? Contact Dermatitis 44:248

58. Leyden JJ, Kligman AM (1979) Contact dermatitis to neomycin sulfate. JAMA 242:1276–1278

59. Levy C, Hanau D, Foussereau J (1980) Contact dermatitis in children. Contact Dermatitis 6:260–262

60. Fisher AA (1995) Cosmetic dermatitis in childhood. Cutis 55:15–16

61. Fisher AA (1994) Allergic contact dermatitis and patch testing in childhood. Cutis 54:230–232

62. Andersen KE, Hjorth N, Menne T (1984) The baboon syndrome: systemically induced allergic contact dermatitis. Contact Dermatitis 10:97–100

63. Moreno-Ramirez D, Garcia-Bravo B, Rodriguez Pichardo A, Peral Rubio F, Camacho Martinez F (2004) Baboon syndrome in childhood: easy to avoid, easy to diagnose, but the problem continues. Pediatr Dermatol 21:250–253

64. Goossens C, Sass U, Song M (1997) Baboon syndrome. Dermatology 194:421–422

65. Torinuki W (1990) Generalized erythema-multiforme-like eruption following allergic contact dermatitis. Contact Dermatitis 23:202–203

66. Jappe U, Hausen BM, Petzoldt D (2001) Erythema-multiforme-like eruption and depigmentation following allergic contact dermatitis from a paint-on henna tattoo, due to para-phenylenediamine contact hypersensitivity. Contact Dermatitis 45:249–250

67. Baldari U, Alessandrini F, Raccagni AA (1999). Diffuse erythema multiforme-like contact dermatitis caused by disperse blue 124 in a 2 year old child. J Eur Acad Dermatol Venerol 12:180–181

68. Kütting B, Brehler R, Traupe H (2004) Allergic contact dermatitis in children – strategies of prevention and risk management. Eur J Dermatol 14:80–85

69. Lembo G, Balato N, Patruno C, Pini D, Ayala F (1987) Lichenoid contact dermatitis due to aminoglycoside antibiotics. Contact Dermatitis 17:122–123

70. Ho VC, Johnston MM (1986) Nickel dermatitis in infants. Contact Dermatitis 15:270–273

71. Schultz E, Mahler V (2002) Prolonged lichenoid reaction and cross-sensitivity to para-substituted amino-compounds due to temporary henna tattoo. Int J Dermatol 41:301–303

72. Bowling JC, Groves R (2002) Clinical picture: an unexpected tattoo. Lancet 23:649

73. Bergfors E, Trollfors B, Inerot A (2003) Unexpectedly high prevalence of persistent itching nodules and delayed hypersensitivity to aluminium in children after the use of adsorbed vaccines from a single manufacturer. Vaccine 22:64–69

74. Caraffini S, Lisi P (1987) Nummular dermatitis-like eruption from ethylenediamine hydrochloride in 2 children. Contact Dermatitis 17:313–314

75. Patrizi A, Rizzoli L, Vincenzi C, Trevisi P, Tosti A (1999) Sensitisation to thimerosal in atopic children. Contact Dermatitis 40:94–97

76. Vogt T, Landthaler M, Stolz W (1998) Generalized eczema in an 18-month-old boy due to phenoxyethanol in DPT vaccine. Contact Dermatitis 38:50–51

77. Kerosuo H, Kanerva L (1997) Systemic contact dermatitis caused by nickel in a stainless steel orthodontic appliance. Contact Dermatitis 36:112–113

78. Akhavan A, Cohen SR (2003) The relationship between atopic dermatitis and contact dermatitis. Clin Dermatol 21:158–162

79. Cohen PR, Cardullo AC, Ruszkowski AM, DeLeo VA (1990) Allergic contact dermatitis to nickel in children with atopic dermatitis. Ann Allergy 65:73–79

80. Pambor M, Winkler S, Bloch Y (1991) Allergic contact dermatitis in children. Contact Dermatitis 24:72–74

81. Motolese A, Manzini BM, Donini M (1995) Patch testing in infants. Am J Contact Dermat 6:153–156

82. De la Cuadra J, Sanz J, Martorell A (1990) Prevalence of positive epicutaneous tests in atopic and non-atopic children without dermatitis. Contact Dermatitis 23:242–243

83. Fisher AA (1991) Nickel dermatitis in children. Cutis 47:19–21

84. Dotterud LK, Falk ES (1994) Metal allergy in north Norwegian schoolchildren and its relationship with ear piercing and atopy. Contact Dermatitis 31:308–313

85. Rystedt I (1985) Contact sensitivity in adults with atopic dermatitis in childhood. Contact Dermatitis 13:1–8

86. Guillet MH, Guillet G (1985) Enquête allergologique chez 251 malades atteints de dermatite atopique modérée ou sévère. Ann Dermatol Venereol (Stockh) 123:157–164

87. Lisi P, Simonetti S (1985) Contact sensitivity in children and adults with atopic dermatitis – a chronological study. Dermatologica 171:1–7

88. Oranje AP, Bruynzeel DP, Stenveld HJ, Dieges PH (1994) Immediate- and delayed-type contact hypersensitivity in children older than 5 years with atopic dermatitis: a pilot study comparing different tests. Pediatr Dermatol 11:209–215

89. Weston WL (1997) Contact dermatitis in children. Curr Opin Pediatr 9:372–376

90. Mallory SB (1995) The pediatric patient. In: Guin JD (ed) Practical contact dermatitis. McGraw-Hill, New York, pp 603–616

91. Röckl H, Müller E, Hiltermann W (1966) Zum Aussagewert positiver Epicutantests bei Säuglingen und Kindern. Arch Klein Exp Dermatol 226:407–419

92. Müller E, Röckl H (1975) Aussagewert von Läppchentests bei Kindern und Jugendlichen. Hautarzt 26:85–87

93. Rietschel RL, Rosenthal LE, North American Contact Dermatitis Group (1990) Standard patch test screening series used diagnostically in young and elderly patients. Am J Contact Dermat 1:53–55

94. Wahlberg JE, Goossens A (2001) Use of patch test concentrations for adults in children and their influence on test reactivity. Occup Environ Dermatol 49:97–101

95. Mortz CG, Andersen KE (1999) Allergic contact dermatitis in children and adolescents. Contact Dermatitis 41:121–130

96. Silverberg NB, Licht J, Friedler S, Sethi S, Laude TA (2002) Nickel contact hypersensitivity in children. Pediatr Dermatol 19:110–113

97. Camarasa JMG, Aspiolea F, Alomar A (1983) Patch tests to metals in children. Contact Dermatitis 9:157–158

98. Van Hoogstraten IMW, Andersen KE, von Blomberg BME, Boden D, Bruynzeel DP, Burrows D, Camarasa JG, Dooms-Goossens A, Kraal G, Lahti A, Menne T, Rycroft RJG, Shaw S, Todd D, Vreeburg KJJ, Wilkinson JD, Scheper RJ (1991) Reduced prevalence of nickel allergy upon oral nickel contact at an early age. Clin Exp Immunol 85:441–445

99. Sharma V, Beyer DJ, Paruthi S, Nopper AJ (2002) Prominent pruritic periumbilical papules: allergic contact dermatitis to nickel. Pediatr Dermatol 19:106–109

100. Byer TT, Morrell DS (2004) Periumbilical allergic contact dermatitis: blue jeans or belt buckles? Pediatr Dermatol 21:223–226

43

101. Veien NK, Hattel T, Justesen O, Norholm A (1986) Why do young girls become nickel sensitive? Contact Dermatitis 15:306–307

102. Räsänen L, Lehto M, Mustikka-Mäki UP (1993) Sensitization to nickel from stainless steel ear-piercing kits. Contact Dermatitis 28:292–294

103. Reiffers J, Hunziker N, Brun R, Vidmar B (1974) Sensibilisations cutanées allergiques peu communes. Dermatologica 148:285–291

104. Jensen CS, Lisby S, Baadsgaard O, Volund A, Menne T (2002) Decrease in nickel sensitization in a Danish schoolgirl population with ears pierced after implementation of the nickel-exposure regulation. Br J Dermatol 146:636–642

105. Schnuch A, Geier J, Lessmann H, Uter W; Informationsverbund Dermatologischer Kliniken (2003) Decrease in nickel sensitization in young patients – successful intervention through nickel exposure regulation? Results of the IVDK, 1992–2001. Hautartz 54:626–632

106. Temesvári E, Rácz I (1988) Nickel sensitivity from dental prosthesis. Contact Dermatitis 18:50–51

107. Veien NK, Borckhorst E, Hattel T, Laurberg G (1994) Stomatitis or systemically-induced contact dermatitis from metal wire in orthodontic materials. Contact Dermatitis 30:210–213

108. De Silva BD, Doherty VR (2000) Nickel allergy from orthodontic appliances. Contact Dermatitis 42:102–103

109. Grimm I (1971) Ungewöhnliche Form einer Kontaktdermatitis durch Kobalt bei einem 11 jährigen Kind. Berufsdermatosen 19:39–42

110. Thomas SE, Tucker WFG, Bleehen SS (1986) Body splint dermatitis in childhood. Contact Dermatitis 14:320–321

111. De la Cuadra J (1993) Sensibilisation cutanée au mercure et à ses composés. Ann Dermatol Venereol (Stockh) 120:37–42

112. Bardazzi F, Vassilopoulos A, Valenti R, Paganini P, Morelli R (1990) Mercurochrome-induced allergic contact dermatitis. Contact Dermatitis 23:381–382

113. Anonide A, Massone L (1996) Periorbital contact dermatitis due to yellow mercuric oxide. Contact Dermatitis 35:61

114. Audicana MT, Munoz D, Dolore del Pozo M, Fernandez E, Gastraminza G, Fernandez de Corres L (2002) Allergic contact dermatitis from mercury antiseptics and derivatives: study protocol of tolerance to intramuscular infections of thimerosal. Am J Contact Dermat 13:3–9

115. Veien NK, Hattel T, Justesen O, Norholm A (1986) Aluminium allergy. Contact Dermatitis 15:295–297

116. Veien NK, Hattel T, Laurberg (1993) Systemically aggravated contact dermatitis caused by aluminium in toothpaste. Contact Dermatitis 28:199–200

117. Kaaber K, Nielsen AO, Veien NK (1990) Aluminium sensitization following vaccination. Contact Dermatitis 23:256

118. O'Driscoll JB, Beck MB, Kesseler ME, Ford G (1991) Contact sensitivity to aluminium acetate eardrops. Contact Dermatitis 24:156–157

119. Kaaber K, Kerusuo H, Kullaa A, Kerusuo E (1992) Vaccination granulomas and aluminium allergy: course and prognostic factors. Contact Dermatitis 26:304–306

120. White IR (2000) Allergic contact dermatitis. In: Harper J, Oranje A, Prose N (eds) Textbook of pediatric dermatology, vol 1. Blackwell Science, Oxford, pp 287–294

121. Boman A, Wahlberg JE (1990) Experimental sensitization with palladium chloride in the guinea pig. Contact Dermatitis 23:256

122. Kanerva L, Kerusuo H, Kullaa A, Kerusuo E (1996) Allergic patch test reactions to palladium chloride in schoolchildren. Contact Dermatitis 34:39–42

123. Hemmer W, Focke M, Wantke F, Götz M, Jarisch R (1996) Contact hypersensitivity to iron. Contact Dermatitis 34:219–220

124. Cockayne SE, Shah M, Messenger AG, Gawkrodger DJ (1998) Foot dermatitis in children: causative allergens and follow-up. Contact Dermatitis 38:203–206

125. Vincenzi C, Peluso AM, Lameli N, Tosti A (1992) Allergic contact dermatitis caused by acyclovir. Am J Contact Dermat 3:105–107

126. Cusano F, Capozzi M, Errico G (1989) Contact dermatitis from dexchlorpheniramine. Contact Dermatitis 21:340

127. Gomez A, Martorell A, de la Cuadra J (1994) Allergic contact dermatitis from fepradinol in a child. Contact Dermatitis 30:44

128. Kabasawa Y, Kanzaki T (1990) Allergic contact dermatitis from ethyl sebacate. Contact Dermatitis 22:226

129. Morren MA, Dooms-Goossens A (1994) Corticosteroid allergy in children: a potential complication of atopic eczema. Eur J Dermatol 4:106–109

130. Shaw DW, Eichenfield LF, Shainhouse T, Maibach HI (2004) Allergic contact dermatitis from tacrolimus. J Am Acad Dermatol 50:962–965

131. Dias M, Conchon I, Vale T (1994) Allergic contact dermatitis from quinine. Contact Dermatitis 30:121–122

132. Pigatto PD, Bigardi A, Fumagalli M, Altomare GF, Riboldi A (1990) Allergic dermatitis from parenteral vitamin K. Contact Dermatitis 22:307–308

133. Balato N, Lembo G, Patruno C, Ayala F (1989) Allergic contact dermatitis from Cerumenex in a child. Contact Dermatitis 21:348–349

134. Svensson A (1988) Allergic contact dermatitis to laureth-4. Contact Dermatitis 18:113–114

135. Lucente P, Iorizzo M, Pazzaglia M (2000) Contact sensitivity to Tween 80 in a child. Contact Dermatitis 43:172

136. Conti A, Motolese A, Manzini BM, Seidenari S (1997) Contact sensitization to preservatives in children. Contact Dermatitis 37:35–36

137. Goulden V, Goodfield MJ (1995) Delayed hypersensitivity reaction to the preservative myristyl picolinium chloride. Contact Dermatitis 33:209–210

138. Osawa J, Kitamura K, Ikezawa Z (1991) A probable role for vaccines containing thimerosal in thimerosal hypersensitivity. Contact Dermatitis 24:178–182

139. Novak M, Kvicalova E, Friedländerova B (1986) Reactions to merthiolate in infants. Contact Dermatitis 15:309–310

140. Trevisan G, Kokelj F (1992) Allergic contact dermatitis due to shoes in children: a 5-year follow-up. Contact Dermatitis 26:45

141. Möller H (1994) All these positive tests to thiomersal. Contact Dermatitis 31:209–213

142. Wantke F, Hemme W, Götz M, Jarisch R (1996) Routine patch testing with thiomersal: why should it be performed? Contact Dermatitis 35:67–68

143. Cox NH, Forsyth A (1988) Thiomersal allergy and vaccination reactions. Contact Dermatitis 18:229–233

144. Aberer W (1991) Vaccination despite thiomersal sensitivity. Contact Dermatitis 24:6–10

145. Aberer W, Kränke B (1996) Reply. Contact Dermatitis 35:67–68

146. Aberer W (1997) Thiomersal-Kontaktallergie und Impfungen mit Thiomersal-konservierten Seren. Dermatosen 45:137

147. Kohl L, Blondeel A, Song M (2002) Allergic contact dermatitis from cosmetics. Dermatology 204:334–337

148. Rastogi SC, Johansen JD, Menné T, Frosch P, Bruze M, Andersen KE, Lepoittevin JP, Wakelin S, White IR (1999) Contents of fragrance allergens in children's cosmetics and cosmetic-toys. Contact Dermatitis 41:84–88

149. Helsing P, Austad J (1991) Contact dermatitis mimicking photodermatosis in a 1-year-old child. Contact Dermatitis 24:140–141

150. Chu CY, Sun CC (2001) Allergic contact dermatitis from triethanolamine in a sunscreen. Contact Dermatitis 44:41

151. Stone N, Varma S, Hughes TM, Stone NM (2002) Allergic contact dermatitis from polyvinylpyrrolidone-1-triacontene copolymer in a sunscreen. Contact Dermatitis 47:49

152. Neri I, Guareschi E, Savoia F, Patrizi A (2002) Childhood allergic contact dermatitis from Henna tattoo. Pediatr Dermatol 19:503–505

153. Brancaccio RR, Brown LH, Chang YT, Fogelman JP, Mafong EA, Cohen DE (2002) Identification and quantification of para-phenylenediamine in a temporary black henna tattoo. Am J Contact Dermat 13:15–18

154. Verhaeghe I, Dooms-Goossens A (1997) Multiple sources of allergic contact dermatitis from parabens. Contact Dermatitis 36:269–270

155. Downs AMR, Sansom JE, Simmons I (1998) Let Rip! Fun Pot dermatitis. Contact Dermatitis 38:234

156. Tosti A, Bassi R, Peluso AM (1990) Contact dermatitis due to a natural plasticine. Contact Dermatitis 22:301–302

157. Rodriguez-Serna M, Molinero J, Febrer I, Aliaga A (2002) Persistent hand eczema in a child. Am J Contact Dermat 13:35–36

158. O'Hagan AH, Bingham EA (2001) Cellist's finger dermatitis. Contact Dermatitis 45:319

159. Rudzki E, Rebandel P (1995) 2 cases of dermatitis from rare sources of sensitization to frequent contactants. Contact Dermatitis 32:361

160. Fowler JF (1990) Case for diagnosis. Am J Contact Dermat 1:71

161. Fisher AA (1994) Contact allergy in children, part 1: rubber allergy. Cutis 54:138–140

162. Castelain M, Castelain PY (1993) Allergic contact dermatitis from cetyl pyridinium chloride in latex gloves. Contact Dermatitis 28:118

163. Placucci F, Vincenzi C, Ghedini G, Piana G, Tosti A (1996) Coexistence of type 1 and type 4 allergy to rubber latex. Contact Dermatitis 34:76

164. Roul S, Ducombs G, Leaute-Labreze C, Labbe L, Taieb A (1996) Footwear contact dermatitis in children. Contact Dermatitis 35:334–336

165. Saha M, Srinivas CR (1993) Footwear dermatitis due to para-fenylenediamine in socks. Contact Dermatitis 28:295

166. Weston JA, Hawkins K, Weston WL (1983) Foot dermatitis in children. Pediatrics 72:824–827

167. Shakelford KE, Belsito DV (2002) The etiology of allergic-appearing foot dermatitis: a 5-year retrospective study. J Am Acad Dermatol 47:715–721

168. Giusti F, Massone F, Bertoni L, Pellacani G, Seidenari S (2003) Contact sensitization to disperse dyes in children. Pediatr Dermatol 20:393–397

169. Vincenzi C, Guerra L, Peluso AM, Zucchelli V (1992) Allergic contact dermatitis due to phenol-formaldehyde resins in a knee-guard. Contact Dermatitis 27:54

170. Shono M, Ezor K, Kaniwa MA, Ikarashi Y, Kojima S, Nakamura A (1991) Allergic contact dermatitis from para-tertiary-butylphenol-formaldehyde resin (PTBP-FR) in athletic tape and leather adhesive. Contact Dermatitis 24:281–288

171. Sood A, Taylor JS, Billock JN (2003) Contact dermatitis to a limb prothesis. Am J Contact Dermat 14:169–171

172. Azurdia RM, King CM (1998) Allergic contact dermatitis due to phenol-formaldehyde resin and benzoyl peroxide in swimming goggles. Contact Dermatitis 38:234–235

173. Stanford D, Georgouras K (1996) Allergic contact dermatitis from benzalkonium chloride in plaster of Paris. Contact Dermatitis 35:371–372

174. Southcott RV, Haegi LAR (1992) Plant hair dermatitis. Med J Aust 156:623–632

175. Rademaker M, Duffill MB (1995) Allergic contact dermatitis to *Toxicodendron succedaneum* (rhus tree): an autumn epidemic. NZ Med J 108:121–123

176. Edwards EK Jr, Edwards EK Sr (1992) Immediate and delayed hypersensitivity to the nettle plant. Contact Dermatitis 27:264–265

177. Wakelin SH, Marren P, Young E, Shaw S (1997) Compositae sensitivity and chronic hand dermatitis in a seven-year-old boy. Br J Dermatol 137:289–291

178. Commens C, McGeogh A, Bartlett B, Kossard S (1984) Bindii (Jo Jo) dermatitis (*Soliva pterosperma* [Compositae]). J Am Acad Dermatol 10:768–773

179. Wood B, Rademaker M (1996) Allergic contact dermatitis from lichen acids. Contact Dermatitis 34:370

180. Tomb RR, Foussereau J, Sell Y (1988) Mini-epidemic of contact dermatitis from gingko tree fruit (*Ginkgo biloba* L.). Contact Dermatitis 19:281–283

181. Kubo Y, Nonaka S, Yoshida H (1988) Allergic contact dermatitis from *Dioscorea batatas* Decaisne. Contact Dermatitis 18:111–112

182. Pazzaglia M, Jorizzo M, Parente G, Tosti A (2000) Allergic contact dermatitis due to avena extract. Contact Dermatitis 42:364

183. Kraus SM, Muselinovic NZ (1991) Pre-employment screening for contact dermatitis among the pupils of a metal industry school. Contact Dermatitis 24:342–344

184. Corazza M, Mantovani L, Bacilieri S, Virgili A (2001) A child with "occupational" allergic contact dermatitis due to MCI/MI. Contact Dermatitis 44:53–54

185. Vigan M, Sauvage C, Adessi B, Girardin P, Meyer JP, Vuitton DA, Laurent R (1994) Pourquoi et comment réaliser une batterie standard chez les enfants? Nouv Dermatol 13:12–15

186. Vigan M, Avenel-Audran M, Blondeel A, Bourrain JL, Castelain M, Dejobert Y, Ducombs G, Flechet ML, Goossens A, Girardin P, Jelen G, Milpied-Homsi B, Pons-Guiraud A, Roul S (1998) Interêt des allergènes de la batterie standard ICDRG pour tester les enfants: étude multicentrique REVIDAL GERDA portant sur 959 enfants. Ann Derm Vénéreol (Stockh) 125(Suppl 3):3S76

43

Chapter 44

Prevention and Therapy

44

Jean-Marie Lachapelle, W. Wigger-Alberti, Anders Boman,
Gunh A. Mellström, Britta Wulfhorst, Meike Bock,
Christoph Skudlik, Swen Malte John, Daniel Perrenoud,
Thierry Gogniat, William Olmstead, Elisabeth Held, Tove Agner

Contents

44.1 Prevention of and Protection from Contact Dermatitis (with Special Reference to Occupational Dermatology)

JEAN-MARIE LACHAPELLE

44.1.1 Introduction: General Principles and Considerations

Preventive dermatology, which is claimed to play a key role in the global management of skin diseases, is not yet accepted as a routine procedure in many aspects of daily life [1]. The prevention of irritant and/or allergic contact dermatitis is briefly and incompletely reviewed in several textbooks on occupational and contact dermatitis [2, 3]. It is therefore imperative to view the prevention of occupational (and nonoccupational) dermatitis as the cornerstone and/or the final aim of many research projects in the field [4].

Various considerations must be borne in mind, particularly in occupational dermatology:

- Contact dermatitis entails both individual aspects (some workers suffer many interruptions to their normal activities over the course of a year due to contact dermatitis) and socioeconomic aspects.
- The subject of prevention is usually divided into two sections: collective (or general) and individual protection measures [2]. There is a general principle: collective prevention and protection measures are usually more effective than individual measures, since the latter depend upon the personal will and constant application of each individual worker. Supervision and surveillance are crucial in this matter.
- The development of occupational medicine has afforded a safer working environment in most industrialized countries than was common a few years ago. Occupational physicians are well aware of general issues such as avoidance (or reduction to an acceptable level) of toxic substances in the working environment, reduction of noise, vibration and/or stress. Nevertheless, they feel less confident when tackling skin problems and seek advice from a dermatologist trained in the management of such situations.

- Some categories of workers are not submitted to regular medical control at work; they may develop dermatitis that is not then treated at an early stage. On the other hand, this situation may differ considerably from one country to another.

In this chapter, the problem of preventing contact dermatitis will be discussed in terms of primary, secondary, and tertiary prevention. This approach permits a better evaluation of the situations encountered in daily life; it is particularly important for preventing and/or controlling outbreaks of irritant and/or allergic contact dermatitis that occur in various circumstances, covered by the areas of topical treatment of skin disease, dermatocosmetology and occupational dermatology.

In the next section we focus on the primary, secondary and tertiary prevention of allergic contact dermatitis. This concept can obviously be adapted for preventing irritant contact dermatitis as well as nonimmunological or immunological contact urticaria.

Core Message

- A general principle: collective measures of prevention and protection are often more efficacious than individual measures, but they are not always applicable.

44.1.2 Primary, Secondary, and Tertiary Prevention of Allergic Contact Dermatitis

Prevention of allergic contact dermatitis can be divided into primary, secondary, and tertiary prevention. It is surprising that this concept and the terms themselves are absent in textbooks of occupational dermatology [2, 3, 5], in view of the fact that the concept is commonly encountered in occupational medicine and public health surveys.

Primary prevention of allergic contact dermatitis focuses on the induction of contact sensitization and on controlling the exposure that eventually leads to contact sensitization. In other words, it includes all measures (collective and/or individual) that are taken before any sign of contact sensitization is observed amongst workers or consumers. These meas-

44

ures are related to the knowledge of a potential risk in the environment.

Secondary prevention is applied when the first clinical signs of allergic contact dermatitis have occurred in a limited number of individuals. This stage of action focuses on a well-defined signal: the early manifestation of the elicitation phase of contact dermatitis.

Tertiary prevention relates to all of the measures used when the condition has developed and is becoming a clear-cut reality and a distressing impairment to the quality of life. This type of prevention is more difficult to manage; indeed, it has to be applied in a suspicious atmosphere, particularly in the field of occupational medicine.

The measures taken for primary and secondary prevention can differ in some respects, but in some cases the exposure assessment performed for secondary prevention can provide the knowledge required to perform primary prevention. Similarly, the measures taken for primary prevention may constitute secondary prevention by preventing new outbreaks in sensitized subjects [6]. The procedures used to eradicate allergic contact dermatitis in preventive dermatology are presented in Tables 1.1–1.3.

Table 1.1. Primary prevention of allergic contact dermatitis

Use of potent haptens in closed systems

Replacement of strongly haptenic chemicals by chemicals of weak or null haptenic potential

Reduction of hapten content in industrial products (such as addition of iron sulfate to cement to reduce the amount of free chromate salts)

Hapten (or allergen) removal, for example in topical drugs and/or cosmetic formulations (monitoring of drugs and cosmetics); checking for hypoallergenicity is a constant aspect of daily life

Specific measures in the work environment, such as automation, ventilation, medicotechnical supervision, and encapsulation of allergic chemicals

Measurements of atmospheric pollution in order to monitor and ultimately reduce the amount of aeroallergens

Initiatives to increase general knowledge of the chemical compositions of end-products

Protective clothing (with special attention to gloves)

Use of "barrier" creams and/or gels before and during work (not very effective compared to preventing irritant contact dermatitis)

Systematic use of moisturizing creams after work, in order to restore the skin barrier function

Labeling of cosmetics, end-products in industry, and so on

Medical education of consumers and workers by means of posters, teaching sessions for people at risk, courses on prevention of skin disorders and skin protection; this has gained more attention in the past few years and is highly recommended

Medical guidelines related to vocational choice (mainly for atopics)

Table 1.2. Secondary prevention of allergic contact dermatitis

Early detection of the incipient clinical signs of allergic contact dermatitis

Careful investigation of anamnestic data, leading to a probable direct link between environmental conditions and clinical signs

Establishment of diagnostic procedures in order to assess the aetiological factors (patch tests, repeated patch tests when needed, prick tests, open tests, semi-open tests, repeated open application tests, use tests, and so on)

In the case of positive allergic reactions, determination of their relevance

Information systems: product labeling, leaflets on product types or occupations, databases

Protective clothing (with special attention to gloves)

Use of appropriate "barrier" creams and/or gels, with awareness of all the limitations linked to the insufficient protective effects of such products

Skin cleansers of low irritant potential

Discussion and conclusions leading to the removal or the reduction of contact with the offending agent(s)

Table 1.3. Tertiary prevention of allergic contact dermatitis

Diagnosis of disabling allergic contact dermatitis

Careful investigation of anamnestic data, leading to a probable direct link between environmental conditions and clinical signs

Establishment of diagnostic procedures in order to confirm the aetiological factors (patch tests, repeated patch tests when needed, prick tests, semi-open tests, open tests, repeated open application tests, use tests, and so on)

Determination of the relevance of positive reactions, using as many approaches as possible

Removal of the allergen(s)

Development of an individual strategy based on reduction of contact, wearing protective clothes

Treatment of allergic contact dermatitis (topical and/or systemic)

In occupational dermatology, registration of the side effects and application of legal measures (which may differ from one country to another)

Alleviation of potential conflicts in the industrial environment

Psychosocial approach to solving the problem

Core Message

■ Strategies used to prevent allergic contact dermatitis can be classified into primary, secondary, and tertiary. Primary prevention is the ultimate goal to reach for all responsible persons: dermato-allergologists, occupational physicians, safety officers, and companies.

44.1.3 Allergies to Dental Acrylates: A Specific Example to Illustrate a Program of Prevention

Occupational allergic contact dermatitis arises in dental surgeons from the use of acrylic resins in composite materials. This provides an example that we can use to illustrate the preventive program. In this type of allergic reaction, fingertip dermatitis is the most common clinical symptom, but as exposure continues, the sides and the backs of the fingers also become involved [7]. The most commonly used acrylates are ethylene glycol dimethacrylate (EGDMA), diethyleneglycol dimethacrylate (DEGDMA), and trimethylpropane trimethacrylate (TMPTMA). Most of the dental composite resin materials are "diluted" with less viscous "difunctional" acrylates. These are the methacrylic monomers, of which EGDMA, DEGDMA, triethyleneglycol dimethacrylate (TREGDMA) and 1,4-butanedioldimethacrylate (BUDMA) are the most extensively used.

To further primary prevention [8], dental products containing acrylics should be delivered in bottles or packaging that allow no-touch techniques to be used for handling. This is currently not the case, and another approach is needed: to educate dentists about the risks that can result from touching dental composite resins and dentin primers without wearing gloves.

Secondary prevention is related exclusively to the use of appropriate gloves. Rubber gloves are readily penetrated by acrylics [9]. Polyvinylchloride, polyethylene, polyvinylacetate and polyvinylalcohol plastic gloves are also inadequate. A new glove material has been introduced, the 4-H glove (Safety 4 AS, Lyngby, Denmark), a laminate made of five layers of polyethylene-ethylenevinylalcohol copolymer – polyethylene (PE/EVOH/PE) – with a thickness of 0.065 mm, and this has been shown to inhibit the penetration of various acrylates [10]. Nevertheless, the 4-H glove does not have a sufficiently close anatomical fit for delicate tasks. It has therefore been suggested that a fingerpiece from the 4-H glove may be used under a disposable glove by dental personnel. Another possibility is to use the fingerpiece outside the disposable latex or vinyl glove [11]. In practice, when manipulations are of short duration, the use of a nitrile glove (N-Dex Best glove; Best Manufacturing, Menlo, Ga., USA) is quite convenient, despite the fact that such a glove can theoretically be penetrated by acrylics.

In the example under consideration, tertiary prevention is very similar to secondary prevention. In some rare instances, fingertip dermatitis does not heal completely and requires long-term topical therapy, including corticosteroid and emollient preparations.

44.1.4 Primary, Secondary, and Tertiary Prevention of Irritant Contact Dermatitis

The major task is to establish a precise diagnosis of irritant contact dermatitis. This implies that allergic contact dermatitis has been ruled out, based on a careful investigation including some of the various procedures mentioned in Tables 1.1–1.3.When an accurate diagnosis of irritant contact dermatitis has been reached, measures of primary, secondary and tertiary prevention are clearly delineated. In many respects, they are comparable to those applied in allergic contact dermatitis.

Two points deserve special attention:

■ Removal of the irritant(s) is usually optional. Measures leading to the reduction of the offending contacts in terms of frequency, concentration, and so on are usually sufficient. For example, reducing the daily number of shampoos by young hairdressers prevents severe irritant contact dermatitis. Another example concerns the use of biocides that are sometimes added "wildly" to cutting oils in certain plants.
■ The use of "barrier" creams and/or gels before and during work is more effective against irritation than against allergy (see later). This is also true for protective clothing, particularly gloves.

There is still a high prevalence of irritant contact dermatitis in various sectors of activity. Therefore, the

44

current experience puts an emphasis on its careful prevention, particularly in terms of worker's education and teaching programs.

Core Message

■ Measures taken for primary, secondary and tertiary prevention of irritant contact dermatitis are one of the most important challenges in environmental dermatology.

44.1.5 An Overview of Applicable Collective Measures of Prevention and Protection

Various procedures can be used to achieve an efficient program of prevention and/or protection. The strategy of prevention is not limited to occupational life, but extends to all activities of daily life that imply contacts with either irritants or allergens. The various measures are intended to reduce contact with irritants and/or allergens.

44.1.5.1 Use of Potent Allergens in Closed Systems

It is absolutely essential that very potent allergens are kept in "closed systems"; any contact with intact or damaged skin of workers must be avoided. For instance, 2,4-dinitro-1-chlorobenzene (DNCB) has been used extensively as an algicide in air-conditioning cooling systems [12]. It is clearly kept in a closed system; nevertheless, maintenance or repair activities involve "insidious" occasional contact between some categories of workers and the allergen. This can provoke epidemics of contact dermatitis involving such workers. A similar situation can occur with various plasticizers and other additives in synthetic polymers [13].

44.1.5.2 Automation

Automation is the only practical means of avoiding some epidemics of contact dermatitis in industry. There are many examples of industrial airborne irritant contact dermatitis that could not be resolved by individual measures of protection. Automation of the industrial procedure has been advised in several such cases. This is especially true when dust particles are responsible for skin irritation [14]. An epidemic of slag dermatitis was reported [15] in a metallurgic plant where permanent mold casting techniques had been introduced. At one stage of production, workers poured slag (a mixture of silicium oxide and calcium oxide powders) into ingot molds. Dust, penetrating through protective clothes or between sleeves and gloves, accumulated in the flexures and on the extensor aspects of the thighs and arms. Subjective and objective skin symptoms were similar to those of fiberglass dermatitis. Scratch marks, papules and pustules were sometimes present. Microscopic examination of powder particles revealed that some were oblong and sharp-edged (length: ±10–80 µm). The dermatitis was considered to have arisen due to mechanical irritation of the skin by sharp-edged particles. We reviewed the problem and dispersed several samples of different slag particles in distilled water. The pH of the supernatant measured between 8 and 12. Slag dermatitis was therefore caused not only by the roughness of the particles, but also was also due to irritation by alkali. This large-scale occupational problem demanded effective measures and has been solved by complete automation.

Among photographers, the problem of allergic contact dermatitis from color developers has been solved almost completely in Scandinavian countries with the widespread use of automated procedures [16, 17]. Nevertheless, some cases are still observed among technicians who use "artistic" (nonautomated) procedures. The drawback of automation is also related to maintenance and repair, during which workers may be caught off-guard.

The recent switch from cameras based on photographic film to digital cameras provides a good illustration of the continuously changing nature of occupational dermatology. This example, a significant problem discussed in former editions of the book, is insignificant these days.

44.1.5.3 Allergen Replacement or Removal

Allergen replacement (or removal) is a possible solution to many problems from allergic contact dermatitis. Some of the following examples are difficult to apply, whereas others are simple:

■ Replacement of epoxy resins by other types of resins [13]. Theoretical; not easy in practice.
■ Use of epoxy resins with a molecular weight greater than 1 kDa [18]. Theoretical; not easy in practice.

- Substitution of a catalyst or curing agent in an epoxy resin system [13]. Can be discussed and realized in practice.
- Replacement of accelerators and antioxidants in rubber factories. Conceivable in practice.
- Addition of ferrous sulfate to cement. Cement causes dermatitis not only in areas directly exposed to the dust but also in areas covered with dust-impregnated clothing. Premixed cement delivered wet to the workplace eliminates the dust hazard to some extent. The addition of ferrous sulfate to cement immediately before mixing reduces the hexavalent chromium to the trivalent state and may thus prevent dermatitis. In some countries, ferrous sulfate is available in sacks to be added to cement (Melstar, marketed in the Netherlands). Its use is not always possible in practice for various reasons. Follow-up of workers, in order to evaluate the efficacy of such a preventive measure, has shown the value of adding ferrous sulfate, but it is nonetheless difficult to evaluate its precise impact, since automation has also played an important role in reducing the number of affected workers [19].
- Removal of chromate from household and/or industrial products is essential. Calnan has emphasized that "chromate sensitization produces such a chronic and recalcitrant dermatitis that dermatologists should always try to limit its use in materials or fluids, which may contaminate the skin, even in low concentrations" [20]. The presence of sodium dichromate in eau de Javel is no longer justified, either as a coloring agent or a stabilizer. The decision to remove sodium dichromate from eau de Javel by the French Trade Society of producers in Paris was a notable example of such an effort in preventive dermatology. In this case, one of the arguments in favor of removal was the fear raised by the medical authorities of provoking and/or perpetuating allergic contact dermatitis from chromate among users. It is interesting to note that this measure is not only important for preventing housewives' dermatitis but also for occupational dermatology, since eau de Javel is used on a large scale for cleaning or antiseptic purposes [21].
- Replacement of a biocide as an additive in many industrial products such as soluble oils. This is a fairly common problem, relatively easy to solve in practice.

The removal of irritants or allergens can also be achieved, at least in part, with general local exhaust ventilation.

In the field of dermatocosmetology, the example of Kathon CG is rewarding in many respects. The biocide Cl+Me-isothiazolinone (Kathon CG; Rohm and Haas, Philadelphia, Pa., USA) provoked outbreaks of allergic contact dermatitis among consumers of cosmetic products in the 1980s and early 1990s. Most of the cases occurred when Kathon CG was incorporated into "leave-on" formulations, at a concentration of 15 ppm. Removal of the biocide was necessary due to many complaints from consumers and dermatologists. It was decided to maintain Kathon CG as a biocide in "rinse-off" formulations, such as in shampoos, at a concentration of 7.5 ppm. Such shampoos are well tolerated by patients who had previously experienced allergic problems with "leave-on" preparations containing Kathon CG at 15 ppm. In this example, the risk analysis process for a microbiocide with broad applications as well as varied human exposure patterns involves assiduous planning, along with development and implementation of appropriate actions to monitor and reduce risk levels [22].

44.1.5.4 Measures Promoting the Proper Use of Industrial Irritants or Allergens

One very important measure to be applied in factories is the proper use of many chemicals. It is noteworthy that some products are not used as advised by the manufacturer. Two examples serve to illustrate this situation.

Biocides are very often used at excessively high concentrations in industrial fluids. Workers attempt to "rejuvenate" solutions by reducing bacterial contamination with unacceptable amounts of biocides. Increased concentrations of biocides can be responsible for outbreaks of irritant or allergic contact dermatitis.

Glutaraldehyde solutions are used to disinfect rooms in hospitals. Cases of allergic contact dermatitis can be observed among staff members when glutaraldehyde solutions are sprayed, for instance, over radiators, the vapors being responsible for airborne contact dermatitis.

44.1.5.5 Visit of the Dermatologist to the Workplace

Occasionally, when a difficult dermatological issue arises in a factory, a more in-depth investigation of the (presumable) occupational dermatosis requires a factory visit [5].

Indeed, the worker's conditions cannot be fully appreciated in the office by the dermatologist, even when he (or she) is well acquainted with occupational problems [3]. A visit to the workplace makes it easier to gain insight into the work environment.

Questions related to the workplace would probably include [3]:

- The nature of each chemical used (with its complete formulation)
- All steps and/or procedures involved in the manufacturing process
- Occupational positions at different stages of work
- The protective and cleaning measures used by the workers (see later)
- The psychological "atmosphere" at the workplace and, more generally, in the factory

Independently from the visit to the workplace, the organization of a joint meeting in the factory may play a useful role. All plant representatives should ideally be present: manager, industrial hygienist (safety officer), occupational physician, occupational nurse (if any!), and trade unions representatives.

Following the visit, the skin investigation of the worker should be performed at the clinic or the private office, where the worker is "reconsidered to be a patient". Testing at the factory is a last resort that is not usually advisable.

Core Message

- Visiting factories or other work facilities is very rewarding; it can provide useful information on many aspects of occupational life.

References

1. San Marco JL (1997) Prevention. In: Grob JJ, Stern RS, Mac Kie RM, Weinstock WA (eds) Epidemiology, causes and prevention of skin diseases. Blackwell Science, Oxford, pp 16–26
2. Lachapelle JM, Frimat P, Tennstedt D, Ducombs G (1992) Précis de dermatologie professionnelle et de l'environnement. Masson, Paris, pp 273–288
3. Marks JG Jr, Elsner P, de Leo V (2002) Contact and occupational dermatology, 3nd edn. Mosby, St Louis, Mo., pp 323–338
4. Lachapelle JM (1997) Prevention of allergic contact dermatitis. In: Grob JJ, Stern RS, Mac Kie RM, Weinstock WA (eds) Epidemiology, causes and prevention of skin diseases. Blackwell Science, Oxford, pp 318–323
5. Funke U (2000) Risk management of occupational hazards at the workplace. In: Kanerva L, Elsner P, Wahlberg JE, Maibach HI (eds) Handbook of occupational dermatology. Springer, Berlin Heidelberg New York, Ch 45, pp 367–370
6. Lachapelle JM (1999) Preventive measures in allergic contact dermatitis. In: Dyall-Smith D, Marks R (eds) Dermatology at the millennium. Parthenon, New York, pp 234–238
7. Kanerva L, Henriks-Eckerman ML, Estlander T (1994) Occupational allergic contact dermatitis and composition of acrylates in dentin bounding systems. J Eur Acad Dermatol 3:157–168
8. Kanerva L, Estlander T, Jolanki R, Tarvainen K (1995) Statistics on allergic patch test reactions caused by methacrylate. Am J Contact Dermat 6:1–4
9. Pegum JS, Medhurst FA (1971) Contact dermatitis by acrylic monomer. Br Med J 2:141
10. Roed-Petersen J (1989) A new glove material protective against epoxy and acrylate monomer. In: Frosch P, Dooms-Goossens A, Lachapelle JM, Rycroft RJG (eds) Current topics in contact dermatitis. Springer, Berlin Heidelberg New York, pp 603–606
11. Kanerva L, Turjanmaa K, Estlander T, Jolanki R (1991) Occupational allergic contact dermatitis from 2-hydroxyethyl methacrylate (2-HEMA) in a new dentin adhesive. Am J Contact Dermat 2:24–30
12. Malten KE (1974) DNCB in cooling water. Contact Dermatitis Newsletter 15:466
13. Björkner B (2000) Plasticizers and other additives in synthetic polymers. In: Kanerva L, Elsner P, Wahlberg JE, Maibach HI (eds) Handbook of occupational dermatology, chap 85. Springer, Berlin Heidelberg New York, pp 688–690
14. Lachapelle JM (1987) Industrial airborne irritant contact dermatitis due to dust particles. Boll Dermatol Allerg Prof 2:83–89
15. Lachapelle JM (1984) Occupational airborne irritant contact dermatitis to slag. Contact Dermatitis 10:315–316
16. Lidén C, Brehmer-Andersson E (1988) Occupational dermatoses from colour developing agents. Clinical and histopathological observations. Acta Derm Venereol (Stockh) 68:514–522
17. Lidén C, Sollenberg J, Hansen L, Arvidson A (1989) Contact allergy to colour developing agents. Analysis of test preparations, bulk chemicals and tank solutions by high-performance liquid chromatography. Derm Beruf Umwelt 37:47–52
18. Thorgeirsson A, Fregert S, Fammas O (1978) Sensitization capacity of epoxy resin oligomers in the guinea pig. Acta Derm Venereol (Stockh) 58:17–21

19. Avnstrop C (1989) Follow-up of workers from the prefabricated concrete industry after the addition of ferrous sulphate to Danish cement. Contact Dermatitis 20:365–371
20. Calnan CD (1978) Chromate in colorant water of gramophone record presses. Contact Dermatitis 4:246–247
21. Lachapelle JM, Lauwerys R, Tennstedt D, Andanson J, Benezra C, Chabeau G, Ducombs G, Foussereau J, Lacroix M, Martin P (1980) Eau de Javel and prevention of chromate allergy in France. Contact Dermatitis 6:107–110
22. Frosch PJ, Lahti A, Hannuksela M et al (1995) Chloromethylisothiazolinone/methylisothiazolinone (CMI/MI) use test with a shampoo on patch-test-positive subjects: results of a multicenter double-blind crossover trial. Contact Dermatitis 32:210–217

44.2 Skin Protection and Skin Care

W. Wigger-Alberti

44.2.1 Introduction

Contact dermatitis, particularly that of the hands, remains the most prevalent occupational skin disease in the industrialized world, resulting in individual morbidity and impacting economically on the community. Since the course may be chronic, leading to disability, and since treatment is frequently of limited efficacy, prevention should be emphasized in order to reduce the incidence and prevalence of both irritant contact dermatitis (ICD) and allergic contact dermatitis (ACD). The incidence of ICD therefore closely correlates with exposure to skin-damaging materials and to wet work conditions [69]. Apart from total elimination of cutaneous contact with hazardous substances and the use of gloves or protective clothing, protective creams/gels (PC), or so-called "barrier creams," are one of the classical means of protecting skin on the hands against low-grade hazards from the environment.

The search for protective creams started in 1915, when a general practitioner from Wigan, England, Dr R. Prosser White, wrote that it was necessary that men's clothes and skin should be protected by overalls and suitable covering. Any cutaneous surfaces that were soiled were to be cleansed as soon as possible. To assist in this, it was advised that a bland, insoluble ointment was to be rubbed into the exposed surfaces prior to work. The quantity used was not to be large, but enough to block up the stomata of the skin [13]. In general, this concept is still true for the use of PCs at the workplace. However, we must bear in mind that skin protection products cannot offer the same level of protection as gloves. Preparations marketed as being an "invisible glove" may encourage workers at risk to be careless upon contact with irritants. On the other hand, they often remain the only practical preventative measure that can be used in occupations that require a good sense of touch, finger mobility, or when working at rotating machines.

Basically, the dermatological principle behind the use of an integrative skin protection in the workplace consists of pre-exposure PCs designed to prevent skin damage due to irritant contact, mild skin cleansers that remove aggressive substances from the skin, and post-exposure skin care products such as emollients or moisturizers that restore the natural barrier function and increase skin hydration and skin smoothing (Table 2.1) [42, 78]. It is debatable as to whether a strict distinction between skin care products used before and after work is justified, since emollients alone have been shown to treat and prevent ICD [63]. Moreover, the benefit of an integrated skin protection based on different products has only rarely been validated [7]. However, it should be kept in mind that a strict and easily understandable separation into pre-exposure PCs, mild skin cleansers and post-exposure skin care products might be necessary to increase the acceptance and appreciation of skin care at the workplace. Most manufacturers offer special plans to pursue this aim. This chapter reviews essential work on the benefits of pre-exposure PCs.

Table 2.1. Dermatological skin protection in the workplace

Type of product	Time of application	Formulations
Pre-exposure protective creams	Before and during work	o/w emulsions, w/o emulsions, multiple w/o/w emulsions, tanning agents, aluminum chlorohydrate, zinc oxide, talcum, perfluorpolyethers, chelating agents, quarternium-18 bentonite, UV absorbers
Cleansing products	During and after work	Detergents, solvents, natural and synthetic grits
Post-exposure skin care	Mainly after work	Emollients, moisturizers, humactants (including glycerol, sorbitol, urea), lipids

Core Message

■ Protective creams are not intended to replace other personal protection measures. They are recommended in conjunction with technical measures and upon the use substances that are less irritating to the skin.

44

44.2.2 Protection Principles

During recent years the prevailing opinion on PCs has been that they are effective in a purely physical way, since their composition enables a diffusion barrier against the offending irritant to be built up to prevent penetration. Hazardous substances with similar physico-chemical properties are grouped together (for example water-miscible or non-water-miscible) to simplify the process of choosing a product [13, 42]. In agreement with this common principle, water-in-oil (W/O) emulsions should provide benefit against hydrophilic and water-soluble irritants such as detergents, acids, alkalis, metal working fluids, and even plain water. Oil-in-water (O/W) emulsions are recommended against hydrophobic irritants such as oils, varnishes and organic solvents. However, the theory that the product builds up a physical barrier between the skin and the irritant, and that the formulation remains unchanged after the product has been applied to the skin, may be incorrect [21]. Additionally, in many workplaces skin contact with both water-miscible and non-water-miscible irritants is unavoidable, and a simple formulation may not prevent against both types of irritants. Moreover, it must be pointed out that the efficacy of a skin protection product cannot be judged theoretically on the basis of the formulation concept alone; it has to be examined individually in sufficient test models.

Special investigations have been undertaken to develop preparations with dual modes of action, combining the different effect of hydrophilic ingredients such as propylene glycol, glycerol and sorbitol with those of lipophilic ingredients such as stearic acid and dimethylpolysilicane. However, a foamy skin protector ("invisible glove") that was claimed to form a two-dimensional network of crystalline stearic acid that was impermeable to hydrophilic agents failed a repetitive irritation test involving the anionic detergent sodium lauryl sulfate (SLS) and the solvent toluene (TOL) [20]. Other preparations are supposed to build up a firm second layer on the skin, which prevents penetration of various agents in a steric manner, including a fatty amine amide acetate that binds to negatively charged carboxyl groups of keratin, and a positive fatty ammonium ion that binds firmly to the negative charge of the epidermis [21].

Some products are claimed to have special protective properties due to tanning agents that are used to generate a hardening effect on the skin surface, increasing the resistance of the skin to mechanical hazards or irritants. Tanning agents are also contained in PCs recommended for use under occlusive gloves to reduce skin maceration due to occlusion [1, 37, 94, 95].

The decreased swelling is caused by direct binding of the tanning substance to keratin. Aluminum chlorohydrate in combination with glycerol was experimentally demonstrated to be more effective at countering skin irritation than glycerol alone [28], and was additionally found to reduce the increased sweating of the hands induced by wearing gloves [9].

Perfluorpolyethers are chemically unreactive liquid polymers with special physico-chemical properties that have recently shown promise as protective preparations in the prevention of ICD [17, 66]. Zinc oxide has a shielding effect. Some products include additional ingredients to counter artificial and natural UV light. Chelating agents, or other substances that can bind metal ions or reduce the penetration through the skin have also been intensively investigated [65]. Although the model formulations were shown to have some benefit in sensitized individuals under experimental conditions [8, 70], their use in the prevention of ACD has been disappointing under practical conditions. However, some publications indicate a benefit from some PCs used as "active" creams to prevent ACD, from using complexing agents against nickel allergy, or from using quaternium-18 bentonite against poison ivy/oak ACD [23, 25, 31, 34, 53, 56, 64, 89]. Recently, a new approach with natural vegetable fats has been presented to investigate their abilities to suppress ICD in the foodstuffs industry, due to their special requirements and problems regarding the taste and smell of products [67].

Core Message

■ The complex interaction between a cream formulation and the specific irritant must be examined individually in sufficient test models.

44.2.3 Proof of Efficacy

Much effort has been undertaken to develop valid methods for evaluating the actual protective properties of PCs. Of course, intervention studies in factories are required for proper assessment, but double-blinded, placebo-controlled, randomized clinical tests of PCs are still missing due to methodological difficulties, ethical doubts, and the enormous expenditure directed towards the tests in relation to the preventative benefit of PCs in practice. Publications on real intervention studies of PCs in a workplace setting are scarce [6, 22, 30, 58]. In most studies the interpretation is difficult due to the small sample size, or because of the short follow-up. The observed effect is a combination of the intervention effect being measured, and a number of disturbing variables reflecting the organizational complexity of such studies [12]. Therefore, the potential effect of PCs in the prevention of work-related hand eczema has mostly been documented in a laboratory setting and on experimentally damaged skin. The majority of information available is based on these experiments.

Since Suskind introduced the "slide test" to evaluate PCs in the 1950s [71], various in vitro studies using penetration, diffusion and absorption models along with excised human skin or reconstructed epidermis have been performed to investigate both the effects of irritants on skin barrier function and the benefit of PCs under highly experimental conditions [10, 14, 15, 18, 26, 27, 32, 33, 41, 47, 51, 52, 54, 62, 72–75, 77, 90, 92, 96]. However, all of these studies are not considered close enough to real workplace situations. Promising results from investigations using the isolated perfused bovine udder skin model have been presented recently and compared to human in vivo data [40, 61]. Patterson et al [57] evaluated the ability of a commercially available PC to reduce irritation against SLS in a repeated patch test, while Fowler [17] demonstrated improvement of hand dermatitis after using the cream for six weeks in a non-placebo-controlled study.

In 1994, Frosch and Kurte introduced the repetitive irritation test (RIT), with cumulative irritation over a two-week period by standard irritants such as SLS, sodium hydroxide, lactic acid and TOL [21]. A specific profile of PC efficacy could be demonstrated by quantifying irritant cutaneous reactions by non-invasive measurements. In recent years, this model has been used in many laboratories as a routine procedure, as it is considered to be suitable for comparing results from the use of PCs simultaneously with a non-pretreated control site on the volunteers' back. However, manufacturers of skincare products prefer easy study protocols that provide valid data in a short time with few restrictions on the volunteers. Therefore, the short duration and easy application associated with a one-week test using the forearms of healthy volunteers was highly desirable.

In a next step, a repetitive irritation test on based on the RIT was developed to optimize the concentration of irritants against which PCs are tested and to evaluate the necessary cumulative application time [83, 84]. Using a set of various irritants modified in terms of their different concentrations and their application to volunteers' ventral forearms, it could be demonstrated that a one-week period was sufficient to evaluate the efficacy of PCs against most irritants, even if lower concentrations of irritants were used. Based on the RIT, a national multi-center study was subsequently designed to standardize a test procedure for the evaluation of skin protective products. A repeated short-time occlusive irritation test (ROIT) was evaluated in two parts (12 day and 5 day protocols) in four and six skilled centers, respectively. Using two irritants (SLS and TOL, each applied twice daily for 30 min twice a day for 30 min) and three different cream bases with different hydrophilicities, the evaluation showed that significant results could be readily achieved with the 5-day protocol. Furthermore, the ranking of the vehicles regarding reduction of the irritant reaction was consistent in all centers [68].

Despite promising data, one criticism is that in all models presented, the investigation of PC efficacy has been limited to exposure to only a single irritant. Skin exposure in the occupational setting can be very complex. Hydrophilic and hydrophobic irritants such as the anionic surfactant SLS and the organic solvent TOL have mainly been used in studies, but repetitive contact to both hydrophilic and hydrophobic substances together or, more commonly, one after the other, occurs regularly in the workplace setting. For instance, workers in the metalworking industry are repeatedly exposed to water-based metal working fluids, neat oils, detergents and organic solvents. Therefore, interactions between irritant chemicals have significant practical consequences. Indeed, concurrent application of SLS and TOL was shown to induce significantly stronger reactions than those caused by twice daily application of each irritant on its own [85]. This additive effect of mixed irritant application impacts upon the use of PCs in practice and upon the way that PCs should be tested. In a recent study, the benefit from a commercially-available PC compared to non-pretreated control sites was tested against the sequential application of two irritants in the so-called tandem repeated irritation test (TRIT). A significant protective effect from the PC was obtained against treatment combinations SLS/SLS and SLS/TOL [87]. Interaction of further irritants should be investigated with attention to professions where a multitude of hazardous substances may cause ICD.

We should note here that some authors found that the PC gave no protection, or even aggravated ICD. A foamy "skin protector" was not convincing in a guinea pig model, and it also caused an aggravating effect on the existing irritation due to NaOH [20]. Also using a guinea pig model, it was shown that treatment with PC can increase skin irritated by cutting oil fluids [29]. Boman and Mellström showed that the absorption of butanol through stripped skin treated with PC was higher than the absorption through untreated skin [11]. A PC was shown to amplify the inflammation from TOL [83], and its protective properties against the systemic absorption of solvents were less than adequate [10, 41, 46].

Besides not being very effective against irritants or even amplifying barrier damage, the creams themselves may induce ICD or ACD [35, 60]. Preservatives, cream bases such as wool alcohols, emulsifiers and fragrances have an irritant and allergic potential of their own, and should be chosen with care.

Core Message

■ Relevant irritants must be included in standardized test designs. In vitro methods may help to discriminate between different formulations. Repetitive irritation tests in humans are more closely related to actual situation in the workplace.

44.2.4 Usage and Application

The cosmetic acceptance of PCs must be sufficient, because their use is often avoided in cases where a tight grip of tools and small objects is necessary. Additionally, PCs are not intended for use on diseased skin; only on mainly intact skin. They should be applied before contact with irritants, and reapplied after every break or after a certain period of time (half a work shift according to manufacturers' claims). Before the product is reapplied, the skin must be cleaned and dried properly to avoid increased penetration of any remaining irritants on the skin surface [42].

It is clear that the effectiveness of a PC is also influenced by the application itself. They must be applied not only frequently enough but also in adequate amounts and to all skin areas that need protection. In particular, the PC should be applied properly into the interdigital spaces. Studies with a fluorescent-marked PC have indicated that the application of PC was the worst for different professional groups and patients with hand eczema, especially in the dorsum of the hands and the interdigital spaces, excluding the space between the index finger and the thumb [79–81]. This method is now covered by many worker education programs and programs to evaluate product application and acceptance [3, 5]. A simple device with a fluorescent source (a Dermalux checkbox) can be used as a training tool in critical occupational working conditions to visualize and teach the proper use of a PC, giving direct feedback about the most

commonly unprotected regions [39]. This experience, rather than anonymous instructive brochures given to the workers, can initiate changes in behavior [48, 81].

Core Message

■ Even the best product is of little, if any, benefit when insufficiently applied.

44.2.5 Strategies

Though PCs are one of the common measures employed to prevent ICD, their actual benefit in the workplace remains controversial [36, 44] and is debated in recent reviews [2, 45, 50, 82, 86, 93]. It has recently been suggested that, in analogy to the sun protection factor, a standardized testing method could be used to specify (irritant-specific) "skin protection factors" for each PC. Reasons for a lack of protection in practice are obviously inefficient products [20], products that are effective against a special irritant but that aggravate reactions from to other irritants [83], or insufficient application of products on exposed skin areas [79]. Data from in vitro and in vivo tests underline the importance of careful selection of PCs for specific workplaces. Choosing the wrong preparation may well worsen the effect of an irritant.

PCs are still not perfect. Much effort is needed to develop products that will give more protection and fewer side-effects. Efficacy and cosmetic acceptance are both important qualities of skin care products that provide protection in the workplace, but knowledge of how they are correctly used is critical. It goes without saying that their ability to prevent ICD and ACD must be evaluated in reliable studies. Results from animal experiments may not be valid for humans, particularly when dealing with irritants, in view of their complex action mechanisms and the high inter-individual variability of the susceptibility of human skin [91]. Considering the various models used to investigate the efficacy of skin care products, the validation of a sensitive, standardized and widely accepted model proved by interlaboratory standardization or controlled clinical studies in the workplace still seems to be necessary. Clearly, studies performed both under experimental conditions and in the workplace are needed before a rational recommendation about whether a product is safe and effective for skin protection can be made. Up to now, it has been largely unclear whether the various in vitro and in vivo methods used are suitable for simulating real workplace conditions, and whether these test results can be related to real occupational exposure. Further studies, especially under daily working conditions evaluating the contribution of each single element of the skincare program (products, frequency of application and education programme) are needed to produce evidence-based recommendations for skin protection [44]. However, repetitive studies in humans – even if they are experimental – are still the gold standard. Supplementary test methods can be used as screening tests but they must be compared to in vivo methods such as ROIT that are more closely linked to real life situations [40].

Due to the wide range of potential irritants at the workplace, standard irritants are often used to examine the effectiveness of products in relation to groups of irritants (for example detergents). This is permissible if the manufacturer states the fact that the examination was performed using a model. Whenever protection against an individual substance, groups of working materials or other substances hazardous to skin is claimed, it must be proven that the skin protection was examined against these substances. If the use of PCs is recommended against a combination of irritants, models with this combination of irritants should be used [87]. The same is true for the benefits from an integrative skin protection concept and the interactions of protection, skin cleansing and regeneration [7, 49].

The majority of investigation takes place in healthy volunteers exposed with standardized and relevant irritants. Additionally, prospective cohort studies and intervention studies [4, 16, 24, 38, 76] or randomized and controlled studies with the inclusion of a placebo [6, 55, 58] may contribute important knowledge when examining the relevance of the experimental data and evaluating the actual use of the skin protection product in a concrete situation. Both model investigations and cohort or intervention studies need proper statistical analysis and a sufficient number of volunteers in order to reach significant differences between intervention and control. Correct biometric methods should be applied [43]. Recommendations for evaluating the efficacies of PCs have recently been published [88].

Core Message

■ Product claims must be based on relevant test methods. Human in vivo studies are still the gold standard.

Besides the use of products with proven efficacy, periodical training and motivation of individuals at risk is of utmost importance, because the best preventative measures have no effect when they are used irregularly and insufficiently. Special emphasis needs to be placed on educating the individual during apprenticeship. It is easier to train a preclinical student nurse in the correct use of protective products than to attempt to change their behavior after several years of work [48]. Up-to-date, informal academic presentations should be used to educate young people in professional training schools [59, 81]. In the end, general education and training of exposed workers in the use of PCs and preventative measures will have the most impact on the prevention of occupational contact dermatitis. With the words of Maria Montesori in mind, we ask people that say that education is too expensive: what is the cost of ignorance [81]?

Core Message

■ Education is the basis of all prevention.

Suggested Reading

1. Frosch PJ, Kurte A (1994) Efficacy of skin barrier creams (IV). The repetitive irritation test (RIT) with a set of four standard irritants. Contact Dermatitis 31:161–168
   The first standardized test in humans with a set of four relevant irritants. In contrast to previously published procedures, the back (instead of the forearm) and a total of four irritants were used. Different formulations could be simultaneously compared to the control field, which received the irritant only, without pretreatment with PC. The irritants sodium lauryl sulfate, sodium hydroxide, lactic acid and undiluted toluene were applied occlusively for 30 min, over 2 weeks. The PCs tested were applied 30 min before contact with the irritants. Irritant cutaneous reactions were quantified by four parameters: erythema score, transepidermal water loss, blood flow volume and stratum corneum hydration by measuring capacitance. The main conclusion was that the accepted notion that oil-in-water emulsions against lipophilic irritants, and water-in-oil emulsions are primarily effective against hydrophilic irritants needs to be re-evaluated.
   These observations still hold true after many years. The interaction between the skin, the formulation and the irritant is complex and must be evaluated in humans. Most repetitive test designs used nowadays are based on the RIT.
2. Schnetz E, Diepgen TL, Elsner P, Frosch PJ, Klotz AJ, Kresken J, Kuss O, Merk H, Schwanitz HJ, Wigger-Alberti W, Fartasch M (2000) Multicentre study for the development of an in vivo model to evaluate the influence of topical formulations on irritation. Contact Dermatitis 42:336–343

This was the first national multi-center study performed to establish a standardized test procedure for the evaluation of skin protective products. Based on the RIT, a repeated short-time occlusive irritation test (ROIT) was evaluated in six skilled centers. The skin reaction was induced by two irritants (sodium lauryl sulfate and toluene). The irritation was monitored by bioengineering means (transepidermal water loss measurement, colorimetry) and by clinical scoring. The evaluation showed that significant results could be achieved with a five-day protocol. Furthermore, despite the expected inter-center variations due to the heterogeneity of the individual thresholds of irritation, interpretation of clinical scores, and inter-instrumental variability, the ranking of the PCs in terms of reduction of the irritant reaction was consistent in all centers.

It was of the utmost importance that the reproducibility of this test was demonstrated. By using a set of different bioengineering methods, three standard formulations were ranked in terms of their ability to prevent skin irritation caused by sodium lauryl sulfate.

3. Wigger-Alberti W, Maraffio B, Wernli M, Elsner P (1997) Self-application of a protective cream: pitfalls of occupational skin protection. Arch Dermatol 133:861–864

One hundred and fifty healthy workers in several occupations were recruited for a questionnaire interview and for typical self-application of a PC. Precisely how the workers applied the PC at the workplace was monitored and quantified by a fluorescence technique. Many areas were skipped when viewed under Wood light. The PC was incompletely applied, especially on the dorsal aspects of the hands and in the interdigital spaces.

Despite promising experimental data demonstrating the efficacy of protective creams (PC), their practical value is still viewed with scepticism. However, lack of protection could simply be caused by uneven or spotty application of these products. Individuals should be made aware of the most commonly missed regions in order to ensure complete skin protection. This simple method is a useful way to assess self-application and should be included in worker education.

References

1. Allmers H (2001) Wearing test with 2 different types of latex gloves with and without the use of skin protection cream. Contact Dermatitis 44:30–33
2. Alvarez MS, Brown LH, Brancaccio RR (2001) Are barrier creams actually effective? Curr Allergy Asthma Rep 1: 337–341
3. Bankova L, Lindenau S, Fuchs S, Tittelbach J, Fischer TW, Elsner P (2002) Influence of the galenic form of a skin-protective preparation on the application pattern assessed by a fluorescence method. Exog Dermatol 1:313–318
4. Bauer A, Kelterer D, Stadeler M, Schneider W, Kleesz P, Wollina U, Elsner P (2001) The prevention of occupational hand dermatitis in bakers, confectioners and employees in the catering trades: preliminary results of a skin protection program. Contact Dermatitis 44:85–88
5. Bauer A, Kelterer D, Bartsch R, Pearson J, Stadeler M, Kleesz P, Elsner P, Williams H (2002) Skin protection in bakers' apprentices. Contact Dermatitis 46:81–85
6. Berndt U, Wigger-Alberti W, Gabard B, Elsner P (2000) Efficacy of a barrier cream and its vehicle as protective measures against occupational irritant contact dermatitis. Contact Dermatitis 42:77–80
7. Berndt U, Gabard B, Schliemann-Willers S, Wigger-Alberti W, Zitterbart D, Elsner P (2002) Integrated skin protection from work place irritants: a new model for efficacy assessment. Exog Dermatol 1:45–48
8. Blanken R, Nater JP, Veenhoff E (1987) Protective effect of barrier creams and spray coatings against epoxy resins. Contact Dermatitis 16:79–83
9. Bock M, Wulfhorst B, Gabard B, Schwanitz HJ (2001) Okklusionseffekt von Schutzhandschuhen/Effizienz einer Aluminiumchlorhydrat-haltigen Hautschutzcreme. Derm Beruf Umwelt 49:85–87
10. Boman A, Wahlberg JE, Johansson G (1982) A method for the study of the effect of barrier creams and protective gloves on the percutaneous absorption of solvents. Dermatologica 164:157–160
11. Boman A, Mellström GA (1989) Percutaneous absorption of 3 organic solvents in the guinea pig (III). Effect of barrier creams. Contact Dermatitis 21:134–140
12. Coenraads PJ, Diepgen TL (2003) Problems with trials and intervention studies on barrier creams and emollients at the workplace. Int Arch Occup Environ Health 76: 362–366
13. Cronin E (1985) Barrier creams. In: Griffith WAD, Wilkinson S (eds) Essentials of industrial dermatology. Blackwell Science, Oxford, pp 106–110
14. De Fraissinette A, Picarles V, Chibout S, Kolopp M, Medina J, Burtin P, Ebelin ME, Osborne S, Mayer FK, Spake A, Rosdy M, de Wever B, Ettlin RA, Cordier A (1999) Predictivity of an in vitro model for acute and chronic skin irritation (SkinEthic) applied to the testing of topical vehicles. Cell Biol Toxicol 15:121–135
15. De Fine Olivarius F, Brinch Hansen A, Karlsmark T, Wulf HC (1996) Water protective effect of barrier creams and moisturizing creams: a new in vivo test method. Contact Dermatitis 35:219–225
16. Diepgen TL (1999) Epidemiological intervention study of skin protection for occupational-stressed skin. 12th International Contact Dermatitis Symposium, 15–18 October 1999, San Francisco, Calif.
17. Elsner P, Wigger-Alberti W, Pantini G (1998) Perfluoropolyethers in the prevention of irritant contact dermatitis. Dermatology 197:141–145
18. Eun HC, Nam C (2003) Alternative methods for evaluating skin irritation using three-dimensional cultures. Exog Dermatol 2:1–5
19. Fowler JF (2000) Efficacy of a skin-protective foam in the treatment of chronic hand dermatitis. Am J Contact Dermat 33:165–169
20. Frosch P, Schulze-Dirks A, Hoffmann M, Axthelm I (1993) Efficacy of skin barrier creams (II). Ineffectiveness of a popular "skin protector" against various irritants in the repetitive irritation test in the guinea pig. Contact Dermatitis 29:74–77
21. Frosch PJ, Kurte A (1994) Efficacy of skin barrier creams (IV) The repetitive irritation test (RIT) with a set of 4 standard irritants. Contact Dermatitis 31:161–168
22. Frosch PJ, Peiler D, Grunert V, Grunenberg B (2003) Efficacy of barrier creams in comparison to skin care products in dental laboratory technicians – a controlled trial. JDDG 1:547–557
23. Fullerton A, Menné T (1995) In vitro and in vivo evaluation of the effect of barrier gels in nickel contact allergy. Contact Dermatitis 32:100–106
24. Funke U, Fartasch M, Diepgen TL (2001) Incidence of work-related hand eczema during apprenticeship: first results of a prospective cohort study in the car industry. Contact Dermatitis 44:166–172

25. Gawkrodger DJ, Healy J, Howe AM (1995) The prevention of nickel contact dermatitis. A review of the use of binding agents and barrier creams. Contact Dermatitis 32: 257–265

26. Gehring W, Dördelmann C, Gloor M (1994) Effektivitätsnachweis von Hautschutzpräparaten. Allergologie 17: 97–101

27. Gehring W (2004) Das Stratum corneum in vitro – ein Modell zur Entwicklung von Hautschutzpräparaten mit entquellenden Eigenschaften auf die Hornschicht. Derm Beruf Umwelt 52:139–145

28. Gloor M, Gabard B, Fluhr JW, Lehmacher W (2001) Action of an aluminium chlorohydrate and glycerol containing skin protection cream in experimental skin irritation produced by sodium laurylsulfate and solvents. Derm Beruf Umwelt 49:76–70

29. Goh CL (1991) Cutting oil dermatitis on guinea pig skin (I). Cutting oil dermatitis and barrier cream. Contact Dermatitis 24:16–21

30. Goh CL, Gan SL (1994) Efficacies of a barrier cream and an afterwork emollient cream against cutting fluid dermatitis in metalworkers: a prospective study. Contact Dermatitis 31:176–180

31. Grevelinck SA, Murrell DF, Olsen EA (1992) Effectiveness of various barrier preparations in preventing and/or ameliorating experimentally produced *Toxicodendron* dermatitis. J Am Acad Dermatol 27:182–188

32. Grunewald A, Gloor M, Gehring W, Kleesz P (1995) Efficacy of skin barrier creams. In: Elsner P, Maibach HI (eds) Irritant dermatitis: new clinical and experimental aspects. Karger, Basel, pp 187–197

33. Guillemin M, Murset JC, Lob M, Riquez J (1974) Simple method to determine the efficiency of a cream used for skin protection against solvents. Br J Ind Med 31:310–316

34. Guin JD (2001) Treatment of *Toxicodendron* dermatitis (poison ivy and poison oak). Skin Therapy Lett 6:3–5

35. Gupta BN, Shanker R, Viswanathan PN et al (1987) Safety evaluation of a barrier cream. Contact Dermatitis 17:10–12

36. Hogan DJ, Dannaker CJ, Lal S, Maibach HI (1990) An international survey on the prognosis of occupational contact dermatitis of the hands. Derm Beruf Umwelt 38:143–147

37. Jepsen JR, Sparre-Jorgensen A, Kyst A (1985) Hand protection for car-painters. Contact Dermatitis 13:317–320

38. John SM, Uter W, Schwanitz HJ (2000) Relevance of multiparametric skin bioengineering in a prospectively-followed cohort of junior hairdressers. Contact Dermatitis 43:161–168

39. Kelterer Kelterer D, Fluhr JW, Elsner P (2003) Application of protective creams: use of a fluorescence-based training system decreases unprotected areas on the hands. Contact Dermatitis 49:159–160

40. Klotz A, zur Mühlen A, Thörner B, Kietzmann M, Holtmann W, Pittermann W (2003) Testing the efficacy of skin protection products in-vivo and in-vitro. SÖFW J 129: 10–16

41. Korinth G, Geh S, Schaller KH, Drexler H (2003) In vitro evaluation of the efficacy of skin barrier creams and protective gloves on percutaneous absorption of industrial solvents. Int Arch Occup Environ Health 76:382–386

42. Kresken J, Klotz A (2003) Occupational skin-protection products – a review. Int Arch Occup Environ Health 76: 355–358

43. Kuss O, Diepgen TL (1998) Proper statistical analysis of transepidermal water loss (TEWL) measurements in bioengineering studies. Contact Dermatitis 39:64–67

44. Kutting B, Drexler H (2003) Effectiveness of skin protection creams as a preventive measure in occupational dermatitis: a critical update according to criteria of evidence-based medicine. Int Arch Occup Environ Health 76: 253–259

45. Lachapelle JM (1996) Efficacy of protective creams and/or gels. In: Elsner P, Lachapelle JM, Wahlberg J, Maibach HI (eds) Prevention of contact dermatitis. Current problems in dermatology. Karger, Basel, pp 182–192

46. Lauwerys RR, Dath T, Lachapelle JM, Buchet JP, Roels H (1978) The influence of two barrier creams on the percutaneous absorption of *m*-xylene in man. J Occup Med 20: 17–20

47. Lodén M (1986) The effect of 4 barrier creams on the absorption of water, benzene, and formaldehyde into excised human skin. Contact Dermatitis 14:292–296

48. Löffler H, Effendy I (2002) Prevention of irritant contact dermatitis. Eur J Dermatol 12:4–9

49. Löffler H, Effendy I (2002) Hautschutz- oder Hautregenerationscreme? Der Halbseitenversuch in der Bewertung eines hautpflegenden Externums. Z Hautkr 77:234–238

50. Lushniak B, Mathias CG, Taylor JS (2003) Barrier creams: fact or fiction? Am J Contact Dermat 14:97–99

51. Mahmoud G, Lachapelle JM, van Neste D (1984) Histological assessment of skin damage by irritants: its possible use in the evaluation of a 'barrier cream'. Contact Dermatitis 11 :179–185

52. Mahmoud G, Lachapelle JM (1985) Evaluation of the protective value of an antisolvent gel by laser Doppler flowmetry and histology. Contact Dermatitis 13:14–19

53. Marks JG Jr, Fowler JF Jr, Sheretz EF, Rietschel RL (1995) Prevention of poison ivy and poison oak allergic contact dermatitis by quaternium-18 bentonite. J Am Acad Dermatol 33:212–216

54. Marks R, Dykes PJ, Hamami I (1989) Two novel techniques for the evaluation of barrier creams. Br J Dermatol 120: 655–660

55. McCormick RD, Buchmann TL, Maki DG (2000) Double-blind, randomized trial of scheduled use of a novel barrier cream and an oil-containing lotion for protecting the hands of health care workers. Am J Infect Control 28: 302–310

56. Menné T (1995) Prevention of nickel dermatitis. Allergologie 18:447

57. Patterson SE, Williams JV, Marks JG Jr (1999) Prevention of sodium lauryl sulfate irritant contact dermatitis by Pro-Q aerosol foam skin protectant. J Am Acad Dermatol 40: 783–785

58. Perrenoud D, Gallezot D, van Melle G (2001) The efficacy of a protective cream in a real-world apprentice hairdresser environment. Contact Dermatitis 45:134–138

59. Perrenoud D, Gogniat T, Olmstedt W (2001) Importance of education with appropriate material for the prevention of occupational dermatitis. Derm Beruf Umwelt 49:88–90

60. Pinola A, Estlander T, Jolanki R, Tarvainen K, Kanerva L (1993) Occupational allergic contact dermatitis due to coconut diethanolamide (cocamide DEA). Contact Dermatitis 29:262–265

61. Pittermann W, Holtmann W, Kietzmann M (2003) Prävention gegen lipophile Noxen durch Hautschutzprodukte. Arbeitsmed Sozialmed Umweltmed 38:435–442

62. Ponec M, Gibbs S, Pilgram G, Boelsma E, Koerten H, Bouwstra J, Mommaas M (2001) Barrier function in reconstructed epidermis and its resemblance to native human skin. Skin Pharmacol Appl Skin Physiol 14 [Suppl 1]: 63–71

63. Ramsing DW, Agner T (1997) Preventive and therapeutic effects of a moisturizer. An experimental study of human skin. Acta Dermato Venereol (Stockh) 77:335–337

44

64. Romaguera C, Grimalt F, Vilaplana J et al (1985) Formulation of a barrier cream against chromate. Contact Dermatitis 12:49–52

65. Schliemann S, Wigger-Alberti W, Elsner P (1999) Prevention of allergy by protective skin creams: possibilities and limits. Schweiz Med Wochenschr 129:996–1001

66. Schliemann-Willers S, Wigger-Alberti W, Elsner P (2001) Efficacy of a new class of perfluoropolyethers in the prevention of irritant contact dermatitis. Acta Derm Venereol (Stockh) 81:392–394

67. Schliemann-Willers S, Wigger-Alberti W, Kleesz P, Grieshaber R, Elsner P (2002) Natural vegetable fats in the prevention of irritant contact dermatitis. Contact Dermatitis 46:6–12

68. Schnetz E, Diepgen TL, Elsner P, Frosch PJ, Klotz AJ, Kresken J, Kuss O, Merk H, Schwanitz HJ, Wigger-Alberti W, Fartasch M (2000) Multicentre study for the development of an in vivo model to evaluate the influence of topical formulations on irritation. Contact Dermatitis 42:336–343

69. Schwanitz HJ, Uter W (2000) Interdigital dermatitis: sentinel skin damage in hairdressers. Br J Dermatol 142:1011–1012

70. Schuppli R, Ziegler G (1967) Neue Möglichkeiten des Hautschutzes gegen Metalle. Z Haut Geschlechtskrankh 42:345–348

71. Suskind RR (1955) The present status of silicone protective creams. Indust Med Surg 24:413–416

72. Treffel P, Gabard B, Juch R (1994) Evaluation of barrier creams: an in vitro technique on human skin. Acta Derm Venereol (Stockh) 74:7–11

73. Tronnier H (1964) Über Hautschutzsalben. 1. Mitteilung: Untersuchungen über die Diffusion von Schadstoffen durch Hautschutzsalben. Berufsdermatosen 12:241–281

74. Tronnier H (1993) Methodische Ansätze zur Prüfung von Hautschutzmitteln. Dermatosen 41:100–107

75. Ursin C, Hansen CM, van Dyk JW, Jensen PO, Christensen IJ, Ebbehoej J (1995) Permeability of commercial solvents through living human skin. Am Ind Hyg Assoc J 56:651–660

76. Uter W, Pfahlberg A, Gefeller O, Schwanitz HJ (1999) Hand dermatitis in a prospectively-followed cohort of hairdressing apprentices: final results of the POSH study. Prevention of occupational skin disease in hairdressers. Contact Dermatitis 41:280–286

77. Voss H (1998) Definition und Messung eines Hautschutzfaktors. SÖFW J 124:60–71

78. Wigger-Alberti W, Elsner P (1997) Preventive measures in contact dermatitis. Clin Dermatol 15:661–665

79. Wigger-Alberti W, Maraffio B, Wernli M, Elsner P (1997) Self-application of a protective cream: pitfalls of occupational skin protection. Arch Dermatol 133:861–864

80. Wigger-Alberti W, Maraffio B, Elsner P (1997) Anwendung von Hautschutpräparaten durch Patienten mit Berufsdermatosen: Notwendigkeit einer verbesserten Verhaltensprävention. Schweiz Med Wochenschr 127:899–904

81. Wigger-Alberti W, Maraffio B, Elsner P (1997) Training workers at risk for occupational contact dermatitis in the application of protective creams: efficacy of a fluorescence technique. Dermatology 195:129–133

82. Wigger-Alberti W, Elsner P (1998) Do barrier creams and gloves prevent or provoke contact dermatitis? Am J Contact Dermat 9:100–106

83. Wigger-Alberti W, Rougier A, Richard A, Elsner P (1998) Efficacy of protective creams in a modified repeated irritation test (RIT): methodological aspects. Acta Derm Venereol (Stockh) 78:270–273

84. Wigger-Alberti W, Caduff L, Burg G, Elsner P (1999) Experimentally-induced irritant contact dermatitis to evaluate the efficacy of protective creams in vivo. J Am Acad Dermatol 40:590–596

85. Wigger-Alberti W, Krebs A, Elsner P (2000) Experimental irritant contact dermatitis due to cumulative epicutaneous exposure to sodium lauryl sulphate and toluene: single and concurrent application. Br J Dermatol 143:551–556

86. Wigger-Alberti W, Elsner P (2000) Barrier creams and emollients. In: Kanerva L, Elsner P, Wahlberg JE, Maibach HI (eds) Handbook of occupational dermatology. Springer, Berlin Heidelberg New York, pp 490–496

87. Wigger-Alberti W, Spoo J, Schliemann-Willers S, Klotz A, Elsner P (2002) The tandem repeated irritation test: a new method to assess prevention of irritant combination damage to the skin. Acta Derm Venereol (Stockh) 82:94–97

88. Wigger-Alberti W, Diepgen TL, Elsner P, Korting HC, Kresken J, Schwanitz HJ (2003) Beruflicher Hautschutz. Gemeinsame Richtlinie der Arbeitsgemeinschaft für Berufs- und Umweltdermatologie (ABD) in der Deutschen Dermatologen Gesellschaft (DDG) und der Gesellschaft für Dermopharmazie e. V. (GD). Derm Beruf Umwelt 51:15–21

89. Wohrl S, Kriechbaumer N, Hemmer W, Focke M, Brannath W, Gotz M, Jarisch R (2001) A cream containing the chelator DTPA (diethylenetriaminepenta-acetic acid) can prevent contact allergic reactions to metals. Contact Dermatitis 44:224–228

90. Zhai H, Maibach HI (1996) Percutaneous penetration (dermatopharmacokinetics) in evaluating barrier creams. In: Elsner P, Lachapelle JM, Wahlberg J, Maibach HI (eds) Prevention of contact dermatitis. Current problems in dermatology. Karger, Basel, pp 193–205

91. Zhai H, Maibach HI (1996) Effect of barrier creams: human skin in vivo. Contact Dermatitis 35:92–96

92. Zhai H, Willard P, Maibach HI (1998) Evaluating skin-protective materials against contact irritants and allergens. Contact Dermatitis 38:155–158

93. Zhai H, Maibach HI (2000) Barrier creams (skin protective creams). Cosmet Toiletries 115:30–34

94. Zhai H, Maibach HI (2001) Effects of skin occlusion on percutaneous absorption: an overview. Skin Pharmacol Appl Skin Physiol 14:1–10

95. Zhai H, Schmidt R, Levin C, Klotz A, Maibach HI (2001) Prevention and therapeutic effects of a model emulsion on glove-induced irritation and dry skin in man. Derm Beruf Umwelt 50:134–138

96. Zur Mühlen A, Klotz A, Weimans S, Veeger M, Thorner B, Diener B, Hermann M (2004) Using skin models to assess the effects of a protection cream on skin barrier function. Skin Pharmacol Physiol 17:167–175

44.3 Protective Gloves

Anders Boman, Gunh A. Mellström

44.3.1 Introduction

At the beginning of the 1990's, new directives and regulations concerning the use of and safety requirements for protective gloves came in to force in Europe. Since then the occupational use of protective gloves has increased tremendously, as has the interest in their ability to protect against harmful chemicals and blood-borne infections (such as hepatitis and HIV). In the last few years, the risk of biological/chemical warfare agents being released by terrorists has also increased significantly, and so equipment for protecting against and destroying these types of agents are attracting increased interest.

In order to select, purchase and use protective gloves, it is necessary to obtain information on current quality standards, the nature of the hazard(s) encountered, performance data, the acceptable level of exposure to the hazard(s), and any potential adverse effects caused by rubber or plastic protective gloves. Initially, information on the performance of protective gloves could be found in a selection of test reports in the literature. Today, such information is still reported in the literature, but most performance data are now available on the internet, on the websites of glove manufacturers, related authorities and organizations.

44.3.2 Intended Use of Gloves

44.3.2.1 Protective Gloves

In Europe, gloves intended to protect the user are referred to as *personal protective equipment*, and they are covered by the Personal Protective Equipment Directive 89/686/EEC. The EEC Directive states the general requirements for all personal protective equipment, and the requirements for each type of glove have been described previously [23].

Protective gloves are classified into three categories according to the *intended use* and validation procedures:

- Category I: Gloves of a simple design – for minimal risk applications
- Category II: Gloves of an intermediate design (not simple or complex) for intermediate risk
- Category III: Gloves of a complex design – for irreversible/mortal risks

The requirements for EC-type certification for all categories of gloves are:

- A declaration of conformity
- A technical documentation file
- An affixed CE mark.

For categories II and III there are additional requirements:

- EC-type examination testing by approved laboratories, certified by approved notified bodies
- Manufacture under a formal EC quality assurance system
- Labeling requirements with pictograms

General requirements for most kinds of protective gloves are defined in the European Standard EN 420. Key aspects are fitness of purpose, nontoxicity, good construction, storage, sizing, adequate glove hand dexterity, and good product information and labeling.

44.3.2.2 Medical Gloves

Gloves intended for use in the medical field to protect patients and users from cross-contamination are referred to as *medical devices* and are covered by the Council Directive 93/42/EEC concerning such medical devices [23]. A survey of the US rules, regulations and standards concerning the use of protective and medical gloves has been presented by Henry [12].

They are classified into categories:

- Surgical gloves
- Examination gloves (sterile or nonsterile)
- Foil film gloves

44.3.3 Selection Procedure

44.3.3.1 Selecting Gloves to Protect Against Chemicals

Several factors need to be taken into account when selecting a glove for a particular application. The selection process and the factors to be considered in the selection process, such as the work activity and classification of the chemicals encountered, have

44

been described for gloves used to protect against chemicals [15, 30]. The selection procedure, adapted to the EN requirements and standards for protective gloves, is briefly presented in Table 3.1.

44.3.3.2 Selecting Gloves to Protect Against Microorganisms

The selection process and the use of gloves by health care personnel in different working situations has been described by Burman and Fryklund [7] and Ransjö [32]. A scheme for this selection process is presented in Table 3.2. It is based on purpose, working procedure, type of glove (medical gloves or protective gloves), and the risk of exposure to infection or microorganism.

44.3.4 Glove Materials and Manufacturing

Today the materials used to manufacture protective gloves are natural rubber, synthetic rubber, textile fibers, leather and several polymeric materials. A survey of glove materials used for protective (PG) and medical gloves (MG) is presented in Table 3.3. Mellström and Boman [22] have presented detailed descriptions of the materials used for glove manufacturing as well as different manufacturing methods and glove types.

The protective effects of different glove materials against hazardous chemicals is dependent on the following factors:

- *Thickness*: the breakthrough time increases as the thickness of the glove material increases (in a nonlinear fashion, however) [13, 35].
- *Material composition*: chemical resistance capacities vary, even for the same generic material produced by different manufacturers, due to variations in polymer formulation. The barrier effects of different generic materials vary. Each combination of chemical and protective glove material must be considered [27, 33]. The quality and protective effects of gloves made from the same material can differ due to different manufacturing processes, additives and quality control [22, 31].

Table 3.1. Glove selection: protective gloves

Gloves needed and requirements	Degree of exposure	Chemical classification and risk of skin injury
Cat. I	Risk of exposure, possible splashing	Mainly contact with chemicals classified as toxic, harmful or irritant
No testing of the protective effect is required	Occasional, repeated and expected exposure *Minimal risk only of slight injuries*	
Cat. II	Occasional, repeated and expected exposure	Mainly contact with chemicals classified as toxic, harmful or irritant
Breakthrough time (BT) and/or permeation rate (PR) is required	Continuous exposure at certain times, expected or accidental *Intermediate risk of moderate, reversible injuries*	
Cat. III	Continuous exposure at certain times, expected or accidental	Mainly contact with chemicals classified as highly toxic, highly corrosive, corrosive, and with agents causing cancer, sensitization, or those absorbed through the skin
Breakthrough time (BT) and/or permeation rate (PR) are required	*High risk of severe or irreversible injuries*	
In addition, also test results from performing the glove task		

Table 3.2. Glove selection: medical gloves

Protection of personnel from hepatitis (A, B, C), HIV, HTLV	Protection of personnel and patients from various viruses and bacteria	Protection of patients from hepatitis, HIV and other viruses and bacteria
Surgical glove: surgery	*Protective gloves*: handling of feces, urine, vomit, and so on	*Surgical glove*: surgery
Examination gloves, nonsterile: dentistry, risk of contact with blood procedures		*Examination gloves, sterile*: invasive
Protective gloves (such as domestic gloves): risk of contact with blood		*Examination gloves, nonsterile*: dentistry, isolation, barrier nursing
		Protective gloves: isolation, handling of feces, urine, vomit, and so on

Table 3.3. Survey of glove materials used for protective and medical gloves (*PG* protective glove, *MG* medical glove for single use)

Material name/Trade name(s)	Intended use
Natural rubber (Latex)	PG and MG
Synthetic rubber materials	
Polyisoprene	MG
Butyl rubber	PG
Chloroprene / Neoprene	PG and MG
Fluor rubber / Viton	PG
Nitrile rubber / Nitrilite, N-Dex	PG
Styrene-butadiene	MG
Styrene-ethylene-butadiene	MG
Plastic polymeric materials	
Polyisocyanate urethane	PM and MG
EMA (ethylene-methylacrylate)	PG and MG
Polyethylene, polythene (PE)	PG and MG
Polyvinyl chloride (PVC)	PG and MG
PE/EVAL/PE, laminate / 4H/Silver Shield glove	PG
Leather	PG
Textile:	PG
Cotton, nylon, jersey	PG, inner gloves
Fiber materials / Kevlar, Lycra and Spectra fiber	Used in jersey surgical inner gloves, cut resistant

44.3.5 Testing the Protective Glove Barrier

If protective gloves and medical gloves intended for single use are required to give an adequate level of protection, their properties must be tested and evaluated.

44.3.5.1 Standard Test Methods

The most relevant standard test methods for protective gloves and medical gloves are presented in Tables 3.4 and 3.5. Standard test methods are revised on a regular basis, and some former EN standards have now become EN-ISO standards.

In Europe, the testing is performed in a standardized way, by approved laboratories, certified by approved and notified bodies. The test results should be compared with others performed in a similar way. The standard test procedure is not supposed to illustrate the working situation.

When testing gloves in a nonstandardized way, in order to illustrate a certain working situation or extreme working conditions, approved test laboratories, glove manufacturers and consulting companies in the field can give advice and/or design and perform an appropriate testing procedure.

Table 3.4. Relevant standard test methods for gloves that protect against chemicals (*EN* European Standard from the European Committee for Standardization, *ASTM* American Society of Testing and Materials)

Document number	Title
ASTM F 739	Standard test methods for resistance of protective clothing materials to *permeation* by liquids and gases under conditions of *continuous contact*
ASTM F 1383	Standard test method for resistance of protective clothing materials to *permeation* by liquids and gases under conditions of *intermittent contact*
ASTM F 903	Standard test method for resistance of protective clothing materials to *penetration* by liquids
EN 420	General requirements for gloves
EN 374	Protective gloves against *chemicals and microorganisms*:
Part 1	Terminology and performance requirements
Part 2	Determination of resistance to *penetration*
Part 3	Determination of resistance to *permeation* by chemicals

Table 3.5. Relevant standard test methods for medical gloves (*EN* European Standard from the European Committee for Standardization, *ASTM* American Society of Testing and Materials)

Document number	Title
ASTM D 3577	Standard specification for rubber surgical gloves
ASTM D 3578	Standard specification for rubber examination gloves
ASTM D 5151	Standard test method for *detection of holes* in medical gloves
ASTM D 5250	Standard specification for polyvinyl chloride gloves for medical application
ASTM D 5712	Standard test method for analysis of *protein in natural rubber* and its products
EN 455	Medical gloves for single use:
Part 1	Requirements and testing for *freedom from holes*
Part 2	Requirements and testing for *physical properties*
Part 3	Requirements and testing for *biological evaluation*

Physical Properties

In the EN and ASTM standard specifications, requirements and test methods are given, such as sampling and selection of test pieces, physical dimensions with length, strength and thickness, load for breaking before and after accelerated ageing. The barrier effect is also affected by the *storage conditions*, and this is particularly important for medical gloves made of natural rubber latex.

Penetration (Leakage)

Penetration of chemicals and/or microorganisms is a process which can be defined as the flow through closures, porous materials, seams and pinholes or other imperfections in a protective or medical glove material, at a nonmolecular level. Leakage can lead to uncontrolled contact with hazardous chemicals or infectious materials; especially in the healthcare field. Penetration test methods for protective gloves and leakage testing for medical gloves have been described by Mellström et al [26]. As a rule, leakage tests include a random sampling procedure where a certain number of gloves are filled with a specified volume of water or air. These are pass or fail tests, and the number of gloves allowed to fail per number of gloves tested is dependent upon the batch or lot size. The sampling procedure for inspection by attributes defined by the International Organization for Standardization (ISO 2859 should be used.

There are several standardized leakage test methods designed for medical gloves that have been evaluated, and all test methods have inherent limitations [8–10]. In an overview, Schroeder et al [36] presented standard quality control testing and virus penetration. The standard tests used for glove integrity and virus penetration through used and intact gloves are discussed, as well as those used to test penetration through punctures in gloves. Tests used to evaluate the barrier integrity fall into two categories:

- Those intended to ensure quality during and after manufacturing
- Those tests that challenge the barrier with viral or chemical agents.

They concluded that latex gloves provided significant barrier protection against very small viruses, and that apparent barrier integrity cannot ensure safety, but current quality control protocols ensure that medical gloves provide significant protection.

Permeation

The permeation is usually described as the process by which a chemical migrates through the protective clothing material on a molecular level, including sorption, diffusion and desorption processes. The principle of permeation standard testing is a flow-through system where a two-compartment permeation cell of standard dimensions is used. The test specimen acts as barrier between the first compartment of the cell, which contains the test chemical, and the second compartment through which a stream of the collecting medium (gas or liquid) is passed. The collecting medium will collect the diffused molecules of the test chemical or its component chemicals for analysis. The standard methods defined in EN-374:3 and those of the corresponding ASTM F-739 standard have now been harmonized and are considered equivalent.

The key parameters measured for permeability are usually:

- *Breakthrough time* (BT, min): in the ASTM and EN standard test methods, the breakthrough time is defined as the time when a specified permeation rate is reached
- *Permeation rate* (PR): the mass of test chemical permeating the material per unit time per unit area ($\mu g \cdot min^{-1} \cdot cm^{-2}$)
- *Steady-state permeation* (SP): a state that is reached when the permeation rate becomes virtually constant.
  In the European Standard for gloves used to protect against chemicals and microorganisms, one of the requirements is that the protective effect of a particular combination of protective glove/test chemical should be presented as a *protection index*. The protection index is based on the breakthrough time measured for *constant* contact with the test chemical (European Standard EN 374–1). See Table 3.6.

Table 3.6. Index based on breakthrough times determined during constant contact with the test chemical described in European Standard EN 374–3

Protection Index	Measured breakthrough time (min)
Class 1	> 10
Class 2	> 30
Class 3	> 60
Class 4	>120
Class 5	>240
Class 6	>480

Biocompatibility

Over the last few years, the number of severe adverse reactions caused by latex products (such as latex proteins in gloves) in health care workers has risen significantly. Adverse reactions due to rubber chemicals, powder, lubricants, endotoxins and pyrogens are well known and are more frequent than reactions to proteins. In Europe, the requirements and test methods for biological evaluations of medical gloves have been defined and the EN 455 standard (Medical gloves for single use. Part 3: *Requirements and testing for biological evaluation*) is now in force. Results from the test and applied test methods are to be made available on request.

44.3.5.2 In Vivo Testing

Additional information on the protective efficacy of gloves can be derived from in vivo testing in man or in experimental animals [38]. For screening, an animal model can be used for comparative investigation of the protective effects of gloves [5, 6].. In work-related studies, the effects of exposure to potentially hazardous chemicals used in the workplace are studied. Protective effects and side effects of gloves can be studied by patch testing contact allergic individuals with the specific allergen together with pieces of glove [2, 3, 16].

44.3.6 Protective Effects of Gloves

44.3.6.1 Protection Against Microorganisms

A number of studies of the barrier effect of gloves against microorganisms, performed using various test methods during the period 1976–1993, have been reviewed by Hamann and Nelson [11]. Their conclu-

44

sions were that the barrier effect of the gloves is dependent on a complex interaction of several factors:

- Type and brand of glove (latex or plastic materials)
- Condition of use (unused, stimulated use or in actual clinical situations)
- Sensitivity of the assay (water-, air-, dye-leak tests, bacterial or viral penetration)

They also concluded that some trends could be seen in the data, such as:

- The material is an important determinant of the glove barrier
- The brand of glove influences the outcome of barrier testing
- The quality of a glove is more closely related to the manufacturer than to the glove material
- Leakage rates are related to the level of use a glove receives
- The efficacy of the glove barrier varies with the sensitivity of the testing procedure

44.3.6.2 Protection Against Some Chemical Agents Hazardous to the Skin

In both Europe and in the US there are comprehensive guides, with classifications of hazardous chemicals of all kinds. The risk codes and safety phrases are usually given in the safety data sheets for the actual chemical, and this sheet should always be made available by the supplier of the chemical.

Disinfectants

Disinfectants are generally used to clean surfaces and objects and for the cold sterilization of instruments. The use of different kinds of disinfectants is frequent for the preoperative skin disinfection of patients and in working situations where there is a risk of acquiring blood-borne infections. In these circumstances it is important to use gloves, both to protect the skin against infections and to avoid contact with disinfectants harmful to the skin. Some of these agents are known to cause allergic and/or irritant reactions after contact with the skin; for example ethanol, isopropyl alcohol, chlorocresol and glutaraldehyde. The influence of four disinfectant products on six different brands of medical gloves, evaluated by measuring the permeation and through SEM (Scanning Elec-

tronic Microscopy) studies of the exposed glove material surfaces, has been described by Mellström et al [24]. They found that gloves made from latex, PVC and polyethylene gave acceptable protection from contact with *p*-chloro-*m*-cresol (Blifacid) and glutaraldehyde (Cidex) containing products for at least 60 min, but did not provide acceptable protection from contact with isopropanol and ethanol. Recent studies also show that they provide inadequate protection from formaldehyde [17, 20, 21].

Pharmaceuticals

Pharmaceutical preparations of drugs, e.g., cytostatic agents have very heterogeneous mechanism of action, they have potent pharmacological properties and it is well known that they can cause acute skin injuries in cases of accidental exposure [14]. The extent of health hazard due to chronic exposure to small amounts of cytostatic drugs by personnel is still not completely known and therefore it is necessary to minimize the exposure. In order to minimize the risk of contact when preparing, dispensing and administrating these drugs, a standard procedure, appropriate technique together with personal protective equipment, e.g., gloves should be used. However, there are no requirements or criteria for evaluating medical glove quality for this purpose of use [25]. Several cytostatic drugs penetrated latex gloves [17, 37].

Composite Materials (Bone Cement, Dental Filling Materials)

The increased use of acrylic compounds as a substitute for amalgam by dentists, dental nurses and dental technicians has resulted in an increased frequency of hand eczema for these groups. This is a serious problem because there are currently no commercially available gloves that have the required dexterity but that also provide sufficient protection for the skin. Standard procedures, appropriate techniques, and packaging design together with adjusted personal protective gloves are urgently required. In several studies of the permeability of medical gloves to methacrylates in resinous dental material, no gloves were impervious, but nitrile and chloroprene showed a little more resistance than other glove materials [4, 17, 18, 28, 29]. However, it is important to note that the use of acetone as a solvent in a bonding material may reduce the protective effect markedly. The combined use of latex gloves with 4H/Silver Shield gloves as an inner glove may be useful in some working situations. The protective efficacies of seven different nonlatex gloves against a dental bonding product containing 2-HEMA were evaluated on eight patients with a test-verified contact allergy to 2-HEMA. Gloves made of neoprene gave the best protection, and gloves made of polyethylene gave comparable results to the positive control (no gloves) [2, 3].

Solvents

Alcohol and other aliphatic and aromatic organic solvents have a degreasing and irritating effect on the skin, and can be absorbed through the skin into the blood. For splashes or very short contact times (10–30 min), gloves made of natural rubber, PE or PVC can be useful for protecting against these solvents. For occasional (30–60 min) and intentional exposure, gloves made of nitrile rubber, natural rubber or neoprene rubber can be useful, while for intentional exposure for extended periods (>60 min), 4H/Silver Shield-gloves, Viton or butyl rubber should be used.

Corrosive Agents

Short repeated exposures or an extended exposure to small amounts of corrosive substances and oxidizing/reducing agents, acids, bases and concentrated salt solutions can cause severe irritation to the skin. Glove materials suitable for protecting from brief exposure (10–30 min) to this kind of hazardous chemical are natural rubber, PE and PVA. Occasional but intentional exposure (for 30–60 min) requires gloves made of neoprene, natural rubber or nitrile rubber. Intentional exposure for extended periods (>60 min) necessitates butyl rubber, Viton or 4H/Silver Shield gloves.

Detergents, Surfactants, Cleansers

Washing-up liquids, cleaning agents and soaps are usually water-based and cause only mild effects to the skin when used in recommended concentrations; however, when used at high concentrations they can cause skin injuries. Sometimes organic solvents like white spirit or isopropanol are added. For splashes or very short contact times (10–30 min), gloves made of EMA, PE or PVC are useful. For occasional but intentional (30–60 min) exposure, gloves made of natural rubber, neoprene or PVC are useful, while extended exposure (>60 min) necessitates gloves made of natural rubber, neoprene or PVC. If organic solvent is added, then gloves made of nitrile rubber should be used.

Oils, Cutting Fluids, Lubricant Oils

These agents often contain anticorrosive agents, bactericides and antioxidants. Oils can contain small amounts of chromium, nickel and cobalt. For splashes or very short contact times (10–30 min), gloves made of natural rubber or PVC gloves can be useful. Occasional but intentional (30–60 min) exposure requires industrial gloves made of nitrile rubber, natural rubber or neoprene, while intentional exposure for extended periods (>60 min) necessitates 4H/Silver Shield gloves or nitrile rubber gloves.

Warning! When working at machinery with rotating and moving parts, using gloves can increase the risk of tear injuries and so they should be used with caution.

44.3.7 Information Sources

44.3.7.1 Internet

The easiest way to get information on the performance of protective gloves intended for use when working with hazardous chemicals is to search on the internet. Most glove manufacturers have a selection guide/selection procedure and performance data for gloves of all categories on their websites. Related authorities and organizations, and universities, have useful information on standards, test reports, and links to, for example, glove–chemical compatibility guides. Below are some website addresses that may be useful during the selection procedure. Since the Web is a dynamic source of information, these URLs may change, so it may be necessary to make use of search engines to find the data required.

Glove Manufacturer Websites

- AnsellPro Gloves (http://www.ansell-edmont.com)
- Ansell Healthcare (http://www.ansellhealthcare.com)
- Best Gloves (http://www.bestglove.com)
- Comasec (http://www.comasec.com)
- Mapa Gloves (http://www.mapaglove.com)
- Marigold Industrial (http://www.marigoldindustrial.com)
- North Safety Products (http://www.northsafety.com)

44

Websites of Some Related Authorities andOrganizations

- ASTM International (http://www.astm.org)
- European Committee for Standardisation (http://www.cenorm.be)
- National Institute for Occupational Safety and Health (http://www.cdc.gov/niosh)
- OSCHA (http://www.oscha.gov)
- AIHA Laboratory Health and Safety Committee (http://www2.umdnj.edu/eohssweb/aiha/technical/ppe.htm)
- Eurofins Scientific (http://www.eurofins.com)

44.3.7.2 Bibliographic Data

Useful and relevant information is also still available in scientific journals (many of which are on the internet), handbooks and guide books, as well as in test reports.

44.3.8 Limitations on Use Due to Side-Effects, and Therapeutic Alternatives

Allergic reactions to gloves can be caused by, for example, rubber chemicals, organic pigments, and latex proteins. *Irritant reactions* to gloves are caused by, say,. mechanical stress, endotoxins, ethylene dioxide and glove powder. *Side effects* can also occur from contact with glove powder, such as starch-induced adhesions and granulomas following surgery.

Risks and side effects from the use of gloves are described in detail in other chapters in this book.

44.3.8.1 Gloves Made From Synthetic Materials

The use of gloves made from polymer materials is necessary both when treating patients and when employees have a known allergy to latex proteins, in order to reduce the risk of contact dermatitis caused by rubber additives as well as of contact urticaria from latex proteins. Gloves made from polymer materials are also needed by employees with known allergies to the chromate in leather gloves.

44.3.8.2 Double Gloving

- Using natural rubber latex gloves with inner gloves made from plastic material, nylon or cotton reduces the risk of contact dermatitis and urticaria caused by latex rubber gloves
- Using natural rubber latex gloves with synthetic fiber gloves reduces the risk of cut and puncture injuries
- Using natural rubber latex gloves with latex or plastic gloves reduces the risk of blood-borne infections and/or chemical permeation

44.3.8.3 Powder-Free Gloves

Powder-free gloves should be used to reduce the risk of symptoms from rhinitis, conjunctivitis, urticaria and asthma caused by glove powder contaminated by latex proteins.

44.3.9 Conclusions

Important factors that should be considered during the selection procedure include:

- Nature of the work task and risk of exposure
- Length of work
- Mechanical quality of the glove material (tensile strength, dexterity, cut, tear and puncture resistance).
- Resistance to penetration and permeation of hazardous chemicals and microorganisms
- Risk of adverse effects when using a specific glove (allergic contact dermatitis, contact urticaria, irritation, itching, and so on)
- Function (using the gloves must not create another risk or be a hindrance)
- Comfort, fit, "wearability"
- Quality (and whether the quality is maintained for every glove), price

The large number of factors suggests that the selection procedure can be rather complicated!

References

1. Andersson T, Bruze M (1999) In vivo testing of the protective efficacy of gloves against allergen-containing products using an open chamber system. Contact Dermatitis 41:260–263
2. Andersson T, Bruze M, Björkner B (1999) In vivo testing of the protection of gloves against acrylates in dentin-bonding systems on patients with known contact allergy to acrylates. Contact Dermatitis 41:254–259
3. Andersson T, Bruze M, Gruvberger B, Björkner B (2000) In vivo testing of the protection provided by nonlatex gloves against a 2-hydoxyethyl methacrylate-containing acetone-based dentin-bonding product to acrylates. Acta Derm Venereol (Stockh) 80:435–437
4. Andreasson H, Boman A, Johnsson S, Karlsson S, Barregård L. (2003) On permeability of methyl methacrylate, 2-hydroxyethyl methacrylate and triethyleneglycol dimethacrylate through protective gloves in dentistry. Eur J Oral Sci 111:529–535
5. Boman AS, Mellström GA (1989) Percutaneous absorption of three organic solvents in the guinea pig. IV. Effect of protective gloves. Contact Dermatitis 21:260–266
6. Boman AS, Mellström GA (1994) Percutaneous absorption studies in animals. In: Mellström GA, Wahlberg JE, Maibach HI (eds) Protective gloves for occupational use. CRC Press, Boca Raton, FL, pp 91–107
7. Burman LG, Fryklund B (1994) The selection and use of gloves by health care professionals. In: Mellström GA, Wahlberg JE, Maibach HI (eds) Protective gloves for occupational use. CRC, Boca Raton, Fla., pp 283–292
8. Carey R, Herman W, Herman B, Casamento J (1989) A laboratory evaluation of standard leakage tests for surgical and examination gloves. J Clin Eng 14:133–143
9. Douglas AA, Neufeld PD, Wong RKW (1992) An interlaboratory comparison of standard test methods for medical gloves. In: McBriarty JP, Henry N (eds) Performance of protective clothing, vol 4. ASTM STP 1133, American Society for Testing and Materials, Philadelphia, pp 99–113
10. Douglas A, Simon TR, Goddard M (1997) Barrier durability of latex and vinyl medical gloves in clinical settings. Am Ind Hyg Assoc J 58:672–676
11. Hamann CP, Nelson JR (1993) Permeability of latex and thermoplastic elastomer gloves to the bacteriophage Phi X 174. Am J Infect Control 21:289–296
12. Henry NW III (2004) US rules, regulations and standards for protective gloves for occupational use. In: Boman A, Estlander T, Wahlberg JE, Maibach HI (eds) Protective gloves for occupational use, 2nd edn. CRC, Boca Raton, Fla., pp 35–41
13. Jencen DA, Hardy JK (1989) Effect of glove material thickness on permeation characteristics. Am Ind Hyg Assoc J 50:623–626
14. Knowles RS, Virden JE (1980) Occasional review. Handling of injectable antineoplastic agents. Br Med J 30:589–591
15. Leinster P (1994) The selection and use of gloves against chemicals. In: Mellström GA, Wahlberg JE, Maibach HI (eds) Protective gloves for occupational use. CRC, Boca Raton, Fla., pp 269–281
16. Lidén C, Wrangsjö K (1994) Protective effect of gloves illustrated by patch test testing-practical aspects. In: Mellström GA, Wahlberg JE, Maibach HI (eds) Protective gloves for occupational use. CRC, Boca Raton, Fla., pp 207–212
17. Mäkelä E A, Jolanki R (2004) Chemical permeation through disposable gloves. In: Boman A, Estlander T, Wahlberg JE, Maibach HI (eds) Protective gloves for occupational use, 2nd edn. CRC, Boca Raton, Fla., pp 299–314
18. Mäkelä EA et al (1992)
19. Mäkelä EA, Väänänen V, Alanko K, Jolanki R, Estlander T, Kanerva L (1999) Resistance of disposable gloves to permeation by 2-hydroxymethacrylate and triethylene glycol-dimethacrylate. Occup Hyg 582:121–129
20. Mäkelä EA, Vainiotalo S, Peltonen K (2003a) The permeability of surgical gloves to seven chemicals commonly used in hospitals. Ann Occup Hyg 47:313–323
21. Mäkelä EA, Vainiotalo S, Peltonen K (2003b) Permeation of 70% isopropyl alcohol through surgical gloves: comparison of the standard methods ASTM F739 and EN 374. Ann Occup Hyg 47:305–312
22. Mellström GA, Boman A (2004) Gloves: types, materials, and manufacturing. In: Boman A, Estlander T, Wahlberg JE, Maibach HI (eds) Protective gloves for occupational use use, 2nd edn. CRC, Boca Raton, Fla., pp 15–28
23. Mellström G A, Carlsson B (2004) European Standards on protective gloves. In: Boman A, Estlander T, Wahlberg JE, Maibach HI (eds) Protective gloves for occupational use, 2nd edn. CRC, Boca Raton, Fla., pp 29–33
24. Mellström GA, Lindberg M, Boman A (1992) Permeation and destructive effects of disinfectants on protective gloves. Contact Dermatitis 26:163–170
25. Mellström GA, Wrangsjö K, Wahlberg JE, Fryklund B (1996) The value and limitation on gloves in medical health service, part II. Dermatol Nursing 8:287–295
26. Mellström GA, Carlsson B, Boman A (2004) Testing of protective effect against liquid chemicals. In: Boman A, Estlander T, Wahlberg JE, Maibach HI (eds) Protective gloves for occupational use, 2nd edn. CRC, Boca Raton, Fla., pp 71–87
27. Mickelsen RL, Hall RC (1987) A breakthrough time comparison of nitrile and neoprene glove materials produced by different glove manufacturers. Am Ind Hyg Assoc J 48:941–947
28. Munksgaard EC (1992) Permeability of protective gloves to (di) methacrylates in resinous dental materials. Scand J Dent Res 100:189–192
29. Munksgaard EC (2000) Permeability of protective gloves by HEMA and TEGDMA in the presence of solvents. Acta Odontol Scand 58:57–62
30. Packham CL, Packham HE (2004) Practical considerations when selecting and using gloves for chemical protection in a workplace. In: Boman A, Estlander T, Wahlberg JE, Maibach HI (eds) Protective gloves for occupational use, 2nd edn. CRC, Boca Raton, Fla., pp 255–285
31. Perkins JL, Pool B (1997) Batch lot variability in permeation trough nitrile gloves Am Ind Hyg Assoc J 58:474–479
32. Ransjö U (2004) Gloves as protection against microbial contamination. In: Boman A, Estlander T, Wahlberg JE, Maibach HI (eds) Protective gloves for occupational use, 2nd edn. CRC, Boca Raton, Fla., pp 315–320
33. Sansone EB, Tewari YB (1980) Differences in the extent of solvent penetration through natural rubber and nitrile gloves from various manufacturers. Am Ind Hyg Assoc J 41:527–528
34. Schwope AD, Costas PP, Jackson JO, Weitzman JO (1985) Guidelines for the selection of protective clothing. American Conference of Governmental Industrial Hygienists, Cincinnati
35. Schwope AD, Costas PP, Mond CR, Nolen RL, Conoley M, Garcia DB, Walters DB, Prokopetz AT (1988) Gloves for protection from aqueous formaldehyde: permeation resistance and human factors analysis. Appl Ind Hyg 3:167–176
36. Schroeder LW, Walsh DL, Schwerin MR, Richardson DC, Kisielewski RW, Cyr WH (2004) In: Boman A, Estlander T, Wahlberg JE, Maibach HI (eds) Protective gloves for occupational use, 2nd edn. CRC, Boca Raton, Fla., pp 89–109

44

37. Sessink PJM, van de Kerkhof MCA, Anzion RB, Bos RP (1994) Environmental contamination and assessment of exposure to antineoplastic agents by determination of Cyclophosphamide in urine of exposed pharmacy technicians: Is skin absorption an important exposure route? Arch Environ Health 4:165–169
38. Svedman C, Bruze M (2004) In vivo testing of the protective effect of gloves. In: Boman A, Estlander T, Wahlberg JE, Maibach HI (eds) Protective gloves for occupational use, 2nd edn. CRC, Boca Raton, Fla., pp 111–119

44.4 Worker Education and Teaching Programs

44.4.1 The German Experience

Britta Wulfhorst, Meike Bock,
Christoph Skudlik, Swen Malte John[1]

44.4.1.1 Introduction

The number of work-related skin disorders has decreased in the last few years. However, despite the detailed knowledge available on their pathogenesis, diagnosis and therapy, they remain extraordinarily common, necessitating continual care for employees in "wet work" jobs, since they are a high-risk group for work-related skin disorders and allergies [24, 28, 32].

In this chapter we describe a range of interdisciplinary prevention strategies for work-related skin disorders, comprising both medical and educational measures. This integrative approach was developed using a framework of different projects investigating primary, secondary and tertiary prevention of occupational skin disorders. The theoretical basis for these projects was predominantly the World Health Organization's definition of health promotion [33]. In order to meet the requirements of the WHO for health promotion, including self-determination, autonomy, and the social responsibilities of the individual and the social environment, it is necessary to design preventive strategies concerning work-place conditions at an individual level [29, 20]. The efficacy of such measures is evaluated using the example of affected skin. In addition to adequate dermatological diagnosis and therapy for acute and chronic skin changes, the task of prevention also includes clarifying, for those at risk, the correlation between health risks and their own ability to act in order to protect themselves. This knowledge should then lead to individual empowerment [33].

---

[1] This chapter is dedicated to our highly respected academic teacher Professor Hans Joachim Schwanitz

44.4.1.2 Primary Prevention of Occupational Contact Dermatitis

Hairdressers belong to an occupational group that is commonly affected by occupational skin disease. Occupational contact dermatitis predominantly affects apprentices [28, 31]. In order to prevent occupational skin changes in hairdressing trainees, an intervention study was performed between 1996 and 1999. Comprising medical and educational intervention, this study was based upon interdisciplinary concepts [23].

Methods

The study concentrated on hairdressers' apprentices who started their vocational training in 1996. The participants of the intervention group were pupils of a vocational school in Osnabrück, while participants of the matched control group were pupils of a vocational school in Hannover (both schools were in Lower Saxony, Germany). During their vocational training, all of the participants were examined four times by a dermatologist. Their skin conditions were recorded using standardized scores [31]. Participants of the intervention group participated in six seminars (15 hours of lessons), held by professional educators. Therefore, these participants were specifically trained in skin care management and the prevention of occupational contact dermatitis. Moreover, they were supplied with the necessary skin care products, such as gloves and specific protective creams. Consultations about their work environments were also offered and given. Using written questionnaires, knowledge and attitudes concerning skin care management were checked in both the interventional group and the control group at the beginning and end of their second "school year". Statistically significant differences ($p<0.05$) in skin conditions were analyzed using the Wilcoxon Signed-Rank Test for grouped data. Statistically significant results gained from questionnaires on the attitudes, knowledge and behavior regarding skin care were analyzed using Mann-Whitney and Wilcoxon U-tests.

Results

The incidence of occupational contact dermatitis in both groups was comparable in the year 1997 (Table 4.1). In 1998 90% of the participants from the interventional group and 75% of those from the control group had no skin changes (Table 4.1). These differences were significant ($p<0.05$). At the end of the training program 80% of the intervention group and 66% of the control group had encountered no skin

Table 4.1. Results of the Osnabrück Intervention Study 1996 (*I* Interventions group, *C* Control group, *0* nothing, *1* mild, *2* moderate, *3* severe)

Parameter	Response	1996				1997				1998				1999			
		I	%	C	%	I	%	C	%	I	%	C	%	I	%	C	%
(*n*)		73		112		50		73		39		48		41		56	
Skin changes	0	63	86.3	81	72.3	28	56	41	56.2	35	90	36	75	33	80.5	37	66.1
Severity	1	10	13.7	26	23.3	19	38	22	30.1	4	10	8	16.7	7	19.5	11	19.6
	2	0		2	1.8	2	4	5	6.8	0		3	2.1	0		7	12.5
	3	0		3	2.7	1	2	5	6.8	0		1	6.3	0		1	1.8

changes (Table 4.1). Concerning the severity of skin changes, no statistical significant differences were observed in either the intervention or the control group at the beginning (1996) of the study (Table 4.1). Furthermore, the incidence of OCD of both groups was comparable in 1997 (Table 4.1). 90% of the participants from the interventional group and 75% from the control group had encountered no skin changes in 1998 (Table 4.1). These differences were significant ($p<0.05$). At the end of the training program (1999), 80% of the participants from the intervention group and 66% from the control group had encountered no skin changes (Table 4.1).

44.4.1.3 Secondary Prevention of Occupational Contact Dermatitis

Secondary Prevention Project for Hairdressers

A job-specific secondary prevention program was created to enable hairdressers to remain at work despite their skin problems. Again, an interdisciplinary and integrative approach comprising both medical and educational measures, using the concept of an intervention study, was developed.

Methods

A group of measures were used that built on each other. These consisted of, on the one hand, continuous dermatological diagnosis and therapy (Table 4.2). On the other hand, pre-existing and behavior-influencing attitudes to the emergence and the course of the illness were determined within the framework of health education intervention [9, 15]. An exploration of basic attitudes towards personal health and illness as well as towards the determinants of these attitudes (social environment, motivation, and so on) took place during the first consultation, which was recorded on a semi-standardized inter-

view sheet. This was repeated in a modified form when each participant completed the project. Other measures included a theoretical and practical seminar on skin protection that went into the causes and forms of work-related skin disorders. This also elaborated on the skin protection measures that could be implemented. The material learned could be directly put into practice in a practical session. This meant that, for example, cutting hair whilst wearing gloves was practiced directly. All workers and barber-shop owners took part in work consultations carried out after the seminars. The causes of work-related skin disorders and ways to prevent them by applying adequate skin protection techniques were also discussed during the work consultations. A recap seminar was given for the participants at the end of the project. Difficulties encountered when putting the skin protection techniques learned into practice were discussed and solution strategies were worked out together [27]. Altogether 215 participants were enrolled in the project, and it was completed by 150 participants.

The project was evaluated according to its structure, process and results [5, 12]. This contribution will concentrate on just the results from it. In this regard, the whole evaluation process proceeded by comparing the participants' group with an unsupervised

Table 4.2. Secondary prevention of occupational dermatoses: project phases and measures

Phase 1:	Dermatological examination, first consultation, exploratory interview
Phase 2:	Skin protection seminar: *Theory and practice of skin disorders and skin protection in the hairdressing trade*, dermatological examination
Phase 3:	Consultations in the participants' salons
Phase 4:	Final seminar/final consultation, dermatological examination

control group. Moreover, an instrument of evaluation was developed for each individual measure in order to rate the level of success for each measure. Each individual investigative instrument, which will be elaborated on when the results are presented, comprised both qualitative and quantitative methods. Qualitative measures were seen as complementary to quantitative methods, especially when considering subject-oriented data [3].

Results

■ **Subjective Attitudes and Changes in Attitude.** The significance of subjective concepts to the willingness to implement preventative changes in behavior was demonstrated. Occupational socialization can influence behavioral patterns. This becomes clear from the fact that at the beginning of the project 46.7% (*n*=70) of the participants agreed with the statement that slightly reddened or rough hands were quite normal in the hairdressing trade. By the end of the project (final consultation), only 26% (*n*=39) considered slightly reddened and rough hands as being "normal."

■ **Seminars.** The following results emerged from the theoretical and practical seminars (173 affected hairdressers took part in small groups). The results are based on the answers given by the participants to questionnaires filled out after each seminar. In addi-

tion to the presentation of basic skin care information (which in most cases was not previously known by the participants) on the topics "skin disorders – causes, forms and course of illness", "trade associations" and "skin protection", the exchange of experiences among the participants was of particular significance. Participants stressed again and again that discussing experiences with people in similar situations helped enormously (for example "no one laughed", "…it helped a great deal to see that others have the same problems…"). The practical exercises in skin protection also proved to be effective, enabling initially skeptical attitudes about carrying out some hairdressing activities with gloves to be reduced.

■ **Overall Evaluation/Control Group.** In conclusion, 150 participants completed the project, 121 (81%) of them successfully, meaning that the OCD had healed to an extent that allowed them to continue to work as hairdressers. A follow-up survey of the participants carried out 3 months after completion of the project at the earliest showed that 79.9% had been able to remain in work, as opposed to a rate of 60% in the control group that had been under *medical* supervision alone (Fig. 4.1). A five-year follow-up recently revealed that the difference between the two groups was even more pronounced: 65% of the intervention group were still at work but only 29% of the controls remained (unpublished observations).

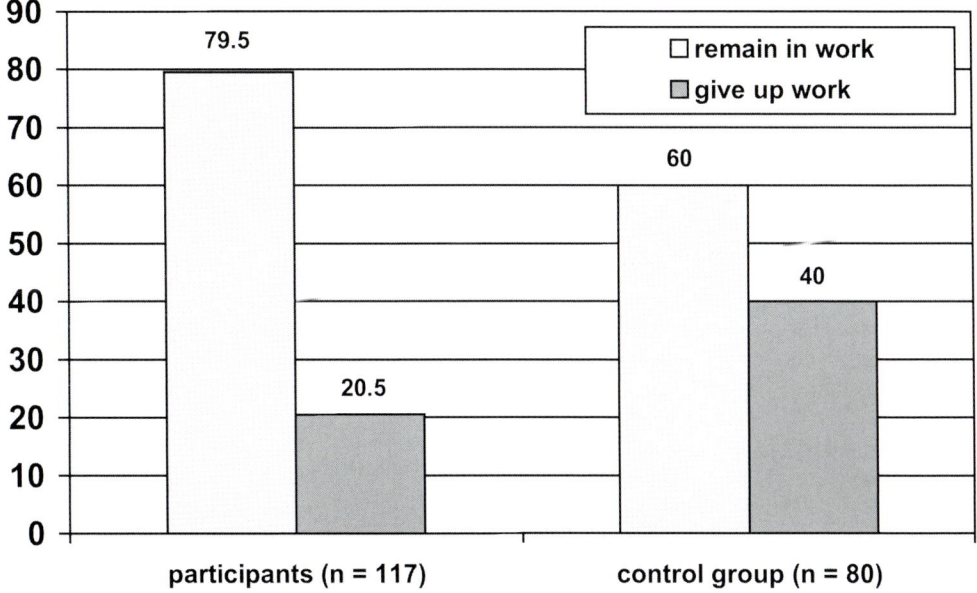

Fig. 4.1. Frequency of those remaining in work among the participants and the control group in the secondary prevention project for hairdressers, data in percent

■ **Workplace Interventions.** During the course of the Secondary Prevention project for hairdressers, an additional workplace consultation was offered to each of the 215 participants who attended the intervention program. Therefore, workplace consultations were carried out consecutively in 103 salons, provided consent was given by the salon-owners. In these 103 salons a total of 652 hairdressers (including the participants of the intervention study, their employers and colleagues) received detailed information on the pathogenesis and epidemiology of OCD, skin protection and legal regulations. Three months after this workplace intervention, a questionnaire-based, anonymous survey amongst the participants ($n=625$) was performed.

■ **Skin Changes in Hairdressers.** The importance of the additional – and unique – workplace intervention described above is made clear if we note the number of "hidden" cases of OCD revealed by the colleagues and employers of the hairdressers who initially attended our seminars. Of the 625 questionnaires given out, 134 (21.4%) were returned. Seventy-three (54.4%) participants stated that they had suffered from skin changes at the workplace, such as dryness, scaling, reddening, vesicles, oozing, and fissures.

Another result of this questionnaire-based study was that the use of protective gloves increased considerably after the consultations. For example, the number of workers that wore gloves when washing hair increased from 26.9% before to 51.5% after the workplace consultations. In total, 60.4% of the 134 participants claimed to have significantly improved their skin protection behavior after the workplace consultations.

Secondary Prevention Project for Geriatric Nurses

The design of the intervention study described above for hairdressers was subsequently used to investigate OCD in geriatric nurses. One hundred two affected geriatric nurses completed all elements of the intervention (see "Secondary Prevention Project for Hairdressers" section). A control group of 107 geriatric nurses was observed, who all received dermatological outpatient treatment. After 3 months, significant differences were observed, indicating that the intervention group achieved better results (Chi-square test). Ninety-six percent of the intervention group were still working as geriatric nurses, compared to 86% in the control group ($p=0.019$). Fifty-three percent of the intervention group complained of occupational skin disorders, in comparison to 82% in the control group ($p<0.001$). The use of gloves during patient washing increased by 22% in the intervention group while no change occurred in the control group. The results underline the advantages of this interdisciplinary dermatological and pedagogical intervention, and its transferability to other high-risk professions [16].

44.4.1.4 Tertiary Prevention of Occupational Contact Dermatitis in High-Risk Professions

A pilot-study, treating patients with *severe* OCD as inpatients, took place between 1994 and 1999 at the University of Osnabrück [27, 30]. This study focused on the tertiary prevention of skin disorders, as well as on their optimized rehabilitation, with the aim of maintaining the profession.

Methods

Participants were only allowed a two-to-three-week inpatient treatment if they suffered from OCD that was resistant to standard outpatient treatments, and so job loss was a strong possibility. After the inpatient phase, treatment was continued by the local dermatologist on an outpatient basis for another two to three weeks. The employee did not work during the resulting complete intervention period of 4–6 weeks. This long work leave is recommended because a perturbed epidermal barrier in humans requires at least four weeks for complete recovery, and frequently even longer [7]. During the inpatient phase, specifically trained dermatologists offered optimized diagnostic and therapeutic strategies as well as an individualized skin protection program. These medical interventions were complemented by educational interventions on many different interacting levels. In order to keep the individual employee in the workplace, one-to-one consultations, group seminars, practical training, ergotherapy and psychological advice was offered.

In order to determine the quality of this intervention, the patients, local dermatologists and social insurance companies were interviewed one year after admittance to the hospital [27].

Results

Four hundred ninety questionnaires were sent out to the participants, of which 352 (71.8%) were returned. Figure 4.2 reveals that 65.9% ($n=232$) of these people were able to maintain their profession, 23% ($n=81$) were unable to work due to OCD, 8.5% ($n=30$) ceased working due to other reasons, and 1.1% ($n=4$)

Fig. 4.2.
Tertiary prevention (inpatient program) from 1994–1999 (n=352): 332 (65.9% "Yes") of the participants in the secondary prevention project for hairdressers still in their profession a year after hospitalization (23% "No, due to OCD", 8.1% "No, due to other reasons" and 1.1% "No, for unknown reasons")

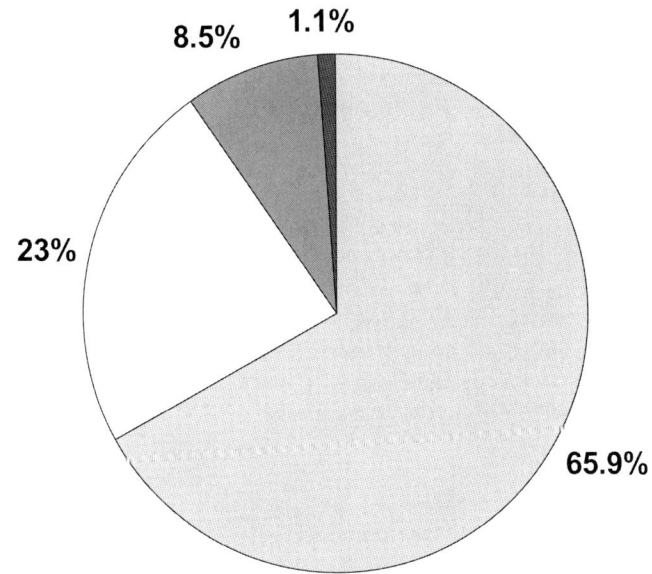

□ Yes □ No due to OCD ▨ No due to other reasons ■ No, unknown reasons

stopped working for unknown reasons. While 81.3% (n=286) continued using improved skin protection as advised, 6.8% (n=24) did not, and 11.9% (n=42) did not comment. Of the employees questioned, 55.7% (n=96) stated that their employer provided protective gloves, 18.2% (n=64) did not receive gloves from their employer, 9.9% (n=35) did not comment on that question, and 16.2% (n=57) of the answers could not be analyzed.

Discussion

■ **Primary Prevention.** The above-mentioned intervention study demonstrates the importance of including skin care and protection management in the education of trainees in high-risk professions. If this is done, the incidence of OCD can be reduced significantly. The improved outcome seen for the intervention group is probably due to improved behavioral patterns resulting from the educational intervention and the supply of skin care and protective products. In conclusion, intervention proved to be effective in this context. Early introduction of trainees to prevention measures appears to be necessary to avoid bad habits which may then become a matter of routine [11, 18].

■ **Secondary Prevention.** The main result from the intervention project on secondary prevention of OCD in hairdressers was that 80% of the project participants remained in work in comparison to just 60% of those in the control group. By investigating

existing attitudes to the emergence of the skin disorder and the willingness to intervene autonomously in the course of the illness, it was possible to work out and successfully implement ways of motivating people to change attitudes and behavioral patterns. For example, the answers given to the question regarding the acceptance of slight skin changes as being an obligatory characteristic of the profession shed light on the significance of occupational socialization, which is partly based on old traditions [13]. The realization that we cannot expect the affected hairdressers to see a causal link between their illness and work-related skin disorders illustrates the need for theoretical material on the emergence of skin disorders in the hairdressing trade to be presented in the seminars. Explanatory and motivating strategies are two examples of such interventions [14, 21]. First of all, the teaching of theory in the seminars made it possible to achieve a positive effect by increasing knowledge about this illness. It is known from the training of patients, such as those with rheumatic diseases, that improved knowledge of the illness leads to an improvement in functional capacity. Similarly, positive therapeutic effects can be achieved by means of groups led by psychologists, supportive and clarifying conversations between patients and experts, as well as by means of an exchange of both experiences and emotional stress between the patients themselves [19]. Ehlers et al also point to the greater effectiveness of preventive measures when psychological approaches are included [6]. These remarks correspond to the results from the seminars carried out in the above-mentioned project. It has been known for a long time that skin disorders, and in this case hand eczema in particular, are particularly stressful (on a psychosocial level) for those affected [25, 26, 29]. In some cases, each group of seminar participants became similar to a self-help group. The educational supervision, however, facilitates professional help, for example in relation to the categorization of everyday theories and lay ideas. This therefore corresponds to the requirement that any attempts by experts to intervene by preventing or rehabilitating illness should take the psychosocial level into consideration and so pay attention to the attitudes of so-called "laymen" to health and illness.

■ **Workplace Interventions.** The role of employers in the successful implementation of preventive measures was made particularly apparent during the workplace consultations. The employer is often the only contact workers can turn to in matters of health and safety, particularly in small businesses. External regulations are more often ignored in small businesses than in larger ones, effective support from an occupational physician often does not exist in such cases. The results from the workplace consultations add weight to the call for formalized supervision structures [1, 8, 11, 13].

The measures developed in Osnabrück have been placed in general use by the German Trade Association for the Health Service and Welfare Care, the responsible statutory accident insurer in the hairdressing trade. Between 1997 and 2002, a total of 2437 hairdressers participated in the secondary prevention program. Complete data are available for 635 hairdressers (26%). This fraction is partly due to the fact that the evaluation is restricted to certain regions in Germany. The percentage of hairdressers with severe skin symptoms dropped from 49% at the start of the rehabilitation program to 11% after completion of the program. The proportion of hairdressers using gloves and applying skin care techniques doubled. The rehabilitation program therefore appears to be a successful way of helping hairdressers to cope with skin problems [22].

The success of the project described above underlines the need to establish further measures in the field of health and safety. In this context, health educational concepts were developed for other professions at high risk of OCD [16]. Recent studies on the prevention of OCD in apprentices in various high-risk professions, like bakers, catering trade, nurses and metalworkers, confirm these conclusions [2, 4, 10, 11].

■ **Tertiary Prevention.** Patients with OCD resistant to standardized outpatient care, that had been admitted to hospital, were interviewed (questionnaire) about the status of their skin and their situation at the workplace one year after hospital release. The majority of the participants had remained in their professions and practiced the advised skin care strategies. Considering the remarkable success rates of these interdisciplinary tertiary prevention programs, they should be recommended as a standard procedure whenever employees are at risk of having to leave their professions due to severe, recalcitrant OCD [30].

Core Message

■ It is possible to verify the efficacy of various educational programs, for example by controlled intervention studies. The results underline the necessity for even more pronounced implementation of health pedagogical interventions in joint interdisciplinary initiatives for prevention of OCD. Of course, health pedagogical measures must be evidence-based; continuous quality management and long-term evaluations are crucial.

References

1. Agner T, Held E (2002) Skin protection programmes. Contact Dermatitis 47:253–256
2. Bauer A, Kelterer D, Bartsch R, Pearson J, Stadeler M, Kleesz P, Elsner P, Williams H (2002) Skin protection in bakers' apprentices. Contact Dermatitis 46:81–85
3. Berg M (1991) Evaluation of a questionnaire used in dermatological epidemiology. Discrepancy between self-reported symptoms and objective signs. Acta Derm Venereol (Stockh) 156:13–17
4. Berndt U, Hinnen U, Iliev D, Elsner P (2000) Hand eczema in metalworker trainees – an analysis of risk factors. Contact Dermatitis 43:327–332
5. Donabedian A (1968) Promoting quality through evaluating the process of patient care. Med Care 6:181–202
6. Ehlers A, Gieler U, Stangier U (1995) Treatment of atopic dermatitis: a comparison of psychological and dermatological approaches to relapse prevention. J Consult Clin Psychol 63:624–635
7. Fartasch M (1995) Human barrier formation and reaction to irritation. In: Elsner P, Maibach HI (eds) Irritant dermatitis. New clinical and experimental aspects. Current problems in dermatology. Karger, Basel, pp 95–103
8. Geraut C, Tripodi D (2002) Prevention of occupational dermatitis. Rev Prat 52:1446–1450
9. Graziani C, Rosenthal MP, Diamond JJ (1999) Diabetes education program use and patient-perceived barriers to attendance. Family Med 31:358–363

10. Held E, Wolff C, Gyntelberg F, Agner T (2001) Prevention of work-related skin problems in student auxiliary nurses: an intervention study. Contact Dermatitis 44:297–303

11. Held E, Mygind K, Wolff C, Gyntelberg F, Agner T (2002) Prevention of work related skin problems: an intervention study in wet work employees. Occup Environ Med 59:556–561

12. Heron RJL (1997) Worker education in the primary prevention of occupational dermatoses. Occup Med 47:407–410

13. Jensen LK, Kofoed LB (2002) Musculoskeletal disorders among floor layers: is prevention possible? Appl Occup Environ Hyg 17:797–806

14. Kalimo K, Kautiainen H, Niskanen T, Niemi L (1999) 'Eczema school' to improve compliance in an occupational dermatology clinic. Contact Dermatitis 41:315–319

15. Kanzler MH, Gorsulowsky DC (2002) Patients' attitudes regarding physical characteristics of medical care providers in dermatologic practices. Arch Dermatol 138:463–466

16. Klippel U, Schürer NY, Schwanitz HJ (2004) Sekundäre Individualprävention von Handekzemen in der Altenpflege: Perspektive der Gesundheitspädagogik. Derm Beruf Umwelt 52:106–112

17. Lee A, Nixon R (2001) Occupational skin disease in hairdressers. Australas J Dermatol 42:1–6

18. Löffler H, Effendy I (2002) Prevention of irritant contact dermatitis. Eur J Dermatol 12:4–9

19. Lorish CD, Boutaugh ML (1997) Patient education in rheumatology. Curr Opin Rheumatol 9:106–111

20. Napalkov N (1995) The role of the World Health Organization in promoting patient education with emphasis on chronic diseases. In: Assal J-P, Golay A, Visser AP (eds) New trends in patient education. Elsevier, Amsterdam, pp 5–7

21. Nevitt GJ, Hutchinson PE (1996) Psoriasis in the community: prevalence, severity and patients beliefs and attitudes towards the disease. Br J Dermatol 135:533–537

22. Nienhaus A, Rojahn K, Skudlik C, Wulfhorst B, Dulon M, Brandenburg S (2004) Sekundäre Individualprävention bei FriseurInnen mit arbeitsbedingten Hauterkrankungen. Gesundheitswesen 66:759–764

23. Riehl U (2000) Interventionsstudie zur Prävention von Hauterkrankungen bei Auszildenden des Friseurhandwerks. Rasch, Osnabrück

24. Rycroft RJG (2001) Occupational contact dermatitis. In: Rycroft RJG, Menné T, Frosch PJ, Lepoittevin JP (eds) Textbook of contact dermatitis, 3rd edn. Springer, Berlin Heidelberg New York, pp 555–580

25. Schmid-Ott G, Jaeger B, Kuensebeck HW, Ott R, Lamprecht F (1996) Dimension of stigmatisation in patients with psoriasis in a "Questionnaire on experience with skin complaints". Dermatology 193:304–310

26. Schwanitz HJ (1988) Atopic palmoplantar eczema. Springer, Berlin Heidelberg New York

27. Schwanitz HJ, Riehl U, Schlesinger T, Bock M, Skudlik C, Wulfhorst B (2003) Skin care management: educational aspects. Int Arch Occup Environ Health 76:374–381

28. Schwanitz HJ, Uter W (2000) Interdigital dermatitis: sentinel skin damage in hairdressers. Br J Dermatol 142:1011–1012

29. Schwanitz HJ, Wulfhorst B (2000) Workers education. In: Kanerva L, Elsner P, Wahlberg JE et al (eds) Handbook of occupational dermatology. Springer, Berlin Heidelberg New York, pp 441–443

30. Skudlik C, Schwanitz HJ (2004) Tertiary prevention of occupational skin diseases. JDDG 2:424–433

31. Uter W, Pfahlberg A, Gefeller O, Schwanitz HJ (1998) Prevalence and incidence of hand dermatitis in hairdressing apprentices: results of the POSH study. Prevention of occupational skin disease in hairdressers. Int Arch Occup Environ Health 71:487–492

32. Van der Walle HB, Brunsveld VM (1994) Dermatitis in hairdressers (I). The experience of the past four years. Contact Dermatitis 30:217–221

33. World Health Organization (WHO) (1986) Ottawa Charta for Health Promotion. WHO, Geneva

34. Wulfhorst B (2002) Theorie der Gesundheitspädagogik. Legitimation, Aufgabe und Funktionen von Gesundheitserziehung. Reihe Grundlagentexte Gesundheitswissenschaft. Juventa, Weinheim

44.4.2 The Swiss Experience: www.2hands.ch

Daniel Perrenoud, Thierry Gogniat, William Olmstead

44.4.2.1 Introduction

The idea for a national campaign for the prevention of work-related contact dermatitis began in 1997 when informal conversations with teachers in professional training schools were initiated. In Switzerland about a quarter of all occupational disability claims handled by the Swiss Accident Insurance Fund (SUVA) involve skin disease, and more than half of these are hand-related. This being the case, it seemed appropriate to begin with those most at risk: apprentices.

We started with some basic ideas which we modified as our campaign evolved. The campaign was to be based on a kit that would be a complete self-contained unit that would place the teacher at the center of the presentation.

We distributed our first kits in September 1999. By early 2000, 300 kits had been distributed to teachers of apprentices all over Switzerland. Since 2003, all our material has been made available on the internet.

44.4.2.2 The Beginning

We started by studying the material available.

We found illustrations in the style familiar to all medical students, showing the complex anatomy of the skin of a hand. We also found a number of professionally-made videos from Sweden, each focusing on one particular problem by using a short story involving different groups of young people.

Neither of these approaches were suited to our purposes. The drawback we found was that they were too complex for the audience we were targeting.

We also realized that our audience of apprentices and young workers might have negative reactions to overly formal academic presentations. In addition, we wanted the teachers to be the presenters – the conduit through which our material would be delivered.

44.4.2.3 Developing New Material

To break through the negative expectations of "just another lecture on hand care," we decided to start our presentation with a very lively MTV-style music video.

This two-and-a-half-minute video was about hands, but there was only music and mostly unintelligible voices – a disco scene.

The result we hoped for was that the audience would be intrigued and involved – they would ask themselves "What is this? It's clearly not a typical documentary-style presentation!". This was one of our basic ideas: to establish a rapport with the audience.

When the video stops the teacher takes center stage. The teacher presents a series of overheads, adapted to the audience. Overheads were preferred to slides. With overheads, the teacher looks at the audience and is the messenger. With a slide presentation the presenter fades into the background in a usually dimly-lit room.

This was another of our basic ideas: to make sure that it's the teacher who delivers the information. Our whole kit is designed to ensure this – it gives the teacher everything required.

Our kit includes 23 transparencies accompanied by a set of notes with suggestions for discussion and in-depth treatment, as well as a great deal of supplementary material.

We created many graphic images. Two typical ones are reminiscent of Malten's famous review paper, *Thoughts on Irritant Contact Dermatitis*, published in Contact Dermatitis in 1981 [1]. We show the mechanism of skin irritation and then distinguish between acute and cumulative irritation (Figs. 4.3, 4.4).

The contrast is made between viruses and allergens, in terms of their relationship with the immune system. Different professions and their specific dangers are profiled in turn. Irritation is then presented as opening the door to allergy.

The point is then made that once an allergy happens the young apprentice may have to change professions.

All this is presented as graphically and as simply as possible (Fig. 4.5). We wanted to make a presentation that would be very graphic in nature and thus something that a nonspecialist teacher could comfortably present with just a few supporting notes, and whose message an unsophisticated audience could grasp. Aside from simplicity, another advantage of a graphically-oriented presentation is the ease with which it can be adapted to other languages.

44.4.2.4 A Graphical Course for the Workplace

After we had already started our first campaign, we were asked by the Swiss Accident Insurance Fund (SUVA) to develop a graphic educational course to be used in the metalworking industry workplace [2]. This required that we simplify the graphic message

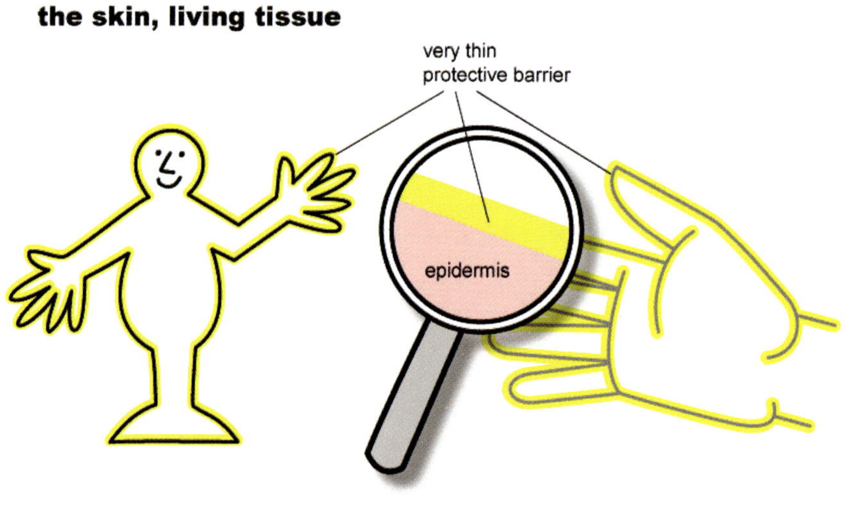

Fig. 4.3.
Skin irritation allows environmental chemicals to penetrate the skin and induce inflammation

44

Fig. 4.4.
Acute and cumulative irritation result in comparable effects on the skin, however, weak or moderate irritants are frequently not recognized as harmful

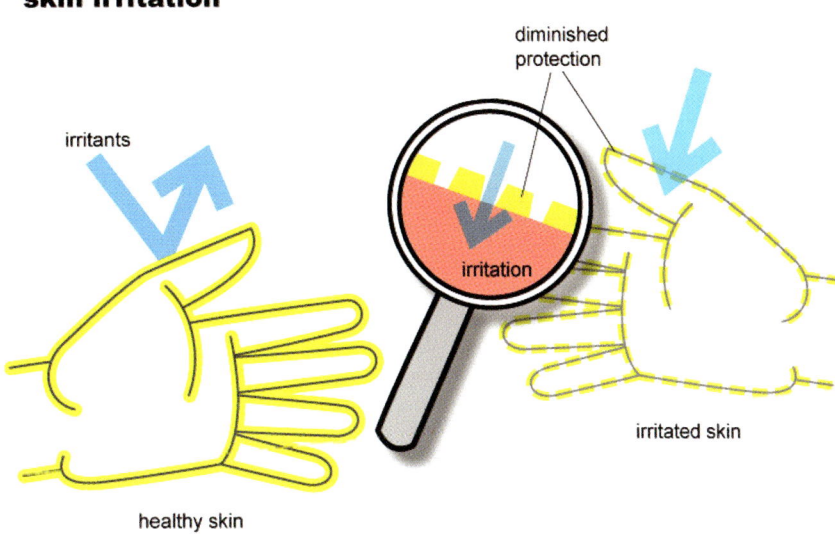

skin irritation

Fig. 4.5.
A good drawing is worth a thousand words: keep the message simple!

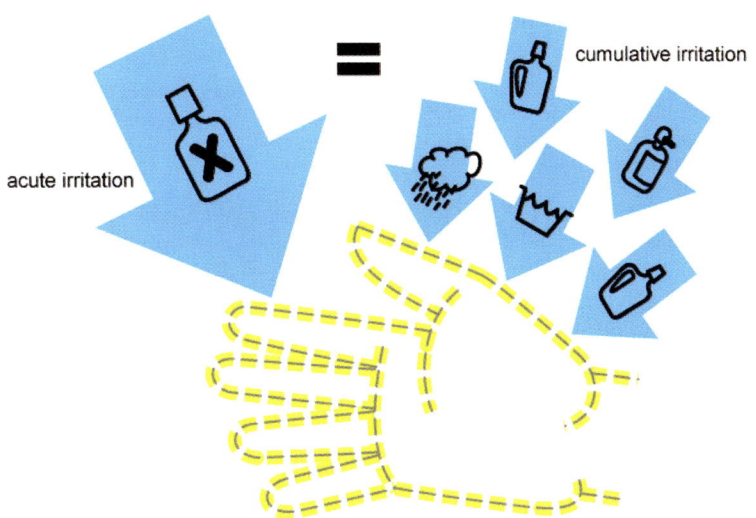

the 2 kinds of irritation

even further – the text was completely removed. This illustrates a basic principle we follow: adapt the presentation of the information to the audience and the circumstances.

Lastly, we tried to ensure that what we produced would be used fully: we made a complete kit. A point now about the kit being a complete solution. We offer information in the hope of changing attitudes and eventually behavior. We think that it's important to actually practice the desired behavior in the classroom or at the workplace sessions. Therefore, we give each participant a sample of handcream and then instruct them on how to ensure that no areas of the skin are missed. Just like any other prophylactic, it must be used each time you are exposed, and used properly.

We put all of the material into a box that can be easily transported, stored, and even mailed through the regular post.

Teachers rapidly embraced the kit thanks to its simplicity and ease of use. Feedback was also gratifyingly high among those outside the teaching profession per se: health professionals, safety engineers and others involved in skin disease prevention, even outside Switzerland.

44.4.2.5　The 2hands.ch Website

Since 2003, all of our material has been available on the Internet. As a matter of fact, we took the opportunity to redesign both the course and the educational text material completely. We also translated all of the material into English, making the content of our website available in four languages. We also introduced new themes, such as "How to find the right gloves for the right occupation". This chapter was deliberately an easy-to-use tool for end users: students, teachers, workers, housewives, and any person interested in skin care and protection. We developed it with the support of, and in close co-operation with, the SUVA and its department that sells safety products, called Sapros, online [4].

At present, occupational schools that are using our kit are now switching to using our material in electronic format; it is available in Acrobat PDF format on our website [3]. Putting the material on the Web increased the interest from Swiss industry in our material on the prevention of skin disease in the workplace. On average, our website currently gets over 120 hits daily – well beyond our initial expectations.

44.4.2.6　Making the Knowledge Available Where Needed

We close with a quote from an article called *Strong Inference* [5]: "We speak piously of taking measurements and making small studies that will 'add another brick to the temple of science'. Most such bricks just lie around the brickyard."

In other words, aside from doing good research and publishing the results, aside from designing good education material and prevention campaigns, aside from developing better protective creams and gloves, we must take the extra step of fulfilling our social responsibility to ensure that all of the material ("all of the bricks") – are used to make something useful to the world at large.

■ **Acknowledgements.** We warmly thank Dr Hanspeter Rast, Dr Rudolf Schütz, Ms Désirée Schibig and all their colleagues at the SUVA in Lucerne, who have believed in and continuously supported our work since the beginning.

References

1. Malten KE (1981) Thoughts on irritant contact dermatitis. Contact Dermatitis 7:238–247
2. Suva (2005) Module d'apprentissage Protection de la peau. Notice de formation pour l'industrie de la métallurgie. Suva, Lucerne (réf 88803, see http://www.suva.ch)
3. Perrenoud D, Gogniat T (2005) 2hands.ch websites. (See http://www.2hands.ch, http://www.2mains.ch, http://www.2haende.ch, and http://www.2mani.ch)
4. Sapros (2005) Sapros homepage. See (http://www.sapros.ch)
5. Platt JR (1964) Strong inference. Science 146:347–353

44.4.3　The Danish Experience: Prevention of Skin Problems in Wet Work Employees

ELISABETH HELD, TOVE AGNER

In Denmark, hand eczema (HE) is the most commonly recognized occupational disease, accounting for about 40% of all recognized cases [1]. Wet work is considered to be the most important risk factor for the development of chronic HE. It is important to prevent HE, since the disease often becomes chronic or even disabling. Important preventive measures include exposure control, employee education and use of personal protective equipment such as gloves and moisturizers. Intervention studies in the workplace are, however, necessary to determine the effectiveness of such preventive measures.

44.4.3.1　Intervention Studies

Using the concept of an intervention study, it is possible to demonstrate whether a given intervention is possible and whether it will have the intended effect [2]. Employee education is an important preventive measure and should preferably result in increased knowledge about the function of the skin, awareness of symptoms due to occupational hazards and an understanding of managing hazards and the correct use of moisturizers and gloves. Organizational support is, however, also important, and written policies on work procedures should also be implemented at the workplace [3].

In the following, the experiences gained from some Danish intervention programs will be discussed. Two intervention studies were conducted with wet work employees: one in student auxiliary nurses (study I) [4] who were having their first apprentice period, and one study in wet work employees in nursing homes (study II) [5]. An intervention

44

group and a matched control group were included in both studies, and the intervention group was exposed to an *educational program* including a *skin protection program* before or during the intervention period. The educational program provided information about normal and diseased skin, leading to increased awareness and early recognition of skin symptoms due to wet work. One of the prerequisites was for the participants to understand recommendations regarding wet work procedures (skin protection program). The skin protection program [6] was a series of practical instructions about skin protection that included updated evidence-based recommendations about wet work procedures and the use of protective measures (for ten actions that can help prevent hand eczema, refer to Chap 19).

44.4.3.2 Student Auxiliary Nurses (I)

The intervention group included 61 students (three classes) from one school and the control group included 46 students (three classes) from another school, both located in the County of Copenhagen, and they were both followed during the first ten weeks of their first practical training in county hospitals. The intervention group was given an educational program just before the students had their first practical training. In each intervention class, a 2×2 h course was given with the sessions separated by an interval of 14 days. The course was conducted by two teachers and included an informative video and a booklet, which students were asked to read in between the two teaching sessions. The educational program was an interactive dialog based on the student's own experiences of wet work and included an introduction to the physiology of normal and diseased skin and to allergic and irritant contact dermatitis. As part of the intervention, the students were exposed to the evidence-based skin protection program and all participants in the intervention group were given a moisturizer (100 g), with a documented positive effect on irritant contact dermatitis [7, 8].

To evaluate the participants, they were each given a questionnaire to fill in, a clinical hand examinations and patch testing, and their transepidermal water loss (TEWL) was measured, both before and after the 10 weeks of practical training.

Of the 107 student auxiliary nurses included in the study, 13 participants dropped out during the training period (seven in the intervention group and six in the control group).

After the practical training, where the student auxiliary nurses were exposed to wet work, there was a significant increase in the number of participants

with skin problems ($p<0.0005$) as judged by clinical examination (48% in the intervention group and 58% in the control group; $p>0.05$). Aggravation of skin problems was associated with having doctor-diagnosed atopic dermatitis (odds ratio: 4.89, confidence interval: 1.16–20.64, $p=0.027$). Three students with atopic dermatitis (all belonging to the control group) developed severe vesiculous hand eczema during the training. Patch testing revealed that 25% of those in the intervention group and 38% of those in the control group had nickel allergies ($p=0.35$).

A significant increase in TEWL, indicating a defect in the skin barrier function, was seen in the control group but not in the intervention group after ten weeks of practical training. High basal TEWL was not associated with occurrence of skin symptoms during the practical training, as evaluated by clinical examination.

44.4.3.3 Wet Work Employees (Nursing Homes) (II)

Three hundred seventy-five wet-work employees were included in a prospective randomized controlled trial, allocated to either intervention ($n=207$) or control ($n=168$). The study period was 5 months. The study population was recruited from employees (nursing, kitchen and cleaning) of seven old peoples homes in the City of Copenhagen. Three nursing homes were chosen at random for the intervention group and four for the control group. A formalized educational program was given to a team of frontline employees (10–20 persons) called the "participatory team" in each intervention workplace. This team included employees willing to undergo an educational program and willing to teach and instruct other employees. The team included at least one person from management, one from the local safety board, and one from each working sector (nursing, kitchen and cleaning). After the training the participatory team passed the information on to their colleagues. As part of the intervention, a skin protection policy (including written instructions) was established in each workplace. Moisturizers [7, 8] and cotton gloves were freely available for all employees.

The intervention and control groups completed questionnaires on behavior and symptoms and underwent clinical examination of their hands before and after the five-month period, as well as answering a test quiz.

Three-quarters (156/207) of the intervention group and slightly more (78%; 131/168) of the control group completed the study. No difference was found between the intervention and the control group at baseline with respect to clinical symptoms or behavior. Evaluation after the five-month intervention period revealed significantly more knowledge of skin protection techniques in the intervention group as compared to the control group ($p=0.003$), a significant change in wet work behavior in the intervention group but not in the control group, and significantly fewer skin symptoms as evaluated clinically for the intervention group ($p<0.0001$) but not for the control group ($p=1.00$). The significant change in behavior included fewer hours spent with wet hands, fewer rings worn on fingers, and increased use of cotton gloves. Ninety percent of the participants in the intervention group agreed that they had received information about good skin protection during the 5 months of intervention. Ninety-seven percent of the employees had received moisturizers that were freely provided, and 79% had received cotton gloves. Seventy-four percent (116/156) of the intervention group and 55% (72/131) of the control group accepted patch testing. Nickel allergy was confirmed in 29% of the patch-tested participants in the intervention group and in 32% of the control group ($p>0.05$).

44.4.3.4 Discussion

Study I confirmed that atopic dermatitis is a significant risk factor for skin problems or aggravation of already existing skin problems when exposed to wet work for a ten-week period. This is supported by numerous previous findings [9–11], and it highlights the fact that a history of atopic dermatitis and wet work are often noncompatible factors. Some studies have shown that skin irritation often occurs early in the professional career [12, 13]. The present study confirms this, indicating that clinical examination of the hands (pre-employment screening) may be advantageous for trainees. In study I, that included student auxiliary nurses, the clinical examination did not reveal any statistically significantly difference between the intervention group and the control group after the ten-week period of training. This was either a true negative finding or one related to the small number of participants included. A possible explanation is that the intervention strategy used in this study targeted at an individual level, so no organizational support was included. Bioengineering measuring methods for predicting skin susceptibility have been found to be useful in experimental studies, but their relevance in field studies is still debated. Some experimental studies have shown that high baseline TEWL may be a good predictor of skin susceptibility [14, 15]. Significant increases in TEWL in the exposed skins of the student auxiliary nurses were seen in the

control group after 10 weeks of training, perhaps indicating subclinical skin irritation, but baseline TEWL failed to predict the development of skin symptoms.

In study II, including wet work employees from nursing homes, the behavioral changes prescribed in the skin protection program for the intervention group were achieved for some measurable activities, such as an increased use of cotton gloves, and fewer hours spent with wet hands. The success of the intervention may be related to the fact that the behavioral changes were limited to small practical changes during work hours and that positive changes in skin symptoms due to altered behavior can be followed closely, thereby motivating the employee to continue the skin protection program. A methodological problem in clinical studies is that subjects suffering from skin problems are more likely to use protective measures and preventive measures will then be associated with the outcome variable hand eczema, as stated by Diepgen and Coenraads [16].

In the field of prevention of work-related HE, particular attention has been paid to the effect of moisturizers. In the intervention studies presented here, a moisturizer that had proved efficient for treating irritant skin reactions in experimental studies was available to all participants in the intervention group. In both studies, no differences were observed in the use of moisturizer between the intervention and the control group, neither before nor after the intervention. Most of the participants (93%) were already using a moisturizer before they began the study (II). A similar high percentage of moisturizer use has been found in other studies in health care workers [13].

In both intervention studies (I and II), a high percentage ($>25\%$) of the participants had nickel allergy (confirmed by patch testing), but any statistically significant correlation between nickel allergy and skin problems/HE was not confirmed.

Participatory action research implies that the employees take an active role in all phases of the intervention [2]. This approach has proven effective in the prevention of musculoskeletal disorders among health care workers [17]. A similar method was used in study II, where a group of frontline employees first underwent a training program, then developed written procedures and subsequently introduced the messages to their colleagues.

In conclusion, an educational program, including an evidence-based skin protection program with recommendations on wet work procedures and the use of preventive measures, was tested in student auxiliary nurses and in wet work employees. In study II, the intervention had a positive influence on wet work behavior, on knowledge, as well as on clinical skin

44

problems, whereas study I failed to show any statistically significantly influence on the number of clinical skin problems. In study II, the focus was on prevention at both the individual and the organizational level. Both strategies are important, but intervention at an organizational level ("policy making") ensures that preventive measures are integrated as a part of the daily routine after the intervention period has stopped, ensuring a continuous learning process [18].

It is important that recommendations in skin protection programs undergo evaluation at regular intervals in order to include the latest evidence from both clinical and experimental studies.

44.4.3.5 Important Messages

- Intervention at the workplace should improve employee knowledge, wet-work behavior and clinical skin conditions.
- Involvement at an organizational level is necessary to obtain successful prevention.
- Intervention studies are necessary to document the effects of preventive measures.

References

1. National Board of Industrial Injuries in Denmark (2005) Website (see http://www.ask.dk)
2. Kristensen TS (2000) Workplace intervention studies. Occup Med 15:293–305
3. Goldenhar LM, Schulte PA (1994) Intervention research in occupational health and safety. J Occup Med 36:763–775
4. Held E, Wolff C, Gyntelberg F, Agner T (2001) Prevention of work-related skin problems in student auxiliary nurses. An intervention study. Contact Dermatitis 44:297–303
5. Held E, Mygind K, Wollf C, Gyntelberg F, Agner T (2002) Prevention of work related skin problems. An intervention study in wet-work employees. Occcup Environ Med 59:556–561
6. Agner T, Held E (2002) Skin protections. Contact Dermatitis 47:253–256
7. Ramsing DW, Agner T (1997) Preventive and therapeutic effects of a moisturizer. An experiment study on human skin. Acta Derm Venereol (Stockh) 77:35–37
8. Held E, Agner T (1999) Comparison between two test models in evaluating the effect of a moisturizer on irritated human skin. Contact Dermatitis 40:261–268
9. Brisman J, Meding B, Järvholm B (1998) Occurrence of self reported hand eczema in Swedish bakers. Occup Environ Med 55:750–754
10. Rystedt I (1985) Hand eczema and long-term prognosis in atopic dermatitis (thesis). Acta Derm Venereol (Stockh) 117:1–59
11. Tacke J, Schmidt A, Fartasch M, Diepgen TL (1995) Occupational contact dermatitis in bakers, confectioners and cooks: a population-based study. Contact Dermatitis 33:112–117
12. Bauer A, Bartsch R, Stadeler M, Schneider W, Grieshaber R, Wollina U, Gebhardt M (1998) Development of occupational skin diseases during vocational training in baker and confectioner apprentices: a follow-up study. Contact Dermatitis 39:307–311
13. Hansen KS (1983) Occupational dermatoses in hospital cleaning woman. Contact Dermatitis 9:343–351
14. Pinnagoda J, Tupker RA, Coenraads PJ, Nater JP (1989) Prediction of susceptibility to an irritant response by transepidermal water loss. Contact Dermatitis 20:341–346
15. John SM, Uter W, Schwanitz HJ (2000) Relevance of multi-parametric skin bioengineering in a prospectively-followed cohort of junior hairdressers. Contact Dermatitis 43:161–168
16. Diepgen TL, Coenraads PJ (1997) Inflammatory skin diseases II: contact dermatitis. In: Williams HC, Strachan DP (eds) The challenge of dermato-epidemiology. CRC, Boca Raton, Fla., pp 145–160
17. Evanoff BA, Bohr PC, Wolf LD (1999) Effects of a participatory ergonomics team among hospital orderlies. Am J Ind Med 35:358–365
18. Ford JK, Fisher S (1994) The transfer of safety training in work organizations: a systems perspective to continuous learning. Occup Med 9:241–259

Chapter 45

Legislation

Ian R. White, David Basketter

Contents

45.1 Introduction

Europe has the most highly developed set of legislation regarding contact dermatitis. Rather than catalogue the varying aspects of legislation globally, we have limited the material to a relatively brief consideration of this European perspective, since we believe that it provides a good model. Legislation and regulations regarding chemical substances, preparations, detergents and cosmetics are mentioned, together with information on legislation relating to two very important allergens, nickel and chromate.

45.2 Cosmetics Directive

In Europe, cosmetic safety legislation is governed by the Cosmetics Directive (76/768/EEC) which is then incorporated into the national legislation of the EU member states. DG Enterprise (Unit F3) of the European Commission is responsible for this Directive. The full text is published in English on the website:

http://pharmacos.eudra.org/F3/cosmetic/pdf/vol_1en.pdf.

Regular updates are published in all of the official EU languages: http://pharmacos.eudra.org/F3/cosmetic/Consolidated_dir.htm.

Annex 1 of the Cosmetics Directive provides an illustrative list of cosmetic products. Annex 2 is a list of substances that are prohibited from use in cosmetic products available in Europe. Annex 3 tabulates substances that may be used, but only under certain restrictions (such as for application to hair only, not for oral hygiene). Annexes 6 and 7 are positive lists of preservatives and UV filters.

- Annex 2
  - prohibited
- Annex 3
  - restricted/conditions of use
- Annex 4
  - coloring agents
- Annex 6
  - preservatives
- Annex 7
  - UV filters

In due course it is probable that there will be a positive list of hair dyes (only those substances on the list may be used).

Relatively few ingredients are included in the various annexes. However, the cosmetic industry uses several thousand substances for which there is no specific regulation. The so-called *inventory* of cosmetic ingredients is an indicative but not exhaustive listing of these substances. Again, the inventory is the responsibility of DG Enterprise, which publishes it (see http://pharmacos.eudra.org/F3/cosmetic/cosm_inci_index.htm). Part 1 of the inventory lists general cosmetic ingredients; Part 2 lists fragrance ingredients. The inventory contains the INCI name (International Nomenclature for Cosmetic Ingredients) that must be used for ingredient labeling purposes in the European Union. The INCI system is based on the CTFA nomenclature used in the USA. The important differences between the American (voluntary) system and that used in Europe (legal) are the use of Latin scientific names for biological extracts (rather than common names in the USA), color index numbers (FD&C in the USA) and aqua (water in USA). The prime reason for the differences was to ensure that language was "scientific" and acceptable to all nations, rather than being obviously English.

Ingredient listing was introduced in the sixth amendment of the cosmetic Directive, although a compromise was reached where fragrance compositions in cosmetics would be indicated simply by the word *parfum*. This "fragrance exception" was included because of the lobbying activities of the industry, but identification of 26 "established" fragrance allergens was introduced with the seventh amendment of the Directive. Since March 2005, identification has been required if one of the fragrance substances is present at levels >10 ppm for leave-on products and >100 ppm for rinse off. This should ensure that the great majority of individuals with identified fragrance allergies can adequately avoid exposure. These levels were suggested by the European Parliament as a pragmatic solution, as the "safe" levels for most of the fragrance substances are largely unknown.

Before a cosmetic ingredient is added to one of the annexes in the Cosmetics Directive, there is a requirement that a scientific evaluation of the substance is provided by the independent advisory committee of the European Commission. Until 1997 this was the Scientific Committee for Cosmetology (SCC). From 1997 until 2004 it was the Scientific Committee for Cosmetics and Non-Food Products (SCC NFP), and since 2004 the Scientific Committee for Consumer Products (SCCP). All of the opinions of the SCC NFP are available on the website of DG Sanco (Directorate General for Consumer Safety and Health Protection) http://europa.eu.int/comm/health/ph_risk/committees/sccp/sccp_opinions_en.htm, as are those of the SCCP http://europa.eu.int/comm/health/ph_risk/committees/04_sccp/sccp_opinions_en.htm.

A request for assessment is presented to the advisory committee via DG Enterprise. Requests are made because evaluation is required by the Directive, there is concern raised by a Member State or scientific/clinical data suggests a problem that needs to be evaluated. The information evaluated by the SCCP is normally supplied in a complete dossier (containing the toxicological, chemical, epidemiological data: published, "on file" and "gray" material) of a substance provided by industry, but information may be submitted by others (which happened with methyldibromo glutaronitrile and hydroxyisohexyl 3-cyclo-

Safety assessment versus management

Assessment
- DG SANCO – consumer safety and health protection
- Provides scientific advice
- Scientific committees – SCCP

Management
- DG ENTERPRISE responsible for legal regulation of cosmetics
- Member states

Fig. 1. Safety assessment versus management

hexene carboxaldehyde, where the dermatological community provided the data).

DG Sanco is responsible for assessments of risk, whilst DG Enterprise is concerned with the management of risk (Fig. 1).

The above scientific advisory committees have produced Guidelines for the Safety Evaluation of Cosmetic Ingredients. These guidelines are regularly updated as science and technology progresses and are available from the website.

Although a cosmetic product must comply with all regulatory requirements, it is also a requirement that the safety of each cosmetic product (including that of the ingredients that have not been regulated) be independently assessed by an individual with appropriate expertise – the assessor. Every cosmetic product has an associated dossier containing technical details of the ingredients and a safety (toxicological) assessment (Fig. 2).

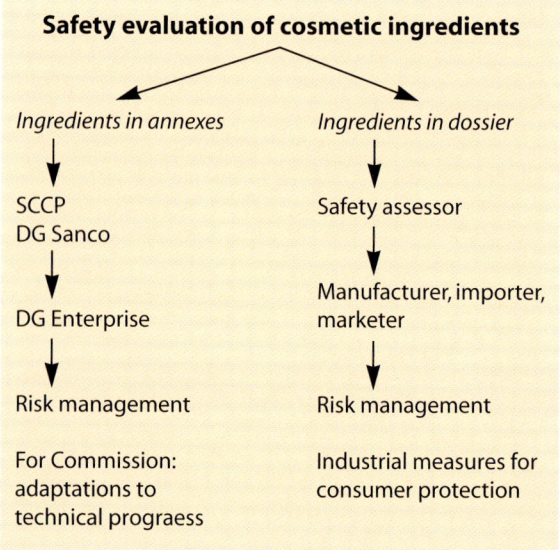

Safety evaluation of cosmetic ingredients

Ingredients in annexes	Ingredients in dossier
SCCP DG Sanco	Safety assessor
DG Enterprise	Manufacturer, importer, marketer
Risk management	Risk management
For Commission: adaptations to technical prograess	Industrial measures for consumer protection

Fig. 2. Safety evaluation of cosmetic ingredients

The seventh amendment also introduced a timeline for the prohibition of animal experiments used to evaluate the safety of cosmetic ingredients that must comply with the requirements of the Directive. There has been prohibition of testing of finished cosmetic products on animals since September 2004. Additionally, with exceptions, there is to be a gradual prohibition of testing of ingredients on animals as alternative validated methods are adopted. There will also be a parallel prohibition of the sale of cosmetics when an ingredient has been tested on animals, within or outside of the EU, to meet the requirements of the Cosmetics Directive after March 2009. The exceptions consist of repeat dose toxicity, toxicokinetics and reprotoxicity, which will be permitted until 2013. The timeline was introduced into the seventh amendment by a process of conciliation, and was politically driven.

There are several steps associated with the process of *risk assessment*:

- Hazard identification
  - In vivo, in vitro tests, QSAR, epidemiology
- Dose-response assessment
  - NOAEL (no observed adverse effect level)
- Exposure assessment
  - Amount, frequency, specific groups
- Risk characterization
  - Margin of safety

As far as dermatological assessments are concerned, the following represents the status (2005) of the validation of and the movement towards the reduction or replacement of animal (in vivo) testing methodologies:

45.2.1 Skin Irritation

- Draize in vivo skin irritation test
  - OECD 404, EC B.4
- Several in vitro skin irritation tests under validation

45.2.2 Skin Corrosivity

- Three validated alternatives:
- TER – Rat Skin Transcutaneous Electrical Resistance Test (draft OECD 430, EC B.40)
- EPISKIN and EpiDerm – reconstructed human epidermal equivalent (draft OECD 431, EC B.40)

45.2.3 Eye Irritation

- No validated alternative to Draize in vivo test (OECD 405, EC B.5)
  ECVAM – the European Centre for Validation of Alternative Methods (http://ecvam.jrc.it/index.htm) – is currently evaluating
- Bovine Cornea Opacity-Permeability test
- Neutral organic chemicals
- Red Blood Cell; Neutral Red Uptake
- Surfactants
- Hen's Egg Test – Chorioallantoic membrane
- Screening finished products

45.2.4 Skin Sensitization

- Magnusson Kligman Guinea Pig Maximization Test (OECD 406, EC B.6)
- Local Lymph Node Assay (OECD draft 429)
  - allows reduction of animal use and refinement of data obtained

45.2.5 Dermal Absorption, Percutaneous Penetration

- In vivo (draft OECD Guideline 427)
- In vitro (draft OECD Guideline 428)
  - isolated human/pig skin

45.2.6 Photoirritation

- 3T3 Neutral Red Uptake Phototoxicity Test (draft OECD 432, EC B.41)
- Expected that chemicals showing photoallergic properties may be positive

45.3 Detergent Regulations

The Detergents Regulations of the European Union came into force in October 2005: http://europa.eu.int/eur-lex/pri/en/oj/dat/2004/l_104/l_10420040408en00010035.pdf.

This regulation requires the listing of preservatives in detergents, household and similar products when present at any concentration in a finished product, and the identification of the presence of any

45

of the fragrance allergens itemized in the Cosmetics Directive and present at >100 ppm (such products are treated as rinse-off cosmetics). The Regulations also require that formulation details are released if needed to investigate an adverse reaction.

45.4 Dangerous Substances Directive (DSD)

The legislation embodied in the DSD deals with all new chemical substances that are being produced in the European Union [1]. Sections consider skin sensitization and skin irritation. Test methods for the identification of skin sensitizers are clearly set out [2, 3], but the legislation also admits a wide range of chemical structure and human evidence in addition.

Where a substance is identified as a skin sensitizer, then it is classified and labeled as *R43: May cause sensitization by skin contact*. Similar strategies apply to the identification of skin irritants, where the classification may be *R38: Irritant*, *R34: Causes burns*, or *R35: Causes severe burns*, depending on the severity of the observed effects. It is unfortunate that, to date, no such categorization of skin sensitizers has been adopted, despite clear proposals from a recent EU expert group [4].

The outcome of classification under the DPD is reflected in the manufacturer's safety data sheet (MSDS) when that substance is supplied, for example to a consumer product manufacturer.

45.5 Dangerous Preparations Directive (DPD)

The legislation contained in the DPD represents, in effect, the consequences for a preparation if a substance in that preparation is classified as irritating or sensitizing [5]. The key consequence is the labeling of the preparation with an appropriate warning, such as: *May cause sensitisation by skin contact*. However, all labeling is subject to largely administrative (not scientifically-based) threshold limits. Thus, for most sensitizing substances, labeling a preparation as carrying a skin sensitization risk is only required when the concentration of the sensitizing substance in the preparation is 1%. The aim here is to protect health by limiting the induction of skin sensitization. To take account of the potential failure of this legislation, such that individuals do become sensitized, additional labeling is shortly to come into force such that, for a concentration between the above labeling threshold and up to a factor of ten lower, the prepar-

ation must be labeled with the name of the sensitizing substance and the words added: *May cause an allergic reaction*.

It might be considered unfortunate that even in the EU, where regulations regarding skin sensitizers and irritants are at their most developed, there is no harmonization between the legislation (for example, to protect those already sensitized, the name of the sensitizer, written in simple language, is clearly sufficient, without any additional wording). It is also most unfortunate that the relative potency of the allergen is not taken into account during labeling (except in rare cases, usually after a considerable clinical problem has arisen).

45.6 Nickel

Nickel is still the most common contact allergen in the EU (and elsewhere). However, in the EU, this is set to change as a result of a relatively recent Directive [6], which arose from action originating in Denmark. The directive limits the allowed release of nickel from metal objects in prolonged contact with the skin to 0.5 $\mu g/cm^2$ per week. The impact of this limit has already paid dividends in Denmark, where a sharp reduction in nickel allergy is now evident [7]. It seems likely that the same will happen elsewhere in Europe.

45.7 Chromate

The European Union has also regulated exposure to chromate in cement. Cement and cement-containing preparations may not be used or placed on the market if they contain, when hydrated, more than 0.0002% (2 ppm) of soluble chromium VI out of the total dry weight of the cement. The Member States of the European Union have been required to meet this limit since January 2005.

References

1. EU (1996) EU dangerous substances directive. 22nd adaptation to technical progress (96/54/EC). Official J Eur Commun L248:199
2. EU (1996) EC Test Method B6. Commission Directive 96/54/EC of 30 July 1996, adapting to technical progress for the twenty-second time Council Directive 67/548/EEC on the approximation of the laws, regulations and administrative provisions relating to the classification, packaging and labelling of dangerous substances. Methods for the determination of toxicity, B6. Acute toxicity skin sensitisation. Official J Eur Commun L248:206–212

3. OECD (2002) Guidelines for testing of chemicals. Guideline no. 429. Skin sensitisation: the local lymph node assay. Organisation for Economic Cooperation and Development, Paris

4. Basketter DA, Andersen KE, Lidén C, van Loveren H, Boman A, Kimber I, Alanko K, Berggren E (2005) Evaluation of the skin sensitising potency of chemicals using existing methods and considerations of relevance for elicitation. Contact Dermatitis 50:39–43

5. EU (1998) EU Council Directive 88/379/EEC of 7 June 1988 on the approximation of the laws, regulations and administrative provisions of the Member States relating to the classification, packaging and labelling of dangerous preparations. Official J Eur Commun L18:14

6. EU (1994) Nickel Directive: European Parliament and Council Directive 94/27/EC of 30 June 1994: amending for the 12th time Directive 76/769/EEC on the approximation of the laws, regulations and administrative provisions of the Member States relating to restrictions on the marketing and use of certain dangerous substances and preparations. Official J Eur Commun L188:1–2

7. Nielsen NH, Linneberg A, Menné T, Madsen F, Frolund L, Dirksen A, Jorgensen T (2002) Incidence of allergic contact sensitization in Danish adults between 1990 and 1998; the Copenhagen Allergy Study, Denmark. Br J Dermatol 147:487–492

8. EU (2003) Cement Directive: Directive 2003/53/EC of the European Parliament and of the Council of 18 June 2003 amending for the 26th time Council Directive 76/769/EEC relating to restrictions on the marketing and use of certain dangerous substances and preparations (nonylphenol, nonylphenol ethoxylate and cement). Official J Eur Commun L 178:24–27

International Comparison of Legal Aspects of Worker Compensation for Occupational Contact Dermatitis

46

Peter J. Frosch, Werner Aberer, Paul J. August, Robert Adams, Tove Agner, Michael H. Beck, Lieve Constandt, L. Conde-Salazar, Matti Hannuksela, Swen M. John, Christophe Le Coz, J. Maqueda, Howard I. Maibach, Haydn L. Muston, Rosemary L. Nixon, Hanspeter Rast, W.I. van Tichelen, Jan Wahlberg

Contents

46.1 Introduction

In a European textbook on contact dermatitis a chapter on legal aspects is entirely appropriate. In many cases an occupational cause is suspected and proven after careful diagnostic procedures. A number of questions then arise that are handled in different ways in different European countries. Faced with the modern enlarged European Union, with its expected labor migration, the occupational physician needs to know and understand the essential differences between the legislation for occupational contact dermatitis in the major countries.

This chapter is largely based upon the feedback from questionnaires sent to members of the European Environmental and Contact Dermatitis Research Group (EECDRG) and other colleagues that are experienced in this field. The underlying concept of handling a case of occupational contact dermatitis in Germany and various other (mainly European) countries, and the probable outcomes for three typical cases are described. Fifteen questions were asked about various aspects of such cases (including institutions involved, report forms, requirements for recognition, retraining, and pension). Due to the nomenclature and country-specific legal rules, it often proved difficult for responders to answer these questions and to make clear statements. Nevertheless, some major differences became apparent.

In the following, the authors have tried to characterize the principle legal characteristics in the various countries. Frequent comparisons are made with the German system; this is only for ease of understanding, and definitely not with any intention of suggesting that this should be regarded as the "standard." In the years to come it will probably be necessary to create more uniform joint legislation in this area, in order to avoid socially unjust decisions.

46

46.2 Occupational Dermatitis in Germany

PETER J. FROSCH, SWEN M. JOHN

In Germany, the legal basis for dealing with occupational diseases is fixed in the seventh book of the State Insurance Code *Sozialgesetzbuch* (SGB 7) and the Decree on Occupational Diseases *Berufskrankheitenverordnung* ("BKV," from 31 October 1997; latest amendment dates from 5 September 2002). Occupational diseases are defined in the official list of recognized occupational diseases; this list is included in the BKV (Anlage zur BKV) and it presently comprises 68 occupational diseases. The two skin diseases in this list are classified under:

- No. 5101: Severe or repeatedly relapsing dermatoses which have clearly necessitated the cessation of all occupational activities which were or could be responsible for causing the disease or its relapse or aggravation
- No. 5102: Cancer or precancer caused by soot, unpurified paraffins, tar, anthracene, pitch or similar substances

The list is updated periodically. The responsibility for dealing with occupational incidents and diseases falls on nonprofit-making statutory insurance institutions, the *Berufsgenossenschaften* (BG). There are 64 BGs, each responsible for a different field of work, such as administrative work and trade, construction, health care (including hairdressing), mechanical engineering and the iron and steel industry, mining, quarrying, transport, wholesale trade and warehousing, food production, agriculture, horticulture, forestry and the wood industry.

Every employee must by law be insured against occupational accidents, injuries and diseases. Only employers have to pay this insurance. The system used to settle claims about occupational accidents and diseases is quite elaborate and has a very "social" feel.

Even when there is only a slight suspicion that a dermatosis case is work-related, a dermatologist's report (*Hautarztbericht*) is filed with the appropriate insurance institution (BG). This report requires the consent of the person concerned. It is based on a detailed examination, including patch tests and atopy screening. It also includes recommendations concerning therapy, protection, skin care, and even changing the workplace. This is an attempt to handle potential occupational dermatoses as quickly and unbureaucratically as possible. If the dermatosis continues, and the suspicion that the disease has an oc-

cupational origin is confirmed, any doctor in contact with the person concerned is obliged *by law* to fill in a special initial report form (the medical report of an occupational disease: *Ärztliche Anzeige über eine Berufskrankheit*). This form is then sent to the relevant BG or to an official government physician dealing with occupational diseases (*Staatlicher Gewerbearzt*). This does not require the consent of the person concerned.

After obtaining the report, the BG investigates the case further, often by sending a specially trained adviser to inspect the workplace. The adviser gives detailed advice to the worker regarding avoidance of irritants and potential allergens, and can recommend the use of barrier creams, gloves and appropriate cleansing agents. These must be provided by the employer. If the patient continues to have skin symptoms he or she is referred to a dermatologist. A detailed work-up is carried out, including patch testing and atopy screening, and the dermatologist's report (*Hautarztbericht*) is sent to the BG. The BG makes a moderate payment for both the initial report and the *Hautarztbericht*. The dermatologist must make a clear statement as to the origin of the disease, including occupational and nonoccupational factors, and provides detailed suggestions for avoidance of occupational risks and recommendations for preventive measures. If all such measures fail (as in the case of the bricklayer given below), the patient must stop working in his or her occupation, and an expert opinion from a dermatologist (usually a different one) is ordered by the BG. This opinion provides the basis for rejecting or recognizing the condition as an occupational skin disease and for payment of compensation and/or retraining.

A copy of the initial report (*Ärztliche Anzeige*) is also sent to an official government physician (*Staatlicher Gewerbearzt*), who can then investigate the case further, order an expert opinion, or decide independently whether the disease is to be classified as occupational or nonoccupational. If the *Gewerbearzt* and the BG disagree on a case, particularly if a monthly pension is at stake, a second or third expert's opinion is obtained. A commission (see below) then makes a decision. If the patient is dissatisfied with the decision, he or she may take the matter to court (*Sozialgericht*). After reviewing the case, the judge often orders another expert opinion from a recognized specialist in occupational dermatology.

According to German law (seventh decree on occupational diseases: *7. Berufskrankheitenverordnung*), to be regarded as a case of occupational contact dermatitis, an eczema must be either "severe" or "repeatedly relapsing," and must have created the need for the insured person to cease all activities that are (or could be) causing the disease, aggravation or relapse of the disease (No. 5101: "*schwere oder wiederholt rückfällige Hauterkrankungen, die zur Unterlassung aller Tätigkeiten gezwungen haben, die für die Entstehung, die Verschlimmerung oder das Wiederaufleben der Krankheit ursächlich waren oder sein können*"). The severity ("*Schwere*") of the dermatitis is based on the clinical picture, on the duration, and on the existence of a sensitization of occupational relevance. The clinical picture is considered severe if the dermatitis is highly vesicular in the acute stage or lichenified with deep fissures in the chronic stage. Further factors are pain, severe pruritus, impairment of mobility, and spreading of the dermatitis beyond the original site. A duration of more than 6 months and a continuous need for medical treatment are important criteria for defining the severity by the course of the disease. Sensitization to an important occupational material that cannot be avoided or replaced is also part of the definition. In the case of a type I allergy, asthma, angioedema or generalized urticaria would qualify as a "severe" degree of occupational origin. Further details are given in the original German publication [7]. "Repeatedly relapsing" (*wiederholt rückfällig*) means that at least three bouts of the disease have occurred. By definition it is also necessary that the disease has healed or at least improved considerably between two bouts.

A further specific term in the German legislation is *Minderung der Erwerbsfähigkeit* (MdE), meaning "diminution of working ability." The physician must estimate, in an abstract manner, the number of occupations in the overall labor market that the patient is unable to work in due to the occupational disease. For instance, a bricklayer who has acquired a chromate allergy and is suffering from severe hand eczema will receive an MdE of 20–30%, which means that he cannot enter about 20–30% of the occupations available in the labor market because chromate is such a ubiquitous allergen. If the estimate is below 20% (for example, 10–15% in the case of a nickel allergy with *slight* hand eczema), the case is still recognized as an occupational disease (*Anerkennung dem Grunde nach,* "basic recognition" or "admission in law"). However, 20% is a critical figure, because a patient with an MdE of 20% or more receives compensation: he or she is paid a pension equivalent to the appropriate percentage of the pension that would have been awarded if he or she were totally disabled (two-thirds of the annual earnings in the year before stopping work). This pension is paid by the insurance institution (BG) for as long as the disability lasts, sometimes for life. Withdrawal of the compensation is difficult, but it can occur if the change in MdE is more than 5% and the new MdE is less than 20%. In

every case, though, once an occupational disease has been legally acknowledged to exist, this acknowledgement can never be withdrawn. Income protection (*Übergangsgeld, Verletztengeld*) during recovery and retraining must always be covered by the BG.

The *Arbeitsgemeinschaft für Berufs- und Umweltdermatologie* [Task Force on Occupational and Environmental Dermatology (ABD) of the German Dermatological Society (DDG)] has published recommendations regarding the degree of MdE based on the presence and severity of skin lesions, the intensity of allergic contact sensitization(s), and the spread (occurrence) of the allergen(s) in daily life. In contrast to earlier recommendations, a severe course of a cumulative irritant dermatitis can also qualify for an MdE of 20% [2].

In the following, three typical examples of occupational "legal cases" are given, as they were handled by the German authorities.

46.2.1 Example A

A bricklayer, aged 35 years, has to stop all occupational activities because of severe hand eczema, which has resulted in at least three sick leaves each of a duration of several weeks. A patch test is strongly positive for dichromate. A further attempt to work with cement of low dichromate content and the use of nitrile gloves did not improve his condition. In the expert's opinion, the dermatologist suggested that he should be retrained, that his disease should be recognized as occupational (*Berufskrankheit* 5101), and that he should be granted a pension of 20%.

The retraining is paid for by the insurance company (BG for construction workers). The retraining program takes two years and costs about 100,000 euros. This procedure is performed according to paragraph 3 of the *Berufskrankheitenverordnung* (BKV), which states that the insurer has to do everything possible to prevent the development, the aggravation or the recurrence of an occupational disease. In general, retraining procedures are not implemented for persons older than 40–45 years.

46.2.2 Example B

A nurse suffers from atopic eczema, which began in childhood. She suffers from hayfever, and when she began her training as a nurse she had slight eczema on the flexures, but not on the hands. After 2 years she developed a hand eczema, which is considered to be irritant because patch tests with occupational allergens are negative. She has had three sick leaves

46

and has occasionally seen a dermatologist. She has voluntarily given up her occupation and wants to be retrained for a clean, dry office job. In the expert's opinion, the physician denies the existence of an occupational skin disease because the patient is suffering from a mild atopic eczema that has been precipitated on the hands by her occupational activities. After stopping nursing she still has skin symptoms on the hands. This is interpreted as the expression of a primarily endogenous skin disease, and not an occupational dermatitis. The physician also recommends retraining, but the costs are not covered by the insurer. In most cases like this the Ministry of Labor will cover part of the costs of retraining.

46.2.2.1 Comment

Cases like this are often difficult to assess. Some dermatologists would recognize this case as occupational because the patient had never had symptoms on her hands before her occupational activity triggered off the eczema at this site. Other dermatologists would recognize the occupational cause of the hand eczema but would argue that, due to the mildness of the disease, there was no objective need to cease all occupational activities. They might, however, recommend measures according to paragraph 3 BKV (therapy, protective measures) in order to prevent relapses of severe hand dermatitis if the patient returned to work as a nurse. This could, in fact, mean that the nurse would be retrained for a new job at the cost of the insurer.

If a patient appeals, the case first has to be taken to a commission at the BG (*Widerspruchsausschuss*), which includes a representative of the employers and a labor union representative. Every detail of the individual case is scrutinized and the opinion of a dermatologist may be heard again.

If the commission's decision is again not accepted by the patient, he or she can appeal and take the insurer to court (*Sozialgericht*). There are no court costs here, and lawyer costs are covered by the patient's labor union, if he or she is a member.

46.2.3 Example C

A surgeon, 40 years of age, develops a contact allergy to rubber gloves. Patch testing confirms that he is allergic to thiurams and must use more expensive, thiuram-free, latex gloves. He is free from symptoms when he uses this type of glove. In the expert opinion the disease is recognized as occupational but the surgeon can continue his work with special precautions.

He does not receive any compensation because he is not obliged to stop working. The costs of the more expensive gloves must be covered by the employer. If the costs are very high, or if the surgeon is self-employed, the insurance institution (BG) will cover all or at least part of it. This is a procedure from paragraph 3 BKV used to keep the surgeon in his occupation.

46.3 Occupational Contact Dermatitis in Other European Countries, Australia and the USA

Table 1 lists the institutions primarily involved in dealing with a case of occupational dermatitis in a number of countries. In nearly all countries except the United Kingdom, where two separate systems exist (see below), such cases are initially handled outside the system of common law. Insurance institutions – private, semiprivate or governmental – deal with the first stage after the case has been reported to them. In most countries this report is filed by the family physician, by a dermatologist or by a company physician, and the suspicion (not the proof) of an occupational cause is sufficient. Further details are discussed below. Most of the institutions listed in Table 1 regularly compile data on occupational skin diseases: the reader may obtain these directly from them.

46.3.1 Australia

Rosemary L. Nixon

All states and territories have slightly different occupational health and safety and workers' compensation legislations. There are also national schemes for government workers and seafarers. Self-employed workers are not covered by workers' compensation in many circumstances.

In the state of Victoria for example, it is the worker who must instigate a claim, except in severe injury circumstances. This requires the worker to complete a three-page claim form, to which they must attach a workers' compensation certificate from their treating doctor.

Claims are classified as standard or minor. A minor claim implies that costs have not exceeded a set dollar amount for that year (indexed annually, and was $A495 in 2004), *and/or* less than 10 days has been lost from work. Costs include medical consultations, diagnostic tests, treatments including pharmaceuti-

Table 1. Institutions primarily involved in the settlement of a case of occupational dermatitis

Country	Institution	Institution collecting data on occupational dermatitis
Australia	Australian Safety and Compensation Council (ASCC) The Allen Woods Building, Level 6, 25 Constitution Avenue Canberra ACT 2601 http://www.ascc.gov.au	
Austria	AUVA (*Allgemeine Unfallversicherung*), *Unfallverhütungsdienst* Webergasse 4, 1203 Vienna, Austria http://www.auva.at HAV@auva.at Court ("*Arbeits- und Sozialgericht*")	AUVA
Belgium	*Fonds voor Beroepsziekten-Fonds des Maladies Professionelles* Ave. de l'Astronomie 1, 1210 Brussels, Belgium http://www.fmp-fbz.fgov.be wouter.vantichelen@fmp-fbz.fgov.be	
Denmark	*Arbeijdsskadestyrelsen* AEbe1Ogade 1, 2100 Copenhagen 0, Denmark	
Finland	Private insurance companies Institute of Occupational Health *Työsuojeluhallitus* (Government Board for Occupational Safety) http://www.occuphealth.fi http://www.mol.fi	Same
France	*Caisse Nationale d'Assurance Maladie des Travailleurs Salariés (CNAMTS)* 50, Avenue du Professeur André Lemierre, 75986 Paris Cedex 20, France http://www.ameli.fr	*Ministère de l'Emploi, du Travail et de la Cohésion Sociale* 127, Rue de Grenelle 75007 Paris http://www.travail.gouv.fr
Germany	*Hauptverband der Gewerblichen Berufsgenossenschaften (HVBG)* Alte Heerstrasse 111, 53757 St. Augustin, Germany info@hvbg.de http://www.hvbg.de *Bundesministerium für Gesundheit und Soziale Sicherung (BMGS)* *Postfach 500,* 53108 Bonn, Germany info@bmgs.bund.de http://www.bmgs.bund.de	Same
Spain	Instituto Nacional de Seguridad e Higiene en el trabajo http://www.mtas.es	Instituto Nacional de Medicina *Seguridad del Trabajo, Corn Evaluac. de Incapacidad* Alcala 56, 28071 Madrid, Spain Private insurance companies
Sweden	National Board of Occupational Safety and Health 17184 Solna, Sweden Labour Market No-Fault Liability Insurance (TFA) 11388 Stockholm, Sweden kundradgivningen@afa.se	Occupational Injury Information System (ISA) arbetsmiljoverket@av.se
Switzerland	SUVA (*Schweiz-Unfallversicherungsanstalt*) *Abteilung Arbeitsmedizin* Postfach, 6002 Luzern, Switzerland Other insurance institutions arbeitsmedizin@suva.ch	SUVA
UK	Department of Work and Pensions http://www.dwp.gov.uk Courts and lawyers (common law action) Private insurance companies	Same HSE: http://www.hse.gov.uk THOR: http://www.coeh.man.ac.uk/thor
USA	State authorities (each state's Division of Occupational Medicine) Private insurance companies	NIOSH, Taft Highway, Cincinnati, Ohio, USA

46

cal prescriptions and travel expenses. The employer must pay these costs as part of their liability. The employer must also pay the worker 95% of their wages for the lost time within their liability of less than ten days. The employer must submit a quarterly report with details of any minor claims that do not affect the cost of their insurance premium.

A standard claim occurs when these expenses are expected to, or have reached, the set dollar amount for that year *and/or* the worker has lost more than 10 days from work. The employer sends the information about the claim to their workers' compensation insurance agent within 10 days of receiving it from the worker, and a decision is made by the agent as to whether to accept the claim or not. If accepted, the agent then pays all further reasonable costs, and 95% of all wages while the employee is off work. Many industrial unions have negotiated workplace agreements that ensure that the employer contributes the missing 5% of pre-injury wage. If the claim is not accepted by the workers' compensation agent, the worker is referred to an independent medical examiner. If the claim is still disputed, a process of conciliation is undertaken.

If a worker remains unable to work and is assessed as having no current work capacity, they will be paid:

- 95% of pre-injury wage to a maximum of $A1,050 (indexed yearly) a week for the first 13 weeks
- After 13 weeks, work capacity is reassessed. If there is still no work capacity, they will be paid 75% of the pre-injury wage up to the maximum, for up to 2 years
- After 2 years, a review takes place and if the worker is still unable to work, they are paid 75% of the pre-injury wage up to the above maximum. This may continue until retirement age, or until a degree of work capacity is shown. If a worker's condition is stable and no further change is anticipated, they may apply for a lump sum payment provided their impairment is 30% or greater, using a formula related to the *American Medical Association's Guide to Permanent Impairment*, Fourth Edition [19].

At any time during the process, the workers' compensation insurer can review the claim and decide to terminate liability, ceasing payments. If the worker is still unable to work, they may apply for a disability pension. If disputation arises, especially with respect to the termination of the claim or the determination of work capacity, the claim is adjudicated by three independent medical practitioners, the "Medical Panel."

Self-employed sole proprietors who do not employ others are not considered "workers" under the scheme and are therefore not covered by workers' compensation. However, if they are hired as a contractor, they may be deemed to be a "worker" and therefore covered in the contract by the employer's workers' compensation insurance. An exception is also made where sole proprietors receive a salary as the director of their own proprietary company and remuneration exceeds $A7,500 per annum.

There is considerable evidence that many Australian workers do not submit claims for occupational skin disease, especially if they do not lose appreciable time from work. As there is a subsidized national health scheme (Medicare), all patients receive a government rebate for a considerable portion of their personal medical expenses, for both general practitioner and specialist expenses. Although patients should not legally claim on Medicare for conditions caused by work, in practice they often prefer the simplicity of this approach, rather than completing the significant amount of paperwork required for a claim, and undergoing the stigma of claiming "compo." Uncertainty surrounding the clinical diagnosis and its work-relatedness often complicates the situation.

In this workers' compensation system, workers rather than medical or other practitioners instigate claims, which is different from the mode of initiating claims utilized in many other countries.

46.3.1.1 Example A

In the Australian system, the bricklayer would be compensated for his time off work. It is the responsibility of the employer to find him suitable duties where possible.

If however he was off work and his skin then improved, the insurance company would pay for some rehabilitation, although this may consist more of assistance with finding a more suitable job, rather than extensive retraining for another career.

In fact, the workers' compensation authority funds an incentive scheme for alternative employers to encourage them to employ people who cannot return to their pre-injury workplace. Support is in the form of a wage subsidy on a sliding scale up to the first 24-weeks and covers training and other relevant costs. However, the worker must have the capacity to work at least 15 h a week. Unfortunately, in reality the bricklayer may not be aware of all possible options and would probably find less-skilled work for himself, if able to do so.

46.3.1.2 Example B

In the Australian system, the nurse would likely be assessed as experiencing *significant* aggravation of her dermatitis at work, so she would receive workers' compensation benefits, and if another job could not be found by her employer, she would most likely be referred to the incentive scheme mentioned above.

46.3.1.3 Example C

In the Australian system, the employing hospital would pay for appropriate gloves for the surgeon. He would not receive workers' compensation benefits, as he remains working. Although his employer could claim the costs of the more expensive gloves from the insurer, this would adversely affect the employer's workers' compensation premium payments, so the hospital would be best advised to pay for the alternative gloves themselves.

46.3.2 Austria

WERNER ABERER

In Austria, the equivalent to the German BGs is the *Allgemeine Unfallversicherungsanstalt* (AUVA), a nonprofit, state-oriented insurance institution that is independent of other health insurers or employers. Every employer must pay a small fee for each of his employees (1.4% of the total income) to be insured by the AUVA. Every physician must report a case of suspected occupational skin disease to the AUVA; the patient's consent is not necessary. The AUVA can then inspect the workplace and will order an expert opinion. The expert will review the case and will make detailed suggestions, in the same way as described for the three German examples. He will also make an estimate of the degree of disability and suggest a pension (for example, 20% for the bricklayer, example A). In general, the main cause of the disease must be occupational in order for it to be judged as a "legal case." A primarily endogenous disease (such as atopic eczema) only qualifies for compensation under special circumstances (such as the first manifestation of the disease due to occupational factors). Cumulative insult dermatitis may be recognized if it is severe, disabling and associated with frequent sick leaves.

Negligence on the part of the employer does not have to be proven. Retraining is available to patients even if they are older than 40 years and costs are met mostly by the AUVA, partly by other state authorities.

The three examples of occupational contact dermatitis given would be handled in a very similar way in Austria to how they would be handled in Germany.

46.3.3 Belgium

LIEVE CONSTANDT, W.I. VAN TICHELEN

In Belgium, occupational skin diseases are handled primarily by the Fund for Occupational Diseases (Fund), which is a public institution with corporate capacity that falls under remit of the Ministry of Social Affairs. It is ruled by a managing committee consisting of a chairman and members nominated by federations of trade unions and employers, respectively. Both sides of the industry have equal representation on the committee.

Every employee must be insured against occupational diseases by law; the social contributions are paid by the employer. Not only employees but also students and apprentices are covered. The law does not apply to civil servants and state railway personnel. For them, other rulings are set out. However, at the request of other governmental insurance institutions (for example the Health Insurance Service for civil servants), the Fund will carry out medical examinations of the patients who claim compensation for an occupational disease. The self-employed are not covered.

Insured persons are entitled to indemnification by the Fund if they can prove that they were exposed to an agent included in the list of those causing occupational diseases and that they suffer from a disease that is related to this kind of exposure. They should be exposed to a much greater extent than the general population. However, the individual causal relationship between the disease and the exposure is legally presumed (presumption of causation). This is the so-called "list system." Practically all cases of occupational skin diseases can be recognized under this system. Compensation for a disease not mentioned in the legal list is possible, but one has to prove the causal relationship between occupation and disease (the so-called "open system").

When an occupational dermatitis is suspected, the company physician is obliged to report the case to the Ministry of Employment and Labor and to the Fund. However, any medical doctor (general practitioner, dermatologist, company physician, physician employed by the mutual sick fund) can initiate the case using a special report form that is forwarded to the Fund. The medical documents that led to the diagnosis need to be supplied. The patient's consent is required before a claim for compensation is filed.

46

The Fund investigates the case. A detailed work-up, including patch testing and atopy screening, is carried out by a specialist in occupational dermatology who is employed by the Fund. He or she recommends recognition or refusal. The final decision is made by the medical superintendent of the Fund, who will estimate the loss of earning capacity. A consulting engineer may inspect the workplace.

After recognition of an occupational skin disease, the worker is not bound to leave his job. Noneconomic loss is generally not compensated. If the patient can continue his work eventually with special precautions, he does not receive any compensation. When he is obliged to stop working due to the occupational dermatitis, he is entitled to a monthly payment (up to 20–30% of his wages, not higher than a defined maximum) – not a lump sum – which is received together with unemployment benefits. Should he be in a position to find alternative work, and if he were to earn less in his new job, he would receive – under certain conditions – financial compensation.

Other benefits provided are the cost of medical treatment in compliance with the rules and after intervention from the sickness insurance, and the cost of special gloves and shoes (up to a certain amount) that do not contain the allergen to which the patient is sensitized. Retraining is paid for by the Fund but is rarely performed.

If the patient is dissatisfied with the decision, he or she is able to appeal to the welfare tribunal. The judge always orders another expert opinion, not necessarily from a recognized specialist in dermatology. The court costs are covered by the Fund.

An allergic contact dermatitis will be recognized providing that the triggering allergen(s) is (are) relevant to the occupation. However, the dermatitis does not have to be wholly occupational to qualify.

A chronic irritant contact dermatitis may be recognized as an occupational disease if its relationship to occupational activities is quite clear. Only medications and protective gloves are paid for by the Fund.

One exception to the rule that noneconomic loss is not compensated is occupational natural rubber latex allergy. Latex-allergic health care workers, cleaning personnel and other workers using latex products will always receive financial compensation (at least 10%), because of the inconvenience and the severe allergic reactions they may experience. Thus, a nurse with latex glove-associated urticaria would receive 10% and additional financial compensation if she had to stop working in her occupation. The cost of latex-free gloves is also covered by the Fund.

46.3.4 Denmark

Tove Agner

In Denmark, either a report can be made to the state authorities (ASK) with the patient's consent, or the case can be reported anonymously. Cases should be reported whenever the slightest suspicion of work-related disease appears. Most cases are reported by general practitioners. Following the report to the ASK, in almost all cases the patient undergoes an examination by a dermatologist, who submits a medical report (expert opinion) on the potentially occupational disease. If 50% or more of the cause of the disease is due to occupational exposure, the disease can be recognized as occupational – even if the disease has disappeared. However, this does not necessarily lead to any financial compensation. Worker's compensation is only paid when the *degree of permanent injury* exceeds 5%, and is proportional to the degree of injury. The degree of permanent injury is determined on the basis of the dermatological medical report. Occupational sensitization to such ubiquitous allergens as nickel, chromate, rubber additives, latex, perfume and formaldehyde acquire a small additional compensation. When the disease is only partially due to the occupation, the compensation will be reduced appropriately. Compensation is paid as a lump sum, and not as a pension or monthly sum. If the degree of injury has worsened after compensation has been paid, the case can be reviewed within 5 years. When retraining is necessary, costs are paid for by the state. In the case where an occupational disease forces a change of job, financial compensation for reduced income can be granted. A fundamental difference between the German and the Danish systems is that worker's compensation can be given to people who are continuing in the same job that caused the damage.

46.3.5 Finland

Matti Hannuksela

In Finland the whole matter of occupational diseases is primarily in the hands of private insurance companies. There is one exception: financial compensation for civil servants comes from government funds, but the principles behind the compensation are the same as in the private systems. Not only the physicians involved but also the patient can initiate an investigation by filling out a special report form. This special report is forwarded to the local Department of Occupational Safety and Health, which usually does not take any action of their own. The insurance company can order an expert opinion, but apparently this is not obligatory in every case.

The reviewing doctor recommends recognition or refusal. The estimate of disability seems, in general, to be higher than in Germany: the bricklayer in example A would receive 20–40%, depending on the severity of the disease. Under Finnish legislation the "inconvenience" and suffering resulting from the occupational disease clearly carry more weight when determining the financial compensation.

Retraining is recommended for patients up to 50 years of age, costs being met by the insurance companies. The lawyer of the insurance company is also involved in the decision about the new occupation for which the patient is to be retrained.

Cumulative insult dermatitis may be recognized as an occupational dermatitis under special circumstances if severe and disabling. It is not accepted as such if endogenous factors clearly predominate. Worsening of nonoccupational diseases for occupational reasons will also be compensated for by the insurance companies.

Otherwise, the three examples of occupational contact dermatitis given above for the German system would be handled in a very similar fashion according to Finnish legislation. The costs of dealing with all suspected and unproven cases of occupational dermatitis are also covered by the private insurance companies.

46.3.6 France

CHRISTOPHE LE COZ

In France, the legal basis for dealing with occupational diseases (OD) is fixed in the *Code de la Sécurité Sociale* and several other statutes, one of which is the *Code Rural* for agriculture.

The French legislation is characterized by the existence of "tables of occupational diseases," which allow recognition and compensation for such conditions. An OD will be recognized only if it is listed in one of the more than 110 tables for the general regimen. These tables are updated periodically, and more than 45 tables concern skin disorders of allergic, irritant, cancerous or infective cause. Each table concerns a particular situation: some tables are devoted to a specific substance (such as table 83, to methyl methacrylate), and other tables concern groups of substances (such as table 51, for epoxy resins and their components) or types of dermatitis (such as table 65, for dermatitis of an allergic mechanism). The tables are divided into three columns. The first one concerns the designation of the diseases with symptoms or lesions, such as "eczematous dermatitis recurring after a new exposure or attested by patch tests" (table 31 for aminoglycosides) or "eczema-like dermatitis" (table 47 for woods) or "dermatitis or chemical burns" (table 32 for fluorine, hydrofluoric acid and salts), or "contact urticaria" (table 95 for latex proteins). The second column, entitled "term of notice" concerns the maximal admissible delay between the last contact with the pathogenic agent and the first medical establishment of the disease: for example, the delay is 7 days in the case of cements (table 8). The third column indicates or enumerates the occupations likely to provoke the disease. There is an indicative (not limited) list of occupations in the main tables. In some cases, however, and mainly for cancerous or infective diseases or in the case of dermatitis due to epoxy resins, there is a limited list of occupations allowing recognition. The procedure is well defined. The medical certificate needed for the declaration is made in triplicate, generally by the dermatologist, sometimes by the patient's practitioner, or even by the occupational physician (art. L. 461–5 of the *Code de la Sécurité Sociale*). The patient will fill in a declaration form and send it with the medical certificate to the *Caisse Primaire d'Assurance Maladie* (CPAM). The CPAM holds a medical and administrative enquiry and then notifies about acceptance or refusal. When the medical, occupational and administrative conditions indicated in the concerned table are fulfilled, a presumption of occupational origin is accorded to the worker and no additional proof is required. So, there is no need for positive tests in suspected allergic dermatitis that relapses after fresh exposure, and no need for recurrence of the dermatitis after new exposure when a patch test is positive, except for latex (table 95). When the dermatitis is recognized as an OD, expenditures related to it are taken care of. If the patient has a permanent disability, compensation can be paid. If this disability is <10%, the patient will receive a lump sum which generally does not exceed 1500 euros. Exceptionally, when the disability is >10%, she or he will receive a monthly pension. When the disease is not recognized as occupational, the patient can refer the *Comité Régional de Reconnaissance des Maladies Professionnelles* (CRRMP).

In some cases, the patient suffers dermatitis described as a "dermatitis with occupational features," listed in complementary tables. For example, an occupational dermatitis due to pyridine or its derivatives is listed under no. 613. Such dermatitis, although of occupational origin, offers no compensation, but must be declared on a special form to the Ministry of

Labour (art. L. 461–6 of *Code de la Sécurité Sociale*). This allows the tables to be extended and updated.

When a patient suffers an occupational dermatitis, the occupational physician usually tries to provide him a new working area. In the case of repeatedly relapsing dermatitis, however, his occupational physician can declare that the patient is unfit to do his job. By law, the employer must find the patient another job in the same company, or must double the redundancy compensation; the option granted partly depends upon the age of the patient. Retraining may be carried out, but is very difficult for many patients.

46.3.6.1 Example A (Bricklayer)

Table no. 8, entitled "diseases due to cements," applies in this case. The OD can be officially recognized, but only if the patient himself makes the notification. A pension will be paid only if there is a residual disease, with a permanent disability that exceptionally exceeds 10%, even with severe lesions. So, occupational physicians are frequently reluctant to declare the patient unfit to do their job, since it means that they will be laid off. This situation is very hard to manage, since a bricklayer often finds it difficult to find another job. Many patients continue to work despite occupational dermatitis. As unfitness only applies to a specific job in a specific work plant, many patients apply for work at other firms, without claiming previous unfitness. For such patients, a declaration to the *Commission Technique d'Orientation et de Reclassement Professionnel* (COTOREP) can be useful, since it can offer routes toward retraining.

46.3.6.2 Example B (Nurse)

If the nurse works in a state hospital, she is considered to be a civil servant. An administrative procedure will be carried out within the hospital. If the affliction corresponds medically and administratively to an entry in one of the tables, an OD will likely be recognized. In practice, the nurse will be rapidly appointed to another post in the same hospital and won't receive any compensation.

46.3.6.3 Example C (Surgeon)

The surgeon must fill in the declaration form, and send it with the medical certificate that indicates an OD corresponding to table 65 (tetramethylthiuram sulfide). The employer will provide adapted gloves but the surgeon won't receive any compensation.

46.3.7 Spain

L. Conde-Salazar, J. Maqueda

In Spain occupational dermatoses are handled by the *Instituto Nacional de Salud Carlor III*, public insurance companies named *Mutuas* associated with the National Health System, and occasionally some workers can be their own occupational managers.

Any dermatologist, occupational physician or general practitioner can report a potential occupational dermatosis case to the National Register System of Occupational Diseases. This notification is mandatory for any dermatitis included in the National List of Occupational Diseases.

Spain's social security system (*Seguridad Social*) reports on whether each case of occupational dermatitis is eligible for economic compensation. Each case must be proven beforehand. The patient must give his consent for this report. The case is then pursued further by a commission from the National Institute for Social Security (*Comisión Técnica Calificadora Seguridad Social*). Medical studies performed in relation to the case fall under the responsibility of the Medical Services for Disability Evaluation, EVI (located at regional or local level).

The EVI takes further action, inspects the workplace, and orders an expert opinion. The reviewing physician does not make any judgments on the disability or the size of compensation.

An important difference from other European countries is that more responsibility is placed on the employer. The company, together with the company's physician, must provide a new working area based on the recommendations of an expert opinion.

If the patient continues to have skin symptoms and suffers from frequent sick leave, after 18 months the National Institute for Social Security can re-evaluate the case for total disability. Meanwhile, workers can also file a claim to the Labor Court.

For skin diseases, a ruling of total disability is rare, and one that is achieved only after a long struggle with lawyers. This is a particular problem with irritant contact dermatitis, which is not included in the National List of Occupational Diseases. Only a court decision can lead to acceptance as an occupational disease, leading to financial compensation to the worker. Examples B and C would be dealt with within the hospital without further intervention from government institutions.

46.3.8 Sweden

Jan Wahlberg

In Sweden a state authority (the National Board of Occupational Safety and Health) is primarily involved in dealing with occupational skin diseases. An injury at work is understood to be an injury incurred in connection with an accident at work, an injury sustained on the way to or from work, or an *occupational disease* contracted as a result of *environmental* conditions at work. A person suffering from an injury at work can receive compensation through statutory social insurance (selected cases) and through labor market insurance. Labor market insurance may pay the injured person for noneconomic loss (for example, for pain and suffering) as well as for disfigurement and permanent disadvantage.

The forms of social insurance primarily concerned with cases of injury at work are those provided through the National Insurance Act (AFL) and the Work Injury Insurance Act (LAF). The LAF was revised in 1993 and has resulted in less compensation compared with previous conditions. The outcome of a recent revision (in 2002) has not yet been evaluated. The labor market insurance, which can give *additional* cover to the cover provided by social insurance, is the Labor Market No Fault Liability Insurance (TFA).

In contrast to most other countries mentioned in this chapter, the employer and the patient report the suspicion of an occupational dermatosis *together*. The special report form (Notification of a Work Injury) is also signed by the patient. Social Health Insurance and the Work Inspectorate review the case; they rarely inspect the workplace but can elicit an expert opinion from a dermatologist. The reviewing doctor examines the case in detail with a careful work-up including patch testing. He makes no estimate regarding the degree of disability or pension. Unfortunately, the frequency of such referrals to dermatologists has decreased in recent years.

When judging whether or not a harmful influence has existed in the work environment of an injured person, different personal factors that are characteristic of the injured person must also be taken into consideration. Examples of such personal factors that may render a person less resistant include previous diseases, congenital weakness or ageing. The principle that a person is insured "in their current condition" is laid down in the legislative material as well as in established practice.

A recognized case of occupational contact dermatitis will lead to retraining if the course is severe, with repeated recurrences. However, the employer is responsible for ensuring that adequate changes of exposure at the workplace, alternative jobs and retraining/education within the plant are considered before rehabilitation is initiated. There is no firm age limit. The decision on the new job is made in cooperation with physicians and Social Health Insurance and, if the injured person requests, union representatives and his/her employer as well. The costs of retraining are covered to some extent by state authorities. However, the current restrictions have unfortunately largely resulted in unemployment among individuals with occupational dermatoses.

A chronic irritant contact dermatitis will be recognized as an occupational disease if the course is severe. The three examples described earlier would be handled differently. The bricklayer would usually be retrained for another occupation with some compensation for economic losses from the LAF and additional costs, not covered by other sources, by the TFA. The nurse's case would be recognized as an occupational disease, because the eczema on her *hands* started after 2 years at work due to occupational contact. More expensive gloves would be provided for the surgeon with an allergy to thiurams, and the cost of this would be covered by the employer and not by an insurance institution. Due to a recession in the Swedish economy, the situation for those with occupational diseases/injuries is no longer as favorable as it used to be.

46.3.9 Switzerland

Hanspeter Rast

The basis for the insurance of accidents and occupational diseases is a law from 1981 (*Unfallversicherungsgesetz*). Recognition, compensation and preventive measures are covered by it. All employees in Switzerland have to be insured. Suva (*Schweizerische Unfallversicherungsanstalt*) is the compulsory insurer for employees in industry, construction, transport, and federal institutions. In addition there are various insurers for small trades and service companies. Only Suva has a staff of technicians for local inspection of companies and medical departments for occupational medicine and rehabilitation. The patient himself and the employer are responsible for reporting the suspicion of an occupational disease. The physician treating the case is asked by the insurer for a medical report. The general rule for recognizing a disease as an occupational one is that the occupational activity must be the sole or overwhelming cause. The government has published a list of substances, exposures, and occupational activities that

46

are the basis for recognition as an occupational disease. If these factors are involved, a causal relationship of more than 50% is sufficient for an individual case to be recognized as an occupational disease. If the disease is caused by other factors not found in the official list, the causal relationship between occupational activity and disease must be at least 75% in order to suffice for recognition. In contrast to other countries, there is no official list of occupational diseases, but rather a compendium of substances and various activities and exposures that have the potential to cause certain diseases. An occupational disease, including a dermatosis, is considered to exist if medical treatment or sick leave has been required. Therefore, no special criteria for severity (as used in Germany, for example) have to be fulfilled for recognition. The insurer pays for the medical treatment and other expenses, including loss of wages. If rehabilitation fails, a pension may be paid. In a case where the employee continues on the job and suffers severe health impairment (such as for spreading contact dermatitis, many recurrences, long sick leaves), Suva is entitled to prohibit certain activities that have proven to be hazardous to the individual (declaration of "unsuitability"). This measure also provides financial security to the employee for up to 4 years. A special state insurance, the *Invalidenversicherung*, is responsible for retraining and occupational rehabilitation.

46.3.9.1 Example A

The bricklayer's condition would be recognized as an occupational disease according to the law. Suva would notify the employee and the employer that all contacts with cement and dichromates must be discontinued. In construction this is actually equivalent to giving up the occupation. The bricklayer would also register with the *Invalidenversicherung* and ask for retraining at his relatively low age. The employee is also entitled to a temporary financial compensation from the insurer in cases of lower wages, unemployment or retraining procedures.

If the disease continues and the patient is considerably handicapped by it, or if rehabilitation measures fail, a permanent pension will be granted. This is covered by several insurances together (*Invalidenversicherung*, accident insurance, pension fund of the former employer). If there is no loss of earnings in the new occupation after retraining, no pension will be paid (in contrast to the German system). If there is a considerable, probably lifelong dermatosis, particularly on the hands and face, an additional lump sum (*Integritätsentschädigung*) is paid once at pension-

able age. Should the worker be dissatisfied with the decision of the insurer, he can appeal to the courts.

46.3.9.2 Example B

If the nurse has contact with substances in the list of occupational hazardous substances, such as aldehydes or rubber accelerators, and these aggravate a pre-existing mild atopic dermatitis in a definite manner, the insurer will cover the case until the previous health status is reattained. The occupational factors must be dominant, at least for some period of time. After that the regular health insurance is liable for all costs. Expert opinions often show discrepancies in such cases of endogenous disease without clear occupational sensitization. If the course of the case is severe and followed by many sick leaves, Suva might declare the "unsuitability" of the person, which usually means giving up the job. The patient can apply to the *Invalidenversicherung* for retraining with or without recognition of an occupational disease.

46.3.9.3 Example C

If the surgeon is employed in a public or a private hospital, the accident insurance under contract (usually a private one) will cover all medical costs, provided that the case is reported at all. In most cases, the hospital will cover additional costs, such as more expensive thiuram-free gloves, for a highly qualified employee. In Switzerland it is the employer's duty to provide all adequate protective measures, including gloves. If special expensive individual procedures have to be installed, the insurer may take care of a part of it.

46.3.10 United Kingdom

Michael H. Beck, Paul J. August,
Hayden L. Muston

In the UK there are two ways of obtaining compensation for occupational dermatoses. Firstly, the Government administers a scheme of National Insurance through the Inland Revenue Service. Employers, the self-employed and employees must make contributions to this central fund. If an individual is unable to work from illness of any kind for longer than 4 days consecutively then they will be entitled to statutory sick pay from their employer for up to 28 weeks. Incapacity benefit is also payable by the state on a longer-term basis for those who are eligible and have been assessed as being incapable of work. Industrial Injuries Disablement Benefit is an additional payment to those suffering from what is known as prescribed industrial disease. Prescribed diseases are divided into:

- A. Conditions due to physical agents
- B. Conditions due to biological agents
- C. Conditions due to chemical agents
- D. Miscellaneous conditions

For dermatologists the most relevant prescribed diseases are:

- A11. Vibration white finger
- B1. Anthrax
- B12. Orf
- C21. Primary carcinoma of the skin from exposure to arsenic or tar-based products or mineral oil or soot
- C25. Occupational vitiligo
- C30. Chrome dermatitis and ulceration of the mucous membranes or epidermis
- D5. Noninfective dermatitis of external origin

It is left to the patient to fill in an application form. The suspicion of an occupational cause is sufficient justification for filing a report to the state. For a claim to succeed, the claimant needs to show that he/she has the prescribed disease and has been in the occupation that caused it. Initially the assessment is made by one or two independent doctors. Definite proof and positive patch tests are not essential in cases of dermatitis. However, a report from a dermatologist will often be the basis for a further decision and patch tests may then be undertaken. In cases of occupational dermatitis, where there have been multifactorial contributions to the skin disorder including constitutional and other nonoccupational factors, the claim will succeed but the assessed percentage disability will be reduced proportionately. Since 1986 the claimant has to be at least 14% disabled to receive any benefit. Establishing this is more difficult than it may sound, because the fact that the person cannot work at his or her own job is not considered disablement, which refers to impairment of everyday life. It must be an exceptionally bad case for a skin complaint to reach 14% disablement, and only a few such cases are currently recorded each year. Disablement Benefit is usually paid as a weekly pension and may be subject to review. The claimant may ask for their case to be reassessed in some circumstances such as ignorance of or a mistake regarding a material fact, as well as deterioration of the condition. A medical

appeals tribunal exists which will examine claims thought to have been administered incorrectly according to the regulations. This tribunal, while set up by the state, is independent of it.

The second way of gaining compensation is for the affected individual to sue the employer for damages through the civil court. Civil actions are brought under a claim for negligence and/or a breach of statutory duty. Statutory duties are encompassed in a number of regulations with which the employer must comply. These include the Control of Substances Hazardous to Health (COSHH) and Personal Protective Equipment at Work Regulations (PPEWR). The regulations together provide a framework to prevent harm to the worker. Regulations ensure that knowledge of the risk, suitable training to avoid the risk, physical protection against the risk, regular review and monitoring of the harmful exposures, health surveillance, plus adequate information are all provided to the worker. In large claims, engineering reports will be obtained to determine whether a breach has occurred, and if it has, the extent of it. The dermatologist must establish the cause of the problem and whether negligence or a breach of the statutory regulations caused the damage.

Every employer in the United Kingdom has to be insured through a private insurance company for what is known as employer liability for common law action. When a claimant sues the firm, a solicitor will be consulted. Since April 1999, new "Woolf Rules" apply to the presentation of expert evidence. In the past each side would instruct its own expert(s), including where necessary a dermatologist. The new rules mean that the court, with the agreement of all the contesting parties, is encouraged to appoint a single independent expert where possible. The expert's duty and report is addressed to the court and is independent of whoever is responsible for the fee. He or she must give an impartial and balanced assessment, and where there may be a range of opinions, this must be documented. The expert is open to questions from all sides. The contesting parties are nevertheless at liberty to appoint their own experts who are required to supply unbiased reports with a range of opinions that would be expected from other dermatological experts in the field. This is more likely in large or complex cases. The experts' duty is again to the court, not to one side or the other. The contesting parties have the choice of whether or not to have the court consider this evidence, in which case all of those involved must discuss the case, and produce a joint report identifying any areas where there is disagreement, thereby providing the court with a condensed view of the issues in question. It is intended that this method will reduce legal expenses and the

46

frequency of court proceedings and attendances by experts. Presently, most cases are settled without going to court.

Unless he or she is in a trade union or has legal expenses insurance, the claimant may have to fund the costs, but many solicitors work on a conditional or "no win, no fee" basis. In successful cases the defendants may be ordered to pay the claimant's expenses. In the past, if the patient did not have sufficient means, the state used to give legal aid, but this has now been withdrawn from such cases.

If the worker is suing for negligence through the courts, the claimant must prove:

- That the skin complaint was contracted at work
- That it was avoidable and foreseeable by a reasonable employer
- That the employer did not take adequate precautions against it

If the claimant is suing for breach (breakdown) of statutory duty, he or she must prove:

- A breach of the statutory regulations occurred
- This breach caused the skin complaint

If the case is accepted as an occupational skin disease, compensation payments will take into account the following:

- Loss of earnings by the person
- Future loss of earnings (including pension)
- Loss of promotion prospects
- Loss of future employment prospects on the open job market
- Pain and suffering
- Loss of amenity in social and domestic activities (for example, if the patient has lost a hand, he or she might be unable to pursue a hobby, such as golf)
- Ongoing treatment costs
- Loss of congenial employment (where relevant)

Following recognition of an occupational skin disease, workers are entitled to stay in the same employment, but if they are unable to fulfil their duties adequately, they may be dismissed or moved to a less well paid post. Retraining in the UK for dermatological cases is not well organized and is rarely done. Even if they are retrained, many people will find it ex-

tremely difficult to get a job because employers are reluctant to take on someone whose skin is vulnerable and who may get skin trouble in the future with the associated worry of possible litigation.

In the UK, the Health and Safety Executive (HSE) has collated statistics for occupational dermatoses from a number of sources. There is no legal requirement for employees or medical personnel to report work-related skin disorders. This means that statistics will not be altogether reliable and probably underestimate those affected.

The HSE have undertaken a study by questionnaire and interview for the years 2001/02 entitled the Self-reported Work-related Illness (SWI) survey. A sample of 96,000 people in England and Wales were contacted. As a result of this survey, it was concluded that there was a prevalence of 39,000 individuals with work related skin disorders at that time (with a 95% confidence interval of 30,000 to 48,000). The best source of information on the incidence of occupational dermatoses in the UK comes from returns made voluntarily by occupational physicians and dermatologists to The Health and Occupation Reporting (THOR) Network based at the Centre for Occupational Health at Manchester University. These schemes are respectively known as OPRA and EPIDERM. In the last 3 years, the estimated number of new cases of occupational dermatosis per year has been between 3000–4000 cases. The vast majority of cases were from suffers of dermatitis. In contrast, an analysis of claims for Industrial Injuries Disablement Benefit for dermatitis confirmed and assessed at more than 1% disability shows the numbers to be in the region of 200 per year for the last 3 years, confirming that a low proportion of those affected make a claim. Another source of occupational skin disease statistics has been from those reported by employers under RIDDOR (Reporting of Injuries, Diseases and Dangerous Occurrences Regulations) to the Health and Safety Executive, but substantial under-reporting occurs. A more detailed account and analysis of these figures can be found on the THOR and HSE websites (http://www.coeh.man.ac.uk/thor/ and http://www.hse.gov.uk/). No formal feedback of any kind is provided by the state or legal system about the outcomes of cases in which dermatologists have provided expert opinions. In the state system this information is also not available on request; in the legal system it will usually be granted, but the dermatologist will rarely know when to ask, since most cases are settled out of court with no further reference to him or her.

Regarding the examples (A, B, and C) described earlier, there is no formal retraining program for such cases in the UK. Any retraining must therefore be undertaken at the affected individual's own expense. The employer should pay statutory sick pay when there is time off work due to dermatitis for up to 28 weeks. Thereafter incapacity benefit would have to be claimed if the affected person is still not working and eligible for the benefit. Some employers may provide income protection insurance. Otherwise it is up to the individual to consider paying for this, but regrettably, many workers fail to obtain insurance cover.

None of the cases is likely to achieve the 14% disablement needed to receive Disablement Benefit as a result of the prescribed disease of dermatitis. The bricklayer and the nurse would both have entered the state disability statistics had they applied for such a pension, but they are unlikely to have done this because of the growing knowledge in the community of the unlikelihood of obtaining such benefit for skin disease. Otherwise it is unlikely that any of these persons would have appeared in official Government statistics. Nevertheless, if they do see a dermatologist or occupational physician who is an active participant in the voluntary reporting scheme (EPIDERM and OPRA), then they will be incorporated into the figures kept by HSE.

The bricklayer could take court action but would need to prove negligence or a breach of statutory duty if he is going to succeed in a claim for damages.

As the nurse has stopped work voluntarily, he or she is unlikely to resort to a civil court action, even though it can be argued that, despite the constitutional background, the condition of the hands would not have arisen if she had not been nursing. Furthermore, the employer should have recognized at the pre-employment medical that there was a foreseeable increased risk of irritant contact dermatitis, bearing in mind the longstanding history of atopic eczema. If she did make a claim and it is shown in court that her employer did not take appropriate action to prevent the dermatitis and act promptly when she did, then she would succeed in a claim for damages. The ongoing nature of her hand problem is a further issue, as the concept of persistent occupational dermatitis is now well recognized.

The surgeon is unlikely to have applied for any form of compensation: if he were directly employed in the National Health Service, the additional expense of his gloves would be met by the employer; if self-employed (as are all dental surgeons, for example), he or she would have to meet the extra cost.

46.3.11 United States

Howard I. Maibach, Robert Adams

Laws establishing worker compensation in the United States were first passed in 1911. In the first decade, coverage was for accidents only. In 1920 illnesses were included, and in recent decades coverage has been extended to disorders caused by cumulative trauma and conditions arising from emotional trauma. As is the case with the laws of most other nations, the basic tenet is *liability without fault*, eliminating the requirement that the worker prove negligence on the part of the employer. The intent was to prevent an adverse climate in the workplace. The system is operated through insurance, which may be a state-supported insurance company, a private insurance company, or self-insurance in the case of large, financially sound companies. Some states permit all methods to be used. Federal employees are covered under a special federal program. Heavy penalties exist for companies that fail to insure their workers. *Medical care* is available without restriction, and may be provided not only by doctors of medicine and osteopathy but also by dentists, podiatrists, optometrists, physical therapists, and chiropractors. In some states Christian Science practitioners and naturopaths are authorized to treat these patients, but only if the employer is notified of this choice prior to injury. While some states provide a free choice of physician, certain states require treatment under a physician designated by the employer for the first 30 days or so, unless the employee makes prior arrangements.

Income protection during recovery is a basic tenet in all states, with a maximum and minimum. The employer assumes the cost through an insurance carrier or, if self-insured, through the company, usually a subsidiary.

Although unusual in dermatology, *death benefit*, when the death is due to illness related to the workplace, is provided with automatic payments to the surviving dependents. Payments usually equal the worker's temporary disability indemnity benefit. Burial expenses are included, with a maximum cost permitted.

Disputes arise in fewer than 10% of cases, but when there is disagreement and *dispute resolution* is necessary, lawyers for the opposing sides may request depositions from the various physicians. Later the case may be presented before a judicial hearing officer (often called a "referee"). The purpose of the hearing is to clarify the issues, with the intent to decide the case fairly and according to the law. If the hearing officer's decision is unacceptable to either

46

party, an appeals board can be requested to hear the case. At that time an *independent medical examiner* is usually appointed to evaluate the case. If there are still unresolved issues, the state appeals court may be petitioned to study the problem; an appellate court is next in line, and finally the state supreme court, but the great majority of cases are settled in the lower courts. An important difference between worker compensation law and ordinary civil law is that the court that originally decided an award may alter its decision if there is reasonable cause, or if the worker's condition changes.

Rehabilitation services are available in most states but are unequal in extent and funding. Job training is available for workers unable to return to their previous work, and is especially important for patients with allergic contact dermatitis in which a workplace allergen has been positively identified.

The following three cases present examples of the way in which compensation would be handled in the United States:

- Rehabilitation training in most states continues indefinitely, even past the normal retirement age of 65. The rating for pension indemnity is based upon the percentage of the workplace from which the worker (the bricklayer in this case) is precluded because of the skin condition. This determination involves a complicated process, requiring the recommendations of rehabilitation specialists, vocational disability experts, and industrial engineers, as well as the examining/reporting physicians.
- The insurance company is required to pay for that period of time in which there was clearly work aggravation of this pre-existing condition (atopic dermatitis for the nurse in this case). Furthermore, if the work appears to have brought a previously inactive condition to clinical activity, which is not uncommon in atopics, the treatment period allowed may be longer. Even if there is no work relationship, rehabilitation services are provided.
- In this case, the contact allergy of the surgeon would be considered work-related, and the cost of the alternative gloves would be paid for by the insurance company. Unfortunately, however, the company (in this case, the hospital) might find other reasons to discharge this surgeon because of the excessive cost of the gloves and the possible increase in insurance premiums, although this more commonly occurs with nonprofessional workers.

46.4 Conclusions and Comment

Profound differences in legislation on occupational skin disease become apparent when the systems used in various European countries are compared. In Germany and Scandinavian countries, recognition of a dermatosis as being occupational is proposed in a relatively easy manner by initiating well-developed and frequently used governmental and insurance pathways. An irritant contact dermatitis or atopic hand eczema will be recognized in most cases if the disease is severe and causes frequent sick leave and if its relationship to occupational activities is quite clear. A patient might receive compensation or retraining for an alternative "clean" job. In a country such as Spain, much more responsibility is placed on the employer to help employees after they have acquired a skin disease in the working environment. The system seems to be less institutionalized and more "privatized."

In most countries, a bricklayer with dichromate allergy would receive financial compensation, but lump sums are preferred to monthly payments. In Germany, retraining is rarely performed after the age of 40 years, while in most other countries the patient can be older than 40. In the questionnaire, the question of the value of retraining and the course of the skin disease was answered by the overwhelming majority in the following way:

- Most patients find a job only with difficulty after retraining
- They continue to have skin problems quite frequently

Regarding the overall evaluation of retraining programs, out of seven responders, three decided it was "very valuable in some cases," two "very valuable," one "of some value" and one "of little value."

These judgments of experienced occupational dermatologists should stimulate further thinking and work. Should we be more restrictive with retraining, because most patients will have problems in finding new satisfying work and will continue to have major skin problems? Are we retraining patients at too late a stage, once the disease has manifested itself and taken on a more endogenous character (see Chaps. 19, 39, and 44)? Is more cooperation necessary between physicians, social workers and specialists in occupational safety, with regard to inspecting the workplace and making far-reaching recommendations for the patient with an occupational skin disease? In every country a striking shortcoming exists:

the workplace is rarely inspected by a physician! Based on many reports in the literature, we know that this is an extremely important aspect of dealing with an occupational disease (see Chaps. 39, 44, 50). The patient inevitably and unintentionally sometimes omits important details from the history that turn out to be diagnostic clues if detected by a trained observer. On visits to dental laboratories, for example, we learned that most technicians are not aware of the risk of sensitization from acrylates and do not avoid frequent direct skin contact [16].

In most countries, the legislation seems to be rather inaccurate and unclear with regard to important aspects and to the definitions of terms such as "severity of disease," "recurrence" and "frequency of relapses." This also holds true for the degree of disability and estimates of the pensionable lump sum for compensation. In connection with the protection of personal data, it seems important to point out that the patient's consent for a report to be made to the insurer or governmental institution is not obligatory in every country. Considering the possibility that the patient may experience retaliation of various kinds in the workplace after the case for compensation has been initiated, the patient's consent to this procedure should be made mandatory.

In order to harmonize the various systems for dealing with occupational dermatoses, we recommend the formation of a committee under the auspices of the European Community.

References

1. Achten G, Oleffe J (1967) Dermatoses professionelles et capacité economique. Arch Belg Dermatol Syphil 23: 280–297
2. Blome O, Bernhard-Klimt C, Brandenburg S, Diepgen T, Dostal W, Drexler H, Frank K, John S, Kleesz P, Schindera I, Schmidt A, Schwanitz H (2003) Begutachtungsempfehlungen für die Berufskrankheit Nr. 5101 der Anlage zur BKV. Dermatol Beruf Umwelt / Occup Environ Dermatol 51: D2–D14
3. Brandenburg S (2003) Unfallversicherungsrechtliche Grundlagen. In: Schwanitz HJ, Wehrmann W, Brandenburg S, John SM (eds) Gutachten Dermatologie. Steinkopff, Darmstadt, pp 139–166
4. Diepgen TL, Schmidt A, Berg A, Plinske W (1996) Berufliche Rehabilitation von hautkranken Beschäftigten. Dtsch Arztebl 93: A31–A40
5. Elsner P, Rast H, Ziegler G (1993) Das Berufskrankheiten-Recht in der Schweiz. Dermatosen 41: 127–132
6. Fabry H, Frosch PJ (2001) Probleme der ärztlichen Begutachtung aus der Dermatologie. In: Fritz E, May B (eds) Die ärztliche Begutachtung. Steinkopf, Darmstadt, pp 893–953
7. Fartasch M, Schmidt A, Diepgen TL (1993) Die Schwere der Hauterkrankung nach BKVO 5101 in der gutachterlichen Beurteilung. Dermatosen 41: 242–245
8. Health and Safety Commission (1999) Health and safety statistics 1998/1999. HSC (HSE), London, ISBN 0-7176-1717-5
9. Schwanitz HJ, John SM, Brandenburg S (2003) Empfehlungen für die Diagnostik von Berufskrankheiten nach BK 5101. In: Korting H, Callies R, Reusch M, Schlaeger M, Sterry W (eds) Dermatologische Qualitätssicherung. Leitlinien und Empfehlungen. Zuckschwerdt, Munich, pp 317–341
10. Lips R, Rast H, Elsner P (1996) Outcome of job change in patients with occupational chromate dermatitis. Contact Dermatitis 34: 268–271
11. Meding B (1995) Skin disease as an occupational injury. Arbeite Och Hälsa Sci Publ Ser 16: 155–169
12. National Board of Occupational Safety and Health, the Swedish Work Environment Fund (ed) (1987) Occupational injuries in Sweden 1983. National Board of Occupational Safety and Health, Solna, Sweden
13. Nauroth E (1989) Hautarztbericht, Berufskrankheitenanzeige, Begutachtung – verwaltungsmäßig/juristische Aspekte. Aktuel Dermatol 15: 347–351
14. Pirilä V, Fregert S, Bandmann H-J et al (1971) Legislation on occupational dermatoses. Acta Derm Venerol (Stockh) 51: 141–145
15. Rast H, Bircher A (2001) Begutachtung von Berufsdermatosen aus Sicht des Unfallversicherungsträgers. Gesetzliche Bestimmungen in der Schweiz. In: Schwanitz J, Szliska C (eds) Berufsdermatosen. Dustri, Deisenhofen, pp 8c.1–8c.10
16. Rustemeyer T, Frosch PJ (1996) Occupational skin diseases in dental laboratory technicians. Contact Dermatitis 34: 125–133
17. Suva (2003) Wegleitung der Suva durch die Unfallversicherung. Schweizerische Unfallversicherung Suva, Luzern (available also in French)
18. Schwanitz HJ (2003) Präventionsmaßnahmen. In: Schwanitz HJ, Wehrmann W, Brandenburg S, John SM (eds) Gutachten Dermatologie. Steinkopff, Darmstadt, pp 17–31
19. AMA (1995) Guides to the evaluation of permanent impairment, 4th edn. American Medical Association, Chicago, Ill.

Chapter 47

Computers in the Management of Contact Dermatitis

47

W. Uter, D. Orton, D. Perrenoud, A. Schnuch

■ **Disclaimer.** No liability is accepted for the continued correctness of URLs. Moreover, the authors disclaim responsibility for the contents of the webpages mentioned, and for the contents of other websites possibly linked to the sites referenced here.

Contents

47.1 Scope

Within a few decades, we have witnessed an overwhelming increase in the rate of technological progress concerning computers. In fact, computers of various kinds have become indispensable in both everyday and professional life. Not only has their sheer number increased, but also their quality in terms of computing power, user-friendliness and versatility. Consequently, the scope of computer applications has become broader and broader, including worldwide connectivity via the Internet. This general trend also applies to the field of medicine. Electronic health records have principal advantages and potential problems, which is an important issue (reviewed in [1]) but one that we will not be addressing here in detail; some important aspects are summarized in Table 1. This chapter will focus on electronic data processing (EDP) applications that can aid the management of patients with contact dermatitis. For instance, computers can be used to retrieve information, such as scientific publications, product compositions or allergen characteristics to aid the diagnostic process and help to advise the patient (see Sect. 47.2, Information Databases). Furthermore, anamnestic and patch test data, along with other clinical or administrative data, can be stored in a structured, computer-based documentation system (see Sect. 47.3, Patient Management Systems). Using such "computerized" patient data, epidemiological and other studies may be performed, again using computers together with appropriate software as a research tool (see Sect. 47.4, Epidemiological Tools). Moreover, computers are increasingly being used in basic research, such as image analysis and bioengineering, and in a variety of other situations (see Sect. 47.5, Further Applications and Perspectives).

Table 1. Some specific potential advantages and dangers of electronic health records

Advantages	Hazards
Availability (in more than one place at a time)	Authenticity as a medical document
Flexible display and report functions	Unauthorized access to data during storage or transfer
Uniform structure	Suitability as a long-term archive (for example, in view of changing data formats)
Readability of written information	Incompatibility of electronic formats in critical situations
Alerts and other dynamic functions	Potentially unclear responsibilities for contents
Rapid communication possible	

47.2 Information Databases

This section refers to data that are not directly related to specific patients, such as allergen and product information, but that may be combined into a database. General considerations regarding all types of databases like this are:

- How precise and how current is the information (is the database updated *regularly*)?
- Who is responsible for the content, as there could be a conflict of interest impairing the validity of data and hence their usefulness?
- Are statements supported by scientific references?
- Is there restricted access to information (access incurs a fee, or only open to user groups) and, if so, is the use of this site cost-effective?

47.2.1 Information on Allergens

Information on the chemical nature of a particular allergen, its biological properties, sources of contact and the clinical pattern of contact dermatitis caused by it is traditionally found in textbooks. In such books, experts in their fields give "state of the art reviews" based on their own results and all relevant literature, thus not only reviewing current information, but also giving a balanced view on potentially conflicting data. The results of such a process could be transferred from print media to electronic media very easily, and indeed more and more textbooks appear in CD-ROM format. Ideally, however, such electronic media should be more than just a copy of the book, enabling users (not termed "readers" anymore) to navigate efficiently through the contents with intelligent tools, such as hyperlink technology, or metathesaurus-based search facilities [2].

New editions of such print media usually appear only every few years, and the production time, including the editing process, is relatively long. Therefore, current knowledge on, in this case, allergens, cannot be incorporated. To access current literature, the clinician (and researcher) must resort to literature databases and retrieval services, the most well known of which is probably Medline, maintained by the US National Library of Medicine. The immediate benefit from consulting Medline on patient care has already been documented [3]; consultation with such databases is part of the structured approach of "Evidence Based Medicine," including "Evidence Based Dermatology" (http://www.ebderm.org). Direct on-line access to Medline is presently possible free of charge via http://www.ncbi.nlm.nih.gov/entrez/. Current Contents and Science Citation Index, published by the Institute for Scientific Information (ISI) (http://www.isinet.com/) and EMBASE (http://www.embase.com) are also popular literature databases, which are also partly available as CD-ROM and as other subscription services. Some of these (commercial) services allow selected entries to be downloaded (which is generally not considered to be a violation of copyright, in contrast to downloading a whole database or major parts of it), which can then be processed further using various commercial reference manager systems. As smaller national journals are sometimes not indexed in the literature databases mentioned, and "gray literature" may be interesting for collection, too, the compilation of an in-house database (examples: [4, 5]) could be considered to be a supplement to external databases such as the ones mentioned. Additional databases dedicated to scientific literature concerning allergens include COSME, INFAL und CDRF [6], which have been recently made available online [7].

If literature databases are used, information on allergens will only be retrieved *indirectly* (the original paper must be retrieved, if the abridged format of the abstract is not sufficiently informative). Allergen databases that directly present details such as synonyms, INCI names, CAS number, chemical formulae, potential sources of contact, and so on, may also be accessed with a computer. For these databases, the issues of constant revision and maintenance raised above are particularly crucial. Table 2 contains a collection of potentially useful websites.

A British website with information on plants relevant to dermatology is still available and has been updated recently [http://bodd.cf.ac.uk/BoDDHomePage.html, R.J. Schmidt (ed.)]. In the course of time this site may disappear, as other valuable sites have, and other sites may be implemented due to the fast pace of development in this field of electronic publishing. The same may hold true for allergen manufacturers that have a presence on the Internet. One manufacturer also offers allergen information in a dictionary format. However, this information is limited and only available in the German language (Hermal/Trolab, Reinbek, Germany, http://www.hautstadt.de/hs/pages/infozentrum_allergie/kontaktallergene.php). Consulting the homepages of national contact dermatitis groups is therefore recommended for advice on allergen sources (see Chapter 48). Information may also be derived using Internet search facilities such as Google (http://www.google.com), Altavista (http://www.altavista.com), Hotbot (http://www.hotbot.com), Yahoo (http://www.yahoo.com) and others.

Table 2. Selected Internet resources regarding information on allergens

URL	Description	Access
http://www.haz-map.com/allergic.htm	A relational database of hazardous chemicals and occupational seases with a description of "chemicals that cause contact allergy"	Free
http://pharmacos.eudra.org/F3/cosmetic/cosm_inci_index.htm	Inventory of INCI names and fragrance compounds	Free
http://chemfinder.cambridgesoft.com/	Information on a broad range of chemicals	Partially Free
http://www.rifm.org/ and http://www.ifraorg.org	Fragrance materials	Free
http://www3.interscience.wiley.com/cgi-bin/mrwhome/104554790/HOME	List of MAK and BAT values (German regulations) for chemicals with scientific statement	Restricted
http://bodd.cf.ac.uk/BoDDHomePage.html	Botanical names and further information on plants	Free, but support appreciated

The Allergen Bank was established in Denmark. Special test materials are stocked in the Bank and made available for dermatologists on request (including plant chemicals, acrylates, animal feed additives, and so on). The Bank's computer system registers several hundred contact allergens in appropriate patch test concentrations as well as patch test results [8]. With a similar aim of supporting patch testing with "uncommon" allergens – in this case cosmetic ingredients – the "IDOK" was established in Germany in November 1997 [9]. Sometimes information on allergenic potential is only available from animal experiments; results from these have previously been compiled in the database "INPRET" [10].

Core Message

- Online (Internet) information resources on allergens differ greatly in terms of the variety of substances covered, the degree of detail, and how current the information is. Their correctness and cost-effectiveness (in case of restricted or paid access) should be evaluated carefully before relying on the information presented.

47.2.2 Product Databases

Many compilations of the ingredients of products are available in print and on electronic media, mostly CD-ROM. For topical drugs, traditional national and international formularies can be regarded as the precursor of modern, computer-based product lists. Since products, or at least brand names, are often specific to a certain country, such lists are primarily of national interest. One example available via the Internet (intended only for Swiss dermatologists) is a Swiss database on the ingredients of topicals [11]. Since Swiss legislation does not require that all ingredients of topical preparations are listed, this database was developed to fill that void. To obtain cooperation from manufacturers in revealing proprietary information, it was agreed that the database would be centralized and accessible only by duly authorized dermatologists. Since computers were used to develop the database and to produce a printed card-file, it was easy to migrate to an on-line file. This was done in 1998 with password protection. Thus all Swiss dermatologists can perform multiple criteria Boolean searches online, including formulations, therapeutic uses and allergenic groups.

In Germany, the compositions of drugs, including topicals, are compiled and available in an almost complete electronic list that is updated yearly ("Rote Liste" [12]). Additional lists were available in the past, such as a compilation of cosmetic products and topicals [13] or ingredients of UV filter-containing cosmetics [14]. Similar databases for local or general use were compiled and reported on quite early in several other countries (for example [4, 15–17]). In the UK, refer to http://www.medicines.org.uk, which lists the excipients of many topical and some oral medicines.

Databases on the ingredients of products can be used to compile a list of products [4] that a patient with a certain contact sensitization can and cannot use – as long as the ingredients are fully (qualitatively) declared. The usefulness of such information has been demonstrated by Edman [16]. Once full declar-

47

ation using a controlled vocabulary regarding ingredients is established – even for only a specific group of products such as cosmetics, as with the INCI declaration [18] – such lists will become unnecessary for patients, although they will still be helpful when estimating the amount of exposure to allergens on the respective market [19]. For other products, such as industrial work materials, full declaration will probably be hard to achieve. In this situation, the maintenance of a central national database containing such information confidentially, with the possibility of accessing a relevant part of it for individual patients, seems a reasonable alternative. The Danish Product Register (PROBAS) is an example of such a database. It is updated on a daily basis and contains information on more than 75,000 (mostly industrial) products, and is notified or updated by producers or importers [20]; however, it is not freely accessible. This database can be used to estimate the extent of exposure in the workplace [21].

One more example of product-related data are systems which monitor adverse effects of, say, cosmetics. Examples of such systems are "IDOK" [9] or the French "Cosmetovigilance" [22].

> ## Core Message
>
> ■ Freely available (online) information on the ingredients of most types of products in terms of potential contact allergens is still scarce, with the exception of information on cosmetics and medicaments.

47.2.3 Other Information

Apart from data on allergens and products, other information may be useful for the management of patients with contact dermatitis.

Protective gloves are a mainstay of primary and secondary prevention of contact dermatitis. While information on the gloves, such as material, size and intended use, is usually readily available from the respective manufacturers or importers, permeability and chemical composition data are often hard to obtain. Different institutions, partly commercial, have tried to meet the need for comprehensive information on gloves by providing EDP databases, although usually without (free) online access:

■ In Sweden, Mellström has compiled a database on protective gloves [23]
■ In the US, a commercial database is available containing information on 321 brands of gloves and protective clothing, tested with 835 different chemicals ("Gloves and CPC Database", compiled by Forsberg and Keith, available from Digital Liaisons, Austin, TX 78731)
■ In Germany, databases concerning the gloves of the respective manufacturer only (KCL, D-36124 Eichenzell, Germany), and another database ("GloSaDa") with 34,000 measurement data on the effects of different chemicals on the six most important glove materials [24], are currently available. A few years ago, a freely accessible online list of potential allergens in protective gloves was created by the occupational liability insurance entity of the construction industry (http://www.gisbau.de: "Aktuelles", in the German language only [25]).

Manufacturers of gloves and other protective materials partly maintain websites, though these mostly contain general and order information only.

Other databases may offer more indirect benefits, such as webpages announcing forthcoming meetings such as those offered by several institutions: for example, the ESCD (http://dermis.multimedica.de/index_e.htm), the Swiss Contact Dermatitis Research Group (http://www.dermacom.ch), the British Contact Dermatitis Society (BCDS) (http://www.bad.org.uk/groups/bcds/), the German Contact Dermatitis Group (http://www.ivdk.gwdg.de/dkg) and others (see Chap. 48). Links to other relevant sites are often included. In the US, DERM-INFONET has provided such facilities with a broad scope for AAD members for many years ([26]; http://www.derm-infonet.com).

Many publishers of scientific journals and books maintain websites of various scopes, which may be used, say, for submitting manuscripts, retrieving articles (sometimes available in full text, for free or on a subscription basis), to get information on products, and so on. Currently, several commercial online providers offer information on scientific facts, pharmaceutical products, political issues in the field of medicine and communication facilities, including closed newsgroups. These services may or may not be regarded as helpful by the individual physician. Benefits and costs should be evaluated before subscribing to any such service; however, a comprehensive in-depth review of these facilities is beyond the scope of this chapter.

Core Message

■ General or detailed information on various issues pertaining to occupational dermatology and contact dermatitis is available, that is sometimes only relevant on a national level. Hence, (national) contact dermatitis societies could establish and maintain online lists of links useful to their members in order to support patient management.

47.3 Patient Management Systems

As already mentioned, electronic patient records are an important area for computer applications (see also Table 1). Despite financial constraints (in some countries) or the conservative attitudes of physicians, computer systems are increasingly used by dermatologists' offices. The potential role of computer systems extends far beyond common applications such as automated billing and other clerical purposes [27], and includes:

■ Immediate access to well-structured patient data
■ Reports for economical or scientific analyses and auditing quality control – both external and internal
■ Output of selected data, for example for medical letters
■ Integration of information databases and communication facilities, as well as transfer of patient data and networking with other offices or health centers.

In the field of contact dermatitis, any computer system needs to store not only the patient's history, but also patch test results. Over the last two decades, different patch test computer systems have been developed in various centers – some of them used locally [28–33], some in national networks of different size [4, 6, 34–38] or in an international network [39]. This list of references is not complete, as many developers and users have not published on their computer system, especially in recent years, during which the use of computers has begun to change from an exception to a rule. The scope of data recorded is mainly determined by local demands, and may range from a "maximum", with the aim of complete, highly individualized documentation of a case, to a "minimum", containing only data considered essential for epidemiological analyses.

In October 1996, the ESSCA working group of the ESCD was established with the aim of continuous international (European) collaboration concerning the collection and analysis of patch test data [40]. As a prerequisite for this, a list of items that should be recorded, in the sense of a "minimal dataset", was first compiled and agreed upon by ESSCA participants. This contained demographic ("patient") data, including date of birth, sex and an identifier (with names stored only on the local system), case data (data which must be recorded for every new consultation because it may change), and actual test data, in other words substances (along with concentration, vehicle and manufacturer) that the "case" had been tested with and all reactions (including doubtful, irritant, and so on) to these allergen preparations, together with a statement as to clinical relevance (current, past or unknown) in the case of *allergic* reactions. This "minimal dataset" has subsequently been amended and is accessible to the public at http://www.ivdk.gwdg.de/essca/doc/minidat8_2003_06.pdf. The document contains the current consensus of the ESSCA network regarding essential and optional data items to be recorded by any patch test software. As far as possible, the catalogs (the lists to choose particular items from, such as allergen names or occupations) should be compatible with internationally used nomenclatures or code numbers. For occupations, the ISCO 88 standard [41], established by the International Labour Organization, should preferably be used [42]. The full details of this 4-digit hierarchical catalogue can be partially collapsed (for various "office workers" for example) or extended by additions to a 5-digit level, as deemed necessary (see http://www.ivdk.gwdg.de/essca/doc/occup_ESSCA_01-02.pdf.

The database used to store this data would be best conceived as a relational database, following the principle of normalization to achieve maximum data integrity, integration of standardized catalogs with well-defined entries, update flexibility and minimum storage requirements [36]. The actual patch test software used to enter and retrieve data should generally be evaluated against the following criteria:

■ How well does the structure and user interface of the computer program follow the stepwise procedures in an allergy department? This is critical for acceptability during routine use.

47

- Is it possible to integrate the computer program into local networks, and into hospital information systems (electronic records) [1] in particular, at least in terms of upgrade flexibility? This may become necessary due to administrative demands. Would it furthermore be possible to integrate data held within the system into a meta-database with health records, for example by employing standardized formats for data exchange such as HTML or XML [43]?
- Is there at least one person in the department or office responsible for daily maintenance, such as back-up, program updates, routine reports?
- Is confidentiality guaranteed (such as password protection)?
- How easily can the program be adapted to local demands, including integration of supplementary anamnestic items and test series and supplementary entries into pre-existing picklists?
- Is historical correctness guaranteed: will it be possible to reconstitute the full and correct set of case data even if the compositions of test series or catalogs have changed in the meantime?
- Can free text be entered where categorical data is inadequate, to individualize documentation?
- How easily can data be exported in a format that can be read by common application programs, or in a "standard" format such as ASCII? This issue might be relevant if more complex analyses are going to be performed locally, or if data is to be passed to a network such as ESSCA.
- Are there any report functions (not just simple download of table contents) to analyze collected data and to print test results, case summaries, and so on, for a given patient? Do these queries require specific knowledge, for example of the structured query language (SQL), or is there a fairly extensive set of predefined reports that only require a few parameters to be entered (such as a time frame, the name of an allergen)? Is there continuous support allowing for the inclusion of new queries? This aspect seems particularly important if export for further analysis into standard application programs is difficult or even impossible.
- Will the computer program be supported by its developers, and if so, how long after initial installation? Is there a hotline for installation or runtime problems? Does the computer program depend on the installation of third party programs or hardware components, and is *their* function and (future) availability guaranteed?

> ## Core Message
>
> - Software used for the electronic registration of patch test results should (1) fulfill certain general quality criteria and (2) include a set of basic data to allow meaningful analyses.

47.4 Epidemiological Tools

The use of a computer program to record patch test results and selected parts of the patient's medical history may be worthwhile for the sake of compact structured storage, and the generation of test results and medical letters. With *online* documentation there may even be minimal or no extra work, compared to conventional records. However, a second, and probably predominant motivation for the use of a computer system – beyond a limited study context – is the ability to analyze the continually growing pool of data, which would not otherwise be possible. This analysis might be retrospective, or prospective, following a certain study objective. Therefore, the report functions mentioned in the above checklist must be deemed essential. This potential has been well recognized for decades [34], and it has been exploited not only for local, but also for multicenter projects and analyses. The special considerations regarding such analyses in terms of clinical epidemiology of contact allergy are outlined in Chapter 10. By continually collecting and analyzing patch test data, a surveillance system for monitoring trends in contact allergies will be established. Additionally, quality control is both a prerequisite for, and an outcome of, such a system [44].

47.4.1 Epidemiological (Multicenter) Surveillance

The monitoring of trends over time, and in particular an increase in the prevalence of sensitization to an allergen, may act as a "sentinel event", serving as a starting point for either targeted research or preventative action. The amalgamation of a large amount of multicenter data allows for more rapid recognition of such trends than the analysis of local data only. This holds especially true for intrinsically small subgroups, such as persons working in a certain occupation [44]. International comparison (within ESSCA for example) may give valuable clues towards determinants of sensitization – if presumed differences in exposure or population characteristics are taken into account. Clearly, a sufficient degree of standardization is a prerequisite for such a task and guidelines for such surveillance systems should be considered [45].

With sufficient structure and process quality, multicenter surveillance may offer considerable benefits: *"We still cling to a traditional research paradigm based on ad hoc studies … despite well recognised limitations (e.g.) … small samples restrict the scope for subgroup analyses and thus the practical value of the results. High quality clinical databases offer an alternative approach, with the potential to bring research closer to practice and audit. The advantages include wide ownership and high generalisability through the participation of many clinicians; relatively low cost for each study, as the expense of data collection is spread over a range of research, audit, and administrative uses; the ability to generate large samples rapidly; the opportunity to study rare conditions or interventions"* [46].

While it is relatively difficult to relate the prevalence of allergen sensitization found in a subgroup of patch-tested patients to the general population (see Chap. 10), the *relative* importance of allergens (such as the preservatives used in cosmetics) can be evaluated based on pooled data, because the average exposure profile can be regarded as reasonably representative (not influenced by local or regional prescriptions or consumer habits or industries). If exposure to different substances (such as preservatives in cosmetics) could be estimated (in this subgroup of test patients), true risk assessment would be possible. However, an estimation of the "exposure denominator" is probably even more difficult than the approximation of a "disease numerator" – except in just a few instances: hairdressers have been exposed both to "alkaline" and "acid" perms (ammonium thioglycolate and glyceryl thioglycolate) quite homogeneously. While the former is apparently a very rare allergen, the latter is known to be one of the most aggressive allergens, with a much higher risk of sensitization under usual working conditions.

47.4.2 Good Clinical Practice in Patch Testing

International groups such as the ICDRG or the ESCD, and many national groups, have devoted much work to the improvement of patch testing. Active participation in such a group must be regarded as essential for participation in a scientific network on contact allergy, such as the IVDK or ESSCA. However, similar to the experience of the NACDG [37], considerable differences (even between members of such specialist groups) were noted upon first analyses of pooled data concerning the interpretation of test reactions; these differences would otherwise not have come to light. As an educational consequence, regular patch test training sessions should be instituted [44].

Furthermore, the composition of patch test series should constantly be adapted to trends in allergen exposure; eliminating allergens which are no longer important, or always cross-react, and introducing new potential allergens. The analysis of a large amount of data greatly supports such decisions, and the addition of allergens presumed to be important (such as bufexamac [47] or hydroxymethyl pentylcyclohexene carboxaldehyde [48] in Austria and Germany) to the standard series for a limited period of time allows rapid estimation of the prevalence of a particular sensitization in the clinical population of patch-tested patients [49]. The analysis of cross-reactivity [50–52] improves when using a large set of data, because statistical estimates such as kappa values, positive predictive values, and so on, are more precise.

Core Message

■ With little extra effort compared to conventional record keeping (and in the case of primary online documentation, without even incurring additional costs), the computerized registration of patch test data, along with selected demographic data, can be exploited for medical letter writing, quality auditing, and clinical epidemiology research.

47

47.5 Further Applications and Perspectives

Beyond the current use of computers in the management of contact dermatitis, the following applications are conceivable, partially realized in experimental settings:

- Composition of a panel of allergens for patch testing according to a certain demographic and occupational profile [53] or even on an *individual* basis (instead of using standard and other series), based on a rule-generating system [54] – commonly termed an "expert system" [55].
- Telemedical applications such as graphical or text-based consultation systems on contact allergies to support daily practice
- Use for image analysis of, for example, ultrasound [56], histological or clinical [57] pictures
- Conception of lecture or self-learning educational material in the field of contact allergy [27]
- Further advances in the use of computers in the search for quantitative structure-activity relationships [58–60].

References

1. Van Bemmel JH, McCray AT (1995) The computer-based patient record. Schattauer, Stuttgart
2. McCray AT, Nelson SJ (1995) The representation of meaning in the UMLS. Methods Inform Med 34:193–201
3. Lindberg DAB, Siegel ER, Rapp BA, Wallingford KT, Wilson SR (1993) Use of MEDLINE by physicians for clinical problem solving. J Am Med Assoc 269:3124–3129
4. Dooms Goossens A, Degreef H, Drieghe J, Dooms M (1980) Computer assisted monitoring of contact dermatitis patients. Contact Dermatitis 6:123–127
5. Ippen H, Schnuch A (1993) Das Göttinger Dokumentations-System (Allphar-Medium). Struktur und Nutzung auf allergologischem Gebiet. Allergologie 16:146–150
6. Goossens A, Drieghe J (1998) Computer applications in contact allergy. Contact Dermatitis 38:51–52
7. Drieghe J, Goossens A (2002) On-line internet facilities for contact allergy software: CDESK/PRO. Contact Dermatitis 47:243
8. Andersen KE, Rastogi SC, Carlsen L (1996) The Allergen Bank: a source of extra contact allergens for the dermatologist in practice. Acta Derm Venereol (Stockh) 76:136–140
9. Uter W, Geier J, Lessmann H, Schnuch A (1999) Unverträglichkeitsreaktionen gegen Körperpflege- und Haushaltsprodukte: was ist zu tun? Dtsch Derm 47:211–214
10. Ziegler V, Richter C, Ziegler B, Haustein UF (1989) INPRET – Database on predictive tests (allergy). Semin Dermatol 8:80–82
11. Perrenoud D, Perroud JP, Grillet JP (1993) Database of topical drugs for Swiss dermatologists. Dermatology 183:229
12. ECV (2004) Rote Liste. ECV, Aulendorf
13. Scheuer B, von Bülow V (1998) Liste Inhaltsstoffe 1998/1. Bits at work, Kiel
14. Schauder S, Schrader A, Ippen H (1996) Göttinger Liste 1996. Sonnenschutzkosmetik in Deutschland. Blackwell, Berlin
15. Rantanen T (1989) INFODERM – a microcomputer database system with Finnish product files. Semin Dermatol 8:94–95
16. Edman B (1988) The usefulness of detailed information to patients with contact allergy. Contact Dermatitis 19:43–47
17. MacEachran JH, Clendenning WE, Gosselin RE (1976) Computer-derived exposure lights for common contact dermatitis antigens. Contact Dermatitis 2:239–246
18. DeGroot AC, Weijland JW (1997) Conversion of common names of cosmetic allergens to the INCI nomenclature. Contact Dermatitis 37:145–150
19. Flyvholm MA (1993) Contact allergens in registered cleaning agents for industrial and household use. Br J Ind Med 50:1043–1050
20. Flyvholm MA, Andersen P, Beck ID, Brandorff NP (1992) PROBAS: the Danish product register database. A national register of chemical substances and products. J Hazard Mat 30:59–69
21. Brandorff NP, Flyvholm MA, Beck ID, Skov T, Bach E (1995) National survey on the use of chemicals in the working environment: estimated exposure events. Occup Environ Med 52:454–463
22. Vigan M (1997) Les nouveaux allergenes des cosmetiques. La cosmetovigilance. Ann Derm Venereol (Stockh) 124:571–575
23. Mellström GA, Lindahl G, Wahlberg JE (1989) DAISY: reference database on protective gloves. Semin Dermatol 8:75–79
24. Geerissen H (1998) Schutzhandschuhe per Datenbank sicher auswählen. Die BG 9:550–554
25. Geier J, Rühl R (2001) Internet-Liste mit Allergenen in Schutzhandschuhen. Derm Beruf Umwelt 49:251
26. Kopf AW, Rigel DS, White R, Rosenthal L, Jordan WP, Carter DM, Everett MA, Moore J (1988) DERM/INFONET: a concept becomes a reality. J Am Acad Dermatol 18:1150–1157
27. Molina CI (1996) Information technology and media in allergy. The Computing Group of the Audiovisual Subcommittee of the European Academy of Allergology and Clinical Immunology. Allergy 51:603–607
28. Beck MH, Hiller V (1989) Computer analysis of patients undergoing contact dermatitis investigation. Semin Dermatol 8:105
29. Gailhofer G (1988) Computerunterstützte Erfassung und Bearbeitung von Epikutantestdaten. Ein Modell. Derm Beruf Umwelt 36:10–12
30. Diepgen T L, Stüben O (1989) ALLDAT: an allergy data system for storage and analysis of test data with regard to epidemiological and occupational dermatology. Semin Dermatol 8:101–102
31. Bahmer FA (1988) Das Homburger Modell zur Erfassung allergologischer Daten mittels EDV. Derm Beruf Umwelt 36:5–9
32. MacFarlane HA, Ross JA (1986) Use of a computer program for contact clinic results. Contact Dermatitis 14:162–164
33. Perrenoud D (1995) Easy management of patch-test data with a new Windows-based software. Dermatology 191:180
34. Fabbri P, Sertoli A (1971) Premesse e programmazione preliminare per l'uso del computer nella diagnostica dermato-allergologica. Folia Allergol 18:138–144

35. Edman B (1989) DALUK: the Swedish computer system for contact dermatitis. Semin Dermatol 8:97–98
36. Uter W, Diepgen TL, Arnold R, Hillebrand O, Pietrzyk PM, Stüben O, Schnuch A (1992) The informational network of departments of dermatology in Germany – a multicenter project for computer-assisted monitoring of contact allergy – electronic data processing aspects. Derm Beruf Umwelt 40:142–149 (published erratum: p 197)
37. Nethercott JR, Holness DL (1989) The compilation of patch test information by the use of computerized databases. J Am Acad Dermatol 21:877–880
38. Richter G (1978) Occupational dermatosis in the Dresden region 1962–1975. Results and problems of computer assisted analysis in Dermatology I. Dermatol Monatsschr 164:36–50
39. Uter W, Arnold R, Wilkinson J, Shaw S, Perrenoud D, Rili C, Vigan M, Ayala F, Krecisz B, Hegewald J, Schnuch A (2003) A multilingual European patch test software concept: WinAlldat/ESSCA. Contact Dermatitis 49:270–271
40. Schnuch A (1997) The European Surveillance System on Contact Allergies (ESSCA) – a new working party of the ESCD. ESCD Newslett 2–3
41. International Labour Organisation (1990) International standard classification of occupations: ISCO-88. ILO, Geneva
42. Uter W (2000) Classification of occupations. In: Kanerva L, Elsner P, Wahlberg J, Maibach HI (eds) Handbook of occupational dermatology. Springer, Berlin Heidelberg New York, pp 27–31
43. McDonald CJ, Overhage JM, Dexter PR, Blevins L, Meeks-Johnson J et al (1998) Canopy computing – using the web in clinical practice. J Am Med Assoc 280:1325–1329
44. Uter W, Schnuch A, Geier J, Frosch PJ (1998) The epidemiology of contact dermatitis. The information network of departments of dermatology (IVDK) in Germany. Eur J Dermatol 8:36–40
45. Schnuch A (2000) Evaluating surveillance systems in contact dermatitis. In: Schwindt DA, Maibach HI (eds) Cutaneous biometrics. Kluwer/Plenum, New York, pp 243–255
46. Black N (1997) Developing high quality clinical databases. BMJ 315:381–382
47. Kränke B, Derhasching J, Komericki P, Aberer W (1996) Bufexamac is a frequent sensitizer. Contact Dermatitis 34:63–64
48. Geier J, Brasch J, Schnuch A, Lessmann H, Pirker C, Frosch PJ (2002) Lyral has been included in the patch test standard series in Germany. Contact Dermatitis 46:295–297
49. Aberer W, Komericki P, Uter W, Hausen BM, Lessmann H, Kranke B, Geier J, Schnuch A (2003) Epidemiologische Überwachung von Kontaktallergenen. Der "Monitorblock" des IVDK. Hautarzt 54:741–749
50. Edman B (1991) Computerized analysis of concomitant contact allergens. Contact Dermatitis 24:110–113
51. Uter W, Gefeller O, Geier J, Schnuch A (2001) Limited concordance between "oakmoss" and colophony in clinical patch testing. J Invest Dermatol 116:478–480
52. Uter W, Lessmann H, Geier J, Becker D, Fuchs T, Richter G (2002) The spectrum of allergic (cross-)sensitivity in clinical patch testing with "para amino" compounds. Allergy 57:319–322
53. Brasch J, Geier J, Schnuch A (1998) Differenzierte Kontaktallergenlisten dienen der Qualitätsverbesserung: Ergebnisse aus der Kooperation von DKG und IVDK (Daten aus 24 Hautkliniken). Hautarzt 49:184–191
54. Albert J, Geier J, Lehmann M, Schoof J (1997) Lernende Klassifizierungssysteme zur fallbasierten Auswertung von Allergietestdaten. Allergo J 6:408
55. Dooms-Goossens A, Drieghe J, Degreff H, Dooms M (1990) The "Codex-E": an expert system for contact dermatitis. Contact Dermatitis 22:180–181
56. Raju BI, Swindells KJ, Gonzalez S, Srinivasan MA (2003) Quantitative ultrasonic methods for characterization of skin lesions in vivo. Ultrasound Med Biol 29:825–838
57. Fullerton A, Rode B, Serup J (2002) Studies of cutaneous blood flow of normal forearm skin and irritated forearm skin based on high-resolution laser Doppler perfusion imaging (HR-LDPI). Skin Res Technol 8:32–40
58. Basketter DA, Scholes EW, Chamberlain M, Barratt MD (1995) An alternative strategy to the use of guinea pigs for the identification of skin sensitization hazard. Food Chem Toxicol 33:1051–1056
59. Smith Pease CK, Basketter DA, Patlewicz GY (2003) Contact allergy: the role of skin chemistry and metabolism. Clin Exp Dermatol 28:177–183
60. Zinke S, Gerner I, Schlede E (2002) Evaluation of a rule base for identifying contact allergens by using a regulatory database: comparison of data on chemicals notified in the European Union with "structural alerts" used in the DEREK expert system. Altern Lab Anim 30:285–298

Chapter 48

Contact Dermatitis Research Groups

48

DERK P. BRUYNZEEL

■ *Australia*   *Contact Dermatitis Committee, Australasian College of Dermatologists*
Chairperson: Susi Freeman
Skin and Cancer Foundation,
277 Bourke Street, Darlinghurst,
New South Wales 2010, Australia
Secretary: Rosemary Nixon
Occupational Dermatology
Research and Education Centre,
PO Box 132, Carlton South,
Victoria 3053, Australia

■ *Austria*   *Arbeitsgruppe Allergologie der Österreichischen Gesellschaft für Dermatologie und Venerologie*
Chairperson: Georg Klein
Department of Dermatology,
Elisabethinen Hospital,
Fadingerstrasse 1, 4020 Linz,
Austria
Secretary: Thomas Hawranek
Department of Dermatology,
Paracelsus Private Medical
University Salzburg, Muellner
Hauptstrasse 48, 5020 Salzburg,
Austria

■ *Belgium*   *Belgian Contact and Environmental Dermatology Group (BCEDG)*
Chairperson: Stefan Kerre
Gijmelse Steenweg 16,
3200 Aarschot, Belgium
Secretary: An Goossens
Dept. of Dermatology –
Contact Allergy Unit, University
Hospital K.U. Leuven,
3000 Leuven, Belgium

■ *Brazil*   *Brazilian Contact Dermatitis Study Group*
Chairperson: Ida Duarte
Rua Diana 820/15 J, São Paulo,
São Paolo 05019–000, Brazil
Secretary: Mario Cezar Pires
Rua Diana 183 AP-63, São Paulo,
São Paolo 05019–000, Brazil

■ *Czech Republic*   *Group for Dermatological Allergology and Occupational Dermatology*
Chairperson: Eliška Dastychová
First Department of
Dermatovenerology,
Faculty Hospital St Anna,
Pekařská 53, 656 91 Brno,
Czech Republic
Secretary: Dagmar Košťálová
Dermatology private practice,
Karlovarská 30, 301 00 Plzeň,
Czech Republic

■ *Denmark*   *Danish Contact Dermatitis Research Group*
Chairperson: Tove Agner
Department of Dermatology KA
1502, Amtssygehuset Gentofte,
2900 Hellerup, Denmark

■ *Europe*   *European Environmental and Contact Dermatitis Research Group (EECDRG)*
Chairperson: Ian White
St. John's Institute of
Dermatology,
St. Thomas's Hospital,
London SE1 7EH,
United Kingdom
Secretary: Margarida Gonçalo,
Department of Dermatology,
University of Coimbra,
Rua Infanta D. Maria,
P-3030 Coimbra,
Portugal

48

■ *Europe*   *European Society of Contact Dermatitis (ESCD)*
Chairperson: Thomas L. Diepgen
University Hospital, Dept. of
Social Medicine, Occupational
and Environmental Dermatology,
Bergheimerstr. 58,
69115 Heidelberg, Germany
Secretary: Pieter-Jan Coenraads
Occupational and Environmental
Dermatology Unit,
University Hospital,
PO Box 30 001,
9700 RB Groningen,
The Netherlands

■ *Finland*   *Finnish Contact Dermatitis Group*
Chairperson: Kristiina Alanko
Finnish Institute of Occupational
Health, Topeliuksenkatu 41 aA,
00250 Helsinki, Finland
Secretary: Taina Hasan
Tampere University Central
Hospital PL 2000, 33521 Tampere,
Finland

■ *France*   *Groupe d'Etude et de Recherches en Dermato-Allergologie (GERDA)*
Chairperson: Michel Castelain
13 Avenue de Montredon,
13008 Marseille, France
Secretary: Gilbert Jelen
92 Grande Rue, 67700 Saverne,
France

■ *Germany*   *Deutsche Kontaktallergie-Gruppe (DKG)*
Chairperson: Detlef Becker
Johannes Gutenberg Universitat,
Dept. of Dermatology,
Langenbeckstr 7, 55101 Mainz,
Germany
Secretary: Vera Mahler
Dermatologische Klinik
mit Poliklinik, Hartmannstr. 14,
91052 Erlangen, Germany

■ *Hungary*   *Hungarian Contact Dermatitis Research Group*
Chairman: Erzsébet Temesvári
National Institute
of Dermato-Venerology,
Mariá u 41, 1085 Budapest,
Hungary
Secretary: Valéria Kohánka
József Fodor National Center of
Public Health, National Institute
of Occupational Health,
Pf 22, 1450 Budapest, Hungary

■   *International Contact Dermatitis Research Group (ICDRG)*
Chairperson: Jean-Marie
Lachapelle
Department of Dermatology,
Louvain University, UCL 3033,
30 Clos Chapelle-aux-Champs,
1200 Brussels, Belgium
Secretary: Hee Chul Eun
Department of Dermatology,
Seoul National University College
of Medicine, 28 Chongo-gu,
Yungon-dong, Seoul 110–744,
Korea

■ *Israel*   *Israeli Contact Dermatitis Society*
Chairperson: Arieh Ingber
Department of Dermatology,
Hadassah University Hospital,
Jerusalem 91120, Israel
Secretary: Akiva Trattner
Department of Dermatology,
Beilinson Medical Center,
Petach Tikva, Israel

■ *Italy*   *Italian Society of Allergologic Occupational and Environmental Dermatology (SIDAPA)*
Chairperson: Paolo Lisi
Dermatologia clinica,
allergologica e venereologica,
Dipartimento di Specialità
medico-chirurgiche,
Università di Perugia,
Policlinico Monteluce,
06100 Perugia, Italy
Secretary: Luca Stingeni
Dermatologia clinica,
allergologica e venereologica,
Dipartimento di Specialità
medico-chirurgiche,
Università di Perugia,
Policlinico Monteluce,
06100 Perugia, Italy

■ Korea   Korean Society for Contact
           Dermatitis and Skin Allergy
           Chairperson: Kea-Jeung Kim
           Dept. of Dermatology, Kangbuk,
           Samsung Hospital,
           School of Medicine,
           Sungkyunkwan University,
           108 Pyung-dong, Chongro-gu,
           Seoul, Korea
           Secretary: Young-Suck Ro
           Dept. of Dermatology,
           Hanyang University College
           of Medicine, 17 Haengdang-dong,
           Sungdong-gu, Seoul, Korea

■ Mexico   Mexican Group for Research
           on Contact and Occupational
           Dermatitis
           Chairperson:
           Armando Ancona-Alayón
           Tonalá 48, Col. Roma,
           Mexico D.F. 06700, Mexico
           Secretary:
           Roberto Blancas-Espinosa
           Tonalá 48, Col. Roma,
           Mexico D.F. 06700, Mexico

■ Netherlands Dutch Contact Dermatitis
               Research Group
               Chairperson: Marcus M.M.
               Meinardi
               Department of Dermatology,
               Academic Medical Centre
               Amsterdam, Meibergdreef 9,
               1105 AZ Amsterdam,
               The Netherlands
               Secretary: Pieter G.M. van der
               Valk
               Department of Dermatology,
               Radboud University Nijmegen
               Medical Centre, PO Box 9101,
               6500 HB Nijmegen,
               The Netherlands

■ North   American Contact Dermatitis
  America   Society
            Chairperson: Kathryn A. Zug
            Dartmouth Medical School,
            Dartmouth Hitchcock Medical
            Center, 1. Medical Center Drive,
            Lebanon, NH, 03756, USA
            Secretariat: 138 Palm Coast
            Parkway NE #333, Palm Coast,
            FL 32137, USA
            Email: info@contactderm.org

■   North American Contact
           Dermatitis Group
           Chairperson: Joseph F. Fowler, Jr
           444 South First Street, Louisville,
           KY, 40202, USA
           Secretary: Kathryn A. Zug
           Dartmouth Medical School,
           Dartmouth Hitchcock Medical
           Center, 1 Medical Center Drive,
           Lebanon, NH, 03756, USA

■ Poland   Allergology Section of the Polish
           Association of Dermatology
           Chairperson: Slawomir Majewski
           Warsaw, Poland
           Secretary

■ Portugal Grupo Português de Estudo das
           Dermites de Contacto (GPEDC)
           Chairperson: Olivia Bordalo
           Centro de Dermatologia,
           Rua José Estevão 135,
           1150–201 Lisboa, Portugal
           Secretary: Raquel Silva
           Serviço de Dermatologia,
           Hospital Santa Maria,
           Av. Prof. Egas Moniz,
           1649–035 Lisboa, Portugal

■ Singapore Environmental and Occupational
           Dermatology Society
           Chairperson: David Koh
           Dept. of Community,
           Occupational and Family
           Medicine, Faculty of Medicine,
           National University of Singapore,
           16 Medical Drive, Singapore
           117597, Republic of Singapore
           Secretary: Anthony Goon
           National Skin Centre,
           1 Mandalay Road,
           Singapore 308205,
           Republic of Singapore

■ South   South American Contact
  America   Dermatitis Research Group
            (DERMOSUR)
            Chairperson: Aliche Alchorne
            Rua Iraúna 469,
            Jardim Novo Mundo,
            SP 04518–060 Sao Paulo, Brasil
            Secretary: S. Iris Ale
            Arazatí 1194, PC 11300
            Montevideo, Uruguay

48

- *Spain*   *Spanish Contact Dermatitis Group (GEIDC)*
Secretary: Begoña García-Bravo
Dept. of Dermatology, Hospital Universitario "Virgen Macarena," Avda. Dr Fedrini 3, 41071 Sevilla, Spain

- *Sweden*   *Swedish Contact Dermatitis Research Group (SCDRG)*
Chairperson: Bernt Sternberg
Department of Dermatology, University Hospital, 901 85 Umeå, Sweden
Secretary: Annica Inerot
Department of Dermatology, Sahlgrenska University Hospital, 413 45 Göteborg, Sweden

- *Switzerland*   *Swiss Contact Dermatitis Research Group (SCDRG)*
Chairperson: Dagmar Simon
Department of Dermatology, University of Bern, 3010 Bern, Switzerland
Secretary: Rita Sigg
Falkenstrasse 3, 6004 Luzern, Switzerland

- *United Kingdom*   *British Contact Dermatitis Group*
Chairperson: David J. Gawkrodger
Department of Dermatology, Royal Hallamshire Hospital, Glossop Road, Sheffield S10 2JF, United Kingdom
Secretary: Barry Statham
Singleton Hospital, Swansea SA2 8QA, United Kingdom

Chapter 49

Patch Test Concentrations and Vehicles for Testing Contact Allergens

49

ANTON C. DE GROOT, PETER J. FROSCH

Patch testing is a relatively safe and reasonably reliable method for identifying contact allergens in patients with contact dermatitis. It has been clearly shown that patch testing is necessary in the majority of patients with eczema [1]. The technique of patch testing is described in Chap. 22.

All patients are tested with the European standard series, containing the most frequent contact allergens in European countries (Table 1). Often, standard series patch testing is not enough, and additional allergens or potential allergens need to be tested, based on the patient's history and clinical examination. Examples are products and chemicals to which the patient is exposed occupationally or in his or her home environment. Test series containing the most frequent allergens in certain products (preservatives, fragrances, dental materials, plastics and glues, medicaments) or in certain occupations (hairdressing, pesticides, oil and cooling fluid) are very helpful. Approximately 510 patch test materials are commercially available from Hermal (Reinbek, Germany, www.hermal.de), Chemotechnique Diagnostics (Malmö, Sweden, www.chemotechnique.se) and Brial Allergen (Greven, Germany, www.brial.com).

For other chemicals and products, the investigator must decide how to apply them as a patch test. Chemicals usually need to be diluted, and it is of the utmost importance to use an appropriate patch test concentration and vehicle to avoid both false-negative and false-positive (irritant) reactions. The most useful reference source for documented test concentrations and vehicles of chemicals, groups of chemicals and products is the book *Patch testing. Test concentrations and vehicles for 3700 chemicals* [2]. Other useful lists are provided in recent textbooks on contact dermatitis [3–6].

Guidelines for testing the patient's own contact materials are provided in Chap. 50.

Table 2 lists alphabetically all chemicals mentioned in this book with their test concentrations and vehicles (sometimes two concentrations are suggested when insufficient data are available) as suggested by the various authors. All allergens commercially available are also listed with their supplier(s), their test concentrations, and vehicles as supplied. It should be appreciated that for a considerable number of allergens, the concentrations vary between suppliers. Table 3 provides a list of test concentrations for groups of chemicals as suggested by various authors in this book. Table 4 finally is an alphabetical listing of commonly used abbreviations and their full chemical synonyms.

References

1. Rycroft RJG (1990) Is patch testing necessary? In: Champion RH, Pye RJ (eds) Recent advances in dermatology, vol 8. Churchill Livingstone, Edinburgh, pp 101–111
2. De Groot AC (1994) Patch testing. Test concentrations and vehicles for 3700 chemicals, 2nd edn. Elsevier, Amsterdam
3. Rietschel RL, Fowler JF Jr (eds) (1995) Fisher's contact dermatitis, 4th edn. Williams and Wilkins, Baltimore, Md.
4. Adams RM (1990) Occupational skin disease, 2nd edn. Saunders, Philadelphia, Pa.
5. De Groot AC, Weijland JW, Nater JP (1994) Unwanted effects of cosmetics and drugs used in dermatology, 3rd edn. Elsevier, Amsterdam
6. Kanerva L, Elsner P, Wahlberg JE, Maibach HI (eds) (2000) Handbook of occupational dermatology. Springer, Berlin Heidelberg New York

Table 1. The European standard series

Chemical		Test concentration and vehicle
Metals	Cobalt chloride	1% pet.
	Nickel sulfate	5% pet.
	Potassium dichromate	0.5% pet.
Rubber chemicals	Thiuram mix	1% pet.
	Dipentamethylenethiuram disulfide (0.25%)	
	Tetramethylthiuram disulfide (0.25%)	
	Tetraethylthiuram disulfide (0.25%)	
	Tetramethylthiuram monosulfide (0.25%)	
	N-Isopropyl-N´-phenyl-p-phenylenediamine	0.1% pet.
	Mercapto mix	2% pet.
	N-Cyclohexylbenzothiazyl sulfenamide (0.5%)	
	Dibenzothiazyl disulfide (0.5%)	
	Mercaptobenzothiazole (0.5%)	
	Morpholinyl mercaptobenzothiazole (0.5%)	
	Mercaptobenzothiazole	2% pet.
Medicaments	Budesonide	0.01% pet.
	Benzocaine	5% pet.
	Neomycin sulfate	20% pet.
	Clioquinol®	5% pet.
	Tixocortol pivalate	0.1% pet.
Cosmetic ingredients	Balsam of Peru (Myroxylon pereirae)	25% pet.
	5-Chloro-2-methylisothiazol-3-one/2-methylisothiazol-3-one (MCI/MI)	0.01% aq.
	Colophonium (rosin)	20% pet.
	Formaldehyde	1% aq.
	Fragrance mix (incl. 5% sorbitan sesquioleate)	8% pet.
	α-Amylcinnamaldehyde (1%)	
	Cinnamal(dehyde) (1%)	
	Cinnamyl alcohol (1%)	
	Eugenol (1%)	
	Geraniol (1%)	
	Hydroxycitronellal (1%)	
	Iso-eugenol (1%)	
	Oak moss absolute (Evernia prunastri) (1%)	
	Paraben mix	16% pet.
	Butylparaben (4%)	
	Ethylparaben (4%)	
	Methylparaben (4%)	
	Propylparaben (4%)	
	p-Phenylenediamine free base	1% pet.
	Quaternium-15	1% pet.
	Wool wax alcohols (lanolin alcohol)	30% pet.
	Hydroxymethylpentylcyclohexenecarboxaldehyde (Lyral®)	5% pet.
Miscellaneous	p-tert-Butylphenol formaldehyde resin	1% pet.
	Epoxy resin	1% pet.
	Primin	0.01% pet.
	Sesquiterpene lactone mix	0.1% pet.
	Alantolactone (0.033%)	
	Dehydrocostus lactone (0.033%)	
	Costunolide (0.033%)	

49

Table 2. Test concentrations, vehicles and commercial availability of contact allergens. [*Alc.* Alcohol, *aq.* water, *DMSO* dimethyl sulfoxide, *Glyc.* glycerine, *MEK* methyl ethyl ketone (butanone), *o.o.* olive oil, *pet.* petrolatum, *prop. glyc.* propylene glycol.] [*icr* Immediate contact reactions reported (Chaps 5 and 26), *de* drug eruption with positive patch test reported (Chap. 24), *fde* fixed drug eruption with positive patch test reported (Chap. 24), *ph* photosensitivity reported (Chaps 6, 17 and 27), *phde* photosensitive drug eruption with positive photopatch test reported (Chaps 6, 17, 24 and 27)]

Allergen	Test Concentration and vehicle	Suppliers		
		Trolab	Chemo	Brial
Abietic acid (icr)	10% pet.	+	+	+
Acebutolol hydrochloride				2% pet.
Aceclofenac	1% pet			
Acetylsalicylic acid (icr)				10% pet.
Achillea millefolium (yarrow extract)	1% pet.	+	+	
Acid black 48 (CI 65005)	1% pet.			
Acid red 14 (azorubine)				0.1% alc.
Acid red 118 (CI 26410)	5% pet.		+	
Acid red 359	5% pet.		+	
Acid violet 17 (CI 42650)	1% pet.			
Acid yellow 36 (CI 13065, metanil yellow)	1% pet.	+	+	+
Acid yellow 61 (CI 18968)			5% pet.	
Actarit (phde)	1% pet			
Aciclovir (fde)	5% pet.			
Alantolactone (icr)			0.33% pet.	
Alclometasone-17,21-dipropionate	1% alc.		1% pet.	
Alcohol, ethyl (icr)	10% aq.			
Alimemazine tartrate	see Trimeprazine tartrate			
Allantoin	0.5% aq.			
Althiazide (phde)	10% pet. or aq.			
Aluminum (icr)			Pure	
Aluminum chloride hexahydrate			2% pet.	
Allylisopropylacetylurea	See Apronalide			
Amalgam		5% pet.		
Amalgam alloying metals	20% pet.	+		+
Amalgam non gamma 2				5% pet.
Amcinonide	1% alc.	0.1% pet.		0.1% pet.
Amerchol ® L-101	See Lanolin alcohol and paraffinum liquidum			
Amethocaine	See Tetracaine hydrochloride			
Amikacin sulfate	20% pet.			
4-Aminoantipyrine	See Ampyrone			
p-Aminoazobenzene (Solvent yellow 1, CI 11000)	0.25% pet	1% pet.	+	1% pet.
ε-Aminocaproic acid	1% aq.			
Amino-4-*N*, *N*-diethylaniline sulfate (TSS Agfa®)				1% pet.
2-2-(Aminoethoxy)ethanol	See Diglycolamine			
Amino-4-*N*-ethyl-*N*-(methanesulfon-aminoethyl)-*m*-toluidine (CD 3)	1% pet.	+	+	
Aminoglycosides (de)	20% pet.			
m-Aminophenol	1% pet.	+	+	+
p-Aminophenol (CI 76550) (icr)	1% pet.	+	+	+
Aminophylline (fde)	10% pet.			
Amitriptyline (phde)	5% pet.			
Amlexanox (fde)	1% pet.			
Ammoniated mercury	1% pet.	+	+	+
Ammonium bituminosulfonate	See Ichthammol			
Ammonium heptamolybdate				1% aq.
Ammonium hexachloroplatinate (icr)	0.1% aq.		+	
Ammonium persulfate (icr)	2.5% pet.	+	+	+
Ammonium tetrachloroplatinate (icr)	0.25% pet.	+	0.25% aq.	+
Ammonium thioglycolate	1% pet., fresh		2.5% aq.	1% pet.
Amorolfine	1% pet.			
Ampicillin (icr)	5% pet.			+
Ampiroxicam (phde)	1% pet.			
Amprolium hydrochloride	10% aq.			
Ampyrone (4-aminoantipyrine) (icr)				10% pet.

Table 2. Continued

Allergen	Test Concentration and vehicle	Suppliers		
		Trolab	Chemo	Brial
α-Amylcinnamaldehyde (icr)	2% pet.	1% pet.	+	1% pet.
Amylocaine hydrochloride	5% pet		+	
Anethole			5% pet.	
Aniline	1% pet.			+
Antazoline	1% pet.			
Anthemis nobilis (chamomilla romana)			1% pet.	
Antipyrine (phenazone) (de)	5% pet.			
Apronalide (allylisopropylacetylurea) (fed)	5% pet.			
Arnica montana (arnica extract)	0.5% pet.	+	+	
Arsanilic acid	10% pet.			
Atenolol (de)	10% pet.			
Atranorin (ph)			0.1% pet.	
Atropine sulfate	1% aq. or pet	+ (aq.)		+ (aq.)
Azathioprine	1% pet.			
Azidamfenicol	2% pet.			
Azodicarbonamide	0.5% pet.			
Azodiisobutyrodinitrile			1% pet.	
Azorubine	See Acid red 14			
Bacitracin (icr)	20% pet.	+	5% pet.	+
Bacitracin zinc	20% pet.			
Balsam of Peru	See *Myroxylon pereirae*			
Balsam of Tolu	See *Myroxylon toluiferum*			
Basic brown 1	See Bismarck Brown R			
Basic red 46			1% pet.	
Beech tar	See *Fagus sylvatica*			
Befunolol	1% aq.			
Benomyl	0.1–1% pet.			
Benoxinate	See Oxybuprocaine			
Benzaldehyde (icr)	5% pet.	+		+
Benzalkonium chloride (BAK)	0.01–0.1% aq.	0.1% pet.	0.1% aq.	0.1% pet.
Benzamine lactate	1% pet.			
2-Benzimidazolethiol (2-mercaptobenzimidazole)				1% pet.
Benzisothiazolinone (BIT) (ph)	0.1% pet.	+	0.05% pet.	+
Benzocaine (icr) (ph)	5% pet.	+	+	+
Benzodiazepines (de)	1–5% aq. or pet.			
Benzoic acid (icr) (ph)			5% pet.	5% pet.; 1% alc./glyc.
Benzoin resin	see *Styrax benzoin*			
Benzophenone-3 (oxybenzone) (ph)	10% pet.	+	+	+
Benzophenone-4 (sulisobenzone) (ph) (icr)	10% pet.	+	+	+
Benzophenone-10 (mexenone) (ph)	10% pet.		+	
IH-Benzotriazole	1% pet.	+	+	+
Benzyl benzoate	5% pet.			
Benzoyl peroxide (icr)	1% pet.	+	+	+
Benzydamine hydrochloride (ph)	5% pet. or aq.			
Benzyl alcohol (icr)	1% pet.	+	+	+
Benzyl cinnamate		5% pet.		
Benzylhemiformal		1% pet.		
Benzyl salicylate	1–5% pet.	1% pet.	2% pet.	1% pet.
Bergamot oil	See *Citrus bergamia*			
Beryllium chloride or sulfate	1% pet.			
Betamethasone dipropionate	1% alc.			
Betamethasone-17-valerate	1% alc.	0.12% pet.	1% pet.	0.12% pet.
Betaxolol hydrochloride	1% aq.			
Betula alba (birch tar)			3% pet.	
BHA (butylated hydroxyanisole) (icr)	2% pet.	+	+	+; 2% alc.
BHT (butylated hydroxytoluene) (icr)	2% pet.	+	+	+; 2% alc.
Bifonazole	1% alc.			

49

Table 2. Continued

Allergen	Test Concentration and vehicle	Suppliers		
		Trolab	Chemo	Brial
Bioban ® CS-1135	1% pet.	+	+	+
Bioban ® CS-1246	1% pet.		+	+
Bioban® P 1487		1% pet.	0.5% pet.	1% pet.
Biocheck 60 ®	0.2% aq.			
Bis(aminopropyl)-lauramine	0.01–0.1–1% aq.			
Bis(dibutyldithiocarbamato) zinc	See Zinc dibutyldithiocarbamate			
Bis(diethyldithiocarbamato) zinc	See Zinc diethyldithiocarbamate			
BIS-EMA	1% pet.		+	
BIS-GMA	2% pet.	+	+	+
BIS-MA	2% pet.		+	
Bismarck Brown (vesuvine brown, basic brown 1, CI 21000)	0.5% pet.	+		+
Bismuth neodecanoate	1% pet.			
Bisphenol A	See 4,4´-isopropylidenediphenol			
Bisphenol A dimethacrylate				2% pet.
Bithionol (ph) (icr)	1% pet.	+	+	+
Black rubber mix (N-isopropyl-N-phenyl-p-phenylenediamine, N-cyclohexyl-N-phenyl-p-phenylenediamine, N, N-diphenyl-p-phenylenediamine)			0.25% pet.	
Boric acid	10% pet.			
Brilliant black				0.1% coca/glyc.
Brilliant lake red R (D&C red 31, CI 15800) (ph) (icr)	1% pet.			
5-Bromo-4´-chlorosalicylanilide (ph)		1% pet.		
2-Bromo-2-nitropropane-1,3-diol (icr)	0.5% pet.	0.25% pet.	0.5% pet.	
Budesonide	0.1% pet.	+	0.01% pet.	+
Bucillamine (de)	1% pet.			
Bufexamac	5% pet.	+		+
Bupivacaine	1% pet.			
Butacaine	5% pet.			
1,4-Butanediol diacrylate (BUDA)	0.1% pet.		+	
1,4-Butanediol dimethacrylate (BUDMA)	2% pet.		+	+
Butethamine hydrochloride	5% pet.			
Butyl acrylate (BA)	0.1% pet.		+	+
Butyl aminobenzoate	5% pet.			
Butylated hydroxyanisole	See BHA			
Butylated hydroxytoluene	see BHT			
4-tert-Butylbenzoic acid			1% pet.	
p-tert-Butylcatechol (PTBC)	0.25% pet		+	1% pet.
Butyl glycidyl ether		0.25% pet.		
t-Butyl hydroquinone	1% pet.	+	+	+
n-Butyl methacrylate (BMA)	2% pet.		+	
Butyl methoxydibenzoylmethane (ph)	10% pet.	+	+	+
Butylparaben (icr)	3% pet.	+	+	+
p-tert-Butylphenol	1% pet.	+	+	+
p-tert-Butylphenolformaldehyde resin (PTBP)	1% pet.	+	+	+
Cadmium chloride (ph)	0.5% pet.		1% aq.	+
Caine mix I (procaine hydrochloride, dibucaine hydrochloride).			3.5% pet	
Caine mix II (dibucaine hydrochloride, lidocaine, tetracaine)			10% pet.	
Caine mix III (benzocaine, dibucaine, tetracaine)			10% pet	
Caine mix IV (amylocaine, lidocaine, prilocaine)			10% pet	
Calcipotriol	2 µg/ml alc.			
Camphor (icr)				1% pet.
Camphoroquinone			1% pet.	
Cananga odorata (cananga oil, ylang-ylang oil)	5% pet.		2% pet.	
Captan	0.5% aq. or pet.		0.5% pet.	

Table 2. Continued

Allergen	Test Concentration and vehicle	Suppliers		
		Trolab	Chemo	Brial
Captopril (de)	0.1–3% pet			
Carbamazepine (de) (fde) (phde)	10% pet. or alc. / 0.01–10% pet.			
Carba mix (*N, N*-diphenylguanidine, zinc dibutyl dithiocarbamate, zinc diethyldithiocarbamate)		3% pet.	3% pet.	
Carbenicillin (de)	5% aq.			
Carprofen	5% pet.			
Carteolol	1% aq.			
Castor oil	Pure			
CD 2 (color developer 2)	See Methyl-3-amino-4-*N, N*-diethyl-aniline			
CD 3 (color developer 3)	See Amino-4-*N*-ethyl-*N*-(methane-sulfonaminoethyl)-*m*-toluidine			
CD 4 (color developer 4)	See 4-(*N*-Ethyl-*N*-2-hydroxyethyl)-2-methylphenylenediamine sulfate			
Cedarwood oil	See *Cedrus atlantica*			
Cedrus atlantica (cedarwood oil) (ph)	10% pet.	+		+
Celecoxib (de)	10% pet.			
Cetalkonium chloride		0.1% pet.		0.1% pet.
Cetrimide	See Cetrimonium bromide			
Cetrimonium bromide (Cetrimide)	0.25% pet.			
Cetyl alcohol (icr)	5% pet.		+	
Cetyl alcohol, stearyl alcohol	20% pet.	+	+	+
Cetylpyridinium chloride	0.1% pet.	+		+
Chamomilla recutita (chamomile extract) (icr)	2.5% pet.			
Chamomilla romana	see *Anthemis nobilis*			
Chlorambucil	2% pet.			
Chloramine-T (icr)	0.05% aq.			
Chloramphenicol (icr)	5% pet.	+	+	10% pet.
Chlorhexidine diacetate (ph, icr)			0.5% aq.	
Chlorhexidine digluconate (ph) (icr)	0.5% aq.	+	+	+
Chlormezanone (fde)	10% pet. or alc.			
Chloroacetamide	0.2% pet.	+	+	+
p-Chloro-*m*-cresol (PCMX) (icr)	1% pet.	+	+	+
5-Chloro-2-methyl-4-isothiazolin-3-one	0.01–0.02% aq.			
5-Chloro-2-methylisothiazol-3-one (MCI), 2-methylisothiazol-3-one (MI)	0.01% aq.	+	+	+
5-Chloro-1-methyl-4-nitroimidazole	0.1% pet.			
Chlorothalonil (icr)	0.001–0.01% acet.			
Chloroxylenol		1% pet.	0.5% pet.	1% pet.
Chlorphenesin	1% pet.			
Chlorpheniramine maleate	5% pet.			+
Chlorpromazine hydrochloride (phde) (icr)	0.1–1% pet. or aq.		0.1% pet.	1% pet.
Chlorquinaldol (ph)	5% pet.	+	+	+
Chlortetracycline hydrochloride	5% pet.			1% pet.
Chromic chloride				1% pet.
Chromic potassium sulfate				2% aq.
Chromic sulfate				0.5% pet.
Chrysanthemum cinerariaefolium (pyrethrum) (icr)	1% pet.		+	
Chrysanthemum parthenium (feverfew flower extract)	1% pet.			
Cimetidine (de)	1% aq.			
Cinchocaine®	See Dibucaine hydrochloride			
Cinnamal (cinnamic aldehyde) (ph) (icr)	1% pet.	+	2% pet.	+
Cinnamic acid (icr)				5% pet.
Cinnamomum cassia (cinnamon oil) (ph)(icr)				0.5% pet.
Cinnamyl alcohol	1–5% pet.	1% pet.	2% pet.	1% pet.
Cinnoxicam	1% pet.			

Table 2. Continued

Allergen	Test Concentration and vehicle	Suppliers		
		Trolab	Chemo	Brial
Ciprofloxacin (fde)	10% pet.			
Citiolone (fde)	10% DMSO			
Citronellal				2% pet.
Citrus aurantium dulcis (neroli oil) (ph)	2% pet.	+		+
Citrus bergamia (bergamot oil) (ph)				2% pet.
Citrus dulcis (orange oil) (ph)		2% pet.		
Citrus limonum (lemon oil) (ph)	2% pet.	+		+
Clioquinol® (icr)	5% pet.	+	+	+
Clarithromycin (fde)	10% aq.			
Clindamycin phosphate (de)	1–20% aq. or pet.			
Clobetasol-17-propionate (icr)	1% alc.	0.25% pet.	1% pet.	0.25% pet.
Clobetasone butyrate	1% alc.			
Clomipramine (phde)	0.1% pet.			
Clonidine	1% pet.			
Cloprednol	1% alc.			
Clotrimazole	5% pet./1% alc.	+ (pet.)		+ (pet)
Clove oil	See *Eugenia caryophyllus*			
Cloxacillin (de) (icr)	Pure			
Coal tar	See Pix ex carbone			
Cobalt chloride (ph) (icr)	1% pet.	+	+	+
Cobaltous sulfate (ph)				2.5% pet.
Cocamide DEA	0.5% pet.	+	+	+
Cocamidopropyl betaine	1% aq.	+	+	1% alc./aq.
Codeine phosphate (de)	0.05% aq.			
Cold cream				Pure
Colophonium (rosin) (ph) (icr)	20% pet.	+	+	+
Compositae mix (*Tanacetum vulgare*, *Arnica montana*, parthenolide, *Chamomilla romana*, *Achillea millefolium*)		6% pet.	5% pet.	5% pet.
Congo red	2% pet.			
Copper oxide	See Cupric oxide			
Copper 8-quinolinate	1% pet.			
Copper sulfate	See Cupric sulfate			
Corticosteroid mix (budesonide, tixocortol pivalate, hydrocortisone-17-butyrate)			2.1% pet.	
Coumarin (ph)				1% pet.
Coumarone indene resin	20% pet.			
p-Cresol	1% aq.			
Cresyl glycidyl ether (icr)	0.25% pet.	+		+
Croconazole	1% alc.			
Cromoglicate sodium	See Cromolyn			
Cromolyn (cromoglicate sodium) (icr)	2% aq.			2% pet.
Crotamiton	3% pet.			
Cupric oxide (copper oxide)			5% pet.	
Cupric sulfate (copper sulfate) (icr)		1% pet.	2% pet.	1% aq.; 2% pet.
Cyclohexanone resin			1% pet.	
Cycloheximide	1% pet.			
N-Cyclohexylbenzothiazyl sulfenamide (CBS)	1% pet.	+	+	+
N-Cyclohexyl-*N*-phenyl-*p*-phenylene-diamine (CPPD)			1% pet.	
Cyclohexyl thiophthalimide	1% pet.	0.5% pet.	+	+
Cyclomethycaine hydrochloride	1% pet.			
Cyclopentolate hydrochloride	0.5% aq.			
Cymbopogon schoenanthus (lemon grass oil) (ph)	2% pet.	+		+
Dandelion	See *Taraxacum officinale*			
Dazomet	0.1% pet.			
D and C red 31	See Brilliant lake red R			
D and C yellow 11	See Solvent yellow 33			

Table 2. Continued

Allergen	Test Concentration and vehicle	Suppliers		
		Trolab	Chemo	Brial
DDT	1% pet. or acet.			
Desketoprofen	1% pet.			
Desonide	1% alc.			
Desoximetasone (ph)	1% alc.			
Dexamethasone				0.5% pet.
Dexamethasone acetate	1% alc.			
Dexamethasone phosphate	1% alc.			
Dexamethasone 21-phosphate disodium salt			1% pet.	
Dexpanthenol	See Panthenol			
Diallyl disulfide	1% -5% pet.		1% pet.	
4,4´-Diaminodiphenylmethane (ph)	0.5% pet.	+	+	+
Diazolidinyl urea	2% pet.	+	+	+
Dibenzothiazyl disulfide (MBTS)	1% pet.	+	+	+
Dibenzthione (sulbentine)	3% pet.			
1,2-Dibromo-2,4-dicyanobutane	See Methyldibromo glutaronitrile			
Dibromosalicylanilide (ph)	1% pet.			
Dibucaine hydrochloride (Cinchocaine ®) (ph)	5% pet.	+	+	+
Dibutyl phthalate	5% pet.	+	+	+
Dibutylthiourea	1% pet.	+	+	+
Dibutyl- and diethylthiourea mix			1% pet.	
Dichlorophene (ph)	0.5% pet.	+	1% pet.	+
Diclofenac sodium	1% pet.			5% pet.
Dicyanodiamide	0.1% aq.			
Dicyclohexylcarbodiimide	0.1% acet. and lower			
Diethanolamine	2% pet.	+		+
Diethyleneglycol diacrylate (DEGDA)	0.1% pet.		+	
Diethylenetriamine (DETA)	1% pet.	0.5% pet.	+	
Di-2-ethylhexyl phthalate (DEHP)	See Dioctyl phthalate			
Diethyl phthalate				5% pet.
Diethylstilbestrol	1% pet.			
Diethylthiourea	1% pet.		+	
Diflorasone diacetate	1% alc.			
Diflucortolone pivalate	1% alc.			
Difolatan	0.1% pet.			
Diglycolamine [2-(2-aminoethoxy)ethanol]	1% pet.			
Dihydroquinidine (de)	Pulverized tablet, pure			
Dihydrostreptomycin	0.1% pet.			
4,4´-Dihydroxydiphenyl		0.1% pet.		0.1% pet.
Diisopropyl carbodiimide	0.1% acet. and lower			
Diltiazem (de)	1% pet.			
Dimethylaminoethyl ether	1% pet.			
N,N-Dimethylaminoethyl methacrylate			0.2% pet.	
Dimethylaminopropylamine			1% aq.	
Dimethylaminopropyl ethyl carbodiimide	0.1% acet. and lower			
Dimethyl dihydroxyethyleneurea			4.5% aq.	
Dimethylol dihydroxyethyleneurea			5% aq.	
4,4-Dimethyloxazolidine/3,4,4,trimethyl-oxazolidine	See Bioban® CS-1135			
N,N´-Dimethyl-p-phenylenediamine		0.25% pet.		
Dimethyl phthalate	5% pet.	+		+
Dimethylol propylene urea	5% aq.			
N,N-Dimethyl-p-toluidine		2% pet.	5% pet.	2% pet.
N,N-di-β-Naphthyl-p-phenylenediamine (DBNPD)			1% pet.	
2,4-Dinitrochlorobenzene (DNCB) (icr)	0.01–0.1% aq. or acet.			
Dioctyl phthalate (di-2-ethylhexyl phthalate) (icr)	5% pet.	+	2% pet.	+
Dipentamethylenethiuram disulfide		0.25% pet.	1% pet.	0.25% pet.
Dipentamethylenethiuram tetrasulfide				0.25% pet.
Dipentene (D-limonene)	2% pet.	+	1% pet.	+
Diperocaine	1% pet.			

Table 2. Continued

Allergen	Test Concentration and vehicle	Suppliers		
		Trolab	Chemo	Brial
Diphenhydramine hydrochloride (ph)	1% pet.		+	
1,3-Diphenylguanidine (DPG) (icr)	1% pet.	+	+	+
Diphenylmethane 4,4-diisocyanate (MDI) (icr)	2% pet.		+	1% pet.
N, N'-Diphenyl-p-phenylenediamine (DPPD)	1% pet.	0.25% pet.	1% pet.	0.25% pet.
Diphenylthiourea (DPTU)	1% pet.	+	+	+
Dipivalyl epinephrine hydrochloride	1% aq.			
Dipyrone (metamizole) (fde) (icr)	10% pet.			1% pet.
Direct black 38 (CI 30235)	1% pet.			
Direct orange 34 (CI 40215)	1% pet.		5% pet.	
Disodium EDTA (edetic acid disodium salt)	1% pet.	+	+	+
Disperse black 1 (CI 11365)	1% pet.			
Disperse black 2 (CI 11255)	1% pet.			
Disperse blue 1 (CI 64500)	1% pet.			+
Disperse blue 3 (CI 61505)	1% pet.	+	+	+
Disperse blue 7 (CI 62500)	1% pet.			
Disperse blue 26 (CI 63305)	1% pet.			
Disperse blue 35 (ph)	1% pet.		+	
Disperse blue 85 (CI 11370)	1% pet.		+	
Disperse blue 102	1% pet.			
Disperse blue 106 (CI 111935)	1% pet.		+	
Disperse blue 124	1% pet.		+	
Disperse blue 153	1% pet.		+	
Disperse blue mix (124/106)	1% pet.	+		+
Disperse brown 1 (CI 11153)	1% pet.		+	
Disperse orange 1 (CI 11080)	1% pet.		+	
Disperse orange 3 (CI 11005)	1% pet.	+	+	+
Disperse orange 13 (CI 26080)	1% pet.			
Disperse orange 76	1% pet.			
Disperse red 1 (CI 11110)	1% pet.	+	+	+
Disperse red 11 (CI 62015)	1% pet.	+		+
Disperse red 17 (CI 11210)	1% pet.	+	+	+
Disperse red 153	1% pet.			
Disperse yellow 1 (CI 10345)	1% pet.			
Disperse yellow 3 (CI 11855)	1% pet.	+	+	+
Disperse yellow 9 (CI 10375)	1% pet.	+	+	+
Disperse yellow 27	1% pet.			
Disperse yellow 39	1% pet.			
Disperse yellow 49	1% pet.			
Disperse yellow 54 (CI 47020)	1% pet.			
Disperse yellow 64 (CI 47023)	1% pet.			
4,4´-Dithiodimorpholine	1% pet.			
Dithranol	0.02% pet.			
Di-o-tolyl biguanidine	1% pet.			
Diurethane dimethacrylate		2% pet.		2% pet.
DMDM hydantoin	2% aq.	+	+	+
Dodecyldi(aminoethyl)glycine (DDAG)	0.5% aq.			
Dodecyl dimethyl ammonium chloride (quaternium-12).	0.01–0.1–1% aq			
Dodecyl gallate (lauryl gallate)		0.3% pet.	0.25% pet.	0.3% pet.
Dodecyl mercaptan	0.1% pet.		+	+
Doxepin	5% pet.			
Doxycycline (phde) (fde)	10% alc. or pet.			
Drometrizole [2-(2´-hydroxy-5´-methyl-phenyl)benzotriazole]			1% pet.	
Echothiophate iodine	1% aq.			
Econazole nitrate	1% alc.		+	
Edetic acid disodium salt	See Disodium EDTA			
Enilconazole	1% alc.			
Eosine (ph)			5% pet.	50% pet.
Ephedrine hydrochloride (de)	5% aq.		1% pet.	

Table 2. Continued

Allergen	Test Concentration and vehicle	Suppliers		
		Trolab	Chemo	Brial
Epichlorohydrin	0.1% pet.			
Epinephrine	1% aq.			
Epoxy acrylate			0.5% pet.	
Epoxy resin (icr)	1% pet.	+	+	+
Epoxy resin, cycloaliphatic			0.5% pet.	
Erythromycin (base and salts) (de)	1% pet.	+		+
Erythrosine (ph)				0.25% pet.; alc./glyc.
Estradiol	2% alc.			
Ethacridine lactate monohydrate (Rivanol®)	2% pet.			
Ethanolamine (monoethanolamine)		2% pet.		2% pet.
Ethenzamide (fde)	20% pet.			
Ethoxyquin (ph)	1% pet.		0.5% pet.	
Ethyl acrylate (EA)	0.1% pet.		+	
Ethyl alcohol	10% aq.			
7-Ethylbicyclooxazolidine	See Bioban® CS-1246			
Ethylbutyl thiourea	1% pet.			
Ethyl cyanoacrylate	5% pet.		10% pet.	
Ethylenediamine dihydrochloride (ph) (icr)	1% pet.	+	+	+
Ethyleneglycol dimethacrylate (EGDMA)	2% pet.	+	+	+
Ethylene thiourea	See 2-Imidazolidinethione			
Ethylene urea	See 2-Imidazolidinone			
Ethyleneurea + melamine-formaldehyde			5% pet.	
2-Ethylhexyl acrylate (EHA)	0.1% pet.		+	+
2-Ethylhexyl-*p*-dimethylaminobenzoate	See Octyl dimethyl PABA			
2-Ethylhexyl-*p*-methoxycinnamate	see Octyl methoxycinnamate			
4-(*N*-Ethyl-*N*-2-hydroxyethyl)-2-methyl-phenylenediamine sulfate (CD 4)	1% pet.	+	+	
Ethyl methacrylate (EMA)	2% pet.		+	
Ethylparaben (icr)	3% pet.	+	+	+
Ethyl sebacate	2% alc.			
N-Ethyl-4-toluenesulfonamide			0.1% pet.	
Etofenamate (icr)	2% pet.			
Eucalyptus globulus (eucalyptus oil)	2% pet.	+		+
Eucerin, anhydrous (lanolin)	Pure			+
Eugenia caryophyllus (clove oil)	2% pet.	+		+
Eugenol (icr) (ph)	2% pet.	1% pet.	+	1% pet.
Euxyl ® K 400		1% pet.	1% pet.	1% pet.
Evernia prunastri (oak moss absolute) (ph)	1% pet.	+	+	+
Evernic acid (ph)			0.1% pet.	
Fagus sylvatica (beech tar)			3% pet.	
Famciclovir	10% aq.			
Feneticillin (de)	Pure			
Fenoprofen	5% pet.			
Fentichlor (ph)			1% pet.	
Fenticonazole	1% alc.			
Feprazone	5% pet.			
Ferrous chloride				2% alc./ glyc.
Ferrous sulfate				5% pet.
Feverfew flower extract	See *Chrysanthemum parthenium*			
Fluazinam	0.5% pet.			
Fludrocortisone acetate	1% alc.			
Flufenamic acid	1% pet.			
Flumethasone acetate	1% alc.			
Fluocinolone acetonide	1% alc.			
Fluocinonide	1% alc.			
Fluocortolone	1% alc.			
Fluorouracil	1% pet.			
Flurbiprofen	5% pet.			

Table 2. Continued

Allergen	Test Concentration and vehicle	Suppliers		
		Trolab	Chemo	Brial
Flutamide (phde)	1–20% acet. or pet.			
Fluticasone propionate	1% alc.			
Folpet	0.1% pet.			
Formaldehyde (ph) (icr)	1% aq.	+	+	+
Formic acid				1% aq.
Fragrance mix (ph) (cinnamic alcohol, cinnamal, hydroxy citronellal, α-amyl-cinnamal, geraniol, eugenol, iso-eugenol, oakmoss absolute)	8% pet.	+	+	+
Framycetin (neomycin B)	20% pet.	10% pet.		
Fusidic acid sodium salt	2% pet.	+		+
Gallium oxide				1% pet.
Ganciclovir	20% aq.			
Gentamicin sulfate (icr)	20% pet.	+	+	+
Geraniol (icr)	2% pet.	1% pet.	1% pet.	1% pet.
Geranium oil, Bourbon			2% pet.	
Glutaral	0.2–0.3% pet.	0.3% pet.	0.2% pet.	0.3% pet.
Glyceryl thioglycolate (icr)	1% pet.	+	+	+
Glyoxal	1% pet./aq.	+ (pet)		+ (pet)
Glyphosate	1–10% aq.			
Gold sodium thiomalate (de) (icr)	5% pet.			
Gold sodium thiosulfate (icr)		0.25% pet.	2% pet.	
Griseofulvin (phde)	1% pet.			
Grotan® BK	See 1,3,5-Tris(2-hydroxyethyl)-hexahydrotriazine			
Halcinonide	1% alc.			
Haloprogin	1% pet.			
Halomethasone	1% alc.			
Hexachlorophene (ph)	1% pet.	+	+	+; 0.5% pet.
Hexamethylene diisocyanate (HDI)	0.1% pet.		+	
Hexamethylenetetramine	See Methenamine			
Hydroxymethylpentylcyclohexene-carboxaldehyde (Lyral®)			5% pet.	
1,6-Hexanediol diacrylate (HDDA)	0.1% pet.		+	
Hexylresorcinol	0.25% pet.	+		+
Homosalate (homomenthyl salicylate)			5% pet.	
Homatropine	1% aq.			
Hydrangenol	0.1% pet.			
Hydrazine sulfate	1% pet.		+	+
Hydroabietyl alcohol	10% pet	+	+	
Hydrochlorothiazide (phde)	1–10% pet.			
Hydrocortisone (ph)	1% alc./pet.	+ (pet.)		+ (pet.)
Hydrocortisone aceponate	1% alc.			
Hydrocortisone acetate	1% alc.			
Hydrocortisone buteprate	1% alc.			
Hydrocortisone-17-butyrate	1% alc.	0.1% pet.	+	0.1% pet.
Hydrogen peroxide			3% aq.	
Hydromorphone (de)	2% aq.			
Hydroquinone (HQ)	1% pet.	+	+	+
Hydroquinone monobenzylether	See Monobenzone			
Hydroxycitronellal (ph)	1–5% pet.	1% pet.	1% pet.	1% pet.
2-Hydroxyethyl acrylate (2-HEA)	0.1% pet		+	+
2-Hydroxyethyl methacrylate (HEMA)	2% pet.	1% pet.	+	1% pet.
Hydroxyisohexyl-3-cyclohexenecarboxaldehyde	See Hydroxymethylpentylcyclo-hexenecarboxaldehyde			
Hydroxylammonium chloride			0.1% aq.	
Hydroxylammonium sulfate			0.1% aq.	
2-Hydroxymethyl-2-nitro-1,3-propanediol	See Tris(hydroxymethyl)nitro-methane			

Table 2. Continued

Allergen	Test Concentration and vehicle	Trolab	Chemo	Brial
2-(2′-Hydroxy-5′-methylphenyl)benzotriazole	See Drometrizole			
Hydroxymethylpentylcyclohexene-carboxaldehyde (Lyral®)		5% pet.		5% pet.
2-Hydroxypropyl acrylate (HPA)	0.1% pet.		+	
2-Hydroxypropyl methacrylate (HPMA)	2% pet.		+	+
2-Hydroxy-4-trifluoromethylbenzoic acid	See Triflusal			
Hypericum perforatum (hypericum oil)				0.5% pet.
Ibuprofen (fde)	5–10% pet.			
Ibuproxam (ph)	2.5% pet.			
Ichthammol (ammonium bituminosulfonate)	10% pet.			+
Idoxuridine	1% pet.			+
2-Imidazolidinethione (ethylene thiourea)	1% pet.			
2-Imidazolidinone (ethylene urea)			1% pet.	
Imidazolidinyl urea	2% pet.	+	+	+
Indium (III) chloride				1% pet.
Indometacin	5% pet.			1% pet.
Iodoform				5% pet.
Iodopropynyl butylcarbamate	0.2% pet.		0.1% pet.	
Isoamyl-*p*-methoxycinnamate (ph)	10% pet.	+		+
Isoconazole nitrate	1% alc.			
Iso-eugenol	2% pet.	1% pet.	+	1% pet.
Isophoronediamine (IPD)	0.1% pet.	0.5% pet.	+	0.5% pet.
Isophorone diisocyanate (IPDI)	1% pet.		+	
Isopropyl dibenzoylmethane (ph)			2% pet.	
4,4′-Isopropylidenediphenol (Bisphenol A)	1% pet.	+		+
Isopropyl myristate		10% pet.	20% pet.	10% pet.
N-Isopropyl-*N*′-phenyl-*p*-phenylenediamine (IPPD)	0.1% pet.	+	+	+
Jasminum officinale (jasmine absolute, synthetic)	5–10% pet.		2% pet.	
Juniperus (juniper tar)			3% pet.	
Kanamycin sulfate	10% pet.	+	+	+
Ketoconazole (icr)	1% alc.			
Ketoprofen (phde) (icr)	1% pet.			
Ketotifen	2.5% pet./0.7% aq.			
Lanette E ®	20% pet.			
Lanette N ®	20% pet.			
Lanoconazole	1% alc.			
Lanolin	Pure			30% pet.
Lanolin alcohol (wool wax alcohols) (icr)	30% pet.	+	+	+
Lanolin alcohol and paraffinum liquidum (Amerchol® L 101)	50% pet.	+	+	+
Laurus nobilis (laurel oil)	2% pet.	+		+
Lauryl gallate	See Dodecyl gallate			
Lavandula angustifolia (lavender, absolute) (ph)			2% pet.	
Lemon grass oil	See *Cymbopogon schoenanthus*			
Lemon oil	See *Citrus limonum*			
Levobunolol hydrochloride	1% aq.			
Lichen acid mix (atranorin, evernic acid, usnic acid)			0.3% pet.	
Lidocaine hydrochloride (icr)	5% pet.	15% pet.	+	15% pet.
D-Limonene	See Dipentene			
Lincomycin hydrochloride	1% aq.			
Lindane (icr)	1% pet.			
Lomefloxacin (phde)	1–10% pet.			
Lyral®	See Hydroxymethylpentylcyclo-hexenecarboxaldehyde			
Mafenide	10% pet.	+		
Malathion	0.5% pet.			
Maneb (ph)	0.5–1% pet.			
Mechlorethamine hydrochloride (icr)	0.02% aq.			

Table 2. Continued

Allergen	Test Concentration and vehicle	Suppliers		
		Trolab	Chemo	Brial
Medroxyprogesterone acetate	1% pet.			
Mefenamic acid (fde)	1–10% pet.			
Melaleuca alternifolia (tea tree oil)			5% pet.	
Melamine formaldehyde			7% pet.	
Mentha piperita (peppermint oil) (icr)	2% pet.	+		+
Menthol (icr)		1% pet.	2% pet.	1% pet.
Mepivacaine	1% pet.			+
Merbromin (mercurochrome)	2% aq. or pet.			
2-Mercaptobenzimidazole	See 2-Benzimidazolethiol			
Mercaptobenzothiazole (MBT) (icr)	2% pet.	+	+	+
Mercapto mix (mercaptobenzothiazole dibenzothiazyl disulfide, morpholinyl mercaptobenzothiazole, *N*-cyclohexyl-benzo-thiazyl sulfenamide)	1% pet.	+	+	+
Mercuric chloride	0.1% pet.		+	
Mercurochrome	See Merbromin			
Mercury (icr)	0.5% pet.		+	+
Mesulfen	5% pet.			
Metamizol	See Dipyrone			
Metanil yellow	See Acid yellow 36			
Methenamine (hexamethylenetetramine)	2% pet	1% pet.	+	1% pet.
Methyl-3-amino-4-*N*, *N*-diethyl-aniline (CD 2)		1% pet.	1% pet.	
p-Methylaminophenol sulfate (Metol®)(icr)		1% pet.	1% pet.	
Methyl anthranilate			5% pet.	
4-Methylbenzylidene camphor (ph)	10% pet.	+	+	+
Methylcoumarin (6-MC) (ph)			1% pet.	
Methyldibromo glutaronitrile (1,2-dibromo-2,4-dicyanobutane)	0.3% pet.	+	+	0.1% pet.
Methyldichlorobenzene sulfonate	0.1% pet.			
N, *N*-Methylenebisacrylamide (MBAA)	1% pet.		+	
Methylene-bis(methyloxazolidine)		1% pet.		
α-Methylene-γ-butyrolactone (tulipalin)	0.001% alc.		0.01% pet.	
Methylhydroquinone (MHQ)			1% pet.	
2-Methyl-4-isothiazolin-3-one	0.01–0.02% aq.			
Methyl methacrylate (MMA)	2% pet.	+	+	+
N-Methylolchloroacetamide			0.1% pet.	
Methyl orange	2% pet.			
Methylparaben (icr)	3% pet.	+	+	+
Methylprednisolone aceponate	1% alc.			
Methylprednisolone acetate	1% alc.			
Methyl salicylate (icr)	2% pet.			+
3-Methyl thiazolidone 2-thion	1% pet.			
Methyl-*p*-toluene sulfonate	0.1% pet.			
Methyl violet				0.5% pet.
Metipranolol	2% aq.			
Metol ®	See *p*-Methylaminophenol sulfate			
Metoprolol (de)	3% aq. / 10% pet.			
Metronidazole (fde)	1% pet., 50% pet.			1% pet.
Mexenone	See Benzophenone-10			
Miconazole nitrate	1% alc.		+	
Minoxidil	5% in aq. + 20% prop. glyc.			
Mitomycin C	0.1% pet.			
Mofebutazone	1% pet.			
Mometasone furoate	1% alc.			
Monobenzone (monobenzylether of hydroquinone)	1% pet.	+	+	+
Monobenzylether of hydroquinone	See Monobenzone			
Monoethanolamine	See Ethanolamine			

Table 2. Continued

Allergen	Test Concentration and vehicle	Suppliers		
		Trolab	Chemo	Brial
2-Monomethylol phenol			1% pet.	
Morpholinyl mercaptobenzothiazole (MOR) (icr)	0.5% pet.	+	1% pet.	1% pet.
Mupirocin	10% pet.			
Musk ambrette (ph)	5% pet.			+
Musk ketone (ph)			1% pet.	
Musk mix (xylene, tibetene, moskene, ketone)			3% pet.	
Musk moskene (ph)			1% pet.	
Musk xylene (ph)			1% pet.	
Myristyl alcohol	5% pet.			
Myroxylon pereirae (balsam of Peru) (ph) (icr)	25% pet.	+	+	+
Myroxylon toluiferum (balsam of Tolu)		20% pet.	10% alc.	20% pet.
Naftifine hydrochloride	5% alc.			
1-Naphthalenethiourea (ANTU)	1% pet.			
Naphthol AS (CI 37505)	1% pet.	+		+
Naphthyl mix (*N, N*-di-β-naphthyl-*p*-phenylene-diamine, *N*-phenyl-2-naphthy-lamine)			1% pet.	
Naproxen	5% pet.			
Narcissus absolute			2% pet.	
Neomycin sulfate (icr)	20% pet.	+	+	+
Neroli oil	See *Citrus aurantium dulcis*			
Neticonazole	1% alc.			
Nickel sulfate (icr)	5% pet.	+	+	+
Nicotine (icr)	10% pet.			
Nifuroxazide (de)	0.001–1% aq./10% pet.			
Nigrosine	1% pet.		+	
Nimesulide (fde)	1–10% pet.			
(Nitrobutyl)morpholine/(ethylnitrotrimethylen) dimorpholine	see Bioban®			
Nitrofurazone	1% pet.		+	+
Nitroglycerin (icr)	1% pet.			
2-Nitro-*p*-phenylenediamine (ONPPD)	1% pet.		+	+
Nonoxynol	5% aq.			
Nordihydroguaiaretic acid	2% pet.			
Norethisterone acetate	1% alc.			
Nystatin (de)	2% pet.	+		+
Oak moss absolute	See *Evernia prunastri*			
Octyl dimethyl PABA (2-ethylhexyl-*p*-dimethyl-aminobenzoate) (ph)	10% pet.	+	+	+
Octyl gallate		0.3% pet.	0.25% pet.	0.3% pet.
Octylisothiazolinone	0.1% pet.	0.025% pet.	+	
Octyl methoxycinnamate (2-ethylhexyl-*p*-methoxycinnamate) (ph)	10% pet.	+	+	+
Octyl phthalate				5% pet.
Octyl triazone (ph)	10% pet.			
Ofloxacin (fde)	20% pet.			
Olaquindox (ph)			1% pet.	
Olea europaea (olive oil)			Pure	
Oleamidopropyl dimethylamine			0.1% aq.	
Oleyl alcohol	30% pet.			
Oligotriacrylate 480	0.1% pet.		+	
Olive oil	See *Olea europaea*			
Orange oil	See *Citrus dulcis*			
Orthocaine	1% pet.			
Oxiconazole	1% alc.			
Oxprenolol (de)	10% pet.			
Oxybenzone	See Benzophenone-3			
Oxybuprocaine (benoxinate)	1% pet.			
Oxyphenbutazone (de) (icr)	1–5% pet.			10% pet.
Oxytetracycline	3% pet.	+		+
PABA (ph)	10% pet.	+	+	+

Table 2. Continued

Allergen	Test Concentration and vehicle	Suppliers		
		Trolab	Chemo	Brial
Palladium chloride (icr)	1% pet.	+	2% pet.	+
Panthenol (dexpanthenol) (icr)	50% aq.	5% pet.		5% pet.
Papain	1% pet.			1% pet.
Paraben mix (butyl, ethyl, methyl, propyl-paraben) (icr).		16% pet.	16% pet.	16% pet
Paracetamol				10% pet.
Paraquat	0.1% pet.			
Paromomycin	10% pet.			
Parthenolide			0.1% pet.	
Pecilocin	1% pet.			
PEG 6 (and) PEG 32 (polyethylene glycol ointment)	Pure	+		+
PEG 400 (icr)				Pure
Penbutolol sulfate	2% aq.			
Penethamate	1% pet.			
D-Penicillamine	1% aq.			
Penicillin G (de) (icr)	100,000 U/g aq. or pet.			
Pentachloronitrobenzene	1% pet.			
Pentaerythritol triacrylate (PETA)	0.1% pet.		+	
Peppermint oil	See *Mentha piperita*			
Perfume mix (cinnamic alcohol, cinnamal, hydroxycitronellal, eugenol, iso-eugenol, geraniol)			6% pet.	
Petrolatum, white (icr)	Pure	+	+	+
Phenacetin				10% pet.
Phenazone	See Antipyrine			
Phenidone ®	See 1-Phenyl-3-pyrazolidinone			
Phenobarbital (de)	1–20% pet.			
Phenol-formaldehyde resin (P-F-R-2)		5% pet.	1% pet.	5% pet.
Phenolphthalein				0.5% pet.
Phenoxyethanol (icr)	1% pet.	+	+	+
Phenyl-azo-2-naphthol (PAN)	0.1% pet.			
Phenylbenzimidazole sulfonic acid (ph)	10% pet.	+	+	+
Phenylbutazone (de) (icr)	1–5% pet.			10% pet.
p-Phenylenediamine dihydrochloride			0.5% pet.	
p-Phenylenediamine free base (ph) (icr)	1% pet.	+	+	+
Phenylephrine hydrochloride	10% aq.	+		10% coca
Phenyl glycidyl ether (icr)	0.25% pet.	0.25% pet.		
Phenylhydrazine	1% pet.			
α-Phenylindole			2% pet.	
Phenyl isocyanate				0.1% pet.
Phenylmercuric acetate (icr)	0.01% aq.	0.05% pet.	+	0.05% pet.
Phenylmercuric borate	0.05% pet.			
Phenylmercuric nitrate (icr)	0.05% pet.			0.01% pet.
Phenyl-β-naphthylamine (PBN)	1% pet.		+	+
o-Phenylphenol (ph) (icr)			1% pet.	
Phenyl-*p*-phenylenediamine				0.25% pet.
1-Phenyl-3-pyrazolidinone (Phenidone®)	1% pet.	+	+	
Phenyl salicylate	1% pet.	+	+	+
Phosphorus sesquisulfide (icr)			0.5% pet.	
Picric acid	1–2% pet.			
Piketoprofen	2.5% pet.			
Pilocarpine hydrochloride (icr)	1% pet.	1% aq.		1% alc./ glyc.
Pindolol				2% pet.
Pinus (pine tar)	3% pet.		+	+
Piperazine (de)	1% pet. or aq.			
Piroxicam (phde) (de)	1–10% pet.			
Pix ex carbone (coal tar) (ph) (icr)	5% pet.		+	+
Polidocanol	3% pet.	+		+

Table 2. Continued

Allergen	Test Concentration and vehicle	Suppliers		
		Trolab	Chemo	Brial
Polyethylene glycol-400	See PEG 400			
Polyethylene glycol ointment	See PEG 6 (and) PEG 32			
Polymyxin B sulfate	3% pet.	+	5% pet.	+
Polyoxyethylene sorbitan monolaurate	See Polysorbate 20			
Polyoxyethylene sorbitan monooleate	See Polysorbate 80			
Polyoxyethylene sorbitan monopalmitate	See Polysorbate 40			
Polysorbate 20 (polyoxyethylene sorbitan monolaurate) (icr)	5% pet.			
Polysorbate 40 (polyoxyethylene sorbitan monopalmitate) (icr)	5% pet.			10% pet.
Polysorbate 80 (polyoxyethylene sorbitan monooleate) (icr)	5% pet.		+	10% pet.
Potassium dichromate (ph)	0.5% pet.	+ & 0.25% pet.	+	+
Potassium dicyanoaurate		0.002% aq.	0.1% aq.	0.002% pet.
Povidone-iodine (icr)	10% aq. or pet.			10% aq.
PPP-HB	5% alc.			
Pramocaine hydrochloride	1% pet.			
Pravastatin (de)	Pulverized tablet pure			
Prednicarbate	1% alc.			
Prednisolone	1% alc.	1% pet.		0.5% pet.
Prilocaine hydrochloride	5% pet.		+	
Primin	0.01% pet.	+	+	+
Pristinamycin (icr) (de)	1–10% pet. or aq.			
Procaine hydrochloride (ph) (icr)	1–2% pet.	2% pet.	1% pet.	2% pet.
Proflavine hydrochloride	1% pet.			
Promethazine hydrochloride (phde) (icr) (fde)	1–10% pet.	0.1% pet.	1% pet.	2% pet.
Propanidid	5% pet.			
Propantheline bromide				5% pet.
Proparacaine (proxymetacaine)	2% pet.			
Propicillin (de)	20% pet.			
Propionic acid			3% pet.	
Propipocaine	1% pet.			
Propolis	10% pet.	+	+	+
Propranolol hydrochloride (de)	10–20% pet.			2% pet.
Propylene glycol (icr)	5% pet. or aq.	5% pet./ 20% aq.	5% pet.	20% aq.
Propylene oxide	0.1–1% alc.			
Propyl gallate	1% pet.	0.5% pet.	1% pet.	0.5% pet.
Propylparaben (icr)	3% pet.	+	+	+
Propyphenazone (icr)				1% pet.
Proxymetacaine	See Proparacaine			
Pyrazinamide (de)	1–10% alc.			
Pyrethrum	See *Chrysanthemum cinerariaefolium*			
Pyridoxine hydrochloride (ph) (de)	10% pet.			
Pyrilamine maleate	2% pet.			
Pyritinol (phde)	20% pet.			
Pyrogallol	1% pet.	+		+
Pyrrolnitrin	1% pet.			
Quaternium-12	See Dodecyl dimethyl ammonium chloride			
Quaternium-15	1% pet.	+	+	+
Quindoxin (ph)	0.1% pet.			
Quinidine sulfate (phde)	1% pet.	+		+
Quinine sulfate (phde)	1% pet.		+	25% pet.
Quinoline mix (clioquinol, chlorquinaldol)			6% pet.	
4-Quinolines (phde)	10% pet.			
Quinoline yellow				0.1% coca

Table 2. Continued

Allergen	Test Concentration and vehicle	Suppliers		
		Trolab	Chemo	Brial
Ranitidine (de)	1% pet.			
Reactive black 5 (CI 20505)			1% pet.	
Reactive blue 21 (CI 18097)			1% pet.	
Reactive blue 238			1% pet.	
Reactive orange 107			1% pet.	
Reactive red 123			1% pet.	
Reactive red 228			1% pet.	
Reactive red 238			1% pet.	
Reactive violet 5 (CI 18097)			1% pet.	
Resorcinol (icr)	1% pet.		+	+
Resorcinol monobenzoate			1% pet.	
Resorcinol/formaldehyde resin				5% pet.
Retinoic acid	0.005% alc.			
Rhodium sulfate (icr)	0.05% aq.			
Ribostamycin	20% pet.			
Rifamycin (icr)	2.5% pet.			
Rivanol®	See Ethacridine lactate monohydrate			
Rosa (rose oil)				0.5% pet.
Rosa centifolia (rose oil, Bulgarian)			2% pet.	
Rosemary (rosemary oil)				0.5% pet.
Rosin	See Colophonium			
Rubidium iodide	1% pet.			
Ruthenium (icr)				0.1% pet.
Salicylaldehyde	2% pet.	+		+
Salicylic acid (icr)	1% pet.			5% pet.
Sandalwood oil	See *Santalum album*			
Santalum album (sandalwood oil) (ph)	10% pet.		2% pet.	
Scopolamine hydrobromide	0.25% aq.			
Sertaconazole	1% alc.			
Sertraline (de)	5–10% alc. or pet.			
Sesamum indicum (sesame oil)	Pure			
Sesquiterpene lactone mix (alantolactone, costunolide, dehydrocostus lactone)	0.1% pet.	+	+	
Silicon tetrachloride	2% pet.			
Silver colloidal				0.1% pet.
Silver nitrate (ph)			1% aq.	
Silver protein				3% pet.
Simvastatin (phde)	10% pet.			
Sisomicin	20% pet.			
Sodium benzoate (icr)	5% pet.	+	+	+
Sodium disulfite				1% pet.
Sodium fusidate	See Fusidic acid sodium salt			
Sodium hypochlorite (icr)	0.5% aq.			
Sodium hyposulfite	1% aq.			
Sodium lauryl sulfate	0.1% aq.			
Sodium metabisulfite		1% pet.		
Sodium nitrite				2% aq./glyc.
Sodium omadine	See Sodium pyrithione			
Sodium pyrithione (sodium omadine)			0.1% aq.	
Sodium thiosulfoaurate		0.25% pet.		0.25% pet.
Sodium valproate (de)	1–5% pet.			
Solvent red 23 (Sudan III)	2% pet.			1% pet.
Solvent red 24 (Sudan IV)	2% pet.			
Solvent yellow 1	See *p*-Aminoazobenzene			
Solvent yellow 33 (D and C yellow 11, CI 47000)	0.1% pet.			
Sorbic acid (icr)	2% pet.	+	+	+; 2% alc./glyc.
Sorbitan laurate (Span® 20) (icr)	5% aq.			

Table 2. Continued

Allergen	Test Concentration and vehicle	Suppliers		
		Trolab	Chemo	Brial
Sorbitan oleate (Span® 80)	5% aq.		5% pet.	
Sorbitan palmitate (Span® 40)	5% aq.			
Sorbitan sesquioleate (icr)	20% pet.	+	2% pet.	+
Spiramycin sulfate (de)	5–10% pet.			
Stannous chloride	1% pet.	0.5% pet.		0.5% pet.
Stearyl alcohol (icr)	30% pet.		+	
Stepronin (de)	18% sol.			
Streptomycin (sulfate) (icr)	1–2.5% pet.			5% pet.
Styrax benzoin (benzoin resin) (icr)			2% pet.	10% alc./ glyc./aq.
Styrenated phenol	1% pet.			
Sudan III	See Solvent red 23			
Sudan IV	See Solvent red 24			
Sulbentine	See Dibenzthione			
Sulconazole nitrate	1% alc.			
Sulfacetamide	5% pet.			
Sulfamethoxazole (de)	Pure			
Sulfanilamide (ph)	5% pet.	+	+	+
Sulfasalazine (fde)	10% pet.			
Sulfur dioxide (icr)				2% aq.
Sulfur, pharmaceutical (precipitated)				10% pet.
Sulindac	1% pet.			
Sulisobenzone	See Benzophenone-4			
Suprofen	0.1% pet.			
Tacalcitol	2 µg/ml alc.			
Tacrolimus	2.5% pet.			
Tanacetum vulgare (tansy extract)	1% pet.	+	+	
Tansy extract	See *Tanacetum vulgare*			
Tantalum				1% pet.
Taraxacum officinale (dandelion)			2.5% pet.	
Tea tree oil	See *Melaleuca alternifolia*			
Tego® 103 G	0.1% aq.			
Tenoxicam (fde)	1–10% pet.			
Terpene phenolic resin	20% pet.			
Testosterone propionate	1% alc.			
Tetracaine hydrochloride (amethocaine)	1% pet.	+	5% pet.	+
Tetrachlorosalicylanilide (TSCA) (ph)			0.1% pet.	
Tetracycline hydrochloride		2% pet.		2% pet.
Tetraethylene glycol dimethacrylate			2% pet.	
Tetraethylthiuram disulfide (TETD)		0.25% pet.	1% pet.	0.25% pet.
Tetrahydrofurfuryl methacrylate (THFMA)	2% pet.		+	
Tetramethylbenzidine			0.1% pet.	
Tetramethyl butanediamine	1% pet.			
Tetramethylol acetylenediurea			5% aq.	
Tetramethylthiuram disulfide (TMTD)		0.25% pet.	1% pet.	0.25% pet.
Tetramethylthiuram monosulfide (TMTM)		0.25% pet.	1% pet.	0.25% pet.
Tetrazepam (phde)	10% pet.			
Thiabendazole	1% pet.			
Thiamphenicol	5% pet.			
Thimerosal (icr)	0.1% pet.	+		+
Thioridazine (phde)	1% pet.			
Thiourea (ph)	0.1% pet.	+	+	+
Thioxolone	0.5% alc.			
Thiram	1% pet.			
Thiuram mix (tetramethylthiuram monosulfide, tetramethylthiuram disulfide, tetraethylthiuram disulfide, dipentamethylenethiuram disulfide)	1% pet.	+	+	+
Tiaprofenic acid (phde)	1% pet.			
Timolol	0.5% aq.			

49

Table 2. Continued

Allergen	Test Concentration and vehicle	Suppliers		
		Trolab	Chemo	Brial
Tin (icr)			50% pet.	
Tinopal CH 3566	1% pet.			
Tiocolchicoside	1% pet.			
Tioconazole	1% alc.			
Tiopronin (de)	0.3–5% pet.			
Titanium-(IV)-oxide				0.1% pet.
Tixocortol pivalate	0.1–1% pet.		0.1% pet.	
Tobramycin (de)	5% aq. or 20% pet.			
α-Tocopherol (vitamin E) (icr)	10% pet.			
Tolazoline	10% aq.			
Tolnaftate	1% pet.			
Toluene-2,5-diamine (*p*-toluenediamine) (PTD)	1% pet.	+	+	+
Toluene diisocyanate (TDI)	2% pet.		+	1% pet.
Toluenesulfonamide/formaldehyde resin	See Tosylamide/formaldehyde resin			
Toluenesulfonhydrazide	0.5% alc.			
4-Tolyldiethanolamine			2% pet.	
Tosylamide/formaldehyde resin (toluene-sulfonamide/formaldehyde resin)	10% pet.	+	+	+
Triamcinolone acetonide	1% alc.	0.1% pet.	1% pet.	0.1% pet.
Tribromsalan (TBS) (ph)	1% pet.		+	
Trichloroethylene	5% o.o.			
(TCC) (ph)	1% pet.		+	+
Triclosan (ph)	2% pet.	+	+	+
Tricresyl phosphate	5% pet.	+	+	+
Triethanolamine	2.5% pet.	+	2% pet.	+
Triethanolamine polypeptide oleate condensate (Xerumenex®)	25% o.o			
Triethyleneglycol diacrylate (TREGDA)	0.1% pet.		+	
Triethyleneglycol dimethacrylate (TREGDMA)	2% pet.	+	+	+
Triethylenetetramine (TETA)	0.5% pet.	+	+	+
Trifluridine	5% pet.			
Triflusal (2-hydroxy-4-trifluoro-methylbenzoic acid) (phde)	1% pet.			
Triglycidyl isocyanurate	0.5% pet.		+	
Trimeprazine tartrate (alimemazine tartrate)				1% pet.
Trimethoprim (de) (fde)	10% alc. or pet.			
2,2,4-Trimethyl-1,2-dihydroquinoline	1% pet.		+	
Trimethylolpropane triacrylate (TMPTA)	0.1% pet.		+	
Tripelennamine	1% pet.			
Triphenyl phosphate	5% pet.	+	+	+
Tripropyleneglycol diacrylate (TPGDA)	0.1% pet.		+	
1,3,5-Tris(2-hydroxyethyl)-hexahydrotriazine (Grotan® BK)		1% pet.	1% aq.	
Tris(hydroxymethyl)nitromethane (tris nitro)	1% pet.	+	+	+
Tris nitro	See Tris(hydroxymethyl)nitro-methane			
Trolamine	See Triethanolamine			
Tromantadine hydrochloride	1% pet.			
Tropicamide (icr)	1% pet.			
TSS Agfa®	See Amino-4-*N*, *N*-diethylaniline sulfate			
Tuberculin (bovine)	10% aq.			
Tulipalin	See α-Methylene-γ-butyrolactone			
Turpentine oil (icr)	10% pet.	+		+; 20% pet.
Turpentine peroxides (icr)			0.3% o.o.	0.3% pet.
Tylosin tartrate	5% pet.			
Undecylenic acid	2% pet.			
Urea formaldehyde resin	10% pet.		+	
Urethane diacrylate (aliphatic)	0.1% pet.		+	

Table 2. Continued

Allergen	Test Concentration and vehicle	Suppliers		
		Trolab	Chemo	Brial
Urethane diacrylate (aromatic)	0.05% pet.		+	
Urethane dimethacrylate (UEDMA)	2% pet.		+	+
Usnic acid (ph)	0.1% pet.	+	+	+
Valaciclovir	10% aq.			
Vanillin (icr)	10% pet.	+	+	+
Vat green 1 (CI 59825)	1% pet.			
Vesuvine brown	See Bismarck Brown			
Virginiamycin (de) (icr)	5% pet.			
Vitamin A acetate	1% pet.			
Vitamin E	See α-Tocopherol			
Vitamin K (K1, K3, K4) (de)	0.1% pet.			
Warfarin	0.5% pet.			
Wood mix (pine, spruce, birch, teak)			20% pet.	
Wood tar mix (pine, beech, juniper, birch) (ph)			12% pet.	12% pet.
Wool wax alcohols	See Lanolin alcohol			
Xerumenex®	See Triethanolamine polypeptide oleate condensate			
Yarrow	See *Achillea millefolium*			
Ylang-ylang oil	See *Cananga odorata*			
Zinc acexamate (de)	5% aq.			
Zinc chloride (icr)			1% pet.	1% pet.
Zinc dibutyldithiocarbamate (ZBC) (icr)	1% pet	+	+	+
Zinc diethyldithiocarbamate (ZDC) (icr)	1% pet.	+	+	+
Zinc dimethyldithiocarbamate (Ziram) (icr)	1% pet.		+	
Zinc ethylenebis(dithiocarbamate)	See Zineb			
Zinc (powder)			2.5% pet.	1% pet.
Zinc pyrithione (ph)	1% pet.		1% pet.	0.1% pet.
Zineb [zinc ethylenebis(dithiocarbamate)] (ph)	1% pet.		+	+
Ziram	See Zinc dimethyldithiocarbamate			
Zirconium oxide				0.1% pet.

49

Table 3. Recommended test concentrations for groups of chemicals. (*acet.* Acetone, *alc.* alcohol, *aq.* water, *pet.* petrolatum.) [*icr* Immediate contact reactions reported (Chaps. 5 and 26), *de* drug eruption with positive patch test reported (Chap. 24), *fde* fixed drug eruption with positive patch test reported (Chap. 24), *ph* photosensitivity reported (Chaps. 6, 17 and 27), *phde* photosensitive drug eruption with positive photopatch test reported (Chaps. 6, 17, 24 and 27)]

Product	Test concentration and vehicle
Acrylates, monoacrylates (icr)	0.1% pet.
Aminoglycosides (de)	20% pet.
Anesthetics, local	0.5–2% aq.
Barbiturates (fde)	10% alc. or pet.
Benzodiazepines (de)	1% aqua; 5–10% pet; 5–20% pet or aq.
Beta-lactam antibiotics (de)	1–20% pet.
Carbowaxes	Pure
Cephalosporins (de) (icr)	10%–20% pet. or 1%–10% aq.
Epoxy resins (DGEBA based)	1% pet.
Epoxy resins (not DGEBA based)	0.25–1% pet.
Epoxy resin hardeners	0.1–1% in pet., acet. or alc.
Epoxy resin reactive diluents	0.1–1% in pet., acet. or alc.
Heparins (de)	Pure
Imidazole antimycotics	1% alc.
Methacrylates, monomers	2% pet.
Penicillins (de)	1–20% pet.
Phenothiazine derivatives (fde)	1–10% pet. or 10% alc.
Phytotherapeutics (de)	Pure and 10%
Polyethylene glycols (icr)	Pure
Quaternary ammonium compounds	0.1% aq.
4-Quinolines (phde)	10% pet.
Sulfonamides (de) (fde)	10% alc. or pet.
Tetracyclines	3% pet.
Triphenylmethane dyes	2% aq.

Table 4. List of abbreviations

ANTU	1-Naphthalenylthiourea	HPMA	2-Hydroxypropyl methacrylate
BA	Butyl acrylate	HQ	Hydroquinone
BAK	Benzalkonium chloride	IBA	Isobornyl acrylate
BIS-EMA	2,2-bis[4-(2-Methacryloxyethoxy)phenyl]propane	IPD	Isophorone diamine
		IPDI	Isophorone diisocyanate
BIS-GA	2,2-bis[4-(2-hydroxy-3-acryloxypropoxy)phenyl]propane (epoxy diacrylate)	IPPD	N-Isopropyl-N′-phenyl-p-phenylenediamine
BIS-GMA	2,2-bis[4-(2-Hydroxy-3-methacryloxypropoxy)phenylpropane]	MBAA	N,N-Methylenebisacrylamid
BIS-MA	2,2-bis[4-(Methacryloxy)phenyl]propane	MBT	Mercaptobenzothiazole
BIT	Benzisothiazolinone	MBTS	Dibenzothiazyl disulfide
BMA	n-Butyl methacrylate	6-MC	Methylcoumarin
BUDA	1,4-Butanediol diacrylate	MCPA	Chloromethylphenoxyacetic acid
BUDMA	1,4-Butanediol dimethacrylate	MDI	Diphenylmethane-4,4-diisocyanate
CBS	N-Cyclohexylbenzothiazyl sulfenamide	MHQ	Methylhydroquinone
CDAA	N,N-Diallyl-2-chloroacetamide	MMA	Methyl methacrylate
CPPD	N-Cyclohexyl-N-phenyl-p-phenylenediamine	MOR	Morpholinyl mercaptobenzothiazole
		ONPPD	2-Nitro-p-phenylenediamine
2,4-D	2,4-Dichlorophenoxyacetic acid	OTA	Oligotriacrylate
2,4-DB	2,4-Dichlorophenoxybutyric acid	PAN	Phenyl-azo-2-naphthol
DBNPD	N,N-Di-β-naphthyl-p-phenylenediamine	PBN	Phenyl-β-naphthylamine
DDAG	Dodecyl di(aminoethyl)glycine	PCMC	p-Chloro-m-cresol
DDT	Dichlorodiphenyltrichloroethane	PCMX	Chloroxylenol
DDVP	Dichlorvos	PCP	Pentachlorophenol
DEGDA	Diethyleneglycol diacrylate	PEA	2-Phenoxyethyl acrylate
DEHP	Di-2-ethylhexyl phthalate (=dioctyl phthalate)	PETA	Pentaerythritol triacrylate
		P-F-R-2	Phenol-formaldehyde resin
DETA	Diethylenetriamine	PPP	Phenylpropylpyridine
DMAEMA	N,N-Dimethylaminoethyl methacrylate	PTBC	p-tert-Butylcatechol
DNCB	2,4-Dinitrochlorobenzene	PTBT	p-tert-Butylphenol-formaldehyde resin
DNOC	4,6-Dinitrocresol	PTD	Toluene-2,5-diamine
DOP	Dioctyl phthalate	2,4,5-T	2,4,5-Trichlorophenoxyacetic acid
DPG	1,3-Diphenylguanidine	TBS	Tribromsalan
DPGDA	Dipropyleneglycol diacrylate	TCA	Sodium thichloroacetate
DPPD	N,N′-Diphenyl-p-phenylenediamine	TCC	Triclocarban
DPTU	Diphenylthiourea	TCSA	Tetrachlorosalicylanilide
EA	Ethyl acrylate	TDI	Toluene diisocyanate
EBADMA	Ethoxylated bisphenol-A dimethacrylate	TETA	Triethylenetetramine
ECA	Ethyl cyanoacrylate	TETD	Tetraethylthiuram disulfide
EDTA	Ethylenediaminetetraacetic acid disodium salt (see disodium EDTA)	TGIC	Tetraglycidyl isocyanurate
		THFMA	Tetrahydrofurfuryl methacrylate
EEA	Ethoxyethyl acrylate	TMPTA	Trimethylolpropane triacrylate
EGDMA	Ethyleneglycol dimethacrylate	TMTD	Tetramethylthiuram disulfide
EHA	2-Ethylhexyl acrylate	TMTM	Tetramethylthiuram monosulfide
EMA	Ethyl methacrylate	TPGDA	Tripropyleneglycol diacrylate
GMA	Glycidyl methacrylate	TREGDA	Triethyleneglycol diacrylate
HCH	Hexachlorocyclohexane	TREGDMA	Triethyleneglycol dimethacrylate
HDDA	1,6-Hexanediol diacrylate	TSS	4-Amino-N,N-dietyhylaniline sulfate
HDI	Hexamethylenediisocyanate	UDA	Urethane diacrylate
2-HEA	2-Hydroxyethyl acrylate	UDMA	Urethane dimethacrylate
HEMA	2-Hydroxyethyl methacrylate	ZBC	Zinc dibutyldithiocarbamate
HPA	2-Hydroxypropyl acrylate	ZDC	Zinc diethyldithiocarbamate

49

Chapter 50

Patch Testing with the Patients' Own Products

50

PETER J. FROSCH, JOHANNES GEIER, WOLFGANG UTER, AN GOOSSENS

Contents

Commercially available patch test kits (standard series and various supplementary series) are the basis of a diagnostic work-up if an allergic contact dermatitis is to be confirmed. However, various investigators have shown that this way of testing is not sufficient. Menné et al. [20] found in a multicenter study that the European Standard Series detects only 37–73% of the responsible allergens in patients with contact dermatitis. The additional and/or separately tested allergens were positive in 5–23%; the authors emphasize the necessity of testing with the products actually used by the patient. In Italy, an analysis of 230 patients referred to a contact clinic because of suspected occupational contact dermatitis showed that the standard series alone detected 69.9% of all cases considered to be of an allergic nature [22]; 26.3% of all allergic cases were positive only to supplementary series. The agents most commonly responsible for allergic contact dermatitis were metals and *para*-phenylenediamine.

In a German study of the IVDK network, the data of 2,460 patients tested between 1989 and 1992 were evaluated [5]. In 208 patients (8.5%) type IV sensitizations were found to a total of 289 materials. In 44% of these cases only the patients' own products were patch test positive and thought to be clinically relevant.

In a subsequent analysis of 1998–2002 data, 8.6% of 3,621 patients had a positive patch test reaction to their own skin-care products additionally patch tested. Of 1,333 patients, 5.3% were tested positive to their own bath and shower products. In about one-third of the patients reacting to either product category, further positive tests to commercial allergens were not observed [1, 29].

The materials most frequently tested are usually topical medications, cosmetics of various types, rubber and leather products.

The group of Kanerva has published an impressive series of papers in which patch testing with the patients' own industrial chemicals has provided the main clue as to the causative agent of allergic contact dermatitis [16]. Various constituents of plastic materials, epoxy glues and paints, reactive dyes, and industrial enzymes were identified after chemical analysis. With regard to isocyanates present in polyurethane resins, for example, it was found that among 22 occupationally related cases, 21 reacted to the isocyanates obtained from the companies involved (13×) or to diaminodiphenylmethane (marker for isocyanate allergy), but only 1 reacted to the commercially available isocyanate, diphenylmethane diisocyanate or MDI (Trolab, Chemotechnique) [11]. Indeed, Frick et al. [7], when analyzing 14 commercial preparations of MDI, found that in most cases its concentration did not match the one stated on the label. Moreover, the isocyanates tested are not always representative of the mixtures used in industry.

Recently, reports were published on contact allergy to the patients' perfume where the current fragrance mix and the commercially available major allergens of perfume remained negative. After repeated testing with various fractions of perfumes the causative allergens were identified: Lilial [9] and coumarin [21]. The experience with perfumes has shown that in this dynamic field, with rapid changes in trendy attractive smells, the consumer is exposed to a wide array of chemicals that may cause sensitization. This subject is reviewed in detail in Chap. 31, Sect. 31.1. Further examples documenting the high value of testing with the patients' own products are published elsewhere [17–19, 28]. In this field and in many industrial areas, patch testing with merely the standard and supplementary series will always be inadequate until new allergens have been identified, their clinical relevance has been confirmed by several study groups, and they are eventually included in a test series.

In the following we want to give guidelines for testing with patients' own materials in order to harmonize this approach in daily practice. Knowledge in this field is often minimal and profound mistakes are made. For example, concentrated biocides or plastic monomers are applied under occlusion in undiluted form causing bullous or ulcerative lesions and possibly active sensitization. In contrast, the material is not infrequently diluted too much or in an inappropriate vehicle resulting in a false-negative reaction.

The guidelines are presented mainly in tables in order to be used at the work bench by technicians. They contain essential information; for more detailed information the reader is referred to other chapters in this book (particularly Chap. 49) and the pertinent references listed at the end.

50.1 Information on the Test Material Before Patch Testing

Never apply coded material obtained from a manufacturer without knowing details about the chemical regarding its toxicity and appropriate test concentration. Major cosmetic manufacturers now have a safety department that will supply this information and often provide the ingredients at adequate dilutions and a vehicle for patch testing. However, some tend to supply the ingredients in dilutions as used in the

products, producing false-negative reactions on patch testing. Unfortunately, this cooperative attitude is rare with manufacturers of industrial products (e.g., metalworking fluids, glues, paints, etc.). The material safety data sheets provide only basic information and do not list all allergologically relevant ingredients. In addition, the producer selling the product is often unaware of contaminants or materials under a different nomenclature (i.e., the manufacturer denies the presence of colophony but admits that abietic acid, the major allergen of colophony, is present in a cooling fluid). In a recent study from Finland on dental restorative materials, a high discrepancy was found between the listing of acrylates/methacrylates in material safety data sheets and the presence of these materials as detected by chemical analytical methods. 2-Hydroxyethyl methacrylate (2-HEMA), bisphenol A glycidyl methacrylate (bis-GMA), ethyleneglycol dimethacrylate (EGDMA), triethylene glycol dimethacrylate (TREGDMA), and (di)urethane dimethacrylate were either omitted completely as ingredients or not listed as often as appropriate. The authors analyzed glues, composite resins, and glass isomers [13].

The German network IVDK has established a model project [27] supporting the breakdown testing of cosmetic products. In cooperation with the manufacturers, the inquiring dermatologist will receive a recommendation on how to test the product ingredients, and which constituents not present in the standard or additional series might be a potential allergen. These are then provided in a test kit supplied by the manufacturer (this service is limited to Germany). Ideally, the test results are fed back to the data center, and are added to the database for the identification of putative "new" allergens – a system similar to the "cosmetovigilance" established in France [30].

50.1.1 Test Method

50.1.1.1 Skin Tests

Methodological details regarding dilution, vehicle, pH measurement, open test, closed patch test, repetitive open application test (ROAT), and use test are dealt with in Chap. 22. In Dortmund we found large Finn chambers (12 mm diameter) useful for testing cosmetics with low irritancy (e.g., moisturizers, lip cosmetics, sunscreens, eye drops [14]; Fig. 1).

The semi-open test as described by Dooms-Goossens [6] is particularly helpful if strong irritancy under occlusion is suspected, e.g., in the case of shampoos, liquid soaps, nail varnish, and also industrial products such as glues, paints, inks, varnishes,

Fig. 1a, b.
Severe cheilitis with eczematous pruritic lesions in the perioral region after long-term use of a lipstick for dry lips (a). The patch test with the lipstick "as is" in a large Finn chamber showed a weak doubtful reaction (b). Breakdown testing with the ingredients provided by the manufacturer revealed a contact allergy to dexpanthenol. The dermatitis cleared rapidly after discontinuance of the lipstick

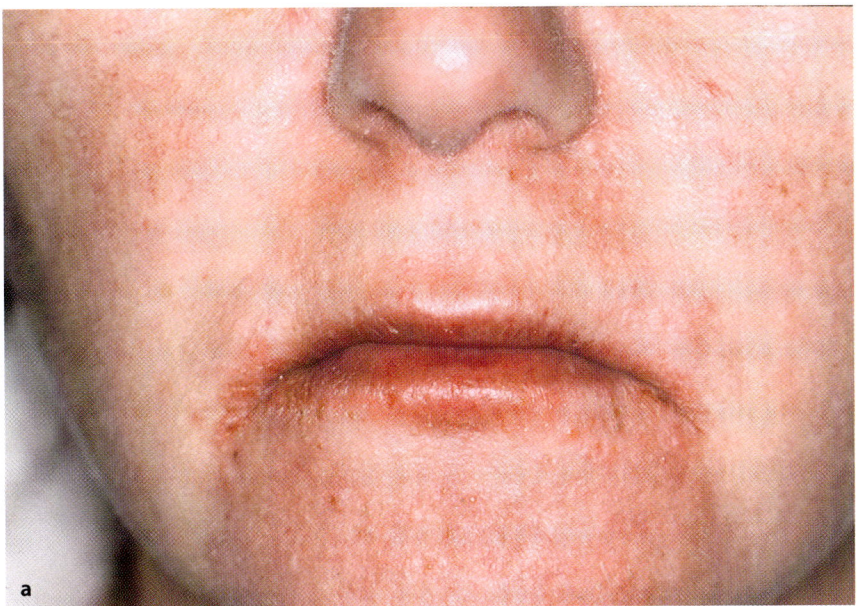

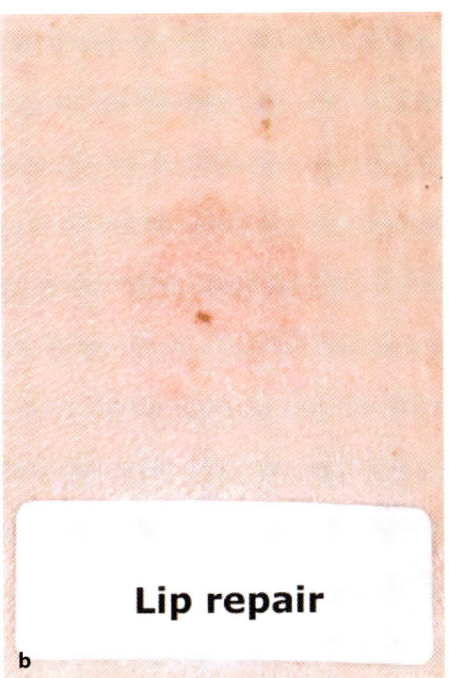

etc. The golden rule is that when a subject comes into direct skin contact with such a product (either on purpose, e.g., cleaning products, or accidentally, e.g., soluble oils, paints), then the product may be tested in this way. Corrosive or other toxic materials (pH <3 or >10) that are normally used in closed systems only or with protection from appropriate clothing are excluded from testing. The material is applied to the skin with a cotton swab (about 15 µl) on a small area (2 × 2 cm), left to dry (possibly dabbing with another Q-tip or tissue), and is then covered with acrylic tape (e.g., Micropore, 3M) (Fig. 2)

50.1.1.2 pH

At pH 4–9, very few irritant reactions are caused by the acidity or alkalinity itself [3]. The buffering solutions listed in Table 1 can be used to dilute water-soluble materials.

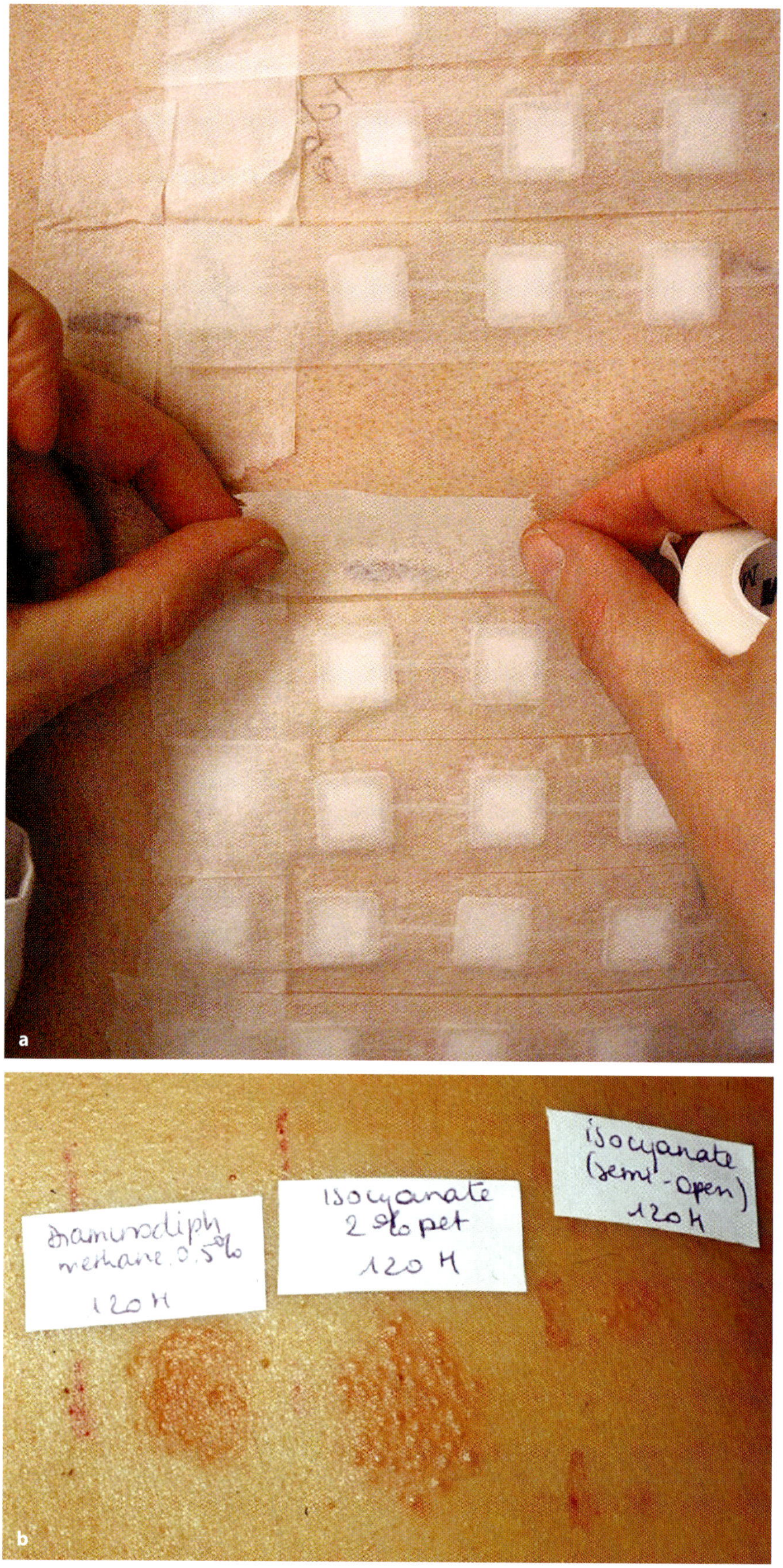

50

Fig. 2a, b.
Semi-open test: after applying the test material with a cotton swab, the completely dried area is covered with acrylic tape (**a**). Comparison of positive reactions obtained with a semi-open test to the patient's own isocyanate solution and a patch test with its dilution at 2% in petrolatum (**b**); there was also a positive reaction to diaminodiphenylmethane as a marker for isocyanate contact allergy

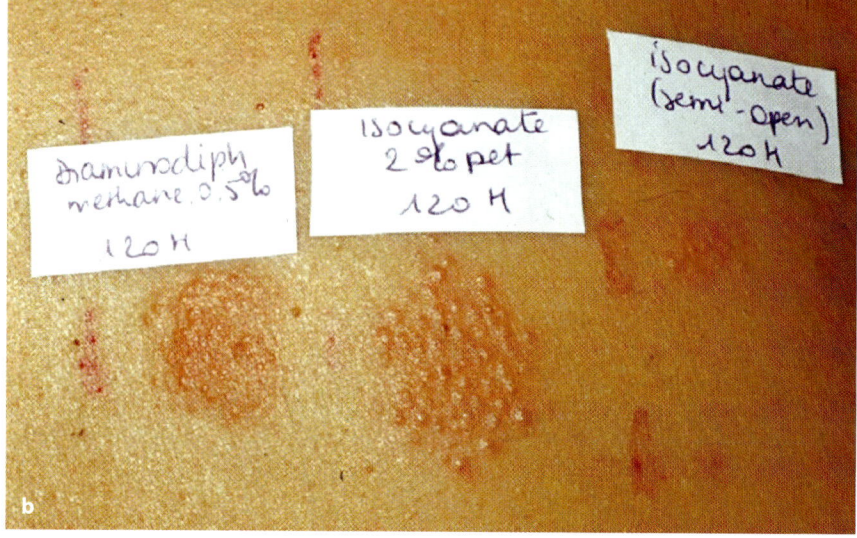

Table 1. Composition of acid buffer solution, pH 4.7, and alkaline buffer solution, pH 9.9 [3]

Compound	Concentration	% of total volume
Acid buffer, pH 4.7		
Sodium acetate	0.1 N (8.2 g CH₃COONa/l aqua)	50
Acetic acid	0.1 N (6.0 g CH₃COOH/l aqua)	50
Alkaline buffer, pH 9.9		
Sodium carbonate	0.1 M (10.6 g Na₂CO₃/l aqua)	50
Sodium bicarbonate	0.1 M (8.4 g NaHCO₃/l aqua)	50

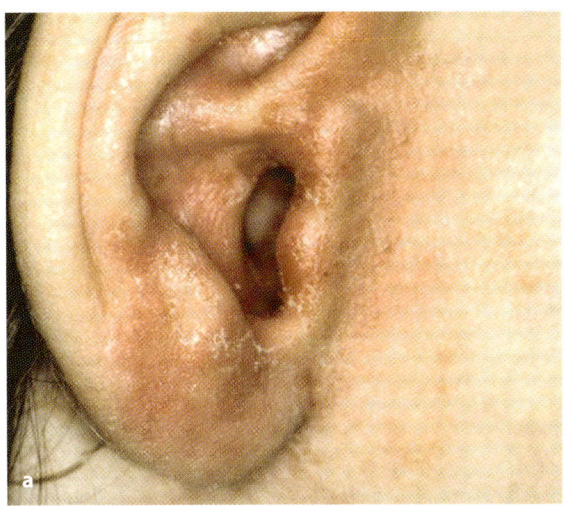

50.1.1.3 Dilution

Solid materials can be tested "as is," placing scrapings or cut pieces in the test chamber, or they can be applied on acrylic tape thus avoiding pressure effects. In this way, positive reactions may be obtained to small pieces of glove, shoes, rubber, or to scrapings of (hard) plastic materials (Fig. 3). However, the reactions often turn out to be false negative because the concentration of the sensitizer is too low or the sensitizer is not released. Alternatively, pressure or friction effects of sharp particles may cause some sort of irritant reaction, which should, however, be clearly identifiable as such. Depending on the material, the sensitizer can be extracted with water or solvents (Table 2; [16]).

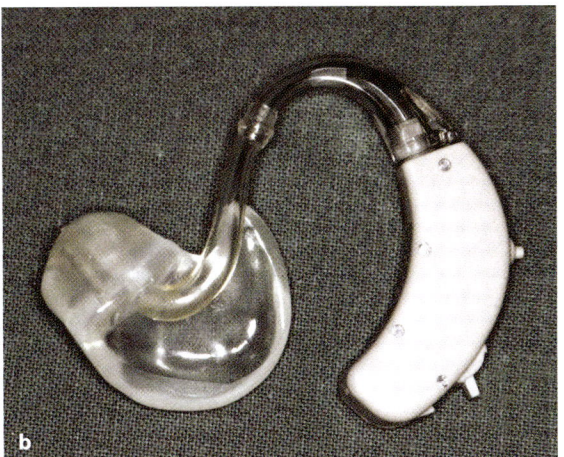

The correct dilution of materials for patch testing often presents a technical problem because the calculation basis is not clear to every technician. Therefore Table 3 provides a practical guideline for diluting liquid materials. For solid materials the dilution is performed based on a weight:volume basis.

Table 2. Materials suitable for extraction and recommended solvents [16]

Material	Solvent
Paper	Ethanol
Plants and wood dusts	Acetone, ether, ethanol or water
Plastics, e.g., gloves	Acetone
Rubber, e.g., gloves	Acetone or water
Textiles	Ethanol

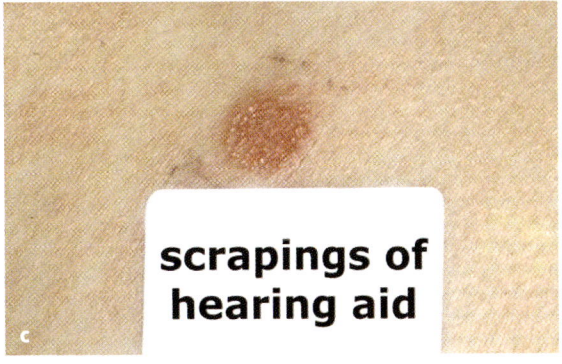

Fig. 3a–c. Contact dermatitis of the ear due to a hearing aid (**a, b**). Patch testing with fine scrapings of the plastic material was strongly positive (**c**). In subsequent testing with the plastic series the patient also showed a positive reaction to 2-hydroxyethyl methacrylate (*2-HEMA*) which was a component of the hearing aid as the manufacturer confirmed

Table 3. Recipe for diluting materials for patch testing [24]

Desired percentage dilution (%)	Quantity (µl) to be mixed in 10 ml of vehicle
0.1	10
0.5	50
1.0	100
2.0	200
5.0	500 (0.5 ml)
10	1000 (1.0 ml)

Table 5. Testing of cleaning products

Product type	Concentration	Comment
Soap bar	1% (w)	Irritation possible; use test
Shampoo	1% (w)	
Shower gel	1% (w)	
Bathing foam	0.1% (w)	
Toothpaste	1% (w)	

Table 4. Testing of decorative cosmetics and sunscreens. Abbreviations for vehicles in the following tables: *ac* acetone, *MEK* methyl ethyl ketone, *oo* olive oil, *pet* petrolatum, *w* water

Cosmetic/sunscreen	Concentration	Comment
Eye make-up		
Eye liner	As is	
Eye shadow	As is	
Mascara	As is	Semi-open test first, allow to dry (solvents)
Make-up cleanser	As is	Semi-open test first, irritation possible (amphoteric or other detergents)
Facial make-up		
Rouge	As is	
Powder	As is	
Foundation	As is	
Lip stick	As is	Photopatch when sunscreens are incorporated
Moisturizers		
Creams, ointments, lotions	As is	Irritation possible; positive patch test reaction should be confirmed by ROAT or use test. Photopatch test when sunscreens present
Bleaching creams	As is	
Sunscreens	As is	Photopatch test including active ingredients as commercially available
Self-tanning creams	As is	
Perfumed products		
Fine fragrances	As is	Allow to dry. Photopatch if clinical findings suggest actinic dermatitis
Eau de Toilette	As is	
After shave	As is	
Deodorants		
Spray, roll on, stick	As is	Allow to dry. Irritation possible. Often false negative, ROAT!
Shaving products		
Cream	1% (w)	Semi-open with product as is first. Irritation possible under occlusion
Soap	1% (w)	

50.1.2 Control Tests

When a reaction to a new material is observed which suggests a contact allergy based on morphology and development over time, control tests on human volunteers should be performed. This procedure is, however, now a great problem in some countries. In most German University departments, for instance, the approval of the ethics committee has to be obtained beforehand and each volunteer has to provide informed consent.

50.2 Product Categories for Patch Testing

50.2.1 Decorative Cosmetics, Sunscreens, Toiletries (Tables 4 and 5)

Many allergens are included in the standard series, the series for vehicles, emulsifiers, and preservatives. Fine fragrances may contain ingredients that are not present in commercially available test compounds. Perfumes in alcoholic solutions can be tested as is – occasionally slight irritant reactions (erythema without infiltration) might occur; the frequency of these reactions can be reduced by allowing the patch to dry before applied to the skin [15].

Many moisturizing creams for the face now contain sunscreens as "anti-aging factors." For details on sunscreens and for photopatch testing see Chap. 27.

The detergents that are active ingredients (sodium lauryl sulfate, lauryl ether sulfates, sulfosuccinic esters, isethionates) are not important allergens. They cause irritant reactions at dilutions at 1–0.5% in most subjects, particularly in patients with sensitive skin. Perfumes and preservatives may be relevant allergens in this category of products [1, 29]). Cocamidopropyl betaine has caused allergic patch test reactions for some time. Now the major allergen (3-dimethy-laminopropylamine) has been identified and removed from this major detergent in shampoos and shower gels.

50.2.2 Hairdressing, Depilatory, and Nail Cosmetics (Table 6)

Major allergens are listed in the standard and supplementary series. However, as the group of Menné has recently shown, not all cases of contact dermatitis from hair dyes are identified by *para*-phenylenediamine (PPD) and derivatives [25]. Therefore individual testing with the patients' own hair dyes might be necessary. To reduce the risk of active sensitization an open test must precede the closed patch test. Recently, an epidemic of allergic contact dermatitis from epilating products in France and Belgium has been elucidated [10]. By testing with the commercial products and the ingredients, it was found that modified colophonium derivatives were the main allergens (although in most patients the colophonium of the standard series was negative); further allergens were methoxy PEG-22/dodecyl glycol copolymer and lauryl alcohol, present in the accompanying skin conditioning tissue.

50.2.3 Topical Medicaments

Most topical medicaments used for dermatological conditions can be tested undiluted. Few contain irritating constituents (benzoyl peroxide, tretinoin, mustard, capsaicin, liquid antiseptic agents such as those containing PVP-iodine and nonoxynol, or quaternary ammonium, etc.) – these must be tested in a dilution series. Chapter 35 on topical drugs lists many chemicals as active ingredients that have been identified as contact allergens by patch testing the material of the patient.

Table 6. Testing of hair dressing products and nail cosmetics

Product	Concentration	Comment
Hair dyes	2% (w)	Active sensitization possible! Semi-open test: 5 drops dye and 5 drops oxidizing agent. If negative after 48 h, closed patch test with 2%
Hair spray	As is	Allow to dry. Irritation possible
Hair gel	As is	Semi-open test first
Depilatory	As is	Semi-open test first. Irritation possible (do not occlude)
Nail lacquer	As is	Always semi-open test only
Nail lacquer remover		Do not test (highly irritating)
Glues for artificial nails	1% and 0.1% (MEK)	Semi-open test as is. Most glues are cured with UV light

50.2.4 Medical Applicances

EKG contact gel	As is
Various aids from plastic materials (prosthesis, hearing aid)	Scrapings, undiluted
Implantations, materials for osteosynthesis	
Metals in standard series	
Methylmethacrylate	2% pet
Palacos® and monomer liquids	Do not test undiluted

Do not test parts of osteosynthesis materials with sharp edges (irritant reactions)

Most patients with a metal allergy (nickel, chromium, cobalt) tolerate implanted metals. Sensitization by implanted materials after a variable latent period of weeks or months, however, has been reported; overall it seems to be rare with modern metal alloys. Predictive testing is not indicated.

50.2.5 Dental Prosthesis and Other Dental Restorative Materials

Fine scrapings of the prosthesis can be tested with a large Finn chamber, physiological saline added. An allergic contact stomatitis caused by these materials is extremely rare. Sensitizations by acrylates may occur, although these are primarily seen in dental technicians on the hands, by daily contacts at work.

50.2.6 Disinfecting Agents

These materials are often irritating under occlusion for 48 h in a patch test. Therefore, a semi-open test should always be performed first (Table 7). Furthermore, it might be necessary to test with the individual constituents of the product to detect a contact allergy (e.g., to hand disinfecting agents).

50.2.7 Clothing

A piece of the suspected material – textiles, gloves, shoes – (2 × 2 cm moistened with saline solution) is applied under occlusion for 48 h on the back.

Textile dyes, formaldehyde resins, and thioureas can be identified by further testing with the supplementary series. Acid dyes may actively sensitize if tested at high concentrations. Therefore, new dyes brought in by the patient must be initially tested at high dilution [see also Chaps. 37 (clothing), 38 and 43 (shoes, textiles and rubber)]. In this context, patch testing with thin-layer chromatograms can serve as an elegant adjunct to quickly identify contact allergy to a certain ingredient of a mixture, such as a textile dye, although the (variable, possibly high) detection limit may yield false-negative results [4].

50.2.8 Pesticides

Most reactions to pesticides are irritant and pose the hazard of systemic toxicity by percutaneous absorption (see Chap. 42). Therefore, we do not recommend patch testing with pesticides unless there is strong evidence for allergic contact dermatitis. Detailed information about toxicity must be obtained before sequential testing (open test, semi-open test, closed patch test).

50.2.9 Detergents for Household Cleaning

General recommendation: 1% and 0.1% (water), semi-open test first, control for pH!

It is usually the additives, such as perfumes, preservatives, dyes etc., that are the sensitizers, rather than the detergents, although the frequency of contact allergy to this type of product is apparently often overestimated [2].

Harsh detergents contain quaternary ammonium compounds, which are highly irritating.

Table 7. Testing of disinfecting agents

Product	Concentration	Comment
Hand disinfection	As is	Semi-open test first. Closed patch test may be irritating. Use test. Test ingredients!
Disinfecting agents for instruments, floors, etc.	1%, 0.1%, 0.01%	Semi-open test first. Often contain strong irritants

50.2.10 Food Stuff

In food handlers and bakers a protein contact dermatitis must be excluded by prick and scratch chamber testing.

50.2.10.1 Scratch Chamber Testing [23]

After four scarifications with a fine needle, the test material is applied under a large Finn chamber for 24 h. Readings are taken after 24 and 48 h. With fruits and vegetables, irritant reactions are quite frequent.

For bakers, the flours used, the spices, and enzymes must be tested in prick and scratch chamber tests (amylase 1% in water).

In rare cases an exposure test with the dough squeezed in the hands for 20 min might confirm a suspected protein contact dermatitis.

50.2.11 Plants

Patch testing with pieces of plants is not recommended in general because irritant reactions are frequent and active sensitization may occur, although direct application on acrylic tape and not occluded by a chamber is less apt to do so. The commercially available and standardized materials for patch testing (sesquiterpene lactone mix, primin, Compositae mix, diallyl sulfide, tulipaline, etc.) are safe and identify most cases of plant dermatitis. In professional gardeners sensitization to various plants might occur. For further details and extraction of allergens, see Chap. 41.

In cases of recalcitrant plant dermatitis and unproductive patch testing with commercially available allergens, it may be worthwhile producing an extract of the suspected plant according to Hausen [12]. The pertinent features are listed in Table 8.

Plant extracts may be highly irritating. Therefore, adequate control tests must be performed in every case. It is self evident that the exact botanical classification is necessary before starting any investigative work.

50.2.12 Woods

Fine wood dust moistened with physiological saline can be patch tested with a Finn chamber or on adhesive acrylic tape. Exotic woods can be strongly irritating and sensitizing (teak, rosewood, Macoré) – these should be diluted to at least 10% in petrolatum

Table 8. The production of a plant extract for patch testing according to Hausen [12]

1. Obtaining a concentrate of the plant juice by cutting, pressing or smashing in a mortar; dilution with water by 1:10 and 1:100
2. Short extraction with diethylether (60–90 s). Working with ether is dangerous because of its explosive nature. If there is no suitable laboratory equipment available (rotation evaporation under an exhaust system), a practical alternative is the use of large open glassware filled with the solvent and the plant, left open in the air for about 1 h
3. Tulips, lilies, alstroemeria and other Liliaceae are extracted more efficiently with ethanol
4. After evaporation of the solvent the extract is incorporated into a suitable vehicle: water, ethanol, methanol, acetone, acidic acid ester, methylethylketone or plant oil. The use of petrolatum is also possible. Dilution series to start with: 1:10, 1:100, 1:1000. The material should be kept in a refrigerator

(sensitization might occur even at lower concentrations in rare cases).

Turpentine and colophony (peroxides) are the major allergens of conifers (pine, spruce, larch).

50.2.13 Office Work

Reactions to paper and cardboard are usually irritant in nature, particularly in atopics. In rare cases sensitizations to colophony or formaldehyde resins may be relevant. A piece of paper (2×2 cm, moistened with physiological saline) is applied occlusively for 2 days. NCR (carbonless) paper can be tested in the same way after rubbing it firmly to release the encapsulated dye. Diethylendiamine and colophony have been identified as allergens in NCR paper [17]. Telefax paper may also contain contact allergens (colophony, Bisphenol A). According to Karlberg and Lidén [31] testing with paper extracts (in acetone or methanol) is more reliable than a patch test with the paper as is.

Other materials that may be relevant to chronic hand eczema in office workers are:

- Rubber articles
- Glues (colophony, various resins)
- Woods (desk tops, handles)
- Metals (nickel in metallic objects such as perforators, pens, etc.)
- Plants
- Liquid soaps, hand creams used at the work place

50.2.14 Construction Materials

- Concrete
- Cement
- Resins for various purposes
- Tile setting materials

Testing with the material as is under occlusion is absolutely contraindicated because of high irritancy. A semi-open test might be indicated in cases with a high suspicion of contact allergy, particularly when resins are involved and testing with the standard and supplementary series remains negative. The main allergen in cement is potassium dichromate, which is present in the standard series. Fast-curing cements contain epoxy resins, which are increasingly recognized as major allergens in the construction industry but also in other industrial areas (painting, metal, electronics, and plastic). The epoxy resin of the standard series is insufficient to detect all cases of relevant epoxy resin allergies, as has been shown by a large German multicenter study [8]. Sometimes acrylic resins may also be present.

50.2.15 Paints, Lacquers

The chemical composition of paints and lacquers is very complex. Acrylates of various types are added for rapid curing. In the so-called biologic paints turpentine and colophony are often present. Isothiazolinones are frequently used in water-based wall paints. Before patch testing is performed with these products detailed information from the manufacturer should be obtained. Semi-open tests can be performed. As a guideline the concentrations as listed in Table 9 can be used.

50.2.16 Greases and Oils

These materials primarily used for lubrication rarely produce an allergic contact dermatitis. They are not very irritating except for hydraulic oils. Table 10 provides the recommended test concentrations.

50.2.17 Metalworking Fluids (MWF)

Metalworking fluids are indispensable for the processing of metal parts. Their chemical composition varies with the purpose and type of metal. Material safety data sheets usually do not contain all relevant allergological information. The most important allergens are rust preventives/emulsifiers, resin acids from distilled tall oil, and biocides. For further details see Chaps. 33 and 39. Table 11 provides guidelines for testing with MWF [26].

The most common mistake when testing water-based MWF is that the concentrate brought in by the

Table 10. Testing of technical greases and oils

Product	Concentration	Comment
Lubricating grease	As is and 20% (pet)	Semi-open test first
Lubricating oils	As is, 50%, 10% (oo)	
Hydraulic oils	1% (oo)	

Table 9. Testing of paints, lacquers and solvents. Semi-open test first for all paints or lacquers

Product	Concentration	Comment
One component (water based, e.g., wall paints)	10–100% (w)	
One component (solvent- or oil-based, e.g., paints for wood, iron, etc.)	1–10% (pet)	
Diisocyanate hardeners of polyurethane paints or lacquers	2–5% (pet)	
Paints containing epoxy, polyesters or acrylics	0.1–1.0% (pet)	Obtain detailed information on chemical composition first. Test conc. may be raised to 10% for some paints (see Chap. 34 on plastics)
Organic solvents		
Aliphatic, cycloaliphatic	1–10% (pet)	
Aromatic	1–5% (pet)	
Chlorinated	0.1–1% (pet)	
Esters	1–10% (pet)	

Table 11. Testing of metalworking fluids (*MWF*) – for details see Chap. 33

Product	Concentration (%)	Comment
Water-based	5 (w)	The usual workplace concentration of fresh MWF is 4–8%. Test a freshly diluted MWF at 5%, the used one as is (provided the concentration at the workplace is less than 8% – otherwise use a dilution of at least 1:1)
Oil-based	50 (oo)	

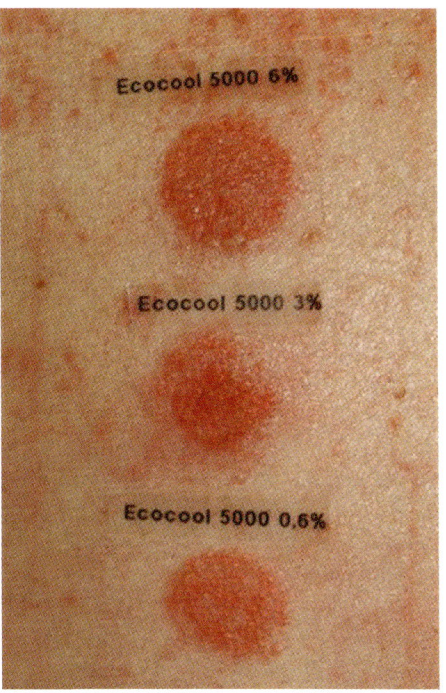

Fig. 4. Strong allergic patch test reactions to a fresh dilution series of a metalworking fluid brought in by a patient with chronic occupational hand eczema (use concentration at the work place was 6% in water). He also showed positive reactions to colophony (2+), abietic acid (3+), monoethanolamine (1+), and 2-(2-aminoethoxy)ethanol (diglycolamine) (1+). These materials are often present in metalworking fluids and may cause relevant sensitizations

patient is patch tested without further dilution. This usually produces severe irritant, sometimes ulcerative, lesions. The concentrate is usually diluted to 4–8% by adding water in the circulatory system of the machine. Metal workers often come into contact with this dilution of the MWF and develop a chronic irritant contact dermatitis (Fig. 4).

Perfumes as "odor masks" are often added and may produce an allergic contact dermatitis. The same holds true for isothiazolinones and other biocides, which are also often added as "system cleaners" in excessive concentrations during the use cycle of a MWF in order to prevent degradation and bad odors. Therefore, testing of both the fresh and the used MWF is obligatory.

50.2.18 Rubber Chemicals

Rubber products can be patch tested as is. This may be particularly worthwhile with protective gloves, rubber masks or other materials with prolonged direct skin contact. Often the usual rubber ingredients available for patch testing remain negative. The isolation of the allergen in rubber products is extremely difficult due to the complex chemical nature and the numerous additives used for maintaining the desired technical features. As a guideline, accelerators, antioxidants, and other materials provided by a cooperative manufacturer can be tested at 1% in petrolatum. Positive reactions require further dilutions and testing on control persons.

50.2.19 Glues and Adhesives

This group of products is nowadays ubiquitous and frequently used at home for production and repairs in various areas. Glues are often irritating in undiluted form. Testing with acrylates in inadequate dilutions can cause active sensitization. The test concentrations as listed in Table 12 provide a guideline only; before patch testing an unknown new material, detailed information from the manufacturer should be obtained. Testing should always start with a semi-open test to avoid strong irritant reactions or active sensitization.

50.2.20 Plastic Materials

Testing with this group of chemicals is recommended with the commercially available substances for patch testing of major manufacturers. These materials have been validated on large groups of patients and the patch test concentrations can be considered as safe and nonsensitizing.

Table 12. Testing of glues and adhesives

Product	Concentration	Comment
Adhesive tapes	As is	
Glues (excluding epoxy, formaldehyde resin and acrylic)		Semi-open test first. Allow to dry when patch testing
Dispersion glues	10–100% (pet or w)	
Solvent-based contact glues	1–10% (pet)	
Cyanoacrylate	2% (pet)	Strong irritant, rare allergen. Semi-open test first

Most patients have contact only with the end product after complete curing and containing no monomers as irritating or sensitizing components. However, as described in detail in Chap. 34 on plastic materials exceptions to this rule do occur and relevant sensitization may only be detected by patch testing fine dust particles of the plastic product or with all ingredients after time-consuming dilution series. Patch testing with a thin-layer chromatogram of a resin of unknown composition may be an interesting option to screen for the causative agent [4].

A few of these materials are carcinogenic and may cause bronchial asthma (for example the group of isocyanates). Therefore, these materials must be handled with great caution.

50.2.21 Do Not Test

In general, the following materials should not be tested because they are known as strong irritants but not as contact allergens (with few exceptions).

Patch testing may be performed only if there is high suspicion of contact allergy by history and clinical findings. Then an open and semi-open test should precede closed patch testing (dilution series from 0.1% to 1%).

- Astringents (e.g., AgNO₃)
- Anti freeze
- Car wax
- Gasoline
- Diesel
- Floor wax
- Lime
- Organic solvents (various types)
- Kerosene
- Metal chips (coarse)
- Rust remover
- White spirit
- Toluene
- Toilet cleaners and other strong caustic cleaning agents
- Cement, concrete

All products that have a strong pungent odor and/or contain organic solvents should be tested for pH (see above). If an open and semi-open test is negative a dilution series starting with a very high dilution can be performed under occlusion (maximum 24 h, locating on the medial aspect of the upper arm, which enables removal by the patient in case pain occurs).

If there is doubt about the nature of the patch test reaction – irritant or allergic – an expert in the field should be consulted before further testing is performed. Active sensitization of volunteers or ulcerative lesions with scar formation may be the risk of further investigative procedures.

References

1. Balzer C, Schnuch A, Geier J, Uter W (2005) Ergebnisse der Epikutantestung mit patienteneigenen Kosmetika und Körperpflegemittel im IVDK, 1998–2002. Dermatol Beruf Umwelt 53 : 8–24
2. Belsito DV, Fransway AF, Fowler JF Jr, Sherertz EF, Maibach HI, Mark JG Jr, Mathias CG, Rietschel RL, Storrs FJ, Nethercott JR (2002) Allergic contact dermatitis to detergents: a multicenter study to assess prevalence. J Am Acad Dermatol 46(2) : 200–2006
3. Bruze M (1984) Use of buffer solutions for patch testing. Contact Dermatitis 10 : 267–269
4. Bruze M, Frick M, Persson L (2003) Patch testing with thin-layer chromatograms. Contact Dermatitis 48 : 278–279
5. Daecke CM (1994) Der Stellenwert patienteneigener Testsubstanzen bei der Epikutantestung. Hautarzt 45 : 292–298
6. Dooms-Goossens A (1995) Patch testing without a kit. In: Guin JD (ed) Practical contact dermatitis. A handbook for the practitioner. McGraw-Hill, Philadelphia, Pa., pp 63–74
7. Frick M, Zimerson E, Karlsson D et al (2004) Poor correlation between stated and found concentration of diphenylmethane-4,4´-diisocyanate (4,4´-MDI) in petrolatum patch-test preparations. Contact Dermatitis 51 : 73–78
8. Geier J, Lessmann H, Hillen U, Jappe U, Dickel H, Koch P et al (2004) An attemt to improve diagnostics of contact allergy due to epoxy resin systems. First results of the multicentre study EPOX 2002. Contact Dermatitis 51 : 263–272
9. Giménez Arnau E, Andersen KE, Bruze M, Frosch PJ, Johansen JD, Menné T, Rastogie SE, White IR, Lepoittevin JP (2000) Identification of Lilial® as a fragrance sensitizer in a perfume by bioassay-guided chemical fractionation and structure-activity relationships. Contact Dermatitis 43 : 351–358

50

10. Goossens A, Armingaud P, Avenel-Audran M et al (2002) An epidemic of allergic contact dermatitis due to epilating products. Contact Dermatitis 46:67–70

11. Goossens A, Detienne T, Bruze M (2002) Occupational allergic contact dermatitis caused by isocyanates. Contact Dermatitis 47:304–308

12. Hausen BM (1988) Allergiepflanzen, Pflanzengifte. Handbuch und Atlas der allergieinduzierenden Wild- und Kulturpflanzen. 1988 Ecomed Verlag, Landsberg Lech

13. Henriks-Eckerman M, Suuronen K, Jolanki R, Alanko K (2004) Methacrylates in dental restorative materials. Contact Dermatitis 50:233–237

14. Herbst RA, Uter W, Pirker C, Geier J, Frosch PJ (2004) Allergic and non-allergic periorbital dermatitis: patch test results of the Information Network of the Departments of Dermatology during a 5-year period. Contact Dermatitis 51:13–19

15. Johansen JD, Frosch PJ, Rastogi SC, Menné T (2001) Testing with fine fragrances in eczema patients. Contact Dermatitis 44:304–307

16. Jolanki R, Estlander T, Alanko K, Kanerva L (2000) Patch testing with a patient's own materials handled at work. In: Kanerva L, Elsner P, Wahlberg JE, Maibach HI (eds) Handbook of occupational dermatology.Springer-Verlag, Berlin Heidelberg New York, pp 375–383

17. Lange-Ionescu S, Bruze M, Gruvberger B, Zimerson E, Frosch PJ (2000) Kontaktallergie durch kohlefreies Durchschlagpapier. Dermat Beruf Umwelt 48:183–187

18. Magerl A, Heiss R, Frosch PJ (2001) Allergic contact dermatitis from zinc ricinoleate in a deodorant and glyceryl ricinoleate in a lipstick. Contact Dermatitis 44:119–121

19. Magerl A, Pirker C, Frosch PJ (2003) Allergisches Kontaktekzem durch Schellack und 1,3-Butylenglykol in einem Eyliner. Journal Deutsch Dermatolog Gesellsch 1:300–302

20. Menné T, Dooms-Goossens A, Wahlberg JE, White IR, Shaw S (1992) How large a proportion of contact sensitivities are diagnosed with the European standard series? Contact Dermatitis 26:201–202

21. Mutterer V, Giménez Arnau E, Lepoittevin JP, Johansen JD, Frosch PJ, Menné T, Andersen KE, Bruze M, Rastogi SC, White IR (1999) Identification of coumarin as the sensitizer in a patient sensitive to her own perfume but negative to the fragrance mix. Contact Dermatitis 40:196–199

22. Nettis E, Marcandrea M, Colonardi MC, Paradiso MT, Ferrannini, Tursi A (2003) Results of standard series patch testing in patients with occupational allergic contact dermatitis. Allergy 58:1304–1307

23. Niinimäki A (1987) Scratch-chamber tests in food handler dermatitis. Contact Dermatitis 16:11–20

24. Sherertz EF, Byers SV (1997) Estimating dilutions for patch testing skin care products: a practical method. Am J Contact Derm 8:181–182

25. Sosted H, Basketter DA, Estrada E, Johansen JD, Patlewicz GY (2004) Ranking of hair dye substances according to predicted sensitization potency: quantitative structure-activity relationships. Contact Dermatitis 51:241–254

26. Tiedemann KH, Zöllner G, Adam M et al (2002) Empfehlungen für die Epikutantestung bei Verdacht auf Kontaktallergie durch Kühlschmierstoffe. 2. Hinweise zur Arbeitsstofftestung. Dermatol Beruf Umwelt 50:180–189

27. Uter W, Geier J, Lessmann H, Schnuch A (1999) Unverträglichkeitsreaktionen gegen Körperpflege- und Haushaltsprodukte: Was ist zu tun? Die Informations- und Dokumentationsstelle für Kontaktallergien (IDOK) des Informationsverbundes Dermatologischer Kliniken (IVDK). Deutsche Dermatologe 47:211–214

28. Uter W, Balzer C, Geier J, Schnuch A, Frosch PJ (2005) Ergebnisse der Epikutantestung mit patienteneigenen Parfüms, Deos und Rasierwässern. Ergebnisse des IVDK 1998–2002. Dermatol Beruf Umwelt 53:25–36

29. Uter W, Balzer C, Geier J, Frosch PJ, Schnuch A (2005) Patch testing with patients' own cosmetics and toiletries – results of the IVDK, 1998–2002. Contact Dermatitis 53:226–233

30. Vigan M (1997) Les nouveaux allergenes des cosmetiques. La cosmetovigilance. Ann Dermatol Venereol 124:571–575

31. Karlberg AT, Lidén C (1992) Colophony (rosin) in newspapers may contribute to hand eczema. Br J Dermatol 126:161–165

Chapter 51

Dictionary of Contact Allergens: Chemical Structures, Sources and References

51

Christophe J. Le Coz, Jean-Pierre Lepoittevin

51.1 Introduction

This chapter has been written in order to familiarize the reader with the chemical structure of chemicals implicated in contact dermatitis, mainly as haptens responsible for allergic contact dermatitis. For each molecule, the principal name is used for classification. We have also listed the most important synonym(s), the Chemical Abstract Service (CAS) Registry Number that characterizes the substance, and its chemical structure. The reader will find one or more relevant literature references. As it was not possible to be exhaustive, some allergens have been omitted since they were obsolete, extremely rarely implicated in contact dermatitis, their case reports were too imprecise or they are extensively treated in other chapters of the textbook. From a practical chemical point of view, acrylates, cyanoacrylates and (meth)acrylates, cephalosporins, and parabens have been grouped together.

1. Abietic acid

CAS Registry Number [514–10–3]

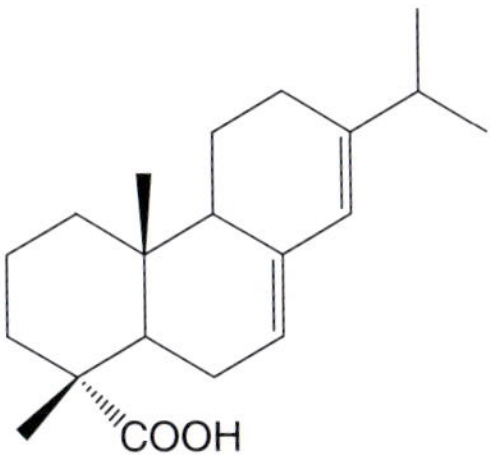

Abietic acid is probably the major allergen of colophony, along with dehydroabietic acid, by way of oxidation products. Its detection in a material indicates that allergenic components of colophony are present.

Suggested Reading

Bergh M, Menné T, Karlberg AT (1994) Colophony in paper-based surgical clothing. Contact Dermatitis 31:332–333

Karlberg AT, Bergstedt E, Boman A, Bohlinder K, Lidén C, Nilsson JLG, Wahlberg JE (1985) Is abietic acid the allergenic component of colophony? Contact Dermatitis 13:209–215

Karlberg AT, Bohlinder K, Boman A, Hacksell U, Hermansson J, Jacobsson S, Nilsson JLG (1988) Identification of 15-hydroperoxyabietic acid as a contact allergen in Portuguese colophony. J Pharm Pharmacol 40:42–47

2. Acetaldehyde

Acetic Aldehyde, Ethanal, Ethylic Aldehyde

CAS Registry Number [75–07–0]

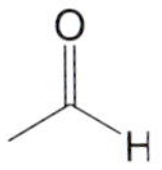

Acetaldehyde, as its metabolite, is responsible for many of the effects of ethanol, such as hepatic or neurological toxicity. A case of contact allergy was reported in the textile industry, where dimethoxane was used as a biocide agent in textiles and its degradation led to acetaldehyde.

Suggested Reading

Eriksson CJ (2001) The role of acetaldehyde in the actions of alcohol (update 2000). Alcohol Clin Exp Res 25 [Suppl 5]:15S–32S
Shmunes E, Kempton RJ (1980) Allergic contact dermatitis to dimethoxane in a spin finish. Contact Dermatitis 6:421–424

3. Acrylamide

CAS Registry Number [79–06–1]

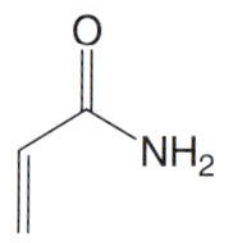

Acrylamide is used in the plastic polymers industry, for water treatments, soil stabilization and to prepare polyacrylamide gels for electrophoresis. This neurotoxic, carcinogenic, and genotoxic substance is known to have caused contact dermatitis in industrial and laboratory workers.

Suggested Reading

Beyer DJ, Belsito DV (2000) Allergic contact dermatitis from acrylamide in a chemical mixer. Contact Dermatitis 42:181–182
Dooms-Goossens A, Garmyn M, Degreef H (1991) Contact allergy to acrylamide. Contact Dermatitis 24:71–72
Lambert J, Mathieu L, Dockx P (1988) Contact dermatitis from acrylamide. Contact Dermatitis 19:65

4. Acrylates, Cyanoacrylate, and Methacrylates

Acrylic Acid and Acrylates

CAS Registry Number [79–10–7]

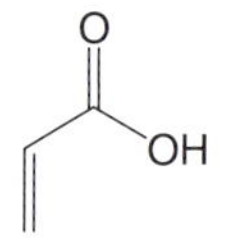

Acrylic acid 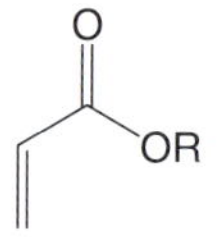   Acrylate

Acrylates are esters from acrylic acid. Occupational contact allergies from acrylates have frequently been reported and mainly concern workers exposed to the glues based on acrylic acid, as well as dental workers and beauticians.

Bisphenol A Diglycidylether Diacrylate

2,2-bis[4-(2-Hydroxy-3-Acryloxypropoxy)phenyl]-Propane (Bis-GA)

CAS Registry Number [8687–94–9]

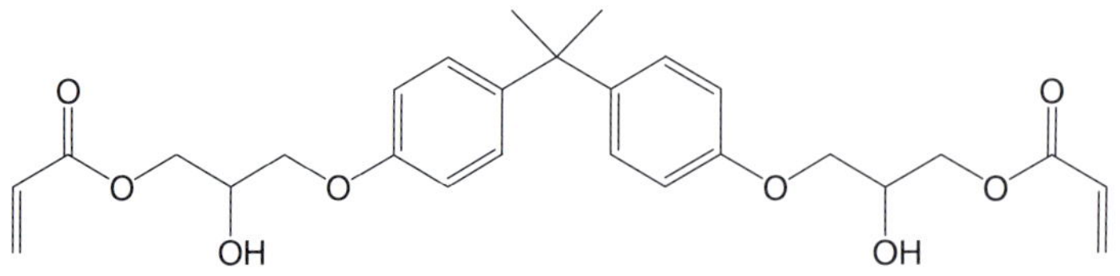

Bis-GA is an epoxy diacrylate. It caused contact dermatitis in a process worker, being contained in ultraviolet-light-curable acrylic paints.

Suggested Reading
Jolanki R, Kanerva L, Estlander T (1995) Occupational allergic contact dermatitis caused by epoxy diacrylate in ultraviolet-light-cured paint, and bisphenol A in dental composite resin. Contact Dermatitis 33:94–99

Bisphenol A Glycidyl Methacrylate

Bis-GMA

CAS Registry Number [1565–94–2]

Bis-GMA is an epoxy-methacrylate. Sensitization occurs in dentists, in beauticians, and in consumers with sculptured photopolymerizable nails.

Suggested Reading
Kanerva L, Estlander T, Jolanki R (1989) Allergic contact dermatitis from dental composite resins due to aromatic epoxy acrylates and aliphatic acrylates. Contact Dermatitis 20:201–211

1,4-Butanediol Diacrylate

CAS Registry Number [1070–70–8]

A positive patch test was observed in a male process worker in a paint factory, sensitized to an epoxy diacrylate contained in raw materials of ultraviolet-light-curable paint. The positive reaction was probably due to a cross-reactivity.

Suggested Reading
Jolanki R, Kanerva L, Estlander T (1995) Occupational allergic contact dermatitis caused by epoxy diacrylate in ultraviolet-light-cured paint, and bisphenol A in dental composite resin. Contact Dermatitis 33:94–99

1,4-Butanediol Dimethacrylate

CAS Registry Number [2082–81–7]

Sensitization to 1,4-butanediol dimethacrylate was reported in dental technicians, with cross-reactivity to methyl methacrylate.

Suggested Reading
Rustemeyer T, Frosch PJ (1996) Occupational skin diseases in dental laboratory technicians. (I). Clinical picture and causative factors. Contact Dermatitis 34:125–133

n-Butyl Acrylate

CAS Registry Number [141–32–2]

Sensitization to n-butyl acrylate can occur in the dental profession.

Suggested Reading

Daecke C, Schaller J, Goos M (1994) Acrylates as potent allergens in occupational and domestic exposures. Contact Dermatitis 30:190–191

Kanerva L, Estlander T, Jolanki R, Tarvainen K (1993) Occupational allergic contact dermatitis caused by exposure to acrylates during work with dental prostheses. Contact Dermatitis 28:268–275

Rustemeyer T, Frosch PJ (1996) Occupational skin diseases in dental laboratory technicians. (I). Clinical picture and causative factors. Contact Dermatitis 34:125–133

tert-Butyl Acrylate

CAS Registry Number [1663–39–4]

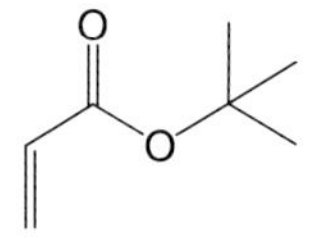

Sensitization may affect dental workers.

Suggested Reading

Kanerva L, Estlander T, Jolanki R, Tarvainen K (1993) Occupational allergic contact dermatitis caused by exposure to acrylates during work with dental prostheses. Contact Dermatitis 28:268–275

51

Cyanoacrylic Acid and Cyanoacrylates

2-Cyanoacrylic Acid

CAS Registry Number [15802–18–3]

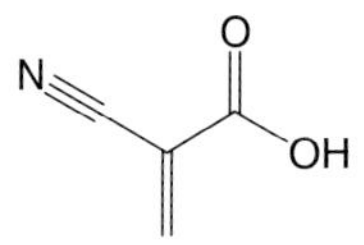

Cyanoacrylic acid 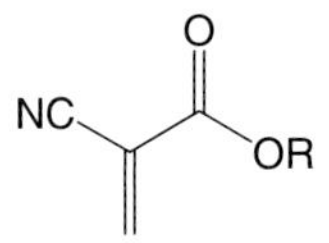   Cyanoacrylate

Cyanoacrylates, particularly 2-ethyl cyanoacrylate, are derived from cyanoacrylic acid. They are used as sealants.

Suggested Reading

Fischer AA (1985) Reactions to cyanoacrylate adhesives: "instant glue". Cutis 35:18, 20, 22

Tarvainen K (1995) Analysis of patients with allergic patch test reactions to a plastics and glue series. Contact Dermatitis 32:346–351

Diethyleneglycol Diacrylate

CAS Registry Number [4074–88–8]

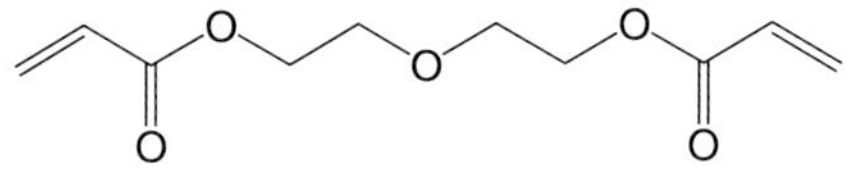

Diethyleneglycol diacrylate was positive in a painter sensitized to his own acrylate-based paint.

Suggested Reading

Nakamura M, Arima Y, Yoneda K, Nobuhara S, Miyachi Y (1999) Occupational contact dermatitis from acrylic monomer in paint. Contact Dermatitis 40:228–229

Ethyl Acrylate

CAS Registry Number [140–88–5]

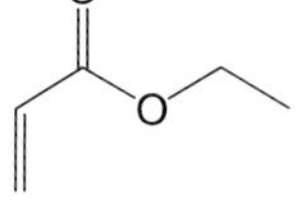

Ethyl acrylate is a sensitizer in the dental profession.

Suggested Reading

Kanerva L, Estlander T, Jolanki R, Tarvainen K (1993) Occupational allergic contact dermatitis caused by exposure to acrylates during work with dental prostheses. Contact Dermatitis 28:268–275

Rustemeyer T, Frosch PJ (1996) Occupational skin diseases in dental laboratory technicians. (I). Clinical picture and causative factors. Contact Dermatitis 34:125–133

Ethyl Cyanoacrylate

Ethyl-2-Cyanoacrylate

CAS Registry Number [7085–85–0]

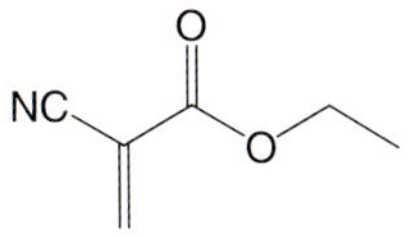

Ethyl cyanoacrylate is contained in instant glues for metal, glass, rubber, plastics, textiles, tissues, and nails. It polymerizes almost instantaneously in air at room temperature and bonds immediately and strongly to surface keratin. Beauticians are exposed to contact dermatitis from nail glues.

Suggested Reading

Bruze M, Björkner B, Lepoittevin JP (1995) Occupational allergic contact dermatitis from ethyl cyanoacrylate. Contact Dermatitis 32:156–159

Fitzgerald DA, Bhaggoe R, English JSC (1995) Contact sensitivity to cyanoacrylate nail-adhesive with dermatitis at remote sites. Contact Dermatitis 32:175–176

Jacobs MC, Rycroft RJG (1995) Allergic contact dermatitis from cyanoacrylate? Contact Dermatitis 33:71

Tomb R, Lepoittevin JP, Durepaire F, Grosshans E (1993) Ectopic contact dermatitis from ethyl cyanoacrylate instant adhesives. Contact Dermatitis 28:206–208

Ethyleneglycol Dimethacrylate

CAS Registry Number [97–90–5]

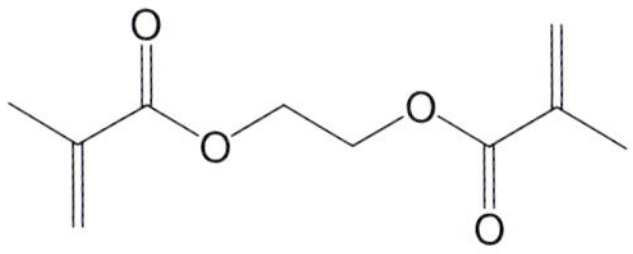

Ethyleneglycol dimethacrylate (EGDMA) is a cross-linking agent of acrylic resins and is employed to optimize the dilution of high-viscosity monomers and to link together the macromolecules constituting the polymer. It caused contact dermatitis in dental technicians and dental assistants. A case was also reported in a manufacturer of car rear-view mirrors.

Suggested Reading

Farli M, Gasperini M, Francalanci S, Gola M, Sertoli A (1990) Occupational contact dermatitis in 2 dental technicians. Contact Dermatitis 22:282–287

Kanerva L, Jolanki R, Estlander T (1995) Occupational allergic contact dermatitis from 2-hydroxyethyl methacrylate and ethylene glycol dimethacrylate in a modified acrylic structural adhesive. Contact Dermatitis 35:84–89

Rustemeyer T, Frosch PJ (1996) Occupational skin diseases in dental laboratory technicians. (I). Clinical picture and causative factors. Contact Dermatitis 34:125–133

Tosti A, Rapacchiale S, Piraccini BM, Peluso AM (1991) Occupational airborne contact dermatitis due to ethylene glycol dimethacrylate. Contact Dermatitis 24:152–153

2-Ethylhexyl Acrylate

2-EHA

CAS Registry Number [1322–13–0]

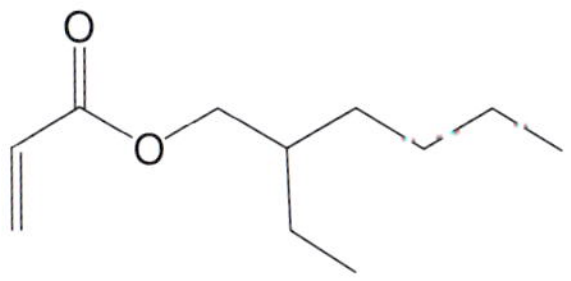

2-EHA was contained in a surgical tape and caused allergic contact dermatitis in a patient.

Suggested Reading

Daecke C, Schaller J, Goos M (1994) Acrylates as potent allergens in occupational and domestic exposures. Contact Dermatitis 30:190–191

Ethyl Methacrylate

CAS Registry Number [97–63–2].

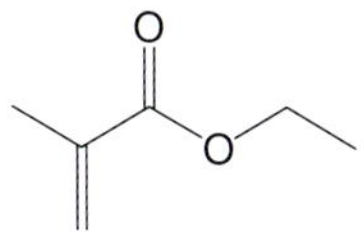

Ethyl methacrylate is used in dental prostheses or in photobonded sculptured nails.

Suggested Reading

Kanerva L, Estlander T, Jolanki R, Tarvainen K (1993) Occupational allergic contact dermatitis caused by exposure to acrylates during work with dental prostheses. Contact Dermatitis 28: 268–275

Kanerva L, Lauerma A, Estlander T, Alanko K, Henriks-Eckerman ML, Jolanki R (1996) Occupational allergic contact dermatitis caused by photobonded sculptured nails and a review of (-meth) acrylates in nail cosmetics. Am J Contact Dermat 7:109–115

Rustemeyer T, Frosch PJ (1996) Occupational skin diseases in dental laboratory technicians. (I). Clinical picture and causative factors. Contact Dermatitis 34:125–133

Glycidyl Methacrylate

CAS Registry Number [106–91–2]

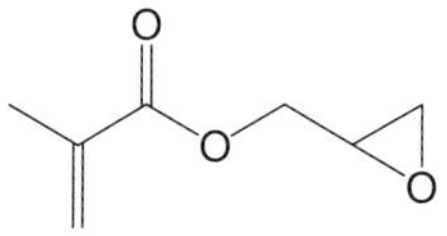

Glycidyl methacrylate was reported as the allergenic component of the anaerobic sealant Sta-Lok.

Suggested Reading

Dempsey KJ (1982) Hypersensitivity to Sta-Lok and Loctite anaerobic sealants. J Am Acad Dermatol 7:779–784

1,6-Hexanediol Diacrylate

Hexamethylene Diacrylate

CAS Registry Number [13048–33–4]

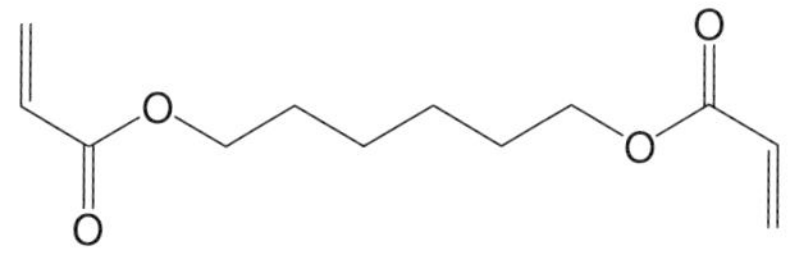

Sensitization occurred after accidental occupational exposure in an employee in the laboratory of a plastic paint factory.

Suggested Reading

Botella-Estrada R, Mora E, de La Cuadra J (1992) Hexanediol diacrylate sensitization after accidental occupational exposure. Contact Dermatitis 26:50–51

2-Hydroxyethyl Acrylate

2-HEA, Ethylene Glycol Acrylate

CAS Registry Number [818–61–1]

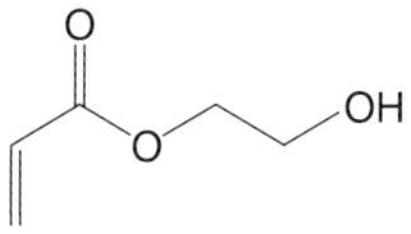

2-HEA is contained in Lowicryl 4KM and K11 M resins. It caused contact dermatitis in workers embedding media for electron microscopy. It may also be contained in UV-cured nail gel used for photobonded, sculptured nails.

Suggested Reading

Kanerva L, Lauerma A, Estlander T, Alanko K, Henriks-Eckerman ML, Jolanki R (1996) Occupational allergic contact dermatitis caused by photobonded sculptured nails and a review of (meth) acrylates in nail cosmetics. Am J Contact Dermat 7:109–115

Tobler M, Wüthrich B, Freiburghaus AU (1990) Contact dermatitis from acrylate and methacrylate compounds in Lowicryl® embedding media for electron microscopy. Contact Dermatitis 23: 96–102

2-Hydroxyethyl Methacrylate

2-HEMA

CAS Registry Number [868–77–9]

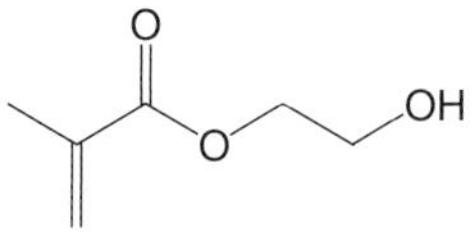

Sensitization to 2-HEMA concerns mainly dental technicians and dentists, but can also occur in other workers such as printers or beauticians or consumers using photopolymerizable sculptured nails.

Suggested Reading

Geukens S, Goossens A (2001) Occupational contact allergy to (meth)acrylates. Contact Dermatitis 44:153–159

Jolanki R, Kanerva L, Estlander T, Tarvainen K (1994) Concomitant sensitization to triglycidyl isocyanurate, diaminodiphenylmethane and 2-hydroxyethyl methacrylate from silk-screen printing coatings in the manufacture of circuit boards. Contact Dermatitis 30:12–15

Kanerva L, Estlander T, Jolanki R, Tarvainen K (1993) Occupational allergic contact dermatitis caused by exposure to acrylates during work with dental prostheses. Contact Dermatitis 28: 268–275

Kanerva L, Jolanki R, Estlander T (1995) Occupational allergic contact dermatitis from 2-hydroxyethyl methacrylate and ethylene glycol dimethacrylate in a modified acrylic structural adhesive. Contact Dermatitis 35:84–89

Rustemeyer T, Frosch PJ (1996) Occupational skin diseases in dental laboratory technicians. (I). Clinical picture and causative factors. Contact Dermatitis 34:125–133

2-Hydroxypropyl Acrylate

CAS Registry Number [999–61–1]

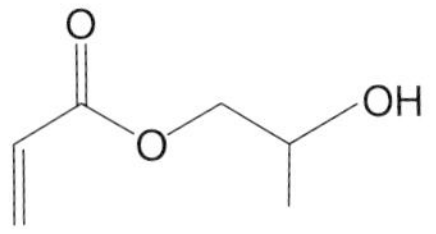

A case of occupational contact dermatitis was reported in industry.

Suggested Reading

Lovell CR, Rycroft RJG, Williams DMJ, Hamlin JW (1985) Contact dermatitis from the irritancy (immediate and delayed) and allergenicity of hydroxypropyl acrylate. Contact Dermatitis 12: 117–118

2-Hydroxypropyl Methacrylate

CAS Registry Number [27813–02–1]

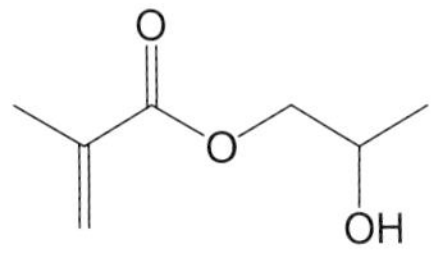

Sensitization to 2-hydroxypropyl methacrylate concerns mainly the dental profession.

Suggested Reading

Kanerva L, Estlander T, Jolanki R, Tarvainen K (1993) Occupational allergic contact dermatitis caused by exposure to acrylates during work with dental prostheses. Contact Dermatitis 28: 268–275

Kanerva L, Estlander T, Jolanki R (1997) Occupational allergic contact dermatitis caused by triacrylic tri-cure glass ionomer. Contact Dermatitis 37:49

Rustemeyer T, Frosch PJ (1996) Occupational skin diseases in dental laboratory technicians. (I). Clinical picture and causative factors. Contact Dermatitis 34:125–133

Methacrylic Acid and Methacrylates

CAS Registry Number [79–41–4]

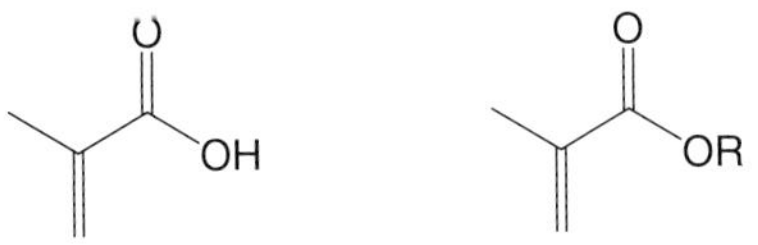

Methacrylic acid

Methacrylate

Methacrylates are derived from methacrylic acid. They are used in the production of a great variety of polymers. As they are moderate to strong sensitizers, sensitization concerns many professions. Dental technicians, assistants, and surgeons are frequently exposed. Methacrylates were reported as occupational allergens in chemically cured or photocured sculptured nails.

Methyl Acrylate

MA

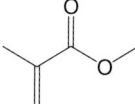

CAS Registry Number [96–33–3].

MA is contained in some nail lacquers.

Suggested Reading

Kanerva L, Estlander T, Jolanki R, Tarvainen K (1993) Occupational allergic contact dermatitis caused by exposure to acrylates during work with dental prostheses. Contact Dermatitis 28:268–275

Kanerva L, Lauerma A, Estlander T, Alanko K, Henriks-Eckerman ML, Jolanki R (1996) Occupational allergic contact dermatitis caused by photobonded sculptured nails and a review of (meth) acrylates in nail cosmetics. Am J Contact Dermat 7:109–115

Methyl Methacrylate and Polymethyl Methacrylate

CAS Registry Numbers [80–62–6] and [9011–14–7]

51

Methyl methacrylate is one of the most common methacrylates. This acrylic monomer, the essential component of the fluid mixed with the powder, causes allergic contact dermatitis mainly in dental technicians and dentists. Cases were also reported following the use of sculptured nails and in ceramic workers. Polymethyl methacrylate is the result of polymerized methyl methacrylate monomers, which are used as sheets, molding, extrusion powders, surface coating resins, emulsion polymers, fibers, inks, and films. This material is also used in tooth implants, bone cements, and hard corneal contact lenses.

Suggested Reading

Farli M, Gasperini M, Francalanci S, Gola M, Sertoli A (1990) Occupational contact dermatitis in 2 dental technicians. Contact Dermatitis 22:282–287

Gebhardt M, Geier J (1996) Evaluation of patch test results with denture material series. Contact Dermatitis 34:191–195

Kanerva L, Estlander T, Jolanki R, Tarvainen K (1993) Occupational allergic contact dermatitis caused by exposure to acrylates during work with dental prostheses. Contact Dermatitis 28:268–275

Kanerva L, Lauerma A, Estlander T, Alanko K, Henriks-Eckerman ML, Jolanki R (1996) Occupational allergic contact dermatitis caused by photobonded sculptured nails and a review of (meth) acrylates in nail cosmetics. Am J Contact Dermat 7:109–115

Kiec-Swierczynska MK (1996) Occupational allergic contact dermatitis due to acrylates in Lodz. Contact Dermatitis 34:419–422

Rustemeyer T, Frosch PJ. Occupational skin diseases in dental laboratory technicians. (I). Clinical picture and causative factors. Contact Dermatitis. 34:125–133

Pentaerythrityl Triacrylate

CAS Registry Numbers [3524–68–3] and others

Pentaerythritol triacrylate is a multifunctional acrylic monomer. It can be contained in photopolymerizable printer's ink or varnishes. Sensitization was described in dental technicians and in a textile fabric printer.

Suggested Reading
Geukens S, Goossens A (2001) Occupational contact allergy to (meth)acrylates. Contact Dermatitis 44:153–159
Kanerva L, Estlander T, Jolanki R, Tarvainen K (1995) Occupational allergic contact dermatitis and contact urticaria caused by polyfunctional aziridine hardener. Contact Dermatitis 33:304–309
Kiec-Swierczynska MK (1996) Occupational allergic contact dermatitis due to acrylates in Lodz. Contact Dermatitis 34:419–422
Rustemeyer T, Frosch PJ (1996) Occupational skin diseases in dental laboratory technicians. (I). Clinical picture and causative factors. Contact Dermatitis 34:125–133

Polyurethane Dimethacrylate

The polyurethane dimethacrylate was contained in Loctite glues of the 300 and 500 series.

Suggested Reading
Dempsey KJ (1982) Hypersensitivity to Sta-Lok and Loctite anaerobic sealants. J Am Acad Dermatol 7:779–784

Tetraethylene Glycol Dimethacrylate

CAS Registry Number [109–17–1]

Tetraethylene glycol dimethacrylate is a crosslinking agent of acrylic resins, employed to optimize the dilution of high-viscosity monomers and to link together the macromolecules constituting the polymer, to make the three-dimensional structure more rigid. Occupational dermatitis was reported in a dental technician.

Suggested Reading
Farli M, Gasperini M, Francalanci S, Gola M, Sertoli A (1990) Occupational contact dermatitis in 2 dental technicians. Contact Dermatitis 22:282–287

Triethylene Glycol Dimethacrylate

CAS Registry Number [109–16–0]

Triethylene glycol dimethacrylate (TREGDMA) is a cross-linking agent of acrylic resins, used in sealants or in dental bonding resins. It is mainly used in dentistry, by dental technicians and dentists.

Suggested Reading

Farli M, Gasperini M, Francalanci S, Gola M, Sertoli A (1990) Occupational contact dermatitis in 2 dental technicians. Contact Dermatitis 22:282–287

Kanerva L, Lauerma A, Estlander T, Alanko K, Henriks-Eckerman ML, Jolanki R (1996) Occupational allergic contact dermatitis caused by photobonded sculptured nails and a review of (-meth) acrylates in nail cosmetics. Am J Contact Dermat 7:109–115

Kiec-Swierczynska MK (1996) Occupational allergic contact dermatitis due to acrylates in Lodz. Contact Dermatitis 34:419–422

Rustemeyer T, Frosch PJ (1996) Occupational skin diseases in dental laboratory technicians. (I). Clinical picture and causative factors. Contact Dermatitis 34:125–133

Trimethylolpropane Triacrylate

CAS Registry Number [15625-89-5]

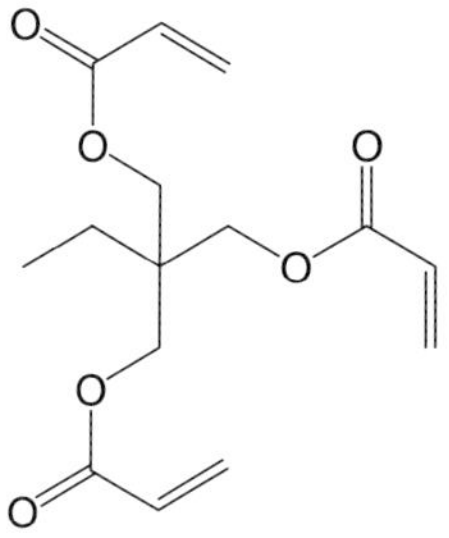

51

Trimethylolpropane triacrylate (TMPTA) is a multifunctional acrylic monomer. It reacts with propyleneimine to form polyfunctional aziridine. Sensitization was observed in a textile fabric printer. Patch tests were positive with the polyfunctional aziridine hardener, but were negative to TMPTA. TMPTA caused contact dermatitis in an optic fibre manufacturing worker and was reported as a sensitizer in a floor top coat or in photopolymerizable inks.

Suggested Reading

Kanerva L, Estlander T, Jolanki R, Tarvainen K (1995) Occupational allergic contact dermatitis and contact urticaria caused by polyfunctional aziridine hardener. Contact Dermatitis 33:304–309

Kiec-Swierczynska MK (1996) Occupational allergic contact dermatitis due to acrylates in Lodz. Contact Dermatitis 34:419–422

Maurice PDL, Rycroft RJG (1986) Allergic contact dermatitis from UV curing acrylate in the manufacture of optical fibres. Contact Dermatitis 15:92–93

Tripropylene Glycol Diacrylate

CAS Registry Number [42978-66-5]

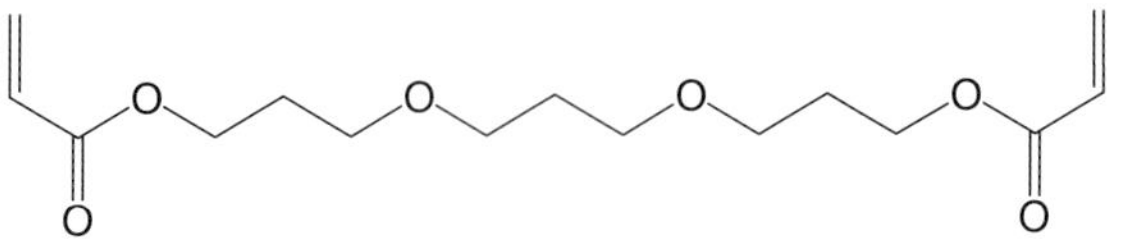

As a cause of occupational contact dermatitis, tripropylene glycol diacrylate was contained in dental resins, in UV-cured inks and in nail cosmetics.

Suggested Reading

Kanerva L, Estlander T, Jolanki R, Tarvainen K (1993) Occupational allergic contact dermatitis caused by exposure to acrylates during work with dental prostheses. Contact Dermatitis 28:268–275

Kanerva L, Lauerma A, Estlander T, Alanko K, Henriks-Eckerman ML, Jolanki R (1996) Occupational allergic contact dermatitis caused by photobonded sculptured nails and a review of (-meth) acrylates in nail cosmetics. Am J Contact Dermat 7:109–115

Urethane Acrylate

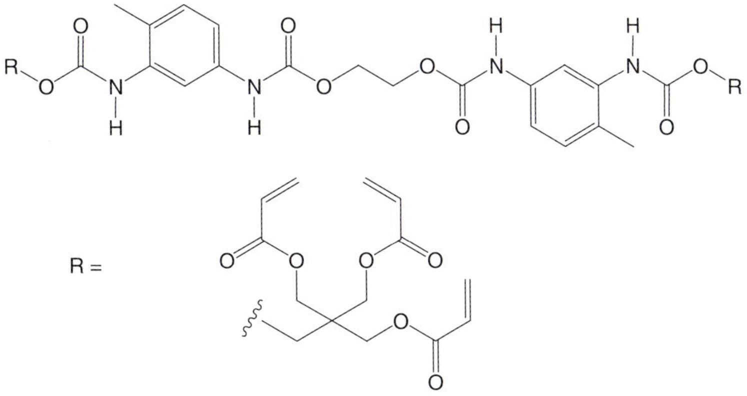

Urethane acrylate gave a positive reaction in a lottery-ticket-coating machine worker sensitized to epoxy acrylate oligomers contained in a UV varnish.

Suggested Reading

Guimaraens D, Gonzalez MA, del Rio E, Condé-Salazar L (1994) Occupational airborne allergic contact dermatitis in the national mint and fiscal-stamp factory. Contact Dermatitis 30:172–173

Kanerva L, Estlander T, Jolanki R, Tarvainen K (1993) Occupational allergic contact dermatitis caused by exposure to acrylates during work with dental prostheses. Contact Dermatitis 28: 268–275

5. Acrylonitrile

2-Propenenitrile

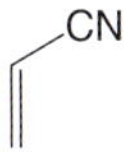

CAS Registry Number [107–13–1]

Acrylonitrile is a raw material used extensively in industry, mainly for acrylic and modacrylic fibres, acrylonitrile-butadiene-styrene and styrene-acrylonitrile resins, adiponitrile used in nylon's synthesis, for nitrile rubber, and plastics. It is also used as an insecticide. This very toxic and irritant substance is also a sensitizer and caused both irritant and allergic contact dermatitis in a production manufacturer.

Suggested Reading

Bakker JG, Jongen SMJ, Van Neer FCJ, Neis JM (1991) Occupational contact dermatitis due to acrylonitrile. Contact Dermatitis 24:50–53

Chu CY, Sun CC (2001) Allergic contact dermatitis from acrylonitrile. Am J Contact Dermat 12:113–114

6. Alachlor®

2-Chloro-2′,6′-Diethyl-N-(Methoxymethyl)-Acetanilide, 2-Chloro-N-(2,6-Diethylphenyl)-N-(Methoxymethyl)Acetamide

CAS Registry Number [15972–60–8]

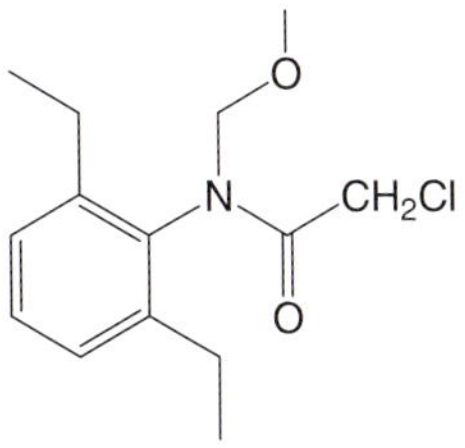

Alachlor® is a herbicide. Occupational contact dermatitis was rarely observed in agricultural workers.

51

Suggested Reading
Won JH, Ahn SK, Kim SC (1993) Allergic contact dermatitis from the herbicide Alachlor®. Contact Dermatitis 28:38–39

7. Alantolactone

CAS Registry Number [546–43–0]

The allergen eudesmanolide sesquiterpene lactone was isolated from elecampane (*Inula helenium* L.). With dehydrocostuslactone and costunolide, it is a component of the (sesquiterpene) lactone mix used to detect sensitization to Compositae–Asteraceae. See also Chap. 41, Plants and Plant Products.

Suggested Reading
Ducombs G, Benezra C, Talaga P, Andersen KE, Burrows D, Camarasa JG, Dooms-Goossens A, Frosch PJ, Lachapelle JM, Menné T, Rycroft RJG, White IR, Shaw S, Wilkinson JD (1990) Patch testing with the "sesquiterpene lactone mix": a marker for contact allergy to Compositae and other sesquiterpene-lactone-containing plants. Contact Dermatitis 22:249–252
Lamminpää A, Estlander T, Jolanki R, Kanerva L (1996) Occupational allergic contact dermatitis caused by decorative plants. Contact Dermatitis 34:330–335

8. Alkyl Glucosides

Alkyl glucosides are copolymers; based on a fatty alcohol and a glucoside polymer, they comprise decyl glucoside, coco glucoside and lauryl (dodecyl) glucoside in cosmetics, and cetearyl glucoside as a surfactant and emulsifying agent because of its higher viscosity. Due to their manufacturing processes, they are blends of several copolymers. For example, coco glucoside contains C_6, C_8, C_{10}, C_{12}, C_{14}, and C_{16} fatty alcohols. Such variations explain uncertainty when searching for the precise CAS Registry Number. Because alkyl glucosides are comparable mixtures, patients sensitive to one alkyl glucoside may also react to others. See also 127. Decyl Glucoside.

Suggested Reading
Goossens A, Decraene T, Platteaux N, Nardelli A, Rasschaert V (2003) Glucosides as unexpected allergens in cosmetics. Contact Dermatitis 48:164–166
Le Coz CJ, Meyer MT (2003) Contact allergy to decyl glucoside in antiseptic after body piercing. Contact Dermatitis 48:279–280

9. Allicin

CAS Registry Number [539–86–6]

Allicin is one of the major allergens in garlic (*Allium sativum* L.). It is responsible for the characteristic flavor of the bulbs, and has immunomodulating and antibacterial properties. See also Chap. 41, Plants and Plant Products.

Suggested Reading
Bruynzeel DP (1997) Bulb dermatitis. Dermatological problems in the flower bulb industries. Contact Dermatitis 37:70–77
Lamminpää A, Estlander T, Jolanki R, Kanerva L (1996) Occupational allergic contact dermatitis caused by decorative plants. Contact Dermatitis 34:330–335

Papageorgiou C, Corbet JP, Menezes-Brandao F, Pecegueiro M, Benezra C (1983) Allergic contact dermatitis to garlic (*Allium sativum L.*). Identification of the allergens: the role of mono-, di- and tri-sulfides present in garlic. A comparative study in man and animal (guinea pig). Arch Dermatol Res 275:229–234

10. Allyl Glycidyl Ether

CAS Registry Number [106–92–3]

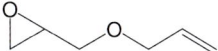

Allyl glycidyl ether is a monoglycidyl derivative, used as a reactive epoxy diluent for epoxy resins. As an impurity, it was considered to be the sensitizing agent in a plastic industry worker allergic to 3-glycidyloxypropyl trimethoxysilane, an epoxy silane compound used as a fixing additive in silicone and polyurethane.

Suggested Reading
Angelini G, Rigano L, Foti C, Grandolfo M, Vena GA, Bonamonte D, Soleo L, Scorpiniti AA (1996) Occupational sensitization to epoxy resin and reactive diluents in marble workers. Contact Dermatitis 35:11–16

Dooms-Goossens A, Bruze M, Buysse L, Fregert S, Gruvberger B, Stals H (1995) Contact allergy to allyl glycidyl ether present as an impurity in 3-glycidyloxypropyltrimethoxysilane, a fixing additive in silicone and polyurethane. Contact Dermatitis 33:17–19

Jolanki R, Kanerva L, Estlander T, Tarvainen K, Keskinen H, Henriks-Eckerman ML (1990) Occupational dermatoses from epoxy resin compounds. Contact Dermatitis 23:172–183

11. Allyl Isothiocyanate

CAS Registry Number [57–06–7]

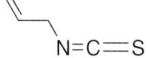

Allyl isothiocyanate is generated by enzymatic hydrolysis of the glucoside sinigrin, present in Cruciferae–Brassicaceae, mainly the oil from black mustard seed (*Brassica nigra* Koch). It may induce irritant and sometimes allergic contact dermatitis, mimicking the "tulip finger" dermatitis. See also Chap. 41, Plants and Plant Products.

Suggested Reading
Ettlinger MG, Lundeen AJ (1956) The structures of sinigrin and sinalbin; an enzymatic rearrangement. J Ann Chem Soc 78:4172–4173

Lerbaek A, Chandra Rastogi S, Menné T (2004) Allergic contact dermatitis from allyl isothiocyanate in a Danish cohort of 259 selected patients. Contact Dermatitis 51:79–83

12. Allylpropyldisulfide

CAS Registry Number [2179–59–1]

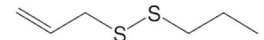

With allicin and diallyl sulfide, allylpropyldisulfide is one of the allergens in garlic (*Allium sativum* L.). See also Chap. 41, Plants and Plant Products.

Suggested Reading
Bruynzeel DP (1997) Bulb dermatitis. Dermatological problems in the flower bulb industries. Contact Dermatitis 37:70–77

13. Alprenolol

CAS Registry Number [13655–52–2]

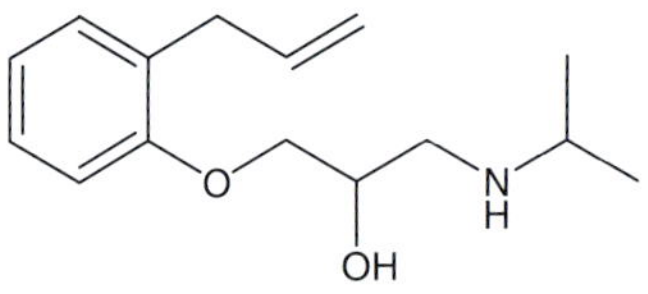

Occupational cases of contact dermatitis were reported in the pharmaceutical industry.

Suggested Reading

Ekenvall L, Forsbeck M (1978) Contact eczema produced by α-adrenergic blocking agent (Alprenolol). Contact Dermatitis 4:190–194

14. Amethocaine

Pantocaine, Tetracaine

CAS Registry Number [136–47–0]

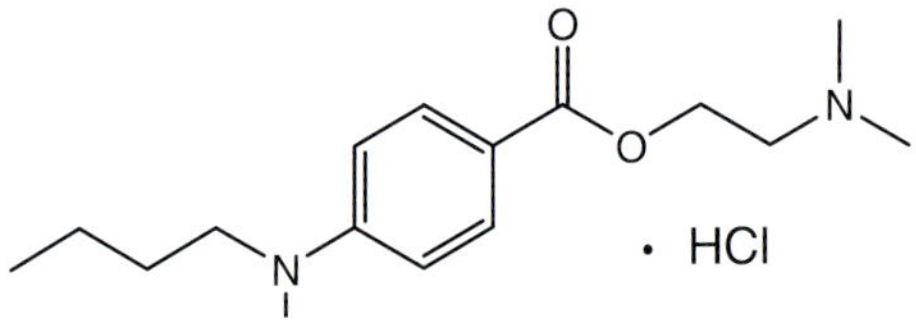

Amethocaine is a local anesthetic used in dental surgery. It was reported as an agent of contact dermatitis in dentists or dental nurses, and in ophthalmologists.

Suggested Reading

Berova N, Stranky L, Krasteva M (1990) Studies on contact dermatitis in stomatological staff. Dermatol Monatschr 176:15–18

Condé-Salazar L, Llinas MG, Guimaraens D, Romero L (1988) Occupational allergic contact dermatitis from amethocaine. Contact Dermatitis 19:69–70

Rebandel P, Rudzki E (1986) Occupational contact sensitivity in oculists. Contact Dermatitis 15:92

15. *p*-Amino-*N,N*-Diethylaniline Sulfate

1,4-Benzenediamine, *N,N-Diethyl-para-Phenylenediamine* Sulfate

CAS Registry Number [6065–27–6]

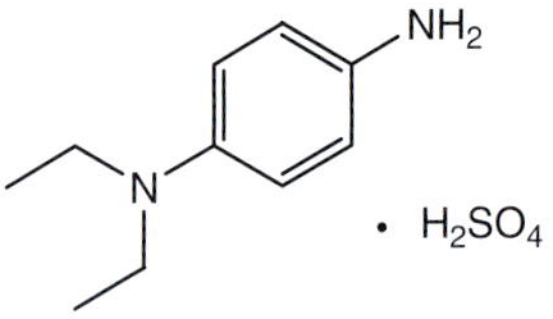

This color developer can induce sensitization in photographers.

Suggested Reading

Aguirre A, Landa N, Gonzalez M, Diaz-Perez JL (1992) Allergic contact dermatitis in a photographer. Contact Dermatitis 27:340–341

16. 4-Amino-3-Nitrophenol

3-Nitro-4-Aminophenol

CAS Registry Number [610–81–1]

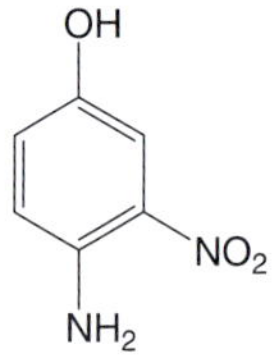

This hair dye used for semi-permanent colors seems to be a rare sensitizer.

Suggested Reading
Sánchez-Pérez J, García del Río I, Alvares Ruiz S, García Diez A (2004) Allergic contact dermatitis from direct dyes for hair coloration in hairdressers' clients. Contact Dermatitis 50:261–262

17. *p*-Aminoazobenzene

Solvent Yellow 1, C.I. 11000, Solvent Blue 7

CAS Registry Number [60–09–3]

This azoic coloring can be reduced in *para*-phenylenediamine (PPD). It can be found in some semi-permanent hair dyes and patch tests are frequently positive (about 30%) in hairdressers with hand dermatitis. Because of hydrolysis of the azo bond, the detection of sensitization to *p*-aminoazobenzene may be assumed by a PPD test.

Suggested Reading
Condé-Salazar L, Baz M, Guimaraens D, Cannavo A (1995) Contact dermatitis in hairdressers: patch test results in 379 hairdressers (1980–1993). Am J Contact Dermat 6:19–23

18. *p*-Aminodiphenylamine (Hydrochloride)

4-Aminodiphenylamine (HCl), CI 76086 (CI 75085)

CAS Registry Number [101–54–2] (CAS Registry Number [2198–59–6])

This substance was formerly used as a hair dye. Sensitization, when detected by patch testing, is relatively low in hairdressers.

Suggested Reading
Frosch PJ, Burrows D, Camarasa JG, Dooms-Goossens A, Ducombs G, Lahti A, Menné T, Rycroft RJG, Shaw S, White IR, Wilkinson JD (1993) Allergic reactions to a hairdresser's series: results from 9 European centres. Contact Dermatitis 28:180–183

19. Aminoethylethanolamine

N-(2-Hydroxyethyl)Ethylenediamine

CAS Registry Number [111–41–1]

Aminoethylethanolamine is a component of colophony in soldering flux, which may cause contact and airborne contact dermatitis in workers in the electronic industry or in cable jointers.

Suggested Reading

Crow KD, Harman RRM, Holden H (1968) Amine-flux sensitization dermatitis in electricity cable jointers. Br J Dermatol 80:701–710

Goh CL (1985) Occupational contact dermatitis from soldering flux among workers in the electronics industry. Contact Dermatitis 13:85–90

Goh CL, Ng SK (1987) Airborne contact dermatitis to colophony in soldering flux. Contact Dermatitis 17:89–91

20. o-Aminophenol

2-Aminophenol, CI 76520

CAS Registry Number [95–55–6]

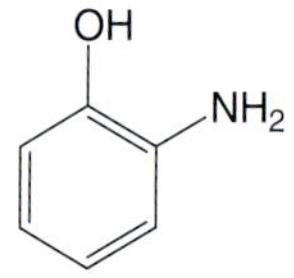

51

It is contained in hair dyes and can cause contact dermatitis in hairdressers and in consumers.

Suggested Reading

Matsunaga K, Hosokawa K, Suzuki M, Arima Y, Hayakawa R (1988) Occupational allergic contact dermatitis in beauticians. Contact Dermatitis 18:94–96

21. p-Aminophenol

4-Aminophenol, Amino-4 Hydroxybenzene, Hydroxy-4 Aniline, CI 76550

CAS Registry Number [123–30–8]

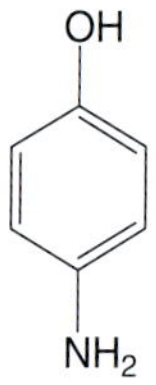

This hair dye is frequently implicated in contact dermatitis in hairdressers, in customers, or in people sensitized to *para*-phenylenediamine, by the way of "black-henna" temporary tattoos.

Suggested Reading

Guerra L, Tosti A, Bardazzi F, Pigatto P, Lisi P, Santucci B, Valsecchi R, Schena D, Angelini G, Sertoli A, Ayala F, Kokeli F (1992) Contact dermatitis in hairdressers: the Italian experience. Gruppo Italiano Ricerca Dermatiti da Contatto e Ambientali. Contact Dermatitis 26:101–107

Le Coz CJ, Lefebvre C, Keller F, Grosshans E (2000) Allergic contact dermatitis caused by skin painting (pseudotattooing) with black henna, a mixture of henna and *p*-phenylenediamine and its derivatives. Arch Dermatol 136:1515–1517

22. Aminophylline

Theophylline Ethylenediamine

CAS Registry Number [317–34–0]

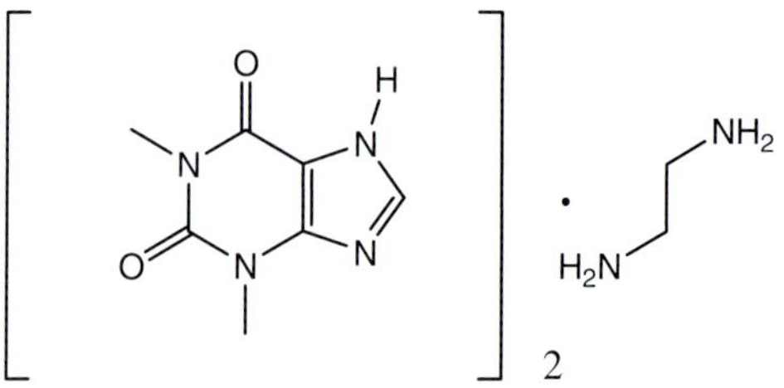

This drug is a 2:1 mixture of the alkaloid theophylline and ethylenediamine (see below). It caused contact dermatitis in industrial plants, in pharmacists, and in nurses. Ethylenediamine is the sensitizer and patch testing is generally positive to both ethylenediamine and aminophylline, and negative to theophylline.

Suggested Reading

Corazza M, Mantovani L, Trimurti L, Virgili A (1994) Occupational contact sensitization to ethylenediamine in a nurse. Contact Dermatitis 31:328–329

Dias M, Fernandes C, Pereira F, Pacheco A (1995) Occupational dermatitis from ethylenediamine. Contact Dermatitis 33:129–130

23. *N,N*-bis-(3-Aminopropyl) Dodecylamine

_N_-(3-Aminopropyl)-_N_-Dodecyl-1,3-Propanediamine

CAS Registry Number [2372–82–9]

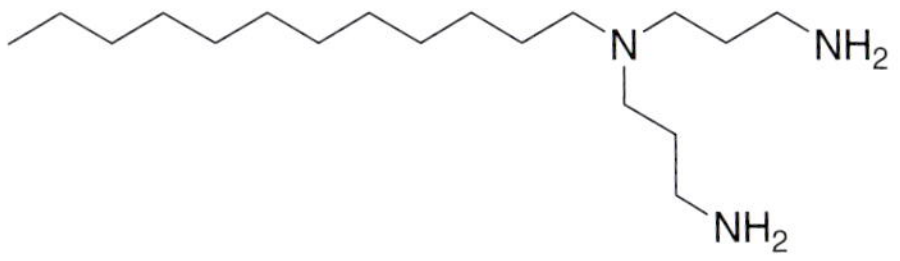

This alkylamine is contained in detergent-disinfectants solutions for medical instruments. It is also contained in association with 3-aminopropyl dodecylamine in liquid laundry disinfectants such as Aset® aqua (Johnson Wax SpA, Rydelle).

Suggested Reading

Dibo M, Brasch J (2001) Occupational allergic contact dermatitis from *N,N*-bis(3-aminopropyl)dodecylamine and dimethyldidecylammonium chloride in two hospital staff. Contact Dermatitis 45:40

24. Ammonium Persulfate

Ammonium Peroxydisulfate

CAS Registry Number [7727–54–0]

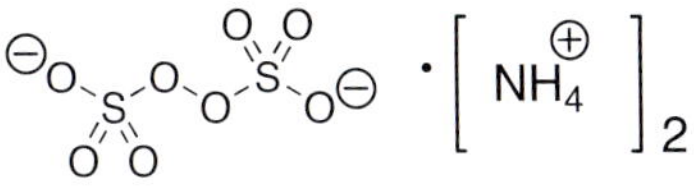

Persulfates are strong oxidizing agents widely used in the production of metals, textiles, photographs, cellophane, rubber, adhesive papers, foods, soaps, detergents, and hair bleaches. Ammonium persulfate is used as a hair bleaching agent. It may induce irritant dermatitis, (mainly) nonimmunologic contact urticaria, and allergic contact dermatitis and represents a major allergen in hairdressers. People reacting to ammonium persulfate also react to other persulfates such as potassium persulfate.

Suggested Reading

Frosch PJ, Burrows D, Camarasa JG, Dooms-Goossens A, Ducombs G, Lahti A, Menné T, Rycroft RJG, Shaw S, White IR, Wilkinson JD (1993) Allergic reactions to a hairdresser's series: results from 9 European centres. Contact Dermatitis 28:180–183

Le Coz CJ, Bezard M (1999) Allergic contact cheilitis due to effervescent dental cleanser: combined responsibilities of the allergen persulfate and prosthesis porosity. Contact Dermatitis 41:268–271

Van Joost T, Roesyanto ID (1991) Sensitization to persulphates in occupational and non-occupational hand dermatitis. Contact Dermatitis 24:376–377

25. Ammonium Thioglycolate

Ammonium Mercaptoacetate

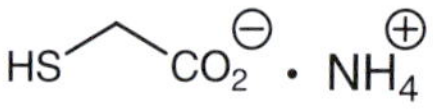

CAS Registry Number [5421–46–5]

This substance is contained in "basic" permanent waves solutions and causes contact dermatitis in hairdressers.

Suggested Reading

Frosch PJ, Burrows D, Camarasa JG, Dooms-Goossens A, Ducombs G, Lahti A, Menné T, Rycroft RJG, Shaw S, White IR, Wilkinson JD (19939 Allergic reactions to a hairdresser's series: results from 9 European centres. Contact Dermatitis 28:180–183

Guerra L, Tosti A, Bardazzi F, Pigatto P, Lisi P, Santucci B, Valsecchi R, Schena D, Angelini G, Sertoli A, Ayala F, Kokeli F (1992) Contact dermatitis in hairdressers: the Italian experience. Gruppo Italiano Ricerca Dermatiti da Contatto e Ambientali. Contact Dermatitis 26:101–107

51

26. Amoxicillin

CAS Registry Number [26787–78–0]

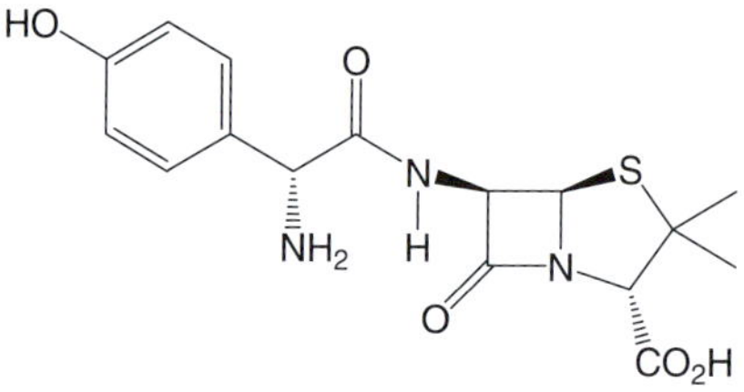

Amoxicillin Trihydrate

CAS Registry Number [61336–70–7]

Amoxicillin Sodium Salt

CAS Registry Number [34642–77–8]

Amoxicillin is both a topical and a systemic sensitizer. Topical sensitization occurs in healthcare workers. Systemic drug reactions are frequent, such as urticaria, maculo-papular rashes, baboon syndrome, acute generalized exanthematous pustulosis, or even toxic epidermal necrosis. Cross-reactivity is common with ampicillin, and can occur with other penicillins.

Suggested Reading

Gamboa P, Jauregui I, Urrutia I (1995) Occupational sensitization to aminopenicillins with oral tolerance to penicillin V. Contact Dermatitis 32:48–49

Rudzki E, Rebandel P (1991) Hypersensitivity to semisynthetic penicillins but not to natural penicillin. Contact Dermatitis 25:192

27. Ampicillin

CAS Registry Number [69–53–4]

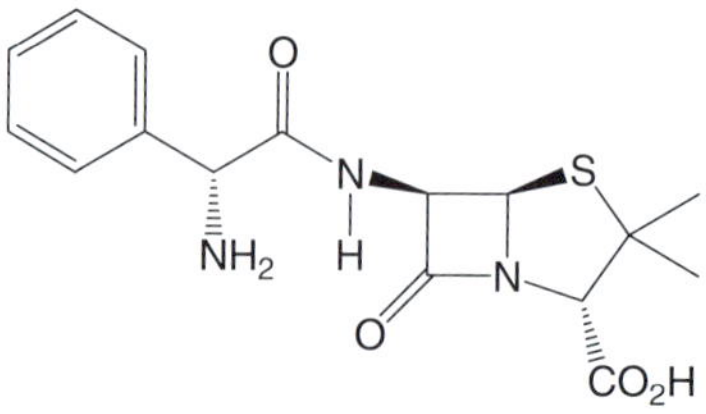

Ampicillin Trihydrate

CAS Registry Number [7177–48–2]

Ampicillin Sodium Salt

CAS Registry Number [69–52–3]

Ampicillin caused contact dermatitis in a nurse also sensitized to amoxicillin (with tolerance to oral phenoxymethylpenicillin), and in a pharmaceutical factory worker. Systemic drug reactions are common. Cross-reactivity is regular with ampicillin, and can occur with other penicillins.

Suggested Reading

Gamboa P, Jauregui I, Urrutia I (1995) Occupational sensitization to aminopenicillins with oral tolerance to penicillin V. Contact Dermatitis 32:48–49

Rudzki E, Rebandel P (1991) Hypersensitivity to semisynthetic penicillins but not to natural penicillin. Contact Dermatitis 25:192

28. Amprolium (Hydrochloride)

CAS Registry Number [121–25–5] (CAS Registry Number [137–88–2])

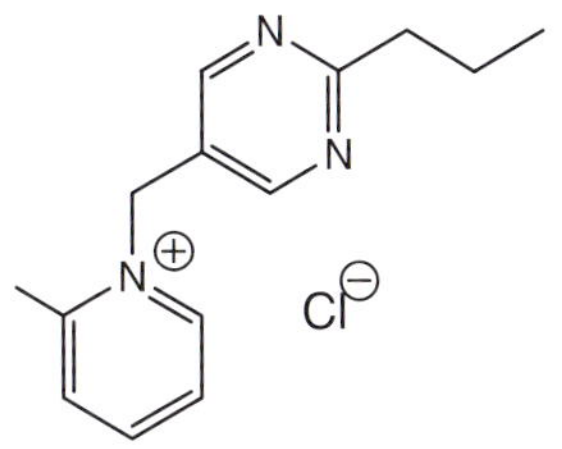

Amprolium is an antiprotozoal agent used for the prevention of coccidiosis in poultry.

Suggested Reading

Mancuso G, Staffa M, Errani A, Berdondini RM, Fabbri P (1990) Occupational dermatitis in animal feed mill workers. Contact Dermatitis 22:37–41

29. Amyl Cinnamyl Alcohol

2-Pentyl-3-Phenylprop-2-en-1-ol, Pentyl-Cinnamic Alcohol, α-Amyl-Cinnamic Alcohol, Buxinol

CAS Registry number [101–85–9]

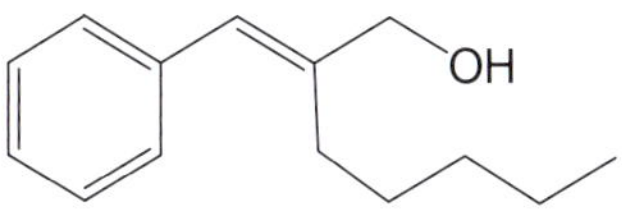

This scented molecule is very close to α-amyl-cinnamic aldehyde. Its presence is indicated by name in cosmetics within the EU.

Suggested Reading

Rastogi SC, Johansen JD, Menné T (1996) Natural ingredients based cosmetics. Content of selected fragrance sensitizers. Contact Dermatitis 34:423–426

30. Amylcinnamaldehyde

α-Amyl Cinnamic Aldehyde, Ammylcinnamal, 2-Benzylideneheptanal, 2-Pentylcinnamaldehyde, Jasminal

CAS Registry Number [122–40–7]

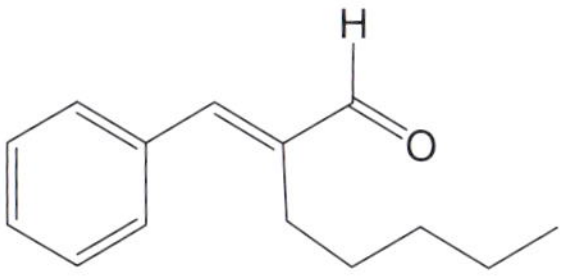

α-Amyl cinnamic aldehyde is an oxidation product of amylcinnamic alcohol, a sensitizing fragrance and one component of the "fragrance mix". It can also be a sensitizer in bakers. It has to be mentioned by name in cosmetics within the EU.

Suggested Reading

Nethercott JR, Holness DL (1989) Occupational dermatitis in food handlers and bakers. J Am Acad Dermatol 21:485–490

31. Anacardic Acids

Anacardic acids are mixture of several analog molecules with alkyl chain (-R) of 13, 15, 17, or 19 carbons, and 0 to 3 unsaturations. They are the main cashew nut shell liquid component with cardol and can cause contact dermatitis in cashew nut workers. See also 405. Urushiol; Chap. 41, Plants and Plant Products.

Suggested Reading
Diogenes MJN, de Morais SM, Carvalho FF (1996) Contact dermatitis among cashew nut workers. Contact Dermatitis 35:114–115

51

32. Anethole

1-Methoxy-4-(1-Propenyl)-Benzene

CAS Registry Number [104–46–1]

Anethole is the main component of anise, star anise, and fennel oils. It is used in perfumes, in the food and cosmetic industries (toothpastes), in bleaching colors, photography, and as an embedding material.

Suggested Reading
Garcia-Bravo B, Pérez Bernal A, Garcia-Hernandez MJ, Camacho F (1997) Occupational contact dermatitis from anethole in food handlers. Contact Dermatitis 37:38

33. Anisyl Alcohol

4-Methoxybenzyl Alcohol, Methoxybenzenemethanol, Anise Alcohol

CAS Registry Number [105–13–5]

Blend of o-, m-, and p-Methoxybenzyl Alcohol

CAS Registry number [1331–81–3]

As a fragrance allergen, anisyl alcohol has to be mentioned by name in cosmetics within the EU.

Suggested Reading

Budavari S, O'Neil MJ, Smith A, Heckelman PE, Kinneary JF (eds) (1996) The Merck Index, 12th edn. Merck, Whitehouse Station, N.J., USA

34. Antimony Trioxide

CAS Registry Number [1309–64–4] Sb_2O_3

This hard shiny metal is often alloyed to other elements. It is used in various industrial fields such as batteries, printing machines, bearing, textile, and ceramics. It caused positive patch test reactions in two workers in the ceramics industry.

Suggested Reading

Motolese A, Truzzi M, Giannini A, Seidenari S (1995) Contact dermatitis and contact sensitization among enamellers and decorators in the ceramics industry. Contact Dermatitis 28 : 59–62

35. Arsenic and Arsenic Salts (Sodium Arsenate)

CAS Registry Number [7440–38–2] and CAS Registry Number [7778–43–0]

As AsO_4H_2Na

Arsenic salts are sensitizers, but most often irritants. They are used in copper or gold extraction, glass, feeds, weedkillers, insecticides, and ceramics. A recent case was reported in a crystal factory worker with positive patch tests to sodium arsenate.

Suggested Reading

Barbaud A, Mougeolle JM, Schmutz JL (1995) Contact hypersensitivity to arsenic in a crystal factory worker. Contact Dermatitis 33 : 272–273

36. Articaine (Hydrochloride)

Carticaine (Hydrochloride)

CAS Registry Number [23964–58–1] (CAS Registry Number [23964–57–0])

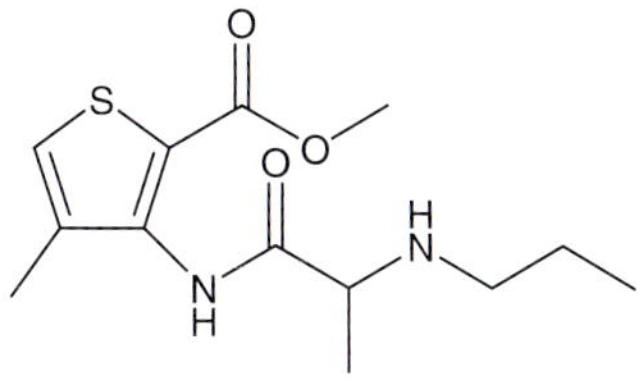

This local amide-type anesthetic is seldom reported as allergenic even in patients sensitized to other amide-type molecules like lidocaine, prilocaine, mepivacaine or bupivacaine.

Suggested Reading

Duque S, Fernandez L (2004) Delayed-type hypersensitivity to amide local anaesthetics. Allergol Immunopathol (Madr) 32 : 233–234

37. Atranol

2,6-Dihydroxy-4-Methyl-Benzaldehyde

CAS Registry number [526–37–4]

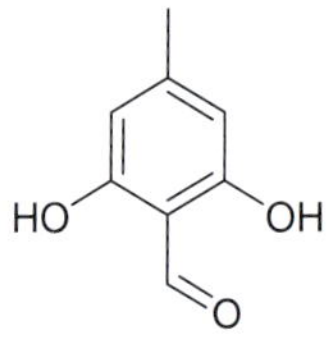

Atranol has been identified as a potent and frequent allergen, occurring from the fragrance material oak-moss absolute, which is of botanical origin.

Suggested Reading

Johansen JD, Andersen KE, Svedman C, Bruze M, Bernard G, Giménez-Arnau E, Rastogi SC, Lepoittevin JP, Menné T (2003) Chloroatranol, an extremely potent allergen hidden in perfumes: a dose response elicitation study. Contact Dermatitis 49:180–184

Rastogi SC, Bossi R, Johansen JD, Menné T, Bernard G, Giménez-Arnau E, Lepoittevin P (2004) Content of oak moss allergens atranol and chloroatranol in perfumes and similar products. Contact Dermatitis 50:367–370

51

38. Azaperone

4′-Fluoro-4-[4-(2-Pyridyl)-1-Piperazininyl]Butyrophenone

CAS Registry Number [1649–18–9]

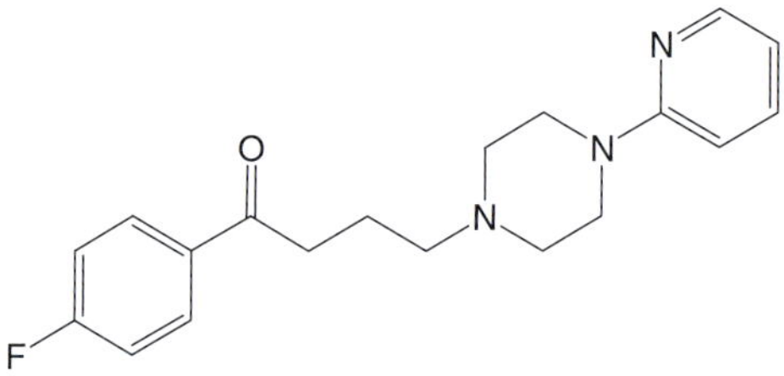

Azaperone is a sedative used in veterinary medicine, to avoid mortality of pigs during transportation. This alternative substance to chlorpromazine is a sensitizer and a photosensitizer.

Suggested Reading

Brasch J, Hessler HJ, Christophers E (1991) Occupational (photo)allergic contact dermatitis from azaperone in a piglet dealer. Contact Dermatitis 25:258–259

39. Azathioprine

6-(1-Methyl-4-Nitroimidazol-5-ylthio)Purine

CAS Registry Number [446–86–6]

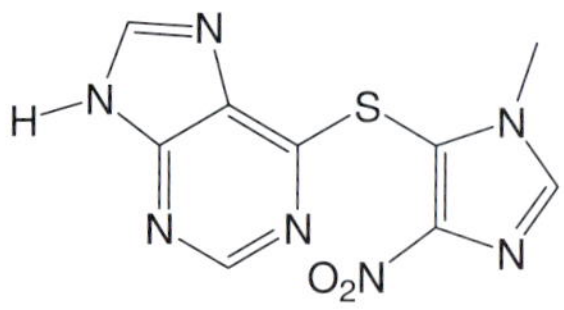

This immunosuppressive and antineoplastic drug is derived from 6-mercaptopurine. It caused allergic contact dermatitis in a mother crushing tablets for her leukemic son, and occupational dermatitis in a pharmaceutical reconditioner of old tablet packaging machines, and in a production mechanic working in packaging for a pharmaceutical company.

Suggested Reading

Burden AD, Beck MH (1992) Contact hypersensitivity to azathioprine. Contact Dermatitis 27: 329–330

Lauerma A, Koivuluhta M, Alenius H (2001) Recalcitrant allergic contact dermatitis from azathioprine tablets. Contact Dermatitis 44:129

Soni BP, Sherertz EF (1996) Allergic contact dermatitis from azathioprine. Am J Contact Dermat 7: 116–117

40. Basic Red 22

Synacril Red 3B

CAS Registry Number [12221–52–2]

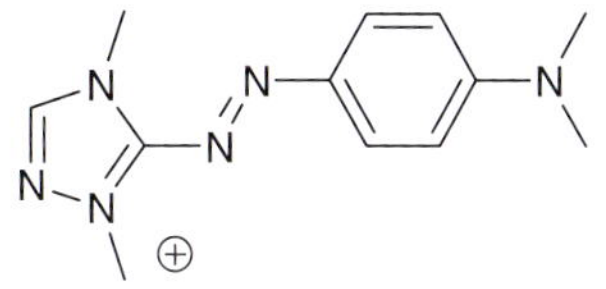

This monoazoic dye was reported as allergenic in a PPD-free hair coloring mousse. See also Chap. 37, Clothing.

Suggested Reading

Salim A, Orton D, Shaw S (2001) Allergic contact dermatitis from Basic Red 22 in a hair-colouring mousse. Contact Dermatitis 45:123

41. Basic Red 46

CAS Registry Number [12221–69–1]

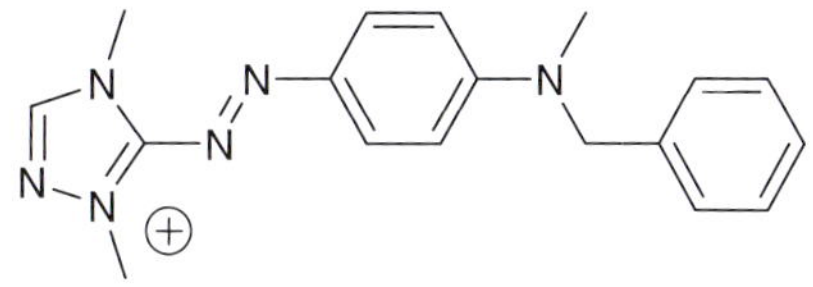

This monoazoic textile dye seems to be an important cause of foot dermatitis, being a frequent allergen in acrylic socks. It caused contact dermatitis in two workers in the textile industry. See also Chap. 37, Clothing.

Suggested Reading

Opie J, Lee A, Frowen K, Fewings J, Nixon R (2003) Foot dermatitis caused by the textile dye Basic Red 46 in acrylic blend socks. Contact Dermatitis 49:297–303

Soni BP, Sherertz EF (1996) Contact dermatitis in the textile industry: a review of 72 patients. Am J Contact Dermat 7:226–230

42. Befunolol

CAS Registry Number [39552–01–7]

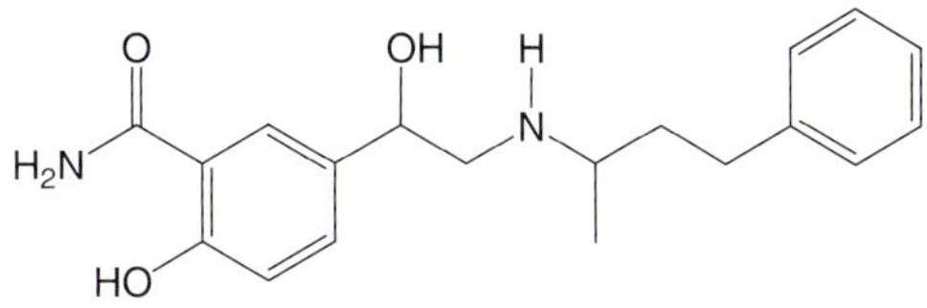

Befunolol was implicated in allergic contact dermatitis due to beta-blocker agents in eye-drops.

Suggested Reading

Giordano-Labadie F, Lepoittevin JP, Calix I, Bazex J (1997) Allergie de contact aux β-bloqueurs des collyres: allergie croisée ? Ann Dermatol Venereol 124:322–324

43. Benomyl

CAS Registry Number [17804–35–2]

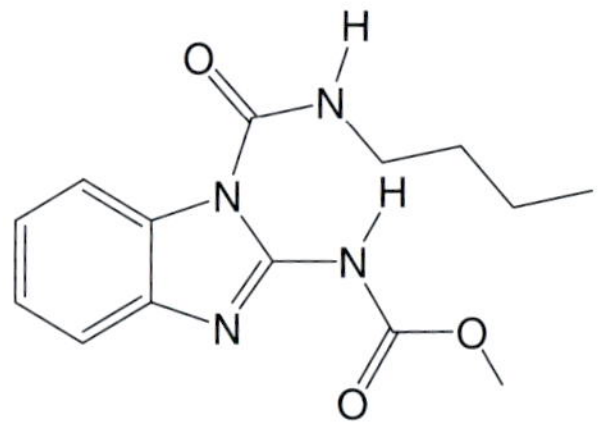

Benomyl is a fungicide, derived from benzimidazole. Cases of sensitization were reported in horticulturists and florists. It is however, at most, a weak sensitizer, with possible false-positive patch reactions, or with cross-reactions after previous exposure to other fungicides.

Suggested Reading

Jung HD, Honemann W, Kloth C, Lubbe D, Pambor M, Quednow C, Ratz KH, Rothe A, Tarnick M (1989) Kontaktekzem durch Pestizide in der Deutschen Demokratischen Republik. Dermatol Monats 175 : 203–214

Larsen AI, Larsen A, Jepsen JR, Jorgensen R (1990) Contact allergy to the fungicide benomyl? Contact Dermatitis 22 : 278–281

O'Malley M, Rodriguez P, Maibach HI (1995) Pesticide patch testing: California nursery workers and controls. Contact Dermatitis 32 : 61–62

44. Benzalkonium Chloride

CAS Registry Number [8001–54–5]

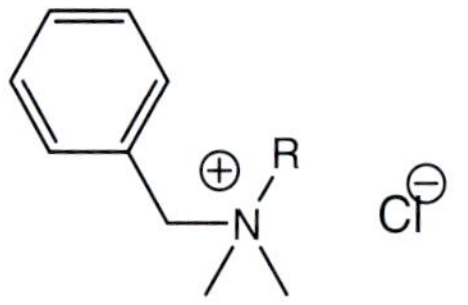

This quaternary ammonium cationic surfactant is a mixture of alkyl, dimethyl, and benzyl ammonium chlorides (-R). It is an irritant rather than a sensitizer, but may cause allergic contact dermatitis from creams, detergents/antiseptics, ophthalmic preparations, and in nursing, veterinary, dental, and medical personnel. Its presence was observed in plaster of Paris.

Suggested Reading

Basketter DA, Marriott M, Gilmour NJ, White IR (2004) Strong irritants masquerading as skin allergens: the case of benzalkonium chloride. Contact Dermatitis 50 : 213–217

Corazza M, Virgili A (1993) Airborne allergic contact dermatitis from benzalkonium chloride. Contact Dermatitis 28 : 195–196

Klein GF, Sepp N, Fritsch P (1991) Allergic reactions to benzalkonium chloride? Do the use test! Contact Dermatitis 25 : 269–270

Stanford D, Georgouras K (1996) Allergic contact dermatitis from benzalkonium chloride in plaster of Paris. Contact Dermatitis 35 : 371–372

45. Benzisothiazolone

1,2-Benzisothiazolin-3-one, BIT, Proxan, Proxel PL

CAS Registry Number [2634–33–5]

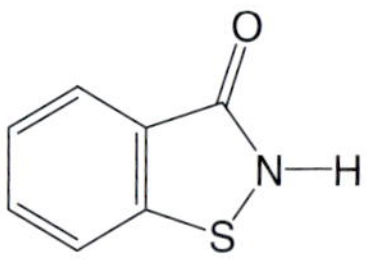

BIT, both an irritant and a skin sensitizer, is widely used in industry as a preservative in water-based solutions such as pastes, paints, and cutting oils. Occupational dermatitis has been reported mainly due to cutting fluids and greases, in paint manufacturers, pottery mold-makers, in acrylic emulsions manufacturers, in plumber, printers and lithoprinters, paper makers, analytical laboratory, rubber factory, and in employees manufacturing air fresheners.

Suggested Reading

Burden AD, O'Driscoll JB, Page FC, Beck MH (1994) Contact hypersensitivity to a new isothiazolinone. Contact Dermatitis 30:179–180

Chew AL, Maibach H (1997) 1,2-Benzisothiazol-3-one (Proxel®): irritant or allergen? A clinical study and literature review. Contact Dermatitis 36:131–136

Dias M, Lamarao P, Vale T (1992) Occupational contact allergy to 1,2-benzisothiazolin-3-one in the manufacture of air fresheners. Contact Dermatitis 27:205–206

Greig DE (1991) Another isothiazolinone source. Contact Dermatitis 25:201–202

Sanz-Gallén P, Planas J, Martinez P, Giménez-Arnau JM (1992) Allergic contact dermatitis due to 1,2-benzisothiazolin-3-one in paint manufacture. Contact Dermatitis 27:271–272

46. Benzophenones

Benzophenone (BZP), and substituted BZP numbered 1–12, trade mark Uvinul®, are photo-screen agents widely used in sunscreens and in cosmetics, such as "anti-aging" creams and hair sprays and shampoos, paints and plastics. The hypolipemiant drug fenofibrate is also a substituted benzophenone.

Benzophenone, Unsubstituted

CAS Registry Number [119–61–9]

Unsubstituted benzophenone is largely used in chemical applications. It acts as a marker for photoallergy to ketoprofen.

Benzophenone 1

Benzoresorcinol, Uvinul 400

CAS Registry Number [131–56–6]

BZP-1 is used in paints, plastics and nail varnishes for example.

Benzophenone-2

2,2′,4,4′-Tetrahydroxybenzophenone

CAS Registry Number [131–55–5]

BZP-2 is widely used in perfumes to prevent their degradation due to light. It can cause allergic contact dermatitis.

Benzophenone-3

Oxybenzone

CAS Registry Number [131–57–7]

BZP-3 is used as a direct sunscreen agent, and in anti-aging creams. Allergic reactions have been reported. Cross reactivity is expected in an average of one in four patients photoallergic to ketoprofen.

Benzophenone-4

Sulisobenzone

CAS Registry Number [4065–45–6]

BZP-4 is widely used in cosmetics, particularly shampoos and hair products. Cross reactivity is rarely expected in patients photoallergic to ketoprofen.

Benzophenone-10

Mexenone

CAS Registry Number [1641–17–4]

BZP-10 is exceptionally positive in ketoprofen-photosensitive patients.

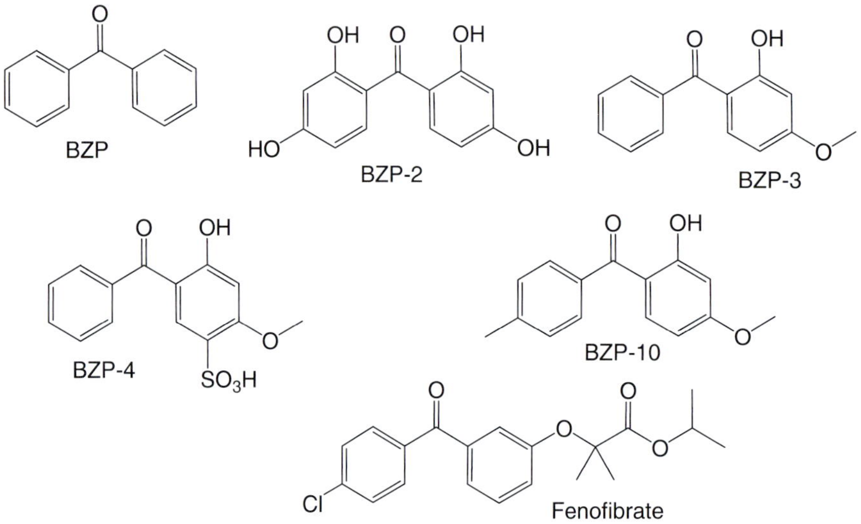

51

BZP   BZP-2   BZP-3

BZP-4   SO₃H   BZP-10

Fenofibrate

Suggested Reading

Alanko K, Jolanki R, Estlander T, Kanerva L (2001) Occupational allergic contact dermatitis from benzophenone-4 in hair-care products. Contact Dermatitis 44:188

Collins P, Ferguson J (1994) Photoallergic contact dermatitis to oxybenzone. Br J Dermatol 131: 124–129

Guin JD (2000) Eyelid dermatitis from benzophenone used in nail enhancement. Contact Dermatitis 43:308–309

Jacobs MC (1998) Contact allergy to benzophenone-2 in toilet water. Contact Dermatitis 39:42

Knobler E, Almeida L, Ruzkowski AM, Held J, Harber L, DeLeo V (1989) Photoallergy to benzophenone. Arch Dermatol 125:801–804

Le Coz CJ, Bottlaender A, Scrivener JN, Santinelli F, Cribier BJ, Heid E, Grosshans EM (1998) Photocontact dermatitis from ketoprofen and tiaprofenic acid: cross-reactivity study in 12 consecutive patients. Contact Dermatitis 38:245–252

Matthieu L, Meuleman L, van Hecke E, Blondeel A, Dezfoulian B, Constandt L, Goossens A (2004) Contact and photocontact allergy to ketoprofen. The Belgian experience. Contact Dermatitis 50:238–241

Ramsay DL, Cohen HJ, Baer RL (1972) Allergic reaction to benzophenone. Simultaneous occurrence of urticarial and contact sensitivities. Arch Dermatol 105:906–908

---

47. Benzoyl Peroxide

CAS Registry Number [94–36–0]

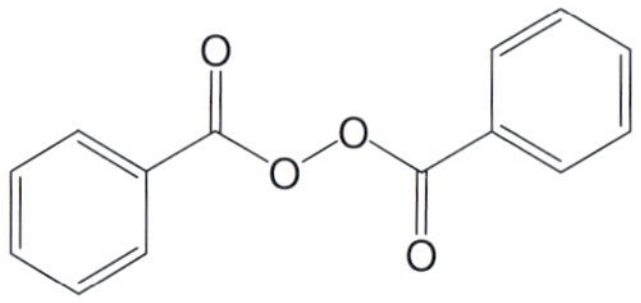

Benzoyl peroxide is an oxidizing agent widely employed in acne topical therapy. It is also used as a polymerization catalyst of dental or industrial plastics, as a decolorizing agent of flours, oils, fats, and waxes. Irritant or allergic dermatitis may affect workers in the electronics and plastics (epoxy resins and catalysts) industries, electricians, ceramic workers, dentists and dental technicians, laboratory technicians, bakers, and acne patients. As it was contained in candles, it also induced contact dermatitis in a sacristan. Patch tests may be irritant.

Suggested Reading
Balato N, Lembo G, Cuccurullo FM, Patruno C, Nappa P, Ayala F (1996) Acne and allergic contact dermatitis. Contact Dermatitis 34: 68–69
Bonnekoh B, Merk H (1991) Airborne allergic contact dermatitis from benzoyl peroxyde as a bleaching agent of candle wax. Contact Dermatitis 24:367–368
Quirce S, Olaguibel JM, Garcia BE, Tabar AI (1993) Occupational airborne contact dermatitis due to benzoyl peroxide. Contact Dermatitis 29:165–166
Rustemeyer T, Frosch PJ (1996) Occupational skin diseases in dental laboratory technicians. (I). Clinical picture and causative factors. Contact Dermatitis 34:125–133

48. Benzydamine Hydrochloride

CAS Registry Number [132–69–4]

It is a nonsteroidal anti-inflammatory drug used both topically and systemically. It has been reported as a sensitizer and a photosensitizer.

Suggested Reading
Foti C, Vena GA, Angelini G (1992) Occupational contact allergy to benzydamine hydrochloride. Contact Dermatitis 27:328–329
Lasa Elgezua O, Egino Gorrotxategi P, Gardeazabal García J, Ratón Nieto JA, Díaz Pérez JL (2004) Photoallergic hand eczema due to benzydamine. Eur J Dermatol 14:69–70

49. Benzyl Alcohol

CAS Registry Number [100–51–6]

Benzyl alcohol is mainly a preservative, mostly used in topical antimycotic or corticosteroid ointments. It is also a component catalyst for epoxy resins, and is contained in the color developer C-22. As a fragrance allergen, it has to be mentioned by name in cosmetics within the EU.

Suggested Reading
Lodi A, Mancini LL, Pozzi M, Chiarelli G, Crosti C (1993) Occupational airborne allergic contact dermatitis in parquet layers. Contact Dermatitis 29:281–282
Scheman AJ, Katta R (1997) Photographic allergens: an update. Contact Dermatitis 37:130
Sestini S, Mori M, Francalanci S (2004) Allergic contact dermatitis from benzyl alcohol in multiple medicaments. Contact Dermatitis 50:316–317

50. Benzyl Benzoate

Benzoic Acid Phenylmethyl Ester

CAS Registry Number [120–51–4]

Benzyl benzoate is the ester of benzyl alcohol and benzoic acid. It is contained in *Myroxylon pereirae* and Tolu balsam. It is used in acaricide preparations against *Sarcoptes scabiei* or as a pediculicide. Direct contact may cause skin irritation but rarely allergic contact dermatitis. As a fragrance allergen, benzyl benzoate has to be mentioned by name in EU cosmetics.

Suggested Reading
Meneghini CL, Vena GA, Angelini G (1982) Contact dermatitis to scabicides. Contact Dermatitis 8: 285–286

51. Benzyl Salicylate

Benzyl-o-Hydroxybenzoate, 2-Hydroxybenzoic Acid Phenylmethyl Ester

CAS Registry Number [118–58–1]

Benzyl salicylate is used as fixer in perfumery and in sunscreen preparations. As a (-weak) perfume sensitizer, it has to be listed by name in cosmetic preparations in the EU.

Suggested Reading
Larsen W, Nakayama H, Lindberg M, Fischer T, Elsner P, Burrows D, Jordan W, Shaw S, Wilkinson J, Marks J Jr, Sugawara M, Nethercott J (1996) Fragrance contact dermatitis: a worldwide multicenter investigation (Part I). Am J Contact Dermat 7:77–83

52. Benzylpenicillin

Penicillin G

CAS Registry Number [61–33–6]

Benzyl penicillin is actually used only intravenously. It was formerly a frequent cause of contact allergy in healthcare workers. Facial contact dermatitis was recently reported in a nurse.

Suggested Reading
Pecegueiro M (1990) Occupational contact dermatitis from penicillin. Contact Dermatitis 23: 190–191

53. BHA

Butylated Hydroxyanisole

CAS Registry Number [25013–16–5]

BHA is an antioxidant widely used in cosmetics and food. Contained in pastry, it can induce sensitization in caterers.

Suggested Reading
Acciai MC, Brusi C, Francalanci Giorgini S, Sertoli A (1993) Allergic contact dermatitis in caterers. Contact Dermatitis 28:48

54. BHT

Butylated Hydroxytoluene, 2,6-di-(tert-Butyl)-p-Cresol

CAS Registry Number [128–37–0]

This antioxidant is contained in food, adhesive glues, industrial oils and greases, including cutting fluids. Sensitization seems very rare.

Suggested Reading
Flyvholm MA, Menné T (1990) Sensitizing risk of butylated hydroxytoluene based on exposure and effect data. Contact Dermatitis 23:341–345

55. Bioban CS-1135

3,4-Dimethyloxazolidine + 3,4,4-Trimethyloxazolidine

CAS Registry Number [81099–36–7] (CAS Registry Number [51200–87–4] +
CAS Registry Number [75673–43–7])

Bioban® CS-1135 is the trade name for the two compounds 3,4-dimethyloxazolidine (74.8%) and 3,4,4-trimethyloxazolidine (2.5%). It is a formaldehyde releaser used as a preservative in latex paints and emulsions, and in cooling fluids. Dimethyl oxazolidine is found in some cosmetics. Bioban® CS-1135 can be a sensitizer per se, in patients without formaldehyde allergy.

Suggested Reading
Brinkmeier T, Geier J, Lepoittevin JP, Frosch PJ (2002) Patch test reactions to Biobans in metalworkers are often weak and not reproducible. Contact Dermatitis 47:27–31
Kanerva L, Estlander T, Jolanki R (1994) Occupational allergic contact dermatitis caused by thiourea compounds. Contact Dermatitis 31:242–248

56. Bioban® CS-1246

Oxazolidine, 5-Ethyl-1-aza-3,7-Dioxa-Bicyclo-3,3,0 Octane

CAS Registry Number [7747–35–5], [504–76–7]

Bioban® CS-1246 is a relatively old formaldehyde releaser, used in cutting oils. Bioban® CS-1248 is a mixture of Bioban® CS-1246 and Bioban® P-1487.

Suggested Reading
Brinkmeier T, Geier J, Lepoittevin JP, Frosch PJ (2002) Patch test reactions to Biobans in metalworkers are often weak and not reproducible. Contact Dermatitis 47:27–31

57. Bioban® P-1487

4-(2-Nitrobutyl)Morpholine + 4,4′-(2-Ethyl-2-Nitrodimethylene)Dimorpholine

**CAS Registry Number [37304–88–4] (CAS Registry Number [2224–44–4] +
CAS Registry Number [1854–23–5]**

51

Bioban® P-1487 is a mixture of 4-(2-nitrobutyl)morpholine CAS Registry Number
[2224–44–4] 70%, and 4,4′-(2-ethyl-2-nitrodimethylene)dimorpholine or 4,4′-(2-
ethyl-2-nitro-1,3-propanediyl)-bis-morpholine CAS Registry Number [1854–23–5]
20%. Both ingredients can be the sensitizers. It is used as a preservative in metalworking cutting fluids. Bioban® CS-1248 is a mixture of Bioban® CS-1246 and Bio-
ban® P-1487.

Suggested Reading
Brinkmeier T, Geier J, Lepoittevin JP, Frosch PJ (2002) Patch test reactions to Biobans in metalworkers are often weak and not reproducible. Contact Dermatitis 47:27–31
Gruvberger B, Bruze M, Zimerson E (1996) Contact allergy to the active ingredients of Bioban P
1487. Contact Dermatitis 35:141–145
Niklasson B, Björkner B, Sundberg K (1993) Contact allergy to a fatty acid ester component of
cutting fluids. Contact Dermatitis 28:265–267

58. Bisphenol A

Diphenylolpropane, Isopropylidene Diphenol

CAS Registry Number [80–05–7]

Bisphenol A is used with epichlorhydrin for the synthesis of epoxy resins bisphenol-
A type, for unsaturated polyester and polycarbonate resins, and epoxy di(meth)ac-
rylates. In epoxy resins, it leads to bisphenol-A diglycidyl ether, which is the
monomer of bisphenol-A-based epoxy resins. Reports of bisphenol-A sensitization
are rare and concern workers at epoxy resin plants, after contact with fiber glass,
semi-synthetic waxes, footwear, and dental materials. It is also a possible sensitizer
in vinyl gloves.

Suggested Reading
Jolanki R, Kanerva L, Estlander T (1995) Occupational allergic contact dermatitis caused by epoxy
diacrylate in ultraviolet-light-cured paint, and bisphenol A in dental composite resin. Contact
Dermatitis 33:94–99
Matthieu L, Godoi AFL, Lambert J, van Grieken R (2004) Occupational allergic contact dermatitis
from bisphenol A in vinyl gloves. Contact Dermatitis 49:281–283
Van Jost T, Roesyanto ID, Satyawan I (1990) Occupational sensitization to epichlorhydrin (ECH)
and bisphenol-A during the manufacture of epoxy resin. Contact Dermatitis 22:125–126

59. Bisphenol A Diglycidyl Ether (DGEBA)

BADGE

CAS Registry Number [1675–54–3]

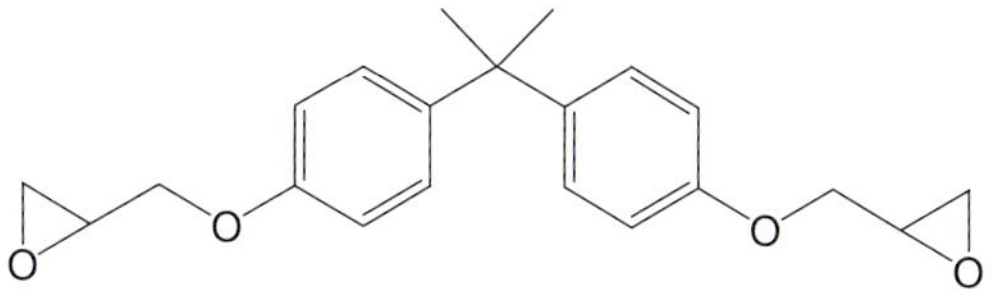

Most epoxy resins result from polymerization of bisphenol A diglycidyl ether (BADGE). Delayed hypersensitivity is caused by the low-molecular-weight monomer BADGE (Mol. Wt. 340 g/mol), the dimer having much a lower sensitization power. This allergen caused contact dermatitis in six workers in a plant producing printed circuits boards made of copper sheets and fiber glass fabric impregnated with a brominated epoxy resin. It can be contained in adhesives.

Suggested Reading

Bruze M, Almgren G (1989) Occupational dermatoses in workers exposed to epoxy-impregnated fiberglass fabric. Dermatosen 37:171–176

Bruze M, Edenholm M, Engenström K, Svensson G (1996) Occupational dermatoses in a Swedish aircraft plant. Contact Dermatitis 34:336–340

Hansson C (1994) Determination of monomers in epoxy resin hardened at elevated temperatures. Contact Dermatitis 31:333–334

60. *o-p′*-Bisphenol F and *p-p′*-Bisphenol F

2,4′-Dihydroxy-Diphenylmethane and 4-4′-Dihydroxy-Diphenylmethane

CAS Registry Number [2467–03–0] and CAS Registry Number [620–92–8]

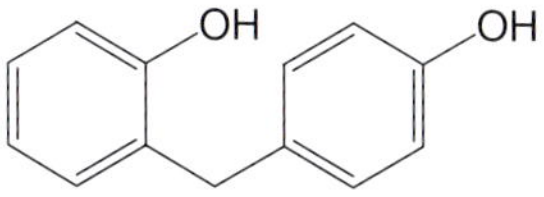

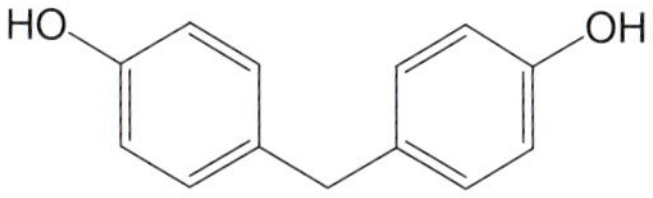

o-p′-Bisphenol F and *p-p′*-bisphenol F are allergenic components of phenol-formaldehyde resins resol-type.

Suggested Reading

Bruze M, Fregert S, Zimerson E (1985) Contact allergy to phenol-formaldehyde resins. Contact Dermatitis 12:81–86

61. Bisphenol F Diglycidyl Ether (DGEBF)

1. *p, p′*-Diglycidyl Ether of Bisphenol F

CAS Registry Number [2095–03–6]

2. *o,p′*-Diglycidyl Ether of Bisphenol F

CAS Registry Number [57469–08–5]

3. *o,o′*-Diglycidyl Ether of Bisphenol F

CAS Registry Number [39817–09–9], [54208–63–8]

Epoxy resins based on Bisphenol F, also called phenolic Novolac, contain bisphenol F diglycidyl ether, which has three sensitizing isomers. DGEBF has a greater resistance than DGEBA. Contact allergy to bisphenol-F based epoxy resins is rarer than that due to bisphenol-A-based resins, and is frequently acquired with flooring materials and putty.

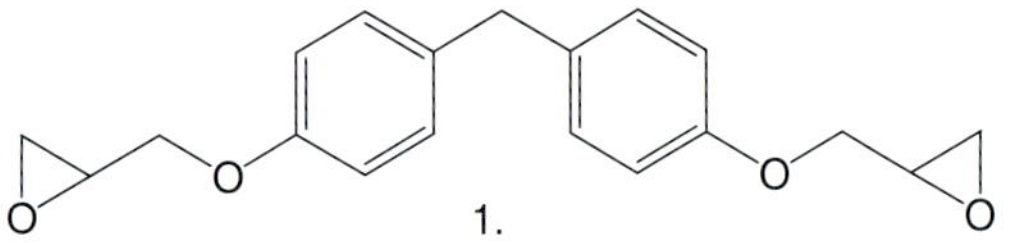

51

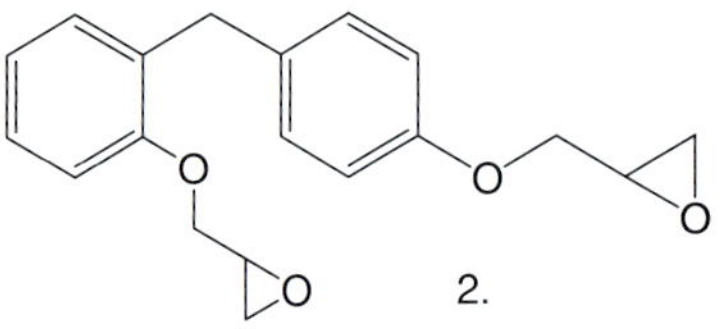

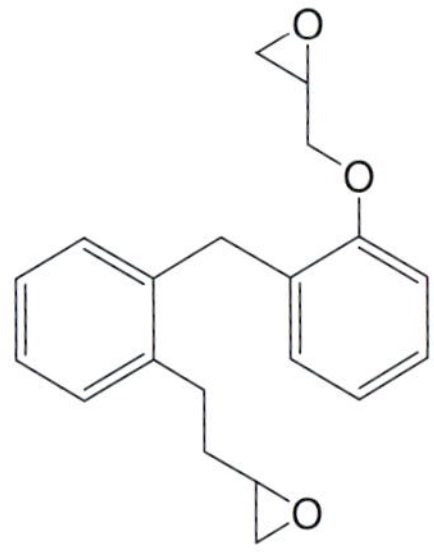

Suggested Reading

Bruze M, Edenholm M, Engenström K, Svensson G (1996) Occupational dermatoses in a Swedish aircraft plant. Contact Dermatitis 34:336–340
Pontén A, Bruze M (2001) Contact allergy to epoxy resin based on diglycidyl ether of Bisphenol F. Contact Dermatitis 44:98–99
Pontén A, Zimerson E, Bruze M (2004) Contact allergy to the isomers of diglycidyl ether of bisphenol F. Acta Derm Venereol (Stockh) 84:12–17

62. Brominated Epoxy Resin

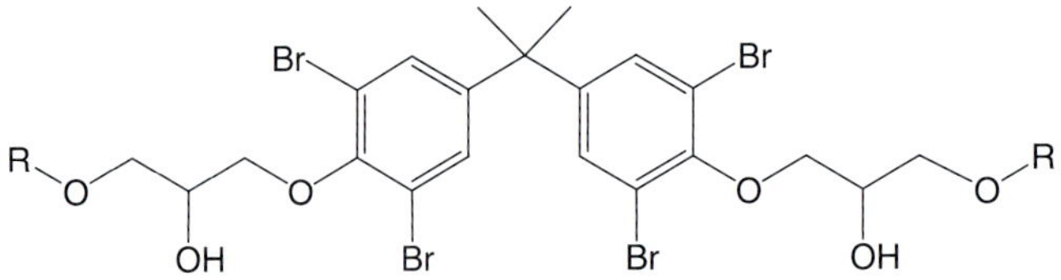

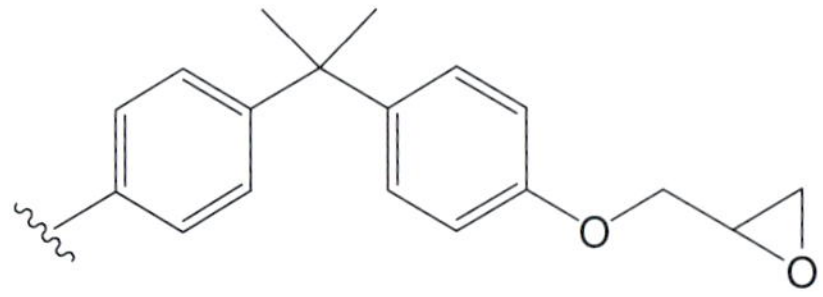

As a component of nondiglycidyl ether of bisphenol A epoxy resins, brominated epoxy resin caused contact dermatitis in a cleaner of worksites in a condenser factory, where condensers were filled with a mixture made of an epoxy resin.

Suggested Reading

Kanerva L, Jolanki R, Estlander T (1991) Allergic contact dermatitis from non-diglycidyl-ether-of-bisphenol-A epoxy resins. Contact Dermatitis 24:293–300

63. 1-Bromo-3-Chloro-5,5-Dimethylhydantoin

Di-Halo, 1-Bromo-3-Chloro-5,5-Dimethyl-2,4-Imidazolidinedione, Agribrom, Slimicide C 77P

CAS Registry Number [16079–88–2]

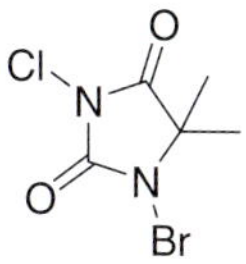

This chlorinated and brominated product is employed in agriculture as a fungicide, for wood preservation. When used to sanitize pools and spas, releasing both chlorine and bromine derivatives, it can induce irritant or allergic contact dermatitis.

Suggested Reading

Rycroft RJG, Penny PT (1983) Dermatoses associated with brominated swimming pools. Br Med J (Clin Res Ed) 287 : 462

Sasseville D, Moreau L (2004) Contact allergy to 1-bromo-3chloro-5, 5-dimethylhydantoin in spa water. Contact Dermatitis 50 : 323–324

64. Bromohydroxyacetophenone

1. 2-Bromo-4′-Hydroxyacetophenone, 1-(4-Hydroxyphenyl)-2-Bromoethanone

CAS Registry Number [2491–38–5]

2. 2-Bromo-2′-Hydroxyacetophenone, (6CI, 7CI, 8CI)

CAS Registry Number [2491–36–3]

3. 5′-Bromo-2′-Hydroxy-Acetophenone (6CI, 7CI, 8CI), 1-(5-Bromo-2-Hydroxyphenyl)Ethanone

CAS Registry Number [1450–75–5]

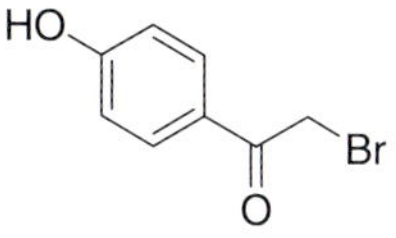

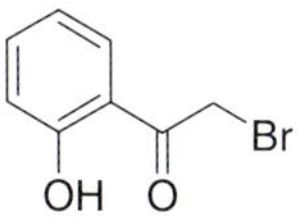

Those substances are biocides used in emulsions, paints, adhesives, waxes, and polishes. They are both irritants and sensitizers. 2-Bromo-4′-hydroxyacetophenone used as a slimicide provoked sensitization after an accidental spillage, and recurrent allergic contact dermatitis at a workplace.

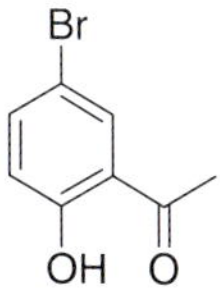

Suggested Reading

Jensen CD, Andersen KE (2003) Allergic contact dermatitis from a paper mill slimicide containing 2-bromo-4′-hydroxyacetophenone. Am J Contact Dermat 14 : 41–43

65. Bronopol

2-Bromo 2-Nitro 1,3-Propanediol

CAS Registry Number [52–51–7]

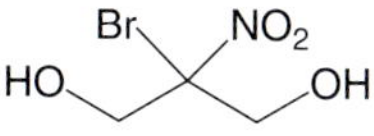

Bronopol is a preservative sometimes considered as a formaldehyde releaser. It was reported to be an allergen in cosmetics, cleaning agents, in dairy workers, and in a lubricant jelly used for ultrasound examination.

Suggested Reading
Grattan CEH, Harman RRM, Tan RSH (1986) Milk recorder dermatitis. Contact Dermatitis 14:
    217–220
Wilson CL, Powell SM (1990) An unusual cause of allergic contact dermatitis in a veterinary sur-
    geon. Contact Dermatitis 23:42–43

66. Budesonide

Budesonide

CAS Registry number [51333–22–3]

R-Budesonide

CAS Registry Number [51372–29–3]

S-Budesonide

CAS Registry Number [51372–28–2]

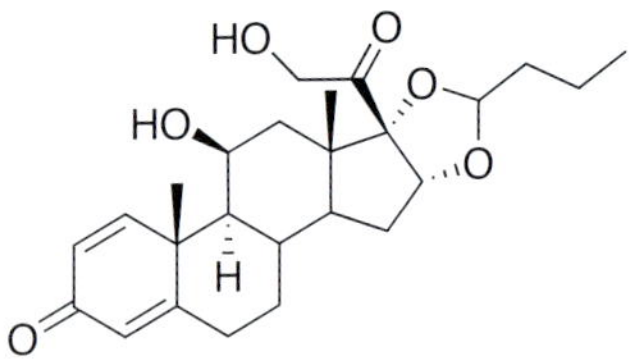

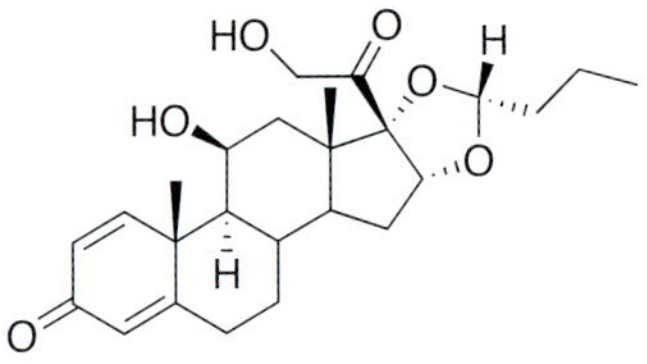

R-Budesonide

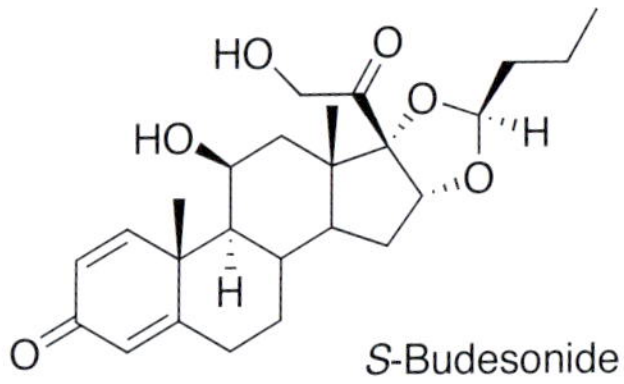

S-Budesonide

Budesonide is a corticosteroid, a blend of two diastereosiomers.

R-Budesonide is a marker of the B group of corticosteroids. Such molecules have a *cis*-diol moiety or an acetal moiety on the C_{16} and C_{17} of the D cycle. One side chain is possible on C_{21}. The B group comprises amcinonide, budesonide, desonide or prednacinolone, flunisolide, fluocinolone and its acetonide, fluocinonide, fluchlorolone and its acetonide, halcinonide, and acetonide, benetonide, diacetate and hexacetonide of triamcinolone.

S-Budesonide is a marker of the D2 group of corticosteroids. Such molecules are nonmethylated in C_{16} and have an ester function in C_{17}. They comprise hydrocortisone 17-butyrate, hydrocortisone-17-valerate, hydrocortisone aceponate, methylprednisolone aceponate, and prednicarbate.

Suggested Reading
Lepoittevin JP, Drieghe J, Dooms-Goossens A (1995) Studies in patients with corticosteroid contact
    allergy. Understanding cross-reactivity among different steroids. Arch Dermatol 131:31–37
Le Coz CJ (2002) Fiche d'éviction en cas d'hypersensibilité aux corticoïdes. Ann Dermatol Vener-
    eol 129:346–347
Le Coz CJ (2002) Fiche d'éviction en cas d'hypersensibilité au 17 butyrate d'hydrocortisone. Ann
    Dermatol Venereol 129:931
Le Coz CJ (2002) Fiche d'éviction en cas d'hypersensibilité au budésonide. Ann Dermatol Venere-
    ol 129:1409–1410

67. 1,4-Butanediol Diglycidyl Ether

CAS Registry Number [2425–79–8]

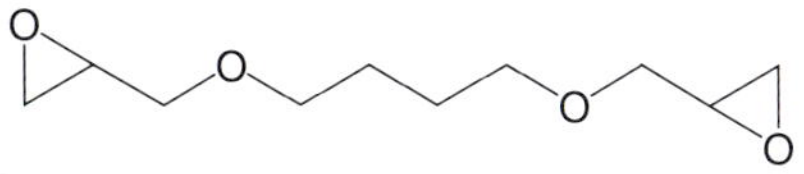

This substance is a reactive diluent in epoxy resins.

Suggested Reading

Jolanki R, Estlander T, Kanerva L (1987) Contact allergy to an epoxy reactive diluent: 1,4-butane-diol diglycidyl ether. Contact Dermatitis 16:87–92

Jolanki R, Kanerva L, Estlander T, Tarvainen K, Keskinen H, Henriks-Eckerman ML (1990) Occu-pational dermatoses from epoxy resin compounds. Contact Dermatitis 23:172–183

68. *N-tert*-Butyl-bis-(2-Benzothiazole) Sulfenamide

CAS Registry Number [3741–80–8]

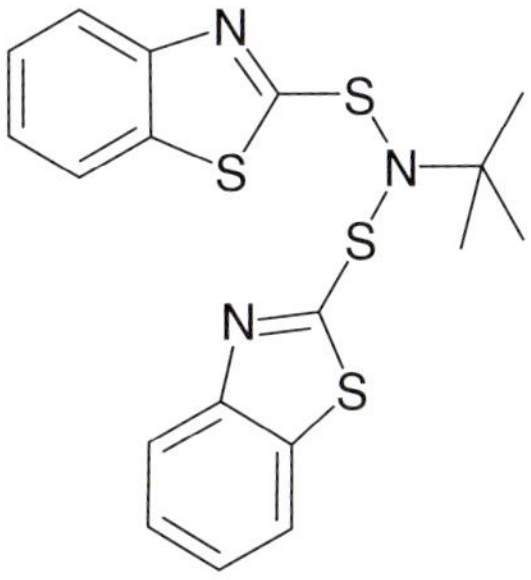

This mercaptobenzothiazole-sulfenamide chemical is used as an accelerator in rub-ber vulcanization.

Suggested Reading

Le Coz CJ (2004) Fiche d'éviction en cas d'hypersensibilité au mercaptobenzothiazole et au mer-capto mix. Ann Dermatol Venereol 131:846–848

69. Butyl Carbitol

Diethylene Glycol Monobutyl Ether

CAS Registry Number [112–34–5]

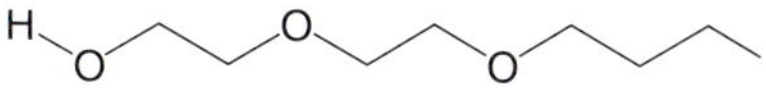

This organic solvent belongs to the carbitols group, and is included in waterbased liquids such as paints, surface cleaners, polishes and disinfectants. It is considered to be an exceptional allergen.

Suggested Reading

Berlin K, Johanson G, Lindberg M (1995) Hypersensitivity to 2-(2-butoxyethoxy)ethanol. Contact Dermatitis 32:54

Schliemann-Willers S, Bauer A, Elsner P (2000) Occupational contact dermatitis from diethylene glycol monobutyl ether in a podiatrist. Contact Dermatitis 43:225

70. *p-tert*-Butyl Catechol

CAS Registry Number [98–29–3]

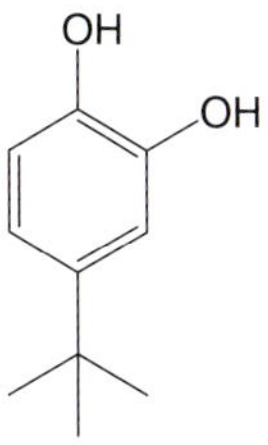

para-tert-Butyl catechol is specially prepared by reacting the impure catechol fraction with tertiary butyl alcohol. It is used for its various properties (inhibitor of polymerization and antioxidizing agent) in the manufacture of rubber, plastics and paints, in the preparation of petrolatum products, and as an anti-oxidant in oils. It may induce vitiligo.

Suggested Reading
Gawkrodger DJ, Cork MJ, Bleehen SS (1991) Occupational vitiligo and contact sensitivity to para-tertiary butyl catechol. Contact Dermatitis 25:200–201

71. *n*-Butyl Glycidyl Ether

CAS Registry Number [2426–08–6]

A reactive diluent used to reduce viscosity of epoxy resins Bisphenol A type.

Suggested Reading
Holness DL, Nethercott JR (1993) The performance of specialized collections of bisphenol A epoxy resin system components in the evaluation of workers in an occupational health clinic population. Contact Dermatitis 28:216–219
Jolanki R, Kanerva L, Estlander T, Tarvainen K, Keskinen H, Henriks-Eckerman ML (1990) Occupational dermatoses from epoxy resin compounds. Contact Dermatitis 23:172–183

72. *tert*-Butyl-Hydroquinone

2-*tert*-Butylhydroquinone, TBHQ

CAS Registry Number [1948–33–0]

This antioxidant has seldom been reported as a sensitizer, mainly in cosmetics (lipsticks, lip-gloss, hair dyes) or in cutting oils. Simultaneous/cross-reactions have been described to butylhydroxyanisole (BHA) and less frequently to butylhydroxytoluene (BHT) but not to hydroquinone.

Suggested Reading
Aalto-Korte K (2000) Allergic contact dermatitis from tertiary-butylhydroquinone (TBHQ) in a vegetable hydraulic oil. Contact Dermatitis 43:303
Le Coz CJ, Schneider GA (1998) Contact dermatitis from tertiary-butylhydroquinone in a hair dye, with cross-sensitivity to BHA and BHT. Contact Dermatitis 39:39–40

73. *p-tert*-Butyl-alpha-Methylhydrocinnamic Aldehyde

**Lilial®, 2-(4-*tert*-Butylbenzyl)Propionaldehyde,
4-(1,1-Dimethylethyl)-α-Methyl-Benzenepropanal,
p-tert-Butyl-α-Methylhydrocinnamaldehyde, Lilestral**

CAS Registry Number [80–54–6]

Lilial® is a synthetic compound listed as a fragrance allergen. Its presence is indicated on cosmetics within the EU.

Suggested Reading
Giménez-Arnau E, Andersen KE, Bruze M, Frosch PJ, Johansen JD, Menné T, Rastogi SC, White IR, Lepoittevin JP (2000) Identification of Lilial as a fragrance sensitizer in a perfume by bioassay-guided chemical fractionation and structure-activity relationships. Contact Dermatitis 43:351–358

74. Butylene Glycol

1,3-Butylene Glycol, 1,3-Butanediol

CAS Registry Number [107–88–0]

This dihydric alcohol is used for its humectant and preservative potentiator properties in cosmetics, topical medicaments and polyurethane, polyester, cellophane, and cigarettes. It has similar properties but is less irritant than propylene glycol. Contact allergies seem to be rare.

Suggested Reading
Diegenant C, Constandt L, Goossens A (2000) Allergic contact dermatitis due to 1,3-butylene glycol. Contact Dermatitis 43:324–235
Matsunaga K, Sugai T, Katoh J, Hayakawa R, Kozuka T, Itoh J, Tsuyuki S, Hosono K (1997) Group study on contact sensitivity of 1,3-butylene glycol. Environ Dermatol 4:195–205

75. *Para-tert*-Butylphenol

CAS Registry Number [98–54–4]

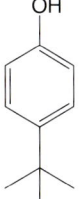

Para-tert-butylphenol is used with formaldehyde to produce the polycondensate *p-tert*-butylphenol formaldehyde resins (PTBPFR). Major occupational sources are neoprene glues and adhesives in industry, in the shoemaking and leather industries or in car production. It is also used as a box preservative in box and furniture manufacture, and in the production of casting molds, car brake linings, insulated electrical cables, adhesives, printing inks, and paper laminates. *Para-tert*-butyl-phenol seems to be the sensitizer.

Suggested Reading
Handley J, Todd D, Bingham A, Corbett R, Burrows D (1993) Allergic contact dermatitis from *para-tertiary*-butylphenol-formaldehyde resin (PTBP-F-R) in Northern Ireland. Contact Dermatitis 29:144–146
Mancuso G, Reggiani M, Berdondini RM (1996) Occupational dermatitis in shoemakers. Contact Dermatitis 34:17–22
Shono M, Ezoe K, Kaniwa MA, Ikarashi Y, Kohma S, Nakamura A (1991) Allergic contact dermatitis from para-tertiary-butylphenol-formaldehyde resin (PTBP-FR) in athletic tape and leather adhesive. Contact Dermatitis 24:281–288
Tarvainen K (1995) Analysis of patients with allergic patch test reactions to a plastics and glue series. Contact Dermatitis 32:346–351

76. Caffeic Acid Dimethyl Allylic Ester

3-Methyl-2-Butenyl-Caffeate

CAS Registry Number [108084–13–7]

This is the major allergen of poplar bud resins and of propolis, the bee glue derived almost exclusively from poplar buds.

Suggested Reading

Lamminpää A, Estlander T, Jolanki R, Kanerva L (1996) Occupational allergic contact dermatitis caused by decorative plants. Contact Dermatitis 34:330–335

Oliwiecki S, Beck MH, Hausen BM (1992) Occupational contact dermatitis from caffeates in poplar bud resin in a tree surgeon. Contact Dermatitis 27:127–128

77. Captafol

CAS Registry Number [2425–06–1]

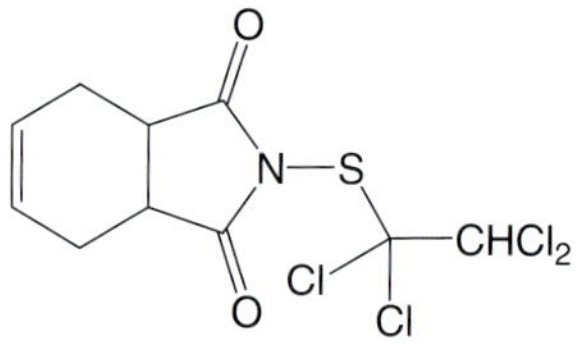

Captafol is a pesticide, belonging to thiophthalimide group. Occupational contact dermatitis was reported in an agricultural worker who had multiple sensitizations.

Suggested Reading

Peluso AM, Tardio M, Adamo F, Venturo N (1991) Multiple sensitization due to bis-dithiocarbamate and thiophthalimide pesticides. Contact Dermatitis 25:327

78. Captan

Captane, *N*-Trichloromethylmercaptotetrahydrophtalimide

CAS Registry Number [133–06–2]

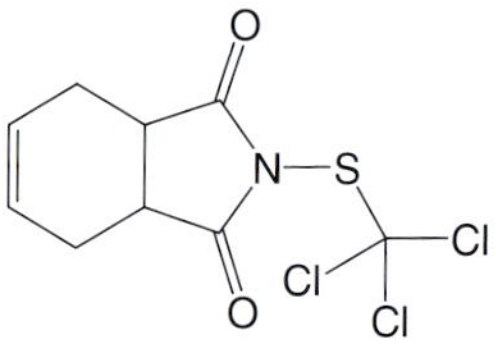

A pesticide, belonging to the thiophthalimide group, mainly affecting agricultural workers. Sensitizer and photosensitizer, it can induce contact urticaria. It is used as a fungicide and a bacteriostatic agent in cosmetics and toiletries, particularly in shampoos. Cases of contact dermatitis were reported in painters, polishers, and varnishers.

Suggested Reading

Aguirre A, Manzano D, Zabala R, Raton JA, Diaz-Perez JL (1994) Contact allergy to captan in a hairdresser. Contact Dermatitis 31:46

Moura C, Dias M, Vale T (1994) Contact dermatitis in painters, polishers and varnishers. Contact Dermatitis 31:51–53

O'Malley M, Rodriguez P, Maibach HI (1995) Pesticide patch testing: California nursery workers and controls. Contact Dermatitis 32:61–62

Peluso AM, Tardio M, Adamo F, Venturo N (1991) Multiple sensitization due to bis-dithiocarbamate and thiophthalimide pesticides. Contact Dermatitis 25:327

Vilaplana J, Romaguera C (1993) Captan, a rare contact sensitizer in hairdressing. Contact Dermatitis 29:107

79. Carbaryl

CAS Registry Number [63–25–2]

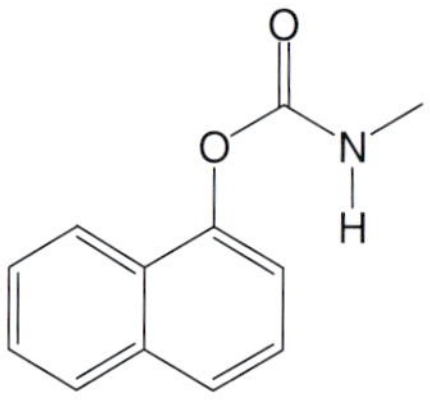

Carbaryl is a pesticide, insecticide, of the carbonate group. It induced sensitization in a farmer.

Suggested Reading
Sharma VK, Kaur S (1990) Contact sensitization by pesticides in farmers. Contact Dermatitis 23: 77–80

80. Carbodiimide

Cyanamide

CAS Registry Number [420–04–2]

Cyanamide and its salts are used in various occasions such as in chemistry, in anti-rust solutions or in a drug (Come®) for treating alcoholism.

Suggested Reading
Goday Bujan JJ, Yanguas Bayona I, Arechavala RS (1994) Allergic contact dermatitis from cyanamide: report of 3 cases. Contact Dermatitis 31:331–332

81. Carbofuran

CAS Registry Number [1563–66–2]

It is a pesticide with insecticide properties, of the carbamate group. It was implicated as a sensitizer in two farmers.

Suggested Reading
Sharma VK, Kaur S (1990) Contact sensitization by pesticides in farmers. Contact Dermatitis 23: 77–80

82. Cardols

Cardols are a mixture of several analog molecules with an alkyl chain (-R) with 13, 15, 17, or 19 carbon and 0–3 unsaturations. One of the main cashew nut shell liquid components, along with anacardic acid. Sensitization occurs in cashew nut workers. See also Chap. 41, Plants and Plant Products.

Suggested Reading
Diogenes MJN, De Morais SM, Carvalho FF (1996) Contact dermatitis among cashew nut workers. Contact Dermatitis 35:114–115

83. Δ-3-Carene

CAS Registry Number [13466–78–9]

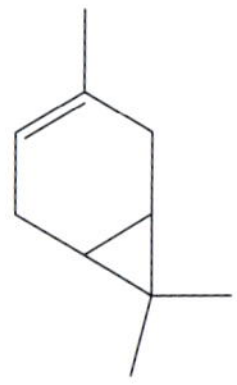

Hydroperoxides of Δ-3-carene are allergens contained in turpentine. Occupational exposure occurs in painters, varnishers, or in ceramic decoration. The percentage of Δ-3-carene is higher in Indonesian than in Portuguese turpentine.

Suggested Reading
Lear JT, Heagerty AHM, Tan BB, Smith AG, English JSC (1996) Transient re-emergence of oil turpentine allergy in the pottery industry. Contact Dermatitis 35:169–172

51

84. Carteolol

CAS Registry Number [51781–06–7]

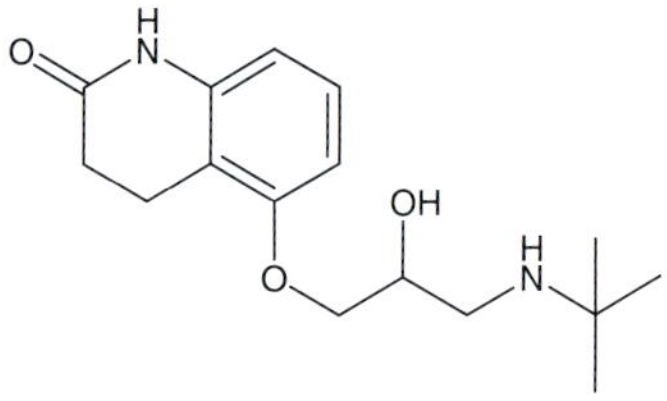

Carteolol was implicated in allergic contact dermatitis due to beta-blockers agents in eye-drops.

Suggested Reading
Giordano-Labadie F, Lepoittevin JP, Calix I, Bazex J (1997) Allergie de contact aux â-bloqueurs des collyres: allergie croisée? Ann Dermatol Venereol 124:322–324

85. CD1

N,N-Diethylparaphenylenediamine Monochlorhydrate

CAS Registry Number [2198–58–5]

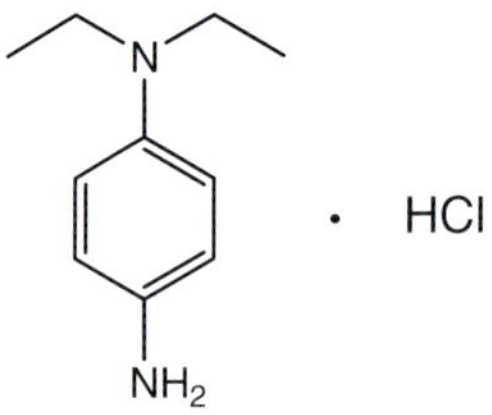

· HCl

A color film developer. It is an allergen and an irritant in photographers. Cross-reactivity is possible with Disperse Blue 124, Disperse Blue 106, and Disperse red 17 but not with *para*-amino compounds.

Suggested Reading
Aguirre A, Landa N, Gonzalez M, Diaz-Perez JL (1992) Allergic contact dermatitis in a photographer. Contact Dermatitis 27:340–341
Galindo PA, Garcia R, Garrido JA, Feo F, Fernandez F (1994) Allergic contact dermatitis from colour developers: absence of cross-sensitivity to para-amino compounds. Contact Dermatitis 30:301
Hansson C, Ahlfors S, Bergendorff O (1997) Concomitant contact dermatitis due to textile dyes and to colour film developers can be explained by the formation of the same hapten. Contact Dermatitis 37:27–31
Lidén C, Brehmer-Andersson E (1988) Occupational dermatoses from colour developing agents. Clinical and histopathological observations. Acta Derm Venereol (Stockh) 68:514–522

86. CD2

4-*N,N*-Diethyl-2-Methyl-1,4-Phenylenediamine (Hydrochloride)

CAS Registry Number [2051–79–8]

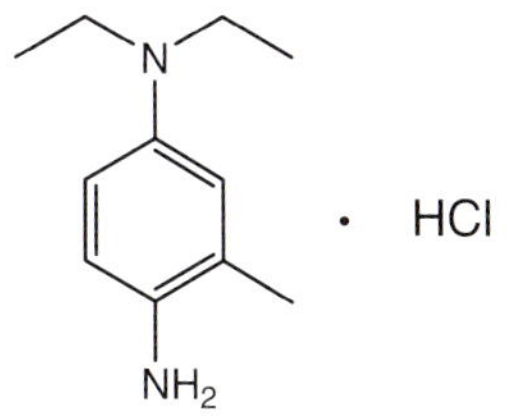

A color film developer. It acts as an allergen and an irritant in photographers. Cross-reactivity is possible with Disperse Blue 124, Disperse Blue 106, and Disperse Red 17 but not to *para*-amino compounds.

Suggested Reading

Aguirre A, Landa N, Gonzalez M, Diaz-Perez JL (1992) Allergic contact dermatitis in a photographer. Contact Dermatitis 27:340–341

Galindo PA, Garcia R, Garrido JA, Feo F, Fernandez F (1994) Allergic contact dermatitis from colour developers: absence of cross-sensitivity to para-amino compounds. Contact Dermatitis 30:301

Hansson C, Ahlfors S, Bergendorff O (1997) Concomitant contact dermatitis due to textile dyes and to colour film developers can be explained by the formation of the same hapten. Contact Dermatitis 37:27–31

Lidén C, Brehmer-Andersson E (1988) Occupational dermatoses from colour developing agents. Clinical and histopathological observations. Acta Derm Venereol (Stockh) 68:514–522

Rustemeyer T, Frosch PJ (1995) Allergic contact dermatitis from colour film developers. Contact Dermatitis 32:59–60

87. CD3

4-(Ethyl-*N*-2-Methan-Sulfonamidoethyl)-2-Methyl-1,4-Phenylenediamine (*1,5H$_2$SO$_4$ *H$_2$O)

CAS Registry Number [25646–71–3]

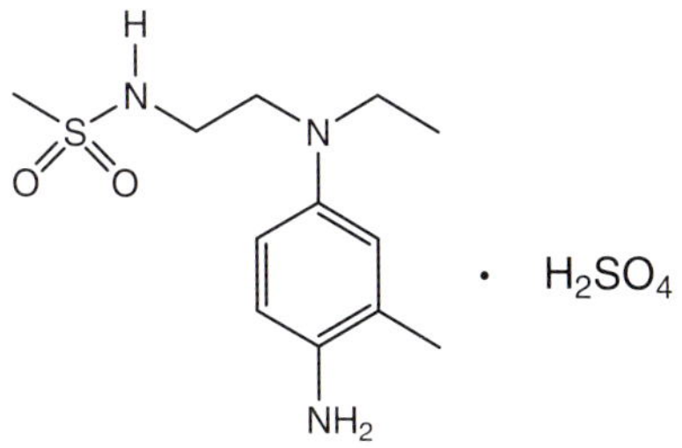

A color film developer. It caused some allergic reactions in photographers. Cross-reactivity is possible with Disperse Blue 124, Disperse Blue 106, and Disperse Red 17

Suggested Reading

Aguirre A, Landa N, Gonzalez M, Diaz-Perez JL (1992) Allergic contact dermatitis in a photographer. Contact Dermatitis 27:340–341

Galindo PA, Garcia R, Garrido JA, Feo F, Fernandez F (1994) Allergic contact dermatitis from colour developers: absence of cross-sensitivity to para-amino compounds. Contact Dermatitis 30:301

Hansson C, Ahlfors S, Bergendorff O (1997) Concomitant contact dermatitis due to textile dyes and to colour film developers can be explained by the formation of the same hapten. Contact Dermatitis 37:27–31

Lidén C, Brehmer-Andersson E (1988) Occupational dermatoses from colour developing agents. Clinical and histopathological observations. Acta Derm Venereol (Stockh) 68:514–522

Rustemeyer T, Frosch PJ (1995) Allergic contact dermatitis from colour developers. Contact Dermatitis 32:59–60

Scheman AJ, Katta R (1997) Photographic allergens: an update. Contact Dermatitis 37:130

88. CD4

4-(Ethyl-*N*-Hydroxyethyl)-2-Methyl-1,4-Phenylenediamine (*H_2SO_4*H_2O)

CAS Registry Number [25646–77–9]

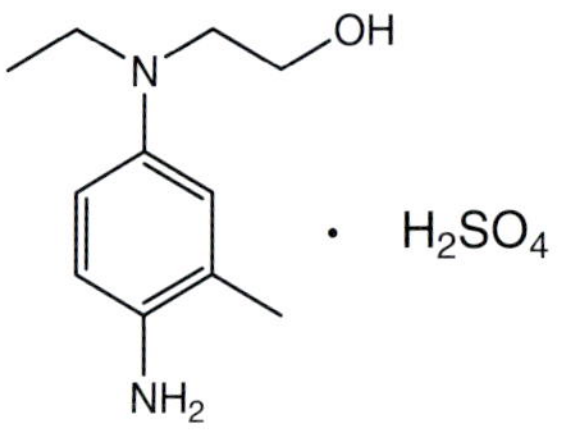

$\cdot \ H_2SO_4$

Color film developer. It is both an allergen and an irritant in photographers. Cross-reactivity is possible with Disperse Blue 124, Disperse Blue 106, and Disperse Red 17.

Suggested Reading

Aguirre A, Landa N, Gonzalez M, Diaz-Perez JL (1992) Allergic contact dermatitis in a photographer. Contact Dermatitis 27:340–341

Galindo PA, Garcia R, Garrido JA, Feo F, Fernandez F (1994) Allergic contact dermatitis from colour developers: absence of cross-sensitivity to para-amino compounds. Contact Dermatitis 30:301

Hansson C, Ahlfors S, Bergendorff O (1997) Concomitant contact dermatitis due to textile dyes and to colour film developers can be explained by the formation of the same hapten. Contact Dermatitis 37:27–31

Lidén C, Brehmer-Andersson E (1988) Occupational dermatoses from colour developing agents. Clinical and histopathological observations. Acta Derm Venereol (Stockh) 68:514–522

Rustemeyer T, Frosch PJ (1995) Allergic contact dermatitis from colour developers. Contact Dermatitis 32:59–60

Scheman AJ, Katta R (1997) Photographic allergens: an update. Contact Dermatitis 37:130

89. CD6

4-Amino-*N*-Ethyl-*N*-(2-Methoxyethyl)-2-Methyl Paraphenylenediamine di-*p*-Toluene Sulfonate

CAS Registry Number [50928–80–8]

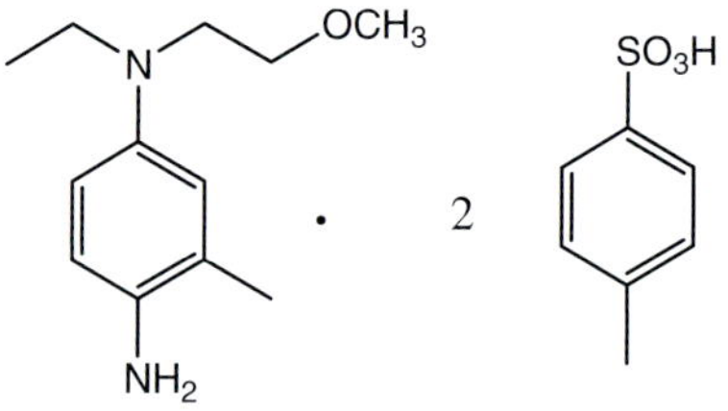

$\cdot \ 2$

This color film developer rarely induced contact dermatitis in photographers.

Suggested Reading

Lidén C (1989) Occupational dermatoses at a film laboratory. Contact Dermatitis 20:191–200

Lidén C, Brehmer-Andersson E (1988) Occupational dermatoses from colour developing agents. Clinical and histopathological observations. Acta Derm Venereol (Stockh) 68:514–522

90. Cefaclor

CAS Registry Number [70356–03–5]

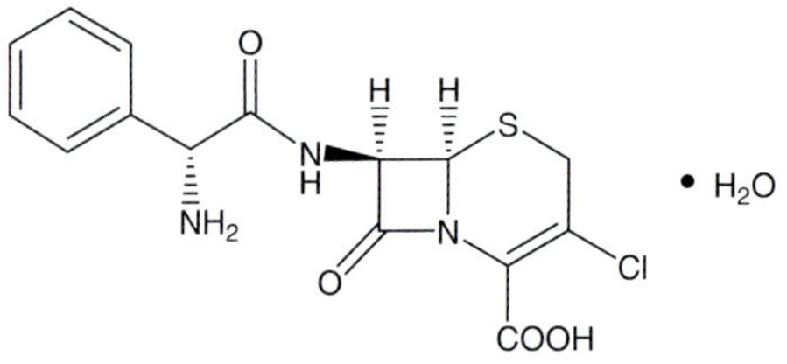

$\cdot \ H_2O$

51

Cefaclor is a semi-synthetic cephalosporin antibiotic, related to cefalexin, and a frequent inducer of serum sickness-like reactions.

Suggested Reading

Hebert AA, Sigman ES, Levy ML (1991) Serum sickness-like reactions from cefaclor in children. J Am Acad Dermatol 25:805–808

91. Cephalosporins

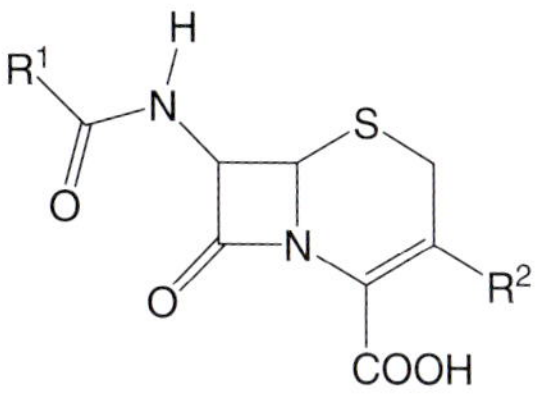

All cephalosporins have a 7-amino-cephalosporanic group (cephem nucleus). They differ by a C_7 and a C_3 substitution. The cause of an allergic reaction to cephalosporins can be the cephem nucleus itself, but this seems to be rare. Allergic contact dermatitis from cephalosporins is uncommon and mainly occurs in healthcare, pharmaceutical, and veterinary professions. Systemic drug reactions are more frequent, and can involve an immuno-allergic mechanism or not. Some of them are severe and life threatening.

Cefaclor is frequently responsible for serum thickness diseases. Cefotaxime, ceftizoxime, ceftazidime, ceftriaxone and cefodizime, several third-generation cephalosporins, caused positive patch reactions in a sensitized nurse. Cefazoline, cefoxitin, ceftriaxone, and ceftazidime were responsible for contact dermatitis in a nurse. Sensitivity to cephalothin, cephamandol and cephazolin, cephalosporins of the first and second generation, was reported in a pharmaceutical laboratory analyst. Ceftiofur sodium, a third-generation veterinary cephalosporin, caused contact dermatitis in two chicken vaccinators. No cross-sensitivity was observed to other cephalosporins. Cephalexin hypersensitivity was reported in three cases, and to cefuroxime in one case with cross-reaction to cephalotin and cephaloridine.

Suggested Reading

Condé-Salazar L, Guimaraens D, Romero LV, Gonzales MA (1986) Occupational dermatitis from cephalosporins. Contact Dermatitis 14:70–71

Filipe P, Soares Almeida RSL, Guerra Rodrigo F (1996) Occupational allergic contact dermatitis from cephalosporins. Contact Dermatitis 34:226

Foti C, Vena GA, Cucurachi MR, Angelini G (1994) Occupational contact allergy from cephalosporins. Contact Dermatitis 31:129–130

Garcia-Bravo B, Gines E, Russo F (1995) Occupational contact dermatitis from ceftiofur sodium. Contact Dermatitis 33:62–63

Romano A, Pietrantonio F, Di Fonso M, Venuti A (1992) Delayed hypersensitivity to cefuroxime. Contact Dermatitis 27:270–271

92. Cetearyl Isononanoate

Cetearyl Hexadecyl Isononanoate

CAS Registry Number [84878–33–1]

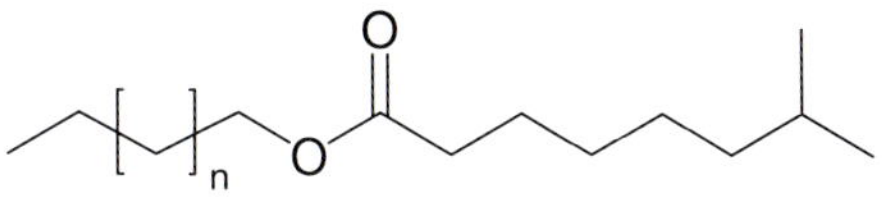

n: 14 to 16

This substance results from esterification of a saturated C_{16} to C_{18} alcohol, namely cetyl or stearyl alcohol, and a branched chain isononanoic acid. It is used as a hair conditioning agent, a skin conditioning agent, and an emollient, and is found in several moisturizing creams.

Suggested Reading

Le Coz CJ, Bressieux A (2003) Allergic contact dermatitis from cetearyl isononanoate. Contact Dermatitis 48:343

93. Chloramphenicol

CAS Registry Number [56–75–7]

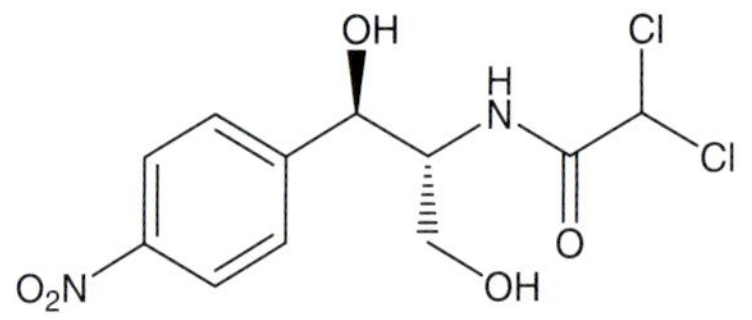

This broad spectrum phenicol group antibiotic has been implicated in allergic contact dermatitis. Cross-sensitivity to thiamphenicol is possible but not systematic.

Suggested Reading

Le Coz CJ, Santinelli F (1998) Facial contact dermatitis from chloramphenicol with cross-sensitivity to thiamphenicol. Contact Dermatitis 38:108–109

94. Chlorhexidine (Digluconate)

CAS Registry Number [55–56–1] (CAS Registry Number [18472–51–0])

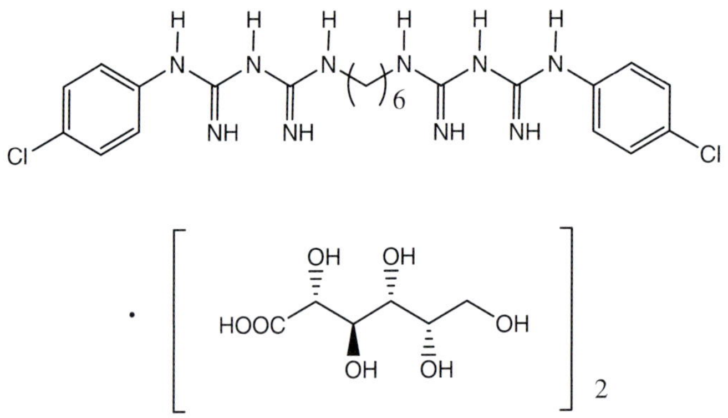

Chlorhexidine is a broad-spectrum antimicrobial agent, a synthetic biguanide antiseptic and disinfectant, available under different forms (diacetate, dihydrochloride, and mostly digluconate). It is also used as a biocide in several topicals and cosmetics. It may cause allergic contact dermatitis, photosensitivity or even fixed drug eruption, mainly after prolonged and repeated applications in health workers, leg ulcer, and leg eczema patients. Immediate-type reactions have been reported: contact urticaria, asthma, and anaphylactic shock.

Suggested Reading

Krautheim AB, Jermann THM, Bircher AJ (2004) Chlorhexidine anaphylaxis: case report and review of the literature. Contact Dermatitis 50:113–116

Rudzki E, Rebandel P, Grzywa Z (1989) Patch tests with occupational contactants in nurses, doctors and dentists. Contact Dermatitis 20:247–250

51

95. 5-Chloro-1-Methyl-4-Nitroimidazole

CAS Registry Number [4897–25–0]

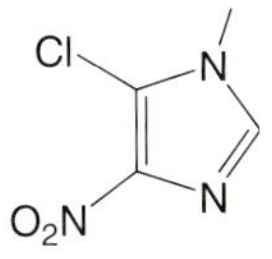

This intermediate in azathioprine synthesis is also present in the end product. It induced contact dermatitis in a man working on azathioprine synthesis. Cross-reactivity is possible with imidazoles tioconazole and econazole.

Suggested Reading

Jolanki R, Alanko K, Pfäffli P, Estlander T, Kanerva L (1997) Occupational allergic contact dermatitis from 5-chloro-1-methyl-4-nitroimidazole. Contact Dermatitis 36:53–54

96. Chloroacetamide

CAS Registry Number [79–07–2]

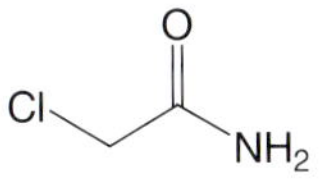

Chloroacetamide is as a preservative used in several applications as in cutting metalworking fluids, in paints or in glues. It can induce contact dermatitis in hairdressers or in shoemakers, being used as a leather preservative.

Suggested Reading

Katsarou A, Koufou B, Takou K, Kalogeromitros D, Papanayiotou G, Vareltzidis A (1995) Patch test results in hairdressers with contact dermatitis in Greece (1985–1994). Contact Dermatitis 33: 347–348

Mancuso G, Reggiani M, Berdondini RM (1996) Occupational dermatitis in shoemakers. Contact Dermatitis 34:17–22

97. Chloroacetophenone

CAS Registry Number [532–27–4]

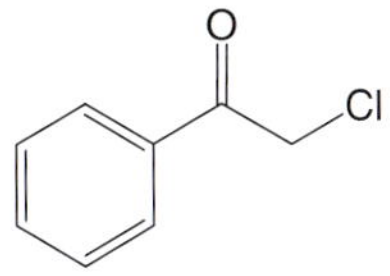

ω-Chloroacetophenone is contained in tear gases (lacrimators). This substance has important irritative potential but can also be a sensitizer.

Suggested Reading

Brand CU, Schmidli J, Ballmer-Weber B, Hunziker T (1995) Lymphozytenstimulationstest, eine mögliche Alternative zur Sicherung einer Cloracetophenon-Sensibilisierung. Hautarzt 46: 702–704

98. Chloroatranol

CAS Registry Number [57074–21–2]

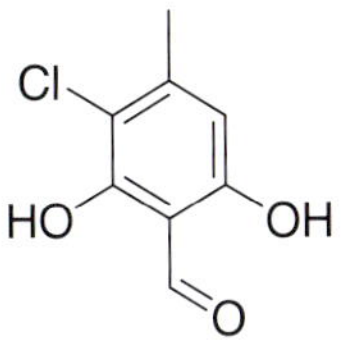

Chloroatranol has recently been identified as a constituent and major allergen in oak moss absolute, a frequent allergen in people sensitized to perfumes. This potent allergen gives reactions with concentrations down to 5 ppm in sensitized patients. It may cross-react with atranol.

Suggested Reading

Bernard G, Giménez-Arnau E, Rastogi SC et al (2003) Contact allergy to oak moss: search for sensitizing molecules using combined bioassay-guided chemical fractionation, GC-MS and structure-activity relationship analysis (part 1). Arch Dermatol Res 295:229–235

Johansen JD, Andersen KE, Svedman C, Bruze M, Bernard G, Giménez-Arnau E, Rastogi SC, Lepoittevin JP, Menné T (2003) Chloroatranol, an extremely potent allergen hidden in perfumes: a dose response elicitation study. Contact Dermatitis 49:180–184

99. Chlorocresol

4-Chloro-3-methylphenol, Parachlorometacresol, 2-Chloro-5-hydroxytoluene

CAS Registry Number [59–50–7]

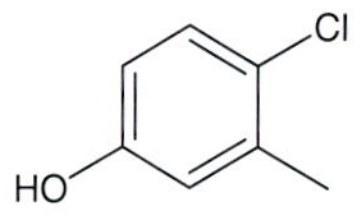

Chlorocresol is a biocide used for its disinfectant and preservative properties, in topicals or in cutting fluid.

Suggested Reading

Le Coz CJ, Scrivener Y, Santinelli F, Heid E (1998) Sensibilisation de contact au cours des ulcères de jambe. Ann Dermatol Venereol 125:694–699

Walker SL, Chalmers RJ, Beck MH (2004) Contact urticaria due to p-chloro-m-cresol. Br J Dermatol 151:936–937

100. Chlorophorin

CAS Registry Number [537–41–7]

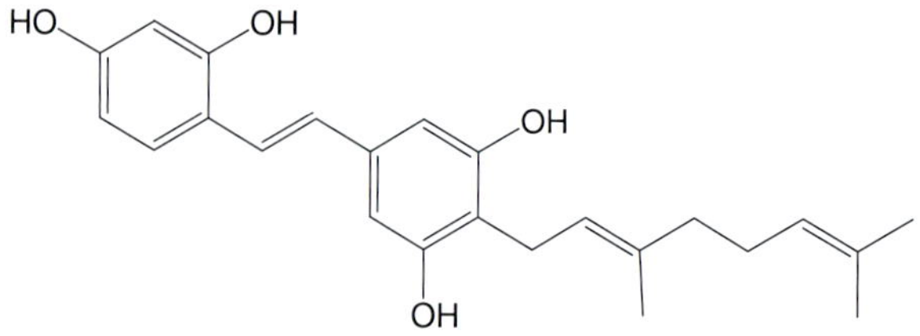

Chlorophorin is the allergen in iroko, kambala (*Chlorophora excelsa*). Occupational dermatitis can occurs in woodworkers. See also Chap. 41, Plants and Plant Products.

Suggested Reading

Lamminpää A, Estlander T, Jolanki R, Kanerva L (1996) Occupational allergic contact dermatitis caused by decorative plants. Contact Dermatitis 34:330–335

101. Chlorothalonil

2,4,5,6–1,3-Tetrachloroisophtalonitrile, 1,3-Dicyano Tetrachlorobenzene, Daconil®

CAS Registry Number [1897–45–6]

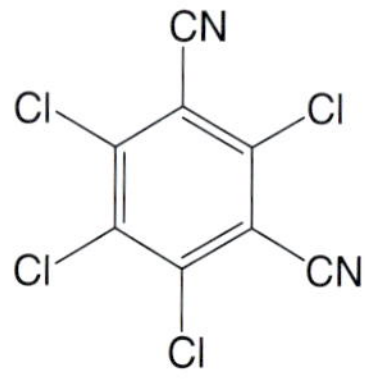

Chlorothalonil is a fungicide widely used in the cultivation of ornamental plants and flowers, rice, and onions. In banana plantations it is used in fumigations by airplanes. It can be used as a preservative of paints and of woods. It can induce contact urticaria, irritant and allergic contact dermatitis, erythema dyschromicum perstans or folliculitis mainly in agricultural workers, wood-related professions or in horticulturists.

Suggested Reading

Boman A, Montelius J, Rissanen RL, Lidén C (2000) Sensitizing potential of chlorothalonil in the guinea pig and the mouse. Contact Dermatitis 43:273–279

Meding B (1986) Contact dermatitis from tetrachloroisophtalonitrile in paint. Contact Dermatitis 15:187

O'Malley M, Rodriguez P, Maibach HI (1995) Pesticide patch testing: California nursery workers and controls. Contact Dermatitis 32:61–62

Penagos H, Jimenez V, Fallas V, O'Malley M, Maibach HI (1996) Chlorothalonil, a possible cause of erythema dyschromicum perstants (ashy dermatitis). Contact Dermatitis 35:214–218

102. Chlorpromazine

CAS Registry Number [50–53–3]

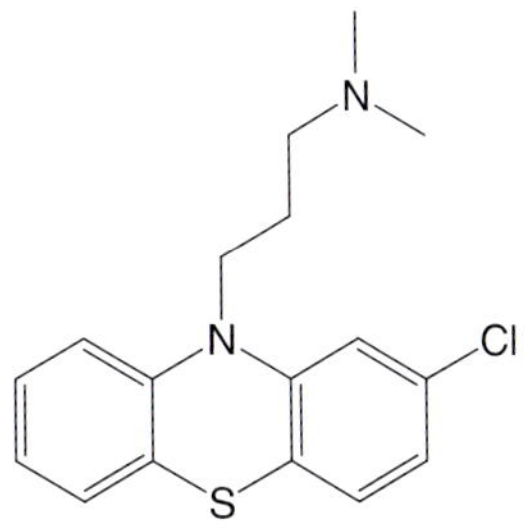

This phenothiazine with sedative properties is used in human medicine and induced contact dermatitis in nurses or those working in the pharmaceutical industry. It is also in veterinary medicine, to avoid mortality of pigs during transportation. It is a sensitizer and a photosensitizer.

Suggested Reading

Brasch J, Hessler HJ, Christophers E (1991) Occupational (photo)allergic contact dermatitis from azaperone in a piglet dealer. Contact Dermatitis 25:258–259

103. Cinnamal

Cinnamic Aldehyde, Cinnamaldehyde, 3-Phenyl-2-Propenal

CAS Registry Number [104–55–2]

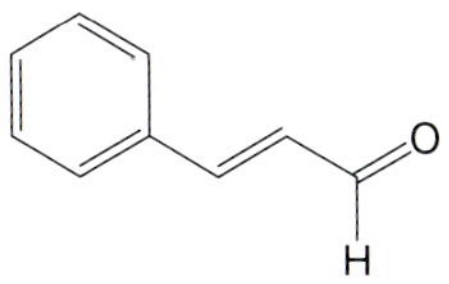

This perfumed molecule is used as a fragrance in perfumes, a flavoring agent in soft drinks, ice creams, dentifrices, pastries, chewing-gum, etc. It can induce both contact urticaria and delayed-type reactions. It can be responsible for dermatitis in the perfume industry or in food handlers. Cinnamic aldehyde is contained in "fragrance mix." As a fragrance allergen, it has to be mentioned by name in cosmetics within the EU.

Suggested Reading

Nethercott JR, Holness DL (1989) Occupational dermatitis in food handlers and bakers. J Am Acad Dermatol 21:485–490

Seite-Bellezza D, El Sayed F, Bazex J (1994) Contact urticaria from cinnamic aldehyde and benzaldehyde in a confectioner. Contact Dermatitis 31:272–273

104. Cinnamyl Alcohol

Cinnamic Alcohol, 3-Phenyl-2-Propenol

CAS Registry Number [104–54–1]

Cinnamyl alcohol occurs (in esterified form) in storax, *Myroxylon pereirae*, cinnamon leaves, and hyacinth oil. It is obtained by the alkaline hydrolysis of storax, and prepared synthetically by reducing cinnamal diacetate with iron filings and acetic acid, and from cinnamaldehyde by Meerwein–Ponndorf reduction with aluminum isopropoxide. Cinnamic alcohol is contained in the "fragrance mix." As a fragrance allergen, it has to be mentioned by name in cosmetics within the EU. Occupational cases of contact dermatitis were reported in perfume industry. Patch tests can be positive in food handlers.

51

Suggested Reading
Gutman SG, Somov BA (1968) Allergic reactions caused by components of perfumery preparations. Vestn Dermatol Venereol 12:62–66

Nethercott JR, Holness DL (1989) Occupational dermatitis in food handlers and bakers. J Am Acad Dermatol 21:485–490

105. Citral

3,7-Dimethyl-2,6-Octadien-1-al, Blend of Neral and Geranial, Blend of (Z)-3,7-Dimethyl-2,6-Octadienal and (E)-3,7-Dimethyl-2,6-Octadienal

CAS Registry Number [5392–40–5]
(CAS Registry Number [141–27–5] +
CAS Registry Number [106–26–3])

Neral   Geranial

Citral is an aldehyde fragrance and flavoring ingredient, a blend of isomers *cis* (Neral) and *trans* (geranial). As a fragrance allergen, citral has to be mentioned by name in cosmetics within the EU.

Suggested Reading
Frosch PJ, Johansen JD, Menné T, Pirker C, Rastogi SC, Andersen KE, Bruze M, Goossens A, Lepoittevin JP, White IR (2002) Further important sensitizers in patients sensitive to fragrances. Contact Dermatitis 47:78–85

106. Citronellol

3,7-Dimethyl-6-Octen-1-ol, Cephrol

CAS Registry Numbers [106–22–9]
and [26489–01–0]

L-Citronellol is a constituent of rose and geranium oils. D-Citronellol occurs in Ceylon and Java citronella oils. As a fragrance allergen, citronellol has to be mentioned by name in cosmetics within the EU.

Suggested Reading

Frosch PJ, Johansen JD, Menné T, Pirker C, Rastogi SC, Andersen KE, Bruze M, Goossens A, Lepoittevin JP, White IR (2002) Further important sensitizers in patients sensitive to fragrances. Contact Dermatitis 47:78–85

107. Clindamycin

Clindamycin

CAS Registry Number [18323–44–9]

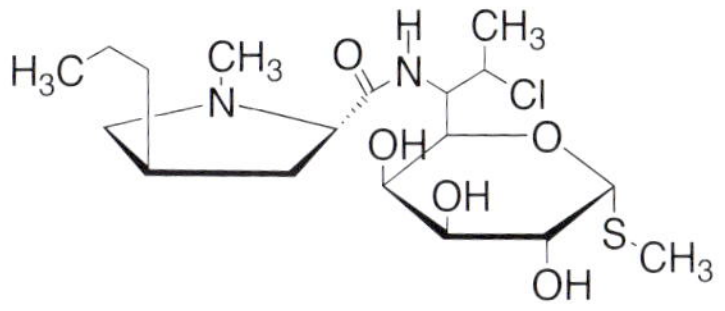

Clindamycin Hydrochloride

CAS Registry Number [21462–39–5]

Clindamycin Phosphate

CAS Registry Number [24729–96–2]

This lincosanide antibiotic is used in topical form for acne, or systemically has been responsible for exanthematous rashes and acute generalized exanthematous pustulosis.

Suggested Reading

Lammintausta K, Tokola R, Kalimo K (2002) Cutaneous adverse reactions to clindamycin: results of skin tests and oral exposure. Br J Dermatol 146:643–648

Valois M, Phillips EJ, Shear NH, Knowles SR (2003) Clindamycin-associated acute generalized exanthematous pustulosis. Contact Dermatitis 48:169

108. Clopidol

Methylchlorpindol, 3,5-Dichloro-2,6-Dimethyl-4-Pyridinol

CAS Registry Number [2971–90–6], [11116–46–4], [68821–99–8]

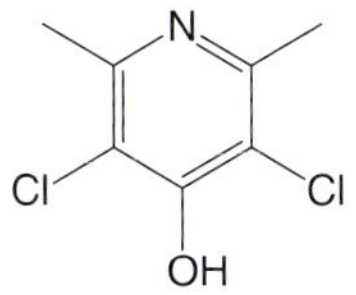

This drug is used for the prevention of coccidiosis in poultry.

Suggested Reading

Mancuso G, Staffa M, Errani A, Berdondini RM, Fabri P (1990) Occupational dermatitis in animal feed mill workers. Contact Dermatitis 22:37–41

Pang GF, Cao YZ, Fan CL, Zhang JJ, Li XM, MacNeil JD (2003) Determination of clopidol residues in chicken tissues by liquid chromatography: collaborative study. J AOAC Int 86:685–693

109. Cloxacillin

CAS Registry Number [61–72–3]

Cloxacillin Sodium Monohydrate

CAS Registry Number: [7081–44–9]

Cloxacillin is a semi-synthetic penicillin close to oxacillin. It induced contact dermatitis in a pharmaceutical factory worker with positive reactions to ampicillin but not to penicillin. In cutaneous drug reactions such as acute generalized exanthematous pustulosis due to amoxicillin, cross-reactivity is frequent to cloxacillin (personal observations).

Suggested Reading
Rudzki E, Rebandel P (1991) Hypersensitivity to semisynthetic penicillins but not to natural penicillin. Contact Dermatitis 25:192

110. Cobalt naphthenate

Naphthenic Acids, Cobalt Salts

CAS Registry Numbers [61789–51–3], [161279–65–8]

Cobalt naphthenate is made by treating cobalt hydroxide or acetate with naphthenic acid. It is an accelerant in rubber, unsaturated polyester, and vinyl ester resins.

Suggested Reading
Shena D, Rosina P, Chieregato C, Colombari R (1995) Lymphomatoid-like contact dermatitis from cobalt naphthenate. Contact Dermatitis 33:197–198
Tarvainen K, Jolanki R, Forsman-Gronholm L, Estlander T, Pfaffli P, Juntunen J, Kanerva L (1993) Exposure, skin protection and occupational skin diseases in the glass-fibre-reinforced plastics industry. Contact Dermatitis 29:119–127

111. Cocamidopropyl Betaine

Cocoamphodipropionate, Cocamidopropyl Dimethyl Glycine, Cocoamphocarboxypropionate, Cocoyl Amide Propylbetaine, N-(2-Aminoethyl)-N-[2-(2-carboxyethoxy)ethyl] beta-Alanine

CAS Registry Numbers [61789–40–0], [83138–08–3], [86438–79–1]

Cocamidopropyl betaine is a pseudo-amphoteric zwitterion detergent derived from long-chain alkylbetaines. It is available from many suppliers under more than 50 trade names (including Tego-betain L7 and Ampholyt JB 130). Exposure occurs via rinse-off products such as liquid soaps, shampoos, and shower gels, but also via leave-on products (for example, roll-on deodorant). Occupational sources are mainly in hairdressing. The first synthesis step consists of the reaction of coconut fatty acids with 3-dimethylaminopropylamine, giving cocamidopropyl dimethylamine. This amido-amine is converted into cocamidopropyl betaine by reaction with sodium monochloroacetate. Both dimethylaminopropylamine and cocamidopropyl dimethylamine are thought to be the sensitizers.

Suggested Reading

Angelini G, Foti C, Rigano L, Vena GA (1995) 3-Dimethylaminopropylamine: a key substance in contact allergy to cocamidopropylbetaine? Contact Dermatitis 32:96–99

De Groot AC, van der Walle HB, Weyland JW (1995) Contact allergy to cocamidopropyl betaine. Contact Dermatitis 33:419–422

McFadden JP, Ross JS, White IR, Basketter DA (2001) Clinical allergy to cocamidopropyl betaine: reactivity to cocamidopropylamine and lack of reactivity to 3-dimethylaminopropylamine. Contact Dermatitis 45:72–74

112. Cocamidopropyl Dimethylamine

N-[3-(Dimethylamino)Propyl]Coco Amides,
1-(N,N-Dimethylamino)-3-(Coconut Oil Amido)-Propane,
Coconut Fatty Acid, Dimethylaminopropylamide

CAS Registry Number [68140–01–2]

This amido amine may be the allergen in cocamidopropyl betaine.

Suggested Reading

McFadden JP, Ross JS, White IR, Basketter DA (2001) Clinical allergy to cocamidopropyl betaine: reactivity to cocamidopropylamine and lack of reactivity to 3-dimethylaminopropylamine. Contact Dermatitis 45:72–74

113. Coconut Diethanolamide

Cocamide DEA, Coconut Oil Fatty Acids Diethanolamide,
N,N-bis(2-Hydroxyethyl)Coco Fatty Acid Diethanolamide,
Cocoyl Diethanolamide

CAS Registry Number [68603–42–9]

Cocamide DEA, manufactured from coconut oil, is widely used in industry and at home as a surface-active agent. It is contained in hand gels, hand washing soaps, shampoos, and dish-washing liquids for its foam-producing and stabilizing properties, and in metalworking fluids and polishing agents as an anticorrosion inhibitor.

Suggested Reading

Fowler JF Jr (1998) Allergy to cocamide DEA. Am J Contact Dermat 9:40–41

Kanerva L, Jolanki R, Estlander T (1993) Dentist's occupational allergic contact dermatitis caused by coconut diethanolamide, N-ethyl-4-toluene sulfonamide and 4-tolydietahnolamine. Acta Derm Venereol (Stockh) 73:126–129

Pinola A, Estlander T, Jolanki R, Tarvainen K, Kanerva L (1993) Occupational allergic contact dermatitis due to coconut diethanolamide (Cocamide DEA). Contact Dermatitis 29:262–265

114. Codeine (Phosphate, Hydrochloride)

Methylmorphine

CAS Registry Number [76–57–3]
(CAS Registry Number [52–28–8],
CAS Registry Number [1422–07–7])

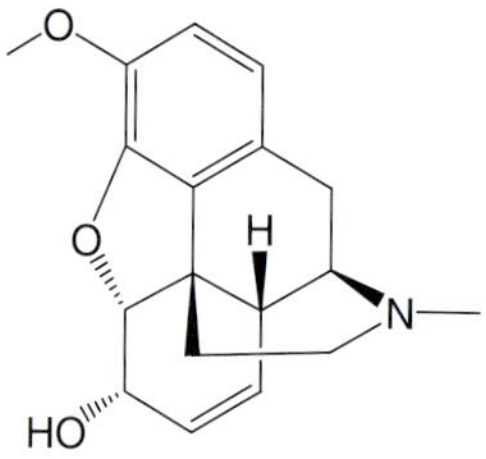

Codeine has been reported as an occupational sensitizer in workers in the production of opium alkaloids. Codeine has been responsible for fixed drug eruptions or generalized dermatitis. Cross-sensitivity is expected to morphine.

Suggested Reading

Condé-Salazar L, Guimaraens D, Gonzalez M, Fuente C (1991) Occupational allergic contact dermatitis from opium alkaloids. Contact Dermatitis 25:202–203

Estrada JL, Alvarez Puebla MJ, Ortiz de Urbina JJ, Matilla B, Rodríguez Prieto MA, Gozalo F (2001) Generalized eczema due to codeine. Contact Dermatitis 44:185

Waclawski ER, Aldridge R (1995) Occupational dermatitis from thebaine and codeine. Contact Dermatitis 33:51

115. Costunolide

CAS Registry Number [553–21–9]

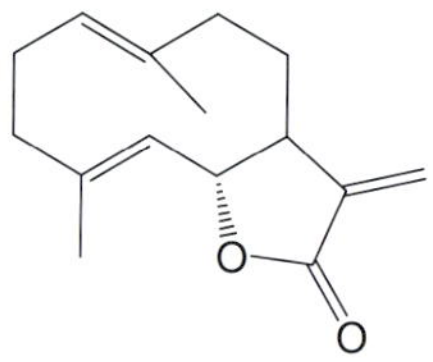

This germacranolide sesquiterpene lactone is extracted from costus oil. With alantolactone and dehydrocostunolide, it is a component of lactone mix used to elicit reactions in patients sensitive to Asteraceae–Compositae. An erythema-multiform-like occupational contact dermatitis case occurred in a chemical student after an accidental exposure to costus oil.

Suggested Reading

Ducombs G, Benezra C, Talaga P, Andersen KE, Burrows D, Camarasa JG, Dooms-Goossens A, Frosch PJ, Lachapelle JM, Menné T, Rycroft RJG, White IR, Shaw S, Wilkinson JD (1990) Patch testing with the "sesquiterpene lactone mix": a marker for contact allergy to Compositae and other sesquiterpene-lactone-containing plants. Contact Dermatitis 22:249–252

Le Coz CJ, Lepoittevin JP (2001) Occupational erythema-multiforme-like dermatitis from sensitization to costus resinoid, followed by flare-up and systemic contact dermatitis from beta-cyclo-costunolide in a chemistry student. Contact Dermatitis 44:310–311

116. Coumarin

1-Benzopyran-2-one, *cis-o*-Coumarinic Acid Lactone

CAS Registry Number [91–64–5]

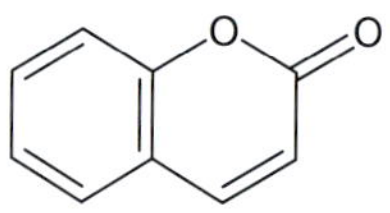

Coumarin is an aromatic lactone naturally occurring in Tonka beans and other plants. As a fragrance allergen, it has to be mentioned by name in cosmetics within the EU.

Suggested Reading

Frosch PJ, Johansen JD, Menné T, Pirker C, Rastogi SC, Andersen KE, Bruze M, Goossens A, Lepoit-
    tevin JP, White IR (2002) Further important sensitizers in patients sensitive to fragrances. Con-
    tact Dermatitis 47:78–85

117. Cresyl Glycidyl Ether

CAS Registry Number [26447–14–3]

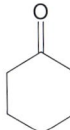

It is a reactive diluent added in epoxy resins Bisphenol A type.

Suggested Reading

Chieregato C, Vincenzi C, Guerra L, Farina P (1994) Occupational allergic contact dermatitis due
    to ethylenediamine dihydrochloride and cresyl glycidyl ether in epoxy resin systems. Contact
    Dermatitis 30:120
Daecke C, Schaller J, Goos M (1994) Acrylates as potent allergens in occupational and domestic ex-
    posures. Contact Dermatitis 30:190–191
Holness DL, Nethercott JR (1993) The performance of specialized collections of bisphenol A epoxy
    resin system components in the evaluation of workers in an occupational health clinic popula-
    tion. Contact Dermatitis 28:216–219
Jolanki R, Kanerva L, Estlander T, Tarvainen K, Keskinen H, Henriks-Eckerman ML (1990) Occu-
    pational dermatoses from epoxy resin compounds. Contact Dermatitis 23:172–183

118. Cyclohexanone

CAS Registry Number [108–94–1]

Used as a polyvinyl chloride solvent, cyclohexanone caused contact dermatitis in a
woman manufacturing PVC fluidotherapy bags. Cyclohexanone probably does not
cross-react with cyclohexanone resin. A cyclohexanone-derived resin used in paints
and varnishes, caused contact dermatitis in painters.

Suggested Reading

Bruze M, Boman A, Bergquist-Karlson A, Björkner B, Wahlberg JE, Woog E (1988) Contact allergy
    to cyclohexanone resin in humans and guinea pigs. Contact Dermatitis 18:46–49
Sanmartin O, de la Cuadra J (1992) Occupational contact dermatitis from cyclohexanone as a PVC
    adhesive. Contact Dermatitis 27:189–190

119. 2-Cyclohexen-1-one

CAS Registry Number [930–68–7]

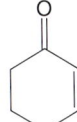

This strong sensitizer has been responsible for chemical burning followed by sensitization in a chemistry student.

Suggested Reading

Goossens A, Deschutter A (2003) Acute irritation followed by primary sensitization to 2-cyclohe-
    nen-1-one in a chemistry student. Contact Dermatitis 48:163–164

120. *N*-Cyclohexyl-2-Benzothiazylsulfenamide

CAS Registry Number [95–33–0]

A rubber accelerator chemical. The most frequent occupational categories are metal industry, homemakers, health services and laboratories, and the building industry.

Suggested Reading

Condé-Salazar L, Del-Rio E, Guimaraens D, Gonzalez Domingo A (1993) Type IV allergy to rubber additives: a 10-year study of 686 cases. J Am Acad Dermatol 29:176–180
Kiec-Swierczynska M (1995) Occupational sensitivity to rubber. Contact Dermatitis 32:171–172
Von Hintzenstern J, Heese A, Koch HU, Peters KP, Hornstein OP (1991) Frequency, spectrum and occupational relevance of type IV allergies to rubber chemicals. Contact Dermatitis 24:244–252

51

121. *N*-Cyclohexyl-*N*′-Phenyl-*p*-Phenylenediamine

N-Phenyl-*N*′-Cyclohexyl-*p*-Phenylenediamine, CPPD

CAS Registry Number [101–87–1]

CPPD is a rubber chemical used as an antioxidant. Cross-reactions are frequently observed with *N*-isopropyl-*N*′-phenylparaphenylenediamine (IPPD).

Suggested Reading

Hervé-Bazin B, Gradiski D, Duprat P, Marignac B, Foussereau J, Cavelier C, Bieber P (1977) Occupational eczema from *N*-isopropyl-*N*′-phenylparaphenylenediamine (IPPD) and *N*-dimethyl-1,3 butyl-*N*′-phenylparaphenylenediamine (DMPPD) in tyres. Contact Dermatitis 3:1–15
Von Hintzenstern J, Heese A, Koch HU, Peters KP, Hornstein OP (1991) Frequency, spectrum and occupational relevance of type IV allergies to rubber chemicals. Contact Dermatitis 24:244–252

122. *N*-Cyclohexyl-Thiophthalimide

CAS Registry Number [17796–82–6]

N-Cyclohexyl-thiophthalimide is a rubber chemical, widely used as a vulcanization retarder. Sensitization sources are often protective gloves.

Suggested Reading

Huygens S, Barbaud A, Goossens A (2001) Frequency and relevance of positive patch tests to cyclohexylthiophthalimide, a new rubber allergen. Eur J Dermatol 11:443–445
Kanerva L, Estlander T, Jolanki R (1996) Allergic patch test reactions caused by the rubber chemical cyclohexyl thiophthalimide. Contact Dermatitis 34:23–26

123. Cymene

Cymol, Methyl-Isopropyl-Benzol

CAS Registry Number [25155–15–1]

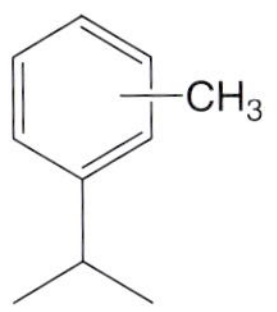

Terpenes, constitutive of essential oils, are hydrocarbons with the general formula $C_{10}H_{16}$. They are structurally related to cymol.

Suggested Reading

Selvaag E, Holm JO, Thune P (1995) Allergic contact dermatitis in an aroma therapist with multiple sensitizations to essential oils. Contact Dermatitis 33:354–355

124. Cymoxanil

2-Cyano-*N*-[(Ethylamino)Carbonyl]-2-(Methoxyimino)Acetamide

CAS Registry Number [57966–95–7]

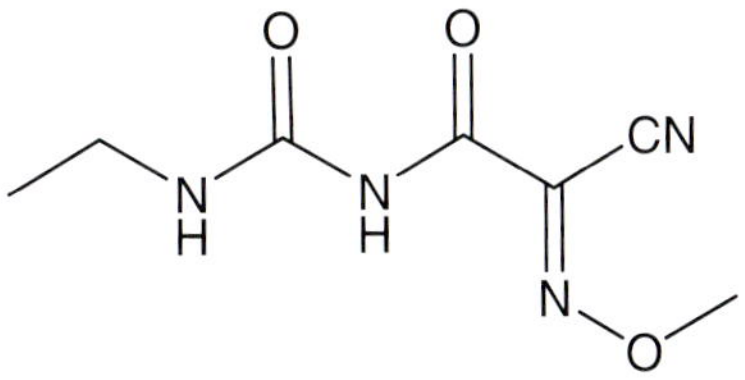

Cymoxanil, an urea derivative, is included (10%) with dithianone (25%) in Aktuan®. It is a fungicide agent, possibly sensitizing agricultural workers.

Suggested Reading

Koch P (1996) Occupational allergic contact dermatitis and airborne contact dermatitis from 5 fungicides in a vineyard worker. Cross-reactions between fungicides of the dithiocarbamate group? Contact Dermatitis 34:324–329

125. Dazomet

3,5-Dimethyltetrahydro-1,3,5(2*H*)Thiadiazine-2-Thione, DMTT

CAS Registry Number [533–74–4]

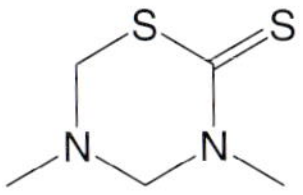

Dazomet is a biocide used to control bacterial and fungal growth in a pulp and paper system, and also in agriculture for soil disinfection. It is contained in Busan 1058, Mylone and Fungicide 974 (Crag™). Sensitization, rarely reported, occurred in a paper mill worker.

Suggested Reading

Warin AP (1992) Allergic contact dermatitis from dazomet. Contact Dermatitis 26:135–136

126. DDT

Dichlorodiphenyltrichloroethane

CAS Registry Number [50–29–3]

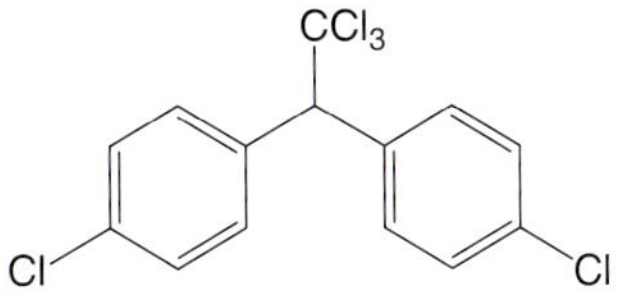

This insecticide was formerly reported as a sensitizer in farmers or agricultural workers.

Suggested Reading
Sharma VK, Kaur S (1990) Contact sensitization by pesticides in farmers. Contact Dermatitis 23 : 77–80

127. Decyl glucoside

CAS Registry Numbers [58846–77–8], [68515–73–1], [141464–42–8], and [54549–25–6]

51

CAS : 54549-25-6   co : 1 to 3

Decyl glucoside or decyl D-glucoside, also named decyl-beta-D-glucopyranoside, belongs to the alkyl glucosides family, and is obtained by condensation of the fatty alcohol decyl alcohol and a D-glucose polymer. This nonionic surfactant and cleansing agent has been widely used for several years, due to its foaming power and good tolerance in rinse-off products such as shampoos, hair dyes and colors, and soaps. Decyl glucoside is also employed in leave-on products such as no-rinsing cleansing milks, lotions and several sunscreen agents, and is contained as a stabilizing surfactant of organic microparticles in sunscreen agent Tinosorb® M.

Suggested Reading
Blondeel A (2003) Contact allergy to the mild surfactant decylglucoside. Contact Dermatitis 49 : 304–305
Le Coz CJ, Meyer MT (2003) Contact allergy to decyl glucoside in antiseptic after body piercing. Contact Dermatitis 48 : 279–280

128. Dehydrocostuslactone

CAS Registry Number [477–43–0]

A guaianolide sesquiterpene lactone extracted from costus oil. It is one of the components of Lactone mix, with costunolide and alantolactone, used to detect Compositae-sensitive patients.

Suggested Reading

Ducombs G, Benezra C, Talaga P, Andersen KE, Burrows D, Camarasa JG, Dooms-Goossens A, Frosch PJ, Lachapelle JM, Menné T, Rycroft RJG, White IR, Shaw S, Wilkinson JD (1990) Patch testing with the "sesquiterpene lactone mix": a marker for contact allergy to Compositae and other sesquiterpene-lactone-containing plants. Contact Dermatitis 22:249–252

129. Deoxylapachol

CAS Registry Number [3568–90–9]

Deoxylapachol is the main allergen identified in teak (*Tectona grandis*). Sensitization often concerns people involved in woodwork. See also Chap. 41 Plants and Plant Products.

Suggested Reading

Lamminpää A, Estlander T, Jolanki R, Kanerva L (1996) Occupational allergic contact dermatitis caused by decorative plants. Contact Dermatitis 34:330–335

Meding B, Ahman M, Karlberg AT (1996) Skin symptoms and contact allergy in woodwork teachers. Contact Dermatitis 34:185–190

130. Diallyl Disulfide

CAS Registry Number [2179–57–9]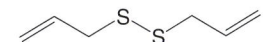

Diallyl disulfide is one of the major allergens in garlic (*Allium sativum*) and onions. Among patients patch-test-positive to garlic, all 13 who were tested had positive reactions to diallyl sulfide 5% pet. See also Chap. 41 Plants and Plant Products.

Suggested Reading

Bruynzeel DP (1997) Bulb dermatitis. Dermatological problems in the flower bulb industries. Contact Dermatitis 37:70–77

Lamminpää A, Estlander T, Jolanki R, Kanerva L (1996) Occupational allergic contact dermatitis caused by decorative plants. Contact Dermatitis 34:330–335

McFadden JP, White IR, Rycroft RJG (1992) Allergic contact dermatitis from garlic. Contact Dermatitis 27:333–334

131. Diaminodiphenylmethane

4,4'-Diaminodiphenylmethane, 4,4'-Methylenedianiline

CAS Registry Number [107–77–9]

4,4'-Diaminodiphenylmethane is an aromatic diamine used as a curing agent in epoxy resins of the bisphenol A type, and in the production of plastics, isocyanates, adhesives, elastomers, polyurethane (elastic and rigid foams, paints, lacquers, adhesives, binding agents, synthetics rubbers, and elastomeric fibres), and butyl rubber. 4,4′-Diaminodiphenylmethane is also a by-product in azo dyes. It is also possibly formed by hydrolysis of diphenylmethane-4,4′-diisocyanate.

Suggested Reading

Bruynzeel DP, van der Wegen-Keijser MH (1993) Contact dermatitis in a cast technician. Contact Dermatitis 28:193–194
Condé-Salazar L, Gonzalez de Domingo MA, Guimaraens D (1994) Sensitization to epoxy resin systems in special flooring workers. Contact Dermatitis 31:157–160
Holness DL, Nethercott JR (1993) The performance of specialized collections of bisphenol A epoxy resin system components in the evaluation of workers in an occupational health clinic population. Contact Dermatitis 28:216–219
Jolanki R, Kanerva L, Estlander T, Tarvainen K, Keskinen H, Henriks-Eckerman ML (1990) Occupational dermatoses from epoxy resin compounds. Contact Dermatitis 23:172–183
Jolanki R, Kanerva L, Estlander T, Tarvainen K (1994) Concomitant sensitization to triglycidyl isocyanurate, diaminodiphenylmethane and 2-hydroxyethyl methacrylate from silk-screen printing coatings in the manufacture of circuit boards. Contact Dermatitis 30:12–15
Kiec-Swierczynska M (1995) Rubber chemical. Occupational sensitivity to rubber. Contact Dermatitis 32:171–172
Mancuso G, Reggiani M, Berdondini RM (1996) Occupational dermatitis in shoemakers. Contact Dermatitis 34:17–22
Tarvainen K (1995) Analysis of patients with allergic patch test reactions to a plastic and glues series. Contact Dermatitis 32:346–351

51

132. Diammonium Hydrogen Phosphate

CAS Registry Number [7783–28–0]

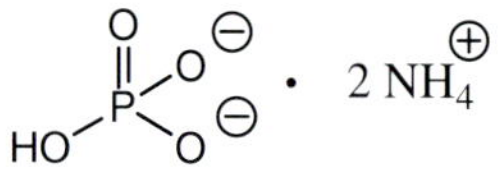

A flame retardant which caused contact dermatitis in surgical personnel. It was due to excessive residual concentrations in surgical garbs.

Suggested Reading

Belsito DV (1990) Contact dermatitis from diammonium hydrogen phosphate in surgical garb. Contact Dermatitis 23:267–268

133. Diazodiethylaniline Chloride

CAS Registry Number [148–90–3]

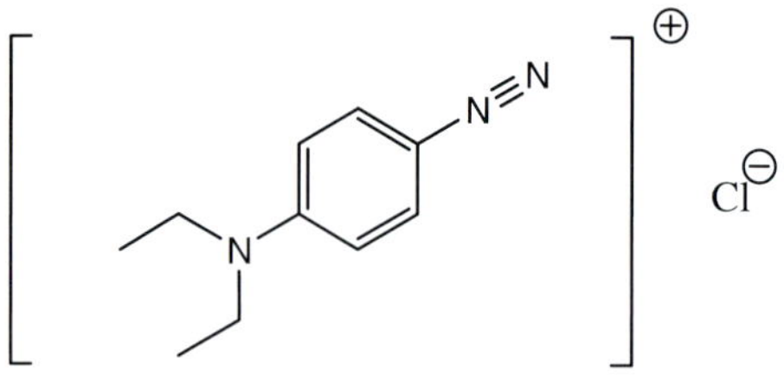

It is a well-known allergen in diazo copy paper. This product is allergenic until exposed to light, and inactivated by UV radiations.

Suggested Reading

Foussereau J, Benezra C (1970) Les eczémas allergiques professionnels. Masson, Paris
Pambor M, Poweleit H (1992) Allergic contact dermatitis due to diazo copy paper. Contact Dermatitis 26:131–132

134. Diazolidinyl Urea

Germall II

CAS Registry Number [78491-02-8]

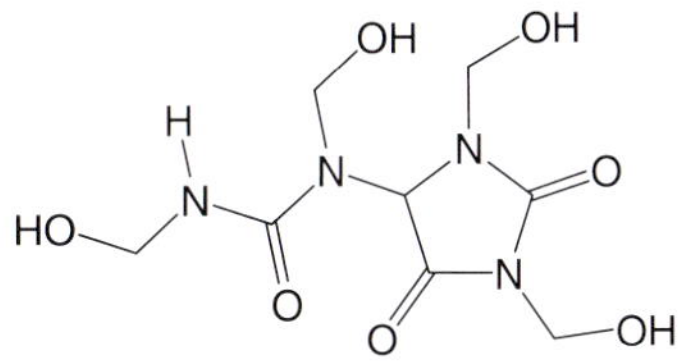

Diazolidinyl urea, a formaldehyde releaser, is contained mainly in cosmetics and toiletries, and can be found in barrier creams.

Suggested Reading

Le Coz CJ (2005) Hypersensibilité à la Diazolidinyl urée et à l'Imidazolidinyl urée. Ann Dermatol Venereol 132 (in press)

Van Hecke E, Suys E (1994) Where next to look for formaldehyde? Contact Dermatitis 31:268

135. Dibenzothiazyl Disulfide

CAS Registry Number [120-78-5]

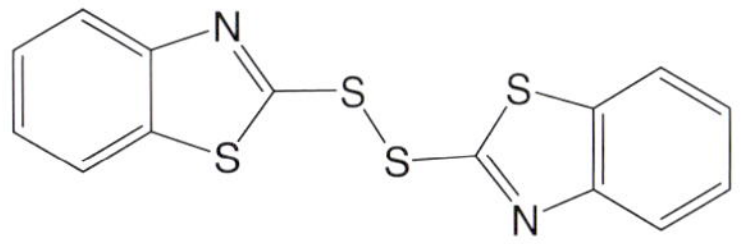

This rubber chemical of the mercaptobenzothiazole group is used as a vulcanization accelerant. The most frequent occupational categories are metal industry, homemakers, health services and laboratories, and the building industry.

Suggested Reading

Condé-Salazar L, Del-Rio E, Guimaraens D, Gonzalez Domingo A (1993) Type IV allergy to rubber additives: a 10-year study of 686 cases. J Am Acad Dermatol 29:176–180

Le Coz CJ (2004) Fiche d'éviction en cas d'hypersensibilité au mercaptobenzothiazole et au mercapto mix. Ann Dermatol Venereol 131:846–848

Von Hintzenstern J, Heese A, Koch HU, Peters KP, Hornstein OP (1991) Frequency, spectrum and occupational relevance of type IV allergies to rubber chemicals. Contact Dermatitis 24:244–252

136. Dibucaine (Hydrochloride)

Cincaine, Cinchocain(e), Percaine, Sovcaine

CAS Registry Number [85-79-0] (CAS Registry Number [61-12-1])

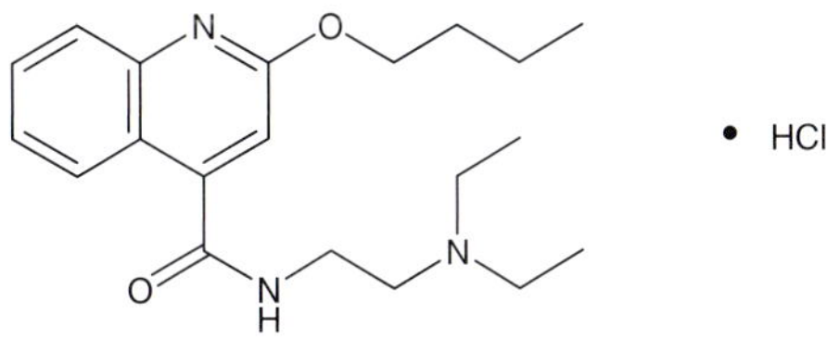

• HCl

Dibucaine hydrochloride is an amide group local anesthetic that can induce allergic contact dermatitis.

Suggested Reading

Erdmann SM, Sachs B, Merk HF (2001) Systemic contact dermatitis from cinchocaine. Contact Dermatitis 44:260–261

Nakada T, Iijima M (2000) Allergic contact dermatitis from dibucaine hydrochloride. Contact Dermatitis 42:283

137. Dibutyl Phthalate

CAS Registry Number [84–74–2]

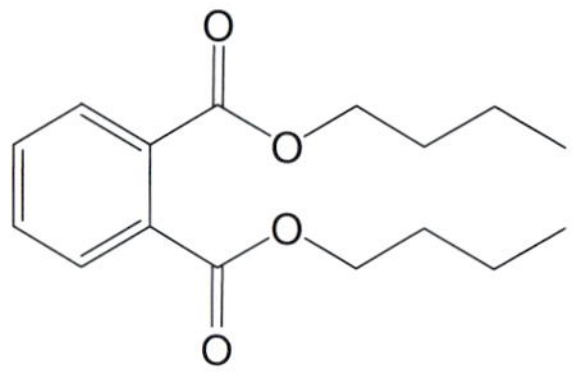

It is mainly used as a nonreactive epoxy diluent.

Suggested Reading

Capon F, Cambie MP, Clinard F, Bernardeau K, Kalis B (1996) Occupational contact dermatitis caused by computer mice. Contact Dermatitis 35:57–58

Chieregato C, Vincenzi C, Guerra L, Farina P (1994) Occupational allergic contact dermatitis due to ethylenediamine dihydrochloride and cresyl glycidyl ether in epoxy resin systems. Contact Dermatitis 30:120

51

138. Dibutylthiourea

1,3-Dibutyl-2-Thiourea

CAS Registry Number [109–46–6]

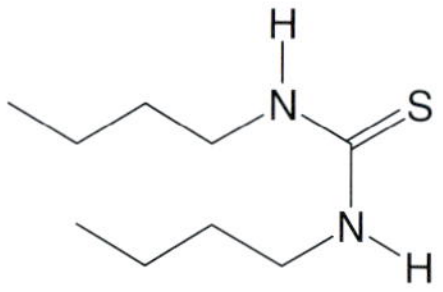

Dibutylthiourea is used in the vulcanization of rubber, in paints and glue removers as an anticorrosive, in phonecards as a component of the thermocoating sprayed over the optically read layer of the card. Cross sensitivity to other thiourea derivatives is possible.

Suggested Reading

Kanerva L, Estlander T, Jolanki R (1994) Occupational allergic contact dermatitis caused by thiourea compounds. Contact Dermatitis 31:242–248

Kiec-Swierczynska M (1995) Occupational sensitivity to rubber. Contact Dermatitis 32:171–172

Schmid-Grendelmeier P, Elsner P (1995) Contact dermatitis due to occupational dibutylthiourea exposure: a case of phonecard dermatitis. Contact Dermatitis 32:308–309

139. 4,5-Dichloro-2-*n*-Octyl-4-Isothiazolin-3-one

Kathon® 930

CAS Registry Number [64359–81–5]

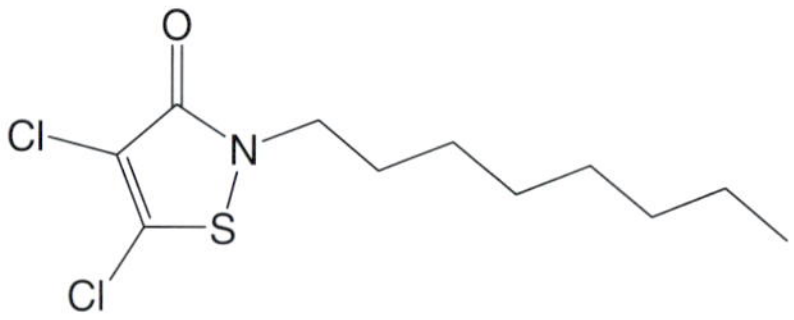

Irritant and sensitizer, Kathon® 930 caused contact dermatitis in employees of a textile finishing factory.

Suggested Reading

Kawai K, Nagakawa M, Sasaki Y, Kawai Y (1993) Occupational contact dermatitis from Kathon® 930. Contact Dermatitis 28:117–118

140. 1,3-Dichloropropene

1,3-Dichloro-1-Prop(yl)ene, 1,3-Dichloro-2-Prop(yl)ene, DD-95

CAS Registry Number [542–75–6]

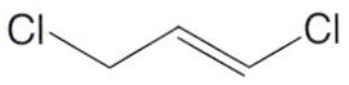

This nematocide is used as a soil fumigant prior to crop cultivation. Farmers and process operators employed at pesticide plants are mainly exposed.

Suggested Reading

Bousema MT, Wiemer GR, van Joost T (1991) A classic case of sensitization to DD-95. Contact Dermatitis 24:132

141. Dichlorvos

CAS Registry Number [62–73–7]

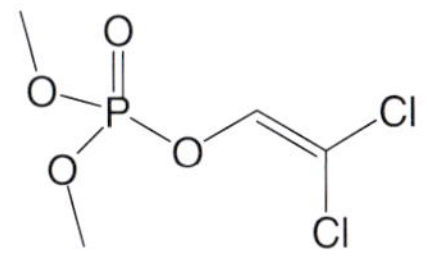

Cases of sensitization to this organophosphorus compound with several commercial names (Benfos, Brevinyl, Chlorvinphos, DDVP, Equigard, Fly fighte, Nogos, and Unifos), were occupationally seen in chrysanthem growers, horticulturists, technicians, and in a chemist.

Suggested Reading

Cleenewerck MB, Martin P (1990) Dermite de contact au Dichlorvos. Rev Fr Allergol 30:38

Mathias CG (1983) Persistent contact dermatitis from the insecticide dichlorvos. Contact Dermatitis 9:217–218

142. *N,N*-Dicyclohexyl-2-Benzothiazole Sulfenamide

CAS Registry Number [4979–32–2]

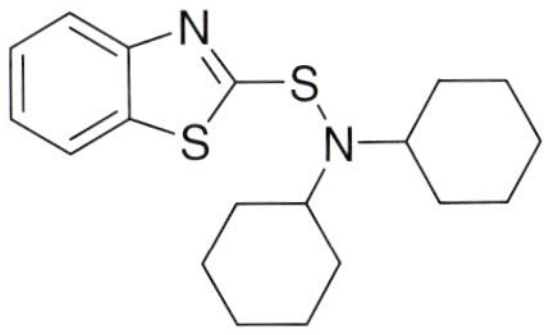

This substance is a rubber accelerator of the mercaptobenzothiazole-sulfenamide group.

Suggested Reading

Le Coz CJ (2004) Fiche d'éviction en cas d'hypersensibilité au mercaptobenzothiazole et au mercapto mix. Ann Dermatol Venereol 131:846–848

143. Dicyclohexyl Carbodiimide

CAS Registry Number [538–75–0]

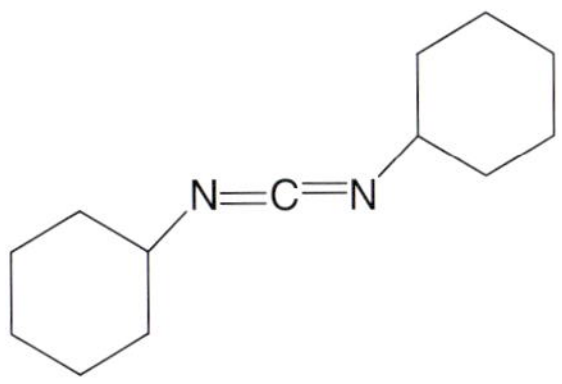

Used in peptide chemistry as a coupling reagent. It is both an irritant and a sensitizer, and has caused contact dermatitis in pharmacists and chemists.

Suggested Reading
Poesen N, de Moor A, Busschots A, Dooms-Goossens A (1995) Contact allergy to dicyclohexyl carbodiimide and diisopropyl carbodiimide. Contact Dermatitis 32:368–369

51

144. Didecyldimethylammonium Chloride

Bardac-22

CAS Registry Number [7173–51–5]

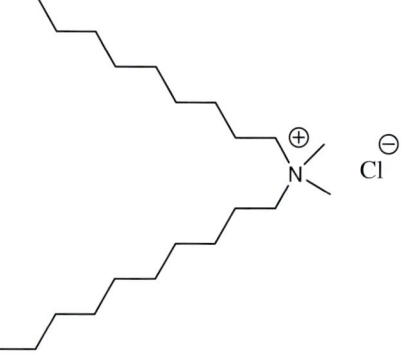

This quaternary ammonium compound is used as a detergent-disinfectant in hospitals, as an algaecide in swimming pools, as a fungicide, and against termites in wood. We recently observed severe contact dermatitis in a slaughterhouse worker using a liquid soap containing this product (personal observation).

Suggested Reading
Dejobert Y, Martin P, Piette F, Thomas P, Bergoend H (1997) Contact dermatitis from didecyldimethylammonium chloride and bis-(aminopropyl)-laurylamine in a detergent-disinfectant used in hospital. Contact Dermatitis 37:95–96

145. Diethanolamine

CAS Registry Number [111–42–2]

Diethanolamine is contained in many products, as a metalworking fluid. Traces may exist in other ethanolamine-containing fluids.

Suggested Reading
Blum A, Lischka G (1997) Allergic contact dermatitis from mono-, di- and triethanolamine. Contact Dermatitis 36:166

146. Diethyl Sebacate

Ethyl Sebacate, Diethyl Decanedioate

CAS Registry Number [110–40–7]

This emulsifier has rarely been reported as a sensitizing agent, mainly in topical treatments.

Suggested Reading
Tanaka M, Kobayashi S, Murata T, Tanikawa A, Nishikawa T (2000) Allergic contact dermatitis from diethyl sebacate in lanoconazole cream. Contact Dermatitis 43:233–234

147. Diethyleneglycol Diglycidyl Ether

Ether, bis[2-(2,3-Epoxypropoxy)Ethyl]

CAS Registry Number [4206–61–5]

Diethyleneglycol diglycidyl ether was contained in a reactive diethyleneglycol-based diluent of epoxy resins and caused contact dermatitis in three workers at a ski factory.

Suggested Reading

Jolanki R, Tarvainen K, Tatar T, Estlander T, Henriks-Eckerman ML, Mustakallio KK, Kanerva L (1996) Occupational dermatoses from exposure to epoxy resin compounds in a ski factory. Contact Dermatitis 34:390–396

148. Diethylenetriamine

CAS Registry Number [111–40–0]

Diethylenetriamine is a hardener in epoxy resins of the Bisphenol A type. It has been reported to be a sensitizer when used in an ultrasonic bath for cleaning jewels, in synthetic lubricants or in carbonless copy paper.

Suggested Reading

Holness DL, Nethercott JR (1993) The performance of specialized collections of bisphenol A epoxy resin system components in the evaluation of workers in an occupational health clinic population. Contact Dermatitis 28:216–219

Jolanki R, Kanerva L, Estlander T, Tarvainen K, Keskinen H, Henriks-Eckerman ML (1990) Occupational dermatoses from epoxy resin compounds. Contact Dermatitis 23:172–183

Kanerva L, Estlander T, Jolanki R (1990) Occupational allergic contact dermatitis due to diethylenetriamine (DETA) from carbonless copy paper and from an epoxy compound. Contact Dermatitis 23:272–273

149. Diethylphthalate

CAS Registry Number [84–66–2]

This plasticizer increases the flexibility of plastics. It is also contained in deodorant formulations, perfumes, emollients, and insect repellents. It can cross react with dimethyl phthalate.

Suggested Reading

Capon F, Cambie MP, Clinard F, Bernardeau K, Kalis B (1996) Occupational contact dermatitis caused by computer mice. Contact Dermatitis 35:57–58

150. Diethylthiourea

Diethylthiocarbamide

CAS Registry Number [105–55–5]

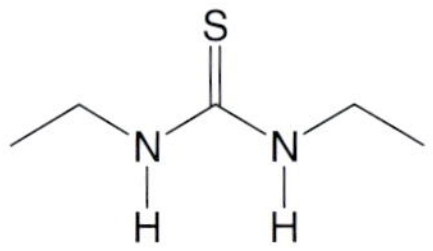

Diethylthiourea, a thiourea derivative, is used mainly as a rubber chemical, particularly in solid neoprene products.

Suggested Reading

Kanerva L, Estlander T, Jolanki R (1994) Occupational allergic contact dermatitis caused by thiourea compounds. Contact Dermatitis 31:242–248

151. Diisopropyl Carbodiimide

51

N,N′-Methanetetraylbis-2-Propanamine

CAS Registry Number [693–13–0]

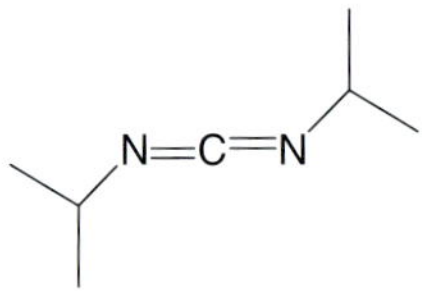

It is used in peptide chemistry as a coupling reagent. It is very toxic and causes contact dermatitis in laboratory workers.

Suggested Reading

Poesen N, de Moor A, Busschots A, Dooms-Goossens A (1995) Contact allergy to dicyclohexyl carbodiimide and diisopropyl carbodiimide. Contact Dermatitis 32:368–369

152. Diisopropylbenzothiazyl-2-Sulfenamide

CAS Registry Number [95–29–4]

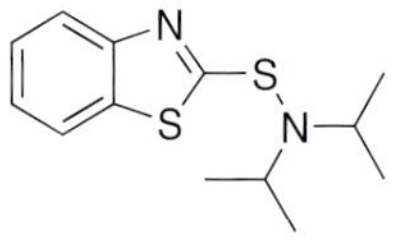

This chemical is a mercaptobenzothiazole-sulfenamide used in rubber vulcanization.

Suggested Reading

Le Coz CJ (2004) Fiche d'éviction en cas d'hypersensibilité au mercaptobenzothiazole et au mercapto mix. Ann Dermatol Venereol 131:846–848

153. 2,5-Dimercapto-1,3,4-Thiadiazole

DMTD

CAS Registry Number [1072–71–5]

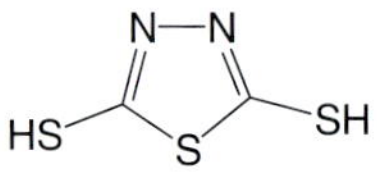

This low-molecular-weight aromatic compound is used in the production of copper corrosion inhibitors for engine oils, flame retardants, and photographic development chemicals. Seven cases of industrial allergic sensitization were reported in a manufacturing plant.

Suggested Reading

O'Driscoll JO, Beck M, Taylor S (1990) Occupational contact allergy to 2,5-dimercapto-1,3,4-thiadiazole. Contact Dermatitis 23:268–269

154. Dimethoate

CAS Registry Number [60–51–5]

This organophosphorus compound is used as a contact and systemic insecticide and acaricide. It induced an erythema-multiform-like contact dermatitis in a warehouseman in an agricultural consortium.

Suggested Reading
Haenen C, de Moor A, Dooms-Goossens A (1996) Contact dermatitis caused by the insecticides omethoate and dimethoate. Contact Dermatitis 35:54–55
Schena D, Barba A (1992) Erythema-multiforme-like contact dermatitis from dimethoate. Contact Dermatitis 27:116–117

155. Dimethoxon

Omethoate

CAS Registry Number [1113–02–6]

Contact dermatitis from omethoate–dimethoxon is rare.

Suggested Reading
De Moor A, Dooms-Goossens A (1996) Contact dermatitis caused by the insecticides omethoate and dimethoate. Contact Dermatitis 35:54–55

156. 2,6-Dimethoxy-1,4-Benzoquinone

CAS Registry Number [530–55–2]

2,6-Dimethoxy-1,4-benzoquinone is an allergen in more than 50 different plants and wood species, e.g., mahogany, macore, sipo, wenge, oak, beech, elms, and poplar. With acamelin, it is one of the allergens of *Acacia melanoxylon*. Sensitization can occur in woodworkers such as carpenters, joiners, and sawyers. See also Chap. 41 Plants and Plant Products.

Suggested Reading
Correia O, Barros MA, Mesquita-Guimaraes J (1992) Airborne contact dermatitis from the woods *Acacia melanoxylon* and *Entandophragma cylindricum*. Contact Dermatitis 27:343–344
Lamminpää A, Estlander T, Jolanki R, Kanerva L (1996) Occupational allergic contact dermatitis caused by decorative plants. Contact Dermatitis 34:330–335

157. (R)-3,4-Dimethoxy-Dalbergione

CAS Registry Number [37555–64–4]

This quinone is the main allergen of *Machaerium scleroxylum* Tul. (Santos rosewood, *Pao ferro*, *Caviuna vermelha*, *Santos palissander*). Occupational sensitization mainly concerns woodworkers. See also Chap. 41 Plants and Plant Products.

Suggested Reading
Chieregato C, Vincenzi C, Guerra L, Rapacchiale S (1993) Occupational airborne contact dermatitis from *Machaerium scleroxylum* (Santos rosewood). Contact Dermatitis 29:164–165
Lamminpää A, Estlander T, Jolanki R, Kanerva L (1996) Occupational allergic contact dermatitis caused by decorative plants. Contact Dermatitis 34:330–335

158. (S)-4,4′-Dimethoxy Dalbergione

CAS Registry Number [4646–87–1]

It is an allergen of *Dalbergia nigra* also contained in *Dalbergia latifolia* Roxb. (East Indian rosewood, palissander). Occupational dermatitis can occur in timberworkers such as carpenters, sawyers, joiners or knifegrinders. See also Chap. 41 Plants and Plant Products.

Suggested Reading
Gallo R, Guarrera M, Hausen BM (1996) Airborne contact dermatitis from East Indian rosewood (*Dalbergia latifolia* Roxb.). Contact Dermatitis 35:60–61

159. 5,8-Dimethoxypsoralen

Isopimpinellin

CAS Registry Number [482–27–9]

Psoralens are natural photoactivable compounds in plants and can cause phototoxic contact dermatitis. For example, *Cachrys libanotis* L., Apiaceae-Umbelliferae family, contains 5,8-dimethoxypsoralen. See also Chap. 41 Plants and Plant Products.

Suggested Reading
Ena P, Cerri R, Dessi G, Manconi PM, Atzei AD (1991) Phototoxicity due to *Cachrys libanotis*. Contact Dermatitis 24:1–5

160. Dimethyl Phthalate

CAS Registry Number [131–11–3]

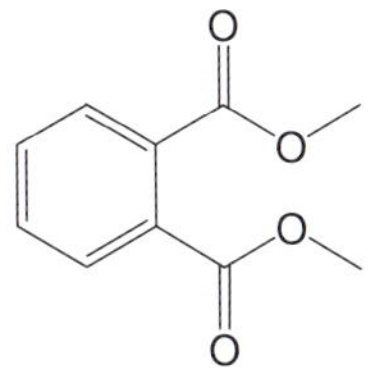

Phthalates are plasticizers, and increase the flexibility of plastics. They are also found in deodorant formulations, perfumes, emollients, and insect repellents.

Suggested Reading

Capon F, Cambie MP, Clinard F, Bernardeau K, Kalis B (1996) Occupational contact dermatitis caused by computer mice. Contact Dermatitis 35:57–58

161. 4-*N,N*-(Dimethylamino) Benzenediazonium Chloride

p-Diazodimethylaniline zinc Chloride Double Salt

CAS Registry Number [100–04–9]

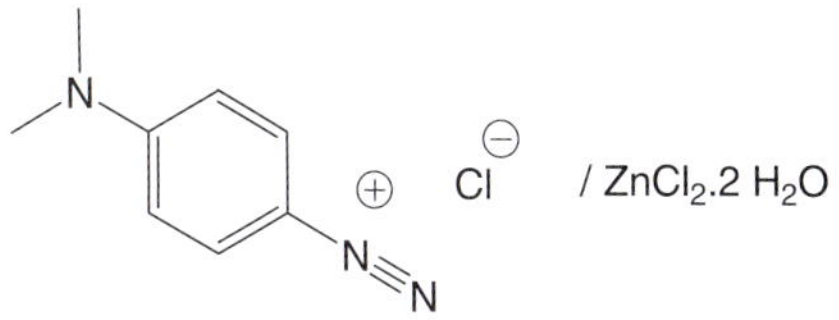

/ ZnCl$_2$.2 H$_2$O

It is a diazo compound found in diazo copy paper. It is allergenic only when unexposed.

Suggested Reading

Geier J, Fuchs T (1993) Contact allergy due to 4-*N,N*-dimethylaminobenzene diazonium chloride and thiourea in diazo copy paper. Contact Dermatitis 28:304–305

162. 3-Dimethylaminopropylamine

CAS Registry Number [109–55–7]

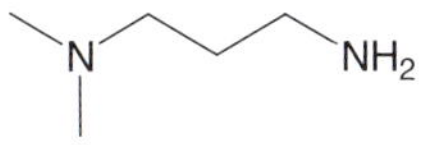

Dimethylaminopropylamine is an aliphatic amine present in amphoteric surfactants such as liquid soaps and shampoos. It is present as a residual impurity thought to be responsible for allergy from cocamidopropylbetaine. It is structurally similar to diethylaminopropylamine. It is also used as a curing agent for epoxy resins and an organic intermediate in chemical synthesises (ion exchangers, additives for flocculants, cosmetics and fuel additives, dyes and pesticides). Patch test has to be carefully interpreted, since the 1% aqueous solution has pH>11 (personal observation).

Suggested Reading

Angelini G, Foti C, Rigano L, Vena GA (1995) 3-Dimethylaminopropylamine: a key substance in contact allergy to cocamidopropylbetaine? Contact Dermatitis 32:96–99

Kanerva L, Estlander T, Jolanki R (1996) Occupational allergic contact dermatitis from 3-dimethylaminopropylamine in shampoos. Contact Dermatitis 35:122–123

Speight EL, Beck MH, Lawrence CM (1993) Occupational allergic contact dermatitis due to 3-dimethylaminopropylamine. Contact Dermatitis 28:49–50

163. Dimethyldiphenylthiuram disulfide

CAS Registry Number [53880–86–7]

This thiuram compound is used as an accelerator for rubber vulcanization.

Suggested Reading
Le Coz CJ (2004) Fiche d'éviction en cas d'hypersensibilité au thiuram mix. Ann Dermatol Venereol 131:1012–1014

164. Dimethylformamide

51

CAS Registry Number [68–12–2]

This is an organic solvent for vinyl resins and acetylene, butadiene and acid gases. It caused contact dermatitis in a technician at an epoxy resin factory, and can provoke alcohol-induced flushing in exposed subjects.

Suggested Reading
Camarasa JG (1987) Contact dermatitis from dimethylformamide. Contact Dermatitis 16:234
Cox NH, Mustchin CP (1991) Prolonged spontaneous and alcohol-induced flushing due to the solvent dimethyl formamide. Contact Dermatitis 24:69–70

165. 2,4-Dimethylol Phenol

CAS Registry Number [2937–60–2]

2,4-Dimethylol phenol in a compound of resins based on phenol and formaldehyde. Cross-reactivity is possible with other phenol derivative molecules.

Suggested Reading
Bruze M, Zimerson E (1997) Cross-reaction patterns in patients with contact allergy to simple methylol phenols. Contact Dermatitis 37:82–86
Bruze M, Zimerson E (1985) Contact allergy to 3-methylol phenol, 2,4-dimethylol phenol and 2,6-dimethylol phenol. Acta Derm Venereol (Stockh) 65:548–551

166. 2,6-Dimethylol Phenol

CAS Registry Number [2937–59–9]

This substance is contained in resins based on phenol and formaldehyde. Cross-reactivity is possible with other phenol derivative molecules.

Suggested Reading

Bruze M, Zimerson E (1985) Contact allergy to 3-methylol phenol, 2,4-dimethylol phenol and 2,6-dimethylol phenol. Acta Derm Venereol (Stockh) 65:548–551

Bruze M, Zimerson E (1997) Cross-reaction patterns in patients with contact allergy to simple methylol phenols. Contact Dermatitis 37:82–86

167. Dimethylthiourea

Dimethylthiocarbamide

CAS Registry Number [534–13–4]

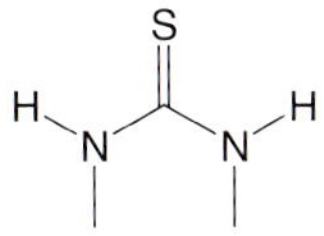

Dimethylthiocarbamide, an antioxygen agent, is responsible for sensitization, when unexposed to light, from diazo papers.

Suggested Reading

Geier J, Fuchs T (1993) Contact allergy due to 4-N,N-dimethylaminobenzene diazonium chloride and thiourea in diazo copy paper. Contact Dermatitis 28:304–305

Kanerva L, Estlander T, Jolanki R (1994) Occupational allergic contact dermatitis caused by thiourea compounds. Contact Dermatitis 31:242–248

168. Dinitrochlorobenzene

DNCB, 2,4-Dinitrochlorobenzene, 2,4-Dinitro-1-Chlorobenzene, 4-Chloro-1,3-Dinitrobenzene, 6-Chloro-1,3-Dinitrobenzene

CAS Registry Number [97–00–7]

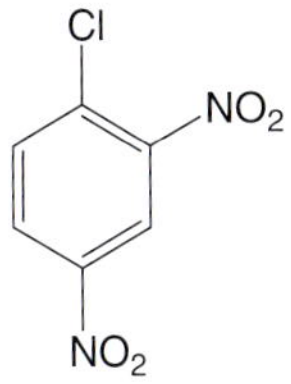

This substance is one of the strongest primary skin irritant known, and a universal contact allergen. Occupational dermatitis has been reported, but current use is decreasing or performed with completely closed systems. DNCB is sometimes used for topical treatment of alopecia areata, severe warts, and cutaneous metastasis of malignant melanoma.

Suggested Reading

Adams RM, Zimmerman MC, Bartlett JB, Preston JF (1971) 1-Chloro-2,4-dinitrobenzene as an algicide. Report of four cases of contact dermatitis. Arch Dermatol 103:191–193

169. Dinitrofluorobenzene

DNFB, FDNB, 2,4-Dinitro-1-Fluorobenzene, Sanger's Reagent

CAS Registry Number [70–34–8]

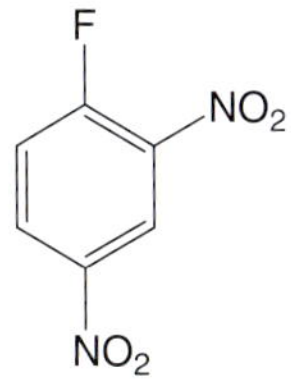

DNFB is a strong skin irritant and a universal contact allergen. It is used as an intermediate in the synthesis of pesticides and pharmaceuticals such as flurbiprofen, a chemical reagent, and as a topical sensitizer for treatment of alopecia areata.

Suggested Reading
Perez A, Narayan S, Sansom J (2004) Occupational contact dermatitis from 2,4-dinitrofluorobenzene. Contact Dermatitis 51:314

170. 2,4-Dinitrotoluene

CAS Registry Number [121–14–12]

Dinitrotoluene induced sensitization in a worker for an explosives manufacturer, also sensitized to nitroglycerin.

Suggested Reading
Kanerva L, Laine R, Jolanki R, Tarvainen K, Estlander T, Helander I (1991) Occupational allergic contact dermatitis caused by nitroglycerin. Contact Dermatitis 24:356–362

171. Dipentamethylenethiuram Disulfide

CAS Registry Number [94–37–1]

A rubber chemical contained in "thiuram mix." The most frequent occupational categories are the metal industry, homemakers, health services and laboratories, and the building industry.

Suggested Reading
Condé-Salazar L, Del-Rio E, Guimaraens D, Gonzalez Domingo A (1993) Type IV allergy to rubber additives: a 10-year study of 686 cases. J Am Acad Dermatol 29:176–180
Condé-Salazar L, Guimaraens D, Villegas C, Romero A, Gonzalez MA (1995) Occupational allergic contact dermatitis in construction workers. Contact Dermatitis 35:226–230
Kiec-Swierczynska M (1995) Occupational sensitivity to rubber. Contact Dermatitis 32:171–172
Von Hintzenstern J, Heese A, Koch HU, Peters KP, Hornstein OP (1991) Frequency, spectrum and occupational relevance of type IV allergies to rubber chemicals. Contact Dermatitis 24:244–252

172. Dipentamethylenethiuram Hexasulfide

CAS Registry Number [971–15–3]

This thiuram compound is used as an accelerator for rubber vulcanization.

Suggested Reading
Le Coz CJ (2004) Fiche d'éviction en cas d'hypersensibilité au thiuram mix. Ann Dermatol Venereol 131:1012–1014

173. Dipentamethylenethiuram Tetrasulfide

CAS Registry Number [120–54–7]

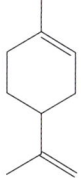

Dipentamethylenethiuram tetrasulfide is a thiuram compound used as an accelerator for rubber vulcanization.

Suggested Reading

Le Coz CJ (2004) Fiche d'éviction en cas d'hypersensibilité au thiuram mix. Ann Dermatol Venereol 131:1012–1014

174. Dipentene

CAS Registry Number [138–86–3]

Dipentene corresponds to a racemic mixture of D-limonene and L-limonene. Dipentene can be prepared from wood turpentine or by synthesis. It is used as a solvent for waxes, rosin and gums, in printing inks, perfumes, rubber compounds, paints, enamels, and lacquers. An irritant and sensitizer, dipentene caused contact dermatitis mainly in painters, polishers, and varnishers.

Suggested Reading

Martins C, Gonçalo M, Gonçalo S (1995) Allergic contact dermatitis from dipentene in wax polish. Contact Dermatitis 33:126–127

Moura C, Dias M, Vale T (1994) Contact dermatitis in painters, polishers and varnishers. Contact Dermatitis 31:51–53

175. Diphencyprone

2,3-Diphenylcyclopropenone

CAS Registry Number [886–38–4]

Diphencyprone is a potent contact allergen used in topical immunotherapy, to treat some severe alopecia areata. It is responsible for occupational contact dermatitis in chemists and dermatology department staff.

Suggested Reading

Sansom JE, Molloy KC, Lovell CR (1995) Occupational sensitization to diphencyprone in a chemist. Contact Dermatitis 32:363

Temesvári E, González R, Marschalkó M, Horváth A (2004) Age dependence of diphenylcyclopropenone sensitization in patients with alopecia areata. Contact Dermatitis 50:381–382

176. *N,N'*-Diphenyl-4-Phenylenediamine

DPPD

CAS Registry Number [74–31–7]

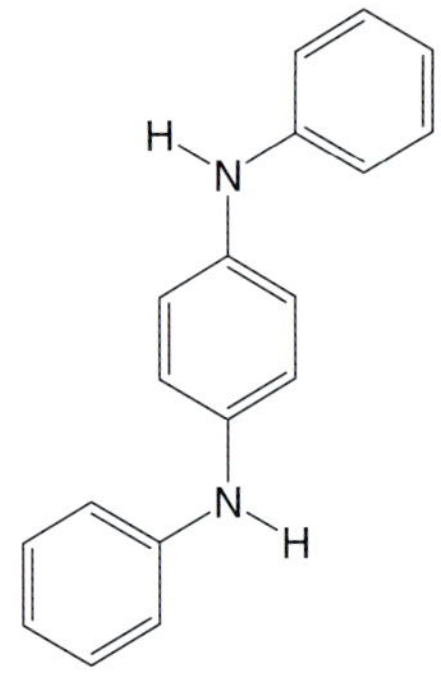

A rubber accelerant, formerly contained in "black-rubber mix." The most frequent occupational categories are in the metal industry, homemakers, health services and laboratories, and the building industry.

Suggested Reading

Condé-Salazar L, Del-Rio E, Guimaraens D, Gonzalez Domingo A (1993) Type IV allergy to rubber additives: a 10-year study of 686 cases. J Am Acad Dermatol 29:176–180

Kiec-Swierczynska M (1995) Occupational sensitivity to rubber. Contact Dermatitis 32:171–172

Von Hintzenstern J, Heese A, Koch HU, Peters KP, Hornstein OP (1991) Frequency, spectrum and occupational relevance of type IV allergies to rubber chemicals. Contact Dermatitis 24:244–252

177. 1,3-Diphenylguanidine

CAS Registry Number [102–06–7]

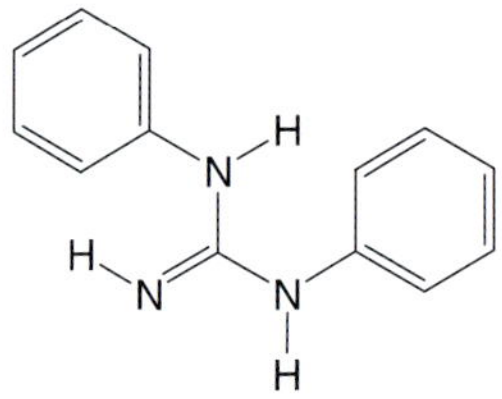

Diphenylguanidine is a rubber sensitizer that can induce immediate-type reactions and delayed-type contact allergy. It was formerly contained in "carba mix." Occupational exposure concerns finished rubber items and the rubber manufacturing industry. The most frequent occupational categories are metal industry, homemakers, health services and laboratories, and the building industry.

Suggested Reading

Bruze M, Kestrup L (1994) Occupational allergic contact dermatitis from diphenylguanidine in a gas mask. Contact Dermatitis 31:125–126

Condé-Salazar L, Del-Rio E, Guimaraens D, Gonzalez Domingo A (1993) Type IV allergy to rubber additives: a 10-year study of 686 cases. J Am Acad Dermatol 29:176–180

Kiec-Swierczynska M (1995) Occupational sensitivity to rubber. Contact Dermatitis 32:171–172

Mancuso G, Reggiani M, Berdondini RM (1996) Occupational dermatitis in shoemakers. Contact Dermatitis 34:17–22

Von Hintzenstern J, Heese A, Koch HU, Peters KP, Hornstein OP (1991) Frequency, spectrum and occupational relevance of type IV allergies to rubber chemicals. Contact Dermatitis 24:244–252

178. 4,4'-Diphenylmethane-Diisocyanate

MDI

CAS Registry Number [101–68–8]

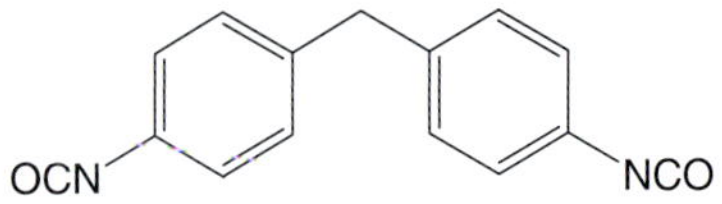

OCN   NCO

51

MDI is used in the manufacture of various polyurethane products: elastic and rigid foams, paints, lacquers, adhesives, binding agents, synthetic rubbers, and elastomeric fibers.

Suggested Reading

Estlander T, Keskinen H, Jolanki R, Kanerva L (1992) Occupational dermatitis from exposure to polyurethane chemicals. Contact Dermatitis 27:161–165

Mancuso G, Reggiani M, Berdondini RM (1996) Occupational dermatitis in shoemakers. Contact Dermatitis 34:17–22

179. Diphenylthiourea

CAS Registry Number [102–08–9]

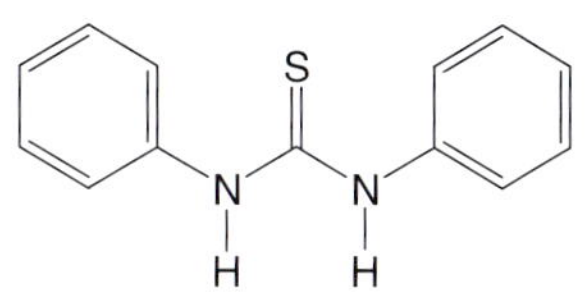

It is a rubber chemical used as an accelerator and stabilizing agent in neoprene.

Suggested Reading

Kanerva L, Estlander T, Jolanki R (1994) Occupational allergic contact dermatitis caused by thiourea compounds. Contact Dermatitis 31:242–248

Kiec-Swierczynska M (1995) Occupational sensitivity to rubber. Contact Dermatitis 32:171–172

180. Disperse Blue 106

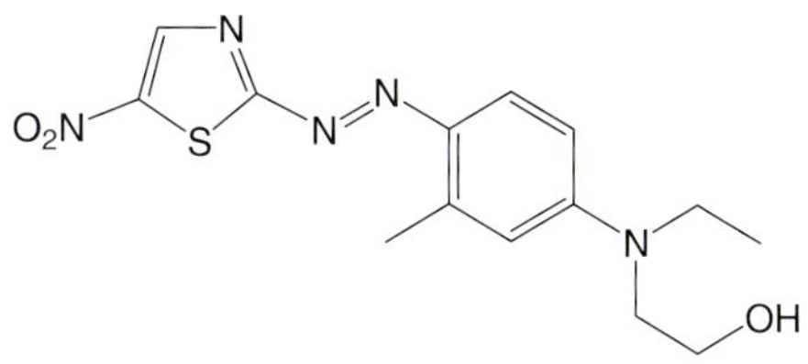

This clothing dye used in synthetic fibers is one of the most potent sensitizers in clothes. Allergic contact dermatitis is relatively frequent in consumers. Occupational textile dye dermatitis was reported in a ready-to-wear shop. Constant concomitant reactions with Disperse Blue 124 are due to their chemical similarities, as with photograph developers CD1, CD2, CD3, and CD4. See also Chap. 37, Clothing.

Suggested Reading

Menezes-Brandão F, Altermatt C, Pecegueiro M, Bordalo O, Foussereau J (1985) Contact dermatitis to Disperse Blue 106. Contact Dermatitis 13:80–84

Mota F, Silva E, Varela P, Azenha A, Massa A (2000) An outbreak of occupational textile dye dermatitis from Disperse Blue 106. Contact Dermatitis 43:235–236

181. Disperse Blue 124

CAS Registry Number [15141–18–1]

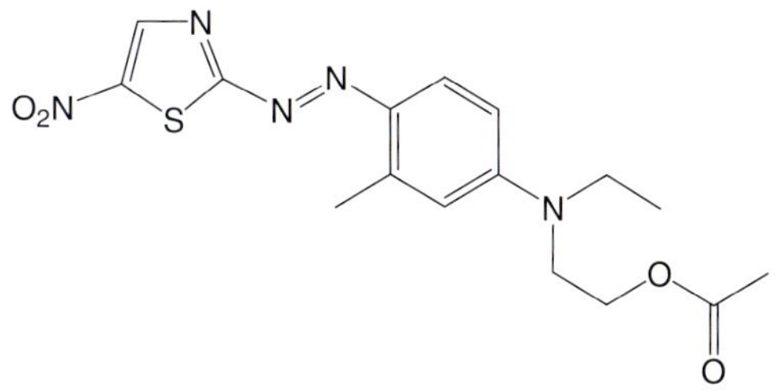

This clothing dye used in synthetic fibers is one of the most potent sensitizers in clothes. It is a textile dye responsible for occupational contact dermatitis in the textile industry. A positive patch test reaction was observed in a painter sensitized to phthalocyanine dyes, with no occupational relevance. Constant concomitant reactions with Disperse Blue 106, and even to photographic developers CD1–4, are due to their chemical similarities. See also Chap. 37, Clothing.

Suggested Reading
Raccagni AA, Baldari U, Righini MG (1996) Airborne dermatitis in a painter. Contact Dermatitis 35:119–120
Soni BP, Sherertz EF (1996) Contact dermatitis in the textile industry: a review of 72 patients. Am J Contact Dermat 7:226–230

182. Disperse Dyes

Disperse dyes are so-called because they are partially soluble in water. These synthetic dyes have either an anthraquinone (disperse anthraquinone dyes) or an azoic structure (disperse azo dyes). They are the most commonly employed dyes, sometimes as hair dyes, but chiefly in the textile industry to color synthetic fibers such as polyester, acrylic and acetate, and sometimes nylon, particularly in stockings. They are not used for natural fibers. These molecules are the main textile sensitizers. See Chap. 37, Clothing.

183. Disperse Orange 3

CI 11005

CAS Registry Number [730–40–5]

Disperse Orange 3 is an azo dye that can induce contact dermatitis in workers in the textile industry. It is positive in a great majority of PPD-positive people, because of hydrolysis in the skin into PPD. Disperse Orange 3 can also be found in some semi-permanent hair dyes. See also Chap. 37, Clothing.

Suggested Reading
Balato N, Lembo G, Patruno C, Ayala F (1990) Prevalence of textile dye contact sensitization. Contact Dermatitis 23:126–127
Condé-Salazar L, Baz M, Guimaraens D, Cannavo A (1995) Contact dermatitis in hairdressers: patch test results in 379 hairdressers (1980–1993). Am J Contact Dermat 6:19–23
Soni BP, Sherertz EF (1996) Contact dermatitis in the textile industry: a review of 72 patients. Am J Contact Dermat 7:226–230

184. Disperse Orange 31

CAS Registry Number [61968-38-5] (and [68391-42-4]?)

The synthetic azo dye Disperse Orange 31 was wrongly substituted by Disperse Orange 3 in patch test materials from Chemotechnique. This situation explains why a relatively low percentage of patients positive to PPD were positive to Disperse Orange 3, although a co-reaction is explained to be very frequent because skin transformation of Disperse Orange 3 into PPD. See also Chap. 37, Clothing.

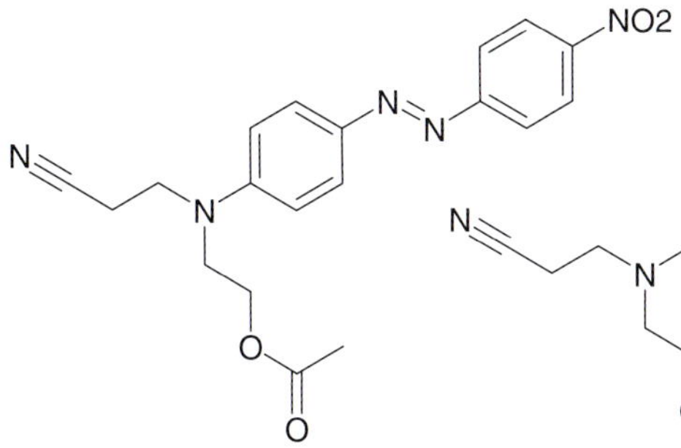

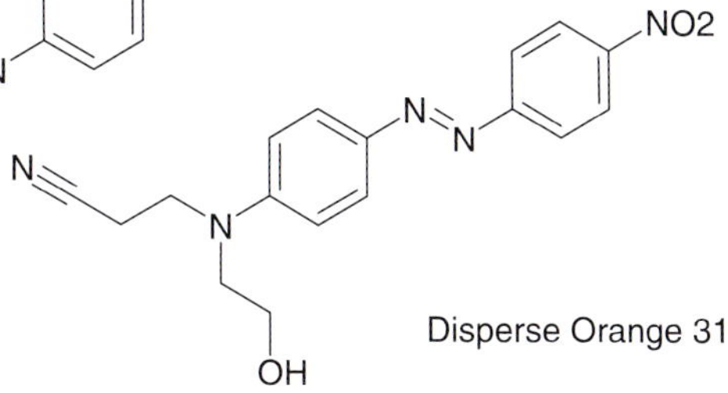

Disperse Orange 31 hydrolyzed

Disperse Orange 31

Suggested Reading

Goon AT, Gilmour NJ, Basketter DA, White IR, Rycroft RJ, McFadden JP (2003) High frequency of simultaneous sensitivity to Disperse Orange 3 in patients with positive patch tests to para-phenylenediamine. Contact Dermatitis 48:248–250

Le Coz CJ, Jelen G, Goossens A, Vigan M, Ducombs G, Bircher A, Giordano-Labadie F, Pons-Guiraud A, Milpied-Homsi B, Castelain M, Tennstedt D, Bourrain JL, Bernard G, GERDA (2004) Disperse (yes), Orange (yes), 3 (no): what do we test in textile dye dermatitis? Contact Dermatitis 50:126–127

185. Disperse Red 11

CI 62015

CAS Registry Number [2872–48–2]

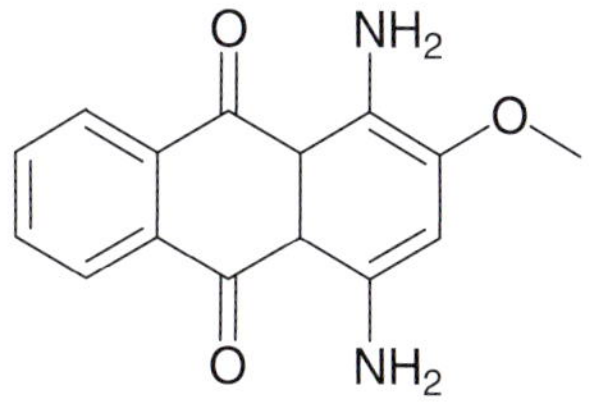

Disperse Red 11 is an example of disperse dye anthraquinone type. See also Chap. 37, Clothing.

Suggested Reading

Cronin E (1980) Contact dermatitis. Churchill Livingstone, Edinburgh, pp 36–92

186. Disperse Yellow 3

CI 11855

CAS Registry Number [2832–40–8]

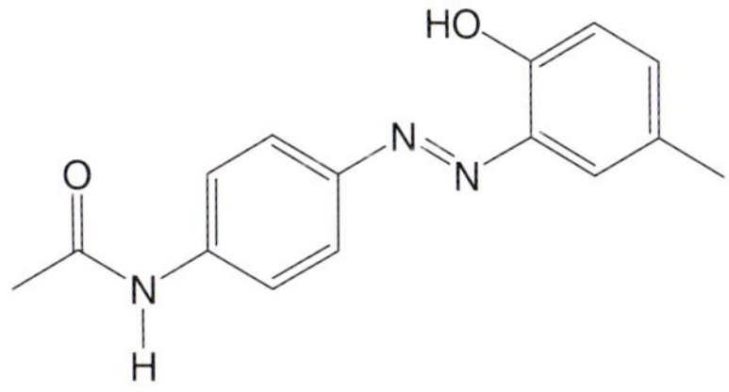

This azoic dye is responsible for textile dermatitis from stockings and occupational contact dermatitis in workers in the textile industry. It can be found in some semi-permanent hair dyes. See also Chap. 37, Clothing.

Suggested Reading

Condé-Salazar L, Baz M, Guimaraens D, Cannavo A (1995) Contact dermatitis in hairdressers: patch test results in 379 hairdressers (1980–1993). Am J Contact Dermat 6:19–23

Soni BP, Sherertz EF (1996) Contact dermatitis in the textile industry: a review of 72 patients. Am J Contact Dermat 7:226–230

187. Dithianone

CAS Registry Number [3347–22–6]

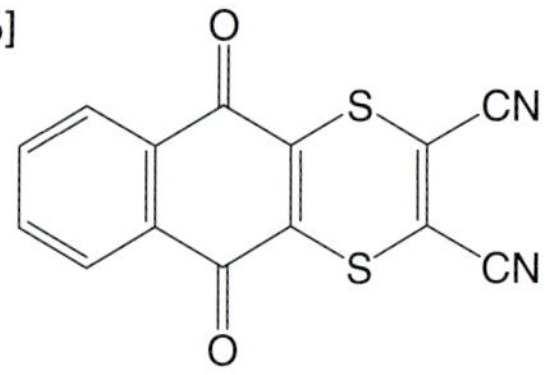

Dithianone is an anthraquinone derivative, used as a fungicide agent. With cymoxanil, it is contained in Aktuan®. Cases in agricultural workers were reported sparsely.

Suggested Reading
Koch P (1996) Occupational allergic contact dermatitis and airborne contact dermatitis from 5
    fungicides in a vineyard worker. Cross-reactions between fungicides of the dithiocarbamate
    group? Contact Dermatitis 34:324–329

51

188. Dodecyl Gallate

Lauryl Gallate

CAS Registry Number [1166–52–5]

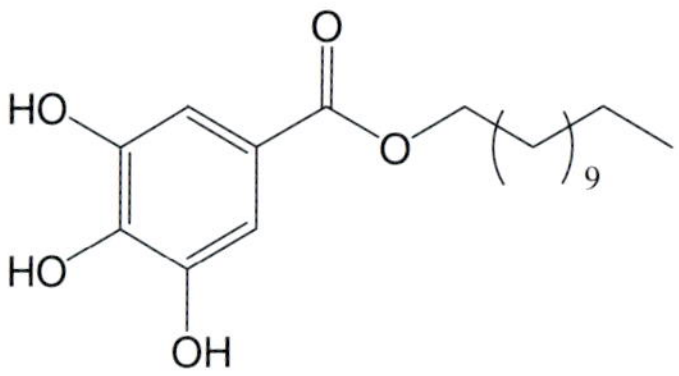

This gallic acid ester (E 310) is an antioxidant added to foods and cosmetics to prevent oxidation of unsaturated fatty acids. Cases were reported in workers of the food industry, gallate being contained in margarine, and from washing powder.

Suggested Reading
De Groot AC, Gerkens F (1990) Occupational airborne contact dermatitis from octyl gallate. Contact Dermatitis 23:184–186
Mancuso G, Staffa M, Errani A, Berdondini RM, Fabri P (1990) Occupational dermatitis in animal
    feed mill workers. Contact Dermatitis 22:37–41

189. Doxepin

CAS Registry Number [1668–19–5]

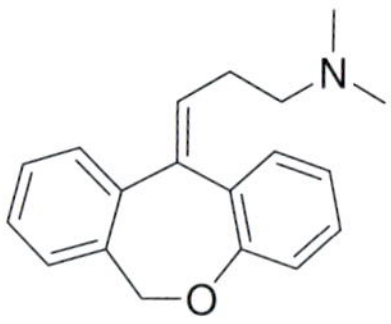

This benzoxepin tricylcic drug has antidepressant, anticholinergic, anti-itching, and antihistamine properties. After oral use, it has been developed as a topical anti-itching agent. Allergic contact dermatitis is not infrequent.

Suggested Reading
Buckley DA (2000) Contact allergy to doxepin. Contact Dermatitis 43:231–232
Taylor JS, Praditsuwan P, Handel D, Kuffner G (1996) Allergic contact dermatitis from doxepin
    cream. One-year patch test clinic experience. Arch Dermatol 132:515–518

190. Epichlorhydrin

1-Chloro-2,3-Epoxypropane

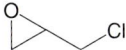

CAS Registry Number [106–89–8]

Epoxy resin of the Bisphenol A type is synthesized from epichlorhydrin and bisphenol A. It leads to bisphenol A diglycidyl ether, which is the monomer of bisphenol-A-based epoxy resins. Sensitization to epichlorhydrin occurs mainly in workers of the epoxy resin industry. Sensitization in individuals not working at epoxy resin plants is rare. It has however been described to occur following exposure to a soil fumigant, due to solvent cement and in a worker in a pharmaceutical plant, in a division of drug synthesis. Epichlorhydrin was used for the production of drugs propranolol and oxprenolol.

Suggested Reading

Holness DL, Nethercott JR (1993) The performance of specialized collections of bisphenol A epoxy resin system components in the evaluation of workers in an occupational health clinic population. Contact Dermatitis 28:216–219

Rebandel P, Rudzki E (1990) Dermatitis caused by epichlorhydrin, oxprenolol hydrochloride and propranolol hydrochloride. Contact Dermatitis 23:199

Van Jost T, Roesyanto ID, Satyawan I (1990) Occupational sensitization to epichlorhydrin (ECH) and bisphenol-A during the manufacture of epoxy resin. Contact Dermatitis 22:125–126

191. Epoxy Resins of the Bisphenol A Type

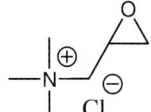

These resins are synthesized from bisphenol A and epichlorhydrin. Hardeners are added, such as amines (ethylenediamine, diethylenetriamine, triethylenetetramine, isophoronediamine, triethylenetriamine and 4,4′-diaminophenylmethane) or acid anhydrides (phthalic anhydride). Reactive diluents may be added, such as allyl glycidyl ether, butanediol diglycidyl ether, n-butyl glycidyl ether, o-cresyl glycidyl ether, hexanediol diglycidyl ether, neopentyl glycol diglycidyl ether, phenyl glycidyl ether, glycidyl ester of synthetic fatty acids, and glycidyl ether of aliphatic alcohols (Epoxide-8).

Suggested Reading

Holness DL, Nethercott JR (1993) The performance of specialized collections of bisphenol A epoxy resin system components in the evaluation of workers in an occupational health clinic population. Contact Dermatitis 28:216–219

Jolanki R, Kanerva L, Estlander T, Tarvainen K, Keskinen H, Henriks-Eckerman ML (1990) Occupational dermatoses from epoxy resin compounds. Contact Dermatitis 23:172–183

192. 2,3-Epoxypropyl Trimethyl Ammonium Chloride

EPTMAC, Glycidyl Trimethyl Ammonium Chloride, Oxiranemethanaminium, N,N, N-Trimethyl Chloride

CAS Registry Number [3033–77–0]

Used in the production of cationic starch for the paper industry, EPTMAC caused contact dermatitis in workers.

Suggested Reading
Estlander T, Jolanki R, Kanerva L (1997) Occupational allergic contact dermatitis from 2,3-epoxy-propyl trimethyl ammonium chloride (EPTMAC) and Kathon R LX in a starch modification factory. Contact Dermatitis 36:191–194

193. Estradiol

17-β-Estradiol, (17β)-Estra-1,3,5(10)-Triene-3.17-diol

CAS Registry Number [50–28–2]

Natural estradiol, used in transdermal systems for hormonal substitution, can induce allergic contact dermatitis, with the risk of systemic contact dermatitis after oral reintroduction.

Suggested Reading
Gonçalo M, Oliveira HS, Monteiro C, Clerins I, Figueiredo A (1999) Allergic and systemic contact dermatitis from estradiol. Contact Dermatitis 40:58–59

194. Ethoxyquin

1,2-Dihydro 6-Ethoxy 2,2,4-Trimethylquinolein, Santoquin®, Santoflex®

CAS Registry Number [91–53–2]

Ethoxyquin is used as an antioxidant in animal feed and caused contact dermatitis in a worker at an animal feed mill.

Suggested Reading
Mancuso G, Staffa M, Errani A, Berdondini RM, Fabri P (1990) Occupational dermatitis in animal feed mill workers. Contact Dermatitis 22:37–41

195. Ethyl Alcohol

Ethanol

CAS Registry Number [64–17–5]

Ethanol is widely used for its solvent and antiseptic properties. It is rather an irritant and sensitization has rarely been reported.

Suggested Reading
Ophaswongse S, Maibach HI (1994) Alcohol dermatitis: allergic contact dermatitis and contact urticaria syndrome. Contact Dermatitis 30:1–6
Patruno C, Suppa F, Sarraco G, Balato N (1994) Allergic contact dermatitis due to ethyl alcohol. Contact Dermatitis 31:124

196. 4-Ethyl-Pyridine

CAS Registry Number [536–75–4]

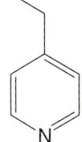

4-Ethyl-pyridine is used as a monomer in polymer chemistry.

Suggested Reading
Sasseville D, Balbul A, Kwong P, Yu K (1996) Contact sensitization to pyridine derivatives. Contact Dermatitis 35:101–102

197. Ethylbutylthiourea

CAS Registry Number [32900–06–4]

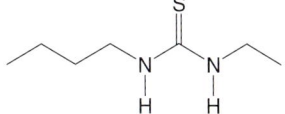

Ethylbutylthiourea is an accelerator used with other thiourea derivatives in the production of neoprene rubber. It is also contained in glues, mainly neoprene type.

Suggested Reading
Bergendorff O, Persson CML, Hansson C (2004) HPLC analysis of alkyl thioureas in an orthopaedic brace and patch testing with pure ethylbutylthiourea. Contact Dermatitis 51:273–277
Kanerva L, Estlander T, Jolanki R (1994) Occupational allergic contact dermatitis caused by thiourea compounds. Contact Dermatitis 31:242–248
Roberts JL, Hanifin JM (1980) Contact allergy and cross-reactivity to substituted thiourea compounds. Contact Dermatitis 6:138–139

198. Ethylene Oxide

CAS Registry Number [75–21–8]

Ethylene oxide is a very strong irritant widely used in the chemical industry, and as a sterilizer of medical supplies, pharmaceutical products, and food. Residues in masks or dressings can produce irritant contact dermatitis.

Suggested Reading
Lerman Y, Ribak J, Skulsky M, Ingber A (1995) An outbreak of irritant contact dermatitis from ethylene oxide among pharmaceutical workers. Contact Dermatitis 33:280–281

199. Ethylenediamine

CAS Registry Number [107–15–3] H_2N ⌣ NH_2

Ethylenediamine is used in numerous industrial processes as a solvent for casein or albumin, as a stabilizer in rubber latex and as a textile lubricant. It can be found in epoxy resin hardeners, cooling oils, fungicides, and waxes. Contact dermatitis from ethylenediamine is almost exclusively due to topical medicaments. Occupational contact dermatitis in epoxy resin systems is rather infrequent. Ethylenediamine can cross-react with triethylenetetramine and diethylenetriamine. Ethylenediamine was found to be responsible for sensitization in pharmacists handling aminophylline suppositories, in nurses preparing and administering injectable theophylline, and in a laboratory technician in the manufacture of aminophylline tablets.

Suggested Reading

Chieregato C, Vincenzi C, Guerra L, Farina P (1994) Occupational allergic contact dermatitis due to ethylenediamine dihydrochloride and cresyl glycidyl ether in epoxy resin systems. Contact Dermatitis 30:120

Corazza M, Mantovani L, Trimurti L, Virgili A (1994) Occupational contact sensitization to ethylenediamine in a nurse. Contact Dermatitis 31:328–329

Jolanki R, Kanerva L, Estlander T, Tarvainen K, Keskinen H, Henriks-Eckerman ML (1990) Occupational dermatoses from epoxy resin compounds. Contact Dermatitis 23:172–183

Mancuso G, Reggiani M, Berdondini RM (1996) Occupational dermatitis in shoemakers. Contact Dermatitis 34:17–22

Sasseville D, Al-Khenaizan S (1997) Occupational contact dermatitis from ethylenediamine in a wire-drawing lubricant. Contact Dermatitis 3:228–229

51

200. Ethylenethiourea

CAS Registry Number [96–45–7]

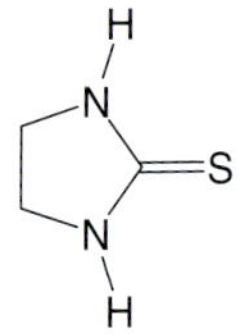

Ethylenethiourea, a thiourea derivative, is a rubber chemical. It caused contact dermatitis mainly in rubber workers.

Suggested Reading

Bruze M, Fregert S (1983) Allergic contact dermatitis from ethylenethiourea. Contact Dermatitis 9:208–212

Kanerva L, Estlander T, Jolanki R (1994) Occupational allergic contact dermatitis caused by thiourea compounds. Contact Dermatitis 31:242–248

201. Ethylhexylglycerin

Octoxyglycerin

CAS Registry Number [70445–33–9]

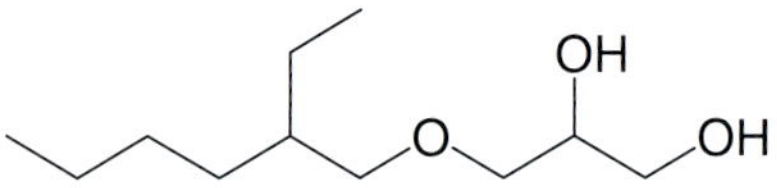

This glycerol monoalkylether is used as a skin conditioning agent, with bactericidal properties against Gram-positive bacteria.

Suggested Reading

Linsen G, Goossens A (2002) Allergic contact dermatitis from ethylhexylglycerin. Contact Dermatitis 47:169

202. Eugenol

CAS Registry Number [97–53–0]

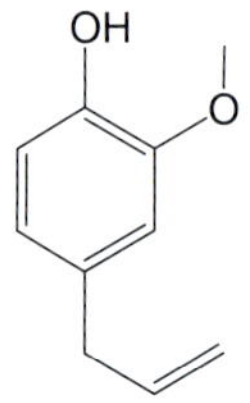

Eugenol is a fragrance allergen obtained from many natural sources. Occupational sensitization to eugenol may occur in dental profession workers. Eugenol is contained in "fragrance mix" and has to be listed by name in cosmetics within the EU.

Suggested Reading

Berova N, Stranky L, Krasteva M (1990) Studies on contact dermatitis in stomatological staff. Dermatol Monatsschr 176:15–18

Rudzki E, Rebandel P, Grzywa Z (1989) Patch tests with occupational contactants in nurses, doctors and dentists. Contact Dermatitis 20:247–250

203. Euxyl®K 400 (see 284. subentry 1,2-Dibromo-2,4-Dicyanobutane and 322. Phenoxyethanol)

Euxyl®K 400 is a mixture of 1,2-dibromo-2,4-dicyanobutane 20% and phenoxyethanol 80%, widely utilized as a preservative in cosmetics, hand creams and toiletries, but also in water-based paints, glues, metalworking fluids, and detergents. Sensitization was reported in masseurs, in a beautician, an offset printer, and a hospital cleaner. We observed four cases of hand contact dermatitis in metalworkers, due to the so-called Euxyl® K 400 contained in barrier creams. No sensitization was observed to phenoxyethanol (personal cases).

Suggested Reading

Aalto-Korte K, Jolanki R, Estlander T, Alanko K, Kanerva L (1996) Occupational allergic contact dermatitis caused by Euxyl K 400. Contact Dermatitis 35:193–194

204. Famotidine

CAS Registry Number [76824–35–6]

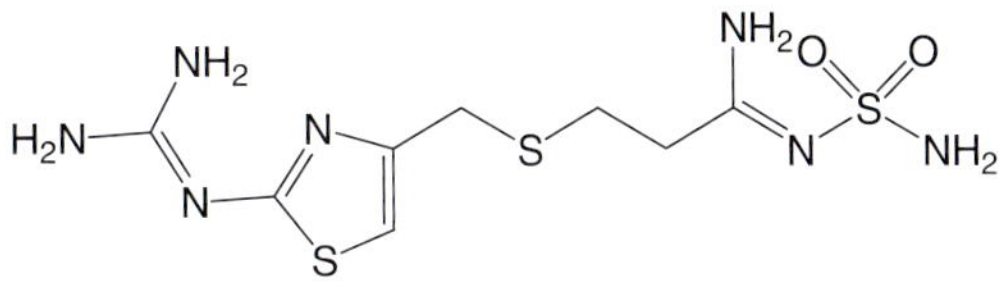

Contact dermatitis in a nurse from famotidine, an H2-receptor agonist, was described. In industry, three cases were reported due to intermediates of the synthesis of 2-diamino-ethylene-amino-thiazolyl-methylenethiourea-dichloride, and 4-chloromethyl-2-guanidinothiazole-nitrochloride.

Suggested Reading

Guimaraens D, Gonzales MA, Condé-Salazar L (1994) Occupational allergic contact dermatitis from intermediate products in famotidine synthesis. Contact Dermatitis 31:259–260

Monteseirin J, Conde J (1990) Contact eczema from famotidine. Contact Dermatitis 22:290

205. Farnesol

3,7,11-Trimethyldodeca-2,6,10-Trienol (Four Isomers)

CAS Registry Numbers [4602–84–0] for the mixture, [106–28–5] for the *trans/trans*, [3790–71–4] for the *cis/trans*, [3879–60–5] for the *trans/cis*, and [16106–95–9] for the *cis/cis*

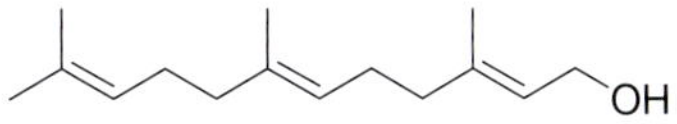

Farnesol is one of the most frequent contact allergens in perfumes. It is contained in small amounts in *Myroxylon pereirae* and in poplar buds. It is a blend of four diastereosiomers *trans/cis*. As a fragrance allergen, farnesol has to be mentioned by name in cosmetics within the EU.

Suggested Reading

Frosch PJ, Johansen JD, Menné T, Pirker C, Rastogi SC, Andersen KE, Bruze M, Goossens A, Lepoittevin JP, White IR (2002) Further important sensitizers in patients sensitive to fragrances. Contact Dermatitis 47:78–85

Schnuch A, Uter W, Geier J, Lessmann H, Frosch PJ (2004) Contact allergy to farnesol in 2021 consecutively patch tested patients. Results of the IVDK. Contact Dermatitis 50:117–121

206. Fenvalerate

CAS Registry Number [51630–58–1]

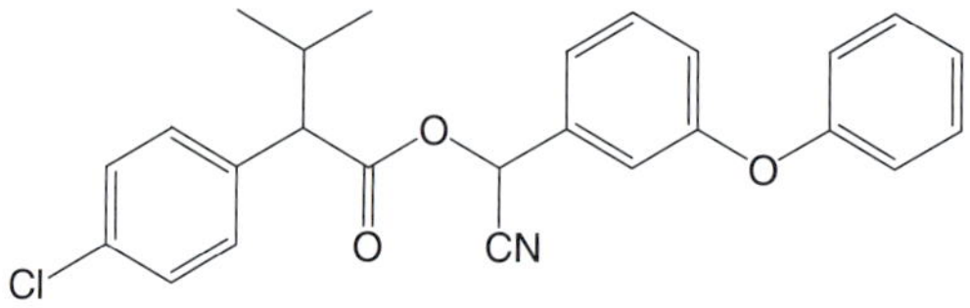

51

Fenvalerate is an insecticide of the synthetic pyrethroid group, which induced sensitization in farmers.

Suggested Reading

Sharma VK, Kaur S (1990) Contact sensitization by pesticides in farmers. Contact Dermatitis 23:
77–80

207. Fluazinam

**Shirlan®, 3-Chloro-*N*-(3-Chloro-5-Trifluoromethyl-2-Pyridyl)-
Trifluoro-2,6-Dinitro-*p*-Toluidine**

CAS Registry Number [79622–59–6]

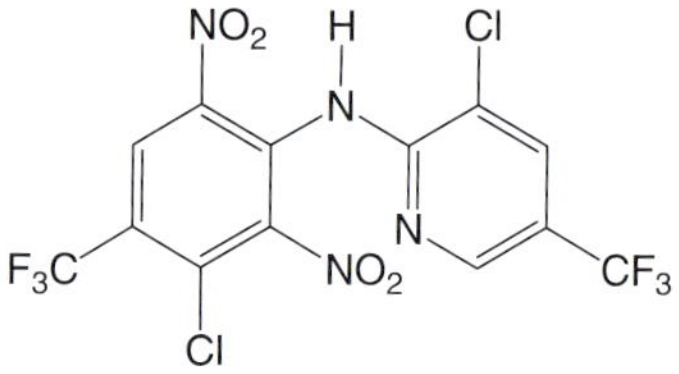

Fluazinam is a pesticide with a broad spectrum of antifungal activity. It caused sensitization in employees in the tulip bulb industry and in farmers. Fluazinam induced
contact dermatitis in a worker in a plant where it was manufactured.

Suggested Reading

Bruynzeel DP, Tafelkruijer J, Wilks MF (1995) Contact dermatitis due to a new fungicide used in the
tulip bulb industry. Contact Dermatitis 33:8–11

Van Ginkel CJW, Sabapathy NN (1995) Allergic contact dermatitis from the newly introduced fungicide fluazinam. Contact Dermatitis 32:160–162

208. Flutamide

**2-Methyl-*N*-[4-Nitro-3-(Trifluoromethyl)Phenyl]Propanamide,
Trifluoro-2-Methyl-4′-Nitro-*m*-Propionotoluidide,
4′-Nitro-3′-Trifluoromethylisobutyranilide, Niftolid**

CAS Registry Number [13311–84–7]

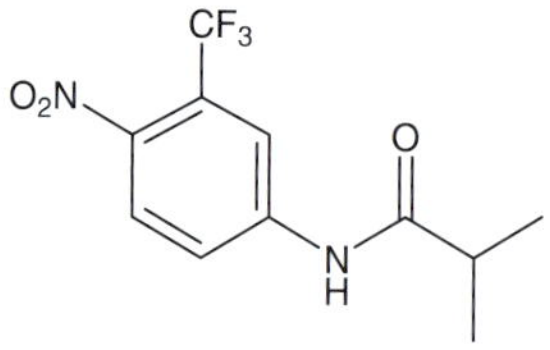

224. Hexanediol Diglycidyl Ether

1,6-Hexanediol Diglycidyl Ether

CAS Registry Number [16096-31-4]

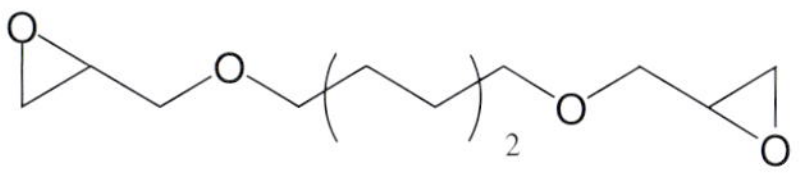

This chemical is a reactive diluent in epoxy resins.

Suggested Reading

Jolanki R, Kanerva L, Estlander T, Tarvainen K, Keskinen H, Henriks-Eckerman ML (1990) Occupational dermatoses from epoxy resin compounds. Contact Dermatitis 23:172–183

225. Hexyl Cinnamic Aldehyde

Hexyl Cinnamaldehyde, Alpha-Hexyl-Cinnamaldehyde, 2-(Phenylmethylene)Octanal, 2-Benzylideneoctanal

CAS Registry Number [101-86-0]

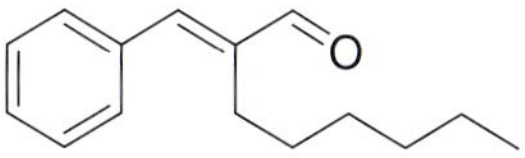

Hexyl cinnamic aldehyde is a fragrance allergen. Its presence has to be mentioned by name in cosmetics within the EU.

Suggested Reading

Frosch PJ, Johansen JD, Menné T, Pirker C, Rastogi SC, Andersen KE, Bruze M, Goossens A, Lepoittevin JP, White IR (2002) Further important sensitizers in patients sensitive to fragrances. Contact Dermatitis 47:78–85

Rastogi SC, Johansen JD, Menné T (1996) Natural ingredients based cosmetics. Content of selected fragrance sensitizers. Contact Dermatitis 34:423–426

226. Hydralazine

CAS Registry Number [86-54-4]

Hydralazine Hydrochloride

CAS Registry Number [304-20-1]

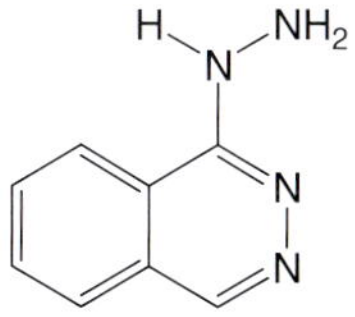

Hydralazine is a hydrazine derivative used as a antihypertensive drug. Skin rashes have been described during treatment. Exposure occurs mainly in the pharmaceutical industry. Cross-sensitivity is frequent with hydrazine, which is considered to be a potent sensitizer.

Suggested Reading

Pereira F, Dias M, Pacheco FA (1996) Occupational contact dermatitis from propranolol, hydralazine, and bendroflumethiazide. Contact Dermatitis 35:303–304

227. Hydrangenol

CAS Registry Number [480-47-7]

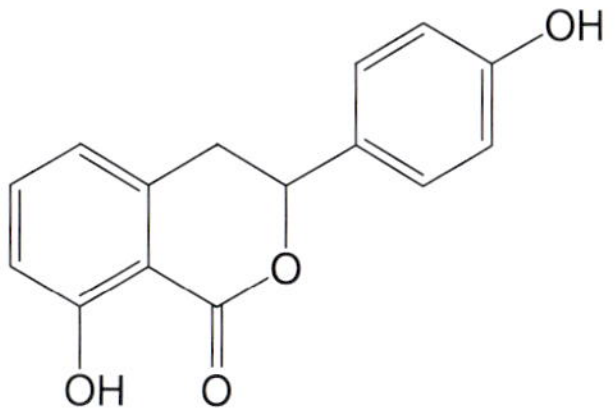

Hydrangenol is the allergen of hydrangea (*Hydrangea macrophylla* Thunb, Hydrangeaceae family). See also Chap. 41, Plants and Plant Products.

Suggested Reading

Avenel-Audran M, Hausen BM, Le Sellin J, Ledieu G, Verret JL (2000) Allergic contact dermatitis from hydrangea – is it so rare? Contact Dermatitis 43:189–191

Kuligowski ME, Chang A, Leemreize JHM (1992) Allergic contact hand dermatitis from hydrangea: report of a 10th case. Contact Dermatitis 26:269–270

228. Hydrazine

CAS Registry Number [302–01–2] $H_2N\text{—}NH_2$

Hydrazine sulphate CAS Registry Number [10034–93–2], dihydrobromide CAS Registry Number [23268–00–0] and hydrochloride {14011–37–1] have been reported as occupational sensitizers, mainly in soldering flux.

Suggested Reading

Frost J, Hjorth N (1959) Contact dermatitis from hydrazine bromide in soldering flux. Acta Derm Venereol (Stockh) 39:82–85

Goh CL, Ng SK (1987) Airborne contact dermatitis to colophony in soldering flux. Contact Dermatitis 17:89–91

Wheeler CE, Penn SR, Cawley EP (1965) Dermatitis from hydrazine hydrobromide solder flux. Arch Dermatol 91:235–239

Wrangsjö K, Martensson A (1986) Hydrazine contact dermatitis from gold plating. Contact Dermatitis 15:244–245

229. Hydrocortisone

Cortisol

CAS Registry Number [50–23–7]

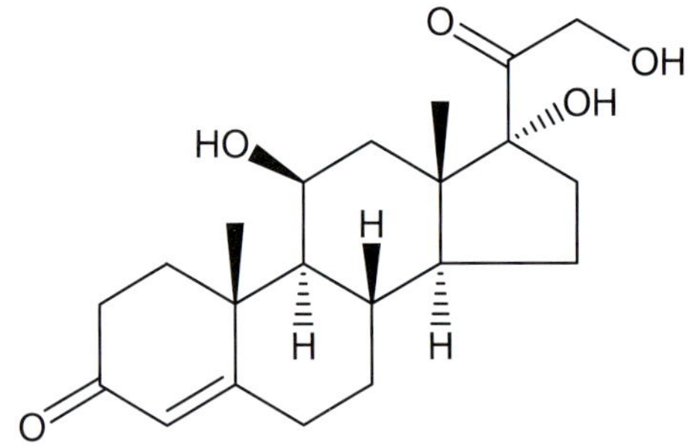

Hydrocortisone is the principal glucocorticoid hormone produced by the adrenal cortex, and is used topically or systemically. It belongs to the allergenic A group. Marker of allergy is tixocortol pivalate.

Suggested Reading

Lepoittevin JP, Drieghe J, Dooms-Goossens A (1995) Studies in patients with corticosteroid contact allergy. Understanding cross-reactivity among different steroids. Arch Dermatol 131:31–37

Le Coz CJ (2002) Fiche d'éviction en cas d'hypersensibilité au pivalate de tixocortol. Ann Dermatol Venereol 129:348–349

230. Hydrocortisone 17-Butyrate

CAS Registry Number [13609–67–1]

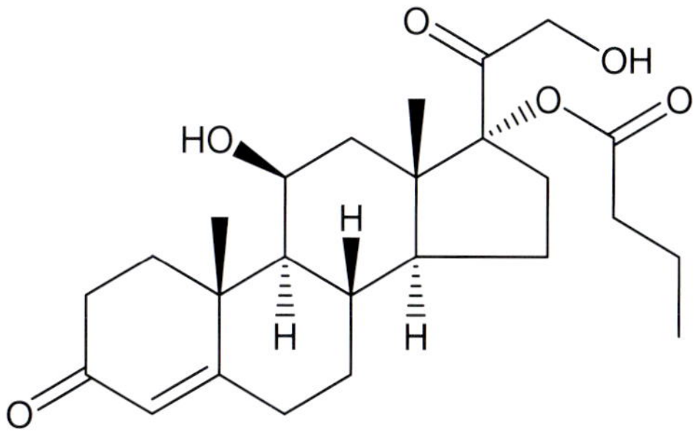

Hydrocortisone 17-butyrate is a C_{17} ester of hydrocortisone. It represents the D2 group of corticosteroids, non C_{16} methylated with a C_{17} ester: hydrocortisone 17-butyrate, hydrocortisone 17-valerate, hydrocortisone aceponate (17-propionate and 21-acetate), methylprednisolone aceponate, and prednicarbate. It is sometimes hydrolyzed in vivo into hydrocortisone, giving allergic reactions to group-A-sensitized people.

Suggested Reading

Le Coz CJ (2002) Fiche d'éviction en cas d'hypersensibilité au 17 butyrate d'hydrocortisone. Ann Dermatol Venereol 129 : 931

Lepoittevin JP, Drieghe J, Dooms-Goossens A (1995) Studies in patients with corticosteroid contact allergy. Understanding cross-reactivity among different steroids. Arch Dermatol 131 : 31–37

231. Hydrogen Peroxide

H_2O_2

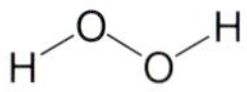

CAS Registry Number [7722–84–1]

Hydrogen peroxide is an oxidizing agent used as a topical antiseptic, and as part of permanent hair-dyes, color-removing preparations, and as a neutralizing agent in permanent waving. The concentration of the hydrogen peroxyde solution is expressed in volume or percentage: 10 volumes correspond to 3%. It is an irritant.

Suggested Reading

Aguirre A, Zabala R, Sanz De Galdeano C, Landa N, Diaz-Perez JL (1994) Positive patch tests to hydrogen peroxide in 2 cases. Contact Dermatitis 30 : 113

232. Hydroquinone

1,4-Benzenediol

CAS Registry Number [123–31–9]

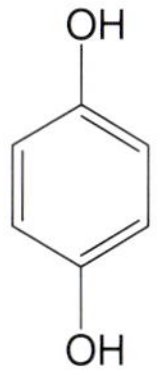

Hydroquinone is used in photography developers (black and white, X-ray, and microfilms), in plastics, in hair dyes as an antioxidant and hair colorant. Hydroquinone is found in many skin bleaching creams.

51

Suggested Reading

Barrientos N, Ortiz-Frutos J, Gomez E, Iglesias L (2001) Allergic contact dermatitis from a bleaching cream. Am J Contact Dermat 12:33–34

Gebhardt M, Geier J (1996) Evaluation of patch test results with denture material series. Contact Dermatitis 34:191–195

Lidén C, Brehmer-Andersson E (1988) Occupational dermatoses from colour developing agents. Clinical and histopathological observations. Acta Derm Venereol (Stockh) 68:514–522

Scheman AJ, Katta R (1997) Photographic allergens: an update. Contact Dermatitis 37:130

233. (S)-4′-Hydroxy 4-Methoxydalbergione

CAS Registry Number [3755–63–3]

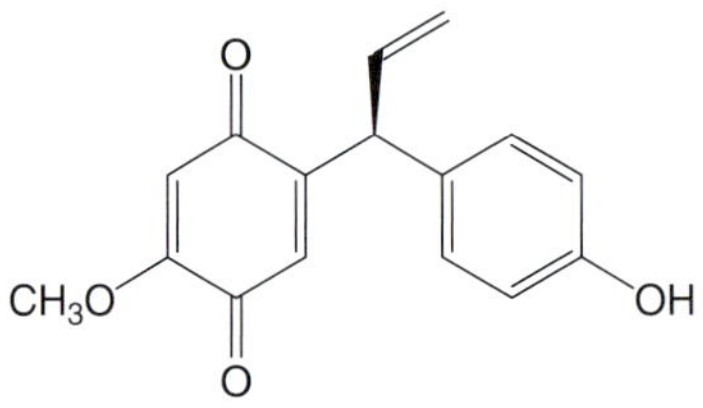

(S)-4′-Hydroxy 4-methoxydalbergione is one of the allergens Brazilian rosewood or Palissander (*Dalbergia nigra* All., Papillionaceae family), cocobolo (*Dalbergia retusa* Hemsl., *Dalbergia granadilla*, and *Dalbergia hypoleuca*) or grenadil (*Dalbergia melanoxylon* Guill. and Perr.). See also Chap. 41, Plants and Plant Products.

Suggested Reading

Hausen BM (1981) Wood injurious to human health. A manual. De Gruyter, Berlin

234. Hydroxycitronellal

7-Hydroxycitronellal, Citronellal Hydrate, Laurine, Muguet Synthetic

CAS Registry Number [107–75–5]

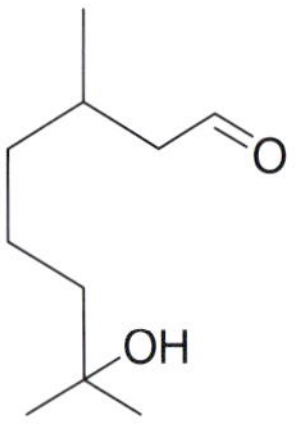

Hydroxycitronellal is a classical fragrance allergen, found in many products. It is contained in "Fragrance Mix." It has to be listed by name in the cosmetics of the EU.

Suggested Reading

Rastogi SC, Johansen JD, Frosch P, Menné T, Bruze M, Lepoittevin JP, Dreier B, Andersen KE, White IR (1998) Deodorants on the European market: quantitative chemical analysis of 21 fragrances. Contact Dermatitis 38:29–35

Svedman C, Bruze M, Johansen JD, Andersen KE, Goossens A, Frosch PJ, Lepoittevin JP, Rastogi S, White IR, Menné T (2003) Deodorants: an experimental provocation study with hydroxycitronellal. Contact Dermatitis 48:217–223

235. Hydroxylamine and Hydroxylammonium Salts

Hydroxylamine

CAS Registry Number [7803–49–8]

Hydroxylammonium Chloride: Hydroxylamine Hydrochloride, Oxammonium Hydrochloride

CAS Registry Numbers [5470–11–1]

Hydroxylammonium Sulfate: Hydroxylamine Sulfate, Oxammonium Sulfate

CAS Registry Number [7803–49–8].

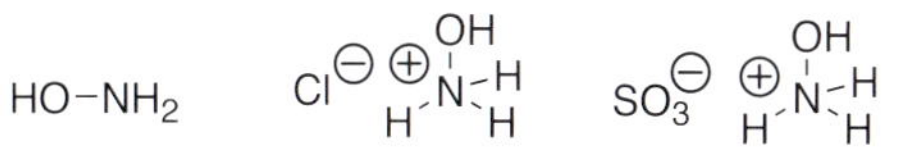

Hydroxylamine and its salts are used in various branches of industry, as reducing agents in color film developers or as reagents in laboratories.

Suggested Reading

Aguirre A, Landa N, Gonzalez M, Diaz-Perez JL (1992) Allergic contact dermatitis in a photographer. Contact Dermatitis 27:340–341

Estlander T, Jolanki T, Kanerva L (1997) Hydroxylammonium chloride as sensitizer in a water laboratory. Contact Dermatitis 36:161–162

Goh CL (1990) Allergic contact dermatitis and onycholysis from hydroxylamine sulphate in colour developer. Contact Dermatitis 22:109

236. Hydroxymethylpentacyclohexenecarboxaldehyde

Lyral®, Hydroxyisohexyl 3-Cyclohexene Carboxaldehyde,
4-(4-Hydroxy-4-Methylpentyl)-3-Cyclohexene-1-Carboxaldehyde,
4-(4-Hydroxy-4-Methylpentyl)Cyclohex-3-ene-Carbaldehyde

CAS Registry Number [31906–04–4]

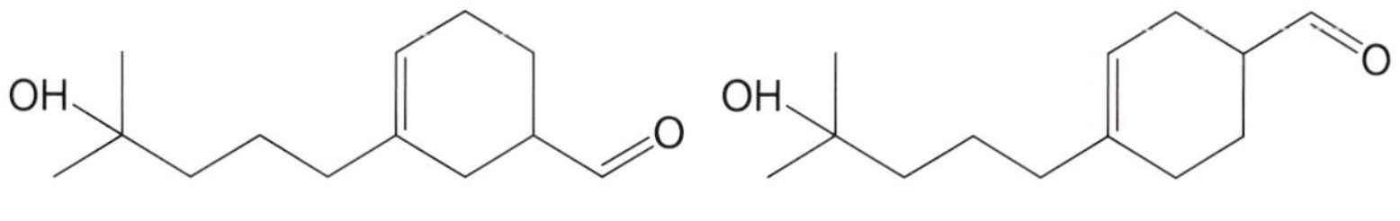

Lyral® is a synthetic blend of two isomers, and one of the most frequently encountered allergen in perfumes. It has to be listed by name in the ingredients of cosmetics in the EU, according to the 7th amendment of the cosmetic directive 76/768/EEC.

Suggested Reading

Johansen JD, Frosch PJ, Svedman C, Andersen KE, Bruze M, Pirker C, Menné T (2003) Hydroxyisohexyl 3-cyclohexene carboxaldehyde – known as Lyral: quantitative aspects and risk assessment of an important fragrance allergen. Contact Dermatitis 48:310–316

237. Hypochlorous Acid and Hypochlorites

Hypochlorous Acid

CAS Registry Number [7790–92–3]

Sodium Hypochlorite

CAS Registry Number [7681–52–9]

Sodium Hypochlorite Hydrate

CAS Registry Number [55248–17–4]

Sodium Hypochlorite Pentahydrate

CAS Registry Number [10022–70–5]

51

Sodium Hypochlorite Heptahydrate

CAS Registry Number [6431–03–9]

Calcium Hypochlorite

CAS Registry Number [7778–54–3]

Calcium Hypochlorite Dihydroxide

CAS Registry Number [12394–14–8]

Calcium Hypochlorite Dihydrate

CAS Registry Number [22464–76–2]

Calcium Sodium Hypochlorite

CAS Registry Number [53053–57–9]

Lithium Hypochlorite

CAS Registry Number [13840–33–0]

Potassium Hypochlorite

CAS Registry Number [7778–66–7]

Hypochlorous acid   Sodium hypochlorite   Calcium hypochlorite

Hypochlorites are derived from hypochlorous acid. They are bleaching agents and have large-spectrum antimicrobial activity. Calcium hypochlorite is used for disinfection in swimming pools and in industrial applications and for pulp and textile bleaching. Sodium hypochlorite is used as household laundry bleach, in commercial laundering, in pulp and paper manufacture, in industrial chemical synthesis, and in the disinfection of drinking water. Lithium hypochlorite is used in swimming pools for disinfection and in household detergents. Hypochlorites have caused hand, diffuse or periulcerous dermatitis, due to bleach settings and detergents, swimming pool water, endodontic treatment solution, or ulcer treatment.

Suggested Reading

Salphale PS, Shenoi SD (2003) Contact sensitivity to calcium hypochlorite. Contact Dermatitis 48: 162

Sasseville D, Geoffrion CT, Lowry RN (1999) Allergic contact dermatitis from chlorinated swimming pool water. Contact Dermatitis 41:347–348

238. Imidazolidinyl Urea

Germall® 115, IMIDUREA®

CAS Registry Number [39236–46–9]

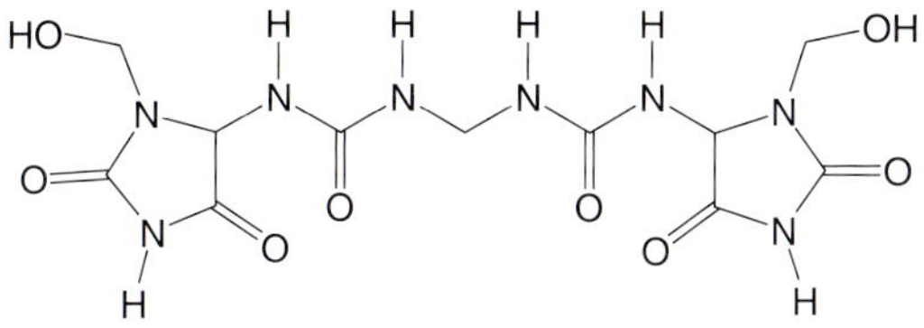

Imidazolidinyl urea, a formaldehyde releaser related to diazolidinyl urea (see above), is used as an antimicrobial agent very active against Gram-positive and Gram-negative bacteria, used as a synergist in combination with parabens. It is used as a preservative in aqueous products, mainly in cosmetics, toiletries, and liquid soaps.

Suggested Reading

Karlberg AT, Skare L, Lindberg I, Nyhammar E (1998) A method for quantification of formaldehyde in the presence of formaldehyde donors in skin-care products. Contact Dermatitis 38:20–28

Lachapelle JM, Ale SI, Freeman S, Frosch PJ, Goh CL, Hannuksela M, Hayakawa R, Maibach HI, Wahlberg JE (1997) Proposal for a revised international standard series of patch tests. Contact Dermatitis 36:121–123

Le Coz CJ (2005) Hypersensibilité à la Diazolidinyl urée et à l'Imidazolidinyl urée. Ann Dermatol Venereol 132:587–588

Van Hecke E, Suys E (1994) Where next to look for formaldehyde? Contact Dermatitis 31:268

239. Iodopropynyl Butylcarbamate

3-Iodo-2-Propynyl-Butyl Carbamate

CAS Registry Number [55406–53–6]

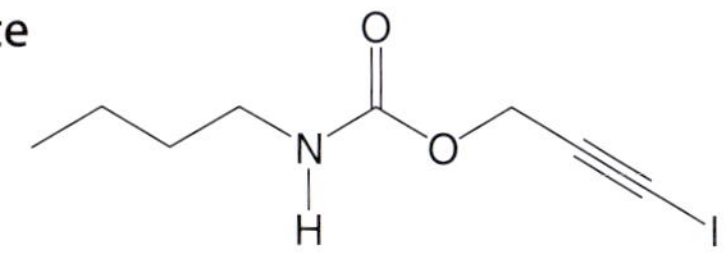

Iodopropynyl butylcarbamate (IPBC) is a broad-spectrum preservative used for years because of its wide field of application, in polymer emulsions and pigment dispersions such as water-based paints and adhesives, cements and inks, as a wood preservative, in metalworking fluids, in household products and in cosmetics. Allergic contact dermatitis to IPBC was reported due to cosmetics, from sanitary wipes, and in metalworkers.

Suggested Reading

Badreshia S, Marks JG Jr (2002) Iodopropynyl butylcarbamate. Am J Contact Dermat 13:77–79

Bryld LE, Agner T, Rastogi SC, Menné T (1997) Iodopropynyl butylcarbamate: a new contact allergen. Contact Dermatitis 36:156–158

Majoie IM, van Ginkel CJW (2000) The biocide iodopropynyl butylcarbamate (IPBC) as an allergen in cutting oils. Contact Dermatitis 43:238–239

240. Isoeugenol

Isoeugenol

CAS Registry Number [97–54–1]

cis-isoeugenol

CAS Registry Number [5912–86–7]

trans-Isoeugenol

CAS Registry Number [5932–68–3]

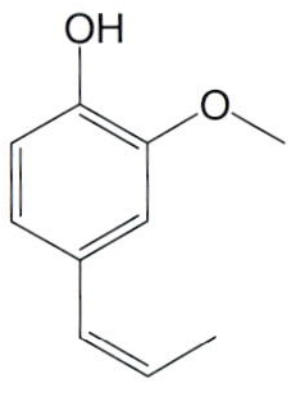

Cis-Isoeugenol

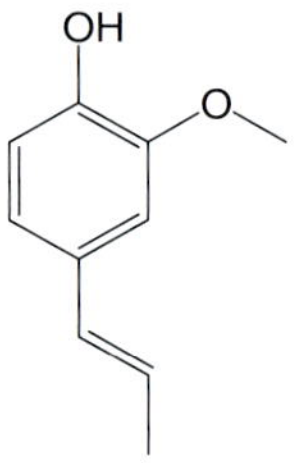

Trans-Isoeugenol

Isoeugenol is a mixture of two *cis* and *trans* isomers. It occurs in ylang-ylang and other essential oils. It is a common allergen of perfumes and cosmetics such as deodorants, and is contained in fragrance mix. Its presence in cosmetics is indicated in the INGREDIENTS series. Substitution by esters such as isoeugenyl acetate (not indicated on the package) does not always resolve the allergenic problem, because of the in vivo hydrolysis of the substitute into isoeugenol.

Suggested Reading

Rastogi SC, Johansen JD, Frosch P, Menné T, Bruze M, Lepoittevin JP, Dreier B, Andersen KE, White IR (1998) Deodorants on the European market: quantitative chemical analysis of 21 fragrances. Contact Dermatitis 38:29–35

Tanaka S, Royds C, Buckley D, Basketter DA, Goossens A, Bruze M, Svedman C, Menné T, Johansen JD, White IR, McFadden JP (2004) Contact allergy to isoeugenol and its derivatives: problems with allergen substitution. Contact Dermatitis 51:288–291

241. Alpha-Isomethylionone

3-Buten-2-one, 3-Methyl-4-(2,6,6-Trimethyl-2-Cyclohexen-1-yl), 3-Methyl-4-(2,6,6-Trimethyl-2-Cyclohexen-1-yl)3-Buten-2-one, Cetone Alpha

CAS Registry Number [127–51–5]

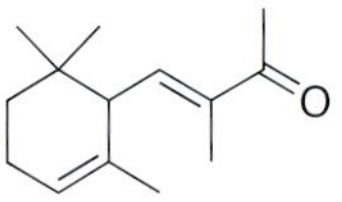

As a fragrance allergen, α-isomethylionone has to be mentioned by name in cosmetics within the EU.

Suggested Reading

Frosch PJ (1998) Are major components of fragrances a problem? In: Frosch PJ, Johansen JD, White IR (eds) Fragrances. Beneficial and adverse effects. Springer, Berlin Heidelberg New York, pp 92–99

242. Isophorone Diamine

**1-Amino-3-Aminomethyl-3,3,5-Trimethylcyclohexane,
3-Aminomethyl-3,5,5-Trimethylcyclohexylamine**

CAS Registry Number [2855–13–2]

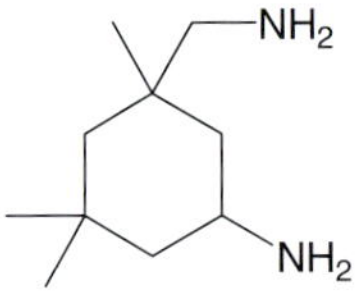

Isophorone diamine is widely used in urethane and epoxy coatings for light-stable, weather-resistant properties. It is used in water proofing and paving concreting, and in the manufacture of diisocyanates and polyamides as an epoxy resin hardener. It is a strong sensitizer and can cause airborne contact dermatitis.

Suggested Reading

Guerra L, Vincenzi, Bardazzi F, Tosti A (1992) Contact sensitization to isophoronediamine. Contact Dermatitis 27:52–53

Kelterer D, Bauer A, Elsner P (2000) Spill-induced sensitization to isophorone diamine. Contact Dermatitis 43:110

Lodi A, Mancini LL, Pozzi M, Chiarelli G, Crosti C (1993) Occupational airborne allergic contact dermatitis in parquet layers. Contact Dermatitis 29:281–282

243. Isopropyl Myristate

Tetradecanoic Acid 1-Methyl Ethyl Ester

CAS Registry Number [110–27–0]

Despite wide use in cosmetics, perfumes, and topical medicaments, isopropyl myristate is a very weak sensitizer and a mild irritant.

Suggested Reading

Uter W, Schnuch A, Geier J, Lessmann H (2004) Isopropyl myristate recommended for aimed rather than routine patch testing. Contact Dermatitis 50:242–244

244. *N*-Isopropyl-*N*-Phenyl-4-Phenylenediamine

IPPD, *N*-Isopropyl-*N*′-Phenyl-*p*-Phenylenediamine, *N*-(1-Methylethyl)-*N*′-Phenyl-1,4-Benzenediamine

CAS Registry Number [101–72–4]

This rubber chemical is used as an antioxidant and anti-ozonant. The main occupational sources are tires.

Suggested Reading

Condé-Salazar L, Del-Rio E, Guimaraens D, Gonzalez Domingo A (1993) Type IV allergy to rubber additives: a 10-year study of 686 cases. J Am Acad Dermatol 29:176–180

Hervé-Bazin B, Gradiski D, Duprat P, Marignac B, Foussereau J, Cavelier C, Bieber P (1977) Occupational eczema from *N*-isopropyl-*N*′-phenylparaphenylenediamine (IPPD) and *N*-dimethyl-1,3 butyl-*N*′-phenylparaphenylenediamine (DMPPD) in tyres. Contact Dermatitis 3:1–15

Von Hintzenstern J, Heese A, Koch HU, Peters KP, Hornstein OP (1991) Frequency, spectrum and occupational relevance of type IV allergies to rubber chemicals. Contact Dermatitis 24:244–252

245. Ketoprofen

CAS Registry Number [22071–15–4]

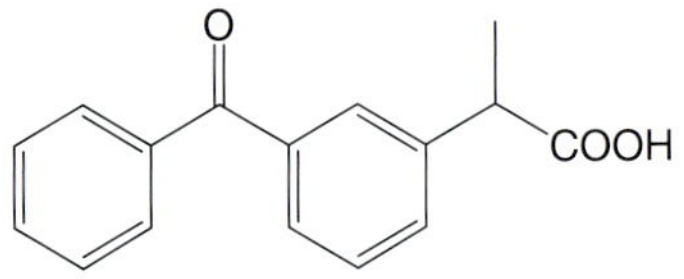

Ketoprofen is an anti-inflammatory drug, used both topically and systemically. It is above all a photoallergen, responsible for photoallergic or photo-worsened contact dermatitis, with sun-induced, progressive, severe, and durable reactions. Recurrent photosensitivity is possible for many years. Photosensitivities are expected to thiophene-phenylketone derivatives such as tiaprofenic acid and suprofen, to ketoprofen esters such as piketoprofen, and to benzophenone derivatives (see above) such as fenofibrate and benzophenone-3. Concomitant photosensitivities – without clinical relevance – have been observed to fenticlor, tetrachlorosalicylanilide, triclosan, tribromsalan, and bithionol.

Suggested Reading

Durbize E, Vigan M, Puzenat E, Girardin P, Adessi B, Desprez P, Humbert P, Laurent R, Aubin F (2003) Spectrum of cross-photosensitization in 18 consecutive patients with contact photoallergy to ketoprofen: associated photoallergies to non-benzophenone-containing molecules. Contact Dermatitis 48:144–149

Le Coz CJ, Bottlaender A, Scrivener JN, Santinelli F, Cribier BJ, Heid E, Grosshans EM (1998) Photocontact dermatitis from ketoprofen and tiaprofenic acid: cross-reactivity study in 12 consecutive patients. Contact Dermatitis 38:245–252

Le Coz CJ, El Aboubi S, Lefèbvre C, Heid E, Grosshans E (2000) Topical ketoprofen induces persistent and recurrent photosensitivity. Contact Dermatitis 42 [Suppl 2]:46

Le Coz CJ, El Aboubi S, Lefèbvre C, Heid E, Grosshans E (2000) Photoallergy from topical ketoprofen: a clinical, allergological and photobiological study. Contact Dermatitis 42 [Suppl 2]:47

246. Labetalol

CAS Registry Number [36894–69–6]

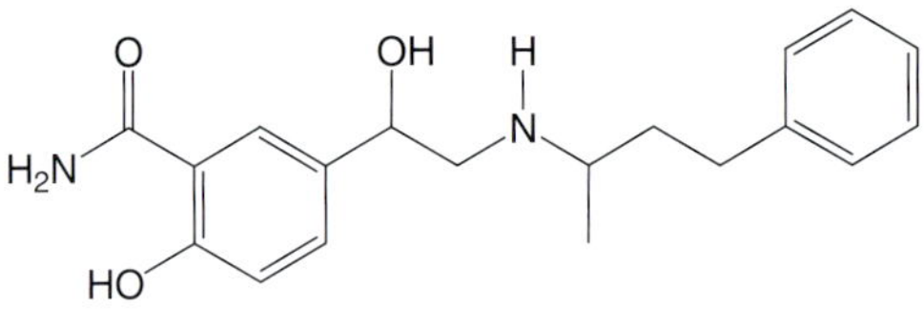

This beta-adrenergic and alpha-1 blocking agent caused contact dermatitis and a contact anaphylactoid reaction during patch testing in a nurse.

Suggested Reading

Bause GS, Kugelman LC (1990) Contact anaphylactoid response to labetalol. Contact Dermatitis 23:51

247. Lactucin

CAS Registry Number [1891–29–8]

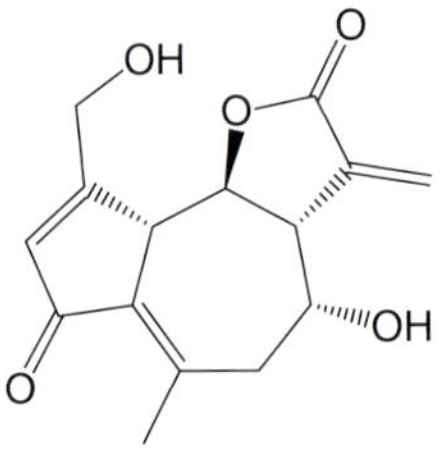

Lactucin, as lactucopicrin, is a sesquiterpene lactone contained in lettuce (*Lactuca sativa* L.).

Suggested Reading

Paulsen E, Andersen KE, Hausen BM (1993) Compositae dermatitis in a Danish dermatology department in one year (I). Results of routine patch testing with the sesquiterpene lactone mix supplemented with aimed patch testing with extracts and sesquiterpene lactones of Compositae plants. Contact Dermatitis 29:6–10

248. Lactucopicrin

Intybin

CAS Registry Number [6466–74–6]

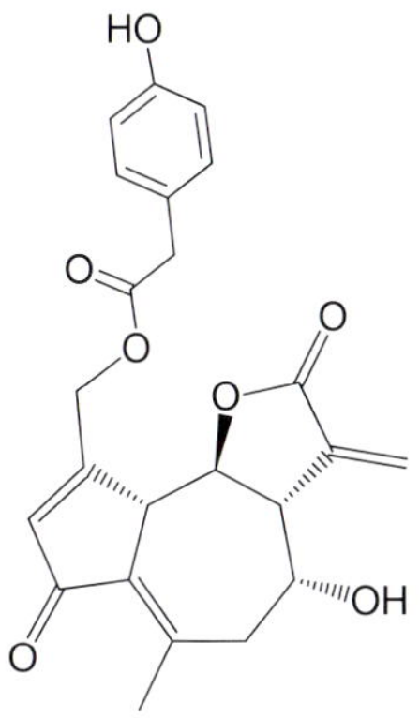

Lactucopicrin, as lactucin, is a sesquiterpene lactone extracted from various *Lactuca* spp. and *Cichorium intybus* L., Asteraceae–Compositae family.

Suggested Reading

Bischoff TA, Kelley CJ, Karchesy Y, Laurantos M, Nguyen-Dinh P, Arefi AG (2004) Antimalarial activity of lactucin and lactucopicrin: sesquiterpene lactones isolated from *Cichorium intybus* L. J Ethnopharmacol 95:455–457

249. Lapachenol

CAS Registry Number [573–13–7]

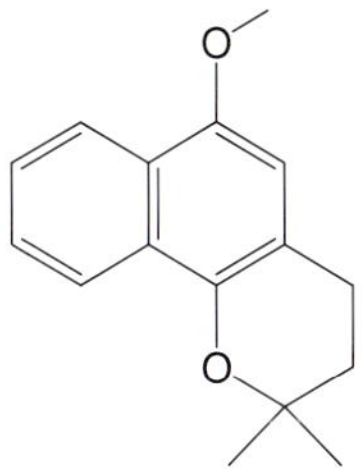

Lapachenol is contained in the heart-wood of Lapacho wood (*Tabebuia avellanedae* Lorentz, Bignoniaceae family). It is a secondary allergen, after lapachol and deoxylapachol, and likely a prohapten transformed in vivo into a quinone hapten. See also Chap. 41, Plants and Plant Products.

Suggested Reading

Hausen BM (1981) Wood injurious to human health. A manual. De Gruyter, Berlin

250. Lapachol

2-Hydroxy-3-(3-Methyl-2-Butenyl)-1,4-Naphthoquinone, CI 75490, CI Natural Yellow 16

CAS Registry Number [84–79–7]

Lapachol, a benzoquinone, is a secondary allergen in teak (*Tectona grandis* L., Verbenaceae family), a wood largely used for various indoor and outdoor applications (doors, windows, etc.) because of its strong durability. It has similar reactivity to deoxylapachol. See also Chap. 41, Plants and Plant Products.

Suggested Reading
Estlander T, Jolanki R, Alanko K, Kanerva L (2001) Occupational allergic contact dermatitis caused by wood dusts. Contact Dermatitis 44:213–217
Lamminpää A, Estlander T, Jolanki R, Kanerva L (1996) Occupational allergic contact dermatitis caused by decorative plants. Contact Dermatitis 34:330–335

251. Lawsone

2-Hydroxy-1,4-Naphthalenedione, Henna

CAS Registry Number [83–72–7]

Henna, prepared by powdering the dried leaves of henna plant (*Lawsonia inermis* L.), is used for coloring and conditioning hair and nails, particularly by Muslims or Hindus. It contains Lawsone, which very rarely induces contact allergy. Most dermatitis caused by "black henna" is due to PPD and derivatives.

Suggested Reading
Le Coz CJ, Lefebvre C, Keller F, Grosshans E (2000) Allergic contact dermatitis caused by skin painting (pseudotattooing) with black henna, a mixture of henna and *p*-phenylenediamine and its derivatives. Arch Dermatol 136:1515–1517
Pasricha JS, Gupta R, Panjwani S (1980) Contact dermatitis to henna (*Lawsonia*). Contact Dermatitis 6:288–290

252. Lidocaine

Lidocaine

CAS Registry Number [137–58–6]

Lidocaine Hydrochloride Monohydrate

CAS Registry Number [6108–05–0]

Lidocaine is an anesthetic of the amide group, like articaine or bupivacaine. Immediate-type IgE-dependent reactions are rare, and delayed-type contact dermatitis is exceptional. Cross reactivity between the different amide anesthetics is not systematic.

Suggested Reading

Duque S, Fernandez L (2004) Delayed hypersensitivity to amide local anaesthetics. Allergol Immunopathol (Madr) 32:233–234

Waton J, Boulanger A, Trechot PH, Schmutz JL, Barbaud A (2004) Contact urticaria from Emla® cream. Contact Dermatitis 51:284–287

253. Lilial®

See 73. *p-tert*-Butyl-alpha-Methylhydrocinnamic Aldehyde

254. Limonene

Limonene: D-**Limonene** + L-**Limonene**

CAS Registry Number [138–86–3]

D-**Limonene:** (+)-**Limonene,** *R*-**Limonene,** α-**Limonene,** (*R*)-*p*-**Mentha-1,8-Diene, Dipentene, Carvene, Citrene**

CAS Registry Number [5989–27–5]

L-**Limonene:** (–)-**Limonene,** *S*-**Limonene,** β-**Limonene,** (4*S*)-1-**Methyl-4-(1-Methylethenyl)-Cyclohexene**

CAS Registry Number [5989–54–8]

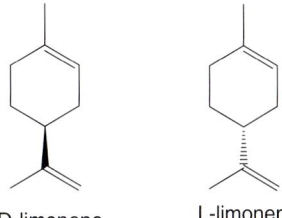

D-limonene   L-limonene

Limonene is a racemic form of D- and L-limonene. D-Limonene is contained in *Citrus* species such as citrus, orange, mandarin, and bergamot. L-Limonene is contained in *Pinus pinea*. The racemic form (D- and L-limonene) is also named dipentene. D-limonene, used as a solvent, may be found in cleansing or in degreasing agents. Its sensitizing potential increases with prolonged air contact, which induces oxidation and leads to oxidation products. The presence of D-limonene has to be mentioned by name in cosmetics of the EU.

Suggested Reading

Karlberg AT, Magnusson K, Nilsson U (1992) Air oxidation of d-limonene (the citrus solvent) creates potent allergens. Contact Dermatitis 26:332–340

Karlberg AT, Dooms-Goossens A (1997) Contact allergy to oxidized d-limonene among dermatitis patients. Contact Dermatitis 36:201–206

Meding B, Barregard L, Marcus K (1994) Hand eczema in car mechanics. Contact Dermatitis 30:129–134

255. Linalool

3,7-Dimethyl-1,6-octadien-3-ol, Linalyl alcohol, 2,6-Dimethyl-2,7-octadien-6-ol

CAS Registry Number [78–70–6]

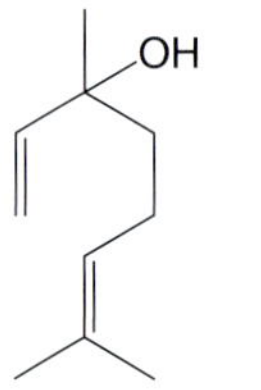

Linalool is a terpene chief constituent of linaloe oil, also found in oils of Ceylon cinnamon, sassafras, orange flower, bergamot, *Artemisia balchanorum*, ylang-ylang. This frequently used scented substance is a sensitizer by the way of primary or secondary oxidation products. As a fragrance allergen, linalool has to be mentioned by name in cosmetics within the EU.

Suggested Reading

Kanerva L, Estlander T, Jolanki R (1995) Occupational allergic contact dermatitis caused by ylang-ylang oil. Contact Dermatitis 33:198–199

Skold M, Borje A, Harambasic E, Karlberg AT (2004) Contact allergens formed on air exposure of linalool. Identification and quantification of primary and secondary oxidation products and the effect on skin sensitization. Chem Res Toxicol 17:1697–1705

256. Lincomycin (Hydrochloride Monohydrate)

Lincomycin

CAS Registry Number [154–21–2]

Lincomycin Hydrochloride Monohydrate

CAS Registry Number [7179–49–9]

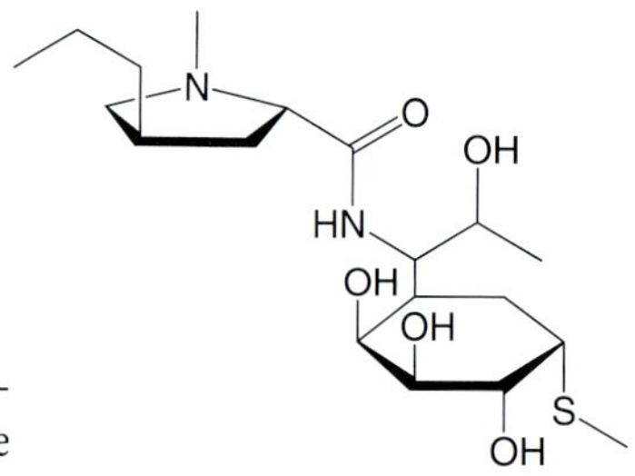

Lincomycin is an antibiotic of the lincosanide group, active against Gram-positive bacteria. Occupational exposure occurs in poultry and pig breeders.

Suggested Reading

Vilaplana J, Romaguera C, Grimalt F (1991) Contact dermatitis from lincomycin and spectinomycin in chicken vaccinators. Contact Dermatitis 24:225–226

257. Lindane

γ-1,2,3,4,5,6-Hexachlorocyclohexane

CAS Registry Number [58–89–9]

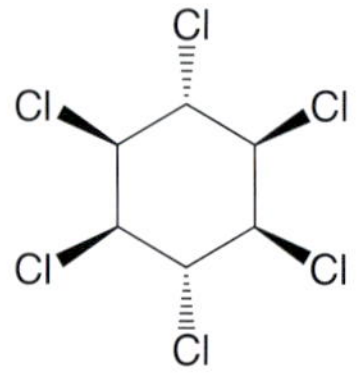

Lindane is a pesticide used for its anti-insect properties in agriculture, wood protection, in anti-insect paints, and veterinary and human medicine against many insects such as spiders, mosquitoes, ticks, scabies, lice, and demodicosis. Its use is controlled, particularly because of neurological toxicity.

Suggested Reading
Anonymous (1992) Fiche toxicologique n°81. Cahiers documentaires de l'INRS
Sharma VK, Kaur S (1990) Contact sensitization by pesticides in farmers. Contact Dermatitis 23:
    77–80

258. Lyral®

See 236. Hydroxymethylpentacyclohexenecarboxaldehyde

259. Malathion

Carbetox, Carbofos, Chemathion, Cimexan, Dorthion, Extermathion, Fosfotion

CAS Registry Number [121–75–5]

This organophosphorus pesticide is used as an insecticide and an acaricide, particularly against head lice. Sensitization was reported in farmers.

Suggested Reading
O'Malley M, Rodriguez P, Maibach HI (1995) Pesticide patch testing: California nursery workers
    and controls. Contact Dermatitis 32:61–62
Sharma VK, Kaur S (1990) Contact sensitization by pesticides in farmers. Contact Dermatitis 23:
    77–80

260. Mancozeb

Zinc Manganese Ethylenebisdithiocarbamate

CAS Registry Number [8018–01–7]

Mancozeb is a fungicide of the ethylene-bis-dithiocarbamate group. It is present in Rondo-M® with pyrifenox. Occupational exposure occurs mainly in agricultural workers, in vineyard workers or in florists.

Suggested Reading
Crippa M, Misquith L, Lonati A, Pasolini G (1990) Dyshidrotic eczema and sensitization to dithio-
    carbamates in a florist. Contact Dermatitis 23:203–204
Iliev D, Elsner P (1997) Allergic contact from the fungicide Rondo-M® and the insecticide Alfa-
    cron®. Contact Dermatitis 36:51
Jung HD, Honemann W, Kloth C, Lubbe D, Pambor M, Quednow C, Ratz KH, Rothe A, Tarnick M
    (1989) Kontaktekzem durch Pestizide in der Deutschen Demokratischen Republik. Dermatol
    Monatsschr 175:203–214
Koch P (1996) Occupational allergic contact dermatitis and airborne contact dermatitis from
    5 fungicides in a vineyard worker. Cross-reactions between fungicides of the dithiocarbamate
    group? Contact Dermatitis 34:324–329

261. Maneb

Ethylenebisdithiocarbamate Manganese

CAS Registry Number [12427–38–2]

Maneb is a pesticide with fungicide properties, belonging to the dithiocarbamate group. Sensitization occurs mainly in farmers and agricultural workers.

Suggested Reading

Crippa M, Misquith L, Lonati A, Pasolini G (1990) Dyshidrotic eczema and sensitization to dithio-carbamates in a florist. Contact Dermatitis 23:203–204

Jung HD, Honemann W, Kloth C, Lubbe D, Pambor M, Quednow C, Ratz KH, Rothe A, Tarnick M (1989) Kontaktekzem durch Pestizide in der Deutschen Demokratischen Republik. Dermatol Monatsschr 175:203–214

Koch P (1996) Occupational allergic contact dermatitis and airborne contact dermatitis from 5 fungicides in a vineyard worker. Cross-reactions between fungicides of the dithiocarbamate group? Contact Dermatitis 34:324–329

O'Malley M, Rodriguez P, Maibach HI (1995) Pesticide patch testing: California nursery workers and controls. Contact Dermatitis 32:61–62

Peluso AM, Tardio M, Adamo F, Venturo N (1991) Multiple sensitization due to bis-dithiocarbamate and thiophthalimide pesticides. Contact Dermatitis 25:327

Piraccini BM, Cameli N, Peluso AM, Tardio M (1991) A case of allergic contact dermatitis due to the pesticide maneb. Contact Dermatitis 24:381–382

Sharma VK, Kaur S (1990) Contact sensitization by pesticides in farmers. Contact Dermatitis 23:77–80

262. Melamine and Melamine-Formaldehyde Resins

Melamine: 2,4,6-Triaminotriazine

CAS Registry Number [108–78–1]

Melamine-formaldehyde resin (MFR) result from condensation of melamine and formaldehyde. It is an active ingredient of strong (reinforced) plasters, such as industrial or some dental plasters used for moulding. It is also used as a textile finish resin. MFR acts as an allergen generally because of formaldehyde releasing (see Chap. 37, Clothing).

Suggested Reading

Aalto-Korte K, Jolanki R, Estlander T (2003) Formaldehyde-negative allergic contact dermatitis from melamine-formaldehyde resin. Contact Dermatitis 49:194–196

Garcia Bracamonte B, Ortiz de Frutos FJ, Iglesias Diez L (1995) Occupational allergic contact dermatitis due to formaldehyde and textile finish resins. Contact Dermatitis 33:139–140

Lewis FM, Cork MJ, McDonagh AJG, Gawkrodger DJG (1993) Allergic contact dermatitis from resin-reinforced plaster. Contact Dermatitis 28:40–41

Rustemeyer T, Frosch PJ (1996) Occupational skin diseases in dental laboratory technicians. (I). Clinical picture and causative factors. Contact Dermatitis 34:125–133

263. Mercaptobenzothiazole

2-Mercaptobenzothiazole, MBT

CAS Registry Number [149–30–4]

MBT is a rubber chemical, accelerant of vulcanization, and contained in "mercapto-mix." The most frequent occupational categories are the metal industry, homemakers, health services and laboratories, the building industry, and shoemakers. It is also used as a corrosion inhibitor in cutting fluids or in releasing fluids in the pottery industry.

Suggested Reading

Condé-Salazar L, Del-Rio E, Guimaraens D, Gonzalez Domingo A (1993) Type IV allergy to rubber additives: a 10-year study of 686 cases. J Am Acad Dermatol 29:176–180

Mancuso G, Reggiani M, Berdondini RM (1996) Occupational dermatitis in shoemakers. Contact Dermatitis 34:17–22

Von Hintzenstern J, Heese A, Koch HU, Peters KP, Hornstein OP (1991) Frequency, spectrum and occupational relevance of type IV allergies to rubber chemicals. Contact Dermatitis 24:244–252

Wilkinson SM, Cartwright PH, English JSC (1990) Allergic contact dermatitis from mercaptobenzothiazole in a releasing fluid. Contact Dermatitis 23:370

264. Mercaptobenzothiazole Salts

Mercaptobenzothiazole, Sodium Salt

CAS Registry Numbers [2492–26–4]

Mercaptobenzothiazole, Zinc Salt

CAS Registry Numbers [155–04–4]

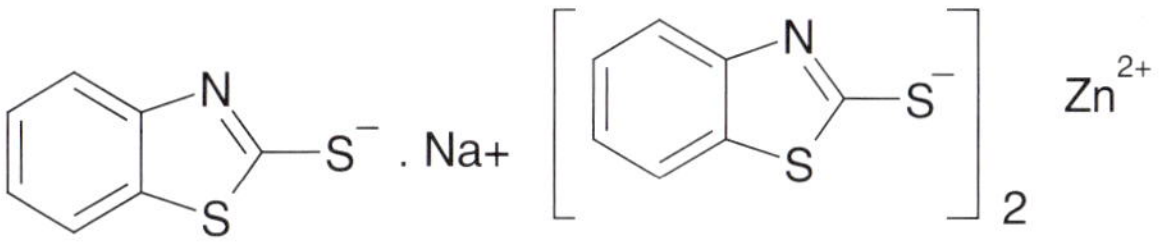

Such mercaptobenzothiazole hydrosoluble salts are used as antioxidants and biocides in cutting fluids and greases, paints or glues.

Suggested Reading

Le Coz CJ (2004) Fiche d'éviction en cas d'hypersensibilité au mercaptobenzothiazole et au mercapto mix. Ann Dermatol Venereol 131:1012–1014

265. MESNA

Sodium 2-Mercaptoethane Sulfonate

CAS Registry Number [19767–45–4]

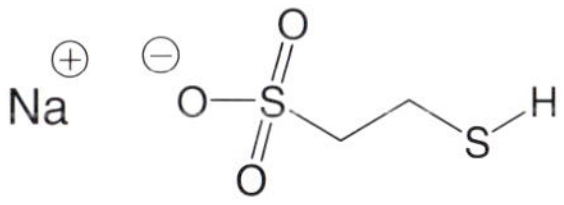

Mesna is used as a mucolytic agent, and as an antidote to chloro-acetyl-aldehyde and acrolein (a bladder toxic metabolite of ifosfamide or cyclophosphamide). It has been reported as a cause of occupational allergic (hand and airborne) dermatitis in nurses.

Suggested Reading

Benyoussef K, Bottlaender A, Pfister HR, Caussade P, Heid E, Grosshans E (1996) Allergic contact dermatitis from mesna. Contact Dermatitis 34:228–229

Kiec-Swierczynska M, Krecisz B (2003) Occupational airborne allergic contact dermatitis from mesna. Contact Dermatitis 48:171

266. Metacresol

3-Cresol, 3-Methylphenol, *m*-Cresol

CAS Registry Number [108–39–4]

Metacresol is contained as a preservative in almost all human insulin. It has been reported as a cause of allergic reaction due to injected insulin.

Suggested Reading
Clerx V, van den Keybus C, Kochuyt A, Goossens A (2003) Drug intolerance reaction to insulin therapy caused by metacresol. Contact Dermatitis 48:162–163

267. Metanil Yellow

Acid Yellow 36, CI 13065

CAS Registry Number [587–98–4]

Metanil yellow is a yellow monoazoic dye. This coloring agent used in leather and wood stains, and was also employed as a food dye in India.

Suggested Reading
Hausen BM (1994) A case of allergic contact dermatitis due to metanil yellow. Contact Dermatitis 31:117–118

268. Methenamine

Hexamethylenetetramine

CAS Registry Number [100–97–0]

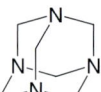

Hexamethylenetetramine is used in the foundry, tire and rubber, and phenol formaldehyde resins industries and in other applications such as a hardener in epoxy resins Bisphenol A type and as an anticorrosive agent. It is an ammonia and formaldehyde releaser sometimes used in topical medicaments and cosmetics.

Suggested Reading
Gonzalez-Perez R, Gonzalez-Hermosa R, Aseginolaza B, Luis Diaz-Ramon J, Soloeta R (2003) Allergic contact dermatitis from methenamine in an antiperspirant spray. Contact Dermatitis 49:266
Holness DL, Nethercott JR (1993) The performance of specialized collections of bisphenol A epoxy resin system components in the evaluation of workers in an occupational health clinic population. Contact Dermatitis 28:216–219

51

269. Methidathion

Somonil, Supracid, Suprathion, Ultracid

CAS Registry Number [950–37–8]

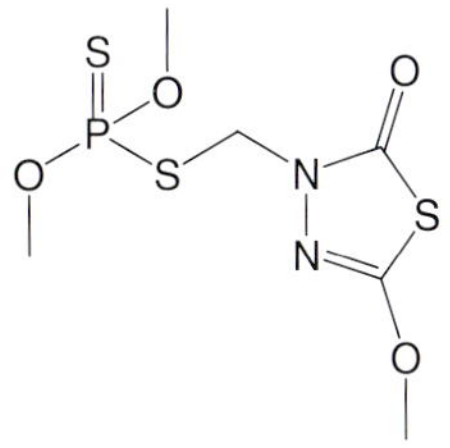

Methidation is an organophosphorus compound used as an insecticide. Cross-sensitivity was described to Dichlorvos.

Suggested Reading

Ueda A, Aoyama K, Manda F, Ueda T, Kawahara Y (1994) Delayed-type allergenicity of triforine (Saprol®). Contact Dermatitis 31:140–145

270. Methiocarb

3,5-Dimethyl-4-(Methylthio)Phenol Methylcarbamate, Mesurol

CAS Registry Number [2032–65–7]

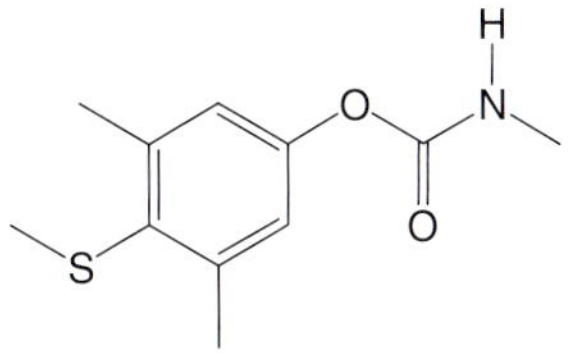

Methiocarb is an insecticide or molluscicide with a cholinesterase inhibiting effect. A case of contact dermatitis was reported in a carnation grower.

Suggested Reading

Willems PWJM, Geursen-Reitsma AM, van Joost T (1997) Allergic contact dermatitis due to methiocarb (Mesurol). Contact Dermatitis 36:270

271. Methomyl

S-Methyl-N-(Methylcarbamoyloxy)-Thioacetimidate, Lannate

CAS Registry Number [16752–77–5]

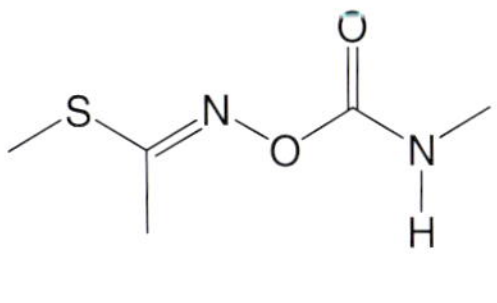

Methomyl is a pesticide agent, a carbamate insecticide with anticholinesterase activity. This mixture of two stereoisomers is used as a foliar spray to control field crops, stables and poultry houses, and in glasshouses on ornamentals and vegetables, or in flypapers. Cases were reported in chrysanthemum growers and in two women working in a plant nursery.

Suggested Reading

Bruynzeel DP (1991) Contact sensitivity to Lannate®. Contact Dermatitis 25:60–61

272. (R)-4-Methoxy Dalbergione

CAS Registry Number [4640–26–0] [28396–75–0]

(R)-4-Methoxy dalbergione is the main allergen of *Dalbergia nigra* All. (Brazilian rosewood, palissander) and *Dalbergia latifolia* Roxb. (East Indian rosewood). Occupational sensitization occurs in timber workers. See also Chap. 41, Plants and Plant Products.

Suggested Reading
Gallo R, Guarrera M, Hausen BM (1996) Airborne contact dermatitis from East Indian rosewood (*Dalbergia latifolia* Roxb.). Contact Dermatitis 35:60–61
Hausen BM (2000) Woods. In: Kanerva L, Elsner P, Wahlberg JE, Maibach HI (eds) Handbook of occupational dermatology. Springer, Berlin Heidelberg New York, pp 771–780

273. Methoxy PEG-17/Dodecyl Glycol Copolymer

CAS Registry Number [88507–00–0]

Methoxy PEG-17/dodecyl glycol copolymer is one of the numerous copolymers recorded in the International Nomenclature of Cosmetics Ingredients (INCI) inventory system. It belongs to the chemical class of alkoxylated alcohols. It is utilized as an emulsion stabilizer, a skin-conditioning and a viscosity-increasing agent in cosmetics.

Suggested Reading
Le Coz CJ, Heid E (2001) Allergic contact dermatitis from methoxy PEG-17/dodecyl glycol copolymer (Elfacos® OW 100). Contact Dermatitis 44:308–309

274. Methoxy-Psoralens

5-Methoxypsoralen, Bergapten(e)

CAS Registry Number [484–20–8]

8-Methoxypsoralen, Methoxsalen, Meladinin, Xanthotoxin

CAS Registry Number [298–81–7]

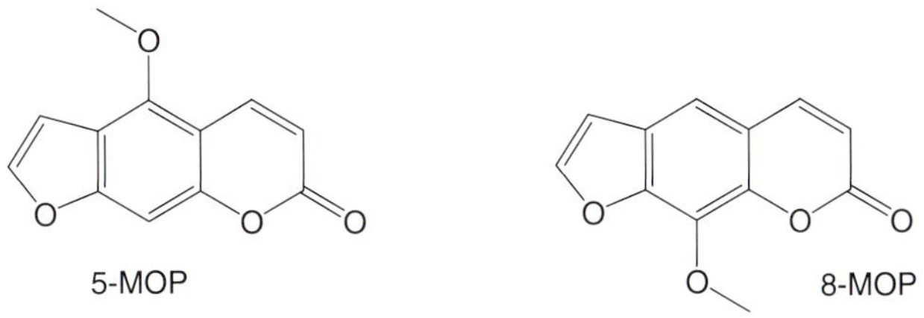

5-MOP   8-MOP

These fur(an)ocoumarins are phototoxic compounds that cause phototoxic dermatitis. Many plants of the Apiaceae–Umbelliferae and most of the Rutaceae family contain 5-methoxypsoralen and 8-methoxypsoralen. Their spectra is in the UVA range (300–360 nm). They are used in combination with UVA to treat various skin disorders such as psoriasis. See also Chap. 41, Plants and Plant Products.

Suggested Reading

Ena P, Camarda I (1990) Phytophotodermatitis from *Ruta corsica*. Contact Dermatitis 22:63

Ena P, Cerri R, Dessi G, Manconi PM, Atzei AD (1991) Phototoxicity due to *Cachrys libanotis*. Contact Dermatitis 24:1–5

275. Methyl 2,3 Epoxy-3-(4-Methoxyphenyl)Propionate

3-(-Methoxyphenyl)Glycidic Acid Methylester,
Methyl 3-(*p*-Methoxyphenyl)Oxirane-2-Carboxylate

CAS Registry Number [42245–42–1]

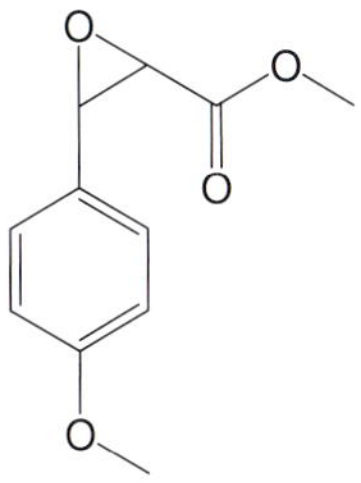

Methyl 2,3 epoxy-3-(4-methoxyphenyl)propionate is an intermediate product in the synthesis of diltiazem hydrochloride. Contact dermatitis was observed in several laboratory technicians.

Suggested Reading

Rudzki E, Rebandel P (1990) Dermatitis from methyl 2,3 epoxy-3-(4-methoxyphenyl)propionate. Contact Dermatitis 23:382

276. Methyl Gallate

CAS Registry Number [99–24–1]

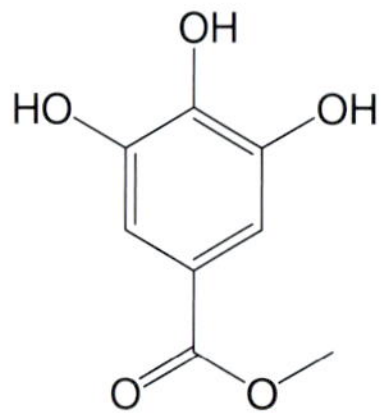

This ester of gallic acid is used as an antioxidant agent. A case was reported by using a reprography paper.

Suggested Reading

Degos R, Lépine J, Akhoundzadeh H (1968) Sensibilisation cutanée due à la manipulation de papier reprographie. Bull Soc Fr Dermatol 75:595–596

51

277. Methyl Heptine Carbonate

Methyl oct-2-ynoate, Folione

CAS Registry Number [111–12–6]

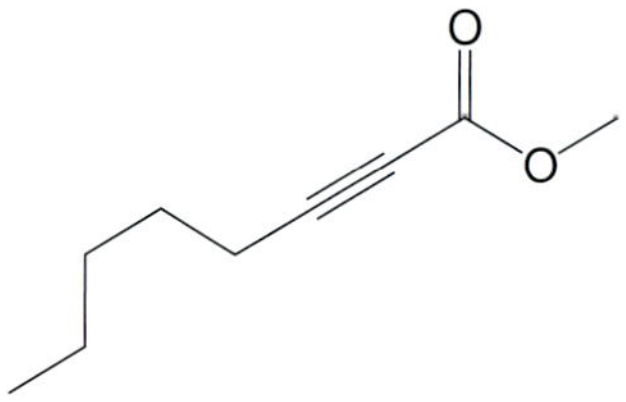

This perfumed molecule belongs to the list of 26 allergens that have to be indicated by name on the ingredients list of cosmetics in the EU.

Suggested Reading

English JS, Rycroft RJ (1988) Allergic contact dermatitis from methyl heptine and methyl octine carbonates. Contact Dermatitis 18:174–175

278. Methyl Octine Carbonate

Methyl non-2-ynoate

CAS Registry Number [111–80–8]

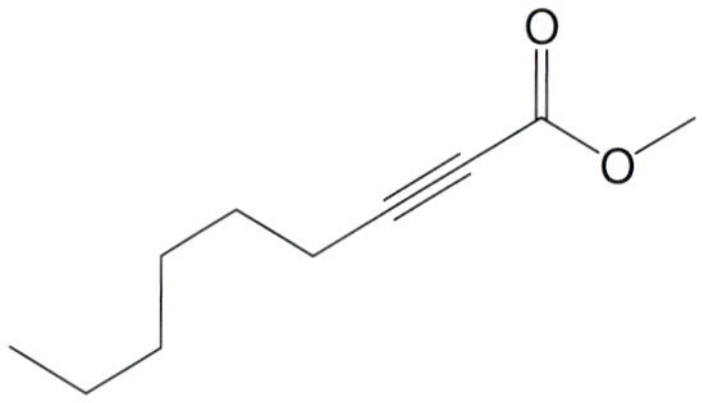

This perfumed molecule is related to methyl heptine carbonate. Cross-reactivity is frequent.

Suggested Reading

English JS, Rycroft RJ (1988) Allergic contact dermatitis from methyl heptine and methyl octine carbonates. Contact Dermatitis 18:174–175

279. Methyl Salicylate

CAS Registry Number [119–36–8]

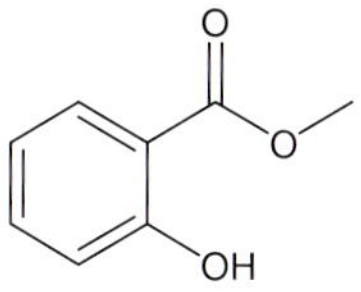

This anti-inflammatory agent is found in a wide number of ointments and can induce allergic contact dermatitis.

Suggested Reading

Hindson C (1977) Contact eczema from methyl salicylate reproduced by oral aspirin (acetyl salicylic acid). Contact Dermatitis 3:348–349

Oiso N, Fulai K, Ishii M (2004) Allergic contact dermatitis due to methyl salicylate in a compress. Contact Dermatitis 51:34–35

280. Methyl-Terpyridine

2,2′:6′,2′′-(4′-Methyl)-*ter*-Pyridine), 4′-Methyl (2,2′,2′′-Terpyridine)

CAS Registry Number for 2,2′,2′′-Terpyridine [1148–79–4]

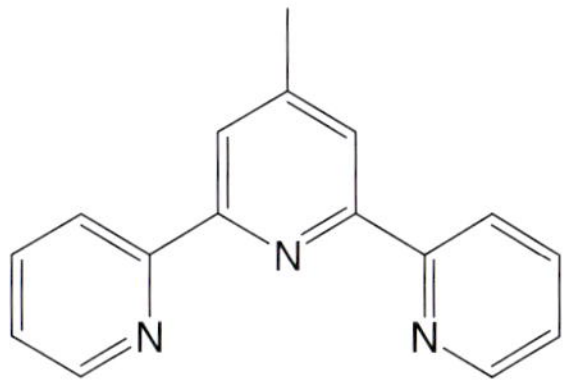

This molecule is a terpyridine with a 4′-methyl substitution. A case of occupational dermatitis was reported in a chemical technician with no cross-reactivity to pyridine derivatives.

Suggested Reading

Le Coz CJ, Caussade P, Bottlaender A (1998) Occupational contact dermatitis from methyl-*ter*-pyridine in a chemistry laboratory technician. Contact Dermatitis 38:214–215

281. 2-Methyl-4,5-Trimethylene-4-Isothiazolin-3-one

CAS Registry Number [82633–79–2]

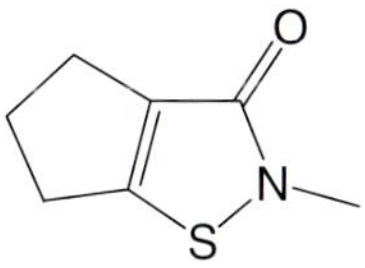

This biocide induced contact dermatitis in a laboratory technician, also sensitive to the other isothiazolinone BIT.

Suggested Reading

Burden AD, O'Driscoll JB, Page FC, Beck MH (1994) Contact hypersensitivity to a new isothiazolinone. Contact Dermatitis 30:179–180

282. Methylchloroisothiazolinone

Chloromethylisothiazolinone, 5-Chloro-2-Methyl-4-Isothiazolin-3-one, MCI

CAS Registry Number [26172–55–4]

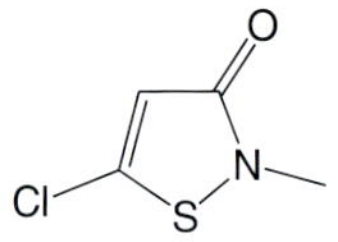

MCI is mainly associated with methylisothiazolinone for its bactericidal and fongis-
tatic properties. It is found in Kathon® CG or derivatives. MCI is found in water-
based products such as cosmetics, paints, and glues. Pure MCI is highly irritant and
may cause active sensitization.

Suggested Reading

Nielsen H (1994) Occupational exposure to isothiazolinones. A study based on a product register.
    Contact Dermatitis 31:18–21
Schubert H (1997) Airborne contact dermatitis due to methylchloro- and methylisothiazolinone
    (MCI/MI). Contact Dermatitis 36:274
Tay P, Ng SK (1994) Delayed skin burns from MCI/MI biocide used in water treatment. Contact
    Dermatitis 30:54–55

283. Methylchloroisothiazolinone + Methylsiothiazolinone (MCI/MI)

CAS Registry Numbers [55965–84–9], [96118–96–6]

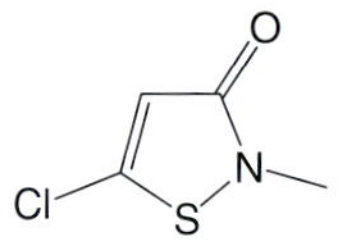

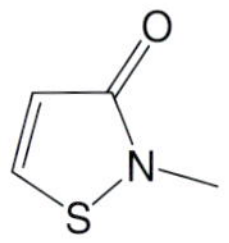

Kathon® CG (CG = Cosmetic Grade) is a 3:1 mixture of CMI and MI, at a 1.5% concentration. It is used for cosmetics and toiletries, metalworking fluids or paints, in
which it can be added only periodically or in color film developers. Kathon® 886
MW (MW = metalworking fluids) is a mixture CMI/MI mixture at a 13.9% concentration, mainly contained in metalworking fluids. Kathon® FP 1.5 contains MCI/MI
at 1.5% concentration in propylene glycol. Kathon® LX (LX = LateX) contains
MCI/MI at a tenfold concentration of Kathon® CG. Kathon® WT (WT = water treatment) is a MCI/MI mixture used in the paper industry. Parmetol® K40, Parmethol®
DF 12 and Parmetol® DF 35, Parmetol® A 23, Parmetol® K50, and Parmetol® DF 18
are other brand names of MCI/MI.

Suggested Reading

Björkner B, Bruze M, Dahlquist I, Fregert S, Gruvberger B, Persson K (1986) Contact allergy to the
    preservative Kathon® CG. Contact Dermatitis 14:85–90
Fernandez de Corres L, Navarro JA, Gastaminza G, del Pozo MD (1995) An unusual case of sensiti-
    zation to methylchloro- and methyl-isothiazolinone (MCI/MI). Contact Dermatitis 33:215
Pazzaglia M, Vincenzi C, Gasparri F, Tosti A (1996) Occupational hypersensitivity to isothiazoli-
    none derivatives in a radiology technician. Contact Dermatitis 34:143–144
Scheman AJ, Katta R (1997) Photographic allergens: an update. Contact Dermatitis 37:130

284. Methyldibromoglutaronitrile

1,2-Dibromo 2,4-Dicyanobutane

CAS Registry Number [35691–65–7]

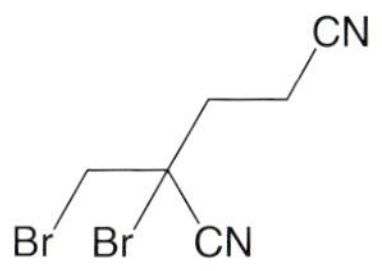

Methyldibromoglutaronitrile is a biocide widely used as a preservative agent in cosmetics, toiletries, and metalworking fluids. It is a potent allergen.

Suggested Reading

Aalto-Korte K, Jolanki R, Estlander T, Alanko K, Kanerva L (1996) Occupational allergic contact dermatitis caused by Euxyl K 400. Contact Dermatitis 35:193–194

Kynemund Pedersen L, Agner T, Held E, Johansen JD (2004) Methyldibromoglutaronitrile in leave-on products elicits contact allergy at low concentration. Br J Dermatol 151:817–822

Le Coz CJ (2005) Hypersensibilité au méthyldibromoglutaronitrile (Dibromodicyanobutane). Ann Dermatol Venereol 132:496–497

285. Methylhexahydrophthalic Anhydride

1,3-Isobenzofurandione, Hexahydromethyl

CAS Registry Numbers [19438–60–9] [39363–62–7], [86403–41–0], [95032–44–3]

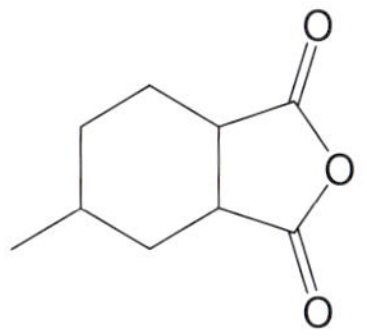

Methylhexahydrophthalic anhydride is an epoxy hardener, irritant to skin and mucous membranes. It is included in non-diglycidyl-ether-of-bisphenol-A epoxy resins. It can induce both allergic contact dermatitis and immunologic contact urticaria. It is structurally close to methyltetrahydrophthalic anhydride, which can also cause sensitization.

Suggested Reading

Kanerva L, Jolanki R, Estlander T (1997) Allergic contact dermatitis from non-diglycidyl-ether-of-bisphenol-A epoxy resins. Contact Dermatitis 36:34–38

Tarvainen K, Jolanki R, Estlander T, Tupasela O, Pfäffli P, Kanerva L (1995) Immunologic contact urticaria due to airborne methylhexahydrophthalic and methyltetrahydrophthalic anhydrides. Contact Dermatitis 32:204–209

286. Methylisothiazolinone

2-Methyl-4-Isothiazolin-3-one, MI

CAS Registry Number [2682–20–4]

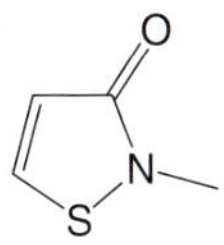

MI is generally associated with MCI, in Kathon® CG, MCI/MI, and Euxyl® K 100. This preservative is currently used in water-based products such as cosmetics, paints, and glues. Skin contact with concentrated solution can cause severe irritant dermatitis.

Suggested Reading

Schubert H (1997) Airborne contact dermatitis due to methylchloro- and methylisothiazolinone (MCI/MI). Contact Dermatitis 36:274

Tay P, Ng SK (1994) Delayed skin burns from MCI/MI biocide used in water treatment. Contact Dermatitis 30:54–55

287. Methylol Phenols

2-Methylol Phenol: 2-Hydroxymethyl-Phenol

CAS Registry Number [90–01–7]

3-Methylol Phenol: 3-Hydroxymethyl-Phenol, 3-Hydroxybenzyl Alcohol

CAS Registry Number [620–24–6]

4-Methylol Phenol: 4-Hydroxymethyl-Phenol

CAS Registry Number [623–05–2]

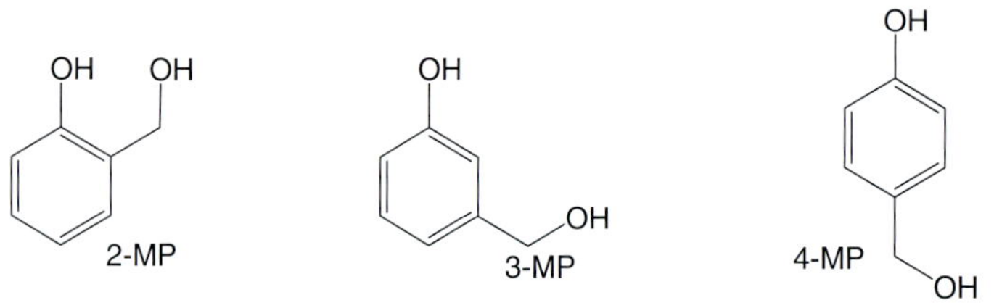

Methylol phenols are sensitizers contained in resins based on phenol and formaldehyde of the resol type. Cross-reactivity is possible with other phenol derivative molecules.

Suggested Reading

Bruze M, Zimerson E (1997) Cross-reaction patterns in patients with contact allergy to simple methylol phenols. Contact Dermatitis 37:82–86

Bruze M, Fregert S, Zimerson E (1985) Contact allergy to phenol-formaldehyde resins. Contact Dermatitis 12:81–86

288. 1-Methylpyrrolidone

N-Methyl-2-Pyrrolidone, 1-Methyl-2-Pyrrolidone

CAS Registry Number [872–50–4].

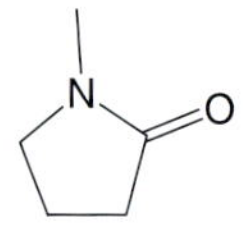

1-Methylpyrrolidone is an aprotic solvent with a wide range of applications: petrochemical processing, surface coating, dyes and pigments, industrial and domestic cleaning compounds, and agricultural and pharmaceutical formulations. It is mainly an irritant, but it can cause severe contact dermatitis due to prolonged contact.

Suggested Reading

Jungbauer FH, Coenraads PJ, Kardaun SH (2001) Toxic hygroscopic contact reaction to N-methyl-2-pyrrolidone. Contact Dermatitis 45:303–304

Leira H, Tiltnes A, Svendsen K, Vetlesen L (1992) Irritant cutaneous reactions to N-methyl-2-pyrrolidone (NMP). Contact Dermatitis 27:148–150

51

289. Metol (Sulfate)

4(Methylamino)Phenol

CAS Registry Number [150–75–4]

4(Methylamino)Phenol Sulfate

CAS Registry Numbers [1936–57–8] (unspecified sulfate), [51–72–9] (sulfate[1 : 1]), [55–55–0] (sulfate[2 : 1])

(. H_2SO_4)

Metol is contained in black and white film developers and caused contact dermatitis in photographers.

Suggested Reading
Liden C, Brehmer-Andersson E (1988) Occupational dermatoses from colour developing agents. Clinical and histopathological observations. Acta Derm Venereol (Stockh) 68 : 514–522
Scheman AJ, Katta R (1997) Photographic allergens: an update. Contact Dermatitis 37 : 130

290. Mevinphos

CAS Registry Number [7786–34–7]

Sensitization to mevinphos (also named Duraphos, Phosdrin, and Phosfene), an organophosphate cholinesterase inhibitor that is used as an insecticide, was rarely reported.

Suggested Reading
Jung HD, Ramsauer E (1987) Akute Pesticid-Intoxication kombiniert mit epicutaner Sensibilisierung durch den organischen Phosphorsäureester Mevinphos (PD5). Aktuel Dermatol 13 : 82–83

291. Mezlocilin

CAS Registry Number [51481–65–3]

Mezlocillin Sodium Salt Monohydrate

CAS Registry Number [59798–30–0]

Mezlocillin is an acylaminopenicillin, which caused both immediate and delayed hypersensitivity in a nurse.

Suggested Reading
Keller K, Schwanitz HJ (1992) Combined immediate and delayed hypersensitivity to mezlocillin. Contact Dermatitis 27 : 348–349

292. Monoethanolamine

Ethanolamine, 2-Aminoethanol

CAS Registry Number [141–43–5]

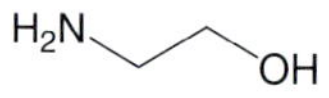

Monoethanolamine is contained in many products, such as metalworking fluids. It is mainly an irritant. Traces may exist in other ethanolamine fluids.

Suggested Reading

Bhushan M, Craven NM, Beck MH (1998) Contact allergy to 2-aminoethanol (monoethanolamine) in a soluble oil. Contact Dermatitis 39:321

Blum A, Lischka G (1997) Allergic contact dermatitis from mono-, di- and triethanolamine. Contact Dermatitis 36:166

293. Morphine (Morphine Hydrochloride, Morphine Tartrate)

CAS Registry Number [57–27–2] (CAS Registry Number [52–26–6], CAS Registry Number [302–31–8])

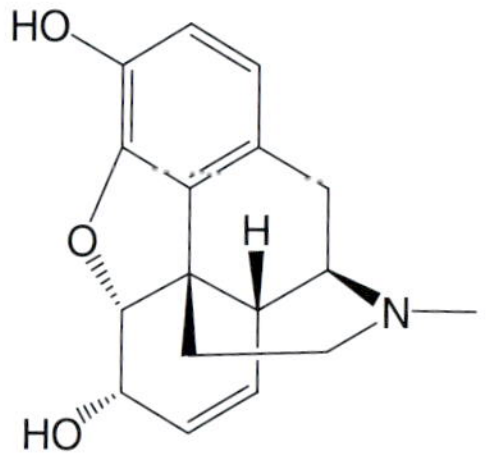

Morphine bitartrate caused contact dermatitis in a worker at a plant producing opium alkaloids. Morphine hydrochloride and morphine bitartrate showed patch-test-positive reactions in another patient with contact dermatitis working in the production of concentrated poppy straw. We observed a concomitant reaction between a morphine base and a codeine base in a patient with drug skin eruption due to codeine.

Suggested Reading

Condé-Salazar L, Guimaraens D, Gonzalez M, Fuente C (1991) Occupational allergic contact dermatitis from opium alkaloids. Contact Dermatitis 25:202–203

294. 4-Morpholinyl-2-Benzothiazyle Disulfide

2-(Morpholinodithio)Benzothiazole, Benzothiazole, 2-(4-morpholinyldithio)

CAS Registry Number [95–32–9]

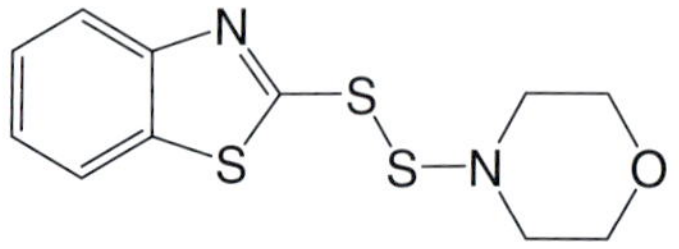

This chemical is a mercaptobenzothiazole-sulfenamide compound, used as moderate accelerator in rubber vulcanization.

Suggested Reading

Le Coz CJ (2004) Fiche d'éviction en cas d'hypersensibilité au mercaptobenzothiazole et au mercapto mix. Ann Dermatol Venereol 131:1012–1014

295. Morpholinyl Mercaptobenzothiazole

2-(4-Morpholinylthiobenzothiazole), 2-Morpholin Benzothiazyl Sulfenamide, Benzothiazole, 2-(4-Morpholinylthio)

CAS Registry Number [102–77–2]

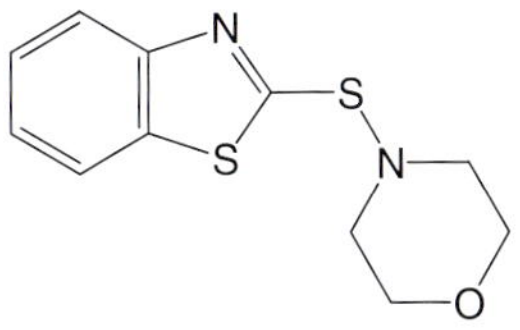

This rubber vulcanization accelerator belongs to the mercaptobenzothiazole-sulfenamide group. It is used as a chemical in the rubber industry, especially in the production of synthetic rubber articles. It is contained in "mercapto mix." As a corrosion inhibitor, it can be found in cutting fluids or in releasing fluids in the pottery industry. It induces mainly delayed-type hypersensitivity, but a case of immediate-type hypersensitivity was reported in a dental assistant.

Suggested Reading

Brehler R (1996) Contact urticaria caused by latex-free nitrile gloves. Contact Dermatitis 34:296

Condé-Salazar L, Del-Rio E, Guimaraens D, Gonzalez Domingo A (1993) Type IV allergy to rubber additives: a 10-year study of 686 cases. J Am Acad Dermatol 29:176–180

Le Coz CJ (2004) Fiche d'éviction en cas d'hypersensibilité au mercaptobenzothiazole et au mercapto mix. Ann Dermatol Venereol 131: 131:846–848

296. Naled

CAS Registry Number [300–76–5]

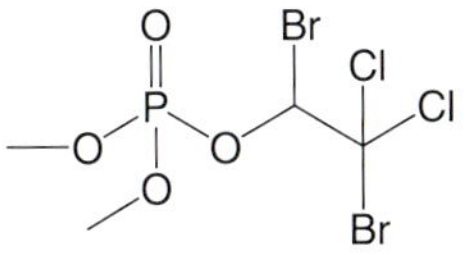

Naled is an organophosphate cholinesterase inhibitor that is used as an insecticide and as an acaricide. Sensitization seems to be very rare.

Suggested Reading

Edmundson WF, Davies JE (1967) Occupational dermatitis from naled. Arch Environ Health 15: 89–91

Mick DL, Gartin TD, Long KR (1970) A case report: occupational exposure to the insecticide naled. J Iowa Med Soc 60:395–396

297. 1-Naphthol

Alpha-Naphthol, CI 76605, CI Oxidation Base 33

CAS Registry Number [90–15–3]

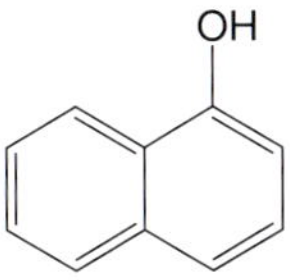

Alpha-naphthol can be used in dye manufacture and is classified as a hair dye. Combined with epichlorhydrin and NaOH to form alpha-naphthyl glycidyl ether, it caused sensitization in one of three workers in a chemical plant.

Suggested Reading

De Groot AC (1994) Occupational contact allergy to alpha-naphthyl glycidyl ether. Contact Dermatitis 30:253–254

298. Naphthol AS

CI 37505, CI Azoic Coupling Component 2

CAS Registry Number [92–77–3]

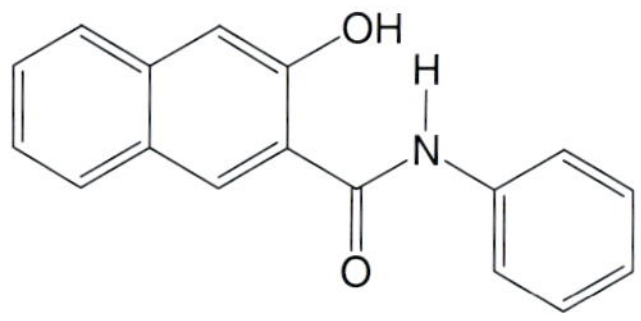

Naphthol AS is a coupling agent in cotton dyeing, inducing occupational dermatitis or contact allergy in consumers in contact with cotton-dyed clothing. It has been indirectly reported as a cause of occupational allergy due to its coupling with Diazo Component 51, or as a cross-sensitizer or sensitizer associated with Pigment Red 23 in red parts of tattoos. Pigmented contact dermatitis is usual in patients with a high phototype.

51

Suggested Reading

Le Coz CJ, Lepoittevin JP (2001) Clothing dermatitis from Naphthol AS. Contact Dermatitis 44: 366–367

Roed-Petersen J, Batsberg W, Larsen E (1990) Contact dermatitis from Naphthol AS. Contact Dermatitis 22:161–163

299. Neomycin (Neomycin B Hydrochloride, Neomycin B Sulfate)

Framycetin, Soframycin®

CAS Registry Number [1404–04–2] (CAS Registry Number [25389–99–5], CAS Registry Number [1405–10–3])

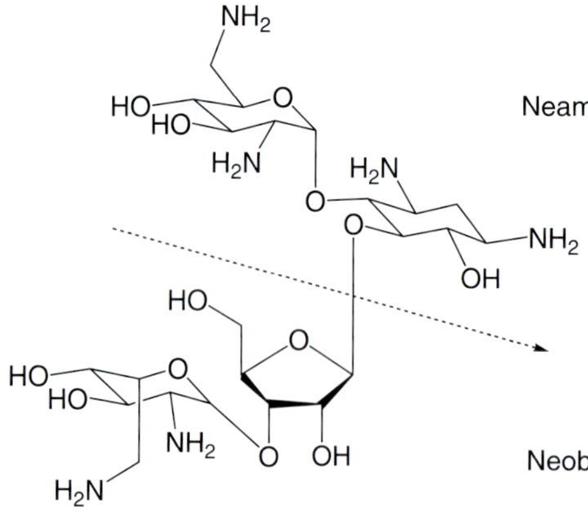

Neomycin is an antibiotic complex of the aminoglycosides group, extracted from *Streptomyces fradiae*. It is composed of neomycin A (neamin) and an isomer neobiosamin, either neomycin B (framycetin or Soframycin®) or neomycin C. Its use has been progressively forbidden in cosmetics and as an additive for animal feed. Occupational contact dermatitis occurs in workers at animal feed mills, in veterinaries or in health workers. Nonoccupational dermatitis mainly concerns patients with chronic dermatitis, leg ulcers or chronic otitis. Cross-sensitivity is usual with other aminoglycosides (amikacin, arbekacin, butirosin, dibekacin, gentamicin, isepamicin, kanamycin, paromomycin, ribostamycin, sisomycin, tobramycin), is rare with netilmicin and streptomycin, but nonexistent with spectinomycin.

Suggested Reading

Le Coz CJ (2001) Fiche d'éviction en cas d'hypersensibilité à la néomycine. Ann Dermatol Venereol 128:1359–1360

Mancuso G, Staffa M, Errani A, Berdondini RM, Fabri P (1990) Occupational dermatitis in animal feed mill workers. Contact Dermatitis 22:37–41

Rebandel P, Rudzki E (1986) Occupational contact sensitivity in oculists. Contact Dermatitis 15:92

300. Nicotine

CAS Registry Number [55-11-5]

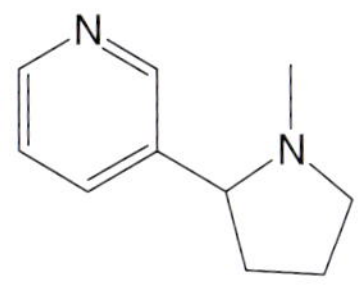

Nicotine is an alkaloid found in tobacco, and is responsible for its pharmacological effects and addiction. Contact dermatitis from nicotine, considered as rare, has been more frequent since its use in transdermal systems. Irritant dermatitis is mainly encountered, as contact urticaria seems to be rare. Allergic contact dermatitis, sometimes generalized, has been reported, with positive patch testing to nicotine base (10% ethanol or petrolatum). No consequences have been reported in patients who start smoking again after skin sensitization.

Suggested Reading

Bircher AJ, Howald H, Rufli T (1991) Adverse skin reactions to nicotine in a transdermal therapeutic system. Contact Dermatitis 25:230–236

Vincenzi C, Tosti A, Cirone M, Guarrera M, Cusano F (1993) Allergic contact dermatitis from transdermal nicotine systems. Contact Dermatitis 29:104–105

301. 3-Nitro-4-Hydroxyethylaminophenol

4-[(2-Hydroxyethyl)Amino]-3-Nitrophenol

CAS Registry Number [65235-31-6]

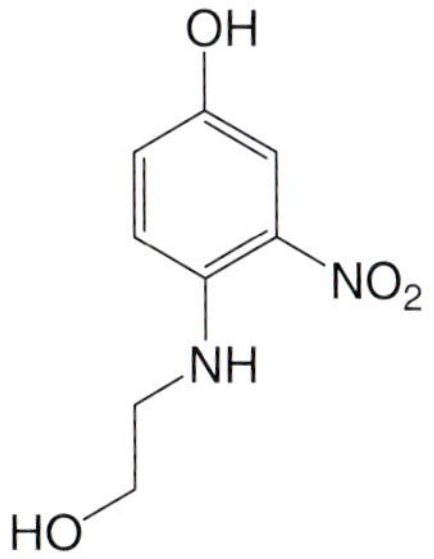

This dye belongs to the aminophenol class and is used as a hair colorant, particularly in semi-permanent hair dye preparations.

Suggested Reading

Le Coz CJ, Kühne S, Engel F (2003) Hair dye allergy due to 3-nitro-*p*-hydroxyethyl-aminophenol. Contact Dermatitis 49:103

302. 2-Nitro-4-Phenylenediamine

o-Nitro-p-Phenylenediamine, ONPD, CI 76070

CAS Registry Number [5307–14–2]

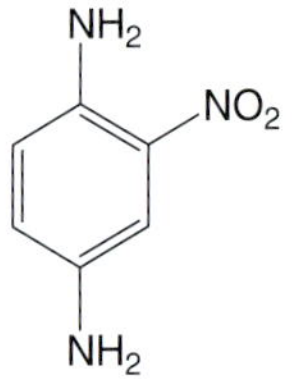

ONPD is a hair dye and a sensitizer in hairdressers and consumers who are generally sensitive to PPD too.

Suggested Reading

Frosch PJ, Burrows D, Camarasa JG, Dooms-Goossens A, Ducombs G, Lahti A, Menné T, Rycroft RJG, Shaw S, White IR, Wilkinson JD (1993) Allergic reactions to a hairdresser's series: results from 9 European centres. Contact Dermatitis 28:180–183

Guerra L, Tosti A, Bardazzi F, Pigatto P, Lisi P, Santucci B, Valsecchi R, Schena D, Angelini G, Sertoli A, Ayala F, Kokelj F (1992) Contact dermatitis in hairdressers: the Italian experience. Gruppo Italiano Ricerca Dermatiti da Contatto e Ambientali. Contact Dermatitis 26:101–107

Van der Walle HB, Brunsveld VM (1994) Dermatitis in hairdressers (I). The experience of the past 4 years. Contact Dermatitis 30:217–220

303. Nitrofurazone

Nitrofural, Nitrozone, Aldomycin

CAS Registry Numbers [59–87–0], [60051–85–6], [8027–71–2]

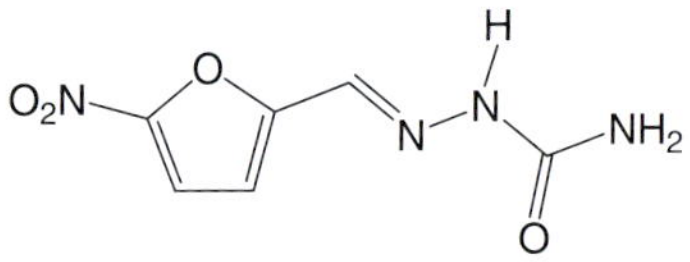

Nitrofurazone is an antibacterial agent used in animal feeds. Occupational dermatitis was reported in cattle breeders or farmers.

Suggested Reading

Condé-Salazar L, Guimaraens D, Gonzalez MA, Molina A (1995) Occupational allergic contact dermatitis from nitrofurazone. Contact Dermatitis 32:307–308

Vilaplana J, Grimalt F, Romaguera C (1990) Contact dermatitis from furaltadone in animal feed. Contact Dermatitis 22:232–233

304. Nitroglycerin

Glyceryl Trinitrate, Glycerol Trinitrate

CAS Registry Number [55–63–0]

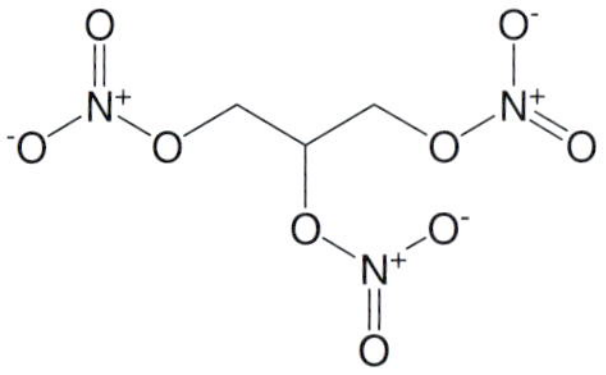

Nitroglycerin is an explosive agent contained in dynamite, and an antianginal and vasodilator treatment available in systemic and topical forms. It is a well known irritant agent in dynamite manufacture. It can also cause allergic reactions in employees of explosives manufacturers, and in the pharmaceutical industry. Transdermal systems are the main source of iatrogenic sensitization. Nitroglycerin can cross-react with isosorbide dinitrate.

Suggested Reading

Aquilina S, Felice H, Boffa MJ (2002) Allergic reactions to glyceryl trinitrate and isosorbide dinitrate demonstrating cross-sensitivity. Clin Exp Dermatol 27:700–702

Kanerva L, Laine R, Jolanki R, Tarvainen K, Estlander T, Helander I (1991) Occupational allergic contact dermatitis caused by nitroglycerin. Contact Dermatitis 24:356–362

Machet L, Martin L, Toledano C, Jan V, Lorette G, Vaillant L (1999) Allergic contact dermatitis from nitroglycerin contained in 2 transdermal systems. Dermatology 198:106–107

305. Nonoxynols

Nonylphenol Ethoxylates, PEG-(n) Nonyl Phenyl Ether, Polyoxyethylene (n) Nonyl Phenyl Ether

CAS Registry Number [26027–38–3] and more than 25 other numbers

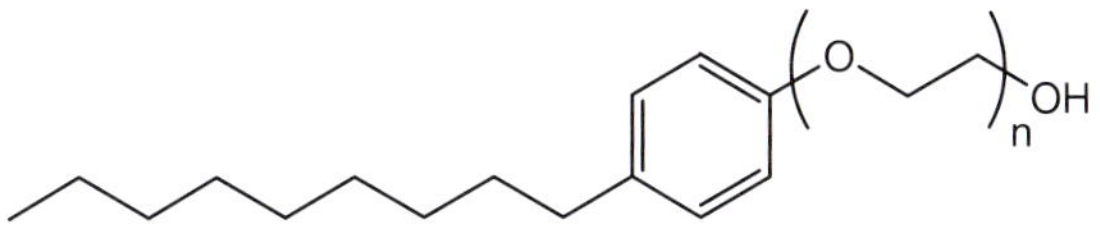

Their general formula is $C_9H_{19}C_6H_4(OCH_2CH_2)_nOH$. Each nonoxynol is characterized by the number (n) of ethylene oxide units repeated in the chain; for example, nonoxynol-9, nonoxynol-14. They are present in detergents, liquid soaps, emulsifiers for creams, fabric softeners, photographic paper additives, hair dyes, lubricating oils, spermicides, and anti-infective agents. They are irritants and sensitizers. Nonoxynol-6 was reported as a sensitizing agent in an industrial hand cleanser and in a crack-indicating fluid in the metal industry. Nonoxynol-9 is the most commonly used, as a preservative in topical antiseptics or in spermicides, acting as a iodophor in PVP-iodine solutions. Nonoxynol-10 was reported as a UVB-photosensitizer. Nonoxynol-12 caused contact dermatitis in a domestic cleaner who used a polish containing it.

Suggested Reading

Dooms-Goossens A, Deveylder H, de Alam AG, Lachapelle JM, Tennstedt D, Degreef H (1989) Contact sensitivity to nonoxynols as a cause of intolerance to antiseptic preparations. J Am Acad Dermatol 21:723–727

Meding B (1985) Occupational contact dermatitis from nonylphenolpolyglycolether. Contact Dermatitis 13:122–123

Nethercott JR, Lawrence MJ (1984) Allergic contact dermatitis due to nonylphenol ethoxylate (nonoxynol-6). Contact Dermatitis 10:235–239

Wilkinson SM, Beck MH, August PJ (1995) Allergic contact dermatitis from nonoxynol-12 in a polish. Contact Dermatitis 33:128–129

306. Octocrylene

Octocrilene

CAS Registry Number [6197–30–4]

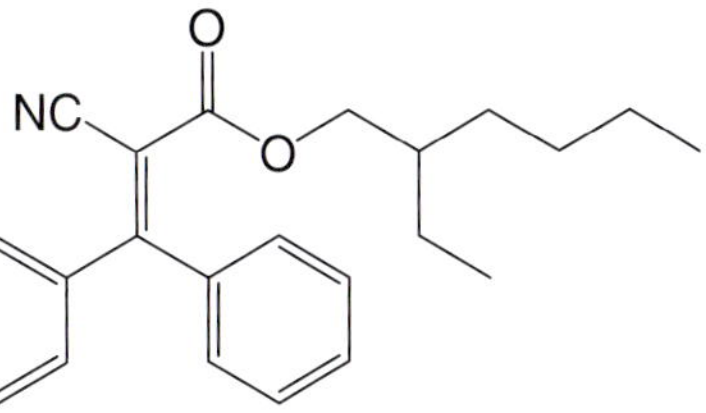

Octocrylene is an anti-UVB filter used in cosmetics that may induce photoallergic contact dermatitis.

Suggested Reading

Carrotte-Lefebvre I, Bonnevalle A, Segard M, Delaporte E, Thomas P (2003) Contact allergy to octocrylene. Contact Dermatitis 48:46–47

307. Octyl Gallate

CAS Registry Number [1034–01–1]

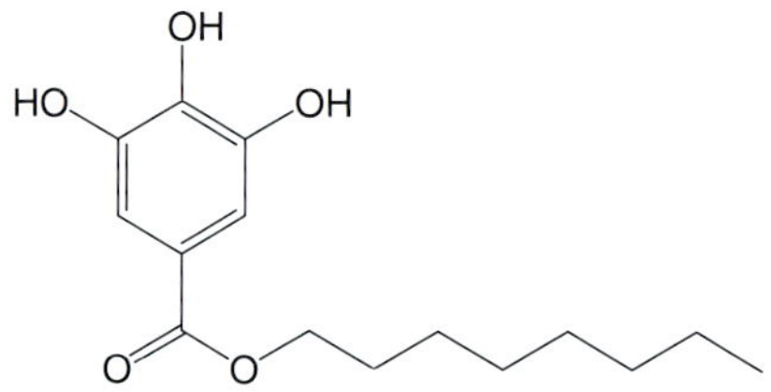

Octyl gallate, a gallate ester (E 311), is an antioxidant added to foods and cosmetics to prevent oxidation of unsaturated fatty acids. Cases were sparsely reported in food industry or from lipsticks. Patch tests are frequently irritant.

Suggested Reading

De Groot AC, Gerkens F (1990) Occupational airborne contact dermatitis from octyl gallate. Contact Dermatitis 23:184–186

Giordano-Labadie F, Schwarze HP, Bazex J (2000) Allergic contact dermatitis from octyl gallate in lipstick. Contact Dermatitis 42:51

308. 2-*n*-Octyl-4-Isothiazolin-3-one

Kathon® LM, Kathon® 4200, Kathon® 893, Pancil, Skane M-8

CAS Registry Number [26530–20–1]

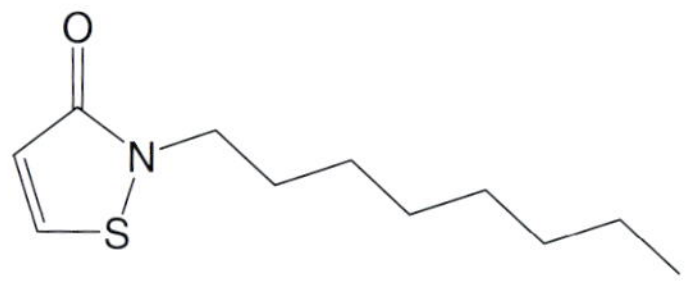

This isothiazolinone, contained in relatively few products compared to other isothiazolinones, is used in cleaning and polishing agents, latex paints, stains, adhesives, wood and leather preservatives, metalworking fluids (cutting oils), and plastic manufacture.

Suggested Reading

Oleaga JM, Aguirre A, Landa N, Gonzalez M, Diaz-Perez JL (1992) Allergic contact dermatitis from Kathon 893. Contact Dermatitis 27:345–346

Young HS, Ferguson JEF, Beck MH (2004) Contact dermatitis from 2-*n*-octyl-4-isothiazoline-3-one in a PhD student. Contact Dermatitis 50:47–48

309. Olaquindox

***N*-(2-Hydroxyethyl)-3-Methyl-2-Quinoxalinecarboxamide 1,4-Dioxide**

CAS Registry Number [23696–28–8]

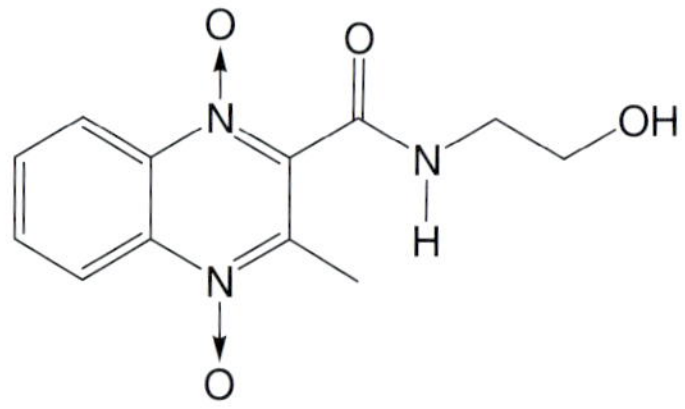

51

Olaquindox is an antibacterial agent derivative of quinoxaline, used as a growth promoter of pigs. It can be found in Bayo-N-Ox® and Proquindox® and numerous other pig feeds. It is a photosensitizer that forms reactive photoproducts on light exposure. It can induce photoallergic contact dermatitis and persistent light reactions.

Suggested Reading

Belhadjali H, Marguery MC, Journe F, Giordano-Labadie F, Lefebvre H, Bazex J (2002) Allergic and photoallergic contact dermatitis to Olaquindox in a pig breeder with prolonged photosensitivity. Photodermatol Photoimmunol Photomed 18:52–53

Kumar A, Freeman S (1996) Photoallergic contact dermatitis in a pig farmer caused by olaquindox. Contact Dermatitis 35:249–250

Schauder S, Schröder W, Geier J (1996) Olaquindox-induced airborne photoallergic contact dermatitis followed by transient or persistent light reactions in 15 pig breeders. Contact Dermatitis 35: 344–354

310. Oxacillin

CAS Registry Number: [66–79–5]

Oxacillin Sodium Salt Monohydrate

CAS Registry Number: [7240–38–2]

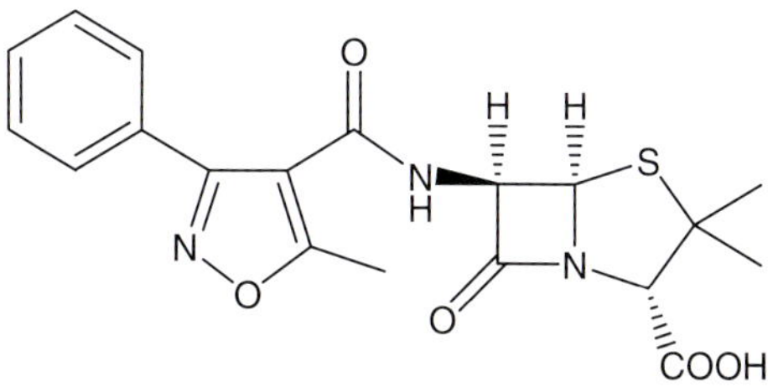

Oxacillin is a semi-synthetic penicillin of the group M. It is closely related to cloxacillin.

Suggested Reading

Budavari S, O'Neil MJ, Smith A, Heckelman PE, Kinneary JF (eds) (1996) The Merck Index, 12th edn. Merck, Whitehouse Station, N.J., USA

311. 7-Oxodehydroabietic Acid

CAS Registry Number [18684–55–4]

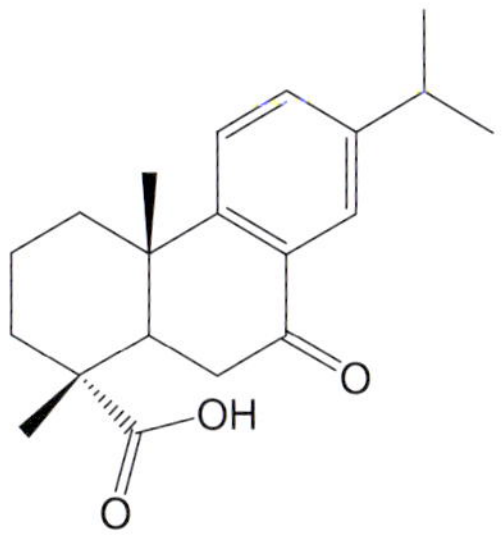

7-Oxodehydroabietic acid is an auto-oxidation product of dehydroabietic acid, and an allergen contained in colophony.

Suggested Reading

Bergh M, Menné T, Karlberg AT (1994) Colophony in paper-based surgical clothing. Contact Dermatitis 31:332–333

312. Oxprenolol

CAS Registry Number [6452–71–7]

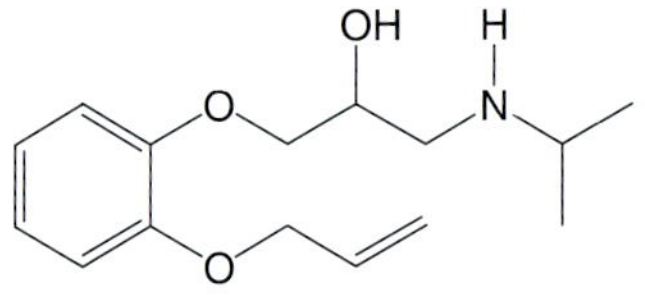

The beta-blocker oxprenolol induced contact dermatitis in a worker at a pharmaceutical plant, in a division for drug synthesis. Epichlorhydrin was also used for the production of drugs propranolol and oxprenolol.

Suggested Reading
Rebandel P, Rudzki E (1990) Dermatitis caused by epichlorhydrin, oxprenolol hydrochloride and propranolol hydrochloride. Contact Dermatitis 23:199

51

313. Pantothenol

2,4-Dihydroxy-*N*-(3-Hydroxypropyl)-3,3-Dimethylbutanamide, Pantothenylol, *N*-Pantoyl-3-Propanolamine, Panthenol, Pantothenyl Alcohol

CAS Registry Number [81–13–0]

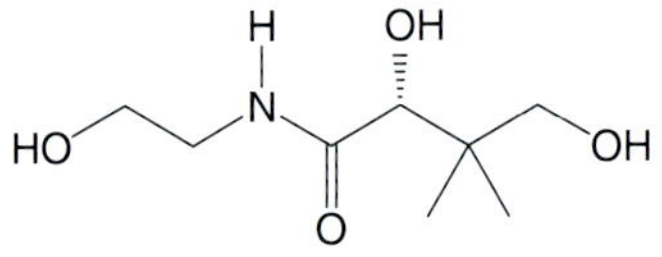

Pan(to)thenol is the alcohol corresponding to pantothenic acid, of the vitamin B5 group. It is used as a food additive, and in skin and hair products as a conditioning agent. Contact dermatitis and urticaria have been reported.

Suggested Reading
Schalock PC, Storrs FJ, Morrison L (2000) Contact urticaria from panthenol in hair conditioner. Contact Dermatitis 43:223

Stables GI, Wilkinson SM (1998) Allergic contact dermatitis due to panthenol. Contact Dermatitis 38:236–237

314. Parabens (Parahydroxybenzoic Acid Esters)

Methylparaben, E218, E219 (Sodium Salt)

CAS Registry Number [99–76–3], E219 (Sodium Salt), CAS Registry Number [5026–62–0]

Ethylparaben, E214, E215 (Sodium Salt)

CAS Registry Number [120–47–8]. E215 (Sodium Salt),
CAS Registry Number [35285–68–8]

Propylparaben, E216, E217 (Sodium Salt)

CAS Registry Number [94–13–3], E217 (Sodium Salt),
CAS Registry Number [35285–69–9]

Isopropylparaben

CAS Registry Number [4191–73–5]

Butylparaben

CAS Registry Number [94–26–8]

Isobutylparaben

CAS Registry Number [4247–02–3]

Phenylparaben

CAS Registry Number [17696–62–7]

Benzylparaben

CAS Registry Number [94–18–8]

Phenoxyethylparaben

CAS Registry Number [55468–88–7]

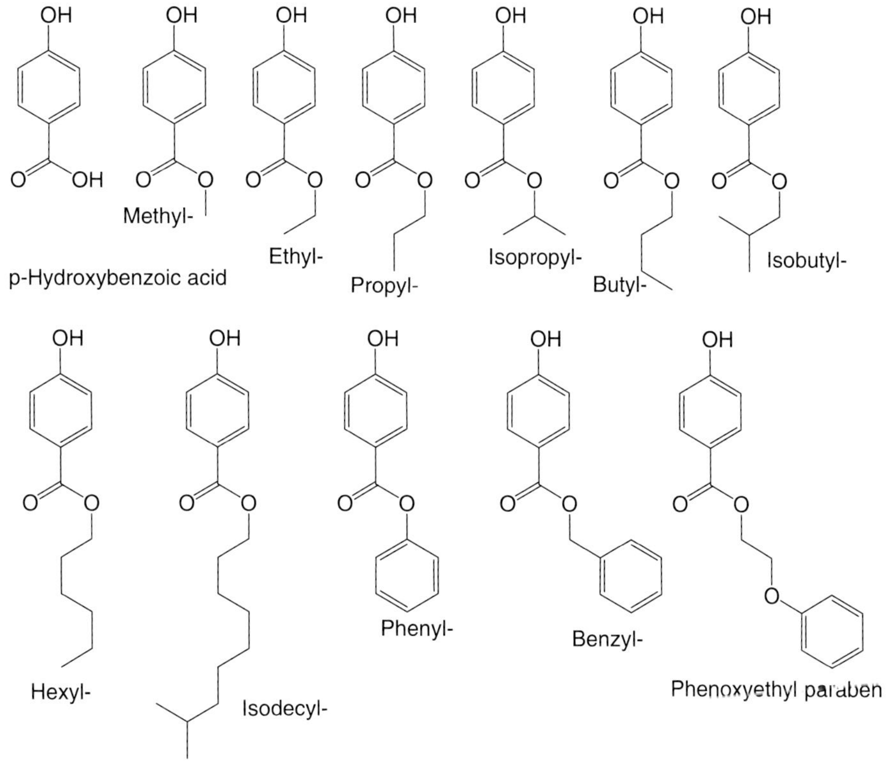

Parabens are esters formed by *p*-hydroxybenzoic acid and an alcohol. They are largely used as biocides in cosmetics and toiletries, medicaments, or food. They have synergistic power with other biocides. Parabens can induce allergic contact dermatitis, mainly in chronic dermatitis and wounded skin.

Suggested Reading

Le Coz CJ (2004) Fiche d'éviction en cas d'hypersensibilité aux esters de l'acide *para*-hydroxybenzoïque (parahydroxybenzoates ou parabens). Ann Dermatol Venereol 131:309–310

315. Paraphenylenediamine

PPD, *p*-Phenylenediamine, 4-Phenylenediamine

CAS Registry Number [106–50–3]

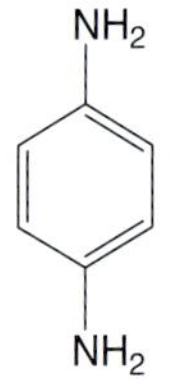

PPD is a colorless compound oxidized by hydrogen peroxide in the presence of ammonia. It is then polymerized to a color by a coupling agent. Although a well-known allergen in hair dyes, PPD can be found as a cause of contact dermatitis in chin rest stains or in milk testers. It is also a marker of group sensitivity to *para* amino compounds such as benzocaine, some azo-dyes and some previous antibacterial sulphonamides.

Suggested Reading

Bork K (1993) Allergic contact dermatitis on a violinist's neck from para-phenylenediamine in a chin rest stain. Contact Dermatitis 28:250–251

Frosch PJ, Burrows D, Camarasa JG, Dooms-Goossens A, Ducombs G, Lahti A, Menné T, Rycroft RJG, Shaw S, White IR, Wilkinson JD (1993) Allergic reactions to a hairdresser's series: results from 9 European centres. Contact Dermatitis 28:180–183

Guerra L, Tosti A, Bardazzi F, Pigatto P, Lisi P, Santucci B, Valsecchi R, Schena D, Angelini G, Sertoli A, Ayala F, Kokelj F (1992) Contact dermatitis in hairdressers: the Italian experience. Gruppo Italiano Ricerca Dermatiti da Contatto e Ambientali. Contact Dermatitis 26:101–107

Le Coz CJ, Lefebvre C, Keller F, Grosshans E (2000) Allergic contact dermatitis caused by skin painting (pseudotattooing) with black henna, a mixture of henna and *p*-phenylenediamine and its derivatives. Arch Dermatol 136:1515–1517

Rebandel P, Rudzki E (1995) Occupational allergy to *p*-phenylenediamine in milk testers. Contact Dermatitis 33:138

316. Paraquat (Dichloride, Methosulfate)

1-1′-Dimethyl-4,4′-Bipyridinium Salt

CAS Registry Numbers [4685–14–7], [116047–10–0] (CAS Registry Number [1910–42–5], CAS Registry Number [2074–50–2])

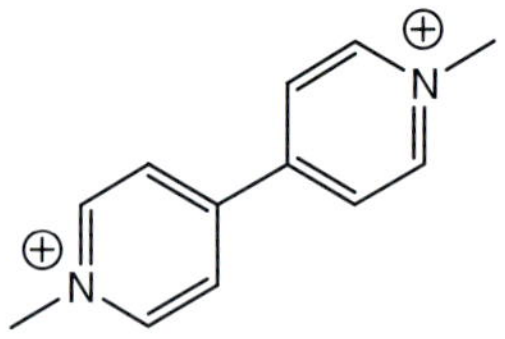

Paraquat is a quaternary ammonium compound with herbicide properties, as diquat. It is contained in Cekuquat® or Dipril®. It can cause contact and phototoxic contact dermatitis, acne, and leukoderma mainly in agricultural workers.

Suggested Reading

Vilaplana J, Azon A, Romaguera C, Lecha M (1993) Phototoxic contact dermatitis with toxic hepatitis due to the percutaneous absorption of paraquat. Contact Dermatitis 29:163–164

317. Parathion

Parathion-Ethyl: Parathion, Ethylparathion, Corothion, Dantion, Folidol

CAS Registry Number [56–38–2]

Paration-Methyl: Methylparathion, Matafos, Paratox, Folidol M

CAS Registry Number [298–00–0]

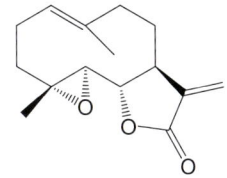

Methyl-Parathion   Ethyl-Parathion

One case was reported of a bullous contact dermatitis due to ethylparathion. A case of sensitization to methyl-parathion was described in a female agricultural worker with multiple sensitization.

Suggested Reading

Jung HD, Holzegel K (1988) Akute Toxisch-bullöse Kontaktdermatitis durch den Phosphorsäurester Parathionethyl im Follidel-Öl. Aktuel Dermatol 14:19–31

Pevny I (1980) Pestizid-Allergie. Dermatosen 28:186–189

318. Parthenolide

CAS Registry Number [20554–84–1]

Parthenolide is a sesquiterpene lactone found Asteraceae–Compositae such as feverfew (*Tanacetum parthenium* Schultz-Bip.) or congress grass (*Parthenium hysterophorus* L.).

Suggested Reading

Hausen BM, Osmundsen PE (1983) Contact allergy to parthenolide in *Tanacetum parthenium* (L.) Schultz-Bip. (feverfew, Asteraceae) and cross-reactions to related sesquiterpene lactone containing Compositae species. Acta Derm Venereol (Stockh) 63:308–314

Lamminpää A, Estlander T, Jolanki R, Kanerva L (1996) Occupational allergic contact dermatitis caused by decorative plants. Contact Dermatitis 34:330–335

Paulsen E, Andersen KE, Hausen BM (1993) Compositae dermatitis in a Danish dermatology department in one year (I). Results of routine patch testing with the sesquiterpene lactone mix supplemented with aimed patch testing with extracts and sesquiterpene lactones of Compositae plants. Contact Dermatitis 29:6–10

319. Penicillins

CAS Registry Number [1406–05–9]

for penicillin

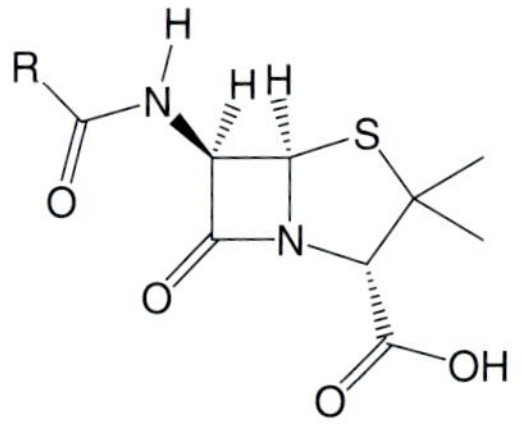

Penicillins can induce contact dermatitis, contact urticaria, and systemic and sometimes severe reactions. Occupational sensitivity to penicillins concerns health workers, workers in the pharmaceutical industry and veterinaries, since these antibiotics
are used by veterinarians and cattle breeders as medications and animal feed antibiotic. All penicillins contain the 6-aminopenicillanic acid moiety. Penicillins of G, V,
A, and M groups are characterized by a specific C_7 side chain. Cross-reactivity is
possible between several penicillins but is not systematic since both immediate- and
delayed-type sensitivity can implicate the 6-aminopenicillanic acid moiety, or be
specific to the 7-side-chain.

Suggested Reading
Guerra L, Venturo N, Tardio M, Tosti A (1995) Airborne contact dermatitis from animal feed anti-
    biotics. Contact Dermatitis 32:61–62
Rudzki E, Rebandel P, Grzywa Z (1989) Patch tests with occupational contactants in nurses, doctors
    and dentists. Contact Dermatitis 20:247–250

320. Pentachloronitrobenzene

Quintozene, PCNB, Brassicol, Terrachlor®

CAS Registry Number [82–68–8]

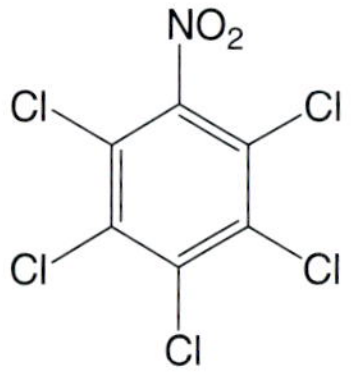

Pentachloronitrobenzene is a pesticide and a fungicide. Sensitization can occur in
farmers or in chemical plants.

Suggested Reading
O'Malley M, Rodriguez P, Maibach HI (1995) Pesticide patch testing: California nursery workers
    and controls. Contact Dermatitis 32:61–62
Sharma VK, Kaur S (1990) Contact sensitization by pesticides in farmers. Contact Dermatitis 23:
    77–80

321. Pentadecylcatechol

3-Pentadecylcatechol, Hydrourushiol, Tetrahydrourushiol

CAS Registry Number [492–89–7]

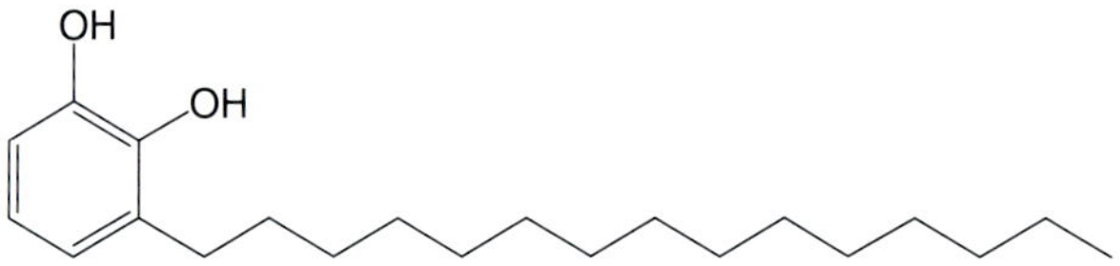

Pentadecylcatechol belongs to the urushiols, and is the main allergen of the Anacardiaceae poison ivy (*Toxicodendron radicans*) and of Poison oak (*Toxicodendron diversiloba, Rhus diversiloba*).

Suggested Reading

Epstein WL (1994) Occupational poison ivy and oak dermatitis. Dermatol Clin 12:511–516

322. Phenoxyethanol

2-Phenoxyethanol

CAS Registry Numbers [122–99–6], [37220–49–8], [56257–90–0]

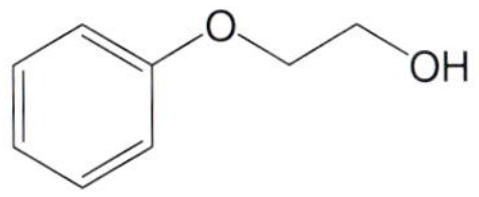

Phenoxyethanol is an aromatic ether-alcohol used mainly as a preservative, mostly with methyldibromoglutaronitrile (in Euxyl® K 400) or with parabens. Sensitization to this molecule is very rare.

Suggested Reading

Vigan M, Brechat N, Girardin P, Adessi B, Meyer JP, Vuitton D, Laurent R (1996) Un nouvel allergène: le dibromodicyanobutane. Etude sur 310 patients de janvier à décembre 1994. Ann Dermatol Venereol 123:322–324

323. Phenyl Glycidyl Ether

CAS Registry Numbers [122–60–1], [66527–93–3]

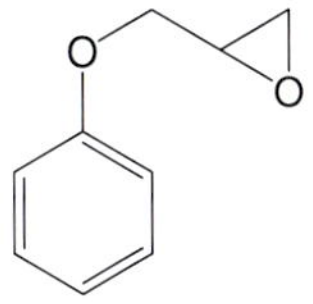

This monoglycidyl derivative is a reactive diluent in epoxy resins Bisphenol A type. It is a component of epoxy paints, epoxy glues, and epoxy resins. Sensitization has been observed in many professions, such as in construction workers, marble workers, ceramic workers, and shoemakers.

Suggested Reading

Angelini G, Rigano L, Foti C, Grandolfo M, Vena GA, Bonamonte D, Soleo L, Scorpiniti AA (1996) Occupational sensitization to epoxy resin and reactive diluents in marble workers. Contact Dermatitis 35:11–16

Condé-Salazar L, Gonzalez de Domingo MA, Guimaraens D (1994) Sensitization to epoxy resin systems in special flooring workers. Contact Dermatitis 31:157–160

Jolanki R, Kanerva L, Estlander T, Tarvainen K, Keskinen H, Henriks-Eckerman ML (1990) Occupational dermatoses from epoxy resin compounds. Contact Dermatitis 23:172–183

Mancuso G, Reggiani M, Berdondini RM (1996) Occupational dermatitis in shoemakers. Contact Dermatitis 34:17–22

Seidenari S, Danese P, di Nardo A, Manzini BM, Motolese A (1990) Contact sensitization among ceramics workers. Contact Dermatitis 22:45–49

Tarvainen K (1995) Analysis of patients with allergic patch test reactions to a plastic and glues series. Contact Dermatitis 32:346–351

324. Phenyl-Alpha-Naphthylamine

Neozone A, CI 44050

CAS Registry Number [90–30–2]

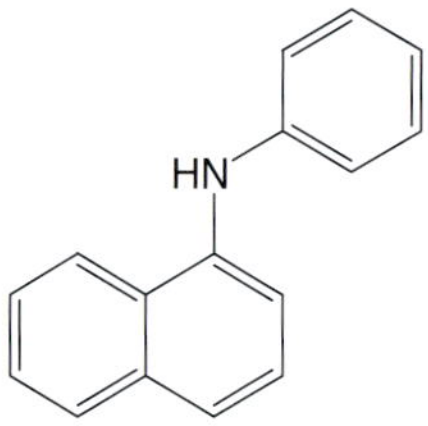

Phenyl-alpha-naphthylamine is contained in some rubbers and oils as an antioxidant of the amine group. It is closely related to phenyl-beta-naphthylamine and to di-beta-naphthyl-*p*-phenylenediamine, but without cross-reactivity.

Suggested Reading

Carmichael AJ, Foulds IS (1990) Isolated naphthylamine allergy to phenyl-alpha-naphthylamine. Contact Dermatitis 22:298–299

Svedman C, Isaksson M, Zimerson E, Bruze M (2004) Occupational contact dermatitis from a grease. Dermatitis 15:41–44

325. Phenyl-Beta-Naphthylamine

N-Phenyl-2-Naphthylamine, Neozone

CAS Registry Numbers [135–88–6], [52907–17–2], [84420–28–0]

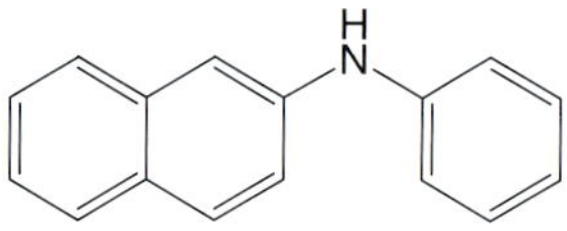

Phenyl-beta-naphthylamine is an amine compound. Sensitization was reported in patients with hypersensitivity from rubber.

Suggested Reading

Condé-Salazar L, Guimaraens D, Romero LV, Gonzalez MA (1987) Unusual allergic contact dermatitis to aromatic amines. Contact Dermatitis 17:42–44

Condé-Salazar L, Del-Rio E, Guimaraens D, Gonzalez Domingo A (1993) Type IV allergy to rubber additives: a 10-year study of 686 cases. J Am Acad Dermatol 29:176–180

Kiec-Swierczynska M (1995) Occupational sensitivity to rubber. Contact Dermatitis 32:171–172

326. Phenylephrine (Hydrochloride)

CAS Registry Number [59–42–7]

Phenylephrine Hydrochloride

CAS Registry Number [61–76–7]

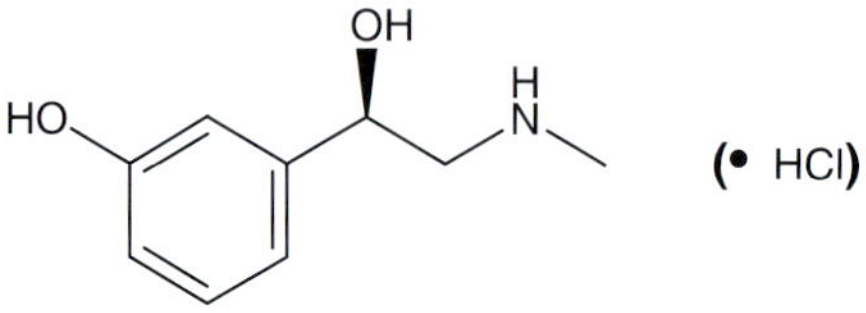

(• HCl)

Phenylephrine hydrochloride is an alpha-adrenergic agonist, used as a mydriatic and decongestant in eyedrops.

Suggested Reading

Narayan S, Prais L, Foulds IS (2002) Allergic contact dermatitis caused by phenylephrine eyedrops. Am J Contact Dermat 13:208–209

51

327. Phenylethyl Caffeate

Caffeic Acid Phenethyl Ester, Capee

CAS Registry Number [104594–70–9]

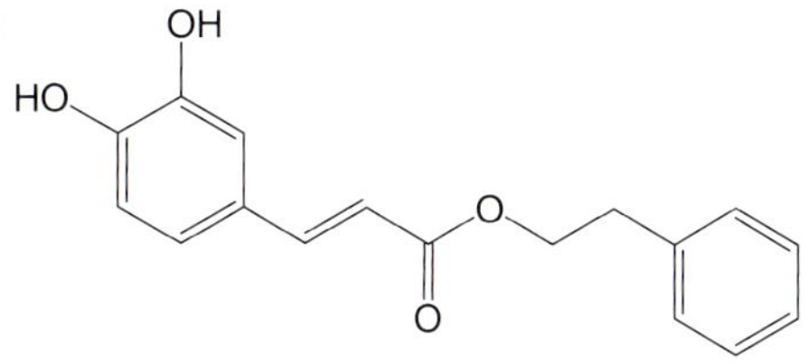

Capee is one of the allergens of propolis (bee glue). It is also contained in poplar bud secretions.

Suggested Reading

Lamminpää A, Estlander T, Jolanki R, Kanerva L (1996) Occupational allergic contact dermatitis caused by decorative plants. Contact Dermatitis 34:330–335

Oliwiecki S, Beck MH, Hausen BM (1992) Occupational contact dermatitis from caffeates in poplar bud resin in a tree surgeon. Contact Dermatitis 27:127–128

328. Phthalic Anhydride

CAS Registry Numbers [85–44–9], [39363–63–8]

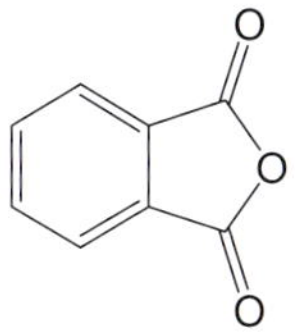

Phthalic anhydride is used in the manufacture of unsaturated polyesters and as a curing agent for epoxy resins. When used as a pigment, it can be responsible for sensitization in ceramic workers. Phthalic anhydride per se is not responsible for the sensitization to the resin used in nail varnishes phthalic anhydride/trimellitic anhydride/glycols copolymer, CAS Registry Number [85–44–9].

Suggested Reading

Seidenari S, Danese P, di Nardo A, Manzini BM, Motolese A (19909 Contact sensitization among ceramics workers. Contact Dermatitis 22:45–49

Tarvainen K, Jolanki R, Estlander T, Tupasela O, Pfäffli P, Kanerva L (1995) Immunologic contact urticaria due to airborne methylhexahydrophthalic and methyltetrahydrophthalic anhydrides. Contact Dermatitis 32:204–209

329. Picric Acid

CI 10305

CAS Registry Number [88–89–1]

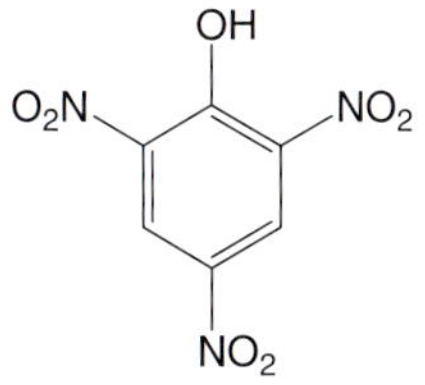

Contact dermatitis occurred primarily in the explosives industry.

Suggested Reading

Aguirre A, Sanz de Galdeano C, Oleaga JM, Eizaguirre X, Diaz Perez JL (1993) Allergic contact dermatitis from picric acid. Contact Dermatitis 28:291

Hausen BM (1994) Letter to the editor. Picric acid. Contact Dermatitis 30:59

330. Alpha-Pinene

CAS Registry Numbers [80–56–8], [2437–95–8]

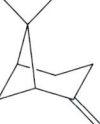

Alpha-pinene is the major constituent of turpentine (about 80%). It exists in levo-gyre form in European turpentine, and in dextrogyre form in turpentine found in North-Americans. Sensitization occurs mainly in painters, polishers, and varnish-ers, and in those in the perfume and in the ceramics industry.

Suggested Reading

Lear JT, Heagerty AHM, Tan BB, Smith AG, English JSC (1996) Transient re-emergence of oil tur-pentine allergy in the pottery industry. Contact Dermatitis 35:169–172

Moura C, Dias M, Vale T (1994) Contact dermatitis in painters, polishers and varnishers. Contact Dermatitis 31:51–53

331. Beta-Pinene

Nopinene, Terebenthene

CAS Registry Number [127–91–3]

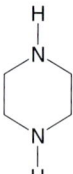

Beta-pinene is a component of turpentine. Concentrations vary with the source, and seem higher in European (Portuguese) than in Asian (Indonesian) turpentine.

Suggested Reading

Lear JT, Heagerty AHM, Tan BB, Smith AG, English JSC (1996) Transient re-emergence of oil tur-pentine allergy in the pottery industry. Contact Dermatitis 35:169–172

332. Piperazine

Diethylenediamine

CAS Registry Number [110–85–0]

Piperazine is contained in pyrazinobutazone, an equimolar salt of piperazine and phenylbutazone. Among occupational cases, most were reported in the pharmaceu-tical industry or laboratory workers, in nurses, and in veterinarians.

Suggested Reading

Dorado Bris JM, Montanes Aragues M, Sols Candela M, Garcia Diez A (1992) Contact sensitivity to pyrazinobutazone (Carudol®) with positive oral provocation test. Contact Dermatitis 26: 355–356

Rudzki E, Rebandel P, Grzywa Z, Pomorski Z, Jakiminska B, Zawisza E (1982) Occupational derma-titis in veterinarians. Contact Dermatitis 8:72–73

51

333. Piroxicam

CAS Registry Number [36332–90–4]

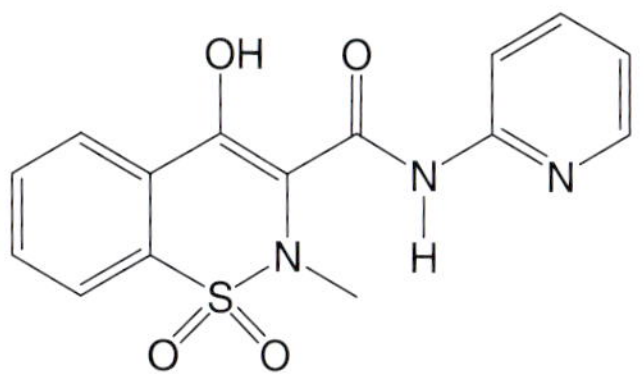

This nonsteroidal anti-inflammatory drug belongs to the oxicam class. It induces photo-allergic contact dermatitis rather than contact allergy. Systemic photosensitivity is frequent, in patients previously sensitized to thiomersal. Thiosalicylic acid, the nonmercurial moiety of thiomersal, is a marker of photoallergy to piroxicam. Reactions are expected with piroxicam β-cyclodextrin but cross-sensitivity is generally not observed to tenoxicam or meloxicam (personal observations).

Suggested Reading

Arévalo A, Blancas R, Ancona A (1995) Occupational contact dermatitis from piroxicam. Am J Contact Dermat 6:113–114

De la Cuadra J, Pujol C, Aliaga A (1989) Clinical evidence of cross-sensitivity between thiosalicylic acid, a contact allergen, and piroxicam, a photoallergen. Contact Dermatitis 21:349–351

334. Pivampicillin

CAS Registry Number [33817–20–8]

Pivampicillin Hydrochloride

CAS Registry Number [26309–95–5]

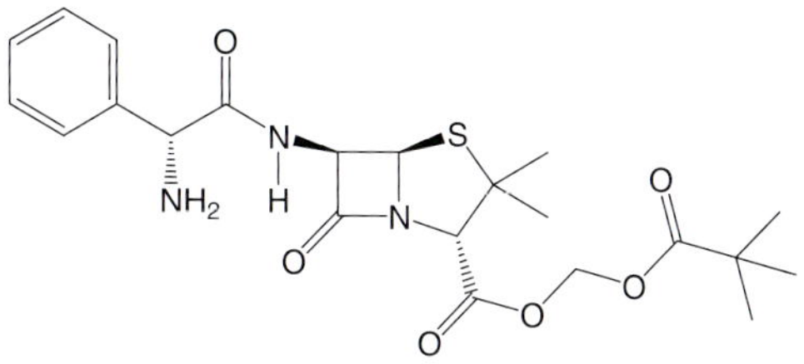

Pivampicillin is a prodrug of ampicillin. It caused sensitization in 56 workers at a penicillin factory. Pivampicillin and pivmecillinam were responsible for contact dermatitis in pharmaceutical production workers. Ampicillin, mecillinam or amdinocillin, penicillin V and penicillin G were also implicated in cross-reactions.

Suggested Reading

Moller NE, von Würden K (1992) Hypersensitivity to semisynthetic penicillins and cross-reactivity with penicillin. Contact Dermatitis 26:351–352

Moller NE, Nielsen B, von Würden K (1990) Changes in penicillin contamination and allergy in factory workers. Contact Dermatitis 22:106–107

335. Potassium Metabisulfite

Sodium Pyrosulfite, Disodium Disulfite, E224

CAS Registry Number [16731–55–8]

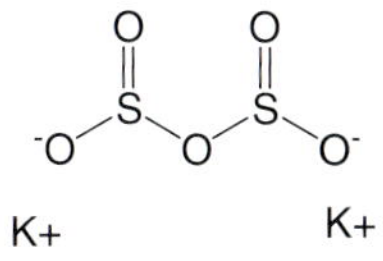

Potassium metabisulfite is an antioxidant used as an antifermentative agent in breweries and wineries, as a preservative of fruits and vegetables, and to bleach straw. Reactions to both sodium and potassium metabisulfite are expected.

Suggested Reading

Budavari S, O'Neil MJ, Smith A, Heckelman PE, Kinneary JF (eds) (1996) The Merck Index, 12th edn. Merck, Whitehouse Station, N.J., USA

336. Povidone-Iodine

Polyvinylpyrrolidone-Iodine, PVP-Iodine

CAS Registry Number [25655–41–8]

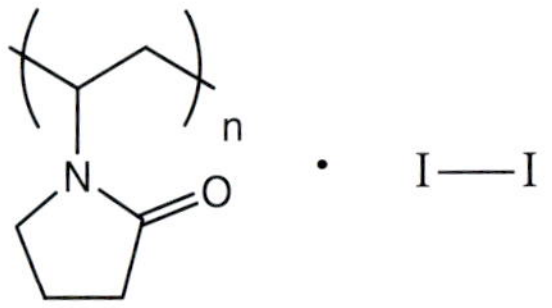

Povidone-iodine is iodophor, used as a topical antiseptic. A 10% povidone-iodine solution contains 1% available iodine, but free-iodine is at 0.1% concentration. Skin exposure causes irritant rather than allergic contact dermatitis. In such a situation however, iodine seems to be the true hapten.

Suggested Reading

Lachapelle JM (2005) Allergic contact dermatitis from povidone-iodine: a re-evaluation study. Contact Dermatitis 52:9–10
Tosti A, Vincenzi C, Bardazzi F, Mariani R (1990) Allergic contact dermatitis due to povidone-iodine. Contact Dermatitis 23:197–198

337. Prilocaine (Hydrochloride)

CAS Registry Number [25655–41–8] (CAS Registry Number [1786–81–8])

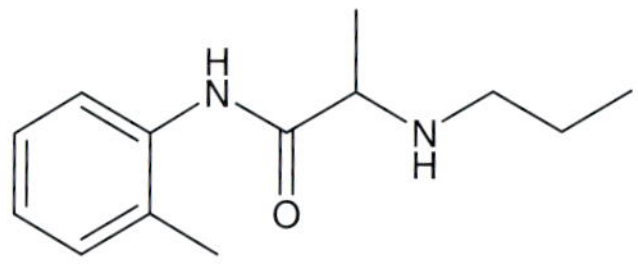

Prilocaine in a local anesthetic of the amide group. It can induce allergic contact dermatitis, particularly from EMLA® cream.

Suggested Reading

Le Coz CJ, Cribier BJ, Heid E (1996) Patch testing in suspected allergic contact dermatitis due to Emla® cream in haemodialyzed patients. Contact Dermatitis 35:316–317

338. Primin

CAS Registry Number [15121–94–5]

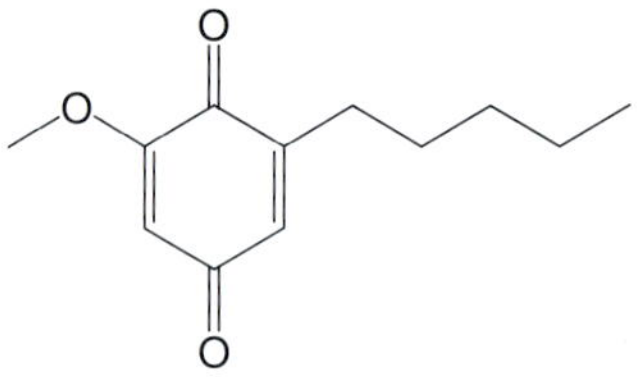

Primin is the major allergen of *Primula obconica* Hance (Primulaceae family). Allergic contact dermatitis is mainly occupational, occurring in florists and horticulturists.

Suggested Reading

Christensen LP, Larsen E (2000) Direct emission of the allergen primin from intact *Primula obconica* plants. Contact Dermatitis 42:149–153
Lamminpää A, Estlander T, Jolanki R, Kanerva L (1996) Occupational allergic contact dermatitis caused by decorative plants. Contact Dermatitis 34:330–335

339. Pristinamycin

Pristinamycin

CAS Registry Number [270076–60–3]

Pristinamycin IA (Streptogramin B, Mikamycin IA, Ostreogrycin B, Vernamycin B$_{alpha}$)

CAS Registry Number [3131–03–1]

Pristinamycin IIA (Mikamycin A, Ostreogrycin A, Pristinamycin II$_A$, Staphylomycin M$_1$, Streptogramin A, Vernamycin A, Virginiamycin M$_1$)

CAS Registry Number [21411–53–0]

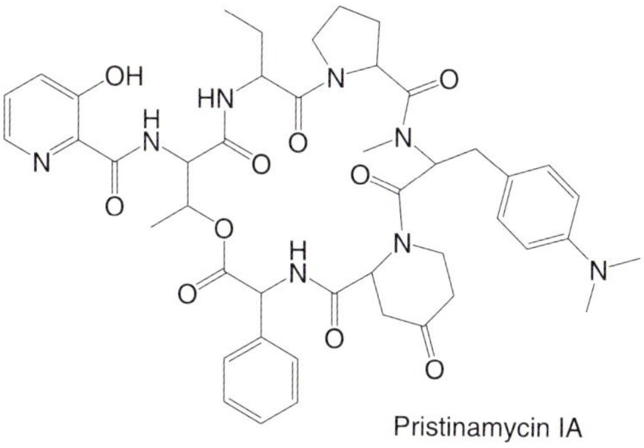

Pristinamycin IA 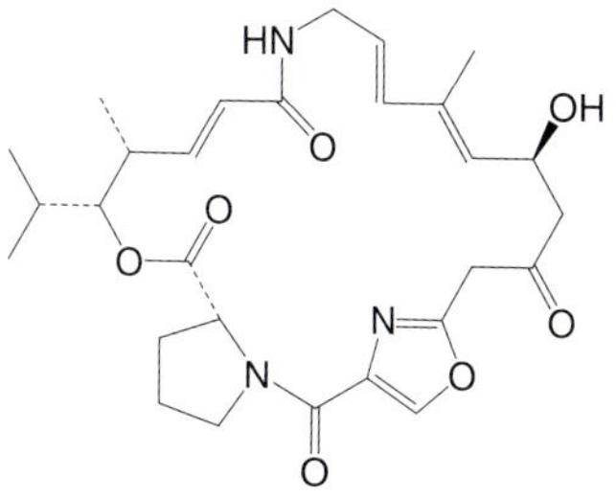   Pristinamycin IIA

Pristinamycin is a systemic antibiotic of the synergistins/streptogramins class, composed of two subunits: pristinamycin IA and pristinamycin IIA. It induces several types of drug reactions such as maculo-papular exanthema, systemic dermatitis or acute generalized exanthematous pustulosis. Some patients have been previously skin-sensitized by virginiamycin (see below). Cross-reactivity is expected to virginiamycin CAS [11006–76–1] and to the associated dalfopristin (CAS [112362–50–2]) and quinupristin (CAS [120138–50–3]).

Suggested Reading

Barbaud A, Trechot P, Weber-Muller F, Ulrich G, Commun N, Schmutz JL (2004) Drug skin tests in cutaneous adverse drug reactions to pristinamycin: 29 cases with a study of cross-reactions between synergistins. Contact Dermatitis 50:22–26

340. Procaine (Hydrochloride)

2-Diethylaminoethyl 4-Aminobenzoate, Novocaine®

CAS Registry Number [59–46–1]

Procaine Hydrochloride

CAS Registry Number [51–05–8]

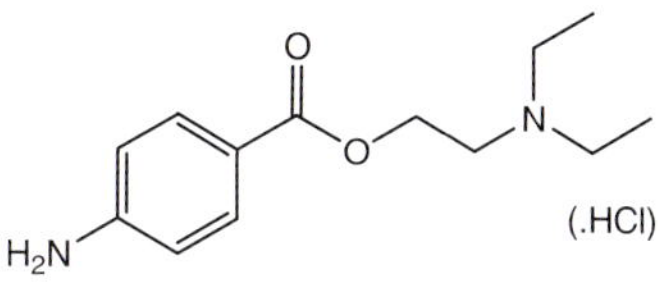

(.HCl)

Procaine is a local anesthetic with *para*-amino function. Sensitization mainly concerns the medical, dental, and veterinary professions.

Suggested Reading

Berova N, Stranky L, Krasteva M (1990) Studies on contact dermatitis in stomatological staff. Dermatol Monatschr 176:15–18

Rudzki E, Rebandel P, Grzywa Z, Pomorski Z, Jakiminska B, Zawisza E (1982) Occupational dermatitis in veterinarians. Contact Dermatitis 8:72–73

341. Propacetamol

4-Acetamidophenyl *N,N*-Diethylglycinate Hydrochloride

CAS Registry Number [66532–85–2]

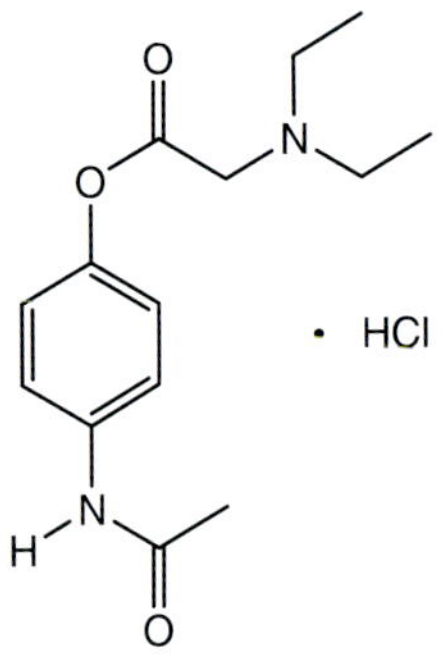

· HCl

51

Propacetamol is a prodrug of paracetamol (acetaminophen) used for intravenous administration. It results from the combination of paracetamol and diethylglycine. It caused contact (hand and airborne) dermatitis in nurses, and acute systemic dermatitis (pompholyx and nummular dermatitis, generalized eczema, urticaria-like eruption) in nurses who had became sick and received intravenous propacetamol. Allergenic properties are due to the *N,N*'-diethylglycine moiety, and not to the paracetamol moiety. Propacetamol is now substituted by a solution of paracetamol in mannitol (Perfalgan®).

Suggested Reading

Barbaud A, Trechot P, Bertrand O, Schmutz JL (1995) Occupational allergy to propacetamol. Lancet 30:902
Berl V, Barbaud A, Lepoittevin JP (1998) Mechanism of allergic contact dermatitis from propacetamol: sensitization to activated *N,N*-diethylglycine. Contact Dermatitis 38:185–188
Le Coz C, Collet E, Dupouy M (1999) Conséquences d'une administration systémique de propacétamol (Pro-Dafalgan®) chez les infirmières sensibilisées au propacétamol. Ann Dermatol Venereol 126 [Suppl 2]:32–33

342. Propargite

Omite®

CAS Registry Number [2312–35–8]

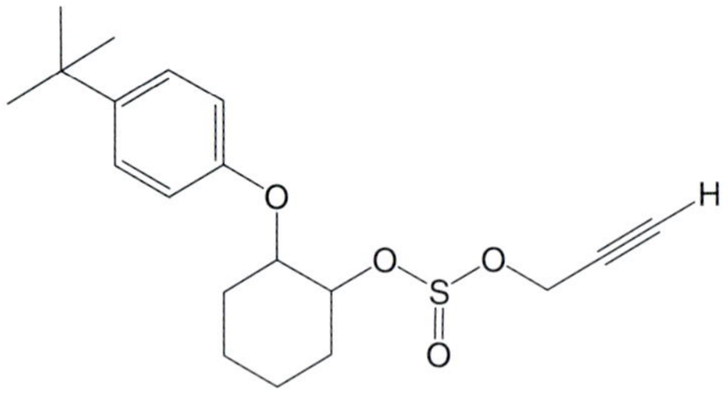

The pesticide omite principally acts as an irritant. Contact dermatitis was reported in 40 of 47 agricultural workers using Omite®.

Suggested Reading

Nishioka K, Kozuka T, Tashiro M (1970) Agricultural miticide (BPPS) dermatitis. Skin Res 12:15
O'Malley M, Rodriguez P, Maibach HI (1995) Pesticide patch testing: California nursery workers and controls. Contact Dermatitis 32:61–62

343. Propranolol

CAS Registry Number [525–66–6]

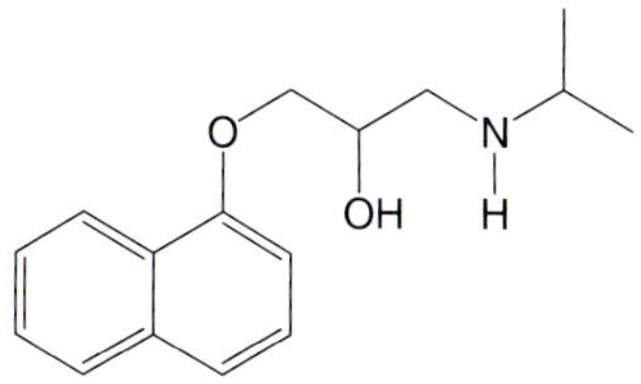

Propranolol is a beta-blocking agent that was responsible for the sensitization of workers in drug synthesis. In one case, epichlorhydrin was used for the production of drugs propranolol and oxprenolol. Cross-reactivity is expected between beta-blockers.

Suggested Reading

Pereira F, Dias M, Pacheco FA (1996) Occupational contact dermatitis from propranolol, hydralazine and bendroflumethiazide. Contact Dermatitis 35:303–304

Rebandel P, Rudzki E (1990) Dermatitis caused by epichlorhydrin, oxprenolol hydrochloride and propranolol hydrochloride. Contact Dermatitis 23:199

344. Propyl Gallate

CAS Registry Number [121–79–9]

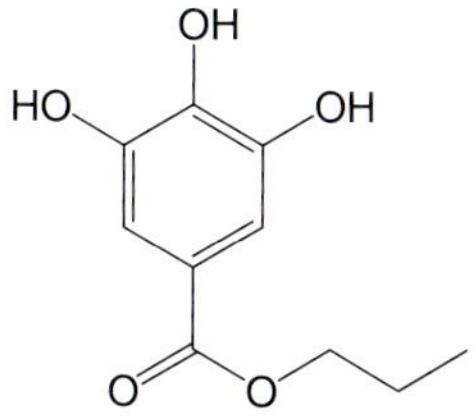

This gallate ester (E 311) is an antioxidant frequently used in the food, cosmetic, and pharmaceutical industries to prevent the oxidation of unsaturated fatty acids into rancid-smelling compounds. It causes cosmetic dermatitis mainly from lipsticks and induced contact dermatitis in a baker, and in a female confectioner, primarily sensitized by her night cream, who fried doughnuts – the margarine probably containing gallates.

Suggested Reading

Bojs G, Niklasson B, Svensson A (1987) Allergic contact dermatitis to propyl gallate. Contact Dermatitis 17:294–298

Marston S (1992) Propyl gallate on liposomes. Contact Dermatitis 27:74–76

Serra-Baldrich E, Puig LL, Gimenez Arnau A, Camarasa JG (1995) Lipstick allergic contact dermatitis from gallates. Contact Dermatitis 32:359–360

345. Propylene Glycol

1,2-Propanediol

CAS Registry Number [57–55–6]

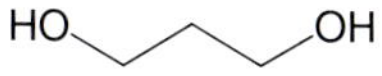

Propylene glycol is used as a solvent, a vehicle for topical medicaments such as corticosteroids or aciclovir, an emulsifier and humectant in food and cosmetics, and as antifreeze in breweries, in the manufactures of resins. It was present as an occupational sensitizer in the color film developer Flexicolor®. Patch tests in aqua are sometimes irritant.

Suggested Reading
Claverie F, Giordano-Labadie F, Bazex J (1997) Eczéma de contact au propylène glycol. Ann Dermatol Venereol 124:315–317
Connoly M, Buckley DA (2004) Contact dermatitis from propylene glycol in ECG electrodes, complicated by medicament allergy. Contact Dermatitis 50:42
Scheman AJ, Katta R (1997) Photographic allergens: an update. Contact Dermatitis 37:130

346. Propylene Oxide

CAS Registry Number [75–56–9]

Propylene oxide is an allergic and irritant agent, used as a solvent and raw material in the chemical industry, as the starting material and intermediate for a broad spectrum of polymers. It can be used as a dehydrating agent for the preparation of slides in electron microscopy. Occupational dermatitis was also reported following the use of a skin disinfectant swab.

Suggested Reading
Steinkraus V, Hausen BM (1994) Contact allergy to propylene oxide. Contact Dermatitis 31:120
Van Ketel WG (1979) Contact dermatitis from propylene oxide. Contact Dermatitis 5:191–192

347. Pseudoephedrine

CAS Registry Number [90–82–4]

Pseudoephedrine Hydrochloride

CAS Registry Number [345–78–8]

Pseudoephedrine Sulfate

CAS Registry Number [7460–12–0]

This sympathomimetic α-adrenergic agonist is found in plants of the genus *Ephedra* (Ephedraceae) and is systemically used as a nasal decongestant. It can induce drug skin reactions such as acute generalized exanthematic pustulosis or generalized eczema.

Suggested Reading
Assier-Bonnet H, Viguier M, Dubertret L, Revuz J, Roujeau JC (2002) Severe adverse drug reactions due to pseudoephedrine from over-the-counter medications. Contact Dermatitis 47:165–182
Padial MA, Alvarez-Ferreira J, Tapia B, Blanco R, Manas C, Blanca M, Bellon T (2004) Acute generalized exanthematous pustulosis associated with pseudoephedrine. Br J Dermatol 150:139–142

348. Pyrethroids

Cypermethrin(e)

CAS Registry Number [52315–07–8]

Permethrin(e)

CAS Registry Number [52645–53–1]

Deltamethrin(e)

CAS Registry Number [52918–63–5]

51

Bioalletrhin(e), Depalethrin(e)

CAS Registry Number [584–79–2]

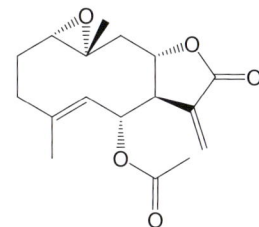

Cypermethrin

Bioallethrin

Permethrin

Deltamethrin

Pyrethroids, also called pyrethrinoids, are neurotoxic synthetic compounds used as insecticides, with irritant properties. Cypermethrin and fenvalerate have been reported as causing positive allergic patch tests, but only fenvalerate was relevant in an agricultural worker.

Suggested Reading

Flannigan SA, Tucker SB, Key MM, Ross CE, Fairchild EJ 2nd, Grimes BA, Harrist RB (1985) Primary irritant contact dermatitis from synthetic pyrethroid insecticide exposure. Arch Toxicol 56: 288–294

Lisi P (1992) Sensitization risk of pyrethroid insecticides. Contact Dermatitis 26:349–350

349. Pyrethrosin

CAS Registry Number [28272–18–6]

Pyrethrosin is an allergen of Asteraceae–Compositae such as *Chrysanthemum cinerariifolium* Vis.

Suggested Reading

Mitchell JC, Dupuis G, Towers GHN (1972) Allergic contact dermatitis from pyrethrum (*Chrysanthemum* spp.). The roles of pyrethrosin, a sesquiterpene lactone, and of pyrethrin II. Br J Dermatol 86:568–573

Paulsen E, Andersen KE, Hausen BM (1993) Compositae dermatitis in a Danish dermatology department in one year (I). Results of routine patch testing with the sesquiterpene lactone mix supplemented with aimed patch testing with extracts and sesquiterpene lactones of Compositae plants. Contact Dermatitis 29:6–10

350. Pyridine

CAS Registry Number [110–86–1]

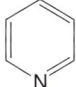

Pyridine (unsubstituted pyridine) and its derivative (substituted pyridines) are widely used in chemistry. Pyridine is a solvent used for many organic compounds and anhydrous metallic salt chemicals. Contained in Karl Fischer reagent, it induced contact dermatitis in a laboratory technician. No cross-sensitivity is observed between those different substances.

Suggested Reading

Knegt-Junk C, Geursen-Reitsma L, van Joost T (1993) Allergic contact dermatitis from pyridine in Karl Fischer reagent. Contact Dermatitis 28:252

351. Pyrithione

Pyrithione, Omadine

CAS Registry Number [1121–30–8]

Sodium Pyrithione, Sodium Omadine

CAS Registry Numbers [1121–30–8], [15922–78–8]

Zinc Pyrithione, Zinc Omadine

CAS Registry Number [13463–41–7] and more than 20 others

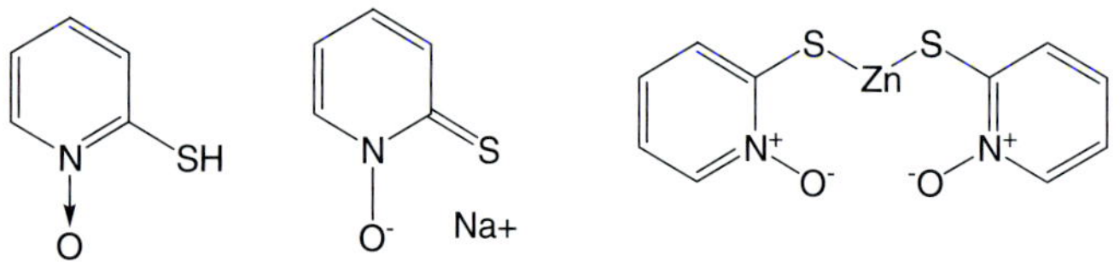

The sodium salt of N-hydroxy-2-pyridinethiones has germicidal activity against yeasts and fungi. Sodium omadine is a 40% aqueous solution of sodium pyrithione. It is used in the metallurgical industry as a component of water-based metalworking fluids, of aceto-polyvinyl lattices, water-based printer's ink, a lubricant for synthetic fibers and anti-dandruff shampoos.

Zinc pyrithione is widely used in anti-dandruff shampoos and is a classic allergen. Concomitant reactions are expected to both zinc and sodium pyrithione.

Suggested Reading

Le Coz CJ (2001) Allergic contact dermatitis from sodium pyrithione in metalworking fluid. Contact Dermatitis 45:58–59

Tosti A, Piraccini B, Brasile GP (1990) Occupational contact dermatitis due to sodium pyrithione. Contact Dermatitis 22:118–119

352. Pyrogallol

1,2,3-Benzenetriol, CI 76515, Pyrogallic Acid

CAS Registry Number [87–66–1]

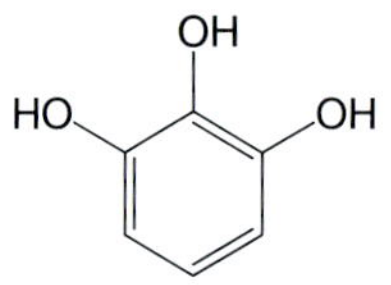

Pyrogallol belongs to the phenols group. It is an old photograph developer and a low sensitizer in hair dyes.

Suggested Reading

Frosch PJ, Burrows D, Camarasa JG, Dooms-Goossens A, Ducombs G, Lahti A, Menné T, Rycroft RJG, Shaw S, White IR, Wilkinson JD (1993) Allergic reactions to a hairdresser's series: results from 9 European centres. Contact Dermatitis 28:180–183

Guerra L, Tosti A, Bardazzi F, Pigatto P, Lisi P, Santucci B, Valsecchi R, Schena D, Angelini G, Serto-li A, Ayala F, Kokelj F (1992) Contact dermatitis in hairdressers: the Italian experience. Gruppo Italiano Ricerca Dermatiti da Contatto e Ambientali. Contact Dermatitis 26:101–107

353. PVP

Polyvinylpyrrolidone, Polyvidone, Povidone, 2-Pyrrolidinone, 1-Ethenyl-, Homopolymer

CAS Registry Number [9003–39–8]

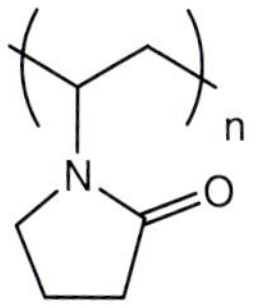

Polyvinylpyrrolidone is widely used as is in cosmetics such as hair care products, and in medical products. It acts as iodophor in iodine-polyvinylpyrrolidone. PVP is an irritant, and has been claimed as the allergen in some cases of dermatitis from iodine-polyvinylpyrrolidone (although iodine is more likely the hapten). It may cause type I contact urticaria or anaphylaxis.

Suggested Reading

Adachi A, Fukunaga A, Hayashi K, Kunisada M, Horikawa T (2003) Anaphylaxis to polyvinylpyr-rolidone after vaginal application of povidone-iodine. Contact Dermatitis 48:133–136

Ronnau AC, Wulferink M, Gleichmann E, Unver E, Ruzicka T, Krutmann J, Grewe M (2000) Anaph-ylaxis to polyvinylpyrrolidone in an analgesic preparation. Br J Dermatol 143:1055–1058

354. PVP/Eicosene Copolymer

Polyvinylpyrrolidone/Eicosene Copolymer

CAS Registry Numbers [28211–18–9], [77035–98–4]

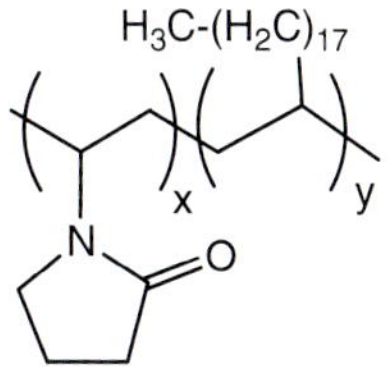

PVP/eicosene copolymer is the polymer of vinylpyrrolidone and of 1-eicosene, and one of the 11 PVP copolymers recorded in the International Nomenclature of Cosmetics Ingredients inventory system. This substance is utilized in cosmetics, in sunscreens to enhance their water resistance, and is an inert ingredient in pesticides. Contact sensitization to a close compound VP/eicosene copolymer was also reported.

Suggested Reading

Gallo R, dal Sacco D, Ghigliotti G (2004) Allergic contact dermatitis from VP/eisosene copolymer (Ganex® V-220) in an emollient cream. Contact Dermatitis 50:261

Le Coz CJ, Lefebvre C, Ludmann F, Grosshans E (2000) Polyvinylpyrrolidone (PVP)/eicosene co-polymer: an emerging cosmetic allergen. Contact Dermatitis 43:61–62

51

355. PVP/Hexadecene Copolymer

CAS Registry Number [32440–50–9]

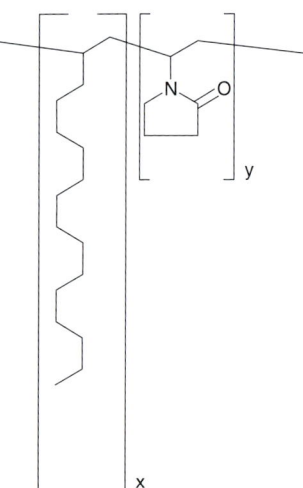

PVP/hexadecene copolymer, another PVP copolymer used for identical applications as PVP/eicosene copolymer, has been rarely implicated in contact dermatitis.

Suggested Reading

De Groot AC, Bruynzeel DP, Bos JD, van der Meeren HL, van Joost T, Jagtman BA, Weyland JW (1988) The allergens in cosmetics. Arch Dermatol 124:1525–1529
Scheman A, Cummins R (1998) Contact allergy to PVP/hexadecene copolymer. Contact Dermatitis 39:201

356. Quaternium-15

N-(3-Chloroallyl)Hexaminium Chloride,
Hexamethylenetetramine Chloroallyl Chloride, Dowicil 200

CAS Registry Numbers [4080–31–3], [103638–29–5], [60789–82–4]

Quaternium-15 is a quaternary ammonium compound, used as a broad-spectrum formaldehyde-releasing bactericide agent. It is contained as a preservative in cosmetics, toiletries, and aqueous products. Allergy is mainly due to formaldehyde and not to Quaternium-15 itself. Occupational case reports concerned hairdressers, a beautician, an engineer working on the maintenance of machinery in a chicken processing plant, and an employee carrying out photocopying tasks.

Suggested Reading

Finch TM, Prais L, Foulds IS (2001) Occupational allergic contact dermatitis from quaternium-15 in an electroencephalography skin preparation gel. Contact Dermatitis 44:44–45
Marren P, de Berker D, Dawber RP, Powell S (1991) Occupational contact dermatitis due to quaternium 15 presenting as nail dystrophy. Contact Dermatitis 25:253–255
O'Reilly FM, Murphy GM (1996) Occupational contact dermatitis in a beautician. Contact Dermatitis 35:47–48
Tosti A, Piraccini BM, Bardazzi F (1990) Occupational contact dermatitis due to quaternium 15. Contact Dermatitis 23:41–42
Zina AM, Fanan E, Bundino S (2000) Allergic contact dermatitis from formaldehyde and quaternium-15 in photocopier toner. Contact Dermatitis 43:241–242

357. Quaternium-22

CAS Registry Numbers [51812–80–7], [82970–95–4]

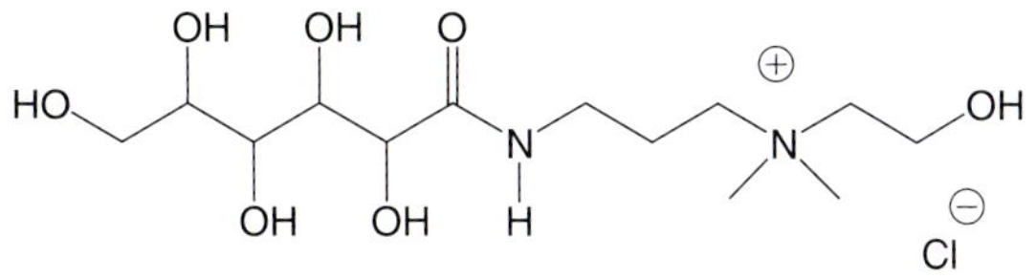

This quaternary ammonium compound, used as a film former and conditioning agent, was reported as a co-sensitizer in eyelid dermatitis due to shellac-based mascara.

Suggested Reading

Le Coz CJ, Leclere JM, Arnoult E, Raison-Peyron N, Pons-Guiraud A, Vigan M, Members of Revidal-GERDA (2002) Allergic contact dermatitis from shellac in mascara. Contact Dermatitis 46: 149–152

Scheman AJ (1998) Contact allergy to quaternium-22 and shellac in mascara. Contact Dermatitis 38:342–343

358. Ranitidine

CAS Registry Number [66357–35–5]

Ranitidine Hydrochloride

CAS Registry Number [66357–59–3]

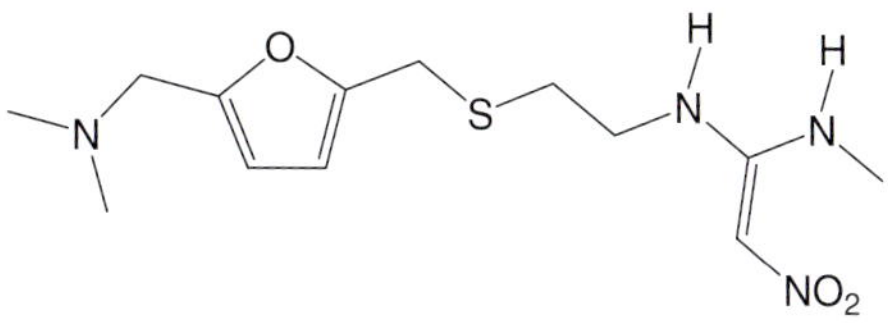

Ranitidine, an H2-receptor antagonist, can cause contact dermatitis within the pharmaceutical industry and in healthcare workers, or may induce systemic drug reactions in patients.

Suggested Reading

Martinez MB, Salvador JF, Aguilera GV, Mas IB, Ramirez JC (2003) Acute generalized exanthematous pustulosis induced by ranitidine hydrochloride. Contact Dermatitis 49:47

Romaguerra C, Grimalt F, Vilaplana J (1988) Epidemic of occupational contact dermatitis from ranitidine. Contact Dermatitis 18:177–178

359. Resorcinol

1,3-Benzendiol, CI 76505

CAS Registry Number [108–46–3]

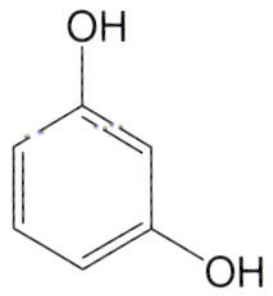

Resorcinol is used in hairdressing as a modifier (or a coupler) of the PPD group of dyes. It is the least frequent sensitizer in hairdressers. It is also used in resins, in skin treatment mixtures, and for tanning. Severe cases of dermatitis due to resorcinol contained in wart preparations have been reported.

Suggested Reading

Barbaud A, Modiano P, Cocciale M, Reichert S, Schmutz JL (1996) The topical application of resorcinol can provoke a systemic allergic reaction. Br J Dermatol 135:1014–1015

Frosch PJ, Burrows D, Camarasa JG, Dooms-Goossens A, Ducombs G, Lahti A, Menné T, Rycroft RJG, Shaw S, White IR, Wilkinson JD (1993) Allergic reactions to a hairdresser's series: results from 9 European centres. Contact Dermatitis 28:180–183

Tarvainen K (1995) Analysis of patients with allergic patch test reactions to a plastics and glue series. Contact Dermatitis 32:346–351

Vilaplana J, Romaguera C, Grimalt F (1991) Contact dermatitis from resorcinol in a hair dye. Contact Dermatitis 24:151–152

360. Silane

Monosilane

CAS Registry Number [7803–62–5] SiH_4

Various silane derivatives are used as bonding agents between glass and the resin used as a coating agent of glass filaments. Organosilanes have been implicated as sensitizers in workers at a glass filament manufactory.

Suggested Reading

Heino T, Haapa K, Manelius F (1996) Contact sensitization to organosilane solution in glass filament production. Contact Dermatitis 34:294

361. Sodium Bisulfite

Sodium Acid Sulfite, E222

CAS Registry Number [7631–90–5]

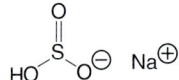

Sodium bisulfite is mainly used as an antioxidant in pharmaceutical products, as a disinfectant or bleach, and in the dye industry. The bisulfite of commerce consists chiefly of metabisulfite, and possesses the same properties as the true bisulfite. So, the allergen to be tested in products containing disulfite is the corresponding metabisulfite.

Suggested Reading

Budavari S, O'Neil MJ, Smith A, Heckelman PE, Kinneary JF (eds) (1996) The Merck Index, 12th edn. Merck, Whitehouse Station, N.J., USA

362. Sodium lauryl sulfate

SLS, Sodium Dodecyl Sulfate

CAS Registry Number [151–21–3]

This anionic detergent is widely used in cosmetics and in industry. As a skin irritant agent, SLS can be used in several dermatological applications. It is also a good indicator of excited skin during patch testing.

Suggested Reading

Geier J, Uter W, Pirker C, Frosch PJ (2003) Patch testing with the irritant sodium lauryl sulfate (SLS) is useful in interpreting weak reactions to contact allergens as allergic or irritant. Contact Dermatitis 48:99–107

363. Sodium Metabisulfite

Sodium Pyrosulfite, Disodium Disulfite, E223

CAS Registry Number [7681–57–4]

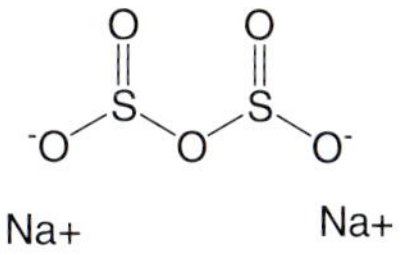

This agent is frequently used as a preservative in pharmaceutical products, in the bread-making industry as an antioxidant, and it can induce contact dermatitis. It can be used as a reducing agent in photography and caused dermatitis in a photographic technician, probably acting as an aggravating irritative factor. Sodium metabisulfite contains a certain amount of sodium sulfite and sodium sulfate.

Suggested Reading

Acciai MC, Brusi C, Francalanci Giorgini S, Sertoli A (1993) Allergic contact dermatitis in caterers. Contact Dermatitis 28:48

Jacobs MC, Rycroft RJG (1995) Contact dermatitis and asthma from sodium metabisulfite in a photographic technician. Contact Dermatitis 33:65–66

Riemersma WA, Schuttelaar ML, Coenraads PJ (2004) Type IV hypersensitivity to sodium metabisulfite in local anaesthetic. Contact Dermatitis 51:148

Vena GA, Foti C, Angelini G (1994) Sulfite contact allergy. Contact Dermatitis 31:172–175

364. Sodium Methyldithiocarbamate

Metham-Na, Carbathion, Sodium-*N*-Methyldithiocarbamate

CAS Registry Number [137–42–8]

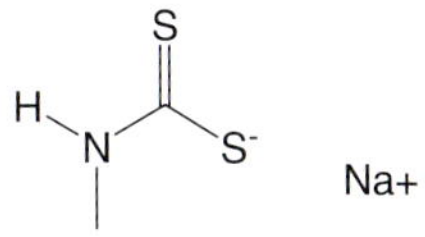

Metham-Na is a fungicide nematocide of the dithiocarbamate group. Sensitization occurs among agricultural workers.

Suggested Reading

Koch P (1996) Occupational allergic contact dermatitis and airborne contact dermatitis from 5 fungicides in a vineyard worker. Cross-reactions between fungicides of the dithiocarbamate group? Contact Dermatitis 34:324–329

Pambor M, Bloch Y (1985) Dimethoat und Dithiocarmabat als berufliche Kontaktallergene bei einer Agrotechnikerin. Dermat Monatsschr 171:401–405

Schubert H (1978) Contact dermatitis to sodium-*N*-methyldithiocarbamate. Contact Dermatitis 4:370–371

Wolf F, Jung HD (1970) Akute Kontaktdermatitiden nach Umgang mit Nematin. Z Ges Hyg 16:423–426

365. Sodium Sulfite

E225

CAS Registry Number [7757–83–7]]

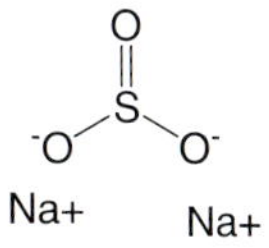

Sodium sulfite is mainly used in photographic developers, for fixing prints, bleaching textile fibers, as a reducer in manufacturing dyes, as a remover of Cl in bleached textiles and paper, and as a preservative in the food industry for meat, egg yolks, and so on.

Suggested Reading
Budavari S, O'Neil MJ, Smith A, Heckelman PE, Kinneary JF (eds) (1996) The Merck Index, 12th
    edn. Merck, Whitehouse Station, N.J., USA
Vena GA, Foti C, Angelini G (1994) Sulfite contact allergy. Contact Dermatitis 31:172–175

366. Solvent Red 23

Sudan III, CI 26100, D and C Red No. 17

CAS Registry Number [85–86–9]

Solvent Red 23 is an oil-soluble red azo-dye used in cosmetic products in Japan. Cases were reported in hairdressers, who also reacted to PPD (the molecule is likely to be hydrolyzed into PPD) and to *p*-aminoazobenzene. One case of contact dermatitis was reported in the metal industry.

Suggested Reading
Fregert S (1967) Allergic contact dermatitis due to fumes from burning alcohol containing an azo-
    dye. Contact Dermatitis Newslett 1:11
Matsunaga K, Hayakawa R, Yoshimura K, Okada J (1990) Patch-test-positive reactions to Solvent
    Red 23 in hairdressers. Contact Dermatitis 23:266

367. Sorbitan Sesquioleate

Sorbitan 9-Octadecenoate (2:3), Arlacel 83, Anhydrohexitol Sesquioleate

CAS Registry Number [8007–43–0], [37318–79–9]

Sorbitan sesquioleate is a mixture of mono and diesters of oleic acid and extol anhydrides derived from sorbitol. It is used as a surfactant and an emulsifier in cosmetics. It acts sometimes as a contact allergen, particularly in leg ulcer patients. It is also responsible for false-positive patch test reactions to haptens, with which some allergen providers emulgated, such as parabens mix, fragrance mix, Amerchol L101, and ethylene-urea /melamine formaldehyde.

Suggested Reading
Orton DI, Shaw S (2001) Sorbitan sesquioleate as an allergen. Contact Dermatitis 44:190–191
Pasche-Koo F, Piletta PA, Hunziker N, Hauser C (1994) High sensitization rate to emulsifiers in pa-
    tients with chronic leg ulcers. Contact Dermatitis 31:226–228

368. Spectinomycin

CAS Registry Number [1695–77–8]

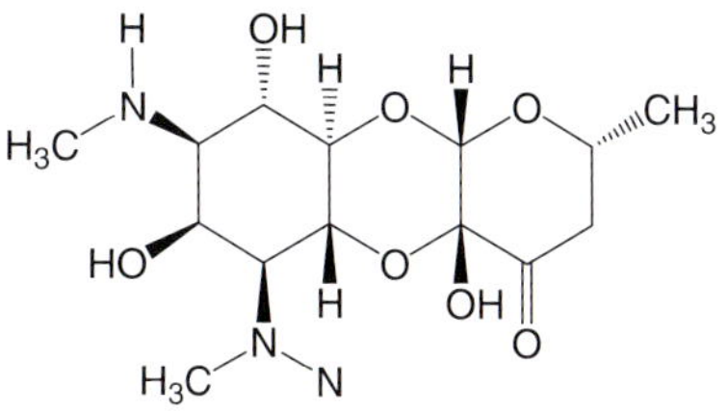

Spectinomycin is an aminocyclitol antibiotic. It is used in human medicine against *Neisseria gonorrhoeae* and in veterinary medicine, especially for poultry, pigs, and cattle. Cases of dermatitis have been reported in veterinary practice.

Suggested Reading

Dal Monte A, Laffi G, Mancini G (1994) Occupational contact dermatitis due to spectinomycin. Contact Dermatitis 31:204–205

Vilaplana J, Romaguera C, Grimalt F (1991) Contact dermatitis from lincomycin and spectinomycin in chicken vaccinators. Contact Dermatitis 24:225–226

369. Tetrabenzylthiuram Disulfide

TBzTD

CAS Registry Number [10591–85–2]

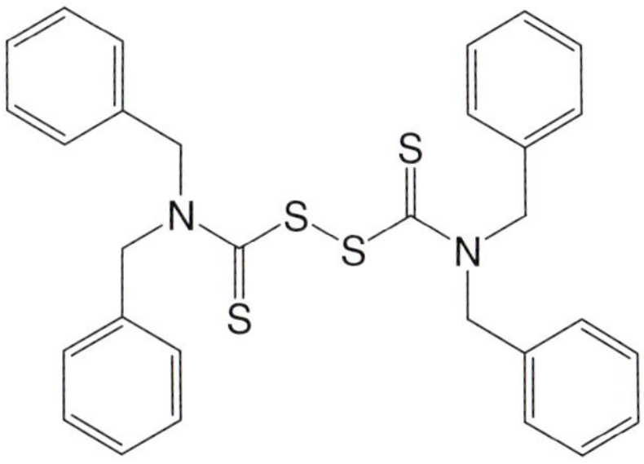

TBzTD is a rubber vulcanization accelerator.

Suggested Reading

Le Coz CJ (2004) Fiche d'éviction en cas d'hypersensibilité au thiuram mix. Ann Dermatol Venereol 131:1012–1014

370. Tetrabutylthiuram Disulfide

TBTD

CAS [1634–02–2]

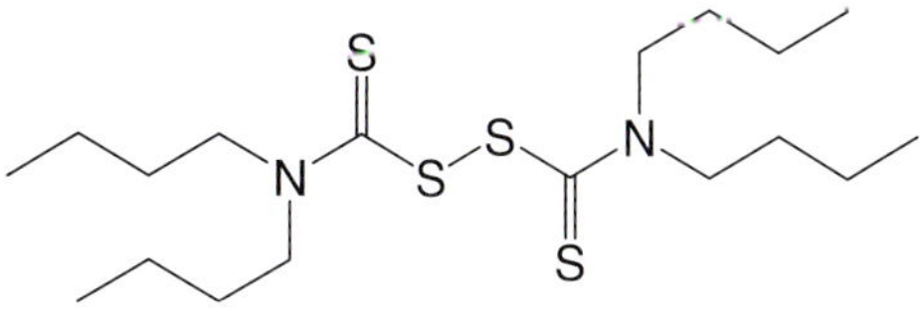

TBTD is a rubber vulcanization accelerator.

Suggested Reading

Le Coz CJ (2004) Fiche d'éviction en cas d'hypersensibilité au thiuram mix. Ann Dermatol Venereol 131:1012–1014

371. Tetrabutylthiuram Monosulfide

TBTM

CAS Registry Number [97–74–5]

TBTM is a rubber vulcanization accelerator.

Suggested Reading

Le Coz CJ (2004) Fiche d'éviction en cas d'hypersensibilité au thiuram mix. Ann Dermatol Venereol 131:1012–1014

372. Tetrachloroacetophenone

CAS Registry Number [39751–78–5]

Tetrachloroacetophone was combined with triethyl phosphate to form an organophosphate insecticide. It induced contact dermatitis in a process operator in an insecticide plant.

Suggested Reading

Van Joost T, Wiemer GR (1991) Contact dermatitis from tetrachloroacetophenone (TCAP) in an insecticide plant. Contact Dermatitis 25:66–67

373. Tetraethylthiuram Disulfide

Disulfiram, TETD, Antabuse, Esperal®

CAS Registry Number [97–77–8]

TETD is a rubber accelerator of the thiuram group, contained in "thiuram mix." It can cross-react with other thiurams, especially TMTD. TETD is used to aid those trying to break their dependence on alcohol. The disulfiram-alcohol reaction is not allergic but due to the accumulation of toxic levels of acetaldehyde. The implanted drug can, however, lead to local or generalized dermatitis, for example ingested disulfiram, mainly in previously rubber-sensitized patients. As an adjunctive treatment of alcoholism, it caused occupational contact dermatitis in a nurse.

Suggested Reading

Condé-Salazar L, Del-Rio E, Guimaraens D, Gonzalez Domingo A (1993) Type IV allergy to rubber additives: a 10-year study of 686 cases. J Am Acad Dermatol 29:176–180

Kiec-Swierczynska M, Krecisz B, Fabicka B (2000) Systemic contact dermatitis from implanted disulfiram. Contact Dermatitis 43(4):246–247

Le Coz CJ (2004) Fiche d'éviction en cas d'hypersensibilité au thiuram mix. Ann Dermatol Venereol 131:1012–1014

Mathelier-Fusade P, Leynadier F (1994) Occupational allergic contact reaction to disulfiram. Contact Dermatitis 31:121–122

Webb PK, Bibbs SC (1979) Disulfiram hypersensitivity and rubber contact dermatitis. JAMP 241:2061

374. Tetraethylthiuram Monosulfide

Sulfiram, TETM, Tetraethylthiodicarbonic Diamide

CAS Registry Number [95–05–6]

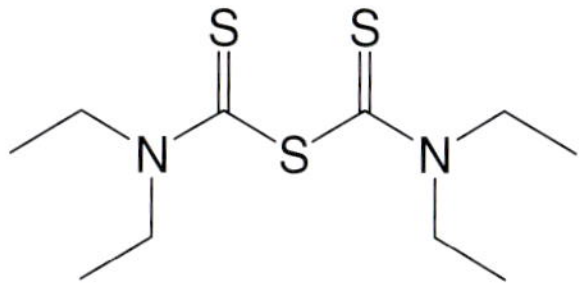

This rubber vulcanization accelerator is also used as an ectoparasiticide against *Sarcoptes scabiei*, louses or in veterinary medicine.

Suggested Reading

Le Coz CJ (2004) Fiche d'éviction en cas d'hypersensibilité au thiuram mix. Ann Dermatol Venereol 131:1012–1014

375. Tetraisobutylthiuram Disulfide

TITD, Thioperoxydicarbonic Diamide, Tetrakis (2-Methylpropyl)

CAS Registry Number [137–26–8]

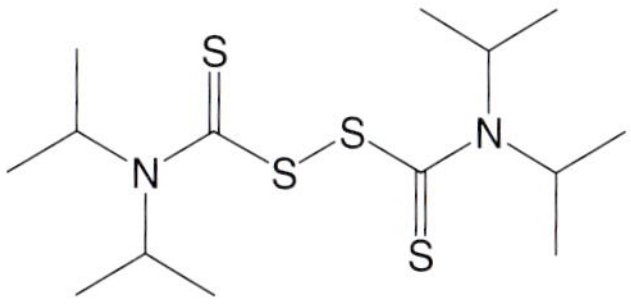

TITD is a rubber vulcanization accelerator.

Suggested Reading

Le Coz CJ (2004) Fiche d'éviction en cas d'hypersensibilité au thiuram mix. Ann Dermatol Venereol 131:1012–1014

376. Tetramethylthiuram Disulfide

Thiram, TMTD

CAS Registry Number [137–26–8]

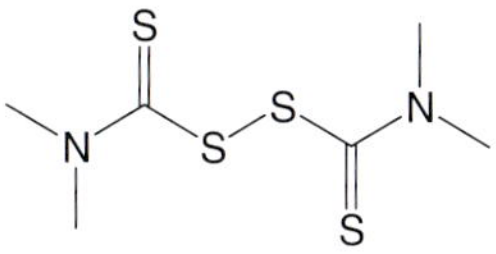

This rubber chemical, accelerator of vulcanization, represents the most commonly positive allergen contained in "thiuram mix." The most frequent occupational categories are the metal industry, homemakers, health services and laboratories, the building industry, and shoemakers. It is also widely used as a fungicide, belonging to the dithiocarbamate group of carrots, bulbs, and woods, and as an insecticide. Thiram is the agricultural name for thiuram.

Suggested Reading

Condé-Salazar L, Guimaraens D, Villegas C, Romero A, Gonzalez MA (1995) Occupational allergic contact dermatitis in construction workers. Contact Dermatitis 35:226–230

Kiec-Swierczynska M (1995) Occupational sensitivity to rubber. Contact Dermatitis 32:171–172

Le Coz CJ (2004) Fiche d'éviction en cas d'hypersensibilité au thiuram mix. Ann Dermatol Venereol 131:1012–1014

Mancuso G, Reggiani M, Berdondini RM (1996) Occupational dermatitis in shoemakers. Contact Dermatitis 34:17–22

Sharma VK, Kaur S (1990) Contact sensitization by pesticides in farmers. Contact Dermatitis 23:77–80

377. Tetramethylthiuram Monosulfide

TMTM

CAS Registry Number [97–74–5]

This rubber accelerator is contained in "thiuram mix." The most frequent occupational categories are the metal industry, homemakers, health services and laboratories, and the building industry.

Suggested Reading

Condé-Salazar L, Del-Rio E, Guimaraens D, Gonzalez Domingo A (1993) Type IV allergy to rubber additives: a 10-year study of 686 cases. J Am Acad Dermatol 29:176–180

Condé-Salazar L, Guimaraens D, Villegas C, Romero A, Gonzalez MA (1995) Occupational allergic contact dermatitis in construction workers. Contact Dermatitis 35:226–230

Le Coz CJ (2004) Fiche d'éviction en cas d'hypersensibilité au thiuram mix. Ann Dermatol Venereol 131:1012–1014

Von Hintzenstern J, Heese A, Koch HU, Peters KP, Hornstein OP (1991) Frequency, spectrum and occupational relevance of type IV allergies to rubber chemicals. Contact Dermatitis 24:244–252

378. Tetrazepam

CAS Registry Number [10379–14–3]

Tetrazepam is a benzodiazepine compound used systemically as a myorelaxant. It may induce skin rashes such as maculo-papular eruption, Stevens–Johnson syndrome or photosensitivity. Occupational sensitization can be observed in pharmaceutical plants. Sensitization generally does not concern other benzodiazepines (personal observations).

Suggested Reading

Barbaud A, Trechot P, Reichert-Penetrat S, Granel F, Schmutz JL (2001) The usefulness of patch testing on the previously most severely affected site in a cutaneous adverse drug reaction to tetrazepam. Contact Dermatitis 44:259–260

Choquet-Kastylevsky G, Testud F, Chalmet P, Lecuyer-Kudela S, Descotes J (2001) Occupational contact allergy to tetrazepam. Contact Dermatitis 44:372

379. Thebaine

CAS Registry Number [115–37–7]

The naturally occurring opiate alkaloid thebaine is present in concentrated poppy straw, and in small concentrations in codeine alkaloid. It is used in the manufacture of other opiate pharmaceuticals, such as buprenorphine and morphine, and caused contact dermatitis in a laboratory worker at an opiates manufacturing pharmaceutical company, also sensitive to codeine.

Suggested Reading
Waclawski ER, Aldridge R (1995) Occupational dermatitis from thebaine and codeine. Contact Dermatitis 33:51

380. Thiabendazole

CAS Registry Number [148–79–8]

This fungicide and vermifuge agent is widely used in agriculture (for example, for citrus fruits), and in medical and veterinary practice as an anthelmintic drug.

Suggested Reading
Izu R, Aguirre A, Goicoechea A, Gardeazabal J, Diaz Perez JL (1993) Photoaggravated allergic contact dermatitis due to topical thiabendazole. Contact Dermatitis 28:243–244
Mancuso G, Staffa M, Errani A, Berdondini RM, Fabri P (1990) Occupational dermatitis in animal feed mill workers. Contact Dermatitis 22:37–41

381. Thimerosal

Thiomersal, Thiomersalate, Merthiolate, Mercurothiolic Acid Sodium Salt

CAS Registry Number [54–64–8]

Thiomersal is an organic mercury salt prepared by reacting ethylmercuric chloride (or ethylmercuric hydroxide) with thiosalicylic acid. It is still used as a disinfectant and a preservative agent, but less commonly than previously, especially in contact lens fluids, eyedrops, and vaccines. The ethylmercuric moiety is the major allergenic determinant, sometimes associated with mercury sensitivity. Thiomersal is an indicator of photosensitivity to piroxicam, through its thiosalicylic moiety.

Suggested Reading
Arévalo A, Blancas R, Ancona A (1995) Occupational contact dermatitis from piroxicam. Am J Contact Dermat 6:113–114
De Groot AC, van Wijnen WG, van Wijnen-Vos M (1990) Occupational contact dermatitis of the eyelids, without ocular involvement, from thimerosal in contact lens fluid. Contact Dermatitis 23:195
Rudzki E, Rebandel P, Grzywa Z, Pomorski Z, Jakiminska B, Zawisza E (1982) Occupational dermatitis in veterinarians. Contact Dermatitis 8:72–73

382. Thiourea

Thiocarbamide

CAS Registry Number [62–56–6]

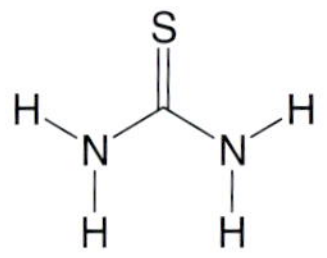

Thiourea is used as a cleaner agent for silver and copper, and as an antioxidant in diazo copy paper. It can induce (photo-)contact dermatitis.

Suggested Reading
Dooms-Goossens A, Debusschère K, Morren M, Roelandts R, Coopman S (1988) Silver polish: another source of contact dermatitis reactions to thiourea. Contact Dermatitis 19:133–135
Geier J, Fuchs T (1993) Contact allergy due to 4-*N,N*-dimethylaminobenzene diazonium chloride and thiourea in diazo copy paper. Contact Dermatitis 28:304–305
Kanerva L, Estlander T, Jolanki R (1994) Occupational allergic contact dermatitis caused by thiourea compounds. Contact Dermatitis 31:242–248

51

383. Thymoquinone

CAS Registry Number [490–91–5]

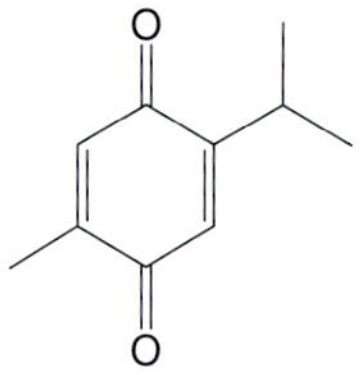

Thymoquinone is an allergen in different cedar species, Cupressaceae family, such as incense cedar (*Calocedrus decurrens* Florin) used for pencils, chests or toys, and western cedar (*Thuja plicata* Donn.) as used for hard realizations such as construction or boats. See also Chap. 41, Plants and Plant Products.

Suggested Reading
Hausen BM (2000) Woods. In: Kanerva L, Elsner P, Wahlberg JE, Maibach HI (eds) Handbook of occupational dermatology. Springer, Berlin Heidelberg New York, pp 771–780
Lamminpää A, Estlander T, Jolanki R, Kanerva L (1996) Occupational allergic contact dermatitis caused by decorative plants. Contact Dermatitis 34:330–335

384. Timolol

CAS Registry Number [26839–75–8]

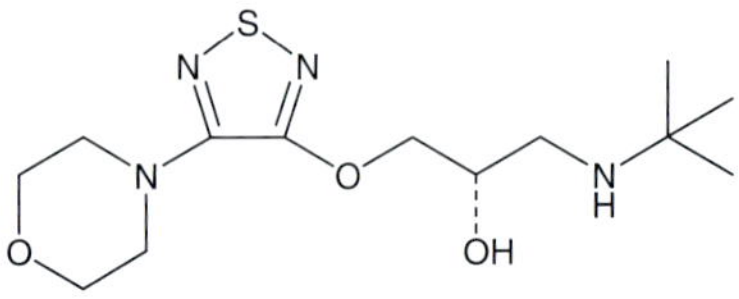

Timolol was implicated in allergic contact dermatitis due to beta-blocker agents in eyedrops.

Suggested Reading
Giordano-Labadie F, Lepoittevin JP, Calix I, Bazex J (1997) Allergie de contact aux â-bloqueurs des collyres: allergie croisée? Ann Dermatol Venereol 124:322–324

385. Tixocortol Pivalate

Tixocortol 21-Pivalate, Tixocortol 21-Trimethylacetate

CAS Registry Number [55560–96–8]

Tixocortol 21-pivalate is a 21-ester of tixocortol, widely used in topical treatments. It can induce severe allergic contact dermatitis. This corticosteroid is a marker of the allergenic A group that includes molecules without major substitution on the D cycle (no C_{16} methylation, no C_{17} side chain). A short-chain C_{21} ester is possible. Molecules are cloprednol, cortisone, fludrocortisone, fluorometholone, hydrocortisone, methylprednisolone, methylprednisone, prednisolone, prednisone, tixocortol, and their C_{21} esters (acetate, caproate or hexanoate, phosphate, pivalate or trimethylacetate, succinate or hemisuccinate, m-sulfobenzoate).

Suggested Reading

Le Coz CJ (2002) Fiche d'éviction en cas d'hypersensibilité au pivalate de tixocortol. Ann Dermatol Venereol 129:348–349

Lepoittevin JP, Drieghe J, Dooms-Goossens A (1995) Studies in patients with corticosteroid contact allergy. Understanding cross-reactivity among different steroids. Arch Dermatol 131:31–37

386. Tocopherol, Tocopheryl Acetate (DL-, D-)

Vitamin E

CAS Registry Number [1406–66–2,]

Vitamin E Acetate DL, Vitamin E Acetate D

CAS Registry Number [7695–91–2], CAS Registry Number [58–95–7]

Tocopherol and tocopheryl acetate are used mainly as antioxidants. Tocopheryl acetate, an ester of tocopherol (vitamin E), can induce allergic contact dermatitis.

Suggested Reading

De Groot AC, Berretty PJ, van Ginkel CJ, den Hengst CW, van Ulsen J, Weyland JW (1991) Allergic contact dermatitis from tocopheryl acetate in cosmetic creams. Contact Dermatitis 25:302–304

Matsumura T, Nakada T, Iijima M (2004) Widespread contact dermatitis from tocopherol acetate. Contact Dermatitis 51:211–212

387. Toluene-2,5-Diamine

p-Toluylenediamine, *p*-Toluenediamine

CAS Registry Number [95–70–5]

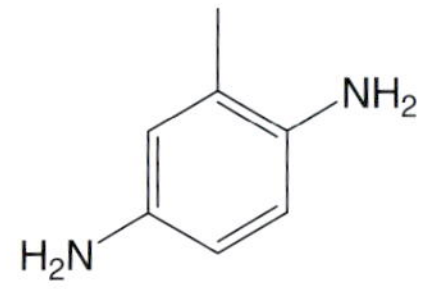

Toluene-2,5-diamine is a permanent hair dye involved in contact dermatitis in hairdressers and consumers. It does not cross-react with PPD, but co-sensitization is frequent.

Suggested Reading

Frosch PJ, Burrows D, Camarasa JG, Dooms-Goossens A, Ducombs G, Lahti A, Menné T, Rycroft RJG, Shaw S, White IR, Wilkinson JD (1993) Allergic reactions to a hairdresser's series: results from 9 European centres. Contact Dermatitis 28:180–183

Guerra L, Tosti A, Bardazzi F, Pigatto P, Lisi P, Santucci B, Valsecchi R, Schena D, Angelini G, Sertoli A, Ayala F, Kokelj F (1992) Contact dermatitis in hairdressers: the Italian experience. Gruppo Italiano Ricerca Dermatiti da Contatto e Ambientali. Contact Dermatitis 26:101–107

Le Coz CJ, Lefebvre C, Keller F, Grosshans E (2000) Allergic contact dermatitis caused by skin painting (pseudotattooing) with black henna, a mixture of henna and *p*-phenylenediamine and its derivatives. Arch Dermatol 136:1515–1517

51

388. Toluene Diisocyanate

Toluene Diisocyanate (Mixture)

CAS Registry Number [26471–62–5]

Toluene 2,4-Diisocyanate

CAS Registry Number [584–84–9]

Toluene 2,6-Diisocyanate

CAS Registry Number [91–08–7]

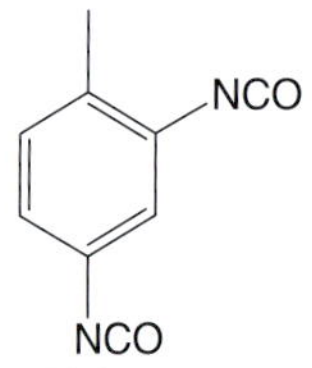

2,4-TDI 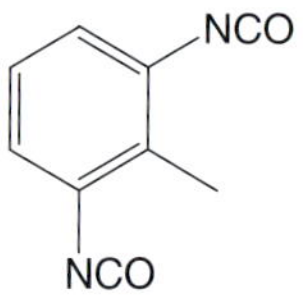   2,6-TDI

Toluene diisocyanate is a mixture of 2,4-TDI and 2,6-TDI. It is used in the manufacture of various polyurethane products: elastic and rigid foams, paints, lacquers, adhesives, binding agents, synthetics rubbers, and elastomeric fibers.

Suggested Reading

Estlander T, Keskinen H, Jolanki R, Kanerva L (1992) Occupational dermatitis from exposure to polyurethane chemicals. Contact Dermatitis 27:161–165

Le Coz CJ, El Aboubi S, Ball C (1999) Active sensitization to toluene di-isocyanate. Contact Dermatitis 41:104–105

389. Tosyl Chloride

p-Toluene Sulfonyl Chloride, *p*-Toluene Sulfochloride

CAS Registry Number [98–59–9].

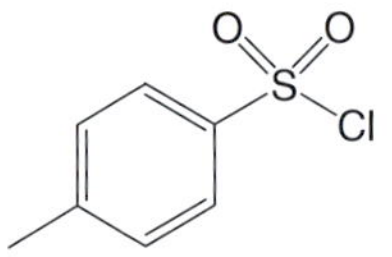

Tosyl chloride is used mainly in the preparation of chemical derivatives in the pharmaceutical, plastics, and organic chemical industries.

Suggested Reading

Watsky KL, Reynolds K, Berube D, Bayer FJ (1993) Occupational contact dermatitis from tosyl chloride in a chemist. Contact Dermatitis 29:211–212

390. Triacetin

Glyceryl Triacetate

CAS Registry Number [102–76–1]

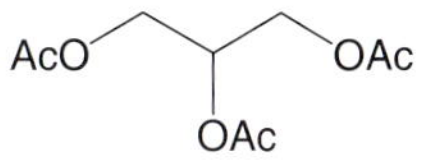

Triacetin is a component of cigarette filters, which induced a contact dermatitis in a worker at a cigarette manufactory.

Suggested Reading
Unna PJ, Schulz KH (1963) Allergisches Kontaktekzem durch Triacetin. Hautarzt 14:423–425

391. Tributyltin Oxide

CAS Registry Number [56–35–9]

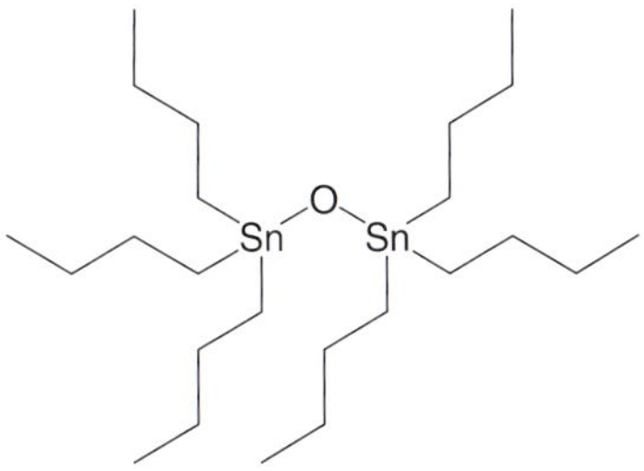

Tributyl tin oxide is used as an antifouling and biocide agent against fungi, algae, and bacteria, particularly in paints. Sometimes used in chemistry, tributyltin oxide is a strong irritant.

Suggested Reading
Goh CL (1985) Irritant dermatitis from tri-*N*-butyl tin oxide in paint. Contact Dermatitis 12:161–163
Grace CT, Ng SK, Cheong LL (1991) Recurrent irritant contact dermatitis due to tributyltin oxide on work clothes. Contact Dermatitis 25:250–251

392. Trichloroethane

1,1,1-Trichloroethane, Methylchloroform

CAS Registry Numbers [71–55–6], [25323–89–1]

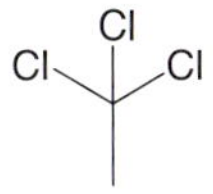

Trichloroethane is a solvent that has wide applications in industry, such as for cold type metal cleaning, and in cleaning plastic molds. It is mainly an irritant but can also provoke allergic contact dermatitis.

Suggested Reading
Mallon J, Tek Chu M, Maibach HI (2001) Occupational allergic contact dermatitis from methyl chloroform (1,1,1-trichloroethane)? Contact Dermatitis 45:107

393. Trichloroethylene

Trilene, Triclene, Trethylene

CAS Registry Number [79–01–6]

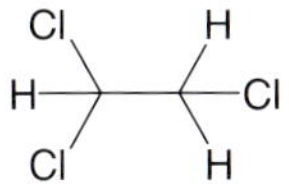

Trichloroethylene is a chlorinated hydrocarbon used as a detergent or solvent for metals, oils, resins, sulfur and as general degreasing agent. It can cause irritant contact dermatitis, generalized exanthema, Stevens–Johnson-like syndrome, pustular or bullous eruption, scleroderma, as well as neurological and hepatic disorders.

Suggested Reading
Goon AT, Lee LT, Tay YK, Yosipovitch G, Ng SK, Giam YC (2001) A case of trichloroethylene hyper-
    sensitivity syndrome. Arch Dermatol 137:274–276
Puerschel WC, Odia SG, Rakoski J, Ring J (1996) Trichloroethylene and concomitant contact der-
    matitis in an art painter. Contact Dermatitis 34:430–431

394. Triethanolamine

Trolamine

CAS Registry Number [102–71–6]

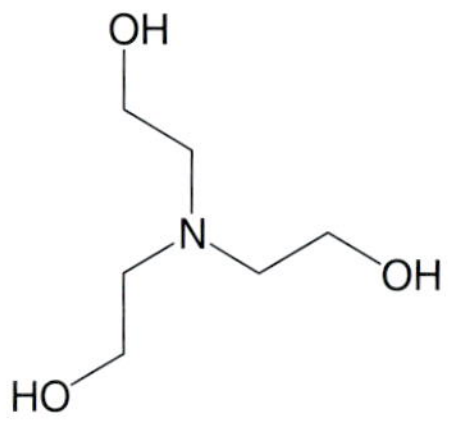

51

This emulsifying agent can be contained in many products such as cosmetics, topical medicines, metalworking cutting fluids, and color film developers. Traces may
exist in other ethanolamines such as mono- and diethanolamine. Contact allergy
seems to be rarer than previously thought.

Suggested Reading
Blum A, Lischka G (1997) Allergic contact dermatitis from mono-, di- and triethanolamine. Con-
    tact Dermatitis 36:166
Le Coz CJ, Scrivener Y, Santinelli F, Heid E (1998) Sensibilisation de contact au cours des ulcères de
    jambe. Ann Dermatol Venereol 125:694–699
Scheman AJ, Katta R (1997) Photographic allergens: an update. Contact Dermatitis 37:130

395. Triethylenetetramine

CAS Registry Number [112–24–3]

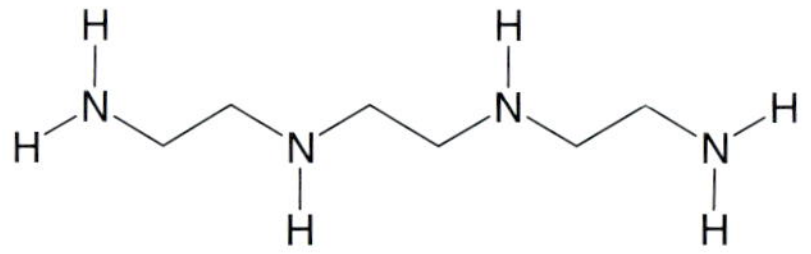

Triethylenetetramine is used as an amine hardener in epoxy resins of the bisphenol A
type. Cross-sensitivity is possible with diethylenetriamine and diethylenediamine.

Suggested Reading
Jolanki R, Kanerva L, Estlander T, Tarvainen K, Keskinen H, Henriks-Eckerman ML (1990) Occu-
    pational dermatoses from epoxy resin compounds. Contact Dermatitis 23:172–183

396. Triforine

Saprol®, 1,4-bis(2,2,2-Trichloro-1-Formamidoethyl)Piperazine

CAS Registry Number [26644–46–2]

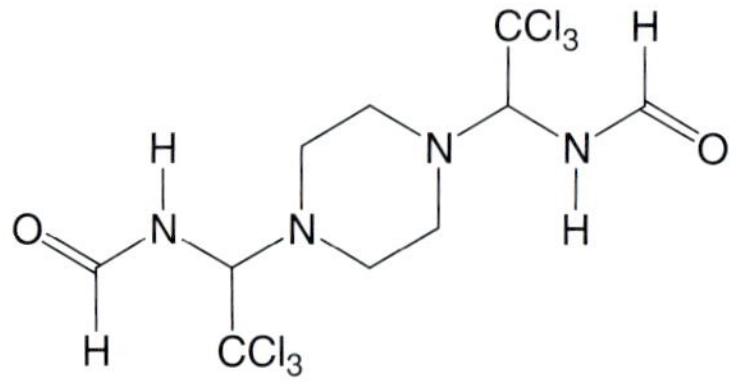

This pesticide is widely used in flower growing. Cross-reactions are expected to
dichlorvos.

Suggested Reading
Ueda A, Aoyama K, Manda F, Ueda T, Kawahara Y (1994) Delayed-type allergenicity of triforine
    (Saprol®). Contact Dermatitis 31:140–145

397. Triglycidyl Isocyanurate

1,3,5-Triglycidyl-*s*-Triazinetrione

CAS Registry Number [2451–62–9]

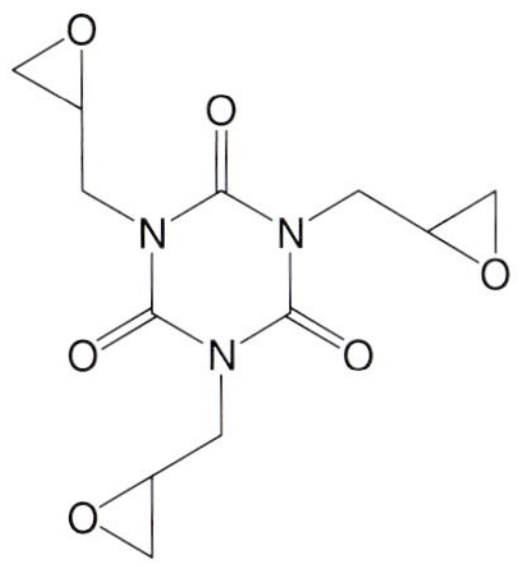

Triglycidyl isocyanurate is a triazine epoxy compound used as a resin hardener in polyester powder paints, in the plastics industry, resin molding systems, inks, and adhesives. Occupational contact dermatitis can occur in people producing this chemical, in those producing the powder coat paint, and in sprayers. Respiratory symptoms have been observed.

Suggested Reading

Erikstam U, Bruze M, Goossens A (2001) Degradation of triglycidyl isocyanurate as a cause of false-negative patch test reaction. Contact Dermatitis 44:13–17

Foulds IS, Koh D (1992) Allergic contact dermatitis from resin hardeners during the manufacture of thermosetting coating paints. Contact Dermatitis 26:87–90

McFadden JP, Rycroft RJG (1993) Occupational contact dermatitis from triglycidyl isocyanurate in a powder paint sprayer. Contact Dermatitis 28:251

Munro CS, Lawrence CM (1992) Occupational contact dermatitis from triglycidyl isocyanurate in a powder paint factory. Contact Dermatitis 26:59

398. *N*-[3-(Trimethoxysilyl)Propyl]-*N′*-(Vinylbenzyl)Ethylenediamine Monohydrochloride

1,2-Ethanediamine, *N*-[(Ethenylphenyl)Methyl]-*N′*-[3-(Trimethoxysilyl)Propyl]-, Monohydrochloride

CAS Registry Number [34937–00–3]

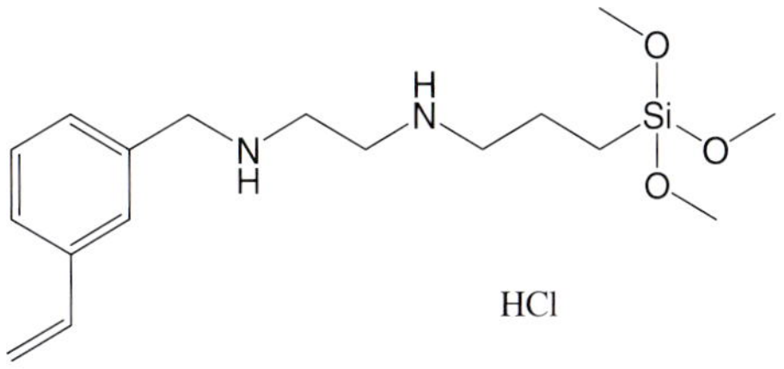

HCl

This amine-functional methoxysilane silane compound, referenced as vinylbenzyl-aminoethyl aminopropyltrimethoxysilane, was implicated in the production of glass filaments.

Suggested Reading

Heino T, Haapa K, Manelius F (1996) Contact sensitization to organosilane solution in glass filament production. Contact Dermatitis 34:294

Toffoletto F, Cortona G, Feltrin G, Baj A, Goggi E, Cecchetti R (1994) Occupational contact dermatitis from amine-functional methoxysilane in continuous-glass-filament production. Contact Dermatitis 31:320–321

399. *N*-(3-Trimethoxysilylpropyl)-Ethylenediamine

Z 6020

CAS Registry Number [1760–24–3]

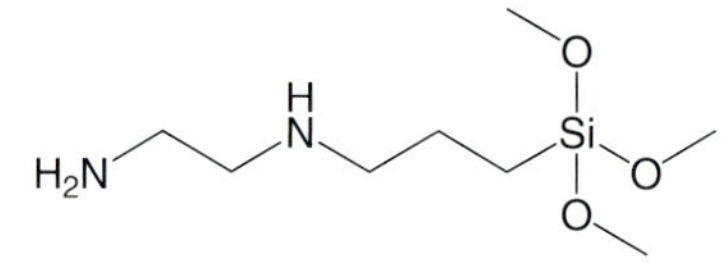

This amine-functional methoxysilane, referenced as aminoethyl aminopropyltrimethoxysilane, was implicated in the production of glass filaments.

Suggested Reading
Heino T, Haapa K, Manelius F (1996) Contact sensitization to organosilane solution in glass filament production. Contact Dermatitis 34:294

400. 2,4,6-Trimethylol Phenol

51

CAS Registry Number [2937–61–3]

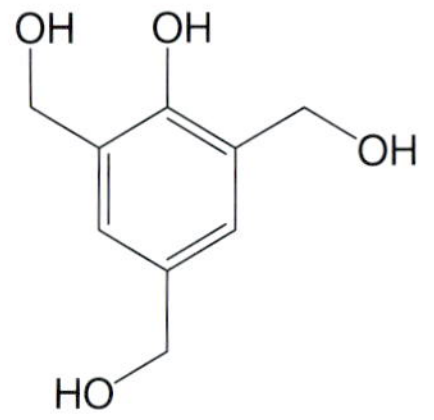

Trimethylolphenol is an allergen in resins based on phenol and formaldehyde. Cross-reactivity is possible with other phenol-derivative molecules.

Suggested Reading
Bruze M, Zimerson E (1997) Cross-reaction patterns in patients with contact allergy to simple methylol phenols. Contact Dermatitis 37:82–86
Bruze M, Fregert S, Zimerson E (1985) Contact allergy to phenol-formaldehyde resins. Contact Dermatitis 12:81–86

401. Trimethylthiourea

CAS Registry Number [2489–77–2]

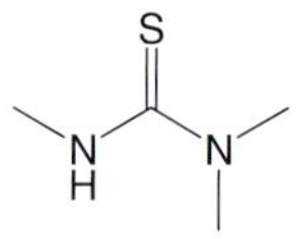

Trimethylthiourea is a thiourea derivative used for polychloroprene (neoprene) rubber vulcanization, for example. Patients sensitized to ethylbutyl thiourea can also react to trimethylthiourea.

Suggested Reading
Kanerva L, Estlander T, Jolanki R (1994) Occupational allergic contact dermatitis caused by thiourea compounds. Contact Dermatitis 31:242–248

402. Tulipalin A and Tulipalin B

α-Methylene-γ-Butyrolactone and β-Hydroxy-α-Methylene-γ-Butyrolactone

CAS Registry Number [547–65–9] and CAS Registry Number [38965–80–9]

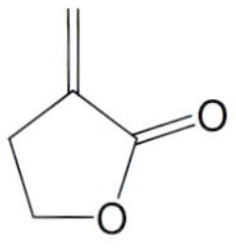

Tulipalin A 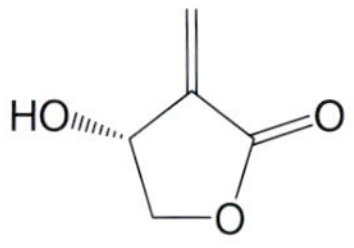   Tulipalin B

Tulipalin A is the unsubstituted α-methylene-γ-butyrolactone contained in the sap of damaged tulips (Liliaceae family) and Alstroemeria (Alstroemeriaceae family). Tulipalin B, due to hydrolysis of tuliposide B, seems to have a weak sensitizing capacity.

Suggested Reading

Bruynzeel DP (1997) Bulb dermatitis. Dermatological problems in the flower bulb industries. Contact Dermatitis 37:70–77

Gette MT, Marks JE (1990) Tulip fingers. Arch Dermatol 126:203–205

403. Tuliposide A

CAS Registry Number [19870–30–5]

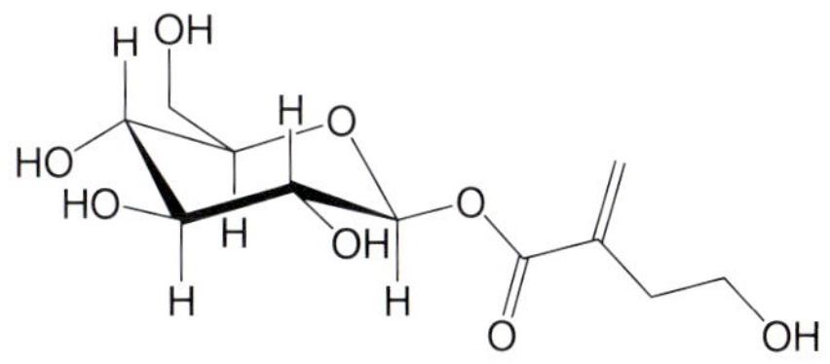

Tuliposide A is a glucoside prohapten contained in tulip bulbs and in Alstroemeria (*Tulipa* spp.; *Alstroemeria* spp.; *Lilium* spp.). It is rapidly hydrolyzed to tulipalin A and represents a common occupational problem among workers in the European tulip industry. Tuliposide can be present as 1-tuliposide A, but is more frequently identified as 6-tuliposide A.

Suggested Reading

Christensen LP, Kristiansen K (1995) A simple HPLC method for the isolation and quantification of the allergens tuliposide A and tulipalin A in *Alstroemeria*. Contact Dermatitis 32:199–203

Gette MT, Marks JE (1990) Tulip fingers. Arch Dermatol 126:203–205

Lamminpää A, Estlander T, Jolanki R, Kanerva L (1996) Occupational allergic contact dermatitis caused by decorative plants. Contact Dermatitis 34:330–335

404. Tylosin

CAS Registry Number [1401–69–0]

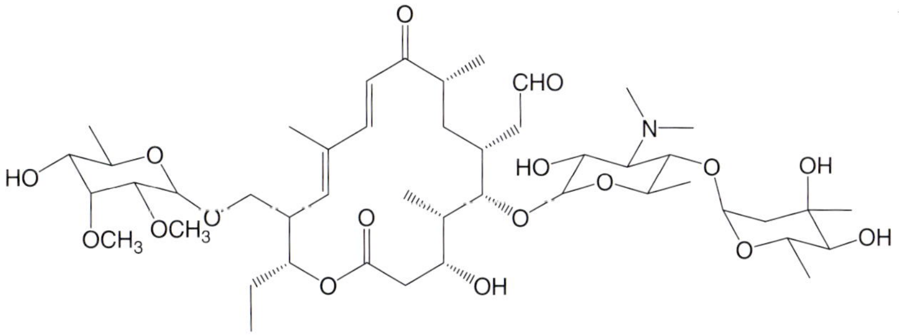

Tylosin is a macrolid antibiotic used in veterinary medicine. Occupational exposure concerns farmers, breeders, animal feed workers, and veterinarians.

Suggested Reading

Barbera E, de la Cuadra J (1989) Occupational airborne allergic contact dermatitis from tylosin. Contact Dermatitis 20:308–309

Carafini S, Assalve D, Stingeni L, Lisi P (1994) Tylosin, an airborne contact allergen in veterinarians. Contact Dermatitis 31:327–328

Guerra L, Venturo N, Tardio M, Tosti A (1991) Airborne contact dermatitis from animal feed antibiotics. Contact Dermatitis 25:333–334

Tuomi ML, Räsänen L (1995) Contact allergy to tylosin and cobalt in a pig-farmer. Contact Dermatitis 33:285

405. Urushiol

CAS Registry Number [492–89–7],
[53237–59–5]

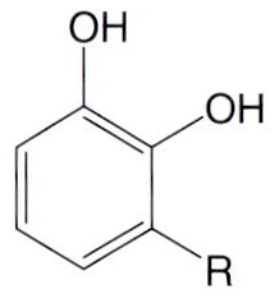

Urushiol is a generic name that indicates a mixture of several close alkylcatechols contained in the sap of the Anacardiaceae family such as *Toxicodendron radicans* Kuntze (poison ivy) or *Anacardium occidentale* L. (cashew nut tree). The R-side chain generally includes 13, 15 or 17 carbons. A urushiol with a C_{15} side chain is named pentadecylcatechol (a term sometimes employed in medical literature for poison ivy urushiol), and a urushiol with a C_{17} side chain is a heptadecylcatechol (mostly encountered in poison oak urushiol).

Suggested Reading

Epstein WL (1994) Occupational poison ivy and oak dermatitis. Dermatol Clin 12:511–516
Kawai K, Nakagawa M, Kawai K, Konishi K, Liew FM, Yasuno H, Shimode Y, Shimode Y (1991) Hyposensitization to urushiol among Japanese lacquer craftsmen. Contact Dermatitis 24:146–147
Kullavanijaya P, Ophaswongse S (1997) A study of dermatitis in the lacquerware industry. Contact Dermatitis 36:244–246

406. Usnic Acid (D-Usnic Acid, L-Usnic Acid)

CAS Registry Number [125–46–2]
(CAS Registry Number [7562–61–0],
CAS Registry Number [6159–66–6])

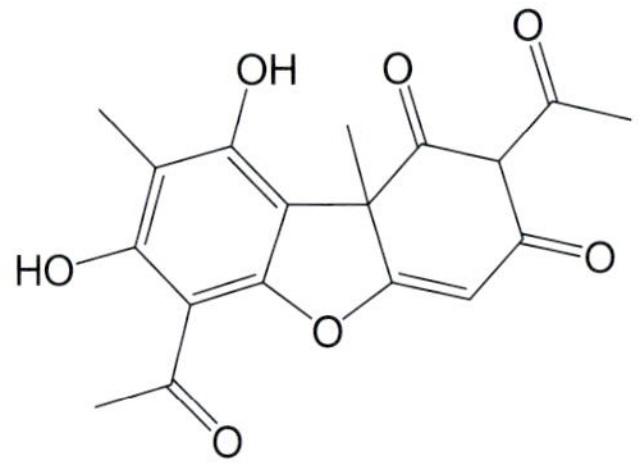

Usnic acid is a component of lichens, also used as a topical antibiotic. Allergic contact dermatitis from lichens occurs mainly occupationally in forestry and horticultural workers, and in lichen pickers.

Suggested Reading

Aalto-Korte K, Lauerma A, Alanko K (2005) Occupational allergic contact dermatitis from lichens in present-day Finland. Contact Dermatitis 52:36–38
Hahn M, Lischka G, Pfeifle J, Wirth V (1995) A case of contact dermatitis from lichens in southern Germany. Contact Dermatitis 32:55–56

407. Vinylpyridine

2-Vinylpyridine

CAS Registry Number [100–69–6]

4-Vinylpyridine

CAS Registry Number [100–43–6]

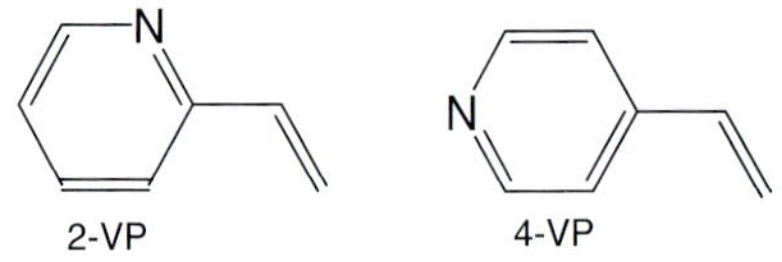

2-VP   4-VP

4-Vinyl pyridine was used as a monomer in polymer chemistry and induced nonimmunological contact urticaria, and allergic contact dermatitis. No cross-reactivity is observed between pyridine derivatives.

Suggested Reading

Bergendorff O, Wallengren J (1999) 4-Vinylpyridine-induced dermatitis in a laboratory worker. Contact Dermatitis 40:280–281

Foussereau J, Lantz JP, Grosshans E (1972) Allergic eczema from vinyl-4-pyridine. Contact Dermatitis Newslett 11:261

Sasseville D, Balbul A, Kwong P, Yu K (1996) Contact sensitization to pyridine derivatives. Contact Dermatitis 35:101–102

408. Virginiamycin

CAS Registry Number [11006–76–1]

Virginiamycin S1: Staphylomycin S

CAS Registry Number [23152–29–6]

Virginiamycin M1: Pristinamycin IIA, Mikamycin A, Ostreogrycin A, Staphylomycin M1, Streptogramin A, Vernamycin A

CAS Registry Number [21411–53–0]

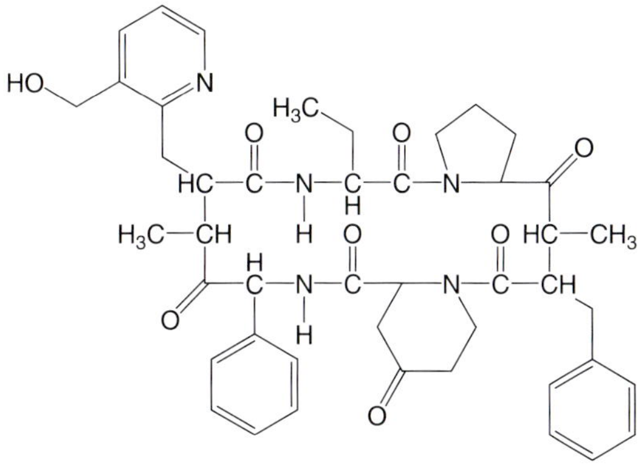

Like the other streptogramin, pristinamycin, virginiamycin is made of two subunits, virginiamycin S1 and virginiamycin M1. Dermatitis was quite common in people using the formerly available topical virginiamycin. Occupational dermatitis was observed in the pharmaceutical industry, in breeders, and in a surgeon who used topical virginiamycin on postoperative wounds (personal observation).

Suggested Reading

Rudzki E, Rebandel P (1984) Contact sensitivity to antibiotics. Contact Dermatitis 11:41–42

Tennstedt D, Dumont-Fruytier M, Lachapelle JM (1978) Occupational allergic contact dermatitis to virginiamycin, an antibiotic used as a food additive for pigs and poultry. Contact Dermatitis 4:133–134

409. Zinc bis-Dibutyldithiocarbamate

Zinc *N,N*-Dibutyldithiocarbamate

CAS Registry Number [136–23–2]

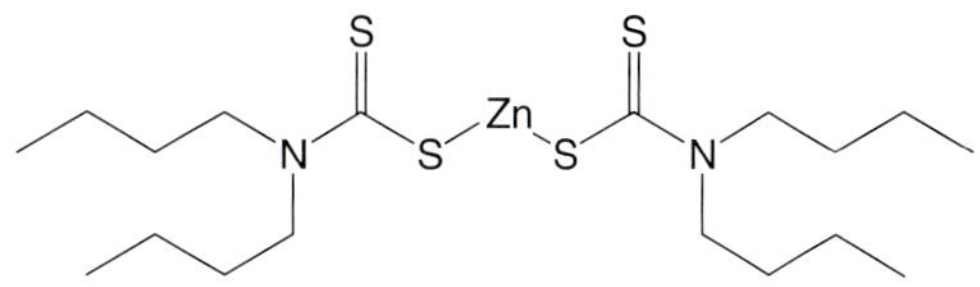

A rubber chemical, used as a vulcanization accelerator. It can also be contained in paints, glue removers, and anticorrosive. It was contained in "carba-mix."

Suggested Reading

Condé-Salazar L, Del-Rio E, Guimaraens D, Gonzalez Domingo A (1993) Type IV allergy to rubber additives: a 10-year study of 686 cases. J Am Acad Dermatol 29:176–180

Condé-Salazar L, Guimaraens D, Villegas C, Romero A, Gonzalez MA (1995) Occupational allergic contact dermatitis in construction workers. Contact Dermatitis 35:226–230

Kiec-Swierczynska M (19959 Occupational sensitivity to rubber. Contact Dermatitis 32:171–172

410. Zinc *bis*-Diethyldithiocarbamate

Zinc *N,N*-Diethyldithiocarbamate, Diethyldithiocarbamic Acid Zinc Salt

CAS Registry Number [14324–55–1]

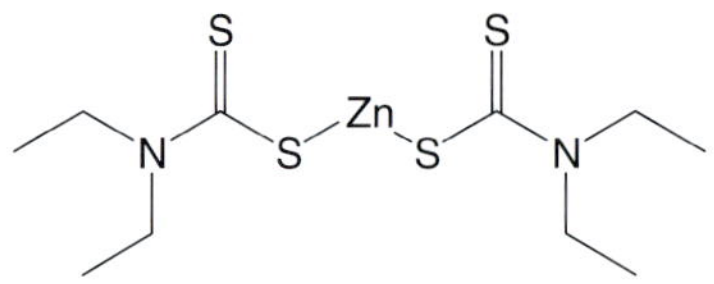

Diethyldithiocarbamate zinc is a rubber component used as a vulcanization accelerator. It can be responsible for rubber dermatitis in health personnel. It was contained in "carba-mix."

Suggested Reading

Condé-Salazar L, Del-Rio E, Guimaraens D, Gonzalez Domingo A (1993) Type IV allergy to rubber additives: a 10-year study of 686 cases. J Am Acad Dermatol 29:176–180

Kiec-Swierczynska M (1995) Occupational sensitivity to rubber. Contact Dermatitis 32:171–172

Vaneckova J, Ettler K (1994) Hypersensitivity to rubber surgical gloves in healthcare personnel. Contact Dermatitis 31:266–267

Von Hintzenstern J, Heese A, Koch HU, Peters KP, Hornstein OP (1991) Frequency, spectrum and occupational relevance of type IV allergies to rubber chemicals. Contact Dermatitis 24:244–252

411. Zinc bis-Dimethyldithiocarbamate

Ziram

CAS Registry Number [137–30–4]

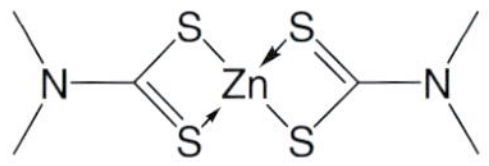

Ziram is a rubber vulcanization accelerator, of the dithiocarbamate group. Sensitization was reported in several patients. Ziram is also used as a fungicide and can cause contact dermatitis in agricultural workers.

Suggested Reading

Kiec-Swierczynska M (1995) Occupational sensitivity to rubber. Contact Dermatitis 32:171–172

Manuzzi P, Borrello P, Misciali C, Guerra L (1988) Contact dermatitis due to Ziram and Maneb. Contact Dermatitis 19:148

412. Zinc Ethylene-bis-Dithiocarbamate

Zineb, Zinc *N,N′*-Ethylenebisdithiocarbamate

CAS Registry Number [12122–67–7]

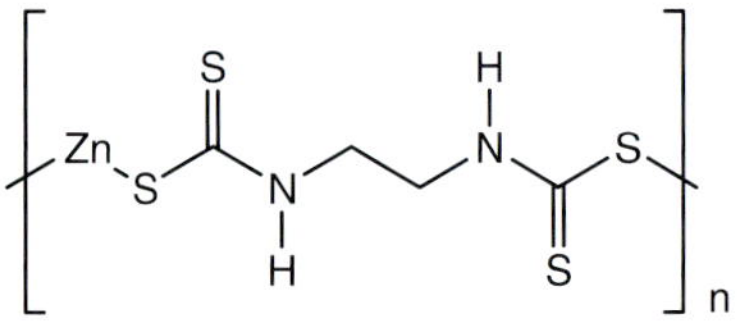

Zineb is a pesticide of the dithiocarbamate group. Sensitization can occur in gardeners and florists.

51

Suggested Reading

Crippa M, Misquith L, Lonati A, Pasolini G (1990) Dyshidrotic eczema and sensitization to dithio-carbamates in a florist. Contact Dermatitis 23:203–204

Jung HD, Honemann W, Kloth C, Lubbe D, Pambor M, Quednow C, Ratz KH, Rothe A, Tarnick M (1989) Kontaktekzem durch Pestizide in der Deutschen Demokratischen Republik. Dermatol Monatsschr 175:203–214

O'Malley M, Rodriguez P, Maibach HI (1995) Pesticide patch testing: California nursery workers and controls. Contact Dermatitis 32:61–62

413. Zinc Propylene-bis-Dithiocarbamate

Propineb, Zinc *N,N'*-Propylene-1,2-bis-Dithiocarbamate

CAS Registry Number [12071–83–9]

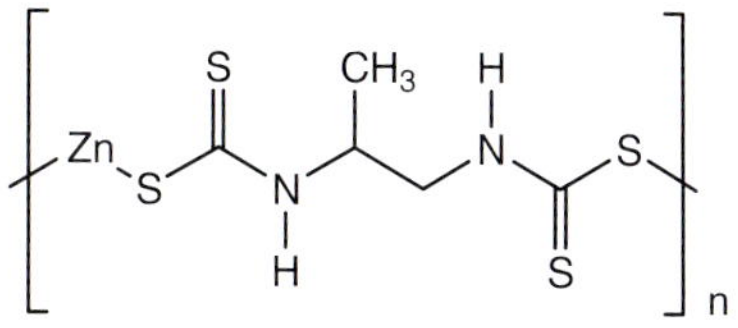

Propineb is a dithiocarbamate compound, which is used as a fungicide. Sensitization was reported in agricultural workers.

Suggested Reading

Jung HD, Honemann W, Kloth C, Lubbe D, Pambor M, Quednow C, Ratz KH, Rothe A, Tarnick M (1989) Kontaktekzem durch Pestizide in der Deutschen Demokratischen Republik. Dermatol Monatsschr 175:203–214

Nishioka K, Takahata H (2000) Contact allergy due to propineb. Contact Dermatitis 43:310

Subject Index

O